Laboratory Test Handbook

3rd Edition

with

Key Word Index

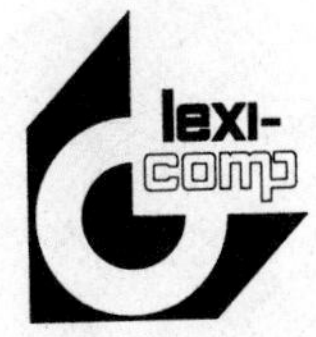

In loving memory of my mother, Harriett Tilzer
— her spirit will always be part of me.

— Lowell Tilzer

Laboratory Test Handbook

3rd Edition

with
Key Word Index

46.50

David S. Jacobs, MD, FACP, FCAP
Editor-in-Chief
Pathologist and Director of Laboratories
Providence Medical Center
Kansas City, Kansas

Wayne R. DeMott, MD, FCAP
Pathologist
Providence Medical Center
Kansas City, Kansas

Paul R. Finley, MD
Chief of Clinical Chemistry
University of Arizona Medical Center
Tucson, Arizona

Rebecca T. Horvat, PhD
University of Kansas Medical Center
Kansas City, Kansas

Bernard L. Kasten, Jr, MD, FCAP
Associate Director of Pathology and Laboratory Services
Bethesda North Hospital
Cincinnati, Ohio

Lowell L. Tilzer, MD, PhD
Editor
Community Blood Center of Greater Kansas City
Kansas City, Missouri

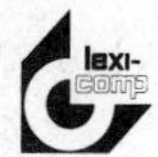

LEXI-COMP INC
Hudson (Cleveland)
1994

Medical Editor: Diane M. Harbart MT(ASCP)

Production Manager: Barbara F. Kerscher

Production Assistants: Jeanne Eads, Julie Kelley, Jacqueline L. Meizer, Jil R. Neuman

Composition Specialist: Alexandra J. Hart

Graphic Designer: Lynn D. Coppinger

Systems Analysts: Jay L. Katzen, Dennis P. Smithers

This manual was produced using the Pathfinder™ Program — a complete publishing service of Lexi-Comp Inc.

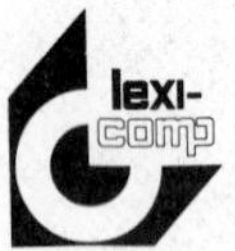

Lexi-Comp Inc
1100 Terex Road
Hudson, Ohio 44236
(216) 650-6506

ISBN 0-916589-12-9 (soft bound)
ISBN 0-916589-13-7 (case bound)

TABLE OF CONTENTS

FOREWORD

The first version of this publication, released in 1984, was an effort by four community-based pathologists to include in a single volume all the routine and many of the more specialized analyses available in a modern clinical laboratory. The next edition represented the efforts of additional authors. The number of contributors to this edition has been considerably expanded. Many are respected authorities in their fields of expertise. It is hoped that this enlarged edition is at once current and more comprehensive.

As in the previous edition, information about each laboratory procedure is presented in a standardized format, including **test name** and **synonyms**, **patient care** recommendations, **specimen requirements**, **reference ranges**, **interpretive** information, **footnotes**, and **references**. Each entry is complete in itself, but the whole work is extensively cross-referenced and indexed. The handbook is intended as a convenient reference resource for clinicians, pathologists, residents, medical and nursing students, medical technologists, ancillary medical personnel, and medical records staff.

We have devoted a great deal of effort to **clinical relevance**. We have been fortunate to have available to us the Lexi-Comp Pathfinder™ system, the Medline® system, and the computer publishing expertise of Lexi-Comp Inc. These assets have made possible extensive internal cross-referencing of entries, the inclusion, even late in the publishing process, of most current references, and the Key Word Index.

The new edition has greatly expanded coverage of laboratory assays directly and indirectly related to molecular pathology; other additions include expanded treatments of clinical virology and therapeutic drug monitoring, and many new entries in the realm of clinical immunology and the other subspecialties of clinical laboratory medicine.

To survive in today's atmosphere of change in healthcare, clinicians must order the **needed** test, obtain reliable and accurate results, and have access to current clinical laboratory information. This book, we hope, will assist with ordering and access. To attain accurate and reliable test results will depend in large measure upon quality attributes of the laboratory performing the analyses.

It is the authors' desire that this newest edition serve as a guide for the clinician and laboratorian, assist in obtaining the appropriate specimen for analysis, and provide avenues toward interpretation and relevance in the interest of optimal patient care.

ACKNOWLEDGMENTS

The *Laboratory Test Handbook with Key Word Index* exists in its present form as the result of the concerted efforts of many individuals. The publisher and president of Lexi-Comp Inc, Robert D. Kerscher, deserves much credit for bringing the concept of such a book to fruition. His dedication to the project, and his support and development of the many unique and innovative features included in the book (eg, format, internal cross-references, comprehensive indexing and Key Word Index) contribute substantially to the content and usefulness of the book.

Other members of the Lexi-Comp staff whose contributions were invaluable and whose patience with the authors' enumerable drafts, revisions, deletions, additions, and enhancements was inexhaustible include Diane M. Harbart, MT(ASCP), medical editor, Barbara F. Kerscher, production manager, Lynn D. Coppinger, graphic designer and illustrator, Alexandra J. Hart, composition specialist, Leonard L. Lance, pharmacist, Jeanne Eads, Julie Kelley, Jil R. Neuman, and Jacqueline L. Meizer, production assistants, Jeff J. Zaccagnini, Jerry M. Reeves, and Brian B. Vossler, sales managers, Edmund A. Harbart, vice-president, custom publishing division, and Jack L. Stones, vice-president, reference publishing division. The complex computer programming required for the typesetting of the book was provided by Dennis P. Smithers, Jay L. Katzen, and David C. Marcus, system analysts, under the direction of Thury L. O'Connor, vice-president, and Alan R. Frasz, vice-president, editorial systems.

The assistance of the medical library staff at Bethesda Hospitals including Michael Douglas, MLS, Joan Dewar, Linda Kittrell, Valerie Ratchford, Elizabeth Curnett, and Zufan Damene is sincerely appreciated. Janet Gates, secretary of Bethesda's Department of Pathology, assisted with correspondence and manuscript drafts.

The editors express their appreciation to Mary McIntyre, MT(ASCP) and Carol Pochler, MT(ASCP) for careful manuscript review and helpful recommendations in the Transfusion Service chapter.

ABOUT THE AUTHORS

Antimo G. Candel, MD

Dr Candel received his BS in chemistry from Grinnell College, Grinnell, Iowa. His postgraduate training was centered at Loyola University Chicago. He received his MD degree from the Loyola Stritch School of Medicine followed by residency training in Anatomic and Clinical Pathology and subspecialty training in Cytopathology at the Medical Center, Maywood, Illinois.

Dr Candel has been active in research, both clinical and basic science, and has contributed numerous publications and presentations during the past 7 years. His primary focus has been on healing and repair, and flow cytometry. He spent a 1-year internship in basic science research studying postsurgical tendon healing.

At present, Dr Candel is an Associate Pathologist at Ingalls Memorial Hospital, Harvey, Illinois. He also holds a Clinical Assistant Professor appointment at Loyola University Medical Center.

Melanie J. Castelli, MD

Dr Castelli received her MD degree from the Loyola Stritch School of Medicine, Chicago, Illinois. She completed an internship in Internal Medicine at Hines Veterans Administration Hospital, Hines, Illinois prior to her combined Anatomic/Clinical Pathology residency training at Loyola Hospital. A 1-year fellowship in Surgical Pathology at Loyola followed.

In 1984 Dr Castelli became Director of Cytopathology at Loyola University Hospital. Development of an active fine needle aspiration service and cytopathology fellowship ensued and remain her primary interests.

Dr Castelli is presently Associate Professor of Pathology at Loyola University Hospital and Medical School. She is board certified in Anatomic and Clinical Pathology with subspecialty certification in Cytopathology. She is a fellow of the College of American Pathologists and the American Society of Clinical Pathologists as well as medical member of the American Society of Cytology and Illinois Society of Cytology.

Wayne R. DeMott, MD

Dr DeMott is a graduate of Reed College (1955) and of the University of Oregon Medical School (1959). He completed his internship at Madigan General Hospital outside Tacoma, Washington. After service in the U.S. Air Force as a General Medical Officer, he completed the pathology residency program at the University of California San Francisco Medical Center (1967). He was certified in Anatomic and Clinical Pathology by the American Board of Pathology in 1968.

As a practicing pathologist at Providence Medical Center since 1968, Dr DeMott has given special attention to the areas of Hematology and Coagulation. He has participated in research activities involving separation of white cells from peripheral blood, measurement of zinc levels in peripheral blood leukocytes utilizing atomic absorption spectrophotometry, and separation of neutrophil enzymes by isoelectric focusing. He was a contributor to the Providence Medical Center (formerly Providence-St Margaret Health Center) School of Medical Technology, is a past president of the medical staff of Providence Medical Center, and is currently chairman or a member of several of the hospital's professional committees, including the Cancer Committee.

Dr DeMott is a member of the American Society of Clinical Pathologists, College of American Pathologists, American Association for Clinical Chemistry, American Medical Association, Kansas Medical Society, Kansas Society of Pathologists, Wyandotte County Medical Society, and Kansas City Society of Pathologists. He is a member of the American Association for the Advancement of Science and the New York Academy of Sciences. He is an Assistant Clinical Professor of Pathology at the University of Kansas Medical Center.

Jaime A. Diaz, MD

Dr Diaz received his MD degree from Javeriana University in Bogota, Columbia. After two rotating internships he completed a 4-year residency in Anatomic Pathology at the University of New York in Buffalo and 2 years of Clinical Pathology at William Beaumont Army Medical Center in El Paso, Texas. Dr Diaz is board certified in Anatomic Pathology, Clinical Pathology, and Dermatopathology. Dr Diaz has 24 years experience in Surgical Pathology and 15 years experience in Renal Pathology.

At the present, he is staff pathologist at Scott and White Clinic in Temple, Texas. His main interests are in Renal Pathology, Dermatopathology, and GYN Pathology. He holds an appointment as Professor of Pathology at Texas A & M Medical School and has received several awards for his teaching ability. Dr Diaz is a member of the American Medical Association, Texas Medical Association, and the College of American Pathologists.

Paul R. Finley, MD

Dr Finley, Professor of Pathology, is chief of Clinical Chemistry at the University Medical Center in Tucson, Arizona. He is responsible for the service, teaching, and research in that division, which includes general clinical chemistry, radioimmunoassay, toxicology, data processing and computer services, information technology, and immunochemistry.

Dr Finley received his MD degree from the University of Minnesota in 1953. His training includes a residency in Clinical and Anatomic Pathology (Minnesota) and a National Institutes of Health postdoctoral fellowship for study at the Royal Postgraduate Medical School in London, England, where he spent 2 years in intensive study of Clinical Chemistry. Dr Finley has published over 100 scientific papers, written chapters in various books, and has assisted in editing of three books in the laboratory field. He is a consultant to many of the most important companies in the biomedical field and plays an active and initial role in the development of instruments and concepts in this critical area. In addition, he carries on research in many diverse areas such as instrumentation and method development, coagulation, toxicology, immunochemistry, drug monitoring, biochemical hematology, multivariate analysis, computer information technology, molecular biology (restriction fragment length polymorphism studies with nucleic acid probe development for genetic disease diagnosis and polymerase chain reaction (PCR) HLA typing and crossmatching), platelet antibody studies by flow cytometry, and interpretive clinical pathology. He is on the editorial board of several recognized journals in the field. He has board certification from the American Board of Pathology in Anatomic and Clinical Pathology, and Radioisotopic Pathology.

Raoul Fresco, MD, PhD

Dr Fresco received his MD degree from Cairo University. He took a rotating internship and Pathology residency at Mount Sinai Hospital of Chicago and was an NIH sponsored trainee in Experimental Pathology at the University of Health Sciences/The Chicago Medical School, from where he earned a PhD degree in Pathology.

Dr Fresco is currently Professor of Pathology and Director of the Diagnostic Electron Microscopy Laboratory at Loyola University Medical Center and consultant to the Laboratory Service of Hines, Illinois, VA Hospital. He has taught Pathology at the Chicago Medical School, Rush Medical College, the Stritch School of Medicine of Loyola University of Chicago, and at the National Center for Advanced Medical Education in Chicago.

Dr Fresco's main interests are in the application of electron microscopy to diagnostic pathology. He has been an active member of numerous professional associations including the American Society of Clinical Pathologists, the International Academy of Pathology, the American Society for Cell Biology, the Society for Ultrastructural Pathology, and the Midwest Society of Electron Microscopists, of which he is a past Director and past President.

Paolo Gattuso, MD

Dr Gattuso received his MD degree from the University of Messina, Sicily. He completed a combined residency in Anatomic and Clinical Pathology at Loyola University Medical Center, Maywood, Illinois. This was followed by a fellowship in cytopathology at Loyola. Dr Gattuso is board certified in Anatomic and Clinical Pathology and also has subspecialty board certification in Cytopathology.

Presently, he is Assistant Professor of Pathology at Loyola University Medical Center and Associate Director of the Pathology Residency Training Program. His main areas of interest are fine needle aspiration biopsy and flow cytometry of solid tumors. Dr Gattuso has published extensively.

Harold J. Grady, PhD

Dr Grady received his PhD from the Department of Biochemistry at St Louis University. He joined the staff of the University of Kansas School of Medicine in 1950 as Assistant Professor and Clinical Chemist to the University of Kansas Medical Center. He became Full Professor of Pathology in 1965. During this period he was a consultant in Clinical Chemistry for several private hospitals in the area.

He left the Medical Center in 1970 to become Director of Clinical Chemistry for Baptist Medical Center. He retired from this position in 1988.

He is currently Full Professor of Pathology at the University of Missouri Kansas City School of Medicine and Director of Clinical Chemistry at the Truman Medical Center.

Dr Grady is a member of the American Association for Clinical Chemistry and the American Chemical Society. He is on the Board of Directors of the American Board of Clinical Chemistry and is certified by that body in Clinical Chemistry and in Toxicological Chemistry.

Larry D. Gray, PhD

Dr Gray received his bachelor's degree from the University of North Carolina at Chapel Hill and his master's and doctorate degrees from Wake Forest University (Bowman Gray School of Medicine). He received his postdoctoral training in Clinical Microbiology and Infectious Diseases at the Mayo Clinic.

Dr Gray has been the Director of Microbiology at Bethesda Hospitals in Cincinnati, Ohio for the last 5 years. He is a Volunteer Associate Professor of Pathology and Laboratory Medicine at the University of Cincinnati College of Medicine, is a Diplomate of the American Board of Medical Microbiology, and is on the editorial board of the *Journal of Clinical Microbiology*. In addition, he is an active member of the American Society for Microbiology, the American Board of Medical Microbiology, and the South Central Association for Clinical Microbiology.

Dr Gray's background includes 12 years of research in the pathogenesis of infectious diseases (ocular and pulmonary bacterial infections, electron microscopy) and the publication of many research, review, chapter, and book publications.

John G. Gruhn, MD

Dr John Gruhn received his MD degree from the Long Island College of Medicine (now the State University of New York) in 1944. After completing training in Internal Medicine and military service, he switched to Pathology in 1949. He is a Diplomate of the American Board of Pathology, certified in Anatomic Pathology in 1953, Clinical Pathology in 1963, and Dermatopathology in 1980.

Dr Gruhn is Associate Professor of Pathology at Rush Medical College in Chicago. He has written four books and over 100 papers. Currently he is Registrar for the Illinois Registry of Pathology and Program Chairman for the Chicago Pathology Society. He has been fascinated by the pathology of the skin for almost 50 years. He teaches Skin Pathology and contributed the section on Skin Biopsies for the *Laboratory Test Handbook*.

Michael S. Handler, MD

Dr Handler was born in Tokyo, Japan and was raised in Jefferson City, MO. He received a BA in biology from Brandeis University in 1975 and his MD degree from Tufts Medical School in 1980. He completed an internship in Internal Medicine at Mt Sinai, Milwaukee, WI and a residency in Pathology at Michael Reese Medical Center in Chicago, IL. He did a Neuropathology fellowship at Columbia-Presbyterian College of Physicians and Surgeons and Mt Sinai Medical Center, both in New York City. He is board certified in Anatomic Pathology (1985) and Neuropathology (1988).

Dr Handler has been an assistant professor of Pathology and Neuropathology at the University of Kansas Medical Center since January 1990. He directs the neuropathology core of the Alzheimer's and Parkinson's Disease Center and lectures on topics in pathology and neuropathology for medical students and residents at the medical schools of the University of Kansas and the University of Missouri.

Rebecca T. Horvat, PhD

Dr Horvat received her doctorate from the University of Kansas Medical Center, Department of Microbiology. After completing her doctorate, Dr Horvat was awarded a postdoctoral fellowship from the American Cancer Society. Subsequent to her postdoctoral fellowship she worked as a Technical Director in the Clinical Laboratories at the University of Kansas Medical Center. In this capacity, she worked with Virology, Microbiology, and Hematology in developing new diagnostic tests based on nucleic acid analysis. Currently Dr Horvat is an Assistant Professor in the Department of Pathology and Laboratory Medicine at the University of Kansas Medical Center in Kansas City, Kansas.

Dr Horvat's research interest involves the investigation of human herpes viruses in the development of leukemias and lymphomas. She is also interested in the diagnostic potential of nucleic acid detection, especially in immunocompromised patients. In her current position, she assists in the administration of the Microbiology and Virology sections of the clinical laboratories. This involves the education and teaching of residents and medical students, developing and instituting new diagnostic technology, and coordinating quality assurance in the Microbiology and Virology sections.

Dr Horvat is a member of the American Association of Immunologists (AAI) and the American Society for Microbiology (ASM).

Douglas W. Huestis, MD

Dr Huestis received his MD degree from McGill University, Montreal, Canada, in 1948 and did postgraduate training in pathology and related fields in Canada, Sweden, England, and the U.S.A. After a few years of general hospital pathology, he began concentrating on the field of blood transfusion and immunohematology in Chicago in 1960 then moved to Tucson to the then new medical school at the University of Arizona in 1969.

His major work while in Chicago was on erythrocyte antigens and antibodies and their relationship to difficulties and complications of blood transfusion. He also did some early work on the development of frozen blood systems, including the use of a unique vaporphase liquid nitrogen storage freezer and a simplified thawing-deglycerolizing system utilizing invert sugar. In Arizona, he developed a procedure for the collection of granulocytes by intermittent flow centrifugation and applied this to the special transfusion support of patients with cancer and leukemia. He has had much to do with the development of technical procedures with blood cell separators for the collection of white blood cells and platelets for transfusion, and for the treatment of leukemic patients with a dangerous excess of white blood cells or platelets. Most recently, he has been increasingly involved in transplantation immunology and in the rapidly developing field of plasma exchange. These various activities have resulted in over 90 scientific articles.

Dr Huestis has served as a director and vice-president of the American Association of Blood Banks and on many of its committees and was editor of two editions of its *Technical Manual*. He received the John Elliott award of that association for such activities. He has been an associate editor of the journal *Transfusion* since 1968. He has served on several advisory committees for the National Institutes of Health, has been a consultant to the U.S. Army and Air Force, and took part in two scientific exchange visits to the Soviet Union under the Soviet-American Health Exchange.

He considers one of his most important achievements to be the textbook *Practical Blood Transfusion*, coauthored with Joseph R. Bove and John Case and published by Little, Brown & Co. The fourth edition of this book appeared in 1988.

Daniel H. Jacobs, MD

Dr Jacobs received an AB in history from Stanford University in 1982, a medical degree from the University of Kansas in 1987, and completed a Neurology residency at the University of Kansas in 1992. Along the journey, Dr Jacobs completed 1 year of Psychiatry at the University of Iowa and a year of Medicine and Neurology at Francis Scott Key Hospital and John Hopkins Hospital.

Currently Dr Jacobs is pursuing research opportunities in higher cortical function and behavioral neurology in the Department of Neurology at the University of Florida College of Medicine in Gainesville. Among his research interests are the role of cholinergic systems in dementia and the neuropsychology of Parkinson's disease.

Dr Jacobs is a member of the American Academy of Neurology, the American Epilepsy Society, and the Kansas Neurological Society.

David S. Jacobs, MD

Dr Jacobs is Director of Laboratories at Providence Medical Center and Clinical Professor at the University of Kansas and the University of Missouri-Kansas City Schools of Medicine. He is a Fellow of the American College of Physicians and of the College of American Pathologists. He is a member of the International Academy of Pathology, the AMA, and the Kansas Medical Society. Dr Jacobs is Secretary of the Wyandotte County Medical Society and past President of the Kansas Society of Pathologists, the Kansas City Society of Pathologists, and of the Medical Staff of the Providence Medical Center (formerly Providence-St Margaret Health Center). He has for many years served as an inspector for both the College of American Pathologists and for the American Association of Blood Banks.

Dr Jacobs' special interests include general pathology, particularly surgical pathology, interpretation of clinical laboratory tests, and transfusion medicine. His publications include items in surgical pathology and the clinical relevance of laboratory testing.

He received premedical education at the University of Michigan. Entering the UM Medical School in the "Letters and Medicine" program, Dr Jacobs remained at Michigan as a general rotating intern, then as a pathology resident. Following service in the U.S. Army Medical Corps as a pathologist with 13 months residency, he returned to Ann Arbor and completed the pathology program under Drs A. J. French and M. R. Abell. He then spent an additional year in Chicago in clinical pathology with Drs Israel Davidsohn and Douglas Huestis.

Bernard L. Kasten Jr, MD

Dr Kasten is a graduate of Miami University, Oxford, Ohio and the Ohio State University College of Medicine. He interned at the University of Miami, Florida and served his residency in Clinical Pathology at the National Institute of Health Clinical Center followed by a fellowship at the National Cancer Institute Laboratory of Pathology. His staff appointments have included service in the Division of Laboratory Medicine at the Cleveland Clinic. For the last 6 years, he has been Associate Director of Pathology and Laboratory Services at Bethesda Hospitals in Cincinnati. Dr Kasten is active as a fellow in the College of American Pathologists, in which he participates in the Inspection and Accreditation Program, Council on Education and Membership Services, Management Resource Committee, and as Chairman of the Publications Committee and contributor and Chairman of the Editorial Board of *CAP Today* since its inception in 1987. He was the recipient of the 1993 Frank W Hartman Award in recognition of his service to the College of American Pathologists.

Dr Kasten was a principle author of the first edition of the *Laboratory Test Handbook* and the author of the *Physicians DRG Handbook*. He has written articles on the use of bar codes in the clinical laboratory. He has presented numerous lectures and seminars on the subjects of improving workflow in the laboratory, total quality management, and the appropriate use of laboratory tests, particularly the rational use of screening tests for prostate-specific antigen. He is a member of the editorial board for Lexi-Comp Inc's medical publishing.

David F. Keren, MS, MD

Dr Keren received his MD degree from the University of Illinois. Subsequently, he spent 5 years in his pathology residency at The Johns Hopkins Hospital in Baltimore, MD. During that time, he developed expertise in the areas of Diagnostic Immunopathology and Mucosal Immunity. For the following 2 years he served as a major in the United States Army, as the Immunopathologist in the Department of Bacterial Diseases at the Walter Reed Army Institute of Research in Washington, DC.

For the next 11 years, Dr Keren served on the faculty of the University of Michigan as the Head of Immunology, Director of the Biochemistry Section in the Department of Pathology. He achieved the rank of Full Professor of Pathology. He held a coappointment in the Department of Microbiology and Immunology at the University of Michigan Medical School.

Dr Keren is the author of several books including *Flow Cytometry and Clinical Diagnosis* (ASCP Press), *Immunology and Immunopathology of the Gastrointestinal Tract* (ASCP Press), *High-Resolution Electrophoresis and Immunofixation* (Butterworths), and *Diagnostic Immunology* (with Jeffrey S. Waffen, MD, Williams & Wilkins). He has also authored over 100 articles in the field of Diagnostic Immunopathology and Mucosal Immunity.

Currently, Dr Keren serves as Director of Warde Medical Laboratory in Ann Arbor, Michigan. He has an appointment at Eastern Michigan University as an Adjunct Professor of Biology. He serves as an advisor to the American Society of Clinical Pathologists, College of American Pathologists, and the American Board of Pathology. He is also a member of the American Association of Pathologists, American Association of Immunologists, American Society of Microbiologists, American Medical Association, American Medical Laboratory Immunologists, and the American Association of Clinical Chemists.

Phillip A. Munoz, MD

Dr Munoz received his MD degree from the University of Kansas Medical Center. He completed his first year of pathology training at Northwestern University and continued his training as a Research Associate in Immunology at the National Institutes of Health. He completed his training in Pathology at the University of Kansas Medical Center, then joined the medical faculty for the next 6 years. During that time, he developed a focus on hybridoma technology and cell marker studies applied to hematopathology and general surgical pathology. He is currently an Associate Pathologist and Director of Hematology and the Cell Marker Laboratories at Research Medical Center, Kansas City, Missouri.

In his current position, Dr Munoz oversees various laboratory aspects of an active hematology/oncology patient population in a large private hospital that serves as the center of a multihospital Kansas City based healthcare network. In addition to general surgical pathology and hematology services, he maintains an integrated immunocytochemistry and flow cytometry laboratory that serves as a reference laboratory for the healthcare system and other hospitals in the Kansas City area.

Dr Munoz is a member of the Kansas City Society of Pathologists, College of American Pathologists, American Society of Clinical Pathologists, American Pathology Foundation, and American Medical Association.

Eugene S. Olsowka, MD, PhD

Dr Olsowka is a pathologist at Providence Medical Center in Kansas City, Kansas and a volunteer Associate Clinical Professor at the University of Kansas School of Medicine. He is a fellow of the College of American Pathologists and the American Society of Clinical Pathologists.

Dr Olsowka studied mathematics as an undergraduate at the University of Chicago. He entered medical school at the University of Illinois in 1977 and was accepted into the MD, PhD program in 1978. He received his MD degree in 1984 and a PhD in Nutritional Sciences from the University of Illinois in 1989. Dr Olsowka was a pathology resident at The McGaw School of Medicine at Northwestern University in Chicago, from 1986 to 1990. He was a fellow in Surgical Pathology at Rush-Presbyterian-St Luke's Medical Center in Chicago from 1990 to 1991. He is board certified in Anatomic and Clinical Pathology and is a fellow of the College of American Pathologists.

Dr Olsowka's interests are general pathology including surgical pathology, chemistry, and cytology.

Christopher J. Papasian, PhD

Dr Papasian received his doctorate in Microbiology from the State University of New York at Buffalo, School of Medicine and completed his postdoctoral training in Medical and Public Health Microbiology at Erie County Medical Center in Buffalo, NY. He is a Board-Certified Diplomate of the American Academy of Microbiology.

Dr Papasian is an Associate Professor of Pathology at the University of Missouri, (Kansas City) School of Medicine and is Director of Diagnostic Microbiology and Immunology Laboratories at Truman Medical Center in Kansas City, Missouri. He emphasizes cost-effective, clinically relevant microbiology in practice and in education, and has authored or coauthored over 40 original articles, book chapters, and abstracts.

Lowell Tilzer, MD, PhD

Dr Tilzer received his medical degree and PhD in a combined medical science program from the Kansas University Medical Center in Kansas City, Kansas. He also did his residency in Anatomic and Clinical Pathology at KU. He is certified in both Anatomic and Clinical Pathology by the American Board of Pathology. Dr Tilzer went on to serve on staff at Kansas University Medical Center in the Department of Pathology in the clinical laboratory. He served as associate Medical Director for 14 years and became Full Professor. He was in charge of Hematology, Blood Bank, Clinical Chemistry, and Lab Computer. His research interests included laboratory computing (especially use of bar codes in specimen management, which he pioneered in the United States) and diagnostic Molecular Biology. He has extensive teaching experience with medical technology students, medical students, graduate students, and pathology residents. In addition, he holds several patents in the molecular biology field and owns his own biotechnology company.

In 1992, Dr Tilzer moved to the Community Blood Center of Greater Kansas City in Kansas City, Missouri. He is Associate Medical Director where he is working on stem cell collection and bone marrow processing.

Dr Tilzer is a member of the American Association of Blood Banks, College of American Pathologists, American Association of Clinical Chemists, American Association for the Advancement of Science, and the Metropolitan Medical Society of Kansas City.

Glen R. Willie, MD

Dr Willie earned his Masters in Biochemistry and Doctor of Medicine at the University of Minnesota with research studying the receptor binding of the antibiotic fusidic acid on the bacterial ribosome. He completed his residency in Internal Medicine at Sinai Hospital of Detroit, and a Nephrology Fellowship at Henry Ford Hospital in Detroit.

Since then, he has held teaching positions as Associate Professor of Medicine at Texas A&M University School of Medicine, teaching in Nephrology and Nutrition. Special areas of interest include nutrition, trace metals, and metabolic bone disease.

Dr Willie is a member of the American College of Physicians, Texas Medical Association, and the International Society of Nephrology.

HOW TO USE THIS HANDBOOK

The *Laboratory Test Handbook with Key Word Index* is arranged alphabetically in chapters by major clinical laboratory disciplines: Anatomic Pathology, Chemistry, Coagulation, Cytopathology, Hematology, Immunology and Serology, Microbiology, Molecular Pathology, Therapeutic Drug Monitoring/Toxicology/Drugs of Abuse, Trace Elements, Transfusion Service (Blood Bank), Urinalysis and Clinical Microscopy, and Virology. A general section, Specimen Collection, precedes the individual chapters. Within each section, the laboratory tests are listed alphabetically and cross-referenced with synonyms referring the user to the actual test name. A brief introduction to each section provides general information.

Each individual test listing is arranged in a consistent format providing five major types of information: Test Name, Patient Care, Specimen, Interpretive, and Footnotes and References.

Test Name

This part gives information pertaining to the **test name.**. Other procedures that contain **related informationthe named entry are listed and cross-referenced by page number. Synonyms** are noted and procedures which are not exact synonyms but have similar instructions, or require similar consideration, are also referred to under the **applies to** heading. Tests **replaced by** a current procedure are noted and a definition of procedures included within the named test is given under **test includes**. The **CPT-4** code is listed for most procedures.

Patient Care

This part contains patient **preparation** and **aftercare** instructions. The patient preparation information includes patient care considerations prior to the collection of specimen or performance of a diagnostic procedure. Aftercare includes patient care considerations following the collection of a specimen or performance of a procedure.

Specimen

This part includes, when appropriate, the specific **specimen** required, the **container, sampling time**, specific **collection** instructions, specimen **storage instructions, causes for rejection** of the specimen by the laboratory, **turnaround time,** and **special instructions** indicating additional pertinent considerations relating to the specimen.

Interpretive

This part contains a discussion of basic information relevant to the clinical application of the test, including **normal** (or reference) **range,** specific **use** of the test, **limitations** of the test method, specific test **methodology** where appropriate, **contraindications** to the test, and **additional information** which may contribute to the interpretation or utilization of a the test.

Footnotes and References

The bibliographic information provided with test listings may include footnotes referring to specific literature quotations, specific points of information, or opinions. Selected general references are provided as sources for the individual test listings.

Acronyms and Abbreviations Glossary

This glossary provides a useful listing of many acronyms and abbreviations commonly associated with laboratory medicine. We offer this glossary not as an exhaustive authoritative list, but more as a guide to assist in interpreting frequently used terminology.

Key Word Index

The Key Word Index is not intended in any way to suggest patterns of physicians' orders, nor is it complete. Rather, it is the intent of the authors and editors to make the information easier to find and utilize in order to support better patient care.

The Key Word Index provides a reference to the test name based on a diagnostic property, disease entity, organ system, or syndrome for which the test is useful. It lists descriptions of specific tests. Some may support possible clinical diagnoses or rule out other diagnostic possibilities.

Each laboratory test relevant to the indexed diagnosis is listed and weighted. Two symbols (••) indicate that the test is diagnostic, that is, it documents the diagnosis if the expected result is found. A single symbol (•) indicates a test frequently used in the diagnosis or management of the particular disease. The other listed tests are useful on a selective basis with consideration of clinical factors and specific aspects of the case.

Diagnoses with *International Classification of Disease—Ninth Revision—Clinical Modification* (ICD-9-CM) codes are indicated within the [ ] symbol.

CPT-4 Index

CPT-4 codes are provided with each test for reference, as a basis for documentation of diagnostic procedures performed and to facilitate financial and patient record keeping. The codes are current. Applications of codes may vary by region of the country and in some instances the application of a specific code to a given procedure is a matter of individual interpretation.

CPT is a listing of descriptive terms and five-digit numeric identifying codes and modifiers for reporting medical services performed by physicians. This presentation includes only CPT descriptive terms, numeric identifying codes and modifiers for reporting medical services, and procedures that were selected by Lexi-Comp Inc for inclusion in this publication.

The most current CPT is available from the American Medical Association.

No fee schedules, basic unit values, relative value guides, conversion factors or scales or components thereof are included in CPT.

Lexi-Comp has selected certain CPT codes and service/procedure descriptions and assigned them to various specialty groups. The listing of a CPT service or procedure description and its code number in this publication does not restrict its use to a particular specialty group. Any procedure or service in this publication may be used to designate the services rendered by any qualified physician.

The AMA assumes no responsibility for the consequences attributable to or related to any use or interpretation of any information or views contained in or not contained in this publication.

Alphabetical Index

The most expedient method for locating a given test is the Alphabetical Index in the last section of this handbook. Test names and synonyms are listed and the page number on which the test description may be found is indicated.

STATISTICS, THE NORMAL RANGE, AND THE ULYSSES SYNDROME

or

A TEST IN SEARCH OF A DISEASE

David S. Jacobs, MD
Eugene S. Olsowka, MD, PhD

During and after the Trojan War, Ulysses was away from home 20 years. While traveling, he was involved in a series of frequently dangerous and sometimes needless adventures. The syndrome[1] was named for Ulysses because patients with it, although healthy at the beginning, journey through clinical investigations and undergo a number of experiences new to them before they once again reach the safe harbor of being considered healthy.

The bottom line of complex clinical, technical, and statistical data leads to a decision — whether or not a given laboratory report is normal for a particular patient.

The College of American Pathologists, in setting standards for their Inspection and Accreditation Program for Clinical Laboratories, indicates that reference values (normal values) for each test should be provided with the report when possible. Two modern laboratory realities must be recognized:

1. A reference range is required for the interpretation of most laboratory tests, and
2. It may not be possible to provide an appropriate reference range in all cases.

It is important to recognize that laboratory methods and types of equipment greatly influence the outcome of any given test. The most relevant reference ranges are those generated by the laboratory performing the assay. Ability of a laboratory to provide meaningful reference ranges is limited by many factors.

Purely statistical approaches are unsatisfactory. For instance, since coronary arterial disease is rampant in present day America, we cannot base "normal" ranges for serum lipids on a Gaussian distribution.

Most tests do not have sharp cutoff points between normal and abnormal. "Normal" curves can be bell shaped, but they are often skewed.

Nominally, "normal" findings may have diagnostic significance in an appropriate setting.[2] Thus, efforts to increase our knowledge of the significance of normal range, and thus narrow the normal range for a given patient, can add value to "normal" results.

The effects of drugs on clinical laboratory tests have been exhaustively reviewed[3] and are therefore not emphasized in this book.

---

[1] Rang M, "The Ulysses Syndrome," *Can Med Assoc J*, 1972, 106:122-3.

[2] Gorry GA, Pauker SG, and Schwartz WB, "The Diagnostic Importance of the Normal Finding," *N Engl J Med*, 1978, 298:486-9.

[3] Young DS, "Effects of Drugs on Clinical Laboratory Tests," *American Association for Clinical Chemistry*, 3rd ed, 1990.

With computers, laboratories can stratify normal ranges by age and sex. We would no more expect a college varsity athlete and a great-grandmother to have the same normal ranges for clinical laboratory examinations, than we would expect them to have the same hat or shoe size. Such stratification is at the fringe of clinical documentation, and relatively few published studies are available which are pertinent to normal ranges for all of the tests done by most laboratories. Clinical input is continually needed to improve available normal ranges.

Special situations in which computer generated normal ranges may be inappropriate, misleading, or nonexistent include the following.

1. **Glucose:** A computer may only be provided with normal ranges for fasting plasma glucose. Blood sugar levels have not been done in years; laboratories use serum and plasma.

2. **Pregnancy:** The well known increases in alkaline phosphatase, decreases in urea nitrogen, and other changes accompanying pregnancy are not always taken into consideration when normal ranges are reported in pregnant individuals. (The laboratory is commonly not aware if an individual is pregnant, and if so, the length of gestation.) Cortisol, alpha$_1$-fetoprotein, alpha$_1$-antitrypsin, amylase, cholesterol, and triglycerides may increase.

3. **Athletes and Exercise:** Athletes are apt to have slight elevations of urea nitrogen and LD, as well as depressions of pulse rate.[4] After physical exercise, significant elevations of total CK are commonplace and creatinine, potassium, uric acid, bilirubin, leukocyte count, haptoglobin, transferrin, and BUN may increase. Exercise increases HDLC, lactate, and may increase aldolase.

4. **The First Month of Life:** Tremendous shifts in normal ranges occur during the first month of life. Some tests ideally should be stratified depending on whether the patient is premature or term, and others (hemoglobin, bilirubin) change significantly during the first month. Many computers cannot stratify in so many intervals. For such tests, a number of normal ranges exist depending upon the age in days in the first month of life, prematurity or term, and other factors.

5. **Posture:** Posture is reported to change the normal range for a number of tests — total protein, albumin, calcium, hemoglobin and hematocrit, plasma renin activity, urinary catecholamines, and perhaps alkaline phosphatase, cholesterol,[5] ALT (SGPT), and iron. Levels of such substances have been described as being higher in an upright position than in a reclining position. Consider that in the reclining individual, interstitial fluid enters the vascular compartment, diluting constituents which the clinical laboratory measures. On standing, the venous pressure in the lower part of the body increases, capillary pressure increases, and some plasma is ultrafiltered into the interstitial space. Cells and constituents such as protein, which do not readily pass the capillary endothelium, increase. So do substances wholly or partly bound to protein (eg, calcium). Urea nitrogen, on the other hand, is so diffusible that patient posture makes no difference.

6. **Body Weight:** Some laboratory computer software makes no allowance for body weight. Creatinine clearance and blood volumes require this data. Posi-

[4] Solomon JG, "Abnormal Laboratory Results in Runners," *JAMA*, 1979, 241:2262, (letter).

[5] Dixon M and Paterson CR, "Posture and the Composition of Plasma," *Clin Chem*, 1978, 24:824:6.

tive weight dependencies are described for uric acid, glucose, and cholesterol, in that many subjects with high concentrations of the analyte are in the high-weight group. Males, but not females, have such body weight associations for creatinine, protein, hemoglobin, and AST (SGOT). Inverse relationships are reported for phosphate and, in females, for calcium.[6]

7. **Topics Requiring Medical Judgment:** The significance of a few red cells in urine depends upon the clinical setting (voided versus catheterized urine, sex, menstruation or not); therefore, some tests cannot be classified as "normal" or "abnormal" by computer, but only by the physician caring for that particular patient.

   Tests having no normals — because **positivity** in any quantity is itself abnormal — include:

   Serum acetone
   Porphobilinogen
   Alcohol and certain other toxins
   Urine glucose, ketones, blood, bile, nitrite
   ART, VDRL, and other serologic tests for syphilis
   Nucleated RBC/100 WBC, blasts, promyelocytes, myelocytes in diff
   LE slide test
   Test for sickling
   Malaria smear

   Laboratory data must always be considered in light of the physician's clinical impression. If the clinician considers acute infarct of myocardium likely, and the laboratory data do not support his initial impression, the patient should be treated as if he indeed had an infarct. (Laboratory data may be normal or inconclusive early in myocardial infarct; this is a particularly good example of the importance of the physician's clinical diagnosis.) When laboratory results are abnormal but not supported by clinical findings, the physician should thoroughly consider the laboratory reports before dismissing them as inconsequential.

   Laboratory data suggest clues to unsuspected disease in about 12% of patients studied in a university hospital series.[7]

8. **Food and Nutrition:** Tests requiring the **fasting state** include fasting blood sugar, lipid profile, iron, iron binding capacity, B_{12}/folate levels, carotene, d-xylose, lactose, and glucose tolerance tests, Schilling test, most insulins, serum bile acids, and gastrin. Serum bile acids are sometimes measured before and after a meal. **Prolonged fasting** may increase serum bilirubin (up to 240% after a 48-hour fast) and cause decreases of plasma glucose and proteins (albumin, transferrin, and complement C_3). Samples for PKU (chemical test), FTA-ABS, and antibodies for virus, fungal, and *Mycoplasma* agents should be clear serum, fasting if necessary.

   Blood drawn immediately after a meal is apt to have elevated potassium and depressed phosphorus and then elevated triglycerides. Alkaline phosphatase may be elevated 2-4 hours after a fatty meal, especially in people who are Lewis-positive secretors of blood type O or B. Increased turbidity in

---

[6] Munan L, Kelly A, PetitClerc C, et al, "Associations With Body Weight of Selected Chemical Constituents in Blood: Epidemiologic Data," *Clin Chem*, 1978, 24:722-7.

[7] Young DS, "Why There Is a Laboratory," *Clin Chem*, Young, Hicks, Nipper, et al, eds, AACC, 1979, 3-22.

postprandial blood can interfere with certain other tests, including bilirubin, LD (LDH), and total protein. Increased turbidity might depress uric acid and BUN, depending on methodology.

High protein diet can elevate BUN, ammonia, and urate. Purines increase uric acid. High intake of **bananas**, **pineapples**, **tomatoes**, and **avocados** may elevate 5-HIAA. **Caffeine** elevates catecholamines, as does **theophylline**.

9. **Drugs: Ethanol** causes immediate increases of uric acid, lactate, and acetone. Intermediate effects include increases of GGT (GGTP) and to a lesser degree ALT (SGPT). Actually, a short-chain carbohydrate, ethanol may induce increases in triglycerides. More chronic alcoholism may be manifested by increases of bilirubin, AST (SGOT), alkaline phosphatase, as well as GGT, and a decrease of folate. Although considerable information is available,[3] a great deal more is needed.

   Oral contraceptives increase T_4 (RIA) and decrease T_3 uptake. They are reported to increase alpha$_1$-antitrypsin (half of alpha$_1$ in serum protein electrophoresis), iron, triglycerides, ALT (SGPT), and GGT; to decrease albumin; and to affect as many as 100 laboratory tests.

10. **Hemolysis** from hemolytic anemia or venipuncture causes increases in LD, bilirubin, AST (SGOT), CK, potassium, ALT (SGPT), magnesium, and acid phosphatase. Hemolysis from traumatic venipuncture may be associated with release of thromboplastins and may invalidate the results of coagulation tests in some cases. Hemolysis has a less marked effect on total protein, alkaline phosphatase, iron, and phosphorus. Hemolysis will mask hemolyzing antibodies in the antibody screen and crossmatch.

11. **Circadian Rhythms:** Circadian (approximately 24-hour) rhythms have implications for physiology, measurement of many laboratory tests, drug excretion (eg, salicylates, sulfonamides), and responses to therapy. Levels fluctuating very significantly during the 24-hour cycle include cortisol (which has different normals for 8 AM and 8 PM), growth hormone, serum acid phosphatase, aldosterone (high 6 AM to 3 PM), transferrin (maximum 4 PM to 8 PM), ACTH, serum iron, serum creatinine (7 PM values 130% of 7 AM concentration), eosinophils (low in afternoon), lymphocytes (maximum early AM), WBC (maximum in early AM), leukocyte function and urine urobilinogen (maximum excretion in afternoon). Urinary excretion of potassium, LH, FSH, TSH, testosterone, and some less commonly ordered hormones have some diurnal variation. Parathyroid hormone is best drawn at 8 AM.

    Triglyceride is higher in the afternoon, as is phosphate, BUN, and the hematocrit. Bilirubin falls, but overnight fasting itself causes bilirubin to increase.[8]

    The waves which characterize circadian rhythms may be square shaped or may occur as a series of pulses. The latter pattern is seen with plasma cortisol concentration, which begins to increase during sleep. A large difference exists between this level and that found in the evening. Still another

---

[8] Pocock SJ, Ashby D, Shaper AG, et al, "Diurnal Variation in Serum Biochemical and Haematological Measurements," *J Clin Pathol*, 1989, 42:172-9.

pattern is a single daily pulse such as occurs with growth hormone secretion.[9]

The magnitude of the effect of circadian rhythms is greater than is generally recognized. Although only 10% variation exists for plasma potassium concentration, urinary potassium excretion can vary fivefold during the day.[10]

Some hormone secretion cycles are longer (infradian) — eg, the menstrual cycle.

12. **Clots** in specimens which should lead to specimen rejection. Tiny clots may go unnoticed and generate misleading results (eg, CBC).

13. **Prolonged contact with the clot**, in the physician's office or in the laboratory, causes glucose to decrease and alkaline phosphatase to change somewhat. Iron, potassium, and LD increase, and AST (SGOT) increases slightly, but ALT (SGPT) and total CK remain constant. The greatest changes are in glucose, potassium, and LD.[11] We have seen some tubes left on a radiator a day or two with characteristic chemistry profile patterns: phosphorus very high, LD high, and no glucose.

14. **Other specimen mishandling** potentially causing misleading results includes blood tube exposure to **sunlight** which can cause misleading increases in white blood cell count, platelet count, and abnormalities in sedimentation rate.[12] Sunlight causes bilirubin to decrease in the test tube as it does in the neonate.

15. **Sampling Problems:** It is best not to draw from an extremity in which there is an I.V. infusion site. Rarely, there is no other place to draw, and such samples are apt to have dilutional changes resulting in invalid test results, especially for electrolytes and glucose, and factitious changes in coagulation parameters. A recommendation to wait 3 minutes after the I.V. has been shut off may lead to misleading results for glucose.[13] Drawing from indwelling venous catheters may present dilutional and many other artifacts.

    A **tourniquet**, with patient clenching and unclenching his hand, will lead to build-up of high potassium and lactic acid from the hand muscles, and pH will decrease. It is best to avoid a tourniquet for electrolytes and lactic acid. Hand clenching is best avoided for such tests.

    Capillary punctures can be done for CBC, differential, platelet count, reticulocyte count, electrolytes, gases, and many chemistry tests but may introduce tissue juices which result in possibly misleading conclusions.

---

[9] Moore-Ede MC, Czeisler CA, and Richardson GS, "Circadian Timekeeping in Health and Disease, Part 1. Basic Properties of Circadian Pacemakers," *N Engl J Med*, 1983, 309:469-76.

[10] Moore-Ede MC, Czeisler CA, and Richardson GS, "Circadian Timekeeping in Health and Disease, Part 2. Clinical Implications of Circadian Rhythmicity," *N Engl J Med*, 1983, 309:530-6.

[11] Laessig RH, Indriksons AA, Hassemer DJ, et al, "Changes in Serum Chemical Values as a Result of Prolonged Contact With the Clot," *Am J Clin Pathol*, 1976, 66:598-604.

[12] O'Bannon RH, "The Effects of Improper Specimen Handling on Lab Tests," *Med Lab Observer*, Nov 1988, 42-7.

[13] Read DC, Viera H, and Arkin C, "Effect of Drawing Blood Specimens Proximal to an In-Place but Discontinued Intravenous Solution," *Am J Clin Pathol*, 1988, 90:702-6.

Arterial specimens, compared to venous, have different normal ranges for lactic acid, pO_2 and oxygen saturation, and only slightly different ranges in the vast majority of well and sick patients for pH and pCO_2.

Unusual sites of venous sampling (other than anticubital veins) may lead to misleading results. Sampling from foot veins, for instance, may lead to results which differ from established levels based on conventional vein draws. With rare exceptions such as drug addicts and obese individuals, foot veins are not accessed. They are saved as a last resort. Such attempts are often unsuccessful.

Inappropriate specimen collection tubes (eg, for trace metals or coagulation tests), incorrect sample collection procedures, and incorrect choice of anticoagulant (eg, as in fibrinopeptide A and beta-thromboglobulin procedures) are potential mistakes inexperienced laboratorians may make.

16. **Lipemic specimens** may present a number of problems.

17. **Instruments:** Some are electronic marvels. Nevertheless, anyone who has ever purchased an automobile, refrigerator, or light bulb is aware that instruments can fail. This phenomenon is best expressed by Murphy's Law, third corollary: "If there is a possibility of several things going wrong, the one that will cause the most damage will be the one to go wrong."[14] Systems are relevant as well.[15]

18. **Genetic variations** exist in how individuals metabolize drugs and major variations occur.

19. **Aging** is accompanied by differences in normal ranges from those established for younger individuals.[16,17]

20. **Other variables** include sex, stress, menstrual cycle, menopause, and altitude.[18]

21. **Normal Range — a Guideline:** The reference or normal ranges in this book are merely guidelines. A great deal of variation exists between methods, instruments, reaction temperatures, and other parameters among laboratories, thus, reported reference ranges vary widely. The most relevant normal ranges for most assays are those developed and reported by the laboratory performing the assay. In situations where the normal range is extremely method dependent, it seemed prudent not to provide a normal range that would differ markedly from that encountered by many readers and thus might be potentially misleading.

---

[14] Block A, *Murphy's Law and Other Reasons Why Things Go Wrong!* Los Angeles, CA: Price/Stern/Sloan Publishers, Inc, 1977.

[15] Gambino R, "Most Laboratory Errors Are System Dependent — Not People Dependent," *Lab Med*, 1989, 123.

[16] Dietz AA, ed, *Aging — Its Chemistry*, Washington, DC: The American Association for Clinical Chemistry, 1980.

[17] Rochman H, *Clinical Pathology in the Elderly*, Basel, Switzerland: Karger, 1988.

[18] Siest G, Henny J, Schiele F, et al, eds, *Interpretation of Clinical Laboratory Tests*, Foster City, CA: Biomedical Publications, 1985.

STATISTICAL REVIEW

Statistics is a branch of mathematics often much maligned by many current day savants. One often hears the incorrect expression, "You can say anything you like by using statistics." Substitution of the word "using" for the more accurate "misusing" corrects an incorrect expression. It is by the misuse of statistics (intentional or otherwise) that facts may be misconstrued. More colloquially, "statistics don't lie, people do." As our common everyday statistics and hypothesis testing are ultimately derived from probabilistic equations, discussion of statistics must necessarily include a discussion of probability. Following are some of the more common definitions and equations that are used daily in laboratory medicine, often hidden from conscious thought.

Sample Space: A collection of objects or outcomes of interest. As an example, in an unbiased single coin toss the sample space consists of the outcome heads or tails.

Relative Frequency: The ratio of the number of times an event occurs to the total number of observations. Relative frequencies are unstable for a small number of observations. For example, the relative frequency of obtaining a heads or a tails in an unbiased coin toss is 50% for a large number of tosses. It may be different for a limited number of tosses — say four.

Probability: The stable (over a large number of observations) relative frequency associated with an event. The probability of event A is usually denoted by the symbol P(A).

Random Variable: Given a sample space S with elements s and a function X, X is called a random variable if it assigns to each element s in the sample space S one and only one real number. Put mathematically, the random function X acting on sample space S is defined by the set of real numbers [x: x=X(s), s is an element of S]. One of the major problems for applied statisticians is to define such functions. As an example: To determine the effect of a diet on development of an animal, we may choose to look at total body weight gain, bone or organ growth, or times to maturation or senescence.

Statistic: A function of the elements of a random sample that does not depend upon any unknown parameters of the sample. Mean, median, mode, range, and variance of a given sample are all statistics.

Median: The middle most number in a data set (assuming set is arranged in ascending or descending order).

Mode: Most frequently occurring result or measurement in a data set.

Population Mean: Usually denoted by the symbol μ.

Population Variance: Usually denoted by the symbol σ^2. Typically μ and σ^2 are unknown and are estimated from $\bar{x}$ and s^2 — the sample mean and variance.

Mean of a Sample: Denoted by:

$$\bar{X} = 1/n\left(\sum_{i=1}^{n} X_i\right)$$

Variance of a Sample: Denoted by:

$$S^2 = (1/n) \sum_{i=1}^{n} (X_i - \overline{X})^2$$

or

$$S^2 = \left((1/n) \sum_{i=1}^{n} X_i^2 \right) - \overline{X}^2$$

Note: Using 1/n yields the variance of the empirical (sample) distribution. Use of 1/n-1 yields the unbiased estimator of σ^2. 1/n+1 yields the minimum mean square error estimator of σ^2. Standard deviation σ is the square root of the variance σ^2

Biased Statistic: A statistic is said to be biased if it is not equal to the parameter it is intended to measure, eg, if the mean $\overline{x}$ of a sampling distribution is not equal to the population mean μ, then the mean $\overline{x}$ is said to be biased. Conversely, if the mean $\overline{x}$ equals the parameter μ, then $\overline{x}$ is said to be unbiased.

Binomial Probability Function: Let p be a probability of success for a certain event, q = 1 – p, n = total number of trials, and x = number of successes in n trials. The probability of a number of successes x in a given number of trials n is given by:

$$P(x) = (n!/x!(n-x)!)\ p^x q^{n-x}$$

Example: If each assay in a particular laboratory has a 1 in 100 chance of being erroneous, find the probability of finding 3 erroneous results in a batch of 10. Here n = 10, x = 3, p = 0.01, and q = 1 - 0.01 = 0.99. Probability of 3 erroneous results in a batch of 10 in this laboratory is given by:

$P(3) = (10!/3!\ (7)!)\ 0.01^3\ 0.99^7$

$P(3) = (3628800/6\ (5040))\ 10^{-6}\ 0.9321$

$P(3) = 120\ (9.321 \times 10^{-7})$

$P(3) = 0.000112$

Example: Under the above error rate assumptions find the probability of an error with a replicate test being made. Here assume tests consists of 5 tests with replicate, for a total of 10 tests. Normally there could be 45 pairs of tests that are in error; (10!/2! 8!) however, we are constrained to 5 combinations of replicate tests. The probability is given by:

$P(\text{error}) = 5\ (0.01^2)\ 0.99^8 = 5\ (10^{-4})\ 0.9227$

$P(\text{error}) = 5\ (9.23 \times 10^{-5}) = 0.0046$

Example: Under current proficiency testing rules, one must either pass all 5 challenges or may miss 1 out of 5, but one may not miss 1 out of 5 twice in a row. CLIA 88 mandates use of a predefined cutoff of $\overline{x} \pm 2SD$ for unregulated analytes and 3 standard deviations (3SD) to pass some challenges for regulated analytes. What is the probability of not successfully passing a challenge for some regulated analytes ($\overline{x} \pm 3SD$) and unregulated analytes ($\overline{x} \pm 2SD$) if given four times a year?

Under proficiency testing guidelines, denote P as 5 successful challenges and I as 1 missed challenge out of 5. The following patterns in the test denote successful outcomes:

a	PPPP
b	IPPP — 4 combinations
c	IPIP — 2 combinations (PIPI)

d IPPI

$$P(P) = \frac{5!}{5!\,0!} (0.05)^0 (0.95)^5 = 0.774$$

$$P(1) = \frac{5!}{4!\,1!} (0.05)^1 (0.95)^4 = 0.204$$

Then probability for a successful outcome is given by:

$$P = P(a) + P(b) + P(c) + P(d)$$

$$\begin{aligned} \text{Probability} = P(a) &= (0.774)^4 = 0.3585 \\ P(b) &= (0.774)^3 (0.204) (4) = 0.3774 \\ P(c) &= (0.77)^2 (0.204)^2 (2) = 0.0497 \\ P(d) &= (0.77)^2 (0.204)^2 = 0.0248 \end{aligned}$$

$$\begin{aligned} \text{Total probability} = P &= 0.3585 + 0.3774 + 0.0497 + 0.0247 \\ P &= 0.8103 \text{ or approximately } 81\% \end{aligned}$$

Probability of not meeting challenge for unregulated analytes is given by:

$1 - P$ or approximately 0.19 (19%)

For some regulated analytes with successful challenge defined as $\bar{x} \pm 3SD$, the probability of not successfully meeting a challenge is given by:

$$P(P) = \frac{5!}{5!\,0!} (0.01)^0 (0.99)^5 = 0.9510$$

$$P(1) = \frac{5!}{4!\,1!} (0.01)^1 (0.99)^4 = 0.0480$$

Then $P = P(a) + P(b) + P(c) + P(d) = 0.8179 + 0.1652 + 0.0042 + 0.0021$
$P = 0.9894$ and $1 - P = 0.0106$ or 1.06%

Thus, for some regulated analytes, the probability of not meeting a successful yearly challenge is 1.06%.

Comment: The above calculations assume a perfectly working unbiased machine. About 1% of the time even perfect machines will fail to successfully meet the yearly challenge. For unregulated analytes using $\bar{x} \pm 2SD$ for cutoffs, the probability of missing a successful challenge assuming a perfect machine is 19%. The College of American Pathologists always cautions in their proficiency survey reports that "proficiency test results are not the sole criteria for judging laboratory performance." One may easily understand this disclaimer when scrutinizing the above calculations. Note that calculations assume that the previous year ended in a pass (P); they do not account for the situation when one gets 4 of 5 analytes correct at the end of the year. In this scenario, probability of passing for the year falls to 0.667 or 66.7% for nonregulated analytes and 0.9439 or 94.4% for some regulated analytes. Thus, probability of not passing a yearly challenge is 33.3% for nonregulated analytes and 5.6% for some regulated analytes if 1 of 5 challenges was missed at the end of the previous year.

Poisson Distribution: A special adaptation of the binomial distribution, given by the formula:

$$P(X = x) = \lambda^x e^{-\lambda} / x!$$

or

$$P(X \leq x) = \sum_{k=0}^{x} \left(\lambda^k e^{-\lambda} / k!\right)$$

where λ is equal to both the mean and the variance of the poisson distribution (the probability of a given event occurring in a short time h must be λh). This distribution may be used to calculate the probabilities of the number of times particular events occur in a given time or on a given object. For example this distribution may be used to calculate the probability of obtaining defective cuvettes over a period of time in a manufacturing process. If a manufacturer of cuvettes expects 2 bad cuvettes every 5 minutes, what is the probability of 5 or more bad cuvettes in 15 minutes? Here, the average number of bad cuvettes in 15 minutes is 6, ie, $\lambda = 6$. If we assume a Poisson process then

$$P(X \geq 5) = 1 - P(X = 4) = \sum_{i=0}^{4} 6^i e^{-6}$$

$$= 1\text{-}0.285 = 0.715 \text{ or } 71\%$$

Normal (Bell-Shaped) Distribution: Let u = mean of the normal random variable, x, σ = standard deviation, π = 3.1416, and e = 2.71828, then the probability density function of a normal distribution is given by the equation:

$$f(x) = \left(1/\sigma\sqrt{2\pi}\right) e^{-\left((x-\mu)^2/2\sigma^2\right)}$$

The z score gives the distance between a measurement and the mean in units equal to the standard deviation, ie, $z = (x - \mu)/\sigma$. The distribution of z scores also known as a standard normal distribution always has a mean of 0 and a standard deviation of 1.

Student's t Distribution: Let Z be a random variable that is normally distributed with mean 0 and variance 1, and let U be a random variable that is chi-square distributed with r degrees of freedom. If Z and U are independent, then

$$T = Z / \sqrt{U / r}$$

has a t distribution with r degrees of freedom. The probability density function is a rather complicated gamma function and the interested reader is encouraged to seek it in more specialized statistical textbooks. Figure 1 compares a normal distribution with mean 0 and variance 1 with a t distribution with 4 degrees of freedom. Note that the t distribution has more extreme probability than the normal distribution.

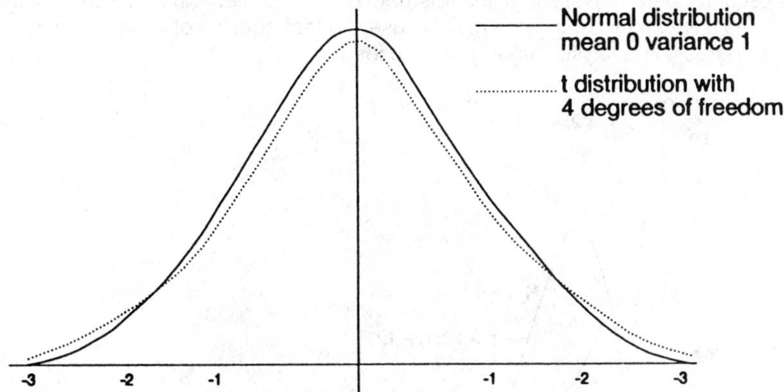

Figure 1. t distribution with 4 degrees of freedom compared with a normal distribution of mean 0 and variance 1

The Gamma Distribution: The random variable X is said to have a gamma distribution if its probability density function is defined by the equation

$$F(x) = \begin{cases} \dfrac{1}{\Gamma(\alpha)\theta^{\alpha}} X^{\alpha-1} e^{-x/\theta} & 0 \leq x < \infty \\ 0 & x < 0 \end{cases}$$

where the gamma function is defined as:

$$\Gamma(t) = \int_0^{\infty} y^{t-1} e^{-y} dy \qquad t > 0$$

The Chi-Square Distribution: Let X have a gamma distribution with $\theta = 2$ and $\alpha = r/2$ where r is a positive integer called the "degrees of freedom. X is chi-square distributed if its probability density function is given by:

$$f(x) = \begin{cases} \dfrac{1}{\Gamma(r/2)2^{r/2}} X^{r/2-1} e^{-x/2} & 0 \leq x < \infty \\ 0 & x < 0 \end{cases}$$

The mean and variance of a chi-square distribution are

$$u = \alpha\theta = r \qquad \text{and} \qquad \sigma^2 = \alpha\theta^2 = 2r$$

ie, the mean is equal to the number of degrees of freedom and the variance is equal to twice the number of the degrees of freedom.

The F Distribution: Let U and V be independent chi-square variables with r1 and r2 degrees of freedom. Then F is said to have an F distribution with r1 and r2 degrees of freedom when defined as:

$$F = \frac{U/r1}{V/r2}$$

The probability density function is complicated and the reader is encouraged to seek out advanced statistical textbooks. Graphs of some typical F distributions are seen in figure 2. Note that this distribution is assymetric and skewed. F distributions have many uses. They may be used to test equality of variances and linearity in regression analysis, among other uses.

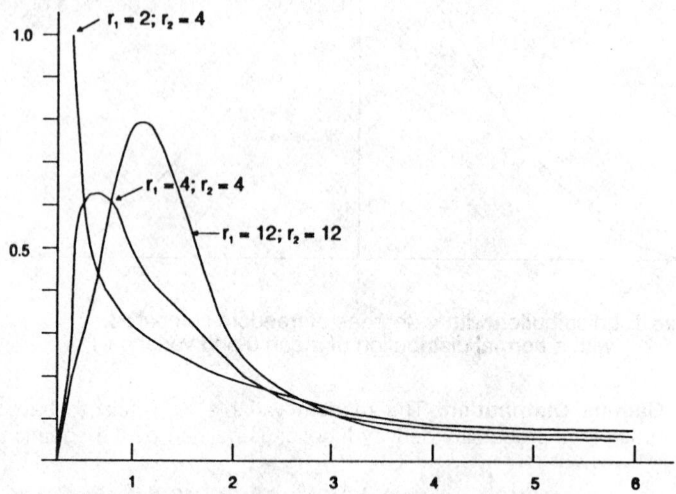

Figure 2. F distribution with r_1 and r_2 degrees of freedom

BRIEF REVIEW OF SIMPLE TESTS OF COMPARISON

t Test: Given two means u_1 with sample size n_1 and u_2 with sample size n_2 and equal variances ($\sigma_1^2 = \sigma_2^2$).

To test null hypothesis that means u_1 and u_2 are equal against the hypothesis that $u_1 - u_2 \neq 0$, use the formula

$$t = \overline{x}_1 - \overline{x}_2 / \sqrt{sp^2 \left(1/n_1 + 1/n_2\right)}$$

This statistic has a t distribution with $n_1 + n_2 - 2$ degrees of freedom. The pooled variance sp^2 may be estimated from the following formula:

$$sp^2 = \left(\sum_{i=1}^{n1} \left(x_{1i} - \overline{x}_1\right)^2 + \sum_{j=1}^{n2} \left(x_{2j} - \overline{x}_2\right)^2 \right) / \left(n_1 + n_2 - 2\right)$$

The t test may be used to answer such questions as to whether mean effects of two treatments are equal. The test may be one tailed or two tailed depending upon the question one is asking.

The F Test: May be used to test the (null) hypothesis that population means do not differ. Let MST be the mean square for a group of k treatments (sum of squares/k-1). Let MSE be the mean square for error given by sum of squares for error/n-k, where n = number of measurements. Then to compare the two sources of variability — source of variability among treatment means with that due to differences within samples, one may use the statistic:

$$F = MST/MSE$$

with k-1 and n-k degrees of freedom. This test assumes that all k populations are normally distributed, the k population variances are equal, and samples are randomly and independently selected. In the case of determining linearity in a single variable regression, the error may be partitioned into that of the regression and residual. An F test defined as:

$$F = MS(regression)/MS(residual)$$

may be used to determine whether there is a true linear effect. Note that as assays become more precise mean square residual error decreases which tends to increase the ratio. Thus as assays become more precise, the F test may appear to magnify subtle departures from linearity. This helps to explain the observation with very precise assays that a clinically acceptable linear assay may not pass a statistical test of linearity. As the F test typically involves a comparison of two sources of variance, procedures utilizing F tests may be referred to as "analysis of variance."

DETECTION OF LABORATORY ERROR

If result of a particular assay is viewed as (blindly) selecting a value from a distribution with a particular mean and variation, then it is expected that one may get a value that is statistically different from that mean. In other words, given the myriads of results a laboratory reports per day, it is expected that a small fraction of these results are erroneous. As some errors are truly random, there is no way to detect them. Can true errors be minimized? Three maneuvers may help to minimize such errors.

1. **Repeat Testing (Replicate):** Such repeat testing is another sampling with the same probability for error. As the probability for two errors is less than for a single error, replicate testing may help to minimize errors.
2. **Analysis of Outliers:** Such maneuvers allow one to discard a result if it is more than a predefined number of standard deviations from a population mean. It is recognized by many that diseases such as metabolic blocks may produce values that are well beyond the population mean (sometimes 10 deviations) . A highly unusual result may attract attention but be a true result. Repeat testing of an outlier may be a good way of minimizing error, but a dilemma exists if the repeat value is markedly different from the first — which is the true result?
3. **Comparison of a Current Value With the Last Value** — the so called delta check. Anyone who has followed serum enzymes for myocardial infarct knows that such a procedure may be misleading. However, one of the authors has had a recent experience in urinalysis where a 1 g/dL urine glucose was properly questioned because the five previous urinalyses had glucose concentrations of 0. Used properly, delta checks may be very helpful. They are not particularly helpful with potentially labile analytes such as serum enzymes, blood gases, or electrolytes.

The above discussion applies to random laboratory error. Errors that are systemic (ie, resulting from faulty technique or equipment) are likely to be picked up by a reasonably good laboratory quality assurance program.

Thus, a wide variety of causes of erroneous or inaccurate laboratory results can cause a patient to begin a journey that may have more than a passing resemblance to Ulysses'.[19]

---

[19] Kasten BL, "Ulysses Comes Home — at Last," *CAP Today*, May 1987.

Laboratory Lament[20]

To the Editor:

Oh, what a tangled web is weavable
When clinical chemistry's not believable.

Digoxin dosage is not titratable.
Coronary risk becomes debatable.

The bottom line will be inscrutable
If based on tests that are disputable!

References

Adrogué HJ, Rashad MN, Gorin AB, et al, "Assessing Acid-Base Status in Circulatory Failure: Differences Between Arterial and Central Venous Blood," *N Engl J Med*, 1989, 320:1312-6.

Creer MH and Ladenson J, "Analytical Errors Due to Lipemia," *Lab Med*, 1983, 14:351-5.

Diamond I, "The Clinical Purposes of Laboratory Testing," *Arch Pathol Lab Med*, 1988, 112:377-8.

Fraser CG, Wilkinson SP, Neville RG, et al, "Biologic Variation of Common Hematologic Laboratory Quantities in the Elderly," *Am J Clin Pathol*, 1989, 92:465-70.

Friedman RB and Young DS, "Effects of Disease on Clinical Laboratory Tests," *Clin Chem*, Washington, DC: AACC Press, 1989.

Gambino R, "Posture and Lab Tests," *Lab Report for Physicians*, 1981, 3:81-2.

Hogg RV and Tanis EA, *Probability and Statistical Inference*, New York, NY: Macmillan Publishing Co Inc, 1977.

Kassirer JP, "Sounding Board: Our Stubborn Quest for Diagnostic Certainty — A Cause of Excessive Testing," *N Engl J Med*, 1989, 320:1489-91.

McClave JT and Dietrich FH, II, *Statistics*, 3rd ed, San Francisco, CA: Dellen Publishing Company, 1985.

Priest JB, Oei TO, and Moorehead WR, "Exercise-Induced Changes in Common Laboratory Tests," *Am J Clin Pathol*, 1982, 77:285-9.

Rosner B, *Fundamentals of Biostatistics*, Boston, MA: Dexbury Press, 1986.

Speicher CE, "All Laboratory Tests Are Not Created Equal," *Arch Pathol Lab Med*, 1985, 109:709-10.

Speicher CE and Smith JW, *Choosing Effective Laboratory Tests*, Philadelphia, PA: WB Saunders Co, 1983.

Valenstein PN, "Evaluating Diagnostic Tests With Imperfect Standards," *Am J Clin Pathol*, 1990, 93:252-8.

Watts NB, "Medical Relevance of Laboratory Tests," *Arch Pathol Lab Med*, 1988, 112:379-82.

Welch MJ and Hertz HS, "The How and Why of an Accuracy Base for Proficiency Testing Programs," *Arch Pathol Lab Med*, 1988, 112:343-5.

Zweig MH, "Evaluation of the Clinical Accuracy of Laboratory Tests," *Arch Pathol Lab Med*, 1988, 112:383-6.

[20] Goldman P, "Laboratory Lament, *New Engl J Med*, 1985, 312:865.

SPECIMEN COLLECTION

Bernard L. Kasten, Jr, MD
Eugene S. Olsowka, MD, PhD

Proper specimen collection is pivotal for provision of meaningful clinical laboratory information.

Although rigorous laboratory quality assurance procedures are required to assure technically accurate results, such techniques cannot safeguard against incorrectly labeled tubes or improperly drawn specimens. If specimen is not representative or has been compromised by improper collection or inappropriate handling, results may be misleading or potentially dangerous. **The laboratory must have an optimum, properly labeled specimen**.

This section includes general information pertaining to the collection of laboratory specimens. Listings for common methods of blood and urine collection are outlined as general considerations. Specimen collection information specific for each individual test is provided with the detailed discussion of the test within the sections of the text. A discussion of the special requirements for collection of specimens for detection of **drugs of abuse and therapeutic drug levels** is presented in the introduction to the Therapeutic Drug Monitoring/Toxicology/Drugs of Abuse chapter, and a typical **chain-of-custody** form is illustrated in the appendix of that chapter. The unique considerations required for the collection of specimens for **trace element** testing are discussed in the introduction of the Trace Elements chapter. Specifically, specimens submitted for trace elements must be submitted in heavy metal-free containers or metal-free Vacutainers®. **Transfusion service** needs are addressed at the beginning of that chapter. Special requirements exist for testing, as described in that chapter.

Overview and Regulatory Considerations

Every healthcare employee, from nurse to housekeeper, has some (albeit small) risk of exposure to HIV and other viral agents such as hepatitis B and Jakob-Creutzfeldt agent. The incidence of HIV-1 transmission associated with a percutaneous exposure to blood from an HIV-1 infected patient is approximately 0.3% per exposure.[1] In 1989, it was estimated that 12,000 United States healthcare workers acquired hepatitis B annually.[2] An understanding of the appropriate procedures, responsibilities, and risks inherent in the collection and handling of patient specimens is necessary for safe practice and is required by Occupational Safety and Health Administration (OSHA) regulations.

The Occupational Safety and Health Administration published its "Final Rule on Occupational Exposure to Bloodborne Pathogens" in the Federal Register on December 6, 1991. OSHA has chosen to follow the Center for Disease Control (CDC) definition of universal precautions. The Final Rule provides full legal force to universal precautions and requires employers and employees to treat blood and certain body fluids as if they were infectious. The Final Rule mandates that healthcare workers must avoid parenteral

[1] Henderson DK, Fahey BJ, Willy M, et al, "Risk for Occupational Transmission of Human Immunodeficiency Virus Type 1 (HIV-1) Associated With Clinical Exposures. A Prospective Evaluation," *Ann Intern Med*, 1990, 113(10):740-6.

[2] Niu MT and Margolis HS, "Moving Into a New Era of Government Regulation: Provisions for Hepatitis B Vaccine in the Workplace, *Clin Lab Manage Rev*, 1989, 3:336-40.

contact and must avoid splattering blood or other potentially infectious material on their skin, hair, eyes, mouth, mucous membranes, or on their personal clothing. Hazard abatement strategies must be used to protect the workers. Such plans typically include, but are not limited to, the following:

- safe handling of sharp items ("sharps") and disposal of such into puncture resistant containers
- gloves required for employees handling items soiled with blood or equipment contaminated by blood or other body fluids
- provisions of protective clothing when more extensive contact with blood or body fluids may be anticipated (eg, surgery, autopsy, or deliveries)
- resuscitation equipment to reduce necessity for mouth to mouth resuscitation
- restriction of HIV- or hepatitis B-exposed employees to noninvasive procedures

OSHA has specifically defined the following terms: **Occupational exposure** means reasonably anticipated skin, eye mucous membrane, or parenteral contact with blood or other potentially infectious materials that may result from the performance of an employee's duties. **Other potentially infectious materials** are human body fluids including semen, vaginal secretions, cerebrospinal fluid, synovial fluid, pleural fluid, pericardial fluid, peritoneal fluid, amniotic fluid, saliva in dental procedures, and body fluids that are visibly contaminated with blood, and all body fluids in situations where it is difficult or impossible to differentiate between body fluids; any unfixed tissue or organ (other than intact skin) from a human (living or dead); and HIV-containing cell or tissue cultures, organ cultures, and HIV- or HBV-containing culture medium or other solutions, and blood, organs, or other tissues from experimental animals infected with HIV or HBV. An **exposure incident** involves specific eye, mouth, other mucous membrane, nonintact skin, or parenteral contact with blood or other potentially infectious materials that results from the performance of an employee's duties.[3] It is important to understand that some exposures may go unrecognized despite the strictest precautions.

A written Exposure Control Plan is required. Employers must provide copies of the plan to employees and to OSHA upon request. Compliance with OSHA rules may be accomplished by the following methods.

- **Universal precautions (UPs)** means that all human blood and certain body fluids are treated as if known to be infectious for HIV, HBV, and other bloodborne pathogens. UPs do not apply to feces, nasal secretions, sputum, sweat, tears, urine, or vomitus unless they contain visible blood.
- **Engineering controls (ECs)** are physical devices which reduce or remove hazards from the workplace by eliminating or minimizing hazards or by isolating the worker from exposure. Engineering control devices include sharps disposal containers, self-resheathing syringes, etc.
- **Work practice controls (WPCs)** are practices and procedures that reduce the likelihood of exposure to hazards by altering the way in which a task is performed. Specific examples are the prohibition of two-handed recapping of needles, prohibition of storing food alongside potentially contaminated material, discouragement of pipetting fluids by mouth, encouraging handwashing after removal of gloves, safe handling of contaminated sharps, and appropriate use of sharps containers.

---

[3] Bruning LM, "The Bloodborne Pathogens Final Rule — Understanding the Regulation," *AORN Journal*, 1993, 57(2):439-40.

- **Personal protective equipment (PPE)** is specialized clothing or equipment worn to provide protection from occupational exposure. PPE includes gloves, gowns, laboratory coats (the type and characteristics will depend upon the task and degree of exposure anticipated), face shields or masks, and eye protection. Surgical caps or hoods and/or shoe covers or boots are required in instances in which gross contamination can reasonably be anticipated (eg, autopsies, orthopedic surgery). If PPE is penetrated by blood or any contaminated material, the item must be removed immediately or as soon as feasible. **The employer must provide and launder or dispose of all PPE at no cost to the employee**. Gloves must be worn when there is a reasonable anticipation of hand contact with potentially infectious material, including a patient's mucous membranes or nonintact skin. Disposable gloves must be changed as soon as possible after they become torn or punctured. Hands must be washed after gloves are removed.

Housekeeping protocols: OSHA requires that all bins, cans, and similar receptacles, intended for reuse which have a reasonable likelihood for becoming contaminated, be inspected and decontaminated immediately or as soon as feasible upon visible contamination and on a regularly scheduled basis. Broken glass that may be contaminated must not be picked up directly with the hands. Mechanical means (eg, brush, dust pan, tongs, or forceps) must be used. Broken glass must be placed in a proper sharps container.

Employers are responsible for teaching appropriate clean-up procedures for the work area and personal protective equipment. A 1:10 dilution of household bleach is a popular and effective disinfectant. It is prudent for employers to maintain signatures or initials of employees who have been properly educated. If one does not have written proof of education of universal precautions teaching, then by OSHA standards, such education never happened.

Pre-exposure and postexposure protocols: OHSA's Final Rule includes the provision that employees, who are exposed to contamination, be offered the hepatitis B vaccine at no cost to the employee. Employees may decline; however, a declination form must be signed. The employee must be offered free vaccine if he/she changes his/her mind. Vaccination to prevent the transmission of hepatitis B in the healthcare setting is widely regarded as sound practice.[4] In the event of exposure, a confidential medical evaluation and follow-up must be offered at no cost to the employee. Follow-up must include collection and testing of blood from the source individual for HBV and HIV if permitted by state law if a blood sample is available. If a postexposure specimen must be specially drawn, the individual's consent is usually required. Some states may not require consent for testing of patient blood after accidental exposure. One must refer to state and/or local guidelines for proper guidance.

The employee follow-up must also include appropriate postexposure prophylaxis, counseling, and evaluation of reported illnesses. The employee has the right to decline baseline blood collection and/or testing. If the employee gives consent for the collection but not the testing, the sample must be preserved for 90 days in the event that the employee changes his/her mind within that time. Confidentiality related to blood testing must be ensured. **The employer does not have the right to know the results** of the testing of either the source individual or the exposed employee.[3]

---

[4] Schaffner W, Gardner P, and Gross PA, "Hepatitis B Immunization Strategies: Expanding the Target," *Ann Intern Med*, 1993, 118(4):308-9.

Hazardous Communication

Communication regarding the dangers of bloodborne infections through the use of labels, signs, information, and education is required. Storage locations (eg, refrigerators and freezers, waste containers) that are used to store, dispose of, transport, or ship blood or other potentially infectious materials require labels. The label background must be red or bright orange with the biohazard design and the word biohazard in a contrasting color. The label must be part of the container or affixed to the container by permanent means.

Education provided by a qualified and knowledgeable instructor is mandated. The sessions for employees must include:[3]

- accessible copies of the regulation
- general epidemiology of bloodborne diseases
- modes of bloodborne pathogen transmission
- an explanation of the exposure control plan and a means to obtain copies of the written plan
- an explanation of the tasks and activities that may involve exposure
- the use of exposure prevention methods and their limitations (eg, engineering controls, work practices, personal protective equipment)
- information on the types, proper use, location, removal, handling, decontamination, and disposal of personal protective equipment)
- an explanation of the basis for selection of personal protective equipment
- information on the HBV vaccine, including information on its efficacy, safety, and method of administration and the benefits of being vaccinated (ie, the employee must understand that the vaccine and vaccination will be offered free of charge)
- information on the appropriate actions to take and persons to contact in an emergency involving exposure to blood or other potentially infectious materials
- an explanation of the procedure to follow if an exposure incident occurs, including the method of reporting the incident
- information on the postexposure evaluation and follow-up that the employer is required to provide for the employee following an exposure incident
- an explanation of the signs, labels, and color coding
- an interactive question-and-answer period

Record Keeping

The OSHA Final Rule requires that the employer maintain both education and medical records. The medical records must be kept confidential and be maintained for the duration of employment plus 30 years. They must contain a copy of the employee's HBV vaccination status and postexposure incident information. Education records must be maintained for 3 years from the date the program was given.

OSHA has the authority to conduct inspections without notice. Penalties for cited violation may be assessed as follows.[3]

Serious violations. In this situation, there is a substantial probability of death or serious physical harm, and the employer knew, or should have known, of the hazard. A violation of this type carries a mandatory penalty of up to $7000 for each violation.

Other-than-serious violations. The violation is unlikely to result in death or serious physical harm. This type of violation carries a discretionary penalty of up to $7000 for each violation.

Willful violations. These are violations committed knowingly or intentionally by the employer and have penalties of up to $70,000 per violation with a minimum of $5000 per violation. If an employee dies as a result of a willful violation, the responsible party, if convicted, may receive a personal fine of up to $250,000 and/or a 6-month jail term. A corporation may be fined $500,000.

Large fines frequently follow visits to laboratories, physicians' offices, and healthcare facilities by OSHA Compliance Safety and Health Offices (CSHOS). Regulations are vigorously enforced. A working knowledge of the final rule and implementation of appropriate policies and practices is imperative for all those involved in the collection and analysis of medical specimens.

Effectiveness of universal precautions in averting exposure to potentially infectious materials has been documented.[5] Compliance with appropriate rules, procedures, and policies, including reporting exposure incidents, is a matter of personal professionalism and prudent self-preservation.

References

Buehler JW and Ward JW, "A New Definition for AIDS Surveillance," *Ann Intern Med*, 1993, 118(5):390-2.

Brown JW and Blackwell H, "Complying With the New OSHA Regs, Part 1: Teaching Your Staff About Biosafety," *MLO*, 1992, 24(4)24-8. Part 2: "Safety Protocols No Lab Can Ignore," 1992, 24(5):27-9. Part 3: "Compiling Employee Safety Records That Will Satisfy OSHA," 1992, 24(6):45-8.

Department of Labor, Occupational Safety and Health Administration, "Occupational Exposure to Bloodborne Pathogens; Final Rule (29 CFR Part 1910.1030)," *Federal Register*, December 6, 1991, 64004-182.

Gold JW, "HIV-1 Infection: Diagnosis and Management," *Med Clin North Am*, 1992, 76(1):1-18.

"Hepatitis B Virus: A Comprehensive Strategy for Eliminating Transmission in the United States Through Universal Childhood Vaccination", *MMWR Morb Mortal Wkly Rep*, 1991, 40(RR-13):1-25.

"Mortality Attributable to HIV Infection/AIDS — United States", *MMWR Morb Mortal Wkly Rep*, 1991, 40(3):41-4.

National Committee for Clinical Laboratory Standards, "Protection of Laboratory Workers From Infectious Disease Transmitted by Blood, Body Fluids, and Tissue," NCCLS Document M29-T, Villanova, PA: NCCLS, 1989, 9(1).

"Nosocomial Transmission of Hepatitis B Virus Associated With a Spring-Loaded Fingerstick Device — California", *MMWR Morb Mortal Wkly Rep*, 1990, 39(35):610-3.

---

[5] Wong ES, Stotka JL, Chinchilli VM, et al, "Are Universal Precautions Effective in Reducing the Number of Occupational Exposures Among Healthcare Workers?" *JAMA*, 1991, 265:1123-8.

Polish LB, Shapiro CN, Bauer F, et al, "Nosocomial Transmission of Hepatitis B Virus Associated With the Use of a Spring-Loaded Fingerstick Device," *N Engl J Med*, 1992, 326(11):721-5.

"Recommendations for Preventing Transmission of Human Immunodeficiency Virus and Hepatitis B Virus to Patients During Exposure-Prone Invasive Procedures," *MMWR Morb Mortal Wkly Rep*, 1991, 40(RR-8):1-9.

"Update: Acquired Immunodeficiency Syndrome — United States", *MMWR Morb Mortal Wkly Rep*, 1992, 41(26):463-8.

"Update: Transmission of HIV Infection During an Invasive Dental Procedure — Florida", *MMWR Morb Mortal Wkly Rep*, 1991, 40(2):21-7, 33.

"Update: Universal Precautions for Prevention of Transmission of Human Immunodeficiency Virus, Hepatitis B Virus, and Other Bloodborne Pathogens in Health-care Settings," *MMWR Morb Mortal Wkly Rep*, 1988, 37(24):377-82, 387-8.

Acquired Immunodeficiency Syndrome Precautions, Specimen Collection *see* Blood and Fluid Precautions, Specimen Collection *on next page*

AIDS Precautions, Specimen Collection *see* Blood and Fluid Precautions, Specimen Collection *on next page*

Allen Test *see* Arterial Blood Collection *on this page*

Arterial Blood Collection

CPT *36600*

Related Information

Blood and Fluid Precautions, Specimen Collection *on next page*
Blood Gases, Arterial *on page 140*
Specimen Identification Requirements *on page 30*

Synonyms Arterial Puncture

Applies to Allen Test

Test Commonly Includes Brachial, radial, or femoral artery puncture by trained personnel to obtain arterial blood most frequently for blood gas analysis

Patient Care **PREPARATION:** The patient should be resting for 20-30 minutes before collection of the specimen. **AFTERCARE:** Direct pressure must be applied to the arterial puncture site and should be maintained for a minimum of 5 minutes. Patients with bleeding tendency due to anticoagulation, platelet deficiency, factor deficiency, or liver disease may bleed excessively and form a hematoma. Such patients should be monitored carefully after the procedure to be sure bleeding has been controlled. Arterial spasm preventing aspiration of the specimen and thrombosis of the punctured artery can occur.

Specimen Arterial blood **CONTAINER:** Heparinized syringe with 21- or 23-gauge needle. Alternatively, a 21- or 23-gauge Butterfly® infusion set may be used. **COLLECTION:** The experienced arterial puncturist should carefully select an appropriate artery. If the radial artery is to be used, Allen's test to assure collateral circulation to the hand from the ulnar artery is performed. To perform the Allen's test, the hand is closed tightly by the patient or by an assistant to form a fist. Pressure is then applied at the wrist, compressing and obstructing both the radial and ulnar arteries. The hand is then opened (but not fully extended), revealing a blanched palm and fingers. The obstructing pressure is next removed from only the ulnar artery while the palm and fingers, including thumb, are observed; they should become flushed within 15 seconds as the blood from the ulnar artery refills the empty capillary bed. If the ulnar artery does not adequately supply the entire hand (a negative Allen test), the radial artery should not be used as a puncture site; an alternate artery should be selected.[1] Recent studies have confirmed the efficacy and usefulness of this test.[2,3] Careful preparation of the puncture site is performed with 70% alcohol (isopropanol). The artery is stabilized by holding with a finger. Take care not to contaminate the puncture site. The artery is punctured at a 30° angle for the radial artery, 45° angle for the brachial, 45° or 90° angle for the femoral. The bevel of the needle or Butterfly® should be pointed toward the direction of blood flow. The syringe should fill spontaneously. Small bore needles or plastic syringes may require gentle slow suction. Be sure no air bubbles are aspirated into the syringe. After adequate sample volume is obtained quickly remove the needle and apply pressure. See Aftercare. Place specimen on ice after sealing the needle into a piece of hard rubber or plastic. Deliver to the laboratory within 15 minutes of collection. **STORAGE INSTRUCTIONS:** Keep the specimen air tight and water tight in a container of ice. This slows the metabolic rate of white cells in the specimen and reduces oxygen consumption. The specimen must be analyzed rapidly. Results are often needed urgently. **CAUSES FOR REJECTION:** Clots in the specimen

Interpretive **USE:** Obtain arterial blood for analysis **LIMITATIONS:** Arterial puncture should be performed by persons familiar with the procedure and the potential complications. Liquid sodium heparin should be used sparingly only to fill the needle and dead space. Excess heparin in the sample will lower the pH and pCO_2, pO_2 may be variably affected, and acid base calculations will be erroneous. Air bubbles in the syringe can greatly alter pO_2. **ADDITIONAL INFORMATION:** The evaluation of alveolar pO_2 is routinely done by assuming that the respiratory gas exchange ratio is equal to 0.8. A recent study of the respiratory gas exchange ratio in patients undergoing arterial puncture revealed that in approximately 25% of cases, there is a transient change in alveolar ventilation associated with arterial puncture that may cause a change in the gas exchange ratio and lead to at least a 10 mm Hg error in estimating alveolar pO_2.[4] Evidently, some patients respond to arterial puncture by transient breath holding or by taking rapid shallow breaths. Arterialized capillary blood is addressed in the listing, Skin Puncture Blood Collection in this chapter.

(Continued)

Arterial Blood Collection *(Continued)*

Footnotes

1. National Committee for Clinical Laboratory Standards, "Percutaneous Collection of Arterial Blood for Laboratory Analysis," Approved Standard, ANSI/NCCLS H11-A-2985, Villanova, PA: National Committee for Clinical Laboratory Standards, 1985.
2. Fuhrman TM, Reilley TE, and Pippin WD, "Comparison of Digital Blood Pressure, Plethysmography, and the Modified Allen's Test as Means of Evaluating the Collateral Circulation to the Hand," *Anaesthesia*, 1992, 47(11):959-61.
3. Choudhury RP and Cleator SJ, "An Examination of Needlestick Injury Rates, Hepatitis B Vaccination Uptake and Instruction on "Sharps" Technique Among Medical Students," *J Hosp Infect*, 1992, 22(2):143-8.
4. Cinel D, Markwell K, Lee R, et al, "Variability of the Respiratory Gas Exchange Ratio During Arterial Puncture," *Am Rev Respir Dis*, 1991, 143(2):217-8.

Arterialized Capillary Blood *see* Skin Puncture Blood Collection *on page 29*

Arterial Puncture *see* Arterial Blood Collection *on previous page*

Bacteriology Specimen Identification *see* Specimen Identification Requirements *on page 30*

Blood and Fluid Precautions, Specimen Collection

See Also Specimen Collection Section Introduction

Related Information

Arterial Blood Collection *on previous page*
Hepatitis B Surface Antigen *on page 688*
Phlebotomist Procedures *on page 28*
Skin Puncture Blood Collection *on page 29*
Venous Blood Collection *on page 32*

Synonyms Acquired Immunodeficiency Syndrome Precautions, Specimen Collection; AIDS Precautions, Specimen Collection; HIV Precautions, Specimen Collection; Isolation Patients, Precautions for Specimen Collection

Patient Care PREPARATION: The Occupational Safety and Health Administration (OSHA) Final Rule requires that the risk to healthcare workers of accidental exposure to infection be minimized. By careful planning and thoughtful attention to detail an appropriate and representative specimen can be safely collected. See Overview and Regulatory Considerations discussed in the introduction of this chapter.

Before entering the isolation room or drawing area:

Put on gloves.

Read the isolation sign on the door or patient's chart. It will explain the type of isolation and what you must wear and do. (**Follow these directions carefully.**)

Check your orders and assemble the equipment needed for this patient. Remember that anything taken into the room must be left there, discarded, or carefully cleansed if taken out of the room.

Find out if it is necessary to take a tourniquet and/or a plastic holder into the room. Many times these items will be there already.

Take in the minimum equipment needed: tourniquet (if one is not in the room); plastic holder (if one is not in the room); evacuated tube needle; alcohol sponges; evacuated blood collection tubes or blood culture media; glass slides (if a blood smear is to be made).

In the room:

Put on gloves.

Place paper towels on table and place your equipment on these towels.

Obtain blood samples in the usual manner, avoiding any unnecessary contact with the patient and the bed.

After obtaining blood samples, leave tourniquet and plastic holder in room and discard needle in proper container.

Wash hands.

Place several clean paper towels on the table, one on top of the other. If the outside of the tubes is contaminated, follow established laboratory decontamination procedures.

If blood smears were made, place smears on two clean paper towels. When ready to leave, wrap smears and tubes in the top paper towel and discard the bottom paper towel.

Label specimens for proper identification (see Specimen Identification Requirements listing) as directed by institutional policy. Label specimens for infectious hazards in a distinctive manner as required by institutional policy. Since the implementation of universal blood and body fluid precautions for **all** patients, special labeling for specific patients may be eliminated, depending upon institutional policies and local regulations. In any case, **universal precautions must be observed.**

Bring specimens to the laboratory.[1]

Specimen SPECIAL INSTRUCTIONS:

Precautions for laboratories: Blood and other body fluids from **all** patients should be considered infective. To supplement the universal blood and body fluid precautions, the following precautions are recommended for healthcare workers in clinical laboratories.

All specimens of blood and body fluids should be put in a well-constructed container with a secure lid to prevent leaking during transport. Care should be taken when collecting each specimen to avoid contamination of the outside of the container and of the laboratory form accompanying the specimen.

All persons collecting and processing blood and body fluid specimens should wear gloves. Masks, protective eyewear, and laboratory coats or gowns should be worn if contact with blood or body fluids is anticipated. Gloves should be changed and hands washed after completion of specimen processing.

For routine procedures, such as histologic and pathologic studies or microbiologic culturing, a biological safety cabinet is not necessary. However, biological safety cabinets (class I or II) should be used whenever procedures are conducted that have a high potential for generating droplets. These include activities such as blending, sonicating, and vigorous mixing. Mechanical pipetting devices should be used for manipulating all liquids in the laboratory. Mouth pipetting must not be done.

Use of needles and syringes should be limited to situations in which there is no alternative, and the recommendations for preventing injuries with needles outlined under universal precautions must be followed.

Laboratory work surfaces should be decontaminated with an appropriate chemical germicide after a spill of blood or other body fluids and when work activities are completed.

Contaminated materials used in laboratory tests should be decontaminated before reprocessing or be placed in bags and disposed of in accordance with institutional policies for disposal of infective waste.

Scientific equipment that has been contaminated with blood or other body fluids should be decontaminated and cleaned before being repaired in the laboratory or transported to the manufacturer.

All persons must wash their hands after completing laboratory activities and should remove personal protective equipment before leaving the laboratory.

Implementation of universal blood and body fluid precautions for **all** patients eliminates the need for warning labels on specimens since blood and other body fluids from all patients should be considered infective. OSHA rules, however, require "Biohazard" labeling or color coding of containers of regulated waste, refrigerators and freezers containing blood or other potentially infectious material, and containers used to store, transport, or ship such materials.

Interpretive ADDITIONAL INFORMATION: Human immunodeficiency virus (HIV), the virus that causes acquired immunodeficiency syndrome (AIDS), is transmitted through sexual contact, exposure to infected blood or blood components, and perinatally from mother to neonate. HIV has been isolated from blood, semen, vaginal secretions, saliva, tears, breast milk, cerebrospinal fluid, amniotic fluid, and urine and is likely to be isolated from other body fluids, secretions, and excretions. However, epidemiologic evidence has implicated only blood, semen, vaginal secretions, and possibly breast milk in transmission.

The increasing prevalence of HIV infection increases the risk that healthcare workers will be exposed to blood from patients infected with HIV, especially when blood and body fluid precautions are not followed for all patients. Thus, The Center for Disease Control (CDC) in its recommendations for prevention of HIV transmission in healthcare settings[2] emphasizes the need for healthcare workers to consider **all** patients as potentially infected with HIV and/or

(Continued)

Blood and Fluid Precautions, Specimen Collection *(Continued)*

other blood-borne pathogens and to adhere rigorously to infection control precautions for minimizing the risk of exposure to blood and body fluids of all patients.

The CDC universal precaution recommendations and the OSHA Final Rule regulations[2,3] have been developed for use in healthcare settings and emphasize the need to treat blood and other body fluids from **all** patients as potentially infective. These same prudent precautions also should be taken in other settings in which persons may be exposed to blood or other body fluids.

Precautions to Prevent Transmission of HIV – Universal Precautions: Since medical history and examination cannot reliably identify all patients infected with HIV or other blood-borne pathogens, blood and body fluid precautions should be consistently used for **all** patients. This approach, previously recommended by CDC and referred to as "universal blood and body fluid precautions" or "universal precautions," must be used in the care of **all** patients as a result of OSHA's Final Rule.[3]

All healthcare workers should routinely use appropriate barrier precautions to prevent skin and mucous membrane exposure when contact with blood or other body fluids of any patient is anticipated. Gloves should be worn for touching blood and body fluids, mucous membranes, or nonintact skin of all patients, for handling items on surfaces soiled with blood or body fluids, and for performing venipuncture and other vascular access procedures. Gloves should be changed after contact with each patient. Masks and protective eyewear or face shields should be worn during procedures that are likely to generate droplets of blood or other body fluids to prevent exposure of mucous membranes of the mouth, nose, and eyes. Laboratory coats, gowns, or aprons should be worn during procedures that are likely to generate splashes of blood or other body fluids.

Hands and other skin surfaces should be washed immediately and thoroughly if contaminated with blood or other body fluids. Hands should be washed immediately after gloves are removed.

All healthcare workers should take precautions to prevent injuries caused by needles, scalpels, and other sharp instruments or devices during procedures; when cleaning used instruments; during disposal of used needles; and when handling sharp instruments after procedures. To prevent needlestick injuries, needles should not be recapped, purposely bent or broken by hand, removed from disposable syringes, or otherwise manipulated by hand. After they are used, disposable syringes and needles, scalpel blades, and other sharp items should be placed in puncture-resistant containers for disposal; the puncture-resistant containers should be located as close as possible to the area of use. Large-bore reusable needles should be placed in a puncture-resistant container for transport to the reprocessing area.

Although saliva has not been implicated in HIV transmission, to minimize the need for emergency mouth-to-mouth resuscitation, mouthpieces, resuscitation bags, or other ventilation devices should be available for use in areas in which the need for resuscitation is predictable.

Healthcare workers who have exudative lesions or weeping dermatitis should refrain from all direct patient care and from handling patient care equipment until the condition resolves.

Pregnant healthcare workers are not known to be at greater risk of contracting HIV infection than healthcare workers who are not pregnant; however, if a healthcare worker develops HIV infection during pregnancy, the infant is at risk of infection resulting from perinatal transmission. Because of this risk, **pregnant healthcare workers should be especially familiar with and strictly adhere to precautions to minimize the risk of HIV transmission.**

Implementation of universal blood and body fluid precautions for **all** patients eliminates the need for use of the isolation category of "Blood and Body Fluid Precautions" previously recommended by CDC for patients known or suspected to be infected with blood-borne pathogens. Isolation precautions (eg, enteric, AFB) should be used as necessary if associated conditions, such as infectious diarrhea or tuberculosis, are diagnosed or suspected.

Environmental Considerations for HIV Transmission: No environmentally mediated mode of HIV transmission has been documented. Nevertheless, the precautions described should be taken routinely in the care of **all** patients.

Sterilization and Disinfection: Standard sterilization and disinfection procedures for patient care equipment currently recommended for use in a variety of healthcare settings, including hospitals, medical and dental clinics and offices, hemodialysis centers, emergency care facilities, and long-term nursing care facilities, are adequate to sterilize or disinfect instruments, devices, or other items contaminated with blood or other body fluids from persons infected with blood-borne pathogens including HIV.

Cleaning and Decontaminating Spills of Blood or Other Body Fluids: Chemical germicides that are approved for use as "hospital disinfectants" and are tuberculocidal when used at recommended dilutions can be used to decontaminate spills of blood and other body fluids. Strategies for decontaminating spills of blood and other body fluids in a patient care setting are different than for spills of cultures or other materials in clinical, public health, or research laboratories. In patient care areas, visible material should first be removed and then the area should be decontaminated. With large spills of cultured or concentrated infectious agents in the laboratory, the contaminated area should be flooded with a liquid germicide before cleaning, then decontaminated with fresh germicidal chemical. In both settings, gloves should be worn during the cleaning and decontaminating procedures.

Studies have shown that HIV is inactivated rapidly after being exposed to commonly used chemical germicides at concentrations that are much lower than used in practice. Embalming fluids (formalin preparations) are similar to the types of chemical germicides that have been tested and found to completely inactivate HIV. Formalin may not rapidly inactivate hepatitis B virus nor quickly kill bacteria. It is a slow-acting antiseptic agent requiring 18 hours or more to kill microorganisms. In addition to commercially available chemical germicides, a solution of sodium hypochlorite (household bleach) prepared daily is an inexpensive and effective germicide. Concentrations ranging from approximately 500 ppm (1:100 dilution of household bleach) sodium hypochlorite to 5000 ppm (1:10 dilution of household bleach) are effective depending on the amount of organic material (eg, blood, mucus) present on the surface to be cleaned and disinfected. Commercially available chemical germicides may be more compatible with certain medical devices that might be corroded by repeated exposure to sodium hypochlorite.

Housekeeping: Environmental surfaces such as walls, floors, and other surfaces are not associated with transmission of infections to patients or healthcare workers. Therefore, extraordinary attempts to disinfect or sterilize these environmental surfaces are not necessary. However, cleaning and removal of soil should be done routinely.

Cleaning schedules and methods vary according to the area of the hospital or institution, type of surface to be cleaned, and the amount and type of soil present. Horizontal surfaces (eg, bedside tables and hard-surfaced flooring) in patient care areas are usually cleaned on a regular basis, when soiling or spills occur, and when a patient is discharged. Cleaning of walls, blinds, and curtains is recommended only if they are visibly soiled. Disinfectant fogging is an unsatisfactory method of decontaminating air and surfaces and is not recommended.

Disinfectant detergent formulations registered by EPA may be used for cleaning environmental surfaces, but the actual physical removal of microorganisms by scrubbing is probably at least as important as any antimicrobial effect of the cleaning agent used. Therefore, cost, safety, and acceptability by housekeepers can be the main criteria for selecting any such registered agent. The manufacturers' instructions for appropriate use should be followed.

Laundry: Although soiled linen has been identified as a source of large numbers of certain pathogenic microorganisms, the risk of actual disease transmission is negligible. Rather than rigid procedures and specifications, hygienic and common sense storage and processing of clean and soiled linen are recommended. Soiled linen should be handled as little as possible with minimum agitation to prevent gross microbial contamination of the air and of persons handling the linen. All soiled linen should be bagged at the location where it was used; it should not be sorted or rinsed in patient care areas. Linen soiled with blood or body fluids must be placed and transported in bags that prevent leakage.

Infective Waste: There is no epidemiologic evidence to suggest that most hospital waste is any more infective than residential waste. Moreover, there is no epidemiologic evidence that hospital waste has caused disease in the community as a result of improper disposal. Therefore, identifying wastes for which special precautions are indicated is largely a matter of judgment about the relative risk of disease transmission. The most practical approach to the management of infective waste is to identify those wastes with the potential for causing infection during handling and disposal and for which some special precautions appear prudent. Hospital wastes for which special precautions are required include microbiology laboratory waste,

(Continued)

Blood and Fluid Precautions, Specimen Collection *(Continued)*

pathology waste, blood specimens or blood products, and other potentially infectious material. Any item that has had contact with blood, exudates, or secretions may be potentially infective. Infective waste, in general, should either be incinerated or should be autoclaved before disposal in a sanitary landfill. Bulk blood, suctioned fluids, excretions, and secretions may be carefully poured down a drain connected to a sanitary sewer. Sanitary sewers may also be used to dispose of other infectious wastes capable of being ground and flushed into the sewer.

Survival of HIV in the Environment: The most extensive study on the survival of HIV after drying involved greatly concentrated HIV samples (ie, 10 million tissue culture infectious doses/mL). This concentration is at least 100,000 times greater than that typically found in the blood or serum of patients with HIV infection. HIV was detectable by tissue culture techniques 1-3 days after drying, but the rate of inactivation was rapid. Studies performed at CDC have also shown that drying HIV causes a rapid (within several hours) 1-2 log (90% to 99%) reduction in HIV concentration. In tissue culture fluid, cell-free HIV could be detected up to 15 days at room temperature, up to 11 days at 37°C (98.6°F), and up to 1 day if the HIV was cell-associated.

When considered in the context of environmental conditions in healthcare facilities, these results do not require any changes in currently recommended sterilization, disinfection, or housekeeping strategies. When medical devices are contaminated with blood or other body fluids, existing recommendations include the cleaning of these instruments followed by disinfection or sterilization, depending on the type of medical device. These protocols assume "worst case" conditions of extreme virologic and microbiologic contamination and whether or not viruses have been inactivated after drying plays no role in formulating these strategies. Consequently, no changes in the published procedures for cleaning, disinfecting, or sterilizing need to be made.

Risk to Healthcare Workers of Acquiring HIV in Healthcare Settings: Healthcare workers with documented percutaneous or mucous membrane exposures to blood or body fluids of HIV-infected patients have been prospectively evaluated to determine the risk of infection after such exposures. The risk of HIV-1 transmission associated with a percutaneous exposure to blood from an HIV-1 infected patient is approximately 0.3% per exposure (95 CI, 0.13% to 0.70%). The risks associated with occupational mucous membrane and cutaneous exposures are likely to be substantially smaller. Universal precautions are widely considered effective in reducing the risk of occupational exposures among healthcare workers,[4] and in a prospective study, physicians on a medical service.[5]

Footnotes

1. Bennett BD, Cox RS, Davis CM, et al, eds, *So You're Going to Collect a Blood Specimen: An Introduction to Phlebotomy*, 5th ed, Northfield, IL: College of American Pathologists, 1992.
2. "Leads From the *MMWR*. Update: Universal Precautions for Prevention of Transmission of Human Immunodeficiency Virus, Hepatitis B Virus, and Other Bloodborne Pathogens in Healthcare Settings," *JAMA*, 1988, 260(4):462-5.
3. Department of Labor, Occupational Safety and Health Administration, "Occupational Exposure to Bloodborne Pathogens; Final Rule (29 CFR Part 1910.1030)," *Federal Register*, 1991, 64004-182.
4. Henderson DK, Fahey BJ, Willy M, et al, "Risk for Occupational Transmission of Human Immunodeficiency Virus Type 1 (HIV-1) Associated With Clinical Exposures – A Prospective Evaluation," *Ann Intern Med*, 1990, 113(10):740-6.
5. Wong ES, Stotka JL, Chinchilli VM, et al, "Are Universal Precautions Effective in Reducing the Number of Occupational Exposures Among Healthcare Workers? A Prospective Study of Physicians on a Medical Service," *JAMA*, 1991, 265(9):1123-8.

References

"Agent Summary Statement for Human Immunodeficiency Viruses (HIVs) Including HTLV-III, LAV, HIV-1, and HIV-2," *MMWR Morb Mortal Wkly Rep*, 1988, 37:1-17.

Blood Collection Tube Information

Related Information

Chain-of-Custody Protocol *on page 952*
Phlebotomist Procedures *on page 28*
Venous Blood Collection *on page 32*

Synonyms Blood Container Description; Vacutainer® Tube Description

Specimen SPECIAL INSTRUCTIONS: **See individual listings throughout this book for particular test requirements.**

Interpretive ADDITIONAL INFORMATION: The following table describes standard color codes, optimum and minimum volumes required, and additives contained in common vacuum draw tubes. **It is important to be certain that a tube is filled with the prescribed minimum volume in order to avoid spurious results due to an inappropriate anticoagulant to specimen ratio.**

Tube Codes

Color	Optimum Volume/Minimum Volume	Additive
Blue	4.5 mL/4.5 mL	Sodium citrate
Blue/navy	7 mL	No additive (for trace metals) Heparin (for trace metals)
Culture (yellow top)	8.3 mL/8.3 mL	SPS
FSP (blue top)	2 mL/2 mL	Thrombin, trypsin inhibitor
Gray	5 mL/5 mL 7 mL/7 mL	Potassium oxalate, sodium fluoride
Green	10 mL/3.5 mL	Heparin
Lavender	7 mL/2 mL	EDTA
Orange	10 mL/NA	Thrombin
Red	10 mL/NA	None
Red/gray (gel)	10 mL/NA	Inert barrier material; clot activator
Yellow	5 mL/NA	ACD
Yellow/black	7 mL	Thrombin
Pediatric Tubes		
Blue	2.7 mL/2.7 mL	Sodium citrate
Culture (yellow top)	3.3 mL/3.3 mL	SPS
Green	2 mL/2 mL	Heparin
Lavender	2 mL/0.6 mL 3 mL/0.9 mL 4 mL/1 mL	EDTA
Red	2 mL/NA 3 mL/NA 4 mL/NA	None

Special needs exist for specimens for coagulation testing. These are addressed in that chapter.

See introduction to the chapter Transfusion Service for specimen requirements.

The introduction to the chapter Trace Metals provides information for specimens drawn for those substances.

See introduction to the chapter Therapeutic Drug Monitoring/Toxicology/Drugs of Abuse and other portions of that chapter for appropriate specimen requirements. It addresses anticonvulsants (antiepileptic drugs), antibiotic and cardiac drug levels, peaks and troughs, as well as collections for drugs of abuse. Chain-of-custody information is provided as a listing and in the Appendix of that chapter.

Blood Collection, Venous *see* Venous Blood Collection *on page 32*

Blood Container Description *see* Blood Collection Tube Information *on previous page*

Blood Specimen Identification *see* Specimen Identification Requirements *on page 30*

Body Fluid Identification *see* Specimen Identification Requirements *on page 30*

Phlebotomist Procedures

Related Information

Blood and Fluid Precautions, Specimen Collection *on page 22*
Blood Collection Tube Information *on page 26*
Skin Puncture Blood Collection *on next page*
Specimen Identification Requirements *on page 30*
Venous Blood Collection *on page 32*

Synonyms Specimen Collection Policy, Phlebotomist

Specimen COLLECTION: Phlebotomists are generally required to adhere to the following procedures. Phlebotomists are only allowed to obtain samples from patients who have been positively identified. See Specimen Identification Requirements listing. Phlebotomists are limited to attempting venipunctures in upper extremities unless so ordered by the physician. Phlebotomists may not perform a venipuncture above an I.V. site or in an arm with a heparin lock or shunt. Only by a physician's order may a trained phlebotomist collect a sample from a fistula or shunt. Phlebotomists should not collect a sample from an arm which is on the same side as a recent mastectomy. Phlebotomists are generally limited to two attempts to obtain a blood sample. After two unsuccessful tries, the phlebotomist must call another phlebotomist or supervisor. If the second phlebotomist is unsuccessful, the physician or responsible nurse will be notified. Phlebotomists are not allowed to force a patient to have blood drawn. If a patient refuses, the phlebotomist will notify the responsible nurse or physician. The phlebotomist will perform skin punctures when ordered by the physician (with some exceptions) or if venipuncture is unsuccessful or prohibited (due to I.V., etc), provided the procedure requested can be performed on a skin puncture specimen. (Dependent on the policy and equipment available in laboratory receiving the specimen.) See Skin Puncture Blood Collection. SPECIAL INSTRUCTIONS: The perception of pain associated with venipuncture in children increases with anxiety and is inversely correlated with the patient's age.[1] Strategies to reduce the child's and parents' distress during venipuncture are important considerations.[2,3] The use of topical anesthetics has also been suggested.[4] More than 33% of adult patients report needle discomfort greater than expected.[5] Every effort should be made to improve patient satisfaction by reducing discomfort from phlebotomy procedures.

Footnotes

1. Lander J, Fowler-Kerry S, and Oberle S, "Children's Venipuncture Pain: Influence of Technical Factors," *J Pain Symptom Manage*, 1992, 7(6):343-9.
2. Manne SL, Redd WH, Jacobsen PB, et al, "Behavioral Intervention to Reduce Child and Parent Distress During Venipuncture," *J Consult Clin Psychol*, 1990, 58(5):565-72.
3. Harrison A, "Preparing Children for Venous Blood Sampling," *Pain*, 1991, 45(3):299-306.
4. Woolfson AD, McCafferty DF, and Boston V, "Clinical Experiences With a Novel Percutaneous Amethocaine Preparation: Prevention of Pain Due to Venipuncture in Children," *Br J Clin Pharmacol*, 1990, 30(2):273-9.
5. Howanitz PJ, Cembrowski GS, and Bachner P, "Laboratory Phlebotomy – College of American Pathologists Q-Probe Study of Patient Satisfaction and Complications in 23,783 Patients," *Arch Pathol Lab Med*, 1991, 115(9):867-72.

References

Bennett BD, Cox RS, Davis CM, et al, eds, *So You're Going to Collect a Blood Specimen: An Introduction to Phlebotomy*, 5th ed, Northfield, IL: College of American Pathologists, 1992.

Phlebotomy, Venous *see* Venous Blood Collection *on page 32*

Rejection Criteria, Specimen *see* Specimen Rejection Criteria *on page 31*

Requisition Information *see* Specimen Identification Requirements *on next page*

Skin Puncture Blood Collection

***CPT** 36415*

Related Information

Blood and Fluid Precautions, Specimen Collection *on page 22*
Phlebotomist Procedures *on previous page*
Specimen Identification Requirements *on next page*

Synonyms Capillary Blood Collection; Fingerstick Blood Collection; Heelstick Blood Collection

Applies to Arterialized Capillary Blood; Peripheral Blood Smear Preparation

Test Commonly Includes Obtaining capillary blood from finger tip of an adult or heel in infants

Patient Care PREPARATION:

Heel puncture: Select a site on the medial or lateral portion of the plantar surface of the foot. Do not puncture greater than 2.4 mm. Do not puncture the posterior curvature of the heel.[1] Do not repuncture previous puncture sites because of the possibility of infection.

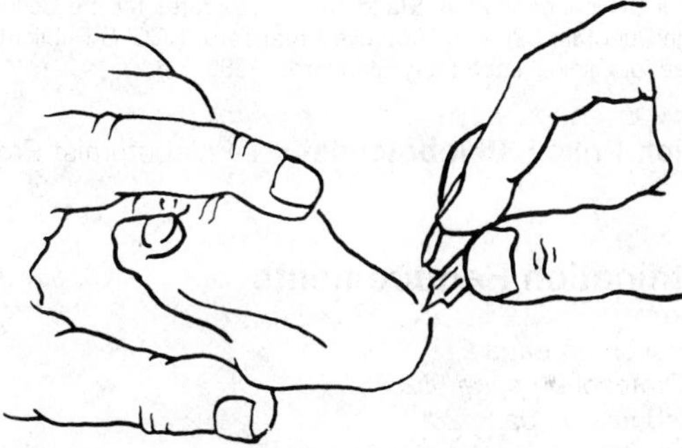

Gloves should be worn when collecting capillary blood specimens. From JD Bauer, *Clinical Laboratory Methods*, 9th ed, St Louis, MO: Mosby-Year Book Inc, 1982, with permission.

Finger puncture: Select a site on the palmar aspect on the center of distal phalanx. Do not puncture the side or tip of the phalanx because the skin is much thinner.

Skin preparation: The skin site selected should be cleaned with 75% alcohol (isopropanol) and dried with sterile gauze. Infection is a frequent complication of fingersticks. Prepare the skin site carefully. Do not use iodine as it interferes with many assays.

Arterialized blood: Warming the site with a moist towel at temperatures not to exceed 42°C produces an increase in blood flow and **arterializes the capillary blood**. pH and blood gas determinations are usually performed on arterialized capillary blood in infants and children.

AFTERCARE: Elevate the site above the body and apply direct pressure to the puncture site with sterile gauze until bleeding stops. Bandaids or bandages are generally not applied because of the risk of skin sensitization to tape and the risk of aspiration, should the bandage come loose.

Specimen Capillary blood or arterialized capillary blood CONTAINER: Capillary tube or microtube COLLECTION: Patient identification: Confirm that the patient being drawn is the correct one by comparing the requisition with the identification wristband. After preparation of the selected site, the skin should be punctured at a slight angle. A disposable skin puncture lancet should be used rather than a surgical blade because a surgical blade may make too deep an incision and damage underlying tissues. The first drop should be wiped away as it may con-

(Continued)

Skin Puncture Blood Collection *(Continued)*

tain tissue fluid. Blood flow will be increased by holding the site downward. Slight pressure may be applied to the surrounding tissue. **Squeezing or milking should not be done.** Tubes should be sealed quickly to avoid exposure to atmospheric oxygen. Specimen identification: The specimen should be labeled with the patient's name, hospital number, room number, date and time of collection, and initials or identification of the person collecting the specimen. SPECIAL INSTRUCTIONS: Avoid injury to the calcaneus (heel bone). Be aware of the volume of specimen being collected from a newborn.

Interpretive USE: Obtain capillary or arterialized capillary blood for analysis. Collection of blood from infants and children, patients who have had repeated venipunctures or whose veins are damaged or inadequate. Procedure of choice for preparing peripheral blood smears for morphologic examinations. LIMITATIONS: Technically, a specimen obtained by skin puncture consists of a mixture of arterial, capillary, and venous blood, and tissue fluid. Specimen volume is limited. Repeat determinations often require repeat blood collection. Finger tips are sensitive; the procedure may be painful. Infection, particularly in debilitated hosts, may occur. Cell counts (ie, RBC, WBC, and platelets) are not accurate on capillary specimens. CONTRAINDICATIONS: Use of surgical blades may create a wound deeper and larger than necessary and are contraindicated. **Finger punctures should not be performed on infants because the distance from the skin to the bone is less than 1.5 mm.** ADDITIONAL INFORMATION: Capillary blood is the specimen of choice for the preparation of peripheral blood smears.

Footnotes

1. Blumenfeld TA, Turi GK, and Blanc WA, "Recommended Sites and Depth of Newborn Heel Skin Punctures Based on Anatomic Measurements and Histopathology," *Lancet*, 1979, 1:230-3.

References

National Committee for Clinical Laboratory Standards, "Procedures for the Collection of Diagnostic Blood Specimens by Skin Puncture," 2nd ed, Approved Standard, NCCLS Publication H4-A2, Villanova, PA: National Committee for Clinical Laboratory Standards, 1986.

Specimen Collection Policy, Phlebotomist *see* Phlebotomist Procedures *on page 28*

Specimen Identification Requirements

Related Information

Arterial Blood Collection *on page 21*
Chain-of-Custody Protocol *on page 952*
Phlebotomist Procedures *on page 28*
Skin Puncture Blood Collection *on previous page*
Urine Collection, 24-Hour *on page 32*
Venous Blood Collection *on page 32*

Synonyms Identification Requirements, Specimen

Applies to Bacteriology Specimen Identification; Blood Specimen Identification; Body Fluid Identification; Cytology Smear Identification; Pathology Specimen Identification; Requisition Information; Spinal Fluid Identification; Urine Specimen Identification

Specimen CAUSES FOR REJECTION: Laboratories reserve the right to refuse improperly labeled specimens. Accurate specimen identification is critical to the provision of accurate results. SPECIAL INSTRUCTIONS: Patient identification: Inpatient: Compare the information on the request form with the patient's identification band and room and bed number. Confirm identification by asking the patient to state his/her full name. If the patient cannot state his/her name, ask a nurse or patient's relative to confirm the patient's identity. Confirm that the specimen label information is identical to the wristband and request form information. Label specimens as indicated below. Outpatient: Confirm identification by asking the patient to state his/her full name. If the patient cannot state his/her name, ask a nurse or patient's relative to confirm the patient's identity. Confirm the specimen label information is identical to the wristband and request form information. The requirements for labeling specimens and requisitions are as follows.

Blood specimens: All blood specimens received by the laboratory must have a permanently attached label with the following information written in black indelible ink: patient's name, hospital number, date and time of collection, initials of person drawing the specimen. Person obtaining blood sample must perform the proper identification check. Draw the sample of blood. Label all the tubes at the patient's bedside. Certain blood tests require special or immediate handling after collection. Consult the individual test listings for specific information and also the Transfusion Service/Blood Bank introductory text for specifics on Blood Bank patient identification.

Urine specimens: All urine specimens received by the laboratory must have the following information fixed to the container (not cover): patient's name, hospital number, date and time of collection. Urine specimens delivered to the laboratory must be placed in the specimen refrigerator. Certain urine tests require special or immediate handling after collection. Consult the individual test listings for specific information.

Cerebrospinal fluids: Each tube submitted must be labeled with the patient's name, hospital number, source of specimen, date and time of collection, tube identification number (1, 2, 3 according to the order of collection). Spinal fluid tests are usually considered to be stat procedures because spinal fluid constituents are unstable. Consequently, spinal fluid must be taken to the laboratory immediately after collection and handed to a technologist or receptionist. Consult the individual test listings for specific information.

Body fluids: All body fluids must be labeled with the patient's name, hospital number, date and time of collection, source of fluid. Body fluid constituents are unstable, and thus, expeditious handling is required. Consult the individual test listings for specific information.

Cytology smears: All slides for cytologic examination should be appropriately and immediately fixed, labeled with the patient's name, and placed in a cardboard folder with the cytology requisition slip containing patient's name, patient information, and physician's name wrapped around it. Further information is provided in the Cytopathology chapter.

Bacteriology specimens: All specimens for bacteriology testing must be labeled with the patient's name, hospital number, date and time of collection, source of material. Bacteriology specimens should be delivered to the laboratory as soon after collection as possible to preserve the viability of bacteria or viruses.

Pathology (surgical) specimens: All specimens for pathology must be labeled with the patient's name, hospital number, name of physician, name of surgeon, and source of specimen. Further information is available in the Anatomic Pathology chapter. For many but not all specimens, the listing Histopathology provides detailed information. Consult individual test listings for specific information pertinent to specimens requiring special handling.

Chain-of-custody specimens: Specimens for drugs of abuse screening and specimens which may be used as legal evidence must be collected according to a chain-of-custody protocol. For further information, see the listing, Chain-of-Custody Protocol, as well as the Appendix in the Therapeutic Drug Monitoring/Toxicology/Drugs of Abuse chapter.

Specimen Rejection Criteria

Synonyms Rejection Criteria, Specimen; Unsatisfactory Specimens Criteria

Specimen CAUSES FOR REJECTION: Criteria for specimen rejection are dependent on individual tests and information may be found under Causes for Rejection in the specimen section under each individual test listings. Generally specimens received by a laboratory are not discarded until the physician ordering the test or responsible nursing unit is notified. Events which may lead to the rejection of a specimen include specimen improperly labeled or unlabeled, specimen improperly collected and/or preserved, specimen submitted without properly completed request form, specimen sample volume not sufficient for requirement of test protocol, outside of container contaminated by specimen (ie, infectious hazard), or patient not properly prepared for test requirements. It is ultimately the responsibility of the ordering physician to make certain that the laboratory is provided with a properly collected and identified specimen for analysis. Communications regarding less than optimal specimens generally should be oriented toward concern for patient welfare and not nonavailability or unwillingness to provide laboratory service.

Spinal Fluid Identification *see* Specimen Identification Requirements *on previous page*

Twenty-Four Hour Urine Collection *see* Urine Collection, 24-Hour *on next page*

Unsatisfactory Specimens Criteria *see* Specimen Rejection Criteria *on this page*

Urine Collection, 12-Hour, 2-Hour, and Timed *see* Urine Collection, 24-Hour *on this page*

Urine Collection, 24-Hour

Related Information

Alcohol, Blood or Urine *on page 936*
Chromium, Urine *on page 1023*
Copper, Urine *on page 1027*
Drugs of Abuse Testing, Urine *on page 962*
Manganese, Urine *on page 1031*
Selenium, Urine *on page 1035*
Specimen Identification Requirements *on page 30*
Zinc, Urine *on page 1038*

Synonyms Twenty-Four Hour Urine Collection

Applies to Urine Collection, 12-Hour, 2-Hour, and Timed

Specimen **COLLECTION:** Twenty-four hour urine collections have always been a problem for both patient and laboratory. A good collection regimen is as follows: Discard first morning specimen on day one. Collect all specimens during the remainder of the day and evening. Collect the first morning specimen on day two. Stop collection. Label specimen with patient's name, hospital number, room number, and date and time of collection. This presumes that time of arising is the same on day one and day two. Alternate regimen: Patient is to empty his/her bladder completely at a designated time (for example, 8 AM). This specimen is discarded. All urine is saved throughout the day and evening. Patient is to empty his/her bladder at the same time on day two as in step 1 above (for example, 8 AM). This specimen is combined with the rest of the collection for the previous 24 hours. Stop collection. Label specimen with patient's name, hospital number, room number, date and time of collection. Normal fluid intake is allowed during 24-hour urine collections. Dietary restrictions are required for some procedures and are specified in the individual test listing. Since results are based on total volume, it is critical that the volume be measured accurately and the information included with the test requisition. Clearance tests require an estimate of body surface area; patient's height and weight must be available to the laboratory or recorded on the requisition whenever a clearance is requested. **SPECIAL INSTRUCTIONS:** See instructions in the particular listings listed above under Related Information for urine collections for trace metals. See specific instructions elsewhere in this book under specific listings for collection procedures for other substances. For information on urine collection procedures for drugs of abuse testing, see the introduction to the Therapeutic Drug Monitoring/Toxicology/Drugs of Abuse chapter.

Interpretive **LIMITATIONS:** Some tests require a critical minimal volume for accuracy. For example, some Schilling test protocols require a minimum of 500 mL/24 hours, and are unreliable for reduced urine volumes. Consult individual test listings for information on critical urine volumes. **ADDITIONAL INFORMATION:** The procedure may be followed for other timed collections (ie, 12-hour, etc) as follows: Discard the initial specimen. Record time. Collect all specimens voided within the requested time frame. Label the specimen with patient's name, hospital number, room number, and date and time of collection.

Urine Specimen Identification *see* Specimen Identification Requirements *on page 30*

Vacutainer® Tube Description *see* Blood Collection Tube Information *on page 26*

Venipuncture, Venous *see* Venous Blood Collection *on this page*

Venous Blood Collection

CPT *36415*

Related Information

Alcohol, Blood or Urine *on page 936*
Blood and Fluid Precautions, Specimen Collection *on page 22*
Blood Collection Tube Information *on page 26*
Chain-of-Custody Protocol *on page 952*
Phlebotomist Procedures *on page 28*
Specimen Identification Requirements *on page 30*

Synonyms Blood Collection, Venous; Phlebotomy, Venous; Venipuncture, Venous

Test Commonly Includes Routine method for obtaining blood when anticoagulants or larger volumes than can be obtained by capillary blood collection are required

Patient Care PREPARATION: Select a suitable site for venipuncture. Prepare the site by scrubbing with 70% alcohol (isopropanol), dry with gauze. Special requirements exist for alcohol levels; see Alcohol, Blood or Urine in the Chemistry chapter. AFTERCARE: Apply pressure to the venipuncture site and elevate the arm until bleeding stops. If bleeding persists, apply a pressure dressing to the site.

Specimen Venous blood CONTAINER: Syringe with a 20- or 21-gauge needle for volumes up to 10 mL, 18-gauge for larger volumes to assure adequate blood flow. Use a Vacutainer® or similar system for multiple specimens or anticoagulants. A 20- or 21-gauge Butterfly® infusion set may be used for difficult draws or blood cultures with multiple tubes. COLLECTION: Cleanly puncture the vein, loosen the tourniquet, and apply gentle suction or insert Vacutainer® tube into holder to fill tubes. Release the tourniquet, remove the needle, and fill the tubes without delay. See figure. **Gently invert tubes 10 times to assure mixing of anticoagulants.**

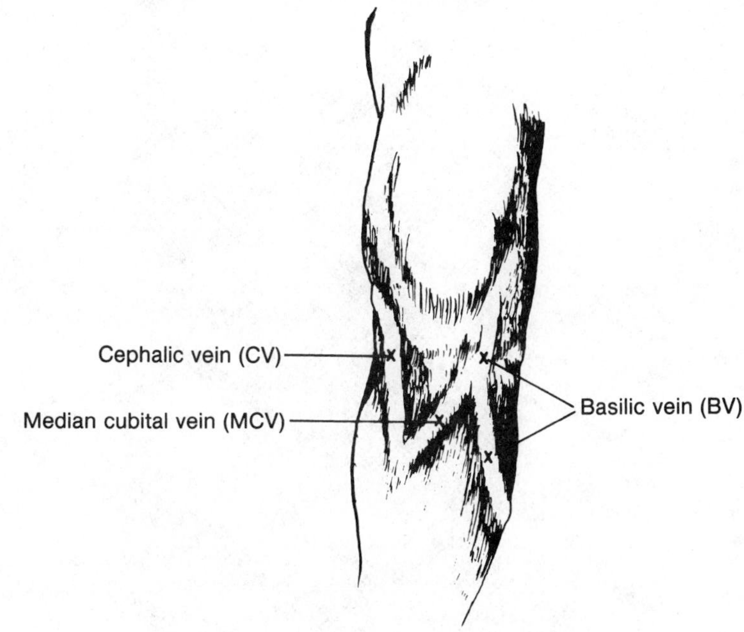

From JD Bauer, *Clinical Laboratory Methods*, 9th ed, St Louis, MO: Mosby-Year Book Inc, 1982, with permission.

CAUSES FOR REJECTION: Samples collected for coagulation studies which have <90% of the expected fill may be rejected. Samples collected for coagulation studies may require additional anticoagulant if the hematocrit is low. Grossly hemolyzed specimens may be rejected depending on tests requested.

Interpretive USE: Obtain venous blood for analysis LIMITATIONS: Venipuncture is technically difficult in obese patients, infants, children, patients with collapsed veins, such as those in shock, and occasionally, other subjects as well. Hemolysis may occur as a result of excessive suction during collection, violent mixing of the specimen, or vigorous transfer of the specimen from syringe to tube. ADDITIONAL INFORMATION: **See individual test listings for specific specimen collection requirements.** To avoid contamination with tissue thromboplastins released by the venipuncture, a two-syringe or two-tube collection technique, in which the first tube is discarded, is required for coagulation specimens (eg, prothrombin time, partial thromboplastin time, etc).

References

Bennett BD, Cox RS, Davis CM, et al, eds, *So You're Going to Collect a Blood Specimen: An Introduction to Phlebotomy*, 5th ed, Northfield, IL: College of American Pathologists, 1992.

(Continued)

Venous Blood Collection *(Continued)*

National Committee for Clinical Laboratory Standards, "Collection, Transport, and Preparation of Blood Specimens for Coagulation Testing and Performance of Coagulation Assays," Approved Guideline, NCCLS Document H21-A, Villanova, PA: National Committee for Clinical Laboratory Standards, 1986.

National Committee for Clinical Laboratory Standards, "Procedures for the Collection of Diagnostic Blood Specimens by Venipuncture," 2nd ed, Approved Standard, NCCLS Publication H3-A2, Villanova, PA: NCCLS, 1984.

National Committee for Clinical Laboratory Standards, "Procedures for the Handling and Processing of Blood Specimens, Approved Guideline," NCCLS Publication H18-A, Villanova, PA: National Committee for Clinical Laboratory Standards, 1990.

ANATOMIC PATHOLOGY

David S. Jacobs, MD
Eugene S. Olsowka, MD, PhD
Phillip A. Munoz, MD

The specialty of anatomic pathology is the morphologic study, both gross and microscopic, of the effects of disease on tissue. It forms the basis of much of our current knowledge on the form and cause of disease. The discipline has been greatly enhanced by increases in sophistication of instruments and technology, including the quality and capabilities of our reagents.

The autopsy is the ultimate quality control procedure in the care of patients. It remains the validator or the invalidator of the results of many of the more recent diagnostic modalities.

As anatomic pathology has become more complex, it has become increasingly difficult for any single pathologist to remain easily familiar with all current information about all of its branches. We have therefore asked a number of other pathologists to help. These contributors and their specialty areas are listed below.

Jaime A. Diaz, MD	Kidney Biopsy
Raoul Fresco, MD	Electron Microscopy
John G. Gruhn, MD	Skin Biopsy
Michael S. Handler, MD	Muscle Biopsy
David F. Keren, MD	Tumor Aneuploidy by Flow Cytometry
Lowell L. Tilzer, MD, PhD	Image Analysis

Alpha Fetoprotein *see* Immunoperoxidase Procedures *on page 60*

Aneuploidy *see* Tumor Aneuploidy by Flow Cytometry *on page 88*

Autopsy

CPT *88000 (necropsy (autopsy), gross examination only without CNS); 88005 (with brain); 88007 (with brain and spinal cord); 88012 (infant with brain); 88014 (stillborn or newborn with brain); 88016 (macerated stillborn); 88020 (necropsy (autopsy), gross and microscopic without CNS); 88025 (with brain); 88027 (with brain and spinal cord); 88028 (infant with brain); 88029 (stillborn or newborn with brain); 88036 (necropsy (autopsy) limited, gross and/or microscopic, regional); 88037 (single organ); 88040 (necropsy (autopsy) forensic examination); 88045 (coroner's call); 88099 (unlisted necropsy (autopsy) procedure)*

Synonyms Necropsy; Postmortem Examination

Applies to Cause of Death; Coroner's Case; Death Certificate; Disease Reporting; Medical Examiner's Case; Quality Assurance in the Practice of Medicine; Vital Statistics

Abstract The expression means to see for oneself, or to see with one's own eyes.

Specimen **SPECIAL INSTRUCTIONS:** **Consent:** A hospital autopsy is not usually performed until the pathologist has, in hand, a properly signed autopsy permit. A valid permit must contain the signature of the highest ranking survivor in the next-of-kin lineage. A commonly used decreasing order of responsibility: spouse, adult children, parents, adult brothers and sisters, relatives, and then anyone who will accept responsibility for the body for purposes of burial. (Check your own state laws.) Witnesses are often required to sign necropsy permits. The topic of consent has been reviewed, with details about some individual state statutes.[1] **It is desirable as well as courteous for the attending physician to discuss the clinical particulars with the pathologist before the dissection is begun.** In regard to physician attendance at autopsy, some of the most important clinicopathologic correlations and in-depth investigations occur in autopsies at which clinicians attend. There are frequently matters discussed which are not in the chart and morphologic findings may provide immediate feedback to a clinician in a way unavailable to him/her from even a long written autopsy report. Clinician attendance at autopsy is always rewarding to everyone involved and improves the quality of the case. It is unfortunate that some nonphysicians and some physicians are unable to recognize the benefits of attendance at autopsy. Particularly in autopsies on nonadmitted individuals, critical clinical facts are likely to be unavailable, fragmentary, or completely unknown. The presence of the attending physician at such autopsies compensates to some degree for the lack of a well worked up chart. It is usually the responsibility of the attending physician to obtain permission for the autopsy from the next-of-kin. Except in coroner's cases, it is usually the responsibility of the attending physician to complete the death certificate.

Interpretive **USE:** Determine cause and manner of death; determine severity of disease; an effort to preserve the quality of medical practice and to support excellence in medicine (quality assurance); enhance medical knowledge and generate sound information needed for research; understand pathogenesis; diagnose hereditary/familial diseases relevant to genetic counseling and possibly pertinent to surviving relatives; diagnose contagious diseases. The autopsy provides valid comparisons between premortem and postmortem diagnoses. It produces valid statistics not otherwise available. Autopsies provide information on effects of environment; document certain environmental or occupational exposures and provide data relevant to the public health and vital statistics. Autopsies yield information on the success or failure of therapy. The autopsy is a teaching instrument of great value and remains a component of good medical care. It has recently been described as a vital clinical quality control measure,[2] a definitive monitor of quality of care given to the patient or by the medical system;[3] *vide infra*. The autopsy may support or provide recognition of new medical entities, such as acquired immunodeficiency syndrome (AIDS), toxic shock syndrome, microbiology of Legionnaires' disease, and sudden infant death syndrome (SIDS). **CONTRAINDICATIONS:** Improperly completed written permission **METHODOLOGY:** Gross organ and microscopic tissue examination with subsequent special procedures as indicated **ADDITIONAL INFORMATION:**

CORONER'S CASES:

In possible medical legal cases, the Coroner's Office or Medical Examiner should be contacted before any suggestion regarding autopsy permission is made to the family of the deceased. Cases falling under the jurisdiction of the coroner usually include all unnatural deaths including sudden unexpected or unexplained death, death due to accident and violence (death following injury immediately or delayed for an indefinite time), cases of suspected homicide or suicide, unusual or suspicious circumstances, and cases falling in the public interest (ie, meningitis or other contagious diseases). The Coroner's Office should be notified in the event of all deaths in which a physician was not recently attending the patient (usually defined as the 48 hours prior to death) or in which the personal physician is unwilling to sign the death certificate. The Coroner's or Medical Examiner's office should be notified of unexpected deaths of children younger than 1 year of age and of all drug deaths, save for anesthetic deaths in most jurisdictions or complications of legitimate therapy. Deaths in custody (jail, psychiatric facilities, and other custodial situations) should elicit notification. Deaths due to abortion, whether self-induced or otherwise, require notification. Deaths related to employment may require notification. Such deaths need not be immediate. Persons who have knowledge of such deaths are usually required to notify the medical examiner or coroner. Failure to do so may be a misdemeanor.

Most adult instances of sudden death are cardiogenic.[4]

The autopsy may resolve insurance questions, including addressing diagnoses of suicide or homicide.

THE AUTOPSY MAY SUPPORT RISK MANAGEMENT:

It may eliminate suspicion and provide reassurance to families; it may provide facts instead of conjecture, and support malpractice defense and reduce medicolegal claims as well as improve the quality of care.[5]

QUALITY ASSURANCE AND THE AUTOPSY:

The declining rate of autopsies is a cause for concern by the Council on Scientific Affairs of the American Medical Association, which emphasizes the lack of change in class I error in spite of better clinical techniques.[6] (Class I error is one in which a different diagnosis before death may have prolonged life.) This *JAMA* paper reports that the House of Delegates of the American Medical Association reaffirmed that autopsies are of fundamental importance in any quality assurance program.[6]

In 1987, the Council on Long Range Planning and Development of the American Medical Association published a paper in which this sentence appears: "Both organized medicine and society at large are in a position to demand autopsy services **in an effort to preserve the quality of medical practice.**"[7]

About 10% of autopsies in a referral hospital revealed a major diagnosis which bears upon therapy and survival. Overreliance on new procedures such as scans, ultrasound, and computerized tomography occasionally leads to missed diagnoses. The value of the autopsy has not been diminished.[8]

A study of 2145 autopsies reported an overall rate of major discrepancies of 29%. The most often misdiagnosed or missed entities in this series included infections and malignancies. The most frequently overlooked immediate causes of death included pulmonary embolism and gastrointestinal hemorrhage.[9] Missed diagnoses of infections include fungal infections.[8,10] Factors influencing discrepancies were extensively studied in 1987.[11]

Cause of death, the death certificate, vital statistics, and disease reporting were discussed in *JAMA*, 1987.[12,13]

In an editorial in *Human Pathology*, Wagner discusses discrepancies between antemortem and postmortem diagnoses. Important discrepancies in 24% to 25% of cases lead Wagner to express skepticism about critical health statistics.[14] This American editorial quotes an epidemiology paper in *Lancet*.[15] This paper, written by Stehbens of New Zealand, observed that Cabot had questioned the accuracy of death certificates in 1912 and that such questions have persisted in the United Kingdom, in the United States, and in a number of other Western countries for very good reasons. He wrote that faith in the validity of mortality statistics in general should not be implicit. He concluded that governmental or health policies based on unreliable data become untenable.

Hill and Anderson discuss the requirements of the Joint Commission on Accreditation of Health Organizations (JCAHO) and that of the Health Care Financing Administration (HCFA). They mention a 1988 *The New York Times* issue which supports Wagner's concerns with regard to flawed national health statistics. Such deficiencies, because of the "astonishing inaccuracy" of death certificates, can lead to "wrong priorities and wrong policies."[16]

Landefeld et al discuss major unanticipated findings in which premortem diagnosis would probably have improved survival in 11% to 12% of cases. They make note of the high level of

(Continued)

Autopsy *(Continued)*

yield of clinically relevant findings and conclude that **it is not currently possible to predict which cases will have high yields.** Of 233 autopsies, 26 patients had class I findings. Fifteen of these were missed because they were not suspected before death and 11 were missed because test results were misleading, inconclusive, misinterpreted, or unavailable at the time of death. Thirty-three of their patients had class II findings, in which diagnosis would not have altered survival. They address the overwhelming data which document conclusively the need for the autopsy in quality assurance.[17]

The autopsy service provides information relevant to quality of care in an institution, the most optimal quality assurance mechanism.

COSTS OF THE AUTOPSY

Friederici, evaluating the autopsy as a postmortem audit, appropriately perceives autopsy information as a gauge of the quality of care of the institution. He observes that third party payors should be interested in auditing, even postmortem, that for which they are asked to pay. He summarizes costs of an autopsy as $900-$2,000.[18]

THE JOINT COMMISSION ON ACCREDITATION OF HEALTHCARE ORGANIZATIONS have published standards.[19] A requirement discussed by Lundberg in the *JAMA*,[20] presently MS. 5.1.8.3 (page 72 of the 1993 JCAHO Manual) is of particular interest: **"The medical staff, with other appropriate hospital staff, develops and uses criteria that identify deaths in which an autopsy should be performed."** The function, in the Medical Staff section, is unchanged from the 1990 manual.

Given the information provided in many of the citations noted in this discussion, the following recommendations might be considered.

- Request autopsy permission whenever cause of death is sufficiently obscure to delay completion of the death certificate (ie, in settings in which there is uncertainty of the credibility of the clinical diagnoses, in an inpatient in a given institution). (Correlational utilization of autopsy data is a cornerstone of quality assurance.)
- Need for autopsy is especially increased when the clinical picture includes the possibility of pulmonary thromboembolism, infection or gastrointestinal bleeding.
- Lundberg emphasizes that "selection bias occurs when one only studies certain cases that seem indicated clinically. To preclude selection bias in quality assessment, autopsy cases need to be randomly chosen, since surprises are, by definition, where you least expect them."[20] This author wholeheartedly concurs with Lundberg! Noteworthy is a published review of 2537 autopsies which disclosed one or more unexpected important findings in 1601 cases (64%). The high incidence of such findings led the authors to conclude that it is fallacious to preselect deaths for a postmortem evaluation.[21]

The College of American Pathologists has published a manual dealing with quality assurance.[22] It provides "Criteria to Decide Whether to Autopsy," intended only as guidelines to underscore situations in which autopsy is most desirable. Such additional guidelines include:

- unanticipated death
- death occurring while the patient is being treated under a new therapeutic trial regime
- intraoperative or intraprocedural death
- death occurring within 48 hours after surgery or an invasive diagnostic procedure
- death related to pregnancy or within 7 days of delivery
- death during a psychiatric admission
- death in admitted infants and children with congenital malformations

Other JCAHO standards include:

- MS. 5.1.8.3.4, 1993 edition: "Findings from autopsies are used as a source of clinical information in quality assessment and improvement activities."
- MR. 2.2.14.4, 1993 edition: "When an autopsy is performed, provisional anatomic diagnoses are recorded in the medical record within 3 days, and the complete protocol is made part of the record within 60 days, unless exceptions for special studies are established by the medical staff."

HAZARDS OF THE AUTOPSY

Ratzan and Schneiderman discuss risk evaluation and risk acceptability. The latter is a subjective assessment of whether a particular risk is worth taking, as they express it.[23] Controversy exists regarding the necessity to perform autopsies in AIDS patients.[24]

Hazards of necropsies include tuberculosis, hepatitis B, acquired immune deficiency syndrome (AIDS), and Jakob-Creutzfeldt disease.[25] Formalin does not kill the etiologic agent of Jakob-Creutzfeldt disease, and it may not kill mycobacteria promptly.

HISTORY

In 1988, Hill and Anderson[26] published on the purposes and ramifications of the autopsy , its costs and its contributions to public policy in the present and future. They discussed the history of the autopsy and its relationship to clinical medicine. This book has stimulated a lively review, in which clinically relevant and timely autopsy reports are urged.[27]

A handbook on death certification is available from the U.S. Department of Health and Human Services.[28] The role of the autopsy in deaths relating to trauma[29] and the emergency departments of hospitals[30] is described.

Footnotes

1. Schmidt S, "Consent for Autopsies," *JAMA*, 1983, 250:1161-4.
2. Scottolini AG and Weinstein SR, "The Autopsy in Clinical Quality Control," *JAMA*, 1983, 250:1192-4.
3. Lundberg GD, "Medical Students, Truth, and Autopsies," *JAMA*, 1983, 250:1199-1200, (editorial).
4. Morales AR, Kulesh M, and Valdes-Dapena M, "Maximizing the Effectiveness of the Autopsy in Cases of Sudden Death," *Arch Pathol Lab Med*, 1984, 108:460-1.
5. Valaske MJ, "Loss Control/Risk Management," *Arch Pathol Lab Med*, 1984, 108:462-8.
6. Council on Scientific Affairs, "Autopsy – A Comprehensive Review of Current Issues," *JAMA*, 1987, 258:364-9.
7. Council on Long Range Planning and Development, "The Future of Pathology," *JAMA*, 1987, 258:370-7.
8. Goldman L, Sayson R, Robbins S, et al, "The Value of the Autopsy in Three Medical Eras," *N Engl J Med*, 1983, 308:1000-5.
9. Stevanovic G, Tucakovic G, Dotlic R, et al, "Correlation of Clinical Diagnosis With Autopsy Findings: A Retrospective Study of 2145 Consecutive Autopsies," *Hum Pathol*, 1986, 17:1225-30.
10. Goldman L, "Diagnostic Advances *vs* the Value of the Autopsy," *Arch Pathol Lab Med*, 1984, 108:501-5.
11. Battle RM, Pathak D, Humble CG, et al, "Factors Influencing Discrepancies Between Premortem and Postmortem Diagnoses," *JAMA*, 1987, 258:339-44.
12. Kircher T and Anderson RE, "Cause of Death – Proper Completion of the Death Certificate," *JAMA*, 1987, 258:349-52.
13. Goodman RA and Berkelman RL, "Physicians, Vital Statistics, and Disease Reporting," *JAMA*, 1987, 258:379-81.
14. Wagner BM, "Mortality Statistics Without Autopsies: Wonderland Revisited," *Hum Pathol*, 1987, 18:875-6.
15. Stehbens WE, "An Appraisal of the Epidemic Rise of Coronary Heart Disease and Its Decline," *Lancet*, 1987, 1:606-11.
16. Hill RB and Anderson RE, "Is a Valid Quality Assurance Program Possible Without the Autopsy?" *Hum Pathol*, 1988, 19(10):1125-6.
17. Landefeld CS, Chren MM, Myers A, et al, "Diagnostic Yield of the Autopsy in a University Hospital and a Community Hospital," *N Engl J Med*, 1988, 318(19):1249-54.
18. Friederici HH, "Reflections on the Postmortem Audit," *JAMA*, 1988, 260(23):3461-5.
19. Joint Commission on Accreditation of Healthcare Organizations: The Joint Commission – Accreditation Manual for Hospitals, Oakbrook Terrace, IL, 1993, 72.
20. Lundberg GD, "Now Is the Time to Emphasize the Autopsy in Quality Assurance," *JAMA*, 1988, 260(23):3488.
21. Friederici HH and Sebastian M, "Autopsies in a Modern Teaching Hospital," *Arch Pathol Lab Med*, 1984, 108:518-21.
22. Travers H, Deppisch LM, and Loring GJ, *Surgical Pathology/Cytopathology Quality Assurance Manual*, Skokie, IL: College of American Pathologists, 1988.
23. Ratzan RM and Schneiderman H, "AIDS, Autopsies, and Abandonment," *JAMA*, 1988, 260(23):3466-9.
24. Frable WJ, *CAP Today*, October, 1987, (letter).
25. Orenstein JM, "Guidelines for High Risk or Potentially High Risk Autopsy Cases," *Pathologist*, 1984, 33-4.
26. Hill RB and Anderson RE, *The Autopsy – Medical Practice and Public Policy*, Boston, MA: Butterworth's Publishers, 1988.
27. Weinstein RS, *Mod Pathol*, 1989, 2:182-3, (book review).
28. "Physicians' Handbook of Medical Certification of Death," Hyattsville, MD: U.S. Department of Health and Human Services, September 1987.
29. Stothert JC Jr, Gbaanador GB, and Herndon DN, "The Role of Autopsy in Death Resulting From Trauma," *J Trauma*, 1990, 30(8):1021-5.
30. Burke MC, Aghababian RV, and Blackbourne B, "Use of Autopsy Results in the Emergency Department Quality Assurance Plan," *Ann Emerg Med*, 1990, 19(4):363-6.

References

Bowman HE and Williams MJ, "Revitalizing the Ultimate Medical Consultation," *Arch Pathol Lab Med*, 1984, 108:437-8.

Brown HG, "Lay Perceptions of Autopsy," *Arch Pathol Lab Med*, 1984, 108:446-8.

Friederici HH and Sebastian M, "An Argument for the Attendance of Clinicians at Autopsy," *Arch Pathol Lab Med*, 1984, 108:522-3.

(Continued)

Autopsy *(Continued)*

Geller SA, "Religious Attitudes and the Autopsy," *Arch Pathol Lab Med*, 1984, 108:494-6.
Hirsch CS, "Talking to the Family After an Autopsy," *Arch Pathol Lab Med*, 1984, 108:513-14.
Hyman AB, "Procedure for Contacting District Coroner," Sedgwick County, Kansas, Office of District Coroner, 1992.
Karwinski B and Hartveit F, "Death Certification: Increased Clinical Confidence in Diagnosis and Lack of Interest in Confirmation by Necropsy Is Not Justified," *J Clin Pathol*, 1989, 42(1):13-7.
King DW, "Potential of the Autopsy," *Arch Pathol Lab Med*, 1984, 108:439-43.
Lundberg GD, "Medicine Without the Autopsy," *Arch Pathol Lab Med*, 1984, 108:449-54.
Lundberg GD, "The Archives of Pathology and Laboratory Medicine and the Autopsy," *JAMA*, 1984, 252:390-2, (editorial).
Michigan Association of Medical Examiners, "The Duties and Organization of Michigan County Medical Examiners," 1993.
Sarode VR, Datta BN, Banerjee AK, et al, "Autopsy Findings and Clinical Diagnoses: A Review of 1000 Cases," *Hum Pathol*, 1993, 24(2):194-8.
Silverberg SG, "The Autopsy and Cancer," *Arch Pathol Lab Med*, 1984, 108:476-8.
Smith RD and Zumwalt RE, "One Department's Experience With Increasing the Autopsy Rate," *Arch Pathol Lab Med*, 1984, 108:455-9.
Svendsen E and Hill RB, "Autopsy Legislation and Practice in Various Countries," *Arch Pathol Lab Med*, 1987, 111:846-50.
Valdes-Dapena M, "The Postautopsy Conference With Families," *Arch Pathol Lab Med*, 1984, 108:497-500.
Wissler RW, "The Value of the Autopsy for Understanding Cardiovascular Disease," *Arch Pathol Lab Med*, 1984, 108:479-83.

Biopsy *see* Histopathology *on page 57*

Biopsy, Breast *see* Breast Biopsy *on this page*

B-Lymphocyte Analysis by Flow Cytometry *see* Immunophenotypic Analysis of Tissues by Flow Cytometry *on page 65*

Brain Biopsy *see* Electron Microscopy *on page 45*

Breast Biopsy

CPT *88305; 88307 (breast, mastectomy – partial/simple); 88309 (breast, mastectomy – with regional lymph nodes)*

Related Information

CA 15-3 *on page 152*
Carcinoembryonic Antigen *on page 167*
Cyst Fluid Cytology *on page 495*
Estrogen Receptor Assay *on page 47*
Estrogen Receptor Immunocytochemical Assay *on page 51*
Fine Needle Aspiration, Superficial Palpable Masses *on page 499*
Frozen Section *on page 54*
Histopathology *on page 57*
Immunoperoxidase Procedures *on page 60*
Immunophenotypic Analysis of Tissues by Flow Cytometry *on page 65*
Nipple Discharge Cytology *on page 505*
Progestogen Receptor Assay *on page 77*
Progestogen Receptor Immunocytochemical Assay *on page 79*
Tumor Aneuploidy by Flow Cytometry *on page 88*

Synonyms Biopsy, Breast

Applies to Cathepsin D; c-erb-B2; DNA; Epidermal Growth Factor Receptor; Flow Cytometry; HER-2/neu; Oncogene Expression; Ploidy; S-Phase

Abstract Breast carcinoma indicators related to good prognosis include tumor size less than 1 cm, low grade, positive estrogen receptors (ER) and progesterone receptors (PR), and negative axillary lymph nodes. Surgical margins, grading, ploidy, S-phase fraction, cathepsin D, epidermal growth factor receptor, and c-erb-B2 are outlined relevant to survival.

Patient Care PREPARATION: Information about the lesion and the patient should be provided with the requisition. Surgical pathologists need clinical details, especially tumor location, particularly for lesions in the area of the nipple that may include florid papillomatosis of nipple. History of prior biopsy may explain fibroplasia that might be mistaken for tumor desmoplasia. History of trauma or current recent pregnancy may be extremely relevant. Whether or not nipple discharge was present and whether the lesion was detected by palpation, mammography, or both should be recorded. For needle localization studies, the original mammograms with x-rays of the needle localization are highly desirable.

Specimen Commonly sent fresh, for immediate evaluation. Open biopsy specimens should be sent to the pathologist intact so that dye can be applied to margins and so that gross characteristics of the lesion can be evaluated. Frozen section of grossly evident tumor can confirm the presence of carcinoma, from which tissue for estrogen and progesterone receptor assays and DNA studies can be retrieved and frozen. Frozen sections of very small tumors should be discouraged, as diagnosis and classification are more important than accessory studies. If needed, receptor and ploidy studies can be performed on paraffin-embedded tissues. Experienced surgeons often recognize benign specimens such as fibroadenomas and fix them in formalin. **CONTAINER:** Fresh specimens of breast tissue should be sent in a clean, dry, labeled container on ice[1] and placed in the hands of a pathologist or histotechnician.

Interpretive **USE:** Establish the presence or absence of carcinoma or of carcinoma *in situ*. Confirm the presence of calcific structures identified in mammograms and characterize them. Specimen radiography is commonly performed to confirm that the biopsied tissue contains the calcific structures, but their etiology can only be evaluated histologically. Since many women presently request breast-conserving surgical procedures, pathological evaluation of the breast tumor specimen has necessarily changed to better evaluate the therapeutic efficacy of the surgical procedure with evaluation of adequacy of margins when possible. Lumpectomy (tylectomy) is presently followed by radiation therapy in many cases. **LIMITATIONS:** Shortcomings of needle biopsies include a great potential for false-negative results related to problems of sampling. Other problems include lack of opportunity to visualize the lesion and its relationship to its environs. Crush artifact may be a serious problem. Needle biopsies are most often used as a guide to open biopsy.[1] Local recurrence may complicate lumpectomy.[2] The margins of resection may be critical, *vide infra*. Foci of carcinoma occur in other quadrants in about 32% of cases.[2] Thus, it may be extremely difficult to assure adequacy of excision despite clear margins from a lumpectomy specimen. **Lobular carcinoma** *in situ* is multifocal.[2] **Multiple foci of carcinoma** are considered contraindications to primary radiation therapy.[3] **METHODOLOGY:** *Vide infra* **ADDITIONAL INFORMATION:** The pathologist determines the orientation of the specimen and the tumor and its relationship to resection margins. Specimen orientation may be desirable for direction of potential further surgery. When the surgeon requires a report reflecting the relationship of the tumor to resection margins, it is necessary to provide surgical sutures as markers (superior, inferior, lateral, medial, deep, superficial) in a combination appropriate for the setting of a given neoplasm. Coating of the specimen surfaces with India ink or other colored marker by the pathologist is desirable in many instances of lumpectomy and of re-excision specimens. It does not interfere with receptor assays, provided that the specimen submitted for receptors is free of ink or dye.[3] Sections can then be taken to provide margin evaluation on microscopy. The complex geometry of lumpectomy margins has been addressed in a variety of ways.[2,3,4] Connolly and others conclude that frozen section evaluation of margins which are grossly free of tumor has no significant role in intraoperative management. It may compromise evaluation of margins in permanent sections. Entry criteria defined in two studies by the National Surgical Adjuvant Breast and Bowel Project (NSABP) required that specimen margins were histopathologically free of tumor. The two studies address receptor-negative and receptor-positive tumors respectively.[5,6]

In up to 33% of instances of breast biopsies done for microcalcifications in which carcinoma is found, the calcifications are in adjacent benign breast tissue and not in the tumor. Therefore, tissue **adjacent** to focal microcalcifications must be included in the biopsy and sampled for microscopy.

Risks of local recurrence in patients treated with conservative surgery and radiation therapy are increased in the presence of extensive intraductal carcinoma coexisting with invasive tumors. Poorly differentiated tumors (high histologic grade), tumor necrosis, vascular invasion, and the presence of infiltrative lobular carcinoma are associated with increased risk of tumor recurrence. Comedocarcinoma is more likely than noncomedo intraductal carcinoma to recur.[4]

Grading of invasive carcinomas of breast is reviewed by Elston[7] and Tavassoli.[8] Bloom and Richardson addressed the relationship between grade and survival. The method Elston describes is based on that of Bloom and Richardson, differing with the report of mitotic rate, an important component.

Histopathologic tumor types include some with more favorable prognosis; pure mucinous (colloid), pure tubular, invasive cribriform carcinoma, and the rare adenoid cystic carcinoma of breast. Metastases from adenoid cystic carcinoma of breast are extremely rare. Inflammatory carcinoma, poorly differentiated carcinomas, and carcinosarcomas are aggressive, with a 5-year survival of only 11% for inflammatory carcinoma.

(Continued)

Breast Biopsy *(Continued)*

Ten year surgical failure is 24% in the absence of axillary lymph node metastases. Immunochemical methods are useful in selected cases for detection of occult lymph node metastases. Primary breast carcinomas larger than 2 cm are more likely to give rise to micrometastases. Vascular invasion is significantly related to recurrence and metastasis, but interobserver variation exists.[8] Immunostains for factor VIII related antigen are sometimes used.

Table 1. Hormone Receptor Status

	Premenopausal	Postmenopausal	Overall
ER+	64%	79%	
PR+	58%	53%	
ER-, PR-			27%
ER-, PR+			2%
ER+, PR-			30%
ER+, PR+			41%

In addition to providing accurate pathological staging information, the pathologist is also becoming increasingly responsible for providing studies of therapeutic and prognostic significance. Estrogen receptor (ER) expression in breast cancer has the unique characteristic of having both prognostic and therapeutic implications. Progesterone receptor (PR) expression has indirect therapeutic implications but may have a more direct bearing on prognosis. The frequency of ER expression tends to increase with age as does the level of ER expression.[9] (See Table 1.) PR expression is induced by estrogen and in part reflects functional integrity of the estrogen regulatory pathway.[10] Accordingly, ER-, PR+ phenotype is very uncommon. Although some conflicting data has been reported, there is consensus that presence of ER is correlated with longer disease-free survival and overall survival. Such differences tend to be most significant at follow-up of 5 years or less. Survival curves tend to merge with longer term follow-up. Stage-matched patients with higher expression of ER tend to follow a more favorable clinical course than do patients with low levels of expression. Generally, both ER and PR expression tend to reflect tumor growth rate rather than metastatic potential.

Although ER expression does not predict response to chemotherapy, it is highly associated with response to endocrine therapy. Tumor-static responses are associated with ER, with the greatest likelihood of response in those with high levels of ER expression and those with coexpression of PR. Some studies have suggested a more favorable course in patients with PR expression while other studies show no added benefit over that associated with ER expression. Patterns of metastasis in ER-positive and ER-negative patients may differ. Patients with ER-negative tumors have a higher rate of visceral involvement while patients with ER-positive tumors have a predilection for bony metastasis.[11]

Estrogen and progesterone receptor assays are provided as separate listings in this section. Expression of both hormone receptors may be measured in several ways. The time honored dextran coated charcoal (DCC) method is based on the binding of radioactive hormone to a cytosol extract of the tumor and does not detect the true intranuclear form of the receptor. More recently, an enzyme immunoassay (EIA) for both hormones has gained favor. Enzyme immunoassays employ monoclonal antibodies to the respective hormone receptors measuring only the cytosol receptor fraction. Receptors are quantitated by a colorimetric enzyme amplified signal. Enzyme immunoassays require less tissue than DCC and are not subject to interference by endogenous or exogenous hormones. When dealing with very small tumors or tissue biopsies, an immunocytochemical stain (ICC) may be employed to qualitatively measure hormone receptor expression. These stains allow direct morphologic correlation of hormone receptor activity with cell type and detect the true intranuclear form of receptor expression. Immunocytochemical studies have demonstrated a surprising degree of heterogeneity in hormone receptor expression, the significance of which is being actively investigated. The relative merits of these assays are summarized in Table 2.

Flow cytometric determination of DNA ploidy and S-phase fraction (SPF) have gained wide acceptance in routine evaluation of breast carcinoma. Such studies may be obtained on tissues submitted for hormone receptor assays or from paraffin blocks. Up to 66% of breast cancers are aneuploid, 30% to 40% are regarded as high SPF tumors. Several studies have demonstrated shorter time to relapse and worse overall survival in stage 1 patients with aneuploid tumors or those with high SPF. Patients with stage 1, low SPF tumors enjoyed a significantly reduced chance for relapse and longer survival.[12,13] When considered separately, tetraploid tumors tend to behave more like diploid tumors than other aneuploid tumors.[14] Aneuploidy and high SPF tumors tend to demonstrate high nuclear grade and are more frequently hormone receptor negative.

Table 2. Relative Merits of Hormone Receptor Assay Techniques

Attribute	DCC/EIA	ICC
Quantitative result	yes	no
Clinically significant cutoff	yes	no
Sample size	larger	smaller
Morphologic correlation	no	yes
Determine heterogeneity	no	yes
Receptor assayed	cytosol	nuclear

Other prognostic markers being actively investigated include **cathepsin D, epidermal growth factor receptor, and c-erb-B2 (HER 2-neu)** oncogene expression. **Cathepsin D** is a ubiquitous lysosomal protease capable of digesting basement membranes and other stromal elements of breast tissue. In normal breast, expression of cathepsin D is estrogen regulated. The possibility that such proteases may serve to promote tumor dissemination has led to studies investigating its prognostic utility. Using tissue extracts assayed by the Western blot procedure in a group of node-negative breast cancer patients, Tandon et al showed a strong correlation with high levels of cathepsin D and shorter disease-free intervals and overall survival.[15] In this study, cathepsin D was correlated with aneuploidy but showed no other significant associations with other clinical and prognostic variables. Another study utilizing immunocytochemical detection of cathepsin D produced conflicting results.[16] Henry et al found an overall increase in mean time to relapse and increased overall survival. In node-negative patients, they found no significant prognostic advantage while node-positive patients showed longer disease-free interval and improved overall survival. Thus, the prognostic significance of cathepsin D remains ambiguous.

Epidermal growth factor receptor (EGFR) is a 170 kD transmembrane glycoprotein with tyrosine kinase activity and is intimately related to proliferation and differentiation of a wide variety of epithelia.[17] Based on an intensive literature review summarizing the results of 40 laboratories, Klijn et al found that about 48% of 5232 breast tumors were regarded as EGFR-positive. Expression of EGFR was correlated with estrogen and progesterone receptor negativity, high grade nuclear morphology, aneuploidy, increased S-phase fraction, and lymph node metastases. Expression in premenopausal patients may be increased. Generally, overall survival and relapse-free survival are significantly worse for patients with increased EGFR expression. Further, EGFR status may identify prognostic subcategories in ER-negative patients.[18] Estrogen receptor-negative, EGFR-positive patients have a relatively poorer prognosis while ER-negative, EGFR-negative patients follow a clinical course more like that of ER-positive patients.

It has also been suggested that the **c-erb-B2 (HER-2/neu)** oncogene has prognostic significance in patients with breast carcinoma. This gene encodes for a transmembrane receptor with tyrosine kinase activity. The exact function of this receptor is unknown but it shares structural similarities with EGFR. A variety of studies have indicated worse overall prognosis in patients with over expression of c-erb-B2. Others have failed to confirm this impression.[19,20,21] There is consensus that overexpression of c-erb-B2 in node-positive patients predicts early relapse and worse overall survival but convincing data in node-negative cases is not yet available.[22,23]

Footnotes

1. Carter D, "Interpretation of Breast Biopsies," *Biopsy Interpretation Series*, 2nd ed, New York, NY: Raven Press, 1990, 14.
2. Carter D, "Margins of "Lumpectomy" for Breast Cancer," *Hum Pathol*, 1986, 17:330-2.
3. Connolly JL and Schnitt SJ, "Evaluation of Breast Biopsy Specimens in Patients Considered for Treatment by Conservative Surgery and Radiation Therapy for Early Breast Cancer," *Pathol Annu*, Part 1, Vol 23, Norwalk, CT: Appleton & Lange, 1988, 1-23.
4. Schnitt SJ and Connolly JL, "Processing and Evaluation of Breast Excision Specimens: A Clinically Oriented Approach," *Am J Clin Pathol*, 1992, 98(1):125-37.
5. Fisher B, Redmond C, Dimitrov NV, et al, "A Randomized Clinical Trial Evaluating Sequential Methotrexate and Fluorouracil in the Treatment of Patients With Node-Negative Breast Cancer Who Have Estrogen-Receptor-Negative Tumors," *N Engl J Med*, 1989, 320(8):473-8.
6. Fisher B, Costantino J, Redmond C, et al, "A Randomized Clinical Trial Evaluating Tamoxifen in the Treatment of Patients With Node-Negative Breast Cancer Who Have Estrogen-Receptor-Positive Tumors," *N Engl J Med*, 1989, 320(8):479-84.
7. Elston CW, "Grading of Invasive Carcinoma of the Breast," *Diagnostic Histopathology of the Breast*, Page DL and Anderson TJ, eds, New York, NY: Churchill Livingstone, 1987, 300-11.
8. Tavassoli FA, *Pathology of the Breast*, New York, NY: Elsevier/North Holland Biomedical Press, 1992, 36-43.

(Continued)

Breast Biopsy *(Continued)*

9. Clark GM, Osborne CK, and McGuire WL, "Correlations Between Estrogen Receptor, Progesterone Receptor, and Patient Characteristics in Human Breast Cancer," *J Clin Oncol*, 1984, 2:1102-9.
10. Osborne CK, "Receptors," *Breast Diseases*, Harris JR, Hellman S, Henderson IC, et al, eds, Philadelphia, PA: JB Lippincott Co, 1991, 210-32.
11. Clark GM, Sledge GW, Osborne CK, et al, "Survival From First Recurrence: Relative Importance of Prognostic Factors in 1015 Breast Cancer Patients," *J Clin Oncol*, 1988, 37:221-6.
12. Dressler LG, Seamer LC, Owens MA, et al, "DNA Flow Cytometry and Prognostic Factors in 1331 Frozen Breast Cancer Specimens," *Cancer*, 1988, 61(3):420-7.
13. Clark GM, Dressler LM, Owens MA, et al, "Prediction of Relapse or Survival in Patients With Node Negative Breast Cancer by DNA Flow Cytometry," *N Engl J Med*, 1989, 320(10):627-33.
14. Witzig TE, Gonchoroff NJ, Therneau T, et al, "DNA Content Flow Cytometry as a Prognostic Factor for Node Positive Breast Cancer. The Role of Multiparameter Ploidy Analysis and Specimen Sonication," *Cancer*, 1991, 68(8):1781-8.
15. Tandon AK, Clark GM, Chamness GC, et al, "Cathepsin D and Prognosis in Breast Cancer," *N Engl J Med*, 1990, 322(5):297-302.
16. Henry JA, McCarthy AL, Angus B, et al, "Prognostic Significance of the Estrogen-Regulated Protein, Cathepsin D, in Breast Cancer," *Cancer*, 1990, 65(2):265-71.
17. Klijn JG, Berns PM, Schmitz PI, et al, "The Clinical Significance of Epidermal Growth Factor Receptor (EGF-R) in Human Breast Cancer: A Review of 5232 Patients," *Endocr Rev*, 1992, 13(1):3-17.
18. Sainsbury JRC, Needham GK, Famdon JR, et al, "Epidermal Growth Factor Receptor Status as a Predictor of Early Recurrence of and Death From Breast Cancer," *Lancet*, 1987, 1:1398-1402.
19. Van de Vijver MJ, Peterse JL, Mooi WJ, et al, "Neu-Protein Overexpression in Breast Cancer," *N Engl J Med*, 1988, 319(19):1239-45.
20. Tandon AK, Clark GM, Chamness GC, et al, "HER-2/Neu Oncogene Protein and Prognosis in Breast Cancer," *J Clin Oncol*, 1989, 7(8):1120-8.
21. Heintz NH, Leslie KD, Rogers LA, et al, "Amplification of the c-erb-B2 Oncogene and Prognosis in Breast Adenocarcinoma," *Arch Pathol Lab Med*, 1990, 114(2):160-3.
22. Wong WW, Vijayakumar S, and Weichselbaum RR, "Prognostic Indicators in Node Negative Early Stage Breast Cancer," *Am J Med*, 1992, 92(5):539-48.
23. Elledge RM, McGuire WL, and Osborne CK, "Prognostic Factors in Breast Cancer," *Semin Oncol*, 1992, 19(3):244-53.

References

Allred DC, Clark GM, Molina R, et al, "Overexpression of HER-2/neu and Its Relationship With Other Prognostic Change During the Progression of *In Situ* to Invasive Breast Cancer," *Hum Pathol*, 1992, 23(9):974-9.

Anderson TJ, "c-erbB-2 Oncogene in Breast Cancer: The Right Target or a Decoy?" *Hum Pathol*, 1992, 23(9):971-3.

Azzopardi JG, "Problems in Breast Pathology," *Major Problems in Pathology*, Vol 11, Philadelphia, PA: WB Saunders Co, 1979.

Bellamy CO, McDonald C, Salter DM, et al, "Noninvasive Ductal Carcinoma of the Breast: The Relevance of Histologic Categorization," *Hum Pathol*, 1993, 24(1):16-23.

Fisher B, Redmond C, Poisson R, et al, "Eight-Year Results of a Randomized Clinical Trial Comparing Total Mastectomy and Lumpectomy With or Without Irradiation in the Treatment of Breast Cancer," *N Engl J Med*, 1989, 320(13):822-8.

Frazier TG, Wong RW, and Rose D, "Implications of Accurate Pathologic Margins in the Treatment of Primary Breast Cancer," *Arch Surg*, 1989, 124(1):37-8.

Frierson HF Jr, "Grade and Flow Cytometric Analysis of Ploidy for Infiltrating Ductal Carcinomas," *Hum Pathol*, 1993, 24(1):24-9.

Lay SF, Crump JM, Frykberg ER, et al, "Breast Biopsy. Changing Patterns During a Five-Year Period," *Am J Surg*, 1990, 56(2):79-85.

Ngai JH, Zelles GW, Rumore GJ, et al, "Breast Biopsy Techniques and Adequacy of Margins," *Arch Surg*, 1991, 126(11):1343-7.

Page DL and Anderson TJ, *Diagnostic Histopathology of the Breast*, New York, NY: Churchill Livingstone, 1987.

Bronchial Biopsy *see* Histopathology *on page 57*

Cancer, Breast *see* Estrogen Receptor Assay *on page 47*

Cardiac Biopsy *see* Electron Microscopy *on next page*

Cathepsin D *see* Breast Biopsy *on page 40*

Cause of Death *see* Autopsy *on page 36*

Cell Sorting Fluorescence Activation *see* Lymph Node Biopsy *on page 72*

c-erb-B2 *see* Breast Biopsy *on page 40*

Chromogranin *see* Immunoperoxidase Procedures *on page 60*

Computerized Interactive Morphometry *see* Image Analysis *on page 58*
Coroner's Case *see* Autopsy *on page 36*
Cytokeratins *see* Immunoperoxidase Procedures *on page 60*
Death Certificate *see* Autopsy *on page 36*
Desmin *see* Immunoperoxidase Procedures *on page 60*
Disease Reporting *see* Autopsy *on page 36*
DNA *see* Breast Biopsy *on page 40*
DNA Content *see* Tumor Aneuploidy by Flow Cytometry *on page 88*
DNA in Tumor Nuclei *see* Image Analysis *on page 58*
DNA Ploidy Studies *see* Immunophenotypic Analysis of Tissues by Flow Cytometry *on page 65*
DNA Synthesis Phase *see* Tumor Aneuploidy by Flow Cytometry *on page 88*

Electron Microscopy

CPT *88348 (diagnostic); 88349 (scanning)*

Related Information

Electron Microscopic Examination for Viruses, Stool *on page 1177*
Fine Needle Aspiration, Deep Seated Lesions *on page 498*
Fine Needle Aspiration, Superficial Palpable Masses *on page 499*
Kidney Biopsy *on page 68*
Muscle Biopsy *on page 75*
Skin Biopsies *on page 84*

Synonyms EM; Transmission Electron Microscopy; Ultrastructural Study

Applies to Brain Biopsy; Cardiac Biopsy

Test Commonly Includes Electron microscopic evaluation of ultrathin sections of a satisfactory specimen

Abstract Ultrastructural examination of tissue.

Specimen Fresh unfixed tissue, blood, bone marrow aspirate **CONTAINER:** Vial containing glutaraldehyde or other appropriate fixative, depending upon institution or reference laboratory. Fresh specimen submitted immediately on a sterile gauze pad moistened with sterile saline is requested by some laboratories. Blood and bone marrow aspirate may be collected in heparinized or EDTA tubes and submitted immediately. **COLLECTION:** Specimen obtained by surgical excision should be cut within 2 minutes of removal from the patient, minced into cubes 1 mm or less, and placed in glutaraldehyde, paraformaldehyde, or other special fixative. Two percent to 4% phosphate or cacodylate-buffered glutaraldehyde is recommended. Formaldehyde-fixed tissue may be used if glutaraldehyde is not available. All EM fixatives, particularly glutaraldehyde, should be refrigerated until used to retard oxidative damage to fixative. Discard if a precipitate forms. **CAUSES FOR REJECTION:** Specimen placed in formalin or not quickly placed in appropriate EM fixative. Lack of appropriate fixative is a relative cause for rejection, depending on the information required. **TURNAROUND TIME:** A report may sometimes be available within 48 hours and within 24 hours in emergent cases.

Interpretive **USE:** A major application of electron microscopy is to define tumor classification, when light microscopy is equivocal and when proper therapy and prognosis depend on accurate diagnosis. In general, poorly differentiated neoplasms may be better defined. When limited material is available, such as fine needle aspiration biopsies, electron microscopy may allow a more precise classification in selected cases.[1,2] Ultrastructural diagnosis is useful especially in endocrine tumors (eg, anterior pituitary tumors, insulinoma), and when neurosecretory granules are found in apudomas. Confirmation of small cell anaplastic carcinoma of neuroendocrine type (oat cell carcinoma) is enhanced, providing distinction from various poorly differentiated nonoat cell carcinomas. Differential diagnosis of small cell tumors of possible Ewing type is supported, especially in the pediatric age range (in which the differential diagnosis includes neuroblastoma, lymphoma/leukemia, embryonal rhabdomyosarcoma). Tumors of the anterior mediastinum and mesothelioma are also sometimes best worked up with electron microscopy. Other important applications include diagnosis of some spindle cell tumors, distinction in occasional instances between carcinoma and sarcoma, and confirmation of amelanotic melanoma, in which it is often possible to identify premelanosomes. Diagnosis of poorly differentiated leukemias, some lymphomas, and of histiocytosis-X is sometimes en-

(Continued)

Electron Microscopy *(Continued)*

hanced by electron microscopy. EM demonstration of platelet peroxidase in the nuclear envelope of the blast cells is essential for the diagnosis of megakaryoblastic leukemias (M7).[3] EM is helpful in differential diagnosis between lymphoma and undifferentiated carcinoma. It may suggest the phenotype of a metastatic tumor.

Electron microscopy is useful in certain viral and other infectious diseases. In AIDS encephalopathy, EM of brain biopsies will help to determine the responsible etiologic agent (ie, HIV, CMV, herpes, JC polyoma - PML, *Toxoplasma*, etc). CNS tumors may sometimes be better characterized by EM as may instances of muscle (eg, mitochondrial myopathies) and peripheral nerve biopsies. No special stain excels EM in sensitivity for identification of amyloid fibrils. Storage/metabolic diseases sometimes are well evaluated with EM. Ceroid lipofuscinoses and Pompe's type II glycogenosis have characteristic inclusions in peripheral blood lymphocytes by EM. Many other lysosomal storage diseases can be identified by EM of skin, conjunctival, or gum biopsies.[4] The immotile cilia syndrome is diagnosed by the absence of one or both dynein arms in cross sections of ciliary microtubules in nasal or bronchial biopsies.[5] Some liver biopsies have lesions in which EM may be useful (eg, Dubin-Johnson syndrome, Rotor's disease). With heart biopsy, EM can reveal Adriamycin® cardiotoxicity.

LIMITATIONS: Sampling errors, expensive, time consuming. Usually not useful in distinction between benignancy and malignancy. Utility is diminished by crushing or drying. The role of electron microscopy has recently been somewhat eroded by rapid advances in immunocytochemistry for the differential diagnosis of tumors. **METHODOLOGY:** Transmission electron microscopy **ADDITIONAL INFORMATION:** A specimen should also be submitted for light microscopic evaluation at the time the specimen is obtained for EM study. Often it is the light microscopic findings which lead to a decision of whether or not EM is indicated (eg, tumors). EM is not a substitute for light microscopy. When renal biopsies are obtained, immunofluorescence studies are recommended, as well as light microscopy. Immunofluorescence and EM are mutually complementary.

Footnotes

1. Strausbauch P, Neill J, Dabbs DJ, et al, "The Impact of Fine Needle Aspiration Biopsy on a Diagnostic Electron Microscopy Laboratory," *Arch Pathol Lab Med*, 1989, 113(12):1354-6.
2. Yazdi HM and Dardick I, "Techniques for Specimen Processing," *Guides to Clinical Aspiration Biopsy, Diagnostic Immunocytochemistry, and Electron Microscopy*, New York, NY: Igaku-Shoin, 1991, 11-25.
3. Koike T, "Megakaryoblastic Leukemia: The Characterization and Identification of Megakaryoblasts," *Blood*, 1984, 64:683-92.
4. Dolman CL, "Diagnosis of Neurometabolic Disorders by Examination of Skin Biopsies and Lymphocytes," *Seminars in Diagnostic Pathology*, 1984, 1:82-97.
5. Afzelius BA, "The Immotile-Cilia Syndrome and Other Ciliary Diseases," *Int Rev Exp Pathol*, 1979, 19:1-43.

References

Azar HA, *Pathology of Human Neoplasms: An Atlas of Diagnostic Electron Microscopy and Immunohistochemistry*, New York, NY: Raven Press, 1988.

Dickersin GR, *Diagnostic Electron Microscopy: A Text/Atlas*, New York, NY: Igaku-Shoin, 1988.

Erlandson RA, *Diagnostic Transmission Electron Microscopy of Human Tumors, The Interpretation of Submicroscopic Structures in Human Neoplastic Cells*, New York, NY: Masson Publishing USA Inc, 1981.

Ghadially FN, *Diagnostic Electron Microscopy of Tumors*, London, UK: Butterworths, 1985.

Ghadially FN, *Ultrastructural Pathology of the Cell and Matrix*, London, UK: Butterworths, 1988.

Henderson DW, Papadimitriou JM, and Coleman M, *Ultrastructural Appearance of Tumors*, New York, NY: Churchill Livingstone, 1986.

Mackay B, *Introduction to Diagnostic Electron Microscopy*, New York, NY: Appleton-Century-Crofts, 1981.

Mackay B, Bruner JM, and Ordonez NG, "Electron Microscopy in Surgical Pathology: I and II," *Lab Med*, 1988, 19:13-7, 78-83.

Trump BJ and Jones RT, *Diagnostic Electron Microscopy*, Vols 1-4, New York, NY: John Wiley and Sons, 1978-1983.

EM *see* Electron Microscopy *on previous page*

Endometrium, Adenocarcinoma *see* Estrogen Receptor Assay *on next page*

Endoscopic Biopsy *see* Histopathology *on page 57*

Epidermal Growth Factor Receptor *see* Breast Biopsy *on page 40*

Epithelial Membrane Antigen (EMA) *see* Immunoperoxidase Procedures *on page 60*

ER *see* Estrogen Receptor Assay *on next page*

Estrogen Receptor Assay

CPT 84233

Related Information

Breast Biopsy *on page 40*
Estrogen Receptor Immunocytochemical Assay *on page 51*
Histopathology *on page 57*
Image Analysis *on page 58*
Immunophenotypic Analysis of Tissues by Flow Cytometry *on page 65*
Progestogen Receptor Assay *on page 77*
Progestogen Receptor Immunocytochemical Assay *on page 79*
Tumor Aneuploidy by Flow Cytometry *on page 88*

Synonyms ER; Estradiol Receptor; Estrogen Binding Protein

Applies to Cancer, Breast; Endometrium, Adenocarcinoma; ER-ICA; Metastatic Neoplasia

Test Commonly Includes Progesterone receptor assay usually included, depending on laboratory. Evaluation of both estrogen receptors (ER) and progesterone receptors (PR) is strongly recommended as both ER and PR provide independent prognostic weight:[1] Thirty percent of breast tumors are discordant with respect to ER/PR receptor (ER+,PR- or ER-,PR+).[2] DNA studies are desirable. They include ploidy (diploid or normal DNA content and aneuploid or abnormal DNA content) and S phase (synthesis phase, estimating proliferative activity of a neoplasm). Such work-up may be done with the ER/PR specimen by flow cytometry.

Abstract Test on fresh tissue to select those breast cancer patients likely to be responsive to endocrine therapy.

Patient Care PREPARATION: Antiestrogen preparations within 2 months may cause false-negative estrogen receptor assays. Exogenous hormones taken for contraceptive purposes, or menopausal estrogens, are related to lower receptor levels. Therefore, hormone use should be discontinued before breast biopsy.[3]

Specimen Receptor assay should be done when possible on all sufficiently large primary breast carcinomas or other tumor types since metastases, should they develop, may not be accessible. Receptor assays may be done on metastases, if accessible, should the primary not have been so analyzed. Send fresh tumor to the laboratory immediately on ice for frozen and permanent sections. Indicate that estrogen/progesterone receptor studies are to be performed with frozen section identification of breast cancer tissue. Generally, 1 g fresh tumor tissue free of fat, necrotic tissue, and free of normal breast tissue is desirable (a mass slightly less than 1 x 1 x 1 cm). It is important that this tissue **not** be formalin (or otherwise) fixed. Rush excised tumor, unfixed, to the laboratory if frozen section was performed on a needle biopsy. The minimal amount of tissue required for assay is laboratory dependent but is in the range of 150 mg. Consult the pathologist regarding proper handling of the specimen prior to surgical removal. CONTAINER: Jar or waxed cardboard container sent in a larger container in which ice has been placed; **no formalin or other fixative.** To be frozen immediately by pathologist. It is imperative that the fresh specimen be kept on ice and sent to the laboratory as quickly as possible; receptor proteins are heat labile.[4] COLLECTION: Container must be labeled at least with patient's name, age, site of specimen (eg, right or left breast), and date. The receptor assay request forms must be completed with patient information. If a dry ice acetone mixture is used for rapid freezing, do not permit tissue to touch this mixture. Rather, first put the tissue in a labeled plastic screw-cap container. Acetone in direct contact with the tissue will denature receptor proteins. Quick freezing can also be done with liquid nitrogen, if available, or in the cryostat. Avoid contact with frozen section embedding media such as O.C.T.®[5] Anecdotal reports exist of pigments such as India ink causing interference with ER assay. If margins are

(Continued)

Estrogen Receptor Assay *(Continued)*

marked with pigments, it may be prudent to trim away such edges of tissue submitted for receptor assay. **STORAGE INSTRUCTIONS:** -70°C freezer or colder. Avoid cyclic temperature fluctuations and prolonged storage. Dry ice is recommended for transportation. **CAUSES FOR REJECTION:** Too little tumor tissue, specimen not malignant or entirely necrotic on frozen section, specimen contaminated by fixatives or cauterized, specimen not brought to Pathology Department immediately **TURNAROUND TIME:** Commonly sent frozen to reference laboratories, most of which can provide turnaround time of less than a week. **SPECIAL INSTRUCTIONS:** Transport **immediately** to Pathology Department as fresh specimen (that is, before wound closure). A delay of even 15 minutes without proper cold packing can alter the results. A frozen section must be performed to document presence of viable breast carcinoma in the tissue to be analyzed. If tumor is sampled away from the frozen section site, then a permanent section of the area adjacent to the sampling site should be processed for permanent (paraffin) sections and designated as such. If the specimen is sent from a small facility, it should be packed in dry ice immediately, kept frozen, and transported promptly while still frozen.

Interpretive **REFERENCE RANGE:** <3 fmol/mg cytosol protein usually indicates no estrogen receptor activity; >10 fmol/mg usually indicates positivity; >100 fmol/mg cytosol protein is strongly positive and the patient is considered a likely candidate for hormonal therapy. Fifty percent to 70% of breast carcinomas are positive for estrogen receptors. **USE:** Patients whose breast carcinomas lack estrogen receptors are often candidates for chemotherapy. Slightly more than 50% of patients having breast carcinomas positive for estrogen receptors respond to endocrine therapy such as tamoxifen. Evidence exists that the incidence of response is enhanced when progesterone receptor is also present.[6] Meningiomas frequently contain progesterone receptors.[7] **LIMITATIONS:** Since the hormone-binding proteins are thermolabile, receptors are destroyed if tissue is not rapidly frozen. Samples that might initially be receptor-positive will then be reported as negative. Tumor heterogeneity for estrogen receptors exists. Sampling errors occur, but are diminished when samples for receptor assay are selected by a pathologist with frozen section control. By virtue of the quantity of tissue required for tissue assay, there still can be admixtures of tumor and undesirably contaminating benign tissue, necrotic tissue, and stroma. Problems exist with very desmoplastic tumors in which there is proportionally more stroma with fewer cancer cells. Similarly, extensively necrotic neoplasms will contain fewer cells per mg of specimen. The volume of tissue required for conventional assays is such that extremely small carcinomas are and should be entirely consumed for tissue diagnosis. For these and probably other reasons, there exists significantly imperfect correlation between receptor positivity and response to endocrine therapy. Estrogen receptor immunocytochemical assay (ERICA) is a reasonable alternative with some advantages compared to conventional cytosolic measurements of estrogen receptors (see listing, Estrogen Receptor Immunocytochemical Assay). **CONTRAINDICATIONS:** Fixed tissue or tissue not quickly frozen **METHODOLOGY:** Biochemical measurement in cytosol fractions of tumor homogenate; dextran-coated charcoal and sucrose gradient assay. Other approaches include fluorescein-labeled estradiol conjugate, immunoperoxidase using tissue sections,[8] enzyme immunoassay (EIA), and *in situ* hybridization.[9] **ADDITIONAL INFORMATION:** Estrogen receptor positivity bears an association with the postmenopausal state, with better histopathologic differentiation, with the disease-free interval, and with longer survival.[10,11,12] About 30% of breast cancer cases have estrogen receptor levels <3 fmol/mg and should be considered negative. Patients with a negative estrogen receptor assay result will have only about an 8% chance of response to endocrine therapy. ER concentration of breast carcinomas appears to predict duration of response but not the response rate to toremifene (nonsteroidal antiestrogen compound).[13] In a multivariate analysis of women with recurrent or metastatic breast cancer, only the ER concentration was significant in predicting the response to tamoxifen.[14]

Presence of significant amounts of blood in the tumor may result in false-negative results, as may lack of tumor in specimen provided. Estrogen receptor results between 5-100 fmol/mg have been reported to have a 46% response rate to hormonal therapy, while cases with ER results >100 fmol/mg have a response rate of 61% to 80%. Although most breast carcinomas responding to endocrine therapy contain receptors, the presence of estrogen receptors does not assure response to endocrine management. Endocrine response is more likely if progesterone receptors are also positive.

Sixteen of 41 specimens of benign breast tissue had estrogen receptor levels >3 fmol/mg protein; 4 were >10 fmol/mg protein.[15]

Additional reports of tumors other than breast carcinoma bearing estrogen receptors appear. Such tissue includes meningiomas, soft tissue tumors,[16] endometrial hyperplasias, carcinomas, and other gynecologic tumors. ER assay is sometimes useful for female patients with metastatic adenocarcinoma of unknown primary site, especially those with axillary lymph node metastases.[17] Meningiomas, adenocarcinomas of lung, and hepatocellular carcinomas are other tissues in which ER assay may be of benefit.[7,18,19,20] ER status may be important in benign entities such as the fibromatoses.[21]

Human tissues may contain a low capacity, high affinity receptor such as may be seen in breast carcinomas. A second binding macromolecule termed type II ER has a lower affinity for estrogen but a higher binding capacity. Type II estrogen receptors have been reported in papillary cystic tumor of the pancreas with control pancreas negative for such receptors.[22] Increased disease-free survival in patients with ER-positive melanomas appears independent of pathologic characteristics of such tumors.[23] Neoplastic proliferation of cervical squamous cells induced by HPV may associated with reduced ER and increased PR expression.[24]

Immunocytochemical assays have been described for frozen and paraffin tissue. Application of monoclonal antibodies to estrogen receptors as an immunocytochemical procedure for frozen sections is described.[12,25,26] Using monoclonal antibodies, estimation of estrogen receptor from paraffin sections is described[27,28] as estrogen receptor immunocytochemical assay (ER-ICA or ERICA).[29] Application of computer assisted image analysis is reported.[30]

Some but not all authors report that ER- and PR-positive ovarian tumors may have a better prognosis,[31] probability of recurrence, and disease-free interval. In Japanese women with breast cancer without nodal metastasis, ER status did not have an effect on relapse-free survival after surgery. However, in Japanese women with four or more positive lymph nodes, ER status appeared to increase postrelapse survival.[32] Many other factors also bear on survival following carcinoma of the breast. Nomura et al report diminution and loss of ER and PR as the malignant state progresses and with endocrine therapy.[32]

Footnotes

1. Chevallier B, Heintzmann F, Mosseri V, et al, "Prognostic Value of Estrogen and Progesterone Receptors in Operable Breast Cancer," *Cancer*, 1988, 62(12):2517-24.
2. Fisher ER, Sass R, and Fisher B, "Pathologic Findings From the National Surgical Adjuvant Breast Project," *Cancer*, 1987, 59:1554-9.
3. Lesser ML, Rosen PP, Senie RT, et al, "Estrogen and Progesterone Receptors in Breast Carcinoma: Correlations With Epidemiology and Pathology," *Cancer*, 1981, 48:299-309.
4. Ellis LM, Wittliff JL, Bryant MS, et al, "Lability of Steroid Hormone Receptors Following Devascularization of Breast Tumors," *Arch Surg*, 1989, 124(1):39-42.
5. Muensch H and Maslow WC, "Interference of O.C.T.® Embedding Compound With Hormone Receptor Assays," *Am J Clin Pathol*, 1984, 82:89-92.
6. Clark GM, McGuire WL, Hubay CA, et al, "Progesterone Receptors as a Prognostic Factor in Stage II Breast Cancer," *N Engl J Med*, 1983, 309:1343-7.
7. Grunberg SM, Weiss MH, Spitz IM, et al, "Treatment of Unresectable Meningiomas With the Antiprogesterone Agent Mifepristone," *J Neurosurg*, 1991, 74(6):861-6.
8. Esteban JM, Kandalaft PL, Mehta P, et al, "Improvement of the Quantification of Estrogen and Progesterone Receptors in Paraffin-Embedded Tumors by Image Analysis," *Am J Clin Pathol*, 1993, 99(1):32-8.
9. Graham DM, Jin L, and Lloyd RV, "Detection of Estrogen Receptor in Paraffin-Embedded Sections of Breast Carcinoma by Immunohistochemistry and *In Situ* Hybridization," *Am J Surg Pathol*, 1991, 15(5):475-85.
10. Mohammed RH, Lakatua DJ, Haus E, et al, "Estrogen and Progesterone Receptors in Human Breast Cancer – Correlation With Histologic Subtype and Degree of Differentiation," *Cancer*, 1986, 58:1076-81.
11. Rochman H, Conniff ES, and Kuk-Nagle KT, "Age and Incidence of Estrogen Receptor Positive Breast Tumors," *Ann Clin Lab Sci*, 1985, 15(2):106-8.
12. King WJ and Weigand RA, "Estrogen Receptor Detection and Measurement Using Monoclonal Antibodies to Human Estrogen Receptor," *Pathologist*, 1986, 40:15-9.
13. Valavaara R, Tuominen J, and Johansson R, "Predictive Value of Tumor Estrogen and Progesterone Receptor Levels in Postmenopausal Women With Advanced Breast Cancer Treated With Toremifene," *Cancer*, 1990, 66(11):2264-9.
14. Bezwoda WR, Esser JD, Dansey R, et al, "The Value of Estrogen and Progesterone Receptor Determinations in Advanced Breast Cancer – Estrogen Receptor Level but Not Progesterone Receptor Level Correlates With Response to Tamoxifen," *Cancer*, 1991, 68(4):867-72.
15. Winek RR, Jiang N-S, and Wold LE, "Estrogen and Progesterone Receptors in Benign Breast Tissue," *Am J Clin Pathol*, 1987, 88:526-7, (abstract).
16. Weiss SW, Langloss JM, Shmookler BM, et al, "Estrogen Receptor Protein in Bone and Soft Tissue Tumors," *Lab Invest*, 1986, 54:689-94.
17. Bhatia SK, Saclarides TJ, Witt TR, et al, "Hormone Receptor Studies in Axillary Metastases From Occult Breast Cancers," *Cancer*, 1987, 59:1170-2.
18. Kobayashi S, Mizuno T, Tobioka N, et al, "Sex Steroid Receptors in Diverse Human Tumors," *Gann*, 1982, 73(9):439-45.

(Continued)

Estrogen Receptor Assay *(Continued)*

19. Beattie CW, Hansen NW, and Thomas PA, "Steroid Receptors in Human Lung Cancer," *Cancer Res*, 1985, 45:4206-14.
20. Nagasue N, Kohno H, Chang Y-C, et al, "Androgen and Estrogen Receptors in Hepatocellular Carcinoma and the Surrounding Liver in Women," *Cancer*, 1989, 63(1):112-6.
21. Lim CL, Walker MJ, Melita RR, et al, "Estrogen and Antiestrogen Binding Sites in Dermoid Tumor," *Eur J Cancer Clin Oncol*, 1986, 22:583-7.
22. Carbone A, Ranelletti FO, Rinelli A, et al, "Type II Estrogen Receptors in the Papillary Cystic Tumor of the Pancreas," *Am J Clin Pathol*, 1989, 92(5):572-6.
23. Walker MJ, Ronan SG, Han MC, et al, "Interrelationship Between Histopathologic Characteristics of Melanoma and Estrogen Receptor Status," *Cancer*, 1991, 68(1):184-8.
24. Konishi I, Fujii S, Nonogaki H, et al, "Immunohistochemical Analysis of Estrogen Receptors, Progesterone Receptors, Ki-67 Antigen, and Human Papillomavirus DNA in Normal and Neoplastic Epithelium of the Uterine Cervix," *Cancer*, 1991, 68(6):1340-50.
25. Hanna W and Mobbs BG, "Comparative Evaluation of ER-ICA and Enzyme Immunoassay for the Quantitation of Estrogen Receptors in Breast Cancers," *Am J Clin Pathol*, 1989, 91(2):182-6.
26. Masood S, "Use of Monoclonal Antibody for Assessment of Estrogen Receptor Content in Fine Needle Aspiration Biopsy Specimen From Patients With Breast Cancer," *Arch Pathol Lab Med*, 1989, 113(1):26-30.
27. Shimada A, Kimura S, Abe K, et al, "Immunocytochemical Staining of Estrogen Receptor in Paraffin Sections of Human Breast Cancer by Use of Monoclonal Antibody: Comparison With That in Frozen Sections," *Proc Natl Acad Sci U S A*, 1985, 82:4803-7.
28. Andersen J, Orntoft T, and Poulsen HS, "Semiquantitative Oestrogen Receptor Assay in Formalin-Fixed Paraffin Sections of Human Breast Cancer Tissue Using Monoclonal Antibodies," *Br J Cancer*, 1986, 53:691-4.
29. Teasdale J, Jackson P, Holgate CS, et al, "Identification of Oestrogen Receptors in Cells of Paraffin-Processed Breast Cancers by IGSS," *Histochemistry*, 1987, 87:185-7.
30. Bacus S, Flowers JL, Press MF, et al, "The Evaluation of Estrogen Receptor in Primary Breast Carcinoma by Computer-Assisted Image Analysis," *Am J Clin Pathol*, 1988, 90(3):233-9.
31. Geisinger KR, Kute TE, Pettenati MJ, et al, "Characterization of a Human Ovarian Carcinoma Cell Line With Estrogen and Progesterone Receptors," *Cancer*, 1989, 63(2):280-8.
32. Nomura Y, Tashiro H, and Shinozuka K, "Changes of Steroid Hormone Receptor Content by Chemotherapy and/or Endocrine Therapy in Advanced Breast Cancer," *Cancer*, 1985, 55:546-51.

References

Allred DC, "Should Immunohistochemical Examination Replace Biochemical Hormone Receptor Assays in Breast Cancer?" *Am J Clin Pathol*, 1993, 99(1):1-3.

Altman E and Cadman E, "An Analysis of 1,539 Patients With Cancer of Unknown Primary Site," *Cancer*, 1986, 57:120-4.

Cohen C, Unger ER, Sgoutas D, et al, "Automated Immunohistochemical Estrogen Receptor in Fixed Embedded Breast Carcinomas - Comparison With Manual Immunohistochemistry on Frozen Tissues," *Am J Clin Pathol*, 1989, 92(5):669-72.

Farley AL, O'Brien T, Moyer D, et al, "The Detection of Estrogen Receptors in Gynecologic Tumors Using Immunoperoxidase and the Dextran-Coated Charcoal Assay," *Cancer*, 1982, 49:2153-60.

Harding M, Cowan S, Hole D, et al, "Estrogen and Progesterone Receptors in Ovarian Cancer," *Cancer*, 1990, 65(3):486-91.

Kaplan FS, Fallon MD, Boden SD, et al, "Estrogen Receptors in Bone in a Patient With Polyostotic Fibrous Dysplasia (McCune-Albright Syndrome)," *Med Intell*, 1989, 319:421-2.

Kiang DT, "The Presence of Steroid Receptors in "Nontarget" Tissues and Its Significance," *Am J Clin Pathol*, 1993, 99(2):120-2.

Nagasue N, Ito A, Yukaya H, et al, "Estrogen Receptors in Hepatocellular Carcinoma," *Cancer*, 1986, 57:87-91.

Nomura Y, Miura S, Koyama H, et al, "Relative Effect of Steroid Hormone Receptors on the Prognosis of Patients With Operable Breast Cancer," *Cancer*, 1992, 69(1):153-64.

Olson JJ, Beck DW, Schlechte J, et al, "Hormonal Manipulation of Meningiomas *In Vitro*," *J Neurosurg*, 1986, 65:99-107.

Pascal RR, Santeusanio G, Sarrell D, et al, "Immunohistologic Detection of Estrogen Receptors in Paraffin-Embedded Breast Cancers: Correlation With Cytosol Measurements," *Hum Pathol*, 1986, 17:370-5.

Paterson DA, Reid CP, Anderson TJ, et al, "Assessment of Oestrogen Receptor Content of Breast Carcinoma by Immunohistochemical Techniques on Fixed and Frozen Tissue and by Biochemical Ligand Binding Assay," *J Clin Pathol*, 1990, 43(1):46-51.

Pierce VE Jr, Rives DA, Sisley JF, et al, "Estradiol and Progesterone Receptors in a Case of Fibromatosis of the Breast," *Arch Pathol Lab Med*, 1987, 111:870-2.

Sabini G, Chumas JC, and Mann WJ, "Steroid Hormone Receptors in Endometrial Stromal Sarcomas - A Biochemical and Immunohistochemical Study," *Am J Clin Pathol*, 1992, 97(3):381-6.

Shintaku IP and Said JW, "Detection of Estrogen Receptors With Monoclonal Antibodies in Routinely Processed Formalin-Fixed Paraffin Sections of Breast Carcinoma," *Am J Clin Pathol*, 1987, 87:161-7.

Tesch M, Shawwa A, and Henderson R, "Immunohistochemical Determination of Estrogen and Progesterone Receptor Status in Breast Cancer," *Am J Clin Pathol*, 1993, 99(1):8-12.

Thornton JG and Wells M, "Oestrogen Receptor in Glands and Stroma of Normal and Neoplastic Human Endometrium: A Combined Biochemical, Immunohistochemical, and Morphometric Study," *J Clin Pathol*, 1987, 40:1437-42.

van Hoeven KH, Menendez-Botet CJ, Strong EW, et al, "Estrogen and Progesterone Receptor Content in Human Thyroid Disease," *Am J Clin Pathol*, 1993, 99(2):175-81.

Wolf RM, Schneider SL, Pontes JE, et al, "Estrogen and Progestin Receptors in Human Prostatic Carcinoma," *Cancer*, 1985, 55:2477-81.

Yokozaki H, Takekura N, Takanashi A, et al, "Estrogen Receptors in Gastric Adenocarcinoma: A Retrospective Immunohistochemical Analysis," *Virchows Archiv [A]*, 1988, 413:297-302.

Estrogen Receptor Immunocytochemical Assay

***CPT** 88342*

Related Information

Breast Biopsy *on page 40*
Estrogen Receptor Assay *on page 47*
Fine Needle Aspiration, Superficial Palpable Masses *on page 499*
Image Analysis *on page 58*
Progestogen Receptor Assay *on page 77*
Progestogen Receptor Immunocytochemical Assay *on page 79*

Synonyms ERICA; ER(ICA); Estradiol Receptor (Immunocytochemical); Estrogen Binding Protein (Immunocytochemical)

Test Commonly Includes Progesterone receptor immunocytochemical assay (PRICA) may be included, depending upon the laboratory. Evaluation of both estrogen and progesterone receptors is strongly recommended as both ER and PR may have independent prognostic weight. DNA studies may be desirable. They include ploidy (diploid aka euploid, normal or aneuploid, abnormal) and S phase (synthesis phase, estimating proliferative activity of a neoplasm). Such work-up may be done with either flow cytometry or image analysis of paraffin-embedded tissue or cytologic smears.

Abstract Evaluation done on paraffin-embedded tissue, frozen sections, or touch preparations to select those breast cancer patients likely to be responsive to endocrine therapy.

Patient Care PREPARATION: The same conditions apply as for determination of estrogen receptor status by cytosolic methods; see listing, Estrogen Receptor Assay.

Specimen ERICA may be done on any primary breast tumor, gynecologic tumor or meningioma, as well as other tissue. Assay may be performed on any paraffin block that is properly fixed, processed, and not subject to temperatures above 60°C. Frozen sections and touch preparations kept at -70°C may also be used. As receptors are quantitated by image analysis (usually), the amount of tissue submitted may be minimal. ERICA is ideal for minimal carcinomas or cases in which only archival material is available. As little as two 4 micron slides for estrogen receptors and two 4 micron slides for progesterone receptors can be used in addition to those needed for conventional light microscopy. Slides should be air dried and unstained. Consult pathologist of laboratory performing assay for proper specimen collection. Tissue sent for assay may be a primary tumor or metastases. Metastases from breast or other primaries, or instances in which the primary is unknown, may be sent along with 4 micron sections of the primary tumor (if available) for comparison, even when estrogen receptor assay by the cytosolic method was previously employed. COLLECTION: Slides must be labeled according to proper surgical pathology procedures. A copy of the surgical pathology report, even if only provisional, should accompany slides or touch preparations to provide proper identification of the slides. Slides may be mailed in any fashion that prevents breakage. STORAGE INSTRUCTIONS: Paraffin-embedded sections should be kept at room temperature below 60°C. Frozen sections and touch preparations should be kept at -70°C. Frozen sections and touch preparations should be mailed on dry ice. Depending upon the technique of the laboratory, touch preparations may be fixed, briefly in formalin. CAUSES FOR REJECTION: Largely necrotic tumor, improper fixation or processing, warming of slides over 60°C, extended thawing of frozen slides TURNAROUND TIME: Commonly sent to reference laboratories. Turnaround time should be less than or equal to 1 week. SPECIAL INSTRUCTIONS: Tumor should be transported to Pathology Department fresh, on ice. The same instructions as for estrogen or progesterone receptor quantitation by the cytosolic method apply.

Interpretive REFERENCE RANGE: Staining of nuclei for estrogen receptors may be semiquantitated visually as none, low, intermediate, or high. Image analysis techniques have been described.[1,2] Use of image analysis techniques may allow for more refined quantitation of receptors using ERICA. ERICA may also be performed on needle aspirates[3] and touch preparations

(Continued)

Estrogen Receptor Immunocytochemical Assay *(Continued)*

or imprints.[4] **USE:** Patients whose breast carcinomas lack estrogen receptors are often candidates for chemotherapy. Slightly more than 50% of patients having breast carcinomas positive for estrogen receptors respond to endocrine therapy such as tamoxifen. **LIMITATIONS:** One disadvantage of ERICA is its semiquantitative nature (*vide infra*). **METHODOLOGY:** Immunoperoxidase procedures utilize monoclonal antiestrogen receptor antibodies. Tissue examined may be paraffin sections, frozen (cryostat) sections, or touch imprints. **ADDITIONAL INFORMATION:** Advantages of ERICA over conventional cytosolic assays include the ability to detect estrogen receptors in minimal breast carcinomas not amenable to receptor quantitation by cytosolic methods.[5] Patients with tumors containing an unusual amount of stroma with few tumor cells may also benefit from ERICA. ERICA does not suffer from method variations in protein concentration determinations as does the cytosolic assay.[6]

Utilizing cytosolic methods, estrogen receptors may be found in benign mammary tissue from mastectomies for breast carcinoma. While most benign ER-positive tissue is associated with ER-positive tumors, the reverse is not true. Benign breast tissue taken from reduction mammoplasty specimens (not for carcinoma) contain ER receptors at a concentration lower than that of benign tissue from resection specimens for breast carcinoma.[7] With immunohistochemical methods 28% to 31% of fibroadenomas, 18% to 28% of epithelial hyperplasias, 30% to 40% of sclerosing adenosis specimens, and 38% to 45% of papillomata demonstrate estrogen receptors.[4] Twenty percent of comedo carcinoma *in situ* specimens demonstrate estrogen receptors compared to >50% of papillary cribriform carcinoma *in situ* specimens.[8]

An early study utilizing fluorescein labeled estradiol demonstrated cytoplasmic staining of breast tumor cells for receptors having good correlation with cytosolic methods.[9] Recently, using receiver operator characteristics, it has been determined that nuclear and not cytoplasmic staining determines the estrogen receptor status for the antiestrogen antibody H222 (Abbott Laboratories, Chicago, Illinois).[10] Comparisons of ERICA on frozen sections with cytosolic methods have generally shown good agreement.[11,12,13,14,15,16] Agreement between the two methods has been as high as 95%. It averages about 85% in the referenced studies, although some investigators have found as little as 79% agreement.[17] Comparisons of paraffin-embedded sections with frozen sections show slightly less agreement, usually between 80% to 85%. Discrepancies may be attributable to presence of normal epithelium adjacent to ERICA negative tumor cells, scant tumor cells in sample, and circulating estrogens occupying receptor sites blocking radioligand (radiolabeled estradiol) from binding to receptor sites in cytosol methods.[15] Fixation of tumors overnight in methacarn (methanol:chloroform:acetic acid 6:3:1) at 4°C may provide optimal agreement with cytosol methods.[16] Paterson et al[16] have reviewed the literature on fixation methods; the choice for the most optimal fixation method is still unclear.

In women with advanced untreated breast cancer, ER-positive patients have a longer median survival (67 vs 32 months) than ER-negative patients. This was an effect of both prolonged disease-free interval (27 vs 17 months) and a prolonged survival after recurrence (41 vs 15 months).[18] In a study of 199 breast cancer patients younger than 50 years of age with node-negative status, 16 of 104 estrogen receptor negative patients versus 1 of 43 estrogen receptor-positive patients developed local or distant recurrence in 44 months of follow-up. Five ER-negative patients died from disease versus 1 ER-positive patient.[19] Breast cancer specimens from a study of 600 women demonstrated that both positive ERICA and PRICA correlate with postmenopausal status. Colloid carcinomas of the breast were most likely to be ERICA and PRICA positive while medullary carcinomas of the breast were most likely to be ERICA and PRICA negative.[20] Positive ERICA was significantly associated with disease-free survival in women with stage I or stage II disease using single variable analysis. Using a Cox proportional hazard model a positive PRICA was the best predictor of survival and disease-free survival.[20] One report describes ERICA on involved lymph nodes in breast cancer patients.[21]

A very modest improvement in response to hormonal therapy has been reported in patients with ER-positive ovarian carcinoma.[22] Progesterone and estrogen receptors correlate with nuclear staining in uterine endometrial adenocarcinomas utilizing immunocytochemical methods.[23,24,25] Histologic grade of such adenocarcinomas correlated with positive ERICA and PRICA status.[23,24] Uterine endometrioid adenocarcinoma had the highest degree of positive ERICA and PRICA status followed by adenosquamous carcinoma, serous carcinoma, and lastly clear cell carcinoma.[24] Sensitivity of ERICA and PRICA compared to cytosolic methods was 78.5% and 58.2% for ER and PR. Survival in uterine endometrial carcinoma was predicted by both positive ERICA and PRICA. Multivariate analysis of this data showed that positive ERICA was the most important predictor of survival.[25]

Footnotes

1. Kommoss F, Bibbo M, Colley M, et al, "Assessment of Hormone Receptors in Breast Carcinoma by Immunocytochemistry and Image Analysis – 1. Progesterone Receptors," *Anal Quant Cytol Histol*, 1989, 11(5):298-306.
2. El-Badawy N, Cohen C, Derose PB, et al, "Immunohistochemical Progesterone Receptor Assay – Measurement by Image Analysis," *Am J Clin Pathol*, 1991, 96(6):704-10.
3. Reiner A, Reiner G, Spona J, et al, "Estrogen Receptor Immunocytochemistry for Preoperative Determination of Estrogen Receptor Status on Fine-Needle Aspirates of Breast Cancer," *Am J Clin Pathol*, 1987, 88:399-404.
4. Helin HJ, Isola JJ, Helin MJ, et al, "Imprint Cytology in Immunocytochemical Analysis of Oestrogen and Progesterone Receptors of Breast Carcinoma," *J Clin Pathol*, 1989, 42(10):1043-5.
5. Russack V, Meurer WT, Viesca T, et al, "Frozen Section Estrogen Receptor Determination in Minimal Breast Tumors," *Surg Pathol*, 1991, 4:113-20.
6. Howanitz PJ, Howanitz JH, Skrodzki CA, et al, "Protein Method Influences on Calculation of Tissue Receptor Concentration," *Am J Clin Pathol*, 1986, 85:37-42.
7. Netto GJ, Cheek JH, Zachariah NY, et al, "Steroid Receptors in Benign Mastectomy Tissue," *Am J Clin Pathol*, 1990, 94(1):14-7.
8. Giri DD, Dundas SA, Nottingham JF, et al, "Oestrogen Receptors in Benign Epithelial Lesions and Intraduct Carcinomas of the Breast: An Immunohistological Study," *Histopathology*, 1989, 15(6):575-84.
9. Hanna W, Ryder DE, and Mobbs BG, "Cellular Localization of Estrogen Binding Sites in Human Breast Cancer," *Am J Clin Pathol*, 1982, 77:391-5.
10. O'Keane JC, Okon E, Moroz K, et al, "Anti-Estradiol Immunoperoxidase Labeling of Nuclei, Not Cytoplasm, in Paraffin Sections, Determines Estrogen Receptor Status of Breast Cancer," *Am J Surg Pathol*, 1990, 14(2):121-7.
11. Esteban JM, Kandalaft PL, Mehta P, et al, "Improvement of the Quantification of Estrogen and Progesterone Receptors in Paraffin-Embedded Tumors by Image Analysis," *Am J Clin Pathol*, 1993, 99(1):32-8.
12. Cudahy TJ, Boeryd BR, Franlund BK, et al, "A Comparison of Three Different Methods for the Determination of Estrogen Receptors in Human Breast Cancer," *Am J Clin Pathol*, 1988, 90(5):583-90.
13. Tesch M, Shawwa A, and Henderson R, "Immunohistochemical Determination of Estrogen and Progesterone Receptor Status in Breast Cancer," *Am J Clin Pathol*, 1993, 99(1):8-12.
14. Ozzello L, DeRosa C, Habif DV, et al, "An Immunohistochemical Evaluation of Progesterone Receptor in Frozen Sections, Paraffin Sections, and Cytologic Imprints of Breast Carcinomas," *Cancer*, 1991, 67(2):455-62.
15. Parl FF and Posey YF, "Discrepancies of the Biochemical and Immunohistochemical Estrogen Receptor Assays in Breast Cancer," *Hum Pathol*, 1988, 19(8):960-6.
16. Paterson DA, Reid CP, Anderson TJ, et al, "Assessment of Oestrogen Receptor Content of Breast Carcinoma by Immunohistochemical Techniques on Fixed and Frozen Tissue and by Biochemical Ligand Binding Assay," *J Clin Pathol*, 1990, 43(1):46-51.
17. Shimada A, Kimura S, Abe K, et al, "Immunocytochemical Staining of Estrogen Receptor in Paraffin Sections of Human Breast Cancer by Use of Monoclonal Antibody: Comparison With That in Frozen Sections," *Proc Natl Acad Sci U S A*, 1985, 82:4803-7.
18. Andersen J and Poulsen HS, "Immunohistochemical Estrogen Receptor Determination in Paraffin-Embedded Tissue – Prediction of Response to Hormonal Treatment in Advanced Breast Cancer," *Cancer*, 1989, 64(9):1901-8.
19. Moot SK, Peters GN, and Cheek JH, "Tumor Hormone Receptor Status and Recurrences in Premenopausal Node Negative Breast Carcinoma," *Cancer*, 1987, 60:382-5.
20. Pertschuk LP, Kim DS, Nayer K, et al, "Immunocytochemical Estrogen and Progestin Receptor Assays in Breast Cancer With Monoclonal Antibodies – Histopathologic, Demographic, and Biochemical Correlations and Relationship to Endocrine Response and Survival," *Cancer*, 1990, 66(8):1663-70.
21. Mori T, Morimoto T, Komaki K, et al, "Comparison of Estrogen Receptor and Epidermal Growth Factor Receptor Content of Primary and Involved Nodes in Human Breast Cancer," *Cancer*, 1991, 68(3):532-7.
22. Fromm G-L, Freedman RS, Fritsche HA, et al, "Sequentially Administered Ethinyl Estradiol and Medroxyprogesterone Acetate in the Treatment of Refractory Epithelial Ovarian Carcinoma in Patients With Positive Estrogen Receptors," *Cancer*, 1991, 68(9):1885-9.
23. Segreti EM, Novotny DB, Soper JT, et al, "Endometrial Cancer: Histologic Correlates of Immunohistochemical Localization of Progesterone Receptor and Estrogen Receptor," *Obstet Gynecol*, 1989, 73(5 Pt 1):780-5.
24. Carcangiu ML, Chambers JT, Voynick IM, et al, "Immunohistochemical Evaluation of Estrogen and Progesterone Receptor Content in 183 Patients With Endometrial Carcinoma – Part I: Clinical and Histologic Correlations," *Am J Clin Pathol*, 1990, 94(3):247-54.
25. Chambers JT, Carcangiu ML, Voynick IM, et al, "Immunohistochemical Evaluation of Estrogen and Progesterone Receptor Content in 183 Patients With Endometrial Carcinoma – Part II: Correlation Between Biochemical and Immunohistochemical Methods and Survival," *Am J Clin Pathol*, 1990, 94(3):255-60.

References

Allred DC, "Should Immunohistochemical Examination Replace Biochemical Hormone Receptor Assays in Breast Cancer?" *Am J Clin Pathol*, 1993, 99(1):1-3.

Briscoe D, Ni K, Wied GL, et al, "Comparison of Estrogen Receptor Immunocytochemical Assay in Frozen and Paraffin Sections," *Anal Quant Cytol Histol*, 1992, 14(2):105-12.

(Continued)

Estrogen Receptor Immunocytochemical Assay *(Continued)*

Cohen C, Unger ER, Sgoutas D, et al, "Automated Immunohistochemical Estrogen Receptor in Fixed Embedded Breast Carcinomas - Comparison With Manual Immunohistochemistry on Frozen Tissues," *Am J Clin Pathol*, 1989, 92(5):669-72.

Graham DM, Jin L, and Lloyd RV, "Detection of Estrogen Receptor in Paraffin-Embedded Sections of Breast Carcinoma by Immunohistochemistry and *In Situ* Hybridization," *Am J Surg Pathol*, 1991, 15(5):475-85.

Helin HJ, Helle MJ, and Helin ML, "Immunocytochemical Detection of Estrogen and Progesterone Receptors in 124 Human Breast Cancers," *Am J Clin Pathol*, 1988, 89:137-42.

Isola JJ, Helle MJ, and Helin HJ, "Immunocytochemical Detection of Progesterone Receptor in Breast Carcinoma. Comparison of Two Monoclonal Antibodies," *Am J Clin Pathol*, 1990, 93(3):378-82.

Kiang DT, "The Presence of Steroid Receptors in "Nontarget" Tissues and Its Significance," *Am J Clin Pathol*, 1993, 99(2):120-2.

Loven D, Rakowsky E, Geier A, et al, "A Clinical Evaluation of Nuclear Estrogen Receptors Combined With Cytosolic Estrogen and Progesterone Receptors in Breast Cancer," *Cancer*, 1990, 66(2):341-6.

Masood S, "Use of Monoclonal Antibody for Assessment of Estrogen Receptor Content in Fine-Needle Aspiration Biopsy Specimen From Patients With Breast Cancer," *Arch Pathol Lab Med*, 1989, 113(1):26-30.

Onetti-Muda A, Crescenzi A, Pujia N, et al, "Demonstration of Oestrogen and Progesterone Receptors in Freeze-Dried, Paraffin-Embedded Sections of Breast Cancer," *Histopathology*, 1991, 18(6):511-6.

Sabini G, Chumas JC, and Mann WJ, "Steroid Hormone Receptors in Endometrial Stromal Sarcomas - A Biochemical and Immunohistochemical Study," *Am J Clin Pathol*, 1992, 97(3):381-6.

Seymour L, Meyer K, Esser J, et al, "Estimation of PR and ER by Immunocytochemistry in Breast Cancer. Comparison With Radioligand Binding Methods," *Am J Clin Pathol*, 1990, 94(4 Suppl 1):S35-40.

van Hoeven KH, Menendez-Botet CJ, Strong EW, et al, "Estrogen and Progesterone Receptor Content in Human Thyroid Disease," *Am J Clin Pathol*, 1993, 99(2):175-81.

Wilbur DC, Willis J, Mooney RA, et al, "Estrogen and Progesterone Receptor Detection in Archival Formalin-Fixed, Paraffin-Embedded Tissue From Breast Carcinoma: A Comparison of Immunohistochemistry With the Dextran-Coated Charcoal Assay," *Mod Pathol*, 1992, 5(1):79-84.

Factor VIII Related Antigen *see* Immunoperoxidase Procedures *on page 60*

Flow Cytometry *see* Breast Biopsy *on page 40*

Flow Cytometry *see* Immunophenotypic Analysis of Tissues by Flow Cytometry *on page 65*

Flow Cytometry of Tumor Aneuploidy *see* Tumor Aneuploidy by Flow Cytometry *on page 88*

Fluorescein-Tagged Antibodies *see* Kidney Biopsy *on page 68*

Fluorescence Activated Cell Sorting *see* Immunophenotypic Analysis of Tissues by Flow Cytometry *on page 65*

Fluorescent Rabies Antibody Test *see* Rabies *on page 82*

Forensic Specimens *see* Histopathology *on page 57*

FRA Test *see* Rabies *on page 82*

Frozen Section

CPT 88331 (single); 88332 (each additional)

Related Information

Breast Biopsy *on page 40*
Histopathology *on page 57*
Lymph Node Biopsy *on page 72*
Virus, Direct Detection by Fluorescent Antibody *on page 1208*

Synonyms FS; Intraoperative Consultation, Pathology; Pathology Operating Room Consultation; Surgical Pathology Consultation

Applies to Intraoperative Rapid Consultation

Test Commonly Includes Gross examination, specimen evaluation, and possible frozen section with interpretation, followed by routine histopathology report. Imprints and smears may be made from fresh tissue. Further studies may be initiated, depending on clinical input, gross observations, and frozen section and/or cytologic findings.

Abstract Provision of intraoperative diagnosis when operative consultation is needed to enhance patient care. Intraoperative consultation may not require a frozen section at all. It is the pathologist's responsibility to discuss the case with the surgeon and do that which is indicated for the best interests of the patient. Tissue freezing may actually be contraindicated. **Rapid diagnosis not leading to enhancement in patient care is not an indication for frozen section.**

Patient Care PREPARATION: A need exists for provision of clinical history to the surgical pathologist.

Specimen Fresh tissue with **no** added fixative or fluid, rapidly submitted in a sterile container CONTAINER: Sterile towel, Petri dish, or jar COLLECTION: Container must be labeled with patient's name, room number, date, operating room, and name of the surgeon requesting frozen section. CAUSES FOR REJECTION: Specimen in fixative

Interpretive USE: Establish rapid histopathologic diagnosis of a pathologic process;[1] occasionally, to ascertain if cultures are indicated and, if so, to provide indication of the type of cultures needed; procure tissue for fat stains; procure tissue for direct immunofluorescent examination (eg, kappa and lambda light chains, bacterial antigens); rapid evaluation for direction of fresh tissues for possible subsequent special studies such as lymphocyte markers, flow cytometry, receptor assays, and/or electron microscopy. Determination of the spread of disease may be accomplished with frozen sections in selected settings; for instance, whether or not the tumor has metastasized beyond a proposed resection field. An example may be given of pelvic lymph node examination prior to radical prostatectomy, one of the applications of frozen sections in which false-negatives from sampling errors occur. Surgeons sometimes request frozen sections to evaluate unanticipated findings (eg, a nodule in the liver). LIMITATIONS: Bone or heavily calcified tissue cannot be cut. Tissues dominated by fat are technically difficult and may not be amenable to frozen section. Fixed tissues are difficult technically to manage for frozen section. Sampling errors occur, leading to false-negative diagnoses.[2,3,4] Some lesions require permanent sections for definitive diagnosis, such as many lymphoid lesions and occasional problematic breast lesions (eg, papillary lesions, instances of lobular and intraductal hyperplasias). In some cases, diagnosis must be delayed for permanent sections. Silverberg recognizes the need for deferral in some cases and recognizes that the frequency of false-positive diagnoses relates inversely to that of deferral of diagnosis.[2,5] Reasons to defer diagnosis at frozen section include need for more extensive sampling, lack of adequate epithelium lining cysts, twisted and infarcted lesions,[3] and need for special stains, immunohistochemistry, and optimal sections.

Sampling errors are important pitfalls in application of frozen sections. Patients usually should not be kept anesthetized while multiple frozen section blocks are processed, cut, stained, and examined when paraffin sections would serve as well, or better. Frozen sections are enormously more useful to provide diagnosis of a visible lesion, than to try to rule out a possibility of an entity of microscopic proportions such as lobular carcinoma *in situ* (LCIS). LCIS, in fact, usually should not be diagnosed on frozen section but only on good quality paraffin sections. False-negative responses are more frequent than false-positive ones.

False-negative frozen section diagnoses relate to the limited sampling possible within the abbreviated time available. Pathologists recognize the potential gravity of false-positive frozen section diagnosis of cancer. In some series a zero incidence of false-positives is reported.[3] The poorest accuracy reported from George Washington University was associated with thyroid and parathyroid glands, related in the former to the ease with which microscopic foci of papillary carcinoma or the presence of capsular or vascular invasion can be missed.[2] Differential diagnosis between reactive gliosis and low grade glioma has been a problem for many experienced surgical pathologists. Differential diagnosis in fact may be difficult on high quality paraffin sections. Silverberg wisely observes that those who publish results of frozen section examinations (false-positives, false-negatives, deferrals) are invariably those who have a great deal of experience with the technique.

Margins of specimens in resections for cancer may be a problem for which surgeons may request frozen section support. Negative margins in tumor resections may be of very limited value, especially when such margins are of substantial size, by virtue of sampling problems. Special problems in the breast are touched upon in the Breast Biopsy listing in this chapter. The presence of fat, the geometry of multiple irregular surfaces in specimens, multiplicity of specimens in some cases, and time limitation while the patient remains under anesthesia all limit the significance of a negative frozen section report of margins. Absence of positive margins does not guarantee local control of the tumor, nor is it in any way a reliable guide to tumor behavior. In Luna's head and neck series, a highly significant relationship between **positive** margins and patient survival exists. If frozen section margins were positive, only 1 of 20 patients lived 2 years.[6]

In addition to sampling errors, Luna recognizes three other types of errors: interpretive, communicative, and technical.[6] Lack of proper clinical information (eg, history of prior irradiation) can lead to interpretive error.

(Continued)

Frozen Section *(Continued)*

The problems of frozen section for thyroid surgery include the differential diagnosis between instances of follicular adenoma versus carcinoma,[7] as well as identification of the occasional relatively small papillary carcinoma.

CONTRAINDICATIONS: Tissue is consumed in the process of frozen section. Tiny critical specimens (for example, possible breast carcinomas less than 5 mm in diameter) are best not risked. Breast specimens not grossly suspicious should not be frozen. The freezing process may distort lymphoid as well as other tissues. Therefore, for suspected lymphoma, it is advisable to await proper fixation of the lymph node and paraffin sections for definitive diagnosis, but frozen sections are commonly utilized for immunohistochemical evaluation of lymphoid lesions. See listing, Lymph Node Biopsy for further details. Frozen section artifact in paraffin sections subsequently processed may make definitive diagnosis inconclusive. If frozen section diagnosis is unnecessary for immediate patient management, Silverberg[5] and many others[4] recognize that it should not be performed. Silverberg comments on the role of the frozen section in provision of instant gratification to the surgeon, observing that charges are made and that information should be of value in patient management. Frozen sections are considered contraindicated when the patient is known to be HIV positive, to avoid contamination of the cryostat.[2] In such instances, imprints and smears can sometimes replace frozen sections.[8] Luna and others include small melanocytic lesions among contraindications to frozen section.[8] **METHODOLOGY:** Liquid nitrogen is better and faster than carbon dioxide. A vacuum bottle containing liquid nitrogen may be kept in the frozen section room. A slice of the specimen on an object holder, placed onto O.C.T.<rf[compound, is lowered into the vacuum bottle with a metal clamp. Cryobaths with a refrigerant such as 3-methyl butane chilled to -70°C also give satisfactory results. The author uses H & E staining. Hematoxylin staining can be abbreviated with a microwave. **ADDITIONAL INFORMATION:** Direct communication between pathologist and surgeon must occur at the time of frozen section diagnosis, according to requirements both of regulatory agencies and of good patient care. Imprints may be stained with H & E, Wright's stain, or by other methods. They sometimes are extremely helpful in interpretation of frozen sections. Occasionally, imprints are more diagnostic than the frozen section. They are especially helpful with lymphoid specimens, occasional breast specimens, and in diagnosis of meningioma.

Footnotes

1. Sawady J, Berner JJ, and Siegler EE, "Accuracy of and Reasons for Frozen Sections: A Correlative, Retrospective Study," *Hum Pathol*, 1988, 19(9):1019-23.
2. Oneson RH, Minke JA, and Silverberg SG, "Intraoperative Pathologic Consultation. An Audit of 1000 Recent Consecutive Cases," *Am J Surg Pathol*, 1989, 13(3):237-43.
3. Obiakor I, Maiman M, Mittal K, et al, "The Accuracy of Frozen Section in the Diagnosis of Ovarian Neoplasms," *Gynecol Oncol*, 1991, 43(1):61-3.
4. Prey MU, Vitale T, and Martin SA, "Guidelines for Practical Utilization of Intraoperative Frozen Sections," *Arch Surg*, 1989, 124(3):331-5.
5. Silverberg SG, *Principles and Practice of Surgical Pathology*, 2nd ed, Vol 1, Chapter 1, New York, NY: Churchill Livingstone, 1990, 1-12.
6. Luna MA, "Uses, Abuses, and Pitfalls of Frozen Section Diagnoses of Diseases of the Head and Neck," *Surgical Pathology of the Head and Neck*, Vol 1, Barnes L, ed, New York, NY: Marcel Dekker Inc, 1985, 7-22.
7. Shaha A, Gleich L, DiMaio T, et al, "Accuracy and Pitfalls of Frozen Section During Thyroid Surgery," *J Surg Oncol*, 1990, 44(2):84-92.
8. Reyes MG, Homsi MF, McDonald LW, et al, "Imprints, Smears, and Frozen Sections of Brain Tumors," *Neurosurgery*, 1991, 29(4):575-9.

References

Fechner RE, "Frozen Section (Intraoperative Consultation)," *Hum Pathol*, 1988, 19:999-1000, (editorial).

Gephardt GN and Rice TW, "Utility of Frozen-Section Evaluation of Lymph Nodes in the Staging of Bronchogenic Carcinoma at Mediastinoscopy and Thoracotomy," *J Thorac Cardiovasc Surg*, 1990, 100(6):853-9.

Nochomovitz L, Sidawy M, Jannotta F, et al, *Intraoperative Consultation: A Guide to Smears, Imprints & Frozen Section*, 1989.

Silva EG and Kraemer BB, *Intraoperative Pathologic Diagnosis: Frozen Sections and Other Techniques*, Baltimore, MD: Williams & Wilkins, 1987.

Zarbo RJ, Hoffman GG, and Howanitz PJ, "Interinstitutional Comparison of Frozen-Section Consultation. A College of American Pathologists Q-Probe Study of 79,647 Consultations in 297 North American Institutions," *Arch Pathol Lab Med*, 1991, 115(12):1187-94.

FS *see* Frozen Section *on page 54*

G_1 Phase *see* Tumor Aneuploidy by Flow Cytometry *on page 88*

Histopathology

CPT *88300 (level I – surgical pathology, gross examination only); 88302 (level II – surgical pathology, gross and microscopic examination of presumptively normal tissue(s) for identification and record purposes); 88304 (level III – surgical pathology, gross and microscopic examination of presumptively abnormal tissue(s) uncomplicated specimen); 88305 (level IV – single complicated or multiple uncomplicated specimens without complex dissection); 88307 (level V – single complicated specimen requiring complex dissection or multiple complicated specimens); 88309 (level VI – complex diagnostic problems with or without extensive dissection)*

Related Information

Aluminum, Bone *on page 1018*
Biopsy or Body Fluid Aerobic Bacterial Culture *on page 778*
Biopsy or Body Fluid Anaerobic Bacterial Culture *on page 778*
Biopsy or Body Fluid Fungus Culture *on page 780*
Biopsy or Body Fluid Mycobacteria Culture *on page 782*
Breast Biopsy *on page 40*
Electron Microscopic Examination for Viruses, Stool *on page 1177*
Estrogen Receptor Assay *on page 47*
Fine Needle Aspiration, Superficial Palpable Masses *on page 499*
Frozen Section *on page 54*
Gene Rearrangement for Leukemia and Lymphoma *on page 911*
Human Papillomavirus DNA Probe Test *on page 916*
Lymph Node Biopsy *on page 72*
Muscle Biopsy *on page 75*
N-myc Amplification *on page 925*
Skin Biopsies *on page 84*
Tumor Aneuploidy by Flow Cytometry *on page 88*
Viral Culture, Tissue *on page 1206*
Virus, Direct Detection by Fluorescent Antibody *on page 1208*

Synonyms Biopsy; Gross and Microscopic Pathology; Pathologic Examination; Pathology; Surgical Pathology; Tissue Examination; Tissue Pathology

Applies to Bronchial Biopsy; Endoscopic Biopsy; Forensic Specimens; Liver Biopsy; Lung Biopsy; Medical Legal Specimens

Test Commonly Includes Gross and microscopic examination and diagnosis. Imprints may be made if the tissue is fresh and unfixed and if indications for imprints exist.

Abstract Surgical pathology has been defined as the discipline which deals with the anatomic pathology of tissues removed from living patients.[1] Smears, aspirates, special stains, immunocytochemistry, flow cytometry, and molecular pathology may be included.

Patient Care PREPARATION: As Silverberg expresses it, it is essential that each specimen be accompanied by an adequate description of what it represents, as well as an appropriate clinical history.[1]

Specimen Fresh tissue, tissue fixed in phosphate buffered formalin or other appropriate fixative. Each specimen container must be labeled to include source as well as patient's name. Each specimen from a different anatomic site must be placed in a separate, correctly labeled container, designated "left," "right," "proximal," "distal," "ventral," "dorsal," and so forth. CONTAINER: Jars of assorted sizes, containing formalin or another appropriate fixative; the neck of

(Continued)

Histopathology *(Continued)*

the container should not be smaller than its diameter. Fresh specimens should be submitted on a sterile gauze pad moistened with sterile saline and should not be left on countertops; they must be placed in the hands of a responsible person. **COLLECTION:** Small biopsy specimens are to be placed immediately in fixative, unless special needs such as frozen section exist. Use approximately 5 to 20 times as much fixative solution as the bulk of the tissue. Small tissues such as those from bronchoscopic biopsy, bladder biopsy, and endometrium can be ruined in a very short time by drying out. **STORAGE INSTRUCTIONS:** Fixation in formalin solution or other appropriate fixative **CAUSES FOR REJECTION:** Mislabeled specimen container, unlabeled specimen **TURNAROUND TIME:** Biopsy reports commonly require a day or more. Need for decalcification or special stains will delay report. **SPECIAL INSTRUCTIONS:** See specific handling instructions in test listings such as those for Muscle Biopsy, Estrogen Receptor Assay, and Frozen Section. Consult the Pathology Department prior to beginning the procedure for specific instructions. Requisition should state operative diagnosis and source of specimen, as well as patient's name, age, sex, room or location, name of surgeon, and names of other physicians who will need a copy of the pathology report.

Interpretive **USE:** Histopathologic diagnosis; evaluate extent of lesions and provision of classification and, when appropriate, grading in the case of tumors **LIMITATIONS:** Tissue fixed in formalin **cannot** be used for bacteriological culture, electron microscopy, conventional estrogen or progesterone receptor assay, certain types of histochemistry, or frozen sections. **ADDITIONAL INFORMATION:** A major advantage of conventional over frozen sections is that extensive sampling of the entire specimen can take place.

Cultures of tissue are best taken in the O.R., where a sterile field exists. A piece of tissue (eg, a curetting of a fistulous tract) should be placed in an appropriate sterile tube with requests for smear, culture, anaerobic culture, AFB, and fungus culture. It should be immediately taken to the Microbiology Laboratory. See Microbiology chapter for Biopsy or Body Fluid Culture, Biopsy or Body Fluid Fungus Culture, and Biopsy or Body Fluid Mycobacteria Culture test listings.

Routine tissues are brought in fixative. Fixative fluids should be picked up prior to the biopsy. Commonly used fixatives include Zenker's fluid (for tiny specimens, eg, endometrial curettage, liver, and other needle biopsies, **not** skin), and formalin (for specimens thicker than 3 mm).

Bullets, shotgun pellets, and other metallic objects require special handling, but no fixative is needed. Of major importance in handling bullets and other specimens of possible forensic significance, including vaginal swabs obtained in rape cases, is the scrupulous maintenance of a chain-of-custody. Specimens must be accurately labeled, and transfer and receipt must be documented. Specimens must be kept under safeguards in the laboratory until turned over to law enforcement officials.

Bone biopsy for metabolic bone disease requires special handling.

Materials sometimes not sent for histopathologic examination, depending on the institution, include bullets, shotgun pellets, neonatal foreskins, grossly unremarkable placentas from uneventful deliveries, and orthopedic appliances. If a specimen is not sent to the Pathology Department, the surgeon should carefully describe the specimen in the operative report.

Footnotes

1. Silverberg SG, *Principles and Practice of Surgical Pathology*, 2nd ed, Vol 1, Chapter 1, New York, NY: Churchill Livingstone, 1990, 1-12.

References

Coulson WF, *Surgical Pathology*, 2nd ed, Vols 1 and 2, Philadelphia, PA: JB Lippincott Co, 1988.

Sternberg SS, Antonioli DA, Carter D, et al, *Diagnostic Surgical Pathology*, Vol 1 and 2, New York, NY: Raven Press, 1989.

HMB-45 *see* Immunoperoxidase Procedures *on page 60*

Image Analysis

CPT 88399

Related Information

Estrogen Receptor Assay *on page 47*
Estrogen Receptor Immunocytochemical Assay *on page 51*
Fine Needle Aspiration, Superficial Palpable Masses *on page 499*

Progestogen Receptor Immunocytochemical Assay *on page 79*
Tumor Aneuploidy by Flow Cytometry *on page 88*

Synonyms Computerized Interactive Morphometry; Image Cytometry

Applies to DNA in Tumor Nuclei; Ploidy; S Phase

Test Commonly Includes Use of computerized imaging system to contribute information which may be useful in determination of prognostic and therapeutic factors of tumors. Such factors may include tumor ploidy, DNA content, oncogene protein content, hormone receptor expression, and cellular proliferative proteins.

Abstract Affordable memory devices with microprocessors and quality cameras make image processing and statistical image analysis practical. Information from optical physics and engineering presently is appearing in pathology journals.[1,2]

Specimen Fresh tissue is the best specimen; 1 cm^2 or less fresh tumor tissue or 1 mL body fluid for concentration by cytospin. Tumor excised at time of surgery made into "touch preps" (tissue touched or spotted lightly on glass slides that allow for release of cells from the connective tissue framework to the slide) for best separation of cells. Frozen section slides and paraffin sections may also be used. Exfoliative cytology specimens and body fluids, concentrated or unconcentrated, may be used. **TURNAROUND TIME:** 2-5 days is needed to prepare the specimen, stain it appropriately, evaluate the cells, interpret the results, and produce a report. Turnaround time may vary with individual laboratories, depending on technical assistance available. Only large hospitals and medical centers may have the equipment and expertise at the time of this writing.

Interpretive **REFERENCE RANGE:** For DNA index, normal is 0.8-1.2 or the diploid state. Normal proliferation index (Ki-67 positivity of tumor cells) is <10%; S phase should be <7%. **USE:** Image analysis is an emerging method which is used to evaluate tumor aggressiveness and patient prognosis. The concept of image analysis holds that the further dedifferentiated a tumor becomes the further it deviates from the normal diploid state. This may be expressed as a tetraploid or aneuploid state according to the amount of DNA in the Feulgen-stained nuclei. In terms of ploidy, this is expressed as a DNA index between 1.0 and 2.0. The amount of cells in the S phase of the cell cycle is also a parameter that can be measured by image analysis. In general, the more cells in S phase (DNA synthesis phase), the more aggressive the tumor.

Image analysis, in combination with immunohistochemistry, may be used to study proteins within tumor cells that are important in cancer prognosis. Estrogen and progesterone receptors[3] may be evaluated with immunochemical staining of breast cancer cells with subsequent study by image analysis. Other proteins such as HER 2-neu, Ki-67, and proliferative antigen have been developed for better prognostication of tumors from many sources. Recently, even gene suppressor gene products have been found to be helpful in evaluation of tumors of the thyroid.[4]

LIMITATIONS: While flow cytometry assays 10,000-20,000 or more nuclei, in image analysis only a few hundred nuclei are counted.[5] **METHODOLOGY:** Microscope, video camera, computer, display screen (cathode ray tube). Reproducibility can be achieved with presently available equipment. Commercial systems are available and personally compiled systems are described.[2] **ADDITIONAL INFORMATION:** Analysis can be restricted to counting only cells of interest (eg, keratin positive cells in instances of epithelial tumors).[5]

Footnotes

1. Wells WA, Rainer RO, and Memoli VA, "Basic Principles of Image Processing," *Am J Clin Pathol*, 1992, 98(5):493-501.
2. Wells WA, Rainer RO, and Memoli VA, "Equipment, Standardization, and Applications of Image Processing," *Am J Clin Pathol*, 1993, 99(1):48-56.
3. El-Badawy N, Cohen C, Derose PB, et al, "Immunohistochemical Progesterone Receptor Assay, Measurement by Image Analysis," *Am J Clin Pathol*, 1991, 96(6):704-10.
4. Figge J, Bakst G, Weisheit D, et al, "Image Analysis Quantitation of Immunoreactive Retinoblastoma Protein in Human Thyroid Neoplasms With a Streptavidin-Biotin-Peroxidase Staining Technique," *Am J Pathol*, 1991, 139(6):1213-9.
5. Robinson RA, "Defining the Limits of DNA Cytometry," *Am J Clin Pathol*, 1992, 98(3):275-7, (editorial).

References

Bosari S, Wiley BD, Hamilton WM, et al, "DNA Measurement by Image Analysis of Paraffin-Embedded Breast Carcinoma Tissue - A Comparative Investigation," *Am J Clin Pathol*, 1991, 96(6):698-703.

Elsheikh TM, Silverman JF, McCool JW, et al, "Comparative DNA Analysis of Solid Tumors by Flow Cytometric and Image Analyses of Touch Imprints and Flow Cell Suspensions," *Am J Clin Pathol*, 1992, 98(3):296-304.

Linder J, "Overview of Digital Imaging in Pathology. The Fifth Wave," *Am J Clin Pathol*, 1990, 94(4 Suppl 1):S30-4.

(Continued)

Image Analysis *(Continued)*

Marchevsky AM, Gil J, and Henreick J, "Computerized Interactive Morphometry in Pathology: Current Instrument and Methods," *Hum Pathol*, 1987, 18:320-31.

Ross DW, "Image Cytometry," *Arch Pathol Lab Med*, 1990, 114(7):734.

Salmon I and Kiss R, "Relationship Between Proliferative Activity and Ploidy Level in a Series of 530 Human Brain Tumors, Including Astrocytomas, Meningiomas, Schwannomas, and Metastases," *Hum Pathol*, 1993, 24(3):329-35.

Image Cytometry *see* Image Analysis *on page 58*

Immunocytochemistry *see* Immunoperoxidase Procedures *on this page*

Immunohistochemistry *see* Immunoperoxidase Procedures *on this page*

Immunomicroscopy *see* Immunoperoxidase Procedures *on this page*

Immunoperoxidase Procedures

CPT 88342

Related Information

Body Fluids Cytology *on page 482*
Breast Biopsy *on page 40*
CA 19-9 *on page 152*
CA 125 *on page 154*
Calcitonin *on page 157*
Carcinoembryonic Antigen *on page 167*
Cerebrospinal Fluid Cytology *on page 490*
Fine Needle Aspiration, Deep Seated Lesions *on page 498*
Fine Needle Aspiration, Superficial Palpable Masses *on page 499*
Gene Rearrangement for Leukemia and Lymphoma *on page 911*
Immunophenotypic Analysis of Tissues by Flow Cytometry *on page 65*
Lymph Node Biopsy *on page 72*
Prostate Specific Antigen, Serum *on page 338*
Skin Biopsies *on page 84*
T- and B-Lymphocyte Subset Assay *on page 750*

Synonyms Immunocytochemistry; Immunohistochemistry; Immunomicroscopy; Immunostains; Peroxidase-Antiperoxidase (PAP)

Applies to Alpha Fetoprotein; Chromogranin; Cytokeratins; Desmin; Epithelial Membrane Antigen (EMA); Factor VIII Related Antigen; GCDFP-15; Glial Fibrillary Acidic Protein; Gross Cystic Disease Fluid Protein-15; hCG; βhCG; HMB-45; Intermediate Filaments; Kappa Light Chains; Ki-67; Lambda Light Chains; Lectins; Leukocyte Common Antigen; Leu M1; Light Chains; Lysozyme; Monoclonal Immunoglobulins; Myoglobin; Myosin; PCNA; Peptide Hormones; Prostate Specific Acid Phosphatase; S100; Synaptophysin; Thyroglobulin; Tissue Antigens; T Lymphocytes; Vimentin

Test Commonly Includes Antigen localization in tissue sections

Abstract Immunocytochemistry is a major diagnostic tool employed in surgical pathology, cytopathology, immunopathology, and hematopathology. Evaluation of tumor with unknown primary site is often expedited by immunocytochemical investigation.

Specimen Blood, bone marrow, or cytology smears; paraffin, plastic or frozen sections; fresh tissue remains important for work-up of possible lymphoma **CONTAINER:** Petri dish ideally containing fresh tissue, immediately delivered to optimize choice of fixatives and to permit the laboratory to snap freeze tissue if indicated. **STORAGE INSTRUCTIONS:** Deliver fresh specimens, not in fixative. **CAUSES FOR REJECTION:** Extensive drying of specimen, very extensive necrosis, tissue left unfixed or unrefrigerated for prolonged periods **SPECIAL INSTRUCTIONS:** Place fresh specimen in the hands of a histotechnician or pathologist.

Interpretive **USE:** Immunoperoxidase techniques are used to identify and localize antigens in tissue sections. The results allow pathologists to determine the major lineage of poorly differentiated neoplasms, document elaboration of tumor associated markers of potential use in monitoring the course of disease, differentiate benign from malignant lymphoid proliferations, subclassify lymphoreticular and hematopoietic neoplasms, and identify or confirm the presence of infectious agents. More recently, new information on oncogene expression has shed insights on molecular mechanisms of tumor biology and offers tools of potential prognostic significance.[1]

Table 1. Characteristic Phenotypic Profile of Neoplasms Based on Histogenesis*

	Intermediate Filaments					Chromgrn	NSE	EMA	S100	LCA	Muscle Actin	A_1ACT
	Cytokeratin	Vimentin	Desmin	NF	GFAP							
Carcinoma, NOS†	+	–/+	–	–	–	–	–/+	+	–/+	–	–	–/+
neuroendocrine§	+/–	–/+	–	–/+	–	+	+	+/–	–	–	–	–
Lymphoma#	–	–/+	–	–	–	–	–/+	–	–	+	–	–
Melanoma•	–	+	–	–	–	–	+/–	–	+	–	–	–/+
Soft tissue tumors fibrous histiocytoma	–	+	–	–	–	–	–	–	–	–	–	+
nerve sheath	–	+	–	–	–	–	–	–	+	–	–	–
muscle	–	+	+	–	–	–	–	–	–	–	+	–
vascular**	–	+	–	–	–	–	–	–	–	–	–	–
Glioma	–	+	–	–	+	–	–	–	+	–	–	–

Abbreviations: NF: neurofilament; GFAP: glial fibrillary acidic protein; Cromgrn: chromogranin A; NSE: neuron specific enolase; EMA: epithelial membrane antigen; LCA: leukocyte common antigen; A_1ACT: alpha$_1$–antichymotrypsin. Designated reactions: +: characteristically positive; +/–: characteristically positive but may be negative; –/+: characteristically negative but may be positive; –: characteristically negative.

Footnotes:
*There are many exceptions to the indicated reactions. The phenotypic profile must always be put into perspective with the light microscopy and other special studies.
†Cytokeratin profile, coexpression of S100 or other tissue specific markers may help identify origin of metastatic carcinoma.
§Expression of various peptide hormones may further aid in the clinicopathologic classification of the neoplasm.
#For additional information, see listing on Lymph Node Biopsy and Immunophenotypic Analysis of Tissues by Flow Cytometry.
•Melanoma associated antigen HMB-45 may help differentiate it from some nerve sheath tumors.
**Many vascular tumors are also positive for factor VIII related antigen and for the lectin UEA-1.

(Continued)

Panel A

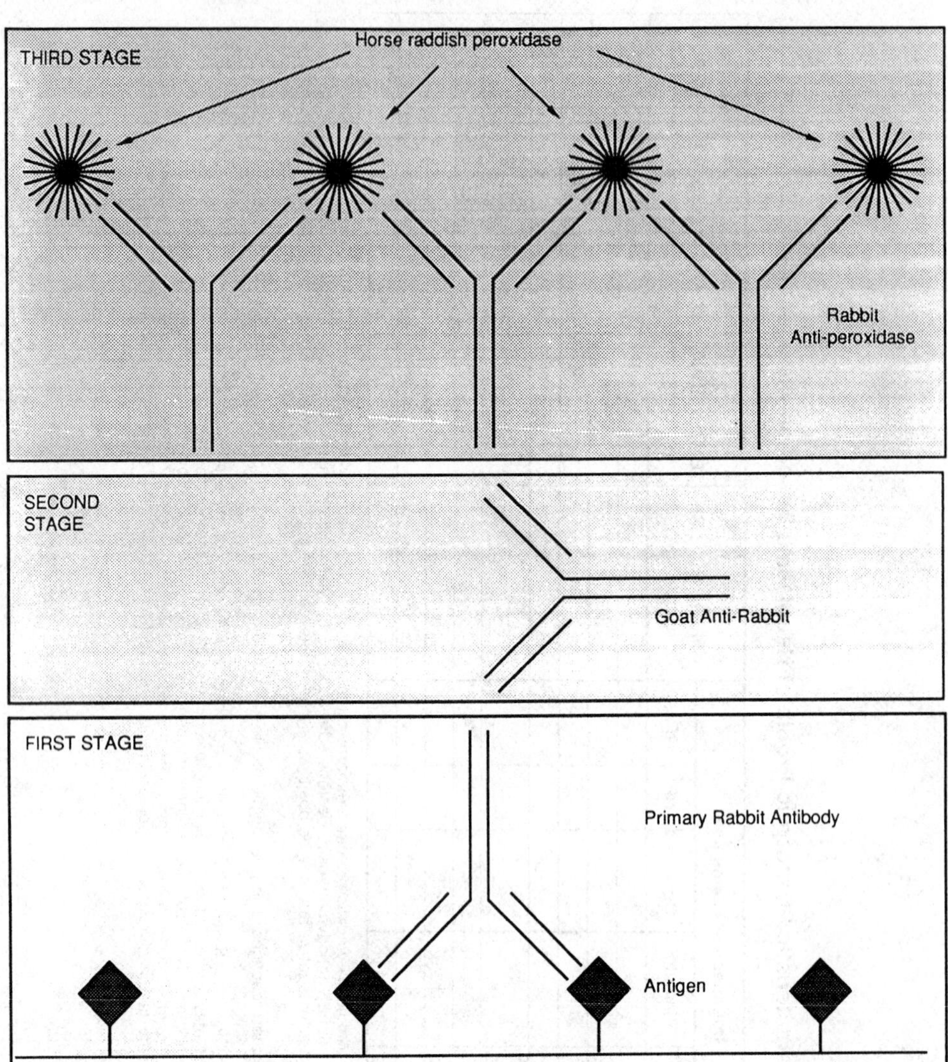

Figure 1. General scheme for performing immunoperoxidase stains: Tissue sections are deparaffinized, hydrated, and blocked to suppress endogenous peroxidase activity and nonspecific protein binding. For some stains (eg, cytokeratin), antigenic determinants are exposed by protease digestion. The first stage, incubation with primary antibody, confers specificity of the stain and is generally similar in both procedures. The PAP procedure (Panel A) employs an unlabeled second stage antibody at dilutions intended to leave one antibody

Panel B

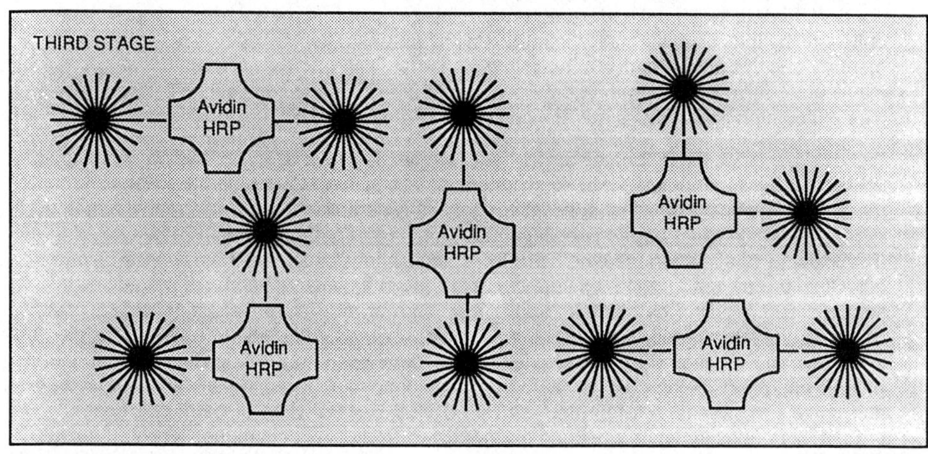

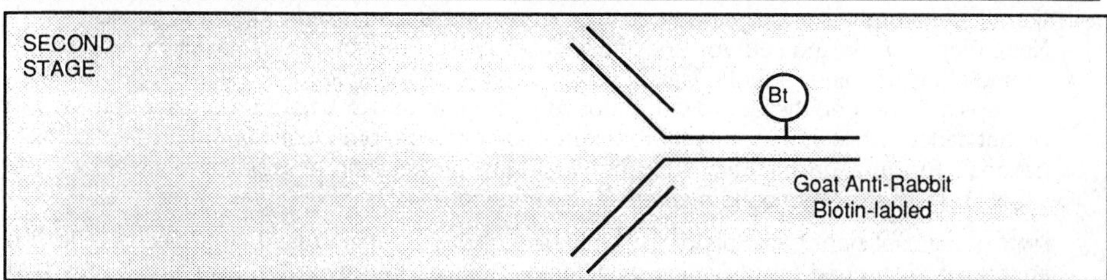

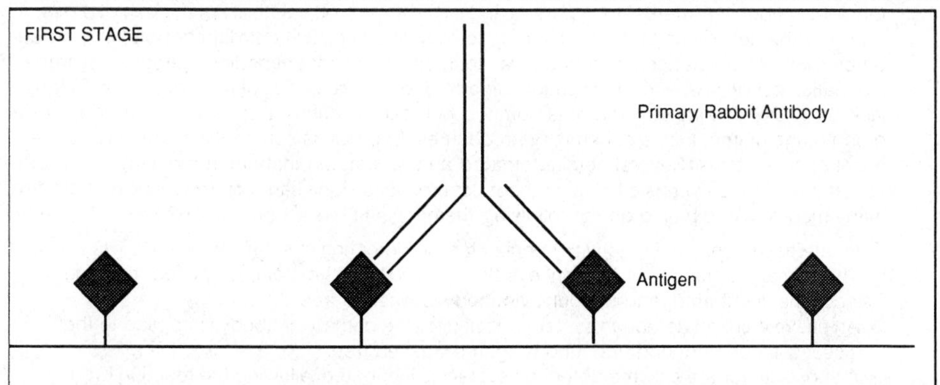

binding site available for the peroxidase antiperoxidase complex. In the third stage, this large soluble immune complex binds to available sites allowing specific localization of multiple peroxidase molecules. In the avidin-biotin system (Panel B), the second stage antibody is covalently labeled with biotin (B complex vitamin) for which avidin has an extraordinarily high affinity. Peroxidase may be covalently coupled to avidin to allow antigenic localization. In general, the avidin-biotin detection system confers stronger staining with cleaner backgrounds than PAP detection systems.

(Continued)

Immunoperoxidase Procedures *(Continued)*

Perhaps among the most common applications is the investigation of the major lineage of poorly differentiated neoplasm based on the phenotypic profile of the tumor. This is most reliably done by the use of a panel of immunostains performed simultaneously to provide complementary positive and negative results. In some situations, the use of overly restricted panels may lead to false interpretation of results (ie, S100 positive carcinomas, as in breast). Examples of common applications are shown in Table 1 on page 61.

Truly, cancer specific antibodies are not yet commercially available, but the potential is highlighted by two antibodies: HMB-45 for melanoma and CA 125 for serous ovarian carcinoma.[2,3,4] The detection of tissue specific antigens may establish the site of origin of a metastatic neoplasm, such as prostate specific antigen (PSA) and prostate specific acid phosphatase (PSAP) for prostatic adenocarcinoma or thyroglobulin for thyroid carcinoma. Gross cystic disease fluid protein (GCDFP-15) has proven useful in confirming carcinoma of breast origin.[5,6] In selected settings, the cytokeratin profile may narrow the differential diagnosis to choices which can be more readily established on a clinical basis.[7,8] Antigens which may be detected in tissues and monitored by serological studies to reflect tumor burden include carcinoembryonic antigen (CEA) in carcinoma, monoclonal immunoglobulins in plasma cell dyscrasias, and some lymphomas, α-fetoprotein and β-hCG for certain types of germ cell tumors, and peptide hormones in neuroendocrine malignancies. The utility of immunostains in the evaluation of lymphoreticular and hematopoietic neoplasms is discussed in the test listing Lymph Node Biopsy. Type and subtype specific antibodies allow detection and classification of viruses and other infectious agents. Markers such as progesterone receptor, c-erb-B2 (HER-2 neu), cathepsin D, and epithelial growth factor receptor may prove useful prognostic markers in breast cancer while estrogen receptor expression has both prognostic and therapeutic implications.[1] Proliferation markers such as Ki-67 and proliferation associated nuclear antigen (PCNA) are useful prognostic markers for a variety of tumors.[9]

LIMITATIONS: Deficient basic histology. Unknown or undesirable cross reactivities of different antibodies. The need for utilization of different fixatives to optimally preserve the broadest range of antigens of interest for a particular case. The intrinsic variability of antigen expression owing to the neoplastic state. Variable specificity and sensitivity of different staining procedures owing to differences in commercial sources of primary antibodies, detection systems, incubation conditions, and modifications adapted to suit the needs of individual labs. Relative lack of quality assurance programs. Limited number of technical personnel are adept in a broad range of immunohistochemistry procedures. Expense is substantial relative to conventional special stains. Several semiautomated and automated instruments may help circumvent many of these intrinsic limitations but cost remains significant. **METHODOLOGY:** There are many modifications based on the following theme (see Figure 1 on page 62.)

- Innate tissue enzymatic activity specific for the detection system is blocked.
- The primary antibody, which conveys the specificity of the stain, is applied to tissue sections, incubated, and unbound antibody is washed free.
- An enzyme-linked detection system specific for the primary antibody is applied to the tissues, incubated, and unbound reagents washed free.
- A substrate for the enzyme detection system is incubated, allowing the reaction product to form an insoluble precipitate, localizing the primary antibody, which is then visualized by light microscopy.

Primary antibodies of diagnostic importance are available from a variety of commercial sources, as monoclonal antibodies derived from mouse or rat, and polyclonal antibodies usually derived from rabbits or goats. Most commercial systems employ a second antibody with specificity for the primary antibody to serve as a link to the enzyme. The two most common detection methods are the peroxidase-antiperoxidase (PAP) technique or the biotin-avidin technique, to specifically introduce the enzyme into the complex. See previous figures.

Specificity and sensitivity of the primary antibody and the detection system should always be verified by testing on a limited library of tissues, which include known positives and negatives. When validated for diagnostic testing, careful attention must be continuously rendered to appropriately fixed control tissues and to internal controls which may be present in the test tissues. A valid positive immunostain will have a clean background and discrete reaction. A negative reaction is equally valid if properly controlled and if it complements a positive reaction for another mutually exclusive antigen.

ADDITIONAL INFORMATION: This method localizes specific antigens for diagnosis of a variety of diseases. Immunofluorescent procedures address similar issues but require a relatively expensive fluorescence microscope, are less sensitive, lack the resolution afforded by light microscopy, and do not produce an archivable slide. However, immunofluorescence is the method of choice for the localization of immunoglobulins, complement, and fibrin in the evaluation of renal biopsies and inflammatory dermatoses. Lectins, plant proteins with specificity for given carbohydrate moieties, are useful for antigen localization and can be used much like a primary antibody. More recently, *in situ* hybridization has been employed to identify nucleic acid sequences in cells. Following procedures generally similar to immunoperoxidase stains, biotin-labeled, genetically-engineered sequences of nucleic acids localize complementary gene sequences to detect viral genes and oncogenes of potential diagnostic significance.

Footnotes

1. Elledge RM, McGuire WL, and Osborne CK, "Prognostic Factors in Breast Cancer," *Semin Oncol*, 1992, 19(3):244-53.
2. Gown AM, Vogel AM, Hoak D, et al, "Monoclonal Antibodies Specific for Melanocytic Tumors Distinguish Subpopulations of Melanocytes," *Am J Pathol*, 1986, 123:195-203.
3. Kabawat SE, Bast RC, Welch WR, et al, "Immunopathologic Characterization of a Monoclonal Antibody That Recognizes Common Surface Antigens of Human Ovarian Tumors of Serous, Endometroid, and Clear Cell Types," *Am J Clin Pathol*, 1983, 79:98-104.
4. Klung TL, Bast RC, Niloff JM, et al, "Monoclonal Antibody Immunoradiometric Assay for an Antigenic Determinant (CA 125) Associated With Human Epithelial Ovarian Carcinomas," *Cancer Res*, 1984, 44:1048-53.
5. Mazoujian G, Parish TH, and Haagensen DE Jr, "Immunoperoxidase Localization of GCDFP-15 With Mouse Monoclonal Antibodies Versus Rabbit Antiserum," *J Histochem Cytochem*, 1988, 36(4):377-82.
6. Wick MR, Lilemoe TJ, Copland GT, et al, "Gross Cystic Disease Fluid Protein-15 as a Marker for Breast Cancer: Immunohistochemical Analysis of 690 Human Neoplasms and Comparison with Alpha-Lactalbumin," *Hum Pathol*, 1989, 20(3):281-7.
7. Cooper D, Schermer A, and Sun TT, "Classification of Human Epithelia and Their Neoplasms Using Monoclonal Antibodies to Keratins: Strategies, Applications, and Limitations," *Lab Invest*, 1985, 52(3):243-56.
8. Kahn HJ, Thorner PS, Yeger H, et al, "Distinct Keratin Patterns Demonstrated by Immunoperoxidase Staining of Adenocarcinomas, Carcinoids, and Mesotheliomas Using Polyclonal and Monoclonal Antikeratin Antibodies," *Am J Clin Pathol*, 1986, 86:566-74.
9. Riley RS, "Cellular Proliferation Markers in the Evaluation of Human Cancer," *Clin Lab Med*, 1992, 12(2):163-99.

References

Battifora H, "Clinical Applications of Immunohistochemistry of Filamentous Proteins," *Am J Surg Pathol*, 1988, 12:24-42.

DeLellis RA and Kwan P, "Technical Considerations in the Immunohistochemical Demonstration of Intermediate Filaments," *Am J Surg Pathol*, 1988, 12:17-23.

Nagle RB, "Intermediate Filaments: A Review of the Basic Biology," *Am J Surg Pathol*, 1988, 12:4-16.

Swanson PE, "Foundations of Immunohistochemistry," *Am J Surg Pathol*, 1988, 90:333-9.

Wolfe HJ, "DNA Probes in Diagnostic Pathology," *Am J Surg Pathol*, 1988, 90:340-4.

Immunophenotypic Analysis of Tissues by Flow Cytometry

CPT *88180 (each cell surface marker); 88182 (cell cycle or DNA analysis)*

Related Information

Body Fluids Cytology *on page 482*
Breast Biopsy *on page 40*
Cerebrospinal Fluid Cytology *on page 490*
Estrogen Receptor Assay *on page 47*
Fine Needle Aspiration, Deep Seated Lesions *on page 498*
Fine Needle Aspiration, Superficial Palpable Masses *on page 499*
Gene Rearrangement for Leukemia and Lymphoma *on page 911*
Immunoperoxidase Procedures *on page 60*
Lymph Node Biopsy *on page 72*
T- and B-Lymphocyte Subset Assay *on page 750*
Terminal Deoxynucleotidyl Transferase *on page 604*
Tumor Aneuploidy by Flow Cytometry *on page 88*

Synonyms Flow Cytometry; Fluorescence Activated Cell Sorting; Lymphocyte Immunophenotyping

Applies to B-Lymphocyte Analysis by Flow Cytometry; DNA Ploidy Studies; Kappa Light Chain Analysis by Flow Cytometry; Lambda Light Chain Analysis by Flow Cytometry; Leukemia Analysis by Flow Cytometry; Light Chain Analysis by Flow Cytometry; Lymphocyte Analysis by Flow Cytometry; Lymphocyte Markers; Lymphoma Analysis by Flow Cytometry; Solid Tumors Analysis by Flow Cytometry; T-Lymphocyte Analysis by Flow Cytometry

(Continued)

Abstract Flow cytometry provides important immunophenotypic and DNA cycle information of both diagnostic and prognostic interest in hematopathology, cytopathology, and general surgical pathology.

Specimen Fresh tissues, fresh frozen tissues, formalin-fixed paraffin-embedded tissue **CONTAINER:** Fresh tissues are best submitted in a Petri dish, test tube, or jar containing saline or tissue culture media. Frozen tissue submitted for DNA ploidy studies should not be embedded in OCT. **STORAGE INSTRUCTIONS:** Fresh tissue submitted for immunophenotypic studies are sufficiently stable to be transported by overnight courier on ice pack to a reference laboratory. Frozen tissue submitted for DNA ploidy studies should be retained frozen during transport to a reference laboratory.

Interpretive **REFERENCE RANGE:** Flow cytometry provides immunophenotypic data and/or DNA cell cycle data, depending on the desired information and processing methodologies. More information on DNA cell cycle studies is available in the Tumor Aneuploidy by Flow Cytometry listing. Immunophenotypic studies are most useful in evaluation of hematologic or lymphoid tissues. In conjunction with immunophenotypic data, information relating to cell size (forward light scatter) and internal complexity (90° light scatter) are obtained. By independently selecting cellular populations for evaluation, immunophenotypic data on respective populations may be extracted without additional preparatory procedures. For example, a lymph node containing populations of small and large lymphoid cells may show a reactive population of small T cells and a monoclonal population of large B cells. Flow cytometry is not well suited for evaluation of nonhematopoietic neoplasms, but lack of CD45 (leukocyte common antigen) expression on a cellular population should be regarded as suspicious for involvement by another process. Approximately 80% of non-Hodgkin's lymphomas are derived from monoclonal B cells. Characteristically, B-cell lymphomas will express at least one of a variety of pan B-cell antigens and express either kappa or lambda immunoglobulin light chains, proving clonality. B-cell lymphomas never express both kappa and lambda light chains, but approximately 5% to 10% of lymphomas are surface immunoglobulin negative.[1] The presence of a significant population of surface immunoglobulin negative B cells is also substantial proof of clonality. Loss of normal pan B-cell antigen expression or acquisition of T-cell antigen expression represents phenotypic aberrancy and satisfies minor criteria for malignancy. B-cell lymphomas which coexpress the T-cell antigen CD5 characterize lymphomas of small lymphocytic and intermediately differentiated (mantle cell) lymphocytic varieties. Expression of CD10 characterizes follicular lymphomas. B-cell lymphomas lacking HLA-Dr expression are thought to represent a poor prognostic group.

Approximately 20% of non-Hodgkin's lymphomas are derived from T cells. For these neoplasms, proof of clonality is more challenging. Clonality may be inferred by documenting abnormal pan T-cell antigen expression, abnormal T-cell subset antigen expression, or expression of thymocyte antigens.[2] For atypical T-cell infiltrates in which flow cytometry cannot prove clonality, use of gene rearrangement studies may be invaluable; see listing, Gene Rearrangement for Leukemia and Lymphoma.

Flow cytometric studies of cases of Hodgkin's disease are generally nondiagnostic. Typically, the majority of cells are reactive mature T cells with variable numbers of polyclonal B cells. This pattern cannot be distinguished from a totally benign reactive hyperplasia. Immunophenotypic verification of Hodgkin's disease is best accomplished in paraffin section using an appropriate panel of antibodies correlated with morphological features of the neoplastic cells.

When considering the possibility of a neoplasm of granulocytic/monocytic precursors, proof of expression of CD13, CD14, or CD33 is usually necessary to some extent. Additionally, expression of CD45 is characteristically weaker than that typically seen in lymphoid neoplasms. Lack of reactivity for other markers of T- or B-cell lineage is also expected. A panel of commonly utilized lymphocyte markers for the evaluation of lymphoma and leukemia is listed in the table.

LIMITATIONS: Flow cytometry is of limited use when nonlymphoid or nonhematopoietic neoplasms are in the differential diagnosis. The nature of the tissue may also confer severe limitations. Generally, endoscopic biopsies are too small to extract sufficient cells for a meaningful evaluation. However, blood, bone marrow, and body fluids are readily suitable for flow cytometric studies. Tissues which are fibrotic or sclerotic such as skin, are frequently too difficult to dissociate. Extraction of enough viable cells for evaluation is difficult. Additionally, necrotic tissues frequently produce poor results. Finally, important diagnostic morphologic and architectural features are lost when single cell suspensions are made. Therefore, the suitability of each biopsy needs to be individually considered before tissues are allocated for special studies beyond that of conventional histopathology. Interpretation of the phenotypic profile

Frequently Used Lymphocyte Differentiation Antigens for Flow Cytometry

Lineage Association	Antigenic Specificity/ Predominate Antigen Distribution
B-cell associated markers	
CD19	Pan B cell
CD20	Pan B cell
CD21	C3d and EBV receptor, resting B cell
CD10	CALLA, follicular center cells
Kappa, lambda	Mature B cells
Ig heavy chains	Mature B cells
T-cell associated antigens	
CD2	Sheep erythrocyte receptor, pan T cell
CD3	T-cell antigen receptor complex, pan T cell
CD5	Pan T cell, B-CLL, B-cell small lymphocytic lymphoma B-cell mantle cell lymphoma
CD7	Pan T cell
CD4	Helper/inducer subset
CD8	Cytotoxic, suppressor subset
CD1	Cortical thymocyte
Myeloid/monocytic antigens	
CD13	Predominately myeloid
CD15	Predominately myeloid, Reed-Sternberg cells
CD14	Predominately monocytic
CD33	Predominately monocytic
Miscellaneous antigens	
CD11c	Predominately granulocytic/monocytic; hairy cell leukemia, some CLL
CD25	IL-2 receptor, activated T cells, hairy cell leukemia
HLA-Dr	Immune response associated antigen, most B cells, activated T cells, early granulocytic and most monocytic cells
Glycophorin A	Erythroid precursors
CDw41	GPIIb/IIIa complex, megakaryocytes

See also a tabular presentation of lymphocyte markers used in paraffin sections in the listing, Lymph Node Biopsy.

must always be correlated with pathological features of individual cases.[3] In those cases in which flow cytometry fails to demonstrate clonality, the use of gene rearrangement studies may be helpful. **METHODOLOGY:** A single cell suspension is required for flow cytometric evaluation. When using tissues, cells are isolated from stromal elements by gentle mechanical dissociation. Most lymphoid tissues release lymphocytes with relative ease while other tissues, such as skin, pose significant difficulties in extracting viable lymphocytes. Isolated lymphocytes are washed and viability may be enriched by density gradient centrifugation. In some specimens, overnight culture is useful to decrease nonspecific staining caused by cytophilic antibody binding mediated by immunoglobulin Fc receptors expressed by lymphoid and other inflammatory cells. However, necrotic tissues and those with high grade neoplasm often lose viable tumor cells and become enriched by reactive T cells. Therefore, discretion is necessary to optimize the preparatory aspects of tissue processing. Ultimately, the single cell suspension is stained with fluorochrome conjugated antibodies, washed, and analyzed on the flow cytometer. Panels of antibodies are utilized to quantitate the numbers of B cells, T cells, and myelomonocytic cells. B-cell clonality is assessed with immunoglobulin light chains while T-cell clonality is inferred by abnormal expression of T-cell antigens.

(Continued)

Immunophenotypic Analysis of Tissues by Flow Cytometry *(Continued)*

Footnotes

1. Little JV, Foucar K, Horvath A, et al, "Flow Cytometric Analysis of Lymphoma and Lymphoma-Like Conditions," *Semin Diagn Pathol*, 1989, 6(1):37-54.
2. Picker LJ, Weiss LM, Medeiros LJ, et al, "Immunophenotypic Criteria for the Diagnosis of Non-Hodgkin's Lymphoma," *Am J Pathol*, 1987, 128:181-201.
3. Foucar K, Chen IM, and Crago S, "Organization and Operation of a Flow Cytometric Immunophenotyping Laboratory," *Semin Diagn Pathol*, 1989, 6(1):13-36.

References

Coon JS and Weinstein RS, *Diagnostic Flow Cytometry*, Baltimore, MD: Williams & Wilkins, 1991.
Keren DF, *Flow Cytometry in Clinical Diagnosis*, Chicago, IL: ASCP Press, 1989.
Knowles DM, *Neoplastic Hematopathology*, Baltimore, MD: Williams & Wilkins, 1992.

Immunostains *see* Immunoperoxidase Procedures *on page 60*
Intermediate Filaments *see* Immunoperoxidase Procedures *on page 60*
Intraoperative Consultation, Pathology *see* Frozen Section *on page 54*
Intraoperative Rapid Consultation *see* Frozen Section *on page 54*
Jones Stain *see* Kidney Biopsy *on this page*
Kappa Light Chain Analysis by Flow Cytometry *see* Immunophenotypic Analysis of Tissues by Flow Cytometry *on page 65*
Kappa Light Chains *see* Immunoperoxidase Procedures *on page 60*
Ki-67 *see* Immunoperoxidase Procedures *on page 60*

Kidney Biopsy

CPT *88305 (surgical pathology); 88307 (kidney, partial/total nephrectomy); 88312 (special stains, each); 88346 (immunofluorescence, each antibody); 88348 (electron microscopy)*

Related Information

Antihyaluronidase Titer *on page 635*
Antineutrophil Cytoplasmic Antibody *on page 636*
Antinuclear Antibody *on page 638*
Creatinine Clearance *on page 201*
Electron Microscopy *on page 45*
Factor B *on page 678*
Glomerular Basement Membrane Antibody *on page 681*
Hemoglobin, Qualitative, Urine *on page 1122*
Kidney Profile *on page 268*
Protein, Quantitative, Urine *on page 1145*
Scleroderma Antibody *on page 745*
Urea Nitrogen, Blood *on page 376*
Urinalysis *on page 1162*

Synonyms Renal Biopsy

Applies to Fluorescein-Tagged Antibodies; Jones Stain; Michael's Solution; PAS Stain; Trichrome Stain; Zeus Fixative

Test Commonly Includes Light microscopy: H & E stain, PAS stain, silver stain, trichrome stain; immunofluorescent studies; electron microscopy

Specimen Fresh kidney tissue obtained by percutaneous needle biopsy or open surgery.

Specimen handling: The core of renal tissue or a wedge obtained by open biopsy is immediately placed in a Petri dish containing physiologic saline solution or sterile culture media to prevent drying. An alternative is wrapping the specimen in saline-moistened gauze. The specimen should be sent to the laboratory within 5-10 minutes. If the specimen cannot be sent to the laboratory within this time frame, it should be divided into three parts and prepared in the appropriate fixative for light microscopy, electron microscopy, and immunofluorescence.

Specimen separation: When dividing the specimen, each part must contain glomeruli. A suggested method is:

A. If an open biopsy or three or more tissue cores are obtained, one core or fragment of the wedge biopsy is submitted for immunofluorescence, one for electron microscopy, and the remainder for light microscopy.

B. If two tissue cores are obtained, one is submitted for light microscopy, and the second core is divided as follows:

- Cut four 1-2 mm fragments with a sharp razor blade. Two from each end of the core. Submit two fragments for electron microscopy and the other two for immunofluorescence. The central portion of the core is submitted for light microscopy (see illustration).

C. If only one tissue core is obtained and it is small (less than 8 mm), submit it for light microscopy. If it is larger than 8 mm, divide it and submit as B. When dividing a small biopsy, priority should be given to: 1) light microscopy, 2) immunofluorescence, and 3) electron microscopy in this order, or at the discretion of the clinician depending on the clinical situation. A hand lens or a dissecting scope can be useful in recognizing the difference between renal cortex and medulla (glomeruli in the cortex appears as red dots, cortex is darker than medulla and is proximal within the needle used for biopsy).

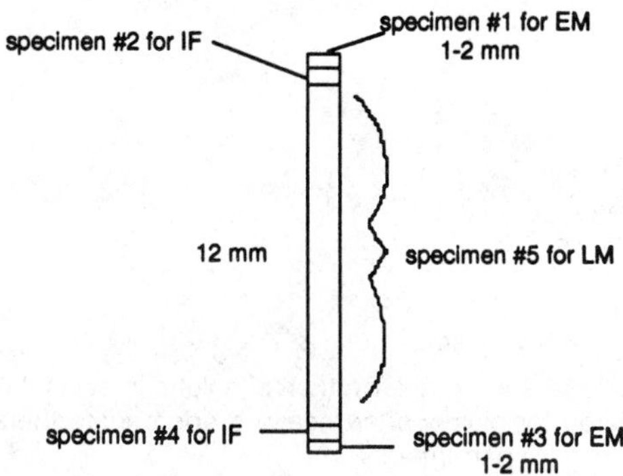

Specimen preparation: Several means of collection may be used. For immunofluorescence studies, one core or portion of a wedge (open biopsy) is placed in a foil or plastic bag, frozen in liquid nitrogen or in a cryostat, shipped on dry ice to the laboratory, and stored at -76°C until processed. The frozen state must be maintained. An alternative method is to immerse the biopsy in a half-saturated ammonium sulfate buffer at room temperature. Some laboratories prefer Michael's solution or Zeus fixative. The tissue should not be held in this fixative for more than 5 days, preferably less. For **light microscopy**, the second core or fragment is fixed in 4% formaldehyde that is 10 times the volume of the tissue. For **electron microscopy**, the third core or fragment is fixed in 2.5% glutaraldehyde fixative.

Possible problems:

- Drying of the specimen. In order to avoid drying, place the specimen, immediately after the biopsy is obtained, in normal saline. Keep it in saline until it is frozen or placed in fixative.
- Absence of cortex. If glomeruli are not identified in the tissue, repeat biopsy is necessary. If glomeruli are only present in the specimen submitted for immunofluorescence or electron microscopy, the remaining tissue may be cut and slides made for light microscopy.
- Too few glomeruli present in the biopsy. A minimum of 8-10 glomeruli is considered to be adequate for proper evaluation of a renal biopsy. This is particularly important in focal glomerular disease. The probability of finding abnormal glomeruli is closely related to the total number of glomeruli present. For evaluation of severity of disease, an adequate number of glomeruli is necessary.[1]

CAUSES FOR REJECTION: Drying of specimen due to lack of fixative **SPECIAL INSTRUCTIONS:** Adequate clinical history, differential diagnosis, and laboratory findings are essential for proper interpretation of renal biopsies and should be received with the specimen.

(Continued)

Kidney Biopsy *(Continued)*

Interpretive USE: There are no absolute indications for renal biopsy. Clinical judgment is required to determine necessity of biopsy. In general, renal biopsy has been found to be useful in the following conditions:

- unresponsive acute renal failure
- asymptomatic proteinuria
- nephrotic syndrome in adults
- unresponsive nephrotic syndrome in children
- acute nephritic syndrome
- hematuria of uncertain etiology
- systemic diseases with renal involvement
- drug toxicity
- transplantation reactions, rejection, or failure

Contraindications:

- bleeding diathesis
- neoplasm
- cystic disease
- obstructive uropathy
- acute pyelonephritis
- abscess
- uncontrolled hypertension
- only one kidney present
- anatomic abnormalities
- pregnancy
- uncooperative patient
- chronic renal disease with very small kidneys

This list of contraindications is more relative than absolute. In several of these situations the patient may be considered for biopsy after receiving appropriate therapy. In some of these cases an open biopsy may be performed.

METHODOLOGY: **Light microscopy**: Specimen is embedded in paraffin, sections are cut at 2-4 microns and stained with H & E, Gomori trichrome, PAS, and silver methenamine (Jones stain). Additional stains such as amyloid, fibrin, and so forth are occasionally needed. In the H & E and PAS stain, the basic pattern of the disease process is determined, and the extent and distribution of morphologic change is noted. Glomeruli, tubules, interstitium, and blood vessels are examined separately and any abnormality noted. The degree of glomerular sclerosis, interstitial fibrosis, tubular atrophy, and vascular changes are quantitatively estimated. Such parameters are important in determination of the degree of chronicity, severity of the renal disease, and overall prognosis. The PAS stain is helpful in studying glomerular and tubular basement membranes and the mesangium. PAS stain highlights hyaline and fibrinoid changes, and the presence of glomerular and arterial sclerosis (all stain red). The trichrome stain is used to determine the presence of interstitial fibrosis and glomerular and vascular sclerosis. It may show immune deposits and fibrin (the collagen stains blue; muscle, immune deposits, and fibrin stain red). The silver stain (Jones stain) is used especially to study the basement membranes. It also stains the mesangium and demonstrates the presence of glomerular sclerosis (all stain black).

Immunofluorescence: The specimen is snap frozen and sectioned. A battery of fluorescein-tagged antibodies against different immunoglobulins and complement is used. The most commonly used are IgG, IgM, IgA, C3, C4, C1q, properdin, and kappa and lambda light chains. Sections are then examined under fluorescence microscopy. Intensity, pattern, and distribution of immunoglobulins are noted. Normal renal biopsy usually shows no immunoglobulin depositions. Immunofluorescence allows for classification of renal disease. One may ascertain the degree of immunologic activity in immune diseases.

Electron microscopy: The specimen is embedded in plastic. Ultrathin sections are treated with osmium. Electron microscopy is useful for localization and quantitation of immune deposits. Abnormalities of the basement membrane and the presence of cellular inclusions may be detected.

Light microscopy, immunofluorescence, and electron microscopy are complementary and necessary in most cases.

ADDITIONAL INFORMATION: Complications of renal biopsy:

- Hematuria. Microscopic hematuria is a common complication seen in most patients. It resolves spontaneously. Gross hematuria is seen in 5% to 9% of the cases and is more common in patients with uncontrolled hypertension or uremia. It usually resolves spontaneously in 2-3 days. In 0.5% of the patients, hematuria will persist for 2-3 weeks, occasionally occurring a few days after the biopsy. Blood transfusions are only necessary in about 1% to 3% of the cases, and nephrectomy for massive or persistent bleeding is necessary in only 1 of 2000-5000 cases.
- Perinephric hematoma is not uncommon, however, only 1% to 2% of patients develop a local mass, hypotension, or diminution in hematocrit. The hematoma usually resolves within a few months.
- Arteriovenous fistula is considered frequent in arteriographic studies. Most cases are clinically silent and resolve spontaneously within 2 years.
- Other complications: Postbiopsy aneurysm appears in <1% of the patients. Other rare complications that have been described are ileus; lacerations of the liver, spleen, pancreas, gallbladder, intestine, visceral and subcostal arteries; pancreatitis; pneumothorax; and dissemination of carcinoma.

In summary, renal biopsy is relatively safe and useful in diagnosis and management of significant renal disease.

Footnotes

1. Madaio MP, "Renal Biopsy," *Kidney Int*, 1990, 38(3):529-43.

References

Alon U, "Hemorrhagic Complications of Kidney Biopsy," *Clin Pediatr (Phila)*, 1991, 30(6):391.

Antonovych TT and Mostofi FK, *Atlas of Kidney Biopsies – Armed Forces Institute of Pathology*, Washington, DC: American Registry of Pathology Armed Forces Institute of Pathology, 1980, 1-5.

Brun and Olsen, *Atlas of Renal Biopsy*, Philadelphia, PA: WB Saunders Co, 1981.

Glassock RJ, Hirschman GH, and Striker GE, "Workshop on the Use of Renal Biopsy in Research on Diabetic Nephropathy: A Summary Report," *Am J Kidney Dis*, 1991, 18(5):589-92.

Jenis EH and Lowenthal DT, *Kidney Biopsy Interpretation*, Philadelphia, PA: FA Davis Co, 1977.

Levison SP, "Renal Disease in the Elderly: The Role of the Renal Biopsy," *Am J Kidney Dis*, 1990, 16(4):300-6.

Mauer SM, Chavers BM, and Steffes MW, "Should There Be an Expanded Role for Kidney Biopsy in the Management of Patients With Type I Diabetes?" *Am J Kidney Dis*, 1990, 16(2):96-100.

McLaughlin J, Gladman DD, Urowitz MB, et al, "Kidney Biopsy in Systemic Lupus Erythematosus. II. Survival Analyses According to Biopsy Results," *Arthritis Rheum*, 1991, 34(10):1268-73.

Rance CP, "When Should Renal Biopsy Be Done?" *Clin Pediatr (Phila)*, 1990, 29(11):653-66.

Silva FG and Pirani CL, "Electron Microscopic Study of Medical Diseases of the Kidney: Update – 1988," *Mod Pathol*, 1988, 1:292-315.

Tisher CC and Brenner BB, *Renal Pathology With Clinical and Functional Correlation*, Philadelphia, PA: JB Lippincott Co, 1989, 1587-98.

Lambda Light Chain Analysis by Flow Cytometry *see* Immunophenotypic Analysis of Tissues by Flow Cytometry *on page 65*

Lambda Light Chains *see* Immunoperoxidase Procedures *on page 60*

Lectins *see* Immunoperoxidase Procedures *on page 60*

Leukemia Analysis by Flow Cytometry *see* Immunophenotypic Analysis of Tissues by Flow Cytometry *on page 65*

Leukocyte Common Antigen *see* Immunoperoxidase Procedures *on page 60*

Leu M1 *see* Immunoperoxidase Procedures *on page 60*

Light Chain Analysis by Flow Cytometry *see* Immunophenotypic Analysis of Tissues by Flow Cytometry *on page 65*

Light Chains *see* Immunoperoxidase Procedures *on page 60*

Liver Biopsy *see* Histopathology *on page 57*

Lung Biopsy *see* Histopathology *on page 57*

Lymph Node Biopsy

CPT *88180 (flow cytometry each cell surface marker); 88305 (surgical pathology); 88307 (lymph nodes, regional resection); 88312 (special stains each); 88342 (immunoperoxidase stains each antibody); 88346 (immunofluorescence each antibody); 88348 (electron microscopy)*

Related Information

bcl-2 Gene Rearrangement *on page 893*
Bone Marrow *on page 524*
Buffy Coat Smear Study of Peripheral Blood *on page 526*
Chromosome Analysis, Blood or Bone Marrow *on page 898*
Complete Blood Count *on page 533*
Epstein-Barr Virus Culture *on page 1179*
Frozen Section *on page 54*
Gene Rearrangement for Leukemia and Lymphoma *on page 911*
Histopathology *on page 57*
Immunoperoxidase Procedures *on page 60*
Immunophenotypic Analysis of Tissues by Flow Cytometry *on page 65*
Infectious Mononucleosis Screening Test *on page 713*
Leishmaniasis Serological Test *on page 717*
Muramidase, Blood and Urine *on page 571*
Peripheral Blood: Differential Leukocyte Count *on page 576*
Skin Biopsies *on page 84*
T- and B-Lymphocyte Subset Assay *on page 750*
Tartrate Resistant Leukocyte Acid Phosphatase *on page 603*
Terminal Deoxynucleotidyl Transferase *on page 604*
White Blood Count *on page 616*

Applies to Cell Sorting Fluorescence Activation; Lymphocyte Markers

Test Commonly Includes Microscopic examination of frozen sections, paraffin and/or plastic sections, and often, touch preparations. Immunoperoxidase studies for immunoglobulin heavy and light chains are best done on snap-frozen cryostat sections rather than paraffin sections.

Specimen Lymph node or other tissues suspected of harboring lymphoma, ideally submitted fresh within minutes of the biopsy **CONTAINER:** Sterile saline moistened sponge or Petri dish **COLLECTION:** Optimal selection of site of biopsy and the lymph nodes to be biopsied enhance ultimate correct diagnosis. Supraclavicular and cervical biopsies will most likely provide diagnostic specimens. The most accessible lymph nodes are not always the best choice.[1] The whole, intact lymph node with its capsule and adjacent fat or other tissue provides an optimal specimen.[1]

Proper initial triage of the tissue is of utmost importance in establishing the correct diagnosis. Usually, sufficient tissue must be available for both permanent sections and for immunophenotypic analysis of frozen sections. Tissues allocated for immunotypic studies are also suitable for genotypic studies if necessary. Routine histopathologic study remains the gold standard in diagnostic hematopathology and optimal histology begins with proper fixation. Fine nuclear detail is best achieved using B5, zinc formalin, or a Zenker's-like fixative. These fixatives are also best for cell marker analysis in paraffin section. An ever expanding selection of antibodies is useful for establishing lineage of hematopoietic cells in paraffin section (see table).[2,3] However, phenotypic indicators of clonal proliferation are most reliably established in frozen section. As morphologic detail in frozen sections is intrinsically limited, every precaution to minimize artifacts must be taken. Snap freezing small, thin slices of tissue using liquid nitrogen-cooled isopentane yields tissues free of freezing artifacts. Special attention to fine details of cryostat sectioning is necessary to yield interpretable results. If a frozen section evaluation is necessary to initiate a "lymphoma protocol," the tissues used for this rapid diagnosis are often unsuitable for immunophenotypic analysis. If the size of biopsy is limiting, a routine frozen section evaluation should be discouraged as freezing distorts lymphoid tissue and may result in errors in final interpretation.

If tissues are to be sent to a reference laboratory for immunotyping, three basic options are available. First, the tissues may be snap frozen and stored at -70°C or colder until such time as immunotyping is considered necessary. If facilities for proper snap freezing and storage are not available, this option should be discouraged. Second, the tissues may be delivered in carrier media or saline-soaked gauze on ice immediately by courier to the reference laboratory, where experienced personnel will process the tissue. Third, tissues may be placed in a carrier media which may circumvent the need for immediate action for 24 hours without significantly compromising the immunologic studies. Primary and reference laboratories should establish a standing agreement upon such options.

Lymphocyte Markers Useful in Paraffin Section*

	LCA CD45	EMA	LN-2 CD71w	L26 CD20	UCHL-1 CD45RO	CD3	Leu-M1 CD15	Mono Ig's	Lysozyme	KP1 CD68	CAE
Non-Hodgkin's lymphoma B-cell lymphomas†	+	-	+	+	-	-	-	+	-	-	-
T-cell lymphomas§	+	-/+	-	-	+	+	-/+	-	-	-	-
Hodgkin's disease (NS, MC, LD)	-	-	+	-	-	-	+	-	-	-	-
Hodgkin's disease, LP	+	+/-	+	+	-	-	-	-	-	-	-
Myeloma/plasmacytoma	-/+	-/+	-	-	-	-	-	+	-	-	-
Granulocytic sarcoma#	+/-	-	-/+	-	-	-	+/-	-	+	+	+
True histiocytic lymphoma#	+/-	-/+	-/+	-	-	-	-	-	+	+	-

Abbreviations: LCA: leukocyte common antigen; EMA: epithelial membrane antigen; Mono Ig's: monoclonal immunoglobulins; CAE: chloroacetate esterase (an enzyme cytochemical stain rather than an immunostain); Hodgkin's disease (NS, MC, LD): nodular sclerosing, mixed cellularity, and lymphocyte depleted subtypes, respectively; Hodgkin's disease, LP: lymphocyte predominate subtype.
Designated reactions: +: characteristically positive; +/-: characteristically positive but may be negative; -/+: characteristically negative but may be positive; -: characteristically negative.

Footnotes:
*Most lymphomas characteristically contain neoplastic and non-neoplastic lymphoid elements in variable proportions. Caution must be exercised in determining the phenotype of the neoplastic cells.
†Monoclonal immunoglobulins are best detected in frozen section. Large cell lymphomas and those with plasmacytic differentiation are more likely to display a convincing staining in paraffin section than other subtypes.
§T-cell clonal proliferation cannot be determined in paraffin section alone. The best phenotypic expression of clonal proliferation is aberrant expression of pan T-cell antigens which can be detected only by frozen section immunohistology, by flow cytometry using cell suspensions, or by gene rearrangement.
#Enzyme cytochemical profile using touch preparations is extremely useful in establishing these diagnoses.

(Continued)

Lymph Node Biopsy *(Continued)*

STORAGE INSTRUCTIONS: Snap frozen tissues should be maintained at -70°C or colder until immunophenotypic analysis can be performed. If frozen tissues are to be transported to a reference laboratory, they should be shipped on dry ice, using an overnight courier if necessary. Tissues placed in carrier media should be maintained on wet ice or at room temperature and packaged in insulated containers to avoid large fluctuations in temperature if sent to a reference laboratory. **CAUSES FOR REJECTION:** Desiccated specimen, formalin exposure, excessive freezing artifact **SPECIAL INSTRUCTIONS:** The specimen should not be placed in fixative if it can be delivered immediately to the laboratory. Diagnostic difficulties in diseases of lymph nodes are compounded by poor fixation and improper handling. Lymph node biopsies should be immediately delivered to the Histology Laboratory uncut in a small sterile jar or Petri dish. Requests for all examinations including bacteriology should accompany the specimen. All such specimens should be brought to the immediate attention of a pathologist. Bone marrow, blood studies sometimes including serologic test for infectious mononucleosis, and clinical information are commonly needed for appropriate work-up.

Interpretive **USE:** Diagnose various lymphadenopathies, including malignant lymphoma and metastatic neoplasia **LIMITATIONS:** Formalin-fixed tissue cannot be used for culture or imprints and is suboptimal for electron microscopy. **METHODOLOGY:** Quality conventional histology is of paramount importance in the evaluation of the lymph node biopsy. Interpretive errors are often due to deficient basic histopathologic procedures.[2] Touch preparations should always be obtained and are often invaluable for final diagnosis. Representative tissues should be allocated for immunotyping, taking the necessary precautions to minimize morphologic artifacts while maintaining maximal antigenicity. Immunoperoxidase stains on paraffin or frozen sections are accomplished according to the general procedures outlined in the test listing Immunoperoxidase Procedures. Immunologic markers on touch preparations and bone marrow smears are often best demonstrated by using an alkaline phosphatase enzyme detection system to minimize background staining. Cultures for infectious agents are sometimes indispensable. **ADDITIONAL INFORMATION:** Correlation with peripheral blood, bone marrow, and other clinical laboratory studies is often desirable and sometimes mandatory. Flow cytometry on dissociated tissues or body fluids is often utilized instead of immunohistology for cell marker analysis. This methodology offers a more quantitative approach to cell markers but only at the critical expense of destruction of immunoarchitecture. In general, immunohistology provides the best approach for typing tissues while flow cytometry is best suited for blood, bone marrow, and other body fluids. Properly acquired and frozen tissue is suitable for gene probe analysis (gene rearrangement studies), which may be necessary to document B- or T-cell clonal proliferation in rare cases.

See also a tabular presentation of frequently used **lymphocyte differentiation antigens** in the listing, Immunophenotypic Analysis of Tissues by Flow Cytometry.

Footnotes

1. Ioachim HL, *Lymph Node Biopsy*, Philadelphia, PA: JB Lippincott Co, 1982, 17-8.
2. Warnke RA and Rouse RV, "Limitations Encountered in the Application of Tissue Section Immunodiagnosis to the Study of Lymphomas and Related Disorders," *Hum Pathol*, 1985, 16:326-31.
3. Chittal SM, Caveriviere P, Schwarting R, et al, "Monoclonal Antibodies in the Diagnosis of Hodgkin's Disease – The Search for a Rational Panel," *Am J Surg Pathol*, 1988, 12(1):9-21.

References

Jaffe ES, "Surgical Pathology of the Lymph Nodes and Related Organs," *Major Problems in Pathology*, Vol 16, Philadelphia, PA: WB Saunders Co, 1985.

Knowles DM, *Neoplastic Hematopathology*, Baltimore, MD: Williams & Wilkins, 1992.

Lymphocyte Analysis by Flow Cytometry *see* Immunophenotypic Analysis of Tissues by Flow Cytometry *on page 65*

Lymphocyte Immunophenotyping *see* Immunophenotypic Analysis of Tissues by Flow Cytometry *on page 65*

Lymphocyte Markers *see* Immunophenotypic Analysis of Tissues by Flow Cytometry *on page 65*

Lymphocyte Markers *see* Lymph Node Biopsy *on previous page*

Lymphoma Analysis by Flow Cytometry *see* Immunophenotypic Analysis of Tissues by Flow Cytometry *on page 65*

Lysozyme *see* Immunoperoxidase Procedures *on page 60*

Medical Examiner's Case *see* Autopsy *on page 36*

Medical Legal Specimens *see* Histopathology *on page 57*

Metastatic Neoplasia *see* Estrogen Receptor Assay *on page 47*

Michael's Solution *see* Kidney Biopsy *on page 68*

Monoclonal Immunoglobulins *see* Immunoperoxidase Procedures *on page 60*

Muscle Biopsy

***CPT** 88305 (surgical pathology); 88312 (special stains each); 88313 (trichrome stain); 88346 (immunofluorescence each antibody); 88348 (electron microscopy)*

Related Information

Aldolase, Serum *on page 103*
Creatine Kinase *on page 196*
Duchenne/Becker Muscular Dystrophy DNA Detection *on page 908*
Electron Microscopy *on page 45*
Histopathology *on page 57*
Myoglobin, Blood *on page 293*
Myoglobin, Qualitative, Urine *on page 1135*
Skeletal Muscle Antibody *on page 747*
Tests for Uncommon Inherited Diseases of Metabolism and Cell Structure *on page 605*
Trichinosis Serology *on page 760*

Synonyms Skeletal Muscle Biopsy

Test Commonly Includes For state-of-the-art muscle biopsy, indeed to make the surgical procedure worthwhile, enzyme histochemistry of the biopsied specimens must be included.

Abstract Diagnosis and classification of muscle disease

Patient Care PREPARATION: Clinical data is required and should include the patient's age and sex; the pattern, severity, and tempo of the muscle involvement; relevant laboratory results (ie, CPK, ESR); electromyographic (EMG) findings; and the presence of significant related conditions (ie, dermatitis, neoplasm, steroid/AZT therapy, AIDS).

Specimen SAMPLING TIME: The biopsy should be performed early in the day as the specimen will immediately require special handling and should arrive when histotechnical personnel are available. The requisition should state a brief clinical history, pertinent laboratory findings, the biopsy site, and the name of the referring internist or neurologist. COLLECTION: **Selection of muscle biopsy site:** The site for muscle biopsy should be one that is familiar to the pathologist (ie, quadriceps, deltoid, biceps, or gastrocnemius). Unusual muscle groups such as oculomotor or pharyngeal muscles should be avoided, as they have several unique and potentially confusing features. Biopsy should be from a muscle that is involved by the disease but has not reached "end-stage" atrophy. EMG/injection sites and sites near the myotendinous junction should be avoided as these biopsies will commonly exhibit artifactual changes.

Surgical technique: Except for children or exceptional adult cases, the procedure is done with local anesthesia. Ideally, the biopsied muscle should not be allowed to contract because this creates severe microscopic artifacts. To achieve an isometric specimen, it is best to use a surgical muscle clamp that prevents contraction. If no clamp is available, the specimen may be pinned to a tongue blade to prevent contraction. A portion of the muscle, in continuity with that held in the clamp, should extend from the clamp so it may be cut off for freezing and histochemistry. A small piece should be placed in 1% glutaraldehyde for electron microscopy. Deliver on a saline-moistened gauze pad immediately to the Pathology Department. Moistened gauze is used to prevent drying. The specimen must not become saturated as this will cause severe ice crystal artifact during snap freezing. **The tissue should not be placed in fixative or frozen**. It should ideally reach the Pathology Laboratory within 30 minutes to retain enzyme activity.

STORAGE INSTRUCTIONS: At least a small portion of the fresh material will be stored deep frozen for possible later use in biochemical assays (eg, quantitation of glycogen, enzymes, or dystrophin levels).

(Continued)

Muscle Biopsy *(Continued)*

Interpretive USE: Evaluate muscle disease in terms of neurogenic atrophy, muscular dystrophies, myositis (infectious and "idiopathic," or autoimmune), endocrine myopathies, and congenital myopathies and enzyme deficiencies. A muscle biopsy may shed light on a systemic condition such as systemic vasculitis in the absence of overt clinical muscle disease. METHODOLOGY: A portion of the clamped muscle is oriented, frozen in isopentane/liquid nitrogen, and transverse sections are obtained for H & E, trichrome, and various histochemical preparations, some of which are listed below.

- Adenosine triphosphate (ATPase): At differing pHs, used to differentiates type I, IIa, and IIb myofibers and reveals abnormal fiber type distributions and diseases that selectively involve certain myofiber types.
- Succinate dehydrogenase (SDH): Stains mitochondria and shows abnormal aggregates or loss. Nicotinamide adenine dinucleotide-tetrazolium reductase (NADH-TR) may be used, but it is less sensitive.
- Oil red O: Stains lipids to detect abnormal accumulations.
- Periodic acid-Schiff (PAS): Used to detect glycogen in glycogenoses (ie, McArdle's disease, Pompe's disease, etc).

Extra frozen sections should be obtained and held in case additional more specific, enzyme preparations are needed (ie, cytochrome C oxidase, phosphofructokinase, phosphorylase). The remaining muscle tissue is formalin-fixed, paraffin-embedded, and stained with H & E and trichrome. Such preparations are used to detect small foci of myositis or vasculitis which may be missed on cryostat-cut sections, which are, of necessity, much smaller.

References

Brooke MH, "Disorders of Skeletal Muscle," *Neurology in Clinical Practice*, Bradley WG, Daroff RB, Fenichel GM, et al, eds, Boston, MA: Butterworth-Heinemann, 1991, 1843-86.

DeGirolami U, Smith TW, Chad D, et al, "Skeletal Muscle," *Principles and Practice of Surgical Pathology*, Silverberg SG, ed, New York, NY: Churchill Livingstone, 1990, 545-92.

Heffner RR Jr, "Muscle Biopsy in Neuromuscular Disorders," *Diagnostic Surgical Pathology*, Sternberg SS, ed, New York, NY: Raven Press, 1989, 119-39.

Heffner RR Jr, "Skeletal Muscle," *Histology for Pathologists*, Sternberg SS, ed, New York, NY: Raven Press, 1992, 81-108.

Plotz PH, "Not Myositis: A Series of Chance Encounters," *JAMA*, 1992, 268(15):2074-7.

Myoglobin *see* Immunoperoxidase Procedures *on page 60*

Myosin *see* Immunoperoxidase Procedures *on page 60*

Necropsy *see* Autopsy *on page 36*

Negri Bodies *see* Rabies *on page 82*

Oncogene Expression *see* Breast Biopsy *on page 40*

PAS Stain *see* Kidney Biopsy *on page 68*

PAS Stain *see* Skin Biopsies *on page 84*

Pathologic Examination *see* Histopathology *on page 57*

Pathology *see* Histopathology *on page 57*

Pathology Operating Room Consultation *see* Frozen Section *on page 54*

PCNA *see* Immunoperoxidase Procedures *on page 60*

Peptide Hormones *see* Immunoperoxidase Procedures *on page 60*

Peroxidase-Antiperoxidase (PAP) *see* Immunoperoxidase Procedures *on page 60*

PgR *see* Progestogen Receptor Assay *on next page*

PgRICA or PgR(ICA) *see* Progestogen Receptor Immunocytochemical Assay *on page 79*

Ploidy *see* Breast Biopsy *on page 40*

Ploidy *see* Image Analysis *on page 58*

Ploidy Analysis of Tumors *see* Tumor Aneuploidy by Flow Cytometry *on page 88*

Postmortem Examination *see* Autopsy *on page 36*

PR *see* Progestogen Receptor Assay *on this page*

PRICA or PR(ICA) *see* Progestogen Receptor Immunocytochemical Assay *on page 79*

Progesterone Binding Protein (Immunocytochemical) *see* Progestogen Receptor Immunocytochemical Assay *on page 79*

Progestogen Receptor Assay

CPT 84234

Related Information

Breast Biopsy *on page 40*
Estrogen Receptor Assay *on page 47*
Estrogen Receptor Immunocytochemical Assay *on page 51*
Progestogen Receptor Immunocytochemical Assay *on page 79*

Synonyms PgR; PR

Test Commonly Includes Performed on same carcinoma specimen on which estrogen receptor is measured.

Abstract Test on fresh tissue to select those breast cancer patients likely to be responsive to endocrine therapy. It may also be applied to uterine, ovarian, and meningioma specimens.

Specimen 1 g (1 x 1 x 1 cm) of tumor biopsy if possible, or excision of tumor from the whole breast if frozen section was performed on needle biopsy. Some laboratories can use as little as 150 mg of tumor tissue, trimmed, for both estrogen and progesterone receptor assays. The test is performed on the same specimen on which estrogen receptor is measured. Please see directions under that test description. Receptor assays may be done on certain tumors other than those of breast (eg, meningioma, especially those of the sphenoid wing and olfactory groove). **CONTAINER:** Jar or waxed cardboard tub, no formalin **COLLECTION:** Immediately transported to Pathology Laboratory fresh, on ice (ie, before wound closure). Container must be labeled with patient's name, location, and date. It is recommended that the container be brought over on ice or the specimen be wrapped in a saline-moistened gauze and placed on ice. **STORAGE INSTRUCTIONS:** Stored at -70°C or colder. Avoid prolonged storage or repeated freezing and thawing. **CAUSES FOR REJECTION:** Less than approximately 0.15 g of tumor tissue, depending on laboratory; some require more neoplastic material. Specimen contaminated by fixatives, specimen not brought to Pathology Laboratory immediately, specimens not kept cold are subject to rejection. **TURNAROUND TIME:** May be as short as several hours, depending upon the laboratory to which the specimen is sent. **SPECIAL INSTRUCTIONS:** Fresh specimen should be **immediately** transported to Pathology Laboratory before wound closure. A delay of even 15 minutes without proper cold packing can alter the results significantly. Please schedule as "FS," as a frozen section should be performed to document presence of viable breast carcinoma. Selected tissue may be kept frozen at -70°C overnight while an adjacent block is processed for permanent section examination to establish diagnosis. If the specimen is sent from an outside facility, it should be packed in dry ice immediately after removal.

Interpretive **REFERENCE RANGE:** <5 fmol/mg protein is negative. A concentration >10 fmol/mg protein (in the 8S fraction of sucrose gradient) is considered positive; >100 fmol/mg is strongly positive **USE:** Progesterone receptor assay helps to predict response to hormonal therapy in patients with breast carcinoma, used in concert with estrogen receptor assay. Use of both assays is widely advocated.[1,2] Especially helpful for patients bearing tumors in which estrogen receptors are <100 fmol/mg. A longer survival in receptor-positive patients may be related to response to endocrine therapy.[3] PR may have some use in prediction of the clinical course of ovarian carcinomas and meningiomas. **LIMITATIONS:** Delay in transport of the specimen may diminish the identification of receptor sites. If tissue is not rapidly frozen, steroid receptors may be destroyed. Samples that might initially have been receptor-positive might then be assayed as negative. It has been shown that PR concentrations are more stable than estrogen and androgen receptors and might be stable for as long as 150 minutes following devascularization of breast tumors.[4] Care must still be taken to deliver the specimen on ice as quickly as possible after excision for rapid freezing to -70°C. Some patients with breast carcinoma characterized by estrogen and progesterone receptor positivity do not respond to endocrine therapy. Progesterone receptor levels varied from not detectable to 95 fmol/mg protein in a series of 41 specimens of benign breast tissue. Nine had >10 fmol/mg protein.[5] Endogenous progestogens may occupy receptors, blocking assay,[6] leading to false-negative results. As in ER, tumors with extensive necrosis or low cellularity may yield misleading low results. **CONTRAINDICATIONS:** Formalin fixation, other fixatives, tissue not promptly frozen **METH-**

(Continued)

Progestogen Receptor Assay *(Continued)*

ODOLOGY: Sucrose density gradient. Cytosol preparation from fresh frozen tumor can be worked up by steroid binding assay or enzyme immunoassay (EIA). Immunohistochemical demonstration of progesterone receptor on cryostat sections is reported[6] and fluorescent cytochemical detection of PR receptors in breast aspirates has been described.[7] **ADDITIONAL INFORMATION:** Up to 75% of estrogen receptor-positive breast carcinomas have progesterone receptor. Estrogen and progesterone assay are both of definite use in evaluation of mammary carcinoma,[2,8] and are of possible use in endometrial, ovarian, and prostatic carcinoma. When in doubt about the possible use of this assay, consultation with a pathologist or oncologist in advance or at the time of surgery may be helpful.

Factors relating to prognosis of breast cancer patients include first the number of positive nodes, extranodal extension of tumor in women with one to three positive lymph nodes, cancer cells in lymph node vessels, tumor size, and presence or absence of favorable breast carcinoma histopathologic type. Progesterone receptor is reported by McGuire and Clark to be the second most critical factor after the number of positive nodes and to be a more significant prognostic factor than the presence or absence of ER,[9] a point with which others concur.[4] Patients whose results of PR remained consistently positive had better prognosis than those whose PR was initially positive but whose PR became negative on second biopsy. Loss of PR was described as ominous. The worst prognosis related to consistent PR negativity.[9]

Two other investigators have reported apparently discrepant results of the prognostic significance of PR receptors in patients with differing clinical stages of disease. In one study of primary breast tumors, independent prognostic factors for survival were tumor size, number of positive lymph nodes, age, PR concentration but not ER concentration.[2] Within this same study, independent prognostic factors for relapse were tumor size, number of positive lymph nodes, age, menopause status, and PR but not ER concentrations. Both PR and ER concentrations contributed to prediction of death rate after metastasis. Patients in this series with tumors containing both PR and ER had the best prognosis. Bezwoda et al reported that in patients with metastatic breast cancer, those with >10 fmol PR/mg of tissue had better responses to tamoxifen than those with <10 fmol/mg.[10] In a multivariate study of these patients using receptors, age, site, and number of metastases, only ER concentration was significant in prediction of the response to treatment with tamoxifen. It appears that presence of occult metastasis (as well as previous tumor therapy) may help to explain sometimes discrepant results between different clinical studies.

Progesterone receptor is described in breast epithelium as a postreceptor marker of functioning estrogen receptors, but occasional breast carcinomas are immunohistochemically positive for progesterone receptor and negative for estrogen receptor. Such tumors are regarded as constitutively progesterone receptor-positive.[6] Such PR-positive tumors apparently are additional to those in which false-negative results for estrogen receptor by radioligand binding assay are encountered, in which endogenous estrogens have saturated available binding sites.[6] Progesterone receptor status provides discrimination for node-negative breast cancer patients with aneuploid tumors.[11]

Footnotes

1. Jiang NS, "Breast Cancer: Estrogen and Progesterone Receptor Assays as a Guide to Therapy," *Mayo Clin Proc*, 1983, 58(1):64.
2. Alexieva-Figusch J, Van Putten WL, Blankenstein MA, et al, "The Prognostic Value and Relationships of Patient Characteristics, Estrogen and Progestin Receptors, and Site of Relapse in Primary Breast Cancer," *Cancer*, 1988, 61(4):758-68.
3. Alanko A, Heinonen E, Scheinin T, et al, "Significance of Estrogen and Progesterone Receptors, Disease-Free Interval, and Site of First Metastasis on Survival of Breast Cancer Patients," *Cancer*, 1985, 56:1696-1700.
4. Ellis LM, Wittliff JL, Bryant MS, et al, "Lability of Steroid Hormone Receptors Following Devascularization of Breast Tumors," *Arch Surg*, 1989, 124(1):39-42.
5. Winek RR, Jiang N-S, and Wold LE, "Estrogen and Progesterone Receptors in Benign Breast Tissue," *Am J Clin Pathol*, 1987, 88:526-7, (abstract).
6. Giri DD, Goepel JR, Rogers K, et al, "Immunohistological Demonstration of Progesterone Receptor in Breast Carcinoma: Correlation With Radioligand Binding Assays and Estrogen Receptor Immunohistology," *J Clin Pathol*, 1988, 41(4):444-7.
7. Masood S and Johnson H Jr, "The Value of Imprint Cytology in Cytochemical Detection of Steroid Hormone Receptors in Breast Cancer," *Am J Clin Pathol*, 1987, 87:30-6.
8. Maass H, Jonat W, Stolzenbach G, et al, "The Problem of Nonresponding Estrogen Receptor-Positive Patients With Advanced Breast Cancer," *Cancer*, 1980, 46:2835-7.
9. McGuire WL and Clark GM, "Role of Progesterone Receptors in Breast Cancer," *J Clin Oncol*, 1984, 2:414-9.

10. Bezwoda WR, Esser JD, Dansey R, et al, "The Value of Estrogen and Progesterone Receptor Determinations in Advanced Breast Cancer – Estrogen Receptor Level but Not Progesterone Receptor Level Correlates With Response to Tamoxifen," *Cancer*, 1991, 68(4):867-72.
11. Clark GM, Dressler LG, Owens MA, et al, "Prediction of Relapse or Survival in Patients With Node-Negative Breast Cancer by DNA Flow Cytometry," *N Engl J Med*, 1989, 320(10):627-33.

References

Allred DC, "Should Immunohistochemical Examination Replace Biochemical Hormone Receptor Assays in Breast Cancer?" *Am J Clin Pathol*, 1993, 99(1):1-3.

Bergqvist A, Ekman R, and Ljungberg O, "Binding of Estrogen and Progesterone to Human Endometrium in the Different Phases of the Menstrual Cycle," *Am J Clin Pathol*, 1985, 83:444-9.

Brustein S, Fruchter R, Greene GL, et al, "Immunocytochemical Assay of Progesterone Receptors in Paraffin-Embedded Specimens of Endometrial Carcinoma and Hyperplasia: A Preliminary Evaluation," *Mod Pathol*, 1989, 2(5):449-55.

Estaban JM, Kandalaft PL, Mehta P, et al, "Improvement of the Quantification of Estrogen and Progesterone Receptors in Paraffin-Embedded Tumors by Image Analysis," *Am J Clin Pathol*, 1993, 99(1):32-8.

Helin HJ, Helle MJ, Helin ML, et al, "Immunocytochemical Detection of Estrogen and Progesterone Receptors in 124 Human Breast Cancers," *Am J Clin Pathol*, 1988, 89:137-42.

Jacobs DH, McFarlane MJ, and Holmes FF, "Female Patients With Meningioma of the Sphenoid Ridge and Additional Primary Neoplasms of the Breast and Genital Tract," *Cancer*, 1987, 60:3080-2.

Kiang DT, "The Presence of Steroid Receptors in 'Nontarget' Tissues and Its Significance," *Am J Clin Pathol*, 1993, 99(2):120-2.

Olson JJ, Beck DW, Schlechte J, et al, "Hormonal Manipulation of Meningiomas *In Vitro*," *J Neurosurg*, 1986, 65:99-107.

Sabini G, Chumas JC, and Mann WJ, "Steroid Hormone Receptors in Endometrial Stromal Sarcomas. A Biochemical and Immunohistochemical Study," *Am J Clin Pathol*, 1992, 97(3):381-6.

Tesch M, Shawwa A, and Henderson R, "Immunohistochemical Determination of Estrogen and Progesterone Receptor Status in Breast Cancer," *Am J Clin Pathol*, 1993, 99(1):8-12.

van Hoeven KH, Menendez-Botet CJ, Strong EW, et al, "Estrogen and Progesterone Receptor Content in Human Thyroid Disease," *Am J Clin Pathol*, 1993, 99(2):175-81.

Progestogen Receptor Cytosolic Assay *replaced by* Progestogen Receptor Immunocytochemical Assay *on this page*

Progestogen Receptor (Immunocytochemical) *see* Progestogen Receptor Immunocytochemical Assay *on this page*

Progestogen Receptor Immunocytochemical Assay

CPT 88342

Related Information

Breast Biopsy *on page 40*
Estrogen Receptor Assay *on page 47*
Estrogen Receptor Immunocytochemical Assay *on page 51*
Fine Needle Aspiration, Superficial Palpable Masses *on page 499*
Image Analysis *on page 58*
Progestogen Receptor Assay *on page 77*

Synonyms PgRICA or PgR(ICA); PRICA or PR(ICA); Progesterone Binding Protein (Immunocytochemical); Progestogen Receptor (Immunocytochemical)

Replaces Progestogen Receptor Cytosolic Assay

Test Commonly Includes Estrogen receptor assay may be included, depending upon the laboratory. Evaluation of both estrogen and progesterone receptors is strongly recommended, as both ER and PR may have independent prognostic weight. DNA studies may be desirable. They include ploidy (diploid, euploid, normal or aneuploid, abnormal) and S phase (synthesis phase, estimating proliferative activity of a neoplasm). Such work-up may be done with either flow cytometry or image analysis of paraffin-embedded tissue.

Abstract Test on paraffin-embedded tissue, frozen sections, or touch preparations to select those breast cancer patients likely to be responsive to endocrine therapy. Useful with certain other tumors, including meningiomas.

Patient Care PREPARATION: Similar conditions apply as those applicable for determination of estrogen or progestogen receptor status by cytosolic methods. Please see individual listings.

Specimen PRICA may be done on any primary breast tumor, gynecologic tumor, or meningioma, as well as any other tissue. Assay may be performed on any paraffin block that is properly fixed, processed, and not subject to temperatures above 60°C. Frozen sections and touch preparations kept at -70°C may also be used. As receptors are quantitated by image analysis

(Continued)

Progestogen Receptor Immunocytochemical Assay *(Continued)*

(usually), the amount of tissue submitted may be minimal. PRICA is ideal for minimal carcinomas or cases where there is only archival material. Minimal amount of tissue may be as little as two 4 micron slides for progestogen receptors and two 4 micron slides for estrogen receptors. Slides should be air dried and unstained. Consult pathologist performing assay for proper specimen collection. Tissue sent for assay may be primary tumor or metastases. Breast and gynecologic metastases may be sent along with 4 micron sections of the primary tumor for comparison, even when estrogen receptor assay by the cytosolic method was previously employed. **COLLECTION:** Slides must be labeled according to proper surgical pathology procedures. A copy of the surgical pathology report, even if only provisional, should accompany slides or touch preparations to ensure proper identification of slides. Slides may be mailed in any fashion that prevents breakage. **STORAGE INSTRUCTIONS:** Paraffin-embedded sections should be kept at room temperature below 60°C. Frozen sections and touch preparations should be kept at -70°C. Frozen sections and touch preparations should be mailed on dry ice. Depending upon the technique of the laboratory, touch preparations may be fixed, briefly in formalin. **CAUSES FOR REJECTION:** Largely necrotic tumor, improper fixation or processing, warming of slides over 60°C, extended thawing of frozen slides **TURNAROUND TIME:** Commonly sent to reference laboratories. Turnaround time should be less than or equal to 1 week. **SPECIAL INSTRUCTIONS:** Tumor should be transported to Pathology Department as a fresh specimen on ice. The same instructions as for estrogen or progesterone receptor quantitation by the cytosolic method apply.

Interpretive **REFERENCE RANGE:** Staining of nuclei for progesterone receptors may be semiquantitated visually as none, low, intermediate, or high. Image analysis techniques have been described.[1,2,3] Use of image analysis techniques may allow for more refined quantitation of receptors using PRICA. ERICA on needle aspirates has been described.[4] This technique also applies to progesterone receptors. PRICA on touch preparations or imprints has also been described.[5,6] **USE:** Progesterone receptor immunocytochemical assay helps to predict response to hormonal therapy in patients with breast carcinoma. Use of both estrogen and progesterone immunocytochemical assay is widely advocated. A longer survival in receptor-positive patients may be related to response to endocrine therapy. PR may have some use in prediction of the clinical course of ovarian carcinomas and meningiomas. **LIMITATIONS:** One disadvantage of PRICA is its only semiquantitative nature (*vide infra*). **METHODOLOGY:** Immunoperoxidase procedures utilize monoclonal antiprogesterone receptor antibodies. Tissues examined may be paraffin sections, frozen (cryostat) sections, or touch imprints. **ADDITIONAL INFORMATION:** Advantages of PRICA over conventional cytosolic assays include the ability to detect estrogen receptors in minimal breast carcinomas not amenable to receptor quantitation by cytosolic methods.[2] Patients with tumors containing an unusual amount of stroma with few tumor cells may also benefit from PRICA. PRICA does not suffer from method variations in protein concentration determinations as does the cytosolic assay.[7]

Utilizing cytosolic methods, progestogen receptors may be found in benign mammary tissue from mastectomies for breast carcinoma. While most benign PR-positive tissue is associated with PR-positive tumors, the reverse is not true. Benign breast tissue taken from reduction mammoplasty specimens (not for carcinoma) contain PR receptors at a concentration lower than that of benign tissue from resection specimens for breast carcinoma.[8] Nuclear and not cytoplasmic staining determines the progestogen receptor status for two antiprogestogen antibodies (mPRi and JZB39).[9] Comparisons of PRICA on frozen sections with cytosolic methods have shown good agreement.[2,3,6,9,10] Agreement between the two methods has been approximately 75% to 80%, a little lower than with ERICA. Some investigators have reported concordance rates as low as 50% for PRICA.[6] Discrepancies as with ERICA may be attributable to presence of normal epithelium adjacent to PRICA-negative tumor cells, scant tumor cells in sample, and circulating progestogens occupying receptor sites blocking radioligand (radiolabeled progestogen) from binding to receptor sites in cytosol methods.[11,12] Fixation of tumors at 4°C may give the most optimal PRICA staining.[13] As fixation appears to influence outcomes more for PRICA than for ERICA, it has been recommended to regard positive stains in paraffin-embedded tissue as evidence for the presence of progesterone receptors but a negative stain in paraffin sections as meaningless.[6]

In a study of 124 primary breast carcinomas, both ER and PR were almost exclusively located in carcinoma cell nuclei. Receptor status was as follows: ER+PR+, 50 patients; ER+PR-, 23 patients; ER-PR-, 26 patients; and ER-PR+, 3 patients.[14] A statistically significant decrease of PR+ tumors (and of ER+PR+ tumors) has been reported in women with more advanced stages of breast cancer. Such findings have led to the speculation that breast carcinomas contain steroid receptors and are hormone dependent from inception.[15]

Breast cancer specimens from a study of 600 women demonstrated that both positive ERICA and PRICA correlate with postmenopausal status. Colloid carcinomas of the breast were most likely to be ERICA and PRICA positive while medullary carcinomas of the breast were most likely to be ERICA and PRICA negative.[16] Positive ERICA was significantly associated with disease-free survival in women with stage I or stage II disease using single variable analysis. Using a Cox proportional hazard model, a positive PRICA was the best predictor of survival and disease-free survival.[16]

A very modest improvement in response to hormonal therapy has been reported in patients with ER-positive ovarian carcinoma.[17] Progesterone and estrogen receptors have also been shown to correlate with nuclear staining in endometrial adenocarcinomas utilizing immunocytochemical methods.[18,19,20] Histologic grade of such adenocarcinomas correlated with positive ERICA and PRICA status.[18,19] Endometrioid adenocarcinoma had the highest degree of positive ERICA and PRICA status followed by adenosquamous carcinoma, serous carcinoma, and lastly clear cell carcinoma.[19] Sensitivity of ERICA and PRICA compared to cytosolic methods was 78.5% and 58.2% for ER and PR. Survival in endometrial carcinoma was predicted by both positive ERICA and PRICA. Multivariate analysis of this data showed that positive ERICA was the most important predictor of survival.[20]

Footnotes

1. Aziz DC, "Quantitation of Estrogen and Progesterone Receptors by Immunocytochemical and Image Analyses," *Am J Clin Pathol*, 1992, 98(1):105-11.
2. El-Badawy N, Cohen C, Derose PB, et al, "Immunohistochemical Progesterone Receptor Assay – Measurement by Image Analysis," *Am J Clin Pathol*, 1991, 96(6):704-10.
3. Kommoss F, Bibbo M, Colley M, et al, "Assessment of Hormone Receptors in Breast Carcinoma by Immunocytochemistry and Image Analysis – 1. Progesterone Receptors," *Anal Quant Cytol Histol*, 1989, 11(5):298-306.
4. Masood S, "Use of Monoclonal Antibody for Assessment of Estrogen Receptor Content in Fine Needle Aspiration Biopsy Specimen From Patients With Breast Cancer," *Arch Pathol Lab Med*, 1989, 113(1):26-30.
5. Helin HJ, Isola JJ, Helin MJ, et al, "Imprint Cytology in Immunocytochemical Analysis of Oestrogen and Progesterone Receptors of Breast Carcinoma," *J Clin Pathol*, 1989, 42(10):1043-5.
6. Ozzello L, DeRosa C, Habif DV, et al, "An Immunohistochemical Evaluation of Progesterone Receptor in Frozen Sections, Paraffin Sections, and Cytologic Imprints of Breast Carcinomas," *Cancer*, 1991, 67(2):455-62.
7. Howanitz PJ, Howanitz JH, Skrodzki CA, et al, "Protein Method Influences on Calculation of Tissue Receptor Concentration," *Am J Clin Pathol*, 1986, 85:37-42.
8. Netto GJ, Cheek JH, Zachariah NY, et al, "Steroid Receptors in Benign Mastectomy Tissue," *Am J Clin Pathol*, 1990, 94(1):14-7.
9. Isola JJ, Helle MJ, and Helin HJ, "Immunocytochemical Detection of Progesterone Receptor in Breast Carcinoma – Comparison of Two Monoclonal Antibodies," *Am J Clin Pathol*, 1990, 93(3):378-82.
10. Esteban JM, Kandalaft PL, Mehta P, et al, "Improvement of the Quantification of Estrogen and Progesterone Receptors in Paraffin-Embedded Tumors by Image Analysis," *Am J Clin Pathol*, 1993, 99(1):32-8.
11. Parl FF and Posey YF, "Discrepancies of the Biochemical and Immunohistochemical Estrogen Receptor Assays in Breast Cancer," *Hum Pathol*, 1988, 19(8):960-6.
12. Wilbur DC, Willis J, Mooney RA, et al, "Estrogen and Progesterone Receptor Detection in Archival Formalin-Fixed, Paraffin-Embedded Tissue From Breast Carcinoma: A Comparison of Immunohistochemistry With the Dextran-Coated Charcoal Assay," *Mod Pathol*, 1992, 5(1):79-84.
13. Paterson DA, Reid CP, Anderson TJ, et al, "Assessment of Oestrogen Receptor Content of Breast Carcinoma by Immunohistochemical Techniques on Fixed and Frozen Tissue and by Biochemical Ligand Binding Assay," *J Clin Pathol*, 1990, 43(1):46-51.
14. Helin HJ, Helle MJ, Helin ML, et al, "Immunocytochemical Detection of Estrogen and Progesterone Receptors in 124 Human Breast Cancers," *Am J Clin Pathol*, 1988, 90(2):137-42.
15. Tinnemans JGM, Beex LVAM, Wobbes T, et al, "Steroid-Hormone Receptors in Nonpalpable and More Advanced Stages of Breast Cancer – A Contribution to the Biology and Natural History of Carcinoma of the Female Breast," *Cancer*, 1990, 66(6):1165-7.
16. Pertschuk LP, Kim DS, Nayer K, et al, "Immunocytochemical Estrogen and Progestin Receptor Assays in Breast Cancer With Monoclonal Antibodies – Histopathologic, Demographic, and Biochemical Correlations and Relationship to Endocrine Response and Survival," *Cancer*, 1990, 66(8):1663-70.
17. Fromm G-L, Freedman RS, Fritsche HA, et al, "Sequentially Administered Ethinyl Estradiol and Medroxyprogesterone Acetate in the Treatment of Refractory Epithelial Ovarian Carcinoma in Patients With Positive Estrogen Receptors," *Cancer*, 1991, 68(9):1885-9.
18. Segreti EM, Novotny DB, Soper JT, et al, "Endometrial Cancer: Histologic Correlates of Immunohistochemical Localization of Progesterone Receptor and Estrogen Receptor," *Obstet Gynecol*, 1989, 73(5 Pt 1):780-5.
19. Carcangiu ML, Chambers JT, Voynick IM, et al, "Immunohistochemical Evaluation of Estrogen and Progesterone Receptor Content in 183 Patients With Endometrial Carcinoma – Part I: Clinical and Histologic Correlations," *Am J Clin Pathol*, 1990, 94(3):247-54.

(Continued)

Progestogen Receptor Immunocytochemical Assay *(Continued)*

20. Chambers JT, Carcangiu ML, Voynick IM, et al, "Immunohistochemical Evaluation of Estrogen and Progesterone Receptor Content in 183 Patients With Endometrial Carcinoma – Part II: Correlation Between Biochemical and Immunohistochemical Methods and Survival," *Am J Clin Pathol*, 1990, 94(3):255-60.

References

Allred DC, "Should Immunohistochemical Examination Replace Biochemical Hormone Receptor Assays in Breast Cancer?" *Am J Clin Pathol*, 1993, 99(1):1-3.

Graham DM, Jin L, Lloyd RV, et al, "Detection of Estrogen Receptor in Paraffin-Embedded Sections of Breast Carcinoma by Immunohistochemistry and *In Situ* Hybridization," *Am J Surg Pathol*, 1991, 15(5):475-85.

Kiang DT, "The Presence of Steroid Receptors in 'Nontarget' Tissues and Its Significance," *Am J Clin Pathol*, 1993, 99(2):120-2.

Onetti-Muda A, Crescenzi A, Pujia N, et al, "Demonstration of Oestrogen and Progesterone Receptors in Freeze-Dried, Paraffin-Embedded Sections of Breast Cancer," *Histopathology*, 1991, 18(6):511-6.

Russack V, Meurer WT, Viesca T, et al, "Frozen Section Estrogen Receptor Determination in Minimal Breast Tumors," *Surg Pathol*, 1991, 4:113-20.

Sabini G, Chumas JC, and Mann WJ, "Steroid Hormone Receptors in Endometrial Stromal Sarcomas. A Biochemical and Immunohistochemical Study," *Am J Clin Pathol*, 1992, 97(3):381-6.

Tesch M, Shawwa A, and Henderson R, "Immunohistochemical Determination of Estrogen and Progesterone Receptor Status in Breast Cancer," *Am J Clin Pathol*, 1993, 99(1):8-12.

van Hoeven KH, Menendez-Botet CJ, Strong EW, et al, "Estrogen and Progesterone Receptor Content in Human Thyroid Disease," *Am J Clin Pathol*, 1993, 99(2):175-81.

Proliferative Indices *see* Tumor Aneuploidy by Flow Cytometry *on page 88*

Prostate Specific Acid Phosphatase *see* Immunoperoxidase Procedures *on page 60*

Quality Assurance in the Practice of Medicine *see* Autopsy *on page 36*

Rabid Animals *see* Rabies *on this page*

Rabies

CPT *88305 (brain/meninges, other than for tumor resection); 88307 (brain biopsy); 88312 (special stains); 88346 (immunofluorescence)*

Related Information

Viral Culture, Central Nervous System Symptoms *on page 1199*

Virus, Direct Detection by Fluorescent Antibody *on page 1208*

Synonyms Rabid Animals

Applies to Fluorescent Rabies Antibody Test; FRA Test; Negri Bodies

Test Commonly Includes Examination of animal brain for Negri bodies or inoculation of mice with suspension of brain tissue

Abstract Rabies has been a recognized disease in humans and animals for more than 25 centuries. Zinke is credited with first demonstrating the virus in 1804. Unlike many other viruses, the rabies virus is capable of infecting a number of different animal species, allowing it to propagate and survive in nature. Individuals with a high risk of contact with rabid animals (veterinarians, animal control officers, etc) should consider vaccination against rabies.

Specimen Head of large animal or entire small animal suspected of rabies. Use gloves and mask when handling an animal carcass suspected of rabies. **CONTAINER:** Sealed container **STORAGE INSTRUCTIONS:** Ideally, animal brain should be examined in the fresh state. Transport using wet ice or place in absorbent material, then in two plastic bags, or, place half the brain in 50% glycerol, half in 10% formalin, depending on instructions from state laboratory. Local state laboratory must be consulted. Rabies virus may also be demonstrated by immunofluorescence in skin biopsies of patients suspected of having rabies (*vide infra*). **CAUSES FOR REJECTION:** Unlabeled or improperly packaged specimen

Interpretive USE: Diagnose rabies;[1] evaluate animal bites **LIMITATIONS:** Negri bodies are found in about 90% of rabid animals. **CONTRAINDICATIONS:** Formalin fixation precludes fluorescent antibody application **METHODOLOGY:** Fluorescent antibody examination (but Negri bodies can be seen in H & E) **ADDITIONAL INFORMATION:** Animals at risk for rabies include skunks, raccoons, dogs, cats, bats, cattle, foxes, and to a lesser extent, jackals, wolves, coyotes, mongooses, weasels, squirrels, and any escaped wild animal. Bites of rabbits, squirrels, hamsters, guinea pigs, gerbils, chipmunks, rats, mice, and other rodents have seldom if ever resulted in human rabies in the United States and are regarded as low risk. High risk species include bats, raccoons, skunks, and foxes among wild carnivorous animals.[2]

Domestic animals should be kept alive if possible, to be quarantined. Animal bites, when unprovoked, are more likely to transmit rabies.[3] Survival of animal for 10 days makes rabies unlikely. Signs of rabies among wild carnivorous animals cannot be reliably interpreted and any such animal that bites or scratches a person should be killed at once and the head submitted for rabies testing.[2]

Rabies is a zoonosis caused by a neurotropic RNA virus which occurs in saliva, central nervous system, urine, and feces. Rabies virus produces Negri bodies (viral inclusions) in neurons.

The geographic area is important. Although a dog bite along the U.S.–Mexican border is considered a rabies exposure until proven otherwise, such bites in New York or Philadelphia are reported not to require prophylaxis.[3] Most Americans dying of rabies were exposed in foreign countries. One patient, bitten by a rabid dog in Kenya, had even had pre-exposure prophylaxis with human diploid cell vaccine. This emphasizes the **necessity for postexposure therapy in appropriate cases.**[4] Almost all rabies follows bite exposure. However, rabies virus can (rarely) enter through nonbite exposure, such as an open wound, or by inhalation of aerosolized bat urine (eg, cave explorers) or by corneal transplantation. The following table lists location of exposure to rabid canine bites and extent of exposure as it relates to mortality rates. The proportion of cases for which the source of exposure is not known has been increasing since 1960.[5,6]

Representative Mortality Rates in Nonvaccinated Individuals Following Exposure to Rabid Canines

Location of Exposure	Extent of Exposure	Mortality (%)
Face	Bites (multiple and severe)	60
Other part of head	Bites (multiple and severe)	50
Face	Bite (single)	30
Fingers/hand	Bite (severe)	15
Face	Bites (multiple and superficial)	10
Hand	Bites (multiple and superficial)	5
Trunk/legs	Scratch	3
Hands/exposed skin	Bleeding and superficial wound	2
Skin covered by clothes	Superficial wound	0.5
Recent wound	Saliva	0.1
Wounds >24 h old	Saliva	0.0

From Whitley RJ and Middlebrooks M, "Rabies," *Infections of the Central Nervous System,* Chapter 7, Scheld WM, Whitley RJ, and Durack DT, eds, New York, NY: Raven Pres, 1991, 134, with permission.

Antemortem rabies virus has been isolated from human saliva, brain tissues, CSF, urine sediment, and tracheal secretions. Rabies virus may also be demonstrated by immunofluorescent rabies antibody staining of skin biopsy tissue. The most reliable and reproducible of the immunofluorescent studies that can aid in patient diagnosis is biopsy of the neck skin. A 6-8 mm full thickness wedge or punch biopsy specimen from the neck containing as many hair follicles as possible should be sampled, snap frozen, and shipped frozen at -70°C to a reference laboratory.[7] Consult with reference laboratory for shipping instructions. False-negative results do occur especially after the development of neutralizing antibodies.[7]

Footnotes

1. Manson-Bahr PE and Apted FI, "Rabies," *Manson's Tropical Diseases*, 18th ed, London, England: Bailliere-Tindall, 1982, 290-5.
2. Center for Disease Control, "Rabies Prevention – United States, 1991 – Recommendations of the Immunization Practices Advisory Committee (ACIP)," *MMWR Morb Mortal Wkly Rep*, 1991, 40(RR-3):1-19.
3. Fishbein DB and Baer GM, "Animal Rabies: Implications for Diagnosis and Human Treatment," *Ann Intern Med*, 1988, 109(12):935-7.
4. Center for Disease Control, "Human Rabies – Kenya," *MMWR Morb Mortal Wkly Rep*, 1983, 32:494-5.
5. Center for Disease Control, "Human Rabies – Oregon," *MMWR Morb Mortal Wkly Rep*, 1989, 38(19):335-7.
6. Smith JS, Fishbein DB, Rupprecht CE, et al, "Unexplained Rabies in Three Immigrants in the United States. A Virologic Investigation," *N Engl J Med*, 1991, 324(4):205-11.

(Continued)

Rabies *(Continued)*

7. Bernard KW and Fishbein DB, "Rabies Virus," *Principles and Practice of Infectious Diseases*, Chapter 140, Mandell GL, Douglas RG Jr, and Bennett JE, eds, New York, NY: Churchill Livingstone, 1990, 1291-1301.

References

Bussereau F, Vincent J, Coudrier D, et al, "Monoclonal Antibodies to Mokola Virus for Identification of Rabies and Rabies-Related Viruses," *J Clin Microbiol*, 1988, 26:2489-94.

Center for Disease Control, "Compendium of Animal Rabies Control, 1990," *MMWR Morb Mortal Wkly Rep*, 1990, 39(RR-4):1-8.

Dietzschold B, Tollis M, Rupprecht CE, et al, "Antigenic Variation in Rabies and Rabies-Related Viruses: Cross-Protection Independent of Glycoprotein-Mediated Virus-Neutralizing Antibody," *J Infect Dis*, 1987, 156:815.

Hefner RR and Strano AJ, "Rabies," *Pathology of Tropical and Extraordinary Diseases*, Washington, DC: Armed Forces Institute of Pathology, 1976, 44-7.

Mrak, RE and Young L, "Rabies Encephalitis in a Patient With No History of Exposure," *Hum Pathol*, 1992, 24(1):109-10.

Reid-Sanden FL, Sumner JW, Smith JS, et al, "Rabies Diagnostic Reagents Prepared From a Rabies N Gene Recombinant Expressed in Baculovirus," *J Clin Microbiol*, 1990, 28:858-63.

Weiner LP and Fleming, "Viral Infections of the Nervous System," *J Neurosurg*, 1984, 61:207-24.

Whitley RJ and Middlebrooks M, "Rabies," *Infections of the Central Nervous System*, Scheld WM, Whitley RJ, and Durack DT, eds, New York, NY: Raven Press, 1991, 134.

Renal Biopsy *see* Kidney Biopsy *on page 68*

S100 *see* Immunoperoxidase Procedures *on page 60*

Skeletal Muscle Biopsy *see* Muscle Biopsy *on page 75*

Skin Biopsies

CPT *88302 (plastic repair); 88304 (cyst/tag/debridement); 88305 (other than cyst/tag/debridement)*

Related Information

Antinuclear Antibody *on page 638*
Electron Microscopic Examination for Viruses, Stool *on page 1177*
Electron Microscopy *on page 45*
Fungus Smear, Stain *on page 813*
Gene Rearrangement for Leukemia and Lymphoma *on page 911*
Gram Stain *on page 815*
Herpes Cytology *on page 502*
Herpes Simplex Virus Antigen Detection *on page 1181*
Histopathology *on page 57*
Immunofluorescence, Skin Biopsy *on page 708*
Immunoperoxidase Procedures *on page 60*
KOH Preparation *on page 825*
Leishmaniasis Serological Test *on page 717*
Lymph Node Biopsy *on page 72*
Oral Cavity Cytology *on page 507*
Pemphigus Antibodies *on page 731*
Skin Fungus Culture *on page 845*
Skin Mycobacteria Culture *on page 846*
Varicella-Zoster Virus Culture *on page 1193*
Varicella-Zoster Virus Serology *on page 761*
Viral Culture *on page 1195*
Viral Culture, Dermatological Symptoms *on page 1201*

Applies to Grocott's-Methanamine Silver Stain; PAS Stain

Abstract This section deals with sampling and procurement techniques and with a selected group of diagnostic skin problems.

Specimen **CONTAINER:** 10% neutral formalin is satisfactory for submission of most specimens, but there are special requirements for immunofluorescence and electron microscopy. See also Histopathology, Electron Microscopy, and Immunoperoxidase Procedures. **COLLECTION:** Techniques for procuring skin specimens:

Shave biopsy: A technique for obtaining superficial samples of predominantly epidermal or projecting lesions by cutting them flush with adjacent skin as illustrated in Figure 1. This technique is usually used for nonmalignant lesions but may be useful for the patch phase of mycosis fungoides. **Since shave biopsy provides the most limited specimen, a serious potential for histopathologic misdiagnosis exists, especially in regard to melanocytic lesions.**

Figure 1. Shave Biopsy

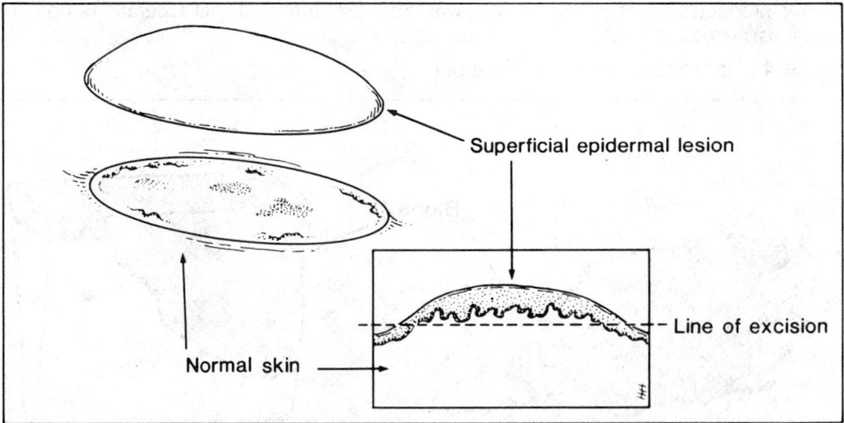

Punch biopsy: Very popular with dermatologists because it can be done easily, quickly, and repetitively at low cost in office practice. Biopsy punches, illustrated in Figure 2, range from 3-6 mm in size. The punch is pressed into the skin and rotated. It yields a plug or core of tissue which is cut from its base by scissors as the punch is withdrawn. It may be difficult to adequately sample subcutanea by punch. Pathologists prefer the largest possible sample.

Figure 2. Punch Biopsy

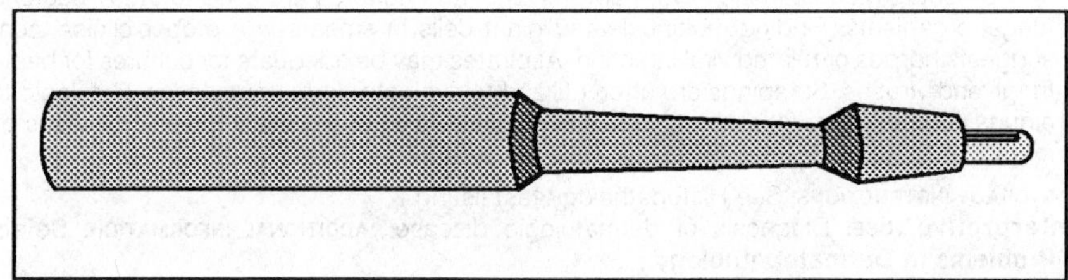

Excisional biopsy: This usually implies total removal of a skin lesion, most commonly a tumor, with a scalpel as illustrated in Figure 3. It is a preferred technique for removal of pigmented lesions and tumors.

Figure 3. Excisional Biopsy by Scalpel

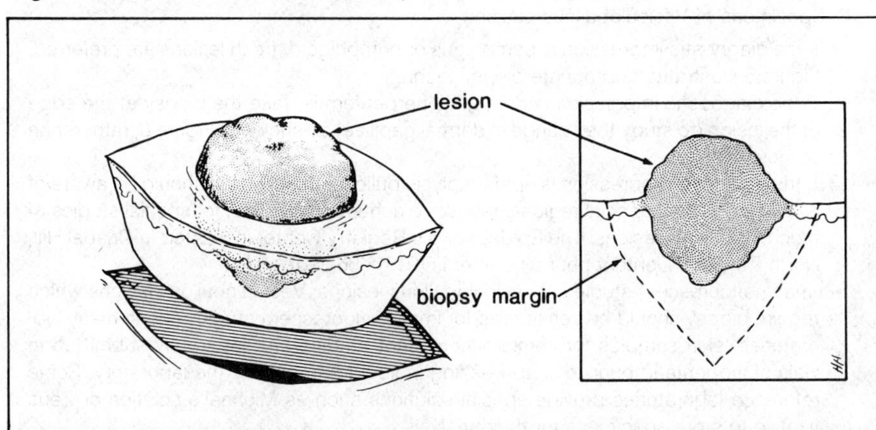

(Continued)

Skin Biopsies *(Continued)*

Incisional biopsy: Removal of a portion of a lesion by scalpel is illustrated in Figure 4. It is performed when a non-neoplastic lesion (ie, necrobiosis lipoidica) is too large to be totally excised but definitive diagnosis mandates a large sample to evaluate overall architectural detail or, in the case of tumors, for which complete excision would require extensive surgery and/or would produce cosmetic deformity that would not be warranted until accurate histopathologic diagnosis is established.

Figure 4. Incisional Biopsy by Scalpel

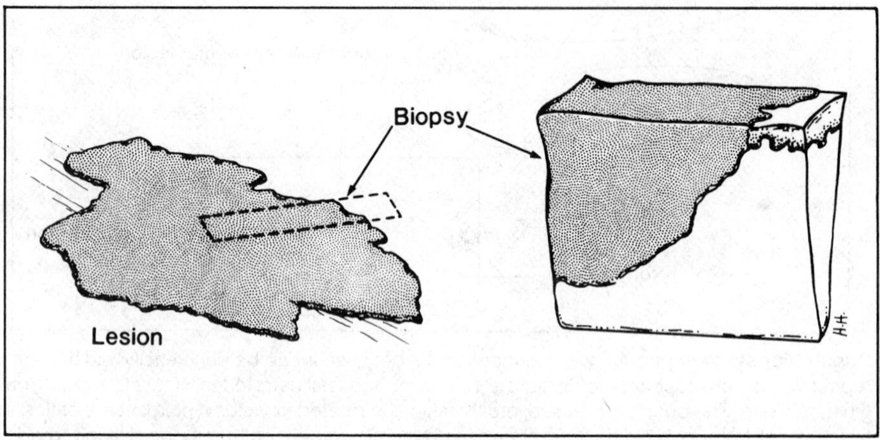

Smears and/or aspirates: Wright or Giemsa type stains may suffice to demonstrate polys or eosinophils (as in toxic erythema or pustular melanosis of newborns). Gram, acid-fast, PAS, and Grocott's-Methenamine-Silver (GMS) stains, and cultures are used to study bacterial or fungal organisms. Finding multinucleated giant cells in smears in a proper clinical context suggests herpes or related viral infection. Aspirates may be adequate for cultures for bacteria, fungi, and viruses. Scrapings are often utilized to evaluate dermatophytoses. Cytologic techniques (Tzanck smears) are rarely used in practice to evaluate acantholytic processes or tumors.

STORAGE INSTRUCTIONS: See Histopathology test listing.

Interpretive USE: Diagnosis of dermatologic disease ADDITIONAL INFORMATION: **Selected Problems in Dermatopathology:**

A. Specimens of Pigmented Lesions and Tumors

1. In general, pigmented lesions and tumors should not be needled, aspirated, curetted, shaved or punched, but should be excised, *in toto*, whenever possible, to permit comprehensive evaluation and measurements appropriate if melanoma.

B. Specimens of Vesiculobullous Lesions

1. If the diagnostic impression is pemphigus or pemphigoid, fresh lesions are preferred. Figure 5 illustrates appropriate biopsy technique.
2. If the diagnostic impression is dermatitis herpetiformis, take the biopsy at the edge of the lesion (to study the change in dermal papillae) as shown in Figure 6, rather than the lesion itself.
3. If the diagnostic impression is epidermolysis bullosa, the clinician should be aware of availability of four special regional reference centers in the USA for special studies of mechanobullous lesions. The Epidermolysis Registry Center is located in Chapel Hill, North Carolina. Contact phone number is (919) 966-2007.
4. Immunofluorescent studies of vesiculobullous lesions: Vesiculobullous lesions which require biopsy should be considered for immunofluorescent studies (IF). In many laboratories, skin samples for immunofluorescent studies are separately submitted in vials of isopentane prior to snap freezing in liquid nitrogen by the laboratory. Some reference laboratories provide special solutions such as Michael's solution or Zeus fixative to store specimens for their analysis.

Figure 5. Punch Biopsy: Pemphigus or Pemphigoid

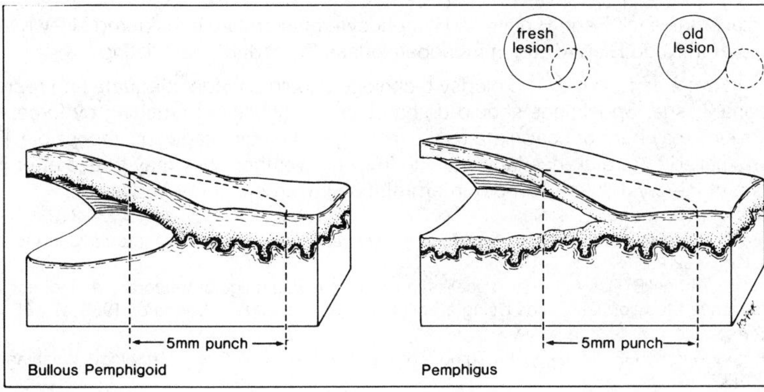

fresh lesion

old lesion

5mm punch

Bullous Pemphigoid

5mm punch

Pemphigus

Figure 6. Punch Biopsy: Dermatitis Herpetiformis

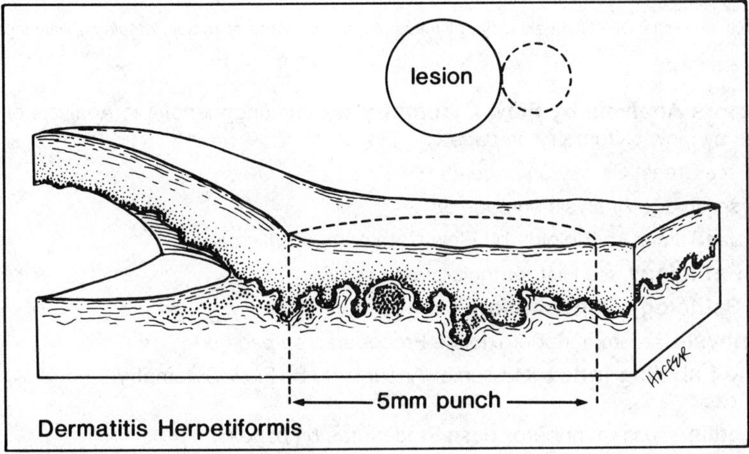

C. Specimens for Lupus Erythematosus (LE)

1. Direct immunofluorescence was first utilized on cutaneous biopsies in LE. The procedure (lupus band test) was widely utilized to study systemic lupus erythematosus (SLE), discoid lupus erythematosus (DLE), and mixed connective tissue disorder (MCTD). Recent data suggests the band test is much less specific and sensitive than previously thought. It is not clinically useful in discrimination of SLE from other connective tissue (CT) disorders or in predicting which patients with undifferentiated CT disease would develop SLE. Serologic evaluation is more sensitive, efficient, and cost effective in discriminating DLE and SLE.[1]

Biopsy Site	SLE	DLE
Lesional Tissue	+	+
Uninvolved, Sun-exposed	+	–

D. Specimens of Epidermolysis Bullosa Acquisita (EBA)

1. Recent studies suggest that from 5% to 10% of patients regarded as bullous pemphigoid by routine direct immunofluorescence can be shown to be EBA based on indirect immunofluorescence on salt-split skin.[2]

(Continued)

Skin Biopsies *(Continued)*

E. Special Studies for Hematopoietic Disorders

1. Special studies for T and B cells and lymphocyte markers are considered elsewhere. See Lymph Node Biopsy and Immunoperoxidase Procedures test listings.

Pitfalls and artifacts to avoid: The biopsy technique should provide adequate and representative lesional tissue. Specimens should be handled gently without crushing by forceps. Cautery of lesions may burn or coagulate tissue making pathologic diagnosis impossible. If specimens are mailed to a reference laboratory in freezing weather, they may freeze after fixation. Formation of ice crystals may render interpretation hazardous if not impossible.

Footnotes

1. Harrist T, *Selected Topics in Cutaneous Immunofluorescence*, Boston, MA: International Academy of Pathology, 1990.
2. Logan RA, Bhogal B, Das AK, et al, "Localization of Bullous Pemphigoid Antibody – An Indirect Immunofluorescence Study of 228 Cases Using a Split-Skin Technique," *Br J Dermatol*, 1987, 17:471.

References

Elder DE and Murphy GF, "Melanocytic Tumors of the Skin," *Atlas of Tumor Pathology*, Washington, DC: AFIP, 1990.

Lever WF and Schaumburg-Lever G, *Histopathology of the Skin*, 7th ed, Philadelphia, PA: JB Lippincott Co, 1990.

Maize JC and Ackerman AB, *Pigmented Lesions of the Skin: Clinicopathologic Correlations*, Philadelphia, PA: Lea & Febiger, 1987.

Murphy GF and Elder DE, "Nonmelanocytic Tumors of the Skin," *Atlas of Tumor Pathology*, Washington, DC: AFIP, 1991.

Solid Tumors Analysis by Flow Cytometry *see* Immunophenotypic Analysis of Tissues by Flow Cytometry *on page 65*

S-Phase *see* Breast Biopsy *on page 40*

S Phase *see* Image Analysis *on page 58*

S Phase *see* Tumor Aneuploidy by Flow Cytometry *on this page*

Surgical Pathology *see* Histopathology *on page 57*

Surgical Pathology Consultation *see* Frozen Section *on page 54*

Synaptophysin *see* Immunoperoxidase Procedures *on page 60*

Thymidine Labeling Index *see* Tumor Aneuploidy by Flow Cytometry *on this page*

Thyroglobulin *see* Immunoperoxidase Procedures *on page 60*

Tissue Antigens *see* Immunoperoxidase Procedures *on page 60*

Tissue Examination *see* Histopathology *on page 57*

Tissue Pathology *see* Histopathology *on page 57*

T-Lymphocyte Analysis by Flow Cytometry *see* Immunophenotypic Analysis of Tissues by Flow Cytometry *on page 65*

T Lymphocytes *see* Immunoperoxidase Procedures *on page 60*

Transmission Electron Microscopy *see* Electron Microscopy *on page 45*

Trichrome Stain *see* Kidney Biopsy *on page 68*

Tumor Aneuploidy by Flow Cytometry

CPT *88358*

Related Information

Body Fluids Cytology *on page 482*
Breast Biopsy *on page 40*
Cerebrospinal Fluid Cytology *on page 490*
Estrogen Receptor Assay *on page 47*
Fine Needle Aspiration, Superficial Palpable Masses *on page 499*
Histopathology *on page 57*
Image Analysis *on page 58*
Immunophenotypic Analysis of Tissues by Flow Cytometry *on page 65*

Urine Cytology *on page 513*

Synonyms Flow Cytometry of Tumor Aneuploidy; Ploidy Analysis of Tumors

Applies to Aneuploidy; DNA Content; DNA Synthesis Phase; G_1 Phase; G_2M; G_0 Phase; Proliferative Indices; S Phase; Thymidine Labeling Index

Test Commonly Includes Assessment of nuclear DNA for aneuploid clones; estimation of percentage of cells in S-phase ("replicating fraction," "S-phase fraction")

Abstract Assessment of ploidy may be helpful to estimate prognosis and to plan therapy for patients from whom tumors have been sampled or excised.

Specimen Portion of tissue, fresh or paraffin-embedded, needle aspiration of neoplasm. Fresh tissue is better than formalin-fixed, paraffin-embedded specimen.[1]

Interpretive REFERENCE RANGE: Almost all specimens of benign, non-neoplastic tissue show a dominant population of diploid nuclei with an amount of stainable DNA designated "2C." There are <10% cells actively synthesizing DNA – "S-phase fraction," and only a small number of premitotic cells with double the normal diploid DNA content – "4C." See diagram. USE: Quantitate nuclear DNA content and replicative activity of neoplastic cells. The presence of aneuploid peaks, representing nuclei with abnormal amounts of DNA and/or an increased percentage of cells actively synthesizing DNA, may be prognostically significant and may be independent of tumor grade and stage, depending on the primary. LIMITATIONS: **This assay is not in itself diagnostic of malignancy.** Results must be interpreted with caution and experience. Results are most meaningful when applied to sample with diagnosis of malignancy already established by histopathology. Neoplasms with diploid cell lines, even if malignant, may be indistinguishable by this technique from benign or normal tissue. Some neoplasms may harbor multiple stem lines, some aneuploid, some not. Some neoplasms have "near-diploid" stem lines which may be difficult or impossible to identify as abnormal. **Some benign adenomas may contain aneuploid cells,** and the DNA content of some carcinomas of the same tissue may be diploid (eg, adrenal cortical adenomas and adenocarcinomas).[2]

Use of poorly fixed blocks or improperly stored blocks may lead to artifacts which may be interpreted as aneuploid peaks. Avoid use of blocks processed with precipitating fixatives such as B-5 or Zenker's, as such fixatives tend to produce poor coefficients of variation and possibly uninterpretable total nuclear protein and light scatter data. If possible, a separate block of tumor should be fixed in nonbuffered formalin.

Flow cytometry from formalin-fixed, paraffin-embedded tissue may not always detect aneuploid cell populations, when compared to analysis of fresh tissue.[3] DNA analysis by flow cytometry, compared to image analysis, has shown high concordance. Discordant results do occur.[4]

METHODOLOGY: Flow cytometry (FC) of tumor cell suspension stained with an intercalating dye which binds quantitatively to DNA (usually ethidium bromide or propidium iodide). The nuclear stain fluoresces when excited by the cytometer's laser, and the emitted light, directly proportional to the amount of nuclear DNA, is detected and quantitated by the instrument's photomultiplier tubes. When sufficient nuclei have been analyzed (usually 5000-10,000), a histogram is generated (see diagrams) plotting the numbers of nuclei with given amounts of DNA. Much the same information can be developed on a quantitative image analysis system (light or fluorescent microscopy with quantitative morphometry and computerized data reduction). Image analysis systems typically gather information on hundreds of cells, rather than thousands. ADDITIONAL INFORMATION: That many cancers have abnormal amounts of nuclear DNA comes as no surprise to anyone who has looked at malignant tissue microscopically. Indeed, this is probably the basis for the prognostic significance of histologic grading systems, in which tumors which "look worse" connote a worse prognosis for the patients from whom the specimen came. If flow cytometry offered no more than quantified confirmation of this phenomenon, it would be only an expensive, elegant redundancy.

Flow cytometry is used to divide tumors into euploid (diploid) or aneuploid types. A tumor is classified as diploid if the DNA distribution has a major proliferation node at the normal diploid DNA value. Such a normal diploid value is typically derived from a cell culture fibroblast line or normal cells processed in the same block as the tumor. DNA measurement by flow cytometry is relatively insensitive, and it is well known that the gain or loss of several chromosomes or minor deletions might go undetected.

The powers of flow cytometric analysis of ploidy are that aneuploid cell lines or increased proliferative capacity can be detected even in some low grade neoplasms. Stage for stage and grade for grade, neoplasms with aneuploid nuclei are generally prognostically worse than

(Continued)

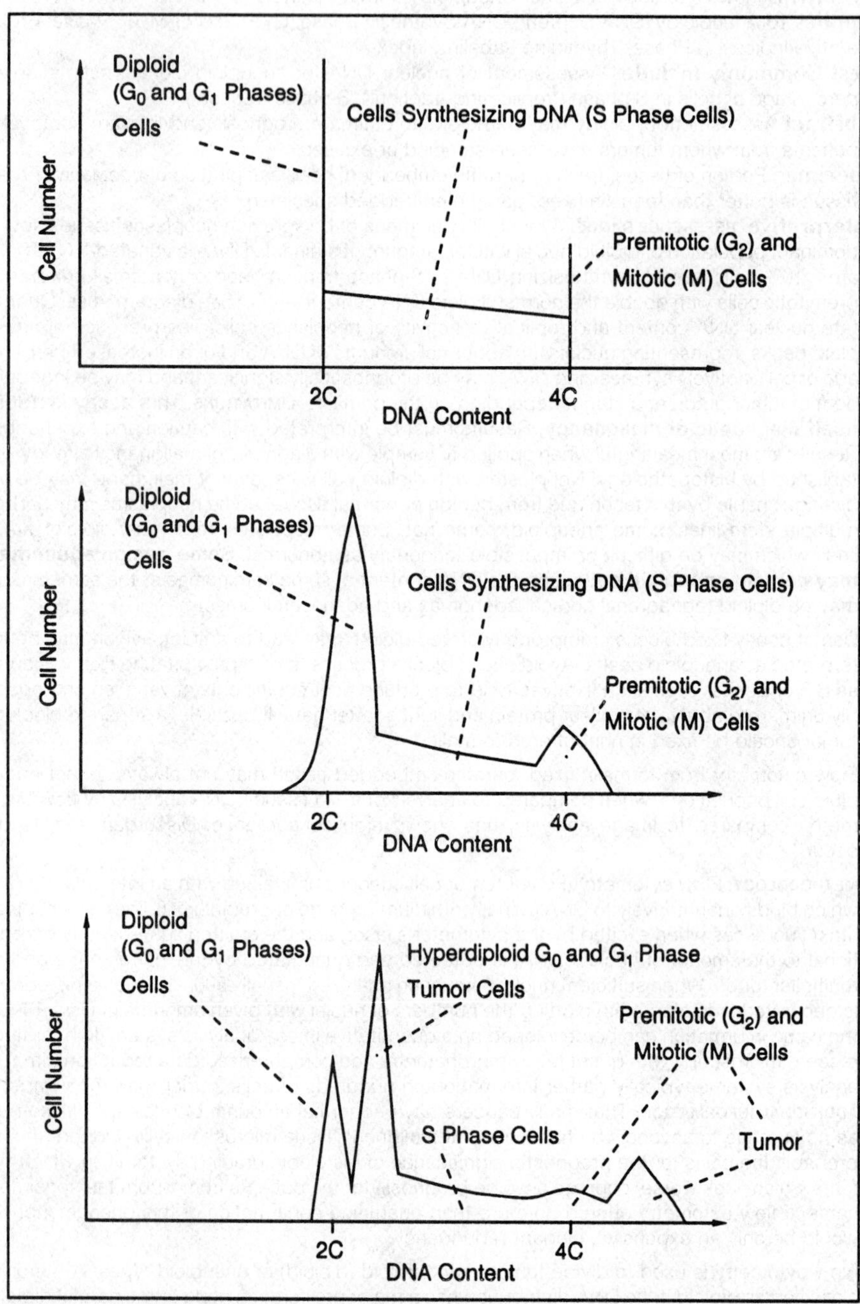

Top: An ideal distribution of DNA content in a cell population. Center: A distribution more typical of those actually obtained by flow cytometry. Bottom: A distribution such as is obtained from a tumor exhibiting DNA aneuploidy.
From Shapiro, "DNA Content," *Arch Pathol Lab Med,* 1989, 113:592, with permission.

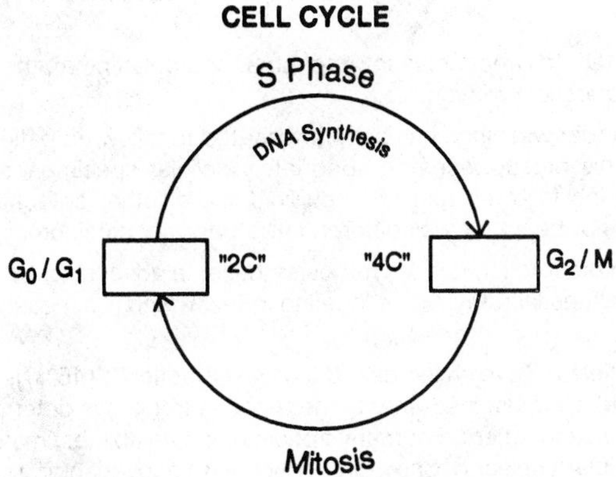
CELL CYCLE
S Phase
DNA Synthesis
G_0 / G_1
"2C"
"4C"
G_2 / M
Mitosis

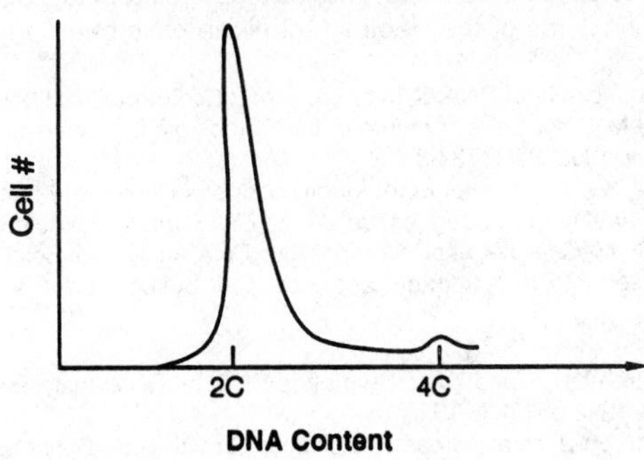
Diploid cells, slowly replicating
Cell #
2C
4C
DNA Content

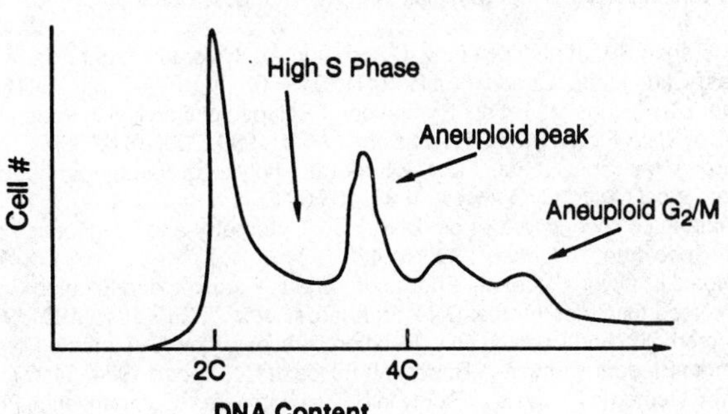
Aneuploid cells, rapid replication
High S Phase
Aneuploid peak
Aneuploid G_2/M
Cell #
2C
4C
DNA Content

(Continued)

Tumor Aneuploidy by Flow Cytometry *(Continued)*

those without. The value of DNA flow cytometry in prediction of tumor prognosis is largely dependent upon tumor type. Predictive value by flow cytometry is most solidly established for cancers of the breast, prostate, and colon. It is less clearly true for cancers of the ovary, lung, and kidney.

For a few neoplasms (acute lymphoblastic lymphoma, neuroblastoma), the presence of aneuploid cell lines is prognostically favorable.

Flow cytometry of bladder washings has been advocated to follow-up patients with transitional cell carcinomas. This presupposes an adequately cellular specimen, and the assurance that the neoplasm being followed had an aneuploid line or other detectable abnormality to begin with. This may not be so for well differentiated papillary carcinomas.

Measurement of S-phase fraction (DNA synthesis phase) is advocated for breast carcinoma. S-phase fraction correlates with thymidine labeling index, which is a measure of cellular proliferation.

Some workers in this field believe an increased "S-phase fraction" (>15%) is itself an indication of an abnormal cell line. On most instruments the S-phase fraction is determined by statistical modeling, not actual measurement. For many specimens a reliable estimate cannot be determined because of cellular/nuclear debris ("dirty specimen") or overlapping of peaks. There are questions how well such modeled S-phase fractions correlate with proliferative indices determined by incorporation of titrated thymidine.

Hedley developed a method of retrieving tissue from paraffin blocks, making possible analysis of archival material. Thus, if a specimen is small, it can be totally processed for microscopy with the assurance that DNA analysis can be done later from the block, if necessary. The Hedley technique also lets one be confident that the material being analyzed indeed represents the cancer. Various modifications of the Hedley technique have been proposed.

Footnotes

1. Robinson RA, "Defining the Limits of DNA Cytometry," *Am J Clin Pathol*, 1992, 98(3):275-7, (editorial).
2. Medeiros LJ and Weiss LM, "New Developments in the Pathologic Diagnosis of Adrenal Cortical Neoplasms," *Am J Clin Pathol*, 1992, 97(1):73-83.
3. Schultz DS and Zarbo RJ, "Comparison of Eight Modifications of Hedley's Method for Flow Cytometric DNA Ploidy Analysis of Paraffin-Embedded Tissue," *Am J Clin Pathol*, 1992, 98(3):291-5.
4. Elsheikh TM, Silverman JF, McCool JW, et al, "Comparative DNA Analysis of Solid Tumors by Flow Cytometric and Image Analyses of Touch Imprints and Flow Cell Suspensions," *Am J Clin Pathol*, 1992, 98(3):296-304.

References

Arber DA, Cook PD, Moser LK, et al, "Variation in Reference Cells for DNA Analysis of Paraffin-Embedded Tissue," *Am J Clin Pathol*, 1992, 97(3):387-92.

Arnerlöv C, Emdin SO, Lundgren B, et al, "Breast Carcinoma Growth Rate Described by Mammographic Doubling Time and S-Phase Fraction. Correlations to Clinical and Histopathologic Factors in a Screened Population," *Cancer*, 1992, 70(7):1928-34.

Babiak J and Poppema S, "Automated Procedure for Dewaxing and Rehydration of Paraffin-Embedded Tissue Sections for DNA Flow Cytometric Analysis Of Breast Tumors," *Am J Clin Pathol*, 1991, 96(1):64-9.

Blomjous EC, Schipper NW, Baak JP, et al, "The Value of Morphometry and DNA Flow Cytometry in Addition to Classic Prognosticators in Superficial Urinary Bladder Carcinoma," *Am J Clin Pathol*, 1989, 91(3):243-8.

Bosari S, Lee AK, Tahan SR, et al, "DNA Flow Cytometric Analysis and Prognosis of Axillary Lymph Node-Negative Breast Carcinoma," *Cancer*, 1992, 70(7):1943-50.

Clark GM, Dressler LG, Owens MA, et al, "Prediction of Relapse or Survival in Patients With Node-Negative Breast Cancer by DNA Flow Cytometry," *N Engl J Med*, 1989, 320(10):627-33.

Danova M, Riccardi A, Mazzini G, et al, "Flow Cytometric Analysis of Paraffin-Embedded Material in Human Gastric Cancer," *Anal Quant Cytol Histol*, 1988, 10:200-6.

Dressler LG, Seamen LC, Owens MA, et al, "DNA Flow Cytometry and Prognostic Factors in 1331 Frozen Breast Cancer Specimens," *Cancer*, 1988, 61:420-7.

Esteban JM, Sheibani K, Owens M, et al, "Effects of Various Fixatives and Fixation Conditions on DNA Ploidy Analysis. A Need for Strict Internal DNA Standards," *Am J Clin Pathol*, 1991, 95(4):460-6.

Farsund T, Hoestmark JG, and Laezum OD, "Relation Between Flow Cytometric DNA Distribution and Pathology in Human Bladder Cancer: A Report on 69 Cases," *Cancer*, 1984, 54:1771-7.

Frierson HF, "Flow Cytometric Analysis of Ploidy in Solid Neoplasms: Comparison of Fresh Tissues With Formalin-Fixed Paraffin-Embedded Specimens," *Hum Pathol*, 1988, 19:290-4.

Frierson HF, "Grade and Flow Cytometric Analysis of Ploidy for Infiltrating Ductal Carcinomas," *Hum Pathol*, 1993, 24(1):24-9.

Fuhr JE, Frye A, Kattine AA, et al, "Flow Cytometric Determination of Breast Tumor Heterogeneity," *Cancer*, 1991, 67(5):1401-5.

Ghali VS, Liau S, Teplitz C, et al, "A Comparative Study of DNA Ploidy in 115 Fresh-Frozen Breast Carcinomas by Image Analysis Versus Flow Cytometry," *Cancer*, 1992, 70(11):2668-72.

Hedley DW, Friedlander ML, Taylor IW, et al, "Method for Analysis of Cellular DNA Content of Paraffin-Embedded Pathological Material Using Flow Cytometry," *J Histochem Cytochem*, 1983, 31:1333-5.

Herbert DJ, Nishiyama RH, Bagwell CB, et al, "Effects of Several Commonly Used Fixatives on DNA and Total Nuclear Protein Analysis by Flow Cytometry," *Am J Clin Pathol*, 1989, 91(5):535-41.

Herman CJ, Hedley D, Wheeless LL, et al, "DNA Cytometry in Cancer Prognosis," *PPO Updates*, 1993, 7(3).

Homburger HA and Wold LE, "College of American Pathologists Conference XV on Analytical Cytology and Immunohistochemistry," *Arch Pathol Lab Med*, 1989, 113:577-683.

Joensun H, Klemi PJ, and Eerola E, "Diagnostic Value of Flow Cytometric DNA Determination Combined With Fine Needle Aspiration Biopsy in Thyroid Tumors," *Anal Quant Cytol Histol*, 1987, 9:328-34.

Jones EC, McNeal J, Bruchovsky N, et al, "DNA Content in Prostatic Adenocarcinoma – A Flow Cytometry Study of the Predictive Value of Aneuploidy for Tumor Volume, Percentage Gleason Grade 4 and 5, and Lymph Node Metastases," *Cancer*, 1990, 66(4):752-7.

Khoo SK, Hurst T, Kearsley J, et al, "Prognostic Significance of Tumor Ploidy in Patients With Advanced Ovarian Carcinoma," *Gynecol Oncol*, 1990, 39(3):284-8.

Landay AL, Ault KA, Bauer KD, et al, eds, *Clinical Flow Cytometry*, Vol 677, New York, NY: The New York Academy of Sciences, 1993.

Lee AK, Wiley B, Loda M, et al, "DNA Ploidy, Proliferation, and Neu-Oncogene Protein Overexpression in Breast Carcinoma," *Mod Pathol* 1992, 5(1):61-7.

Lewis WE, "Prognostic Significance of Flow Cytometric DNA Analysis in Node-Negative Breast Cancer Patients," *Cancer*, 1990, 65(10):2315-20.

Listinsky CM, Bonfiglio TA, and Leary J, "Variable Ploidy of Ovarian Clear Cell Carcinomas," *Anal Quant Cytol Histol*, 1988, 10:21-7.

Look AT, Douglass EC, and Meyer WH, "Clinical Importance of Near-Diploid Tumor Stem Lines in Patients With Osteosarcoma of an Extremity," *N Engl J Med*, 1988, 318:1567-72.

McCarthy RC and Fetterhoff TJ, "Issues for Quality Assurance in Clinical Flow Cytometry," *Arch Pathol Lab Med*, 1989, 113(6):658-66.

Merkel DE, Dressler LG, and McGuire WL, "Flow Cytometry, Cellular DNA Content, and Prognosis in Human Malignancy," *J Clin Oncol*, 1987, 5(10):1690-703.

Meyer JS, Koehm SL, Hughes JM, et al, "Bromodeoxyuridine Labeling for S-Phase Measurement in Breast Carcinoma," *Cancer*, 1993, 71(11):3531-40.

Murphy WM, "DNA Flow Cytometry in Diagnostic Pathology of the Urinary Tract," *Hum Pathol*, 1987, 18:317-9.

Nativ O, Winkler HZ, Raz Y, et al, "Stage C Prostatic Adenocarcinoma: Flow Cytometric Nuclear DNA Ploidy Analysis," *Mayo Clin Proc*, 1989, 64(8):911-9.

Radio SJ, Woodridge TN, and Linder J, "Flow Cytometric DNA Analysis of Malignant Fibrous Histiocytoma and Related Fibrohistiocytic Tumors," *Hum Pathol*, 1988, 19:74-7.

Scott NA, Grande JP, Weiland LH, et al, "Flow Cytometric DNA Patterns From Colorectal Cancers – How Reproducible Are They?" *Mayo Clin Proc*, 1987, 62:331-7.

Stonesifer KJ, Xiang J, Wilkinson EJ, et al, "Flow Cytometric Analysis and Cytopathology of Body Cavity Fluids," *Acta Cytol* 1987, 31:125-30.

Tsushima K, Stanhope CR, Gaffey TA, et al, "Uterine Leiomyosarcomas and Benign Smooth Muscle Tumors: Usefulness of Nuclear DNA Patterns Studied by Flow Cytometry," *Mayo Clin Proc*, 1988, 63:248-55.

van den Ingh HF, Griffioen G, and Cornelisse CJ, "Flow Cytometric Detection of Aneuploidy in Colorectal Adenomas," *Cancer Res*, 1985, 45:3392-7.

Weaver DL, Bagwell CB, Hitchcox SA, et al, "Improved Flow Cytometric Determination of Proliferative Activity (S-Phase Fraction) From Paraffin-Embedded Tissue," *Am J Clin Pathol*, 1990, 94(5):576-84.

Winkler HZ, Rainwater LM, Myers RP, et al, "Stage D1 Prostatic Adenocarcinomas: Significance of Nuclear DNA Ploidy Patterns Studied by Flow Cytometry," *Mayo Clin Proc*, 1988, 63:103-12.

Ultrastructural Study *see* Electron Microscopy *on page 45*

Vimentin *see* Immunoperoxidase Procedures *on page 60*

Vital Statistics *see* Autopsy *on page 36*

Zeus Fixative *see* Kidney Biopsy *on page 68*

CHEMISTRY

Paul R. Finley, MD
Harold J. Grady, PhD
Eugene S. Olsowka, MD, PhD
Lowell L. Tilzer, MD, PhD

Major advances in analytical methods, reagents, and instrumentation have broadened the scope of the clinical chemistry laboratory. Clinical chemistry comprises a variety of methods: chemical, enzymatic, chromatographic (thin-layer, high pressure liquid, gas-liquid), mass spectroscopic, immunoassays, and isotopic assays. Many molecular biology techniques are carried out in clinical chemistry laboratories. (See chapter on Molecular Pathology.) Therapeutic Drug and Toxicology assays are listed in the Therapeutic Drug Monitoring/Toxicology/Drugs of Abuse chapter. Many immunologic assays are listed in the Immunology and Serology chapter.

The terminology used in this chapter has also evolved into a new standard of acceptance. The somewhat ambiguous term "normal range" has been replaced by the more inclusive term "reference range" which can be used for any population provided a description of that population is furnished. The specimen section of each test now reflects the sample analyzed rather than the sample collected (blood vs serum or plasma), and where SI units have gained general acceptance, traditional units have been dropped (mEq/L vs mmol/L).

An extensive review of many of the factors involved in the decision as to whether or not a result is "within the normal range" for a given patient can be found by reading Statistics, the Normal Range, and the Ulysses Syndrome section.

Clinical problems are frequently too complex to allow interpretation of laboratory results without correlation with clinical data. In many instances, a review of the patient's clinical and laboratory findings by an interested and knowledgeable consultant (eg, internist, endocrinologist, nephrologist, clinical pathologist) will increase the usefulness of laboratory determinations and enhance the contribution of the laboratory data to the patient's care.

The careful revisions and new entries in this chapter, as well as in all the other chapters, reflect the rapid increase in knowledge and expertise of the laboratory practioners and their dedication to the implementation of the advances that have been made.

ABGs *see* Blood Gases, Arterial *on page 140*

ACE *see* Angiotensin Converting Enzyme *on page 130*

Acetoacetate *see* Ketone Bodies, Blood *on page 265*

Acetone *see* Ketone Bodies, Blood *on page 265*

Acetylcholinesterase, RBC *see* Acetylcholinesterase, Red Blood Cell *on this page*

Acetylcholinesterase, Red Blood Cell

CPT 82482

Related Information

Alpha$_1$-Fetoprotein, Amniotic Fluid *on page 114*
Alpha$_1$-Fetoprotein, Serum *on page 115*
Dibucaine Number *on page 209*
Pseudocholinesterase, Serum *on page 343*

Synonyms Acetylcholinesterase, RBC; Cholinesterase, Erythrocytic; Erythrocyte Cholinesterase; Red Cell Cholinesterase; True Cholinesterase

Specimen Red blood cells **CONTAINER:** Green top (heparin) tube or heparinized capillary tubes **STORAGE INSTRUCTIONS:** Stable at 4°C to 25°C for 1 week only.

Interpretive REFERENCE RANGE: Not well established, varies with method, age, sex, and use of oral contraceptives.[1] Normally absent in amniotic fluid. **USE:** Erythrocyte cholinesterase is measured to diagnose organophosphate and carbamate toxicity and to detect atypical forms of the enzyme. Cholinesterase is irreversibly inhibited by organophosphate insecticides and reversibly inhibited by carbamate insecticides. Serum or plasma pseudocholinesterase is a better measure of acute toxicity, while erythrocyte levels are better for chronic exposure. (Serum level returns to normal prior to normalizing of red cell level.) Acetylcholinesterase is increased in amniotic fluid in cases of neural tube defect.[1] Persons with an atypical form of the enzyme (with low enzyme activity) exhibit prolonged apnea following the use of certain suxamethonium-type muscle relaxants in anesthesia (succinylcholine sensitivity – AA phenotype). These atypical forms may be detected by the use of fluoride or dibucaine inhibition. In amniotic fluid, is is used for the evaluation of neural tube defects in conjunction with alpha-fetoprotein. **LIMITATIONS:** Values decrease as erythrocytes become senescent. **METHODOLOGY:** Methods are based on determination of result (rate) of hydrolysis of an ester catalyzed by the enzyme acetylcholinesterase and include colorimetry, fluorometry, spectrophotometry based systems. Polyacrylamide gel electrophoresis is used for the qualitative demonstration of acetylcholinesterase in amniotic fluid.[2] Screening methods are available[3] **ADDITIONAL INFORMATION:** The cholinesterase activity in human red cells is highly but not exclusively specific for acetylcholine. It is referred to as true or specific cholinesterase. Cholinesterase activity present in the serum/plasma hydrolyses both choline and aliphatic esters, has a broader range of esterolytic activity and is referred to as "pseudo-" or "nonspecific" cholinesterase. It hydrolyses acetylcholine only slowly. The systematic name for acetylcholinesterase is acetylcholine acetylhydrolase. Systematic name for cholinesterase (serum/plasma) is acylcholine acylhydrolase. The different nature of the cholinesterases was first described in 1940.[4] The plasma enzyme is synthesized by the liver, the red cell enzyme during erythropoiesis.

Cholinesterase activity is low at birth and higher in adult males than females. The enzyme is a large complex protein. There is evidence that it has a multiple subunit structure, four peptide chains that form two dimers. Because of the many constituent amino acids, many molecular variants are possible. The RBC level is **increased** in hemolytic states such as the thalassemias, spherocytosis, hemoglobin SS, and acquired hemolytic anemias. It is **decreased** in paroxysmal nocturnal hemoglobinuria and in relapse of megaloblastic anemia. (It returns to normal with therapy.)

Potent inhibitors of cholinesterase may present important clinical toxicological problems. Systemic insecticides (eg, organophosphates or carbamates) are examples. Both RBC acetylcholinesterase and plasma cholinesterase are usually inhibited. The effect on the plasma enzyme is more marked, however, and serum levels are usually utilized in diagnosis and assessment of recovery. Recovery is best determined by looking for a plateau in erythrocyte cholinesterase activity. Toxic potency may vary, plasma versus red cell cholinesterase, such that in some cases erythrocyte levels may be needed for diagnosis and/or monitoring. If there is suspicion that a decrease in cholinesterase activity may not relate to the inhibitor effect of

(Continued)

Acetylcholinesterase, Red Blood Cell *(Continued)*

an organophosphate then red cell level of acetylcholinesterase should be obtained. If both serum and RBC levels are significantly decreased, findings are those of exogenous toxic effect.

True cholinesterase (acetylcholinesterase RBC cholinesterase) is not normally present in amniotic fluid. Presence of acetylcholinesterase activity and increased levels of alpha-fetoprotein in amniotic fluid are presumptive evidence of an open neural tube defect (eg, anencephaly, open spina bifida, or omphalocele) in the fetus.[5]

Footnotes

1. Tietz NW, *Clinical Guide to Laboratory Tests*, 2nd ed, Philadelphia, PA: WB Saunders Co, 1990, 12-3.
2. Knight GJ, "Maternal Serum Alpha-Fetoprotein Screening," *Techniques in Diagnostic Human Biochemical Genetics*, Hommes FA, ed, New York, NY: Wiley-Liss, 1991, 491-518.
3. Hay DL, Ibrahim GF, and Horacek I, "Rapid Acetylcholinesterase Screening Test for Neural Tube Defect," *Clin Chem*, 1983, 29:1065-9.
4. Alles GA and Hawes RC, "Cholinesterases in the Blood of Man," *J Biol Chem*, 1940, 133:375-90.
5. Wald NJ and Cuckle HS, "Amniotic Fluid Acetylcholinesterase Electrophoresis as a Secondary Test in the Diagnosis of Anencephaly and Open Spina Bifida in Early Pregnancy," *Lancet*, 1981, 2:321-7.

References

King ME, "Cholinesterase," *Methods in Clinical Chemistry*, Pesce AJ and Kaplan LA, eds, St Louis, MO: Mosby-Year Book Inc, 1987, 161-8.

Kobayashi K, Sakoguchi T, and Matsuoka A, "Stimulating Effects of Calcium and Magnesium on Serum Pseudocholinesterase Activity," *Clin Chem*, 1988, 34:173-4.

Whittaker M, "Cholinesterase," *Monographs in Human Genetics*, Vol 11, Beckman L, ed, Basel: Karger, 1986.

Acid-Base Regulation *see* Delta Base, Blood *on page 208*

Acid-Base Status *see* pCO_2, Blood *on page 314*

Acid-Base Status Evaluation *see* Carbon Dioxide, Blood *on page 165*

Acid Phosphatase

***CPT** 84060*

Related Information

Prostate Specific Antigen, Serum *on page 338*

Synonyms *o*-Phosphoric-Monester Phosphohydrolase; PAP; Phosphatase, Acid; Prostatic Acid Phosphatase

Patient Care PREPARATION: Do not order immediately after rectal examination of the prostate, after TUR, or after prostatic massage. Fasting specimen is preferred, as lipemia may interfere.

Specimen Serum or plasma CONTAINER: Red top tube or lavender top (EDTA) tube COLLECTION: Morning collection is recommended, since diurnal variation exists (circadian rhythms). The sample should be drawn in EDTA anticoagulant to provide the proper pH for stabilizing acid phosphatase. Due to the unstable nature of the enzyme, the test should be performed as soon as possible. Serum (red top tube) may also be used although it is possible to lose acid phosphatase activity within 1 hour. STORAGE INSTRUCTIONS: Separate sample and store on ice. Acidify and freeze sample if it cannot be run immediately. Stable frozen at -20°C for 6 months, or at -70°C indefinitely. CAUSES FOR REJECTION: Blood unrefrigerated after collection

Interpretive REFERENCE RANGE: Method dependent; males: ≤5.0 units/L (enzymatic, total); ≤1.2 units/L (enzymatic, prostatic); 2.5-3.7 ng/mL (RIA). USE: Staging of carcinoma of prostate, with other parameters; minimal role in establishing the diagnosis of primary carcinoma of prostate, helpful role in diagnosis of metastatic adenocarcinoma of the prostate and/or extension beyond prostatic capsule; monitor therapy and follow patient's response to treatment. **Not a screening test** for prostatic adenocarcinoma. Used on vaginal material in work-up of alleged rape.[1,2] LIMITATIONS: Specimens stored for any length of time, even at 4°C, will lose activity especially if exposed to air. Acidification to pH 6 will stabilize the enzyme for 1 week at 4°C. When adenocarcinoma is confined within the prostate, acid phosphatase is usually normal. Occasionally in patients with extensive carcinoma of prostate, acid phosphatase levels may be within normal limits. Even immunoassay methods do not detect early carcinomas consistently and, like enzyme methods, there may be false-positives. Acid phosphatase may be **increased** in diseases other than adenocarcinoma of prostate (eg, in infarct).[3] Moderate elevations of total acid phosphatase have been observed also with malignant invasion of bone from nonprostatic primaries, as well as with myelocytic leukemia, Gaucher's disease, and Niemann-Pick disease. However, the thymolphthalein monophosphate method is said to be more specific for prostatic acid phosphatase than are some other chemical substrates. Specimens drawn after recent rectal digital examination, TUR, bladder catheterization, and/or other manipulation of the prostate may have elevated values. The enzyme may be increased with prostatitis and may be increased with urinary retention. Acid phosphatase is increased by radioimmunoassay in up to 27% of patients with benign hypertrophy.[4] Tartrate inhibition is not specific. Acid phosphatase by RIA is not a screening test for carcinoma of the prostate.[4] Acid phosphatase exhibits diurnal variation.[5] **METHODOLOGY:** Immunoassays: Radioimmunoassay (RIA), enzyme immunoassay (EIA), counterimmunoelectrophoresis (CIE); chemical methods: hydrolysis of thymolphthalein monophosphate, alpha naphthylphosphate, other enzymatic methods; tartrate inhibition **ADDITIONAL INFORMATION:** Exacerbations and remissions of adenocarcinoma of prostate are not always correlated with acid phosphatase levels. Other parameters are also needed to follow such patients (eg, serum alkaline phosphatase). The RIA method has little advantage over the enzymatic approach using alpha-naphthyl phosphate substrate. Normal results do not consistently distinguish between localized and more extensive neoplasm. RIA method may not be cost-effective,[6] but it does provide increased sensitivity over enzymatic approaches in following stage D patients.[4,6]

Done chemically, using alpha-naphthyl acid phosphate as substrate, Tavassoli et al reported acid phosphatase increases with bone metastases from nonprostatic primaries. They advocated acid phosphatase as a means of detection of skeletal metastasis.[7]

CK-BB, an isoenzyme of CK, may be detected in the serum of some patients with carcinoma of prostate. It is not a specific test.

Prostate-specific antigen (PSA) is more sensitive than prostatic acid phosphatase, but neither test is specific for adenocarcinoma of the prostate.[8] Neither is 100% sensitive. The organ specificity, sensitivity and diagnostic value of PSA is an advance which should be used with acid phosphatase in staging and follow-up of prostatic carcinoma.[9] Serum PSA is superior to PAP in predicting disease recurrence in stages C and D prostate cancer treated by combination endocrine therapy. The assay of serum PAP does not add significantly to a single measurement of serum PSA alone.[10] Rectal carcinoid tumors may show histochemically positive PAP.[11] Benign prostatic hyperplasia causes definite increase in PAP, whereas intracapsular prostate cancer shows normal levels.[12]

Footnotes

1. Gomez RR, Wunsch CD, Davis JH, et al, "Qualitative and Quantitative Determinations of Acid Phosphatase Activity in Vaginal Washings," *Am J Clin Pathol*, 1975, 64:423-32.
2. Schumann GB, Badawy S, Peglow A, et al, "Prostatic Acid Phosphatase. Current Assessment in Vaginal Fluid of Alleged Rape Victims," *Am J Clin Pathol*, 1976, 66:944-52.
3. Howard PJ Jr and Fraley EE, "Elevation of the Acid Phosphatase in Benign Prostatic Disease," *J Urol*, 1965, 94:687-90.
4. Gittes RF, "Serum Acid Phosphatase and Screening for Carcinoma of the Prostate," *N Engl J Med*, 1983, 309:852-3, (editorial).
5. Brenckman WD, Lastinger LB, and Sedor F, "Unpredictable Fluctuations in Serum Acid Phosphatase Activity in Prostatic Cancer," *JAMA*, 1981, 245:2501-4.
6. Mensink HJ, Marrink J, Hindriks FR, et al, "Prostatic Acid Phosphatase: Comparison of Radioimmunoassay and Enzyme Activity Assay," *J Urol*, 1983, 129:1136-40.
7. Tavassoli M, Rizo M, and Yam LT, "Elevation of Serum Acid Phosphatase in Cancers With Bone Metastasis," *Cancer*, 1980, 45:2400-3.
8. Stamey TA, Yang N, Hay AR, et al, "Prostate-Specific Antigen as a Serum Marker for Adenocarcinoma of the Prostate," *N Engl J Med*, 1987, 317:909-16.
9. Gittes RF, "Prostate-Specific Antigen," *N Engl J Med*, 1987, 317:954-5, (editorial).
10. Dupont A, Cusan L, Gomez JL, et al, "Prostate Specific Antigen and Prostatic Acid Phosphatase for Monitoring Therapy of Carcinoma of the Prostate," *J Urol*, 1991, 146(4):1064-7.
11. Azumi N, Traweek ST, and Battifora H, "Prostatic Acid Phosphatase in Carcinoid Tumors. Immunohistochemical and Immunoblot Studies," *Am J Surg Pathol*, 1991, 15(8):785-90.
12. Salo JO, Rannikko S, and Haapiainen R, "Serum Acid Phosphatase in Patients With Localised Prostatic Cancer, Benign Prostatic Hyperplasia or Normal Prostates," *Br J Urol*, 1990, 66(2):188-92.

References

Heller JE, "Prostatic Acid Phosphatase, Its Current Significance," *J Urol*, 1987, 7:1091-103.

Kaplan LA, Chen IW, Sperling M, et al, "Clinical Utility of Serum Prostatic Acid Phosphatase Measurements for Detection (Screening), Diagnosis, and Therapeutic Monitoring of Prostatic Carcinoma; Assessment of Monoclonal and Polyclonal Enzymes and Radioimmunoassays," *Am J Clin Pathol*, 1985, 84:334-9.

Kroll MH and Nipper H, "Rapid Rise of Serum Acid Phosphatase After Irradiation of Metastatic Carcinoma of Prostate," *Urology*, 1987, 29:650-2.

Maatman TJ, Gupta MK, and Montie JE, "The Role of Serum Acid Phosphatase as a Tumor Marker in Men With Advanced Adenocarcinoma of the Prostate," *J Urol*, 1984, 132:58-63.

(Continued)

Acid Phosphatase *(Continued)*

Seiber PR and Rohner TJ, "Importance of Acid Phosphatase in Response Criteria for Prostate Cancer," *Urology*, 1987, 30:316-7.

ACTH *see* Adrenocorticotropic Hormone *on this page*

ACTH Infusion Test *replaced by* Cosyntropin Test *on page 194*

Actual Base Excess *see* Delta Base, Blood *on page 208*

Adrenocorticotropic Hormone

CPT 82024

Related Information

Calcitonin *on page 157*
Carcinoembryonic Antigen *on page 167*
Cortisol, Blood *on page 191*
Cortisol, Urine *on page 193*
Thorn Test *on page 609*

Synonyms ACTH; Corticotropin

Abstract In Cushing's syndrome, increased ACTH indicates that pituitary ACTH-dependent adrenal cortical hyperplasia or the ectopic ACTH syndrome is present. A battery of adrenal function tests and radiographic procedures are recommended to establish the diagnosis of Cushing's syndrome.[1]

Specimen Plasma **CONTAINER:** Use chilled syringe. Use two lavender top (EDTA) tubes or two green top (heparin) tubes, previously cooled in ice. (Check with laboratory for appropriate container.) **SAMPLING TIME:** ACTH is normally characterized by diurnal variation. Most secretion occurs in the morning. Normal secretion, as well as that in Cushing's disease, is pulsatile and so may require multiple samples. **COLLECTION:** Samples for demonstration of the normal circadian rhythm should be drawn between 6 AM and 10 AM and between 9 PM and 12 PM. Commonly collected simultaneously with cortisol level. **STORAGE INSTRUCTIONS:** Separate plasma in refrigerated centrifuge and freeze immediately. Store frozen at -70°C in plastic tubes. Aprotinin (Trasylol®) 500 kU/mL should be added for long-term storage. **CAUSES FOR REJECTION:** Patient having radioisotopic scan prior to collection of specimen, recently administered radioisotopes, specimen not chilled following collection **SPECIAL INSTRUCTIONS:** Transport specimen **immediately** to the laboratory following collection.

Interpretive **REFERENCE RANGE:** The highest values are normally found between 6 AM and 10 AM: <60 pg/mL (SI: <60 ng/L) but varying among laboratories. Samples drawn between 9 AM and 12 noon have been recommended.[2] Evening samples normally are about one-half to two-thirds of the morning specimens. The normal daily circadian rhythm (periodicity) has diagnostic significance (ie, lack of change is abnormal). **USE:** Evaluate the etiology of Cushing's syndrome; differentiate pituitary from extrapituitary causes of corticosteroid excess and deficiency syndromes; evaluate ectopic ACTH production by neoplasm; examine results of transsphenoidal surgery; follow up patients after bilateral adrenalectomy for diagnosis of Nelson syndrome. (Nelson syndrome is the development of a tumor of the anterior pituitary gland and skin pigmentation following bilateral adrenalectomy.) **LIMITATIONS:** The ACTH level is affected by stress, which may obscure the normal diurnal change. ACTH level must be correlated with cortisol levels. Suppression/stimulation tests are in use.[3] Spurious elevation of immunoreactive ACTH is reported and an extraction is recommended.[1] **METHODOLOGY:** Radioimmunoassay (RIA) after separatory step **ADDITIONAL INFORMATION:** Cortisol excess of any source is "Cushing's syndrome." Increased ACTH from the pituitary, causing the adrenal cortices to produce excessive cortisol, was described by Cushing and called "Cushing's disease." ACTH secretion is stimulated by insulin, metyrapone, and vasopressin and suppressed by dexamethasone. Cushing's disease usually demonstrates suppression of ACTH and cortisol by high-dose dexamethasone, whereas in adrenal adenomas, adrenal carcinomas, and ectopic ACTH-producing tumors. ACTH and cortisol are not suppressed by high-dose dexamethasone. ACTH levels in Cushing's disease may be elevated or in the high normal range (but inappropriately elevated for the patient's plasma cortisol level), with loss of the normal diurnal changes. ACTH levels in ectopic ACTH syndrome are usually very high; whereas in Cushing's syndrome due to adrenal adenoma or carcinoma, ACTH levels are very low to undetectable. Measurement of plasma lipotropin provides an alternative, and possibly better index, than ACTH for diagnosis of Cushing's syndromes and follow-up of treated Cushing's diseases.[4]

In primary adrenal insufficiency (Addison's disease) due to destruction of the glands by tumor, infection or immune mechanisms, ACTH plasma concentrations are elevated and cortisol levels are depressed. ACTH increases are found with congenital adrenal hyperplasia (adrenogenital syndrome). In secondary adrenal insufficiency (secondary to pituitary insufficiency), ACTH and cortisol both are low. For sequential follow-up, ACTH should always be drawn at the same time each day.

ACTH was increased in 30% of patients with oat cell carcinoma and 26% with large cell carcinoma of lung in a series of 110 patients with lung cancer.[5] Ectopic ACTH production may derive from bronchial carcinoids.

Urinary free cortisol is the test of choice for the separation of Cushing's syndrome from entities, including obesity, which mimic it.[6,7]

The increased ACTH of pseudo-Cushing's syndrome does not exhibit normal circadian rhythms and fails to suppress with dexamethasone. Pseudo-Cushing's syndrome is a reversible entity related to alcohol abuse.[6]

Continuous (7-hour) dexamethasone infusion in patients with Cushing's syndrome identifies 100% of patients with ACTH-secreting pituitary adenomas, with a specificity of 90% and diagnostic accuracy of 98%.[8] The corticotropin release hormone (CRH) stimulation test has a 91% sensitivity and a 95% specificity for the pituitary Cushing syndrome.[9]

Footnotes

1. Wickus GG, Pagliara AS, and Caplan RH, "Spurious Elevation of Plasma Immunoreactive Adrenocorticotropic Hormone in Cyclic Cushing's Syndrome," *Arch Pathol Lab Med*, 1989, 113(7):797-9.
2. Leavelle DE, "Adrenocorticotropic Hormone (ACTH), Plasma," *Mayo Medical Laboratories Interpretive Handbook*, Rochester, MN: Mayo Medical Laboratories, 1990, 4.
3. Daniels GH and Martin JB, "Neuroendocrine Regulation and Diseases of the Anterior Pituitary and Hypothalamus," *Harrison's Principles of Internal Medicine*, Chapter 313, 12th ed, Wilson JD, Braunwald E, Isselbacher KJ, et al, eds, New York, NY: McGraw-Hill Inc, 1991, 1655-79.
4. Kuhn JM, Proeschel MF, Seurin DJ, et al, "Comparative Assessment of ACTH and Lipoprotein Plasma Levels in the Diagnosis and Follow-up of Patients With Cushing's Syndrome: A Study of 210 Cases," *Am J Med*, 1989, 86(6 Pt 1):678-84.
5. Gropp C, Havemann K, and Scheuer A, "Ectopic Hormones in Lung Cancer Patients at Diagnosis and During Therapy," *Cancer*, 1980, 46:347-54.
6. Grizzle WE and Dunlap N, "Cushing's Syndrome – Diagnosis of the Atypical Patient," *Arch Pathol Lab Med*, 1989, 113(7):727-8.
7. Flack MR, Oldfield EH, Cutler GB Jr, et al, "Urine Free Cortisol in the High-Dose Dexamethasone Suppression Test for the Differential Diagnosis of the Cushing Syndrome," *Ann Intern Med*, 1992, 116(3):211-7.
8. Biemond P, deJong FH, and Lamberts SW, "Continuous Dexamethasone Infusion for Seven Hours in Patients With the Cushing Syndrome. A Superior Differential Diagnostic Test," *Ann Intern Med*, 1990, 112(10):738-42.
9. Kaye TB and Crapo L, "The Cushing Syndrome: An Update on Diagnostic Tests," *Ann Intern Med*, 1990, 112(6):434-4.

References

Abboud CF, "Endocrine Symposium – Laboratory Diagnosis of Hypopituitarism," *Mayo Clin Proc*, 1986, 61:35-48.

Blunt SB, Sandler LM, Burrin JM, et al, "An Evaluation of the Distinction of Ectopic and Pituitary ACTH Dependent Cushing's Syndrome by Clinical Features, Biochemical Tests and Radiological Findings," *Q J Med*, 1990, 77(283):1113-33.

Carpenter PC, "Cushing's Syndrome: Update of Diagnosis and Management," *Mayo Clin Proc*, 1986, 61:49-58.

Findling JW, "Eutopic or Ectopic Adrenocorticotropic Hormone-Dependent Cushing's Syndrome? A Diagnostic Dilemma," *Mayo Clin Proc*, 1990, 65(10):1377-80.

Findling JW, Kehoe ME, Shaker JL, et al, "Routine Inferior Petrosal Sinus Sampling in the Differential Diagnosis of Adrenocorticotropin (ACTH)-Dependent Cushing's Syndrome: Early Recognition of the Occult Ectopic ACTH Syndrome," *J Clin Endocrinol Metab*, 1991, 73(2):408-13.

Jones KL, "The Cushing Syndromes," *Pediatr Clin North Am*, 1990, 37(6):1313-32.

Lisansky J, Peake GT, Strassman RJ, et al, "Augmented Pituitary Corticotropin Response to a Threshold Dosage of Human Corticotropin-Releasing Hormone in Depressives Pretreated With Metyrapone," *Arch Gen Psychiatry*, 1989, 46(7):641-9.

Siegel SF, Finegold DN, Lanes R, et al, "ACTH Stimulation Tests and Plasma Dehydroepiandrosterone Sulfate Levels in Women With Hirsutism," *N Engl J Med*, 1990, 323(13):849-54.

Stewart PM, Corrie J, Seckl JR, et al, "A Rational Approach for Assessing the Hypothalmo-Pituitary-Adrenal Axis," *Lancet*, 1988, 1:1208-10.

Torosian MH, "The Clinical Usefulness and Limitations of Tumor Markers," *Surg Gynecol Obstet*, 1988, 166:567-79, (review).

AFP *see* Alpha$_1$-Fetoprotein, Serum *on page 115*

AFP, Amniotic Fluid *see* Alpha$_1$-Fetoprotein, Amniotic Fluid *on page 114*

A/G Ratio *see* Albumin/Globulin Ratio *on next page*

ALA *see* Delta Aminolevulinic Acid, Urine *on page 207*

Alanine Aminotransferase

CPT 84460

Related Information

Aspartate Aminotransferase *on page 135*
Donation, Blood *on page 1061*
Lactate Dehydrogenase *on page 269*
Risks of Transfusion *on page 1093*

Synonyms ALT; Glutamic Pyruvate Transaminase; GPT; 2-Oxoglutarate Aminotransferase; SGPT; Transaminase

Applies to Aminotransferases

Replaces Cephalin Flocculation; Isocitric Dehydrogenase; Thymol Turbidity

Abstract Of the aminotransferases, AST and ALT are important, widely used enzymes. Increases over tenfold occur in some cases of hepatitis and shock.

Specimen Serum **CONTAINER:** Red top tube **STORAGE INSTRUCTIONS:** Stable 3 days at 25°C and 1 week at 4°C; refrigeration is preferable to freezing. **CAUSES FOR REJECTION:** Excessive hemolysis

Interpretive **REFERENCE RANGE:** Slightly increased ranges in infancy compared to adult normal range. Typical reference range: 8-45 units/L. Males have slightly higher alanine aminotransferase activity. **USE:** A liver function test, ALT is more sensitive for the detection of hepatocyte injury than for biliary obstruction. ALT is more specific for liver injury than AST (SGOT). Useful for hepatic cirrhosis, and other liver disease. Increased in Reye's syndrome, with AST.[1] Screening test for hepatitis including non-A, non-B hepatitis. Acute hepatitis A or B can be confirmed serologically, as can hepatitis C. Negative serological findings in the presence of hepatitis-like chemistry abnormalities may also suggest acute drug-induced hepatitis, an impression supported by resolution after removal of the offending agent.[2] The combination of increased AST and ALT with negative hepatitis markers occurs in a number of other entities including infectious mononucleosis. Sensitive to heart failure. ALT has been used in combination with anti-HB$_c$ as an indirect screen for non-A, non-B hepatitis in blood donors.[3,4,5] Such assays are still required by the American Association of Blood Banks despite the fact that second generation tests for antibody to hepatitis C provides separation for the vast majority of donors with non-A, non-B hepatitis virus. **LIMITATIONS:** Grossly hemolyzed samples can generate somewhat spurious results. The activity in red cells is six times that of serum. Elevations are reported in trauma to striated muscle, rhabdomyolysis, polymyositis, and dermatomyositis, but the CK (CK-MM fraction) is increased in such patients and it is preferable to consider diseases of skeletal muscle. ALT is less sensitive than is AST to alcoholic liver disease. Increased ALT is found with obesity. **METHODOLOGY:** Spectrophotometry **ADDITIONAL INFORMATION:** Among entities in which AST and ALT increases occur are therapeutic applications of bovine or porcine heparin. LD (LDH) abnormality with elevation of hepatic fractions has also been reported.[6]

In children with acute lymphoblastic leukemia, high ALT activity at diagnosis is associated with rapidly progressive ALL.[7]

A number of drugs, including diphenylhydantoin, heparin therapy, and many others cause ALT increases. Acetaminophen hepatotoxicity may be potentiated in alcoholics, in whom coagulopathy and extremely abnormal aminotransferase levels are described, ALT less than AST.[8]

AST/ALT ratios are highest in alcoholic liver disease but are often above unity in nonalcoholic cirrhosis. AST/ALT ratios are commonly 0.5-0.8 with acute and chronic viral hepatitis.[9] Such ratios may be expected to vary between laboratories by virtue of differences in enzyme methods.

The hepatitis C virion has been detected by polymerase chain reaction and reverse transcriptase of HCV-RNA sequences in patients with elevated ALT and positive anti-HCV.[10]

Footnotes

1. "Diagnosis and Treatment of Reye's Syndrome," (Consensus Conference) *JAMA*, 1981, 246:2441-4.

2. Frank BB and Members of the Patient Care Committee of the American Gastroenterological Association, "Clinical Evaluation of Jaundice – A Guideline of the Patient Care Committee of the American Gastroenterological Association," *JAMA*, 1989, 262(21):3031-4.
3. Biswas R, "Posttransfusion Non-A, Non-B Hepatitis: Significance of Raised ALT and anti-HB_c in Blood Donors" *Vox Sang*, 1989, 56(1):63, (letter).
4. Friedman LS, Dienstag JL, Watkins E, et al, "Evaluation of Blood Donors With Elevated Serum Alanine Aminotransferase Levels," *Ann Intern Med*, 1987, 107:137-44 (published erratum appears in *Ann Intern Med*, 1987, 107:791).
5. Spurling CL and Saxena S, "Controversies in Transfusion Medicine. Alanine Aminotransferase Screening of Blood Donors," *Transfusion*, 1990, 30(4):368-73.
6. Dukes GE Jr, Sanders SW, Russo J, et al, "Transaminase Elevations in Patients Receiving Bovine or Porcine Heparin," *Ann Intern Med*, 1984, 100:646-50.
7. Rautonen J, and Siimes MA, "Elevated Serum Transaminase Activity at Diagnosis Is Associated With Rapidly Progressing Disease in Children With Acute Lymphoblastic Leukemia," *Cancer*, 1988, 61(4):754-7.
8. Seeff LB, Cuccherini BA, Zimmerman HJ, et al, "Acetaminophen Hepatotoxicity in Alcoholics," *Ann Intern Med*, 1986, 104:399-404.
9. Williams AL and Hoofnagle JH, "Ratio of Serum Aspartate to Alanine Aminotransferase in Chronic Hepatitis. Relationship to Cirrhosis," *Gastroenterology*, 1988, 95(3):734-9.
10. Ulrich PP, Romeo JM, Lane PK, et al, "Detection, Semiquantitation, and Genetic Variation in Hepatitis C Virus Sequences Amplified From the Plasma of Blood Donors With Elevated Alanine Aminotransferase," *J Clin Invest*, 1990, 86(5):1609-14.

References

Diehl AM, Goodman Z, and Ishak KG, "Alcohol-Like Liver Disease in Nonalcoholics: A Clinical and Histologic Comparison With Alcohol-Induced Liver Injury," *Gastroenterology*, 1988, 95:1056-62.

Giesen P, Peltenburg HG, and de Zwaan C, "Greater Than Expected Alanine Aminotransferase Activities in Plasma and in Hearts of Patients With Acute Myocardial Infarction," *Clin Chem*, 1989, 35(2):279-83.

Helzberg JH and Spiro HM, "LFTs Test More Than the Liver," *JAMA*, 1986, 256:3006-7.

Klein HG, "Controversies in Transfusion Medicine. Alanine Aminotransferase Screening of Blood Donors: Pro," *Transfusion*, 1990, 30(4):363-7.

Kubo SH, Walter BA, John DHA, et al, "Liver Function Abnormalities in Chronic Heart Failure: Influence of Systemic Hemodynamics," *Arch Intern Med*, 1987, 147:1227-30.

Patwardhan RV, Smith OJ, and Farmelant MH, "Serum Transaminase Levels and Cholescintigraphic Abnormalities in Acute Biliary Tract Obstruction," *Arch Intern Med*, 1987, 147:1249-53.

Saxena S and Korula J, "Donor Alanine Aminotransferase (ALT) Testing: A Review of Guidelines on ALT Testing, Its Interpretation and Donor Notification," *ASCP Check Sample®*, Chicago, IL: The American Society of Clinical Pathologists, 1988.

Saxena S, Korula J, and Shulman IA, "A Review of Donor Alanine Aminotransferase Testing. Implications for the Blood Donor and Practitioner," *Arch Pathol Lab Med*, 1989, 113(7):767-71.

Sherman KE, "Alanine Aminotransferase in Clinical Practice. A Review," *Arch Intern Med*, 1991, 151(2):260-5.

Van Ness MV and Diehl AM, "Is Liver Biopsy Useful in the Evaluation of Patients With Chronically Elevated Liver Enzymes?" *Ann Intern Med*, 1989, 111(6):473-8.

Vincent-Viry M and Delwaide P, "Aspartate Aminotransferase and Alanine Aminotransferase", *Drug Effects on Laboratory Test Results Analytical Interferences and Pharmacological Effects*, Siest G and Galteau MM, eds, Littleton, MA: PSG Publishing Co Inc, 1988, 91-130.

Albs-a *see* Body Fluid *on page 145*

Albumin, Ascites Fluid *see* Body Fluid *on page 145*

Albumin/Globulin Ratio

CPT *84155*

Related Information

Albumin, Serum *on next page*

Synonyms A/G Ratio

Abstract A calculation derived from chemistry profiles.

Specimen Serum **CONTAINER:** Red top tube

Interpretive **REFERENCE RANGE:** ≥1; high ratio is usually clinically insignificant. **USE:** Low A/G ratio is found in cirrhosis and other liver diseases, chronic glomerulonephritis and nephrotic syndromes, myeloma, macroglobulinemia of Waldenström, sarcoidosis and other granulomatous diseases, collagen diseases, severe infections and inflammatory states, cachexia, burns, ulcerative colitis and other chronic inflammatory states. **LIMITATIONS:** More chemically precise A/G ratio is derived from serum protein electrophoresis than from chemical methods, and electrophoresis provides considerably more information. The multilayer-film bromcresol green

(Continued)

Albumin/Globulin Ratio *(Continued)*

method for albumin measurement is significantly inaccurate when albumin/globulin ratio is <0.8.[1] **ADDITIONAL INFORMATION:** A/G ratio, a calculation, is derived from chemistry profiles. Total protein minus albumin equals globulins. Albumin divided by globulins equals the ratio. Some clinicians utilize the combination of the serum total protein and A/G ratio as a screen for determining which patients require a serum protein electrophoresis.

Footnotes

1. Leerink CB and Winckers EK, "Multilayer-Film Bromcresol Green Method for Albumin Measurement Significantly Inaccurate When Albumin/Globulin Ratio Is Less Than 0.8," *Clin Chem*, 1991, 37(5):766-8.

References

Ibrahim K, Zuberi SJ, and Husnain SN, "Serum Total Protein, Albumin, Globulin, and Their Ratio in Apparently Healthy Population of Various Ages and Sex in Karachi," *J Pak Med Assoc*, 1989, 39(1):12-6.

Nandedkar AK, Royal GC Jr, and Nandedkar MA, "Evaluation of Albumin-Globulin Ratio to Confirm the Clinical Stages of Sarcoidosis," *J Natl Med Assoc*, 1986, 78:969-71.

Albumin, Serum

CPT 82040

Related Information

Albumin/Globulin Ratio *on previous page*
Protein Electrophoresis, Serum *on page 734*
Protein, Total, Serum *on page 340*
Zinc, Serum *on page 1036*

Applies to Globulin; Nutritional Status

Specimen Serum **CONTAINER:** Red top tube or capillary tube

Interpretive **REFERENCE RANGE:** 0-1 year: 2.9-5.5 g/dL (SI: 29-55 g/L); 1-31 years: 3.5-5.0 g/dL (SI: 35-50 g/L) with A/G ratio >1. After age 40, the normal range gradually decreases. **POSSIBLE PANIC RANGE:** <1.5 g/dL (SI: <15 g/L) **USE:** Evaluate nutritional status, blood oncotic pressure, renal disease with proteinuria, and other chronic diseases

High albumin may indicate dehydration. Look for increase in hemoglobin, hematocrit in such patients.

Low albumin is found with use of I.V. fluids, rapid hydration, overhydration; cirrhosis, other liver disease, including chronic alcoholism; in pregnancy and with oral contraceptive use; many chronic diseases, including the nephrotic syndromes, neoplasia, protein-losing enteropathies (including Crohn's disease and ulcerative colitis), peptic ulcer, thyroid disease, burns, severe skin disease, prolonged immobilization, heart failure, chronic inflammatory diseases such as autoimmune diseases and other chronic catabolic states.

Starvation, malabsorption, or malnutrition: In the absence of I.V. fluid therapy and in patients without liver or renal disease, low albumin may be regarded as an indication of inadequate body protein reserves. It is described as the most common nutrition-related abnormality in patients with infection.[1] Serum albumin has a half-life of about 18-20 days. Its half-life is decreased in patients with catabolic states: infection and with protein loss through the kidneys (eg, nephrosis), gastrointestinal tract, and skin (eg, burns). Its prognostic application is most useful in patients with weight loss, anorexia, surgical therapy, hemorrhage, and infection. Total iron binding capacity <240 μg/dL (SI: <43 μmol/L)[1] and/or low transferrin levels would support an impression of inadequate protein reserves. Absolute lymphocyte counts of <1500/ mm^3 may also be seen with protein malnutrition.[2] In severe malnutrition, albumin has been reported as <2.5 g/dL (SI: <25 g/L), total lymphocytes as <800/mm^3 and TIBC as <150 μg/dL.[2]

Albumin levels ≤2.0-2.5 g/dL (SI: ≤20-25 g/L) may be the cause of edema (eg, nephrotic syndrome, protein-losing enteropathies).

Albumin, prealbumin, and transferrin are regarded as "negative" acute phase reactants (ie, these proteins decrease with acute inflammatory/infectious processes).

Low albumin values are associated with longer hospital stay.[1]

LIMITATIONS: Bromcresol green somewhat overestimates serum albumin and lacks specificity. Albumin level can decrease (up to 0.5 g/dL) (SI: 5.0 g/L) for patients in supine position. Decreased in highly icteric specimens by HABA method but not by bromocresol green.[3] Ampicillin added *in vitro* interferes with both methods.[3] Salicylates do not interfere with bromcresol green method.[3] Monochromatic measurement of albumin by bromcresol green overestimates albumin in heparinized plasma owing to fibrinogen. The artifact is avoided by using bichromatic wavelengths.[4] Increased albumin-bilirubin complexes (ie, icteric sera) causes an underestimation of albumin in the bromcresol purple method but not in the bromcresol green method.[5] **METHODOLOGY:** Bromcresol green (BCG) is widely used. It measures some alpha-globulins and therefore provides slightly higher figures than does serum protein electrophoresis. **ADDITIONAL INFORMATION:** Twenty-four hour urine collection to measure protein loss is helpful in work-up of some patients with hypoalbuminemia.

Other tests useful in assessment of nutritional status include TIBC, transferrin, iron, absolute lymphocyte count, and vitamin B_{12}/folate levels.

Globulin may be provided as a calculation, total protein minus albumin = globulin. Total protein and albumin are commonly measured on chemistry profiling instruments. Globulins by serum protein electrophoresis, immunoelectrophoresis, or immunofixation, and quantitative IgA, IgM, and IgG are more precise.

Footnotes

1. Anderson CF and Wochos DN, "The Utility of Serum Albumin Values in the Nutritional Assessment of Hospitalized Patients," *Mayo Clin Proc*, 1982, 57:181-4.
2. Shapiro M, Rhodes JB, and Beyer PL, "Malnutrition. Recognition and Correction by Enteral Nutrition," *Kans Med*, 1983, 341-5, 356.
3. Beng CG and Lim KL, "An Improved Automated Method for Determination of Serum Albumin Using Bromcresol Green," *Am J Clin Pathol*, 1973, 59:14-21.
4. Hallbach J, Hoffmann GE, and Guder WG, "Overestimation of Albumin in Heparinized Plasma," *Clin Chem*, 1991, 37(4):566-8.
5. Ihara H, Nakamura H, Aoki Y, et al, "Effects of Serum-Isolated vs Synthetic Bilirubin-Albumin Complexes on Dye-Binding Methods for Estimating Serum Albumin," *Clin Chem*, 1991, 37(7):1269-72.

References

Chu SY and MacLeod J, "Effect of Three-Day Clot Contact on Results of Common Biochemical Tests With Serum," *Clin Chem*, 1986, 32:2100.

Gendler S, "Proteins," *Clinical Chemistry – Theory, Analysis, and Correlation*, 2nd ed, Kaplan LA and Pesce A, eds, St Louis, MO: Mosby-Year Book Inc, 1989, 1029-65.

Herbeth B, Diemert MC, and Galli A, "Albumin," *Drug Effects on Laboratory Test Results Analytical Interferences and Pharmacological Effects*, Siest G and Galteau MM, eds, Littleton, MA: PSG Publishing Co Inc, 1988, 52-66.

ALD *see* Aldolase, Serum *on this page*

Aldolase, Serum

CPT 82085

Related Information

Muscle Biopsy *on page 75*

Synonyms ALD; Fructose Biphosphate Aldolase

Specimen Serum **CONTAINER:** Red top tube **SAMPLING TIME:** Patient should be fasting. **STORAGE INSTRUCTIONS:** Separate serum and freeze immediately. May be stored at -20°C until analysis. The addition of boric acid will stabilize aldolase.[1] **CAUSES FOR REJECTION:** Hemolysis (red cells contain aldolase)

Interpretive **REFERENCE RANGE:** Newborns: up to four times adult levels; pediatrics: 10-24 months: 3.4-11.8 units/L, 25 months to 16 years: 1.2-8.8 units/L (method of Pinto et al[2,3]); adults: 1.7-4.9 units/L **USE:** Evaluate muscle wasting process. High levels are found in progressive Duchenne's muscular dystrophy (MD). Elevations occur in carriers of MD, in limb-girdle dystrophy and other dystrophies, in dermatomyositis, polymyositis, and trichinosis, but not in neurogenic atrophies (eg, multiple sclerosis or in myasthenia gravis). **LIMITATIONS:** As muscle mass diminishes, aldolase decreases. Serum aldolase elevation is not specific for muscle disease (see following discussion). In recent years the assay of creatine kinase (CK) has been preferred for evaluation of muscle disease. It is more specific for skeletal muscle degeneration. **CONTRAINDICATIONS:** Aldolase levels are not frequently needed or ordered. Many laboratories do not offer this test. **METHODOLOGY:** Ultraviolet, kinetic, coupled enzymatic[4] **ADDITIONAL INFORMATION:** In the progressive dystrophies, aldolase levels may be 10 to 15 times normal when muscle mass is relatively intact as in early stages of the disease. When advanced muscle wasting is present, values decline. In the inflammatory myopathies (eg, dermatomyositis) serum aldolase (as well as CK) levels may be applied to monitoring the response to steroid therapy. They are of particular value in guiding tapering of steroid administration.[2]

Aldolase is formed of two subunits. There are three different possible subunits designated A, B, and C, but just four isoenzymes. The molecular form AAAA is the predominant aldolase in

(Continued)

Aldolase, Serum *(Continued)*

skeletal muscle, BBBB predominates in liver, and CCCC in brain and other tissue. A hybrid isoenzyme, AAAC is present in tissues but at a lower concentration.[5] The UV coupled enzymatic methods determine total enzyme activity and thus are not specific for muscle aldolase. Elevated aldolase levels may be found with hepatitis, other liver diseases, myocardial infarction, hemorrhagic pancreatitis, gangrene, delirium tremens, and in some cases of neoplasia. In cases of acute viral hepatitis, increase in serum aldolase tends to parallel ALT (SGPT) levels. A small fraction of cases of measles in young adults have been reported to have significant elevations of serum CK and aldolase.[6,7] Aldolase is an ubiquitous enzyme and is thus not particularly useful in diagnostic work-ups.

Radioimmunoassays for aldolase A, B, and C have been developed but are not widely available. Their clinical utility has not yet been established.[5]

The level of serum aldolase B (RIA method) may be decreased (<20 ng/mL) in some patients with epithelial malignancy (cases studied included esophageal, hepatic, pancreatic, lung, and breast cancers).[8] After successful surgical resection, serum aldolase B levels recovered to normal range (20-60 ng/mL).

Serum aldolase and CK may be elevated in the serum of patients who have taken L-tryptophan and develop eosinophilia-myalgia syndrome.[9]

Footnotes

1. Beardslee R and Owers P, "Stabilization by Boric Acid of Aldolase Activity at Room Temperature," *Clin Chem*, 1976, 22:1543-5.
2. Visnapuu LA, Karlson LK, Dubinsky EH, et al, "Pediatric Reference Ranges for Serum Aldolase," *Am J Clin Pathol*, 1989, 91(4):476-7.
3. Pinto PV, Kaplan A, and VanDreal PA, "II. Spectrophotometric Determination Using an Ultraviolet Procedure," *Clin Chem*, 1969, 15:349-60.
4. Harjanne A, "The Kinetic Measurement of Serum Aldolase," *Clin Chim Acta*, 1979, 92:311-3.
5. Gendler SM, "Aldolase," *Methods in Clinical Chemistry*, Chapter 12, Pesce AJ and Kaplan LA, eds, St Louis, MO: Mosby-Year Book Inc, 1987, 872-5.
6. Leibovici L, Sharir T, Kalter-Leibovici O, et al, "An Outbreak of Measles Among Young Adults: Clinical and Laboratory Features in 461 Patients," *J Adolesc Health Care*, 1988, 9:203-7.
7. Gavish D, Kleinman Y, Morag A, et al, "Hepatitis and Jaundice Associated With Measles in Young Adults," *Arch Intern Med*, 1983, 143:674-7.
8. Asaka M, Kimura T, Nishikawa S, et al, "Decreased Serum Aldolasé B Levels in Patients With Malignant Tumors," *Cancer*, 1988, 62(12):2554-7.
9. Kilbourne EM, Swygert LA, Philen RM, et al, "Interim Guidance on the Eosinophilia-Myalgia Syndrome," *Ann Intern Med*, 1990, 112(2):85-7.

Aldosterone, Blood

***CPT** 82088*

Related Information

Aldosterone, Urine *on page 106*
Potassium, Blood *on page 330*
Renin, Plasma *on page 346*

Abstract Primary aldosteronism is characterized by hypertension with renal potassium wasting. It is found in <1% of subjects with hypertension.

Patient Care **PREPARATION:** No recent radioactive scans or other radioactivity. Diuretics, antihypertensive drugs, cyclic progestogens, estrogens, and licorice should be terminated 2-4 weeks before testing. Patient should be on a normal sodium diet for 2-4 weeks (135 mmol or 3 g sodium/day). Supine sample should be drawn early, before the inpatient arises. If an upright sample is indicated, patient should have been sitting up for 2 hours or more. Replacement of potassium deficit is recommended before samples for aldosterone are taken. **A random measurement of aldosterone is of no diagnostic utility unless plasma renin activity is determined simultaneously**. The diagnosis of hyperaldosteronism requires the demonstration of persistent hyperaldosteronemia in the presence of saline loading or steroid administration.

Specimen Serum or plasma **CONTAINER:** Red top tube, green top (heparin) tube, or lavender top (EDTA) tube **COLLECTION:** Specify exact source of specimen. Specify patient's position. Renin levels are often indicated in the same clinical settings requiring measurement of aldosterone; consider obtaining sufficient blood for both assays. **STORAGE INSTRUCTIONS:** Transport on ice. Freeze serum or plasma in a plastic vial as soon as possible after sampling. **CAUSES FOR REJECTION:** Patient not prepared properly, insufficient sample, specimen did not arrive on ice, specimen not stored properly, recently administered radioisotopes **SPECIAL INSTRUCTIONS:** Transport at once to the laboratory on ice.

Interpretive REFERENCE RANGE: Varies with sodium intake, with time of day, source of specimen (eg, peripheral vein, adrenal vein), and with posture (upright posture is accompanied by higher aldosterone values). Reference ranges differ with laboratory, but vary from 4-30 ng/dL (SI: 111-832 pmol/L) in upright individuals, on unrestricted salt intake, peripheral venous blood. Prolonged heparin therapy decreases serum levels. Aldosterone may be low in diabetics. Aldosterone decreases with higher altitudes and with pre-eclampsia.[1] USE: The principal use for aldosterone measurements is in the diagnosis of primary hyperaldosteronism, which is most commonly caused by a specific type of adrenal adenoma. Primary aldosteronism caused by adrenal tumor is Conn's syndrome. Secondary aldosteronism is more common. Work-up is especially indicated in the younger patient with hypertension and hypokalemia not induced by diuretic agents. Beeler and Catrou use criteria of serum potassium <3.5 mmol/L, 24-hour urine potassium ≥ 50 mmol/L, to begin work-up of a hypertensive patient for aldosteronism.[2] Low plasma renin activity suggests primary aldosteronism and provides indication for aldosterone measurement in a hypertensive subject with renal potassium wasting.[3] High resolution CT is highly accurate for detection of aldosterone-producing adenoma, but results must be correlated with endocrine studies.[4] Secondary aldosteronism may occur in congestive heart failure, cirrhosis with ascites, nephrosis, potassium loading, sodium-depleted diet, toxemia of pregnancy and other states of contraction of plasma volume, and Bartter's syndrome. Renin is high in secondary aldosteronism, low in primary aldosteronism. LIMITATIONS: Decreased perfusion of the kidneys leads to increased aldosterone and renin. Aldosterone may be falsely elevated in chronic renal failure when assayed by direct RIA.[5] METHODOLOGY: Radioimmunoassay (RIA), chemiluminescence assay (CIA)[6] ADDITIONAL INFORMATION: Aldosterone is a mineralocorticoid hormone produced in the adrenal zona glomerulosa under complex control by the renin-angiotensin system. Its action is on the renal distal tubule where it increases resorption of sodium and water at the expense of increased potassium excretion. Thus, syndromes of primary aldosterone excess show hypokalemia. Conversely, increased serum potassium levels act to increase aldosterone output. Renin also acts to increase aldosterone secretion through a feedback loop including angiotensins I and II.

Footnotes

1. August P, Lenz T, Ales KL, et al, "Longitudinal Study of the Renin-Angiotensin-Aldosterone System in Hypertensive Pregnant Women: Deviations Related to the Development of Superimposed Pre-eclampsia," *Am J Obstet Gynecol*, 1990, 163(5 Pt 1):1612-21.
2. Beeler MF and Catrou PG, "Interpretations in Clinical Chemistry. A Textbook Approach to Chemical Pathology," Chicago, IL: American Society of Clinical Pathologists, 1983.
3. Watts NB and Keffer JH, "Renin-Angiotensin-Aldosterone," *Practical Endocrinology*, 4th ed, Philadelphia, PA: Lea & Febiger, 1989, 130-5.
4. Radin DR, Manoogian C, and Nadler JL, "Diagnosis of Primary Hyperaldosteronism: Importance of Correlating CT Findings With Endocrinologic Studies," *AJR Am J Roentgenol*, 1992, 158(3):553-7.
5. Koshida H, Miyamori I, Miyazaki R, et al, "Falsely Elevated Plasma Aldosterone Concentration by Direct Radioimmunoassay in Chronic Renal Failure," *J Lab Clin Med*, 1989, 114(3):294-300.
6. Stabler TV and Siegel AL, "Chemiluminescence Immunoassay of Aldosterone in Serum," *Clin Chem*, 1991, 37(11):1987-9.

References

Alpern RJ and Toto RD, "Hypokalemic Nephropathy – A Clue to Cystogenesis?" *N Engl J Med*, 1990, 322(6):398-9.

Brands MW and Freeman RH, "Aldosterone and Renin Inhibition by Physiological Levels of Atrial Natriuretic Factor," *Am J Physiol*, 1988, 254:1011-6.

Bravo EL, "Physiology of the Adrenal Cortex," *Urol Clin North Am*, 1989, 16(3):433-7, (review).

Bravo EL, "Primary Aldosteronism," *Urol Clin North Am*, 1989, 16(3):481-6.

Chattoraj SC and Watts BH, "Endocrinology," *Textbook of Clinical Chemistry*, Tietz NW, ed, Philadelphia, PA: WB Saunders Co, 1986, 997-1171.

Cuche JL, "Dopaminergic Control of Aldosterone Secretion. State-of-the-Art Review," *Fundam Clin Pharmacol*, 1988, 2:327-39, (review).

Garcia-Robles R and Ruilope LM, "Pharmacological Influences on Aldosterone Secretion," *J Steroid Biochem*, 1987, 27:947-51, (review).

Kotchen TA and Guthrie GP Jr, "Effects of Calcium on Renin and Aldosterone," *Am J Cardiol*, 1988, 62:416-26, (review).

McKenna TJ, Sequeira SJ, Heffernan A, et al, "Diagnosis Under Random Conditions of All Disorders of the Renin-Angiotensin-Aldosterone Axis, Including Primary Hyperaldosteronism," *J Clin Endocrinol Metab*, 1991, 73(5):952-7.

McLeod MK, Thompson NW, Gross MD, et al, "Idiopathic Aldosteronism Masquerading as Discrete Aldosterone-Secreting Adrenal Cortical Neoplasms Among Patients With Primary Aldosteronism," *Surgery*, 1989, 106(6):1161-7.

Miyamoto S, Shimokawa H, Sumioki H, et al, "Circadian Rhythm of Plasma Atrial Natriuretic Peptide, Aldosterone, and Blood Pressure During the Third Trimester in Normal and Pre-eclamptic Pregnancies," *Am J Obstet Gynecol*, 1988, 158:393-9.

(Continued)

Aldosterone, Blood *(Continued)*

Muller J, "Regulation of Aldosterone Biosynthesis. Physiological and Clinical Aspects," *Monogr Endocrinol*, 1987, 29:1-364, (review).

Quinn SJ and Williams GH, "Regulation of Aldosterone Secretion," *Annu Rev Physiol*, 1988, 50:409-26, (review).

Tait JF and Tait SA, "A Steroids Memoir. A Decade (or More) of Electrocortin (Aldosterone)," *Steroids*, 1988, 51:213-50, (review).

Torres VE, Young WF Jr, Offord KP, et al, "Association of Hypokalemia, Aldosteronism, and Renal Cysts," *N Engl J Med*, 1990, 322(6):345-51.

Young DB, "Quantitative Analysis of Aldosterone's Role in Potassium Regulation," *Am J Physiol*, 1988, 255:F811-22, (review).

Young WF Jr, Hogan MJ, Klee GG, et al, "Primary Aldosteronism: Diagnosis and Treatment," *Mayo Clin Proc*, 1990, 65(1):96-110.

Aldosterone, Urine

CPT 82088

Related Information

Aldosterone, Blood *on page 104*
Electrolytes, Urine *on page 213*
Potassium, Blood *on page 330*
Renin, Plasma *on page 346*

Patient Care PREPARATION: Diuretics, antihypertensive drugs, cyclic progestogens, estrogens, and licorice should be terminated for at least 2 weeks and preferably 4 weeks prior to testing. Patient should be on a diet containing 135 mmol (3 g) sodium/day for at least 2 weeks and preferably 30 days prior to testing. No recent radioactive scans. Potassium deficiencies should be corrected before specimen is collected.[1]

Specimen 24-hour urine CONTAINER: Plastic urine container COLLECTION: Boric acid preservative is used by some laboratories. Other laboratories require 20 mL of 33% acetic acid or hydrochloric acid added to the container prior to starting the collection. Check with laboratory. Instruct the patient to void at 8 AM and discard the specimen. Then collect all urine including the final specimen voided at the end of the 24-hour collection period (ie, 8 AM the next morning). Refrigerate during collection. Label with patient's name, date and time collection started, and date and time collection finished. STORAGE INSTRUCTIONS: Freeze CAUSES FOR REJECTION: 12-hour or random specimen, preservative not added to container, recently administered radioisotopes, inadequate preparation of patient SPECIAL INSTRUCTIONS: A 24-hour urine collection or an aliquot from same, indicating total volume is required.

Interpretive REFERENCE RANGE: Reference ranges vary at different laboratories; approximately 2-26 μg/24 hours (SI: 6-72 nmol/day) in a normal individual on normal salt intake. Salt loading in a normal individual will decrease aldosterone secretion. Black children secrete less aldosterone.[2] USE: Diagnose hyperaldosteronism: The two major causes of primary aldosteronism are aldosterone-producing adenoma and idiopathic hyperaldosteronism.[3] LIMITATIONS: Urinary aldosterone measurements alone are of limited value in the diagnosis of hyperaldosteronism. Elevated levels mandate further investigation. METHODOLOGY: Radioimmunoassay (RIA) following extraction

Footnotes

1. Watts NB and Keffer JH, "Renin-Angiotensin-Aldosterone," *Practical Endocrinology*, 4th ed, Philadelphia, PA: Lea & Febiger, 1989, 130-5.
2. Pratt JH, Jones JJ, Miller JZ, et al, "Racial Differences in Aldosterone Excretion and Plasma Aldosterone Concentrations in Children," *N Engl J Med*, 1989, 321(17):1152-7.
3. Arteaga E, Klein R, and Biglieri EG, "Use of the Saline Infusion Test to Diagnose the Cause of Primary Aldosteronism," *Am J Med*, 1985, 79:722-8.

References

Garcia-Zozaya JL, Padilla-Viloria M, and Castro A, "Essential Arterial Hypertension: Plasma and Urinary Aldosterone Alterations," *South Med J*, 1987, 80:1224-7.

Weaver DK and Glenn GC, "The Urine Chemistry Survey – Series 2: 5 Years Experience With an Interlaboratory Comparison Program," *Arch Pathol Lab Med*, 1989, 113(7):713-22.

Alkaline Phosphatase, Heat Stable

CPT 84078

Related Information

Alkaline Phosphatase Isoenzymes *on next page*
Alkaline Phosphatase, Serum *on page 109*

Gamma Glutamyl Transferase *on page 230*

Synonyms Fractionated Alkaline Phosphatase; Heat Stable Alkaline Phosphatase; Heat Stable ALP; Thermostable Alkaline Phosphatase

Test Commonly Includes Total alkaline phosphatase and heat stable alkaline phosphatase as a percent of total

Patient Care PREPARATION: Patient should be fasting.

Specimen Serum CONTAINER: Red top tube STORAGE INSTRUCTIONS: Refrigerate serum.

Interpretive REFERENCE RANGE: In nonpregnant subjects, percent residual activity >25% favors hepatic origin; <10% favors bone origin. USE: Differentiate liver and bone diseases in patients with increased alkaline phosphatase LIMITATIONS: Sometimes misleading. Prolonged storage at room temperature can increase alkaline phosphatase activity. Hemolysis causes false elevation of alkaline phosphatase. If intestinal ALP or other more heat stable isozymes (eg, placental) of ALP are present, percentage of liver fraction may be falsely increased. Serum GGT, leucine aminopeptidase, and 5' nucleotidase may be more helpful in differentiating between osseous and hepatic etiologies of elevated alkaline phosphatase. CONTRAINDICATIONS: Total alkaline phosphatase not elevated METHODOLOGY: Heat inhibition at 56°C. Liver fraction is more resistant to heat and urea inactivation than is the bone isoenzyme. The bone fraction is very heat labile, while placental and cancer (Regan, Nagao) isoenzymes are extremely stable to heat (90% stable).[1] Heating serum at 65°C for 5 minutes results in loss of activity of all ALP fractions with the exception of placental ALP. Heating 56°C for 10 minutes results in 20% loss of intestinal fraction activity, 60% loss of hepatic fraction, and 80% loss of bone ALP activity. Heat inactivation, when used alone, is an inferior technique, since sharp demarcations of the heat stability of the ALP isoenzymes do not occur. The presence of very heat-stable forms (Regan) may give unusually high half-life values. Extremely close temperature control is required. The preferred method is electrophoresis in polyacrylimide gel or high resolution agarose.[2] ADDITIONAL INFORMATION: Heat stable alkaline phosphatase provides an alternative to alkaline phosphatase electrophoresis. Postmenopausal females generally have slightly elevated total alkaline phosphatase and a low percentage of heat stable fraction, indicating osseous origin.

Footnotes

1. Wolf PL, "Clinical Significance of an Increased or Decreased Serum Alkaline Phosphatase Level," *Arch Pathol Lab Med*, 1978, 102:497-501.
2. Day AP, Saward S, Royle CM, et al, "Evaluation of Two New Methods for Routine Measurement of Alkaline Phosphatase Isoenzymes," *J Clin Pathol*, 1992, 45(1):68-71.

References

Chapman JF, Woodard LL, and Silverman LM, "Alkaline Phosphatase Isoenzymes," *Methods in Clinical Chemistry*, Chapter 139, Pesce AJ and Kaplan LA, eds, St Louis, MO: Mosby-Year Book Inc, 1987, 1081-92.

Goldberg DM, "Diagnostic Enzymology," *Applied Biochemistry of Clinical Disorders*, 2nd ed, Chapter 3, Gornall AG, ed, Philadelphia, PA: JB Lippincott Co, 1986, 36-9.

Alkaline Phosphatase Isoenzymes

***CPT** 84080*

Related Information

Alkaline Phosphatase, Heat Stable *on previous page*
Alkaline Phosphatase, Serum *on page 109*
Gamma Glutamyl Transferase *on page 230*

Synonyms ALP Isoenzymes; Isoenzymes of Alkaline Phosphatase; Isozymes of Alkaline Phosphatase

Test Commonly Includes Total ALP level with or without neuraminidase and with or without pretreatment by monoclonal antibody to intestinal fraction ALP. May include combinations of heat and/or L-phenylalanine inactivation with or without electrophoretic differentiation.

Patient Care PREPARATION: Patient should be fasting.

Specimen Serum CONTAINER: Red top tube TURNAROUND TIME: Method dependent, ordinarily at least 2-3 days

Interpretive USE: Evaluate contribution of liver, bone, placental, and Regan isoenzymes to total alkaline phosphatase. Bone fraction is increased in Paget's disease of bone. In the usual chemistry panel, marked isolated increase of alkaline phosphatase in a nonpregnant, older patient who has no healing fracture, with other tests within normal range, is likeliest to indicate Paget's disease of bone. Osteoblastic tumor can also cause increased alkaline phosphatase. LIMITATIONS: For evaluation of biliary tract, the alternatives of GGT, LAP (leucine aminopepti-

(Continued)

Alkaline Phosphatase Isoenzymes *(Continued)*

dase), and 5' nucleotidase as well as radiologic imaging techniques are generally preferred, rather than alkaline phosphatase isoenzymes.[1] **CONTRAINDICATIONS:** Normal total alkaline phosphatase level **METHODOLOGY:** Differential susceptibility of alkaline phosphatase to inhibition by L-phenylalanine and inactivation by heat. Intestinal and placental ALP are inhibited by L-phenylalanine. Skeletal and intestinal ALP are sensitive to inactivation by heat.[2] Polyacrylamide gel electrophoresis with or without pretreatment of sample with neuraminidase and/or monoclonal antibody to the intestinal fraction of ALP (I-ALP). Intestinal fraction can be measured using a method involving sequestration of I-ALP by a monoclonal antibody.[3] Partial digestion with neuraminidase enhances subsequent electrophoretic separation of bone and liver fractions. Pretreatment of samples with monoclonal antibody to I-ALP will retard movement of the latter, allowing for separation of the bone fraction.[4] Isoelectric focusing over a pI range of 3.01-4.86 has separated ALP isoenzymes into 12 bands reflecting at least 12 cellular components. It is claimed that the availability and application of this methodology to clinical problems will render the above manipulations unnecessary.[5,6] **ADDITIONAL INFORMATION:** Virtually any patient with an elevation of serum total alkaline phosphatase (T-ALP) is a candidate for ALP isoenzyme study. In the majority of such cases, however, the elevation in T-ALP is reasonably well defined on the basis of other already established clinical-pathologic findings. The usually more readily available LD (LDH) isoenzyme fractionation frequently serves to define the clinical problem sufficiently that recourse to ALP separation is not necessary. In a minority of patients, elevation of T-ALP resists explanation. Here, application of ALP isoenzyme studies may indicate whether T-ALP is increased on the basis of contributions from liver, bone, intestinal, placental, endothelial cell, or pathologic (tumor markers Regan and Nagao) fractions.

Total liver and bone ALP are increased in hyperthyroid patients. B-ALP is most commonly and significantly increased. I-ALP is not elevated in the hyperthyroid state.[7] Thyroid hormone has a direct stimulatory action on osteoblasts.[8]

T-ALP may be elevated in rheumatic diseases (30% to 50% of cases) (eg, rheumatoid arthritis and ankylosing spondylitis).[9] Osteoarthritis and inactive RA are nearly always associated with normal T-ALP. A few cases of RA have increase in liver AP. Increase in T-ALP and in bone fraction has been shown to correlate with disease activity and the number of involved joints.[9]

Cobalamin (vitamin B_{12}) deficient patients have reduced bone ALP. The degree of megaloblastic anemia has been found to correlate with the decrease in enzyme level.[10] T-ALP level, however, is usually within normal range in B_{12} deficient patients.

A number of ALP isoenzymes have been described (rarely) in association with carcinoma. They are most commonly seen with hepatocellular cancer or carcinoma metastatic to liver. They include Regan, Magoo, Regan variant, Kashahara, fetal intestinal, and Timperley types. The Regan isoenzyme, which is similar to placental ALP, is seen in 1% to 3% of carcinomas (varying in primary site of origin) metastatic to liver.

Footnotes

1. Lum G, Catrou P, Liuzza G, et al, "Clinical Assessment of the Electrophoretic Separation of Alkaline Phosphatase Isoenzymes," *Am J Clin Pathol*, 1983, 80:682-5.
2. Farley JR, Chesnut CH, and Baylink DJ, "Improved Method for Quantitative Determination in Serum of Alkaline Phosphatase of Skeletal Origin," *Clin Chem*, 1981, 27:2002-7.
3. Brock DJH, Barron L, Bedgood D, et al, "Prenatal Diagnosis of Cystic Fibrosis Using a Monoclonal Antibody Specific for Intestinal Alkaline Phosphatase," *Prenat Diagn*, 1984, 4:421-6.
4. Tibi L, Collier A, Patrick AW, et al, "Plasma Alkaline Phosphatase Isoenzymes in Diabetes Mellitus," *Clin Chim Acta*, 1988, 177:147-55.
5. Griffiths J and Black J, "Separation and Identification of Alkaline Phosphatase Isoenzymes and Isoforms in the Serum of Healthy Persons by Isoelectric Focusing," *Clin Chem*, 1987, 33:2171-7.
6. Griffiths J, "Alkaline Phosphatases: Newer Concepts in Isoenzymes and Clinical Applications," *Clin Lab Med*, 1989, 9(4):717-30.
7. Tibi L, Patrick AW, Leslie P, et al, "Alkaline Phosphatase Isoenzymes in Plasma in Hyperthyroidism," *Clin Chem*, 1989, 35(7):1427-30.
8. Sato K, Han DC, Fujii Y, et al, "Thyroid Hormone Stimulates Alkaline Phosphatase Activity in Cultured Rat Osteoblastic Cells (ROS 17/2.8) Through 3,5,3'-Triiodo-L-Thyronine Nuclear Receptors," *Endocrinology*, 1987, 120:1873-81.
9. Siede WH, Seiffert UB, Merle S, et al, "Alkaline Phosphatase Isoenzymes in Rheumatic Diseases," *Clin Biochem*, 1989, 22(2):121-4.
10. Carmel R, Lau, KH, Baylink DJ, et al, "Cobalamin and Osteoblast-Specific Proteins," *N Engl J Med*, 1988, 319(2):70-5.

References

Domar U, Danielsson A, Hiramo K, et al, "Alkaline Phosphatase Isozymes in Nonmalignant Intestinal and Hepatic Diseases," *Scand J Gastroenterol*, 1988, 23:793-800.

Fisken J, Leonard RC, Shaw G, et al, "Serum Placental-Like Alkaline Phosphatase (PLAP): A Novel Combined Enzyme Linked Immunoassay for Monitoring Ovarian Cancer," *J Clin Pathol*, 1989, 42(1):40-5.

Panteghini M and Pagani F, "Reference Intervals for Two Bone-Derived Enzyme Activities in Serum: Bone Isoenzyme of Alkaline Phosphatase (ALP) and Tartrate-Resistant Acid Phosphatase (TR-ACP)," *Clin Chem*, 1989, 35(1):180-1.

Schreiber WE and Sadro LC, "Agarose Gel Patterns of ALkaline Phosphatase Isoenzymes Before and After Treatment With Neuraminidase," *Am J Clin Pathol*, 1988, 90:181-6.

Seabrook RN, Bailyes EM, Price CP, et al, "The Distinction of Bone and Liver Isoenzymes of Alkaline Phosphatase in Serum Using a Monoclonal Antibody," *Clin Chim Acta*, 1988, 172:261-6.

Alkaline Phosphatase, Serum

***CPT** 84075*

Related Information

Alkaline Phosphatase, Heat Stable *on page 106*
Alkaline Phosphatase Isoenzymes *on page 107*
Gamma Glutamyl Transferase *on page 230*
Kidney Stone Analysis *on page 1129*
Leucine Aminopeptidase *on page 276*
5' Nucleotidase *on page 297*

Synonyms ALP; Phosphatase, Alkaline

Replaces BSP

Abstract Serum alkaline phosphatase (ALP) activity normally originates from liver and bone. ALP is excreted in bile. Serum total ALP level provides a useful but nonspecific indication of liver or bone disease. With biliary tract obstruction, the rise in ALP parallels increase in serum bilirubin. Heating serum at 56°C causes significant inactivation of ALP of bone origin.

Patient Care PREPARATION: Patient should be fasting.

Specimen Serum CONTAINER: Red top tube or capillary tube STORAGE INSTRUCTIONS: Refrigerate. Serum alkaline phosphatase increases slowly with storage. Increases of 5% to 10% can be expected after less than 4 hours storage at 4°C. For this reason, it is best to analyze on the day of collection.

Interpretive REFERENCE RANGE: Normal values are higher for pediatric patients and in pregnancy. Levels are two to three or more times adult range in children and are increased in puberty compared to adult range. During episodes of very rapid growth, levels as high as 1000 units/L may be normal. The high level of ALP in childhood results from increase in bone fraction. Post-puberty, serum ALP is mostly of liver origin. Adult normal range is approximately 35-100 units/L. Values in adult males are slightly higher than in adult females. With menopause and after, values in women increase, are similar to or higher than those in men, and are higher than in younger subjects. USE: Causes of **high alkaline phosphatase** include nonfasting specimen; elevations occur especially 2-4 hours after a fatty meal, especially in people who are Lewis positive secretors of blood type O or B. (See Additional Information.) Standing of blood specimen before analysis; up to 30% increase with storage of serum. Bone growth, healing fracture, acromegaly, osteogenic sarcoma, liver or bone metastases, leukemia, myelofibrosis, and rarely myeloma. Alkaline phosphatase is used as a tumor marker.[1,2]

In rickets and osteomalacia, serum calcium and phosphorus are low to normal; and alkaline phosphatase may be normal or increased.

Hypervitaminosis D may cause elevations in alkaline phosphatase.

In Paget's disease of bone, there is often isolated elevation of serum alkaline phosphatase. Some of the highest levels of serum ALP are seen in Paget's disease.

Hyperthyroidism, by its effects upon bone, may elevate alkaline phosphatase. There is evidence that thyroid hormone (T_3) acts to stimulate bone alkaline phosphatase activity through an osteoblast nuclear receptor-mediated process.[3]

Hyperparathyroidism, in some patients.

Pseudohyperparathyroidism.

Chronic alcohol ingestion (in chronic alcoholism, alkaline phosphatase may be normal or increased, but often with high AST (SGOT) and/or high bilirubin and especially with high GGT; MCV may be high).

Biliary obstruction (tenfold increase may be seen with carcinoma of the head of pancreas, choledocholithiasis); cholestasis; GGT also high. Cholecystitis with cholangitis. (In most patients with cholecystitis and cholangitis who do not have a common duct stone, alkaline phos-

(Continued)

Alkaline Phosphatase, Serum *(Continued)*

phatase is within normal limits or only slightly increased.) Sclerosing cholangitis (eg, with ulcerative colitis), although importantly, 3% of cases of symptomatic sclerosing cholangitis may have normal serum ALP.[4] Endoscopic retrograde cholangiography might be considered then in patients with diseases known to be associated with primary sclerosing cholangitis and with appropriate symptomatology even though ALP level is normal. With primary or metastatic tumor in the liver, there may be a marked increase in alkaline phosphatase and GGT. Only three laboratory markers were consistently abnormal, in screening for metastatic carcinoma of breast, prior to clinical detectability of metastases: these were alkaline phosphatase, GGT, and CEA.[2]

Cirrhosis, especially in primary biliary cirrhosis, in which fivefold or more increases are seen.

Gilbert's syndrome: Increase in intestinal alkaline phosphatase is seen.[5]

Hepatitis: Moderate increases in alkaline phosphatase occur in viral hepatitis, but greater elevations of the transaminases (AST (SGOT), ALT (SGPT)) are usually found.

Fatty metamorphosis of liver (moderate increase occurs in acute fatty liver).

Diabetes mellitus, diabetic hepatic lipidosis.

Infiltrative liver diseases (eg, sarcoid, TB, amyloidosis, abscess).

Sepsis and certain viral diseases including infectious mononucleosis and cytomegalovirus infections.

Postoperative cholestasis – pancreatitis, carcinoma of pancreas, cystic fibrosis.

Pulmonary infarct (1-3 weeks after embolism. Healing infarcts in other organs, including kidney, may also cause increased alkaline phosphatase); other situations in which angiofibroplasia occurs, such as healing in a large decubitus ulcer.

Tumors, especially hypernephroma; neoplastic ectopic production (Regan, Nagao isoenzymes).

Fanconi syndrome.

Peptic ulcer, erosion; intestinal strangulation or obstruction, or ulcerative lesion; steatorrhea, malabsorption (from bone, secondary to vitamin D deficiency); ulcerative colitis with pericholangitis, other erosive lesions of colon.

Congestive heart failure.

Parenteral hyperalimentation of glucose, intravenous albumin administration.

Familial hyperphosphatasemia.

Idiopathic.

Drugs – estrogens (large doses), birth control agents, methyltestosterone, phenothiazines, oral hypoglycemic agents, erythromycin, or any drug producing hypersensitivity or toxic cholestasis. Many commonly and uncommonly used drugs elevate alkaline phosphatase, and tenfold increases may be seen with drug cholestasis.

Causes of **low alkaline phosphatase** are said to include: Hypothyroidism – but most hypothyroid patients have normal alkaline phosphatase.

Pernicious anemia – in very few patients.

Hypophosphatasia: Very low alkaline phosphatase values are found in the presence of normocalcemia or hypocalcemia. This diagnosis may be confirmed by quantitation of urinary phosphoethanolamine.

Malnutrition has been reported to relate to low values, but in practice, diseases causing malnutrition relate often to high alkaline phosphatase results (eg, disseminated neoplasia).

Some drugs (clofibrate, azathioprine, estrogens and estrogens in combination with androgens) lower serum ALP activity.

LIMITATIONS: Normal ranges dependent upon methodology, age, and sex. Used alone, alkaline phosphatase may be misleading. **METHODOLOGY:** Some original spectrophotometric methods and their modifications (eg, King-Armstrong, described in 1934 and using the substrate phenylphosphate[6]) have been largely supplanted by more recent end point, kinetic spectrophotometric or fluorescent procedures. Most current assays use *p*-nitrophenyl phosphate (pNPP) as substrate (eg, Bessay-Lowry-Brock). More recent techniques utilize chromogenic substrates (eg, methylumbelliferyl phosphate) and improved buffer systems with resultant increased sensitivity. A reference method using pNPP as substrate has been proposed by the American Association of Clinical Chemistry.[7] **ADDITIONAL INFORMATION:** Serum alkaline phosphatase is a member of a family of zinc metalloprotein enzymes that function to split off a terminal phosphate group from an organic phosphate ester. This enzyme functions in an alkaline environment (optimum pH of 10). Active center of ALP enzymes includes a serine residue. Magnesium and zinc ions are required for minimal activity. Enzyme activity is localized in the brush border of the proximal convoluted tubule of the kidney, intestinal mucosal epithelial cells, hepatic sinusoidal membranes, vascular endothelial cells, and osteoblasts of bone. There are distinctive forms of ALP in the placenta and small intestine; hepatic, renal, and osteoblast (bone) ALP are similar molecules.

Serum ALP activity of intestinal origin occurs only in individuals of ABO blood type O or A. They are secretors of ABH RBC antigens and also carry the Lewis red cell antigen. Serum intestinal ALP level increases in these individuals about 2 hours following consumption of a fatty meal.

Liver alkaline phosphatase is increased in cholestasis and inflammatory liver disease as well as in infiltrative liver disease. The enzyme is sensitive to obstructive biliary processes, even small secondary bile duct obstruction, and thus may be increased in those patients when the bilirubin is normal due to compensatory bilirubin excretion by the rest of the liver. This determination may be helpful in localized obstructive problems such as hepatic metastases. An electrophoretically slow moving isoenzyme with high relative mass may occur in some patients with bile duct obstruction and hepatic metastases and may result in false elevation of CK-MB.[8]

To confirm biliary abnormality, an additional useful test is GGT. GGT is elevated in hepatobiliary disease, not in uncomplicated bone disease.

Serum ALP is increased during pregnancy. Marked decline of high ALP of pregnancy is seen with placental insufficiency and imminent fetal demise.

Footnotes

1. Narayanan S, "Alkaline Phosphatase as Tumor Marker," *Ann Clin Lab Sci*, 1983, 13:133-6.
2. Coombes RC, Powles TJ, Gazet JC, et al, "Screening for Metastases in Breast Cancer: An Assessment of Biochemical and Physical Methods," *Cancer*, 1981, 48:310-5.
3. Sato K, Han DC, Fujii Y, et al, "Thyroid Hormone Stimulates Alkaline Phosphatase Activity in Cultured Rat Osteoblastic Cells (ROS 17/2.8) Through 3,5,3'-Triiodo-L-Thyronine Nuclear Receptors," *Endocrinology*, 1987, 120:1873-81.
4. Cooper JF and Brand EJ, "Symptomatic Sclerosing Cholangitis in Patients With a Normal Alkaline Phosphatase: Two Case Reports and a Review of the Literature," *Am J Gastroenterol*, 1988, 83(3):308-11.
5. Lieverse AG, van Essen GG, Beukeveld GJ, et al, "Familial Increased Serum Intestinal Alkaline Phosphatase: A New Variant Associated With Gilbert's Syndrome," *J Clin Pathol*, 1990, 43(2):125-8.
6. King EJ and Armstrong AR, "A Convenient Method for Determining Serum and Bile Phosphatase Activity," *Can Med Assoc J*, 1934, 31:376-81.
7. Tietz NW, Burtis CA, Duncan P, et al, "A Reference Method for Measurement of Alkaline Phosphatase Activity in Human Serum," *Clin Chem*, 1983, 29:751-61.
8. Butch AW, Goodnow TT, Brown WS, et al, "Stratus Automated Creatine Kinase - MB Assay Evaluated: Identification and Elimination of Falsely Increased Results Associated With High-Molecular-Mass Form of Alkaline Phosphatase," *Clin Chem*, 1989, 35(10):2048-53.

References

Batsakis JG, "Serum Alkaline Phosphatase. Refining an Old Test for the Future," *Diagn Med*, 1982, 25-33.

Epstein S, "Serum and Urinary Markers for Bone Remodeling: Assessment of Bone Turnover," *Endocr Rev*, 1988, 9:437-49.

Kazmierczak SC and Lott JA, "Alkaline Phosphatase," Chapter 138, *Methods in Clinical Chemistry*, Pesce AJ and Kaplan LA, eds, St Louis, MO: Mosby-Year Book Inc, 1987.

Kihn L, Dinwoodie A, and Stinson RA, "High-Molecular-Weight Alkaline Phosphatase in Serum Has Properties Similar to the Enzyme in Plasma Membranes of the Liver," *Am J Clin Pathol*, 1991, 96(4):470-8.

Reichling JJ and Kaplan MM, "Clinical Use of Serum Enzymes in Liver Disease," *Dig Dis Sci*, 1988, 33:1601-4.

Van Hoof VO, Hoylaerts MF, Geryl H, et al, "Age and Sex Distribution of Alkaline Phosphatase Isoenzymes by Agarose Electrophoresis," *Clin Chem*, 1990, 36(6):875-8.

Vincent-Viry M and Galteau MM, "Alkaline Phosphatases," *Drug Effects on Laboratory Test Results Analytical Interferences and Pharmacological Effects*, Siest G and Galteau MM, eds, Littleton, MA: PSG Publishing Co Inc, 1988, 67-90.

Wilson JW, "Inherited Elevation of Alkaline Phosphatase Activity in the Absence of Disease," *N Engl J Med*, 1979, 301:983-4.

Allergen Profile *see* Allergen Specific IgE Antibody *on this page*

Allergen Specific IgE Antibody

CPT 86421 (up to 5 antigens); 86422 (6 or more antigens)

Synonyms Allergen Profile; Allergy Screen; IgE Allergen Specific; Radioallergosorbent Test; RAST®

Test Commonly Includes *Alternaria tenuis*, bermuda grass, cat epithelium, common ragweed, *Dermatophagoides farinae*, dog epithelium, egg white, English plantain, house dust, maple, oak, timothy, or specific mini panels of grasses, foods, animal danders, etc

Patient Care PREPARATION: No isotopes administered 24 hours prior to venipuncture.

Specimen Serum CONTAINER: Red top tube STORAGE INSTRUCTIONS: Separate serum and refrigerate. CAUSES FOR REJECTION: Recently administered radioisotopes TURNAROUND TIME: 1 week (test is commonly performed by a reference laboratory)

Interpretive REFERENCE RANGE: Each allergen scored from 0-4, 0 meaning no IgE detected, 1 meaning a borderline result, and 2-4 increasing IgE against allergen USE: Detect possible allergic responses to various substances in the environment such as animals, antibiotics, foods, grasses, house dust, mites, insects, insulin, molds, smuts, trees, and weeds. Evaluate hay fever, extrinsic asthma, atopic eczema, respiratory allergy.

RAST® is indicated when:

- specific allergic sensitivity is needed to allow immunotherapy ("desensitization shots") to be initiated
- testing for food or chemical sensitivity, where skin testing is unreliable
- there is a history of severe allergic reaction to skin testing
- testing infants
- evaluating patients who refuse skin tests or who are unable to have them because of dermatopathic conditions
- immunotherapy or other therapeutic measures based on skin testing results have not led to a satisfactory remission of symptoms

LIMITATIONS: RAST® results should be interpreted in the context of all available clinical and laboratory findings. False-negative results are possible and may reflect the timing of the blood sample relative to the previous adverse reaction. High levels of total IgE (>3000 IU/mL as may be seen due to parasitic infestation) may result in nonspecific binding and thus, false-positive RAST® results. Total quantitative IgE level must usually be ordered separately. Not all IgE allergens can be tested at this time. Levels less than the geometric mean of IgE probably will not have significant RAST® results. CONTRAINDICATIONS: Recently administered radioisotopes will interfere with this test, causing spurious results.

RAST® is contraindicated when:

- all skin tests are negative
- the patient has only mild symptoms or can be successfully treated with medication and avoidance
- IgE levels are <10 IU/mL unless there is strong clinical suggestion of allergic disease
- patients have successfully responded to immunotherapy
- evaluating non-IgE mediated disease, such as certain drug and food reactions

METHODOLOGY: Radioallergosorbent test (a radioimmunoassay); in this procedure specific allergen is adsorbed on a paper disk; immunospecific IgE, if present in the test (patient's) serum will bind to the disk; detection is effected by radiolabeled anti-IgE. Different scoring systems comparing test results with the absolute binding of a negative control are in use. Commonly, the Fadal/Nalebuff modified RAST® procedure is followed with overnight incubation and resultant greater sensitivity.[1] Monoclonal anti-IgE techniques are useful in the detection of specific IgE in serum.[2] Also, multi-allergen dipstick screening test has been introduced recently.[3] ADDITIONAL INFORMATION: IgE is elevated 4 to 30 times normal in various diseases, among which atopic disorders and parasitic infections are most prominent. The principal limitation of this test is the wide and overlapping range of IgE values between atopic and nonatopic disease states. A positive value is usually meaningful; a negative value is equivocal. RAST® test is valuable on patients who do not respond to environmental control or conservative medical management and where skin tests are contraindicated.

Over 20 years have passed since RAST® testing has been available. Identification of allergen or allergens in patients with atopic disease may be approached clinically by history, avoidance of the offender, by skin testing and/or by RAST® studies. Numerous reports comparing skin testing and RAST® have accumulated in the literature, generally to assess which method has the better sensitivity/specificity. The results appear to vary with the allergen, that is, the relative performance of the two different methods is allergen-dependent.[4] This finding has provided the stimulus for expanded allergen specific comparison studies in the decade of the eighties. A brief summary of a subset of such studies follows:

- With dog and cat as allergens, sensitivity/specificity are similar but negative predictive value of either skin test or RAST® is much greater than positive predictive value.[5]
- Sensitivity of skin test vs RAST® in studies of shrimp allergens is somewhat comparable. There are apparent species-specific shrimp allergens possibly explaining intermittent nature of symptoms in some patients. Test sensitivity may be increased by use of extracts from more than one species of shrimp.[6]
- A comparison of fresh food skin prick tests and RAST® for a variety of vegetables, fruits, and nuts in patients with oral allergy syndrome showed generally variable specificity but better sensitivity with skin testing. RAST® showed better sensitivity only with hazelnut.[7]
- A comparison of RAST® with skin prick testing results in wasp venom allergy found systemic reaction to correlate with a positive paper RAST®. There was relatively good specificity with paper RAST® and skin prick testing, nearly all patients with a systemic reaction had positive paper RAST®.[8]

New assays for the detection of specific IgE are of recent development and include RIA, EIA, and immunofluorometric based systems.[9]

Footnotes

1. King WP, "Efficacy of a Screening Radioallergosorbent Test," *Arch Otolaryngol Head Neck Surg*, 1982, 108:781-6.
2. Duc J, Peitrequin R, and Pecoud AR, "Clinical Evaluation of a New Enzymo-Assay for Allergen Specific IgE," *Ann Allergy*, 1989, 62(6):503-6.
3. Twiggs JT, Gray RL, Pichler K, et al, "Evaluation of Multi-Allergen Dipstick Screening Test," *Ann Allergy*, 1989, 63(3):225-8.
4. Wittig HJ and Blaiss MS, "How Helpful Is the Radioallergosorbent Test in the Diagnosis of Allergic Disease?" *South Med J*, 1982, 75:820-3.
5. Ferguson AC and Murray AB, "Predictive Value of Skin Prick Tests and Radioallergosorbent Tests for Clinical Allergy to Dogs and Cats," *Can Med Assoc J*, 1986, 134:1365-8.
6. Morgan JE, O'Neil CE, Daul CB, et al, "Species-Specific Shrimp Allergens: RAST® and RAST®-Inhibition Studies," *J Allergy Clin Immunol*, 1989, 83(6):1112-7.
7. Ortolani C, Ispano M, Pastorello EA, et al, "Comparison of Results of Skin Prick Tests (With Fresh Foods and Commercial Food Extracts) and RAST® in 100 Patients With Oral Allergy Syndrome," *J Allergy Clin Immunol*, 1989, 83(3):683-900.
8. Heinig JH, Mosbech H, Engel T, et al, "A Comparison of Two RAST® Methods and Skin Prick Testing in the Diagnosis of Wasp Venom Allergy," *Allergy*, 1989, 44(4):260-3.
9. Gueant JL, Moneret-Vautrin DA, Dejardin G, et al, "Comparative Evaluation of RAST® and FAST for 11 Allergens in 288 Patients," *Allergy*, 1989, 44(3):204-8.

References

AMA Council on Scientific Affairs, "*In Vitro* Testing for Allergy," *JAMA*, 1987, 258:1639-43.

AMA Council on Scientific Affairs, "*In Vivo* Diagnostic Testing and Immunotherapy for Allergy," Part I, *JAMA*, 1987, 258:1363-7.

AMA Council on Scientific Affairs, "*In Vivo* Diagnostic Testing and Immunotherapy for Allergy," Part II, *JAMA*, 1987, 258:1505-7.

Canadian Paediatric Society, Allergy Section, "Blood Tests for Allergy in Children," *Can Med Assoc J*, 1990, 142(11):1207-8.

Kelso JM, Sodhi N, Gosselin VA, et al, "Diagnostic Performance Characteristics of the Standard Phadebas RAST®, Modified RAST®, and Pharmacia CAP System Versus Skin Testing," *Ann Allergy*, 1991, 67(5):511-4.

Nadelbuff DJ and Fadel RG, "RAST®-Based Immunotherapy," *Rhinology*, 1984, 22:11-9.

Ownby DR, "Allergy Testing: *In Vitro* Versus *In Vivo*," *Pediatr Clin North Am*, 1988, 35:995-1009.

Shearer WT, "Specific Diagnostic Modalities: IgE, Skin Tests, and RAST®," *J Allergy Clin Immunol*, 1989, 84(6 Pt 2):1112-6.

Van Arsdel PP Jr and Larson EB, "Diagnostic Tests for Patients With Suspected Allergic Disease," *Ann Intern Med*, 1989, 110(4):304-12.

Yunginger JW, "Allergens: Recent Advances," *Pediatr Clin North Am*, 1988, 35:981-93.

Allergy Screen *see* Allergen Specific IgE Antibody *on previous page*

ALP *see* Alkaline Phosphatase, Serum *on page 109*

Alpha$_1$-Fetoprotein, Amniotic Fluid

CPT 82106

Related Information

Acetylcholinesterase, Red Blood Cell *on page 95*
Alpha$_1$-Fetoprotein, Serum *on next page*
Amniotic Fluid, Chromosome and Genetic Abnormality Analysis *on page 891*
Chromosome *In Situ* Hybridization *on page 901*
Cystic Fibrosis DNA Detection *on page 903*
Duchenne/Becker Muscular Dystrophy DNA Detection *on page 908*

Synonyms AFP, Amniotic Fluid

Applies to Amniotic Fluid Acetylcholinesterase

Abstract Alpha-fetoprotein (AFP) is a glycoprotein. Amniotic fluid AFP testing is done following positive maternal screening, but it is also done when the maternal or family history is positive for neural tube defect.

Patient Care PREPARATION: Since interpretation depends on gestational age, diagnostic ultrasound is more desirable than calculated gestational age.[1] (Ultrasound may also delineate other important information, eg, twins.)

Specimen Amniotic fluid CONTAINER: Sterile syringe COLLECTION: The optimal time to collect amniotic fluid for AFP is between the 16th and 18th week of gestation. Include the gestational age on the requisition. If the amniotic fluid is traumatic (bloody), a maternal blood specimen should also be submitted. One or two drops of blood in amniotic fluid can give false-positive results. CAUSES FOR REJECTION: Sample determined not to be amniotic fluid; contamination of amniotic fluid with maternal or fetal blood; recently administered radioisotopes; urine urea nitrogen (UUN) of maternal urine >100 g/day, that of normal amniotic fluid is much less.

Interpretive REFERENCE RANGE: Interlaboratory differences exist. Ranges are stratified by weeks of gestation, decreasing with increasing maturity. It is essential that the reference ranges supplied by the laboratory performing the assay be used to interpret results, which are expressed as "multiples of the median" (MOM) and are generally <2.5 MOM and >0.5 MOM. Most authorities, however, regard MOM >2.0 as abnormal until proven otherwise. MOM is **not** corrected for maternal race, maternal weight, and maternal insulin-dependent diabetes mellitus. Amniotic fluid AFP peak differs from that of maternal serum. USE: Analyze midtrimester amniotic fluid for detection of neural tube defects: anencephaly, spina bifida, myelocele, hydrocephaly LIMITATIONS: Amniotic fluid alpha-fetoprotein may also be increased in nonneural tube anomalies (such as congenital nephrosis, esophageal atresia, duodenal atresia) and fetal bleeding into the amniotic space. The Kleihauer-Betke stain can detect fetal blood contamination of the tap but requires that fetal intact red cells be present. Fetal serum contains mg/mL levels of AFP. Closed neural tube defects are generally not detected by alpha-fetoprotein testing. When an amniotic fluid alpha-fetoprotein level is elevated, confirmatory testing, such as high resolution ultrasonography and measurement of amniotic fluid acetylcholinesterase, should be undertaken to confirm the neural tube defect. Acetylcholinesterase is independent of gestational age and is not affected by fetal blood contamination. METHODOLOGY: Immunoassay, solid-phase and enzyme-labeled monoclonal antibody directed to different epitopes ADDITIONAL INFORMATION: Levels of amniotic fluid AFP >3.0 MOM are generally regarded as abnormally high. (Many use >2.0).

When evaluating amniotic fluid AFP and acetylcholinesterase levels in twin gestations in which only one fetus is affected, placental anatomy appears to be important.[1] With diamniotic-dichorionic twin placentas, amniotic fluid AFP and acetylcholinesterase are within normal range for the unaffected fetus, and elevated in the affected fetus. With diamniotic-monochorionic twin placentas, the unaffected twin may demonstrate elevated amniotic fluid AFP and acetylcholinesterase levels, presumably due to diffusion across the amnion bilayer membrane from the affected site.

Fetal status can be assessed by ultrasound (high-resolution) and chorionic villous sampling by the end of the first trimester. The finding that determination of AFP (coupled with "cautious" interpretation of acetylcholinesterase) has application to detection of neural tube defects during this period has important value.[2] The expected level of α-fetoprotein in amniotic fluid between 11 and 15 weeks should not be determined by extrapolation backward from medians of later gestational age.[3,4] The laboratory must establish its own database for MOMs. The calculation is based on a smoothed weighted log-linear regression. The amniotic fluid MOM is uncorrected, whereas the serum MOM must be corrected for weight, race, and insulin-dependent diabetes.

AFP in amniotic fluid is of two sources, one from the fetal liver, the other originating from the fetal yolk sac. These two forms show varying affinity for concanavalin-A. As gestation advances, the yolk sac contribution to amniotic fluid decreases. The decrease in AFP in amniotic fluid surrounding fetuses with trisomy 21 involves proportionately equal reduction in the yolk sac subfraction and total AFP. No advantage in diagnostic efficiency has been found, therefore, in differential determination of the yolk sac subfractions.[5]

AFP levels in Down syndrome overlap normal values.[6] An excellent review is relatively recent.[7]

Footnotes

1. Stiller RJ, Lockwood CJ, Belanger K, et al, "Amniotic Fluid Alpha-Fetoprotein Concentrations in Twin Gestations: Dependence on Placental Membrane Anatomy," *Am J Obstet Gynecol*, 1988, 158(5):1088-92.
2. Drugan A, Syner FN, Greb A, et al, "Amniotic Fluid Alpha-Fetoprotein and Acetylcholinesterase in Early Genetic Amniocentesis," *Obstet Gynecol*, 1988, 72(1):35-8.
3. Crandall BF, Hanson FW, Tennant F, et al, "Alpha-Fetoprotein Levels in Amniotic Fluid Between 11 and 15 Weeks," *Am J Obstet Gynecol*, 1989, 160(5 Pt 1):1204-6.
4. Brumfield CG, Cloud GA, Davis RO, et al, "The Relationship Between Maternal Serum and Amniotic Fluid Alpha-Fetoprotein in Women Undergoing Early Amniocentesis," *Am J Obstet Gynecol*, 1990, 163(3):903-6.
5. Jones SR, Evans SE, and Gillan L, "Amniotic Fluid Alpha-Fetoprotein Subfractions in Fetal Trisomy 21 Affected Pregnancies," *Br J Obstet Gynaecol*, 1988, 95(4):327-9.
6. Wenk RE and Rosenbaum JM, "Analyses of Amniotic Fluid," *Todd-Sanford-Davidsohn Clinical Diagnosis and Management by Laboratory Methods*, 18th ed, Henry JB, ed, Philadelphia, PA: WB Saunders Co, 1991, 482-96.
7. Bock JL, "Current Issues in Maternal Serum Alpha-Fetoprotein Screening," *Am J Clin Pathol*, 1992, 97(4):541-54.

References

American Society of Human Genetics, "Maternal Serum Alpha-Fetoprotein Screening Programs and Quality Control for Laboratories Performing Maternal Serum and Amniotic Fluid Alpha-Fetoprotein Assay," *Can Med Assoc J*, 1987, 136:1253-6.

Brumfield CG, Cloud GA, Finley SC, et al, "Amniotic Fluid Alpha-Fetoprotein Levels and Pregnancy Outcome," *Am J Obstet Gynecol*, 1987, 157:822-5.

Drugan A, Syner FN, Belsky R, et al, "Amniotic Fluid Acetylcholinesterase: Implications of an Inconclusive Result," *Am J Obstet Gynecol*, 1988, 159:469-74.

Hogge WA, Thiagarajah S, Ferguson JE 2d, et al, "The Role of Ultrasonography and Amniocentesis in the Evaluation of Pregnancies at Risk for Neural Tube Defects," *Am J Obstet Gynecol*, 1990, 163(3):520-3.

Knight GJ, "Maternal Serum Alpha-Fetoprotein Screening," *Techniques in Diagnostic Human Biochemical Genetics*, Hommes FA, ed, New York, NY: Wiley-Liss, 1991, 491-518.

Richards DS, Seeds JW, Katz VL, et al, "Elevated Maternal Serum Alpha-Fetoprotein With Oligohydramnios: Ultrasound Evaluation and Outcome," *Obstet Gynecol*, 1988, 72:337-41, (review).

Stephens JD, "Amniotic Fluid Alpha-Fetoprotein and Acetylcholinesterase in Early Genetic Amniocentesis," *Obstet Gynecol*, 1989, 73(1):141-2, (letter).

Alpha$_1$-Fetoprotein, Serum

***CPT** 82105*

Related Information

Acetylcholinesterase, Red Blood Cell *on page 95*
Alpha$_1$-Fetoprotein, Amniotic Fluid *on previous page*
Body Fluid *on page 145*
CA 19-9 *on page 152*
Carcinoembryonic Antigen *on page 167*
Cyst Fluid Cytology *on page 495*
Human Chorionic Gonadotropin, Serum *on page 254*

Synonyms AFP

Abstract A major protein of normal fetal plasma. Very low levels are found in the serum of nonpregnant adults. It is increased in hepatic disorders attended by hepatocyte regenerative activity, in hepatoma, and in various germ cell derived tumors. With some neural tube congenital (developmental) defects (eg, spina bifida), it is elevated in amniotic fluid and therefore in the serum of the gravid woman. With some fetal chromosomal abnormalities (Down syndrome, trisomy 21, trisomy 18), it is relatively low in the maternal serum.

Patient Care PREPARATION: Avoid recent isotope scan.

Specimen Serum CONTAINER: Red top tube SAMPLING TIME: The optimal time to draw **maternal serum** for AFP, for prenatal screening, is between the 16th week and 18th week of gestation.[1] Repeat 1 week or more later if a high result is found. Maternal serum can be collected be-

(Continued)

Alpha$_1$-Fetoprotein, Serum *(Continued)*

tween the 15th and 22nd weeks. **STORAGE INSTRUCTIONS:** Refrigerate **CAUSES FOR REJECTION:** Recently administered radioisotopes **SPECIAL INSTRUCTIONS:** Include maternal age, gestational age, maternal weight, race, and diabetic status on requisition.

Interpretive **REFERENCE RANGE:** Normal adults: 2-16 ng/mL (SI: 2-16 μg/L) serum. Interlaboratory differences exist. The level in maternal serum increases to a maximum of 550 ng/mL (SI: 550 μg/L) during the third trimester of pregnancy. Normal values for maternal serum may vary from laboratory to laboratory. Normal is considered 0.5-2.5 multiples of the median (MOM), although some authorities recommend 0.5-2.0 MOM recently.[1] The MOM is always corrected for maternal weight, maternal race, and maternal insulin-dependent diabetes mellitus. **USE:** Diagnose **hepatocellular carcinoma:** With sensitive RIA procedures, elevation of AFP will occur in 90% of patients with hepatocellular carcinoma. Values in excess of 1000 ng/mL (SI: >1000 μg/L) are almost always secondary to hepatocellular carcinoma. However, overlap with AFP elevations caused by nonmalignant chronic liver diseases is widely recognized.

Gonadal and extragonadal germinal tumor types include endodermal sinus tumor (yolk sac tumor), embryonal carcinoma, teratocarcinoma, and choriocarcinoma. AFP increases occur as well from extragonadal locations, retroperitoneum, and mediastinum.

Monitor therapy with antineoplastic drugs, in patients being treated for hepatoma or germinal neoplasm.

Differential diagnosis of **neonatal hepatitis** versus biliary atresia in newborns.

Useful in **intrauterine** screening. Elevated values are found in anencephaly, spina bifida, myelomeningocele, and other open neural tube defects; fetal death; esophageal atresia; congenital nephrosis; diagnose multiple pregnancy; oligohydramnios; abruptio placentae; and preeclampsia.[2] Increased values of AFP in maternal serum can result from underestimated gestational age or from contamination with fetal plasma. Low values may be associated with chromosomal abnormalities including trisomy 21 and trisomy 18.

LIMITATIONS: High in some cases of nonmalignant liver disease (eg, massive hepatic necrosis, acute hepatitis, alcoholic cirrhosis, and chronic active hepatitis). American instances of hepatocellular carcinoma are not as consistently AFP rich, as are many cases from overseas.

Pure **seminomas, dysgerminomas, and teratomas** do not produce AFP, and increased AFP in a subject with seminoma by histology suggests nonseminomatous elements such as embryonal carcinoma, or hepatic metastasis.[3]

Elevations have been described in tyrosinemia, ataxia telangiectasia, and congenital nephrotic syndrome. A low incidence of elevations occurs in a variety of tumors, especially carcinoma of stomach, pancreas, and biliary tract.

Some maternal serum samples from women carrying fetuses with closed **neural tube defects** have normal levels of AFP. False-positives for prenatal diagnosis of neural tube defects have been reported. Increased AFP in maternal serum can occur with twins, incorrect gestational age, any blockage of fetal gastrointestinal tract, fetal death, and other conditions.[4]

CONTRAINDICATIONS: Recently administered radioisotopes may interfere with the RIA test. **METHODOLOGY:** Radioimmunoassay (RIA), enzyme immunoassay (EIA) **ADDITIONAL INFORMATION:** AFP is a major glycoprotein of fetal plasma, structurally similar to albumin with molecular weight of about 65,000. In the embryo it is synthesized by the yolk sac and later by the fetal liver. During the 6th week of gestation, AFP appears in fetal serum. It achieves peak concentration in fetal serum and amniotic fluid at 14 weeks gestation. In the maternal circulation, AFP is about 10 ng/mL (SI: 10 μg/L) at the 8th week, 100 ng/mL (SI: 100 μg/L) at 20 weeks and undergoes further rise to term.

Maternal screening for presence of open neural tube defects (eg, spina bifida) is based on the finding of elevated AFP in a maternal serum specimen ideally taken at the 16th to 18th week of gestation. The findings must be confirmed by amniotic fluid acetylcholinesterase study and ultrasound study of the fetal spine to detect the possibility of false-positive resulting from inaccurate dating, twins, threatened abortion, congenital nephrosis, and other causes.

Unexplained increase in maternal serum AFP with second trimester oligohydramnios is associated with an especially poor prognosis. There is evidence that serial ultrasound evaluations of amniotic fluid volume can assist in predicting pregnancy outcome.[5] With severe decrease in amniotic fluid (eg, severe oligohydramnios or no amniotic fluid), the majority (essentially all) of cases will have pulmonary hypoplasia, Potter deformities, renal developmental abnormalities (such as polycystic kidney), or neonatal death. Genetic testing may be indicated in cases of low values for correct gestational age.

AFP levels may be increased in cases of hepatic parenchymal regeneration (eg, following traumatic injury, associated with the viral hepatitides, and following recovery from exposure to hepatotoxins).

Extremely high AFP levels are found with endodermal sinus tumors (yolk sac tumors).[3] Such neoplasms occur in testis, ovary, and in extragonadal sites. Typically they occur in young subjects.

While some hepatocarcinomas are associated with very high AFP levels (>10,000 µg/L), there is evidence that tumors with such high levels are decreasing in prevalence while tumors with lower levels are becoming more common.[6] For size-matched cases of hepatocellular carcinoma, prognosis has been found to relate importantly to serum AFP levels. Patients with low levels of AFP (≤20 µg/L) had two- to threefold increase in survival as compared with patients having the highest (>10,000 µg/L) levels.[6]

Low levels are found in mothers with Down syndrome (trisomy 21) pregnancies. However, the test to screen for this condition has poor predictive value. Maternal serum AFP levels are decreased in other examples of fetal chromosomal abnormalities (trisomy 18).[7] Recently, the combination of maternal serum AFP with maternal serum human chorionic gonadotropin (hCG) and unconjugated estriol (UE_3) have been advocated to improve the predictive value of screening for Down syndrome.[8] This "triple test" can detect 60% to 75% of Down syndrome cases with a false-positive rate of about 6%. Some sources suggest that the UE_3 is not essential for the screen. Others have advocated the use of a free beta-hCG assay to improve predictive value. National surveys by the CAP found that larger laboratories tend to make the clinically important adjustments for maternal weight, race, and diabetic status more often than smaller laboratories.

AFP testing is useful in the detection of pregnancy complications such as intrauterine growth retardation, fetal distress, fetal demise, or in the presence of severe maternal pregnancy-induced hyperpertension. In all these instances, the serum AFP was increased >2.0 MOM. The use of this test was found to be more valuable in detecting these complications than in detecting neural tube defects.[1]

Forty percent of patients with nonseminomatous germ cell tumor present with increased levels of hCG. Approximately 7% to 18% of patients with pure seminoma present or develop an elevated hCG in the course of their disease. Assay of hCG is useful in post-treatment prediction of survival. Pretreatment levels are also useful in prognosis and response to treatment.[3]

Footnotes

1. Lenke RR, Guerrieri J, Nemes JM, et al, "Elevated Maternal Serum Alpha-Fetoprotein Values: How Low Is High?" *J Reprod Med*, 1989, 34(8):511-6.
2. Milunsky A, Jick SS, Bruell CL, et al, "Predictive Values, Relative Risks, and Overall Benefits of High and Low Maternal Serum α-Fetoprotein Screening in Singleton Pregnancies: New Epidemiologic Data," *Am J Obstet Gynecol*, 1989, 161(2):291-7.
3. Bajorin DF and Bosl GJ, "The Use of Serum Tumor Markers in the Prognosis and Treatment of Germ Cell Tumors," *Principles and Practice of Oncology*, 1992, 6:1-11.
4. Cunningham FG and Gilstrap LC, "Maternal Serum Alpha-Fetoprotein Screening," *N Engl J Med*, 1991, 325(1):55-7, (editorial).
5. Richards DS, Seeds JW, Katz VL, et al, "Elevated Maternal Serum Alpha-Fetoprotein With Oligohydramnios: Ultrasound Evaluation and Outcome," *Obstet Gynecol*, 1988, 72(3 Pt 1):337-41, (review).
6. Nomura F, Ohnishi K, and Tanabe Y, "Clinical Features and Prognosis of Hepatocellular Carcinoma With Reference to Serum Alpha-Fetoprotein Levels," *Cancer*, 1989, 64(8):1700-7.
7. Clinical Pathology Rounds, "Trisomy 18 Detected by MSAFP Screening," *Lab Med*, 1991, 22:605-7.
8. MacDonald ML, Wagner RM, and Slotnick RN, "Sensitivity and Specificity of Screening for Down Syndrome With Alpha-Fetoprotein, hCG, Unconjugated Estriol, and Maternal Age," *Obstet Gynecol*, 1991, 77(1):63-8.

References

Bock JL, "Current Issues in Maternal Serum Alpha-Fetoprotein Screening," *Am J Clin Pathol*, 1992, 97(4):541-54.

Bosl GJ, Lange PH, Nochomovitz LE, et al, "Tumor Markers in Advanced Nonseminomatous Testicular Cancer," *Cancer*, 1981, 47:572-6.

Chen DS and Sung JL, "Serum Alpha-Fetoprotein in Hepatocellular Carcinoma," *Cancer*, 1977, 40:779-83.

Curtin JP, Rubin SC, Hoskins WJ, et al, "Second-Look Laparotomy in Endodermal Sinus Tumor: A Report of Two Patients With Normal Levels of Alpha-Fetoprotein and Residual Tumor at Reexploration," *Obstet Gynecol*, 1989, 73(4):893-5.

Eckfeldt JH and Long TA, "Influence of Laboratory Test Volume and Geographic Location on Maternal Alpha-Fetoprotein Results," *Arch Pathol Lab Med*, 1991, 115(7):647-53.

Macri JN, "Critical Issues in Prenatal Maternal Serum Alpha-Fetoprotein Screening for Genetic Abnormalities," *Am J Obstet Gynecol*, 1986, 155:240-6.

(Continued)

Alpha$_1$-Fetoprotein, Serum *(Continued)*

Sato Y, Nakata K, Kato Y, et al, "Early Recognition of Hepatocellular Carcinoma Based on Altered Profiles of Alpha-Fetoprotein," *N Engl J Med*, 1993, 328(25):1802-6.

Upton K, "Fetal Monitoring," *Clinical Laboratory Science: Strategies for Practice*, Chapter 41, Davis BG, Bishop ML, and Mass D, eds, Philadelphia, PA: JB Lippincott Co, 1989, 493-508.

Virji MA, Mercer DW, and Herberman RB, "Tumor Markers in Cancer Diagnosis and Prognosis," *CA*, 1988, 38:105-26.

Wu JT, "Serum Alpha-Fetoprotein and Its Lectin Reactivity in Liver Diseases: A Review," *Ann Clin Lab Sci*, 1990, 20(2):98-105.

Alpha$_1$ Lipoprotein Cholesterol *see* High Density Lipoprotein Cholesterol *on page 249*

Alpha-Hydroxybutyric Dehydrogenase (HBDH) *replaced by* Cardiac Enzymes/Isoenzymes *on page 170*

Alpha-Hydroxybutyric Dehydrogenase, Serum *replaced by* Lactate Dehydrogenase Isoenzymes *on page 271*

Alpha Tocopherol *see* Vitamin E, Serum *on page 389*

ALP Isoenzymes *see* Alkaline Phosphatase Isoenzymes *on page 107*

ALT *see* Alanine Aminotransferase *on page 100*

Amino Acid Screen *see* Amino Acid Screen, Qualitative, Urine *on page 120*

Amino Acid Screen, Plasma

CPT 82128

Related Information

Amino Acid Screen, Qualitative, Urine *on page 120*
Ammonia, Blood *on page 120*
Phenylalanine, Blood *on page 317*

Synonyms Inborn Errors of Metabolism Screen; Metabolic Screen for Amino Acids

Test Commonly Includes Screening for the presence of all amino acids

Patient Care **PREPARATION:** Infants: 4-hour fast; children and adults: 12-hour fast. Protein intake does not affect diurnal variation, but it influences absolute concentrations of amino acids in blood or urine. One day of fasting will decrease the excretion by 50%.

Specimen Plasma **CONTAINER:** Green top (heparin) tube **COLLECTION:** Routine venipuncture **STORAGE INSTRUCTIONS:** Centrifuge. Transfer plasma to plastic vial and freeze within 1 hour of collection. Stable frozen for 2-4 weeks, analysis within 1 week is preferable.

Interpretive **REFERENCE RANGE:** Established by each laboratory **USE:** Screen for inborn errors of metabolism of amino acids **LIMITATIONS:** Amphetamines, antihistamines, and phenothiazines are known to interfere with this assay. Patient should not take these drugs for at least 72 hours prior to specimen collection. **METHODOLOGY:** Plasma screen by single dimension thin-layer chromatography (TLC), amino acid analyzer (ion-exchange chromatography), gas chromatography (GC), and high performance liquid chromatography (HPLC) may have clinical application[1,2,3] **ADDITIONAL INFORMATION:** Amino acid concentrations show a significant circadian rhythm with plasma level variation of 30%. Values are highest in midafternoon and lowest in the early morning. A variety of inherited metabolic disorders result in aminoacidemia/aminoaciduria. **Cystinuria** has an autosomal recessive mode of inheritance, is a disorder of amino acid transport involving renal tubules/GI tract and should be suspect in cases of urinary stone disease. It is characterized by the formation of radiopaque stones and by the presence of characteristic hexagonal crystals in the urine. **Lysinuric protein intolerance** is another disorder of membrane transport. As in some cases of cystinuria, cationic amino acids (lysine, arginine and ornithine) are involved. Lysine is present in large amounts in the urine but is normal or decreased in plasma. Patients have poor appetite, fail to thrive, develop hepatosplenomegaly, hypotonia, sparse hair, osteoporosis, mental retardation, and a variety of other problems. In **Hartnup disease**, there is impaired neutral amino acid transport involving the kidneys and small intestine. It is characterized clinically by pellagra-like features, mental retardation and/or psychotic behavior, intermittent ataxia and is inherited as an autosomal recessive. A comprehensive review of these and other amino acidurias is provided in the text edited by Scriver et al.

The usual approach is to screen urine for amino acids. However, urinary levels are variable: plasma is more definitive. In all cases in which an amino acid is elevated in blood, it will also be elevated in urine. CSF amino acids are useful in the diagnosis of nonketotic hyperglycinemia. See table.

Congenital Disorders of Amino Acid Metabolism

Name	Enzyme or Metabolic Pathways	Clinical Findings	Laboratory Findings
Classic phenylketonuria and variants	Phenylalanine hydroxylase	Mental retardation (untreated)	Plasma phenylalanine >15 mg/dL
Benign hyperphenylalaninemia	Phenylalanine hydroxylase	Asymptomatic	Elevated plasma phenylalanine <15 mg/dL
Neonatal tyrosinemia	*p*-Hydroxyphenylacetic acid hydroxylase	Asymptomatic (newborn)	Transient elevated plasma tyrosine
Hereditary tyrosinemia	*p*-Hydroxyphenylacetic acid hydroxylase	Hepatic cirrhosis, renal tubular dysfunction	Increased plasma tyrosine
Histidinemia	Histidine ammonia lyase	Usually mental retardation	Plasma and urine histidine increased
Branched-chain hyperaminoacidemia (maple syrup urine disease)	Branched-chain α-keto-acid oxidase	Seizures, ketosis, mental retardation (variants exist)	Increased branched-chain amino acids in plasma and metabolites in urine
Homocystinuria	Serinehydrolase (cystathionine synthase)	Mental retardation, thromboembolism, skeletal abnormalities	Methionine, homocystine, and derivatives in blood and urine
Cystathioninuria	Homoserine hydrolase (cystathionase)	Asymptomatic	Cystathionine in blood and urine
Hyperglycinemias Ketotic form	Propionyl-CoA-carboxylase	Ketosis, neutropenia, mental retardation	Glycine and propionic acid in blood and urine
Nonketotic form	Glycine decarboxylase	Developmental retardation	Glycine in blood and urine
Urea cycle abnormalities	Carbamoylphosphate synthase, ornithine-carbamoyltransferase, citrulline aspartate lyase, argininosuccinate arginine-lyase	Vomiting, lethargy, protein intolerance, seizures, and hepatomegaly—with variation by disease	Ammonia in plasma; glutamine, citrulline, or argininosuccinic acid in blood and urine, depending on disorder
Cystinuria (types I-III)	Renal transport system for cystine and dibasic amino acids	Cystine stones (severity varies with disorder)	Urine cystine and dibasic amino acids
Glycinuria	Renal transport system for glycine and imino acids	Asymptomatic	Urine glycine, proline, and hydroxyproline
Hartnup disease	Renal transport system for neutral amino acids	Variable—may have ataxia, rashes, retardation	Urine neutral amino acids
Fanconi's syndrome	General renal transport deficiency	Acidosis and rickets	General aminoaciduria, glycosuria, phosphaturia

Adapted from *Gradwohl's Clinical Laboratory Methods and Diagnosis,* 8th ed, St Louis, MO: Mosby-Year Book Inc, 1980, with permission.

*Compounds mentioned are present in increased concentrations.

Footnotes

1. Gamerith G, "Analysis of Amino Acids as Their N-TFA n-Propyl Esters," *Amino Acid Analysis by Gas Chromatography*, Vol II, Chapter 5, Zumwalt RW, Kuo KCT, and Gehrke CW, eds, Boca Raton, FL: CRC Press Inc, 1987, 117-39.
2. Desgrès J and Padieu P, "Gas-Liquid Chromatographic Analysis of Amino Acids as Isobutyl Esters, N(O)-Heptafluorobutyrate Derivatives: Applications to Clinical Biology," *Amino Acid Analysis by Gas Chromatography*, Vol I, Chapter 5, Gehrke CW, Kuo KCT, and Zumwalt RW, eds, Boca Raton, FL: CRC Press Inc, 1987, 119-42.
3. Hancock WS and Harding DRK, "Review of Separation Conditions," and Ishimitsu S, Fujimoto S, and Ohara K, "m- and O-Tyrosine," *CRC Handbook of HPLC for the Separation of Amino Acids, Peptides, and Proteins*, Vol I, Hancock WS, ed, Boca Raton, FL: CRC Press Inc, 1984, 235-62, 263-73.

References

Cleary MA and Wraith JE, "Antenatal Diagnosis of Inborn Errors of Metabolism," *Arch Dis Child*, 1991, 66(7 Spec No):816-22.

Forman DT, "Role of the Laboratory in Diagnosis of Organic Acidurias," *Ann Clin Lab Sci*, 1991, 21(2):85-93.

National Academy of Clinical Biochemistry 14th Annual Symposium, "Diagnosis and Treatment of Inborn Errors of Metabolism," *Clin Biochem*, 1991, 24(4):289-381.

Rutledge JC and Rudy J, "HPLC Qualitative Amino Acid Analysis in the Clinical Laboratories," *Am J Clin Pathol*, 1987, 87:614-8.

Scriver CR, "Amino Acids," Part 4 and "Membrane Transport Systems," Part 15, *The Metabolic Basis of Inherited Disease*, 6th ed, Scriver CR, Beaudet AL, Sly WS, et al, eds, New York, NY: McGraw-Hill Inc, 1989, 495-771, 2479-580.

(Continued)

Amino Acid Screen, Plasma *(Continued)*

Shih VE, "Detection of Hereditary Metabolic Disorders Involving Amino Acids and Organic Acids," *Clin Biochem*, 1991, 24(4):301-9.

Slocum RH and Cummings JG, "Amino Acid Analysis of Physiological Samples," *Techniques in Diagnostic Human Biochemical Genetics*, Hommes FA, ed, New York, NY: Wiley-Liss, 1991, 87-126.

Verjee ZH, "Amino Acid Screen," *Methods in Clinical Chemistry*, Chapter 22, Pesce AJ and Kaplan LA, eds, St Louis, MO: Mosby-Year Book Inc, 1987, 146-53.

Amino Acid Screen, Qualitative, Urine

***CPT** 82128*

Related Information

Amino Acid Screen, Plasma *on page 118*

Phenylalanine, Blood *on page 317*

Synonyms Amino Acid Screen; Inborn Errors of Metabolism Screen; Metabolic Screen for Amino Acids

Test Commonly Includes Glycine, hydroxyproline, isoleucine, leucine, methionine, ornithine, phenylalanine, proline, tyrosine, valine

Specimen Urine **CONTAINER:** Plastic urine container, no preservative **COLLECTION:** Random specimen acceptable. Morning urine preferred. **STORAGE INSTRUCTIONS:** Freeze **CAUSES FOR REJECTION:** Specific gravity of the urine must be $\geq$1.010

Interpretive **REFERENCE RANGE:** Subjective interpretation based on comparison of patient, normal, and control urines of comparable age. Interpretation is age dependent. **USE:** Screen for "inborn errors of metabolism" of amino acids, Fanconi syndrome, and Wilson's disease **LIMITATIONS:** Dilute urines cannot be run. Must have concentrated urine. Amphetamines, norepinephrine, levodopa, and all antibiotics have been reported to interfere chemically with this test. Amino acid concentrations in urine are physiologically increased by aspirin, bismuth, hydrocortisone, insulin, lead poisoning, and triamcinolone. **METHODOLOGY:** Thin-layer chromatography (TLC) **ADDITIONAL INFORMATION:** Excretion of certain amino acids is increased in several specific aminoacidurias, such as phenylketonuria and maple syrup urine disease. Aminoaciduria may also be seen in a variety of other disorders, including viral hepatitis, multiple myeloma, rickets, hyperparathyroidism, and chronic renal failure. A positive test should be followed up with quantitation on a 24-hour collection.

References

Coe FL and Kathpalia S, "Hereditary Tubular Disorders," *Harrison's Principles of Internal Medicine*, 12th ed, Chapter 231, Wilson JD, Braunwald E, Isselbacher KJ, et al, eds, New York, NY: McGraw-Hill Inc, 1991, 1196-202.

Rosenberg LE, "Inherited Disorders of Amino Acid Metabolism," *Harrison's Principles of Internal Medicine*, 12th ed, Chapter 334, Wilson JD, Braunwald E, Isselbacher KJ, et al, eds, New York, NY: McGraw-Hill Inc, 1991, 1868-75.

Slocum RH and Cummings JG, "Amino Acid Analysis of Physiological Samples," *Techniques in Diagnostic Human Biochemical Genetics*, Hommes FA, ed, New York, NY: Wiley-Liss, 1991, 87-126.

Aminolevulinic Acid *see* Delta Aminolevulinic Acid, Urine *on page 207*

Aminoterminal Propeptide of Type III Procollagen *see* CA 125 *on page 154*

Aminotransferases *see* Alanine Aminotransferase *on page 100*

Aminotransferases *see* Aspartate Aminotransferase *on page 135*

Ammonia, Blood

***CPT** 82140*

Related Information

Amino Acid Screen, Plasma *on page 118*

Cerebrospinal Fluid Glutamine *on page 177*

Valproic Acid *on page 1008*

Synonyms NH_3, Blood

Applies to Ammonia, Cerebrospinal Fluid

Patient Care **PREPARATION:** Patient should avoid smoking prior to sampling.

Specimen Plasma **CONTAINER:** Green top (sodium or lithium heparin) tube or lavender top (EDTA) tube. One author, however, suggests that heparin will produce false low results.[1] **COLLECTION:** Tube must be filled completely and kept tightly stoppered at all times. Specimen must be placed on ice immediately and rotated, then centrifuged at 4°C. Plasma should be very promptly separated from the cells. Test must be performed within 20 minutes of the venipuncture, or the plasma frozen immediately. Concentration rapidly increases on standing. Never freeze whole blood. **STORAGE INSTRUCTIONS:** Ammonia is stable for several days at -70°C. **CAUSES FOR REJECTION:** Improper collection tube, not stoppered, delayed delivery to the laboratory **SPECIAL INSTRUCTIONS:** Avoid hemolysis, which increases plasma ammonia.

Interpretive **REFERENCE RANGE:** Variations of reference ranges between laboratories exist for ammonia. See table for approximate ranges. Ammonia level in cerebrospinal fluid is about 33% to 50% of that in arterial blood. **USE:** Ammonia is elevated in liver disease, urinary tract infection with distention and stasis, Reye's syndrome, inborn errors of metabolism including deficiency of enzymes in the urea cycle, HHH syndrome (hyperornithinemia, hyperammonemia-homocitrullinuria), some normal neonates (usually returning to normal in 48 hours), total parenteral nutrition, ureterosigmoidostomy, and sodium valproate therapy. Ammonia determination is indicated in neonates with neurological deterioration, subjects with lethargy and/or emesis not explained, and in patients with possible encephalopathy.

Ammonia, Blood

Age	μmg/dL	SI: μmol/L
Neonate	90–150	64–107
<2 wk	79–129	56–92
Children	29–70	21–50
Adults	15–45	11–32

Note: Values are somewhat higher in capillary blood.

The diagnostic utility of ammonia measurements is limited. They are mainly of use in the diagnosis of urea cycle deficiencies (any neonate with unexplained nausea, vomiting, or neurological deterioration appearing after first feeding); and they play an important part in the detection of Reye's syndrome.

In Reye's syndrome, threefold increases in AST, ALT, and serum ammonia are required for diagnosis with/or the diagnostic liver biopsy findings. Ammonia levels increase characteristically early; serum ammonia ≥100 μg/dL (SI: ≥59 μmol/L) reflects severe hepatic changes. Prothrombin time is increased in essentially all patients, prototypically three seconds longer than the control. Bilirubin is usually normal. Glucose should be monitored; hypoglycemia may develop. Hyperosmolality and acid-base imbalance may develop, lactate may increase, CK may increase and CK-MB may be elevated. Uric acid may increase.[2,3] Increased ammonia and prolonged prothrombin time provide indicators of disease progression.[4]

LIMITATIONS: The correlation between blood ammonia levels and hepatic coma is poor. Ammonia determinations are not reliable predictors of impending hepatic coma. Ammonia levels are not always high in all patients with urea cycle disorders. High protein diet may cause increased levels.[5] Ammonia levels may also be elevated with gastrointestinal hemorrhage. If portal hypertension develops with cirrhosis, hepatic blood flow is altered, leading to elevated blood ammonia levels. **METHODOLOGY:** Laboratory contamination by NH_4OH, tobacco smoke, urine, formaldehyde must be avoided.[6] Ion-selective electrode (ISE) methods are preferred; Ektachem® dry film method is also recommended. A number of methods for ammonia are found in standard texts. Many are in use. Some are obsolete. A recommendation to soak glassware in hypochlorite, 52.5 g/L and to then rinse it thoroughly with deionized water is provided to Paramax™ users. **ADDITIONAL INFORMATION:** Ammonia and alpha-ketoglutarate with NADH yield glutamate; glutamate and ammonia yield glutamine. Cerebrospinal fluid glutamine levels are useful in hepatic encephalopathy and with Reye's syndrome.[7] In the HHH syndrome hyperammonemia is intermittent; it presents in infancy often, but symptoms can be delayed.[8]

Footnotes

1. Dorwart WV and Saner M, "Heparinized Plasma Is an Unacceptable Specimen for Ammonia Determination," *Clin Chem*, 1992, 38(1):161, (letter).
2. Bakerman S and Bakerman P, "Reye Syndrome: Laboratory and Clinical Features," *Lab Management*, August 1986, 25-8.
3. Meythaler JM and Varma RR, "Reye's Syndrome in Adults: Diagnostic Considerations," *Arch Intern Med*, 1987, 147:61-4.
4. Heubi JE and Daugherty CC, "Grade 1 Reye's Syndrome: Outcome and Predictors of Progression to Deeper Coma States," *N Engl J Med*, 1984, 311:1539-42.
5. Glasgow AM, "Clinical Application of Blood Ammonia Determinations," *Lab Med*, 1981, 12:151-7.
6. Ladenson JH, "Nonanalytical Sources of Variation in Clinical Chemistry Results," *Gradwohl's Clinical Laboratory Methods and Diagnosis*, 8th ed, Sonnenwirth AC and Jarett L, eds, St Louis, MO: Mosby-Year Book Inc, 1980, 149-92.

(Continued)

Ammonia, Blood *(Continued)*

7. Romshe CA, "Laboratory Diagnosis of Reye's Syndrome," *Reye's Syndrome*, Pollack JD, ed, New York, NY: Grune and Stratton Inc, 1975, 15-26.
8. Valle D and Simell O, "The Hyperornithinemias," *The Metabolic Basis of Inherited Disease*, 6th ed, Chapter 19, Scriver CR, Beaudet AL, Sly WS, et al, eds, New York, NY: McGraw-Hill Inc, 1989, 599-627.

References

Cascino GD, Jensen JM, Nelson LA, et al, "Periodic Hyperammonemic Encephalopathy Associated With a Ureterosigmoidostomy," *Mayo Clin Proc*, 1989, 64(6):653-6.

Diamond DA, Blight A, Samuell CT, et al, "Ammonia Levels in Paediatric Ureterosigmoidostomy Patients: A Screen for Hyperammonaemia?" *Br J Urol*, 1991, 67(5):541-4.

Fine P, Adler K, and Gerstenfeld D, "Idiopathic Hyperammonemia After High-Dose Chemotherapy," *Am J Med*, 1989, 86(5):629, (letter).

Fishman RA, *Cerebrospinal Fluid in Diseases of the Nervous System*, 2nd ed, Philadelphia, PA: WB Saunders Co, 1992, 238-9.

Gambino R, "When and How Should Ammonia Be Measured?" *Lab Report for Physicians*,™ 1988, 10:78-80.

Giacoia GP and Padilla-Lugo A, "Severe Transient Neonatal Hyperammonemia," *Am J Perinatol*, 1986, 3:249-54.

Green A, "When and How Should We Measure Plasma Ammonia?" *Ann Clin Biochem*, 1988, 25:199-204.

Hurwitz ES, "Reye's Syndrome," *Epidemiol Rev*, 1989, 11:249-53.

Ammonia, Cerebrospinal Fluid *see* Ammonia, Blood *on page 120*

Amniotic Fluid Acetylcholinesterase *see* Alpha$_1$-Fetoprotein, Amniotic Fluid *on page 114*

Amniotic Fluid Analysis for Erythroblastosis Fetalis

CPT *82143*

Related Information

Amniotic Fluid, Chromosome and Genetic Abnormality Analysis *on page 891*
Cord Blood Screen *on page 1057*
Prenatal Screen, Immunohematology *on page 1085*

Synonyms Amniotic Fluid Analysis for Hemolytic Disease of the Newborn; Amniotic Fluid Spectral Analysis; Liley Test; OD 450 Method; Spectral Analysis, Amniotic Fluid

Replaces Amniotic Fluid Bilirubin

Test Commonly Includes Delta OD 450 spectral analysis, creatinine and total bilirubin

Abstract Amniocentesis is performed in selected instances, in the presence of a maternal antibody which may cause severe hemolytic disease of the newborn.

Patient Care AFTERCARE: If the amniotic tap of an Rh negative pregnant woman is bloody, draw a maternal blood specimen an hour later for a Kleihauer test, to ascertain need for RhIG.

Specimen Amniotic fluid, 5-10 mL CONTAINER: Brown sterile plastic or glass container which is put in a larger, opaque container. Alternatively, a glass container can be wrapped with opaque tape or aluminum foil. COLLECTION: Amniocentesis performed by physician, usually after 30 weeks. Protect from light throughout. If possible collect on ice in order to allow an L/S determination, if ordered, on the same specimen. STORAGE INSTRUCTIONS: Centrifuge promptly and filter supernatant in the dark. Protect supernatant from light at 4°C. SPECIAL INSTRUCTIONS: Protect collected specimen from the light. Requisition should state date and length of pregnancy to date.

Interpretive REFERENCE RANGE: Dependent on gestational age. The useful range is only clearly defined for Rh incompatibility and is only of use in the first sensitized pregnancy. OD at 450 nm (Delta 450) of 0.0-0.20 corresponds to Freda classification of 1+, normal or only slightly affected. POSSIBLE PANIC RANGE: Delta 450 of 0.3-0.70, Freda 3+, indicates severe fetal distress and danger; >0.70, Freda 4+, indicates impending fetal death.[1] USE: Evaluate fetal jeopardy in fetal-maternal irregular antibody incompatibility (in hemolytic disease of the newborn or erythroblastosis fetalis) LIMITATIONS: False-negatives and false-positives occur. Amniotic fluid contaminated with meconium can have significant elevations due to bilirubin content. Trends from sequential determinations are used (single results may be misleading). Amniotic fluid contaminated with maternal blood can give incorrect results. Maternal urine can be aspirated instead of amniotic fluid, but urinary urea nitrogen (UUN) and creatinine of maternal urine would be many times that of amniotic fluid. Diamniotic twin pregnancies contain two sacs; each should be sampled. Hazards exist for the fetus, but in experienced hands they are limited. METHODOLOGY: Spectral analysis of centrifuged amniotic fluid using a scanning spectrophotometer. The peak at 450 nm relates to bilirubin. ADDITIONAL INFORMATION: The spectral analysis is based on the quantity of free bilirubin in amniotic fluid, which bears a relationship to the degree of hemolysis present in the fetus.[2] Useful figures are published by Huestis, Bove, and Case.[3] Amniotic fluid creatinine is useful for estimation of fetal age. The delta optical density measurement at 450 nm may be unreliable in patients with sickle cell disease.[4,5]

In the past, most cases of erythroblastosis fetalis caused by maternal antibody reacting with fetal erythrocytes were due to anti-D. With the widespread utilization of Rh immune globulin, the incidence of anti-D caused erythroblastosis fetalis has decreased. This has lead to a **relative** increase in the incidence of other antibodies, particularly other Rh antibodies and anti-Kell, as causes of hemolytic disease of the newborn. Liley curves are not as reliable in those instances.

Footnotes

1. Bauer JD, "Examination of Biologic Fluids, Sputum, and Pus," *Clinical Laboratory Methods*, 9th ed, St Louis, MO: Mosby-Year Book Inc, 1982, 750-79.
2. Dito WR, "Amniotic Fluid and Maternal Serum Assessment in Pregnancies at Risk," *Gradwohl's Clinical Laboratory Methods and Diagnosis*, 8th ed, Sonnenwirth AC and Jarett L, eds, St Louis, MO: Mosby-Year Book Inc, 1980, 469-77.
3. Huestis DW, Bove JR, and Case J, *Practical Blood Transfusion*, 4th ed, Boston, MA: Little, Brown and Co, 1988.
4. Hadi HA, Fadel HE, Nelson GH, et al, "The Unreliability of Amniotic Fluid Bilirubin Measurements in Isoimmunized Pregnancies in Sickle Cell Disease Patients," *Obstet Gynecol*, 1985, 65:758-60.
5. Lindsay MK and Lupo VR, "Nonpredictive Value of Measurements of Delta Optical Density at 450 nm in SS Disease," *Am J Obstet Gynecol*, 1985, 153:75-6.

References

Ananth U and Queenan JT, "Does Midtrimester ΔOD_{450} of Amniotic Fluid Reflect Severity of Rh Disease?" *Am J Obstet Gynecol*, 1989, 161(1):47-9.

Ananth U, Warsof SL, Coulehan JM, et al, "Midtrimester Amniotic Fluid Delta Optical Density at 450 nm in Normal Pregnancies," *Am J Obstet Gynecol*, 1986, 155:664-6.

Horger EO III and Moody LO, "Use of Indigo Carmine for Twin Amniocentesis and Its Effect on Bilirubin Analysis," *Am J Obstet Gynecol*, 1984, 150:858-60.

Kiltz RJ, Burke MS, and Porreco RP, "Amniotic Fluid Glucose Concentration as a Marker for Intra-amniotic Infection," *Obstet Gynecol*, 1991, 78(4):619-22.

Liley AW, "Liquor Amnio Analysis in the Management of the Pregnancy Complicated by Rhesus Sensitization," *Am J Obstet Gynecol*, 1961, 82:1359-70.

McDonald OL and Watts MT, "Use of Commercially Prepared Control Sera as Quality Control Materials for Spectrophotometric Bilirubin Determinations in Amniotic Fluid," *Am J Clin Pathol*, 1985, 84:513-7.

Reece EA, Cole SW, Romero R, et al, "Ultrasonography Versus Amniotic Fluid Spectral Analysis: Are They Sensitive Enough to Predict Neonatal Complications Associated With Isoimmunization?" *Obstet Gynecol*, 1989, 74(3 Pt 1):357-60.

Wenk RE and Rosenbaum JM, "Analyses of Amniotic Fluid," *Todd-Sanford-Davidsohn Clinical Diagnosis and Management by Laboratory Methods*, 18th ed, Henry JB, ed, Philadelphia, PA: WB Saunders Co, 1991, 482-96.

Amniotic Fluid Analysis for Hemolytic Disease of the Newborn *see* Amniotic Fluid Analysis for Erythroblastosis Fetalis *on previous page*

Amniotic Fluid Bilirubin *replaced by* Amniotic Fluid Analysis for Erythroblastosis Fetalis *on previous page*

Amniotic Fluid Creatinine

***CPT** 82565*

Related Information

Amniotic Fluid, Chromosome and Genetic Abnormality Analysis *on page 891*

Synonyms Creatinine, Amniotic Fluid

Specimen Amniotic fluid **CONTAINER:** Brown sterile plastic or glass bottle **STORAGE INSTRUCTIONS:** Keep on ice, protect from light. **SPECIAL INSTRUCTIONS:** Correlation of maternal serum and amniotic fluid creatinine levels is recommended.

Interpretive **REFERENCE RANGE:** >2 mg/dL (SI: >177 μmol/L) at 37th to 38th week; results >2 mg/dL indicate maturity. Concentrations of 1.6-1.8 mg/dL (SI: 141-159 μmol/L) are found at 36th week. **POSSIBLE PANIC RANGE:** Creatinine in amniotic fluid <1.6 mg/dL (SI: <141 μmol/L) bears an implication that the fetus is immature or premature,[1] <2500 g. **USE:** Estimate fetal age in concert with other parameters. Creatinine of 2 mg/dL (SI: 177 μmol/L) is an indication of maturity. This test is rarely performed. **LIMITATIONS:** Oligohydramnios, related to fetal urinary tract obstruction or to renal agenesis, or polyhydramnios, may alter the usual amniotic

(Continued)

Amniotic Fluid Creatinine *(Continued)*

fluid criteria set forth above.[1] Elevation of maternal creatinine may cause increases in the amniotic fluid creatinine level. Complications of amniocentesis may occur. **CONTRAINDICATIONS:** Fetal age must be estimated from more than a single facet. **METHODOLOGY:** Colorimetry, Jaffé reaction **ADDITIONAL INFORMATION:** Fetal lung and kidney development are related, and normal lung development is dependent on the normal development of the kidneys. Estimation of fetal kidney maturity by measuring amniotic fluid creatinine, therefore, provides an indirect assessment of fetal lung maturity. In addition to creatinine, amniotic fluid urea nitrogen has been suggested as a marker for fetal renal maturity and as a predictor of respiratory distress syndrome.[2]

Amniotic fluid protein decreases with advancing maturity: a level ≤180 mg/dL (SI: ≤1.8 g/L) supports fetal age of 36 weeks or more. Uric acid in amniotic fluid can be used to project maturity and predict the Lesch-Nyhan syndrome.[1] Amniotic fluid C-peptide has been proposed as a parameter of intrauterine growth. Most laboratories utilize amniotic fluid phosphatidylglycerol and lecithin/sphingomyelin ratio as the primary tests for assessing fetal lung maturity and do not use the creatinine measurement.

Footnotes

1. Dito WR, "Amniotic Fluid and Maternal Serum Assessment in Pregnancies at Risk," *Gradwohl's Clinical Laboratory Methods and Diagnosis*, 8th ed, Sonnenwirth AC and Jarett L, eds, St Louis, MO: Mosby-Year Book Inc, 1980, 469-77.
2. Almeida OD and Kitay DZ, "Amniotic Fluid Urea Nitrogen in the Prediction of Respiratory Distress Syndrome," *Am J Obstet Gynecol*, 1988, 159(2):465-8.

References

Darling RE and Zlatnik FJ, "Comparison of Amniotic Fluid Optical Density, L/S Ratio and Creatinine Concentration in Predicting Fetal Pulmonary Maturity," *J Reprod Med*, 1985, 30:460-4.

Raghav M, Vijay G, Chowdhary DR, et al, "Amniotic Fluid Amino Acids, Urea, Creatinine in Normal and Toxemic Pregnancies," *Indian J Med Sci*, 1985, 39:291-3.

Troccoli R, Stella C, Pachi A, et al, "Hydroxyproline and Creatinine Levels in Normal Amniotic Fluid," *Ric Clin Lab*, 1986, 16:37-41.

Tyden O, Eriksson U, Agren H, et al, "Estimation of Fetal Maturity by Amniotic Fluid Cytology, Creatinine, Lecithin/Sphingomyelin Ratio and Phosphatidylglycerol," *Gynecol Obstet Invest*, 1983, 16:317-26.

Amniotic Fluid Foam Test *see* Amniotic Fluid Pulmonary Surfactant *on page 126*

Amniotic Fluid Lecithin/Sphingomyelin Ratio and Phosphatidylglycerol

CPT *83661 (L/S ratio); 84081 (phosphatidylglycerol)*

Related Information

Amniotic Fluid, Chromosome and Genetic Abnormality Analysis *on page 891*
Amniotic Fluid Cytology *on page 482*
Amniotic Fluid Pulmonary Surfactant *on page 126*
Nile Blue Fat Stain *on page 505*

Synonyms Lecithin/Sphingomyelin Ratio; L/S Ratio

Applies to Phosphatidylglycerol; Phosphatidylinositol

Test Commonly Includes L/S ratio; may include qualitative determination of phosphatidylglycerol (PG).

Abstract Test for assessment of fetal lung maturity to attempt to ascertain the probability of development of respiratory distress syndrome.

Patient Care **AFTERCARE:** Kleihauer-Betke should be done on maternal blood after amniocentesis on Rh negative patients. If result is increased, Rh immune globulin (human) (RhIG) is recommended. Others bypass the Kleihauer-Betke after amniocentesis on Rh negative patients and directly give RhIG.

Specimen Amniotic fluid, 10 mL **CONTAINER:** Sterile brown plastic or glass tube protected from light; aluminum foil is useful **STORAGE INSTRUCTIONS:** Specimen may be light sensitive, a point for which documentation is obscure. Record color and, if present, any mucus or heavy precipitate. Centrifuge specimen only at low speed for 10 minutes and transfer supernatant to a clean glass tube. It can be stored at 4°C for up to 10 days, and it can be stored frozen indefinitely. **SPECIAL INSTRUCTIONS:** Send sample to the laboratory **immediately** after collection.

Interpretive **REFERENCE RANGE:** Mature lung: L/S ratio >2.0; borderline: L/S ratio 1.5-1.9 with risk of respiratory distress syndrome (RDS). The L/S ratio is 1.0 at 32 weeks and reaches 2.0

by 35 weeks. While sphingomyelin tends to decrease from the 32nd week, lecithin increases. Caution is necessary in interpretation of results from the diabetic patient, in whom misleading evidence for pulmonary maturity has been reported.[1] Presence of phosphatidylglycerol (PG) is evidence that the fetus is within 2-6 weeks of full-term. The incidence of respiratory distress syndrome (RDS) is very low when the L/S ratio is >2.0, in the presence of PG. **POSSIBLE PANIC RANGE:** Immature lung: L/S ratio <1.5. This level predicts RDS on delivery and bears an implication of 34 weeks or less gestation. **USE:** Attempt to prevent respiratory distress syndrome (RDS) from low surfactant in early delivery, by evaluation of fetal pulmonary maturation. Amniotic fluid test for fetal maturity; indicator to determine optimal time for obstetrical intervention in cases of possible fetal distress: maternal diabetes, toxemia, hemolytic disease of the newborn (erythroblastosis fetalis), postmaturity. **LIMITATIONS:** False-negative results (L/S <2.0 but no lung disease) occur in 5% of cases; false-positive results occur in 0.6% of cases. Fifty percent of the false-positive results occur in diabetics. Measurement of PG improves diagnostic accuracy. Maternal blood contamination of the specimen decreases the ratio. Fetal plasma contains a large amount of lecithin, and fetal blood falsely elevates the L/S ratio. Heavy contamination by meconium distorts the ratio. However, fluid contaminated by blood or meconium can still be analyzed for PG. The L/S ratio is labor intensive. Results are less objective than are many other laboratory tests and require experience in interpretation. **METHODOLOGY:** Thin-layer chromatography (TLC). PG may also be measured by immunologic and enzymatic assays.[2] **ADDITIONAL INFORMATION:** Repeat sampling weekly or in 2 weeks, as clinically indicated, when the L/S ratio indicates transitional phase of maturation (ratio 1.5-1.9). Lecithin increases sharply in amniotic fluid during the last weeks of gestation. PG appears at about 35 weeks. Phosphatidylinositol is found in amniotic fluid before phosphatidylglycerol, usually by the middle of the third trimester.[3] The following factors may increase surfactant production: maternal diabetes, toxemia, hypertension, malnutrition, placenta previa, drug addiction, premature rupture of membranes, intrauterine growth retardation, female fetus, and hemoglobinopathy. The following factors may decrease surfactant production: anemia, polyhydramnios, hypothyroidism, male fetus, twins, isoimmune disease, liver disease, renal disease, advanced maternal age, syphilis, and toxoplasmosis. A fluorescence polarization assay (TDx analyzer, Abbott Laboratories) may represent an alternate means of assessing fetal lung maturity comparable to the L/S ratio.[4,5,6] A fairly current review article is available.[6]

Footnotes

1. Ojomo EO and Coustan DR, "Absence of Evidence of Pulmonary Maturity at Amniocentesis in Term Infants of Diabetic Mothers," *Am J Obstet Gynecol*, 1990, 163(3):954-7.
2. Eisenbrey AB, Epstein E, Zak B, et al, "Phosphatidylglycerol in Amniotic Fluid. Comparison of an "Ultrasensitive" Immunologic Assay With TLC and Enzymatic Assay," *Am J Clin Pathol*, 1989, 91(3):293-7.
3. Kisabeth RM, *Mayo Medical Laboratories Test Catalog*, Rochester, MN: Mayo Medical Laboratories, 1993.
4. Ashwood ER, Tait JF, Foerder CA, et al, "Improved Fluorescence Polarization Assay for Use in Evaluating Fetal Lung Maturity. III. Retrospective Clinical Evaluation and Comparison With the Lecithin/Sphingomyelin Ratio," *Clin Chem*, 1986, 32:260-4.
5. Talt JF, Foerder CA, Ashwood ER, et al, "Prospective Clinical Evaluation of an Improved Fluorescence Polarization Assay for Predicting Fetal Lung Maturity," *Clin Chem*, 1987, 33:554-8.
6. Dubin SB, "The Laboratory Assessment of Fetal Lung Maturity," *Am J Clin Pathol*, 1992, 97(6):836-49.

References

Darling RE and Zlatnik FJ, "Comparison of Amniotic Fluid Optical Density, L/S Ratio and Creatinine Concentration in Predicting Fetal Pulmonary Maturity," *J Reprod Med*, 1985, 30:460-4.

Garite TJ, Freeman RK, and Nageotte MP, "Fetal Maturity Cascade: A Rapid and Cost-Effective Method for Fetal Lung Maturity Testing," *Obstet Gynecol*, 1986, 67:619-22.

Hallman M, Arjomaa P, Mizumoto M, et al, "Surfactant Proteins in the Diagnosis of Fetal Lung Maturity. I. Predictive Accuracy of the 35 kD Protein, the Lecithin/Sphingomyelin Ratio, and Phosphatidylglycerol," *Am J Obstet Gynecol*, 1988, 158:531-5.

Jobe A, "Amniotic Fluid Tests of Fetal Lung Maturity," *Maternal-Fetal Medicine: Principles and Practice*, 2nd ed, Creasy RK and Resnik R, eds, Philadelphia, PA: WB Saunders Co, 1989, 426-33.

Nugent CE, Ayers JW, and Menon KM, "Comparison of Amniotic Fluid Desaturated Phosphatidylcholine and the Lecithin-Sphingomyelin Ratio in the Prediction of Fetal Lung Maturity," *Obstet Gynecol*, 1986, 68:541-5.

Parker CR Jr, Leveno KJ, Milewich L, et al, "Lecithin-Sphingomyelin Ratios in Amniotic Fluid of Pregnancies With an Anencephalic Fetus," *Obstet Gynecol*, 1986, 68:546-9.

Saad SA, Fadel HE, Fahmy K, et al, "The Reliability and Clinical Use of a Rapid Phosphatidylglycerol Assay in Normal and Diabetic Pregnancies," *Am J Obstet Gynecol*, 1987, 157:1516-20.

Shaver DC, Spinnato JA, Whybrew D, et al, "Comparison of Phospholipids in Vaginal and Amniocentesis Specimens of Patients With Premature Rupture of Membranes," *Am J Obstet Gynecol*, 1987, 156:454-7.

Teng SH, Andrews AG, and Horacek I, "Rapid Enzyme Analysis of Amniotic Fluid Phospholipids Containing Choline: A Comparison With the Lecithin to Sphingomyelin Ratio in Prenatal Assessment of Fetal Lung Maturity," *J Clin Pathol*, 1985, 38:1304-8.

(Continued)

Amniotic Fluid Lecithin/Sphingomyelin Ratio and Phosphatidylglycerol *(Continued)*

Towers CV and Garite TJ, "Evaluation of the New Amniostat-FLM Test for the Detection of Phosphatidylglycerol in Contaminated Fluids," *Am J Obstet Gynecol*, 1989, 160(2):298-303.

Amniotic Fluid Pulmonary Surfactant

CPT 84999

Related Information

Amniotic Fluid, Chromosome and Genetic Abnormality Analysis *on page 891*
Amniotic Fluid Lecithin/Sphingomyelin Ratio and Phosphatidylglycerol *on page 124*
Cystic Fibrosis DNA Detection *on page 903*

Synonyms Pulmonary Surfactant; Shake Test

Applies to Amniotic Fluid Foam Test

Test Commonly Includes Semiquantitative estimate of pulmonary surfactant and fetal maturity

Abstract The assessment of fetal lung maturity is to determine the probability of development of respiratory distress syndrome, if the fetus was presently delivered. A low prevalence exists for this clinical entity.

Specimen Amniotic fluid **CONTAINER:** Clean glass or plastic tube

Interpretive **USE:** Evaluate fetal lung maturity, newborn risk for respiratory distress syndrome (hyaline membrane disease of newborn); manage high risk pregnancies, such as intrauterine growth retardation, maternal diabetes **LIMITATIONS:** Contamination of specimen with blood or meconium can falsely increase results. Falsely decreased results can occur; negative tests occur with normal lungs.[1] Although the test generally correlates with the L/S ratio, **the shake test has serious limitations**. Interpretation is subjective; blood, meconium, and vaginal fluid may interfere, and the ratio of false-negatives is high (50%). **METHODOLOGY:** Dilutions of amniotic fluid are mixed with ethanol and then shaken.[1] **ADDITIONAL INFORMATION:** The surfactant complex lowers surface tension in alveoli. It moves into amniotic fluid, a sample of which can provide projections of fetal lung maturity. An article discussed the theoretical effects of amniotic fluid volume changes on surfactant measurements.[2] Chronic oligohydramnios/polyhydramnios had minimal effect on the surfactant concentration measurement in the amniotic fluid. Acute oligohydramnios/polyhydramnios may significantly affect the amniotic fluid surfactant measurement if the acute change in volume is due to decreased/increased volume of inflow. Acute oligohydramnios/polyhydramnios due to increased/decreased volume of outflow had much less effect on the amniotic fluid surfactant measurement.

Footnotes

1. Jobe A, "Amniotic Fluid Tests of Fetal Lung Maturity," *Maternal-Fetal Medicine: Principles and Practice*, 2nd ed, Creasy RK and Resnik R, eds, Philadelphia, PA: WB Saunders Co, 1989, 426-33.
2. Nelson GH and Nelson SJ, "Theoretical Effects of Amniotic Fluid Volume Changes on Surfactant Concentration Measurements," *Am J Obstet Gynecol*, 1985, 152:870-8.

References

Dubin SB, "The Laboratory Assessment of Fetal Lung Maturity," *Am J Clin Pathol*, 1992, 97(6):836-49.

Nakamura Y, Yamamoto I, Funatsu Y, et al, "Decreased Surfactant Level in the Lung With Oligohydramnios: A Morphometric and Biochemical Study," *J Pediatr*, 1988, 112:471-4.

Sher G, Statland B, and Freer DE, "Clinical Evaluation of the Quantitative Foam Stability Index Test," *Obstet Gynecol*, 1980, 55:617-20.

Statland BE and Sher G, "Reliability of Amniotic Fluid Surfactant Measurements," *Am J Clin Pathol*, 1985, 83:382-4.

Amniotic Fluid Spectral Analysis *see* Amniotic Fluid Analysis for Erythroblastosis Fetalis *on page 122*

AMP, Cyclic, Plasma *see* Cyclic AMP, Plasma *on page 204*

AMP, Cyclic, Urine *see* Cyclic AMP, Urine *on page 204*

Amylase, Body Fluid *see* Body Fluid Amylase *on page 148*

Amylase/Creatinine Ratio *see* Amylase, Urine *on page 129*

Amylase, Peritoneal Fluid *see* Body Fluid Amylase *on page 148*

Amylase, Pleural Fluid *see* Body Fluid Amylase *on page 148*

Amylase, Serum

CPT 82150

Related Information

Amylase, Urine *on page 129*
Body Fluid Amylase *on page 148*
Lipase, Serum *on page 277*

Synonyms 1,4-α-D Glucanohydrolase, Serum

Abstract Amylase is a group of enzymes (hydrolases) from the exocrine pancreas.

Specimen Serum **CONTAINER:** Red top tube **COLLECTION:** Anticoagulants other than heparin diminish amylase activity **STORAGE INSTRUCTIONS:** Amylase is stable for 1 week at 25°C and 2 months at 4°C. **SPECIAL INSTRUCTIONS:** Dilution of lipemic sera may cause amylase values to increase.

Interpretive **REFERENCE RANGE:** 23-85 units/L. Method dependent. Newborns' serum shows little amylase activity. Much of this activity is apparently of salivary origin. Children up to 2 years of age have virtually no pancreatic isoamylase. Markedly low values may not rise to adult values until the end of the second year of life. **POSSIBLE PANIC RANGE:** Over three times the upper limit of normal for a given method probably indicates a significant increase. **USE:** Work up abdominal pain, epigastric tenderness, nausea, and vomiting. Such findings characterize acute pancreatitis as well as acute surgical emergencies such as gastrointestinal perforation (eg, peptic ulcer with perforation) or bowel infarct. Amylase is used in the differential diagnosis of acute or chronic pancreatitis, which may or may not in an individual be related to alcoholism. Hypercalcemia related to pancreatitis is described with hyperparathyroidism and other entities. About 80% of subjects with acute pancreatitis have increased serum amylase within 24 hours.[1] **LIMITATIONS:** Poor specificity. Oxalate or citrate depress results. Lipemic sera (hypertriglyceridemia) may contain inhibitors which falsely depress results. About 20% of patients with acute pancreatitis have abnormal lipids. Normal serum amylase may occur in pancreatitis, especially relapsing and chronic pancreatitis. (Subjects in whom pseudocysts complicate chronic pancreatitis often do have elevations of the pancreatic enzymes.) The entire pancreas can be destroyed in pancreatitis; in such cases serum amylase will derive from other structures (eg, the salivary glands). Urinary amylase increases often persist longer than do those of serum. High levels in alcoholics, in pregnancy, and in diabetic ketoacidosis are of salivary rather than pancreatic origin. Salivary type amylase makes up about 60% of the enzyme, while it is the pancreatic fraction that is of clinical interest.[2] The expression "salivary amylase" includes other nonpancreatic sources of the enzyme. Serum amylase is cleared by renal excretion. Serum amylase may increase one to two times upper limit of normal in renal failure without diagnostic significance. In such cases, urine amylase is normal or low. **METHODOLOGY:** Amyloclastic, saccharogenic, chromolytic; up to 200 methods exist **ADDITIONAL INFORMATION:** Causes of **high serum amylase** include acute pancreatitis, pancreatic pseudocyst, pancreatic ascites, pancreatic abscess, neoplasm in or adjacent to pancreas, trauma to pancreas, and common duct stones.

Nonpancreatic causes of hyperamylasemia include inflammatory salivary lesions (eg, mumps), perforated peptic ulcer involving pancreas or not, intestinal obstruction and infarction, afferent loop syndrome, biliary tract disease including stones, aortic aneurysm, peritonitis, acute appendicitis, cerebral trauma, burns and traumatic shock, the postoperative state (with and without pancreatitis), diabetic ketoacidosis, and extrapancreatic carcinomas (especially of esophagus, lung, ovary). Amylase levels more than 25-fold the upper limit of normal are often found when metastatic tumors produce ectopic amylase. Such levels are higher than those usually found in cases of pancreatitis.[3] In renal insufficiency amylase is usually not more than three times the upper limit of normal. Moderate increases may be reported in normal pregnancy. Increases may be found with tubo-ovarian abscess, ruptured ectopic pregnancy, macroamylasemia, and with a substantial number of drugs, including morphine. Relationships between pancreatitis and hyperlipidemias types I, IV, and V are described. Amylasemia may be associated with hyperparathyroidism.

Macroamylase is a high molecular weight material, normal amylase complexed to high molecular weight protein such as immunoglobulin. It is characterized by high serum amylase and low to normal urine amylase. Macroamylase occurs in normal as well as abnormal subjects.[4]

Other tests: In **pancreatitis**, varying percentages of patients have the following other abnormalities in varying combinations: elevation of triglyceride, alkaline phosphatase, AST (SGOT), total bilirubin, white blood cell count, left shift. Calcium levels should be followed in fulminant pancreatitis, since extremely low serum calcium levels can evolve. **Serum lipase and 2-hour**

(Continued)

Amylase, Serum *(Continued)*

urine amylase may both be extremely valuable. Although determination of serum methemalbumin has been advocated as a test for acute hemorrhagic pancreatitis, it is cumbersome and is not done in many American laboratories.

Isoenzymes of amylase exist: pancreatic and salivary type, as noted under Limitations. They can be separated by polyacrylamide gel or agarose film electrophoresis, isoelectric focusing, ion exchange chromatography, and plant isoamylase inhibitors. A monoclonal antibody approach is described.[3,5] Amylase isoenzymes are separated in few laboratories. Where available the procedure is an expensive one. It is useful in assessing the decrease of pancreatic function in cystic fibrosis, in children older than 5 years of age, who may be candidates for enzyme replacement.

Footnotes

1. McNeely MD, "Pancreatic Function," *Clinical Chemistry Theory, Analysis, and Correlation*, 2nd ed, Kaplan LA and Pesce AJ, eds, St Louis, MO: Mosby-Year Book Inc, 1989, 390-7.
2. Ellis C, Koehler DF, Eckfeldt JH, et al, "Evaluation of an Inhibitor Assay to Determine Serum Isoamylase Distribution," *Dig Dis Sci*, 1982, 27:897-901.
3. Eckfeldt JH and Levitt MD, "Diagnostic Enzymes for Pancreatic Disease," *Clin Lab Med*, 1989, 9(4):731-43.
4. Van Gossum A, "Macroamylasemia: A Biochemical or Clinical Problem?" *Dig Dis*, 1989, 7(1):19-27.
5. Warshaw AL and Hawboldt MM, "Puzzling Persistent Hyperamylasemia, Probably Neither Pancreatic Nor Pathologic," *Am J Surg*, 1988, 155(3):453-6.

References

Aderka D, Tene M, Graff E, et al, "Amylase-Creatinine Clearance Ratio: A Simple Test to Predict Gentamicin Nephrotoxicity," *Arch Intern Med*, 1988, 148:1093-6.

Agarwal N, Pitchumoni CS, and Sivaprasad AV, "Evaluating Tests for Acute Pancreatitis," *Am J Gastroenterol*, 1990, 85(4):356-66.

Barnett JL and Wilson JA, "Alcoholic Pancreatitis and Parotitis: Utility of Lipase and Urinary Amylase Clearance Determinations," *South Med J*, 1986, 79:832-5.

Borgström A and Bohe M, "Severe Acute Pancreatitis and Normal Serum Amylase Activity Due to Pancreatic Isoamylase Deficiency," *Dig Dis Sci*, 1989, 34(4):644-6.

Clavien PA, Burgan S, and Moossa AR, "Serum Enzymes and Other Laboratory Tests in Acute Pancreatitis," *Br J Surg*, 1989, 76(12):1234-43.

Dougherty SH, Saltzstein EC, Peacock JB, et al, "Rapid Resolution of High Level Hyperamylasemia as a Guide to Clinical Diagnosis and Timing of Surgical Treatment in Patients With Gallstones," *Surg Gynecol Obstet*, 1988, 166:491-6.

Dubick MA, Conteas CN, Billy HT, et al, "Raised Serum Concentrations of Pancreatic Enzymes in Cigarette Smokers," *Gut*, 1987, 28:330-5.

Eckfeldt JH and Kershaw MJ, "Hyperamylasemia Following Methyl Alcohol Intoxication: Source and Significance," *Arch Intern Med*, 1986, 146:193-4.

Feintuch TA, "Amylase: Review of Methods," *ASCP Check Sample®*, Chicago, IL: American Society of Clinical Pathologists, 1986, 2:1-12.

Gumaste VV, Dave PB, Weissman D, et al, "Lipase/Amylase Ratio. A New Index That Distinguishes Acute Episodes of Alcoholic From Nonalcoholic Acute Pancreatitis," *Gastroenterology*, 1991, 101(5):1361-6.

Hayakawa T, Kameya A, Mizuno R, et al, "Hyperamylasemia With Papillary Serous Cystadenocarcinoma of the Ovary," *Cancer*, 1984, 54:1662-5.

Humphries LL, Adams LJ, Eckfeldt JH, et al, "Hyperamylasemia in Patients With Eating Disorders," *Ann Intern Med*, 1987, 106:50-2.

Kleinman DS and O'Brien JF, "Macroamylase," *Mayo Clin Proc*, 1986, 61:669-70.

Lott JA and Lu CJ, "Lipase Isoforms and Amylase Isoenzymes: Assays and Application in the Diagnosis of Acute Pancreatitis," *Clin Chem*, 1991, 37(3):361-8.

Moss DW, Henderson AR, and Kachmar JF, "Enzymes," Tietz NW, ed, *Fundamentals of Clinical Chemistry*, 3rd ed, Philadelphia, PA: WB Saunders Co, 1987, 346.

Rattner DW, Gu Z-Y, Vlahakes GJ, et al, "Hyperamylasemia After Cardiac Surgery – Incidence, Significance, and Management," *Ann Surg*, 1989, 209(3):279-83.

Ruzena S, "Normal Serum Amylase in Acute Pancreatitis," *Dig Dis Sci*, 1989, 34(6):960-1, (letter).

Spechler ST, "How Much Can We Know About Acute Pancreatitis?" *Ann Intern Med*, 1985, 102:704-5.

Steinberg WM, Goldstein SS, Davis ND, et al, "Diagnostic Assays in Acute Pancreatitis: A Study of Sensitivity and Specificity," *Ann Intern Med*, 1985, 102:576-80.

Tietz NW and Shuey DF, "Determination of P-Type Amylase in Serum Using a Selective Inhibitor," *Lab Med*, 1986, 17:739-41.

Wilson C and Imrie CW, "Amylase and Gut Infarction," *Br J Surg*, 1986, 73:219-21.

Amylase, Urine

CPT 82150

Related Information

Amylase, Serum *on page 127*
Body Fluid Amylase *on page 148*
Lipase, Serum *on page 277*

Synonyms 1,4-α-D Glucanohydrolase, Urine

Applies to Amylase/Creatinine Ratio; Trypsin, Immunoreactive

Specimen 2-hour urine specimen is preferred **CONTAINER:** Plastic urine container, no preservative **COLLECTION:** Collect timed specimen. Instruct the patient to void at the beginning of the collection period and discard the specimen. Collect all urine including the final specimen voided at the end of the collection period. Centrifugation to provide optically clear specimen is desirable. **STORAGE INSTRUCTIONS:** Keep refrigerated. **SPECIAL INSTRUCTIONS:** Requisition should include date and time collection started, date and time collection finished.

Interpretive **REFERENCE RANGE:** 4-30 units/2 hours. Method dependent. Normals for random urine specimens have not been established. **USE:** Work up abdominal pain, epigastric tenderness, nausea, and vomiting. An enzyme with molecular weight of 45,000-55,000 daltons, increased urinary amylase is useful in the differential diagnosis of pancreatitis. It is also elevated in about 25% of patients with carcinoma of the pancreas. It is very useful in diagnosis of pseudocyst of the pancreas, in which the urine amylase may remain elevated for weeks after the serum amylase has returned to normal, after a bout of acute pancreatitis. **METHODOLOGY:** Maltopentose, other methods also available **ADDITIONAL INFORMATION:** Macroamylasemia is characterized by high serum amylase but normal urine amylase. The **amylase/creatinine ratio** remains useful for the diagnosis of macroamylasemia, but its nonspecificity has otherwise left it with few other applications. In macroamylasemia the clearance is very low.[1] Unlike serum amylase, urine amylase levels are normal with renal failure. While serum amylase usually returns to normal within 3-5 days, without complications urine amylase is increased longer than serum amylase in acute pancreatitis. Two-hour collections are more practical and provide results sooner than longer collections. The major test for pancreatitis additional to serum and urine amylase is serum lipase. It has good specificity and its laboratory analysis is greatly improved from the 1960s. Also, some patients with pancreatitis have very high triglyceride levels. **Immunoreactive trypsin** is not available stat and is not widely available at all.

Footnotes

1. Eckfeldt JH and Levitt MD, "Diagnostic Enzymes for Pancreatic Disease," *Clin Lab Med*, 1989, 9(4):731-43.

References

Bertholf RL, Winn-Deen ES, and Bruns DE, "Amylase in Urine as Measured by a Single-Step Chromolytic Procedure," *Clin Chem*, 1988, 34:754-7.

Androstenedione, Serum

CPT 82157

Related Information

Dehydroepiandrosterone Sulfate *on page 206*
Testosterone, Free and Total *on page 358*

Abstract An androgen precursor for peripheral conversion to testosterone and dihydrotestosterone.

Patient Care **PREPARATION:** Fasting morning specimen is preferred. Collect 1 week before or after menstrual period.

Specimen Serum **CONTAINER:** Red top tube **STORAGE INSTRUCTIONS:** Freeze serum. **CAUSES FOR REJECTION:** Recently administered radioisotopes

Interpretive **REFERENCE RANGE:** Male: 1-3 months: 20-45 ng/dL (SI: 0.7-1.6 nmol/L), 3-5 months: 10-40 ng/dL (SI: 0.3-1.4 nmol/L), adults: 75-125 ng/dL (SI: 2.6-4.4 nmol/L); female: 1-3 months: 15-25 ng/dL (SI: 0.5-0.9 nmol/L), 3-5 months: 10-15 ng/dL (SI: 0.3-0.5 nmol/L), adults: 110-190 ng/dL (SI: 3.8-6.6 nmol/L)[1] **POSSIBLE PANIC RANGE:** $>$1000 ng/dL (SI: $>$34.9 nmol/L) suggests a virilizing tumor **USE:** Evaluate androgen production in hirsute females; less useful in evaluation of other aspects of virilization. Very elevated in congenital adrenal hyperplasia due to C_{21}-hydroxylase deficiency. **LIMITATIONS:** Poor correlation of plasma levels with clinical severity **METHODOLOGY:** Radioimmunoassay (RIA) **ADDITIONAL INFORMATION:** Androstenedione is a major precursor in the biosynthesis of androgens and estrogens. It serves as prohormone for testosterone and estrone, particularly in menopausal females. Androstenedione is a weak testosterone produced in equal amounts by adrenal glands and ovaries in normal women.[2] The

(Continued)

Androstenedione, Serum *(Continued)*

predominant androgens in the female are androstenedione and dehydroepiandrosterone. Androstenedione is increased in cases of hirsutism, including Stein-Leventhal syndrome, and in other virilizing conditions as well as in congenital adrenal hyperplasia, Cushing's syndrome, ectopic ACTH-producing tumor, and ovarian hyperplasia of tumor. About 60% of cases of female hirsutism will show elevations of androstenedione. A marked diurnal variation exists, with a peak around 7 AM and a nadir around 4 PM. Levels rise sharply after puberty to peak at about 20 years of age. An abrupt decline occurs after menopause.

Footnotes

1. Watts NB and Keffer JH, "Adrenal Cortex," *Practical Endocrinology*, 4th ed, Philadelphia, PA: Lea & Febiger, 1989, 91-120.
2. Lipsett MB, "Androgens in the Female," *Gynecologic Endocrinology*, 3rd ed, Gold JJ and Josimovich JB, eds, Hagerstown, MD: Harper & Row Publishers, 1980, 587-93.

References

Gompel A, Wright F, Kuttenn F, et al, "Contribution of Plasma Androstenedione to 5 Alpha-Androstanediol Glucuronide in Women With Idiopathic Hirsutism," *J Clin Endocrinol Metab*, 1986, 62:441-4.

Holdaway M, Croxson MS, Frengley PA, et al, "Clinical and Biochemical Evaluation of Patients With Hirsutism," *Aust N Z J Obstet Gynaecol*, 1984, 24:23-9.

Mahlck CG, Backstrom T, Kjellgren O, et al, "Plasma Progesterone and Androstenedione in Relation to Changes in Tumor Volume and Recurrence in Women With Ovarian Carcinoma," *Gynecol Obstet Invest*, 1986, 22:157-64.

Speroff L, Glass RH, and Kase NG, *Clinical Gynecologic Endocrinology and Infertility*, 4th ed, Baltimore, MD: Williams & Wilkins, 1989.

Ylikorkala O, Stenman UH, and Halmesmaki E, "Testosterone, Androstenedione, Dehydroepiandrosterone Sulfate, and Sex-Hormone-Binding Globulin in Pregnant Alcohol Abusers," *Obstet Gynecol*, 1988, 71:731-5.

Androsterone *see* 17-Ketosteroids Fractionation, Urine *on page 267*

Angiotensin *see* Renin, Plasma *on page 346*

Angiotensin Converting Enzyme

***CPT** 82164*

Synonyms ACE; Angiotensin-I-Converting Enzyme

Applies to Angiotensin Converting Enzyme, CSF; Cerebrospinal Fluid Angiotensin Converting Enzyme

Patient Care PREPARATION: Patient need not be fasting.

Specimen Serum or plasma CONTAINER: Red top tube or green top (heparin) tube STORAGE INSTRUCTIONS: Separate serum (or plasma) immediately. Stable 1 week at 4°C, 6 months at -20°C.

Interpretive REFERENCE RANGE: 20-50 units/L USE: **High** in sarcoidosis, more often when the disease is active. Of value in assessing the response of sarcoidosis to corticosteroid therapy. Changes in serum ACE correlate with clinical status and results of gallium scans (which reflect presence and activity of inflammatory granulomatous lesions). Falling ACE level is a favorable prognostic sign. Rising levels may reflect activity uncontrolled by therapy. LIMITATIONS: Test lacks specificity and sensitivity for diagnosis of sarcoidosis. Elevations have been reported in about 35% to 80% of cases of sarcoidosis (see reference by Jordan et al for entry to the somewhat older literature on this subject). ACE levels are less likely to be increased with chronic sarcoidosis. Different admixtures of acute and chronic cases may explain some of the apparent variation in reported incidence of elevation in sarcoidosis. Elevations have been found in patients with diabetes mellitus, Gaucher's disease and leprosy. Twenty-five percent of 86 patients with acute histoplasmosis had elevated levels.[1] Increased in some patients with primary biliary cirrhosis, amyloidosis, myeloma, Melkersson-Rosenthal syndrome, some alpha$_1$-antitrypsin variants, and hyperthyroidism. It has been found increased in some cases of hyperparathyroidism and in some instances of oncogenic hypercalcemia. Thus, it is not a specific marker for the diagnosis of sarcoidosis.[2] Positives are also reported in patients with extrinsic allergic alveolitis, coccidioidomycosis, beryllium disease, asbestosis, silicosis, and alcoholic liver disease.[3] ACE activity is decreased during starvation, independent of the level of thyroid activity (as monitored by T_3 levels).[4] ACE is physiologically decreased by administration of captopril, enalapril, and lisinopril. Hemolysis and lipemia interfere with these methods. METHODOLOGY: Spectrofluorometric or radioimmunoassay (RIA), spectrophotometric utilizing synthetic substrates ADDITIONAL INFORMATION: **Other abnormalities found in**

some sarcoidosis patients include elevations of serum alkaline phosphatase, calcium, gamma globulin with polyclonal gammopathy, and hypercalciuria. Serum angiotensin converting enzyme is elevated in half of the cases of sarcoidosis but not in cases of active tuberculosis or Hodgkin's disease. Increases are less frequent when sarcoidosis is inactive.[2] Some 80% to 90% of patients with demonstrably active sarcoidosis have elevated serum ACE. Angiotensin converting enzyme activity is also increased in sarcoid lymph node homogenate. The diagnosis of sarcoidosis is an histopathologic/clinical complex. Noncaseating granulomas must be proven not to be caused by tuberculosis, histoplasmosis, or other microbiologic entities. Berylliosis is a very rare cause of such granulomas.

ACE is a dipeptidyl carboxypeptidase. It functions to split dipeptides from the free carboxy end of a variety of polypeptides including angiotensin I and bradykinin. It is especially known for its generation of the octapeptide angiotensin II by releasing the dipeptide histidyl-leucine from angiotensin I. The major site of ACE production is the pulmonary bed of endothelial cells.

Thyroid hormone may modulate ACE activity. Both patients with low T_3 levels (and clinical hypothyroidism) and patients with anorexia nervosa with associated findings of hypothyroidism may have low serum ACE activity.[5,6] Monitoring of ACE levels may have application in assessing risk of pulmonary damage due to use of some antineoplastic agents, in particular bleomycin.[7] Serum ACE is decreased in some patients with bronchogenic carcinoma. With response to chemotherapy/radiation therapy the ACE level has been noted to normalize.[8] Cerebrospinal fluid ACE is useful in patients with neurosarcoidosis.

Elevated serum ACE levels in a case of the uncommon entity, Melkersson-Rosenthal syndrome, probably relate to the sarcoid-like noncaseating granulomas that are found in this condition. ACE levels normalized after successful (clinical management) therapy with methotrexate.[9]

Serum ACE abnormality has been reported in 20% to 30% of alpha$_1$-antitrypsin variants (MZ, ZZ, and MS Pi types) but in only about 1% of individuals with normal MM Pi type.[10] There is evidence that paraquat poisoning (because of its effect on pulmonary capillary endothelium) is associated with elevated serum ACE.[11]

Footnotes

1. Ryder KW, Jay SJ, Kiblawi SO, et al, "Serum Angiotensin Converting Enzyme Activity in Patients With Histoplasmosis," *JAMA*, 1983, 249:1888-9.
2. Lufkin EG, DeRemee RA, and Rohrbach MS, "The Predictive Value of Serum Angiotensin Converting Enzyme Activity in the Differential Diagnosis of Hypercalcemia," *Mayo Clin Proc*, 1983, 58:447-51.
3. Studdy PR, Lapworth R, and Bird R, "Angiotensin Converting Enzyme and Its Clinical Significance – A Review," *J Clin Pathol*, 1983, 36:938-47.
4. Butkus NE, Burman KD, and Smallridge RC, "Angiotensin-Converting Enzyme Activity Decreases During Fasting," *Horm Metab Res*, 1987, 19:76-9.
5. Matsubayashi S, Tamai H, Kobayashi N, et al, "Angiotensin Converting Enzyme and Anorexia Nervosa," *Horm Metab Res*, 1988, 20:761-4.
6. Smallridge RC, Rogers J, and Verma PS, "Serum Angiotensin Converting Enzyme: Alterations in Hyperthyroidism, Hypothyroidism, and Subacute Thyroiditis," *JAMA*, 1983, 250:2489-93.
7. Nussinovitch N, Peleg E, Yaron A, et al, "Angiotensin Converting Enzyme in Bleomycin-Treated Patients," *Int J Clin Pharmacol Ther Toxicol*, 1988, 26:310-3.
8. Schweisfurth H, Schmidt M, Brugger E, et al, "Alterations of Serum Carboxypeptidases N and Angiotensin-I-Converting Enzyme in Malignant Diseases," *Clin Biochem*, 1985, 18:242-6.
9. Leicht S, Youngberg G, and Modica L, "Melkersson-Rosenthal Syndrome: Elevations in Serum Angiotensin Converting Enzyme and Results of Treatment With Methotrexate," *South Med J*, 1989, 82(1):74-6.
10. Lieberman J and Sastre A, "Serum Angiotensin Converting Enzyme Levels in Patients With Alpha$_1$-Antitrypsin Variants," *Am J Med*, 1986, 81:821-4.
11. Hollinger MA, Potwell SW, Zuckerman JE, et al, "Effect of Paraquat on Serum Angiotensin Converting Enzyme," *Am Rev Respir Dis*, 1980, 121:795-8.

References

Beneteau-Burnat B, Baudin B, Morgant G, et al, "Serum Angiotensin-Converting Enzyme in Healthy and Sarcoidotic Children: Comparison With the Reference Interval for Adults," *Clin Chem*, 1990, 36(2):344-6.

Jordan DR, Anderson RL, Nerad JA, et al, "The Diagnosis of Sarcoidosis," *Can J Ophthalmol*, 1988, 23:203.

Kessler G, "Angiotensin Converting Enzyme," *Methods in Clinical Chemistry*, Chapter 123, Pesce AJ and Kaplan LA, eds, St Louis, MO: Mosby-Year Book Inc, 1987, 935-43.

Lieberman J, "Enzymes in Sarcoidosis: Angiotensin Converting Enzyme (ACE)," *Clin Lab Med*, 1989, 9(4):745-55.

Sharma OP, "Sarcoidosis," *Dis Mon*, 1990, 36(9):469-535.

Seidman MD, Lewandowski CA, Sarpa JR, et al, "Angioedema Related to Angiotensin-Converting Enzyme Inhibitors," *Otolaryngol Head Neck Surg*, 1990, 102(6):727-31.

Silverstein F, Fierst SM, Simon MR, et al, "Angiotensin Converting Enzyme in Crohn's Disease and Ulcerative Colitis," *Am J Clin Pathol*, 1981, 75:175-8.

(Continued)

Angiotensin Converting Enzyme *(Continued)*

Thomas PD and Hunninghake GW, "Current Concepts of the Pathogenesis of Sarcoidosis," *Am Rev Respir Dis*, 1987, 135:747-60.

Thompson AB, Cale WF, and Lapp NL, "Serum Angiotensin-Converting Enzyme Is Elevated in Association With Underground Coal Mining," *Chest*, 1991, 100(4):1042-5.

Angiotensin Converting Enzyme, CSF *see* Angiotensin Converting Enzyme *on page 130*

Angiotensin-I-Converting Enzyme *see* Angiotensin Converting Enzyme *on page 130*

Anion Gap

CPT *84999*

Related Information

Alcohol, Blood or Urine *on page 936*
Chloride, Serum *on page 182*
Electrolytes, Blood *on page 212*
Ethylene Glycol *on page 965*
HCO_3, Blood *on page 248*
Ketone Bodies, Blood *on page 265*
Ketones, Urine *on page 1128*
Lactic Acid, Blood *on page 273*
Osmolality, Calculated *on page 299*
pH, Blood *on page 315*
Salicylate *on page 999*
Sodium, Blood *on page 349*
Urinalysis *on page 1162*
Volatile Screen *on page 1010*

Synonyms Electrolyte Gap; Gap; Ion Gap

Applies to Urinary Anion Gap

Test Commonly Includes A calculation from electrolytes, sodium, potassium, HCO_3^-, and chloride to ascertain quantities of unmeasured cations and anions

Abstract The anion gap is useful in evaluation of patients with acid-base abnormalities. The sum of anions and cations must be equal in the blood.

Specimen Serum **CONTAINER:** Red top tube

Interpretive **REFERENCE RANGE:** 6-16 mmol/L (SI: 6-16 mmol/L); slight differences may be established in different laboratories. Electrolytes until recently were done mostly by flame photometry. As ion-selective electrodes have come into wider use, reference ranges for anion gap will probably change.[1] **USE:** Extensively used for quality control in the laboratory, the widest clinical application of the anion gap is in the diagnosis of types of metabolic acidosis. Unmeasured cations include Ca^{2+} and Mg^{2+}. Unmeasured anions include protein, PO_4^{3-}, SO_4^{2-}, and organic acids.[2] Organic acidosis includes lactic acidosis and ketoacidosis.

A marked elevation of anion gap, >30 mmol/L, bears a strong implication of metabolic acidosis.[3] Increased anion gaps are found in states such as renal failure and toxic ingestions. Above 30 mmol/L gap increase is commonly secondary to lactic acidosis or ketoacidosis but can be caused also by rhabdomyolysis or nonketotic hyperglycemic coma.

In diabetic ketoacidosis plasma glucose is high, often much >300 mg/dL (SI: >16.7 mmol/L), pH is <7.3, and ketones are found in blood and urine. Increased serum osmolality and increased calculated osmolality (osmolar gap) are found, and serum sodium is often decreased.

In alcoholic ketoacidosis glucose may be increased, normal or low, but a high alcohol level may be found, and amylase and uric acid may be increased.

LIMITATIONS: Minor differences in formula are used by different laboratories. A spurious increase may follow excessive exposure of the sample to room air as well as underfilling the Vacutainer® tube.[4] Some gaps remain unexplained. All metabolic abnormalities are not detected by abnormal gaps (eg, isopropanol ingestion is accompanied by normal gap, but ketone bodies are positive). There are a number of causes of normal anion gap acidosis associated with hyperchloremia. Anion gap is unsuitable as a quick screen for lactic acidosis. Still useful, the anion gap should not replace assay for lactate, creatinine, ketone bodies, or osmolality. In one study, only 66% of patients with an anion gap of 20-29 mmol/L could be proven to have an organic acidosis.[1] **METHODOLOGY:** Calculation: (Na^+ + K^+) – (Cl^- + HCO_3^-) or Na^+ – (Cl^- + HCO_3^-) = anion gap; actually determined by the difference between concentrations of anions and cations. **ADDITIONAL INFORMATION:** Anion gap represents approximately the sum of the unmeasured anions charges of which with Cl^- and HCO_3^-, balance Na^+. (Measured anions are chloride and bicarbonate. Measured cations are sodium.)

Anion gap high ("unmeasured anions"): With **pH high:** extracellular volume contraction; massive transfusion (with renal failure and/or volume contraction); carbenicillin, penicillin (large doses), salts of organic acids such as citrate. With **pH low:** uremia: most common cause; abnormal anion gap in uremia is usually seen only when creatinine is >4.0 mg/dL (SI: >354 μmol/L). Uremic acidosis is rare without hyperphosphatemia. Nonketotic hyperglycemic coma and rhabdomyolysis may cause high anion gap metabolic acidosis. Lactic acidosis and diabetic or alcoholic ketoacidosis characteristically fall into this group. With **normal osmolal gap**: salicylate and paraldehyde toxicity; with **increased osmolal gap**: methanol and ethylene glycol toxicity.

High anion gap metabolic acidosis without elevated lactic acid or acetone; consider: ketoacidosis with negative or slightly positive "acetone" if patient is hypoxic and/or has alcoholic ketoacidosis, such ketoacidosis may be life-threatening;[3] salicylate toxicity; methanol toxicity (paint thinners); ethylene glycol toxicity (antifreeze) – urinary sediment contains abundant calcium oxalate and/or hippurate crystals; paraldehyde intoxication (may have positive ketone reactions); toluene toxicity[5] (transmission fluid, paint thinner inhalation or sniffing).

Anion gap low: Caused by retained unmeasured anions. Most common cause is hypoalbuminemia (eg, in nephrosis, cirrhosis), dilution, hypernatremia, very marked hypercalcemia, very severe hypermagnesemia, IgG myeloma and polyclonal gamma globulin increases[6] – hyperviscosity with certain lab instruments, lithium toxicity, bromism (low anion gap may not be present). Decreased anion gap with spurious hyperchloremia and with hyponatremia is reported in hyperlipidemia.[7] Dilution of extracellular fluid may cause a decreased gap.[8] The finding of a low anion gap is perceived as an unreliable diagnostic parameter and may indicate potential laboratory error.[1]

Normal anion gap may occur with **metabolic acidosis,** causes have been published.[3] They include diarrhea, renal tubular acidosis, hyperalimentation, ureteroileostomy, ureterosigmoidostomy, external drainage of pancreaticobiliary fluids, NH_4Cl and other drugs.

The urinary anion gap is used in the diagnosis of hyperchloremic metabolic acidosis[9] and evaluation of renal potassium wasting.[10]

Footnotes

1. Badrick T and Hickman PE, "The Anion Gap: A Reappraisal," *Am J Clin Pathol*, 1992, 98(2):249-52.
2. Oh MS and Carroll HJ, "The Anion Gap," *N Engl J Med*, 1977, 297:814-7.
3. Emmett M and Narins RG, "Clinical Use of the Anion Gap," *Medicine (Baltimore)*, 1977, 56:38-54.
4. Herr RD and Swanson T, "Pseudometabolic Acidosis Caused by Underfill of Vacutainer® Tubes," *Ann Emerg Med*, 1992, 21(2):177-80.
5. Fischman CM and Oster JR, "Toxic Effects of Toluene: A New Cause of High Anion Gap Metabolic Acidosis," *JAMA*, 1979, 241:1713-5.
6. Keshgegian AA, "Anion Gap and Immunoglobulin Concentration," *Am J Clin Pathol*, 1980, 74:282-4.
7. Graber ML, Quigg RJ, et al, "Spurious Hyperchloremia and Decreased Anion Gap in Hyperlipidemia," *Ann Intern Med*, 1983, 98:607-9.
8. Preuss HG, "Fundamentals of Clinical Acid-Base Evaluation," *Clin Lab Med*, 1993, 13(1):103-16.
9. Batlle DC, Hizon M, Cohen E, et al, "The Use of the Urinary Anion Gap in the Diagnosis of Hyperchloremic Metabolic Acidosis," *N Engl J Med*, 1988, 318(10):594-9.
10. Oster JR, Perez GO, and Materson BJ, "Use of the Anion Gap in Clinical Medicine," *South Med J*, 1988, 81(2):229-37.

References

Adams SL, "Alcoholic Ketoacidosis," *Emerg Med Clin North Am*, 1990, 8(4):749-60.

Baker RJ, "Biochemical Gaps: Osmolal and Anion," *Curr Surg*, 1987, 44:378-81.

Cembrowski GS, Westgard JO, and Kurtycz DF, "Use of the Anion Gap for the Quality Control of Electrolyte Analyzers," *Am J Clin Pathol*, 1983, 79:688-96.

Hertford JA, McKenna JP, and Chamovitz BN, "Metabolic Acidosis With an Elevated Anion Gap," *Am Fam Physician*, 1989, 39(4):159-68.

Holroyd K and Brown E, *N Engl J Med*, 1988, 319:586, (letter).

Rothenberg DM, Berns AS, Barkin R, et al, "Bromide Intoxication Secondary to Pyridostigmine Bromide Therapy," *JAMA*, 1990, 263(8):1121-2.

Wrenn K, "The Delta (Delta) Gap: An Approach to Mixed Acid-Base Disorders," *Ann Emerg Med*, 1990, 19(11):1310-3.

(Continued)

Anion Gap *(Continued)*

Wrenn KD, Slovis CM, Minion GE, et al, "The Syndrome of Alcoholic Ketoacidosis," *Am J Med*, 1991, 91(2):119-28.

Wrong OM, "Urinary Anion Gap in Hyperchloremic Metabolic Acidosis," *N Engl J Med*, 1988, 319:585-6, (letter).

Apo A-I *see* Apolipoprotein A and B *on this page*

Apo B *see* Apolipoprotein A and B *on this page*

Apolipoprotein A and B

CPT *82172*

Related Information

Cholesterol *on page 185*
High Density Lipoprotein Cholesterol *on page 249*
Lipid Profile *on page 278*
Lipoprotein (a) *on page 280*
Low Density Lipoprotein Cholesterol *on page 284*
Triglycerides *on page 370*

Synonyms Apo A-I; Apo B; Apolipoprotein A-I

Patient Care **PREPARATION:** Patient must be fasting 12-14 hours.

Specimen Serum **CONTAINER:** Red top tube **STORAGE INSTRUCTIONS:** Separate serum and refrigerate. **Do not freeze.** Stable 1 week at 4°C. **CAUSES FOR REJECTION:** Specimen from nonfasting patient, frozen specimen

Interpretive **REFERENCE RANGE:** Apolipoprotein A: male: 66-151 mg/dL, female: 75-170 mg/dL; apolipoprotein B: male: 49-123 mg/dL, female: 26-119 mg/dL **USE:** Evaluate the risk of coronary artery disease **METHODOLOGY:** Nephelometry (preferred), turbidimetry. Apo A and Apo B have recently been standardized, and all commercial assays should conform to the new calibrator standards.[1] The precision of the nephelometric assays is superior (2% to 3% CV). **ADDITIONAL INFORMATION:** Apolipoprotein is the protein component of a lipoprotein complex. Apolipoprotein A is the main component of HDL, chylomicrons, and VLDL. Measurement of apolipoprotein A is more useful than the measurement of HDL in predicting patients with high risk of coronary artery disease. Levels of apolipoprotein A are inversely correlated with the risk of premature coronary artery disease. Apolipoprotein B is the major component of low density lipoproteins. The relative proportion of apolipoprotein B to apolipoprotein A is more effective in differentiating those with or without ischemic heart disease than the measurement of lipid or lipoprotein cholesterol. An adverse Apo B/Apo A profile at a young age is potentially a marker for coronary heart disease.

Footnotes

1. Albers JJ and Marcovina SM, "Standardization of Apolipoprotein B and A-I Measurements," *Clin Chem*, 1989, 35(7):1357-61.

References

Boerwinkle E, Brown SA, Rohrbach K, et al, "Role of Apolipoprotein E and B Gene Variation in Determining Response of Lipid, Lipoprotein, and Apolipoprotein Levels to Increased Dietary Cholesterol," *Am J Hum Genet*, 1991, 49(6):1145-54.

Genest JJ Jr, Bard JM, Fruchart JC, et al, "Plasma Apolipoprotein A-I, A-II, B, E, and C-III Containing Particles in Men With Premature Coronary Artery Disease," *Atherosclerosis*, 1991, 90(2-3):149-57.

Paulweber B, Friedl W, Krempler F, et al, "Association of DNA Polymorphism at the Apolipoprotein B Gene Locus With Coronary Heart Disease and Serum Very Low Density Lipoprotein Levels," *Arteriosclerosis*, 1990, 10(1):17-24.

Shephard MD, Hester J, Walmsley RN, et al, "Variation in Plasma Apolipoprotein A-1 and B Concentrations Following Myocardial Infarction," *Ann Clin Biochem*, 1990, 27(Pt 1):9-14.

Walmsley TA, Grant S, and George PM, "Effect of Plasma Triglyceride Concentrations on the Accuracy of Immunoturbidimetric Assays of Apolipoprotein B," *Clin Chem*, 1991, 37(5):748-53.

Williams KJ, Petrie KA, Brocia RW, et al, "Lipoprotein Lipase Modulates Net Secretory Output of Apolipoprotein B *In Vitro*. A Possible Pathophysiologic Explanation for Familial Combined Hyperlipidemia," *J Clin Invest*, 1991, 88(4):1300-6.

Young SG, "Recent Progress in Understanding Apolipoprotein B," *Circulation*, 1990, 82(5):1574-94.

Apolipoprotein A-I *see* Apolipoprotein A and B *on this page*

Arterial-Ascitic Fluid pH Gradient *see* Body Fluid pH *on page 150*

Arterial Blood Gases *see* Blood Gases, Arterial *on page 140*

Arylamidase *see* Leucine Aminopeptidase *on page 276*
Arylamidase Naphthylamidase *see* Leucine Aminopeptidase *on page 276*
Ascitic Fluid Analysis *see* Body Fluid *on page 145*

Ascorbic Acid, Blood

CPT 82180

Synonyms Vitamin C

Patient Care PREPARATION: Patient should be fasting.

Specimen Plasma, serum, or leukocytes, or urine following a loading test; Lee et al write that the fundamental question is what ought to be measured.[1] CONTAINER: Green top (heparin) tube preferred; red top tube, lavender top (EDTA) tube, or gray top (sodium fluoride) tube also acceptable; check with the laboratory. COLLECTION: Draw blood in chilled tube. Keep specimen on ice. STORAGE INSTRUCTIONS: Freeze separated plasma (serum). Stable 30 minutes at 25°C. Stable 4 days at -20°C. CAUSES FOR REJECTION: Specimen not frozen

Interpretive REFERENCE RANGE: Plasma or serum: 0.6-2.0 mg/dL (SI: 34-114 μmol/L); leukocytes: 20-50 μg/10^8 WBC CRITICAL VALUES: <0.3 mg/dL (SI: <17 μmol/L) in plasma provides evidence for least the risk of deficiency and <0.2 mg/dL (SI: <11 μmol/L) indicates deficiency USE: Evaluate vitamin C deficiency CONTRAINDICATIONS: Ascorbic acid therapy METHODOLOGY: High performance liquid chromatography (HPLC), acidic 2,4-dinitrophenylhydrazine[2] ADDITIONAL INFORMATION: Plasma or serum levels of vitamin C are an adequate measurement of clinical status, although leukocyte levels are superior but more difficult to obtain. Vitamin C is a cofactor for protocollagen hydroxylase; it promotes the conversion of tropocollagen to collagen.[3] Low values occur in scurvy, malabsorption, alcoholism, pregnancy, hyperthyroidism, and renal failure. Smokers have lower levels than nonsmokers. Patients with scurvy have values <0.2 mg/dL (SI: <11 μmol/L). Principal clinical findings in scurvy include bleeding gums, petechiae, follicular hyperkeratosis, perifollicular hemorrhages beginning on the lower thighs, muscle aches, easy fatiguability, and emotional changes.

Footnotes

1. Lee W, Davis KA, Rettmer RL, et al, "Ascorbic Acid Status: Biochemical and Clinical Considerations," *Am J Clin Nutr*, 1988, 48(2):286-90.
2. Leavelle DE, *Mayo Medical Laboratories Interpretive Handbook*, Rochester, MN: Mayo Medical Laboratories, 1990.
3. McCormick DB, "Vitamins," *Fundamentals of Clinical Chemistry*, 3rd ed, Tietz NW, ed, Philadelphia, PA: WB Saunders Co, 1987, 497-516.

References

Basu J, Vermund SH, Mikhail M, et al, "Plasma Reduced and Total Ascorbic Acid in Healthy Women: Effects of Smoking and Oral Contraception," *Contraception*, 1989, 39(1):85-93.

Garry PJ, Vanderjagt DJ, and Hunt WC, "Ascorbic Acid Intakes and Plasma Levels in Healthy Elderly," *Ann N Y Acad Sci*, 1987, 498:90-9.

Henson DE, Block G, and Levine M, "Ascorbic Acid: Biologic Functions and Relation to Cancer," *J Natl Cancer Inst*, 1991, 83(8):547-50.

Jacob RA, Otradovec CL, Russell RM, et al, "Vitamin C Status and Nutrient Interactions in a Healthy Elderly Population," *Am J Clin Nutr*, 1988, 48:1436-42.

Levine M, Dhariwal KR, Washko PW, et al, "Ascorbic Acid and In Situ Kinetics: A New Approach to Vitamin Requirements," *Am J Clin Nutr*, 1991, 54(6 Suppl):1157S-1162S.

Schorah CJ, Bishop N, Wales JK, et al, "Blood Vitamin C Concentrations in Patients With Diabetes Mellitus," *Int J Vitam Nutr Res*, 1988, 58:312-8.

Vanderjagt DJ, Garry PJ, and Bhagavan HN, "Ascorbic Acid Intake and Plasma Levels in Healthy Elderly People," *Am J Clin Nutr*, 1987, 46:290-4.

Zilva JF and Pannall PR, *Clinical Chemistry in Diagnosis and Treatment*, 4th ed, Chicago, IL: Year Book Medical Publishers Inc, 1985, 451-3.

Aspartate Aminotransferase

CPT 84450

Related Information

Alanine Aminotransferase *on page 100*
Lactate Dehydrogenase *on page 269*

Synonyms AST; Glutamic Oxaloacetic Transaminase, Serum; GOT; L-Aspartate: 2-Oxoglutarate Aminotransferase; SGOT; Transaminase

Applies to Aminotransferases

Replaces Cephalin Flocculation; Thymol Turbidity

(Continued)

Aspartate Aminotransferase *(Continued)*

Specimen Serum **CONTAINER:** Red top tube **STORAGE INSTRUCTIONS:** Stable 3 days at 25°C and 1 week at 4°C; fairly stable refrigerated or frozen. **CAUSES FOR REJECTION:** Hemolysis

Interpretive **REFERENCE RANGE:** Levels in infancy are two to three times those found in adults. Ranges decrease during childhood years. Typical adult reference range: 8-45 units/L. AST reference values are higher in males. **USE:** A wide range of disease entities alters AST (SGOT), with origin from many organs. When an increased AST is from the liver, it is more likely to relate to disease of the hepatocyte. Other enzymes, including alkaline phosphatase and GGT, are more sensitive indicators of biliary obstruction.

Causes of low AST: uremia, vitamin B_6 deficiency (this can be corrected), metronidazole, trifluoperazine.

Causes of high AST: chronic alcohol ingestion, not limited to overt chronic alcoholism; cirrhosis. In alcoholic hepatitis, AST values usually are <300 units/L. In viral hepatitis, look for high AST/LD (LDH) ratio, >3, and very high AST peaking at 500-3000 units/L in acute viral hepatitis (ie, in clinical acute viral hepatitis the transaminases may be increased ten times or more above their upper limits of normal). AST increases are found in other types of liver disease, including earlier stages of hemochromatosis and chemical injury, (eg, necrosis related to toxins such as carbon tetrachloride). Some instances of cholecystitis cause increased AST.

AST and ALT (SGPT) are increased in Reye's syndrome.[1,2] In infectious mononucleosis, LD (LDH) is commonly considerably higher than AST. Trauma (including head trauma and including surgery) and other striated muscle diseases, including dystrophy, dermatomyositis, trichinosis, polymyositis, and gangrene cause AST increases. Both AST and ALT elevations are found with Duchenne's muscular dystrophy. Look for high CK in myositis, high LD_5 (or isomorphic pattern in some instances of polymyositis) on LD isoenzymes.

In myocardial infarction AST peaks about 24 hours after infarct and returns to normal 3-7 days later. In acute MI without shock or heart failure, ALT is not apt to increase significantly. AST increases in congestive failure with centrilobular liver congestion, in which high LD_5 on LD isoenzymes is found, and in pericarditis, myocarditis, pancreatitis, and other inflammatory states including Legionnaires' disease. In renal infarction LD is usually high, out of proportion to AST.[3] Lung infarction and other disease entities leading to necrosis including large, necrotic tumors cause increased AST; LD is commonly also increased in such instances. Shock (LD also usually increased); hypothyroidism (LD and/or CK not infrequently increased in myxedema); hemolytic anemias (LD high with increased LD_1) and certain CNS diseases may increase AST.

Very high AST levels usually are caused by liver disease and/or by shock.

Drugs: A large number of commonly used drugs have been reported to elevate AST: isoniazid, phenothiazines, erythromycin, progesterone, anabolic-androgenic steroids, halothane, methyldopa, opiates, indomethacin, salicylates in children, and other drugs. Hepatotoxicity from drugs may cause high aminotransferase activity with elevation of AST/ALT ratio.[4]

Acetaminophen hepatotoxicity deserves special mention. In alcoholics, apparently moderate doses of the analgesic have caused severe hepatotoxicity. Doses of 2.6-16.5 g/24 hours are reported with total bilirubin 1.3-23.9 mg/dL (SI: 22-409 μmol/L), AST 1,960-29,700 units/L, and ALT 12,000-12,550 units/L. The characteristic pattern included mild to severe coagulopathy and AST greater than ALT by a considerable margin.[5]

Macroenzyme causing unexplained increase of AST is described with normal levels of CK and ALT.[6]

LIMITATIONS: Only gross hemolysis may cause falsely high values. **METHODOLOGY:** Spectrophotometry, kinetic assay, malate dehydrogenase; like ALT, AST can be measured at 25°C, 30°C, 32°C, and 37°C.[4] **ADDITIONAL INFORMATION:** AST has origin from heart, liver, skeletal muscle, kidney, pancreas, spleen, and lung. Very high values, >500 units/L, usually suggest hepatitis or other kinds of hepatocellular necrosis but can also be found with large necrotic tumors, other types of necrosis or extensive hypoxia, congestive failure, and shock. Unexplained AST elevations should first be investigated with ALT and GGT. Mitochondrial AST (m-AST) may be useful in the diagnosis of alcoholic liver disease; it is reviewed by Rej.[4]

Footnotes

1. Lichtenstein PK, Heubi JE, Daugherty CC, et al, "Grade I Reye's Syndrome. A Frequent Cause of Vomiting and Liver Dysfunction After Varicella and Upper Respiratory Tract Infection," *N Engl J Med*, 1983, 309:133-9.
2. DeVivo DC, "How Common Is Reye's Syndrome?" *N Engl J Med*, 1983, 309:179-81, (editorial).

3. Winzelberg GG, Hull JD, Agar JW, et al, "Elevation of Serum Lactate Dehydrogenase Levels in Renal Infarction," *JAMA*, 1979, 242:268-9.
4. Rej R, "Aminotransferase in Disease," *Clin Lab Med*, 1989, 9(4):667-87.
5. Seeff LB, Cuccherini BA, Zimmerman HJ, et al, "Acetaminophen Hepatotoxicity in Alcoholics," *Ann Intern Med*, 1986, 104:399-404.
6. Litin SC, O'Brien JF, Pruett S, et al, "Macroenzyme as a Cause of Unexplained Elevation of Aspartate Aminotransferase," *Mayo Clin Proc*, 1987, 62:681-7.

References

Faulkner WR, "Best First Tests for Reye Syndrome," *Lab Report for Physicians*, 1987, 9:76-8.

Rosenthal P and Haight M, "Aminotransferase as a Prognostic Index in Infants With Liver Disease," *Clin Chem*, 1990, 36(2):346-8.

Rotenberg Z, Weinberger I, Davidson E, et al, "Does Determination of Serum Aspartate Aminotransferase Contribute to the Diagnosis of Acute Myocardial Infarction?" *Am J Clin Pathol*, 1989, 91(1):91-4.

Schölmerich J, Gross V, Johannesson T, et al, "Detection of Biliary Origin of Acute Pancreatitis. Comparison of Laboratory Tests, Ultrasound, Computed Tomography, and ERCP," *Dig Dis Sci*, 1989, 34(6):830-3.

Vincent-Viry M and Delwaide P, "Aspartate Aminotransferase and Alanine Aminotransferase," *Drug Effects on Laboratory Test Results Analytical Interferences and Pharmacological Effects*, Siest G and Galteau MM, eds, Littleton, MA: PSG Publishing Co Inc, 1988, 91-130.

Williams AL and Hoofnagle JH, "Ratio of Serum Aspartate to Alanine Aminotransferase in Chronic Hepatitis. Relationship to Cirrhosis," *Gastroenterology*, 1988, 95:734-9.

AST *see* Aspartate Aminotransferase *on page 135*

AST/ALT Ratio *see* Cardiac Enzymes/Isoenzymes *on page 170*

Baby Bilirubin *see* Bilirubin, Neonatal *on next page*

Base Excess *see* Delta Base, Blood *on page 208*

Beta-Carotene *see* Carotene, Serum *on page 172*

Beta-Hydroxybutyrate *see* Ketone Bodies, Blood *on page 265*

Beta Lipoproteins *see* Low Density Lipoprotein Cholesterol *on page 284*

Beta Subunit, hCG *see* Human Chorionic Gonadotropin, Serum *on page 254*

Beta-Subunit Human Chorionic Gonadotropin Urine or Serum *see* Pregnancy Test *on page 333*

Beutler Test *see* Galactose Screening Tests for Galactosemia *on page 228*

Bicarbonate *see* HCO_3, Blood *on page 248*

Bilirubin, Conjugated *see* Bilirubin, Direct *on this page*

Bilirubin, Direct

CPT *82250*

Related Information

Bile, Urine *on page 1111*

Urobilinogen, 2-Hour Urine *on page 1167*

Synonyms Bilirubin, Conjugated; Direct Bilirubin

Specimen Serum **CONTAINER:** Red top tube, red top Microtainer™ for babies **COLLECTION:** Pediatrics: Blood drawn from a heelstick **STORAGE INSTRUCTIONS:** Store in refrigerator. **Protect from light**. **CAUSES FOR REJECTION:** Specimen not protected from light, gross hemolysis **SPECIAL INSTRUCTIONS:** Transport promptly.

Interpretive **REFERENCE RANGE:** Newborns: varies with age in days, prematurity vs maturity; adults: ≤0.4 mg/dL (SI: ≤7 μmol/L) **USE:** Evaluate liver and biliary disease. Increased direct bilirubin occurs with biliary diseases, including both intrahepatic and extrahepatic lesions. Hepatocellular causes of elevation include hepatitis, cirrhosis, and advanced neoplastic states. Increased with cholestatic drug reactions, Dubin-Johnson syndrome, and Rotor syndrome. In the latter two syndromes, the level is usually <5 mg/dL. **LIMITATIONS:** Cord blood samples may yield elevated values. Visibly hemolyzed samples may yield spurious results. **CONTRAINDICATIONS:** Measurement of direct bilirubin is usually not necessary when the total bilirubin is <1.2 mg/dL (SI: <21 μmol/L). **METHODOLOGY:** Diazo reaction, high performance liquid chromatography (HPLC) **ADDITIONAL INFORMATION:** Theoretically, direct bilirubin should not be increased in hemolytic anemias, in which bilirubin increase should be in the indirect bilirubin fraction in the absence of complications. In practice, some increase in the direct fraction may be encountered in patients with hemolytic anemia in whom complications have not been proven. Some

(Continued)

Bilirubin, Direct *(Continued)*

methods have shown the direct bilirubin to be spuriously high. This may be due to different concentrations of sodium nitrite, which may convert some of the unconjugated bilirubin to conjugated bilirubin.[1,2] Direct bilirubin is the water soluble fraction. When conjugated bilirubin is increased in serum, bilirubin should become positive in the urine. Physiologic jaundice, occurring 2-4 days after birth, is due to lack of liver glucuronyl transferase.

Footnotes

1. Chan KM, Scott MG, Wu TW, et al, "Inaccurate Values for Direct Bilirubin With Some Commonly Used Direct Bilirubin Procedures," *Clin Chem*, 1985, 31:1560-3.
2. Mair B and Klempner LB, "Abnormally High Values for Direct Bilirubin in the Serum of Newborns as Measured With the Du Pont aca®," *Am J Clin Pathol*, 1987, 87:642-4.

References

Franquemont DW, Sutphen JL, Herold DA, et al, "Characterization of Sulfasalazine's Interference in the Measurement of Conjugated Bilirubin by the Ektachem® Slide Method," *Clin Chem*, 1989, 35(8):1760-2.

Newman TB, Hope S, and Stevenson DK, "Direct Bilirubin Measurements in Jaundiced Term Newborns. A Reevaluation," *Am J Dis Child*, 1991, 145(11):1305-9.

Rosenthal P, Keefe MT, Henton D, et al, "Total and Direct-Reacting Bilirubin Values by Automated Methods Compared With Liquid Chromatography and With Manual Methods for Determining Delta Bilirubin," *Clin Chem*, 1990, 36(5):788-91.

Bilirubin, Neonatal

***CPT** 82250*

Related Information

Antiglobulin Test, Indirect *on page 1051*

Cord Blood Screen *on page 1057*

Hemolytic Disease of the Newborn, Antibody Identification *on page 1070*

Synonyms Baby Bilirubin; Microbilirubin; Total Bilirubin, Neonatal

Specimen Serum **CONTAINER:** Microbilirubin tube **COLLECTION:** Draw blood from heel using capillary pipette. **STORAGE INSTRUCTIONS:** Protect sample from light; bilirubin is photosensitive.

Interpretive REFERENCE RANGE: Normal range depends on whether baby is premature or term, and age in days. See table. **POSSIBLE PANIC RANGE:** >15.0 mg/dL (SI: >257 μmol/L) in term infants, 10.0-15.0 mg/dL (SI: 171-257 μmol/L) in premature babies **USE:** Monitor erythroblastosis fetalis (hemolytic disease of the newborn), which usually causes jaundice in the first 2 days of life.[1] Other causes of neonatal jaundice include physiologic jaundice, hematoma/hemorrhage, hypothyroidism, Crigler-Najjar syndrome, and obstructive jaundice. Time sequences and differential diagnosis have been outlined.[1] **LIMITATIONS:** Only total bilirubin is measured with "neonatal bilirubin." Procedure is not utilized for patients older than 10 days of age due to formation of endogenous carotenoids. Ten percent fat emulsion has been reported to interfere with neonatal bilirubin measurement.[2] **CONTRAINDICATIONS:** Request regular total bilirubin for infants older than 10 days of age. **METHODOLOGY:** Spectrophotometric, direct (bichromatic) **ADDITIONAL INFORMATION:** Erythroblastosis fetalis occurs from Rh_o(D), other Rh antibodies, ABO incompatibility, and antibodies involving additional blood groups (including Kidd, Kell, Duffy, and others).

Bilirubin, Neonatal
Upper Reference Limit (mg/dL)

Age	Premature	Full-Term
Cord	2.9	2.5
<24h	8.0	6.0
<48 h	12.0	10.0
3–5 d	15.0	12.0
7 d	15.0	10.0

Note: At 7 days, occasional premature infants may develop kernicterus at 10.0–12.0 mg/dL of bilirubin.

Causes of neonatal jaundice also include galactosemia, sepsis, syphilis, toxoplasmosis, cytomegalovirus, and rubella. Red cell enzyme problems include G-6-PD and pyruvate kinase deficiencies. Spherocytosis can lead to neonatal icterus.[3]

Drugs may displace bilirubin from albumin. It is the so-called "free" form of bilirubin, thus displaced, which crosses the blood-brain barrier.[4]

Jaundice may also be seen in babies who are breast feeding. Mothers sometimes want to stop breast feeding because of such jaundice. They should not be encouraged to cease breast feeding prematurely.[5]

Phototherapy reduces the need for exchange transfusions in premature babies who are Coombs' negative. In infants who weigh more than 2500 g and who are Coombs' positive, phototherapy was not significantly beneficial over control babies, and did not reduce the need for exchange transfusions.[6]

Footnotes

1. Thaler MM, "Jaundice in the Newborn," *Using the Clinical Laboratory in Medical Decision-Making*, Lundberg GD, ed, Chicago, IL: American Society of Clinical Pathologists, 1983, 33-9.
2. Moore JJ, Sax SM, and DeFranc S, "Liposyn® Interference With Neonatal Bilirubin Measurements," *Clin Chem*, 1982, 28:2334-5, (letter).
3. Polesky HF, "Diagnosis, Prevention, and Therapy in Hemolytic Disease of the Newborn," *Clin Lab Med*, 1982, 2:107-22.
4. Walker PC, "Neonatal Bilirubin Toxicity: A Review of Kernicterus and the Implication of Drug-Induced Bilirubin Displacement," *Clin Pharmacokinet*, 1987, 13:26-50.
5. Kemper K, Forsyth B, and McCarthy P, "Jaundice, Terminating Breast Feeding, and the Vulnerable Child," *Pediatrics*, 1989, 84(5):773-8.
6. Maurer HM, Kirkpatrick BV, McWilliams NB, et al, "Phototherapy for Hyperbilirubinemia of Hemolytic Disease of the Newborn," *Pediatrics*, 1985, 75(Suppl):407-12.

References

Benaron DA and Bowen FW, "Variation of Initial Serum Bilirubin Rise in Newborn Infants With Type of Illness," *Lancet*, 1991, 338(8759):78-81.

Cashore WJ, "Neonatal Hyperbilirubinemia," *N Y State J Med*, 1991, 91(11):476-7.

Graziani LJ, Mitchell DG, Kornhauser M, et al, "Neurodevelopment of Preterm Infants: Neonatal Neurosonographic and Serum Bilirubin Studies," *Pediatrics*, 1992, 89(2):229-34.

Newman TB and Maisels MJ, "Bilirubin and Brain Damage: What Do We Do Now?" *Pediatrics*, 1989, 83(6):1062-5.

Scheidt PC, Graubard BI, Nelson KB, et al, "Intelligence at Six Years in Relation to Neonatal Bilirubin Levels: Follow-Up of the National Institute of Child Health and Human Development Clinical Trial of Phototherapy," *Pediatrics*, 1991, 87(6):797-805.

Seidman DS and Stevenson DK, "Neonatal Bilirubin," *Lancet*, 1992, 339(8784):65-6, (letter).

Bilirubin, Total

***CPT** 82250*

Related Information

Bile, Urine *on page 1111*
Gamma Glutamyl Transferase *on page 230*
Liver Profile *on page 282*
Urobilinogen, 2-Hour Urine *on page 1167*

Synonyms Total Bilirubin

Specimen Serum **CONTAINER:** Red top tube; capillary tube for babies **COLLECTION:** Blood drawn from a heelstick for babies. **STORAGE INSTRUCTIONS:** Protect sample from light. **CAUSES FOR REJECTION:** Grossly hemolyzed specimen, specimen not protected from light

Interpretive **REFERENCE RANGE:** Newborns: see table under Bilirubin, Neonatal; adults: 0.3-1.0 mg/dL (SI: 5-17 μmol/L) **USE:** Causes of **high bilirubin:** Liver disease: hepatitis, cholangitis, cirrhosis, other types of liver disease (including primary or secondary neoplasia); alcoholism (usually with high AST (SGOT), GGT, MCV, or some combination of these findings); biliary obstruction (intrahepatic or extrahepatic); infectious mononucleosis (look also for increased LD (LDH), lymphocytosis); Dubin-Johnson syndrome; Gilbert's disease[1] (familial hyperbilirubinemia) is encountered as a moderate elevation with otherwise unremarkable chemistries.

Anorexia or prolonged fasting: 36 hours or more may cause moderate rise.

Pernicious anemia, hemolytic anemias, erythroblastosis fetalis, other neonatal jaundice, hematoma and following a blood transfusion, especially if several units are given in a short time.

Pulmonary embolism and/or infarct, congestive heart failure.

Drugs: A large number of drugs can cause jaundice by *in vivo* action or by chemistry methodology. Drugs causing cholestasis and/or hepatocellular damage include diphenylhydantoin, azathioprine, phenothiazines, erythromycin, penicillin, sulfonamides, oral contraceptives, anabolic-androgenic steroids, halothane, aminosalicylic acid, isoniazid, methyldopa, indomethacin, pyrazinamide, and others.

LIMITATIONS: Differential diagnosis of liver diseases requires total and direct bilirubin values, as well as other tests. Visibly hemolyzed sera and lipemia can produce erroneous results. **METHODOLOGY:** Diazo reaction for adults, differential spectrophotometry for neonates **ADDITIONAL INFORMATION:** Total bilirubin is commonly available in chemistry multitest profiling instruments, in

(Continued)

Bilirubin, Total *(Continued)*

which it is a useful parameter. Interpretation of increased bilirubin is greatly enhanced by other chemistry results. In acute viral hepatitis with jaundice, for instance, the transaminases ALT (SGPT) and AST (SGOT) are consistently increased, while an isolated elevation of bilirubin is seen in Gilbert's disease.[1] **Obstruction** causes increases in bilirubin and alkaline phosphatase greater than and out of proportion to the transaminases.[2] Amylase and lipase are useful in differential diagnosis of obstructive jaundice. In **intrahepatic cholestasis,** the transaminases are not as increased, relative to bilirubin, as they are in hepatitis.[3] Work-up of jaundice has been outlined.[4,5]

Nicotinic acid increases the formation of bilirubin in the spleen, leading to a rise in unconjugated bilirubin. This can be used as a test for Gilbert's disease[1] in which there is a decreased hepatic clearance of unconjugated bilirubin. Although the indirect bilirubin level is increased in normal controls when nicotinic acid is given, the increase is much greater in patients with Gilbert's disease. In the Crigler-Najjar syndrome type I, the unconjugated bilirubin is >20 μg/dL. In type II, the level is <20 μg/dL.

Footnotes

1. Ohkulo H and Okuda K, "The Nicotinic Acid Test in Constitutional Conjugated Hyperbilirubinemia and the Effects of Steroids," *Hepatology*, 1984, 4:1206-8.
2. Scharschmidt BF, Goldberg HI, and Schmid R, "Current Concepts in Diagnosis. Approach to the Patient With Cholestatic Jaundice," *N Engl J Med*, 1983, 308:1515-9.
3. Goldberg DM, Spooner RJ, Ellis G, et al, "Biochemical Features of Intrahepatic Cholestasis," *Am J Clin Pathol*, 1979, 71:557-63.
4. Ostrow JD, "Jaundice in Older Children and Adults," *Using the Clinical Laboratory in Medical Decision Making*, Lundberg GD, ed, Chicago, IL: American Society of Clinical Pathologists, 1983, 41-8.
5. Fischer MG, Gelb AM, and Weingarten LA, "Cholestatic Jaundice in Adults," *Using the Clinical Laboratory in Medical Decision Making*, Lundberg GD, ed, Chicago, IL: American Society of Clinical Pathologists, 1983, 49-54.

References

Adachi Y, Katoh H, Fuchi I, et al, "Serum Bilirubin Fractions in Healthy Subjects and Patients With Unconjugated Hyperbilirubinemia," *Clin Biochem*, 1990, 23(3):247-51.

Donnachie EM, Seccombe DW, Urquhart NI, et al, "Indocyanine Green Interference in the Kodak Ektachem® Determination of Total Bilirubin," *Clin Chem*, 1989, 35(5):899-900, (letter).

Frank BB, "Clinical Evaluation of Jaundice – A Guideline of the Patient Care Committee of the American Gastroenterological Association," *JAMA*, 1989, 262(21):3031-4.

Helzberg JH and Spiro HM, "LFTs Test More Than the Liver," *JAMA*, 1986, 256:3006-7.

Lepage L and Trivin F, "Total Bilirubin," *Drug Effects on Laboratory Test Results Analytical Interferences and Pharmacological Effects*, Siest G and Galteau MM, eds, Littleton, MA: PSG Publishing Co Inc, 1988, 131-47.

Westwood A, "The Analysis of Bilirubin in Serum," *Ann Clin Biochem*, 1991, 28(Pt 2):119-30.

Biotin *see* Lactic Acid, Blood *on page 273*

Blood Gases, Arterial

***CPT** 82803*

Related Information

Arterial Blood Collection *on page 21*
Carbon Dioxide, Blood *on page 165*
Carboxyhemoglobin *on page 165*
HCO_3, Blood *on page 248*
Methemoglobin *on page 290*
Oxygen Saturation, Blood *on page 305*
pCO_2, Blood *on page 314*
pH, Blood *on page 315*
Phlebotomy, Therapeutic *on page 1075*

Synonyms ABGs; Arterial Blood Gases; Gases, Arterial

Applies to Oxygen Content; Oxygen Saturation; pCO_2; pH; pO_2

Test Commonly Includes Measured results include pH, pCO_2 ($PaCO_2$), pO_2 (PaO_2), hematocrit, and may also include electrolytes, and ionized calcium. Calculated values include total carbon dioxide (TCO_2), bicarbonate (HCO_3^-), oxygen saturation, oxygen content, base excess, alveolar-arterial (A-a) gradient, and P_{50} offered by some laboratories. Standard bicarbonate concentration (SBc), base excess of extracellular fluid, carboxyhemoglobin, methemoglobin, normalized calcium, hemoglobin content, and anion gap and osmolality (if electrolytes measured) may also be provided as calculations.

Patient Care **PREPARATION:** Patient should be supine, relaxed. The patient's temperature should be recorded. **AFTERCARE:** Watch for bleeding, hematoma. Ideally, extremity punctured should be kept up for 10 minutes with pressure applied to the puncture site if the patient is not on anticoagulants. If patient is receiving heparin, pressure must be applied to puncture site for a minimum of 15 minutes. Arterial puncture may be especially hazardous in the anticoagulated patient. However, there is frequently simultaneous need for arterial blood gases and for anticoagulation.

Specimen Whole blood **CONTAINER:** Heparinized syringe or through an indwelling arterial line **COLLECTION:** Very small diameter needles are used, usually 25-gauge. Specimen is drawn into air-free heparinized syringe, then stoppered. The radial artery is commonly used, utilizing the Allen test. The Allen test is used to assess the presence of normal collateral circulation. The brachial artery is the second choice. **All specimens should be on ice and brought to the laboratory immediately.** Mode of oxygen delivery or room air must be indicated. Rapid changes may occur if collected immediately after exercise.[1] Avoid excessive heparin. Strict anaerobiosis must be maintained. Blood drawn from a vein or capillary can provide helpful information including pH, pCO_2, and, occasionally, pO_2 **STORAGE INSTRUCTIONS:** Place on ice. The following *in vitro* changes occur in blood gas parameters:[2] pH, 0.001/10 minutes at 4°C, pCO_2, 0.1 mm Hg/10 minutes at 4°C, pO_2, 3 mm Hg/10 minutes at 4°C. No difference exists between glass and newer plastic syringes. **CAUSES FOR REJECTION:** Specimen **not** received on ice, air bubbles or clots in syringe **SPECIAL INSTRUCTIONS:** Sample obtained just after a change in FiO_2 (eg, room air or quantity of therapeutic oxygen delivered) is apt to generate confusing results.

Interpretive **REFERENCE RANGE:** Arterial: pH 7.35-7.45, TCO_2: 23-29 mmol/L, pCO_2: 35-45 mm Hg, pO_2: adult: 80-95 mm Hg, newborn: 60-70 mm Hg, O_2: 95% to 99% saturation. Such normal ranges must be interpreted in light of the FiO_2 and other parameters. **POSSIBLE PANIC RANGE:** pH <7.2, >7.55; pCO_2 <20 mm Hg, >60 mm Hg; pO_2 <40 mm Hg **USE:** Evaluate oxygen and carbon dioxide gas exchange, respiratory function including hypoxia, and acid-base status. Assess asthma, chronic obstructive pulmonary disease (COPD), and other types of lung disease,[3] embolism including fat embolism, and coronary arterial bypass surgical cases.

ARTERIAL BLOOD GAS QUALITY ASSURANCE AND APPROPRIATENESS REVIEW:

In the following lists, clinical judgment is required. Many of the clinical entities listed do not necessarily require blood gas analysis.

Criteria:

Severe cardiorespiratory disturbances:

- shock
- cardiac arrest
- coma
- acute respiratory failure
- acute infarct, myocardium with complications
- severe congestive heart failure
- pulmonary edema
- serious disturbances of cardiac rhythm
- unexplained right heart failure
- suspected R-L shunt evaluation
- evaluate V/Q abnormality

Investigate cardiorespiratory, metabolic, central nervous system disturbances:

- shortness of breath by history, if indicated
- unexplained tachypnea, if indicated
- unexplained dyspnea, if indicated
- lung disease, if indicated
- decompensated established lung disease
- deep vein thrombus
- pulmonary embolism, including fat embolism
- pneumonia
- unexplained polycythemia, erythrocytosis
- unexplained mental status abnormalities
- cyanosis
- smoke inhalation, possibly with CO intoxication
- toxin ingestion (CN, ASA, methanol, ethylene glycol)

(Continued)

Blood Gases, Arterial *(Continued)*

- rule out carboxyhemoglobinemia or methemoglobinemia
- monitor oxygen therapy as medically needed
- home oxygen management, selected instances
- exercise, oxygen therapy
- fracture
- metabolic acidosis and alkalosis, selected instances
- electrolyte disturbances (abnormal bicarbonate level, anion gap), selected cases
- change in patient's clinical status
- rest and exercise pulmonary function testing
- sleep disorder work-up

Miscellaneous medical/surgical conditions:

- change in ventilatory settings, if indicated
- contemplated prolonged anesthesia
- contemplated major abdominal surgery, if indicated
- contemplated pulmonary resection
- chest pain, pleurisy, if indicated
- abnormal chest x-ray with clinical indications
- follow-up abnormal ABG, if indicated
- follow O_2 prescription if needed
- during surgery, if indicated
- abnormal oxygen saturation, if indicated
- during dialysis, if needed
- after prescription of $NaHCO_3$ or Na citrate, if indicated
- Kussmaul respirations
- uncontrolled diabetes with suspected acidosis as medically indicated
- previous pH <7.35 or 7.30, if indicated
- renal failure (creatinine >4 mg/dL (SI: >353 μmol/L) or creatinine clearance <25 mL/min), if indicated
- profuse diarrhea, if indicated
- history of renal tubular acidosis (RTA), if indicated
- ureterosigmoidostomy, if indicated
- pancreatic, small bowel or biliary drainage, if indicated
- nausea/vomiting, if indicated
- nasogastric drainage, if indicated
- hypokalemia, if indicated
- diuretic use, if indicated

In ill adults who are stable, blood gas analysis is considered when a change in clinical management is considered or when an alteration in the patient's clinical status develops.

LIMITATIONS: Arterial puncture may be extremely difficult in some individuals. O_2 saturation is calculated on assumption of 100% A hemoglobin. Reported value may be misleading when hemoglobins with different dissociation curves are present. Calculations commonly assume body temperature of 37°C.

When hemoglobin is reported with blood gases, it usually is a screening hemoglobin, which is less reliable than a conventional hemoglobin ordered as such.

Variability of results occurs;[3] changes in pO_2 in isolated reports must be interpreted cautiously and in light of data trends, oxygen delivery, and the patient's clinical appearance. Such variation occurs without change in FiO_2 or the patient's clinical status.

Correlation of arterial gases with pulmonary function testing in asthma was reported as poor.[4] Correlation with severity of asthma is suboptimal.

ABGs are of little value in treatment decisions for carbon monoxide poisoning.[5]

Complications of arterial puncture potentially include hematoma, bleeding, arterial occlusion, infection, and, very rarely, gangrene.

Although normal pO_2 diminishes the likelihood of pulmonary embolism, the former does not rule out the latter. (Alveolar-arterial gradient usually is widened in pulmonary embolism.)

METHODOLOGY: Specific electrodes **ADDITIONAL INFORMATION:** The pH, pCO_2 and pO_2 are measured directly while the hemoglobin, carboxyhemoglobin, and methemoglobin are measured and calculated using spectrophotometric analysis at specific wavelengths and electronic representation of mathematical relationships. It is assumed that largely normal A hemoglobin is present (most importantly that there are no significant levels of fetal hemoglobin.) Methemoglobin levels <10% are subject to about a 1% error; but with methemoglobin levels >10%, the error is at about the 10% level. High serum bilirubin levels do not contribute to error. Methylene blue (used in treatment of some forms of methemoglobinemia) may interfere and result in nonrepresentative methemoglobin and other hemoglobin measurements. Sulfhemoglobin is a cause of spectral interference.

"Hypoxemia" can be defined as pO_2 <80 mm Hg, but other, more sophisticated definitions are available.[6]

Raffin points out that few studies are available to indicate how many arterial samples are actually indicated. He observes that a complete list of clinical settings involving ill patients in whom blood gas studies might be indicated would include much of the tables of contents of general medicine texts.[6]

The combination of pH values <7.25 without elevation of pCO_2, may indicate need for a lactic acid determination.

Nonsurvivors in a group of COPD patients had lower arterial oxygen tension and higher carbon dioxide tension.[7,8]

Assessment of acid-base status of tissues in patients in circulatory failure may be misleading if only arterial blood gas data is available. Adrogué presents data supporting the need for information on mixed venous as well as arterial gases in care of critically ill patients.[9]

Footnotes

1. Ries AL, Fedullo PF, and Clausen JL, "Rapid Changes in Arterial Blood Gas Levels After Exercise in Pulmonary Patients," *Chest*, 1983, 83:454-6.
2. Bruegger BB and Sherwin JE, "Blood Gas Analysis and Oxygen Saturation," *Methods in Clinical Chemistry*, Pesce AJ and Kaplan LA, eds, St Louis, MO: Mosby-Year Book Inc, 1987, 54-66.
3. Thorson SH, Marini JJ, Pierson PJ, et al, "Variability of Arterial Blood Gas Values in Stable Patients in the ICU," *Chest*, 1983, 84:14-8.
4. Nowak RM, Tomlanovich MC, Sarkar DD, et al, "Arterial Blood Gases and Pulmonary Function Testing in Acute Bronchial Asthma. Predicting Patient Outcomes," *JAMA*, 1983, 249:2043-6.
5. Myers RA and Britten JS, "Are Arterial Blood Gases of Value in Treatment Decisions for Carbon Monoxide Poisoning?" *Crit Care Med*, 1989, 17(2):139-42.
6. Raffin TA, "Indications for Arterial Blood Gas Analysis," *Ann Intern Med*, 1986, 105:390-8.
7. Kawakami Y, Kishi F, Yamamoto H, et al, "Relation of Oxygen Delivery, Mixed Venous Oxygenation, and Pulmonary Hemodynamics to Prognosis in Chronic Obstructive Pulmonary Disease," *N Engl J Med*, 1983, 308:1045-9.
8. Bergofsky EH, "Tissue Oxygen Delivery and Cor Pulmonale in Chronic Obstructive Pulmonary Disease," *N Engl J Med*, 1983, 308:1092-4, (editorial).
9. Adrogué HJ, Rashad MN, Gorin AB, et al, "Assessing Acid-Base Status in Circulatory Failure: Differences Between Arterial and Central Venous Blood," *N Engl J Med*, 1989, 320(20):1312-6.

References

Anderson S, "ABGs. Six Easy Steps to Interpreting Blood Gases," *Am J Nurs*, 1990, 90(8):42-5.

Courtney SE, Weber KR, Breakie LA, et al, "Capillary Blood Gases in the Neonate. A Reassessment and Review of the Literature," *Am J Dis Child*, 1990, 144(2):168-72.

Eichhorn JH, "Performance Characteristics for Devices Measuring pO_2 and pCO_2 in Blood Samples," *National Committee for Clinical Laboratory Standards*, 1989.

Hansen JE, "Arterial Blood Gases," *Clin Chest Med*, 1989, 10(2):227-37.

Hibbard JU, Hibbard MC, and Whalen MP, "Umbilical Cord Blood Gases and Mortality and Morbidity in the Very Low Birth Weight Infant," *Obstet Gynecol*, 1991, 78(5 Pt 1):768-73.

Meyer BA, Dickinson JE, Chambers C, et al, "The Effect of Fetal Sepsis on Umbilical Cord Blood Gases," *Am J Obstet Gynecol*, 1992, 166(2):612-7.

Pierson DJ, "Pulse Oximetry Versus Arterial Blood Gas Specimens in Long-Term Oxygen Therapy," *Lung*, 1990, 168(Suppl):782-8.

Ribbert LS, Snijders RJ, Nicolaides KH, et al, "Relation of Fetal Blood Gases and Data From Computer-Assisted Analysis of Fetal Heart Rate Patterns in Small for Gestation Fetuses," *Br J Obstet Gynaecol*, 1991, 98(8):820-3.

Blood Gases, Capillary

***CPT** 82803*

Related Information

Carbon Dioxide, Blood *on page 165*

pCO_2, Blood *on page 314*

(Continued)

Blood Gases, Capillary *(Continued)*

pH, Blood *on page 315*

Synonyms Capillary Blood Gases

Test Commonly Includes Measured results include pH, pCO_2 ($PaCO_2$), pO_2 (PaO_2), hematocrit, and may also include electrolytes, and ionized calcium. Calculated values include total carbon dioxide (TCO_2), bicarbonate (HCO_3), oxygen saturation, oxygen content, base excess, alveolar-arterial (A-a) gradient, and P_{50} offered by some laboratories. Standard bicarbonate concentration (SBc), base excess of extracellular fluid, carboxyhemoglobin, methemoglobin, normalized calcium, hemoglobin content, and anion gap and osmolality (if electrolytes measured) may also be provided as calculations.

Patient Care PREPARATION: Nursing staffs have traditionally, in many hospitals, prewarmed the heel. However, *vide infra*. The puncture should be deep enough to allow a free flow of blood. Blood is then collected in heparinized capillary tubes, which should be filled as much as possible, capped and mixed well. AFTERCARE: Apply pressure on site for 5-10 minutes, apply bandaid.

Specimen Whole blood CONTAINER: Two heparinized 250 μL capillary tubes capped tightly with internal mixing flea COLLECTION: Fill both tubes completely excluding any air bubbles, mix immediately with heparin to avoid clotting. A 2.5 mm x 1.5 mm microlancet may be used for skin punctures. STORAGE INSTRUCTIONS: Immediately put in iced water. CAUSES FOR REJECTION: No heparin, sample clotted, specimen not received on ice

Interpretive REFERENCE RANGE: pH: 7.35-7.45, pO_2: >90 mm Hg, pCO_2: 26.4-41.2 mm Hg, O_2 saturation: 95% to 99% USE: Acid base balance. McLain et al conclude that although capillary blood is satisfactory for most purposes for pH and pCO_2, the role of capillary pO_2 is limited to exclusion of hypoxia.[1] Capillary blood sampling is less likely to cause complications than is arterial puncture. METHODOLOGY: Specific electrodes ADDITIONAL INFORMATION: Warming the heel, a traditional practice, made no difference in a study from Leeds.[1]

Footnotes

1. McLain BI, Evans J, Dear PR, et al, "Comparison of Capillary and Arterial Blood Gas Measurements in Neonates," *Arch Dis Child*, 1988, 63(7 Spec No):743-7.

References

Couriel JM, "Interpretation of Blood Gas Analysis," *Indian J Pediatr*, 1988, 55:656-60.

Dong SH, Liu HM, Song GW, et al, "Arterialized Capillary Blood Gases and Acid-Base Studies in Normal Individuals From 29 Days to 24 Years of Age," *Am J Dis Child*, 1985, 139:1019-22.

Blood Gases, Venous

CPT 82803

Related Information

Carbon Dioxide, Blood *on page 165*

pH, Blood *on page 315*

Synonyms Venous Blood Gases

Applies to Central Venous Blood

Test Commonly Includes Measured results include pH, pCO_2 ($PaCO_2$), pO_2 (PaO_2), hematocrit, and may also include electrolytes, and ionized calcium. Calculated values include total carbon dioxide (TCO_2), bicarbonate (HCO_3^-), oxygen saturation, oxygen content, base excess, alveolar-arterial (A-a) gradient, and P_{50} offered by some laboratories. Standard bicarbonate concentration (SBc), base excess of extracellular fluid, carboxyhemoglobin, methemoglobin, normalized calcium, hemoglobin content, and anion gap and osmolality (if electrolytes measured) may also be provided as calculations.

Abstract Determination of pH and pCO_2 can be done reliably from venous blood in most clinical situations.

Patient Care PREPARATION: The patient should be supine, relaxed.

Specimen Whole blood CONTAINER: Heparinized syringe, green top (heparin) tube COLLECTION: Draw specimen into air-free heparinized syringe or green top vacuum blood collection tube. If a vacuum blood collection tube is used, it must be removed from needle before needle is removed from patient's arm. Keep sample on ice. Indicate specimen source (ie, venous) and mode of oxygen delivery or room air if applicable on requisition. STORAGE INSTRUCTIONS: Keep specimen on ice. CAUSES FOR REJECTION: Specimen **not** received on ice, specimen clotted

Interpretive REFERENCE RANGE: Venous pH: 7.32-7.43, TCO_2: 23-30 mmol/L, pCO_2: 38-50 mm Hg, pO_2 should be about 40 mm Hg, O_2 saturation should be about 75%. USE: Evaluate cellular hypoxia, acid-base balance. A major use is to obtain pH in infants, children, and adults in whom oxygen parameters are not needed, without arterial puncture. In many metabolic situations a venous pH is adequate for pH, and arterial puncture is unnecessary. Both arterial and central venous blood samples play a role in assessment of acid-base status in subjects in critical hemodynamic compromise. With severe hypoperfusion central venous blood better detects hypercapnia and acidemia.[1] The pO_2, pCO_2, and pH from pulmonary arterial samples correlate with central venous specimens.[2] **LIMITATIONS:** In hypotensive subjects with severe circulatory failure, Adrogué et al describe substantial differences between mean arterial and central venous pH and pCO_2.[1] **METHODOLOGY:** Specific electrodes **ADDITIONAL INFORMATION:** The arteriovenous pH difference is usually extremely small (0.01-0.03), except in patients in congestive heart failure and in shock. The differences in pH and pCO_2 widen only slightly with moderate cardiac failure.[1] Total CO_2 values are slightly higher in venous blood than in arterial blood. Arterial blood, however, must be used to accurately measure pO_2 and oxygen saturation.

Footnotes

1. Adrogué HJ, Rashad MN, Gorin AB, et al, "Assessing Acid-Base Status in Circulatory Failure: Differences Between Arterial and Central Venous Blood," *N Engl J Med*, 1989, 320(20):1312-6.
2. Eichhorn JH, "Accuracy and Comparisons in Blood Gas Measurements," *Chest*, 1988, 94(1):1-2, (editorial).

Blood Gas P-50 *see* P-50 Blood Gas *on page 307*

Blood Lactate *see* Lactic Acid, Blood *on page 273*

Blood pH *see* pH, Blood *on page 315*

Blood Spot Screen for Galactose/Galactose-1-Phosphate *see* Galactose Screening Tests for Galactosemia *on page 228*

Blood Sugar, Fasting *see* Glucose, Fasting *on page 238*

Blood Urea Nitrogen *see* Urea Nitrogen, Blood *on page 376*

Body Fluid

***CPT** 89051 (cell count with differential)*

Related Information

Alpha$_1$-Fetoprotein, Serum *on page 115*
Biopsy or Body Fluid Aerobic Bacterial Culture *on page 778*
Biopsy or Body Fluid Anaerobic Bacterial Culture *on page 778*
Biopsy or Body Fluid Fungus Culture *on page 780*
Biopsy or Body Fluid Mycobacteria Culture *on page 782*
Body Fluid Amylase *on page 148*
Body Fluid Glucose *on page 148*
Body Fluid Lactate Dehydrogenase *on page 149*
Body Fluid pH *on page 150*
Body Fluids Analysis, Cell Count *on page 523*
Body Fluids Cytology *on page 482*
CA 15-3 *on page 152*
CA 19-9 *on page 152*
CA 125 *on page 154*
Carcinoembryonic Antigen *on page 167*
Viral Culture, Body Fluid *on page 1198*
Washing Cytology *on page 515*

Synonyms Ascitic Fluid Analysis; Fluid, Peritoneal; Fluid, Pleural; Paracentesis Fluid Analysis; Pericardial Fluid Analysis; Peritoneal Fluid Analysis; Pleural Fluid Analysis; Thoracentesis Fluid Analysis

Applies to Albs-a; Albumin, Ascites Fluid; CEA, Body Fluid; Cyst Fluid Chemistry; Lactic Acid, Body Fluid; LD, Body Fluid; Rheumatoid Factor, Body Fluid; Serum-Ascites Albumin Difference

Patient Care **PREPARATION:** Usual aseptic aspiration procedure

Specimen Body fluid (ie, ascitic fluid, pleural fluid, etc) **CONTAINER:** Red top tube, lavender top (EDTA) tube, and green top (heparin) tube; sterile container for microbiologic cultures **COLLECTION:** Body fluids are usually worked up in several laboratory sections. A common error is not to provide sufficient quantity of fluid for adequate examinations. A simultaneous blood specimen drawn for serum chemistry can be useful.

(Continued)

Body Fluid *(Continued)*

Interpretive REFERENCE RANGE: Pathologic fluids: When such fluids as pleural or peritoneal transudates or exudates are examined, no normal ranges exist because such fluids by their very nature are not normal. USE: Evaluate effusions; diagnose transudate versus exudate. Transudates are watery to yellow, clear, and do not clot. Exudates may be opaque to purulent, contain fibrinogen, and may clot (thus, green top tubes are needed for cytology). Causes of **transudates** include congestive heart failure, hepatic cirrhosis, and the nephrotic syndromes. **Exudates** are caused by various types of infection including TB, esophageal or other hollow viscus rupture, abscess such as subphrenic or liver abscess, neoplasia, the rheumatoid arthritis state, pancreatitis, embolization or lung infarct, trauma, and systemic LE.[1] ADDITIONAL INFORMATION: Tests commonly helpful in work-up of a fluid include cell count and differential, hemoglobin/hematocrit, fluid and serum analysis by multichemistry panel, specific gravity, amylase and pH. Protein quantitation, as in the table, is somewhat useful for pleural fluid but is less reliable for peritoneal fluid. Cultures are commonly indicated, require a sterile specimen, and generally are ordered for routine, anaerobic, TB and fungi.

Cytology is often critically important. Lung and breast carcinoma are the two most common tumors causing pleural effusion. CEA, CA 15-3, and CA 19-9 may be useful, additional to exfoliative cytology, in work-up for cancer.[2] Additionally, CA 125 can be helpful in selected cases.

Other tests sometimes helpful include pH, especially in chest fluids. Urea nitrogen (BUN) is helpful if a question of bladder content versus ascitic fluid exists.

Test green fluids for bilirubin; if positive, consider perforated intestine, peptic ulcer, or gallbladder

Bloody fluids, if not caused by traumatic tap, are generally exudates. TB as well as infarct or cancer must be considered. Hematocrit of the fluid is useful for diagnosis of hemothorax or hemoperitoneum (eg, trauma).

Pericardial fluid specimens are usually exudates (Such fluids are selected by having been tapped. Pericarditis related to the uremic state is not usually sampled, for instance.)

Chylous fluids appear milky. Chylous effusion contains chylomicrons and has very high triglycerides. Such effusions relate to trauma and lymphoma; carcinoma and tuberculosis also are reported to cause chylous effusion.[1]

High levels of **rheumatoid factor** in a pleural fluid support a diagnosis of rheumatoid effusion, while in SLE, rheumatoid factor titers are apt to be only about 1:40.[3]

Peritoneal and pleural fluid **lactic acid** is increased with infection. In uninfected ascites, ascitic fluid lactate was 15 ± 5 mg/dL (SI: 1.7 ± 0.6 mmol/L), while in bacterial peritonitis, 14 patients ranged 45 ± 37 mg/dL (SI: 5.0 ± 4.1 mmol/L). A cutoff >25 mg/dL (SI: >2.8 mmol/L) is suggested.[4] Lactic acid may also be increased in malignant disease in body fluids.

The differential diagnosis of ascites includes cancer and hepatic cirrhosis. The ratio of LD (LDH) in serum to that of ascitic fluid is helpful. Ratios of less than unity occur with malignant disease, while ratios >1 are reported mostly with cirrhosis, when these two groups are compared.[5] However, a few instances of cancer have ratios greater than unity.[5] The LD of the ascitic fluid of cirrhosis is usually $<60\%$ that of serum.[6]

Albumin in body fluids is the main determinant of oncotic pressure. The gradient between serum and ascites is expressed as **"Albs-a"**, referring to albumin concentration. It correlates with the pressure gradient between the portal capillaries and the peritoneal cavity.[7,8] It is ≥ 1.1 g/dL (SI: 11 g/L) in the presence of portal hypertension, and less without. Ascites in subjects with portal hypertension (Albs-a ≥ 1.1 g/dL) **is usually caused by** cirrhosis, right ventricular failure or constrictive pericarditis.[6] Serum/ascites albumin gradient is greater in transudates (1.6 ± 0.5 g/dL) than exudates (0.6 ± 0.4 g/dL).[1]

Ascites not associated with portal hypertension (Albs-a <1.1 g/dL) is caused by leaking thoracic, pancreatic or biliary ducts, malignant disease, tuberculosis, myxedema, SLE, certain ovarian diseases and severe hypoalbuminemia.[6,7] "High protein ascites," >2.5 g total protein/dL (SI: >25 g/L), is found in 15% to 20% of subjects who have hepatic disease, while a similar fraction of patients with malignant disease have "low protein ascites."[7]

Cholesterol levels have been studied in pleural[9] and ascitic[10] fluids and may prove useful in differential diagnosis of body fluids. See table.

Malignant tumors give rise to fluids commonly more similar to **exudates** than to **transudates.** However, cytology is more useful than chemistry for tumor diagnosis.

Body Fluid

	Transudate	Exudate
WBC/mm	<100/mm^3	>1000/mm^3
Specific gravity	<1.016	>1.016
Total protein	<2.5–3.0 g/dL	>3.0 g/dL
LD (LDH)	Similar to serum LD or lower	Fluid LD to serum LD ratio >0.6 or LD >200 units/L
Glucose		Low — especially in rheumatoid effusion
Cholesterol pleural	<60 mg/dL (SI: <1.55 mol/L)	>60 mg/dL (SI: >1.55 mol/L)
Cholesterol ascitic	<46 mg/dL (SI: <1.19 mol/L)	>46 mg/dL (SI: >1.19 mol/L)

The separation between transudate and exudate is blurring; Albs–a (serum–ascites albumin difference) provides useful information — see text.

Tumor markers are also useful in body fluids, including CEA[11] and CA 125.[11,12] CEA increases occur with many carcinomas primary in the gastrointestinal tract, breast, and lung. CEA level is normal with lymphoma and mesothelioma. CA 125 increased without high CEA is consistent with primary carcinoma of ovary, fallopian tube or endometrium, but may occur with stage III or IV endometriosis.[12] CEA is commonly negative in müllerian carcinomas but positive with mucinous cystadenocarcinoma of ovary.[11] (Adenocarcinoma primary in the endocervix is often CEA positive.) Normal CEA and CA 125 in malignant fluids suggest possible mesothelioma, melanoma, or lymphoma.[11] Leucine aminopeptidase is reported high in malignant ascites.[13]

Footnotes

1. Kjeldsberg CR and Knight JA, *Body Fluids – Laboratory Examination of Amniotic, Cerebrospinal, Seminal, Serous, and Synovial Fluids*, 3rd ed, Chicago, IL, ASCP Press, 1993, 159-253, 186-7.
2. Couch WD, "Combined Effusion Fluid Tumor Marker Assay, Carcinoembryonic Antigen (CEA) and Human Chorionic Gonadotropin (hCG), in the Detection of Malignant Tumors," *Cancer*, 1981, 48:2475-9.
3. Dines DE, "Studies on Pleural Fluid," *Mayo Clin Proc*, 1981, 56:460.
4. Garcia-Tsao G, Conn HO, and Lerner E, "The Diagnosis of Bacterial Peritonitis: Comparison of pH, Lactate Concentration and Leukocyte Count," *Hepatology*, 1985, 5:91-6.
5. Greene LS, Levine R, Gross MJ, et al, "Distinguishing Between Malignant and Cirrhotic Ascites by Computerized Step-Wise Discriminant Functional Analysis of Its Biochemistry," *Am J Gastroenterol*, 1978, 70:448-54.
6. Rector WG Jr, "An Improved Diagnostic Approach to Ascites," *Arch Intern Med*, 1987, 147:215, (editorial).
7. Marshall JB and Vogele KA, "Serum-Ascites Albumin Differences in Tuberculous Peritonitis," *Am J Gastroenterol*, 1988, 83(11):1259-61.
8. Rector WG and Reynolds TB, "Superiority of the Serum-Ascites Albumin Difference Over the Ascites Total Protein Concentration in Separation of "Transudative" and "Exudative" Ascites," *Am J Med*, 1984, 77:83-5.
9. Hamm H, Brohan U, Bohmer R, et al, "Cholesterol in Pleural Effusions: A Diagnostic Aid," *Chest*, 1987, 92:296-302.
10. Prieto M, Gómez-Lechón MJ, Hoyos M, et al, "Diagnosis of Malignant Ascites: Comparison of Ascitic Fibronectin, Cholesterol, and Serum-Ascites Albumin Difference," *Dig Dis Sci*, 1988, 33(7):833-8.
11. Pinto MM, Bernstein LH, Brogan DA, et al, "Immunoradiometric Assay of CA 125 in Effusions: Comparison With Carcinoembryonic Antigen," *Cancer*, 1987, 59:218-22.
12. Dawood MY, Khan-Dawood FS, and Ramos J, "Plasma and Peritoneal Fluid Levels of CA 125 in Women With Endometriosis," *Am J Obstet Gynecol*, 1988, 159(6):1526-31.
13. Cohn EM, "Ascites," *Gastroenterology*, Vol 1, 4th ed, Berk JE, ed, Philadelphia, PA: WB Saunders Co, 1985, 177-90.

References

Desai SD and Sackett DL, "Ratios of Pleural Fluid to Serum Immunoglobulins in Malignant Pleural Effusions," *Cancer*, 1983, 52:2151-5.

Kiltz RJ, Burke MS, and Porreco RP, "Amniotic Fluid Glucose Concentration as a Marker for Intra-amniotic Infection," *Obstet Gynecol*, 1991, 78(4):619-22.

Paavonen T, Liippo K, Aronen H, et al, "Lactate Dehydrogenase, Creatine Kinase, and Their Isoenzymes in Pleural Effusions," *Clin Chem*, 1991, 37(11):1909-12.

Rocco VK and Ware AJ, "Cirrhotic Ascites," *Ann Intern Med*, 1986, 105:573-85.

(Continued)

Body Fluid *(Continued)*

Rodriguez-Panadero F and Lopez-Mejias J, "Low Glucose and pH Levels in Malignant Pleural Effusions. Diagnostic Significance and Prognostic Value in Respect to Pleurodesis," *Am Rev Respir Dis*, 1989, 139(3):663-7.

Body Fluid Amylase

CPT 82150

Related Information

Amylase, Serum *on page 127*
Amylase, Urine *on page 129*
Body Fluid *on page 145*
Body Fluids Analysis, Cell Count *on page 523*
Body Fluids Cytology *on page 482*
Lipase, Serum *on page 277*

Synonyms Amylase, Body Fluid; Amylase, Peritoneal Fluid; Amylase, Pleural Fluid

Abstract High pleural fluid amylase is found with pancreatitis and its complications, rupture of the esophagus and with tumors, especially adenocarcinoma of lung and ovary. Peritoneal fluid work-up may resolve diagnostic issues.

Specimen Body fluid (ie, ascitic fluid, pleural fluid, etc); simultaneously drawn serum for amylase **CONTAINER:** Clean container, no preservative **COLLECTION:** Peritoneal fluid may be obtained by peritoneal lavage.[1] Centrifugation is desirable. **STORAGE INSTRUCTIONS:** Amylase is fairly stable at normal levels.

Interpretive **REFERENCE RANGE:** Elevation of fluid amylase bears an implication of an increase above the serum limits or 1.5 or more increase greater than that of the serum level.[2] **USE:** Pancreatitis with or without pseudocyst formation or pancreatic pleural fistula is the most common cause of amylase elevation in pleural fluid. Rupture of the esophagus is the second most common group and malignant effusion is the third.[3] Other causes include pancreatic ascites and pancreatic duct trauma. Defect in the wall of the gastrointestinal tract (eg, perforated peptic ulcer) will allow pancreatic secretion to enter the peritoneal cavity. Similarly, peritoneal fluid amylase elevations may be found in the presence of necrotic bowel. Peritoneal fluid, containing such amylase, can find its way into a pleural space. **LIMITATIONS:** In collection of ascitic fluid, the localization of the catheter is likely to affect the chemistry result.[1] Oxalate or citrate depress results. Lipemic sample may contain inhibitors which falsely depress results. Benign ovarian cyst fluids may have significant amylase activity. In about 10% of the instances of pancreatic disease, ascitic fluid, as well as serum amylase, may be within normal limits.[2] **ADDITIONAL INFORMATION:** Most patients with pancreatic ascites have high peritoneal fluid amylase as well as amylase elevations in serum and urine. Pancreatitis may present with pleural effusion. Of 34 patients who had high amylase in pleural fluid associated with neoplasms, 18 had carcinoma of lung. Other tumors were gynecologic, gastrointestinal, lymphoma, breast, and malignancy of unknown origin.[3]

Footnotes

1. Robert JH, Meyer P, and Rohner A, "Can Serum and Peritoneal Amylase and Lipase Determinations Help in the Early Prognosis of Acute Pancreatitis?" *Ann Surg*, 1986, 203:163-8.
2. Kjeldsberg CR and Knight JA, *Body Fluids – Laboratory Examination of Amniotic, Cerebrospinal, Seminal, Serous, and Synovial Fluids*, 3rd ed, Chicago, IL: ASCP Press, 1993, 159-222.
3. Kramer MR, Saldana MJ, Cepero RJ, et al, "High Amylase Levels in Neoplasm-Related Pleural Effusion," *Ann Intern Med*, 1989, 110(7):567-9.

Body Fluid GGT *see* Gamma Glutamyl Transferase *on page 230*

Body Fluid Glucose

CPT 82947

Related Information

Body Fluid *on page 145*
Body Fluid pH *on page 150*
Body Fluids Analysis, Cell Count *on page 523*
Body Fluids Cytology *on page 482*
Carcinoembryonic Antigen *on page 167*
Cerebrospinal Fluid Glucose *on page 176*
Glucose, Fasting *on page 238*

Synovial Fluid Analysis *on page 1158*

Synonyms Glucose, Body Fluid

Abstract Decreased pleural fluid glucose may be found in bacterial infection, tuberculosis, rheumatoid effusion, and with malignant disease.

Specimen Body fluid; simultaneously drawn plasma glucose **CONTAINER:** Sterile container

Interpretive **REFERENCE RANGE:** Fluid glucose concentration is usually similar to plasma glucose concentration. Levels <60 mg/dL or 40 mg/dL less than the plasma level drawn simultaneously, are decreased.[1] **USE:** Decreased fluid glucose concentration is usually associated with septic or inflammatory processes; in pleural effusion, very low glucose is a facet of rheumatoid effusion: pleural fluid glucose <50 mg/dL (SI: <2.8 mmol/L) characterizes rheumatoid effusion. It is often much less. In contrast, fluid glucose in SLE is usually >60 mg/dL. Pleural fluid glucose levels <60 mg/dL indicate rheumatoid effusion or grossly purulent parapneumonic effusion. Pericardial effusions with decreased glucose are reported with malignant disease and with bacterial endocarditis.[1] Ascitic fluid glucose is often decreased in tuberculous peritonitis and with malignant disease but is usually normal with cirrhosis or congestive failure. **LIMITATIONS:** Garcia-Tsao et al found glucose the least reliable of the tests they evaluated for the diagnosis of bacterial peritonitis; ascitic fluid glucose in their series ranged from 0-418 mg/dL (SI: 0-23 mmol/L). They also found poor correlation with blood glucose levels. This group recognized the more consistent glucose decrease found in smaller, sequestered fluid collections such as those of meningitis (cerebrospinal fluid) and empyema (pleural fluid).[2] **METHODOLOGY:** Enzymatic, colorimetric **ADDITIONAL INFORMATION:** Potts et al describe loculated effusions or empyemas with low glucose and low pH. Low glucose is found with empyema, tuberculosis, neoplasia, and rheumatoid effusion.[3] In cases of malignant pleural effusions, when there is low pleural fluid glucose, <60 mg/dL (SI: <3.3 mmol/L), and pH <7.30, a probability of 90% that the cytologic yield will be positive was reported.[4]

Footnotes

1. Kjeldsberg CR and Knight JA, *Body Fluids – Laboratory Examination of Amniotic, Cerebrospinal, Seminal, Serous, and Synovial Fluids*, 3rd ed, Chicago, IL: ASCP Press, 1993, 159-222.
2. Garcia-Tsao G, Conn HO, and Lerner E, "The Diagnosis of Bacterial Peritonitis: Comparison of pH, Lactate Concentration and Leukocyte Count," *Hepatology*, 1985, 5:91-6.
3. Potts DE, Taryle DA, and Sahn SA, "The Glucose-pH Relationship in Parapneumonic Effusions," *Arch Intern Med*, 1978, 138:1378-80.
4. Rodriguez-Panadero F and Lopez-Mejias JL, "Low Glucose and pH Levels in Malignant Pleural Effusions. Diagnostic Significance and Prognostic Value in Respect to Pleurodesis," *Am Rev Respir Dis*, 1989, 139(3):663-7.

Body Fluid Lactate Dehydrogenase

CPT 83615

Related Information

Body Fluid *on page 145*
Body Fluid pH *on next page*
Body Fluids Analysis, Cell Count *on page 523*
Body Fluids Cytology *on page 482*
Cerebrospinal Fluid LD *on page 179*
Synovial Fluid Analysis *on page 1158*

Synonyms Lactate Dehydrogenase, Variable; LD, Fluid; LD Variable

Abstract Elevated body fluid LD levels are higher than serum levels in malignant effusions, unlike cases of benign effusions. Elevations are found in inflammatory states.[1]

Specimen Body fluid; simultaneously drawn serum **CONTAINER:** Sterile container **STORAGE INSTRUCTIONS:** Transport specimen to the laboratory as soon as possible. **SPECIAL INSTRUCTIONS:** Requisition must state type of fluid and source.

Interpretive **REFERENCE RANGE:** Fluid LD activity is normally much less than the plasma LD activity **USE:** Differential diagnosis of effusions, includes work-up for rheumatoid effusion and classification as transudate or exudate; aid in differential diagnosis of traumatic tap vs central nervous system (CNS) hemorrhage in newborns **LIMITATIONS:** This test has limited usefulness due to its nonspecificity. **METHODOLOGY:** Lactate to pyruvate monitored at 340 nm **ADDITIONAL INFORMATION:** Lactate dehydrogenase (LD) is a normal component of CSF. LD_1 and LD_2 are decreased in lavage fluid in pulmonary alveolar proteinosis.[2] See Body Fluid listing for more information.

Footnotes

1. Kjeldsberg CR and Knight JA, *Body Fluids – Laboratory Examination of Amniotic, Cerebrospinal, Seminal, Serous, and Synovial Fluids*, 3rd ed, Chicago, IL: ASCP Press, 1993, 159-222.

(Continued)

Body Fluid Lactate Dehydrogenase *(Continued)*

2. Hoffman RM and Rogers RM, "Serum and Lavage Lactate Dehydrogenase Isoenzymes in Pulmonary Alveolar Proteinosis," *Am Rev Respir Dis*, 1991, 143(1):42-6.

Body Fluid Lipase *see* Lipase, Serum *on page 277*

Body Fluid pH

***CPT** 83986*

Related Information

Biopsy or Body Fluid Aerobic Bacterial Culture *on page 778*
Biopsy or Body Fluid Anaerobic Bacterial Culture *on page 778*
Biopsy or Body Fluid Fungus Culture *on page 780*
Biopsy or Body Fluid Mycobacteria Culture *on page 782*
Body Fluid *on page 145*
Body Fluid Glucose *on page 148*
Body Fluid Lactate Dehydrogenase *on previous page*
Body Fluids Analysis, Cell Count *on page 523*
Body Fluids Cytology *on page 482*

Applies to Arterial-Ascitic Fluid pH Gradient; Peritoneal Fluid pH; pH Body Fluid; Pleural Fluid pH; Thoracentesis Fluid pH

Abstract Among tests done on pleural and peritoneal fluids, a role exists for determination of pH.

Specimen Pleural fluid **CONTAINER:** Sample should be collected anaerobically. A green top (lithium heparin) tube to prevent clotting should be used, especially if the syringe has not been rinsed with heparin. Keep on ice and promptly analyze for pH. **COLLECTION:** A syringe rinsed with 0.2 mL of heparin, 1:1000 may be used; collect anaerobically. **STORAGE INSTRUCTIONS:** Keep the specimen refrigerated. **SPECIAL INSTRUCTIONS:** If the specimen is collected in a syringe, all air should be expelled and needle sealed and capped. The pH should be measured anaerobically without delay.

Interpretive **REFERENCE RANGE:** Serous fluid pH about 7.4-7.64; since body fluid accumulations are themselves abnormal, provision of a digital "range" would be misleading. **USE:** Determine pH of body fluid to work up diagnosis (eg, pleuritis, empyema, bacterial peritonitis, rheumatoid effusion, carcinoma, esophageal rupture) **METHODOLOGY:** pH meter **ADDITIONAL INFORMATION:** pH of pleural fluid <6.0 is highly suggestive of rupture of esophagus.[1] Pleural fluid amylase is very helpful for this diagnosis as well. pH <7.3 relates to exudates: in empyema and in loculated effusions pleural fluid pH is <7.2-7.3.[1,2]

The pH is often <7.2 and consistently <7.3[1] in rheumatoid pleural effusion, which is characterized by low glucose, high LD (LDH), and high rheumatoid factor titer. pH >7.3 is in general a feature of transudates. Low pH and low glucose together are found with loculated effusion or with empyema.[3] Effusions related to lupus erythematosus generally have a pH >7.35.[1]

Effusions of tuberculosis usually have pH <7.3,[1] usually with increased lymphocytes. In the single patient with proven tuberculous peritonitis in the series of Garcia-Tsao et al, ascitic fluid pH was 7.33.[4]

In bacterial peritonitis pH is decreased: cutoff of <7.35 is useful, especially with PMNs >500/mm^3. The mean pH of infected ascitic fluid is reported as 7.24. The **arterial-ascitic fluid pH gradient** >0.10 with >500 PMNs is described as virtually diagnostic of bacterial peritonitis.[4]

Reduction of pH and in some, but not all, series increments of PMN counts may be found also with peritoneal metastases.[4,5] Low pleural fluid pH with negative cytologic examination may indicate lack of recognizable malignant cells in a sample of malignant effusion but may point to tuberculosis or rheumatoid effusion. Differences in survival exist between patients with low pH and normal pH in malignant pleural effusions, a significant inverse relationship.[5]

A transudative low pH (<7.30) pleural fluid in which the pleural fluid/serum creatinine ratio is >1 points toward urinothorax, a possibility to be considered in patients with obstructive uropathy.[6]

Footnotes

1. Kjeldsberg CR and Knight JA, *Body Fluids – Laboratory Examination of Amniotic, Cerebrospinal, Seminal, Serous, and Synovial Fluids*, 3rd ed, Chicago, IL: ASCP Press, 1993, 186-7.
2. Dines DE, "Studies on Pleural Fluid," *Mayo Clin Proc*, 1981, 56:460.
3. Potts DE, Taryle DA, and Sahn SA, "The Glucose-pH Relationship in Parapneumonic Effusions," *Arch Intern Med*, 1978, 138:1378-80.

4. Garcia-Tsao G, Conn HO, and Lerner E, "The Diagnosis of Bacterial Peritonitis: Comparison of pH, Lactate Concentration, and Leukocyte Count," *Hepatology*, 1985, 5:91-6.
5. Sahn SA and Good JT, "Pleural Fluid pH in Malignant Effusions: Diagnostic, Prognostic, and Therapeutic Implications," *Ann Intern Med*, 1988, 108(3):345.
6. Miller KS, Wooten S, and Sahn SA, "Urinothorax: A Cause of Low pH Transudative Pleural Effusions," *Am J Med*, 1988, 85(3):448-9.

References

el-Touny M, Osman L, Abd-el-Hamid T, et al, "Re-evaluation of the Value of Ascitic Fluid pH Lactate Dehydrogenase and Total Proteins in the Diagnosis of Spontaneous Bacterial Peritonitis (SBP)," *J Trop Med Hyg*, 1989, 92(1):6-9.

Halla JT, Schrohenloher RE, and Volanakis JE, "Immune Complexes and Other Laboratory Features of Pleural Effusions: A Comparison of Rheumatoid Arthritis, Systemic Lupus Erythematosus, and Other Diseases," *Ann Intern Med*, 1980, 92:748-52.

Bovine ACTH *replaced by* Cosyntropin Test *on page 194*

Bromism *see* Chloride, Serum *on page 182*

BSP *replaced by* Alkaline Phosphatase, Serum *on page 109*

BSP *replaced by* Gamma Glutamyl Transferase *on page 230*

BSP *replaced by* 5' Nucleotidase *on page 297*

BUN *see* Urea Nitrogen, Blood *on page 376*

BUN/Creatinine Ratio

***CPT** 82565 (creatinine); 84520 (BUN)*

Related Information

Creatinine, Serum *on page 202*

Urea Nitrogen, Blood *on page 376*

Test Commonly Includes Serum creatinine and urea nitrogen

Specimen Serum

Interpretive REFERENCE RANGE: 6-20; mean about 10 USE: **High BUN/creatinine ratio** is found in overproduction or lowered excretion of urea nitrogen.[1] High ratios occur with prerenal azotemia,[2] decreased renal perfusion, shock, hypotension, and dehydration. Often the BUN/creatinine ratio is greatly elevated in gastrointestinal bleeding and with swallowed blood from the upper airway. A BUN/creatinine ratio >36 suggests upper gastrointestinal bleeding, whereas a ratio <36 is not helpful in locating the source of the bleeding.[3] It may be increased with high protein diet, with ileal conduit, with catabolic states, and rarely with urinary tract obstruction.[4] It may also be increased with tetracyclines or steroids.

Low BUN/creatinine ratio may be found in low protein diet, malnutrition, pregnancy, liver disease, rhabdomyolysis, prolonged I.V. fluid therapy, ketosis (acetoacetic acid interferes with and falsely elevates creatinine), repeated hemodialysis, inappropriate secretion of antidiuretic hormone, with drugs which increase creatinine but not BUN (eg, cimetidine, trimethoprim), and with tetracycline use (antianabolic effect).

LIMITATIONS: Patients' variability in protein intake and mass of voluntary muscle can cause this ratio to be misleading.[2] METHODOLOGY: Calculation

Footnotes

1. Maher JF, "Disparity in BUN and Plasma Creatinine Test Results in Patient," *JAMA*, 1977, 237:2535.
2. Beck LH, "Hypouricemia in the Syndrome of Inappropriate Secretion of Antidiuretic Hormone," *N Engl J Med*, 1979, 301:528-30.
3. Richards RJ, Donica MB, and Grayer D, "Can the Blood Urea Nitrogen/Creatinine Ratio Distinguish Upper From Lower Gastrointestinal Bleeding?" *J Clin Gastroenterol*, 1990, 12(5):500-4.
4. Dossetor JB, "Creatininemia Versus Uremia: The Relative Significance of Blood Urea Nitrogen and Serum Creatinine Concentrations in Azotemia," *Ann Intern Med*, 1966, 65:1287-99.

References

Lindeman RD, "Assessment of Renal Function in the Old: Special Considerations," *Clin Lab Med*, 1993, 13(1):269-77.

Olsen LH and Andreassen KH, "Stools Containing Altered Blood-Plasma Urea: Creatinine Ratio as a Simple Test for the Source of Bleeding," *Br J Surg*, 1991, 78(1):71-3.

CA 15-3

CPT 86316

Related Information

Body Fluid *on page 145*
Breast Biopsy *on page 40*
CA 19-9 *on this page*
CA 125 *on page 154*
Carcinoembryonic Antigen *on page 167*

Synonyms Carbohydrate Antigen 15-3

Applies to TAG 72, Placental Alkaline Phosphatase

Test Commonly Includes CA 19-9, CEA, TAG 72

Abstract The measurement of CA 15-3 has greatest utility in monitoring recurrent carcinoma of the breast.

Specimen Serum **CONTAINER:** Red top tube **STORAGE INSTRUCTIONS:** Refrigerate serum. Stable at 4°C for 2 weeks.

Interpretive **REFERENCE RANGE:** <25-30 U/mL (SI: <25-30 kU/L) **USE:** Monitor patients for systemic recurrence of breast carcinoma.[1] With CEA, CA 15-3 is helpful to monitor therapeutic response. It is **not** suitable as a screening test. Ninety-six percent of patients with combined local and systemic disease had increased CA 15-3 levels.[1] **LIMITATIONS:** Like CEA, CA 15-3 fails as a reliable marker for early breast cancer. It lacks specificity for primaries of breast. **ADDITIONAL INFORMATION:** The use of CA 15-3 in the evaluation of pelvic masses in women is less effective than the measurement of CA 125, CA 15-3, and TAG 72. The employment of all three markers facilitates the separation of benign from malignant masses.[2] In a large study comparing CEA and CA 15-3 in the diagnosis and monitoring of breast cancer, it was found that CA 15-3 was more sensitive than CEA in detection of recurrent tumor. There was good correlation of CA 15-3 levels with tumor stage of breast cancer, and CA 15-3 was better than CEA in detection of metastases.[3]

Footnotes

1. Geraghty JG, Coveney EC, Sherry F, et al, "CA 15-3 in Patients With Locoregional and Metastatic Breast Carcinoma," *Cancer*, 1992, 70(12):2831-4.
2. Soper JT, Hunter VJ, Daly L, et al, "Preoperative Serum Tumor-Associated Antigen Levels in Women With Pelvic Masses," *Obstet Gynecol*, 1990, 75(2):249-54.
3. Safi F, Kohler I, Rottinger E, et al, "The Value of the Tumor Marker CA 15-3 in Diagnosing and Monitoring Breast Cancer. A Comparative Study With Carcinoembryonic Antigen," *Cancer*, 1991, 68(3):574-82.

References

Dnistrian AM, Schwartz MK, Greenberg EJ, et al, "CA 15-3 and Carcinoembryonic Antigen in the Clinical Evaluation of Breast Cancer," *Clin Chim Acta*, 1991, 200(2-3):81-93.

Ferroni P, Szpak C, Greiner JW, et al, "CA 72-4 Radioimmunoassay in the Diagnosis of Malignant Effusions. Comparison of Various Tumor Markers," *Int J Cancer*, 1990, 46(3):445-51.

Jacobs IJ, Oram DH, and Bast RC Jr, "Strategies for Improving the Specificity of Screening for Ovarian Cancer With Tumor-Associated Antigens CA 125, CA 15-3, and TAG 72.3," *Obstet Gynecol*, 1992, 80(3 Pt 1):396-9.

Kiang DT, Greenberg LJ, and Kennedy BJ, "Tumor Marker Kinetics in the Monitoring of Breast Cancer," *Cancer*, 1990, 65(2):193-9.

Robertson JF, Pearson D, Price MR, et al, "Objective Measurement of Therapeutic Response in Breast Cancer Using Tumour Markers," *Br J Cancer*, 1991, 64(4):757-63.

Shinozaki T, Chigira M, and Kato K, "Multivariate Analysis of Serum Tumor Markers for Diagnosis of Skeletal Metastases," *Cancer*, 1992, 69(1):108-12.

CA 19-9

CPT 86316

Related Information

Alpha$_1$-Fetoprotein, Serum *on page 115*
Body Fluid *on page 145*
CA 15-3 *on this page*
CA 125 *on page 154*
Carcinoembryonic Antigen *on page 167*
Immunoperoxidase Procedures *on page 60*

Synonyms Carbohydrate Antigen 19-9

Applies to CA 50; CA 242; SPan-1; Tissue Polypeptide Antigen; TPA

Abstract CA 19-9 is a carbohydrate antigen, a monosialoganglioside. Its widest use has been work-up for and monitoring of carcinoma of the pancreas. Small carcinomas of the pancreas may be detected with CA 19-9, SPan-1, and imaging.[1]

Specimen Serum **CONTAINER:** Red top tube **STORAGE INSTRUCTIONS:** Freeze to ship. **CAUSES FOR REJECTION:** Inadequate specimen identification

Interpretive **REFERENCE RANGE:** <37 U/mL. This value is arbitrary and statistically derived. **USE:** Useful for monitoring gastrointestinal cancers, head and neck tumors, and gynecologic tumors; predict the recurrence of stomach, pancreatic, liver, and colorectal malignancies **LIMITATIONS:** CA 19-9 has so far been evaluated in highly selected populations. It is described as inferior to CEA as a marker for colorectal carcinoma.[2] Tissue polypeptide antigen (TPA) has been found to provide a closer relationship to clinical status than CEA or CA 19-9 in subjects with bronchogenic carcinoma.[3] False-positive CA 19-9 and alpha-fetoprotein (AFP) assays are described with hepatic cirrhosis. CA 19-9 is described as inferior to AFP in detection of carcinoma arising in cirrhosis.[4] Its sensitivity and specificity in other settings needs to be established. It is **not** a screening test. **METHODOLOGY:** Immunoradiometric assay (IRMA). Like CEA, it is used immunocytochemically as well. **ADDITIONAL INFORMATION:** CA 19-9, a carbohydrate antigen, is related to Lewis blood group antigen. Individuals who are Lewis (a-b-) phenotype (6% of the population) cannot synthesize CA 19-9, CA 50, and CA 195; and this may account for the lesser diagnostic value of these markers compared to CEA, in the diagnosis of colorectal cancer.[5] It has been shown to be elevated in sera of some patients with gastrointestinal tumors. CA 19-9, as a tumor marker, is helpful in post-therapeutic monitoring to determine success of therapy or development of recurrence when used serially. CA 19-9 has been reported as positive in 70% to 80% of pancreatic carcinomas, 50% to 60% of gastric cancers, 60% of hepatobiliary cancers, 30% of colorectal cancers, and few lung, breast, renal cell, or prostate cancers. Serum levels may differentiate pancreatic cancer from pancreatitis. The test may also be positive in patients with nonneoplastic disease, particularly inflammatory disease of the bowel, cirrhosis, and autoimmune conditions including rheumatoid arthritis (33%), systemic lupus erythematosus (32%), and scleroderma (33%). The prognostic value of serum CA 19-9 levels in histologically proven pancreatic adenocarcinoma was recently studied.[6] Levels were significantly lower in patients with tumors less than 5 cm in diameter than in those with tumors greater than 5 cm. Average survival time was longer in those patients whose levels returned to normal after resection than in those whose level decreased but did not return to normal. In those who underwent resection, recurrent elevation of CA 19-9 preceded changes detected by computed tomography or clinical examination by 2-9 months. In those patients who died of pancreatic carcinoma, 65% had a definite rise in CA 19-9 levels before death.

CA 19-9 and CA 50 are useful in distinguishing hepatocellular carcinoma from cholangiocarcinoma. CA 19-9 and CA 50 antigens are normal constituents of bile ducts. In a small series of cases, 9 out of 10 cholangiocarcinomas stained (immunoperoxidase) for CA 50 and 8 out of 10 for CA 19-9. Eleven cases of hepatocellular carcinomas were negative for both markers by immunoperoxidase technique.[7]

A study of 54 patients with pancreatic adenocarcinoma and 27 patients with chronic pancreatitis showed that serum levels of CA 19-9 were less accurate than CT-guided pancreatic fine-needle aspiration biopsy and ultrasound in distinguishing the two entities.[8]

In a large study of carcinoma of the gallbladder in a high-risk population in Mexico and Bolivia, it was found that serum levels of CA 19-9 had superior sensitivity (79.4%) than serum CEA levels (50.0%). Using the tests in parallel did not improve results.[9]

A new marker, CA 242, shows great promise as a marker for colorectal, pancreatic, and hepatobiliary carcinoma. Its sensitivity and specificity exceeds that of CEA, CA 19-9, and CA 50.[10,11]

Footnotes

1. Satake K, Chung YS, Umeyama K, et al, "The Possibility of Diagnosing Small Pancreatic Cancer (Less Than 4.0 cm) by Measuring Various Serum Tumor Markers," *Cancer*, 1991, 68(1):149-52.
2. Quentmeier A, Möller P, Schwarz V, et al, "Carcinoembryonic Antigen, CA 19-9, and CA 125 in Normal and Carcinomatous Human Colorectal Tissue," *Cancer*, 1987, 60:2261-6.
3. Buccheri GF, Ferrigno D, Sartoris AM, et al, "Tumor Markers in Bronchogenic Carcinoma – Superiority of Tissue Polypeptide Antigen to Carcinoembryonic Antigen and Carbohydrate Antigenic Determinant 19-9," *Cancer*, 1987, 60:42-50.
4. Fabris C, Basso DA, Leandro G, et al, "Serum CA 19-9 and Alpha-Fetoprotein Levels in Primary Hepatocellular Carcinoma and Liver Cirrhosis," *Cancer*, 1991, 68(8):1795-8.
5. van der Schouw YT, Verbeek AL, Wobbes T, et al, "Comparison of Four Serum Tumour Markers in the Diagnosis of Colorectal Carcinoma," *Br J Cancer*, 1992, 66(1):148-54.
6. Tian F, Appert HE, Myles J, et al, "Prognostic Value of Serum CA 19-9 Levels in Pancreatic Adenocarcinoma," *Ann Surg*, 1992, 215(4):350-5.
7. Haglund C, Lindgren J, Roberts PJ, et al, "Difference in Tissue Expression of Tumour Markers CA 19-9 and CA 50 in Hepatocellular Carcinoma and Cholangiocarcinoma, " *Br J Cancer*, 1991, 63(3):386-9.

(Continued)

CA 19-9 *(Continued)*

8. DelMaschio A, Vanzulli A, Sironi S, et al, "Pancreatic Cancer Versus Chronic Pancreatitis: Diagnosis With CA 19-9 Assessment, US, CT, and CT-Guided Fine-Needle Biopsy," *Radiology*, 1991, 178(1):95-9.
9. Strom BL, Maislin G, West SL, et al, "Serum CEA and CA 19-9: Potential Future Diagnostic or Screening Tests for Gallbladder Cancer?" *Int J Cancer*, 1990, 45(5):821-4.
10. Nilsson O, Johansson C, Glimelius B, et al, "Sensitivity and Specificity of CA 242 in Gastrointestinal Cancer. A Comparison With CEA, CA 50, and CA 19-9," *Br J Cancer*, 1992, 65(2):215-21.
11. Kuusela P, Haglund C, and Roberts PJ, "Comparison of A New Tumour Marker CA 242 With CA 19-9, CA 50, and Carcinoembryonic Antigen (CEA) in Digestive Tract Diseases," *Br J Cancer*, 1991, 63(4):636-40.

References

Barillari P, Sammartino P, Cardi M, et al, "Gastrointestinal Cancer Follow-Up: The Effectiveness of Sequential CEA, TPA, and CA 19-9 Evaluation in the Early Diagnosis of Recurrences," *Aust N Z J Surg*, 1991, 61(9):675-80.

Beretta E, Malesci A, Zerbi A, et al, "Serum CA 19-9 in the Postsurgical Follow-Up of Patients With Pancreatic Cancer," *Cancer*, 1987, 60:2428-31.

Collazos J, "Serum CA 19-9 and Alpha-Fetoprotein Levels in Primary Hepatocellular Carcinoma and Liver Cirrhosis," *Cancer*, 1992, 70(5):1202-3.

Konishi I, Fujii S, Nanbu Y, et al, "Mucin Leakage Into the Cervical Stroma May Increase Lymph Node Metastasis in Mucin-Producing Cervical Adenocarcinomas," *Cancer*, 1990, 65(2):229-37.

Kouri M, Pyrhönen S, and Kuusela P, "Elevated CA 19-9 as the Most Significant Prognostic Factor in Advanced Colorectal Carcinoma," *J Surg Oncol*, 1992, 49(2):78-85.

Loy TS, Sharp SC, Andershock CJ, et al, "Distribution of CA 19-9 in Adenocarcinomas and Transitional Cell Carcinomas – An Immunohistochemical Study of 527 Cases," *Am J Clin Pathol*, 1993, 99:726-8.

Lucarotti ME, Habib NA, Kelly SB, et al, "Clinical Evaluation of Combined Use of CEA, CA 19-9, and CA 50 in the Serum of Patients With Pancreatic Carcinoma," *Eur J Surg Oncol*, 1991, 17(1):51-3.

Mercer DW, "Immunoassays for the Detection of Tumor-Associated Antigens," *Manual of Clinical Laboratory Immunology*, Chapter 118, Rose NR, Friedman H, and Fahey JL, eds, Washington, DC: American Society for Microbiology, 791-5.

Pleskow DK, Berger HJ, Gyves J, et al, "Evaluation of a Serologic Marker, CA 19-9, in the Diagnosis of Pancreatic Cancer," *Ann Intern Med*, 1989, 110(9):704-9.

Richter JM, Christensen MR, Rustgi AK, et al, "The Clinical Utility of the CA 19-9 Radioimmunoassay for the Diagnosis of Pancreatic Cancer Presenting as Pain or Weight Loss – A Cost-Effective Analysis," *Arch Intern Med*, 1989, 149(10):2292-7.

Satake K, Kanazawa G, Kho I, et al, "Evaluation of Serum Pancreatic Enzymes, Carbohydrate Antigen 19-9, and Carcinoembryonic Antigen in Various Pancreatic Diseases," *Am J Gastroenterol*, 1985, 80:630-6.

Shimomura C, Eguchi K, Kawakami A, et al, "Elevation of a Tumor-Associated Antigen CA 19-9 Levels in Patients With Rheumatic Diseases," *J Rheumatol*, 1989, 16(11):1410-5.

Steinberg W, "The Clinical Utility of the CA-19-9 Tumor-Associated Antigen," *Am J Gastroenterol*, 1990, 85(4):350-5.

Torosian MH, "The Clinical Usefulness and Limitations of Tumor Markers," *Surg Gynecol Obstet*, 1988, 166:567-9.

Warshaw AL and Fernández-del Castillo C, "Pancreatic Carcinoma," *N Engl J Med*, 1992, 326(7):455-64.

Wobbes T, Thomas CM, Segers MF, et al, "Evaluation of Seven Tumor Markers (CA 50, CA 19-9, CA 19-9 TruQuant, CA 72-4, CA 195, Carcinoembryonic Antigen, and Tissue Polypeptide Antigen) in the Pretreatment Sera of Patients With Gastric Carcinoma," *Cancer*, 1992, 69(8):2036-41.

CA 50 *see* CA 19-9 *on page 152*

CA 125

***CPT** 86316*

Related Information

Body Fluid *on page 145*
Body Fluids Analysis, Cell Count *on page 523*
Body Fluids Cytology *on page 482*
CA 15-3 *on page 152*
CA 19-9 *on page 152*
Carcinoembryonic Antigen *on page 167*
Cyst Fluid Cytology *on page 495*
Immunoperoxidase Procedures *on page 60*

Synonyms Cancer Antigen 125

Applies to Aminoterminal Propeptide of Type III Procollagen; PIIINP; TAG 72

Abstract The antigen CA 125 is recognized by a monoclonal antibody, OC-125. It is increased in most patients with advanced, nonmucinous (serous) ovarian cancer. It is advocated preoperatively for prognostic information. When measured serially, it may be useful in detection of relapse and as a monitor of patient response to chemotherapeutic agents.

Specimen Serum **CONTAINER:** Red top tube **STORAGE INSTRUCTIONS:** Refrigerate within 2 hours of collection. Freeze at -20°C for long-term storage. **CAUSES FOR REJECTION:** Inadequate specimen identification

Interpretive **REFERENCE RANGE:** <35 U/mL (SI: <35 kU/L); levels >35 U/mL (SI:>35 kU/L) are highly correlated with malignancy **USE:** Tumor marker for monitoring disease progression in nonmucinous common epithelial neoplasms of the ovary. It may be found in patients with adenocarcinoma and adenosquamous carcinoma of the cervix. It may prove to be useful in detection of advanced, extrauterine carcinoma of endometrium. **LIMITATIONS:** CA 125 is not specific for tumors of the ovary and cannot distinguish benign from malignant tumors. It is **not** a screening test. False-positive CA 125 values have been reported in patients who developed antibodies against mouse immunoglobulins when monoclonal-based double determinant immunoradiometric assays are used. The interference can be removed by affinity chromatography on columns designed to remove human IgG. Lack of elevation of CA 125 results does not provide reliable information that a patient is tumor-free, but rising levels do indicate poor prognosis. Hysterectomy and menopausal status effect levels.[1] Fifty percent of the patients with stage I ovarian cancer have normal levels of CA 125, although most subjects with advanced stage tumor have elevations. Elevations bear correlation with tumor stage, but normal levels are reported with large volume tumors.[2] High levels are described with peritonitis and with hepatic cirrhosis.[3] **METHODOLOGY:** Enzyme immunoassay (EIA), radioimmunoassay (RIA); immunohistochemical methods are in use **ADDITIONAL INFORMATION:** CA 125 is a 220 kD glycoprotein expressed by more than 80% of nonmucinous ovarian epithelial neoplasms. It is also expressed by other coelomic epithelial derivatives and other gynecologic neoplasms such as endometrial and fallopian tube carcinoma, and some tumors of the pancreas, liver, colon, breast, and lung (in smaller percentages). It can also be detected in pregnancy, abruptio placentae, tubo-ovarian abscess, advanced endometriosis, and benign teratomas (dermoids).

Levels >65 units/mL are associated with malignancy in over 90% of cases with pelvic masses.

CA 125 is most useful in monitoring progression or recurrence in cases of known ovarian carcinoma. For this purpose, levels >35 IU/mL may be significant; although a lower level does not replace a second-look operation. About 25% of patients have CA 125 levels <35 IU/mL before a second-look laparotomy despite the presence of residual tumor. However, some patients with a negative second-look procedure reverted to a positive CA 125 within 1 month. Therefore, CA 125 remains a useful tool to follow these patients.

A long-term (3-7 years) follow-up study of 33 patients with advanced nonmucinous epithelial ovarian carcinoma after primary treatment, using monthly determination of CA 125, showed a sensitivity of 95% in detecting early recurrence.[4] A similar study showed that serial monitoring was useful, and the elevations in progressive disease preceded clinical diagnosis by a median time of 6 months.[5]

Because of the high frequency of false-positive results associated with common benign conditions, CA 125 is not useful as a screening test for ovarian carcinoma. Some of these benign conditions are menstruation, pregnancy, benign pelvic tumors, pelvic inflammatory disease, ovarian hyperstimulation syndrome, and peritonitis.[6]

The preoperative evaluation of endometrial carcinoma using CA 125, TAG 72, and CA 15-3 was of limited use in predicting extent of disease and presence of distant metastases.[7] However, a favorable report of the use of CA 125 to monitor endometriosis in infertile women has appeared.[8]

Use of additional markers, such as CA 15-3, TAG 72, and placental alkaline phosphatase, with CA 125 has been advocated to enhance specificity.[9]

In effusion fluids, elevation of CA 125 without increases of CEA are in keeping with a primary in ovary, fallopian tube, or endometrium. Increased CEA without elevation of CA 125 may be found with mucinous adenocarcinoma of lung, breast, gastrointestinal tract, as well as ovary.[10]

CA 125 is advocated as a monitor of the course of advanced carcinoma of the endometrium only with aminoterminal propeptide of type III procollagen (PIIINP).[11]

Footnotes

1. Grover S, Quinn MA, Weideman P, et al, "Factors Influencing Serum CA 125 Levels in Normal Women," *Obstet Gynecol*, 1992, 79(4):511-4.
2. Patsner B, Orr JW Jr, Mann WJ Jr, et al, "Does Serum CA 125 Level Prior to Second-Look Laparotomy for Invasive Ovarian Adenocarcinoma Predict Size of Residual Disease?" *Gynecol Oncol*, 1990, 38(3):373-6.

(Continued)

CA 125 *(Continued)*

3. Ruibal A and Siuriana R, "Evidence of A Relationship Between High Serum CA 125 and Liver Failure Pattern in Cirrhotic Patients Without Ascites and Jaundice," *Int J Biol Markers*, 1989, 1(1):55-6.
4. Hogberg T and Kagedal B, "Long-Term Follow-Up of Ovarian Cancer With Monthly Determinations of Serum CA 125," *Gynecol Oncol*, 1992, 46(2):191-8.
5. Sevelda P, Rosen A, Denison U, et al, "Is CA 125 Monitoring Useful in Patients With Epithelial Ovarian Carcinoma and Preoperative Negative CA 125 Serum Levels?" *Gynecol Oncol*, 1991, 43(2):154-8.
6. Daoud E and Bodor G, "CA 125 Concentrations in Malignant and Nonmalignant Disease," *Clin Chem*, 1991, 37(11):1968-74.
7. Soper JT, Berchuck A, Olt GJ, et al, "Preoperative Evaluation of Serum CA 125, TAG 72, and CA 15-3 in Patients With Endometrial Carcinoma," *Am J Obstet Gynecol*, 1990, 163(4 Pt 1):1204-9.
8. Pittaway DE, "The Use of Serial CA 125 Concentrations to Monitor Endometriosis in Infertile Women," *Am J Obstet Gynecol*, 1990, 163(3):1032-7.
9. Bast RC Jr, Knauf S, Epenetos A, et al, "Coordinate Elevation of Serum Markers in Ovarian Cancer but Not in Benign Disease," *Cancer*, 1991, 68(8):1758-63.
10. Rudolph RA, Pinto MM, and Bernstein LH, "Measuring Decision Values for CEA and CA 125 in Effusions," *Lab Med*, 1990, 21(9):574-8.
11. Tomás C, Penttinen J, Risteli J, et al, "Serum Concentrations of CA 125 and Aminoterminal Propeptide of Type III Procollagen (PIIINP) in Patients With Endometrial Carcinoma," *Cancer*, 1990, 66(11):2399-406.

References

Averette HE, Steren A, and Nguyen HN, "Screening in Gynecologic Cancers," *Cancer*, 1993, 72:1043-9.

Bast RC , Hunter V, and Knapp RC, "Pros and Cons of Gynecologic Tumor Markers," *Cancer*, 1987, 60:1984-92.

Bergmann JF, Bidart JM, George M, et al, "Elevation of CA 125 in Patients With Benign and Malignant Ascites," *Cancer*, 1987, 59:213-7.

Bersinger NA and Rageth JC, "A Comparison Between Pregnancy-Associated α_2-Glycoprotein (α_2-PAG), Carcin-Embryonic Antigen (CEA), CA 125, and CA 15-3 as Tumor Markers in Breast Cancer," *Eur J Gynaecol Oncol*, 1990, 11(2):135-9.

Brand E and Lidor Y, "The Decline of CA 125 Level After Surgery Reflects the Size of Residual Ovarian Cancer," *Obstet Gynecol*, 1993, 81(1):29-32.

Buller RE, Berman ML, Bloss JD, et al, "CA 125 Regression: A Model for Epithelial Ovarian Cancer Response," *Am J Obstet Gynecol*, 1991, 165(2):360-7.

Cruickshank DJ, Paul J, Lewis CR, et al, "An Independent Evaluation of the Potential Clinical Usefulness of Proposed CA 125 Indices Previously Shown to Be of Prognostic Significance in Epithelial Ovarian Cancer," *Br J Cancer*, 1992, 65(4):597-600.

Diez M, Cerdàn FJ, Ortega MD, et al, "Evaluation of Serum CA 125 as a Tumor Marker in Non-Small Cell Lung Cancer," *Cancer*, 1991, 67(1):150-4.

Duk JM, De Bruijn HW, Groenier KH, et al, "Adenocarcinoma of the Uterine Cervix – Prognostic Significance of Pretreatment Serum CA 125, Squamous Cell Carcinoma Antigen, and Carcinoembryonic Antigen Levels in Relation to Clinical and Histopathologic Tumor Characteristics," *Cancer*, 1990, 65(8):1830-7.

Fedele L, Vercellini P, Arcaini L, et al, " CA 125 in Serum, Peritoneal Fluid, Active Lesions and Endometrium of Patients With Endometriosis," *Am J Obstet Gynecol*, 1988, 158:166-70.

Finkler NJ, Benacerraf B, Lavin PT, et al, "Comparison of Serum CA 125, Clinical Impression, and Ultrasound in the Preoperative Evaluation of Ovarian Masses," *Obstet Gynecol*, 1988, 72:659-64.

Gadducci A, Ferdighini M, Ceccarini T, et al, "A Comparative Evaluation of the Ability of Serum CA 125, CA 19-9, CA 15-3, CA 50, CA 72-4, and TATI Assays in Reflecting the Course of Disease in Patients With Ovarian Carcinoma," *Eur J Gynaecol Oncol*, 1990, 11(2):127-33.

Ghazizadeh M, Sasaki Y, Oguro T, et al, "Combined Immunohistochemical Study of Tissue Polypeptide Antigen and Cancer Antigen 125 in Human Ovarian Tumours," *Histopathology*, 1990, 17(2):123-8.

Helzisouer KJ, Bush TL, Alberg AJ, et al, "Prospective Study of Serum CA 125 Levels as Markers of Ovarian Cancer," *JAMA*, 1993, 269(9):1123-6.

Hising C, Anjegard IM, and Einhorn N, "Clinical Relevance of the CA 125 Assay in Monitoring of Ovarian Cancer Patients," *Am J Clin Oncol*, 1991, 14(2):111-4.

Hosono MN, Endo K, Sakahara H, et al, "Different Antigenic Nature in Apparently Healthy Women With High Serum CA 125 Levels Compared With Typical Patients With Ovarian Cancer," *Cancer*, 1992, 70(12):2851-6.

Hunter VJ, Daly L, Helms M, et al, "The Prognostic Significance of CA 125 Half-Life in Patients With Ovarian Cancer Who Have Received Primary Chemotherapy After Surgical Cytoreduction," *Am J Obstet Gynecol*, 1990, 163(4 Pt 1):1164-7.

Jacobs IJ, Oram DH, and Bast RC Jr, "Strategies for Improving the Specificity of Screening for Ovarian Cancer With Tumor-Associated Antigens CA 125, CA 15-3, and TAG 72.3," *Obstet Gynecol*, 1992, 80(3 Pt 1):396-9.

Kamiya N, Mizuno K, Kawai M, et al, "Simultaneous Measurement of CA 125, CA 19-9, Tissue Polypeptide Antigen, and Immunosuppressive Acidic Protein to Predict Recurrence of Ovarian Cancer," *Obstet Gynecol*, 1990, 76 (3 Pt 1):417-21.

Motoyama T, Watanabe H, Takeuchi S, et al, "Cancer Antigen 125, Carcinoembryonic Antigen, and Carbohydrate Determinant 19-9 in Ovarian Tumors," *Cancer*, 1990, 66(12):2628-35.

O'Shaughnessy A, Check JH, Nowroozi K, et al, "CA 125 Levels Measured in Different Phases of the Menstrual Cycle in Screening for Endometriosis," *Obstet Gynecol*, 1993, 81(1):99-103.

Podczaski E, Whitney C, Manetta A, et al, "Use of CA 125 to Monitor Patients With Ovarian Epithelial Carcinomas," *Gynecol Oncol*, 1989, 33(2):193-7.
Richardson GS, "Ovarian Cancer," *JAMA*, 1993, 269(9):1163, (editorial).
Tseng PC, Sprance HE, Carcangiu ML, et al, "CA 125, NB/70K, and Lipid-Associated Sialic Acid in Monitoring Uterine Papillary Serous Carcinoma," *Obstet Gynecol*, 1989, 74(3 Pt 1):384-7.
Turpeinen U, Lehtovirta P, Alfthan H, et al, "Interference by Human Anti-Mouse Antibodies in CA 125 Assay After Immunoscintigraphy: Anti-Idiotypic Antibodies Not Neutralized by Mouse IgG but Removed by Chromatography," *Clin Chem*, 1990, 36(7):1333-8.
van Nagell JR Jr, "Ovarian Cancer Screening," *Cancer*, 1991, 68(4):679-80.
Witt BR, Miles R, Wolf GC, et al, "CA 125 Levels in Abruptio Placentae," *Am J Obstet Gynecol*, 1991, 164(5 Pt 1):1225-8.
Zurawski VR Jr, Sjovall K, Schoenfeld DA , et al, "Prospective Evaluation of Serum CA 125 Levels in a Normal Population, Phase I: The Specificities of Single and Serial Determinations in Testing for Ovarian Cancer," *Gynecol Oncol*, 1990, 36(3):299-305.

CA 242 *see* CA 19-9 *on page 152*
Ca, Blood *see* Calcium, Serum *on page 160*

Calcitonin

CPT 82308

Related Information

Adrenocorticotropic Hormone *on page 98*
Catecholamines, Fractionation, Plasma *on page 172*
Catecholamines, Fractionation, Urine *on page 174*
Immunoperoxidase Procedures *on page 60*
Phosphorus, Urine *on page 322*

Synonyms CT; HCT; Human Calcitonin; Thyrocalcitonin

Abstract A polypeptide made by the normal C cells (parafollicular cells) of the thyroid gland, by tumors of the C cells, medullary carcinoma of thyroid, and by certain other neoplasms (lung, breast, pancreas).

Patient Care **PREPARATION:** Patient should fast overnight.

Specimen Serum or plasma **CONTAINER:** Red top tube or green top (heparin) tube **STORAGE INSTRUCTIONS:** Collect into chilled tube. Process within 10 minutes of collection. Separate in a refrigerated centrifuge. Separate serum (plasma) into plastic tube and freeze. **CAUSES FOR REJECTION:** Patient not fasting, stored specimen not frozen, recent isotope scan or other radioactivity, hemolyzed specimen

Interpretive **REFERENCE RANGE:** <19 pg/mL (SI: <19 ng/L) basal, depending on the assay. Normal ranges for calcium/pentagastrin stimulation tests are available.[1] **POSSIBLE PANIC RANGE:** Elevated levels are not diagnostic of medullary carcinoma of the thyroid (MCT). However, some patients with MCT have values >500 pg/mL. **USE:** Detect and confirm C-cell hyperplasia (the precursor of medullary carcinoma of thyroid) as well as a tumor marker for diagnosis and management of **medullary carcinoma of the thyroid** gland. Preoperative serum calcitonin is reported to roughly correlate with tumor weight or extent of disease; therefore, postoperative levels also have prognostic application. The doubling time of serum levels correlates with recurrence.[2] Multiple endocrine neoplasia (MEN) type II includes medullary carcinoma of the thyroid, hyperparathyroidism, and pheochromocytoma. This is Sipple's syndrome. MEN type IIB includes medullary carcinoma of the thyroid, pheochromocytoma, mucosal neuromas, marfanoid habitus, and intestinal ganglioneuromatosis.

An important use of calcitonin assay is in the follow-up of patients with medullary carcinoma and the work-up of their families to detect early, subclinical cases. Indications for calcitonin assay include family history of unspecified type of thyroid cancer, calcified thyroid mass, thyroid tumor associated with hypercalcemia and/or pheochromocytoma, amyloid-containing metastatic carcinoma with unknown primary site and the presence of mucosal neuromas.

LIMITATIONS: In numbers of patients with medullary carcinoma of the thyroid (especially those with familial medullary carcinoma of thyroid) the baseline calcitonin may be normal; however, an abnormally large calcitonin response may follow provocative infusion of calcium and/or pentagastrin.[3] Most subjects with microscopic medullary carcinoma and all with C-cell hyperplasia have normal basal calcitonin levels; provocative testing is needed.

Occasional spurious high results are encountered. Hemolysis can cause spurious high levels. The purity of standards may vary and antibodies in various assays may lack uniform specificities. Calcitonin in patients' sera lacks immunoreactive uniformity.

(Continued)

Calcitonin *(Continued)*

METHODOLOGY: Radioimmunoassay (RIA), immunoradiometric assay (IRMA)[4] **ADDITIONAL INFORMATION:** High concentrations of calcitonin occur not only in patients with malignant parafollicular or C-cell tumors (medullary thyroid carcinoma), but also in many patients with carcinomas of the lung; in some individuals with carcinoma of breast, carcinoids, islet cell tumors, apudomas, in patients with pancreatitis, thyroiditis, and in renal failure. Hypergastrinemia may account for calcitonin elevations in the Zollinger-Ellison syndrome and in pernicious anemia. Medullary carcinoma arises from thyroid C cells (parafollicular cells). C-cell hyperplasia is a preneoplastic state in patients with MEN. Provocative tests that may be used for diagnosis of medullary thyroid carcinoma are pentagastrin and calcium infusion. A combined calcium pentagastrin test is described. These tests are much more useful than random plasma levels of calcitonin for the diagnosis of MCT. Early diagnosis of medullary carcinoma of thyroid is needed; total thyroidectomy is curative if the tumor is treated early.[1]

Calcitonin was increased in 48% of patients with oat cell carcinoma in a study of 110 patients with lung cancer.

Recently, calcitonin gene-related peptide (CGRP) has been suggested as a useful test together with calcitonin, as tumor markers in MEN type II.[5]

CEA is next most useful, after calcitonin, as a marker for medullary carcinoma. CEA generates less fluctuation than calcitonin in calculation of doubling time.[2] Medullary carcinomas may produce other substances, including ACTH and serotonin. Such ectopic ACTH secretion may cause Cushing's syndrome.

If there are preoperative findings to suggest medullary carcinoma (eg, family history of unspecified type of thyroid cancer) in a patient with a thyroid mass, then calcitonin level, metanephrines, catecholamines, and CAT scan of the adrenals for pheochromocytoma should be considered. Medullary carcinomas of the thyroid gland have a variable histologic picture. Correlation between serum calcitonin levels and immunoperoxidase staining of the neoplastic thyroid tissue for calcitonin may assist in confirming the diagnosis in difficult cases.

The direct manifestation of high calcitonin levels is secretory diarrhea in 30% of patients with medullary thyroid carcinoma.

Footnotes

1. Leshin M, "Multiple Endocrine Neoplasia," *Williams Textbook of Endocrinology*, 7th ed, Wilson JD and Foster DW, eds, Philadelphia, PA: WB Saunders Co, 1985, 1274-89.
2. Miyauchi A, Matsuzuka F, Kuma K, et al, "Evaluation of Surgical Results and Prediction of Prognosis in Patients With Medullary Thyroid Carcinoma by Analysis of Serum Calcitonin Levels," *World J Surg*, 1988, 12:610-5.
3. Guilloteau D, Perdrisot R, Calmettes C, et al, "Diagnosis of Medullary Carcinoma of the Thyroid (MCT) by Calcitonin Assay Using Monoclonal Antibodies: Criteria for the Pentagastrin Stimulation Test in Hereditary MCT," *J Clin Endocrinol Metab*, 1990, 71(4):1064-7.
4. Perdrisot R, Bigorgne JC, Guilloteau D, et al, "Monoclonal Immunoradiometric Assay of Calcitonin Improves Investigation of Familial Medullary Thyroid Carcinoma," *Clin Chem*, 1990, 36(2):381-3.
5. Schifter S, "Calcitonin Gene-Related Peptide and Calcitonin as Tumour Markers in MEN 2 Family Screening," *Clin Endocrinol (Oxf)*, 1989, 30(3):263-70.

References

Boultwood J, Wynford-Thomas D, Richards GP, et al, "*In Situ* Analysis of Calcitonin and CGRP Expression in Medullary Thyroid Carcinoma," *Clin Endocrinol (Oxf)*, 1990, 33(3):381-90.

Carter WB, Taylor RL, Kao PC, et al, "Determination of Plasma Calcitonin Gene-Related Peptide Concentrations by a New Immunochemiluminometric Assay in Normal Persons and Patients With Medullary Thyroid Carcinoma and Other Neuroendocrine Tumors," *J Clin Endocrinol Metab*, 1991, 72(2):327-35.

Fraser D, Jones G, Kooh SW, et al, "Calcium and Phosphate Metabolism," *Textbook of Clinical Chemistry*, Tietz NW, ed, Philadelphia, PA: WB Saunders Co, 1986, 1356.

Ghillani PP, Motte P, Troalen F, et al, "Identification and Measurement of Calcitonin Precursors in Serum of Patients With Malignant Diseases," *Cancer Res*, 1989, 49(23):6845-51.

Hansen M, Hammer M, and Hummer L, "ACTH, ADH, and Calcitonin Concentrations as Markers of Response and Relapse in Small Cell Carcinoma of the Lung," *Cancer*, 1980, 46:2062-7.

Rougier P, Calmettes C, LaPlanche A, et al, "The Values of Calcitonin and Carcinoembryonic Antigen in the Treatment and Management of Nonfamilial Medullary Thyroid Carcinoma," *Cancer*, 1983, 51:855-62.

Sanchez GJ, Venkataraman PS, Pryor RW, et al, "Hypercalcitoninemia and Hypocalcemia in Acutely Ill Children: Studies in Serum Calcium, Blood Ionized Calcium, and Calcium-Regulating Hormones," *J Pediatr*, 1989, 114(6):952-6.

Calcitriol *see* Vitamin D_3, Serum *on page 387*

Calcium, Ionized

CPT 82330

Related Information

Kidney Stone Analysis *on page 1129*

Kidney Stone Analysis on page 1129

Synonyms Ionized Calcium

Patient Care PREPARATION: Patient should be recumbent for 30 minutes prior to collection.

Specimen Whole blood (preferred), serum, or plasma CONTAINER: Green top (heparin) tube if whole blood or plasma is used or red top tube COLLECTION: Collect anaerobically, leave stoppers in; do not use tourniquet. Heparin syringe is best; 1 unit of heparin/mL of blood lowers ionized calcium 0.01 mmol/L. The use of dry, electrolyte balanced heparin virtually eliminates the heparin interference.[1] STORAGE INSTRUCTIONS: Store anaerobically. Such specimens can be stored 48 hours at 4°C. SPECIAL INSTRUCTIONS: Controversy exists over the ideal specimen for ionized calcium determination. Concern exists that ionized calcium values may be altered by clotting (serum) or by heparin binding of calcium (plasma). However, serum and plasma have been found to give generally similar values, while whole blood is 1% to 2% higher.

The procedure of calculating ionized calcium may become redundant in large laboratories with availability of instruments that measure it directly on small volumes of blood. Adjusting pH to 7.4 is not necessary if blood is collected anaerobically.

Interpretive REFERENCE RANGE: See table. USE: Evaluate nonbound calcium; a measure of physiologically active calcium fraction. Ionized calcium is increased with hyperparathyroidism, ectopic parathyroid hormone-producing neoplasms, and with excessive vitamin D.

Patients with renal failure and/or transplantation, in whom problems include secondary hyperparathyroidism; balance in dialysis patients.

Ill premature infants with hypoproteinemia and acidosis. Occasionally useful when hypercalcemia coexists with abnormal protein state such as myeloma, in disturbances of acid base balance; in cirrhosis.

Calcium, Ionized

Age	Reference Range	
	Conventional units (mg/dL)	SI units (mmol/L)
Cord blood	5.20–5.84	1.30–1.46
3–24 h	4.32–5.12	1.08–1.28
24–48 h	4.00–4.72	1.00–1.18
Adults	4.48–5.28	1.12–1.32

Low in hypoparathyroidism, vitamin D deficiency, pseudohypoparathyroidism.

A role for ionized calcium levels may exist in patients having cardiac arrest.[2] It is widely used in cardiac thoracic surgery and heart transplantation.

LIMITATIONS: Total calcium remains the first line test for evaluation of calcium abnormality. METHODOLOGY: Ion-selective electrode (ISE) ADDITIONAL INFORMATION: Calcium in serum exists ionized, bound to organic anions such as phosphate and citrate, and bound to proteins (mainly albumin). Of these, ionized calcium is the physiologically important form.

Measurement of serum ionized calcium provides insight into the effect of total protein and albumin on serum calcium levels. A patient can have high total calcium, with normal ionized calcium and increased total protein and/or albumin, as in dehydration or in myeloma.

Women have greater circadian variation of ionized calcium and intact PTH than men.[3]

There is an inverse relationship between ionized calcium and phosphate concentration.[4]

Footnotes

1. Toffaletti J, Ernst P, Hunt P, et al, "Dry Electrolyte-Balanced Heparinized Syringes Evaluated for Determining Ionized Calcium and Other Electrolytes in Whole Blood," *Clin Chem*, 1991, 37:(10 Pt 1)1730-3.
2. Urban P, Scheidegger D, Buchmann B, et al, "Cardiac Arrest and Blood Ionized Calcium Levels," *Ann Intern Med*, 1988, 109(2):110-3.
3. Calvo MS, Eastell R, Offord KP, et al, "Circadian Variation in Ionized Calcium and Intact Parathyroid Hormone: Evidence for Sex Differences in Calcium Homeostasis," *J Clin Endocrinol Metab*, 1991, 72(1):69-76.
4. Lehmann M and Mimouni F, "Serum Phosphate Concentration. Effect on Serum Ionzied Calcium Concentration *In Vitro*," *Am J Dis Child*, 1989, 143(11):1340-1.

References

Cooper RS, et al, "Ionized Serum Calcium in Black Hypertensives: Absence of a Relationship With Blood Pressure," *J Clin Hypertens*, 1987, 3:514-9.

Engel K, Pedersen KO, Nielsen SP, et al, "Ionized Calcium Workshop No 1," *Scand J Clin Lab Invest*, 1983, 165(Suppl):1-126.

(Continued)

Calcium, Ionized *(Continued)*

Forman DT and Lorenzo L, "Ionized Calcium: Its Significance and Clinical Usefulness," *Ann Clin Lab Sci*, 1991, 21(5):297-304.

Fraser D, Jones G, Kooh SW, et al, "Calcium and Phosphate Metabolism," *Textbook of Clinical Chemistry*, Tietz NW, ed, Philadelphia, PA: WB Saunders Co, 1986, 705-28.

Loughead JL, Mimouni F, and Tsang RC, "Serum Ionized Calcium Concentrations in Normal Neonates," *Am J Dis Child*, 1988, 142:516-8.

Rasmussen N, Frolich A, Hornnes PJ, et al, "Serum Ionized Calcium and Intact Parathyroid Hormone Levels During Pregnancy and Postpartum," *Br J Obstet Gynaecol*, 1990, 97(9):857-9.

Roelofsen JM, Berkel GM, Uttendorfsky OT, et al, "Urinary Excretion Rates of Calcium and Magnesium in Normal and Complicated Pregnancies," *Eur J Obstet Gynecol Reprod Biol*, 1988, 27:227-36.

Rosen IB and Pollard A, "Ionized Calcium in Monitoring Effective Parathyroidectomy: A Preliminary Report," *World J Surg*, 1988, 12:630-4.

Thode J, Holmegaard SN, Transbol I, et al, "Adjusted Ionized Calcium (at pH 7.4) and Actual Ionized Calcium (at Actual pH) in Capillary Blood Compared for Clinical Evaluation of Patients With Disorders of Calcium Metabolism," *Clin Chem*, 1990, 36(3):541-4.

Wu AH, Bracey A, Bryan-Brown CW, et al, "Ionized Calcium Monitoring During Liver Transplantation," *Arch Pathol Lab Med*, 1987, 111:935-8.

Calcium Oxalate, Urine *see* Oxalate, Urine *on page 303*

Calcium, Serum

CPT 82310

Related Information

Aluminum, Bone *on page 1018*
Aluminum, Serum *on page 1019*
Calcium, Urine *on page 163*
Concentration Test, Urine *on page 1115*
Cyclic AMP, Urine *on page 204*
Kidney Stone Analysis *on page 1129*
Magnesium, Serum *on page 287*
Parathyroid Hormone *on page 311*
Phosphorus, Serum *on page 319*
Phosphorus, Urine *on page 322*
Potassium, Blood *on page 330*

Synonyms Ca, Blood; Total Calcium, Serum

Applies to Chloride/Phosphorus Ratio

Test Commonly Includes Disorders of calcium metabolism are initially evaluated with measurements of serum phosphorus, alkaline phosphatase, albumin, chloride, total protein and commonly, parathormone assays as well as serum and often 24-hour urine calcium levels.

Abstract The two most common causes of hypercalcemia (beyond slight increases from dehydration) are primary hyperparathyroidism and malignancy.

Specimen Serum **CONTAINER:** Red top tube **SAMPLING TIME:** Morning, fasting sample is desirable, since some diurnal variation exists (which may reflect postural changes). **COLLECTION:** Pediatric: Blood drawn from heelstick for capillary. Since about half of serum calcium is bound to proteins, there is variation with posture. Venous stasis in sampling causes misleading results. **STORAGE INSTRUCTIONS:** Refrigerate in stoppered vials, not in sample cups. **CAUSES FOR REJECTION:** Gross hemolysis

Interpretive **REFERENCE RANGE:** Infant to 1 month: 7.0-11.5 mg/dL (SI: 1.75-2.87 mmol/L); 1 month to 1 year: 8.6-11.2 mg/dL (SI: 2.15-2.79 mmol/L) normal range slowly descends. Up to 30 years: 8.2-10.2 mg/dL (SI: 2.05-2.54 mmol/L). It decreases slightly in older years. **POSSIBLE PANIC RANGE:** $<$7.0 mg/dL (SI: $<$1.75 mmol/L) may lead to tetany. Calcium $>$12.0 mg/dL (SI: $>$2.99 mmol/L) may induce coma, although some patients tolerate higher levels. Possibly life-threatening levels: $\leq$6.0 mg/dL (SI: $\leq$1.50 mmol/L), $\geq$14.0 mg/dL (SI: $\geq$3.49 mmol/L). Extremely high levels may be found with primary parathyroid carcinomas, which are very uncommon. **USE:** Work-up for coma, pancreatitis and other gastrointestinal problems, nephrolithiasis, polydipsia, polyuria, azotemia, multiple endocrine adenomatosis.

Causes of high calcium:

- Hyperparathyroidism – look also for high ionized calcium, measured or calculated. Hyperparathyroidism may coexist with other endocrine tumors (multiple endocrine adenomatosis syndromes).

- Carcinoma, with or without bone metastases. Humoral hypercalcemia of malignancy (HHM), (tumor induced hypercalcemia) is seen especially in primary squamous cell carcinoma of lung, head and neck, but other important tumors include primaries in the kidney, liver, bladder, and ovary. It is probably caused by parathormone-like peptides. The most common solid tumors causing bone metastases are primaries in the breast and lung. Other neoplasms may also cause hypercalcemia. Differences between HPT and humoral hypercalcemia of malignancy include low dihydroxyvitamin D, reduced calcium absorption,[1] and the presence of a nonparathyroid tumor. Hypercalcemia with alkaline phosphatase more than twice its upper limit is more suggestive of **cancer** than of hyperparathyroidism. Especially if there is only a brief duration of symptoms, anemia, hypoalbuminemia, and other findings suggestive of malignant disease, chloride/phosphorus ratio <29 mmol/L, chloride <100 mmol/L, high serum LD (LDH) and/or phosphorus, think first of malignant neoplasm.[2] **The chloride/phosphorus ratio** is predominantly of value when it is <29 mmol/L, to provide evidence **against** a diagnosis of primary hyperparathyroidism.[2] Laboratory results which would favor malignancy include anemia, increased LD and alkaline phosphatase, decreased serum albumin and chloride, and chloride/phosphorus ratio <29 mmol/L. **Parathyroid hormone-related protein** was recently purified and identified by molecular cloning as a 141-amino acid peptide with limited homology to PTH itself. Both peptides activate the PTH receptor to produce hypercalcemia. PTH-related protein is now recognized as the cause of hypercalcemia in most solid tumors, particularly squamous, and renal carcinomas.[3]
- Myeloma
- Leukemia, lymphoma; especially T-cell[4] lymphoma/leukemia and Burkitt's lymphoma.
- Dehydration is an extremely common cause of slight increases of calcium.
- Sarcoidosis (a fraction of patients have high serum calcium; usually without low serum phosphorus). More have hypercalciuria.
- Chronic hypervitaminosis D. Vitamin A intoxication, isotretinoin (a vitamin A derivative).[5]
- Prolonged immobilization (probably uncommon), in patient with increased bone turnover (eg, Paget's disease of bone, malignancy, children).
- TB, histoplasmosis, coccidioidomycosis, berylliosis
- Milk-alkali syndrome: prolonged use of calcium-containing materials and alkali, eg, $CaCO_3$ or other absorbable alkali ulcer remedies with high milk intake (now rare).
- Idiopathic hypercalcemia of infancy (uncommon)
- Endocrine: hyperthyroidism; Addison's disease; acromegaly; pheochromocytoma (rare cause of hypercalcemia)
- Advanced chronic liver disease
- Bacteremia
- Familial hypocalciuric hypercalcemia[6] (dominant inheritance); the best test for familial benign hypercalciuria (FBH) is a plot of fasting serum PTH against fasting urine calcium excretion[7]
- Aluminum induced renal osteomalacia
- Rhabdomyolysis
- Several commonly used drugs cause *in vivo* elevation, including calcium salts, lithium, thiazide/chlorthalidone therapy, other diuretics; vitamins D and A and estrogens (rapid increase in patients with breast carcinoma).

In any case of hypercalcemia, it is desirable to measure magnesium and potassium levels. A helpful mnemonic for the differential diagnosis of the more common causes of hypercalcemia is DCHIMPS (drugs, cancer, hyperparathyroidism, intoxication with vitamin D or A, milk alkali syndrome, Paget's disease of bone, sarcoidosis).[1]

Causes of low calcium:

- Low albumin and low total protein relate to common, usually slight decreases of calcium. The routine method measures **total** calcium, about half of which is bound to plasma proteins. Since the metabolically active form of calcium is the ionized state, the patient's serum protein level should be considered when interpreting a calcium result. For example, a patient's ionized calcium may be normal when the total calcium is elevated in the presence of elevated proteins and, conversely, may also be normal when the total calcium is low and the proteins are low.
- High phosphorus: renal insufficiency, hypoparathyroidism, pseudohypoparathyroidism

(Continued)

Calcium, Serum *(Continued)*

- Vitamin D deficiency, rickets, osteomalacia (Alkaline phosphatase is a screening test for osteomalacia. Calcium, phosphorus, and alkaline phosphatase can all be normal in osteomalacia.)
- Milkman's syndrome
- Malabsorption or malnutrition with interference with vitamin D and/or calcium absorption
- Renal tubular acidosis
- Pancreatitis, acute
- Dilutional: I.V. fluids
- Bacteremia
- Hypomagnesemia
- Anticonvulsants and other common drugs, most by *in vivo* action, can depress calcium. Barbiturates in elderly may cause calcium decrease; other drugs including calcitonin, corticosteroids, gastrin, glucagon, glucose, insulin, magnesium salts, methicillin, and tetracycline in pregnancy.

The differential diagnosis is shown in a graph presented in the listing Parathyroid Hormone, in which PTH is plotted against calcium.

LIMITATIONS: Sodium citrate, EDTA, and NaF potassium oxalate interfere. Gross hemolysis falsely elevates results. **METHODOLOGY:** Cresolphthalein complexone; complexone is required to minimize effect of hemolysis[8]; atomic absorption (AA) is not used extensively, but remains the reference method. **ADDITIONAL INFORMATION:** In the differential diagnosis of hypercalcemia serum calcium should be measured on at least three occasions. In **primary hyperparathyroidism** (HPT), parathyroid hormone, serum chloride, and urine calcium are increased. Rarely, in HPT the hypercalcemia is accompanied by a low-normal PTH.[9] In HPT, calcium rises, then phosphorus falls, then alkaline phosphatase rises. Alkaline phosphatase is usually not more than twice its upper limit in HPT. Measured ionized calcium and calculated ionized calcium may be helpful.

Twenty-four hour urinary calcium is increased in HPT, low in **familial hypocalciuric hypercalcemia** (FHH) which is characterized by hypercalcemia and hypocalciuria. An autosomal dominant, it apparently has no complications. Ratio of renal calcium clearance to creatinine clearance <0.01 suggests this genetic disease. The calcium/creatinine clearance ratio is said to discriminate between FHH and hyperparathyroidism.[2] Family studies are highly desirable.

Hypocalcemia, then hypercalcemia occur with rhabdomyolysis - induced acute renal failure.[10,11]

Footnotes

1. Watts NB and Keffer JH, "The Parathyroid Glands, Kidney Stones and Osteoporosis," *Practical Endocrinology*, 4th ed, Chapter 8, Philadelphia, PA: Lea & Febiger, 1989.
2. Wong ET and Freier EF, "The Differential Diagnosis of Hypercalcemia. An Algorithm for More Effective Use of Laboratory Tests," *JAMA*, 1982, 247:75-80.
3. Strewler GJ and Nissenson RA, "Hypercalcemia in Malignancy," *West J Med*, 1990, 153(6):635-40.
4. Sirianni SR, Mora ME, Sands AM, et al, "Malignant Lymphoma Presenting With Severe Hypercalcemia," *N Y State J Med*, 1989, 89(9):533-5.
5. Valentic JP, Elias AN, and Weinstein GD, "Hypercalcemia Associated With Oral Isotretinoin in the Treatment of Severe Acne," *JAMA*, 1983, 250:1899-900.
6. Marx SJ, "Familial Hypocalciuric Hypercalcemia," *N Engl J Med*, 1980, 303:810-1, (editorial).
7. Gunn IR and Wallace JR, "Urine Calcium and Serum Ionized Calcium, Total Calcium and Parathyroid Hormone Concentrations in the Diagnosis of Primary Hyperparathyroidism and Familial Benign Hypercalcaemia," *Ann Clin Biochem*, 1992, 29(Pt 1):52-8.
8. Corns CM, "Interference by Haemoglobin With the Cresolphthalein Complexone Method for Serum Calcium Measurement," *Ann Clin Biochem*, 1990, 27(Pt 2):152-5.
9. Hollenberg AN and Arnold A, "Hypercalcemia With Low-Normal Serum Intact PTH: A Novel Presentation of Primary Hyperparathyroidism," *Am J Med*, 1991, 91(5):547-8.
10. Llach F, Felsenfeld AJ, and Haussler MR, "The Pathophysiology of Altered Calcium Metabolism in Rhabdomyolysis-Induced Acute Renal Failure, Interactions of Parathyroid Hormone, 25-Hydroxycholecalciferol, and 1,25-Dihydroxycholecalciferol," *N Engl J Med*, 1981, 305:117-23.
11. Knochel JP, "Serum Calcium Derangements in Rhabdomyolysis," *N Engl J Med*, 1981, 305:161-3, (editorial).

References

Aderka D, Schwartz D, Dan M, et al, "Bacteremic Hypocalcemia: A Comparison Between the Calcium Levels of Bacteremic and Nonbacteremic Patients With Infection," *Arch Intern Med*, 1987, 147:232-6.

Balland M and Trivin F, "Total Calcium," *Drug Effects on Laboratory Test Results Analytical Interferences and Pharmacological Effects*, Siest G and Galteau MM, eds, Littleton, MA: PSG Publishing Co Inc, 1988, 148-64.

Bourke E and Delaney V, "Assessment of Hypocalcemia and Hypercalcemia," *Clin Lab Med*, 1993, 13(1):157-81.
Broadus AE, Mangin M, Ikeda K, et al, "Humoral Hypercalcemia of Cancer: Identification of a Novel Parathyroid Hormone-Like Peptide," *N Engl J Med*, 1988, 319:556-63.
Budayr AA, Nissenson RA, Klein RF, et al, "Increased Serum Levels of a Parathyroid Hormone-like Protein in Malignancy-Associated Hypercalcemia," *Ann Intern Med*, 1989, 111(10):807-12.
Cadeau BJ and MacKay JS, "Serum Calcium: Review of Methods," *ASCP Check Sample®*, Chicago, IL: American Society of Clinical Pathologists, 1988.
Chasan SA, Pothel LR, and Huben RP, "Management and Prognostic Significance of Hypercalcemia in Renal Cell Carcinoma," *Urology*, 1989, 33(3):167-70.
Gerhardt A, Greenberg A, Reilly JJ Jr, et al, "Hypercalcemia: A Complication of Advanced Chronic Liver Disease," *Arch Intern Med*, 1987, 147:274-7.
Gibbs WN, Lofters WS, Campbell M, et al, "Non-Hodgkin Lymphoma in Jamaica and Its Relation to Adult T Cell Leukemia-Lymphoma," *Ann Intern Med*, 1987, 106:361-8.
Jayabose S, Iqbal K, Newman L, et al, "Hypercalcemia in Childhood Renal Tumors," *Cancer*, 1988, 61:788-91.
Klee GG, Kao PC, and Heath H III, "Hypercalcemia," *Endocrinol Metab Clin North Am*, 1988, 17:573-600.
Law WM Jr and Heath H III, "Familial Benign Hypercalcemia (Hypocalciuric Hypercalcemia)," *Ann Intern Med*, 1985, 102:511-9.
Law WM Jr, Wahner HW, and Heath H III, "Bone Mineral Density and Skeletal Fractures in Familial Benign Hypercalcemia (Hypocalciuric Hypercalcemia)," *Mayo Clin Proc*, 1984, 59:811-5.
Lobaugh B, Neelon FA, Oyama H, et al, "Circadian Rhythms for Calcium, Inorganic Phosphorus, and Parathyroid Hormone in Primary Hyperparathyroidism: Functional and Practical Considerations," *Surgery*, 1989, 106(6):1009-16.
Samaan NA, Ouais S, Ordonez NG, et al, "Multiple Endocrine Syndrome Type I: Clinical, Laboratory Findings, and Management in Five Families," *Cancer*, 1989, 64(3):741-52.
Sanchez GJ, Venkataraman PS, Pryor RW, et al, "Hypercalcitoninemia and Hypocalcemia in Acutely Ill Children: Studies in Serum Calcium, Blood Ionized Calcium, and Calcium-Regulating Hormones," *J Pediatr*, 1989, 114(6):952-6.
Walter RM Jr and Greenberg BR, "Hypercalcemia in the Accelerated Phase of Chronic Myelogenous Leukemia," *Cancer*, 1980, 46:1174-8.
Zaloga GP, Chernow B, and Eil C, "Hypercalcemia and Disseminated Cytomegalovirus Infection in the Acquired Immunodeficiency Syndrome," *Ann Intern Med*, 1985, 102:331-3.

Calcium, Urine

***CPT** 82340*

Related Information

Calcium, Serum *on page 160*
Kidney Stone Analysis *on page 1129*
Magnesium, Urine *on page 289*
Parathyroid Hormone *on page 311*
Phosphorus, Urine *on page 322*
Uric Acid, Urine *on page 380*
Vitamin D_3, Serum *on page 387*

Patient Care **PREPARATION:** In stone evaluation, urinary calcium results are more meaningful if the patient initially is on his/her usual diet for 3 days prior to urine collection. Drugs affecting mineral metabolism include antacids, phosphates, glucocorticoids, carbonic anhydrase inhibitors, anticonvulsants, and diuretics including thiazides. Thiazides are used therapeutically to lower urine calcium excretion. If the patient is on a stone prevention regime and test is for follow-up, then medications should **not** be stopped for the test.

Specimen 24-hour urine **CONTAINER:** Plastic urine container or acid-washed glass bottle **COLLECTION:** Instruct the patient to void at 8 AM and discard the specimen. Then collect all urine including the final specimen voided at the end of the 24-hour collection period (ie, 8 AM the next morning). Container must be labeled with patient's name, date and time collection started and finished.

Interpretive **REFERENCE RANGE:** Varies with diet; based on average calcium intake of 600-800 mg/24 hours (SI: 15-20 mmol/day): excretion may be 100-250 mg/24 hours (SI: 2.5-6.2 mmol/day). On a diet of 400-800 mg/24 hours of calcium daily (SI: 10-20 mmol/day), others set the upper limit at 200 mg/24 hours of calcium (SI: 5 mmol/day) in a 24-hour urine collection.[1] More than 4 mg/kg is associated with increased prevalence of stone formation. Low calcium diet: <150 mg/24 hours (SI: <3.7 mmol/day) excreted. High calcium diet: 250-300 mg/24 hours (SI: 6.2-7.5 mmol/day) excreted. Hypercalciuria has been defined as calcium excretion in excess of 250 mg/24 hours (SI: 6.2 mmol/day) for women, 300 mg/24 hours (SI: 7.5 mmol/day) for men.[2] Calcium excretion, like other laboratory results, must be related to the individual pa-

(Continued)

Calcium, Urine *(Continued)*

tient. The rate of calcium excretion can also be expressed as a calcium/creatinine ratio. In healthy individuals with constant muscle mass, urinary calcium (mg/dL)/creatinine (mg/dL) is <0.14 (SI: calcium (mmol/L)/creatinine (mmol/L) is <0.40). Values >0.20 (mg/dL) or >0.57 (mmol/L units) suggest hypercalciuria. **USE:** Reflects intake, rates of intestinal calcium absorption, bone resorption, and renal loss. Those processes relate to parathyroid hormone and vitamin D levels. Evaluate bone disease, calcium metabolism, renal stones (nephrolithiasis)[3]; idiopathic hypercalciuria[4], and especially, parathyroid disorders. Follow up patients on calcium therapy for osteopenia.

High in 30% to 80% of instances of primary hyperparathyroidism, but urinary calcium excretion does not consistently, reliably distinguish hyperparathyroidism from other entities. High in sarcoidosis.[5] Increased with immobilization, with steroid therapy, with Paget's disease of bone, and in primary (idiopathic) hypercalciuria.[6] Increased with entities causing high ultrafiltrable calcium: ectopic hyperparathyroidism, some cases of renal tubular acidosis, Fanconi syndrome, increased calcium intake, vitamin D intoxication, hyperthyroidism, diabetes mellitus, acromegaly, glucocorticoid excess, some cases of Crohn's disease and ulcerative colitis, myeloma, some instances of leukemia and lymphoma, and carcinoma metastatic to bone. Reported relationship to hematuria in children.[7]

Low in familial hypocalciuric hypercalcemia, for which urine calcium measurements are mandatory; low with thiazide diuretics, vitamin D deficiency, renal osteodystrophy, vitamin D resistant rickets, hypoparathyroidism, pseudohypoparathyroidism and pre-eclampsia.[8]

LIMITATIONS: Decreased in patients on oral contraceptives. Lacks specificity for hyperparathyroidism when increased. Five percent of the population have hypercalciuria.[6] **METHODOLOGY:** Cresolphthalein complexone, atomic absorption (AA) **ADDITIONAL INFORMATION:** Twenty percent to 25% of patients who form calcium stones have hyperuricosuria. Urinary calcium reflects in part the relation between GFR and tubular reabsorption.

Footnotes

1. Beeler MF and Catrou PG, "Disorders of Calcium Metabolism," *Interpretations in Clinical Chemistry. A Textbook Approach to Chemical Pathology*, 2nd ed, Chicago, IL: American Society of Clinical Pathologists, 1983, 34-44.
2. Palmieri GM, "Calcium, Phosphate, and Magnesium Metabolism," *The Laboratory in Clinical Medicine. Interpretation and Application*, 2nd ed, Halsted JA and Halsted CH, eds, Philadelphia, PA: WB Saunders Co, 1981, 688-96.
3. Silverberg SJ, Shane E, Jacobs TP, et al, "Nephrolithiasis and Bone Involvement in Primary Hyperparathyroidism," *Am J Med*, 1990, 89(3):327-34.
4. Lemann J Jr and Gray RW, "Idiopathic Hypercalciuria," *J Urol*, 1989, 141(3 Pt 2):715-8.
5. Scully RE, ed, "Case Records of the Massachusetts General Hospital. Weekly Clinicopathological Exercises. Case 50-1981. A 76 Year Old Woman With Intermittent Hypercalcemia," *N Engl J Med*, 1981, 305:1457-64.
6. Erickson SB, "Hypercalciuria," *Mayo Clin Proc*, 1981, 56:579.
7. Stark H, Tieder M, Eisenstein B, et al, "Hypercalciuria as a Cause of Persistent or Recurrent Haematuria," *Arch Dis Child*, 1988, 63(3):312-3.
8. Taufield PA, Ales KL, Resnick LM, et al, "Hypocalciuria in Pre-eclampsia," *N Engl J Med*, 1987, 316:715-8.

References

Friedman RB and Young DS, *Effects of Disease on Clinical Laboratory Tests*, Washington, DC: American Association of Clinical Chemistry Press, 1989.

Gunn IR and Wallace JR, "Urine Calcium and Serum Ionized Calcium, Total Calcium and Parathyroid Hormone Concentrations in the Diagnosis of Primary Hyperparathyroidism and Familial Benign Hypercalcaemia," *Ann Clin Biochem*, 1992, 29(Pt 1):52-8.

Lemann J Jr, Pleuss JA, Gray RW, et al, "Potassium Administration Reduces and Potassium Deprivation Increases Urinary Calcium Excretion in Healthy Adults," *Kidney Int*, 1991, 39(5):973-83.

Lemann J Jr, Worcester EM, and Gray RW, "Hypercalciuria and Stones," *Am J Kidney Dis*, 1991, 17(4):386-91.

Marx SJ, Stock JL, Attie MF, et al, "Familial Hypocalciuric Hypercalcemia: Recognition Among Patients Referred After Unsuccessful Parathyroid Exploration," *Ann Intern Med*, 1980, 92:351-6.

Sanchez-Ramos L, Jones DC, and Cullen MT, "Urinary Calcium as an Early Marker for Pre-eclampsia," *Obstet Gynecol*, 1991, 77(5):685-8.

cAMP, Plasma *see* Cyclic AMP, Plasma *on page 204*

cAMP, Urine *see* Cyclic AMP, Urine *on page 204*

Cancer Antigen 125 *see* CA 125 *on page 154*

Capillary Blood Gases *see* Blood Gases, Capillary *on page 143*

Carbohydrate Antigen 15-3 *see* CA 15-3 *on page 152*

Carbohydrate Antigen 19-9 *see* CA 19-9 *on page 152*

Carbon Dioxide, Blood

***CPT** 82374*

Related Information

Blood Gases, Arterial *on page 140*
Blood Gases, Capillary *on page 143*
Blood Gases, Venous *on page 144*
Chloride, Serum *on page 182*
Electrolytes, Blood *on page 212*
HCO_3, Blood *on page 248*
Kidney Stone Analysis *on page 1129*
pCO_2, Blood *on page 314*
pH, Blood *on page 315*

Synonyms CO_2 Content; CO_2T; tCO_2

Applies to Acid-Base Status Evaluation

Specimen Whole blood **CONTAINER:** Green top (heparin) tube **COLLECTION:** Specimen should be kept tightly closed, as CO_2 will diffuse out, causing erroneous values. This loss may amount to 6 mmol/hour.[1] Anaerobic conditions are best.

Interpretive **REFERENCE RANGE:** Infancy to 2 years: 18-28 mmol/L (SI: 18-28 mmol/L); 2 years and older: arterial: 23-29 mmol/L (SI: 23-29 mmol/L); venous: 22-26 mmol/L (SI: 22-26 mmol/L)[1] **POSSIBLE PANIC RANGE:** <15 mmol/L (SI: <15 mmol/L), >50 mmol/L (SI: >50 mmol/L) **USE:** Evaluate the total carbonate buffering system in the body, acid-base balance. High results may represent respiratory acidosis with CO_2 retention, or metabolic alkalosis (eg, prolonged vomiting). Low value may indicate respiratory alkalosis as in hyperventilation or metabolic acidosis, (eg, diabetes with ketoacidosis). **LIMITATIONS:** Interpretation requires clinical information and the other electrolytes. **METHODOLOGY:** Colorimetry, enzyme assay, or pCO_2 electrode. Organic acids interfere (positively) in the total carbon dioxide as measured on the Kodak Ektachem® 700.[2,3] **ADDITIONAL INFORMATION:** "Total carbon dioxide" consists of CO_2 in solution or bound to proteins, HCO_3^-, CO_3^{2-}, and H_2CO_3. In practice, 80% to 90% is present as bicarbonate (HCO_3^-). "Hypercapnia" means excessive carbon dioxide in the blood. Impaired elimination of CO_2 reflects interaction of abnormalities in respiratory drive, the muscles of respiration, and the function of the lung. Elimination of carbon dioxide from the lung involves alveolar ventilation but not dead-space ventilation. Partitioning of these spaces is expressed as a ratio between dead space and total volume per breath: the tidal volume. The tidal volume normally is <0.30. These and other aspects of pulmonary gas exchange, ventilation and their consequences are addressed as the partial pressure of arterial carbon dioxide, $PaCO_2$, a part of arterial blood gases.[4]

Footnotes

1. Tietz NW, Pruden EL, and Siggaard-Andersen O, "Electrolytes, Blood Gases, and Acid-Base Balance," *Textbook of Clinical Chemistry*, Tietz NW, ed, Philadelphia, PA: WB Saunders Co, 1986, 1172-253.
2. Rifai N, Hyde J, Iosefsohn M, et al, "Organic Acids Interfere in the Measurement of Carbon Dioxide Concentration by the Kodak Ektachem® 700," *Ann Clin Biochem*, 1992, 29(Pt 1):105-8.
3. O'Leary TD and Langton SR, "Calculated Bicarbonate or Total Carbon Dioxide?" *Clin Chem*, 1989, 35(8):1697-700.
4. Weinberger SE, Schwartzstein RM, and Weiss JW, "Hypercapnia," *N Engl J Med*, 1989, 321(18):1223-31.

References

Henneman PL, Gruber JE, Marx JA, et al, "Development of Acidosis in Human Beings During Closed-Chest and Open-Chest CPR," *Ann Emerg Med*, 1988, 17:672-5.

McLain BI, Evans J, Dear PR, et al, "Comparison of Capillary and Arterial Blood Gas Measurements in Neonates," *Arch Dis Child*, 1988, 63:743-7.

Carbonic Anhydrase III *see* Myoglobin, Blood *on page 293*

Carbon Monoxide *see* Carboxyhemoglobin *on this page*

Carboxyhemoglobin

***CPT** 82375*

Related Information

Blood Gases, Arterial *on page 140*
(Continued)

Carboxyhemoglobin *(Continued)*

Synonyms Carbon Monoxide; CO; COHb

Test Commonly Includes COHb is sometimes included in Blood Gases, but may be ordered as a separate test.

Patient Care PREPARATION: In suspected carbon monoxide poisoning, the specimen should be collected immediately.

Specimen Whole blood CONTAINER: Green top (heparin) tube or lavender top (EDTA) tube, depending upon laboratory SAMPLING TIME: Draw before the patient is started on oxygen if possible. COLLECTION: Keep tube capped STORAGE INSTRUCTIONS: Refrigerate immediately after collection. Do not remove cap. Carboxyhemoglobin is stable 4 months in filled, well-capped tube.

Interpretive REFERENCE RANGE: Nonsmokers: <2%; smokers: 1-2 packs/day: 4% to 5%, >2 packs/day: 8% to 9%. Carboxyhemoglobin in the **newborn** may run to 10% to 12%. Carbon monoxide is a metabolic product of hemoglobin catabolism. The increased turnover of hemoglobin in the newborn together with decreased efficiency of the infant's respiratory system may and does lead to higher levels of carboxyhemoglobin. CRITICAL VALUES: Toxic concentration is 20%; lethal is >50% POSSIBLE PANIC RANGE: Disturbance of judgment, headache, and dizziness occur at 10% to 30%; coma at 50% to 60%; fatality occurs at 60% or more, and rapid death at level of 80%. USE: Determine the extent of carbon monoxide poisoning, toxicity. Check on effect of smoking on the patient; work up headache, irritability, nausea, vomiting, vertigo, dyspnea, collapse, coma, convulsions. Work up persons exposed to fires and smoke inhalation. LIMITATIONS: Carbon monoxide levels are of limited value in screening for smoking, since it is cleared rapidly. The half-life of carboxyhemoglobin in individuals with normal cardiopulmonary function is 1-2 hours. Urinary nicotine, if available, is preferable as a screening test for tobacco use. Arterial blood gases may be of limited value in treatment decisions for carbon monoxide poisoning.[1] METHODOLOGY: Spectrophotometric, gas-liquid chromatography (GLC), pulse oximetry[2] ADDITIONAL INFORMATION: Carboxyhemoglobin is useful in judging the extent of carbon monoxide toxicity and in considering the effect of smoking on the patient. A direct correlation has been claimed between CO level and symptoms of atherosclerotic diseases, intermittent claudication, angina, and myocardial infarction. Exposure may occur not only from smoking but also from garage exposure and from various engines. This test may be included when blood gases are ordered, when there is sufficient sample, and when such instrumentation is available.

A danger of missed diagnosis of CO intoxication is continued exposure of the patient and others to a toxic environment.[3] The cherry red color of CO poisoning is not consistently seen.[4] CO intoxication may contribute to the risk of myocardial infarction.[4,5]

A strong correlation is present between carboxyhemoglobin levels and psychometric testing abnormalities.[1] Psychometric testing measures actual neurologic disability and may therefore better define carboxyhemoglobin poisoning severity than blood CO level. The half-life with O_2 administration is 80 minutes. With O_2 at three atmospheres, the half-life is 24 minutes.

Footnotes

1. Myers RA and Britten JS, "Are Arterial Blood Gases of Value in Treatment Decisions for Carbon Monoxide Poisoning," *Crit Care Med*, 1989, 17(2):139-42.
2. Vegfors M and Lennmarken C, "Carboxyhaemoglobinaemia and Pulse Oximetry," *Br J Anaesth*, 1991, 66(5):625-6.
3. Crawford R, Campbell DG, and Ross J, "Carbon Monoxide Poisoning in the Home: Recognition and Treatment," *BMJ*, 1990, 301(6758):1161.
4. Grace TW and Platt FW, "Subacute Carbon Monoxide Poisoning. Another Great Imitator," *JAMA*, 1981, 246:1698-700.
5. Kaufman DW, Helmrich SP, Rosenberg L, et al, "Nicotine and Carbon Monoxide Content of Cigarette Smoke and the Risk of Myocardial Infarction in Young Men," *N Engl J Med*, 1983, 308:409-13.

References

Dolan MC, Haltom TL, Barrows GH, et al, "Carboxyhemoglobin Levels in Patients With Flu-Like Symptoms," *Ann Emerg Med*, 1987, 16:782-6.

Fechner GG and Gee DJ, "Study on the Effects of Heat on Blood and on the Postmortem Estimation of Carboxyhemoglobin and Methaemoglobin," *Forensic Sci Int*, 1989, 40(1):63-7.

Heckerling PS, Leikin JB, Maturen A, et al, "Screening Hospital Admissions From the Emergency Department for Occult Carbon Monoxide Poisoning," *Am J Emerg Med*, 1990, 8(4):301-4.

Krantz T, Thisted B, Strøm J, et al, "Acute Carbon Monoxide Poisoning," *Acta Anaesthesiol Scand*, 1988, 32:278-82.

Thom SR and Keim LW, "Carbon Monoxide Poisoning: A Review Epidemiology, Pathophysiology, Clinical Findings, and Treatment Options Including Hyperbaric Oxygen Therapy," *J Toxicol Clin Toxicol*, 1989, 27(3):141-56.

Variend S and Forrest AR, "Carbon Monoxide Concentrations in Infant Deaths," *Arch Dis Child*, 1987, 62:417-8.

Zijlstra WG, Buursma A, and Meeuwsen-van-der-Roest WP, "Absorption Spectra of Human Fetal and Adult Oxyhemoglobin, Deoxyhemoglobin, Carboxyhemoglobin, and Methemoglobin," *Clin Chem*, 1991, 37(9):1633-8.

Carcinoembryonic Antigen

***CPT** 82378*

Related Information

Adrenocorticotropic Hormone *on page 98*
Alpha$_1$-Fetoprotein, Serum *on page 115*
Body Fluid *on page 145*
Body Fluid Glucose *on page 148*
Body Fluids Analysis, Cell Count *on page 523*
Body Fluids Cytology *on page 482*
Breast Biopsy *on page 40*
CA 15-3 *on page 152*
CA 19-9 *on page 152*
CA 125 *on page 154*
Cyst Fluid Cytology *on page 495*
Immunoperoxidase Procedures *on page 60*

Synonyms CEA

Patient Care PREPARATION: Avoid radioisotope scan prior to collection of specimen (if radioisotope based procedure is used or if method by which CEA is to be determined is unknown).

Specimen Serum or plasma, effusion fluid, bronchoalveolar lavage[1] CONTAINER: Red top tube or lavender top (EDTA) tube, avoid heparin anticoagulant SAMPLING TIME: Preoperative; approximately 4 weeks postoperative and subsequently STORAGE INSTRUCTIONS: Separate serum (or plasma) from cells and refrigerate if assayed within 24 hours. For longer storage, freeze at -20°C.

Interpretive REFERENCE RANGE: Adult: nonsmoker: $<$2.5 ng/mL (SI: $<$2.5 μg/L), smoker: $\leq$5.0 ng/mL (SI: $\leq$5.0 μg/L) USE: CEA is most useful as a chemical monitor of recurrence and of therapy in patients with gastrointestinal carcinomas, especially colorectal neoplasms, to follow postoperative patients regardless of whether or not preoperative CEA was increased. Increase bears an implication of treatment failure or recurrence and is a possible signal for second-look procedures. Detection of locally recurrent carcinoma, lung or hepatic metastasis, especially from colorectal primaries, may lead to resection of recurrent or metastatic carcinoma for cure. The highest levels occur with metastases to liver or bone. Marker for monitoring effectiveness of therapy. CEA is also useful for other primary carcinomas of entodermal origin, such as stomach and pancreas. Significant elevations may be found with primaries of breast, lung, and ovary. High CEA occurs with medullary carcinoma of thyroid. Increases have been reported with giant cell carcinomas of thyroid and with neuroblastoma. Work-up of effusion fluids for carcinoma. LIMITATIONS: CEA levels are elevated in smokers; patients with inflammation including infections, inflammatory bowel disease, and pancreatitis; some patients with hypothyroidism; cirrhosis; and in some patients with noncolorectal neoplasms especially gastric, pancreatic, breast, and ovarian (CA 15-3 is a better marker than CEA in breast cancer).[2] CEA is **not** a screening test for occult cancer. Many negatives occur in patients with early carcinoma. Doubtful cost-effectiveness for many patients. Negative in some patients with even metastatic colorectal and other neoplasms: a minority of such patients do not have high CEA levels. CEA testing may be less sensitive with poorly differentiated tumors. Correlation between tumor burden and CEA level is imperfect, especially with lung primaries. Hepatotoxicity of antineoplastic drugs, as well as tumor cell necrosis or membrane damage may permit escape of CEA into the circulation and cause CEA increase; simultaneous evaluation of liver-related tests has been advocated for the former. Radiation therapy may also induce a transient rise in CEA. As patients are followed, CEA testing should be repeated by the same laboratory. Benign diseases usually do not cause CEA levels $>$5-10 ng/mL (SI: $>$5-10 μg/L). METHODOLOGY: Radioimmunoassay (RIA), enzyme immunoassay (EIA). Patients who received diagnostic presurgical radioimmunoscintography with ^{111}In-labeled anti-CEA murine monoclonal antibody and who had no clinical evidence of disease after resection showed an increase in CEA concentrations. In these cases, CEA was measured with a double-antibody enzyme immunoassay. This increase, in many cases, is an artifact, and the artifact can be eliminated by adding polyclonal IgG or a mixture of IgG_1, IgG_{2a}, and IgG_{2b} monoclonal antibodies before assay. This correction is critical in the follow-up of patients who receive murine monoclonal antibodies for diagnosis or treatment. The role of antimurine antibody (HAMA) should

(Continued)

Carcinoembryonic Antigen *(Continued)*

be considered in all such cases.[3,4] **ADDITIONAL INFORMATION:** CEA is an oncofetal glycoprotein antigen. It is present in embryonic tissues and certain epithelial malignancies as described above. Chemical heterogeneity in the carbohydrate portion of the CEA molecule is the basis for a family of molecules varying in immunologic specificity. CEA may vary in different tissues and individuals. Progressive elevations of CEA may herald tumor recurrence 3-36 months before clinical evidence of metastases. A small rise may signal local recurrence, a large rise hepatic metastasis. Important monitors for breast and colon cancer patients include GGT, alkaline phosphatase, and CEA. CEA is not specific for any one type of cancer; however, values >20 ng/mL (SI: >20 μg/L) are most significantly correlated with metastatic disease and/or with primary pancreatic and colorectal carcinoma.

CEA is more sensitive to recurrence of colonic than rectal primaries.[5] It is positive in about 63% of patients having a colorectal carcinoma; about 20% of patients with Dukes A, 58% with Dukes B, 68% with Dukes C.[6]

Hepatic scans have become positive months after a rise in CEA; lack of sensitivity of liver scans for early, resectable metastases is widely recognized. Similarly, serum alkaline phosphatase has been disappointing, but its value may be enhanced in concert with GGT and CEA. Monthly testing for these three is desirable for the first 1-2 years after resection, followed by progressively less frequent testing until 5 years have elapsed.

Shorter time delays between confirmed CEA increase and second look procedure relate to resectability rate for cure. Mean time delays for resectable cases were 1.4 months, and 4.5 months for unresectable patients, in a Memorial Sloan-Kettering series.[7]

Although 37 of 118 tumor-free patients had CEA false-positive at >5 ng/mL (SI: >5 μg/L) on at least one occasion, CEA was described as the most sensitive means to detect recurrent colon cancer, short of the history. CEA may be more sensitive to distant metastasis of colon cancer than to local recurrence.[8]

Of a relatively small group of patients with detectable recurrence who are resectable, 30% to 50% survive 5 years after resection.[8]

A study of 1774 patients from 63 hospitals indicates that the preoperative level of serum CEA can be used as a prognostic indicator (of survival) in patients with colorectal cancer, independent of stage of disease at diagnosis.[9]

On the other hand, an immunocytochemistry study of 180 primary breast carcinomas utilizing antisera to CEA and CEA/NCA (nonspecific cross reacting antigen) showed no correlation between positivity of CEA immunocytochemistry and histologic grade, lymph node stage, disease-free interval or patient survival.[10] As concerns circulating levels of CA 15-3 and CEA, a study of 173 patients with advanced breast carcinoma found that elevated CEA levels correlated with extent of disease but not with survival.[11]

Earlier studies have shown that plasma CEA is elevated in 60% to 70% of patients with metastatic breast cancer and that CEA level tends to reflect tumor burden.[12] Disparate conclusions, however, have been reached concerning prognostic significance.[12,13,14] Measurement of CEA levels in nipple discharge from patients with nonpalpable breast cancer has been reported to have value in separating malignant from benign disease. Cases of breast cancer generally had nipple discharge levels >100 ng/mL (SI: >100 μg/L).[15]

There is active continuing interest in improving the sensitivity/specificity performance of CEA and other tumor antigen or tumor associated tests in the detection/evaluation of colorectal and other carcinomas.

CEA is one of a number of oncofetal antigens (adenocarcinoma-associated antigens) to which radiolabeled monoclonal antibodies have been prepared and utilized in the radioimmunodetection and therapy of colorectal cancer.[16,17,18,19]

Rule provides an excellent review of the molecular nature of CEA, its heterogeneity and important aspects of RIA analytic methodology.[20] As the measurement of CEA and other oncofetal antigens has not been useful in screening for presence of colon cancer, attention is currently focused on utilization of molecular biologic techniques and genotypic markers.[19] The familial adenomatous polyposis syndrome (Gardner syndrome) as well as some sporadic colorectal carcinomas have 5q chromosome defects (Gardner's interstitial deletion of 5q13-q22). Possibly, other genotypic markers for human colorectal carcinoma (cancer susceptibility genes) will be identified allowing application of DNA hybridization technology to presymptomatic diagnosis and screening.[21]

Footnotes

1. deDiego A, Compte L, Sanchis J, et al, "Usefulness of Carcinoembryonic Antigen Determination in Bronchoalveolar Lavage Fluid. A Comparative Study Among Patients With Peripheral Lung Cancer, Pneumonia, and Healthy Individuals," *Chest*, 1991, 100(4):1060-3.
2. Safi F, Kohler I, Rottinger E, et al, "The Value of the Tumor Marker CA 15-3 in Diagnosing and Monitoring Breast Cancer. A Comparative Study With Carcinoembryonic Antigen," *Cancer*, 1991, 68(3):574-82.
3. Price T, Beatty BG, Beatty JD, et al, "Human Anti-Murine Antibody Interference in Measurement of Carcinoembryonic Antigen Assessed With a Double-Antibody Enzyme Immunoassay," *Clin Chem*, 1991, 37(1):51-7.
4. Hardman N, Gill LL, DeWinter RF, et al, "Generation of a Recombinant Mouse-Human Chimaeric Monoclonal Antibody Directed Against Human Carcinoembryonic Antigen," *Int J Cancer*, 1989, 44(3):424-33.
5. Welch CE and Malt RA, "Abdominal Surgery (Second of Three Parts)," *N Engl J Med*, 1983, 308:685-95.
6. Martin EW Jr, James KK, Hurtubise PE, et al, "The Use of CEA as an Early Indicator for Gastrointestinal Tumor Recurrence and Second-Look Procedures," *Cancer*, 1977, 39:440-6.
7. Attiyeh FF and Stearns MW Jr, "Second-Look Laparotomy Based on CEA Elevations in Colorectal Cancer," *Cancer*, 1981, 47:2119-25.
8. Beart RW Jr and O'Connell MJ, "Postoperative Follow-Up of Patients With Carcinoma of the Colon," *Mayo Clin Proc*, 1983, 58:361-3.
9. Sener SF, Imperato JP, Chmiel J, et al, "The Use of Cancer Registry Data to Study Preoperative Carcinoembryonic Antigen Level as an Indicator of Survival in Colorectal Cancer," *CA*, 1989, 39(1):50-7.
10. Robertson JFR, Ellis IO, Bell J, et al, "Carcinoembryonic Antigen Immunocytochemistry in Primary Breast Cancer," *Cancer*, 1989, 64(8):1638-45.
11. Colomer R, Ruibal A, and Salvador L, "Circulating Tumor Marker Levels in Advanced Breast Carcinoma Correlate With the Extent of Metastatic Disease," *Cancer*, 1989, 64(8):1674-81.
12. Waalkes TP, Enterline JP, Shaper JH, et al, "Biological Markers for Breast Carcinoma," *Cancer*, 1984, 53:644-51.
13. Mansour EG, Hastert M, Park CH, et al, "Tissue and Plasma Carcinoembryonic Antigen in Early Breast Cancer: A Prognostic Factor," *Cancer*, 1983, 51:1243-8.
14. Cohen C, Sharkey FE, Shulman G, et al, "Tumor-Associated Antigens in Breast Carcinomas: Prognostic Significance," *Cancer*, 1987, 60:1294-8.
15. Inaji H, Yayoi E, Maeura Y, et al, "Carcinoembryonic Antigen Estimation in Nipple Discharge as an Adjunctive Tool in the Diagnosis of Early Breast Cancer," *Cancer*, 1987, 60:3008-13.
16. Murray JL and Unger MW, "Radioimmunodetection of Cancer With Monoclonal Antibodies: Current Status, Problems, and Future Directions," *Crit Rev Oncol Hematol*, 1988, 8:227-53.
17. Schlom J, "Innovations in Monoclonal Antibody Tumor Targeting: Diagnostic and Therapeutic Implications," *JAMA*, 1989, 261(5):744-6.
18. Dillman RO, "Monoclonal Antibodies for Treating Cancer," *Ann Intern Med*, 1989, 111(7):592-603.
19. Kaplan EH, "New Perspectives in Large Bowel Cancer: The Diagnostic and Therapeutic Use of Monoclonal Antibodies in Colorectal Cancer," *Hematol Oncol Clin North Am*, 1989, 3:125-31.
20. Rule AH, "Carcinoembryonic Antigens," *Methods in Clinical Chemistry*, Chapter 90, Pesce AJ and Kaplan LA, eds, St Louis, MO: Mosby-Year Book Inc, 1987, 702-13.
21. Moore M, Jones DJ, Schofield PF, et al, "Current Status of Tumor Markers in Large Bowel Cancer," *World J Surg*, 1989, 13(1):52-9.

References

Bhayana V and Diamandis EP, "A Double Monoclonal Time-Resolved Immunofluorometric Assay of Carcinoembryonic Antigen in Serum," *Clin Biochem*, 1989, 22(6):433-8.

Goslin RH, Skarin AT, and Zamcheck N, "Carcinoembryonic Antigen. A Useful Monitor of Therapy of Small Cell Lung Cancer," *JAMA*, 1981, 246:2173-6.

Greiner JW, Guadagni F, Goldstein D, et al, "Evidence for the Elevation of Serum Carcinoembryonic Antigen and Tumor-Associated Glycoprotein-72 Levels in Patients Administered Interferons," *Cancer Res*, 1991, 51(16):4155-63.

Kiang DT, Greenberg LJ, and Kennedy BJ, "Tumor Marker Kinetics in the Monitoring of Breast Cancer," *Cancer*, 1990, 65(2):193-9.

Klee GG and Go VL, "Serum Tumor Markers," *Mayo Clin Proc*, 1982, 57:129-32.

Koch M and McPherson TA, "Carcinoembryonic Antigen Levels as an Indicator of the Primary Site in Metastatic Disease of Unknown Origin," *Cancer*, 1981, 48:1242-4.

Kudo R, Sasano H, Koizumi M, et al, "Immunohistochemical Comparison of New Monoclonal Antiody 1C5 and Carcinoembryonic Antigen in the Differential Diagnosis of Adenocarcinoma of the Uterine Cervix," *Int J Gynecol Pathol*, 1990, 9(4):325-36.

Kuhajda FP, Offutt LE, and Mendelsohn G, "The Distribution of Carcinoembryonic Antigen in Breast Carcinoma. Diagnostic and Prognostic Implications," *Cancer*, 1983, 52:1257-64.

Norton JA, "Carcinoembryonic Antigen. New Applications for an Old Marker," *Ann Surg*, 1991, 213(2):95-7.

Primus FJ, Newell KD, Blue A, et al, "Immunological Heterogeneity of Carcinoembryonic Antigen: Antigenic Determinants on Carcinoembryonic Antigen Distinguished by Monoclonal Antibodies," *Cancer Res*, 1983, 43:686-92.

Rocklin MS, Senagore AJ, and Talbott TM, "Role of Carcinoembryonic Antigen and Liver Function Tests in the Detection of Recurrent Colorectal Carcinoma," *Dis Colon Rectum*, 1991, 34(9):794-7.

Shahangian S, Fritsche HA, and Hughes JI, "Carcinoembryonic Antigen in Serum of Patients With Colorectal Polyps: Correlation With Histology and Smoking Status," *Clin Chem*, 1991, 37(5):651-5.

(Continued)

Carcinoembryonic Antigen *(Continued)*

Steele G Jr, Zamcheck N, Wilson R, et al, "Results of CEA-Initiated Second-Look Surgery for Recurrent Colorectal Cancer," *Am J Surg*, 1980, 139:544-8.
Tatsuta M, Iishi H, Ichii M, et al, "Diagnosis of Gastric Cancers With Fluorescein-Labeled Monoclonal Antibodies to Carcinoembryonic Antigen," *Lasers Surg Med*, 1989, 9(4):422-6.
Theriault RL, Hortobagyi GN, Fritsche HA, et al, "The Role of Serum CEA as a Prognostic Indicator in Stage II and III Breast Cancer Patients Treated With Adjuvant Chemotherapy," *Cancer*, 1989, 63(5):828-35.
Torosian MH, "The Clinical Usefulness and Limitations of Tumor Markers," *Surg Gynecol Obstet*, 1988, 166:567-79, (review).

Cardiac Enzymes/Isoenzymes

CPT *82550 (CK); 83615 (LD); 84450 (AST); 84460 (ALT)*

Related Information

Creatine Kinase *on page 196*
Creatine Kinase Isoenzymes *on page 197*
Lactate Dehydrogenase *on page 269*
Lactate Dehydrogenase Isoenzymes *on page 271*
Myoglobin, Blood *on page 293*
Troponin *on page 375*

Applies to AST/ALT Ratio; CK Isoenzymes; LD Isoenzymes; Myocardial Infarct Panel

Replaces Alpha-Hydroxybutyric Dehydrogenase (HBDH)

Test Commonly Includes CK with isoenzymes, LD (LDH) with isoenzymes; some recommend that AST (SGOT) remain included with cardiac enzymes, especially for diagnosis of patients who present subsequent to the CK-MB peak. In this setting AST supports evidence of abnormal LD isoenzymes.

Specimen Serum **CONTAINER:** Red top tube **SAMPLING TIME:** Samples are usually taken on admission, at 12, 24, and 48 hours, depending on clinical history, initial results, and perceptions of the attending physician. Further information on timing is provided in the listing Creatine Kinase Isoenzymes. A case is made for sampling on admission and at 16 hours after onset for CK-MB peak.[1] Some patients seek medical attention hours or even a day or more following onset. **COLLECTION:** Avoid hemolysis, which causes false increase of LD and may cause false LD_1:LD_2 inversion. **STORAGE INSTRUCTIONS:** Separate serum; freeze serum for CK isoenzymes (but store LD isoenzymes at room temperature) if not done same day. **CAUSES FOR REJECTION:** Hemolysis **SPECIAL INSTRUCTIONS:** Isoenzymes should be run, if acute MI is suspected, even if total enzyme(s), CK and/or LD, are within normal limits[2], unless they are so low that a given laboratory does not feel that attempted separation is practical.

Interpretive **REFERENCE RANGE:** Decision limits are extensively discussed in the literature. They are method dependent. Each laboratory should evaluate its own methods and experience in concert with cardiologists and with active chart review. Problems relevant to decision limits in cardiac enzymes and isoenzymes are shared with many other laboratory tests, as problems of sensitivity versus specificity. Arguments which claim that in many patients the diagnosis of AMI is missed include cases of fatal AMI.[1] **USE:** Diagnosis of acute infarct of myocardium (acute MI, or AMI) **LIMITATIONS:** At onset of acute infarction of myocardium, all enzymes and isoenzymes are normal. It is desirable to draw cardiac enzymes at onset for a baseline. LD_1:LD_2 flip (inversion) and CK-MB elevation have been reported during marathon training with increases of total LD and CK.[3] Elevations of total CK with increased CK-MB and CK-BB, was found with necrotic intestine in experimental animals.[4] Myositis, various myopathies, rhabdomyolysis, and Reye's syndrome are reported to cause elevations of CK-MB. Thus, the test is not entirely specific for AMI, and confirmation by LD isoenzyme studies may be indicated.[5] High LD occurs in a variety of diseases. LD isoenzyme separations greatly improve the diagnostic specificity of an elevated LD value. **METHODOLOGY:** Isoenzymes have been done mostly by electrophoretic separation. Other techniques such as immunoassays and immunoinhibition have been introduced which are more rapid, sensitive, and specific than electrophoresis (to CK-MB in particular).[6] **ADDITIONAL INFORMATION:** **Acute MI:** CK and CK-MB (CK_2 MB) have been widely considered to peak about 1 day following onset, as does AST in usual hospital practice. However, see Sampling Time in Creatine Kinase Isoenzymes listing. LD_1 usually peaks at second day, when LD_1:LD_2 inversion (flip) is most commonly found. CK and CK isoenzymes can be discontinued after MB returns to normal. LD isoenzymes can be stopped after LD_1:LD_2 flip with elevation of LD_1 is found.

CK-MB, LD_1, LD_1:LD_2 ratio, total CK and total LD classically increase with acute MI. CK-MB and LD_1 increase in percentage and absolutely (each isoenzyme percent times the respective total enzyme), peak, then decrease. More information is provided in the individual test listings.

New investigational tests which may allow for much earlier detection of acute myocardial injury include CK-MM and CK-MB isoforms,[7,8,9] quantitation of human ventricular myosin light chains in the blood, and an assay of troponin. These newer tests may have particular value in determining candidates for and monitoring response to thrombolytic therapy (tissue plasminogen activator, streptokinase).[10]

The literature continues to call attention to the poor sensitivity of the ECG for acute myocardial infarction.[1]

The use of AST (SGOT) in diagnosis of AMI includes its application with ALT (SGPT). Myocardial injury can generate an AST/ALT ratio ≥3.1, or a twofold increase in this ratio. Only certain kinds of hepatocellular injury can also cause such AST/ALT ratio abnormality; they include acetaminophen or ethanol toxicity, hepatoma or metastatic carcinoma to liver, marked hepatocellular congestion, cirrhosis, and severe injury to striated muscle.[1] Further, AST and ALT are usually available on a stat basis.

AST (aspartate aminotransferase) with LD and LD isoenzymes is advocated when the patient reaches medical attention 48-72 hours after onset of a possible acute myocardial infarct.[11,12]

Footnotes

1. Pappas NJ Jr, "Enhanced Cardiac Enzyme Profile," *Clin Lab Med*, 1989, 9(4):689-716.
2. Scottolini AG, Zaim MT, and Bhagavan NV, "Acute Myocardial Infarction With Normal Total Cardiac Enzymes and Specific Isoenzyme Patterns," *Prac Cardiol*, 1983, 9:193-202.
3. Apple FS and McGue MK, "Serum Enzyme Changes During Marathon Training," *Am J Clin Pathol*, 1983, 79:716-9.
4. Graeber GM, O'Neill JF, Wolf RE, et al, "Elevated Levels of Peripheral Serum Creatine Phosphokinase With Strangulated Small Bowel Obstruction," *Arch Surg*, 1983, 118:837-40.
5. Wolf PL, "Common Causes of False-Positive CK-MB Test for Acute Myocardial Infarction," *Clin Lab Med*, 1986, 6:577-82.
6. Gibler WB, Lewis LM, Erb RE, et al, "Early Detection of Acute Myocardial Infarction in Patients Presenting With Chest Pain and Nondiagnostic ECGs: Serial CK-MB Sampling in the Emergency Department," *Ann Emerg Med*, 1990, 19(12):1359-66.
7. Puleo PR, Blick D, Guadagno PA, et al, "Early Diagnosis of Myocardial Infarction Using a Newly Developed Rapid Assay for MB Creatine Kinase Subforms," *American Heart Association Meeting*, 1988, (abstract).
8. Puleo PR, Guadagno P, Scheel M, et al, "Diagnostic Accuracy of a Rapid MB-CK Subform Assay in the Early Hours of Myocardial Infarction," *Clin Chem*, 1989, 35:1119.
9. Wu AH, Gornet TG, Wu VH, et al, "Early Diagnosis of Acute Myocardial Infarction by Rapid Analysis of Creatine Kinase Isoenzyme-3 (CK-MM) Subtypes," *Clin Chem*, 1987, 33:358-62.
10. Apple FS, Sharkey SW, Werdick M, et al, "Analyses of Creatine Kinase Isoenzymes and Isoforms in Serum to Detect Reperfusion After Myocardial Infarction," *Clin Chem*, 1987, 33:507-11.
11. Rotenberg Z, Weinberger I, Davidson E, et al, "Does Determination of Serum Aspartate Aminotransferase Contribute to the Diagnosis of Acute Myocardial Infarction?" *Am J Clin Pathol*, 1989, 91(1):91-4.
12. Faulkner WR, "Aspartate Aminotransferase and Acute Myocardial Infarction," *Lab Report for Physicians*, 1989, 11:92-3.

References

de Leon AC Jr, Farmer CA, King G, et al, "Chest Pain Evaluation Unit: A Cost-Effective Approach for Ruling Out Acute Myocardial Infarction," *South Med J*, 1989, 82(9):1083-9.

Galbraith LV, Leung FY, Jablonsky G, et al, "Time-Related Changes in the Diagnostic Utility of Total Lactate Dehydrogenase, Lactate Dehydrogenase Isoenzyme-1, and Two Lactate Dehydrogenase Isoenzyme-1 Ratios in Serum After Myocardial Infarction," *Clin Chem*, 1990, 36(7):1317-22.

Jensen AE, Reikvam A, Nordgard S, et al, "Diagnostic Accuracy of Kodak Creatine Kinase MB, Stratus Creatine Kinase MB, and Lactate Dehydrogenase Isoenzyme 1 in Serum After Acute Myocardial Infarction," *Clin Chem*, 1990, 36(10):1847-8.

Karagounis L, Moreno F, Menlove RL, et al, "Effects of Early Thrombolytic Therapy (Anistreplase Versus Streptokinase) on Enzymatic and Electrocardiographic Infarct Size in Acute Myocardial Infarction. Team-2 Investigators," *Am J Cardiol*, 1991, 68(9):848-56.

Lee TH, Juarez G, Cook EF, et al, "Ruling Out Acute Myocardial Infarction. A Prospective Multicenter Validation of A 12-Hour Strategy for Patients at Low Risk," *N Engl J Med*, 1991, 324(18):1239-46.

Lott JA and Abbott LB, "Creatine Kinase Isoenzymes," *Clin Lab Med*, 1986, 6:547-76, (review).

Manzo V, Sun T, and Lien YY, "Misdiagnosis of Acute Myocardial Infarction," *Ann Clin Lab Sci*, 1990, 20(5):324-8.

Reis GJ, Kaufman HW, Horowitz GL, et al, "Usefulness of Lactate Dehydrogenase and Lactate Dehydrogenase Isoenzymes for Diagnosis of Acute Myocardial Infarction," *Am J Cardiol*, 1988, 61:754-8.

Remaley AT and Wilding P, "Macroenzymes: Biochemical Characterization, Clinical Significance, and Laboratory Detection," *Clin Chem*, 1989, 35(12):2261-70.

Wright LT, "Changes in Cardiac-Enzyme Analysis in Diagnosis of Acute Myocardial Infarction," *Clin Lab Sci*, 1988, 1:355-7.

β-Carotene *see* Carotene, Serum *on this page*

Carotene, Serum

***CPT** 82380*

Related Information

Vitamin A, Serum *on page 385*

Synonyms Beta-Carotene; β-Carotene

Abstract The use of the test is controversial. Precursors of vitamin A, carotenes when measured do not often provide high levels of diagnostic information. Beta-carotene is a retinoid found in fresh fruits and vegetables. Beta-carotene is a fat-soluble provitamin.

Patient Care **PREPARATION:** Patient must fast a minimum of 8 hours.

Specimen Serum **CONTAINER:** Red top tube **STORAGE INSTRUCTIONS:** Separate serum from clot. Freeze in plastic vial. Prevent exposure to light. **CAUSES FOR REJECTION:** Patient not fasting, hemolysis

Interpretive **REFERENCE RANGE:** 50-250 μg/dL (SI: 0.9-4.6 μmol/L); varies with diet and between laboratories (*vide infra*). The levels vary in infancy and childhood.[1] **USE:** Confirm the diagnosis of carotenoderma; screen for fat malabsorption, depressed carotene levels may be found in cases of steatorrhea **LIMITATIONS:** High levels are useful to rule out steatorrhea but lower values lack specificity. There is poor sensitivity. High in the serum of those ingesting large amounts of vegetables. The gold standard for confirmation of a diagnosis of malabsorption remains fat measurement of a 72-hour stool specimen. Variability of reference ranges and poor technical precision at lower levels, which are the decision levels, have led to recommendations to discontinue use of this test. **METHODOLOGY:** High performance liquid chromatography (HPLC), colorimetry with extraction step to eliminate other carotenoids **ADDITIONAL INFORMATION:** Vitamin A serum levels do not correlate well with liver stores. Carotenemia may be confused with jaundice. It is also reported high with some cases of diabetes mellitus, myxedema, chronic nephritis, nephrotic syndrome,[2,3] liver disease, hypothyroidism, type I, IIA, and IIB hyperlipoproteinemia, and in a group of amenorrheic hypogonadotropic women.[2] An inverse relationship between serum beta-carotene and the risk of bronchogenic squamous cell carcinoma is reported.[4] The highest carotene levels are found in the serum of faddists ingesting large amounts of vegetables.[5] Oral leukoplakia responds well to beta-carotene therapy.[6] Low beta-carotene levels are associated with oral contraceptives and smoking.[7]

Footnotes

1. Leung AK, Siu TO, Chiu AS, et al, "Serum Carotene Concentrations in Normal Infants and Children," *Clin Pediatr (Phila)*, 1990, 29(10):575-8.
2. Kemmann E, Pasquale SA, and Skaf R, "Amenorrhea Associated With Carotenemia," *JAMA*, 1983, 249:926-9.
3. McNeely MD, "Gastrointestinal Function," *Gradwohl's Clinical Laboratory Methods and Diagnosis*, 8th ed, Sonnenwirth AC and Jarett L, eds, St Louis, MO: Mosby-Year Book Inc, 1980, 517-36.
4. Menkes MS, Comstock GW, Vuilleumier JP, et al, "Serum Beta-Carotene, Vitamins A and E, Selenium, and the Risk of Lung Cancer," *N Engl J Med*, 1986, 315:1250-4.
5. Gerard SK, "Serum Carotene: A Screening Test for Malabsorption," *Pathologist*, April 1986, 36-7.
6. Garewal HS, Meyskens FL Jr, Killen D, et al, "Response of Oral Leukoplakia to Beta-Carotene," *J Clin Oncol*, 1990, 8(10):1715-20.
7. Palan PR, Romney SL, Vermund SH, et al, "Effects of Smoking and Oral Contraception on Plasma Beta-Carotene Levels in Healthy Women," *Am J Obstet Gynecol*, 1989, 161(4):881-5.

References

Heinonen PK, Kuoppala T, Koskinen T, et al, "Serum Vitamins A and E and Carotene in Patients With Gynecologic Cancer," *Arch Gynecol Obstet*, 1987, 241:151-6.

Leung AK, "Carotenemia," *Adv Pediatr*, 1987, 34:223-48, (190 ref).

Catecholamines *see* Metanephrines, Total, Urine *on page 289*

Catecholamines, Fractionation, Plasma

***CPT** 82383 (total); 82384*

Related Information

Calcitonin *on page 157*
Homovanillic Acid, Urine *on page 253*
Metanephrines, Total, Urine *on page 289*
Vanillylmandelic Acid, Urine *on page 382*

Synonyms Pressor Amines

Applies to Clonidine Suppression Test; Plasma Neuropeptide Y

Test Commonly Includes Plasma catecholamines, total and fractionated (epinephrine, norepinephrine, dopamine)

Patient Care PREPARATION: Patient should be fasting for 4 or more hours without smoking. Walnuts, bananas, and alpha methyldopa (Aldomet®) should be avoided for a week prior to sampling. Other drug interference may occur, including epinephrine and epinephrine-like drugs (eg, nosedrops, sinus and cough preparations, bronchodilators, appetite suppressants). Test is unreliable in subjects on levodopa or methenamine mandelate. It is best to communicate with the laboratory which will do the test with regard to other sources of interference, including drug interference. Avoid exposure to radioactivity (eg, scans) if laboratory will use a radioenzymatic procedure. Avoid patient stress.[1] See Limitations.

Specimen Plasma CONTAINER: EDTA-sodium metabisulfite tube. Some laboratories request a green top (heparin) tube, which is reported to enhance stability.[2] COLLECTION: An indwelling heparinized venous catheter is advocated, since venipuncture can cause an increase in the substances for which testing is being done. Patient should remain supine in quiet surroundings for at least 30 minutes. Some laboratories require a chilled, special container; invert to mix blood with preservatives and place in an ice bath. STORAGE INSTRUCTIONS: Spin blood in a refrigerated centrifuge. Chill carriers if a refrigerated centrifuge is not available. Separate plasma into a plastic vial and freeze in an upright position at -70°C. Do not let specimen thaw during transit.[3] Others report considerable stability for catecholamines.[4] CAUSES FOR REJECTION: Sample not drawn in correct tube, inadequate patient preparation

Interpretive REFERENCE RANGE: Reference ranges vary among laboratories. Values for specimens taken when the subject is standing are higher than the ranges for supine posture for norepinephrine and epinephrine but not for dopamine. Depending on cutoff levels of epinephrine and norepinephrine, the diagnostic efficacy in diagnosing pheochromocytoma ranges from 85% to 95% (sensitivity) and 95% to 98% (specificity). USE: Diagnose pheochromocytoma and those paragangliomas which may secrete epinephrine, norepinephrine or both. Such tumors may cause paroxysmal or persistent hypertension. Investigation of hypertensive patients, especially younger individuals, particularly when hypertension is paroxysmal, suggesting pheochromocytoma. Plasma catecholamines with urinary metanephrines and VMA are a recommended test battery for pheochromocytoma.[5] Others recommend plasma catecholamines when urinary collections are not diagnostic. Work-up of multiple endocrine adenomatosis, type II. Used also in diagnosis of disorders related to the nervous system and in assessment of resuscitation.[2] LIMITATIONS: Plasma levels are useful if elevated, especially during or immediately following an episode of hypertension, but false-negatives occur when the specimen is drawn during an uneventful period. Normotensive pheochromocytoma has been reported.[6] False-positive results are common. Epinephrine secretion increases in response to cold and hypoglycemia. Depending on methods, drugs which may affect plasma norepinephrine levels include alpha- and beta-adrenergic blockers, vasodilators, clonidine, bromocriptine, theophylline, phenothiazine, tricyclic antidepressants, labetalol, calcium channel blockers, converting enzyme inhibitors, bromocriptine, chlorpromazine, haloperidol, and cocaine. Plasma catecholamines are less sensitive than are urinary catecholamines.[3] In general, urinary fractionated catecholamines result in values more consistent than those from plasma. METHODOLOGY: High performance liquid chromatography (HPLC) with electrochemical detection is the method of choice.[7] Other methods include high performance liquid chromatography (HPLC) with fluorometric or spectrophotometric detection, radioimmunoassay (RIA), and radiochemical assays.[8] ADDITIONAL INFORMATION: The adrenal medullary catecholamines (epinephrine, norepinephrine, and their precursor, dopamine) are rapidly metabolized materials with intense vasoactivity, among many other properties. They can be synthesized by extra-adrenal cells or neoplasms of the APUD system. They are pathogenic in the episodic hypertension of pheochromocytoma, and will be elevated during and immediately after such a paroxysm. However, levels may be normal during asymptomatic intervals. Urine catecholamines, metanephrines, VMA and HVA provide additive information. Extra-adrenal pheochromocytomas may represent 15% of adult and 30% of childhood pheochromocytomas; the most common location is the superior para-aortic region between the diaphragm and lower renal poles.[9]

A clonidine-suppression test has been described; failure to suppress plasma catecholamines with clonidine supports the diagnosis.[10,11,12]

Plasma neuropeptide Y, a 36 amino acid peptide, is a marker for nervous system tissue. Its value remains to be established. Plasma levels can be assayed by immunoradiometric methods. Increased levels have been found with pheochromocytomas, neuroblastomas, and in some subjects with other neuroendocrine tumors such as carcinoids, medullary carcinoma of thyroid, and small cell carcinoma of lung.[13]

(Continued)

Catecholamines, Fractionation, Plasma *(Continued)*

Footnotes

1. Sheps SG, Jiang N-S, Klee GG, et al, "Recent Developments in the Diagnosis and Treatment of Pheochromocytoma," *Mayo Clin Proc*, 1990, 65(1):88-95.
2. D'Alesandro MM, Reed HL, Robertson R, et al, "Simplified Method of Collecting and Processing Whole Blood for Quantitation of Plasma Catecholamines," *Lab Med*, 1990, 26-9.
3. Rumley AG, "The *In Vitro* Stability of Catecholamines in Whole Blood," *Ann Clin Biochem*, 1988, 25(Pt 5):585-86.
4. Weir TB, Smith CCT, Round JM, et al, "Stability of Catecholamines in Whole Blood, Plasma, and Platelets," *Clin Chem*, 1986, 32:882-3.
5. Knight JA and Wu JT, "Catecholamines and Their Metabolites: Clinical and Laboratory Aspects," *Lab Med*, 1987, 18:153-8.
6. Feldman JM, Blalock JA, Zern RT, et al, "Deficiency of Dopamine-β-hydroxylase. A New Mechanism for Normotensive Pheochromocytomas," *Am J Clin Pathol*, 1979, 72:175-85.
7. Koller M, "Results for 74 Substances Tested for Interference With Determination of Plasma Catecholamines by "High Performance" Liquid Chromatography With Electrochemical Detection," *Clin Chem*, 1988, 34(5):947-9.
8. Moyer TP, Jaing NS, Tyce GM, et al, "Analysis for Urinary Catecholamines by Liquid Chromatography With Amperometric Detection: Methodology and Clinical Interpretation of Results," *Clin Chem*, 1979, 25:256-63.
9. Whalen RK, Althausen AF, and Daniels GH, "Extra-adrenal Pheochromocytoma," *J Urol*, 1992, 147(1):1-10.
10. Bravo EL, Tarazi RC, Fouad FM, et al, "Clonidine-Suppression Test: A Useful Aid in the Diagnosis of Pheochromocytoma," *N Engl J Med*, 1981, 305:623-6.
11. Landsberg L and Young JB, "Pheochromocytoma," *Harrison's Principles of Internal Medicine*, Braunwald E, Isselbacher KJ, Petersdorf RG, et al, eds, New York, NY: McGraw-Hill Inc, 1987, 1775-8.
12. Bravo EL and Gifford RW Jr, "Pheochromocytoma: Diagnosis, Localization, and Management," *N Engl J Med*, 1984, 311:1298-303.
13. Grouzmann E, Comoy E, and Bohuon C, "Plasma Neuropeptide Y Concentrations in Patients With Neuroendocrine Tumors," *J Clin Endocrinol Metab*, 1989, 68(4):808-13.

References

Bouloux PM, Perrett D, and Besser GM, "Methodology Considerations in the Determination of Plasma Catecholamines by "High Performance" Liquid Chromatography With Electrochemical Detection," *Ann Clin Biochem*, 1985, 22:194-203.

Elliott WJ, Murphy MB, Straus FH 2d, et al, "Improved Safety of Glucagon Testing for Pheochromocytoma by Prior α-Receptor Blockade," *Arch Intern Med*, 1989, 149(1):214-6.

Leavelle DE, *Mayo Medical Laboratories Interpretive Handbook*, Rochester, MN: Mayo Medical Laboratories, 1990.

Rogers PJ, Tyce GM, Weinshilboum RM, et al, "Catecholamine Metabolic Pathways and Exercise Training. Plasma and Urine Catecholamines, Metabolic Enzymes, and Chromogranin-A," *Circulation*, 1991, 84(6):2346-56.

Tyce GM, Ahlskog JE, Carmichael SW, et al, "Catecholamines in CSF, Plasma, and Tissue After Autologous Transplantation of Adrenal Medulla to the Brain in Patients With Parkinson's Disease," *J Lab Clin Med*, 1989, 114(2):185-92.

Yoshino K, Takahashi K, Shirai T, et al, "Changes in Plasma Catecholamines and Pulsatile Patterns of Gonadotropin Release in Subjects With a Normal Ovulatory Cycle and With Polycystic Ovary Syndrome," *Int J Fertil*, 1990, 35(1):34-9.

Catecholamines, Fractionation, Urine

***CPT** 82382 (total); 83835 (metanephrines); 84585 (VMA)*

Related Information

Calcitonin *on page 157*
Homovanillic Acid, Urine *on page 253*
Metanephrines, Total, Urine *on page 289*
Vanillylmandelic Acid, Urine *on page 382*

Synonyms Free Catecholamine Fractionation, Urine

Applies to Dopamine, Urine; Epinephrine, Urine; Norepinephrine, Urine

Replaces Total Urinary Catecholamines

Patient Care PREPARATION: Avoid patient stress, exercise, smoking, and pain. Many drugs (reserpine and α-methyldopa, levodopa, monoamine oxidase inhibitors, and sympathomimetic amines) may interfere and should be discontinued 2 weeks prior to specimen collection. Nose drops, sinus and cough medicines, bronchodilators and appetite suppressants, α_2-agonists, calcium channel blockers, converting enzyme inhibitors, bromocriptine, phenothiazine, tricyclic antidepressants, alpha and beta blockers, labetolol may interfere.[1] Mandelamine® interferes, but thiazides do not. Caffeine products should be avoided before and during collection. The patient should not be subjected to hypoglycemia or exertion. Increased intracranial pressure and clonidine withdrawal can also cause false-positive results.[1,2]

Specimen 24-hour urine CONTAINER: Brown urine container. Adjust to pH 4 with acetic or hydrochloric acid. COLLECTION: 24-hour urine collection STORAGE INSTRUCTIONS: Refrigerate during and after collection.

Interpretive REFERENCE RANGE: Adults: approximate range, urine: epinephrine: 0-20 μg/24 hours (SI: 0-118 nmol/day); norepinephrine: 15-80 μg/24 hours (SI: 89-473 nmol/day); dopamine: 65-400 μg/24 hours (SI: 384-2364 nmol/day). Ranges given here are not identical among all laboratories. CRITICAL VALUES: >50 μg/24 hours (SI: >297 nmol/day) of epinephrine secretion may be the only abnormality in subjects who have the multiple endocrine adenomatosis syndrome.[2] USE: Work up neuroblastoma; diagnose pheochromocytoma. Pheochromocytomas and occasional paragangliomas may cause persistent or paroxysmal hypertension. Work up of palpitation, severe headache, diaphoresis. Urine collections are preferred to blood sampling when there is suspicion for tumor (eg, family history of MEA II) when hypertension is not paroxysmal. Evaluate possible multiple endocrine adenomatosis type II. LIMITATIONS: False-negatives and false-positives occur. Many interfering substances exist for fluorometric assays. Urine collections for metanephrines are among the best screening tests for pheochromocytoma.[3] Sheps et al use urinary catecholamine fractionation as confirmation, following a metanephrine screen.[1] Neuroblastoma is better worked up with urinary collections for HVA and VMA. MHPG (3-methoxy-4-hydroxyphenylethylene glycol) is a major metabolite of norepinephrine in the central nervous system; it is a metabolite of some neuroblastomas. METHODOLOGY: High performance liquid chromatography (HPLC) with electrochemical detection, trihydroxyindole methods after boric acid elution or resin exchange column extraction. Alumina absorption methods displayed the poorest intralaboratory precision in a CAP urine chemistry survey.[4] ADDITIONAL INFORMATION: The expression "free" in free catecholamine fractionation means unconjugated. This assay is of most value for pheochromocytoma when specimen is collected during a hypertensive episode. Since a 24-hour urine collection represents a longer sampling time than a random, or symptom-directed serum sample, and because catecholamine secretion by pheochromocytomas is intermittent, the urine test may detect some cases missed by a blood level.

Footnotes

1. Sheps SG, Jiang N-S, Klee GG, et al, "Recent Developments in the Diagnosis and Treatment of Pheochromocytoma," *Mayo Clin Proc*, 1990, 65(1):88-95.
2. Landsberg L and Young JB, "Pheochromocytoma," *Harrison's Principles of Internal Medicine*, Braunwald E, Isselbacher KJ, Petersdorf RG, et al, eds, New York, NY: McGraw-Hill Inc, 1987, 1775-8.
3. Knight JA and Wu JT, "Catecholamines and Their Metabolites: Clinical and Laboratory Aspects," *Lab Med*, 1987, 18:153-8.
4. Weaver DK and Glenn GC, "The Urine Chemistry Survey - Series 2: 5 Years Experience With and Interlaboratory Comparison Program," *Arch Pathol Lab Med*, 1989, 113(7):713-22.

References

"Case Records of the Massachusetts General Hospital. Weekly Clinicopathological Exercises. Case 45-1989. A 48 Year-Old Woman With Acute Respiratory Failure and a Left Suprarenal Mass," *N Engl J Med*, 1989, 321(19):1316-29.

Cleland JG and Dargie HJ, "Arrhythmias, Catecholamines and Electrolytes," *Am J Cardiol*, 1988, 62:55A-9A, (review).

Davidson DF, "Urinary Free Catecholamines-Diagnostic Application of an HPLC Technique to the Investigation of Neural Crest Tumors," *Ann Clin Biochem*, 1987, 24:494-9.

Graham-Pole J, Salmi T, Anton AH, et al, "Tumor and Urine Catecholamines (CATs) in Neurogenic Tumors. Correlations With Other Prognostic Factors and Survival," *Cancer*, 1983, 51:834-9.

Rosano TG, Swift TA, and Hayes LW, "Advances in Catecholamine and Metabolite Measurements for Diagnosis of Pheochromocytoma," *Clin Chem*, 1991, 37(10 Pt 2):1854-67.

Weinkove C, "Measurement of Catecholamines and Their Metabolites in Urine," *J Clin Pathol*, 1991, 44(4):269-75.

CEA *see* Carcinoembryonic Antigen *on page 167*

CEA, Body Fluid *see* Body Fluid *on page 145*

Central Venous Blood *see* Blood Gases, Venous *on page 144*

Cephalin Flocculation *replaced by* Alanine Aminotransferase *on page 100*

Cephalin Flocculation *replaced by* Aspartate Aminotransferase *on page 135*

Cerebrospinal Fluid Angiotensin Converting Enzyme *see* Angiotensin Converting Enzyme *on page 130*

Cerebrospinal Fluid Glucose

CPT *82947*

Related Information

Bacterial Antigens, Rapid Detection Methods *on page 775*
Body Fluid Glucose *on page 148*
Cerebrospinal Fluid Analysis *on page 527*
Cerebrospinal Fluid Culture *on page 798*
Cerebrospinal Fluid Fungus Culture *on page 800*
Cerebrospinal Fluid Lactic Acid *on page 178*
Cerebrospinal Fluid LD *on page 179*
Cerebrospinal Fluid Mycobacteria Culture *on page 801*
Cerebrospinal Fluid Protein *on page 659*
Glucose, Fasting *on page 238*
Gram Stain *on page 815*
Viral Culture, Central Nervous System Symptoms *on page 1199*

Synonyms Glucose, Cerebrospinal Fluid

Abstract For diagnosis of meningitis, culture and then Gram staining have priority over all other testing, when only a small quantity of cerebrospinal fluid (CSF) is available. Cell count with differential deserve the next priority, followed by glucose and protein.

Patient Care PREPARATION: Blood (ie, plasma) glucose is needed also. Ideally, it should be drawn 2 hours before the lumbar puncture, the equilibration time.

Specimen Cerebrospinal fluid CONTAINER: Clean, sterile CSF tube COLLECTION: Tubes should be labeled with patient's name, hospital number, date, time of collection, and with numbers indicating the sequence in which tubes were obtained. SPECIAL INSTRUCTIONS: A plasma glucose should be drawn.

Interpretive REFERENCE RANGE: 50-80 mg/dL (SI: 2.8-4.4 mmol/L) in fasting patients, should be interpreted with plasma glucose. Values may be somewhat higher in children, 45-100 mg/dL (SI: 2.5-5.6 mmol/L).[1] CSF glucose should be 60% to 70% of plasma glucose. However, equilibration between plasma and CSF glucose levels may require several hours. In premature and newborn infants, CSF glucose may be 80% or more of plasma glucose, possibly due to greater permeability of the blood-brain barrier and/or increased rate of cerebral blood flow. POSSIBLE PANIC RANGE: <40 mg/dL (SI: <2.2 mmol/L), especially with increased cells and/or protein USE: Evaluate viral, bacterial, tuberculous, and other types of meningitis; neoplastic involvement of meninges; other neurological disorders. Diagnose of neuroglycopenia, even in presence of normal plasma glucose. While the finding of glucose in clear nasal discharge has in past years been considered indicative of CSF rhinorrhea,[2] studies have shown that glucose may be present in non-CSF nasal fluids.[3,4] LIMITATIONS: Falsely decreased levels may result due to cellular and bacterial utilization of glucose if the test is not performed immediately. Visibly xanthochromic samples may give misleading results. The sensitivity of CSF glucose for bacterial meningitis was only 72% in a series from Rochester, New York, inferior to the sensitivity of the nucleated blood cell count.[5] Bloody taps cause falsely increased glucose, since there is more glucose in blood. METHODOLOGY: Same procedures as used for blood glucose (eg, glucose oxidase, hexokinase reactions); a reagent strip and a handheld analyzer method have been reported as reliable for use in the bedside determination of CSF glucose.[6] ADDITIONAL INFORMATION: Elevation implies hyperglycemia 2-4 hours earlier. Significantly decreased cerebrospinal fluid glucose levels are <40 mg/dL (SI: <2.2 mmol/L) in fasting patient with normal plasma glucose. The frequency of low CSF glucose in bacterial meningitis varies somewhat between series; a major textbook of pediatrics points out that acute viral meningitis is often differentiated from acute bacterial meningitis, because the latter is characterized by a CSF glucose <30 mg/dL, a CSF glucose-to-blood glucose ratio of <0.2-0.3 as well as a protein >200 mg/dL, a CSF PMN count >1000/mm^3, and an 80% to 90% likelihood of positive Gram stain in an illness often occurring during the winter in a child younger than 2 years of age.[7] The magnitude of the seasonal curves for viral versus bacterial meningitis (the former more frequent in the summer) is greater than most clinicians appreciate.[8] In 134 Gram stain positive cases, CSF glucose was 14.4/30.6/50.4 mg/dL, 25th/percentile median/75th percentile.[8] **The gold standard for the diagnosis of bacterial meningitis is the culture,**[5,9] which is fundamental to appropriate diagnosis and treatment.[10] Decreased CSF glucose is characteristically but not invariably found in tuberculous, fungal, and amebic meningitis (*Naegleria*) as well as in bacterial meningitis. Glucose is usually normal in viral meningitis, but in herpes or mumps meningoencephalitis, lymphocytic choriomeningitis, and with enterovirus infection, glucose may be low. Sarcoidosis and neurosyphilis are reported causes of low CSF glucose. Other very uncommon causes of low CSF glucose include meningeal cysticercosis, trichinosis, and with the chemical meningitis which accompanies intrathecal therapy. Low CSF glucose may also occur in subarachnoid hemorrhage and neoplasia (eg, medulloblastoma). Low CSF glucose may be found in CNS leukemia. Decrease has led to the diagnosis of insulinoma presenting with CNS symptoms. Rheumatoid meningitis and lupus myelopathy may cause low CSF glucose.[10] CSF glucose levels ≤20 mg/dL are highly correlated with bacterial meningitis.[11]

Lactic acid may be useful in the diagnosis of bacterial meningitis, but values overlap those found with viral meningitis (aseptic meningitis).[10]

Footnotes

1. Knight JA, Dudek SM, and Haymond RE, "Early (Chemical) Diagnosis of Bacterial Meningitis-Cerebrospinal Fluid Glucose, Lactate, and Lactate Dehydrogenase Compared," *Clin Chem*, 1981, 27:1431-4.
2. Beckhardt RN, Setzen M, and Carras R, "Primary Spontaneous Cerebrospinal Fluid Rhinorrhea," *Otolaryngol Head Neck Surg*, 1991, 104(4):425-32.
3. Hull HF and Morrow G, "Glucorrhea Revisited: Prolonged Promulgation of Another Plastic Pearl," *JAMA*, 1975, 234:1052-3.
4. Steedman DJ and Gordon M, "CSF Rhinorrhoeae: Significance of the Glucose Oxidase Strip Test," *Injury*, 1987, 18:327-8.
5. Rodewald LE, Woodin KA, Szilagyi PG, et al, "Relevance of Common Tests of Cerebrospinal Fluid in Screening for Bacterial Meningitis," *J Pediatr*, 1991, 119(3):363-9.
6. Slovis CM, Negus RA, Amerson SM, et al, "Bedside Cerebrospinal Fluid Glucose Analysis," *Ann Emerg Med*, 1989, 18(9):931-3.
7. Behrman RE, Kliegman RM, Nelson WE, et al, *Nelson Textbook of Pediatrics*, 14th ed, Philadelphia, PA: WB Saunders Co, 1992, 683-91.
8. Spanos A, Harrell FE Jr, and Durack DT, "Differential Diagnosis of Acute Meningitis. An Analysis of the Predictive Value of Initial Observations," *JAMA*, 1989, 262(19):2700-7.
9. Smith AL, "Bacterial Meningitis," *Pediatr Rev*, 1993, 14(1):11-8.
10. Fishman RA, *Cerebrospinal Fluid in Diseases of the Nervous System*, 2nd ed, Philadelphia, PA: WB Saunders Co, 1992, 219-21.
11. Greenlee JE, "Approach to Diagnosis of Meningitis - Cerebrospinal Fluid Evaluation," *Infect Dis Clin North Am*, 1990, 4(4):583-98.

References

Avery GM, "Measurement of Glucose in Cerebrospinal Fluid With Reagent Strips and a Reflectance Photometer," *Clin Chem*, 1991, 37(4):590-1, (letter).

Bonadio WA and Smith D, "Cerebrospinal Fluid Changes After 48 Hours of Effective Therapy for *Haemophilus influenzae* Type B Meningitis," *Am J Clin Pathol*, 1990, 94(4):426-8.

Brumback RA, "Collecting Cerebrospinal Fluid: Chemistry," *The Cerebrospinal Fluid*, Chapter 4, Herndon RM and Brumback RA, eds, Boston, MA: Kluwer Academic Publishers, 1989, 222-6.

Gray LD and Fedorko DP, "Laboratory Diagnosis of Bacterial Meningitis," *Clin Microbiol Rev*, 1992, 5(2):130-45.

Cerebrospinal Fluid Glutamine

***CPT** 82975*

Related Information

Ammonia, Blood *on page 120*

Synonyms CSF Glutamine; Glutamine, Spinal Fluid

Abstract Ammonia is toxic to the nervous system. It combines with alpha-ketoglutarate to yield glutamine. Such glutamine formation serves to protect the nervous system.[1]

Specimen Cerebrospinal fluid **CONTAINER:** Clean, sterile CSF tube **COLLECTION:** Tube should be labeled with the number indicating the sequence in which tubes were obtained. **STORAGE INSTRUCTIONS:** With immediate ethanol deproteinization CSF samples may be stored for 9 months at -80°C.[2] **CAUSES FOR REJECTION:** Samples contaminated with red blood cells **SPECIAL INSTRUCTIONS:** Specimen must be transported **immediately** to the laboratory.

Interpretive **REFERENCE RANGE:** 6-15 mg/dL (SI: 411-1026 μmol/L) enzymatic, infants: 24-193 mg/L (SI: 164-1321 μmol/L)[3] (note the units in which the authors have expressed the range). Isotachophoresis method (adults): 20-100 mg/L (SI: 137-685 μmol/L)[4] **USE:** Evaluate hepatic encephalopathy and aid in assessment of its severity; evaluate coma; increased in many instances of Reye's syndrome (20 of 27 cases);[5] work up hyperammonemic encephalopathies. Levels from 25-95 mg/dL are seen with hepatic coma. Values >35 mg/dL are almost always related to encephalopathy.[1] **LIMITATIONS:** Higher levels are reported with parenteral nutrition, meningitis, and in cerebral hemorrhage.[2] **METHODOLOGY:** Enzymatic, amino acid analyzer, high performance liquid chromatography (HPLC), capillary-isotachophoresis.[4] Glutamine/glutamate levels vary widely with different methods and in particular with specimen handling

(Continued)

Cerebrospinal Fluid Glutamine *(Continued)*

and preparation prior to analysis. This may be due importantly to *in vitro* hydrolysis of glutamine to glutamate. Immediate deproteinization of CSF with ethanol may circumvent this problem.[2] **ADDITIONAL INFORMATION:** Glutamine is the most prominent amino acid in CSF. CSF glutamine levels are used with blood ammonia determinations in diagnosis of hepatic encephalopathy. In hepatic encephalopathy, plasma glutamine values correlate better with the clinical course than do values for blood ammonia but imperfect correlation exists with CSF ammonia levels.[1] There is evidence that CSF glutamine levels are within normal range in a variety of infectious, inflammatory, degenerative and metabolic neurologic disorders.[4] Levels are increased in some cases of meningitis and associated with CSF pleocytosis. Elevated CSF total protein (>40 mg/dL (SI: >0.4 g/L)), in which some examples of loss of integrity of the blood-brain-CSF would be expected, is not accompanied by increase in CSF glutamine unless cell count is also increased. With response of meningitis to therapy (and fall in CSF cell count), CSF glutamine also declines.[4] Increase in CSF glutamine relating to pleocytosis is of a much lesser magnitude than the high levels occurring in cases of hepatic coma.

Footnotes

1. Fishman RA, *Cerebrospinal Fluid in Diseases of the Nervous System*, 2nd ed, Philadelphia, PA: WB Saunders Co, 1992, 238-9.
2. Alfredsson G, Wiesel FA, and Lindberg M, "Glutamate and Glutamine in Cerebrospinal Fluid and Serum From Healthy Volunteers - Analytical Aspects," *J Chromatogr*, 1988, 424:378-84.
3. Boeckx RL, Iosefsohn M, and Hicks JM, "Reference Values for Cerebrospinal Fluid Glutamine Concentration in Infants," *Clin Chem*, 1980, 26:601-3.
4. Hiraoka A, Miura I, Tominaga I, et al, "Capillary-Isotachophoretic Determination of Glutamine in Cerebrospinal Fluid of Various Neurological Disorders," *Clin Biochem*, 1989, 22(4):293-6.
5. Romshe CA, "Laboratory Diagnosis of Reye's Syndrome," *Reye's Syndrome*, Pollack JD, ed, New York, NY: Grune and Stratton Inc, 1975, 15-26.

References

Fernstrom MH and Fernstrom JD, "Rapid Measurement of Free Amino Acids in Serum and CSF Using High Performance Liquid Chromatography," *Life Sci*, 1981, 29:2119-30.

Kjeldsberg CR and Knight JA, *Body Fluids: Laboratory Examination of Cerebrospinal, Synovial and Serous Fluids: A Textbook Atlas*, 2nd ed, Chicago, IL: ASCP Press, 1982.

Mizock BA, Sabelli HC, Dubin A, et al, "Septic Encephalopathy. Evidence for Altered Phenylalanine Metabolism and Comparison With Hepatic Encephalopathy," *Arch Intern Med*, 1990, 150(2):443-9.

Cerebrospinal Fluid Lactic Acid

***CPT** 83605*

Related Information

Cerebrospinal Fluid Analysis *on page 527*
Cerebrospinal Fluid Culture *on page 798*
Cerebrospinal Fluid Glucose *on page 176*
Cerebrospinal Fluid Protein *on page 659*
Gram Stain *on page 815*
Viral Culture, Central Nervous System Symptoms *on page 1199*

Synonyms Lactic Acid, Cerebrospinal Fluid

Abstract Interest in CSF lactic acid has related to increases in bacterial meningitis and partially treated bacterial meningitis, in contrast to the usual finding of normal lactic acid with viral meningitis. However, overlapping concentrations in tuberculous, other bacterial and viral meningitis have limited its diagnostic value.[1,2]

Specimen Cerebrospinal fluid **CONTAINER:** Clean, sterile CSF tube **STORAGE INSTRUCTIONS:** Unstable at room temperature[3]

Interpretive **REFERENCE RANGE:** Increased in first 2 weeks of life. Control group with no CNS disease: 10-20 mg/dL (SI: 1.1-2.2 mmol/L).[1] Amperometric lactate analyzer, CSF from patients without neurologic disease: 9.9-21.6 mg/dL (SI: 1.1-2.4 mmol/L)[4] **POSSIBLE PANIC RANGE:** Values ≥25.2 mg/dL (SI: ≥2.8 mmol/L) are suggestive of bacterial meningitis. Values up to 35.1 mg/dL (SI: 3.9 mmol/L) may be equivocal, but others have reported that lactic acid >30.1 mg/dL (SI: >3.34 mmol/L) in essentially all instances of bacterial meningitis, inversely related to CSF glucose. Lower results are reported in partially treated bacterial meningitis. **USE:** The role of CSF lactic acid determinations is controversial. CSF lactic acid has been used in differentiation of bacterial and nonbacterial meningitis. Rutledge et al reported that with equivocal clinical and spinal fluid findings, CSF lactic acid failed to distinguish between bacterial and nonbacterial infections.[5] CSF lactate must not be used in place of the traditional laboratory evaluation of meningitis. CSF lactate was elevated in all patients (group of 21) with culture proven tuberculous meningitis.[6] It was also elevated in cases of biopsy proven Creutzfeldt-Jakob disease (CJD) and has been suggested as a biochemical marker of that disease.[7] CSF lactic acid increase is a characteristic finding of acute infarct of cerebrum. Increased levels are found with cerebral hemorrhage, subarachnoid hemorrhage, primary CSF acidosis, malignant hypertension, hepatic encephalopathy, diabetes mellitus, hypoglycemia coma, and in the first 3 days following head injury.[1] An entity of developmental delay with infantile seizures and with depressed CSF glucose and lactate levels is noteworthy, because it responds to a special diet.[1] **LIMITATIONS:** Increases must be interpreted in light of the clinical setting and in concert with conventional parameters of meningitis work-up (glucose, protein, cell count, Gram stain, and culture). Slight increases have been described with craniocerebral trauma, stroke, seizures (up to 81.1 mg/dL (9.0 mmol/L)), and brain tumor. Results from neurosurgical cases must be interpreted cautiously. It is reported as elevated in fungal infections,[1] but levels have been reported to be erratic in cryptococcal meningitis. *Staphylococcus epidermidis* meningitis after shunt installation and very early neonatal bacterial meningitis have been described without increased lactic acid levels. Overlapping results limit the value of lactate levels in differential diagnosis between viral meningitis, partially treated bacterial meningitis, and tuberculous meningitis. The assay for lactic acid has not been shown to contribute to accuracy of diagnosis in instances of possible meningitis.[1] **METHODOLOGY:** Enzymatic, gas-liquid chromatography (GLC), amperometric utilizing a lactate-sensitive electrode[3] **ADDITIONAL INFORMATION:** A linear increase in CSF lactate in relation to lactate producing inflammatory cells with high levels at cell counts $>350/mm^3$ has been noted.[8] It is implied that increase in CSF lactate results from CSF pleocytosis. Antimicrobial therapy given prior to collection of spinal fluid may decrease reliability of the usual diagnostic tests (Gram stain, culture, protein, and glucose levels). Equivocal results of tests in some instances of aseptic meningitis may lead to an erroneous diagnosis of bacterial etiology. The Gram stain may be negative in as many as 25% of culture-proven bacterial meningitides. Lactate determination may provide an indicator of the presence or absence of bacterial meningitis. Lactic acid in viral meningitis will occasionally fall between 2.78-3.34 mmol/L. Relapse has been detected by lactic acid assay, which may be of value in calibration of therapeutic response. In early stage of tuberculous meningitis, elevated CSF lactate persists even with adequate antituberculous therapy.[8] Spinal fluid lactate levels are said to be independent of plasma levels.

Footnotes

1. Fishman RA, *Cerebrospinal Fluid in Diseases of the Nervous System*, 2nd ed, Philadelphia, PA: WB Saunders Co, 1992.
2. Feigin RD, "Bacterial Meningitis Beyond the Newborn Period," *Principles and Practice of Pediatrics*, Oski FA, DeAngelis CD, Feigin RD, et al, eds, Chapter 54, Philadelphia, PA: JB Lippincott Co, 1990, 1028-35.
3. Brook I, "Stability of Lactic Acid in Cerebrospinal Fluid Specimens," *Am J Clin Pathol*, 1982, 77:213-6.
4. Wandrup J, Tvede K, Grinsted J, et al, ""Stat" Measurements of L-Lactate in Whole Blood and Cerebrospinal Fluid Assessed," *Clin Chem*, 1989, 35(8):1740-3.
5. Rutledge J, Benjamin D, Hood L, et al, "Is the CSF Lactate Measurement Useful in the Management of Children With Suspected Bacterial Meningitis?" *J Pediatr*, 1981, 98:20-4.
6. Tang LM, "Serial Lactate Determinations in Tuberculous Meningitis," *Scand J Infect Dis*, 1988, 20:81-3.
7. Awerbuch G, Peterson P, and Sandyk R, "Elevated Cerebrospinal Fluid Lactic Acid Levels in Creutzfeldt-Jakob Disease," *Int J Neurosci*, 1988, 42:1-5.
8. Kolmel HW and von Maravic M, "Correlation of Lactic Acid Level, Cell Count and Cytology in Cerebrospinal Fluid of Patients With Bacterial and Nonbacterial Meningitis," *Acta Neurol Scand*, 1988, 78:6-9.

Cerebrospinal Fluid LD

***CPT** 83615*

Related Information

Body Fluid Lactate Dehydrogenase *on page 149*
Cerebrospinal Fluid Analysis *on page 527*
Cerebrospinal Fluid Culture *on page 798*
Cerebrospinal Fluid Cytology *on page 490*
Cerebrospinal Fluid Glucose *on page 176*
Cerebrospinal Fluid Protein *on page 659*

Synonyms Cerebrospinal Fluid LDH; Lactate Dehydrogenase, Cerebrospinal Fluid

Applies to Lactic Acid Dehydrogenase, Fluid

Abstract Lactate dehydrogenase (LD) is a normal component of cerebrospinal fluid (CSF). Overlapping values between cases of bacterial and viral meningitis limit the usefulness of CSF LD in differential diagnosis of meningitis.

Specimen Cerebrospinal fluid **CONTAINER:** Clean, sterile CSF tube

Interpretive **REFERENCE RANGE:** CSF LD (LDH) activity is normally much less than the plasma

(Continued)

Cerebrospinal Fluid LD *(Continued)*

LD activity. Normal spinal fluid LD levels are about 10% of serum values. In children normal range is 0-23.5 units/L.[1] **USE:** A high fluid LD activity, nearly equal to the serum activity is usually associated with inflammatory processes. Increased amounts may occur in association with ischemic necrosis, meningitis, leukemia, metastatic cancer of the CNS, and lymphoma. High fluid LD level, greater than the serum level, is found with neoplasm and with inflammation. Spinal fluid LD has been used by some to identify bacterial meningitis,[1] but overlapping with results in cases of viral meningitis is recognized.[2] CSF lactate, LD (LDH), and LD isoenzymes do not provide definitive data for a diagnosis of bacterial meningitis in childhood.[3]

With CK and AST (SGOT), cerebrospinal fluid LD has been advocated to distinguish cortical from lacunar stroke. These three enzymes are increased in cases of cortical stroke. While CK and AST are not increased with lacunar stroke, LD is only slightly elevated. CSF LD is increased in patients with severe brain injury but is not useful (as is CK-BB) in assessing the degree of injury or in monitoring outcome.[4]

Another application of LD measurement is the differential diagnosis of intracranial hemorrhage in neonates versus traumatic tap. Lactate dehydrogenase is elevated in proportion to severity of CNS hemorrhage, but unchanged by traumatic tap. CSF LDH is higher in stroke than in transient ischemic attack.[5]

LIMITATIONS: This test has very limited usefulness alone due to its nonspecificity. **ADDITIONAL INFORMATION:** A tabulation of CSF enzymes in neurological diseases is available.[2]

Footnotes

1. Knight JA, Dudek SM, and Haymond RE, "Early (Chemical) Diagnosis of Bacterial Meningitis-Cerebrospinal Fluid Glucose, Lactate, and Lactate Dehydrogenase Compared," *Clin Chem*, 1981, 27:1431-4.
2. Fishman RA, *Cerebrospinal Fluid in Diseases of the Nervous System*, 2nd ed, Philadelphia, PA: WB Saunders Co, 1992, 215-6.
3. Castro-Gago M, Couce ML, Losada MC, et al, "C-Reactive Protein, Lactate, and LDH Isoenzymes in the Cerebrospinal Fluid in the Diagnosis in Childhood Meningitis," *An Esp Pediatr*, 1988, 28:31-3.
4. Paşaoğlu A and Paşaoğlu H, "Enzymatic Changes in the Cerebrospinal Fluid as Indices of Pathological Change," *Acta Neurochir*, 1989, 97(1-2):71-6.
5. Lampl Y, Paniri Y, Eshel Y, et al, "Cerebrospinal Fluid Lactate Dehydrogenase Levels in Early Stroke and Transient Ischemic Attacks," *Stroke*, 1990, 21(6):854-7.

References

Donnan GA, Zapf P, Doyle AE, et al, "CSF Enzymes in Lacunar and Cortical Stroke," *Stroke*, 1983, 14:266-9.

Lampl Y, Paniri Y, Eshel Y, et al, "LDH Isoenzymes in Cerebrospinal Fluid in Various Brain Tumours," *J Neurol Neurosurg Psychiatry*, 1990, 53(8):697-9.

Cerebrospinal Fluid LDH *see* Cerebrospinal Fluid LD *on previous page*

Ceruloplasmin

CPT 82390

Related Information

Copper, Serum *on page 1024*

Copper, Urine *on page 1027*

Specimen Serum **CONTAINER:** Red top tube **COLLECTION:** Draw in chilled tube. Keep specimen on ice. Prolonged storage at room temperature leads to decreased levels. **STORAGE INSTRUCTIONS:** Separate serum and freeze.

Interpretive **REFERENCE RANGE:** Neonatal levels are lower than adults. Adult levels are reached 3-6 months after birth. Adults: 20-40 mg/dL (SI: 1.26-2.52 μmol/L). Ranges depend on methods, but <10 mg/dL (SI: <0.63 μmol/L) is strong evidence for Wilson's disease. **USE:** Decreased in most instances of Wilson's disease (hepatolenticular degeneration); hence, ceruloplasmin is used in evaluation of chronic active hepatitis, cirrhosis and other liver disease. In Wilson's disease, there is decreased ability to incorporate copper into apoceruloplasmin. As a result, free copper levels in plasma and in tissue, especially liver and brain, are greatly increased.

Should be considered in cases of central nervous system disease of obscure etiology. Neurological symptoms include problems of coordination.

Ceruloplasmin is **low** in Menkes' kinky hair syndrome (in Menkes' syndrome the defect is secondary to poor absorption and utilization of dietary copper), and with protein loss such as the nephrotic syndromes, malabsorption, and with some cases of advanced liver disease in which decreases of serum proteins have occurred.

Ceruloplasmin is **high** in a variety of neoplastic and inflammatory states, since it behaves as an acute phase reactant, although levels rise more slowly than "acute phase reactants". Increases are described with carcinomas, leukemias, Hodgkin's disease, primary biliary cirrhosis, and with SLE and rheumatoid arthritis. High levels occur in pregnancy, with estrogens, and with oral contraceptive use when the agent contains estrogen as well as progesterone. Increased with copper intoxication.

LIMITATIONS: A normal ceruloplasmin does not rule out Wilson's disease. Serum copper should be measured in addition. Discrepancies occur between immunologic and enzymatic assays in serum of patients with Wilson's disease. **METHODOLOGY:** Spectrophotometric, nephelometric, radial immunodiffusion. Multiplying ceruloplasmin level (mg/L) by three gives the binding protein's contribution to serum copper (μg/L). This may be as great as 90% to 95% of total serum copper. Performing this maneuver allows the clinician to exert a measure of quality control on the laboratory results. **ADDITIONAL INFORMATION:** Ceruloplasmin is an α_2-globulin containing copper. About 70% or more of total serum copper is associated with ceruloplasmin, 7% with a high MW protein, transcuprein, 19% with albumin, and 2% with amino acids.[1]

Laboratory parameters of Wilson's disease include decreased serum ceruloplasmin, decreased serum copper concentration, increased 24-hour urine copper excretion, increased liver copper concentration, and abnormal liver function studies. Demonstration of failure to incorporate radiolabeled copper into ceruloplasmin is the definitive test for Wilson's disease. Liver and CNS manifestations of Wilson's disease need not both be present. Kayser-Fleischer rings are extremely helpful findings.

Excessive therapeutic zinc may lead to block of intestinal absorption of copper and a copper deficiency syndrome characterized by hypochromic microcytic anemia with leukopenia/neutropenia and zero level of ceruloplasmin. A prolonged period of time may be required to eliminate the excess zinc, overcome the block of intestinal copper absorption, and obtain increase in serum copper and ceruloplasmin levels.[2]

Footnotes

1. Barrow L and Tanner MS, "Copper Distribution Among Serum Proteins in Pediatric Liver Disorders and Malignancies," *Eur J Clin Invest*, 1988, 18:555-60.
2. Hoffman HN II, Phyliky RL, and Fleming CR, "Zinc-Induced Copper Deficiency," *Gastroenterology*, 1988, 94(2):508-12.

References

Danks DM, "Disorders of Copper Transport," *The Metabolic Basis of Inherited Disease*, 6th ed, Scriver CR, Beaudet AL, Sly WS, et al, eds, New York, NY: McGraw-Hill Inc, 1989, 1411-31.

Lockitch G, Halstead AC, Quigley G, et al, "Age and Sex Specific Pediatric Reference Intervals: Study Design and Methods Illustrated by Measurement of Serum Proteins With the Behring LN Nephelometer," *Clin Chem*, 1988, 34:1618-21.

Menkes JH, "Kinky Hair Disease: Twenty-Five Years Later," *Brain Dev*, 1988, 10:77-9.

Scheinberg IH and Sternlieb I, *Wilson's Disease*, Philadelphia, PA: WB Saunders Co, 1984.

Chemistry Profile

***CPT** 80012 (12 tests)*

Applies to Health Fairs; Wellness Programs

Test Commonly Includes The tests present in the Chemistry Profile vary widely among laboratories. Often included are total protein, albumin, calcium, phosphorus, glucose, urea nitrogen (BUN), uric acid, creatinine, total bilirubin, alkaline phosphatase, LD (LDH), AST (SGOT), electrolytes (often, but not always), and calculated ionized calcium (occasionally). A/G ratio may be provided as a calculation. Other calculations which may be offered include BUN/creatinine ratio and globulins. Chemistry profiles may be done by a variety of instruments and include a variable number of tests. The previous list is one of a large number of possible configurations. Such chemistry profiles should be significantly less expensive than when the same tests are individually carried out.

Patient Care **PREPARATION:** 8- to 12-hour fast is preferred.

Specimen Serum **CONTAINER:** Red top tube **STORAGE INSTRUCTIONS:** Separate serum promptly and refrigerate. **CAUSES FOR REJECTION:** Gross hemolysis

Interpretive **USE:** Multiple organ system survey **LIMITATIONS:** More meaningful results are obtained if the specimen is collected after an 8- to 12-hour fast. Lipemia will interfere with some tests. This battery of tests may be or may have been intended for screening, but many laboratories operate their chemistry profiles as definitive tests. **ADDITIONAL INFORMATION:** Additional tests can be ordered if indicated. The tests listed are those which the author feels are desirable, inclusive of creatinine. Provision of chemistry profile with rapid turnaround on hospital

(Continued)

Chemistry Profile *(Continued)*

patients enhances good care and cost-containment. In many institutions, chemistry profiles are cost-effective; we agree that fewer tests may increase overall hospital costs[1] by prolonging hospitalization prior to diagnosis. In wellness programs and health fairs, cholesterol and glucose are often selected. A case for ferritin and thyroid testing can be made.[2]

Footnotes

1. Horvath B, Pecci J, and Gay W, "Fewer Tests May Cost More," *N Engl J Med*, 1985, 312:1645-6, (letter).
2. Witte DL, Angstadt DS, and Schweitzer JK, "Chemistry Profiles in "Wellness Program": Test Selection and Participant Outcomes," *Clin Chem*, 1988, 34(7):1447-50.

References

Berwick DM, "Screening in Health Fairs – A Critical Review of Benefits, Risks, and Costs," *JAMA*, 1985, 254:1492-8.

Collen MF, Dales LG, Friedman GD, et al, "Multiphasic Check-Up Evaluation Study. 4. Preliminary Cost Benefit Analysis for Middle-Aged Men," *Prev Med*, 1973, 2:236-46.

Ring AM, "Multiphasic Screening: Panacea or Diagnostic Nightmare?" *JAMA*, 1985, 254:1499.

Speicher CE, "So Duplicate Chemistry Profiles Correlate With Multiple Physicians: Let's Not Blame the Doctors," *Arch Pathol Lab Med*, 1988, 112:235-6.

Young DS, "Why There Is a Laboratory," *Clin Chem*, Young DS, Hicks J, Nipper H, et al, eds, Washington, DC: American Association of Clinical Chemistry, 1979.

Chloride/Phosphorus Ratio *see* Calcium, Serum *on page 160*

Chloride, Serum

CPT 82435

Related Information

Anion Gap *on page 132*
Bromide, Serum *on page 948*
Carbon Dioxide, Blood *on page 165*
Electrolytes, Blood *on page 212*
Kidney Stone Analysis *on page 1129*
Potassium, Blood *on page 330*
Sodium, Blood *on page 349*

Synonyms Cl, Serum

Applies to Bromism

Specimen Serum **CONTAINER:** Red top tube. Green top (heparin) tube is acceptable, but use of anticoagulants other than heparin may alter electrolyte composition. **COLLECTION:** Pediatric: Blood drawn from heelstick for capillary. **STORAGE INSTRUCTIONS:** Refrigerate

Interpretive **REFERENCE RANGE:** Premature: 95-110 mmol/L (SI: 95-110 mmol/L); full-term: 96-106 mmol/L (SI: 96-106 mmol/L); children and adults: 97-107 mmol/L (SI: 97-107 mmol/L) **POSSIBLE PANIC RANGE:** <80 mmol/L (SI: <80 mmol/L), >115 mmol/L (SI: >115 mmol/L) **USE:** Electrolyte evaluation; acid-base balance; water balance. Chloride generally increases and decreases with plasma or serum sodium.

Chloride is **increased** in dehydration, with ammonium chloride administration, with renal tubular acidosis (hyperchloremic metabolic acidosis), and with excessive infusion of normal saline. Differential diagnosis of acidemias and alkalemias. Chloride is higher in hyperparathyroidism than in some of the other causes of hypercalcemia, but a great deal of overlap exists.

Chloride is **decreased** with overhydration, congestive failure, syndrome of inappropriate secretion of ADH, vomiting, gastric suction, chronic respiratory acidosis, Addison's disease, salt-losing nephritis, burns, metabolic alkalosis, and in some instances of diuretic therapy.

An important use of chloride is in application of the anion gap. Consult that listing for more information.

LIMITATIONS: Interference from bromide occurs in hospital patients, in some of whom bromide concentrations are detectable.[1,2] Chloride is not used independently, but only with sodium, commonly with potassium and a measurement of carbon dioxide. **METHODOLOGY:** Coulometry, colorimetry, mercuric thiocyanate, ion-specific electrode (ISE) **ADDITIONAL INFORMATION:** Like other electrolytes, chloride cannot be interpreted without clinical knowledge of the patient. A diagnostic approach to the evaluation of hyperchloremic metabolic acidosis includes use of the urinary anion gap in conjunction with measurement of plasma potassium and urinary pH.[3]

Footnotes

1. Wenk RE, Lustagarten JA, Pappas NJ, et al, "Serum Chloride Analysis, Bromide Detection, and the Diagnosis of Bromism," *Am J Clin Pathol*, 1976, 65:49-57.

2. Rehak NN and Andersen TE, "Evaluation of Gilford Chemistry Control Interference With the Chloride Method in the Beckman Synchron CX3 System Analyzer: Cumulative Effect of Bromide on Chloride Results," *Clin Chem*, 1989, 35(7):1538.
3. Batlle DC, Hizon M, Cohen E, et al, "The Use of the Urinary Anion Gap in the Diagnosis of Hyperchloremic Metabolic Acidosis," *N Engl J Med*, 1988, 318(10):594-9.

References

Koch SM and Taylor RW, "Chloride Ion in Intensive Care Medicine," *Crit Care Med*, 1992, 20(2):227-40.
Lowe RA, Wood AB, Burney RE, et al, "Rational Ordering of Serum Electrolytes: Development of Clinical Criteria," *Ann Emerg Med*, 1987, 16:260-9.
McCleane GJ, "Urea and Electrolyte Measurement in Preoperative Surgical Patients," *Anaesthesia*, 1988, 43:413-5.
Rothenberg DM, Berns AS, Barkin R, et al, "Bromide Intoxication Secondary to Pyridostigmine Bromide Therapy," *JAMA*, 1990, 263(8):1121-2.
Wrenn KD, Slovis CM, Minion GE, et al, "The Syndrome of Alcoholic Ketoacidosis," *Am J Med*, 1991, 91(2):119-28.

Chloride, Sweat

***CPT** 82435 (analysis); 89360 (collection)*

Related Information

Cystic Fibrosis DNA Detection *on page 903*

Tryptic Activity, Stool *on page 1161*

Synonyms Cystic Fibrosis Sweat Test; Iontophoresis; Sweat, Chloride

Applies to Sodium, Sweat

Test Commonly Includes Sodium level may also be measured.

Specimen Sweat

Interpretive REFERENCE RANGE: 5-40 mmol/L (SI: 5-40 mmol/L). Sweat chloride and sodium levels >70 mmol/L are essentially diagnostic of cystic fibrosis in children, but all values must be interpreted with the family history and clinical presentation to include the presence of chronic obstructive pulmonary disease or documentation of pancreatic exocrine insufficiency.[1] Intermediate range is 40-60 mmol/L.[1] Adult values up to 50 mmol/L may be normal. In adults, >70 mmol/L is diagnostic,[2] and >60 mmol/L is diagnostic when other criteria are present.[1] CRITICAL VALUES: More than 60 mmol/L is considered diagnostic up to about 20 years of age. In adults, >70 mmol/L was diagnostic.[2] USE: Establish the diagnosis of cystic fibrosis (mucoviscidosis); evaluate frequent and/or foul stools, diarrhea, malabsorption, pancreatic insufficiency, history of meconium ileus, neonatal intestinal obstruction, rectal prolapse, infant celiac disease, other chronic problems of gastrointestinal tract and/or lung disease in children; work up chronic obstructive pulmonary disease, asthma, chronic cough, mucoid *Pseudomonas*, and other bronchitis in children;[3] work up children for failure to thrive and of young adult males for aspermia[3] LIMITATIONS: Duplicate tests should always be done. Skin covered by rashes or lesions will cause higher chloride levels. Elevations have been reported in adrenal insufficiency, ectodermal dysplasia, hereditary nephrogenic diabetes insipidus, hypothyroidism, malnutrition, fucosidosis, glucose-6-phosphatase deficiency, mucopolysaccharidosis and other entities. Shwachman and Mahmoodian emphasize that in some of the diseases listed, sweat chloride and sodium elevations lack the constancy that is found in cystic fibrosis,[2] and Rosenstein et al point out the different clinical facets of such entities. False low results have been described with edema, hypoproteinemia, and excessive sweating. Results are highly variable in adults, especially women in whom sweat chloride levels vary with the menstrual cycle. Sweat chloride levels in adults must be interpreted cautiously: false-positives and negatives may occur.

Borderline tests must be repeated.[4] Even negative tests should be repeated if the clinical picture suggests mucoviscidosis. Warwick and Hansen are among those who advocate subsequent confirmation of positives.[5] Sweat chloride test does not identify carriers (heterozygotes). Reliability in the first weeks of life is questionable.[1]

Standards for sweat electrolytes are not widely available as standards are for other chemistry assays, but can be made locally. One percent to 2% of cystic fibrosis patients do not have diagnostic sweat chloride patterns.[1,3] The measurement of sodium and the determination of the Na/Cl ratio may be useful.

An application of evolving pathology involves isolation of DNA with amplification utilizing the polymerase chain reaction. See Cystic Fibrosis DNA Detection in the Molecular Pathology chapter.

CONTRAINDICATIONS: Dermatitis. Do not collect sweat from the palm of the hand, or from any site following excessive sweating such as following high temperature or heavy exercise. Im-

(Continued)

Chloride, Sweat *(Continued)*

proper placement of pad or electrode can cause skin burn.[3] **METHODOLOGY:** Chloride in sweat from the forearm by pilocarpine-ionotophoresis.[1] It may be necessary in infants to use the upper back. Measurement by an ion-specific electrode (ISE). Schales and Schales method, Cotlove titration are acceptable. At least 50 mg of sweat must be collected for test validity.[1] Usual collections, using proper equipment producing exactly 1.5 ma, range from 100-400 mg of sweat. The recent introduction of the Cystic Fibrosis Indicator System™ (Medtronic) may be promising.[6] **ADDITIONAL INFORMATION:** Meconium ileus, very strongly associated with cystic fibrosis, is a separate entity from the meconium plug syndrome.

Other laboratory abnormalities in cystic fibrosis may include low total protein, prolongation of prothrombin time and abnormalities which may relate to evolving hepatic cirrhosis.

Normal sweat **sodium** level is 5-40 mmol/L. Sweat sodium >80 mmol/L also is evidence for cystic fibrosis. High sweat sodium may be found in Addison's disease, ectodermal dysplasia, hereditary nephrogenic diabetes insipidus, glucose-6-phosphatase deficiency, hypothyroidism, hypoparathyroidism, familial cholestasis,, pancreatitis, mucopolysaccharidoses, fucosidosis, and malnutrition.[1] Low sodium may be found with sodium depletion and in hyperaldosteronism.

Testing of stool samples for decreased trypsin activity (due to pancreatic exocrine dysfunction) has also been used as a screening test for cystic fibrosis in infants and young children. However, testing for stool trypsin activity is less reliable than the sweat chloride test and should not be used in its place. Assay of serum immunoreactive trypsinogen may be a useful test in cystic fibrosis screening programs.[7] Molecular recombinant DNA diagnostic techniques may ultimately be the best way to diagnose the disease and the carrier states.

Footnotes

1. Behrman RE, Kliegman RM, and Nelson WE, *Nelson Textbook of Pediatrics*, 14th ed, Philadelphia, PA: WB Saunders Co, 1992, 1108-9.
2. Hall SK, Stableforth DE, and Green A, "Sweat Sodium and Chloride Concentrations – Essential Criteria for the Diagnosis of Cystic Fibrosis in Adults," *Ann Clin Biochem*, 1990, 27(Pt 4):318-20.
3. Schwachman H and Mahmoodian A, "The Sweat Test and Cystic Fibrosis," *Diagn Med*, 1982, 61-77.
4. Stern RC, Boat TF, Abramowsky CR, et al, "Intermediate-Range Sweat Chloride Concentration and *Pseudomonas* Bronchitis. A Cystic Fibrosis Variant With Preservation of Exocrine Pancreatic Function," *JAMA*, 1978, 239:2676-80.
5. Warwick WJ and Hansen L, "Measurement of Chloride in Sweat With the Chloride-Selective Electrode," *Clin Chem*, 1978, 24:2050-3.
6. Warwick WJ, Hansen LG, and Werness ME, "Quantification of Chloride in Sweat With the Cystic Fibrosis Indicator System," *Clin Chem*, 1990, 36(1):96-8.
7. Hammond KB, Abman SH, Sokol RJ, et al, "Efficacy of Statewide Neonatal Screening for Cystic Fibrosis by Assay of Trypsinogen Concentrations," *N Engl J Med*, 1991, 325(11):769-74.

References

Meites S, *Pediatric Clinical Chemistry: Reference (Normal) Values*, 3rd ed, Washington, DC: American Association of Clinical Chemistry Press, 1989, 244-7.

Waters DL, Dorney SFA, Gaskin KJ, et al, "Pancreatic Function in Infants Identified as Having Cystic Fibrosis in a Neonatal Screening Program," *N Engl J Med*, 1990, 322(5):303-8.

Chloride, Urine

***CPT** 82436*

Related Information

Electrolytes, Urine *on page 213*
Potassium, Blood *on page 330*
Potassium, Urine *on page 332*
Sodium, Blood *on page 349*
Sodium, Urine *on page 351*

Synonyms Cl, Urine; Urine Cl

Specimen Timed or random urine **CONTAINER:** Plastic urine container, no preservative

Interpretive **REFERENCE RANGE:** 110-250 mmol/24 hours (SI: 110-250 mmol/day) in adults, lower values in infancy and childhood. Results depend on ingestion of chloride. **USE:** Evaluate electrolyte composition of urine, acid-base balance studies. Distinguish whether or not a case of metabolic alkalosis is chloride-responsive (salt responsive). Sherman and Eisinger[1,2] discuss bicarbonate excretion, blood volume, potassium depletion, and the differential diagnosis of metabolic alkalosis with loss of gastric juice (emesis, intubation) and after diuretics. Chloride depleted patients excrete urine with low chloride, <10 mmol/L. Such patients are chloride-responsive (ie, they respond to chloride sufficient to return body stores to normal). Metabolic alkalosis with low urine chloride is also found with villous tumors of the colon.

Endogenous or exogenous corticosteroids produce urine chloride values in excess of 20 mmol/L. Such patients are chloride resistant. The finding of chloride resistant metabolic alkalosis may provide a stimulus to identify an ACTH or aldosterone producing neoplasm (eg, Cushing's syndrome or Conn's syndrome). In Bartter's syndrome with metabolic alkalosis, there is usually increased urine chloride. The complex relationships of chronic pulmonary disease with metabolic alkalosis are mentioned by Sherman and Eisinger.

LIMITATIONS: Halogens other than chloride (bromide), which are also present in urine, may erroneously elevate the chloride result. Isolated urine chloride, without urine sodium or potassium or without serum or plasma electrolytes, can provide misleading information. Discussion of electrolyte balance is beyond the scope of this manual (eg, effect of profound potassium depletion on impairment of chloride reabsorption). Fetal urinary electrolytes are an unreliable guide to evaluate fetal renal function.[3] **METHODOLOGY:** Coulometric titration, ion-specific electrode (ISE) **ADDITIONAL INFORMATION:** Urine chloride is often ordered with sodium and potassium as a timed urine. The urinary anion gap $[Na^+ - (Cl^- + HCO_3^-)]$ or $[(Na^+ + K^+) - (Cl^-)]$ is useful in the initial evaluation of hyperchloremic metabolic acidosis.[4] In metabolic alkalosis, spot urine chloride in the presence of hypertension can provide important information.[5]

Footnotes

1. Sherman RA and Eisinger RP, "The Use (and Misuse) of Urinary Sodium and Chloride Measurements," *JAMA*, 1982, 247:3121-4.
2. Sherman RA and Eisinger RP, "Urinary Sodium and Chloride During Renal Salt Retention," *Am J Kidney Dis*, 1983, 3:121-3.
3. Elder JS, O'Grady JP, Ashmead G, et al, "Evaluation of Fetal Renal Function: Unreliability of Fetal Urinary Electrolytes," *J Urol*, 1990, 144(2 Pt 2):574-8.
4. Batlle DC, Hizon M, Cohen E, et al, "The Use of the Urinary Anion Gap in the Diagnosis of Hyperchloremic Metabolic Acidosis," *N Engl J Med*, 1988, 318(10):594-9.
5. Preuss HG, "Fundamentals of Clinical Acid-Base Evaluation," *Clin Lab Med*, 1993, 13(1):103-16.

References

Anderson FP and Miller WG, "Chloride," *Methods in Clinical Chemistry*, Pesce AJ and Kaplan LA, eds, St Louis, MO: Mosby-Year Book Inc, 1987, 73-7.

Harrington JT and Cohen JJ, "Measurement of Urinary Electrolytes – Indications and Limitations," *N Engl J Med*, 1975, 293:1241-3.

Jeffery RW, Mullenbach VA, Bjornson-Benson WM, et al, "Home Testing of Urine Chloride to Estimate Dietary Sodium Intake: Evaluation of Feasibility and Accuracy," *Addict Behav*, 1987, 12:17-21.

Kamel KS, Magner PO, Ethier JH, et al, "Urine Electrolytes in the Assessment of Extracellular Fluid Volume Contraction," *Am J Nephrol*, 1989, 9(4):344-7.

Cholecalciferol (25-OH D_3) *see* Vitamin D_3, Serum *on page 387*

Cholesterol

CPT 82465

Related Information

Apolipoprotein A and B *on page 134*
High Density Lipoprotein Cholesterol *on page 249*
Lipid Profile *on page 278*
Lipoprotein Electrophoresis *on page 281*
Low Density Lipoprotein Cholesterol *on page 284*
Triglycerides *on page 370*

Patient Care **PREPARATION: To support proper interpretation of lipid analysis:**

- For optimum patient condition at the time of blood drawing: no change in diet for 3 weeks, stable body weight, and fasting (no food, except water and possibly black coffee without sugar in the morning) for 12 hours.
- Posture may be a significant factor: cholesterol values may be 10% to 15% lower after 20 minutes in a recumbent position. From standing to a sitting position values are about 6% lower after 20 minutes.
- Increases of 2% to 5% in cholesterol may be seen if tourniquet is applied for 2 minutes during sampling. Emotional and physical stress may also be factors influencing cholesterol levels.
- Abstinence from alcohol for 72 hours may be desirable, but only inconclusive information is available.

Specimen Serum **CONTAINER:** Red top tube

Interpretive **REFERENCE RANGE:** Sharp inconsistencies are obvious when one studies pub-

(Continued)

Cholesterol *(Continued)*

lished normal ranges of serum cholesterol in the United States through the 1970s and much of the 1980s. Cholesterol levels have decreased from 1980 to 1987 in a study by the Minnesota Heart Survey.[1]

Cord blood cholesterol: <100 mg/dL (SI: <2.59 mmol/L); >100 mg/dL (SI: >2.59 mmol/L) is indicative of type II hyperlipoproteinemia. 0-1 month: 45-100 mg/dL (SI: 1.16-2.59 mmol/L). Adults, 20 years and older: Although 100-210 mg/dL (SI: 2.59-5.43 mmol/L) would be regarded as a low normal range for American adults, an increase between ages 25 and 45 of about 25 mg/dL (SI: 0.65 mmol/L) is recognized.[2] Levels >180 mg/dL (SI: >4.65 mmol/L) are not desirable,[3] but are commonplace in the United States. Percentile values are provided in a LRC report.[4]

Cholesterol <115 mg/dL (SI: <2.97 mmol/L) in youthful subjects is in the 5th percentile for males, <119 mg/dL (SI: <3.08 mmol/L) for females 0-19 years. Cholesterol levels <50 mg/dL (SI: <1.29 mmol/L) are found in the Bassen-Kornzweig syndrome with triglycerides <30 mg/dL. Cholesterol levels <100 mg/dL are found in Tangier disease without low triglycerides. Each is an autosomal recessive disease. Severe liver disease, severe acute illness, and abetalipoproteinemia may lower cholesterol dramatically.

Cholesterol >240 mg/dL (SI: >6.21 mmol/L) may indicate need for dietary or other intervention.[2,5] This level is excessive for young adults and even 220 mg/dL (SI: 5.69 mmol/L) is somewhat high for young adults, depending on LDL, HDL, family history, and other factors.

A national effort is underway to identify patients at risk for coronary heart disease due to elevated cholesterol levels. A key facet is standardization of cholesterol measurements traceable to the National Reference System for Cholesterol, rather than the customary instrument/method dependent "reference ranges." NBS (National Bureau of Standards) Standard Reference Material for Cholesterol in Human Serum was released to general laboratories in the first half of 1988 and has been valuable.[6] A collaborative study between the CAP and CDC to evaluate reference materials has been of great utility in the effort to determine specific instrument bias.[7]

Plasma cholesterol values are up to 10% lower than serum values. This difference should be considered when comparing patient values to published reference tables.

USE: Evaluate risk of coronary arterial occlusion, atherosclerosis, myocardial infarction, and complications including the demise of the patient. **Increased** in primary hypercholesterolemia, secondary hyperlipoproteinemias including nephrotic syndrome, hypothyroidism, primary biliary cirrhosis, and some cases of diabetes mellitus. **Low levels** have been found in cases of malnutrition, malabsorption, hyperthyroidism, myeloma, macroglobulinemia of Waldenström, polycythemia vera, myeloid metaplasia, myelofibrosis, chronic myelocytic leukemia, analphalipoproteinemia (Tangier disease), abetalipoproteinemia (Bassen-Kornzweig syndrome) (acanthocytosis), and in some individuals who subsequently present with carcinoma. Levy points out that the weak inverse relationship with cancer, mostly colon carcinoma, is limited to cholesterol levels <190 mg/dL (SI: <4.91 mmol/L) and is limited to men.[8] Hypocholesterolemia may occur with sideroblastic anemia or in the thalassemias.

Cholesterol relates to coronary heart disease risk.[4] Since premature mortality from coronary arterial disease is rampant and since cholesterol levels are available as a test which can detect a modifiable risk factor, serum cholesterol remains a critical and genuinely newsworthy topic and an important screening test. Effective intervention is available when cholesterol studies identify subjects likely to benefit, asymptomatic persons as well as those with recognized coronary disease. A report of the Lipid Research Clinics (LRC) is available with reference ranges.[4]

LIMITATIONS: Other risk factors for coronary arterial disease include hypertension, family history of premature coronary arterial disease, use of cigarettes, obesity, physical inactivity, low HDLC, diabetes mellitus, prior myocardial infarct, prior cerebrovascular or occlusive peripheral vascular disease, *vide infra*. Many heart attacks occur at levels of cholesterol considered "within normal limits." In fact, a majority of cases of heart disease are found in persons whose cholesterol levels are not worse than moderately elevated. The curves of those without and those with a coronary event heavily overlap when plotted against cholesterol levels. Random testing of TC, HDLC, and LDLC may fail to detect wide fluctuations in these levels (±20%). Variations of more than ±20% were seen in 75%, 65%, and 95% of a tested group.

Cholesterol values are altered by weight loss, pregnancy and (like HDL and apolipoproteins) acute illness, as well as by acute myocardial infarct. Inconsistencies exist between the serum cholesterol, the proportion of younger individuals who experience coronary occlusion, and the severity of atherogenesis. Nevertheless, cholesterol determinations done in good, well-standardized laboratories on samples from well subjects provide reliable information. The serum total cholesterol is insufficient as a screening tool for detection of elevated levels of low-density lipoprotein cholesterol in children and adolescents.[9]

METHODOLOGY: Enzymatic, ferric chloride-sulfuric acid, Leibermann-Burchardt reaction **ADDITIONAL INFORMATION:** About 50% to 80% of plasma/serum cholesterol is carried as low density lipoprotein cholesterol (LDLC) (β-lipoprotein). Much of the remainder is found in HDL, with small quantities as VLDL and as chylomicrons. Cholesterol is a component of cell membranes and organelles. It is the precursor of steroid hormones.

Cholesterol is included in lipid profiles. For optimal prediction of coronary atherosclerosis, some do not regard cholesterol alone as an adequate evaluation of all adults' blood lipids. However, relationships have been shown between diet, serum cholesterol, and long-term risk of death from coronary arterial disease in middle-aged American men. Rifkind and Segal point out that male subjects in the upper quintile of cholesterol levels had more than 50% of excessive coronary events related to high cholesterol.[4] Hyperlipoproteinemia type II (hypercholesterolemia) is recognizable at any age and can be recognized at birth from cord blood cholesterol. Cholesterol levels should not be drawn immediately after a myocardial infarct has occurred.

The National Cholesterol Education Program (NCEP) has defined a classification based on cholesterol. Unfortunately, this program did not provide age-adjusted normal ranges. Palumbo, reacting to the NCEP recommendations, wrote his opinions regarding the data and the recommendations. He went on to discuss the disconcerting lack of data on older persons.[10] Palumbo, writing the Mayo editorial, compares proposals of the NCEP with those of the Consensus Conference of 1985 for serum cholesterol levels. Dr. Palumbo recommends that "...the most prudent advice seems to be to adhere to the recommendations of the Consensus Conference of 1985"[11] and use the 75th and 90th percentile for serum cholesterol levels based on age as guidelines. See table. Palumbo's editorial should itself be read through. He writes that there is no quibble that hyperlipidemia, especially hypercholesterolemia, is associated with an increased risk for cardiovascular morbidity and mortality and that treatment of hypercholesterolemia will reduce such risks.

"Hyperlipoproteinemia" indicates increased cholesterol and/or triglyceride. Intervention levels from the Lipid Research Clinics Data were presented by Kuske and Feldman.[12] See table.

Intervention Levels for Serum Cholesterol by Sex and Age*

Males					Females				
Age	Percentile				Age	Percentile			
	75th		90th			75th		90th	
0–19 y	170	(4.40)	185	(4.80)	0–19 y	175	(4.50)	190	(4.90)
20–24 y	185	(4.80)	205	(5.30)	20–24 y	190	(4.90)	215	(5.55)
25–29 y	200	(5.15)	225	(5.80)	25–34 y	195	(5.05)	220	(5.70)
30–34 y	215	(5.55)	240	(6.20)	35–39 y	205	(5.30)	230	(5.95)
35–39 y	225	(5.80)	250	(6.45)	40–44 y	215	(5.55)	235	(6.05)
40–44 y	230	(5.95)	250	(6.45)	45–49 y	225	(5.80)	250	(6.45)
45–69 y	235	(6.05)	260	(6.70)	50–54 y	240	(6.20)	265	(6.85)
70+ y	230	(5.95)	250	(6.45)	55+ y	250	(6.45)	275	(7.10)

*From the Lipid Research Clinics Data, with permission. Values are given in mg/dL (mmol/L). *Arch Intern Med,* 1987, 147:357–60.

Palumbo, writing an editorial in *JAMA*, emphasizes that for individuals older than 60 years intervention should be based on the judgment of the physician and patient preference.[13] Calculating 24 million Americans eligible for antilipid medications, he discusses costs and benefits. Sempos et al also examine prevalence and project about 60 million Americans' candidacy for medical advice and intervention.[14]

(Continued)

Cholesterol *(Continued)*

Classification Based on Total Cholesterol

<200 mg/dL	(SI: <5.17 mmol/L)	Desirable blood cholesterol
200-239 mg/dL	(SI: 5.17-6.18 mmol/L)	Borderline-high blood cholesterol
≥240 mg/dL	(SI: ≥6.21 mmol/L)	High blood cholesterol

- The total blood cholesterol level is the basis for initial patient classification.
- All blood cholesterol levels >200 mg/dL (SI: >5.17 mmol/L) should be confirmed by repeat measurements, with the average used to guide clinical decisions.
- Other CHD risk factors should be taken into account in selecting appropriate follow-up measures for patients with borderline-high cholesterol levels.
- All patients with a level ≥240 mg/dL (SI: 6.21 mmol/L), which is classified as high blood cholesterol, should receive a lipoprotein analysis. Patients with borderline-high blood cholesterol levels 200-239 mg/dL (SI: 5.17-6.18 mmol/L), who in addition have definite CHD or two other CHD risk factors, should also have a lipoprotein analysis performed.
- CHD risk factors as defined in the report include:
  - male sex
  - family history of premature CHD (definite myocardial infarction or sudden death before age 55 in a parent or sibling)
  - cigarette smoking (currently more than 10 cigarettes per day)
  - hypertension
  - low HDL cholesterol concentration (mg/dL (SI: <0.91 mmol/L) confirmed by repeat measurement)
  - diabetes mellitus
  - history of definite cerebrovascular or occlusive peripheral vascular disease
  - Severe obesity (≥30% overweight)
- In public screening programs, all patients with a level >200 mg/dL (SI: >5.17 mmol/L) should be referred to their physician for remeasurement and evaluation.

"National Cholesterol Education Program, Adult Treatment Panel Report 1987," National Cholesterol Education Program, National Heart, Lung and Blood Institute, National Institutes of Health, C-200, Bethesda, MD 20892, 1987.
Compare to the following table.
Note lack of age stratification. Some authorities suggest that stratification should be maintained.

Values for Selecting Adults at Moderate and High Risk Requiring Treatment

Age	Moderate Risk		High Risk	
	mg/dL	SI: mmol/L	mg/dL	SI: mmol/L
20–29 y	>200	5.17	>220	5.69
30–39 y	>220	5.69	>240	6.21
≥40 y	>240	6.21	>260	6.72

From "Lowering Blood Cholesterol to Prevent Heart Disease," *JAMA,* 1985, 253:2080–6, with permission.

Portable chemistry analyzers have appeared in places such as shopping malls. A relevant paper addresses a perceived need for further evaluation of the instruments as well as recommendation for training of the personnel who use them regarding maintenance and quality assurance procedures.[15] A Health and Human Services inspector general's report was reiterated by Rep Ron Wyden (D, Oregon), that the accuracy and usefulness of public cholesterol screening may be compromised by need for quality assurance, improved on site counseling and referral to a physician when appropriate, according to American Medical News.[16] In 1993, the FDA approved a "home" cholesterol test.

Footnotes

1. Burke GL, Sprafka JM, Folsom AR, et al, "Trends in Serum Cholesterol Levels From 1980 to 1987. The Minnesota Heart Survey," *N Engl J Med*, 1991, 324(14):941-6.
2. Hulley SB and Lo B, "Choice and Use of Blood Lipid Tests. An Epidemiologic Perspective," *Arch Intern Med*, 1983, 143:667-73.
3. Carleton RA, "Criterion for Cholesterol Norms – Healthy or Statistical?" *Am J Clin Pathol*, 1983, 79:402, (editorial).
4. Rifkind BM and Segal P, "Lipid Research Clinics Program Reference Values for Hyperlipidemia and Hypolipidemia," *JAMA*, 1983, 250:1869-72.
5. "National Cholesterol Education Program, Adult Treatment Panel Report 1987," National Cholesterol Education Program, National Heart, Lung and Blood Institute, National Institutes of Health, 1987, C-200, Bethesda, MD 20892.
6. Bock JL, "Accuracy of Cholesterol Measurements," *Arch Intern Med*, 1991, 151(8):1677, (letter).
7. Myers GL, Schap D, Smith SJ, et al, "College of American Pathologists – Centers for Disease Control Collaborative Study for Evaluating Reference Materials for Total Serum Cholesterol Measurements," *Arch Pathol Lab Med*, 1990, 114(12):1199-205.
8. Levy RI, "Cholesterol and Disease – What Are the Facts?" *JAMA*, 1982, 248:2888-90, (editorial).
9. Dennison BA, Kikuchi DA, Srinivasen SR, et al, "Serum Total Cholesterol Screening for the Detection of Elevated Low-Density Lipoprotein in Children and Adolescents: The Bogalusa Heart Study," *Pediatrics*, 1990, 85(4):472-9.
10. Palumbo PJ, "National Cholesterol Education Program: Does the Emperor Have Any Clothes?" *Mayo Clin Proc*, 1988, 63(1):88-90.
11. Office of Medical Applications of Research, National Institutes of Health, Bethesda, MD: Consensus Conference, "Lowering Blood Cholesterol to Prevent Heart Disease," *JAMA*, 1985, 253:2080-6.
12. Kuske TT and Feldman EB, "Hyperlipoproteinemia, Atherosclerosis Risk, and Dietary Management," *Arch Intern Med*, 1987, 147:357-60.
13. Palumbo PJ, "Cholesterol Lowering for All: A Closer Look," *JAMA*, 1989, 262(1):91-2.
14. Sempos C, Fulwood R, Haines C, et al, "The Prevalence of High Blood Cholesterol Levels Among Adults in the United States," *JAMA*, 1989, 262(1):45-52.
15. Naito HK, Hutchison JD, Bowers GN Jr, et al, "Current Status of Blood Cholesterol Management in Clinical Laboratories in the United States: A Report From the Laboratory Standardization Panel of the National Cholesterol Education Program," *Clin Chem*, 1988, 34:193-201.
16. Jones L, "Fried Eggs or Oat Bran? House Panel Delves Into Cholesterol Debate," *American Medical News*, 1989, December 22/29, 2.

References

American Academy of Pediatrics Committee on Nutrition, "Indications for Cholesterol Testing in Children," *Pediatrics*, 1989, 83(1):141-2.

Anderson KM, Castelli WP, and Levy D, "Cholesterol and Mortality: 30 Years of Follow-Up From the Framingham Study," *JAMA*, 1987, 257:2176-80.

Austin GE, Hollman J, Lynn MJ, et al, "Serum Lipoprotein Levels Fail to Predict Postangioplasty Recurrent Coronary Artery Stenosis," *Cleve Clin J Med*, 1989, 56(5):509-14.

Bak AA and Grobbee DE, "The Effect on Serum Cholesterol Levels of Coffee Brewed by Filtering or Boiling," *N Engl J Med*, 1989, 321(21):1432-7.

Benfante R and Reed D, "Is Elevated Serum Cholesterol Level a Risk Factor for Coronary Heart Disease in the Elderly?" *JAMA*, 1990, 263(3):393-6.

Borhani NO, "Prevention of Coronary Heart Disease in Practice: Implications of the Results of Recent Clinical Trials," *JAMA*, 1985, 254:257-62.

Bowers GN Jr, "Accuracy and Blood Cholesterol Measurements," *Clin Chem*, 1988, 34:192.

Bradford RH and Rifkind BM, "Lowering Blood Cholesterol to Reduce Coronary Heart Disease Risk," *Clin Lab Med*, 1989, 9(1):1-6.

Christenson RH, Roeback JR Jr, Watson TE, et al, "Improving the Reliability of Total and High-Density Lipoprotein Cholesterol Measurements. Four Testing Strategies Compared in a High-Risk Population," *Arch Pathol Lab Med*, 1991, 115(12):1212-6.

Copeland BE, "Serum Cholesterol Methodology: 100 Years of Development," *Ann Clin Lab Sci*, 1990, 20(1):1-11.

Garber AM, "Where to Draw the Line Against Cholesterol," *Ann Intern Med*, 1989, 111(8):625-7.

Garber AM, Sox HC Jr, and Littenberg B, "Screening Asymptomatic Adults for Cardiac Risk Factors: The Serum Cholesterol Level," *Ann Intern Med*, 1989, 110(8):622-39.

Goodman DS, "New Guidelines for Lowering Blood Cholesterol," *Clin Lab Med*, 1989, 9(1)17-27.

(Continued)

Cholesterol *(Continued)*

Goodman DS, Bradford RH, Brewer HB Jr, et al, "AHA Conference Report on Cholesterol. Diagnosis, Evaluation, and Treatment: Current Status and Issues," *Circulation*, 1989, 80(3):735-8.
Grundy SM, "Cholesterol and Coronary Heart Disease: A New Era," *JAMA*, 1986, 256:2849-58.
Harlan WR and Stross JK, "An Educational View of a National Initiative to Lower Plasma Lipid Levels," *JAMA*, 1985, 253:2087-90.
Isles CG, Hole DJ, Gillis CR, et al, "Plasma Cholesterol, Coronary Heart Disease, and Cancer in the Renfrew and Paisley Survey," *Br Med J [Clin Res]*, 1989, 298(6678):920-4.
Iso H, Jacobs DR Jr, Wentworth D, et al, "Serum Cholesterol Levels and Six-Year Mortality From Stroke in 350,977 Men Screened for the Multiple Risk Factor Intervention Trial," *N Engl J Med*, 1989, 320(14):904-10.
Koch DD, Hassemer DJ, Wiebe DA, et al, "Testing Cholesterol Accuracy: Performance of Several Common Laboratory Instruments," *JAMA*, 1988, 260:2552-7.
Kronmal RA, "Commentary on the Published Results of the Lipid Research Clinics Coronary Primary Prevention Trial," *JAMA*, 1985, 253:2091-3.
Laemmle P, Unger L, McCray C, et al, "Cholesterol Guidelines, Lipoprotein Cholesterol Levels, and Triglyceride Levels: Potential for Misclassification of Coronary Heart Disease Risk," *J Lab Clin Med*, 1989, 113(3):325-33.
Lipid Research Clinics Program Investigators, "Reply to Commentary by Richard Kronmal," *JAMA*, 1985, 254:263-4.
Marshall WJ and Ballantyne FC, "Clinical Topics: Current Clinical Laboratory Practice: Investigation of Plasma Lipids - Which Tests and When?" *Br Med J [Clin Res]*, 1986, 292:1652-4.
McManus BM, "Reference Ranges and Ideal Patient Values for Blood Cholesterol," *Arch Pathol Lab Med*, 1986, 110:469-73.
McManus BM, Toth AB, Engel JA, et al, "Progress in Lipid Reporting Practices and Reliability of Blood Cholesterol Measurement in Clinical Laboratories in Nebraska," *JAMA*, 1989, 262(1):83-8.
Naito HK, "Cholesterol: Review of Methods," *ASCP Check Sample®*, Chicago, IL: American Society of Clinical Pathologists, 1988, 4:1-20.
Naito HK, "The Need for Accurate Total Cholesterol Measurement: Recommended Analytical Goals, Current State of Reliability, and Guidelines for Better Determinations," *Clin Lab Med*, 1989, 9(1):37-60.
Schucker B, Wittes JT, Cutler JA, et al, "Change in Physician Perspective on Cholesterol and Heart Disease," *JAMA*, 1987, 258:3521-6.
Shekelle RB, Shryock AM, Paul D, et al, "Diet, Serum Cholesterol, and Death From Coronary Heart Disease. The Western Electric Study," *N Engl J Med*, 1981, 304:65-70.
Stamler J, Wentworth D, and Neaton JD, "Is Relationship Between Serum Cholesterol and Risk of Premature Death From Coronary Heart Disease Continuous and Graded?" *JAMA*, 1986, 256:2823-8.
Steinmetz J, Jouanel P, and Delattre J, "Total Cholesterol," *Drug Effects on Laboratory Test Results Analytical Interferences and Pharmacological Effects*, Siest G and Galteau MM, eds, Littleton, MA: PSG Publishing Co Inc, 1988, 165-84.
Vanderlinde RE, Bowers GN Jr, Schaffer R, et al, "The National Reference System for Cholesterol," *Clin Lab Med*, 1989, 9(1):89-104.
Wilson PWF, Christiansen JC, Anderson KM, et al, "Impact on National Guidelines for Cholesterol Risk Factor Screening: The Framingham Offspring Study," *JAMA*, 1989, 262(1):41-4.

Cholinesterase, Erythrocytic *see* Acetylcholinesterase, Red Blood Cell *on page 95*

Cholinesterase Inhibition by Dibucaine *see* Dibucaine Number *on page 209*

Cholinesterase, Serum *see* Pseudocholinesterase, Serum *on page 343*

Chorionic Somatomammotropin *see* Placental Lactogen, Human *on page 324*

Chylomicrons *see* Triglycerides *on page 370*

CK *see* Creatine Kinase *on page 196*

CK Isoenzymes *see* Cardiac Enzymes/Isoenzymes *on page 170*

CK Isoenzymes *see* Creatine Kinase Isoenzymes *on page 197*

CK Isoforms *see* Creatine Kinase Isoenzymes *on page 197*

CK-MB and Total CK *see* Creatine Kinase Isoenzymes *on page 197*

Clomid® Test *see* Clomiphene Test *on this page*

Clomiphene Test

CPT *83001 (follicle stimulating hormone); 83002 (luteinizing hormone)*

Related Information

Follicle Stimulating Hormone *on page 222*

Luteinizing Hormone, Blood or Urine *on page 286*

Synonyms Clomid® Test

Test Commonly Includes FSH analysis, post-clomiphene LH

Abstract Clomiphene is a very weak nonsteroidal antiestrogenic agent which competes with estradiol at the hypothalamus, thereby blocking the negative feedback of the endogenous gonadal steroids on the hypothalamus. In the presence of an intact hypothalamic-pituitary-gonadal axis, administration of clomiphene leads to increased secretion of LH and FSH, inducing ovulation in many anovulatory patients.

Patient Care PREPARATION: Four weeks of basal body temperatures are recorded. Ascertain that the patient is not pregnant and that the ovaries are not enlarged. No isotopes administered 24 hours prior to venipuncture. Females initially take 50 mg clomiphene orally daily for 5 days beginning on the fifth day of the induced or spontaneous menstrual cycle.

Specimen Serum CONTAINER: Red top tube COLLECTION: Females: draw 5-9 days after last oral dose. STORAGE INSTRUCTIONS: Refrigerate serum. LH and FSH stable at least 7 days in refrigerated serum. CAUSES FOR REJECTION: Recently administered radioisotopes SPECIAL INSTRUCTIONS: State on slip if post-clomiphene sample(s).

Interpretive REFERENCE RANGE: FSH and LH are expected to peak 5-9 days after completing Clomid®. Ovulation assessed by basal body temperature or serum progesterone 2 weeks after last clomiphene dose. USE: Clomiphene may be used to evaluate the integrity of the hypothalamic-pituitary-gonadal axis and to enhance fertility in anovulatory patients with normal ovarian function. CONTRAINDICATIONS: In females, observation hyperstimulation of ovaries but unusual on dose less than 200 mg, and there is a small risk of multiple pregnancies, about 5%. METHODOLOGY: Radioimmunoassay (RIA)

References

Blankstein J and Quigley MM, "The Anovulatory Patient. An Orderly Approach to Evaluation and Treatment," *Postgrad Med*, 1988, 83:97-102.

Check JH, Chase JS, Nowroozi K, et al, "Empirical Therapy of the Male With Clomiphene in Couples With Unexplained Infertility," *Int J Fertil*, 1989, 34(2):120-2.

Cunha GR, Taguchi O, Namikawa R, et al, "Teratogenic Effects of Clomiphene, Tamoxifen, and Diethylstilbestrol on the Developing Human Female Genital Tract," *Hum Pathol*, 1987, 18:1132-43.

Dickey RP, Olar TT, Taylor SN, et al, "Relationship of Follicle Number and Other Factors to Fecundability and Multiple Pregnancy in Clomiphene Citrate-Induced Intrauterine Insemination Cycles," *Fertil Steril*, 1992, 57(3):613-9.

Fedele L, Brioschi D, Dorta M, et al, "Prediction and Self-Prediction of Ovulation in Clomiphene Citrate-Treated Patients," *Eur J Obstet Gynecol Reprod Biol*, 1988, 28:297-303.

Keenan JA, Herbert CM, Bush JR, "Diagnosis and Management of Out-of-Phase Endometrial Biopsies Among Patients Receiving Clomiphene Citrate for Ovulation Induction," *Fertil Steril*, 1989, 51(6):964-7.

Clonidine Suppression Test *see* Catecholamines, Fractionation, Plasma *on page 172*

Cl, Serum *see* Chloride, Serum *on page 182*

Cl, Urine *see* Chloride, Urine *on page 184*

CO *see* Carboxyhemoglobin *on page 165*

CO_2 Content *see* Carbon Dioxide, Blood *on page 165*

CO_2T *see* Carbon Dioxide, Blood *on page 165*

COHb *see* Carboxyhemoglobin *on page 165*

Compound F *see* Cortisol, Blood *on this page*

Connecting Peptide Insulin *see* C-Peptide *on page 195*

Coproporphyrins *see* Porphyrins, Quantitative, Urine *on page 327*

Coronary Heart Disease Risk Index *see* Lipid Profile *on page 278*

Corticotropin *see* Adrenocorticotropic Hormone *on page 98*

Cortisol, Blood

***CPT** 82533*

Related Information

Adrenocorticotropic Hormone *on page 98*

Cosyntropin Test *on page 194*

17-Hydroxycorticosteroids, Urine *on page 256*

(Continued)

Cortisol, Blood *(Continued)*

17-Ketogenic Steroids, Urine *on page 265*
Metyrapone Test *on page 292*
Thorn Test *on page 609*

Synonyms Compound F; Hydrocortisone, Serum

Applies to Dexamethasone Suppression Test

Specimen Serum or plasma **CONTAINER:** Red top tube or green top (heparin) tube **SAMPLING TIME:** AM and PM levels **COLLECTION:** Blood may be drawn at 8 AM and 4 PM to evaluate baseline diurnal variation. (Some prefer the evening draw at 11 PM.) Morning specimen is often ordered with ACTH level. **STORAGE INSTRUCTIONS:** Stable 7 days at 4°C to 25°C. **SPECIAL INSTRUCTIONS:** Dexamethasone suppression test requires administration of high-dose or low-dose dexamethasone and subsequent measurement of cortisol levels.

Interpretive **REFERENCE RANGE:** AM: 5-25 μg/dL (SI: 138-690 nmol/L), PM: 2-9 μg/dL (SI: 55-248 nmol/L) depending on test, assay **USE:** Low cortisol is found with adrenogenital syndrome, primary adrenocortical insufficiency (Addison's disease), and with hypopituitarism. High cortisol occurs in adrenocortical hypersecretion due to either adrenal hyperplasia or adrenal adenoma (Cushing's syndrome) and with excess pituitary ACTH (Cushing's disease) or ectopic ACTH. **Not useful for following dosage of exogenous, synthetic corticosteroids.** **LIMITATIONS:** Random serum cortisol may be misleading because of circadian variation in secretion. Method may have a high cross reaction with corticosterone and with 11-deoxycortisol (compound S). Cortisol is physiologically increased in patients with hypoglycemia, stress, and in pregnancy. False-negatives occur. **CONTRAINDICATIONS:** Single samples taken under uncontrolled conditions for cortisol assays are worthless.[1] **METHODOLOGY:** Immunoassay **ADDITIONAL INFORMATION:** Cortisol is the major adrenal glucocorticoid steroid hormone and is normally under feedback control by pituitary ACTH and the hypothalamus. The physiologic effects of cortisol are beyond the scope of this book.

Causes of **low cortisol** include pituitary destruction or failure, with resultant loss of ACTH to stimulate the adrenal, and metabolic errors or destruction of the adrenal gland itself (adrenogenital syndromes, tuberculosis, histoplasmosis). The diagnosis of hypoadrenalism generally requires confirmation with ACTH stimulation, due to the circadian rhythms of cortisol and other factors. Causes of **increased cortisol**, which may present initially simply as loss of normal diurnal variation, include pituitary overproduction of ACTH, production of ACTH by a tumor (notably oat cell carcinomas), adrenal adenomas, and carcinomas.

Dexamethasone suppression test helps distinguish among causes of elevated cortisol.[2] Dexamethasone is a synthetic steroid which will suppress ACTH secretion. Under normal circumstances decreased cortisol levels follow. Suppressibility of elevated cortisol shows that feedback regulation is intact, and usually rules out Cushing's syndrome. If there is no suppression overnight after 1 mg of dexamethasone, higher doses and longer times may suppress ACTH production by a pituitary adenoma, but will not suppress an adrenal adenoma. Measurement of ACTH may also be informative. For the diagnosis of adrenocortical insufficiency, the cosyntropin test is recommended. The corticotropin-releasing hormone (CRH) stimulation test (1 μg/kg ovine CRH by I.V. administration) works well as the standard high-dose dexamethasone suppression test in distinguishing pituitary Cushing's disease from ectopic ACTH secretion. The test is less time consuming and can be an outpatient test. Cortisol in ACTH response is measured at timed intervals. A positive response (four times baseline) occurs in pituitary Cushing's disease, and a negative response is seen in ectopic ACTH-secreting tumor. There is a 97% positive predictive value. Cushing's is excluded in only 70% if there is nonresponse, however when both tests (dexamethasone suppression and CRH stimulation) show no response, there is a 100% predictive value for ectopic ACTH-secreting tumor. The stimulation test should not be used in hypoadrenalism. For the diagnosis of Cushing's syndrome (hypercortisolism), the urinary free cortisol is the test of choice.

The dexamethasone suppression test (DST) is abnormal in many psychiatric illnesses. The sensitivity of the DST in major depression is approximately 40% to 50%, but is higher (60% to 70%) in severe (especially psychotic) affective disorders.[3] False-positive results occur with alcoholism and with stress (eg, hospitalization). In critically ill subjects, transient decreases of corticotropin may occur. Cortisol <15 μg/dL provides indication of adrenal cortisol insufficiency.[4]

Footnotes

1. Watts NB and Keffer JH, *Practical Endocrine Diagnosis*, 4th ed, Philadelphia, PA: Lea & Febiger, 1989.

2. Weiner MF, "Age and Cortisol Suppression by Dexamethasone in Normal Subjects," *J Psychiatr Res*, 1989, 23(2):163-8.
3. "The Dexamethasone Suppression Test: An Overview of Its Current Status in Psychiatry," The APA Task Force on Laboratory Tests in Psychiatry, *Am J Psychiatry*, 1987, 144:1253-62.
4. Kidess AI, Caplan RH, Reynertson RH, et al, "Transient Corticotropin Deficiency in Critical Illness," *Mayo Clin Proc*, 1993, 68(5):435-41.

References

Bravo EL, "Physiology of the Adrenal Cortex," *Urol Clin North Am*, 1989, 16(3):433-7, (review).
Brien TG, "Pathophysiology of Free Cortisol in Plasma," *Ann N Y Acad Sci*, 1988, 538:130-6, (review).
Dam H, "Dexamethasone Suppression Test," *Acta Psychiatr Scand Suppl*, 1988, 345:38-44, (review).
Davidson M, Bastiaens L, Davis BM, et al, "Endocrine Changes in Alzheimer's Disease," *Neurol Clin*, 1988, 6:149-57, (review).
Guechot J, Lepine JP, Cohen C, et al, "Simple Laboratory Test of Neuroendocrine Disturbance in Depression: 11 PM Saliva Cortisol," *Neuropsychobiology*, 1987, 18:1-4.
Kirkman S and Nelson DH, "Alcohol-Induced Pseudo-Cushing's Disease: A Study of Prevalence With Review of the Literature," *Metabolism*, 1988, 37:390-4, (review).
Macro M, Reznik Y, Leymarie P, et al, "The Effect of Intrathecal Dexamethasone Injection on Plasma Cortisol Level," *Br J Rheumatol*, 1991, 30(3):238, (letter).
Nierenberg AA and Feinstein AR, "How to Evaluate a Diagnostic Marker Test. Lessons From the Rise and Fall of Dexamethasone Suppression Test," *JAMA*, 1988, 259:1699-702, (review).
Weller EB and Weller RA, "Neuroendocrine Changes in Affectively Ill Children and Adolescents," *Neurol Clin*, 1988, 6:41-54, (review).

Cortisol Response to Cosyntropin *see* Cosyntropin Test *on next page*

Cortisol, Urine

***CPT** 82533*

Related Information

Adrenocorticotropic Hormone *on page 98*
17-Ketogenic Steroids, Urine *on page 265*
Metyrapone Test *on page 292*
Thorn Test *on page 609*

Synonyms Urinary Free Cortisol; Urine Cortisol

Test Commonly Includes Creatinine concentration and total volume, to support adequacy of collection

Abstract The diagnosis of Cushing's syndrome requires evidence of autonomous, inappropriate secretion of cortisol.

Patient Care PREPARATION: Patient should avoid spironolactone or quinacrine. Avoid patient stress.

Specimen 24-hour urine CONTAINER: Plastic urine container, kept on ice. 20 mL of 33% acetic acid or 1 g boric acid added before start of the collection may be required. If this is used, it is not necessary to refrigerate during collection. COLLECTION: Instruct the patient to void at 8 AM and discard the specimen. Then collect all urine including the final specimen voided at the end of the 24-hour collection period (ie, 8 AM the next morning). Keep urine sample refrigerated during collection. A normal diurnal rhythm exists with highest levels in the morning, but this circadian rhythm is lost in Cushing's syndrome.[1] STORAGE INSTRUCTIONS: Refrigerate during collection if preservative not used. Stable 7 days at 4°C if preservative used.

Interpretive REFERENCE RANGE: 30-100 μg/24 hours (SI: 83-276 nmol/day) (normal adult); lower in infants and children as a function of decreased cortisol production CRITICAL VALUES: <10 μg/24 hours (SI: <28 nmol/day) in general excludes Cushing's syndrome[2] USE: Evaluate adrenal cortical function, especially hyperfunction. Evaluate obese or hypertensive subjects with glucose intolerance, plethora, round face, hirsutism, striae, backache, irregular menses in various combinations, most of whom do not have Cushing's syndrome;[3] elevation of urinary free cortisol in a properly collected specimen in the unstressed patient is sufficient to diagnose Cushing's syndrome, and a normal result is strong evidence against that diagnosis. This is the screening test of choice for the diagnosis of Cushing's syndrome. Urinary free cortisol is a more accurate reflection of cortisol secretion than a single serum specimen.[2] It is sensitive and specific.[1,2] LIMITATIONS: Low values do not necessarily mean adrenal hypofunction. Vagaries of improper urine collection or renal disease may lead to misleading results. Avoid stressing the patient during collection; this physiologically raises cortisol. Increased in pregnancy and with oral contraceptives. METHODOLOGY: Radioimmunoassay (RIA) after extraction, high performance liquid chromatography (HPLC) ADDITIONAL INFORMATION: Urinary cortisol re-

(Continued)

Cortisol, Urine *(Continued)*

flects the portion of serum-free cortisol filtered by the kidney, freely filtered. It correlates with cortisol secretion rate. Cushing's syndrome is caused by an endocrine tumor of pituitary or adrenal cortex; ectopic production of ACTH includes that of small cell carcinomas of lung, thymomas, carcinoids, and medullary thyroid carcinomas.[2] The dexamethasone suppression test is useful as well.[1,2,3] Recently a new test was described, corticotropin-releasing hormone stimulation following low-dose dexamethasone administration. The test was more accurate in distinguishing Cushing's syndrome from pseudo-Cushing's states.[4]

Footnotes

1. Dunlap NE, Grizzle WE, and Siegel AL, "Cushing's Syndrome: Screening Methods in Hospitalized Patients," *Arch Pathol Lab Med*, 1985, 109:222-9.
2. Watts NB and Keffer JH, "Adrenal Cortex," *Practical Endocrinology*, 4th ed, Philadelphia, PA: Lea & Febiger, 1989, 91-120.
3. Oxley DK, "Cushing's Syndrome," *Arch Pathol Lab Med*, 1985, 109:221, (editorial).
4. Yanovski JA, Cutler GB, Chrousos GP, et al, "Corticotropin-Releasing Hormone Stimulation Following Low-Dose Dexamethasone Administration. A New Test to Distinguish Cushing's Syndrome From Pseudo-Cushing's States," *JAMA*, 1993, 269(17):2232--8.

References

Bondy PK, "Disorders of the Adrenal Cortex," *Williams Textbook of Endocrinology*, 8th ed, Wilson JD, Foster DW, eds, Philadelphia, PA: WB Saunders Co, 1985, 816-90.

Bravo EL, "Physiology of the Adrenal Cortex," *Urol Clin North Am*, 1989, 16(3):433-7, (review).

Flack MR, Oldfield EH, Cutler GB Jr, "Urine Free Cortisol in the High-Dose Dexamethasone Suppression Test for the Differential Diagnosis of the Cushing Syndrome," *Ann Intern Med*, 1992, 116(3):211-7.

Gwirtsman HE, Kaye WH, George DT, et al, "Central and Peripheral ACTH and Cortisol Levels in Anorexia Nervosa and Bulimia," *Arch Gen Psychiatry*, 1989, 46(1):61-9.

Howanitz JH, Howanitz PJ, and Henry JB, "Evaluation of Endocrine Function," Henry JB, ed, *Todd-Sanford-Davidsohn Clinical Diagnosis and Management by Laboratory Methods*, 18th ed, Henry JB, ed, Philadelphia, PA: WB Saunders Co, 1991, 308-48.

Weaver DK and Glenn GC, "The Urine Chemistry Survey – Series 2: 5 Years Experience With an Interlaboratory Comparison Program," *Arch Pathol Lab Med*, 1989, 113(7):713-22.

Yeh J and Barbieri RL, "Twenty-Four Hour Urinary Free Cortisol in Premenopausal Cigarette Smokers and Nonsmokers," *Fertil Steril*, 1989, 52(6):1067-9.

Zis AP, Remick RA, Clark CM, et al, "Evening Urine Cortisol Excretion and DST Results in Depression and Anorexia Nervosa," *J Psychiatr Res*, 1989, 23(3-4):251-5.

Cortrosyn® Test *see* Cosyntropin Test *on this page*

Cosyntropin Test

***CPT** 82536 (cortisol, each sample)*

Related Information

Cortisol, Blood *on page 191*
Metyrapone Test *on page 292*
Thorn Test *on page 609*

Synonyms Cortisol Response to Cosyntropin; Cortrosyn® Test; Rapid ACTH Test

Replaces ACTH Infusion Test; Bovine ACTH

Test Commonly Includes Baseline level and levels 30 and 60 minutes after cosyntropin stimulation

Patient Care PREPARATION: Patient should fast a minimum of 10 hours. Baseline serum cortisol is drawn. AFTERCARE: Additional serum cortisol levels are collected after injection of cosyntropin. Failure of postinjection cortisol levels to increase is abnormal and must lead to further work-up.

Specimen Serum CONTAINER: Red top tube COLLECTION: Test should begin with 8 AM baseline cortisol level. Cosyntropin, 250 μg, is injected I.M., and samples are drawn at 30 and 60 minutes. These are assayed for cortisol. STORAGE INSTRUCTIONS: Separate serum and freeze.

Interpretive REFERENCE RANGE: Normal baseline cortisol. Increase in serum cortisol after cosyntropin injection >7 μg/dL (SI: >193 nmol/L) or peak response >18 μg/dL (SI: >497 nmol/L). USE: A test for adrenal insufficiency to determine the response of the adrenals to ACTH. LIMITATIONS: Response may be abnormal after prolonged steroid therapy. METHODOLOGY: Immunoassay ADDITIONAL INFORMATION: Cosyntropin (Cortrosyn®) is a synthetic 1-24 amino acid ACTH and does not produce anaphylaxis as bovine ACTH may. If the adrenal glands are physically intact, and normally responsive to ACTH, cortisol will rise significantly after administration of cosyntropin. Absence of such a rise is evidence for primary adrenal insufficiency. If the adrenals can respond to exogenous ACTH (cosyntropin), then a metyrapone test can evaluate the integrity of the pituitary-adrenal axis. Adrenocortical sensitivity to cosyntropin may be enhanced in patients with depression.[1,2,3] A new test involving pretreatment with low-dose dexamethasone followed by corticotropin-releasing hormone stimulation and measurement of plasma cortisol 15 minutes later, successfully separated all patients with mild Cushing's syndrome from those with pseudo-Cushing's states.[4]

Footnotes

1. Amsterdam JD, Maislin G, Berwish N, et al, "Enhanced Adrenocortical Sensitivity to Submaximal Doses of Cosyntropin (Alpha 1-24 Corticotropin) in Depressed Patients," *Arch Gen Psychiatry*, 1989, 46(6):550-4.
2. Jaeckle RS, Kathol RG, Lopez JF, et al, "Enhanced Adrenal Sensitivity to Exogenous Cosyntropin (ACTH Alpha 1-24) Stimulation in Major Depression. Relationship to Dexamethasone Suppression Test Results," *Arch Gen Psychiatry*, 1987, 44:233-40.
3. Clayton RN, "Diagnosis of Adrenal Insufficiency," *BMJ*, 1989, 298(6669):271-2.
4. Yanovski JA, Cutler GB, Chrousos GP, et al, "Corticotropin-Releasing Hormone Stimulation Following Low-Dose Dexamethasone Administration. A New Test to Distinguish Cushing's Syndrome From Pseudo-Cushing's States," *JAMA*, 1993, 269(17):2232-8.

References

Watts NB and Keffer JH, *Practical Endocrine Diagnosis*, 4th ed, Philadelphia, PA: Lea & Febiger, 1989.

C-Peptide

CPT *84681*

Related Information

Glucose, Fasting *on page 238*
Glucose Tolerance Test *on page 241*
Insulin Antibody, Serum *on page 260*
Insulin, Blood *on page 260*

Synonyms Connecting Peptide Insulin; Insulin C-Peptide; Proinsulin C-Peptide

Test Commonly Includes Glucose is usually needed at the time a C-peptide specimen is drawn.

Abstract Proinsulin is cleaved into insulin and a biologically inactive protein. The latter is C-peptide.

Patient Care PREPARATION: Patient should fast for a minimum of 10 hours for basal values. No recent scans or other radioactivity.

Specimen Serum CONTAINER: Red top tube COLLECTION: Date and time must be absolutely correct. Draw in chilled tube. Keep specimen on ice. Trasylol® (2000 units/mL) may be added to prevent degradation. STORAGE INSTRUCTIONS: Spin in centrifuge at 4°C. Take off serum. Freeze immediately in a plastic tube. CAUSES FOR REJECTION: Stored specimen not frozen, recent injection of radioactive material

Interpretive REFERENCE RANGE: Fasting: 0.5-2.5 ng/mL (SI: 0.17-0.83 nmol/L). Varies between laboratories. USE: The principal use of C-peptide is in the evaluation of hypoglycemia. Patients with insulin-secreting neoplasms have high levels of both C-peptide and endogenous insulin; in contrast, patients with factitious hypoglycemia will have low C-peptide levels in the presence of elevated (exogenous) serum insulin. C-peptide is also useful in evaluating residual beta cell function in insulin-dependent diabetics, many of whom have antibodies that interfere with insulin assays. Glucagon-stimulated C-peptide concentration has been shown to be a good discriminator between insulin-requiring and noninsulin-requiring diabetic patients.[1,2] The diagnosis of islet cell tumor is supported by elevation of C-peptide when plasma glucose is ≤40 mg/dL (SI: ≤2.2 mmol/L). LIMITATIONS: C-peptide levels are increased with renal failure. (C-peptide is normally excreted by the kidneys.) Instances of insulinoma have been described in which proinsulin was increased but insulin and C-peptide were not. METHODOLOGY: Radioimmunoassay (RIA)[3] ADDITIONAL INFORMATION: Because of its longer half-life, the molar ratio of C-peptide to insulin is approximately 5:1.

Footnotes

1. Koskinen PJ, Viikari JS, and Irjala KM, "Glucagon-Stimulated and Postprandial Plasma C-Peptide Values as Measures of Insulin Secretory Capacity," *Diabetes Care*, 1988, 11:318-22.
2. Laakso M, Sarlund H, Korhonen T, et al, "Stopping Insulin Treatment in Middle-Aged Diabetic Patients With High Postglucagon Plasma C-Peptide. Effect on Glycaemic Control, Serum Lipids and Lipoproteins," *Acta Med Scand*, 1988, 223:61-8.
3. Myrick JE, Gunter EW, Maggio VL, et al, "An Improved Radioimmunoassay of C-Peptide and Its Application in a Multiyear Study," *Clin Chem*, 1989, 35(1):37-42.

References

Argoud GW, Schade DS, Eaton RP, et al, "C-Peptide Suppression Test and Recurrent Insulinoma," *Am J Med*, 1989, 86(3):335-7.

(Continued)

C-Peptide *(Continued)*

Beer SF, Parr JH, Temple RC, et al, "The Effect of Thyroid Disease on Proinsulin and C-Peptide Levels," *Clin Endocrinol (Oxf)*, 1989, 30(4):379-83.
Bonora E, Rizzi C, Lesi C, et al, "Insulin and C-Peptide Plasma Levels in Patients With Severe Chronic Pancreatitis and Fasting Normoglycemia," *Dig Dis Sci*, 1988, 33:732-6.
Fukuda M, Tanaka A, Tahara Y, et al, "Correlation Between Minimal Secretory Capacity of Pancreatic Beta Cells and Stability of Diabetic Control," *Diabetes*, 1988, 37:81-8.
Karjalainen J, Salmela P, Ilonen J, et al, "A Comparison of Childhood and Adult Type I Diabetes Mellitus," *N Engl J Med*, 1989, 320(14):881-6.
Service FJ, "Hypoglycemias," *West J Med*, 1991, 154(4):442-54.
Watts NB and Keefer JH, "Diabetes Mellitus and Hypoglycemia," *Practical Endocrinology*, 4th ed, Philadelphia, PA: Lea & Febiger, 1989, 161-86.

CPK *see* Creatine Kinase *on this page*
CPK Isoenzymes *see* Creatine Kinase Isoenzymes *on next page*

Creatine Kinase

CPT 82550

Related Information

Cardiac Enzymes/Isoenzymes *on page 170*
Creatine Kinase Isoenzymes *on next page*
Lactate Dehydrogenase *on page 269*
Muscle Biopsy *on page 75*
Myoglobin, Blood *on page 293*
Myoglobin, Qualitative, Urine *on page 1135*
Skeletal Muscle Antibody *on page 747*
Troponin *on page 375*

Synonyms CK; CPK; Creatine Phosphokinase, Total, Serum

Patient Care **PREPARATION:** Avoid exercise before venipuncture. Increases may be anticipated in the immediate postoperative period following surgical procedures involving incision through muscle.

Specimen Serum **CONTAINER:** Red top tube **STORAGE INSTRUCTIONS:** Separate serum from red cells. Store in refrigerator. Avoid hemolysis.[1] **CAUSES FOR REJECTION:** Hemolyzed specimen

Interpretive **REFERENCE RANGE:** Method dependent, but usually 0-250 units/L. Females have levels 20% to 25% less than males. Infants to 1 year of age may have levels two times adult. On average, black females have higher levels than white males. **USE:** Test for acute myocardial infarct and for skeletal muscular disease or damage; elevated in some patients with myxedema (hypothyroidism); elevated in patients with malignant hyperthermia syndrome. Elevated in muscular dystrophy: CK is a marker for Duchenne's muscular dystrophy, with elevations of 20 to 200 times normal.[2] CK is increased in female carriers of this X-linked disease, and in muscular stress, in polymyositis, dermatomyositis, and with muscle trauma. Elevated in myocarditis. Documentation of postictal state (recent grand mal seizure). Extremely high values are seen in some instances of myositis and in the postictal state. CK may be elevated in a number of entities, including the eosinophilia-myalgia syndrome.[3] Marked increases occur with rhabdomyolysis including that with cocaine intoxication.[4] CK is sometimes increased with cerebrovascular accident. Malignancy (advanced) may show increased CK.[5] Cardioversion with multiple shocks may release CK-MB and may result in a false-positive diagnosis of myocardial infarction.[6] Low CK may reflect decreased muscle mass. It has been reported with a number of entities, including metastatic neoplasia, patients with steroid therapy, with alcoholic liver disease[7] and with connective tissue diseases.[8] Overnight bedrest may lower CK 10% to 20%. **LIMITATIONS:** Intramuscular injections increase serum CK activity. Elevated following exercise. Increases in CK and CK-MB must be interpreted cautiously during the peripartum period.[9] **Normal at onset of acute MI** unless the subject has been exercising or doing physical work. Elevation of CK following acute MI may not be observed until 6 or more hours after onset. CK returns to normal early in approximately 48-72 hours after acute MI. Total CK can be normal early in acute MI, when CK-MB is increased. Newer tests (CK isoforms, human ventricular myosin light chains and Troponin A) may allow for earlier detection of myocardial injury/infarction than routine CK and CK-MB measurements.[10,11] Low CK does not rule out myositis in patients with the connective tissue diseases.[7] Decreased with pregnancy. **METHODOLOGY:** Kinetic – UV spectrophotometric **ADDITIONAL INFORMATION:** High CK is found after trauma, surgery, and exercise; these entities are not accompanied by elevation of CK-

MB. To distinguish myoglobinuria from hemoglobinuria, serum CK and LD may be helpful. CK is normal with uncomplicated hemolysis but LD and LD_1 usually are increased. When myoglobin is released, 40-fold elevation of CK may be anticipated with only moderate increase in serum LD and increased LD_5.[12]

Footnotes

1. Greenson JK, Farber SJ, and Dubin SB, "The Effect of Hemolysis on Creatine Kinase Determination," *Arch Pathol Lab Med*, 1989, 113(2):184-5.
2. Rosalki SB, "Serum Enzymes in Disease of Skeletal Muscle," *Clin Lab Med*, 1989, 9(4):767-81.
3. Kilbourne EM, Swygert LA, Philen RM, et al, "Interim Guidance on the Eosinophilia-Myalgia Syndrome," *Ann Intern Med*, 1990, 112(2):85-7.
4. Roth D, Alarcón FJ, Fernandez JA, "Acute Rhabdomyolysis Associated With Cocaine Intoxication," *N Engl J Med*, 1988, 319(11):673-7.
5. Eng C, Skolnick AE, and Come SE, "Elevated Creatine Kinase and Malignancy," *Hosp Pract [Off]*, 1990, 25(12):123, 126, 129-30.
6. O'Neill PG, Faitelson L, Taylor A, et al, "Time Course of Creatine Kinase Release After Termination of Sustained Ventricular Dysrhythmias," *Am Heart J*, 1991, 122(3 Pt 1):709-14.
7. Nanji AA and Blank D, "Low Serum Creatine Kinase Activity in Patients With Alcoholic Liver Disease," *Clin Chem* 1981, 27:1954.
8. Wei N, Pavlidis N, Tsokos G, et al, "Clinical Significance of Low Creatine Phosphokinase Values in Patients With Connective Tissue Diseases," *JAMA*, 1981, 246:1921-3.
9. Leiserowitz GS, Evans AT, Samuels SJ, et al, "Creatine Kinase and Its MB Isoenzyme in the Third Trimester and the Peripartum Period," *J Reprod Med*, 1992, 37(11):910-6.
10. Wu AH, Gornet TG, Wu VH, et al, "Early Diagnosis of Acute Myocardial Infarction by Rapid Analysis of Creatine Kinase Isoenzyme-3 (CK-MM) Sub-Types," *Clin Chem*, 1987, 33:358-62.
11. Apple FS, Sharkey SW, Werdick M, et al, "Analyses of Creatine Kinase Isoenzymes and Isoforms in Serum to Detect Reperfusion After Myocardial Infarction," *Clin Chem*, 1987, 33:507-11.
12. Faulkner WR, "Update on Myoglobinurias," *Lab Report for Physicians*, 1989, 11:91-2.

References

Beek AM, Verheugt FW, and Meyer A, "Usefulness of Electrocardiographic Findings and Creatine Kinase Levels on Admission in Predicting the Accuracy of the Interval Between Onset of Chest Pain of Acute Myocardial Infarction and Initiation of Thrombolytic Therapy," *Am J Cardiol*, 1991, 68(13):1287-90.

Crisp DE, Ziter FA, and Bray PF, "Diagnostic Delay in Duchenne's Muscular Dystrophy," *JAMA*, 1982, 247:478-80.

Leung FY, Griffith AP, Jablonsky G, et al, "Comparison of the Diagnostic Utility of Timed Serial (Slope) Creatine Kinase Measurements With Conventional Serum Tests in the Early Diagnosis of Myocardial Infarction," *Ann Clin Biochem*, 1991, 28(Pt 1):78-82.

Lott JA, "Serum Enzyme Determinations in the Diagnosis of Acute Myocardial Infarction," *Hum Pathol*, 1984, 15:706-16.

Creatine Kinase Isoenzymes

***CPT** 82552*

Related Information

Cardiac Enzymes/Isoenzymes *on page 170*
Creatine Kinase *on previous page*
Lactate Dehydrogenase Isoenzymes *on page 271*
Myoglobin, Blood *on page 293*
Troponin *on page 375*

Synonyms CK Isoenzymes; CK Isoforms; CK-MB and Total CK; CPK Isoenzymes; Creatine Phosphokinase-MB Isoenzyme and Total Creatine Phosphokinase, Serum

Test Commonly Includes Separation of enzyme CK into its isoenzymes

Specimen Serum **CONTAINER:** Red top tube **SAMPLING TIME: CK is most commonly elevated in** acute myocardial infarction (AMI) in which it has its greatest usefulness. Collection of specimen at onset of symptoms to establish baseline values is needed. A patient at onset of acute myocardial infarction (AMI) will have normal results, but some patients reach medical attention at or beyond CK peak. To support the diagnosis of AMI, three CK isoenzyme determinations have classically been recommended, one on admission, a second 12 hours after admission, a third 24 hours after admission. Another at 48 hours may be needed. The new mass concentration assays have improved sensitivity over the more cumbersome electrophoretic assays, and some have suggested sampling times at 0, 3, 6, and 12 hours, to detect the rise of CK-MB.[1] The same sampling times should be used to assess the effective myocardial reperfusion after thrombolytic therapy. In this case the CK and CK-MB rise very early and very high compared to patients not reperfused.[2] CK-MB usually peaks between 15-20 hours after the onset of a myocardial infarction. Pappas summarizes current literature regarding timing as follows. In non-Q wave, incomplete occlusion, nontransmural MI, CK-MB peaks on the average 15

(Continued)

Creatine Kinase Isoenzymes *(Continued)*

hours from onset. In Q wave (complete occlusion) (transmural) infarction, CK-MB average peak is 17-20 hours after onset of symptoms. He emphasizes the importance of a sample for CK-MB drawn 16 hours after onset.[3] When increased CK-MB values have returned to normal, CK isoenzyme determinations are usually no longer required. **STORAGE INSTRUCTIONS:** Separate serum from red cells and freeze. **CAUSES FOR REJECTION:** Gross hemolysis

Interpretive **REFERENCE RANGE:** Method dependent. CK-MB normally is less than 6% of total CK. In many laboratories normal range of MB is zero. The most common cause of elevation of MB is acute infarct of myocardium. Most normal individuals have only MM. **USE:** Diagnose myocardial infarction (MI). Three fractions normally may be found. Each is an isoenzyme.

- MM is present in normal serum.
- MB is the myocardial fraction associated with MI and occurs in certain other states. MB can be used in estimation of infarct size.

A study using the chemiluminescence mass concentration assay for CK-MB showed that a CK-MB ≥10 ng/mL and %MB ≥3% (ng/mL CK-MB per unit CK x 100) gave these results: sensitivity = 1.00; specificity = 0.97; positive predictive value = 1.00; diagnostic efficiency = 0.97.[4]

MB increases have been reported with other entities which cause damage to the myocardium, such as myocarditis, some instances of cardiomyopathy, and with extensive rhabdomyolysis, Duchenne's muscular dystrophy, malignant hyperthermia, polymyositis, dermatomyositis, mixed connective tissue disease, myoglobinemia, Rocky Mountain spotted fever, Reye's syndrome, and rarely in rheumatoid arthritis with high titer RF.[5] CK-MB does not generally abruptly rise and fall in such nonacute MI settings, as it does in acute myocardial infarct (AMI).

- BB is rarely present. BB has been described as a marker for adenocarcinoma of the prostate, breast, ovary, colon, adenocarcinomas of gastrointestinal tract, and for small cell anaplastic carcinoma of lung. BB has been reported with severe shock and/or hypothermia, infarction of bowel,[6] brain injury, stroke, as a genetic marker in some families with malignant pyrexia, and with MB in alcoholic myopathy.

LIMITATIONS: Exercise, intramuscular injections, myxedema, grand mal seizures, prior trauma or surgery, and acute MI very early or late lead to the combination of increased total CK but usually normal CK-MB. Increased CK-MB has been described in marathon runners without MI.[7] CK isoenzyme analysis is not usually practical when the total CK is very low, although in elderly people with low muscle mass, the use of sensitive mass concentration assays may be useful. A single CK isoenzyme examination may be misleading. One should look for a pattern in serial CK isoenzyme analyses and seek confirmation with the isoenzymes of LD (LDH), ideally beginning with onset to establish the baseline. LD isoenzyme 1:2 flip is most consistently found about 2 days after onset of acute infarction of myocardium. **The diagnosis of myocardial injury should not be based solely on MB isoenzyme, but rather should be supported by clinical findings, ECG, and often other laboratory parameters (ie, confirmation by LD isoenzymes).**[3] AST/ALT ratio is mentioned in the listing Cardiac Enzymes/Isoenzymes. Most laboratories are able to do electrophoresis for CK isoenzymes only once daily. **CONTRAINDICATIONS:** CK-MB is increased with cardiac surgery. **METHODOLOGY:** Electrophoresis with densitometry is commonly used to separate isoenzymes of CK. The advent of monoclonal CK-MB antibody has allowed the use of sensitive immunoassays, including microparticulate fluorescence,[8] enhanced luminescence, fluorescence, and chemiluminescence. These all measure mass concentration rather than enzyme activity. A very rapid test is that of Hybritech®, which uses the immunocentration format (ICON™). **ADDITIONAL INFORMATION:** CK-MB is found in much higher concentrations in cardiac muscle than in ordinary skeletal muscle.

CK-MB is usually not elevated in exercise (total CK elevated); myxedema (total CK elevated in about half of cases); injections into muscle (total CK elevated); strokes, CVA, and other brain disorders in which total CK may be increased; pericarditis; pneumonias or other lung diseases; pulmonary embolus; seizures (CK may be very high but no great MB increase, if any). Although CK-MB is not usually increased in angina, some CK-MB elevations are recognized in angina patients, depending partly on laboratory methodology.

Atypical forms of CK occur. **Macro-CK** migrates between MM and MB and is composed of immunoglobulin complexes of normal isoenzymes. This is found mainly in elderly women and is of no clinical significance. **Mitochondrial-CK** migrates cathodal to MM and is found in seriously ill patients, especially those with metastatic carcinoma. Its presence is a poor prognostic sign.

CK-MM and CK-MB isoforms are currently being evaluated to detect their potential value for early detection of acute myocardial infarction and for assessing myocardial reperfusion following AMI. (An isoform is a subtype of an individual isoenzyme.)[2,3,9,10,11,12] The disadvantage of this type of assay is that there is only one commercially available instrument for this measurement (Helena Laboratories).[13,14]

Footnotes

1. Marin MM and Teichman SL, "Use of Rapid Serial Sampling of Creatine Kinase MB for Very Early Detection of Myocardial Infarction in Patients With Acute Chest Pain," *Am Heart J*, 1992, 123(2):354-61.
2. Lott JA and Stang JM, "Differential Diagnosis of Patients With Abnormal Serum Creatine Kinase Isoenzymes," *Clin Lab Med*, 1989, 9(4):627-42.
3. Pappas NJ Jr, "Enhanced Cardiac Enzyme Profile," *Clin Lab Med*, 1989, 9:689-716.
4. Pearson JR and Carrea F, "Evaluation of the Clinical Usefulness of a Chemiluminometric Method for Measuring Creatine Kinase MB," *Clin Chem*, 1990, 36(10):1809-11.
5. Wolf PL, "Common Causes of False-Positive CK-MB Test for Acute Myocardial Infarction," *Clin Lab Med*, 1986, 6:577-82.
6. Fried MW, Murthy UK, Hassig SR, et al, "Creatine Kinase Isoenzymes in the Diagnosis of Intestinal Infarction," *Dig Dis Sci*, 1991, 36(11):1589-93.
7. Seigel AJ, Silverman LM, and Evans WJ, "Elevated Skeletal Muscle Creatinine Kinase MB Isoenzyme Levels in Marathon Runners," *JAMA*, 1983, 250:2835-7.
8. Brandt DR, Gates RC, Eng KK, et al, "Quantifying the MB Isoenzyme of Creatine Kinase With the Abbott "IMx" Immunoassay Analyzer," *Clin Chem*, 1990, 36(2):375-8.
9. Apple FS, Sharkey SW, Werdick M, et al, "Analyses of Creatine Kinase Isoenzymes and Isoforms in Serum to Detect Reperfusion After Myocardial Infarction," *Clin Chem*, 1987, 33:507-11.
10. Puleo PR, Guadagno P, Scheel M, et al, "Diagnostic Accuracy of a Rapid MB-CK Subform Assay in the Early Hours of Myocardial Infarction," *Clin Chem*, 1989, 35:1119.
11. Wu AH, Gornet TG, Wu VH, et al, "Early Diagnosis of Acute Myocardial Infarction by Rapid Analysis of Creatine Kinase Isoenzyme-3 (CK-MM) Sub-types," *Clin Chem*, 1987, 33:358-62.
12. Apple FS, "Diagnostic Use of CK-MM and CK-MB Isoforms for Detecting Myocardial Infarction," *Clin Lab Med*, 1989, 9(4):643-54.
13. Puleo PR, Guadagno PA, Roberts R, et al, "Early Diagnosis of Acute Myocardial Infarction Based on Assay for Subforms of Creatine Kinase-MB," *Circulation*, 1990, 82(3):759-64.
14. Abendschein DR, "Rapid Diagnosis of Myocardial Infarction and Reperfusion by Assay of Plasma Isoforms of Creatine Kinase Isoenzymes," *Clin Biochem*, 1990, 23(5):399-407.

References

Ahrenholz DH, Schubert W, and Solem LD, "Creatine Kinase as a Prognostic Indicator in Electrical Injury," *Surgery*, 1988, 104:741-7.

Bark CJ, "Mitochondrial CK – A Poor Prognostic Sign," *JAMA*, 1980, 243:2058-60.

Brush JE Jr, Brand DA, Acampora D, et al, "Relation of Peak Creatine Kinase Levels During Acute Myocardial Infarction to Presence or Absence of Previous Manifestations of Myocardial Ischemia (Angina Pectoris or Healed Myocardial Infarction)," *Am J Cardiol*, 1988, 62:534-7.

Coolen RB, Pragay DA, Nosanchuk JS, et al, "Elevation of Brain-Type Creatine Kinase in Serum From Patients With Carcinoma," *Cancer*, 1979, 44:1414-8.

Cox DA, Stone PH, Muller JE, et al, "Prognostic Implications of an Early Peak in Plasma MB Creatine Kinase in Patients With Acute Myocardial Infarction," *J Am Coll Cardiol*, 1987, 10:979-90.

Davidson E, Weinberger I, Rotenberg Z, et al, "Elevated Serum Creatine Kinase Levels," *Arch Intern Med*, 1988, 148:2184-6.

Devries SR, Jaffe AS, Geltman EM, et al, "Enzymatic Estimation of the Extent of Irreversible Myocardial Injury Early After Reperfusion," *Am Heart J*, 1989, 117(1):31-6.

Gulbis B, Unger P, Lenaers A, et al, "Mass Concentration of Creatine Kinase MB Isoenzyme and Lactate Dehydrogenase Isoenzyme 1 in Diagnosis of Perioperative Myocardial Infarction After Coronary Bypass Surgery," *Clin Chem*, 1990, 36(10):1784-8.

Hood D, Van Lente F, and Estes M, "Serum Enzyme Alterations in Chronic Muscle Disease. A Biopsy-Based Diagnostic Assessment," *Am J Clin Pathol*, 1991, 95(3):402-7.

King DT, Fu PC, and Wishon GM, "Persistent Creatine Kinase MB Isoenzyme Without Cardiac Disease," *Arch Pathol Lab Med*, 1978, 102:481-2.

Lang H, ed, *Creatine Kinase Isoenzymes, Pathophysiology and Clinical Application*, New York, NY: Springer-Verlag, 1981.

Lee RT, Lee TH, Poole WK, et al, "Rate of Disappearance of Creatine Kinase-MB After Acute Myocardial Infarction: Clinical Determinants of Variability," *Am Heart J*, 1988, 116:1493-9.

Lewis BS, Ganz W, Laramee P, et al, "Usefulness of a Rapid Initial Increase in Plasma Creatine Kinase Activity as a Marker of Reperfusion During Thrombolytic Therapy for Acute Myocardial Infarction," *Am J Cardiol*, 1988, 62:20-4.

Lott JA, "Serum Enzyme Determinations in the Diagnosis of Acute Myocardial Infarction," *Hum Pathol*, 1984, 15:706-16.

Nidorf SM, Thompson PL, Byrne A, et al, "The Creatine Kinase Ratio: A Useful Means of Detecting Early Peaking of the Creatine Kinase Curve After Acute Myocardial Infarction," *Am J Cardiol*, 1988, 62:961-3.

Nidorf SM, Thompson PL, de Klerk NH, et al, "Prognostic Significance of an Early Rise to Peak Creatine Kinase After Acute Myocardial Infarction," *Am J Cardiol*, 1988, 61:1178-80.

(Continued)

Creatine Kinase Isoenzymes *(Continued)*

Piérard LA, Dubois C, Albert A, et al, "Prognostic Significance of a Low Peak Serum Creatine Kinase Level in Acute Myocardial Infarction," *Am J Cardiol*, 1989, 63(12):792-6.

Quale J, Kimmelstiel C, Lipschik G, et al, "Use of Sequential Cardiac Enzyme Analysis in Stratification of Risk for Myocardial Infarction in Patients With Unstable Angina," *Arch Intern Med*, 1988, 148:1277-9.

Sharkey SW, Apple FS, Elsperger KJ, et al, "Early Peak of Creatine Kinase-MB in Acute Myocardial Infarction With a Nondiagnostic Electrocardiogram," *Am Heart J*, 1988, 116:1207.

Silverman LM, Dermer GB, Zweig MH, et al, "Creatine Kinase BB: A New Tumor-Associated Marker," *Clin Chem*, 1979, 25:1432-5.

Swaroop A, "CK Isoenzyme Variants in Electrophoresis," *Lab Med*, 1989, 20:305-10.

Thompson WG, Mahr RG, Yohannan WS, et al, "Use of Creatine Kinase MB Isoenzyme for Diagnosing Myocardial Infarction When Total Creatine Kinase Activity Is High," *Clin Chem*, 1988, 34:2208-10.

Vaidya HC, Maynard Y, Dietzler DN, et al, "Direct Measurement of Creatine Kinase-MB Activity in Serum After Extraction With a Monoclonal Antibody Specific to the MB Isoenzyme," *Clin Chem*, 1986, 32:657-63.

Wu AH, Gornet TG, Harker CC, et al, "Role of Rapid Immunoassays for Urgent ("Stat") Determinations of Creatine Kinase Isoenzyme MB," *Clin Chem*, 1989, 35(8):1752-6.

Creatine Phosphokinase-MB Isoenzyme and Total Creatine Phosphokinase, Serum *see* Creatine Kinase Isoenzymes *on page 197*

Creatine Phosphokinase, Total, Serum *see* Creatine Kinase *on page 196*

Creatinine, 12- or 24-Hour Urine

CPT *82570*

Related Information

Creatinine Clearance *on next page*

Uric Acid, Urine *on page 380*

Synonyms Urine Creatinine

Test Commonly Includes Urine creatinine in mg/dL and mg/24 hours or mg/12 hours

Abstract Timed urine collection is a portion of creatinine clearance.

Specimen 12- or 24-hour urine **CONTAINER:** Plastic urine container **COLLECTION:** If the specimen is a 24-hour collection, instruct the patient to void at 8 AM and discard the specimen. Then collect all urine including the final specimen voided at the end of the 24-hour collection period (ie, 8 AM the next morning). Keep specimen on ice during collection. Container must be labeled with patient's name, date, and time collection started and date and time collection finished. **STORAGE INSTRUCTIONS:** Refrigerate **CAUSES FOR REJECTION:** Incomplete collection

Interpretive **REFERENCE RANGE:** Children: 2-3 years: 6-22 mg/kg/24 hours (SI: 52.8-193.6 μmol/kg/day), older than 3 years: 12-30 mg/kg/24 hours (SI: 105.0-264.0 μmol/kg/day); adults: male: 1-2 g/24 hours (SI: 8.8-17.7 mmol/day), female: 0.8-1.8 g/24 hours (SI: 7.1-15.9 mmol/day). Creatinine excretion decreases with advanced age as muscle mass diminishes. Normal age-adjusted values for anticipated creatinine excretion stratified for each sex by height are published. These tables assume ideal weight.[1] **USE:** Renal function test when used as part of creatinine clearance; crude marker for completeness of 24-hour urine collections when collected for other purposes **LIMITATIONS:** Complete urine collections require vigilance on the part of nursing personnel. Ingestion of meat may increase creatinine values of urine collections as well as serum creatinine values. Application of urine creatinine excretion as a marker for complete collection is questioned.[2] **Drugs** interfering with tubular creatinine secretion include cimetidine, trimethoprim, and probenecid. Creatinine **reabsorption** occurs with very low urine flow rates. Entities in which reabsorption occurs include severe congestive heart failure, uncontrolled diabetes mellitus, and acute renal failure.[3] **METHODOLOGY:** Jaffé reaction (alkaline picrate) **ADDITIONAL INFORMATION:** Urine creatinine is not ordered alone. Creatinine clearance, which requires a serum creatinine, offers useful renal function data. Serum creatinine alone is not an adequate index of glomerular filtration rate.[3]

Footnotes

1. Walser M, "Creatinine Excretion as a Measure of Protein Nutrition in Adults of Varying Age," *J Parenter Enteral Nutr*, 1987, 11:73S-78S.
2. Duarte CG, Elveback LR, and Liedeke RR, "Creatinine," *Renal Function Tests. Clinical Laboratory Procedures and Diagnosis*, Duarte CG, ed, Boston, MA: Little, Brown and Co, 1980, 1-28.
3. Levey AS, Perrone RD, and Madias NE, "Serum Creatinine and Renal Function," *Annu Rev Med*, 1988, 39:465-90.

References

Schwab SJ, Christensen RL, Dougherty K, et al, "Quantitation of Proteinuria by the Use of Protein-to-Creatinine Ratios in Single Urine Samples," *Arch Intern Med*, 1987, 147:943-4.

Creatinine, Amniotic Fluid *see* Amniotic Fluid Creatinine *on page 123*

Creatinine Clearance

***CPT** 82575*

Related Information

Creatinine, 12- or 24-Hour Urine *on previous page*
Creatinine, Serum *on next page*
Kidney Biopsy *on page 68*
Kidney Stone Analysis *on page 1129*

Applies to GFR

Replaces Urea Clearance; Urea Nitrogen Clearance

Test Commonly Includes Serum creatinine, urine creatinine

Abstract The most common test for evaluation of renal function is creatinine; the next is creatinine clearance.

Patient Care PREPARATION: Avoid cephalosporins. If possible, drugs should be stopped beforehand. Have patient drink water before the clearance is begun and continue good hydration throughout the clearance.

Specimen 24-hour urine and serum; test can be done for shorter periods CONTAINER: Plastic urine container and red top tube COLLECTION: Instruct the patient to void at 8 AM and discard the specimen. Then collect all urine including the final specimen voided at the end of the 24-hour collection period (ie, 8 AM the next morning). Keep specimen on ice during collection. Bottle must be labeled with patient's name, date and time for a 24-hour collection. Especially for creatinine clearance, accuracy and precision of collection are important. Complete, carefully timed (usually 24-hour) collection is needed; 4- and 12-hour collections are acceptable. STORAGE INSTRUCTIONS: Refrigerate CAUSES FOR REJECTION: No blood creatinine ordered, urine specimen not timed SPECIAL INSTRUCTIONS: Blood creatinine should be ordered at the same time. Requisition should state date and time collection started, date and time collection finished, patient's age, height, and weight.

Interpretive REFERENCE RANGE: Children: 70-140 mL/min/1.73 m^2 (SI: 1.17-2.33 mL/s/1.73 m^2); adults: male: 85-125 mL/min/1.73 m^2 (SI: 1.42-2.08 mL/s/1.73 m^2), female: 75-115 mL/min/1.73 m^2 (SI: 1.25-1.92 mL/s/1.73 m^2) USE: Renal function test to estimate glomerular filtration rate (GFR); evaluate renal function in small or wasted subjects; follow possible progression of renal disease; adjust dosages of medications in which renal excretion is pivotal (eg, aminoglycosides, methotrexate, cisplatin). LIMITATIONS: Exercise may cause increased creatinine clearance. The glomerular filtration rate is substantially increased in pregnancy. Ascorbic acid, ketone bodies (acetoacetate), hydantoin, numerous cephalosporins[1,2] and glucose may influence creatinine determinations. Trimethoprim, cimetidine, quinine, quinidine, procainamide reduce creatinine excretion. Icteric samples, lipemia and hemolysis may interfere with determination of creatinine. Since tubular secretion of creatinine is fractionally more important in progressing renal failure, the creatinine clearance overestimates GFR with high serum creatinine levels. While ingestion of meats may cause some increase in creatinine excretion, in practice this seems to make little difference. Intraindividual variation in creatinine clearance is about 15%. Males excrete more creatinine and have slightly higher clearance than females. METHODOLOGY: Jaffé reaction (alkaline picrate). The calculation for corrected creatinine clearance in mL/minute = [(urine volume per minute x urine creatinine)/serum creatinine] x (1.73/surface area of body in square meters). Body surface area is obtained from nomograms which require age, height, and weight. ADDITIONAL INFORMATION: Glomerular filtration rate declines about 10% per decade after 50 years of age. Some patients with significant impairment of glomerular filtration rate have only slightly elevated serum creatinine.[3] Creatinine clearance is calculated on the basis of the surface area of the patient. The estimated error of determining creatinine clearance utilizing serum and 24-hour urine collection has been found to be in the range of 10% to 15%. Any test requiring a 24-hour urine collection may also be run on this specimen (eg, protein, quantitative, 24-hour urine).

Footnotes

1. Swain RR and Briggs SL, "Positive Interference With the Jaffé Reaction by Cephalosporin Antibiotics," *Clin Chem*, 1977, 23:1340-2.
2. Levey AS, Perrone RD, and Madias NE, "Serum Creatinine and Renal Function," *Annu Rev Med*, 1988, 39:465-90.
3. Klahr S, "The Modifications of Diet in Renal Disease Study," *N Engl J Med*, 1989, 320(13):864-6.

References

Duarte CG and Preuss HG, " Assessment of Renal Function: Glomerular and Tubular," *Clin Lab Med*, 1993, 13(1):33-52.

(Continued)

Creatinine Clearance *(Continued)*

Luke DR, Halstenson CE, Opsahl JA, et al, "Validity of Creatinine Clearance Estimates in the Assessment of Renal Function," *Clin Pharmacol Ther*, 1990, 48(5):503-8.

Payne RB, "Biological Variation of Serum and Urine Creatinine and Creatinine Clearance," *Ann Clin Biochem*, 1989, 26(Pt 6):565-6.

Van Lente F and Suit P, "Assessment of Renal Function by Serum Creatinine and Creatinine Clearance: Glomerular Filtration Rate Estimated by Four Procedures," *Clin Chem*, 1989, 35(12):2326-30.

Creatinine, Serum

***CPT** 82565*

Related Information

Amikacin *on page 938*
Amphotericin B *on page 942*
BUN/Creatinine Ratio *on page 151*
Creatinine Clearance *on previous page*
Digoxin *on page 959*
Gentamicin *on page 970*
Kidney Stone Analysis *on page 1129*
Lactic Acid, Blood *on page 273*
Tobramycin *on page 1004*
Urea Nitrogen, Blood *on page 376*
Uric Acid, Serum *on page 378*

Patient Care **PREPARATION:** Fasting may be desirable. Certain cephalosporins, especially cefoxitin, cause misleading (high) results.[1]

Specimen Serum **CONTAINER:** Red top tube **COLLECTION:** Pediatrics: Blood drawn from heelstick. **CAUSES FOR REJECTION:** Hemolysis

Interpretive **REFERENCE RANGE:** Children: 1-5 years: 0.3-0.5 mg/dL (SI: 27-44 μmol/L), 5-10 years: 0.5-0.8 mg/dL (SI: 44-71 μmol/L); adults: male: up to 1.2 mg/dL (SI: 106 μmol/L), female: up to 1.1 mg/dL (SI: 97 μmol/L).[2] Variation between sources for serum creatinine normal ranges is perhaps greater than for many other important tests. There are slight differences between the sexes with males higher, since the range relates to the amount of muscle mass present. The glomerular filtration rate increases in pregnancy; thus, serum creatinine should be slightly less during that period. In older patients, decrease of muscle mass must be considered in interpretation of results; the elderly have reduced creatinine generation. Similarly, other patients may have creatinine levels in which muscle abnormalities must be considered, including long-term corticosteroid therapy, hyperthyroidism, muscular dystrophy and paralysis, and dermatomyositis and polymyositis. **USE:** The most common clinical renal function test, providing a rough approximation of glomerular filtration.

Causes of high creatinine include renal diseases and insufficiency with decreased glomerular filtration (uremia or azotemia if severe); urinary tract obstruction; reduced renal blood flow including congestive heart failure, shock and dehydration; rhabdomyolysis causes high serum creatinine, which may be elevated out of proportion to BUN, or to the reduction in renal function.

Causes of low creatinine include small stature, debilitation, decreased muscle mass, some complex cases of severe hepatic disease. In advanced liver disease, low creatinine may result from decreased hepatic production of creatinine and inadequate dietary protein as well as reduced muscle mass.[1]

Index of fetal maturity in amniotic fluid analysis.

LIMITATIONS: With reduced renal blood flow, creatinine rises less quickly than urea nitrogen. Concentration of creatinine only becomes abnormal when about half or more of the nephrons have stopped functioning in chronic progressive renal disease.

Increased serum creatinine results may occur from noncreatinine substances, including meat ingestion, glucose, pyruvate, uric acid, fructose, guanidine, ketonemia (acetoacetate), hydantoin, ascorbic acid, and numerous cephalosporin antibiotics, especially cefoxitin. Cefoxitin levels fall in patients with normal kidney function, such that a sample can be drawn 2 hours after a dose but preferably, 4 hours or more afterwards.[3] With severe renal disease, creatinine is not reliable in the presence of cefoxitin therapy. There is less interference reported from the cephalosporins cephalothin, cephaloridine, cephadrile sodium, and cephaloglycin dihydrate.[4] Cephazolin and cefamandole may cause increased colorimetric values.[5] Cephapirin and moxalactam are described as not causing interference.[6] Differences in the interference of such cephalosporins between assay systems are published.[4,6]

Methyldopa and trimethoprim may increase serum creatinine levels.[7] Lipemia, hemolysis, and bilirubin may interfere.[8,9] High creatinine in serum has been reported with methanol intoxication.[10]

An antifungal drug, 5-flucytosine, and glucose interfere with the imidohydrolase method.[5]

Tagamet® interferes with creatinine excretion in the renal tubule, causing a rise in creatinine without reduction in renal function. It may also cause an allergic nephritis with reduced renal function.

Moderate variation of results exists between chemistry analyzer systems.

Serum creatinine is only a crude guide to the progress of renal disease.[5] Moderate changes in the glomerular filtration rate (GFR) may not be detected by serum creatinine levels. Levey et al and others emphasize that the serum creatinine does **not** provide an adequate estimate of GFR.[5] A fraction of urine creatinine is from tubular secretion. Such tubular secretion increases with declining renal function.

METHODOLOGY: Alkaline picrate (Jaffé reaction), *o*-nitrobenzaldehyde (Sakaguchi reaction), imidohydrolase (Ektachem®). Many interference problems are still unresolved in the Jaffé reaction.[11] **ADDITIONAL INFORMATION:** Serum creatinine level is proportional to lean body muscle mass. It is unaffected by most diet or activity and is freely filtered by the glomerulus. Both BUN and creatinine are often ordered to follow renal problems. Creatinine overall is the more reliable index, but each has pitfalls. As creatinine increases in chronic renal failure, the hematocrit decreases, total carbon dioxide and bicarbonate fall, and serum phosphate and BUN increase.[12] When serum creatinine increases postoperatively, a group of patients may be identified who are at risk for more severe renal failure. Creatinine clearances have a role in such investigations.[13] Serum creatinine has a role in determination of dosages of some drugs (eg, the aminoglycosides and digoxin), especially in elderly subjects.[14]

Footnotes

1. Takabatake T, Ohta H, Ishida Y, et al, "Low Serum Creatinine Levels in Severe Hepatic Disease," *Arch Intern Med*, 1988, 148(6):1313-5.
2. Savory DJ, "Reference Ranges for Serum Creatinine in Infants, Children, and Adolescents," *Ann Clin Biochem*, 1990, 27(Pt 2):99-101.
3. Durham SR, Bignell AH, and Wise R, "Interference of Cefoxitin in the Creatinine Estimation and its Clinical Relevance," *J Clin Pathol*, 1979, 32:1148-51.
4. Saah AJ, Koch TR, and Drusano GL, "Cefoxitin Falsely Elevates Creatinine Levels," *JAMA*, 1982, 247:205-6.
5. Levey AS, Perrone RD, and Madias NE, "Serum Creatinine and Renal Function," *Annu Rev Med*, 1988, 39:465-90.
6. Kirby MG, Gal P, Baird HW, et al, "Cefoxitin Interference With Serum Creatinine Measurement Varies With the Assay System," *Clin Chem*, 1982, 28:1981, (letter).
7. Porter GA and Bennett WM, "Toxic Nephropathies," *The Kidney*, 2nd ed, Brenner BM and Rector FC Jr, eds, Philadelphia, PA: WB Saunders Co, 1981, 2045-108.
8. Bowers CD and Wong ET, "Kinetic Serum Creatinine Assays: A Critical Evaluation and Review," *Clin Chem*, 1980, 26:555-61.
9. Soldier SJ, Henderson L, and Hill JG, "The Effect of Bilirubin and Ketones on Reaction Rate Methods for the Measurement of Creatinine," *Clin Biochem*, 1978, 11:82-6.
10. Wu AHB, Stout R, and McComb RB, "Falsely High Serum Creatinine Concentration Associated With Severe Methanol Intoxication," *Clin Chem*, 1983, 29:205-8.
11. Weber JA and van Zanten AP, "Interferences in Current Methods for Measurements of Creatinine," *Clin Chem*, 1991, 37(5):695-700.
12. Hakim RM and Lazarus JM, "Biochemical Parameters in Chronic Renal Failure," *Am J Kidney Dis*, 1988, 11(3):238-47.
13. Charlson ME, MacKenzie CR, Gold JP, et al, "Postoperative Changes in Serum Creatinine: When Do They Occur and How Much Is Important?" *Ann Surg*, 1989, 209(3):328-33.
14. Lindeman RD, "Assessment of Renal Function in the Old: Special Considerations," *Clin Lab Med*, 1993, 13(1):269-77.

References

Abuelo JG, "Benign Azotemia of Long-Term Hemodialysis: Increase in Blood Urea Nitrogen and Serum Creatinine Concentrations After the Initiation of Dialysis," *Am J Med*, 1989, 86(6 Pt 1):738-9.

Duarte CG and Preuss HG, "Assessment of Renal Function: Glomerular and Tubular," *Clin Lab Med*, 1993, 13(1):33-52.

Lemann J, Bidani AK, Bain RP, et al, "Use of the Serum Creatinine to Estimate Glomerular Filtration Rate in Health and Early Diabetic Nephropathy. Collaborative Study Group of Angiotensin Converting Enzyme Inhibition in Diabetic Nephropathy," *Am J Kidney Dis*, 1990, 16(3):236-43.

Lepage L and Galimany R, "Creatinine," *Drug Effects on Laboratory Test Results Analytical Interferences and Pharmacological Effects*, Siest G and Galteau MM, eds, Littleton, MA: PSG Publishing Co Inc, 1988, 198-210.

(Continued)

Creatinine, Serum *(Continued)*

Narayanan S, "Creatinine: Review of Methods," *ASCP Check Sample®*, Gambino SR and Batsakis JG, eds, Chicago, IL: American Society of Clinical Pathologists, 1988, 4:1-10.

CSF Glutamine *see* Cerebrospinal Fluid Glutamine *on page 177*

CT *see* Calcitonin *on page 157*

3', 5'-Cyclic Adenosine Monophosphate, Plasma *see* Cyclic AMP, Plasma *on this page*

Cyclic Adenosine Monophosphate, Urine *see* Cyclic AMP, Urine *on this page*

3', 5'-Cyclic Adenosine Monophosphate, Urine *see* Cyclic AMP, Urine *on this page*

Cyclic AMP, Plasma

***CPT** 82030*

Related Information

Parathyroid Hormone *on page 311*

Synonyms AMP, Cyclic, Plasma; cAMP, Plasma; 3', 5'-Cyclic Adenosine Monophosphate, Plasma

Applies to Nephrogenous Cyclic AMP

Patient Care **PREPARATION:** Avoid radioisotope scan prior to collection of specimen.

Specimen Plasma **CONTAINER:** Lavender top (EDTA) tube; do not use heparin or citrate tube **COLLECTION:** Stable 1 hour in plasma at 25°C, specimen should then be frozen[1] if longer storage is anticipated **STORAGE INSTRUCTIONS:** Separate plasma and freeze **immediately** upon receipt of the specimen. **SPECIAL INSTRUCTIONS:** Transport specimen to the laboratory **immediately** following collection.

Interpretive **REFERENCE RANGE:** 5.6-10.9 ng/mL (SI: 17-33 nmol/L) **USE:** Differential diagnosis of hypercalcemia of hyperparathyroidism; calculate nephrogenous cAMP **LIMITATIONS:** Used with urine cAMP **METHODOLOGY:** Immunoassay or high performance liquid chromatography (HPLC) **ADDITIONAL INFORMATION:** Serum and 2-hour urine collection for cAMP and creatinine in the recumbent, prepared patient are sometimes used in the differential diagnosis of hyperparathyroidism. In hyperparathyroidism and hypercalcemia of malignancy there are increased values for nephrogenous cyclic AMP. Utilization of cAMP in the diagnosis of hyperparathyroidism has been de-emphasized in recent years.[2] In patients with primary hyperparathyroidism, the loss of circadian rhythm of intact PTH and nephrogenous cyclic AMP occurs.[3]

Footnotes

1. Tietz NW, ed, *Clinical Guide to Laboratory Tests*, Philadelphia, PA: WB Saunders Co, 1983, 156-7.
2. Watts NB and Keffer JH, "The Parathyroid Glands," *Practical Endocrine Diagnosis*, 4th ed, Philadelphia, PA: Lea & Febiger, 1989, 137-46.
3. Logue FC, Fraser WD, Gallacher SJ, et al, "The Loss of Circadian Rhythm for Intact Parathyroid Hormone and Nephrogenous Cyclic AMP in Patients With Primary Hyperparathyroidism," *Clin Endocrinol (Oxf)*, 1990, 32(4):475-83.

References

Aurbach GD, Marx SJ, and Spiegel AM, "Parathyroid Hormone, Calcitonin, and the Calciferols," *Williams Textbook of Endocrinology*, 7th ed, Wilson JD and Foster DW, eds, Philadelphia, PA: WB Saunders Co, 1985.

Levitzki A, "From Epinephrine to Cyclic AMP," *Science*, 1988, 241:800-6.

Cyclic AMP, Urine

***CPT** 82030*

Related Information

Calcium, Serum *on page 160*

Parathyroid Hormone *on page 311*

Synonyms AMP, Cyclic, Urine; cAMP, Urine; Cyclic Adenosine Monophosphate, Urine; 3', 5'-Cyclic Adenosine Monophosphate, Urine

Applies to Nephrogenous Cyclic AMP

Patient Care **PREPARATION:** Avoid radioisotope scan prior to collection of specimen. PTH or ADH may be administered as a provocative test.

Specimen Random urine **CONTAINER:** Plastic urine container **STORAGE INSTRUCTIONS:** Acidify to below pH 4 and freeze.

Interpretive REFERENCE RANGE: 112-188 μg/L (SI: 340-570 nmol/L) creatinine, (3-5 μmol/g creatinine), 6.6-15.5 μg/L (SI: 20-47 nmol/L) glomerular filtrate. Nephrogenous cAMP: <9.9 μg/L (SI: <30 nmol/L) glomerular filtrate USE: Differential diagnosis of hyperparathyroidism. In hyperparathyroidism there is increased cAMP in 24-hour urine specimens, also in humoral hypercalcemia of malignancy and vitamin D deficiency. The plasma concentrations of immunoreactive parathyroid hormone-related protein correlate with levels of excreted cyclic AMP.[1] LIMITATIONS: There is some overlap between results of patients with hyperparathyroidism and those of normal subjects. Not all patients with hyperparathyroidism have abnormal urinary cAMP results. Urinary cAMP is reported increased in hypercalcemic cancer patients. METHODOLOGY: Radioimmunoassay (RIA) ADDITIONAL INFORMATION: Please see prior listing with citations. There is a role for cAMP excretion measurement in the evaluation of Zollinger-Ellison syndrome and differentiation of sporadic cases from those of multiple endocrine neoplasia type I.[2] Assay of nephrogenous cyclic AMP has been applied to the monitoring of calcium intake in cases of osteoporosis.[3]

A target of parathyroid hormone (PTH) action is the renal tubule. The result is release of cAMP into the urine. Cyclic AMP output in the urine is thus an indirect measure of parathyroid action. PTH utilizes cyclic AMP to exert its effect on cells. Upon binding of PTH to its receptor, the latter undergoes a confirmational change which increases its affinity (through a second binding site) for a linking protein (Ns) which also binds guanosine triphosphate.

Type I pseudohypoparathyroidism (autosomal dominant inheritance), mimics hypoparathyroidism with hypocalcemia resistant to vitamin D and high serum phosphate and PTH levels. This condition appears to be due to a defect in linking protein (Ns) structure. Type I is characterized by defective renal tubular response to PTH and increased circulating and urinary cyclic AMP. Type II pseudohypoparathyroidism (autosomal dominant inheritance) has a normal cyclic AMP response.[4]

The level of urinary cAMP is the result of cAMP released by PTH, action of other hormones and plasma cAMP filtered by the renal glomerulus. "Nephrogenous cAMP" is the urinary excretion of cAMP minus that filtered by the glomerulus and correlates best with the results of plasma PTH levels.[5]

Footnotes

1. Burtis WJ, Brady TG, Orloff JJ, et al, "Immunochemical Characterization of Circulating Parathyroid Hormone-Related Protein in Patients With Humoral Hypercalcemia of Cancer," *N Engl J Med*, 1990, 322(16):1106-12.
2. Mignon M and Bonfils S, "Diagnosis and Treatment of Zollinger-Ellison Syndrome," *Baillieres Clin Gastroenterol*, 1988, 2:677-98.
3. Licata A, Gall D, and Gupta M, "Monitoring Calcium Intake in Osteoporosis by Assay of Nephrogenous Cyclic AMP," *Am J Clin Nutr*, 1988, 47(6):1022-4.
4. Anderson DC and Braidman IP, "Hormone Receptor Disorders," *Subcellular Pathology of Systemic Disease*, Chapter 12, Peters TJ, ed, London, England: Chapman and Hall, 1987, 229-47.
5. Pollard A, Pritzker KPH, and Grynpas MD, "Disorders of Calcium, Magnesium, and Bone Metabolism," *Applied Biochemistry of Clinical Disorders*, 2nd ed, Chapter 17, Gornall AG, ed, Philadelphia, PA: JB Lippincott Co, 1986, 408-10.

References

Arnaud CD, "The Parathyroid Glands, Hypercalcemia, and Hypocalcemia," *Cecil Textbook of Medicine*, 19th ed, Vol 1, Wyngaarden JB, Smith LH Jr, and Bennett JC, eds, Philadelphia, PA: WB Saunders Co, 1992.

Cysteine, Qualitative *see* Cystine, Qualitative *on this page*

Cyst Fluid Chemistry *see* Body Fluid *on page 145*

Cystic Fibrosis Sweat Test *see* Chloride, Sweat *on page 183*

Cystine, Qualitative

CPT 82615

Related Information

Kidney Stone Analysis *on page 1129*

Urinalysis *on page 1162*

Applies to Cysteine, Qualitative; Homocysteine, Qualitative

Test Commonly Includes Homocystine, cysteine

Abstract Cystinuria is an inherited disease. Patients with cystine stones face recurrent urolithiasis (33% recurrence rate) and repeated urinary tract infections.

(Continued)

Cystine, Qualitative *(Continued)*

Patient Care PREPARATION: Penicillamine (a chelating agent) can cause false-negative results.

Specimen Random urine CONTAINER: Urine container COLLECTION: Random urine or 24-hour collection for quantitation STORAGE INSTRUCTIONS: Acidify to pH 2-3 or freeze specimen at -20°C, or 20 mL toluene can be added to the container prior to the start of a 24-hour collection.

Interpretive REFERENCE RANGE: Negative USE: Detect cystinuria, homocystinuria and other diseases related to the sulfur-containing amino acids. Work up nephrolithiasis.[1,2,3] Cystine stones account for 1% to 3% of renal calculi.[4] Early age at onset, positive family history, and recurrence of urolithiasis are features suggestive of cystine lithiasis.[5] LIMITATIONS: **Cystinosis,** a different entity from **cystinuria,** is not detected by this test. A majority of patients with infantile nephropathic **cystinosis** have neurologic deficits; becoming apparent in infancy; there is failure to thrive and renal dysfunction.[6] METHODOLOGY: Nitroprusside screening test is positive with cystine or homocystine; high performance liquid chromatography (HPLC), ion exchange chromatography ADDITIONAL INFORMATION: Procedure is to be used as a screening technique for excessive concentrations of cystine or homocystine. A positive test should be followed up by a quantitative procedure for cystine. In cystinosis, plasma cystine is usually normal, but increased cystine may be found in tissues. Therapy for cystinuria includes hydration, diet, urinary alkalinization (pH of urine maintained >7.5), chelation, surgery, and chemolysis. Cystine stones appear to be more resistant to shock wave destruction than most stones.[4] Percutaneous ultrasonic lithotripsy is described for such patients.[5]

Footnotes

1. Wilson DM, "Clinical and Laboratory Approaches for Evaluation of Nephrolithiasis," *J Urol*, 1989, 141(3 Pt 2):770-4.
2. Pak CY, "Etiology and Treatment of Urolithiasis," *Am J Kidney Dis*, 1991, 18(6):624-37.
3. Sakhaee K, Poindexter JR, and Pak CY, "The Spectrum of Metabolic Abnormalities in Patients With Cystine Nephrolithiasis," *J Urol*, 1989, 141(4):819-21.
4. Singh A, Marshall FF, and Chang R, "Cystine Calculi: Clinical Management and *In Vitro* Observations," *Urology*, 1988, 31:207-10.
5. Knoll LD, Segura JW, Patterson DE, et al, "Long-Term Follow-up in Patients With Cystine Urinary Calculi Treated by Percutaneous Ultrasonic Lithotripsy," *J Urol*, 1988, 140(2):246-8.
6. Trauner DA, Chase C, Scheller J, et al, "Neurologic and Cognitive Deficits in Children With Cystinosis," *J Pediatr*, 1988, 112(6):912-4.

References

Singer A and Das S, "Cystinuria: A Review of the Pathophysiology and Management," *J Urol*, 1989, 142(3):669-73.

Cytochrome b_5 Reductase *see* Methemoglobin *on page 290*

Dehydroepiandrosterone *see* 17-Ketosteroids Fractionation, Urine *on page 267*

Dehydroepiandrosterone, Serum *see* Dehydroepiandrosterone Sulfate *on this page*

Dehydroepiandrosterone Sulfate

CPT *82627*

Related Information

Androstenedione, Serum *on page 129*
17-Ketosteroids, Total, Urine *on page 267*
Testosterone, Free and Total *on page 358*

Synonyms DHEA-S; DHEAS

Applies to Dehydroepiandrosterone, Serum; DHEA

Abstract DHEA and its sulfate, DHEA-S, are the major precursors of 17-ketosteroids. DHEA-S is predominantly an adrenal androgen. DHEA-S is the most abundant circulating C19 steroid. It is a precursor of dehydroepiandrosterone (DHEA).

Specimen Serum or plasma CONTAINER: Red top tube or green top (heparin) tube STORAGE INSTRUCTIONS: Separate within 1 hour of collection. Serum or plasma stable 24 hours at 4°C. Freeze for longer storage.[1] CAUSES FOR REJECTION: Recently administered radioisotopes SPECIAL INSTRUCTIONS: Commonly ordered in work-up for hirsutism and/or infertility in women; related tests include testosterone and 3-α-androstanediol glucuronide.

Interpretive REFERENCE RANGE: Normal range varies between laboratories. Adult ranges may be approximate. See table. Infants and children have lower values. USE: Work up women with infertility, amenorrhea, or hirsutism, to identify the source of excessive androgen. Aid in evaluation of androgen excess (hirsutism and/or virilization), including Stein-Leventhal syndrome and adrenocortical diseases, including congenital adrenal hyperplasia and adrenal tumor.

DHEA-S is not increased with hypopituitarism. It is low in Addison's disease. **METHODOLOGY:** Radioimmunoassay (RIA) or gas chromatography/mass spectrometry (GC/MS) **ADDITIONAL INFORMATION:** DHEA is the major steroid of the fetal adrenal. DHEA is the principal adrenal androgen and is secreted together with cortisol under the control of ACTH and prolactin. DHEA-S is elevated with hyperprolactinemia.

Dehydroepiandrosterone, Serum

DHEA	ng/mL	SI: nmol/L
Male	1.7–4.2	6–15
Female	2.0–5.2	7–18
DHEA–S	**μg/mL**	**SI: μmol/L**
Male	2.0–3.4	5.2–8.7
Female		
premenopausal	0.8–3.4	2.1–8.8
postmenopausal	0.1–0.6	0.3–1.6
term pregnancy	0.2–1.2	0.6–3.0

Elevated levels may be found in the adrenogenital syndrome[2] or adrenocortical neoplasms or hyperplasias. In females and children, DHEA excess causes masculinization.

Increased 3-α-androstanediol glucuronide indicates excessive androgen in peripheral tissues. Persistent anovulation, the polycystic ovary or Stein-Leventhal syndrome is characterized by increases of circulating levels of testosterone, androstenedione, dehydroepiandrosterone and DHEA-S. 17-hydroxyprogesterone and DHEA-S are only mildly increased compared to cases of adrenal hyperplasia. Patients with androgen-producing adrenal tumors also have moderate increases of 17-KS.

Testosterone is derived from ovaries, adrenals, and the peripheral tissues. Increased DHEA-S with normal testosterone provides evidence for an adrenal cause of excessive androgen. Low levels are found in amniotic fluid in Down syndrome.[3]

Footnotes

1. Fody EP, Bennett BP, Richardson LD, et al, *Clinical Laboratory Handbook for Patient Preparation and Specimen Handling: Fascicle V, Endocrinology/Metabolism*, Skokie, IL: College of American Pathologists, 1989.
2. Pintor C, Genozanni AR, Carboni G, et al, "Adrenal Androgens and Pubertal Development in Physiological and Pathological Conditions," *Adrenal Androgens*, Genozanni AR, Thiossen JHH, and Seiteri PK, eds, New York, NY: Raven Press, 1985, 816-90.
3. Cuckle HS, Wald NJ, Densem JW, et al, "Second Trimester Amniotic Fluid Oestriol, Dehydroepiandrosterone Sulphate, and Human Chorionic Gonadotropin Levels in Down Syndrome," *Br J Obstet Gynaecol*, 1991, 98(11):1160-2.

References

Droegemueller W, Herbst AL, Mishell DR, et al, *Comprehensive Gynecology*, St Louis, MO: Mosby-Year Book Inc, 1987.

Leavelle DE, *Mayo Medical Laboratories Interpretive Handbook*, Rochester, MN: Mayo Medical Laboratories, 1990.

Meites S, *Pediatric Clinical Chemistry: Reference (Normal) Values*, 3rd ed, Washington, DC: American Association of Clinical Chemistry Press, 1989, 119-20.

Pang SY, Legido A, Levine LS, et al, "Adrenal Androgen Response to Metyrapone, Adrenocorticotropin, and Corticotropin-Releasing Hormone Stimulation in Children With Hypopituitarism," *J Clin Endocrinol Metab*, 1987, 65:282-9.

Siegel SF, Finegold DN, Lanes R, et al, "ACTH Stimulation Tests and Plasma Dehydroepiandrosterone Sulfate Levels in Women With Hirsutism," *N Engl J Med*, 1990, 323(13):849-54.

Speroff L, Glass RH, and Kase NG, *Clinical Gynecologic Endocrinology and Infertility*, 4th ed, Baltimore, MD: Williams & Wilkins, 1989.

Weykamp CW, Penders TJ, Schmidt NA, et al, "Steroid Profile for Urine: Reference Values," *Clin Chem*, 1989, 35(12):2281-4.

Delta-ALA *see* Delta Aminolevulinic Acid, Urine *on this page*

Delta Aminolevulinic Acid, Urine

CPT *82135*

Related Information

Lead, Blood *on page 976*
Lead, Urine *on page 977*
Porphobilinogen, Qualitative, Urine *on page 325*
Porphyrins, Quantitative, Urine *on page 327*
Protoporphyrin, Free Erythrocyte *on page 341*
Protoporphyrin, Zinc, Blood *on page 342*
(Continued)

Delta Aminolevulinic Acid, Urine *(Continued)*

Synonyms ALA; Aminolevulinic Acid; Delta-ALA

Abstract ALA is a precursor of the porphyrins, uroporphyrin, coproporphyrin, and protoporphyrin

Specimen 24-hour urine **CONTAINER:** Dark urine container, kept on ice **COLLECTION:** Acidify with acetic acid to pH 3-4.5; other laboratories use 2 g barbituric acid as a preservative. Sodium bicarbonate is appropriate as a preservative also for porphyrins and porphobilinogen. **STORAGE INSTRUCTIONS:** Protect from light and freeze.

Interpretive **REFERENCE RANGE:** Normal: up to approximately 7 mg/24 hours urine (SI: 53 μmol/day), depending on method and laboratory **POSSIBLE PANIC RANGE:** >20 mg/24 hours (SI: >153 μmol/day) **USE:** Diagnose porphyrias: delta-ALA may be increased in attacks of acute intermittent porphyria, hereditary coproporphyria, and porphyria variegata; evaluate certain neurological problems with abdominal pain; diagnose lead or mercury poisoning. Urinary delta-ALA is not a sensitive indicator of lead poisoning in children because it does not increase until blood lead concentration is 40 μg/dL, well above the recommended level of <15 μg/dL. ALA is increased also in tyrosinemia.[1,2] **Porphobilinogen and delta aminolevulinic acid are the tests of choice for acute intermittent porphyria**. Recently the molecular lesions have been identified in a severely affected homozygote with delta aminolevulinate dehydratase deficient porphyria.[3] **LIMITATIONS:** ALA may be normal during latent period of acute intermittent porphyria, hereditary coproporphyria, porphyria variegata. For the diagnosis of lead poisoning, measurement of blood and urine lead, and free erythrocyte protoporphyrin are other available options. **METHODOLOGY:** Ion-exchange resin columns, colorimetry **ADDITIONAL INFORMATION:** Conversion of ALA to porphobilinogen is inhibited by lead and mercury; thus, **lead poisoning** causes increased urinary delta-ALA as well as increases of coproporphyrin and of free erythrocyte protoporphyrin.

Footnotes

1. Labbe RF and Lamon JM, "Porphyrins and Disorders of Porphyrin Metabolism," *Fundamentals of Clinical Chemistry*, 3rd ed, Tietz NW, ed, Philadelphia, PA: WB Saunders Co, 1987, 825-41.
2. "Hereditary Tyrosinaemia," *Lancet*, 1990, 335(8704):1500-1.
3. Plewinska M, Thunell S, Holmberg L, et al, "Delta-Aminolevulinate Dehydratase Deficient Porphyria: Identification of the Molecular Lesions in a Severely Affected Homozygote," *Am J Hum Genet*, 1991, 49(1):167-74.

References

Bird TD, Wallace DM, and Labbe RF, "The Porphyria, Plumbism, Pottery Puzzle," *JAMA*, 1982, 247:813-4.

Bloomer JR and Bonkovsky HL, "The Porphyrias," *Dis Mon*, 1989, 35(1):1-54.

Elder GH, Smith SG, and Smyth SJ, "Laboratory Investigation of the Porphyrias," *Ann Clin Biochem*, 1990, 27(Pt 5):395-412.

Delta Base, Blood

CPT 84999

Related Information

pH, Blood *on page 315*

Synonyms Actual Base Excess; Base Excess

Applies to Acid-Base Regulation

Abstract An expression of metabolic imbalance.

Interpretive **REFERENCE RANGE:** -3 to +3 **USE:** A measure with which to assess abnormalities of metabolic or acute respiratory acidosis or alkalosis. **LIMITATIONS:** The validity of delta base is questioned by some. **METHODOLOGY:** Calculated from a Siggaard-Andersen curve nomogram or can be read directly from blood gas instruments which have computer calculation capabilities. Delta base represents deviation from normal buffer base. **ADDITIONAL INFORMATION:** Delta base is the difference in concentration of strong base in whole blood and in the same blood titrated with strong acid or base to pH 7.40 at pCO_2 40 mm Hg and 37°C. This is an *in vitro* expression used mainly to describe situations with metabolic imbalance. Delta base below -3 indicates deficiency of fixed base or excess of acid (ie, metabolic acidosis). Delta base more than +3 indicates excess fixed base or deficit of nonvolatile acid (ie, metabolic alkalosis). Clinically, therapy is usually not given until -5 or +5 is reached. Umbilical cord blood gases do not predict morbidity in very low birth weight infants (500-1500 g).[1]

Footnotes

1. Hibbard JU, Hibbard MC, and Whalen MP, "Umbilical Cord Blood Gases and Mortality and Morbidity in the Very Low Birth Weight Infant," *Obstet Gynecol*, 1991, 78(5 Pt 1):768-73.

References

Burbea ZH, Gullans SR, and Ben-Yaakov S, "Delta Alkalinity: A Simple Method to Measure Cellular Net Acid-Base Fluxes," *Am J Physiol*, 1987, 253:C525-34.

Dickinson JE, Eriksen NL, Meyer BA, et al, "The Effect of Preterm Birth on Umbilical Cord Blood Gases," *Obstet Gynecol*, 1992, 79(4):575-8.
Dunham CM, Siegel JH, Weireter L, et al, "Oxygen Debt and Metabolic Acidemia as Quantitative Predictors of Mortality and the Severity of the Ischemic Insult in Hemorrhagic Shock," *Crit Care Med*, 1991, 19(2):231-43.
Economides DL, Johnson P, and MacKenzie IZ, "Does Amniotic Fluid Analysis Reflect Acid-Base Balance in Fetal Blood?" *Am J Obstet Gynecol*, 1992, 166(3):970-3.

11-Deoxycortisol *see* Metyrapone Test *on page 292*
Dexamethasone Suppression Test *see* Cortisol, Blood *on page 191*
1,4-α-D Glucanohydrolase, Serum *see* Amylase, Serum *on page 127*
1,4-α-D Glucanohydrolase, Urine *see* Amylase, Urine *on page 129*
DHEA *see* Dehydroepiandrosterone Sulfate *on page 206*
DHEA-S *see* Dehydroepiandrosterone Sulfate *on page 206*
DHEAS *see* Dehydroepiandrosterone Sulfate *on page 206*

Dibucaine Number

CPT 82638

Related Information

Acetylcholinesterase, Red Blood Cell *on page 95*
Pseudocholinesterase, Serum *on page 343*

Synonyms Cholinesterase Inhibition by Dibucaine; Pseudocholinesterase Inhibition

Applies to Fluoride Inhibition of Cholinesterase

Specimen Serum or plasma **CONTAINER:** Red top tube or green top (heparin) tube **COLLECTION:** Do not collect within 24 hours of administration of muscle relaxant. **STORAGE INSTRUCTIONS:** Serum cholinesterase (pseudocholinesterase) is stable and may be stored at 0°C to 4°C or at room temperature for 1 year or more and may be frozen/thawed a number of times without changing activity of the enzyme.[1]

Interpretive **REFERENCE RANGE:** Normal individuals have normal (high) amounts of serum cholinesterase (pseudocholinesterase) activity which can be inhibited by dibucaine. Approximately 70% to 86% inhibition is normal; atypical enzyme shows resistance to inhibition, at about the level of only 20%. See normal range of laboratory doing the test. **POSSIBLE PANIC RANGE:** Homozygotes for abnormal cholinesterase activity have low results in assay for serum cholinesterase (pseudocholinesterase), not inhibited by dibucaine. Administration of succinylcholine by anesthesiologist may pose a risk to patients with abnormal pseudocholinesterase. **USE:** Assess presence of homozygous or heterozygous "atypical" cholinesterase variant in patients who have low result of serum cholinesterase assay and may be at risk of apnea when given succinylcholine muscle relaxant **LIMITATIONS:** No single simple test currently exists that can detect all enzyme variants. **METHODOLOGY:** Hydrolysis of propionylthiocholine or butyrylthiocholine with and without dibucaine at 20°C to 40°C; fluoride inhibition at 25°C.[2,3,4,5] **ADDITIONAL INFORMATION:** The degree of serum cholinesterase inhibition produced by dibucaine (and fluoride) is under genetic control. Sensitivity to succinylcholine is dependent upon at least four allelic genes. The most widely accepted system of classification (Motulsky) designates E_1 as the first locus for plasma cholinesterase (see table). The E_1^u gene codes for the most common form of the plasma enzyme. The E_1^a gene is responsible for the atypical enzyme which resists inhibition by dibucaine, E_1^f gene for the enzyme that is fluoride resistant, and the E_1^s (silent) gene results in an enzyme with little or no activity.[6] An international gene nomenclature conference has proposed a system designating the four alleles as "CHE1*U," "CHE1*A," "CHE1*F," and "CHE1*QO." Single quantitative cholinesterase determinations may not be reliable in detecting sensitivity to succinyl choline as variant enzymes exhibit qualitative and quantitative differences in substrate specificity. Another common phenotypic designation (of the 15 different phenotypes known) is those at risk, AF; FS and FF (moderate risk); and AA, AS, and SS (severe risk).

Dibucaine Number

Genotype	Phenotype	Previous Term
E_1^u E_1^u	U	Usual
E_1^u E_1^a	I	Intermediate
E_1^a E_1^a	A	Atypical
E_1^u E_1^s	U	Usual
E_1^s E_1^s	S	Silent
E_1^u E_1^f	UF	
E_1^f E_1^f	F	

(Continued)

Dibucaine Number *(Continued)*

Dibucaine and fluoride numbers indicate the percent inhibition of enzyme activity by these agents when a serum sample is tested under standard conditions (inhibition expressed as a percent). This approach to screening for presence of serum cholinesterase variants does not entirely avoid the problem of variation in reactivity with some atypical enzymes. Individuals with the genotype E_1^u, E_1^f show resistance to fluoride inhibition (low fluoride number) but do not show resistance to dibucaine inhibition (the normal situation with high dibucaine number). This variant was published almost 30 years ago by Harris and Whittaker.[7] Prolonged apnea following hemodilutional cardiopulmonary bypass has been reported in a patient whose admission (preoperative) plasma cholinesterase level was slightly below the normal range.[8]

Footnotes

1. Huizenga JR, van der Belt K, Gips CH, "The Effect of Storage at Different Temperatures on Cholinesterase Activity in Human Serum," *J Clin Chem Clin Biochem*, 1985, 23:283-5.
2. Abernethy MH, George PM, Herron JL, et al, "Plasma Cholinesterase Phenotyping With Use of Visible-Region Spectrophotometry," *Clin Chem*, 1986, 32:194-7.
3. Abernethy MH, George PM, and Melton VE, "A New Succinylcholine-Based Assay of Plasma Cholinesterase," *Clin Chem*, 1984, 30:192-5.
4. Evans RT and Wroe J, "Is Serum Cholinesterase Activity a Predictor of Succinyl Choline Sensitivity? An Assessment of Four Methods," *Clin Chem*, 1978, 24:1762-6.
5. Rostron P and Higgins T, "Serum Pseudocholinesterase and Dibucaine Numbers as Measured With the Technicon™ RA-1000 Analyzer," *Clin Chem*, 1988, 34(9):1924-5.
6. Motulsky AG, "Pharmacogenetics," *Prog Med Genet*, Vol 3, Chapter 2, Steinberg AG and Bearn AG, eds, New York, NY: Grune & Stratton, 1964, 49-52.
7. Harris H and Whittaker M, "Differential Inhibition of Human Serum Cholinesterase With Fluoride: Recognition of Two New Phenotypes," *Nature*, 1961, 496-8.
8. Jackson SH, Bailey GWH, and Stevens G, "Reduced Plasma Cholinesterase Following Haemodilutional Cardiopulmonary Bypass," *Anaesthesia*, 1982, 37:319-20.

References

Kambam JR, Horton B, Parris WC, et al, "Pseudocholinesterase Activity in Human Cerebrospinal Fluid," *Anesth Analg*, 1989, 68(4):486-8.

King ME, "Cholinesterase," *Methods in Clinical Chemistry*, Pesce AJ and Kaplan LA, eds, St Louis, MO: Mosby-Year Book Inc, 1987, 161-8.

Whittaker M, "Cholinesterase," *Monographs in Human Genetics*, Vol 11, Beckman L, ed, Basel: Karger, 1986.

1,25-Dihydroxy Vitamin D_3 *see* Vitamin D_3, Serum *on page 387*

Direct Bilirubin *see* Bilirubin, Direct *on page 137*

Dopamine, Urine *see* Catecholamines, Fractionation, Urine *on page 174*

2,3-DPG *see* Oxygen Saturation, Blood *on page 305*

2,3-DPG *see* P-50 Blood Gas *on page 307*

d-Xylose Absorption Test

CPT 84620

Related Information

Folic Acid, RBC *on page 544*

Reducing Substances, Stool *on page 1149*

Synonyms Xylose Absorption Test; Xylose Tolerance Test

Abstract d-Xylose is a five-carbon monosaccharide. It can be absorbed by the normal duodenum and jejunum, by a mechanism different from the absorption of other monosaccharides. It is used as a screening test for carbohydrate malabsorption by the mucosa of the proximal small intestine.

Patient Care PREPARATION: Urea nitrogen, creatinine, and first morning urinalysis should be normal. Patient must fast a minimum of 8 hours prior to administration of d-xylose. Pediatric patients must be fasting for at least 4 hours. Patient must remain in supine position for duration of test. No food is permitted during the test. This substance, d-xylose, is a pentose. Patient should refrain from eating foods containing pentose. These include fruits, jams, jellies, and pastries. Many medications, including aspirin, indomethacin, other nonsteroidal anti-inflammatory drugs, neomycin, glipizide, or atropine interfere. These and preferably all medications should be discontinued for 24 hours prior to the test. No water restriction; in fact, patient should be encouraged to drink during the fasting period and during test. Start test at 8 AM. Instruct patient to void completely. Discard this urine. Draw fasting blood specimen.

Administer d-xylose: Adults, 25 g dose; for children under 12 years, a 5 g oral dose is recommended.[1] Others use weight-based dosage of d-xylose for children, oral administration: 0.5 g/kg body weight up to a maximum of 25 g, dissolved in water 10% (w/v) with a maximum of 250 mL. Have patient drink entire amount. Fill cup with 250 mL of water and have patient drink this also. Have patient drink another cup with 250 mL of water after 1 hour. Collect urine for 5 hours after administration of d-xylose.

Specimen Craig and Atkinson recommend a 25 g d-xylose absorption test with a 5-hour urine collection and a 1-hour serum specimen for adults, and the 1-hour serum test only for subjects with intermediate renal insufficiency. Others, for 5-hour urine: blood specimens drawn at fasting, 30, 60, and 120 minutes in red top tubes. A 1-hour draw is also done, for infants and children in some institutions. **CONTAINER:** Brown urine container, red top tube **COLLECTION:** Container must be labeled with patient's name, date, and time. **STORAGE INSTRUCTIONS:** Refrigerate urine during collection. **SPECIAL INSTRUCTIONS:** A 5-hour urine specimen is collected on patients 12 years of age or older as part of the test.

Interpretive **REFERENCE RANGE:** Absorption and excretion of d-xylose increase with age; in geriatric patients the serum test is preferable. Renal excretion diminishes in patients older than 60 years of age.

Mean 5-hour urine excretion (% of load): pediatrics: Craig and Atkinson urge that urine tests be abandoned for children. Others have also stated the test is not useful in children.[2] Some recommend 10% to 33% of dose ingested.

Older than 10 years: >16% (4 g) of a 25 g dose should be excreted; this criterion is widely used by Craig, Atkinson, and others.

Still others use ≥23% of a 5 g dose excreted over 5 hours as a criterion of normality. If <3 g is excreted, the diagnosis is most likely to be enterogenous malabsorption. In adults, the 5-hour urine collection was said to be more accurate in detecting intestinal malabsorption than the 1-hour blood test.[3]

Blood: A level of blood d-xylose between 20-40 mg/dL (SI: 1.3-2.7 mmol/L) should be reached in 30-60 minutes and maintained for a further 60 minutes. Craig and Atkinson recognize a lower limit for adults of 25 mg/dL (SI: 1.7 mmol/L) for the 1-hour serum specimen and 20 mg for patients with intermediate renal insufficiency. For 1-hour sample, subjects up to 12 years of age: >20 mg/dL (SI: >1.3 mmol/L) following a 5 g oral d-xylose dose.

In malabsorption syndromes, the highest level in blood may be <20 mg/dL (SI: <1.3 mmol/L), following a 5 g oral d-xylose dose. Blood levels are especially important in older patients and in those with renal disease, liver disease with ascites and with delayed gastric emptying.

USE: Use of the d-xylose test is mostly to work up gluten enteropathy, tropical sprue, and celiac disease. In general it is to evaluate possible enterogenous malabsorption syndromes; a test for functional integrity of the jejunum. Classically decreased in tropical and nontropical sprue (gluten-induced enteropathy, celiac disease). It may be abnormal in amyloidosis, lymphoma, small bowel ischemia, Whipple's disease, eosinophilic gastroenteritis, Zollinger-Ellison syndrome, radiation enteritis, scleroderma, following massive resection, bacterial overgrowth, and with certain parasitic infestations. **LIMITATIONS:** Poor renal function, vomiting, decreased or very rapid gastric emptying, hypomotility, intestinal stasis syndromes (eg, surgical blind loops), dehydration/hypovolemia, and certain drugs may cause low urine values **not** secondary to intestinal malabsorption. Normal results have been described with celiac disease. Renal function may present a problem in geriatric and other patients. The usefulness of the test has been somewhat controversial. Krawitt and Beeken studied urine excretion without blood levels and concluded in 1975 that no reason exists to do such d-xylose testing, when jejunal biopsies are available.[4]

Application of both blood and urine examination makes d-xylose considerably more reliable. Availability of small bowel mucosal biopsy by endoscopy must be considered, especially when results of blood and urine tests are inconsistent and before patient is committed to gluten-free diet.

It is not easy to reliably and accurately collect urine in children, leading Craig et al to prefer the 1-hour serum level after 5 g of d-xylose.[1]

Causes of low absorption: Small intestinal bacterial overgrowth, *Giardia lamblia* infestation, hookworm, schistosomiasis, viral gastroenteritis as well as recognized diseases causing malabsorption. Urinary tests without blood levels have been shown to be misleading. The test may cause mild diarrhea.

(Continued)

d-Xylose Absorption Test *(Continued)*

METHODOLOGY: Colorimetry **ADDITIONAL INFORMATION: Normal renal function is necessary if urine values alone are determined.** BUN and creatinine serum levels should be measured to exclude patients with renal impairment, resulting in poor xylose excretion and elevated blood xylose levels. Low blood and urine xylose levels indicate malabsorption. For this reason at least a 1- or 2-hour blood specimen is recommended. Elderly individuals with normal intestinal absorption may have elevated blood xylose levels and decreased urine xylose levels due to mild (subclinical) renal impairment. The [^{14}C] d-xylose breath test, if available, is useful for identifying malabsorption due to small intestinal bacterial overgrowth.[1] Pancreatic enzymes are not required for absorption of d-xylose. The d-xylose test is normal in the chronic nonspecific diarrhea syndrome of infancy.

Footnotes

1. Craig RM and Atkinson AJ Jr, "D-xylose Testing: A Review," *Gastroenterology*, 1988, 95(1):223-31.
2. Lifschitz CH and Polanco I, "The D-xylose Test in Pediatrics: Is It Useful?" *Gastroenterology*, 1989, 97(1):246-7.
3. Peled Y, Doron O, Laufer H, et al, "D-xylose Absorption Test. Urine or Blood?" *Dig Dis Sci*, 1991, 36(2):188-92.
4. Krawitt EL and Beeken WL, "Limitations of the Usefulness of the d-Xylose Absorption Test," *Am J Clin Pathol*, 1975, 63:261-3.

References

Ehrenpreis ED, Gulino SP, Patterson BK, et al, "Kinetics of D-xylose Absorption in Patients With Human Immunodeficiency Virus Enteropathy," *Clin Pharmacol Ther*, 1991, 49(6):632-40.

Hommes FA, ed, *Techniques in Diagnostic Human Biochemical Genetics*, New York, NY: Wiley-Liss, 1991.

Labib M, Gama R, and Marks V, "Predictive Value of D-xylose Absorption Test and Erythrocyte Folate in Adult Coeliac Disease: A Parallel Approach," *Ann Clin Biochem*, 1990, 27(Pt 1):75-7.

E_2, Unconjugated *see* Estradiol, Serum *on page 216*

Ecto-5'NT *see* 5' Nucleotidase *on page 297*

Electrolyte Gap *see* Anion Gap *on page 132*

Electrolytes, Blood

CPT 80004

Related Information

Anion Gap *on page 132*
Carbon Dioxide, Blood *on page 165*
Chloride, Serum *on page 182*
HCO_3, Blood *on page 248*
Kidney Stone Analysis *on page 1129*
Osmolality, Calculated *on page 299*
Osmolality, Serum *on page 300*
Potassium, Blood *on page 330*
Sodium, Blood *on page 349*

Synonyms Plasma Electrolytes; Serum Electrolytes

Test Commonly Includes Sodium, potassium, chloride; often total CO_2, but in some laboratories pH and pCO_2 are measured and bicarbonate (HCO_3), and CO_2T calculated. Anion gap is reported with electrolytes by some laboratories.

Specimen Serum or plasma **CONTAINER:** Red top tube or green top (heparin) tube **COLLECTION:** Best to collect without tourniquet if possible. Do **not** allow patient to clench-unclench his/her hand. **STORAGE INSTRUCTIONS:** Do not freeze.

Interpretive USE: Monitor electrolyte status, screen water balance, diagnose respiratory and metabolic acid-base balance; evaluate hydrational status, diarrhea, dehydration, ketoacidosis in diabetes mellitus and other disorders; evaluate alcoholism and other toxicity states **LIMITATIONS:** Hemolysis and prolonged contact of serum with cells produces elevation of potassium. The usual order for "electrolytes" does not include magnesium, osmolality, phosphorus, or lactic acid. **METHODOLOGY:** Ion-selective electrodes (ISE) or flame photometry are used for sodium and potassium. Sodium and potassium may also be measured by inductively-coupled plasma emission spectrometry.[1] **ADDITIONAL INFORMATION:** May be performed on heparinized plasma but not on EDTA plasma. Knowledge of pertinent clinical criteria allows for more cost effective ordering of blood electrolytes in patients in whom the information will be clinically significant.[2] The anion gap, calculated $Na^+ - (Cl^- + HCO_3^-)$, provides useful information for interpreting acid-base disorders and may be useful for establishing a differential diagnosis in some conditions.[3]

Footnotes

1. Melton LA, Tracy ML, and Moller G, "Screening Trace Elements and Electrolytes in Serum by Inductively-Coupled Plasma Emission Spectrometry," *Clin Chem*, 1990, 36(2):247-50.
2. Lowe RA, Wood AB, Burney RE, et al, "Rational Ordering of Serum Electrolytes: Development of Clinical Criteria," *Ann Emerg Med*, 1987, 16:260-9.
3. Oster JR, Perez GO, and Materson BJ, "Use of the Anion Gap in Clinical Medicine," *South Med J*, 1988, 81(2):229-37.

References

Cleland JG and Dargie HJ, "Arrhythmias, Catecholamines and Electrolytes," *Am J Cardiol*, 1988, 62:55A-9A, (review).

Ford HC, Lim WC, Chisnall WN, et al, "Renal Function and Electrolyte Levels in Hyperthyroidism: Urinary Protein Excretion and the Plasma Concentrations of Urea, Creatinine, Uric Acid, Hydrogen Ion, and Electrolytes," *Clin Endocrinol (Oxf)*, 1989, 30(3):293-301.

Graber M and Corish D, "The Electrolytes in Hyponatremia," *Am J Kidney Dis*, 1991, 18(5):527-45.

Kapsner CO and Tzamaloukas AH, "Understanding Serum Electrolytes. How to Avoid Mistakes," *Postgrad Med*, 1991, 90(8):151-4, 157-8, 161.

Lowe RA, Arst HF, and Ellis BK, "Rational Ordering of Electrolytes in the Emergency Department," *Ann Emerg Med*, 1991, 20(1):16-21.

McCleane GJ, "Urea and Electrolyte Measurement in Preoperative Surgical Patients," *Anaesthesia*, 1988, 43:413-5.

Olshaker JS and Mason JD, "The Usefulness of Serum Electrolytes in the Evaluation of Acute Adult Gastroenteritis," *Ann Emerg Med*, 1989, 18(3):258-60.

Shanbhogue LK, Sikdar T, Jackson M, et al, "Serum Electrolytes and Capillary Blood Gases in the Management of Hypertrophic Pyloric Stenosis," *Br J Surg*, 1992, 79(3):251-3.

Electrolytes, Serum or Plasma *see* Potassium, Blood *on page 330*

Electrolytes, Urine

***CPT** 80003*

Related Information

Aldosterone, Urine *on page 106*
Chloride, Urine *on page 184*
Kidney Stone Analysis *on page 1129*
Osmolality, Urine *on page 302*
Potassium, Urine *on page 332*
Renin, Plasma *on page 346*
Sodium, Urine *on page 351*

Synonyms Urine Electrolytes

Test Commonly Includes Sodium, potassium, and chloride on random or timed collections. Osmolality must be ordered as such.

Specimen Random, 12-, or 24-hour urine **CONTAINER:** Clean urine container **COLLECTION:** Specify whether random or timed collection. **CAUSES FOR REJECTION:** Blood in urine **SPECIAL INSTRUCTIONS:** Urine osmolality may be ordered with urine electrolytes, usually it must be specifically ordered.

Interpretive **REFERENCE RANGE:** Please see individual listings. There is a large diurnal variation in range for spot samples. Na/K ratio: 0.90-3.88. Borderline Na/K ratio: 0.3-6.0 **USE:** Monitor kidney function, fluid and electrolyte balance, water balance, acid-base balance; evaluate electrolyte composition of urine, correlation with renin and aldosterone studies. Urine sodium levels are appropriate in patients with volume depletion, with acute oliguria, and with decreased plasma sodium. Urine potassium levels are needed in work-up of hypokalemia of unknown etiology, eg, possible Conn's syndrome (primary aldosteronism), adrenal hyperplasia, Bartter's syndrome, renal tubular acidosis, Fanconi's syndrome. Urine chloride is helpful to work up metabolic alkalosis in patients who are not on diuretics; assess dietary salt restriction. Urine electrolytes are used in work-up with aldosterone and renin assays. **ADDITIONAL INFORMATION:** If a 24-hour timed specimen is collected, other tests which may be ordered simultaneously include Protein, Quantitative, 24-hour Urine and/or Creatinine Clearance, (all of which can be collected together). Aldosterone and other adrenocortical steroids enhance reabsorption of sodium and promote excretion of potassium. In subjects with hyponatremia, normal blood volume, and urine Na and Cl >40 mmol/L, the differential diagnosis includes hypothyroidism and the syndrome of inappropriate secretion of antidiuretic hormone. See Osmolality, Urine listing. Metabolic alkalosis, urinary chloride excretion, and relationships to Cushing's, Conn's, and Bartter's syndromes are discussed in the references following. Fetal (amniotic fluid) electrolytes are not predictive of ultimate renal function.[1]

(Continued)

Electrolytes, Urine *(Continued)*

Footnotes

1. Elder JS, O'Grady JP, Ashmead G, et al, "Evaluation of Fetal Renal Function: Unreliability of Fetal Urinary Electrolytes," *J Urol*, 1990, 144(2 Pt 2):574-8.

References

Kamel KS, Ethier JH, Richardson RM, et al, "Urine Electrolytes and Osmolality: When and How to Use Them," *Am J Nephrol*, 1990, 10(2):89-102.

Kamel KS, Magner PO, Ethier JH, et al, "Urine Electrolytes in the Assessment of Extracellular Fluid Volume Contraction," *Am J Nephrol*, 1989, 9(4):344-7.

Knuiman JT, van Poppel G, Burema J, et al, "Multiple Overnight Urine Collections May Be Used for Estimating the Excretion of Electrolytes and Creatinine," *Clin Chem*, 1988, 34(1):135-8.

Sherman RA and Eisinger RP, "The Use (and Misuse) of Urinary Sodium and Chloride Measurements," *JAMA*, 1982, 247:3121:4.

Epinephrine, Urine *see* Catecholamines, Fractionation, Urine *on page 174*

EPO *see* Erythropoietin, Serum *on this page*

Erythrocyte Cholinesterase *see* Acetylcholinesterase, Red Blood Cell *on page 95*

Erythrocyte Porphobilinogen Deaminase *see* Uroporphyrinogen-I-Synthase *on page 381*

Erythrocyte Uroporphyrinogen-I-Synthase *see* Uroporphyrinogen-I-Synthase *on page 381*

Erythropoietin, Serum

CPT 82668

Related Information

Blood Volume *on page 522*
Ferritin, Serum *on page 220*
Hemoglobin *on page 554*
Iron and Total Iron Binding Capacity/Transferrin *on page 262*
Phlebotomy, Therapeutic *on page 1075*
Red Cell Count *on page 594*
Red Cell Mass *on page 595*
Viscosity, Blood *on page 610*
Vitamin B_{12} Unsaturated Binding Capacity *on page 615*

Synonyms EPO; S-Epo

Test Commonly Includes Serum iron

Abstract A glycoprotein formed mainly in the kidney, erythropoietin (EP) has been purified and the gene cloned. The gene is found on chromosome 7. It stimulates erythropoiesis. Hypoxia increases erythropoietin production; bilateral nephrectomy drastically reduces erythropoietin synthesis and thereby inhibits erythropoiesis. Cloning has led to the production of erythropoietin by recombinant technology, now available therapeutically.

Specimen Serum **CONTAINER:** Red top tube **SPECIAL INSTRUCTIONS:** Done only by a few laboratories

Interpretive **REFERENCE RANGE:** Radioimmunoassay: 5-36 mU/mL[1] (SI: 5-36 IU/L); immunoassay: negative: <10 mU/mL (SI:<10 IU/L), equivocal: 11-48 mU/mL (SI: 11-48 IU/L), positive: >48 mU/mL (SI: >48 IU/L). Reference values in children have been published.[2] **USE:** Investigate obscure anemias and the anemia of end-stage renal disease. Certain tumors may produce erythropoietin, giving rise to otherwise unexplained polycythemia (eg, hemangioblastoma of cerebellum, pheochromocytoma, hepatoma, nephroblastoma, and rarely leiomyomas, renal cysts, and renal adenocarcinoma). It may be used to differentiate types of polycythemia. **LIMITATIONS:** Increased with pregnancy. **Hazards:** Therapeutic administration of erythropoietin has been associated with vascular thrombosis. Serum erythropoietin levels may be increased by phlebotomy, androgens, TSH, ACTH, angiotensin, epinephrine, and growth hormone levels. Transfusions and estrogens may lower erythropoietin levels. **METHODOLOGY:** The development of recombinant erythropoietin[3] has made available assays from clinical specimens using radioimmunoassay (RIA) and immunoassays.[4,5] Thus, the estimation of erythropoietin may now become part of the hematological investigation in certain anemias.[6] **ADDITIONAL INFORMATION:** Winearls et al[7] report 10 patients with end stage renal disease, all of whom responded with a good increase in their hemoglobin levels. Erythropoietin was given three times a week with increasing doses. Two patients developed thrombosis at the site of vascular access. One patient developed hypertensive encephalopathy. Treatment lasted 12 weeks. The dose schedule may not have been ideal. Eschbach et al treated 25 patients with end-stage renal disease.[8] Eighteen had been previously treated with blood transfusions. Twelve of these 18 patients no longer needed blood transfusion. At a dosage of 50 units/kg three times a week of erythropoietin the hematocrit rose to normal levels in all patients. Iron therapy was also needed. Four patients developed hypertension. Two developed hyperkalemia, one of whom died. The Ad Hoc Committee of the National Kidney Foundation has also reviewed the use of erythropoietin.[9] Erythropoietin and other growth factors have recently been reviewed by Metcalf.[10,11]

In the anemia of renal disease the serum erythropoietin level is generally lower than expected. Plasma erythropoietin is inappropriately low in adult nephrotic syndrome mostly because of renal/urinary loss of the protein and this contributes to the anemia.[12] In chronic iron deficiency the level of erythropoietin is increased, but the increase may not be as high as expected for the degree of anemia.

The effectiveness of recombinant erythropoietin in the treatment in other types of refractory anemia is under evaluation.

The anemia of AIDS[13] did not respond to zidovudine. This was not due to a low serum immunoreactive erythropoietin, which sometimes increased tenfold during the zidovudine treatment. The hemoglobin level fell.

Erythropoietin has been used to improve the yield of autologous units of blood before orthopedic surgery. Erythropoietin was given twice a week for 21 days, 600 units/kg, intravenously.[14]

Erythropoietin response to anemia (excluding renal disease and pregnancy) in older subjects is similar to that of younger subjects.[15]

S-Epo was below its reference range in 34 of 36 patients with polycythemia vera, elevated in cases of secondary polycythemia, and normal in all but one of the cases of relative polycythemia.[16]

Footnotes

1. Goldwasser E and Sherwood JB, "Radioimmune Assay of Erythropoietin," *Br J Haematol*, 1981, 48:359-63.
2. Pressac M, Morgant G, Farnier MA, et al, "Enzyme Immunoassay of Serum Erythropoietin in Healthy Children: Reference Values," *Ann Clin Biochem*, 1991, 28(Pt 4):345-50.
3. Egrie JC, Cotes PM, Lane J, et al, "Development of Radioimmunoassays for Human Erythropoietin Using Recombinant Erythropoietin as Tracer and Immunogen," *J Immunol Methods*, 1987, 99:235-41.
4. Widness JA, Schmidt RL, Veng-Pedersen P, et al, "A Sensitive and Specific Erythropoietin Immunoprecipitation Assay: Application to Pharmacokinetic Studies," *J Lab Clin Med*, 1992, 119(3):285-94.
5. Mason-Garcia M, Beckman BS, Brookins JW, et al, "Development of a New Radioimmunoassay for Erythropoietin Using Recombinant Erythropoietin," *Kidney Int*, 1990, 38(5):969-75.
6. Schlageter MH, Toubert ME, Podgorniak MP, et al, "Radioimmunoassay of Erythropoietin: Analytical Performance and Clinical Use in Hematology," *Clin Chem*, 1990, 36(10):1731-5.
7. Winearls CG, Oliver DO, Pippard MJ, et al, "Effect of Human Erythropoietin Derived From Recombinant DNA on the Anemia of Patients Maintained by Chronic Haemodialysis," *Lancet*, 1986, ii:1175-7.
8. Eschbach JW, Egrie JC, Downing MR, et al, "Correction of the Anemia of End-Stage Renal Disease With Recombinant Erythropoietin," *N Engl J Med*, 1987, 316:73-8.
9. Ad Hoc Committee for the National Kidney Foundation, "Statement on the Clinical Use of Recombinant Erythropoietin in Anemia of End-Stage Renal Disease," *Am J Kidney Dis*, 1989, 14(3):163-9, (review).
10. Metcalf D, "Haemopoietic Growth Factors 1," *Lancet*, 1989, 1(8642):825-7.
11. Metcalf D, "Haemopoietic Growth Factors 2: Clinical Applications," *Lancet*, 1989, 1(8643):885-7, (review).
12. Vaziri ND, Kaupke CJ, Barton CH, et al, "Plasma Concentration and Urinary Excretion of Erythropoietin in Adult Nephrotic Syndrome," *Am J Med*, 1992, 92(1):35-40.
13. Spivak JL, Barnes DC, Fuchs E, et al, "Serum Immunoreactive Erythropoietin in HIV-Infected Patients," *JAMA*, 1989, 261(21):3104-7.
14. Goodnough LT, Rudnick S, Price TH, et al, "Increased Preoperative Collection of Autologous Blood With Recombinant Human Erythropoietin Therapy," *N Engl J Med*, 1989, 321(17):1163-8.
15. Powers JS, Krantz SB, Collins JC, et al, "Erythropoietin Response to Anemia as a Function of Age," *J Am Geriatr Soc*, 1991, 39(1):30-2.
16. Birgegard G and Wide L, "Serum Erythropoietin in the Diagnosis of Polycythaemia and After Phlebotomy Treatment," *Br J Haematol*, 1992, 81(4):603-6.

References

"Erythropoietin Reaches the Pharmacy," *Lancet*, 1989, 2(8674):1252-4, (editorial).

Eschbach JW and Adamson JW, "Guidelines for Recombinant Human Erythropoietin Therapy," *Am J Kidney Dis*, 1989, 14(2 Suppl 1):2-8.

(Continued)

Erythropoietin, Serum *(Continued)*

Groopman JE, Molina JM, and Scadden DT, "Hematopoietic Growth Factors. Biology and Clinical Applications," *N Engl J Med*, 1989, 321(21):1449-59.
Hubbard JD and Wheeler DJ, "Erythropoietin Measurement by EIA," *Lab Med*, 1989, 20:849-54.
Johnson GR, "Erythropoietin," *Br Med Bull*, 1989, 45(2):506-14.
Jones EH, "Recombinant Human Erythropoietin," *Am J Hosp Pharm*, 1989, 46(11 Suppl 2):S20-3.
Paganini EP, Latham D, and Abdulhadi M, "Practical Considerations of Recombinant Human Erythropoietin Therapy," *Am J Kidney Dis*, 1989, 14(2 Suppl 1):19-25.
Spivak JL, "Erythropoietin," *Blood Rev*, 1989, 3(2):130-5.
Zanjani ED and Ascensao JL, "Erythropoietin," *Transfusion*, 1989, 29(1):46-57.

Estradiol, Serum

***CPT** 82670*

Synonyms E_2, Unconjugated

Abstract Estradiol is the most active estrogen. It is derived from ovaries, testes, and placentas.[1]

Specimen Serum **CONTAINER:** Red top tube **SAMPLING TIME:** In females, the portion of the menstrual cycle may be needed for interpretation. **COLLECTION:** Separate serum and freeze within 1 hour.[1] **CAUSES FOR REJECTION:** Recent radioactive scan

Interpretive **REFERENCE RANGE:** Children: <10 pg/mL (SI: <37 pmol/L);[2] males: 10-50 pg/mL (SI: 37-184 pmol/L); females: premenopausal: 30-400 pg/mL (SI: 110-1468 pmol/L), postmenopausal: 0-30 pg/mL (SI: 0-110 pmol/L) **USE:** Estradiol is useful to evaluate infertility, menstrual irregularities and sexual precocity in females. Other conditions causing elevations include the polycystic ovary syndrome and feminizing tumors of the ovary or adrenals. Ovarian failure causes decreased levels. In males, estradiol may be useful to evaluate feminizing states. Liver disease may cause increases. Oral contraceptives lower estradiol levels and clomiphene will increase them. **LIMITATIONS:** In menopausal females, order **estrogens** rather than estradiol. Estradiol increases with hepatic cirrhosis. Oral contraceptives increase serum levels. **CONTRAINDICATIONS:** Should not be used in pregnant females or to evaluate fetal well-being because **it does not measure estriol.** Estriol comprises >90% of maternal estrogens. However, Guillaume et al reports the use of estradiol in the effective diagnosis of ectopic pregnancy (low values are seen).[3] **METHODOLOGY:** Radioimmunoassay (RIA) following extraction; noncompetitive immunoassay[4] **ADDITIONAL INFORMATION:** Estradiol measurements, in conjunction with gonadotropin levels, can be used to categorize amenorrhea syndromes, including anorexia nervosa. Estradiol levels are very low in gonadal dysgenesis, and may be very high in hormonally active ovarian neoplasms. Estradiol augments the amplitude of prolactin pulsatile secretion. Very high serum estradiol levels are not detrimental to clinical outcome of *in vitro* fertilization.[5]

Footnotes

1. Leavelle DE, "Estradiol, Serum," *Mayo Medical Laboratories Interpretive Handbook*, Rochester, MN: Mayo Medical Laboratories, 1990, 74.
2. Veldhuis JD, Evans WS, and Stumpf PG, "Mechanisms That Subserve Estradiol's Induction of Increased Prolactin Concentrations: Evidence of Amplitude Modulation of Spontaneous Prolactin Secretory Bursts," *Am J Obstet Gynecol*, 1989, 161(5):1149-58.
3. Guillaume J, Benjamin F, Sicuranza BJ, et al, "Serum Estradiol as an Aid in the Diagnosis of Ectopic Pregnancy," *Obstet Gynecol*, 1990, 76(6):1126-9.
4. Barnard G and Kohen F, "Idiometric Assay: Noncompetitive Immunoassay for Small Molecules Typified by the Measurement of Estradiol in Serum," *Clin Chem*, 1990, 36(11):1945-50.
5. Chenette PE, Sauer MV, and Paulson RJ, "Very High Serum Estradiol Levels Are Not Detrimental to Clinical Outcome of *In Vitro* Fertilization," *Fertil Steril*, 1990, 54(5):858-63.

References

Darne J, McGarrigle HH, and Lachelin GC, "Saliva Oestriol, Oestradiol, Oestrone, and Progesterone Levels in Pregnancy: Spontaneous Labour at Term Is Preceded by a Rise in the Saliva Oestriol:Progesterone Ratio," *Br J Obstet Gynaecol*, 1987, 94:227-35.
Kicklighter EJ and Norman RJ, "The Gonads," *Clinical Chemistry – Theory, Analysis, and Correlation*, 2nd ed, Kaplan LA and Pesce AJ, eds, St Louis, MO: Mosby-Year Book Inc, 1989, 650-63.
Kiel DP, Baron JA, Plymate SR, et al, "Sex Hormones and Lipoproteins in Men," *Am J Med*, 1989, 87(1):35-9.
Phillips GB, Yano K, and Stemmerman GN, "Decrease in Serum Estradiol Values With Storage," *N Engl J Med*, 1984, 311:1635.
Pont A, Goldman ES, Sugar AM, et al, "Ketoconazole-Induced Increase in Estradiol-Testosterone Ratio," *Arch Intern Med*, 1985, 145:1429-31.
Segal KR, Dunaif A, Gutin B, et al, "Body Composition, Not Body Weight, Is Related to Cardiovascular Disease Risk Factors and Sex Hormone Levels in Men," *J Clin Invest*, 1987, 80:1050-5.
Stewart MO, Whittaker PG, Persson B, et al, "A Longitudinal Study of Circulating Progesterone, Oestradiol, hCG and hPL During Pregnancy in Type 1 Diabetic Mothers," *Br J Obstet Gynaecol*, 1989, 96(4):415-23.

Studd J, Savvas M, Waston N, et al, "The Relationship Between Plasma Estradiol and the Increase in Bone Density in Postmenopausal Women After Treatment With Subcutaneous Hormone Implants," *Am J Obstet Gynecol*, 1990, 163(5 Pt 1):1474-9.

Estriol, Unconjugated, Pregnancy, Blood or Urine

CPT *82677*

Synonyms Unconjugated Estriol, Pregnancy

Abstract Estriol is the major estrogen of pregnancy, but it is generally no longer considered very useful for the detection of fetal distress.

Specimen Serum or plasma, urine **CONTAINER:** Red top tube or green top (heparin) tube for blood; 24-hour urine container **COLLECTION:** Since circadian rhythms exist, serum estriol should be drawn at the same time of day on each visit. **CAUSES FOR REJECTION:** Recently administered radioisotopes

Interpretive **REFERENCE RANGE:** **Urine** concentrations of estriol increase with gestation, from 2 mg/24 hours (SI: 7 nmol/day) at 16 weeks gestation to 10-40 mg/24 hours (SI: 35-139 nmol/day) at term.[1,2] A wide normal range exists. **Serum** levels in the tables do not represent reference ranges for all laboratories. Different assays lead to wide differences of estriol in the same sample.

Normal Serum or Plasma Unconjugated Estriol Values[2,3,4] (Fetal Well-Being)

Weeks of Gestation	µg/L	SI: nmol/L
25	3.5–10.0	12–35
28	4.0–12.5	14–43
30	4.5–14.0	16–49
32	5.0–16.0	17–55
34	5.5–18.5	19–64
36	7.0–25.0	24–87
37	8.0–28.0	28–97
38	9.0–32.0	31–111
39	10.0–34.0	35–118
40	5.0–40.0	17–139

Note: This table is to be used to monitor fetal being.

Serum Unconjugated Estriol Medians for Risk Prediction of Fetal Chromosomal Abnormalities

Weeks of Gestation	Median µg/L	Median SI: nmol/L
15	0.82	2.83
16	1.16	4.01
17	1.45	5.02
18	1.73	5.98
19	2.06	7.13
20	2.36	8.16
21	2.70	9.34

Note: Data courtesy of Dr Linda Bradley, Director, Biochemical Genetics, Vivigen, Santa Fe, NM. (Every laboratory should establish their own reference data.)

POSSIBLE PANIC RANGE: Value of urinary estriol <4 mg/24 hours or 40% below mean of three prior values demands immediate evaluation of fetal well-being. **USE:** Serial estriol values, depending upon the integrity of the fetal-placental-maternal unit, have been thought to assess fetal well-being and placental function in later pregnancy, especially in high risk settings.[1,2] Estriol decreases in fetal adrenal aplasia or hypoplasia and anencephaly,[2] and increases with

(Continued)

Estriol, Unconjugated, Pregnancy, Blood or Urine *(Continued)*

high fetal adrenocortical activity (eg, congenital adrenal hyperplasia).[3] LIMITATIONS: Single values are almost impossible to interpret; trends in a series of measurements are much more important. May be low in case of placental sulfatase deficiency in the presence of a healthy baby. Other causes of decreased estriol levels include subjects living at high altitudes, on penicillin or related drugs, corticosteroids, dexamethasone, betamethasone, diuretics, Mandelamine®, probenecid, estrogens, phenazopyridine, meprobamate, phenolphthalein, cascara, senna, and glutethimide.[2] It is decreased with anemia and severe liver disease.[2] Estriol may be increased with multiple pregnancy[2] and with oxytocin.[3] It is not reliable in the presence of renal disease.[2,3] Use of the test has become controversial.[2] It is no longer done in a number of laboratories. **Few feel that a role for estriol remains with other more accurate and reliable means to monitor fetal well-being available**. METHODOLOGY: Radioimmunoassay (RIA) or high performance liquid chromatography (HPLC) ADDITIONAL INFORMATION: Estriol, E_3, is synthesized in the placenta from 16-α-hydroxydehydroepiandrosterone of fetal origin. Thus, normal production can serve as a measure of the integrity of the fetoplacental unit. Sequential monitoring of estriol in high risk pregnancy has made possible early intervention and fetal salvage. Chronically low estriol values are found in intrauterine growth retardation but also are sometimes seen in normal pregnancy. A decreasing trend is indicative of fetal distress. The sensitivity and specificity of this test for detecting fetal distress are very poor; **thus its use for this purpose has been largely abandoned**.

Since estriol comprises approximately 90% of the estrogen in the maternal urine in later pregnancy, many laboratories measure total urinary estrogen levels instead of estriol.

Combined evaluation of unconjugated serum estriol, maternal serum hCG, maternal serum AFP, and maternal age has value in predicting risk for fetal chromosomal abnormalities during pregnancy. The use of maternal serum AFP, hCG, and estriol predicts 65% of Down syndrome, as opposed to 28% if only serum AFP is used.[4,5,6] An opposing view of unconjugated estriol use is presented by Macri et al.[7]

Estriol/creatinine ratios have been advocated for evaluation of urinary estriol excretion. Total and unconjugated estriol levels by RIA are the most used plasma estriol assays.[8]

Footnotes

1. Knuppel RA and Goodlin RC, "Maternal-Placental-Fetal Unit; Fetal & Early Neonatal Physiology," *Current Obstetric & Gynecologic Diagnosis & Treatment 1987*, Pernoll ML and Benson RC, eds, Norwalk, CT: Appleton & Lange, 1987, 135-60.
2. Catanzarite VA, Perkins RP, and Pernoll ML, "Assessment of Fetal Well-Being," *Current Obstetric & Gynecologic Diagnosis & Treatment 1987*, Pernoll ML and Benson RC, eds, Norwalk, CT: Appleton & Lange, 1987, 279-302.
3. Speroff L, Glass RH, and Kase NG, *Clinical Gynecologic Endocrinology and Infertility*, 4th ed, Baltimore, MD: Williams & Wilkins, 1989.
4. White RS 3d, "Down Syndrome: Current Screening Technique," *South Med J*, 1989, 82(12):1483-6.
5. Heyl PS, Miller W, and Canick JA, "Maternal Serum Screening for Aneuploid Pregnancy by Alpha-Fetoprotein, hCG, and Unconjugated Estriol," *Obstet Gynecol*, 1990, 76(6):1025-31.
6. MacDonald ML, Wagner RM, and Slotnick RN, "Sensitivity and Specificity of Screening for Down Syndrome with Alpha-Fetoprotein, hCG, Unconjugated Estriol, and Maternal Age," *Obstet Gynecol*, 1991, 77(1):63-8.
7. Macri JN, Kasturi RV, Krantz DA, et al, "Maternal Serum Down Syndrome Screening: Unconjugated Estriol Is Not Useful," *Am J Obstet Gynecol*, 1990, 162(3):672-3.
8. Ray DA, "Biochemical Fetal Assessment," *Clin Obstet Gynecol*, 1987, 30:887-98.

Estrogens, Nonpregnant, Urine

CPT 82672

Synonyms Total Urinary Estrogens

Test Commonly Includes Urine volume, creatinine concentration and concentration of estradiol (E2), estrone (E1), estriol (E3), and estetrol (E4), unconjugated

Abstract In the normal cycle, estrogen increase begins in the middle of the proliferative phase.

Specimen 24-hour urine CONTAINER: Plastic urine container, no preservative COLLECTION: Instruct the patient to void at 8 AM and discard the specimen. Then collect all urine including the final specimen voided at the end of the 24-hour collection period (ie, 8 AM the next morning). Keep specimen on **ice** during collection. Container must be labeled with patient's name, date, and time.

Interpretive **REFERENCE RANGE:** Children: <10 μg/24 hours (SI: <35 μmol/day); male: 15-40 μg/24 hours (SI: 52-139 μmol/day); female: menstruating: 15-80 μg/24 hours (SI: 52-277 μmol/day), postmenopausal: <20 μg/24 hours (SI: <69 μmol/day) (values at Mayo Medical Laboratories) **USE:** Predict ovulation; the increase of estrogen occurs before that of LH and progesterone;[1] evaluate hyperestrogenic and hypoestrogenic states, including hypopituitarism, hypogonadism, adrenal hyperplasia, neoplasms, anorexia nervosa, and stress **CONTRAINDICATIONS:** This test is not used to assess fetal well-being. **METHODOLOGY:** Extraction and separation of estrogens, quantitation by spectroscopy or fluorometry. A method of estimation of urinary estrogen by competitive latex agglutination inhibition is described.[1] **ADDITIONAL INFORMATION:** Urinary estrogens may be increased in adrenal hyperplasia and in functional ovarian neoplasms. Estrogens are excreted throughout pregnancy in increasing amounts. Estrogens are decreased in primary or secondary ovarian failure, with forms of gonadal dysgenesis, and with normal menopause. The use of this test is generally the same as that of serum or plasma estradiol. With the advent of specific hormone immunoassays, total estrogen measurements have largely been replaced by more specific methods.

Footnotes

1. Ishikawa M, Hoshiai H, Tozawa H, et al,"Monitoring Follicular Maturation Through Measurement of Urinary Estrogen Excretion by Latex Agglutination Inhibition Reaction," *Fertil Steril*, 1987, 48:688-90.

References

Avioli LV, "Hyperparathyroidism, Estrogens, and Osteoporosis," *Hosp Pract Off Ed*, 1991, 26(1):115-22, 127-8, 133-4.

Bartelsmeyer JA and Petrie RH, "Erythema Nodosum, Estrogens, and Pregnancy," *Clin Obstet Gynecol*, 1990, 33(4):777-81.

Goldin BR and Gorbach SL, "Effect of Diet on the Plasma Levels, Metabolism, and Excretion of Estrogens," *Am J Clin Nutr*, 1988, 48:787-90.

Longcope C, Goldfield SR, Brambilla DJ, et al, "Androgens, Estrogens, and Sex Hormone-Binding Globulin in Middle-Aged Men," *J Clin Endocrinol Metab*, 1990, 71(6):1442-6.

Longcope C, Herbert PN, McKinlay SM, et al, "The Relationship of Total and Free Estrogens and Sex Hormone-Binding Globulin With Lipoproteins in Women," *J Clin Endocrinol Metab*, 1990, 71(1):67-72.

Silberstein SD and Merriam GR, "Estrogens, Progestins, and Headache," *Neurology*, 1991, 41(6):786-93.

Stampfer MJ, "Smoking, Estrogen, and Prevention of Heart Disease in Women," *Mayo Clin Proc*, 1989, 64(12):1553-7.

Etiocholanolone *see* 17-Ketosteroids Fractionation, Urine *on page 267*

Fast Hemoglobins *see* Glycated Hemoglobin *on page 244*

Fasting Blood Sugar *see* Glucose, Fasting *on page 238*

Fat, Quantitative, 72-Hour Stool Collection *see* Fecal Fat, Quantitative, 72-Hour Collection *on this page*

FBS *see* Glucose, Fasting *on page 238*

Fe and TIBC *see* Iron and Total Iron Binding Capacity/Transferrin *on page 262*

Fecal Fat, Quantitative, 72-Hour Collection

***CPT** 82710*

Related Information

Fat, Semiquantitative, Stool *on page 1118*
Meat Fibers, Stool *on page 1133*

Synonyms Fat, Quantitative, 72-Hour Stool Collection; Quantitative Fecal Fat, 72-Hour Collection; Stool Fat, Quantitative

Abstract Nonspecific test for investigation of malabsorption and steatorrhea.

Patient Care **PREPARATION:** 80-100 g/day fat diet for 3 days

Specimen 72-hour stool collection, usually in the fourth, fifth, and sixth days of the 100 g/day fat diet **CONTAINER:** Plastic stool container, preweighed **SAMPLING TIME:** 72 hours; shorter collection periods are not usually acceptable **COLLECTION:** Specimen should be refrigerated during its collection. A dietary fat intake of 50-150 g/day for at least 2 days before and during the collection period. **STORAGE INSTRUCTIONS:** Freeze on dry ice if analysis is not to be done promptly. **CAUSES FOR REJECTION:** Improper container (ie, paper cartons, coffee cans, plastic bags, etc), foreign matter other than feces inside of container (ie, spoons, tongue depressors, plastic bags, toilet paper, etc), patient not on special diet, not 72-hour collection, inadequate labeling of container or requisition **SPECIAL INSTRUCTIONS:** Requisition must state date and time collection started, date and time collection finished.

(Continued)

Fecal Fat, Quantitative, 72-Hour Collection *(Continued)*

Interpretive REFERENCE RANGE: 2-6 g/24 hours (SI: 2-6 g/day); <20% of total solids USE: Diagnose the presence of steatorrhea, supporting a diagnosis of one of the malabsorption syndromes, including nontropical sprue, Crohn's disease, chronic pancreatitis, cystic fibrosis, Whipple's disease LIMITATIONS: Fecal fat collection does not provide a diagnostic explanation for the presence of steatorrhea. Stool fat collection is an unpleasant experience for the patient as well as others. It may be within normal limits in the presence of advanced loss of pancreatic parenchyma. Fecal fat measurement is regarded as unnecessary for investigation of pancreatic insufficiency.[1] CONTRAINDICATIONS: Patient taking mineral oil METHODOLOGY: Extraction and titration of long chain fatty acids by sodium hydroxide. Fatty acids represent 60% to 80% of total fecal lipids. ADDITIONAL INFORMATION: Identification of types of stool fat (eg, free fatty acids, triglycerides, neutral fats, phospholipids) is of little value. Fecal fat excretion >6 g/day is abnormal but nonspecific. Small intestinal, pancreatic or hepatobiliary diseases may cause such increased excretion. Increased fecal fat levels do not differentiate between pancreatic and intestinal steatorrhea.[2]

Footnotes

1. Holmes GK and Hill PG, "Do We Still Need to Measure Faecal Fat?" *Br Med J [Clin Res]*, 1988, 296(6636):1552-3.
2. Bai JC, Andrush A, Matelo G, et al, "Fecal Fat Concentration in the Differential Diagnosis of Steatorrhea," *Am J Gastroenterol*, 1989, 84(1):27-30.

References

Colombo C, Maiavacca R, Ronchi M, et al, "The Steatocrit: A Simple Method for Monitoring Fat Malabsorption in Patients With Cystic Fibrosis," *J Pediatr Gastroenterol Nutr*, 1987, 6:926-30.

"Dietary Fat Intake, 72-Hour Excretion, and Sudan Stain for Fecal Fat," *Gastroenterology*, 1989, 97(2):550-1.

Simko V and Michael S, "Absorptive Capacity for Dietary Fat in Elderly Patients With Debilitating Disorders," *Arch Intern Med*, 1989, 149(3):557-60.

Sokol RJ, Reardon MC, Accurso FJ, et al, "Fat-Soluble-Vitamin Status During the First Year of Life in Infants With Cystic Fibrosis Identified by Screening of Newborns," *Am J Clin Nutr*, 1989, 50(5):1064-71.

Wright TL and Heyworth MF, "Maldigestion and Malabsorption," *Gastrointestinal Disease*, Sleisenger MH and Fordtran JS, eds, Philadelphia, PA: WB Saunders Co, 1989, 263-82.

FEP *see* Protoporphyrin, Free Erythrocyte *on page 341*

Ferritin, Serum

CPT *82728*

See Also Anemia Flowchart in the Hematology Appendix

Related Information

Complete Blood Count *on page 533*
Erythropoietin, Serum *on page 214*
Hemoglobin *on page 554*
Iron and Total Iron Binding Capacity/Transferrin *on page 262*
Iron Stain, Bone Marrow *on page 562*
Protoporphyrin, Zinc, Blood *on page 342*
Red Cell Count *on page 594*
Transferrin *on page 369*

Patient Care PREPARATION: No recent radioactive scans or other radioactivity if laboratory uses RIA for ferritin.

Specimen Serum CONTAINER: Red top tube STORAGE INSTRUCTIONS: Separate serum from clot and freeze immediately in plastic vial.

Interpretive REFERENCE RANGE: 1 ng/mL of serum ferritin in normal subjects corresponds to approximately 8 mg of storage iron. Ferritin increases in adulthood in men to about the fifth decade and in women after the menopause. Typical reference range: male: 33-236 ng/mL (SI: 33-236 μg/L); female: younger than 40 years: 11-122 ng/mL (SI: 11-122 μg/L), older than 40 years: 12-263 ng/mL (SI: 12-263 μg/L).[1] USE: Diagnose hypochromic, microcytic anemias. Decreased in iron deficiency anemia and increased in iron overload. Ferritin levels correlate with and are useful in evaluation of total body storage iron. In hemochromatosis, both ferritin and iron saturation are increased. Ferritin levels in hemochromatosis may be >1000 ng/mL (SI: >1000 μg/L). LIMITATIONS: Ferritin escapes from necrotic hepatocytes. In the presence of liver disease, with inflammation such as rheumatoid arthritis, with malignancy or with iron therapy, iron deficiency may not be reflected by low serum ferritin. Ferritin determinations are not reliable in infants on iron therapy. Bone marrow aspiration may be needed in some settings, such as low-normal ferritin and low serum iron in the presence of apparent anemia of chronic disease, low-normal ferritin in the presence of liver disease.[1] **METHODOLOGY:** Radioimmunometric, radioimmunoassay (RIA), enzyme-linked immunosorbent assay (ELISA), fluoroenzymoimmunometric assay, colorimetric, immunoenzymometric[2] **ADDITIONAL INFORMATION:** The serum ferritin is, other than a bone marrow examination, the most reliable indicator of total body iron stores. When combined with the serum iron and percent saturation of iron binding capacity/transferrin, it can usually differentiate the microcytic hypochromic anemias into iron deficiency anemia (ferritin low, iron low, saturation low, TIBC high, transferrin high), the anemia of chronic disease (ferritin normal or high, iron low, normal to low transferrin or TIBC), or thalassemia (ferritin normal or high). In iron deficiency, the red cell distribution width is increased, while it is normal with heterozygous alpha or beta thalassemia trait. The MCV is reduced in iron deficiency and alpha or beta thalassemia trait; each is normal with lead poisoning. Ferritin is low with combined iron deficiency and thalassemia. **In adults**, serum ferritin level $\leq$10 ng/mL indicates iron deficiency. High serum ferritin levels may be associated with inflammation, liver disease, megaloblastic anemia, hemolytic anemia, sideroblastic anemia, thalassemia, iron overload (hemochromatosis, hemosiderosis), and malignant diseases. The later include leukemia and malignant lymphoma. Very high levels indicate iron overload. Oral and injected iron increase ferritin levels. Increased serum ferritin may be a risk factor in primary hepatocellular carcinoma.[3]

Primary hemochromatosis is inherited in an autosomal recessive manner with preliminary evidence that the involved gene is linked to the A locus of the histocompatibility complex on chromosome 6. Inappropriate increase in iron absorption and parenchymal tissue deposition may eventuate in hepatic cirrhosis, diabetes, testicular atrophy, and fine, soft, bronze to slate gray skin and very high serum ferritin levels (usually >1000 ng/mL).

Red cell ferritin in conjunction with plasma ferritin may be useful in distinguishing iron deficiency from iron overload in patients who have β-thalassemia.[4]

The decline in serum ferritin occurring during adolescence has been shown to be due to the onset of menarche rather than as a result of the accompanying growth spurt.[5]

Elevated serum ferritin levels in patients with cancer is associated with a poor prognosis which may be due in part to deleterious biological effects of tumor ferritins on lymphocyte and granulocyte function.[6] Extensive data is accumulating on the nature of isoferritins and their association with and possible utilization in the evaluation of malignant neoplasia.[7]

An immunoassay utilizing calibrated mixtures of anti-H and anti-L ferritin subunit monoclonal antibodies has been shown to recognize intermediate isoferritins but was not found to have significant application to tumor monitoring.[8]

Footnotes

1. Sheehan RG, Newton MJ, and Frenkel EP, "Evaluation of a Packaged Kit Assay of Serum Ferritin and Application to Clinical Diagnosis of Selected Anemias," *Am J Clin Pathol*, 1978, 70:79-84.
2. Ramm GA, Duplock LR, Powell LW, et al, "Sensitive and Rapid Colorimetric Immunoenzymometric Assay of Ferritin in Biological Samples," *Clin Chem*, 1990, 36(6):837-40.
3. Hann HW, Kim CY, London WT, et al, "Increased Serum Ferritin in Chronic Liver Disease: A Risk Factor for Primary Hepatocellular Carcinoma," *Int J Cancer*, 1989, 43(3):376-9.
4. Van Der Weyden MB, Fong H, Hallam LJ, et al, "Red Cell Ferritin and Iron Overload in Heterozygous Beta-Thalassemia," *Am J Hematol*, 1989, 30(4):201-5.
5. Kagamimori S, Fujita T, Naruse Y, et al, "A Longitudinal Study of Serum Ferritin Concentration During the Female Adolescent Growth Spurt," *Ann Hum Biol*, 1988, 15:413-9.
6. Hann HW, Stahlhut MW, Lee S, et al, "Effects of Isoferritins on Human Granulocytes," *Cancer*, 1989, 63(12):2492-6.
7. Albertini A, Arosio P, Chiancone E, et al, "Ferritins and Isoferritins as Biochemical Markers," *Proceeds of Advanced Course on Ferritins and Isoferritins as Biochemical Markers*, Amsterdam, Holland: Elsevier/North Holland Biomedical Press, 1984.
8. Cozzi A, Levi S, Bazzigaluppi E, et al, "Development of an Immunoassay for All Human Isoferritins, and Its Application to Serum Ferritin Evaluation," *Clin Chim Acta*, 1989, 184(3):197-206.

References

Bothwell TH, Charlton RW, and Motulsky AG, "Hemochromatosis," *The Metabolic Basis of Inherited Disease*, 6th ed, Scriver CR, Beaudet AL, Sly WS, et al, eds, New York, NY: McGraw-Hill Inc, 1989, 1433-62.

Brittenham GM, Cohen AR, McLaren CE, et al, "Hepatic Iron Stores and Plasma Ferritin Concentration in Patients With Sickle Cell Anemia and Thalassemia Major," *Am J Hematol*, 1993, 42(1):81-5.

Conrad ME and Umbreit JN, "A Concise Review: Iron Absorption – The Mucin-Mobilferrin-Integrin Pathway. A Competitive Pathway for Metal Absorption," *Am J Hematol*, 1993, 42(1):67-73.

Dawson DW, Fish DI, and Shackleton P, "The Accuracy and Clinical Interpretation of Serum Ferritin Assays," *Clin Lab Haematol*, 1992, 14(1):47-52.

(Continued)

Ferritin, Serum *(Continued)*

Halliday CE, Halliday JW, and Powell LW, "The Clinical Manifestations of Chronic Iron Overload," *Baillieres Clin Haematol*, 1989, 2(2):403-21.

Hann HW, Lange B, Stahlhut MW, et al, "Prognostic Importance of Serum Transferrin and Ferritin in Childhood Hodgkin's Disease," *Cancer*, 1990, 66(2):313-6.

Oski FA, "Iron Deficiency in Infancy and Childhood," *N Engl J Med*, 1993, 329(3):190-3.

Stacy DL and Han P, "Serum Ferritin Measurement and the Degree of Agreement Using Four Techniques," *Am J Clin Pathol*, 1992, 98(5):511-5.

Vernet M, Revenant MC, Bied A, et al, "Rapid Determination of Ferritin in Serum by the "Stratus" Fluoroenzymoimmunometric Assay," *Clin Chem*, 1989, 35(4):672-3.

Fluid, Peritoneal *see* Body Fluid *on page 145*

Fluid, Pleural *see* Body Fluid *on page 145*

Fluoride Inhibition of Cholinesterase *see* Dibucaine Number *on page 209*

Follicle Stimulating Hormone

CPT 83001

Related Information

Clomiphene Test *on page 190*
Luteinizing Hormone, Blood or Urine *on page 286*
Testosterone, Free and Total *on page 358*

Synonyms Follitropin; FSH

Abstract LH and FSH are gonadotropic hormones. They are glycoproteins. The alpha subunits of LH, FSH, TSH, and hCG are identical and specificity resides in the beta subunits.

Specimen Serum or plasma, urine **CONTAINER:** Red top tube or green top (heparin) tube; plastic urine container with boric acid **COLLECTION:** Refrigerate urine during collection. **STORAGE INSTRUCTIONS:** Separate and freeze serum or plasma; avoid hemolysis. FSH is stable 4 hours at 4°C to 25°C, 2 weeks at -20°C, 3 months at -70°C. In urine, stable 3 months at -20°C.[1,2] **CAUSES FOR REJECTION:** Recently administered radioisotopes **SPECIAL INSTRUCTIONS:** For females, date of last menstrual period is necessary for evaluation.

Interpretive **REFERENCE RANGE:** Normal ranges for FSH will vary among laboratories and are dependent upon which international is used. Serum: prepubertal children: <10 mIU/L (SI: <10 IU/L), adults: male: <22 mIU/L (SI: <22 IU/L); adults: female: nonmidcycle: <20 mIU/L (SI: <20 IU/L), midcycle surge: <40 mIU/L (SI: <40 IU/L), (ovulatory midcycle peak about twice the basal level) postmenopause: 40-160 mIU/L (SI: 40-160 IU/L).

Urine: male: 0-8 years of age: <5 mIU/24 hours (SI: <5 IU/day), older than 9 years: <22 mIU/24 hours (SI: <22 IU/day); female: 0-8 years: <5 mIU/24 hours (SI: <5 IU/day), 9-15 years: <22 mIU/24 hours (SI: <22 IU/day), older than 15 years: <30 mIU/24 hours (SI: <30 IU/day), postmenopausal: two to three times cycling level

USE: Excessive FSH and LH are found in hypogonadism, anorchia, gonadal failure,[3] complete testicular feminization syndrome, menopause, Klinefelter's syndrome, alcoholism, castration. FSH and LH are pituitary products, useful to distinguish primary gonadal failure from secondary (hypothalamic/pituitary) causes of gonadal failure, menstrual disturbances and amenorrhea. Useful in defining menstrual cycle phases in infertility evaluation of women and testicular dysfunction in men. FSH is commonly used with LH, which also is a gonadotropin. Both are low in pituitary or hypothalamic failure. FSH and LH levels are high following menopause. Urinary collections for FSH escape the problems of pulsatile, episodic secretion. They are used mainly for children being worked up for precocious puberty and for cycles for *in vitro* fertilization. **LIMITATIONS:** Secretion of both LH and FSH are pulsatile, in response to the normal intermittent release of gonadotropin releasing hormone (GnRH). In addition, in females both FSH and LH vary over the course of the menstrual cycle, with peaks at time of ovulation. Thus, interpretation of a single determination may be difficult. It has been suggested that samples be obtained at 15- to 30-minute intervals and equal volumes of serum be pooled to decrease the effect of pulsatile excretion. **METHODOLOGY:** Radioimmunoassay (RIA) **ADDITIONAL INFORMATION:** FSH and LH are under complex regulation by hypothalamic GnRH and by gonadal sex hormones, estrogen and progesterone in females, and testosterone. On the simplest level, FSH and LH are high in conditions in which sex hormones cannot be elaborated, and low in conditions of primary pituitary dysfunction. FSH acts on granulosa cells of the ovary and the Sertoli cells of testis. LH acts on Leydig (interstitial) cells of the gonads. Normally FSH increase occurs at an early stage of puberty, 2-4 years before LH reaches the same levels.

FSH **is high** in Klinefelter's syndrome and in some subjects with precocious puberty. It is decreased with precocious puberty related to adrenal tumors or congenital adrenal hyperplasia. Normal FSH in an adult nonovulating female, represents dysfunction at the central nervous system hypothalamic/pituitary level, and a "normal" value should in such a setting be considered pseudonormal.

High LH/FSH ratio (>1.5) is found in the polycystic ovary syndrome.[4]

Footnotes

1. Kubasik NP, Ricotta M, Hunter T, et al, "Effect of Duration and Temperature of Storage on Serum Analyte Stability – Examination of 14 Selected Radioimmunoassay Procedures," *Clin Chem*, 1982, 28:164-5.
2. Livesey JH, Hodgkinson SC, Roud MR, et al, "Effect of Time, Temperature, and Freezing on the Stability of Immunoreactive LH, FSH, TSH, Growth Hormone Prolactin and Insulin in Plasma," *Clin Biochem*, 1980, 13:151-5.
3. Layman LC, Wilson JT, Huey LO, et al, "Gonadotropin-Releasing Hormone, Follicle-Stimulating Hormone Beta, Luteinizing Hormone Beta Gene Structure in Idiopathic Hypogonadotropic Hypogonadism," *Fertil Steril*, 1992, 57(1):42-9.
4. Watts NB and Keffer JH, *Practical Endocrine Diagnosis*, 4th ed, Philadelphia, PA: Lea & Febiger, 1989.

References

Jaakkola T, Ding YQ, Kellokumpu-Lehtinen P, et al, "The Ratios of Serum Bioactive/Immunoreactive Luteinizing Hormone and Follicle-Stimulating Hormone in Various Clinical Conditions With Increased and Decreased Gonadotropin Secretion: Reevaluation by a Highly Sensitive Immunometric Assay," *J Clin Endocrinol Metab*, 1990, 70(6):1496-505.

Follitropin *see* Follicle Stimulating Hormone *on previous page*

Follitropin *see* Luteinizing Hormone, Blood or Urine *on page 286*

Fractionated Alkaline Phosphatase *see* Alkaline Phosphatase, Heat Stable *on page 106*

Free Catecholamine Fractionation, Urine *see* Catecholamines, Fractionation, Urine *on page 174*

Free Erythrocyte Protoporphyrin *see* Protoporphyrin, Free Erythrocyte *on page 341*

Free T_4 *see* Thyroxine, Free *on page 368*

Free Thyroxine *see* Thyroxine, Free *on page 368*

Free Thyroxine Index

CPT 84999

Related Information

T_3 Uptake *on page 355*
Thyroid Antimicrosomal Antibody *on page 755*
Thyroid Antithyroglobulin Antibody *on page 756*
Thyrotropin-Receptor Antibody *on page 756*
Thyroxine Binding Globulin *on page 366*
Thyroxine, Free *on page 368*
Triiodothyronine *on page 373*

Synonyms FT_4I; FT_4 Index; FTI

Test Commonly Includes T_3 uptake and T_4

Abstract The free thyroxine index may be calculated as the product of T_3 resin uptake (RT_3U) and total T_4 level; it is usually proportional to actual FT_4. It is an imperfect measure but provides acceptable results with pregnant subjects and in a variety of other settings. A tendency exists for the free thyroxine index to provide low results in assays of subjects with nonthyroidal illness. In euthyroid elderly people, low FTIs may be found; and this may be due to a resetting of threshold of thyrotropin feedback suppression.[1]

Patient Care PREPARATION: No recent administration of radioactive substances (eg, no recent scans). Schedule scans, if necessary, **after** thyroid profile is drawn. FT_4I may be increased with radiologic contrast agents, propranolol, amiodarone, and heparin.[2]

Specimen Serum CONTAINER: Red top tube STORAGE INSTRUCTIONS: Separate within 48 hours; separated serum stable 1 week at 25°C

Interpretive REFERENCE RANGE: 10 years to adult: normal: 5.5-10.0, borderline low: 4.9-5.4, low: ≤4.8, borderline high: 10.1-13.9, high: ≥14.0. Normal ranges will differ somewhat between laboratories. To prevent confusion with serum T_4 or T_3, units are omitted or expressed as "index

(Continued)

Free Thyroxine Index *(Continued)*

units."[3] **USE:** In the basic thyroid work-up, the FT_4 index is a physiologic index of metabolic activity which generally correlates with free thyroxine. Costs of each should be compared. **LIMITATIONS:** Nelson and Tomel conclude that no free T_4 index based on T_3 binding to serum proteins (eg, T_3 uptake) is reliable when decreased serum thyroxine is caused by decreased thyroid hormone binding to thyroxine binding globulin (ie, the value of the free thyroxine index in the differential diagnosis of low total T_4 is minimal). Although these authors conclude that the free thyroxine index and the T_4:TBG ratio are not a substitute for measurement of free T_4.[4] **CONTRAINDICATIONS:** Recent radioactive scan **METHODOLOGY:** Calculation from results of T_3 uptake and T_4. The FTI = (T_3U(%) of patient/T_3U(%) normal control mean) x T_4 **ADDITIONAL INFORMATION:** Calculation includes the T_4 and T_3 uptake values. T_3 uptake and T_4 are influenced by pregnancy, contraceptive pills, abnormalities of serum proteins and other factors, mostly in opposite directions. The free thyroxine index permits meaningful interpretation by balancing out most nonthyroidal factors.[5] For example, a pregnant euthyroid patient would have an increased T_4, but the FTI would be normal. An euthyroid patient with nephrotic syndrome may have a decreased T_4 (due to decreased levels by binding proteins), but the FTI would be normal. Wilke described the FTI to be equal to the thyroid hormone/TBG ratio in hyperthyroidism and a better index in pregnancy, in thyroid binding globulin deficiency and in hypothyroidism.[6] The FT_4I is increased with levothyroxine.[2]

Footnotes

1. Lewis GF, Alessi CA, Imperial JG, et al, "Low Serum Free Thyroxine Index in Ambulating Elderly Is Due to a Resetting of the Threshold of Thyrotropin Feedback Suppression," *J Clin Endocrinol Metab*, 1991, 73(4):843-9.
2. Wartofsky L and Ingbar SH, "Diseases of the Thyroid," *Harrison's Principles of Internal Medicine*, 12th ed, Wilson JD, Braunwald E, Isselbacher KJ, et al, eds, New York, NY: McGraw-Hill Inc, 1991, 1692-712.
3. Larsen PR, Alexander NM, Chopra IJ, et al, "Revised Nomenclature for Tests of Thyroid Hormones and Thyroid-Related Proteins in Serum," *Arch Pathol Lab Med*, 1987, 111:1141-5
4. Nelson JC and Tomei RT, "Dependence of the Thyroxine/Thyroxine-Binding Globulin (TBG) Ratio and the Free Thyroxine Index on TBG Concentrations," *Clin Chem*, 1989, 35(4):541-4.
5. Nusynowitz ML, "Free Thyroxine Index," *JAMA*, 1975, 232:1050.
6. Wilke TJ, "Free Thyroid Hormone Index, Thyroid Hormone/Thyroxine-Binding Globulin Ratio, Triiodothyronine Uptake, and Thyroxine-Binding Globulin Compared for Diagnostic Value Regarding Thyroid Function," *Clin Chem*, 1983, 29:74-9.

References

Grund FM and Niewoehner CB, "Hyperthyroxinemia in Patients Receiving Thyroid Replacement Therapy," *Arch Intern Med*, 1989, 149(4):921-4.

Helfand M and Crapo LM, "Screening for the Thyroid Disease," *Ann Intern Med*, 1990, 112(11):840-9.

Mandel SJ, Larsen PR, Seely EW, et al, "Increased Need for Thyroxine During Pregnancy in Women With Primary Hypothyroidism," *N Engl J Med*, 1990, 323(2):91-6.

Fructosamine

***CPT** 82985*

Related Information

Glucose, Fasting *on page 238*
Glucose, Quantitative, Urine *on page 1120*
Glycated Hemoglobin *on page 244*

Synonyms Glycated Albumin

Abstract A fructose-amine follows glucose linking covalently with albumin or other proteins, producing a glycated product, a stable ketoamine.

Specimen Serum **CONTAINER:** Red top tube **STORAGE INSTRUCTIONS:** Refrigerate. Freeze sample if assay is not done within 2 hours.

Interpretive **REFERENCE RANGE:** Normal ranges vary considerably according to method. Nondiabetics: 1.5-2.7 mmol/L; diabetics: ≥2.0-5.0 mmol/L depending on the degree of control. **USE:** Evaluate diabetic control, reflecting diabetic control over a shorter time period (2-3 weeks) than that represented by glycated hemoglobin (hemoglobin A_{1c}) (4-8 weeks). Indicated as an index of longer term control than glucose levels, especially in diabetic subjects with abnormal hemoglobins, patients with gestational diabetes,[1] and in type I diabetes in children.[2] Fructosamine levels may be useful in screening geriatric populations.[3] Glycated albumin, because of its short half-life, lends itself as a test to monitor and control gestational diabetes.[1] **LIMITATIONS:** Fructosamine, like Hb A_{1c}, is probably not a useful test for screening for diabetes mellitus. **METHODOLOGY:** Colorimetry or affinity chromatography. Methods suitable for automated analyzers have been described.[4] **ADDITIONAL INFORMATION:** Fructosamine is found in the plasma of both normal and diabetic individuals. "Fructosamine" is the term used to describe proteins that have been glycated (ie, are derivatives of the nonenzymatic reaction product of glucose and albumin). Recently it has been advocated as an alternative test to hemoglobin A_{1c} for the monitoring of long-term diabetic control. Fructosamine and hemoglobin A_{1c} do not measure exactly the same thing, since fructosamine has a shorter half-life and probably is somewhat more sensitive to short-term variations in glucose levels. However, this is not necessarily a disadvantage. Much of the development of fructosamine has occurred outside the United States. Although the tests are not exactly identical, probably one or the other is sufficient in routine diabetic patients for the assessment of long-term control of hyperglycemia. It is not necessary to order both tests in all patients, although this may be a value in selective problem patients. Fructosamine is clearly superior in patients with abnormal hemoglobins because of the interference of abnormal hemoglobins in the anion-exchange chromatography methods for Hb A_{1c}. Recently, an ion-capture immunoassay (Abbott Laboratories) can measure Hb A_{1c} in the presence of abnormal hemoglobins.

Footnotes

1. Narayanan S, "Laboratory Monitoring of Gestational Diabetes," *Ann Clin Lab Sci*, 1991, 21(6):392-401.
2. Cefalu WT, Mejia E, Puente GR, et al, "Correlation of Serum Fructosamine Activity in Type I Diabetic Children," *Am J Med Sci*, 1989, 297(4):244-6.
3. Croxson SC, Absalom S, and Burden AC, "Fructosamine in Diabetes Screening of the Elderly," *Ann Clin Biochem*, 1991, 28(Pt 3):279-82.
4. Hill RP, Hindle EJ, Howey JE, et al, "Recommendations for Adopting Standard Conditions and Analytical Procedures in the Measurement of Serum Fructosamine Concentration," *Ann Clin Biochem*, 1990, 27(Pt 5):413-24.

References

Allgrove J and Cockrill BL, "Fructosamine or Glycated Haemoglobin as a Measure of Diabetic Control?" *Arch Dis Child*, 1988, 63:418-22.

Comtois R, Desjarlais F, Nguyen M, et al, "Clinical Usefulness of Estimation of Serum Fructosamine Concentration as Screening Test for Gestational Diabetes," *Am J Obstet Gynecol*, 1989, 160(3):651-4.

Daubresse JC, Laurent E, Ligny C, et al, "The Usefulness of Fructosamine Determination in Diabetic Patients and Its Relation to Metabolic Control," *Diabete Metab* Paris, 1987, 13:217-21.

Desjarlais F, Comtois R, Beauregard H, et al, "Technical and Clinical Evaluation of Fructosamine Determination in Serum," *Clin Biochem*, 1989, 22(4):329-35.

Faulkner WR, "Fructosamine in the Assessment of Glycemic Control," *Lab Report for Physicians*, 1988, 10:1-5.

Gebhart SS, Wheaton RN, Mullins RE, et al, "A Comparison of Home Glucose Monitoring With Determinations of Hemoglobin A_{1c}, Total Glycated Hemoglobin, Fructosamine, and Random Serum Glucose in Diabetic Patients," *Arch Intern Med*, 1991, 151(6):1133-7.

Jerntorp P, Sundkvist G, Fex G, et al, "Clinical Utility of Serum Fructosamine in Diabetes Mellitus Compare With Hemoglobin A_{1c}," *Clin Chim Acta*, 1988, 175:135-42.

Kaufman HW, "Screening for Gestational Diabetes Mellitus," *Am Fam Physician*, 1989, 40(6):109-11.

Lapolla A, Poli T, Barison A, et al, "Fructosamine Assay: An Index of Medium-Term Metabolic Control Parameters in Diabetic Disease," *Diabetes Res Clin Pract*, 1988, 4:231-5.

Lloyd DR, Nott M, and Marples J, "Comparison of Serum Fructosamine With Glycosylated Serum Protein (Determined by Affinity Chromatography) for the Assessment of Diabetic Control," *Diabetic Med*, 1985, 2:474-8.

Negoro H, Morley JE, and Rosenthal MJ, "Utility of Serum Fructosamine as a Measure of Glycemia in Young and Old Diabetic and Nondiabetic Subjects," *Am J Med*, 1988, 85:360-4.

Roberts AB, Baker JR, James AG, et al, "Fructosamine in the Management of Gestational Diabetes," *Am J Obstet Gynecol*, 1988, 159:66-71.

Salemans THB, Van Dieijen-Visser MP, and Brombacher PJ, "The Value of Hb A_1 and Fructosamine in Predicting Impaired Glucose Tolerance – Alternative to OGTT to Detect Diabetes Mellitus or Gestational Diabetes," *Ann Clin Biochem*, 1987, 24:447-52.

Swai ABM, Harrison K, Chuwa LM, et al, "Screening for Diabetes: Does Measurement of Serum Fructosamine Help?" *Diabetic Med*, 1988, 5:648-52.

Fructose Biphosphate Aldolase *see* Aldolase, Serum *on page 103*

FSH *see* Follicle Stimulating Hormone *on page 222*

FT_4 *see* Thyroxine, Free *on page 368*

FT_4I *see* Free Thyroxine Index *on page 223*

FT_4 Index *see* Free Thyroxine Index *on page 223*

FTI *see* Free Thyroxine Index *on page 223*

Galactokinase, Blood

CPT 82759

Related Information

Galactose Screening Tests for Galactosemia *on page 228*

Applies to RBC Galactokinase

Specimen Whole blood **CONTAINER:** Green top (heparin) tube **COLLECTION:** Send blood immediately (on ice, not frozen) to the laboratory. **STORAGE INSTRUCTIONS:** Red blood cells must be washed repeatedly immediately after receipt in laboratory, therefore, transportation to the laboratory is critical. **CAUSES FOR REJECTION:** Specimen collected in the wrong container, quantity not sufficient, not on ice, too long in transit **SPECIAL INSTRUCTIONS:** Communicate with laboratory, as this test is not routinely available and may require referral.

Interpretive **REFERENCE RANGE:** Children: 0-2 years: 11-150 mU/g Hgb (levels in infants are 3 to 4 times those of adults,[1]) 2-18 years: 11-53.6 mU/g Hgb; adults: 12.1-39.7 mU/g Hgb **USE:** Establish the diagnosis of galactokinase-deficiency galactosemia. Galactosemia may also be caused by a deficiency of galactose-1-phosphate uridyl transferase and uridine diphosphoglucose 4-epimerase.[2] **METHODOLOGY:** Radioisotopic: RBCs are hemolyzed and the hemolysate is incubated with radiolabeled galactose. The 1-^{14}C-galactose-1-phosphate is quantitated after binding to DEAE chromatography paper.[1] **ADDITIONAL INFORMATION:** This condition should enter into the differential consideration of any child with cataracts.[3] It is an autosomal recessive inherited enzyme deficiency, 0.2% of the population is heterozygous for the defect. Homozygotes have a form of galactosemia that is associated with cataracts but usually do not suffer mental retardation or liver disease. Heterozygotes are at risk for the development of cataracts in young adult life. In each of the different forms of galactosemia, an alternative route of galactose metabolism is utilized. Reduction (of galactose) to galactitol and oxidation to galactonate occurs. Galactitol accumulates in the lens, produces osmotic imbalance resulting in cataract formation. An incidence of 6.9% of galactokinase deficiency has been found in a group of idiopathic cataract patients 50 years of age or younger.[4] Heterozygotes have about 50% of the normal enzyme activity. Galactokinase deficiency is in the differential consideration of patients with pseudotumor cerebri.[5] Therapy, as for transferase deficiency, consists of galactose restriction.

Footnotes

1. Beutler E, Paniker NV, and Trinidad F, "The Assay of Red Cell Galactokinase," *Biochem Med Metab Biol*, 1971, 5:325-32.
2. Beutler E, "Galactosemia: Screening and Diagnosis," *Clin Biochem*, 1991, 24(4):293-300.
3. Stevens RE, Datiles MB, Srivastava SK, et al, "Idiopathic Presenile Cataract Formation and Galactosaemia," *Br J Ophthalmol*, 1989, 73(1):48-51.
4. Elman MJ, Miller MT, and Matalon R, "Galactokinase Activity in Patients With Idiopathic Cataracts," *Ophthalmology*, 1986, 93:210-5.
5. Litman N, Kanter A, and Finberg L, "Galactokinase Deficiency Presenting as Pseudotumor Cerebri," *J Pediatr*, 1975, 86:410-2.

References

Applegarth DA, Dimmick JE, and Toone JR, "Laboratory Detection of Metabolic Disease," *Pediatr Clin North Am*, 1989, 36(1):49-65.

Segal S, "Disorders of Galactose Metabolism: Galactokinase Deficiency Galactosemia," *The Metabolic Basis of Inherited Disease*, 6th ed, Chapter 13, Scriver CR, Beaudet AL, Sly WS, et al, eds, New York, NY: McGraw-Hill Inc, 1989, 469-71.

Galactokinase Deficiency *see* Galactose-1-Phosphate Uridyl Transferase, Erythrocyte *on next page*

Galactose-1-Phosphate

CPT 84999

Related Information

Galactose Screening Tests for Galactosemia *on page 228*

Specimen Whole blood **CONTAINER:** Green top (heparin) tube **STORAGE INSTRUCTIONS:** Store at 4°C. **CAUSES FOR REJECTION:** Specimen more than 3 hours old

Interpretive **REFERENCE RANGE:** Usually <1 mg/dL galactose-1-phosphate/100 mL lysed packed red blood cells **USE:** Monitor galactosemic patients on a galactose-free diet **LIMITATIONS:** Analysis is offered by only a few specialized laboratories. Monitoring of galactose-free diet may be more simply achieved and less costly by using whole blood filter paper spot tests. **METHODOLOGY:** Enzymatic rate reaction (absorbance of NADH); normal red cells used as a source of galactose-1-phosphate uridyltransferase; galactose-1-phosphate of patient's red cells is limiting factor to which rate of reduction of NAD is proportional.[1] A method to detect galactose and galactose-1-phosphate from dried blood has recently been described.[2] **ADDITIONAL INFORMATION:** Galactosemia, the result of an inherited cellular deficiency of galactokinase or uridine diphosphate galactose-4-epimerase, is characterized by galactosuria and increased red cell galactose-1-phosphate. The level of galactose in the blood relates to the dietary intake of lactose (as present in milk but also in foods containing lactose but not so labeled, ie, candy, breads, frankfurters, etc). Patients with congenital galactosemia maintained on a milk-free diet should have level of galactose-1-phosphate <2 mg/100 mL lysed packed red cells. If such patients are ingesting lactose (eg, drinking milk), levels of 9-20 mg/100 mL packed red cell lysate will be obtained.[1] A range of characteristic abnormalities result from galactose toxicity including failure to thrive, vomiting, abnormal liver function with resultant cirrhosis, and mental retardation.[3] Signs and symptoms (including even cataracts) will regress under the influence of a galactose-free diet. An increased frequency of hypergonadotropic hypogonadism in females (decreased or absent ovarian tissue) has been reported[4] and occurs especially in subjects in whom diet therapy was delayed.

Footnotes

1. O'Brien D, Ibbott FA, and Rodgerson DO, *Laboratory Manual of Pediatric Micro-Biochemical Techniques*, 4th ed, New York, NY: Hoeber, 1968, 149-52.
2. Diepenbrock F, Heckler R, Schickling H, et al, "Colorimetric Determination of Galactose and Galactose-1-Phosphate From Dried Blood," *Clin Biochem*, 1992, 25(1):37-9.
3. Segal S, "Disorders of Galactose Metabolism," *The Metabolic Basis of Inherited Disease*, 6th ed, Scriver CR, Beaudet AL, Sly WS, et al, eds, New York, NY: McGraw-Hill Inc, 1989, 453-80.
4. Kaufman FR, Kogut MD, Donnell GN, et al, "Hypergonadotropic Hypogonadism in Female Patients With Galactosemia," *N Engl J Med*, 1981, 304:994-8.

References

Applegarth DA, Dimmick JE, and Toone JR, "Laboratory Detection of Metabolic Disease," *Pediatr Clin North Am*, 1989, 36(1):49-65.

Beutler E, "Galactosemia: Screening and Diagnosis," *Clin Biochem*, 1991, 24(4):293-300.

Reichardt JK, Packman S, and Woo SL, "Molecular Characterization of Two Galactosemia Mutations: Correlation of Mutations With Highly Conserved Domains in Galactose-1-Phosphate Uridyl Transferase," *Am J Hum Genet*, 1991, 49(4):860-7.

Galactose-1-Phosphate Uridyl Transferase, Erythrocyte

***CPT** 82775*

Applies to Galactokinase Deficiency; UDP Galactose-4-Epimerase Deficiency

Specimen Erythrocytes **CONTAINER:** Green top (heparin) tube, lavender top (EDTA) tube **STORAGE INSTRUCTIONS:** Stable 14 days at room temperature, 4 weeks at 4°C; do not freeze. **SPECIAL INSTRUCTIONS:** Always include a blood sample from a control individual.

Interpretive **REFERENCE RANGE:** 17-37 units (μmol/hour/g hemoglobin) **USE:** Diagnose galactosemia (galactose-1-phosphate uridyl transferase deficiency). Two other enzyme deficiencies cause galactosemia, galactokinase, and UDP galactose-4-epimerase. **METHODOLOGY:** Radioactive with ^{14}C-galactose-1-phosphate as the substrate; colorimetric (dried blood)[1] **ADDITIONAL INFORMATION:** Galactosemia is an autosomal recessive disorder of galactose metabolism most often caused by a deficiency of galactose-1-phosphate uridyl transferase, rarely by a deficiency of galactokinase or UDP galactose-4-epimerase. Molecular genetic studies have revealed molecular heterogeneity which is related to the variable clinical outcome observed in this disorder.[2] The resulting accumulation of galactitol and/or galactose-1-phosphate can result in juvenile cataracts, liver failure, failure to thrive, and mental retardation in galactose-1-phosphate uridyl transferase deficiency. Dietary restriction of galactose is a very effective treatment, and liver and lens changes are reversible. Quantitative assays, in addition to diagnosing transferase deficiency, can identify heterozygous transferase deficient carriers and homozygous transferase variants (Duarte variants). Blood for galactosemia screening should be obtained as early in life as possible (less than 3-4 days) so that effective therapy can be instituted.

Footnotes

1. Diepenbrock F, Heckler R, Schickling H, et al, "Colorimetric Determination of Galactose and Galactose-1-Phosphate From Dried Blood," *Clin Biochem*, 1992, 25(1):37-9.
2. Reichardt JK, Packman S, and Woo SL, "Molecular Characterization of Two Galactosemia Mutations: Correlation of Mutations With Highly Conserved Domains in Galactose-1-Phosphate Uridyl Transferase," *Am J Hum Genet*, 1991, 49(4):860-7.

References

Kelley RI and Segal S, "Evaluation of Reduced Activity Galactose-1-Phosphate Uridyl Transferase by Combined Radioisotopic Assay and High-Resolution Isoelectric Focusing," *J Lab Clin Med*, 1989, 114(2):152-6.

(Continued)

Galactose-1-Phosphate Uridyl Transferase, Erythrocyte *(Continued)*

Lagrou K and Declercq PE, "Simplified Assay of Galactose-1-Phosphate Uridyltransferase," *Clin Chem*, 1991, 37(12):2157-8.

Galactose Screening Tests for Galactosemia

CPT *82760*

Related Information

Galactokinase, Blood *on page 226*
Galactose-1-Phosphate *on page 226*
T_4 Newborn Screen *on page 357*

Synonyms Beutler Test; Blood Spot Screen for Galactose/Galactose-1-Phosphate; Paigen Test (*E. coli* Bacteriophage Resistance to Lysis Assay)

Test Commonly Includes Combinations of screening tests for red cell galactose/galactose-1-phosphate (increase) and red cell galactose-1-phosphate uridyltransferase (absence)

Abstract Effective screening test/tests for three inherited disorders causing galactosemia. Prompt treatment can reverse the potential for nutritional failure, mental retardation, cataracts, and liver disease attendant upon these conditions.

Specimen Whole blood, dried as a spot on filter paper; may use heparinized whole blood **SAMPLING TIME:** Screening should be performed within the first 3 days of life but may be method/diet dependent. **COLLECTION:** Drop of whole blood soaked into provided filter paper. See Phenylalanine, Blood test listing for collection details. **STORAGE INSTRUCTIONS:** Avoid exposure to high temperature during transit to the laboratory (eg, especially during heat of summer) (applies primarily to Beutler test).[1] **CAUSES FOR REJECTION:** Insufficient or improper application of blood to filter paper spot, excessive exposure to heat, specimen paper without proper label/identification, blood collected in acid-citrate-dextrose or EDTA in some cases[2]

Interpretive **REFERENCE RANGE:** Normal neonates: blood galactose <1 mg/dL (SI: <0.06 mmol/L) in 88%, 1-5 mg/dL (SI: 0.06-0.28 mmol/L) in 12% of cases. Galactosemic infants usually have blood galactose >20 mg/dL (SI: >1.11 mmol/L) (Paigen test);[3] presence of galactose transferase is the normal condition (Beutler-Baluda test).[2] **USE:** Detect galactosemia; monitor dietary therapy of galactosemia **LIMITATIONS:** Antibiotics present in the sample have not yet been reported to result in a false-negative in the Paigen test (*E. coli* bacteriophage resistance to lysis), see following information. The Beutler-Baluda test will detect transferase deficient cases of galactosemia only (galactose kinase and epimerase deficiencies although uncommon, would be missed). The Paigen screen for increased RBC galactose/galactose-1-phosphate, if positive, should be followed by a transferase screen (eg, Beutler test) which, if negative, would indicate a different cause for the galactosemia (eg, galactose kinase or epimerase deficiency, see following information). A galactose screening test that is not sensitive also to galactose-1-phosphate will require that the newborn have ingested milk prior to testing or a false-positive result may be obtained. **Transfusion may result in a false-negative Beutler-Baluda test for as long as 2-3 months.** **METHODOLOGY:** Urine can be screened for galactosuria by reagents usually commonly available in the Urinalysis and/or Chemistry sections of most clinical laboratories. Specimen is first tested for reducing substances by a cupric ion reduction method (eg, Benedict's Test, Clinitest® tablets). If positive, a glucose oxidase specific method is applied. If the specific test for glucose is negative, but a reducing substance is present, there is presumptive evidence for one of the three forms of galactosemia.

Screening programs for galactosemia have been established by most states in the United States and many countries of the world. Ease of specimen transport to high volume reference laboratories favors dried blood spot over urine testing. A variety of applicable tests utilizing whole blood samples spotted on filter paper have been described.[4]

The Beutler test has a fluorescent end point, tests for deficiency of galactose-1-phosphate uridyltransferase, and can be performed rapidly. Fluorescence may be delayed, however, in infants with partial enzyme deficiency (eg, heterozygotes for transferase deficiency or with the Duarte variant).[2]

The Paigen assay screens for increase in galactose and galactose-1-phosphate. It is the most effective **single** test available for all forms of galactosemia.[4] The procedure uses a strain of *E. coli* that resists C21 bacteriophage lysis in the presence of galactose. Thus, bacterial growth occurs around filter paper blood spots in cases of galactosemia. In the absence of galactose (normal nongalactosemic newborn), no growth occurs as the bacteria are killed by the phage. The diameter of the growth zone is proportional to the concentration of galactose.[3]

An enzymatic centrifugal analyzer chemical method has been developed. Galactose is determined by measuring the change in absorbance of reduced NADH at 340 nm after addition of galactose dehydrogenase.[5] A presumptive positive is defined as a blood galactose plus galactose-1-phosphate level of >0.30 mmol/L. Each presumptive positive is also screened with a Beutler spot test to assess transferase activity. This method for galactosemia screening is rapid, sensitive and may be the method of choice for mass screening.[5] A microplate fluorometric method based on the GADH-NAD^+/NADH system has similar advantages to the Manitoba system noted above, is rapid, reliable, and applicable to routine screening of newborns.[6]

Third generation cephalosporin antibiotics may cause false-positive results in *E. coli* W5 based tests (in which presence of galactose inhibits bacterial growth).[7] Presence of galactosemia, however, is not excluded, until another sample is appropriately tested by a different method.

ADDITIONAL INFORMATION: Galactosemia may occur with any of three metabolic abnormalities but is usually the result of an inherited deficiency of galactose-1-phosphate uridyltransferase activity. This condition, if undetected and untreated, is characterized clinically by failure to thrive, vomiting, cataracts, mental retardation, liver disease, and death. Incidence, generally is about 1:60,000 but estimates worldwide have ranged from 1:18,000 to 1:180,000. A number of starch gel electrophoretic variants have been defined of which the Duarte and Los Angeles variants are the most common (see reference by Segal). The Duarte variant is characterized by intermediate levels of transferase (higher than those of the classical deficiency) and by an electrophoretically distinctive enzyme. Duarte form appears clinically benign. The Indiana variant is an unstable electrophoretically distinct enzyme. Individuals with Los Angeles variant do not have abnormal galactose metabolism.

Deficiency of cellular galactokinase results in a galactose toxicity that is usually milder and limited to development of cataracts.

The third cause of galactosemia, uridine diphosphate galactose-4-epimerase deficiency, occurs in two forms. One involves only red and white blood cells and is benign. The second form is unusual and requires care in dietary management. It manifests as does transferase deficiency and responds to dietary restriction of galactose. A low level of galactose must be maintained in the diet, however, since epimerase is involved in supplying UDP-galactose for complex carbohydrate, galactolipid and galactoprotein synthesis. While estimates of incidence of galactokinase and epimerase deficiencies have been in the 1:20,000 to 1:40,000 range, very few clinically deficient cases have been reported as compared to cases of transferase deficiency. The enzyme deficiencies responsible for galactosemia have an autosomal recessive mode of inheritance.

Galactose is present normally in blood and urine but in very low concentration, serum, 0.70 mg/dL (SI: 0.04 mmol/L); urine, 4 mg/dL (SI: 0.22 mmol/L). Urine from normal newborns may have levels of galactose as high as 60 mg/dL (SI: 3.33 mmol/L) urine (physiologic melituria); in premature infants this may occur over the first 2 weeks of life.[8] High level of milk intake may also produce galactosuria.[9] In cases of galactosemia, galactosuria may be intermittent (partly relating to the intake of milk) and may be missed if urine is very dilute. A screening program based on a copper reduction test, then, may result in false-negatives. Early identification and treatment of the infant with galactosemia is critical as cataracts, mental retardation, liver disease with hepatosplenomegaly, and death due to septicemia (in particular, *E. coli* septicemia) may occur in the untreated individual. Specific enzyme assays should be employed to define abnormalities detected by screening tests.

Footnotes

1. American Academy of Pediatrics, Committee on Genetics, "Newborn Screening Fact Sheets: Galactosemia," *Pediatrics*, 1989, 83:458-60.
2. Beutler E and Baluda MC, "A Simple Spot Screening Test for Galactosemia," *J Lab Clin Med*, 1966, 68:137-41.
3. Paigen K, Pacholec F, and Levy HL, "A New Method of Screening for Inherited Disorders of Galactose Metabolism," *J Lab Clin Med*, 1982, 88:895-907.
4. Levy HL and Hammersen G, "Newborn Screening for Galactosemia and Other Galactose Metabolic Defects," *J Pediatr*, 1978, 92:871-7.
5. Greenberg CR, Dilling LA, Thompson R, et al, "Newborn Screening for Galactosemia: A New Method Used in Manitoba," *Pediatrics*, 1989, 84(2):331-5.
6. Yamaguchi A, Fukushi M, Mizushima Y, et al, "Microassay for Screening Newborns for Galactosemia With Use of a Fluorometric Microplate Reader," *Clin Chem*, 1989, 35(9):1962-4.
7. Schunk JP, Bradley JS, Buist NR, et al, "Interference by Third Generation Cephalosporins With Neonatal Screening for Galactosemia," *J Pediatr*, 1988, 112(5):842, (letter).

(Continued)

Galactose Screening Tests for Galactosemia *(Continued)*

8. Dahlquist A and Svenningsen NW, "Galactose in the Urine of Newborn Infants," *J Pediatr*, 1969, 75:454.
9. Holl WK, Cravey CE, Chen PT, et al, "An Evaluation of Galactosuria," *J Pediatr*, 1970, 77:625.

References

Applegarth DA, Dimmick JE, and Toone JR, "Laboratory Detection of Metabolic Disease," *Pediatr Clin North Am*, 1989, 36(1):49-65.

Berry HK and Croft CC, "Reagent That Restores Galactose-1-Phosphate Uridyltransferase Activity in Dry Blood Spots," *Clin Chem*, 1987, 33:1471-2.

Kirby LT, Norman MG, Applegarth DA, et al, "Screening of Newborn Infants for Galactosemia in British Columbia," *Can Med Assoc J*, 1985, 132:1033-5.

Segal S, "Disorders of Galactose Metabolism," *The Metabolic Basis of Inherited Disease*, 6th ed, Scriver CR, Beaudet AL, Sly WS, et al, eds, New York, NY: McGraw-Hill Inc, 1989, 453-80.

Sokol RJ, McCabe ER, Kotzer AM, et al, "Pitfalls in Diagnosing Galactosemia: False-Negative Newborn Screening Following Red Blood Cell Transfusion," *J Pediatr Gastroenterol Nutr*, 1989, 8(2):266-8.

Gamma Glutamyl Transferase

***CPT** 82977*

Related Information

Alkaline Phosphatase, Heat Stable *on page 106*
Alkaline Phosphatase Isoenzymes *on page 107*
Alkaline Phosphatase, Serum *on page 109*
Bilirubin, Total *on page 139*
Leucine Aminopeptidase *on page 276*
5' Nucleotidase *on page 297*

Synonyms Gamma Glutamyl Transpeptidase; GGT; GGTP; Glutamyl Transpeptidase; GT; GTP

Applies to Body Fluid GGT

Replaces BSP

Patient Care **PREPARATION:** The patient ideally should fast for 8 hours prior to collection of the specimen. Since elevations may occur with phenytoin or phenobarbital therapy, one of the alternate tests, leucine aminopeptidase (LAP) or 5' nucleotidase, is preferable in such patients.

Specimen Serum **CONTAINER:** Red top tube **STORAGE INSTRUCTIONS:** Hemolysis and prolonged contact with erythrocytes do not interfere. Stable 1 month at 4°C and 1 year at -20°C.[1]

Interpretive **REFERENCE RANGE:** Varies between laboratories. The following is appropriate only for some laboratories: higher in newborns, in first 3-6 months; male, 6 months and older: 15-85 units/L; female, 6 months and older: 5-55 units/L. Values in adult males are 25% higher than adult females. **USE:** A biliary enzyme that is especially useful in the diagnosis of obstructive jaundice, intrahepatic cholestasis, and pancreatitis.[2] GGT is more responsive to biliary obstruction than are aspartate aminotransferase (AST) (SGOT) and alanine aminotransferase (ALT) (SGPT).

Increased in hepatoma and carcinoma of pancreas. Useful in diagnosis of metastatic carcinoma in the liver. Increasing levels in carcinoma patients relate to tumor progression and diminishing levels to response to treatment.[3] CEA, alkaline phosphatase, and GGT used together are useful markers for hepatic metastasis from breast and colon primaries. GGT is elevated in some instances of seminoma.

Useful in diagnosis of chronic alcoholic liver disease, but some heavy drinkers do not have GGT increases. Serial determinations of serum GGT, AST, and ALT levels can distinguish recovering alcoholics who resume drinking from those who remain abstinent.[4,5] Increase in body mass is positively correlated with increased GGT levels.[6] With MCV of red cells, GGT is useful as a screen for alcoholism.

GGT is the test for cholestasis during or immediately following pregnancy. Commonly elevated in cirrhosis and hepatitis. The transaminases, AST and ALT rise higher in acute viral hepatitis; these tests with GGT and other parameters are best used together in work-up of liver disease.

Increased in systemic lupus erythematosus.[3] Very high levels are common in primary biliary cirrhosis. High GGT is found in infants with biliary atresia. It is increased with hyperthyroidism and decreased in those with hypothyroidism.[7] GGT is comparable in many ways to two other biliary tests, LAP and 5' nucleotidase. In some cases, five tests (including alkaline phosphatase and bilirubin) are necessary to evaluate the biliary tract. GGT usually is the most sensitive.

In **ascitic fluid**, very high GGT is increased in some, but not all cases of hepatoma, as opposed to cirrhosis or liver metastases. As in serum, it is high in the ascitic fluid of those with alcoholic cirrhosis.[8]

LIMITATIONS: Acetaminophen toxicity has been reported to cause an *in vivo* increase. The combination of high alkaline phosphatase and normal GGT does not rule out liver disease completely. Activity is not significantly increased in sera of patients with lymphoma (unless there is hepatic involvement by the lymphoma). Baden et al concluded that as a preoperative screening test for metastasis with colorectal carcinoma, GGT is unsatisfactory.[9] As part of a screening battery for carcinoma patients, 19% of GGT results from patients with progressive disease were not abnormal, and 4% of values from patients without evidence of tumor were high.[3] **METHODOLOGY:** Kinetic **ADDITIONAL INFORMATION:** GGT is helpful to work up elevated alkaline phosphatase values. GGT is a biliary excretory enzyme which is more specific for hepatic disease than is alkaline phosphatase. It is normal in most instances of renal failure.[10] GGT has no origin in bone or placenta, unlike alkaline phosphatase, and age beyond infancy does not influence GGT levels. Activity of GGT is highest in obstructive liver disease. It is commonly elevated in patients with infectious mononucleosis. When GGT and alkaline phosphatase are both high, but one is disproportionately elevated, suspect the possibility of drug-induced cholestasis (including alcoholism if it is GGT which is much higher). GGT, postprandial glucose, and triglyceride bear some correlation in certain groups of patients, including alcoholism and diabetes mellitus. Treatment of hypertriglyceridemia may also lead to decreased GGT. **GGT is normal** in normal children, adolescents, and in pregnant women. Unlike AST, it is not elevated in skeletal muscle disease.

Footnotes

1. Tietz NW, *Clinical Guide to Laboratory Tests*, Tietz NW, ed, Philadelphia, PA: WB Saunders Co, 1990, 262.
2. Stein TA, Burns GP, and Wise L, "Diagnostic Value of Liver Function Tests in Bile Duct Obstruction," *J Surg Res*, 1989, 46(3):226-9.
3. Sahm DF, Murray JL, Munson PL, et al, "Gamma Glutamyl Transpeptidase Levels as an Aid in the Management of Human Cancer," *Cancer*, 1983, 52:1673-8.
4. Irwin M, Baird S, Smith TL, et al, "Use of Laboratory Tests to Monitor Heavy Drinking by Alcoholic Men Discharged From a Treatment Program," *Am J Psychiatry*, 1988, 145(5):595-9.
5. Frimpong NA and Lapp JA, "Effects of Moderate Alcohol Intake in Fixed or Variable Amounts on Concentration of Serum Lipids and Liver Enzymes in Healthy Young Men," *Am J Clin Nutr*, 1989, 50(5):987-91.
6. Robinson D and Whitehead TP, "Effect of Body Mass and Other Factors on Serum Liver Enzyme Levels in Men Attending for Well Population Screening," *Ann Clin Biochem*, 1989, 26(Pt 5):393-400.
7. Schaffner F, "Tests Related to the Liver," *Gastroenterology*, 4th ed, Berk JE, ed, Vol 1, Philadelphia, PA: WB Saunders Co, 1985, 410-26.
8. Kjeldsberg CR and Knight JA, *Body Fluids – Laboratory Examination of Amniotic, Cerebrospinal, Seminal, Serous, and Synovial Fluids*, 3rd ed, Chicago, IL: ASCP Press, 1993, 235.
9. Baden H, Andersen B, Augustenborg G, et al, "Diagnostic Value of Gamma Glutamyl Transpeptidase and Alkaline Phosphatase in Liver Metastases," *Surg Gynecol Obstet*, 1971, 133:769-73.
10. Lum G and Gambino SR, "Serum Gamma Glutamyl Transpeptidase Activity as an Indicator of Disease of Liver, Pancreas, or Bone," *Clin Chem*, 1972, 18:358-62.

References

Artur Y and Gouy D, "Gamma Glutamyltransferase," *Drug Effects on Laboratory Test Results Analytical Interferences and Pharmacological Effects*, Siest G and Galteau MM, eds, Littleton, MA: PSG Publishing Co Inc, 1988, 224-40.

Brotman B and Prince AM, "Gamma Glutamyltransferase as a Potential Surrogate Marker for Detection of the Non-A, Non-B Carrier State," *Vox Sang*, 1988, 54:144-7.

Gjerde H, Amundsen A, Skog OJ, et al, "Serum Gamma Glutamyltransferase: An Epidemiological Indicator of Alcohol Consumption?" *Br J Addict*, 1987, 82:1027-31.

Gamma Glutamyl Transpeptidase *see* Gamma Glutamyl Transferase *on previous page*

Gap *see* Anion Gap *on page 132*

Gases, Arterial *see* Blood Gases, Arterial *on page 140*

Gastric Analysis

***CPT** 82926 (gastric acid, free and total single specimen); 89135 (gastric intubation aspiration and fractional collections, 1 hour); 89136 (2 hours); 89140 (2 hours with gastric stimulation, eg, pentagastrin); 89141 (3 hours with gastric stimulation)*

Related Information

Gastrin, Serum *on page 234*
Helicobacter pylori Urease Test and Culture *on page 820*
Intrinsic Factor Antibody *on page 714*
Parietal Cell Antibody *on page 730*

Synonyms Pentagastrin Stimulation Test; Peptavlon® Stimulation Test

Replaces Gastric Analysis, Nocturnal Acid Output; Histalog™ Stimulation Test; Tubeless Gastric Analysis

Test Commonly Includes Basal and four poststimulation specimens for pH, volume, and acid output

Patient Care PREPARATION: Antacids and H_2-receptor antagonists should not be given to patient for 24-48 hours prior to testing. Drugs that affect gastric acid secretion, such as tricyclic antidepressants, anticholinergics, reserpine, and so forth should be discontinued overnight to 72 hours prior to testing. The patient must fast after the evening meal on the day prior to the test day, but may have water up to 1 hour before the test. After pentagastrin has been administered, medical supervision should be maintained since side reactions may occur.

Specimen Gastric secretions, four 15-minute basal and four 15-minute poststimulation collections. Entire volume collected. Longer periods are sometimes used (eg, 24-hour measurement) but are not well standardized and may be dangerous. CONTAINER: Clean containers, no preservative COLLECTION: A cold lubricated gastric (Levine) tube is inserted orally or nasally while the patient is in a sitting or reclining position on his/her left side. The tube must have a radiopaque tip. Nasal intubation is used if the patient has a hyperactive gag reflex. It should be positioned in the stomach so that the tip is opposite the angularis or "re-entrant angle" in the most dependent portion of the stomach. In a patient who has had a subtotal gastrectomy, the tube should be placed well within the lumen of the stomach, below the fundus and above the anastomosis. Proper positioning of the tube is confirmed by fluoroscopy or x-ray. Wait 10-15 minutes for the patient to adjust to the tube. The patient should be in a sitting position. Gentle constant suction is needed, except for brief intervals when a small quantity of air can be injected to clear the tube. The first two or three specimens immediately following intubation (the first 15-30 minutes) should not be utilized as basal secretion as they do not accurately reflect the basal state. Give no liquids to the patient during the test and request that the patient expectorate saliva. The basal specimen is obtained by continuous aspiration of the gastric fluid with a Toomey syringe for 60 minutes as four 15-minute specimens. These are the BAO (basal acid output). After the basal sample has been collected, pentagastrin is injected (6 μg/kg body weight) subcutaneously with a tuberculin syringe (see package insert). The collection of the poststimulation specimens must begin immediately. The gastric content is continuously aspirated for the next 60 minutes, during which time the gastric contents obtained from each of four 15-minute periods are collected into separate plastic containers labeled poststimulation number 1, 2, 3 and 4 respectively. (Some institutions use six 15-minute samples.) Securely fasten the lids on the containers and send the eight specimens (four basal and four poststimulation) to the laboratory. The containers must identify the order in which the specimens were collected. STORAGE INSTRUCTIONS: Refrigerate if test delayed more than 4 hours. CAUSES FOR REJECTION: Contamination of specimens with duodenal contents, indicated by the yellow color of bile

Interpretive REFERENCE RANGE: Normal gastric juice may be clear or contain some bile. If red or black, test for blood.

Normal BAO is up to 10.5 mmol/hour (men) and 5.6 mmol/hour (women). BAO represents gastric acid secretion in the absence of stimulation. It follows circadian rhythm and is highest from 2-11 PM. Brady et al define basal hypersecretion as basal acid output >11 mmol/hour (men) and 6 mmol/hour (women). They describe features of patients with *Helicobacter pylori* (*Campylobacter pylori*) according to acid secretory status.[1]

Normal MAO (maximal acid output) is up to 48 mmol/hour (men) and 30 mmol/hour (women). MAO is the sum of four 15-minute collections following pentagastrin.

Normal PAO (peak and output) is 11-60 mmol/hour (men) and 8-40 mmol/hour (women).

Normal BAO to PAO is 0.29 (men) and 0.23 (women).

USE: Evaluate gastric function. Support the diagnosis of pernicious anemia: work up gastric mucosal atrophy, recurrent peptic ulcer, Zollinger-Ellison (Z-E) syndrome, Ménétrier's disease. Ménétrier's disease is not sharply defined in terms of surgical pathology. **Gastrinoma/ Zollinger-Ellison syndrome** can lead to peptic ulcer with massive acid secretion. The Zollinger-Ellison syndrome is characterized by the presence of nonbeta neuroendocrine tumors which secrete gastrin. The diagnosis of the Zollinger-Ellison syndrome is established by demonstration of gastric acid hypersecretion, basal acid secretion $>$15 mmol/hour in an unoperated subject with peptic ulcer, with fasting gastrin level $>$1000 pg/mL (SI: $>$1000 ng/L).[2]

Pernicious anemia: Anacidity has been an essential component for the diagnosis of PA. High gastrin levels are found, *vide infra*.

Gastritis: Severe gastritis with mucosal atrophy is associated with anacidity or is thought to produce progressive loss of secretory ability. Availability of superior endoscopy has diminished indications for gastric analysis for gastritis.

Gastric carcinoma: Few if any cases clinically, endoscopically and/or radiologically considered to be carcinoma, presently have gastric analysis. Gastric carcinoma and gastric polyps, classically, have often been associated with decreased-to-absent hydrochloric acid. Of course, carcinoma occurs without anacidity and anacidity occurs without carcinoma. The demonstration of complete anacidity to maximal stimulation in the presence of a gastric ulcer supports (but does not prove) a diagnosis of malignancy. Patients with gastric ulcers generally show low to normal basal and maximum acid output.

LIMITATIONS: Tube not in proper place for aspiration, incomplete volume collection. Losses of gastric juice into the duodenum occur, especially in patients who have had pyloroplasty or gastroenterostomy.

Gastric analysis itself is insufficient for the diagnosis of gastrinoma. Substantial overlap exists between patients with gastrinoma, with common duodenal ulcer and normal subjects in rates of gastric acid output.[2] Gastric analysis is time consuming, uncomfortable for the patient and it is expensive.

CONTRAINDICATIONS: Gastric intubation is contraindicated for patients with esophageal varices, diverticula, stenosis, malignant neoplasm of the esophagus, aortic aneurysm, severe gastric hemorrhage, and congestive heart failure. It is not necessary for the usual duodenal ulcer patient in whom the Zollinger-Ellison is not suspected.

Patient must not receive medication that influences gastric secretion; such contraindications include antacids, anticholinergic drugs, reserpine, alcohol, adrenergic blocking agents, and adrenocorticosteroids.

Histalog™ is contraindicated in patients with a history of asthma or paroxysmal hypertension, but asthmatics, severely hyperallergenic problems are thought not to be contraindications when pentagastrin is used as the stimulant (see package insert). Hypersensitivity or idiosyncrasy to pentagastrin is described. Histalog™ should not be given if the patient's systolic pressure is $<$110 mm Hg.

METHODOLOGY: Volume measurement, pH measurement by pH meter. Do not use pH paper.[3] Peak acid output (PAO) is a calculation, in which the two highest 15-minute MAO specimens are combined and multiplied by 2. **ADDITIONAL INFORMATION:** "Anacidity" is regarded as pH $>$6 following stimulation. If specimens become grossly bloody, physician should be contacted to ascertain if procedure should be continued. Confirm if indicated with a test for hemoglobin.

Basal gastric analysis: Specimens should be collected at 15-minute intervals for 1 hour, labeled basal 1, basal 2, etc, and sent to the laboratory.

Maximal stimulation gastric analysis: This measures the response to maximal stimulation by pentagastrin, 6 μg/kg body weight, given subcutaneously, with a tuberculin syringe. This material is administered after collection of the basal specimens. Thirty minutes after administration of pentagastrin, four to six 15-minute specimens of gastric juice are aspirated as described, labeled "Max 1", "2", etc, and sent to the laboratory. The patient should be observed regularly, preferably by the physician. With proper precautions, side effects are rare.

Availability of assays for gastrin diminish the need for gastric analysis.

Contemporary work-up for pernicious anemia (PA) includes vitamin B_{12}/folate assays, Schilling test and sometimes, testing for antibodies to intrinsic factor and to parietal cells.

Of 36 subjects with *Helicobacter pylori* (*Campylobacter pylori*) who underwent gastric analysis, 25 were normochlorhydric and 11 were hypochlorhydric. Nineteen normochlorhydric pa-

(Continued)

Gastric Analysis *(Continued)*

tients had ulcers (10 gastric and 9 duodenal). Two hypochlorhydric patients had gastric ulcers. These authors were unable to identify a consistent relationship between *Helicobacter pylori* (*Campylobacter pylori*) and acid secretion.[1] Several studies showed that *H. pylori* is not a major contributing factor in duodenal ulcer associated with Z-E syndrome.[4,5]

Footnotes

1. Brady CE 3d, Hadfield TL, Hyatt JR, et al, "Acid Secretion and Serum Gastrin Levels in Individuals With *Campylobacter pylori*," *Gastroenterology*, 1988, 94(4):923-7.
2. Wolfe MM, "Diagnosis of Gastrinoma: Much Ado About Nothing?" *Ann Intern Med*, 1989, 111(9):697-9.
3. Caballero GA, Ausman RK, Quebbeman EJ, et al, "Gastric Secretion pH Measurement: What You See Is Not What You Get!" *Crit Care Med*, 1990, 18(4):396-9.
4. Saeed ZA, Evans DJ Jr, Evans DG, et al, "*Helicobacter pylori* and Zollinger-Ellison Syndrome," *Dig Dis Sci*, 1991, 36(1):15-8.
5. Fich A, Talley NJ, Shorter RG, et al, "Zollinger-Ellison Syndrome. Relation to *Helicobacter pylori*-Associated Chronic Gastritis and Gastric Acid Secretion," *Dig Dis Sci*, 1991, 36(1):10-4.

References

Andersen DK, "Current Diagnosis and Management of Zollinger-Ellison Syndrome," *Ann Surg*, 1989, 210(6):685-703.

Berg CL and Wolfe MM, "Zollinger-Ellison Syndrome," *Med Clin North Am*, 1991, 75(4):903-21.

Dooley CP, Cohen H, Fitzgibbons PL, et al, "Prevalence of *Helicobacter pylori* Infection and Histologic Gastritis in Asymptomatic Persons," *N Engl J Med*, 1989, 321(23):1562-6.

Feldman M, "Gastric Secretion in Health and Disease," *Gastrointestinal Disease: Pathophysiology Diagnosis Management*, 4th ed, Sleisenger MH and Fordtran JS, eds, Philadelphia, PA: WB Saunders Co, 1989, 713-34.

Fraker DL and Norton JA, "The Role of Surgery in the Management of Islet Cell Tumors," *Gastroenterol Clin North Am*, 1989, 18(4):805-30.

Malagelada JR, Davis CS, O'Fallon WM, et al, "Laboratory Diagnosis of Gastrinoma. 1. A Prospective Evaluation of Gastric Analysis and Fasting Serum Gastrin Levels," *Mayo Clin Proc*, 1982, 57:211-8.

Pisegna JR, Norton JA, Slimak GG, et al, "Effects of Curative Gastrinoma Resection on Gastric Secretory Function and Antisecretory Drug Requirement in the Zollinger-Ellison Syndrome," *Gastroenterology*, 1992, 102(3):767-78.

Segal HL, "Clinical Measurements of Gastric Secretion: Significance and Limitations," *Ann Intern Med*, 1960, 53:447.

Soybel DI and Modlin IM, "Sustained Suppression of Gastric Secretion and the Risk of Neoplasia in the Gastric Mucosa," *Am J Gastroenterol*, 1991, 86(12):1713-9.

Sparberg ME and Kersner JB, "Gastric Secretory Activity With Reference to HCl," *Arch Intern Med*, 1964, 114:508.

Gastric Analysis, Nocturnal Acid Output *replaced by* Gastric Analysis *on page 232*

Gastrin, Serum

CPT 82941

Related Information

Gastric Analysis *on page 232*
Helicobacter pylori Urease Test and Culture *on page 820*
Schilling Test *on page 598*
Vitamin B_{12} *on page 612*

Abstract Gastrin is normally produced by cells in the gastric antral mucosa.

Patient Care PREPARATION: The patient must be fasting overnight, preferably 12 hours or more. Protein meal can cause a marked increase in serum gastrin. No recent radioactive isotopes. Gastrin may be increased following gastroscopy.

Specimen Serum CONTAINER: Red top tube COLLECTION: Transport specimen immediately to the laboratory following collection. Postprandial specimens should be so indicated. STORAGE INSTRUCTIONS: Separate in a refrigerated centrifuge and freeze immediately. Stable 4 hours at 4°C and 30 days at -20°C. CAUSES FOR REJECTION: Avoid anticoagulated tubes for this assay.

Interpretive REFERENCE RANGE: Fasting: up to 100 pg/mL (SI: 47.7 pmol/L) (up to 200 pg/mL (SI: 95.3 pmol/L) in some laboratories). Postprandial: 95-140 pg/mL (SI: 45.3-66.7 pmol/L) usually under 250 pg/mL (SI: 119.2 pmol/L). Secretin stimulation is positive if the serum gastrin rises 200 pg/mL (SI: 95.3 pmol/L) or more anytime following secretin administration.[1] USE: Diagnose Zollinger-Ellison (Z-E) syndrome; diagnose gastrinoma. Gastrin >1000 pg/mL (SI: >476.6 pmol/L) with gastric acid hypersecretion (basal acid secretion over 15 mmol/hour in a patient with peptic ulcer who has not had surgery) establishes unequivocally the diagnosis of the Zollinger-Ellison syndrome.[2] Antral G-cell hyperplasia may relate to high gastrin levels and duodenal ulcer. **LIMITATIONS:** Gastric hyperacidity must be documented. Gastric ulcer, chronic renal failure, hyperparathyroidism, pyloric obstruction, carcinoma of stomach,[3] vagotomy without gastric resection, retained gastric antrum and short bowel syndrome have been reported with moderate elevations of gastrin levels. Gastrin levels are increased with pernicious anemia. H_2-receptor blockers (cimetidine) may result in elevated levels. Overlap of serum gastrin values between gastrinoma and other states occurs. Up to 40% of Z-E patients have fasting gastrin values between 100-500 pg/mL (SI: 47.7-238.3 pmol/L), while a few patients with gastric or duodenal ulcer without gastrinoma, have results in this range. At least half of patients with the Z-E syndrome lack diagnostic serum gastrin levels, although in nearly all, fasting serum gastrin levels are increased.[2] One report describes a patient with Z-E syndrome with a normal screening gastrin level.[4] **METHODOLOGY:** Radioimmunoassay (RIA) **ADDITIONAL INFORMATION:** Gastrin is secreted by antral G cells and stimulates gastric acid production, antral motility, and secretion of pepsin and intrinsic factor. The principle forms of gastrin in blood are G-34 (big gastrin, half-life 5 minutes) and G-14 (minigastrin, half-life 5 minutes). Each of these polypeptides circulates in nonsulfated (I) or sulfated (II) forms. Instilling acid into the stomach normally inhibits gastrin secretion. Elevated gastrin levels should be interpreted in light of gastric acid secretion and other parameters. The neuroendocrine tumors associated with the Zollinger-Ellison syndrome are characterized by elevated rates of gastric HCl secretion and upper gastrointestinal ulcer disease. Gastrin levels >500-600 pg/mL (SI: >238-286 pmol/L) in a patient with basal acid hypersecretion often indicates gastrinoma, but antral G-cell hyperplasia cases can have gastrin levels >500 pg/mL and hyperchlorhydria. If gastrinoma is likely but fasting gastrin level is not diagnostic, the secretin test is the provocative test of choice. Absolute increase in serum gastrin level above the basal figure is preferred to percent change.[2] I.V. secretin normally diminishes gastrin, but serum gastrin increases in gastrinoma patients. Wolfe provides an explanation for this paradoxical effect.[2] Calcium infusion also stimulates gastrin release but does not distinguish other causes of ulcer as well as the secretin test. Protocols for stimulation tests are published.[5]

Fifteen percent to 26% of Z-E patients have evidence of Werner's syndrome (multiple endocrine neoplasia type 1). It may include hyperparathyroidism, islet cell tumors of the pancreas, pituitary tumors, Cushing's syndrome (adrenal glands), and hyperparathyroidism.[6] Gastrinoma are malignant in 62% of cases, and 44% of patients have metastases.

No consistent relationship has been established between *Helicobacter pylori* (*Campylobacter pylori*) and gastric acid secretion or serum gastrin levels.[1]

Features of gastrinoma additional to those of peptic ulcer may include diarrhea and steatorrhea.

Gastrinomas are usually found in the pancreas but they may be primary in the duodenum. A few cases in which a gastrinoma was primary in the stomach have been reported. The morphology is that of foregut carcinoids.[7]

Somatostatin inhibits the expression of gastrin mRNA.[8]

Footnotes

1. Brady CE 3d, Hadfield TL, Hyatt JR, et al, "Acid Secretion and Serum Gastrin Levels in Individuals With *Campylobacter pylori*," *Gastroenterology*, 1988, 94(4):923-7.
2. Wolfe MM, "Diagnosis of Gastrinoma: Much Ado About Nothing?" *Ann Intern Med*, 1989, 111(9):697-9.
3. Rakic S and Milicevic MN, "Serum Gastrin Levels in Patients With Intestinal and Diffuse Type of Gastric Cancer," *Br J Cancer*, 1991, 64(6):1189.
4. Yanda RJ, Ostroff JW, Ashbaugh CD, et al, "Zollinger-Ellison Syndrome in a Patient With Normal Screening Gastrin Level," *Dig Dis Sci*, 1989, 34(12):1929-32.
5. Malagelada JR, Glanzman SL, and GO VLW, "Laboratory Diagnosis of Gastrinoma. II. A Prospective Study of Gastrin Challenge Tests," *Mayo Clin Proc*, 1982, 57:219-26.
6. Jensen RT, Gardner JD, Raufman JP, et al, "Zollinger-Ellison Syndrome: Current Concepts and Management," *Ann Intern Med*, 1983, 98:59-75.
7. Wilander E, "Endocrine Cell Tumours," *Gastrointestinal and Oesophageal Pathology*, Whitehead R, ed, New York, NY: Churchill Livingstone, 1989, 629-41.
8. Karnik PS, Monahan SJ, and Wolfe MM, "Inhibition of Gastrin Gene Expression by Somatostatin," *J Clin Invest*, 1989, 83(2):367-72.

References

den Hartog G, van der Meer JWM, Jansen JBMJ, et al, "Decreased Gastrin Secretion in Patients With Late-Onset Hypogammaglobulinemia," *N Engl J Med*, 1988, 318:1563-7.

Fraker DL and Norton JA, "The Role of Surgery in the Management of Islet Cell Tumors," *Gastroenterol Clin North Am*, 1989, 18(4):805-30.

Green DW, Gomez G, and Greeley GH Jr, "Gastrointestinal Peptides," *Gastroenterol Clin North Am*, 1989, 18(4):695-733.

(Continued)

Gastrin, Serum *(Continued)*

Malagelada JR, Davis CS, O'Fallon WM, et al, "Laboratory Diagnosis of Gastrinoma. I. A Prospective Evaluation of Gastric Analysis and Fasting Serum Gastrin Levels," *Mayo Clin Proc*, 1982, 57:211-8.
McQuaid KR, "Much Ado About Gastrin," *J Clin Gastroenterol*, 1991, 13(3):249-54.
Solcia E, Capella C, Fiocca R, et al, "The Gastroenteropancreatic Endocrine System and Related Tumors," *Gastroenterol Clin North Am*, 1989, 18(4):671-93.
Warburton R and Close JR, "The *In Vitro* Stability of Gastrin in Serum and Whole Blood," *Ann Clin Biochem*, 1987, 24:320-1.
Wolfe MM, Jain DK, and Edgerton JR, "Zollinger-Ellison Syndrome Associated With Persistently Normal Fasting Serum Gastrin Concentrations," *Ann Intern Med*, 1985, 103:215-7.

Gestational Diabetes Screening Test *see* Glucose Tolerance Test *on page 241*

GFR *see* Creatinine Clearance *on page 201*

GGT *see* Gamma Glutamyl Transferase *on page 230*

GGTP *see* Gamma Glutamyl Transferase *on page 230*

GH *see* Growth Hormone *on page 245*

GHB *see* Glycated Hemoglobin *on page 244*

Globulin *see* Albumin, Serum *on page 102*

Globulin *see* Protein, Total, Serum *on page 340*

Glucagon *see* Vasoactive Intestinal Polypeptide *on page 384*

Glucagon, Plasma

CPT 82943

Related Information

Vasoactive Intestinal Polypeptide *on page 384*

Abstract A single chain polypeptide, glucagon is secreted, responding to hypoglycemia. Glucagonoma is a rare endocrine tumor reported in MEN I.[1]

Patient Care **PREPARATION:** Overnight fasting for basal levels. If diabetic, patient should be in good control before specimen is drawn.

Specimen Plasma **CONTAINER:** Draw blood into a chilled lavender top (EDTA) tube. Deliver to the laboratory immediately. **STORAGE INSTRUCTIONS:** Freeze. Stable 2 months at -20°C. **CAUSES FOR REJECTION:** Recent radioactive tracer (eg, for radioactive scan) **SPECIAL INSTRUCTIONS:** Mix the blood immediately and centrifuge in a refrigerated centrifuge.

Interpretive **REFERENCE RANGE:** $\leq$60 pg/mL (SI: $\leq$60 ng/L) at one laboratory, but other normal ranges are in use **CRITICAL VALUES:** Most patients with glucagonoma have levels >500 pg/mL (SI: >500 ng/L); >1000 pg/mL (SI: >1000 ng/L) is diagnostic.[1] **USE:** Diagnose glucagonoma. Glucagonoma may be present in three different syndromes. The first consists of a characteristic skin rash, necrolytic migratory erythema, diabetes mellitus or impaired glucose tolerance, weight loss, anemia, and venous thrombosis. This form usually shows very high glucagon levels, >1000 pg/mL (SI: >1000 ng/L). The second form is associated with severe diabetes, and the third form with multiple endocrine neoplasia syndrome. This form may have relatively lower glucagon levels. **CONTRAINDICATIONS:** Recent radioactive scan **METHODOLOGY:** Radioimmunoassay (RIA); ethanol extraction removes "big" glucagon, which is not considered biologically active. **ADDITIONAL INFORMATION:** Glucagon is normally secreted by α_2-cells of pancreatic islets, and exerts a counterbalancing effect to insulin in regulation of glucose metabolism. Glucagon exists in "true" form (3500 daltons – biologically active form) and "big" form (160,000 daltons). This form may represent binding of the 3500-dalton glucagon to plasma protein, and rare families have increased amounts of "big" glucagon circulating. Very high levels of glucagon are seen with glucagonomas, and elevations are also seen in diabetic ketoacidosis, stress, uremia, hepatic cirrhosis, hyperosmolality, acute pancreatitis, burns, trauma, surgery, and hypoglycemia. Glucagonoma syndrome is reported with giant cell bronchogenic carcinoma.[2] Decreased values are found in cystic fibrosis, chronic pancreatitis, and in the post-pancreatectomy state. Over 75% of glucagonomas have metastasized at time of diagnosis. After a glucose load, there is no suppression of glucagon in patients with glucagonoma (glucagon suppression test). In glucagon deficiency (cystic fibrosis, chronic pancreatitis) there is a failure of plasma glucagon to rise during arginine infusion.

Footnotes

1. Kaplan LM, "Endocrine Tumors of the Gastrointestinal Tract and Pancreas," *Harrison's Principles of Internal Medicine*, 12th ed, Wilson JD, Braunwald E, Isselbacher KJ, et al, eds, 1991, 1386-93.

2. Hunstein W, Trümper LH, Dummer R, et al, "Glucagonoma Syndrome and Bronchial Carcinoma," *Ann Intern Med*, 1988, 109(11):920-1.

References

Boden G, "Glucagonomas and Insulinomas," *Gastroenterol Clin North Am*, 1990, 18(4):831-45.

Diem P, Redmon JB, Abid M, et al, "Glucagon, Catecholamine, and Pancreatic Polypeptide Secretion in Type I Diabetic Recipients of Pancreas Allografts," *J Clin Invest*, 1990, 86(6):2008-13.

Fraker DL and Norton JA, "The Role of Surgery in the Management of Islet Cell Tumors," *Gastroenterol Clin North Am*, 1989, 18(4):805-30.

Liu D, Moberg E, Kollind M, et al, "A High Concentration of Circulating Insulin Suppresses the Glucagon Response to Hypoglycemia in Normal Man," *J Clin Endocrinol Metab*, 1991, 73(5):1123-8.

Rothe AJ, Young JW, Keramati B, et al, "The Value of Glucagon in Routine Barium Investigations of the Gastrointestinal Tract," *Invest Radiol*, 1987, 22:786-91.

Glucose, 2-Hour Postprandial

***CPT** 82950*

Related Information

Glucose, Quantitative, Urine *on page 1120*
Glucose, Semiquantitative, Urine *on page 1121*
Glycated Hemoglobin *on page 244*
Ketones, Urine *on page 1128*
Microalbuminuria *on page 1134*
Reducing Substances, Urine *on page 1150*

Synonyms 2-Hour PP Glucose; Postprandial Glucose; PP, 2-Hour

Test Commonly Includes Glucose level 2 hours after meal or after measured glucose load

Patient Care PREPARATION: Adequate meal or glucose load 2 hours before "2-hour postprandial glucose," as specified by the patient's physician. Patient is allowed his/her usual meal (breakfast or lunch). Patient must complete meal within 15-20 minutes. Specimen is to be collected 2 hours from beginning of meal. It is preferable to administer 75 g glucose, for work-up for NIDDM, allowing 5 minutes for consumption. Gambino, among others, considers the 2-hour postload (75 g) glucose determination the best single sample for diabetes screening.[1]

Specimen Plasma or serum CONTAINER: Gray top (sodium fluoride) tube or red top tube COLLECTION: Collect in morning after overnight fast and standard meal.

Interpretive REFERENCE RANGE: <140 mg/dL (SI: <7.8 mmol/L) is normal. In an unstressed nonpregnant patient not receiving any medication, a 2-hour postprandial glucose of 140-200 mg/dL (SI: 7.8-11.1 mmol/L) is classified as impaired. A 2-hour result >200 mg/dL, on at least two occasions, supports the diagnosis of diabetes mellitus. For the diagnosis of gestational diabetes mellitus, a plasma glucose >140 mg/dL (SI: >7.8 mmol/L) 1 hour after a 50 g glucose load is an indication for the glucose tolerance test recommended for gestational patients. A 2-hour postprandial glucose <105 mg/dL (SI: <5.8 mmol/L) is desirable. USE: Only a minority of patients with diabetes mellitus have the classic symptoms of polyuria, polyphagia, polydipsia, and weight loss. **The 2-hour postprandial glucose is extensively used to establish the diagnosis of diabetes mellitus**. It may be used along with FBS to follow patients with impaired glucose tolerance. Follow-up of women who had gestational diabetes, of whom most revert after delivery to normal glucose tolerance (up to half ultimately become diabetic). It is used as part of the work-up for impotence, hypertriglyceridemia, neuropathy, retinopathy, gly-

Classification of Diabetes and Related Disorders

Diabetes mellitus (DM)			
Type I	IDDM	Insulin-dependent diabetes mellitus	Formerly called juvenile diabetes
Type II	NIDDM	Noninsulin-dependent diabetes mellitus	Formerly called adult-onset diabetes
Gestational diabetes			
Other types			
Diabetes with acromegaly			
Diabetes with Cushing's syndrome			
Diabetes with pancreatitis			
Diabetes with hemochromatosis			

(Continued)

Glucose, 2-Hour Postprandial *(Continued)*

cosuria and for certain types of renal diseases. Work-up of vulvovaginitis, blurred vision, fatigue, and some instances of urinary tract infections. **Causes of postprandial hypoglycemia** include alimentary type (commonly secondary to prior gastrointestinal surgery); reactive hypoglycemia without prior gastrointestinal surgery – alimentary or spontaneous, functional, idiopathic, indeterminate; some prediabetics; leucine-induced; fructose-induced; galactosemia; indeterminate group. **ADDITIONAL INFORMATION:** Use of fasting and 2-hour postprandial glucose values are recommended to establish the diagnosis of diabetes mellitus. Glycosylated hemoglobin is recommended for monitoring diabetes control. See previous chart.

Footnotes

1. Gambino R, "Criteria for Diagnosis of Diabetes," *Lab Report for Physicians*, 1987, 9:68-9.

References

Home P, "The OGTT: Gold That Does Not Shine," *Diabetic Med*, 1988, 5:313-4.

Jarrett RJ, Keen H, McCartney P, et al, "The Whitehall Study: Ten Year Follow-up Report on New With Impaired Glucose Tolerance With Reference to Worsening to Diabetics and Predictors of Death," *Diabetic Med*, 1984, 1:279-83.

National Diabetes Data Group, "Classification and Diagnosis of Diabetes Mellitus and Other Categories of Glucose Intolerance," *Diabetes*, 1979, 28:1039-57.

Smart LM, Howie AF, Young RJ, et al, "Comparison of Fructosamine With Glycosylated Hemoglobin and Plasma Proteins as Measures of Glycemic Control," *Diabetes Care*, 1988, 11:433-6.

Glucose, Body Fluid *see* Body Fluid Glucose *on page 148*

Glucose, Cerebrospinal Fluid *see* Cerebrospinal Fluid Glucose *on page 176*

Glucose, Fasting

***CPT** 82947*

Related Information

Alcohol, Blood or Urine *on page 936*
Body Fluid Glucose *on page 148*
Cerebrospinal Fluid Glucose *on page 176*
C-Peptide *on page 195*
Fructosamine *on page 224*
Glucose, Quantitative, Urine *on page 1120*
Glucose, Semiquantitative, Urine *on page 1121*
Glucose Tolerance Test *on page 241*
Glycated Hemoglobin *on page 244*
Insulin, Blood *on page 260*
Ketone Bodies, Blood *on page 265*
Microalbuminuria *on page 1134*
pH, Blood *on page 315*
Reducing Substances, Urine *on page 1150*

Synonyms Blood Sugar, Fasting; Fasting Blood Sugar; FBS; Sugar, Fasting

Applies to Tolbutamide Test

Patient Care **PREPARATION:** Patient should be fasting for 8 hours.

Specimen Plasma or serum **CONTAINER:** Gray top (sodium fluoride) tube preferred; red top tube acceptable **COLLECTION:** Neonatal: blood drawn from heelstick **STORAGE INSTRUCTIONS:** Glucose will drop 5-10 mg/dL per hour in unseparated, room temperature blood not collected with sodium fluoride (eg, red top tube).

Interpretive **REFERENCE RANGE:** Premature infants: 40-65 mg/dL (SI: 2.2-3.6 mmol/L), 0-2 years: 60-110 mg/dL (SI: 3.3-6.1 mmol/L), 2 years to adult: 60-115 mg/dL (SI: 3.3-6.4 mmol/L). Normal range increases with age older than 50. Adult results between 115-140 mg/dL (SI: 6.4-7.8 mmol/L) bear re-examination, but if consistent, imply impairment of glucose tolerance. Some recommend oral glucose tolerance test (OGTT) for patients whose FBSs fall in this range, but most would first get additional FBS and 2-hour postprandial glucose. Fasting glucose (after an overnight fast) >140 mg/dL (SI: >7.8 mmol/L) on at least two occasions, indicates diabetes mellitus in the unstressed, ambulatory nonpregnant adult, using conventional methods. **POSSIBLE PANIC RANGE:** Infants: <40 mg/dL (SI: <2.2 mmol/L); adults: male: <50 mg/dL (SI: <2.75 mmol/L), female: <40 mg/dL (SI: <2.2 mmol/L); adults: male and female: >400 mg/dL (SI: >22 mmol/L) **USE:** Establish the diagnosis of diabetes mellitus; evaluate disorders of carbohydrate metabolism, acidosis and ketoacidosis, dehydration, coma, hypoglycemia, and neuroglycopenia; plasma glucose is used to monitor therapy in diabetics; evaluate presence of insulinoma; work up patients with real or apparent alcoholism; investigate polyuria, polydipsia, polyphagia, weight loss, and dehydration **LIMITATIONS:** Mild glucose impairment can exist with fasting glucose within the normal range. Measurement of plasma glucose without spinal fluid glucose can miss neuroglycopenia. To the extent that innovative new methods deviate from reference methods, such alternative techniques may be unreliable for certain patient care needs.[1] Fingerstick glucose determination in shock are lower than venous glucose and are dangerously misleading.[2] **METHODOLOGY:** Plasma (preferably) or serum glucose may be determined by enzyme-based assays, glucose oxidase or hexokinase. Glucose oxidase/oxygen consumption (Astra™ 8, Beckman Instruments), automated serum solid-phase glucose oxidase/peroxidase (Ektachem®, Eastman Kodak), serum solid-phase glucose oxidase/reflectance (Seralyzer®, Ames Co) and whole blood solid-phase glucose oxidase/reflectance (Dextrostix®, Ames Co) have been compared with hexokinase (national reference method) by Gerson and Figoni. These authors express hope that considerations of cost may not be given priority over those of performance and patient care.[1] Portable glucose meters have been studied recently,[3] as well as four types of reagent strips, which performed well except Dextrostix®.[4] A favorable study on a reflectance meter has been published.[5] **ADDITIONAL INFORMATION:** Like a fasting glucose level >140 mg/dL (SI: >7.8 mmol/L), a 2-hour postprandial glucose >200 mg/dL (SI: >11.1 mmol/L) is virtually diagnostic of diabetes mellitus and obviates the need for a glucose tolerance test. An oral glucose tolerance test (OGTT) is not necessary in the setting of sufficiently high fasting and 2-hour postprandial results.

Other causes of **high glucose** (serum or plasma) include nonfasting specimen; recent or current I.V. infusions of glucose; stress states such as myocardial infarct,[6] brain damage, CVA,[7] convulsive episodes, trauma, general anesthesia; Cushing's disease; acromegaly; pheochromocytoma; glucagonoma; severe liver disease; pancreatitis; drugs (thiazide and other diuretics, corticoids, many others are reported to affect glucose).

The danger of **hypoglycemia** (low glucose) is lack of a steady supply of glucose to the brain (neuroglycopenia). Causes of **low glucose:** Excess insulin, including rare insulin autoimmune hypoglycemia, surreptitious insulin injection, and sulfonylurea use; glycolysis in specimens overheated or old; serum permitted to stand on clot in red top tube for chemistry profile. Very prompt removal of plasma and analysis is needed in cases of marked leukocytosis. Hypoglycemia should be confirmed by specimens drawn in fluoride tubes (gray top tubes).

With hypoglycemia, symptoms must be correlated with plasma glucose.

Three major groups of hypoglycemia are defined: reactive, fasting, and surreptitious. The reactive group includes alimentary hyperinsulinism, prediabetic, endocrine deficiency, and idiopathic functional groups.[8] **Postprandial hypoglycemia** may occur after gastrointestinal surgery, and is described with hereditary fructose intolerance, galactosemia, and leucine sensitivity.

Fasting hypoglycemia is likelier to suggest serious organic disease. The overnight fasting glucose level rather than the glucose tolerance test is the optimal test, with glucose drawn during symptoms.

- Pancreatic islet cell tumors (insulinomas) – cause hypoglycemia in fasting individuals or after exercise. Measurement of simultaneous glucose, C-peptide, and insulin levels at the time of spontaneous hypoglycemia help to differentiate insulinoma from other conditions. The glucose/insulin ratio is useful in the diagnosis of insulinoma: insulin levels inappropriately increased for plasma glucose. An intravenous tolbutamide test with plasma glucose and serum insulin determinations may be used for evaluation of insulin-secreting islet cell tumors. The test is positive in approximately 75% of patients with these tumors.[8] Glucagon and leucine stimulation tests are less frequently utilized.
- Extrapancreatic tumors – rare bulky fibromas, sarcomas, mesotheliomas, and carcinomas, including hepatoma and adrenal tumors
- Adrenal insufficiency (Addison's disease), including congenital adrenal hyperplasia
- Hypopituitarism, isolated growth hormone or ACTH deficiency
- Starvation, malabsorption – but starvation does not cause hypoglycemia in normal persons
- Drugs including insulin (see above), oral hypoglycemic agents, and alcoholism, especially with starvation. Ethanolism is a common cause of hypoglycemia. Other drugs can depress glucose levels.

(Continued)

Glucose, Fasting *(Continued)*

- Liver damage, including fulminant hepatic necrosis (hepatitis, toxicity), and severe congestive failure
- Tumor-induced hypoglycemia appears to be caused by increased production of an insulin-like substance (insulin-like growth factor II) by the tumor. This substance induces increased utilization of glucose by the peripheral tissues and the tumor, and impairs the counterregulatory effect of growth hormone by suppressing growth hormone secretion.[9,10]

Infancy and childhood: Infants with tremor, convulsions and/or respiratory distress should have stat glucose, particularly in the presence of maternal diabetes, hemolytic disease of the newborn (erythroblastosis fetalis); babies too large or small for gestational age should also have glucose level measured in the first 24 hours of life. A large number of entities relate to neonatal hypoglycemia, including glycogen storage diseases, galactosemia, hereditary fructose intolerance, ketotic hypoglycemia of infancy, fructose-1,6-diphosphatase deficiency, carnitine deficiency (a treatable disease presenting as Reye's syndrome), and nesidioblastosis.

Footnotes

1. Gerson B and Figoni MA, "Clinical Comparison of Glucose Quantitation Methods," *Arch Pathol Lab Med*, 1985, 109:711-5.
2. Atkin SH, Dasmahapatra A, Jaker MA, et al, "Fingerstick Glucose Determination in Shock," *Ann Intern Med*, 1991, 114:(12)1020-4.
3. Vallera DA, Bissell MG, and Barron W, "Accuracy of Portable Blood Glucose Monitoring. Effect of Glucose Level and Prandial State," *Am J Clin Pathol*, 1991, 95(2):247-52.
4. Cheeley RD and Joyce SM, "A Clinical Comparison of the Performance of Four Blood Glucose Reagent Strips," *Am J Emerg Med*, 1990, 8(1):11-5.
5. Yoo T and Chao J, "Screening for Gestational Diabetes Mellitus. Use and Accuracy of Capillary Blood Glucose Measured With a Reflectance Meter," *J Fam Pract*, 1989, 29(1):41-4.
6. Madsen JK, Haunsoe S, Helquist S, et al, "Prevalence of Hyperglycemia and Undiagnosed Diabetes Mellitus in Patients With Acute Myocardial Infarction," *Acta Med Scand*, 1986, 220:329-32.
7. Berger L and Hakim AM, "The Association of Hyperglycemia With Cerebral Edema in Stroke," *Stroke*, 1986, 17:865-71.
8. Field JB, "Hypoglycemia: A Systematic Approach to Specific Diagnosis," *Hosp Pract*, 1986, 187-94.
9. Daughaday WH, Emanuele MA, Brooks MH, et al, "Synthesis and Secretion of Insulin-Like Growth Factor II by a Leiomyosarcoma With Associated Hypoglycemia," *N Engl J Med*, 1988, 319(22):1434-40.
10. Axelrod L and Ron D, "Insulin-Like Growth Factor II and the Riddle of Tumor-Induced Hypoglycemia," *N Engl J Med*, 1988, 319(22):1477-9, (editorial).

References

Conrad PD, Sparks JW, Osberg I, et al, "Clinical Application of a New Glucose Analyzer in the Neonatal Intensive Care Unit: Comparison With Other Methods," *J Pediatr*, 1989, 114(2):281-7.

Li DF, Wong VC, O'Hoy KM, et al, "Evaluation of the WHO Criteria for 75 g Oral Glucose Tolerance Test in Pregnancy," *Br J Obstet Gynaecol*, 1987, 94:847-50.

Palardy J, Havrankova J, Lepage R, et al, "Blood Glucose Measurements During Symptomatic Episodes in Patients With Suspected Postprandial Hypoglycemia," *N Engl J Med*, 1989, 321(21):1421-5.

Singer DE, Coley CM, Samet JH, et al, "Tests of Glycemia in Diabetes Mellitus. Their Use in Establishing a Diagnosis and in Treatment," *Ann Intern Med*, 1989, 110(2):125-37.

Vassault A and Cloarec A, "Glucose," *Drug Effects on Laboratory Test Results Analytical Interferences and Pharmacological Effects*, Siest G and Galteau MM, eds, Littleton, MA; PSG Publishing Co Inc, 1988, 241-68.

Glucose, Random

***CPT** 82947*

Related Information

Glucose, Quantitative, Urine *on page 1120*
Glucose, Semiquantitative, Urine *on page 1121*
Glycated Hemoglobin *on page 244*
Insulin, Blood *on page 260*
Ketone Bodies, Blood *on page 265*
Ketones, Urine *on page 1128*
Reducing Substances, Urine *on page 1150*

Specimen Plasma or serum **CONTAINER:** Gray top (sodium fluoride) tube preferred; red top tube acceptable **COLLECTION:** Pediatrics: Draw blood from heelstick. **CAUSES FOR REJECTION:** Blood stored overnight on clot

Interpretive **REFERENCE RANGE:** Dependent on time and content of last meal. Glucose of >200 mg/dL (SI: >11.1 mmol/L) in a nonstressed, ambulatory subject supports the diagnosis of diabetes mellitus. Values in term neonates are published.[1] **POSSIBLE PANIC RANGE:** Neonates: <40 mg/dL (SI: <2.2 mmol/L); adults: male: <50 mg/dL (SI: <2.8 mmol/L), >400 mg/dL (SI: >22.2 mmol/L); adults female: <40 mg/dL (SI: <2.2 mmol/L), >400 mg/dL (SI: >22.2 mmol/L) **USE:** Evaluate carbohydrate metabolism, acidosis and ketoacidosis, dehydration; work up alcoholism, or apparent alcoholism; work-up of coma, neuroglycopenia. Hypoglycemia if present should be investigated with insulin levels as well. For the diagnosis of diabetes mellitus in nonpregnant adult subjects, random glucose >200 mg/dL (SI: >11.1 mmol/L) is required. Other criteria exist. Determination of blood glucose on admission in patients who have had an out-of-hospital cardiac arrest can serve as a predictor of neurologic recovery. Higher levels are indicative of more severe brain ischemia and difficult resuscitation.[2] In pregnant women, a value >105 mg/dL usually prompts further investigation. **LIMITATIONS:** Glucose will decrease in samples left on the clot, and in tubes other than fluoride prior to analysis. **METHODOLOGY:** Hexokinase, glucose oxidase, oxygen rate, ortho-toluidine **ADDITIONAL INFORMATION:** Recall that **blood glucose** values are not equivalent to **plasma glucose**. If glucose is >400 mg/dL (SI: >22.2 mmol/L), an acetone (ketone body) examination probably should be done. A fasting and a 2-hour postprandial specimen is preferable to a random specimen for evaluation of possible diabetes mellitus. The incidence of hypoglycemia in hospitalized patients appears to be significant, but may be better controlled if frequent monitoring of glucose levels is employed.[3] Wider utilization of bedside glucose testing may allow for closer patient monitoring, but the establishment of uniform quality control procedures is necessary to ensure valid results from this type of testing.[4,5,6] Evaluation of glycated hemoglobin and self-monitoring of blood glucose are two relatively new means of assessing glycemia which have become widely available.[7]

Footnotes

1. Heck LJ and Erenberg A, "Serum Glucose Levels in Term Neonates During the First 48 Hours of Life," *J Pediatr*, 1987, 110:119-22.
2. Longstreth WT, Diehr P, Cobb LA, et al, "Neurologic Outcome and Blood Glucose Levels During Out-of-Hospital Cardiopulmonary Resuscitation," *Neurology*, 1986, 36:1186-91.
3. Fischer KF, Lees JA, and Newman JH, "Hypoglycemia in Hospitalized Patients: Causes and Outcomes," *N Engl J Med*, 1986, 315:1245-50.
4. Chu SY and Edney-Parker H, "Evaluation of the Reliability of Bedside Glucose Testing," *Lab Med*, 1989, 93-6.
5. Leroux ML and Desjardins PRE, "Establishment and Maintenance of a Hospital Glucose Meter Program," *Lab Med*, 1989, 97-9.
6. Bain OF, Brown KD, Sacher RA, et al, "A Hospital-Wide Blind Control Program for Bedside Glucose Meters," *Arch Pathol Lab Med*, 1989, 113(12):1370-5.
7. Singer DE, Coley CM, Samet JH, et al, "Tests of Glycemia in Diabetes Mellitus – Their Use in Establishing a Diagnosis and in Treatment," *Ann Intern Med*, 1989, 110(2):125-37.

References

Brandt KR and Miles JM, "Relationship Between Severity of Hyperglycemia and Metabolic Acidosis in Diabetic Ketoacidosis," *Mayo Clin Proc*, 1988, 63:1071-4.

Carter PE, Lloyd DJ, and Duffty P, "Glucagon for Hypoglycemia in Infants Small for Gestational Age," *Arch Dis Child*, 1988, 63:1264-6.

Palardy J, Havrankova J, Lepage R, et al, "Blood Glucose Measurements During Symptomatic Episodes in Patients With Suspected Postprandial Hypoglycemia," *N Engl J Med*, 1989, 321(21):1421-5.

Service FJ, "Hypoglycemia and the Postprandial Syndrome," *N Engl J Med*, 1989, 321(21):1472-4.

Weiner CP, Faustich M, Burns J, et al, "The Relationship Between Capillary and Venous Glucose Concentration During Pregnancy," *Am J Obstet Gynecol*, 1986, 155:61-4.

Glucose Tolerance Test

***CPT** 82951 (3 specimens); 82952 (each specimen beyond 3)*

Related Information

C-Peptide *on page 195*
Glucose, Fasting *on page 238*
Glucose, Quantitative, Urine *on page 1120*
Glucose, Semiquantitative, Urine *on page 1121*
Insulin, Blood *on page 260*
Reducing Substances, Urine *on page 1150*

Synonyms GTT; OGTT; Oral Glucose Tolerance Test

Applies to Gestational Diabetes Screening Test

Test Commonly Includes Fasting blood glucose, 30 minutes, first hour, second hour, and hourly thereafter up to time specified (commonly a third hour sample is drawn. A fourth and

(Continued)

Glucose Tolerance Test *(Continued)*

sometimes a fifth hour sample may be ordered.) Many delete the 30-minute specimen, and for noninsulin dependent diabetes mellitus only fasting, 1-hour, and 2-hour glucose is usually needed if GTT is done at all.

Patient Care **PREPARATION:** Patient should not smoke due to glucose stimulation by nicotine. Patient should be active and have had adequate food intake with at least adequate carbohydrates (at least 150 g carbohydrate daily) for 3 days, and then fast 12 hours prior to test. Many drugs interfere. They include steroids, oral contraceptives, diuretics, and antihypertensive drugs including thiazides, furosemide, anticonvulsants, psychoactive drugs, antituberculous agents, and anti-inflammatory drugs including salicylates. Patient should not be stressed. In pregnant subjects, indication for GTT is a positive **gestational diabetes screening test:** 50 g carbohydrate load, sample drawn in 1 hour. A positive usual gestational screening test is glucose >140 mg/dL (SI: >7.8 mmol/L).[1]

Specimen Plasma **CONTAINER:** Gray top (sodium fluoride) tube **COLLECTION:** After fasting blood specimen and urine are obtained, administer oral glucose solution. Weigh patient for proper glucose loading dosage. Children receive 1.75 g/kg body weight up to 75 g. Usual adult dose is 75 g.

100 g is used for possible gestational diabetes mellitus. Then draw blood at 30, 60, 90, and 120 minutes until specified hour. For gestational diabetes, the OGGT is a 3-hour tolerance test, following positive screening test. The screening test for gestational diabetes is not necessarily done fasting.

Collect urine at 1, 2, and 3 hours if urine is to be collected; some delete urines for glucose. During the test, the patient should remain seated and consume nothing but water after the glucose solution is administered. Physical activity should be minimized. Vomiting or diarrhea may alter test results.

CAUSES FOR REJECTION: Time not marked on tubes, patient not appearing in the morning in the fasting state, stressed patient (following surgery, or with infection, or on corticosteroids) should not have GTT

Interpretive **REFERENCE RANGE:** Fasting: 60-115 mg/dL (SI: 3.3-6.4 mmol/L); 1 hour: ≤184 mg/dL (SI: ≤10.2 mmol/L); 2 hours: ≤138 mg/dL (SI: ≤7.7 mmol/L). Many different schemes have been offered to interpret the GTT. Most of these were based on studies in atypical populations and tended to overdiagnose diabetes. The most often used classification currently is the one published by the National Diabetes Data Group, which states: fasting plasma glucose >140 mg/dL (SI: >7.8 mmol/L) or 2-hour postprandial plasma glucose >200 mg/dL (SI: >11.1 mmol/L) → GTT not necessary, patient has diabetes mellitus. GTT, 2-hour plasma glucose >200 mg/dL and at least one other value >200 mg/dL → patient has diabetes mellitus. 2-hour plasma glucose of 140-200 mg/dL and at least one other value >200 mg/dL → patient has **impaired glucose tolerance** but is not clearly diabetic.[2] **USE:** Indications vary somewhat between authorities. Some use the OGTT in individuals whose FBS varies between 115-150 mg/dL (SI: 6.4-8.3 mmol/L) on two or more occasions; others would use further fasting plasma glucose and 2-hour postprandial glucose determinations for such subjects. Some use the GTT infrequently or not at all.

The GTT only establishes the presence of glucose intolerance. It is used in patients with borderline fasting and postprandial glucose to support or rule out the diagnosis of diabetes mellitus. Some use it in unexplained hypertriglyceridemia, neuropathy, impotence, diabetes-like renal diseases, retinopathy, necrobiosis lipoidica diabeticorum, and re-evaluation of prior diagnosis made under substandard conditions. The OGTT is used to work up glycosuria without hyperglycemia (eg, to work up renal glycosuria). It is used to predict perinatal morbidity in pregnancy, to diagnose gestational diabetes. Risks of fetal abnormality and perinatal mortality are increased with abnormal carbohydrate metabolism in pregnancy.[3]

When a glucose <50 mg/dL (SI: <2.8 mmol/L) coincides with symptoms of hypoglycemia, a 6-hour glucose tolerance test is advocated,[4] but many consider the alternatives better. See listings for Insulin, Serum and C-Peptide when patient has symptoms.

Glucose intolerance is due to obesity in some subjects. Abnormal curves may be caused by Cushing's syndrome, pheochromocytoma, or acromegaly.

LIMITATIONS: **Few indications still meet wide acceptance.** Slight hyperglycemic effect is seen in patients on oral contraceptives. Failure to have patient on 3-day high carbohydrate diet may result in a false-positive GGT. Impaired glucose tolerance is **not** equivalent to diabetes mellitus. A normal result does not assure that diabetes will not subsequently develop.

Please see listings Glucose, Fasting and Insulin, Serum for recommendations for work-up of hypoglycemia. **CONTRAINDICATIONS:** FBS >140 mg/dL (SI: >7.8 mmol/L) on two occasions or postprandial blood glucose >200 mg/dL (SI: >11.1 mmol/L) on two occasions are indicative of diabetes mellitus, in the nonstressed subject, and obviate the need for an OGTT. OGTT is contraindicated in the presence of obvious diabetes mellitus. **METHODOLOGY:** Hexokinase, glucose oxidase, oxygen rate, ortho-toluidine **ADDITIONAL INFORMATION:** Emesis is probably an indication to cancel the remainder of a GTT for that day; decision is up to the patient's physician. Excessive growth hormone, adrenocortical and thyroid hormones and catecholamines cause decreased glucose tolerance. Diabetes is much more than glucose intolerance, but until now we have not been able to measure other factors pertinent to prediction of the complications of diabetes. The glucose tolerance test lacks specificity and sensitivity for the complications of diabetes mellitus. Some feel that it only determines glucose intolerance. **Impaired glucose tolerance** is a quasi-entity; 1% to 5% of such patients become overtly diabetic yearly. Such patients have increased risk for cardiovascular disease.

An increased prevalence of idiopathic hemochromatosis exists in the diabetic population compared to the general population.[5]

Criteria for interpretation for gestational diabetes mellitus: two or more of the following must be met. Fasting: ≥105 mg/dL (SI: ≥5.8 mmol/L); 1 hour: ≥190 mg/dL (SI: ≥10.5 mmol/L); 2 hour: ≥165 mg/dL (SI: ≥9.2 mmol/L); 3 hour: ≥145 mg/dL (SI: ≥8.0 mmol/L).[6,7] Pregnant women with an abnormal GTT are at risk for pre-eclampsia/eclampsia and delivering a macrosomic infant.[8,9]

Footnotes

1. Catalano PM, Vargo KM, Bernstein IM, et al, "Incidence and Risk Factors Associated With Abnormal Postpartum Glucose Tolerance in Women With Gestational Diabetes," *Am J Obstet Gynecol*, 1991, 165(4 Pt 1):914-9.
2. National Diabetes Data Group, "Classification and Diagnosis of Diabetes Mellitus and Other Categories of Glucose Intolerance," *Diabetes*, 1979, 28:1039-57.
3. Forest JC, Garrido-Russo M, LeMay A, et al, "Reference Values for the Oral Glucose Tolerance Test at Each Trimester of Pregnancy," *Am J Clin Pathol*, 1983, 80:823-31.
4. Field JB, "Hypoglycemia: A Systematic Approach to Specific Diagnosis," *Hosp Pract*, 1986, 187-94.
5. Phelps G, Chapman I, Hall P, et al, "Prevalence of Genetic Hemochromatosis Among Diabetic Patients," *Lancet*, 1989, 2(8657):233-4.
6. Singer DE, Coley CM, Samet JH, et al, "Tests of Glycemia in Diabetes Mellitus – Their Use in Establishing Diagnosis and in Treatment," *Ann Intern Med*, 1989, 110(2):125-37.
7. Hare JW, "Gestational Diabetes Mellitus. Levels of Glycemia as Management Goals," *Diabetes*, 1991, 40(Suppl 2):193-6.
8. Lindsay MK, Graves W, and Klein L, "The Relationship of One Abnormal Glucose Tolerance Test Value and Pregnancy Complications," *Obstet Gynecol*, 1989, 73(1):103-6.
9. Neiger R and Coustan DR, "The Role of Repeat Glucose Tolerance Tests in the Diagnosis of Gestational Diabetes," *Am J Obstet Gynecol*, 1991, 165(4 Pt 1):787-90.

References

ACOG Technical Bulletin, "Management of Diabetes Mellitus in Pregnancy," 1986, 92:1-5.

Chase HP, Jackson WE, Hoops SL, et al, "Glucose Control and the Renal and Retinal Complications of Insulin-Dependent Diabetes," *JAMA*, 1989, 261(8):1155-60.

de Leacy EA and Cowley DM, "Evidence That the Oral Glucose Tolerance Test Does Not Provide a Uniform Stimulus to Pancreatic Islets in Pregnancy," *Clin Chem*, 1989, 35(7):1482-5.

Gabbe SG, "Gestational Diabetes Mellitus," *N Engl J Med*, 1986, 315:1025-6.

Kritz-Silverstein D, Barrett-Connor E, and Wingard DL, "The Effect of Parity on the Later Development of Non-Insulin-Dependent Diabetes Mellitus or Impaired Glucose Tolerance," *N Engl J Med*, 1989, 321(18):1214-9.

Langer O, Brustman L, Anyaegbunam A, et al, "The Significance of One Abnormal Glucose Tolerance Test Value on Adverse Outcome in Pregnancy," *Am J Obstet Gynecol*, 1987, 157:758-63.

Neiger R and Coustan DR, "Are the Current ACOG Glucose Tolerance Test Criteria Sensitive Enough?" *Obstet Gynecol*, 1991, 78(6):1117-20.

Nelson RL, "Oral Glucose Tolerance Test: Indications and Limitations," *Mayo Clin Proc*, 1988, 63:263-9.

Sacks DA, Abu-Fadil S, Karten GJ, et al, "Screening for Gestational Diabetes With the One-Hour 50 g Glucose Test," *Obstet Gynecol*, 1987, 70:89-93.

Tallarigo L, Giampietro O, Penno G, et al, "Relation of Glucose Tolerance to Complications of Pregnancy in Nondiabetic Women," *N Engl J Med*, 1986, 315:989-92.

Unger RH and Foster DW, "Diabetes Mellitus," *Textbook of Endocrinology*, 7th ed, Wilson JD and Foster DW, eds, Philadelphia, PA: WB Saunders Co, 1985, 1018-80.

Watts NB and Keffer JH, "Diabetes Mellitus and Hypoglycemia," *Practical Endocrinology*, 4th ed, Philadelphia, PA: Lea & Febiger, 1989.

Glutamic Oxaloacetic Transaminase, Serum *see* Aspartate Aminotransferase *on page 135*

Glutamic Pyruvate Transaminase *see* Alanine Aminotransferase *on page 100*

Glutamine, Spinal Fluid *see* Cerebrospinal Fluid Glutamine *on page 177*

Glutamyl Transpeptidase *see* Gamma Glutamyl Transferase *on page 230*

Glycated Albumin *see* Fructosamine *on page 224*

Glycated Hemoglobin

CPT 83036

Related Information

Fructosamine *on page 224*
Glucose, 2-Hour Postprandial *on page 237*
Glucose, Fasting *on page 238*
Glucose, Quantitative, Urine *on page 1120*
Glucose, Random *on page 240*
Glucose, Semiquantitative, Urine *on page 1121*
Microalbuminuria *on page 1134*

Synonyms Fast Hemoglobins; GHB; Hemoglobin A_{1a}, A_{1b}, A_{1c}; Hemoglobin, Glycosylated

Abstract Glycated hemoglobin offers a weighted moving average of prior plasma glucose levels.[1]

Specimen Whole blood (washed erythrocytes or hemolysate) **CONTAINER:** Gray top (sodium fluoride) tube or lavender top (EDTA) tube, the latter for affinity column chromatography **SAMPLING TIME:** Fasting specimens are not required. Testing at 3- to 4-month intervals is suggested for patients with type I diabetes. For patients with type II diabetes, glycated hemoglobins at diagnosis and at 6-month intervals are recommended.[1] **STORAGE INSTRUCTIONS:** Stable 7 days at 4°C.[2]

Interpretive **REFERENCE RANGE:** Dependent upon methodology. Diabetics in good control overlap the normal population. Normal range by affinity columns is reported as 4% to 7%.[3,4] There is no age dependence. **USE:** This is an irreversible glucose-protein bond which extends through the life of an erythrocyte. Glycated hemoglobin values are used to assess long-term glucose control in diabetes, especially in insulin-dependent diabetics whose glucose levels are labile, and in whom blood and urine glucose measurements exhibit significant daily variation. GHB measurements reflect the level of control present over the preceding 100-120 days; more recent levels have greater weight. GHB is especially helpful when renal thresholds are high or low. Glycosylated hemoglobin measurements are less frequently needed in stable diabetics. In such patients, whose fasting glucose concentrations are fairly consistent from day to day, there is a correlation between glycosylated hemoglobin and single fasting glucose levels. Continued high levels of blood glucose are reflected in high GHB concentrations. Glycated hemoglobin has been proposed as a screening test for hemolytic anemia in nondiabetics, since GHB is low with hemolytic anemia.[5] Singer et al suggest a diagnostic approach in which glycated hemoglobin may be substituted for the glucose tolerance test. They advocate it as well as an adjunct in gestational diabetes.[1] It is also useful in evaluation of fetal risk in known type II diabetics who become pregnant. Glycosylated hemoglobin predicts the progression of retinopathy.[6] **LIMITATIONS:** GHB measurements supplement but do not replace conventional urine and blood glucose levels. Chronic blood loss, hemolytic anemia, or other setting for decrease in RBC life span, results in a decrease in the glycated hemoglobin level. Pregnancy may lower glycated hemoglobin. Chronic renal failure with or without dialysis leads to decreased levels of glycated hemoglobin. Misleading high levels of glycated hemoglobin are found by ion exchange resin columns in patients who have elevated levels of fetal hemoglobin (Hb F);[7] high levels of Hb F are found in young children younger than 2 years of age and in some hemoglobinopathies. This is true also for hemoglobins H, I, J and N.[8] Low values derive from blood containing hemoglobin S, G, D, C, or E.[9] Such difficulties with abnormal hemoglobins do not apply to the affinity chromatography method.[4] **CONTRAINDICATIONS:** Not useful more often than at 4- to 6-week intervals. Not widely accepted in diagnosis of diabetes. **METHODOLOGY:** Elution from resin columns, high performance liquid chromatography (HPLC), electrophoresis, isoelectric focusing, affinity chromatography, enzyme immunoassay (EIA).[10] Affinity columns avoid problems of temperature variations and abnormal hemoglobins F, S, C, D, G, and J do not generate misleading data.[3,11] Ion capture immunoassay shows no interference from abnormal hemoglobins. **ADDITIONAL INFORMATION:** A useful test to reassure the patient who is well controlled, and to assess the status of insufficiently controlled patients. If a result does not seem consistent with the clinical findings, ask for a hemoglobin F level. Measurement of glycated hemoglobin by affinity chromatography permits better differentiation of the degree of blood glucose control among diabetics than does hemoglobin A_{1c} or hemoglobin A_1 measurements.[12]

Footnotes

1. Singer DE, Coley CM, Samet JH, et al, "Tests of Glycemia in Diabetes Mellitus – Their Use in Establishing a Diagnosis and in Treatment," *Ann Intern Med*, 1989, 110(2):125-37.
2. Caraway WT and Watts NB, "Carbohydrates," *Fundamentals of Clinical Chemistry*, 3rd ed, Tietz NW, ed, Philadelphia, PA: WB Saunders Co, Philadelphia, 1987, 775-828.
3. Leavelle DE, *Mayo Medical Laboratories Interpretive Handbook*, Rochester, MN: Mayo Medical Laboratories, 1990.
4. Fairbanks VF and Zimmerman BR, "Measurement of Glycosylated Hemoglobin by Affinity Chromatography," *Mayo Clin Proc*, 1983, 58:770-3.
5. Panzer S, Kronik G, Lechner K, et al, "Glycosylated Hemoglobins (GHb): An Index of Red Cell Survival," *Blood*, 1982, 59:1348-50.
6. Klein R, Klein BE, Moss SE, et al, "Glycosylated Hemoglobin Predicts the Incidence and Progression of Diabetic Retinopathy," *JAMA*, 1988, 260(19):2864-71.
7. Bergstrom RW, Kelley JR, and Ward WK, "Fetal Hemoglobin Alters Hemoglobin A_{1c} Measurements," *Ann Intern Med*, 1991, 115(8):656.
8. Krauss JS and Khankhanian NK, "HPLC Determination of Hemoglobin A_{1c} in the Presence of the Fast Hemoglobin I Philadelphia," *Clin Chem*, 1989, 35(3):494-5.
9. Holt GS, Wofford JL, and Velez R, "Hemoglobinopathies Affect Hemoglobin A_{1c} Measurement," *Ann Intern Med*, 1991, 115(1):68-9.
10. Engbaek F, Christensen SE, and Jespersen B, "Enzyme Immunoassay of Hemoglobin A_{1c}: Analytical Characteristics and Clinical Performance for Patients With Diabetes Mellitus, With and Without Uremia," *Clin Chem*, 1989, 35(1):93-7.
11. Gascon F and Molina E, "Precision of Measurement of Glycated Hemoglobin by Affinity Chromatography on Regenerated Columns," *Clin Chem*, 1989, 35(1):191.
12. Teupe B, "Quantitative Determination of Glycated Hemoglobin Using Affinity Chromatography," Symposium Proceedings: The Role of Glycated Hemoglobin in the Management of Diabetes, Akron, OH: Isolab Inc, 1988, 9-16.

References

Allgrove J and Cockrill BL, "Fructosamine or Glycated Haemoglobin as a Measure of Diabetic Control," *Arch Dis Child*, 1988, 63:418-22.

Bunn HF, Gabbay KH, and Gallop PM, "The Glycosylation of Hemoglobin: Relevance to Diabetes Mellitus," *Science*, 1978, 200:21-7.

Cox T, Hess PP, Thompson GD, et al, "Interference With Glycated Hemoglobin by Hemoglobin F May Be Greater Than Is Generally Assumed," *Am J Clin Pathol*, 1993, 99(2):137-41.

Goldstein DE, Little RR, Wiedmeyer HM, et al, "Glycated Hemoglobin: Methodologies and Clinical Application," *Clin Chem*, 1986, 32:B64-B70.

Jerntorp P, Sundkvist G, Fex G, et al, "Clinical Utility of Serum Fructosamine in Diabetes Mellitus Compare With Hemoglobin A_{1c}," *Clin Chim Acta*, 1988, 175:135-42.

Glycolic Acid, Urine *see* Oxalate, Urine *on page 303*

Glyoxylic Acid, Urine *see* Oxalate, Urine *on page 303*

GOT *see* Aspartate Aminotransferase *on page 135*

GPT *see* Alanine Aminotransferase *on page 100*

Growth Hormone

CPT 83003

Related Information

Phosphorus, Urine *on page 322*
Somatomedin-C *on page 354*

Synonyms GH; hGH; Somatotropin

Applies to Somatomedins

Abstract Growth hormone, released by the anterior pituitary, promotes anabolism. Growth is stimulated through somatomedins.

Patient Care PREPARATION: Patient should be fasting and at complete rest for 30 minutes. Patient must not be stressed. Draw from rested patient.

Specimen Serum CONTAINER: Red top tube STORAGE INSTRUCTIONS: Label tube with time and date of collection and identifying data. Separate serum and freeze in plastic container. Stable 4 hours at 25°C and 1 year at -20°C.[1,2] CAUSES FOR REJECTION: Recent radioactive scan SPE-

(Continued)

Growth Hormone *(Continued)*

CIAL INSTRUCTIONS: Physiological state (feeding, fasting, sleep, activity) should be noted on requisition. Stimulation and suppression tests, and somatomedin C levels are often needed. Stimulation tests must be directed by a physician.

Interpretive REFERENCE RANGE: Children: <20 ng/mL (SI: <880 pmol/L); adults: male: ≤5 ng/mL (SI: ≤220 pmol/L), female: <10 ng/mL (SI: <440 pmol/L); Response to oral glucose administration is used in evaluation of acromegaly. Assays using a monoclonal antibody give lower results than those using polyclonal antibodies. USE: Pituitary function test useful in the diagnosis of hypothalamic disorders, hypopituitarism; deficiency leads to dwarfism in children, excess causes gigantism in children and acromegaly in adults. LIMITATIONS: A single fasting GH level is of limited value. Secretion of GH is episodic and pulsatile. GH has a half-life of 20-25 minutes. Testing for growth hormone deficiency in children is best done as part of a dynamic test that involves various stimuli. Patients with dysfunctional thyroids may have abnormal growth hormone release. Patients with GH-producing pituitary tumors often release GH in response to TRH or GnRH. Somatomedin C is used as a screening test for HGH deficiency, but pitfalls exist.[3] METHODOLOGY: Radioimmunoassay (RIA), immunoradiometric assay[4] ADDITIONAL INFORMATION: Growth hormone secretion is influenced by deep sleep, arginine, glucagon, levodopa, low glucose and insulin, exercise and stress, vasopressin. Starvation increases HGH. In obesity, release of GH is reduced; and response of GH to insulin, sleep, or exercise may be impaired. Patients with acromegaly, even those with normal GH levels, will show no suppression of GH by oral glucose and may show a rise. In patients being evaluated for pituitary insufficiency, GH may be assayed after stimulation by administration of insulin, arginine, glucagon, vasopressin, or levodopa.[5] The defined normal response differs among laboratories. With the advent of recombinant growth hormone for treatment of short stature, assays for GH have increased. Somatomedins are produced in response to GH.[3] GH-binding proteins do not interfere significantly in assays commonly employed.[6] In children who are treated with GH and develop GH antibodies, the plasma GH measurement is factitiously elevated whereas the free GH is not.[7] Assays have been developed to measure GH in urine.[8,9]

Footnotes

1. Fody EP, Bennett BD, Richardson LD, et al, *Clinical Laboratory Handbook for Patient Preparation and Specimen Handling: Fascicle V, Endocrinology/Metabolism*, Skokie, IL: College of American Pathologists, 1989.
2. Kabasik NP, Ricotta M, Hunter T, et al, "Effect of Duration and Temperature of Storage on Serum Analyte Stability: Examination of 14 Radioimmunoassay Procedures," *Clin Chem*, 1982, 28:164-5.
3. Watts NB and Keffer JH, "Anterior Pituitary and Hypothalamus," *Practical Endocrinology*, 4th ed, Chapter 2, Philadelphia, PA: Lea & Febiger, 1989, 11-36.
4. Pringle PJ, Jones J, Hindmarsh PC, et al, "Performance of Proficiency Survey Samples in Two Immunoradiometric Assays of Human Growth Hormone and Comparison With Patients' Sample," *Clin Chem*, 1992, 38(4):553-7.
5. Leavelle DE, *Mayo Medical Laboratories Interpretive Handbook*, Rochester, MN: Mayo Medical Laboratories, 1990.
6. Jan T, Shaw MA, and Baumann G, "Effects of Growth Hormone-Binding Proteins on Serum Growth Hormone Measurements," *J Clin Endocrinol Metab*, 1991, 72(2):387-91.
7. Pringle PJ, Hindmarsh PC, DiSilvio L, et al, "The Measurement and Effect of Growth Hormone in the Presence of Growth Hormone-Binding Antibodies," *J Endocrinol*, 1989, 121(1):193-9.
8. Evans AJ and Wood PJ, "Development of an Assay for Human Growth Hormone in Urine Using Commercially Available Reagents," *Ann Clin Biochem*, 1989, 26(Pt 4):353-7.
9. Hourd P and Edwards R, "Measurement of Human Growth Hormone in Urine: Development and Validation of a Sensitive and Specific Assay," *J Endocrinol*, 1989, 121(1):167-75.

References

Baumann G, Shaw MA, and Merimee TJ, "Low Levels of High-Affinity Growth Hormone-Binding Protein in African Pygmies," *N Engl J Med*, 1989, 320(26):1705-9.

Chattoraj SC and Watts NB, "Endocrinology," *Textbook of Clinical Chemistry*, Tietz NW, ed, Philadelphia, PA: WB Saunders Co, 1986, 1021.

Donaldson DL, Pan F, Hollowell JG, et al, "Reliability of Stimulated and Spontaneous Growth Hormone (GH) Levels for Identifying the Child With Low GH Secretion," *J Clin Endocrinol Metab*, 1991, 72(3):647-52.

Golde DW, Bersch N, Kaplan SA, et al, "Peripheral Unresponsiveness to Human Growth Hormone in Laron Dwarfism," *N Engl J Med*, 1980, 303:1156-9.

Grumbach MM, "Growth Hormone Therapy and the Short End of the Stick," *N Engl J Med*, July 1988, 238-41.

Ilondo MM, Vanderschueren-Lodeweyckx M, De Meyts P, et al, "Serum Growth Hormone Levels Measured by Radioimmunoassay and Radioreceptor Assay: A Useful Diagnostic Tool in Children With Growth Disorders?" *J Clin Endocrinol Metab*, 1990, 70(5):1445-51.

Kao PC, Abboud CF, and Zimmerman D, "Laboratory Medicine: Somatomedin C: An Index of Growth Hormone Activity," *Mayo Clin Proc*, 1986, 61:908-9.

Mercado M, Molitch ME, and Baumann G, "Low Plasma Growth Hormone Binding Protein in IDDM," *Diabetes*, 1992, 41(5):605-9.

Rose SR, Ross JL, Uriarte M, et al, "The Advantage of Measuring Stimulated as Compared With Spontaneous Growth Hormone Levels in the Diagnosis of Growth Hormone Deficiency," *N Engl J Med*, 1988, 319:201-7.

GT *see* Gamma Glutamyl Transferase *on page 230*

GTP *see* Gamma Glutamyl Transferase *on page 230*

GTT *see* Glucose Tolerance Test *on page 241*

Guthrie Test *see* Phenylalanine, Blood *on page 317*

HAP *see* Haptoglobin, Serum *on this page*

Haptoglobin, Serum

CPT 83010

See Also Anemia Flowchart in the Hematology Appendix

Related Information

Hemoglobin, Plasma *on page 559*

Myoglobin, Blood *on page 293*

Synonyms HAP; HP; Hp

Specimen Serum **CONTAINER:** Red top tube **CAUSES FOR REJECTION:** Hemolysis from traumatic venipuncture

Interpretive **REFERENCE RANGE:** 40-180 mg/dL (SI: 0.4-1.8 g/L) but method dependent. Newborns reach adult levels at approximately 4 months. **POSSIBLE PANIC RANGE:** Low values, depending on the method, may be <40-50 mg/dL (SI: <0.4-0.5 g/L). **USE:** **Decreased** to absent levels occur more with intravascular than extravascular hemolysis: haptoglobin binds hemoglobin and carries it to the reticuloendothelial system. Thus, haptoglobin is useful in work-up for hemolytic states. It is low in the megaloblastic anemias, which have a hemolytic component. It is decreased in infectious mononucleosis. Decreases can occur with hematoma or tissue hemorrhage. Haptoglobin can be low with liver disease. Congenital absence occurs (small fraction of Blacks/Orientals have ahaptoglobinemia, absence of detectable haptoglobin). Frequently **elevated** as an acute phase reactant, in inflammatory disorders (eg, collagen diseases, infections, tissue destruction), and with advanced malignant neoplasms.[1] Haptoglobin has been used as a genetic marker for forensic paternity exclusion.[2] A variety of α- and β-chain variants have been identified, 20 different α-chain haptoglobin phenotypes have been noted. **LIMITATIONS:** During inflammation or steroid therapy, normal concentrations do not rule out hemolysis; decreased with oral contraceptives; increased with androgens; haptoglobin normally higher in men; methods in use do not necessarily distinguish between haptoglobin phenotypes **METHODOLOGY:** Immunologic methods including radial immunodiffusion (RID), nephelometry, automated immunoprecipitation, hemoglobin binding capacity; in forensic (paternity exclusion) work, starch or acrylamide gel electrophoresis; one-dimensional isoelectric focusing/immunoblotting method has recently been assessed.[2] Differences in size of various haptoglobin phenotypes renders quantitation by RID inaccurate. **ADDITIONAL INFORMATION:** Haptoglobin is a protein which binds free hemoglobin. Part of alpha$_2$ on serum protein electrophoresis, serum haptoglobin is a glycoprotein consisting of two pairs of nonidentical chains, α and β, made by the liver. The subunit structure is represented as $\alpha_2\beta_2$. The haptoglobin bound hemoglobin complex is removed rapidly by the reticuloendothelial system and metabolized to free amino acids and iron in just a few hours. This represents an efficient method for the conservation of iron. Low alpha$_2$ is commonly due to hemolysis and/or liver disease. Serum protein electrophoretic pattern showing low albumin, polyclonal increase in gamma globulin and decrease in alpha$_2$-globulin shown to be due to decreased haptoglobin has been correlated with poor prognosis in severe liver disease.[3] Haptoglobin is decreased for 2-3 days after only 25 mL of blood is lysed.[1] Thus, transfusions, which contain red blood cells which do not all survive in the recipient, can lower the level. The decrease in haptoglobin (after hemolysis) precedes any drop in hemopexin levels or the appearance of methemalbumin in serum or urine.

Myoglobin, unlike hemoglobin, is not bound by haptoglobin.

Immunohistochemical localization and haptoglobin in RNA *in situ* hybridization procedures have been developed.[4]

Fucosylated forms of the beta-chains of haptoglobins have been recently shown to be applicable to the monitoring of tumor burden in cancer patients and differentiating between active and inactive inflammatory (eg, rheumatoid) joint disease.[5] Elevated fucosylated haptoglobin levels, however, are not disease specific.[6]

(Continued)

Haptoglobin, Serum *(Continued)*

Footnotes

1. Peters T Jr, "Proteins," *Chemical Diagnosis of Disease*, Brown SS, Mitchell FL, and Young DS, eds, Amsterdam, Holland: Elsevier/North Holland Biomedical Press, 1979, 311-62.
2. Teige B, Olaisen B, Pedersen L, et al, "Forensic Aspects of Haptoglobin: Electrophoretic Patterns of Haptoglobin Allotype Products and an Evaluation of Typing Procedure," *Electrophoresis*, 1988, 9:384-92.
3. Fitzmaurice M, Valenzuela R, and Winkelman EI, "Serum Protein Electrophoresis Pattern Associated With Decrease Serum Haptoglobin as a Poor Prognostic Indicator in Severe Liver Disease," *Am J Clin Pathol*, 1989, 91:365.
4. Bowman BH, Barnett DR, Lum JB, et al, "Haptoglobin," *Methods Enzymol*, 1988, 163:452-74.
5. Thompson S, Stappenbeck R, and Turner GA, "A Multiwell Lectin-Binding Assay Using *Lotus tetragonolobus* for Measuring Different Glycosylated Forms of Haptoglobin," *Clin Chim Acta*, 1989, 180(3):277-84.
6. Thompson S, Kelly CA, Griffiths ID, et al, "Abnormally-Fucosylated Serum Haptoglobins in Patients With Inflammatory Joint Disease," *Clin Chim Acta*, 1989, 184(3):251-8.

References

Erslev AJ, "Haptoglobin Assay," *Hematology*, 4th ed, Chapter A18, Williams WJ, Beutler E, Erslev AJ, et al, eds, New York, NY: McGraw-Hill Inc, 1990, 1737-8.

Patzelt D, Geserick G, and Schröder H, "The Genetic Haptoglobin Polymorphism: Relevance of Paternity Assessment," *Electrophoresis*, 1988, 9:393-7.

hCG *see* Human Chorionic Gonadotropin, Serum *on page 254*

hCG, Beta Subunit *see* Human Chorionic Gonadotropin, Serum *on page 254*

hCG, Slide Test, Stat *see* Pregnancy Test *on page 333*

hCG, Urine *see* Pregnancy Test *on page 333*

HCO_3, Blood

CPT 82374

Related Information

Anion Gap *on page 132*
Blood Gases, Arterial *on page 140*
Carbon Dioxide, Blood *on page 165*
Electrolytes, Blood *on page 212*
Ketone Bodies, Blood *on page 265*
Osmolality, Calculated *on page 299*
pCO_2, Blood *on page 314*

Synonyms Bicarbonate

Test Commonly Includes Test is part of blood gases panel and electrolytes panel

Specimen Plasma or serum **CONTAINER:** Green top (heparin) tube, red top tube

Interpretive **REFERENCE RANGE:** Newborns and infants: 16-24 mmol/L (SI: 16-24 mmol/L); children and adults: arterial: 21-28 mmol/L (SI: 21-28 mmol/L), venous: 22-29 mmol/L (SI: 22-29 mmol/L) **POSSIBLE PANIC RANGE:** <10 mmol/L, >40 mmol/L **USE:** A measurement in acid-base and electrolyte status, bicarbonate is used in evaluation of fixed base. **Increased** with metabolic alkalosis (and with compensated respiratory acidosis). **Decreased** with metabolic acidosis and with compensated respiratory alkalosis (eg, low in ketoacidosis). **LIMITATIONS:** Calculated arterial bicarbonate was 10 mmol/L lower than directly measured venous bicarbonate, when the former was diluted with excessive heparin. In drawing arterial specimens, only sufficient heparin needed to fill the dead space of the syringe should be used.[1] Inadequate filling of red top Vacutainer® tube will decrease apparent serum bicarbonate levels.[2] **METHODOLOGY:** Calculation is based on the Henderson-Hasselbalch equation when pH and pCO_2 are measured. Total carbon dioxide (TCO_2) (CO_2 content) equals carbonic acid plus bicarbonate. For venous blood electrolytes, methods to measure HCO_3 are widely used. Calculated HCO_3^- concentrations are accurate in pediatric and adult populations. In the vast majority of clinical settings, the calculated HCO_3^- value is comparable to the measured TCO_2 for diagnostic and therapeutic considerations.[3] **ADDITIONAL INFORMATION:** Most pediatric diabetic patients whose initial pH was ≥ 7.20 or whose bicarbonate concentration was ≥ 10 mmol/L had resolution of acidosis, mostly without hospitalization, while most patients whose pH was <7.20 and bicarbonate <10 mmol/L were hospitalized.[4] Other laboratory tests needed in the work-up of diabetic ketoacidosis include the remaining electrolytes, plasma glucose, blood and urine ketone bodies, hematocrit, BUN, and sometimes osmolality.

Footnotes

1. Bloom SA, Canzanello VJ, Strom JA, et al, "Spurious Assessment of Acid-Base Status Due to Dilutional Effect of Heparin," *Am J Med*, 1985, 79:528-30.
2. Herr RD and Swanson T, "Serum Bicarbonate Declines With Sample Size in Vacutainer® Tubes," *Am J Clin Pathol*, 1992, 97(2):213-6.
3. Rivkees SA and Fine BP, "The Reliability of Calculated Bicarbonate in Clinical Practice," *Clin Pediatr (Phila)*, 1988, 27(5):240-2.
4. Bonadio WA, Gutzeit MF, Losek JD, et al, "Outpatient Management of Diabetic Ketoacidosis," *Am J Dis Child*, 1988, 142(4):448-50.

References

Beeler MF, "Disorders of Hydrogen Metabolism," *Interpretations in Clinical Chemistry. A Textbook Approach to Chemical Pathology*, Beeler MF and Catrou PG, eds, Chicago, IL: ASCP Press, 1983, 119-29.

O'Leary TD and Langton SR, "Calculated Bicarbonate or Total Carbon Dioxide?" *Clin Chem*, 1989, 35(8):1697-700.

Yeomans ER, Hauth JC, Gilstrap LC 3d, et al, "Umbilical Cord pH, pCO_2, and Bicarbonate Following Uncomplicated Term Vaginal Deliveries," *Am J Obstet Gynecol*, 1985, 151:798-800.

hCS *see* Placental Lactogen, Human *on page 324*

HCT *see* Calcitonin *on page 157*

HDL *see* High Density Lipoprotein Cholesterol *on this page*

HDLC *see* High Density Lipoprotein Cholesterol *on this page*

HDL Cholesterol *see* High Density Lipoprotein Cholesterol *on this page*

Health Fairs *see* Chemistry Profile *on page 181*

Heat Stable Alkaline Phosphatase *see* Alkaline Phosphatase, Heat Stable *on page 106*

Heat Stable ALP *see* Alkaline Phosphatase, Heat Stable *on page 106*

Hemoglobin A_{1a}, A_{1b}, A_{1c} *see* Glycated Hemoglobin *on page 244*

Hemoglobin, Glycosylated *see* Glycated Hemoglobin *on page 244*

Hemoglobin Saturation, Percent *see* Oxygen Saturation, Blood *on page 305*

hGH *see* Growth Hormone *on page 245*

5-HIAA, Quantitative, Urine *see* 5-Hydroxyindoleacetic Acid, Quantitative, Urine *on page 257*

High Density Lipoprotein Cholesterol

CPT 83718

Related Information

Apolipoprotein A and B *on page 134*
Cholesterol *on page 185*
Lipid Profile *on page 278*
Lipoprotein Electrophoresis *on page 281*
Triglycerides *on page 370*

Synonyms Alpha$_1$ Lipoprotein Cholesterol; HDL; HDLC; HDL Cholesterol

Abstract This is a class of heterogeneous particles of varying sizes and densities, containing lipid and protein. It includes cholesterol esters and free cholesterol, triglycerides, phospholipids, and A, C, and E apoproteins. Two subclasses of HDL predominate: HDL_2 and smaller, denser HDL_3. HDL may function in so-called "reverse transport" of cholesterol to the liver, the significance of which remains to be understood. Nevertheless, an independent, strong, inverse relationship of HDL cholesterol and coronary arterial disease has been essentially confirmed in the industrial world.[1]

Patient Care PREPARATION: Patient ideally should be on a stable diet for 3 weeks and should fast for 12-14 hours prior to collection of specimen. See Preparation in Cholesterol test listing. HDLC is usually done as part of lipid profile.

Specimen Serum CONTAINER: Red top tube COLLECTION: Recent fat intake influences HDL. STORAGE INSTRUCTIONS: Analysis promptly after sampling is best. The specimen can be refrigerated up to several days at 4°C or frozen for several weeks. For long-term storage use -70°C.[2] CAUSES FOR REJECTION: Specimen collected in citrate or heparin anticoagulants

Interpretive REFERENCE RANGE: Male: 15-34 years: 35-65 mg/dL (SI: 0.9-1.7 mmol/L). HDLC levels in men <35 mg/dL (SI: <0.9 mmol/L) represent a coronary risk factor.[1,3] In women, HDLC

(Continued)

High Density Lipoprotein Cholesterol *(Continued)*

<40 mg/dL is a risk factor. The 95th percentile increases to 70 mg/dL at age 45 years; 35-80 mg/dL (SI: 0.9-2 mmol/L) for female subjects. HDL cholesterol values are about 20% of the total cholesterol and may be expressed as a percentage of total cholesterol. HDL after puberty is lower in males. Black Americans have higher HDL than do whites.

USE: A protective substance utilized for prediction of coronary arterial disease, especially useful in individuals with high serum cholesterol levels. Low HDLC is an important predictor of risk of coronary atherosclerosis and coronary heart disease. HDL may act as a protective scavenger molecule (reverse cholesterol transport). The liver is the major site of cholesterol **excretion**. When a slightly increased cholesterol is due to high HDL, therapy is not indicated.[3] **LIMITATIONS:** Increased levels are reported with estrogens and with birth control pills. Clofibrate, Atromid-S® therapy cause increases. There may be interference from very high triglyceride concentrations. Standardization is not as good as that available for cholesterol in 1989 from CDC/NBS, and reliability everywhere may not equal that in published epidemiologic studies. Coefficients of variation are excessive; the problems with lack of desirable levels of accuracy and precision of HDL are widely recognized. Only small mean differences are found between those with coronary arterial disease and those who appear healthy. Bilirubin interferes; icteric specimens lead to underestimation of HDLC. There is a lack of optimal quality control materials. **METHODOLOGY:** Ultracentrifugation; precipitation: heparin and 92 mmol manganese followed by incubation, centrifugation in a refrigerated centrifuge; dextran sulfate and magnesium chloride; each followed by cholesterol analysis; phosphotungstate and magnesium ion also are used. A reflectance photometric technique with prior precipitation has been reported.[4] HDL_2 and HDL_3 cholesterol can be measured by precipitation and ultracentrifugation. Dextran sulfate produces lower results than other precipitating agents. **ADDITIONAL INFORMATION:** Total cholesterol and triglycerides are required as well for determination of lipid risk factors for coronary artery disease. These tests with HDLC and LDLC are the usual lipid profile. HDLC is especially apt to be low in male subjects who are obese and sedentary, in those who smoke cigarettes, and in those who have diabetes mellitus. Uremia is also associated with lower HDLC. Exercise, appropriate diet, and moderate ethanol intake increase HDLC.

HDLC		Coronary Artery Disease Risk (times average)	
mg/dL	SI: mmol/L	Men	Women
25	0.65	2.0	
30	0.78	1.8	
35	0.91	1.5	
40	1.03	1.2	1.9
45	1.16	Average	1.6
50	1.29	0.8	1.3
55	1.42	0.7	Average
60	1.55	0.6	0.8
65	1.68	0.5	0.6
70	1.81		0.5
75	1.94	Longevity	

From Kannel WB, Castelli WP, and Gordon T, "Cholesterol in the Prediction of Atherosclerotic Disease," *Ann Intern Med,* 1979, 90:85, with permission.
Note: Risk is inversely proportional to HDLC.

HDLC is useful with cholesterol in forecasting protection against coronary artery disease in the industrialized countries, possible because of ingestion of high fat diets. LDLC, an excellent predictor, is usually a calculation. Those at least risk for development of coronary arterial disease would have low cholesterol, low triglyceride, and high HDLC.

Thiazides and nonselective beta-adrenergic blocking agents may decrease HDLC.[3]

For risk factors including glucose intolerance, increased systolic blood pressure, cigarette smoking, and left ventricular hypertrophy as well as cholesterol, see Figure 1 of paper of Kannel et al.[5]

Apolipoprotein A-I determination may eventually be shown to be superior to HDLC; increased apoprotein A-I is associated with a diminished risk of atherogenesis. It is measured by RIA[6] and by nephelometry. Apolipoprotein A-I is the major protein of HDL. Problems about apolipoproteins are discussed in the listing Lipid Profile. Essentially, current studies have not yet answered whether or not apoprotein A-I is a better discriminator than HDL.[7] At present, HDL measurement is considered preferable by Gordon and Rifkind.[1]

Factors contributing to decreased HDLC include:

- genetic factors: primary hypoalphalipoproteinemia[8]
- cigarette smoking[9]
- obesity[9]
- hypertriglyceridemia[9]
- lack of exercise
- steroids – androgens, progestogens, anabolic
- thiazides
- beta-adrenergic blockers
- probucol
- neomycin

The rare entity, Tangier disease, is characterized by very low HDL, total cholesterol, and low density lipoprotein cholesterol. Cholesterol esters accumulate in tissues. Severe coronary arterial sclerosis with extremely low HDL (1.4 mg/dL) was reported in a subject with Tangier disease.[10]

Footnotes

1. Gordon DJ and Rifkind BM, "High Density Lipoprotein – The Clinical Implications of Recent Studies," *N Engl J Med*, 1989, 321(19):1311-6.
2. Nanjee MN and Miller NE, "Evaluation of Long-Term Frozen Storage of Plasma for Measurement of High-Density Lipoprotein and Its Subfractions by Precipitation," *Clin Chem*, 1990, 36(5):783-8.
3. Betteridge DJ, "High Density Lipoprotein and Coronary Heart Disease," *BMJ*, 1989, 298(6679):974-5.
4. Ng RH, Sparks KM, and Statland BE, "Direct Measurement of High-Density Lipoprotein Cholesterol by the Reflotron Assay With No Manual Precipitation Step," *Clin Chem*, 1991, 37(3):435-7.
5. Kannel WB, Castelli WP, and Gordon T, "Cholesterol in the Prediction of Atherosclerotic Disease. New Perspectives Based on the Framingham Study," *Ann Intern Med*, 1979, 90:85-91.
6. Maciejko JJ, Holmes DR, Kottke BA, et al, "Apolipoprotein A-1 as a Marker of Angiographically Assessed Coronary Artery Disease," *N Engl J Med*, 1983, 309:385-9.
7. Miller NE, "Associations of High Density Lipoprotein Subclasses and Apolipoproteins With Ischemic Heart Disease and Coronary Atherosclerosis," *Am Heart J*, 1987, 113:589-97.
8. Grundy SM, Goodman DS, Rifkind BM, et al, "The Place of HDL in Cholesterol Management: A Perspective From the National Cholesterol Education Program," *Arch Intern Med*, 1989, 149(3):505-10.
9. Frohlich JJ and Pritchard PH, "The Clinical Significance of Serum High Density Lipoproteins," *Clin Biochem*, 1989, 22(6):417-23.
10. Mautner SL, Sanchez JA, Rader DJ, et al, "The Heart in Tangier Disease. Severe Coronary Atherosclerosis With Near Absence of High-Density Lipoprotein Cholesterol," *Am J Clin Pathol*, 1992, 98(2):191-8.

References

Asayama K, Miyao A, and Kato K, "High-Density Lipoprotein (HDL), HDL2, and HDL3 Cholesterol Concentrations Determined in Serum of Newborns, Infants, Children, Adolescents, and Adults by Use of a Micromethod for Combined Precipitation Ultracentrifugation," *Clin Chem*, 1990, 36(1):129-31.

Blackburn H, "The Meaning of a New Marker for Coronary Artery Disease," *N Engl J Med*, 1983, 309:426-8, (editorial).

Brunner D, Weisbort J, Meshulam N, et al, "Relation of Serum Total Cholesterol and High Density Lipoprotein Cholesterol Percentage to the Incidence of Definite Coronary Events: Twenty Year Follow-Up of the Donolo-Tel Aviv Prospective Coronary Artery Disease Study," *Am J Cardiol*, 1987, 59:1271-6.

Dwyer JH, Rieger-Ndakorerwa GE, Semmer NK, et al, "Low-Level Cigarette Smoking and Longitudinal Change in Serum Cholesterol Among Adolescents: The Berlin-Bremen Study," *JAMA*, 1988, 259:2857-62.

Gambino R, "Physical Exercise & Lipoproteins," *Lab Report for Physicians,™* 1989, 11:43-8.

Gordon DJ, Knoke J, and Probstfield JL, "High-Density Lipoprotein Cholesterol and Coronary Heart Disease in Hypercholesterolemic Men: The Lipid Research Clinics Coronary Primary Prevention Trial," *Circulation*, 1986, 74:1217-25.

Gordon DJ, Probstfield JL, Garrison RJ, et al, "High-Density Lipoprotein Cholesterol and Cardiovascular Disease: Four Prospective American Studies," *Circulation*, 1989, 79(1):8-15.

Gordon T, Castelli WP, Hjortland MC, et al, "High Density Lipoprotein as a Protective Factor Against Coronary Heart Disease. The Framingham Study," *Am J Med*, 1977, 62:707-14.

Grundy SM, "Cholesterol and Coronary Heart Disease: A New Era," *JAMA*, 1986, 256:2849-58.

Kannel WB, "Low High-Density Lipoprotein Cholesterol and What to Do About It," *Am J Cardiol*, 1992, 70(7):810-4, (editorial).

Lavie CJ, O'Keefe JH, Blonde L, et al, "High-Density Lipoprotein Cholesterol. Recommendations for Routine Testing and Treatment," *Postgrad Med*, 1990, 87(7):36-44, 47, 51.

Lees RS and Lees AM, "High Density Lipoproteins and the Risk of Atherosclerosis," *N Engl J Med*, 1982, 306:1546-8, (editorial).

Levin SJ, "High Density Lipoprotein Cholesterol: Review of Methods," *ASCP Check Sample®*, Chicago, IL: The American Society of Clinical Pathologists, 1989, 5:1-9.

Norum RA, Lakier JB, Goldstein S, et al, "Familial Deficiency of Apolipoproteins A-I and C-III and Precocious Coronary Artery Disease," *N Engl J Med*, 1982, 306:1513-9.

Ordovas JM, Schaefer EJ, Salem D, et al, "Apolipoprotein A-1 Gene Polymorphism Associated With Premature Coronary Artery Disease and Familial Hypoalphalipoproteinemia," *N Engl J Med*, 1986, 314:671-7.

(Continued)

High Density Lipoprotein Cholesterol *(Continued)*

Pocock SJ, Shaper AG, and Phillips AN, "Concentrations of High Density Lipoprotein Cholesterol, Triglycerides, and Total Cholesterol in Ischaemic Heart Disease," *Br Med J [Clin Res]*, 1989, 298(6679):998-1002.

Rifkind BM, "High-Density Lipoprotein Cholesterol and Coronary Artery Disease: Survey of the Evidence," *Am J Cardiol*, 1990, 66(6):3A-6A.

Sady SP, Thompson PD, Cullinane EM, et al, "Clinical Investigation: Prolonged Exercise Augments Plasma Triglyceride Clearance," *JAMA*, 1986, 256:2552-5.

Steinmetz J and Delattre J, "High Density Lipoprotein Cholesterol," *Drug Effects on Laboratory Test Results Analytical Interferences and Pharmacological Effects*, Siest G and Galteau MM, eds, Littleton, MA: PSG Publishing Co Inc, 1988, 185-97.

Superko HR, Bachorik PS, and Woods PD, "High Density Lipoprotein Cholesterol Measurements: A Help or Hindrance in Practical Clinical Medicine?" *JAMA*, 1986, 256:2714-7.

Weitzman JB and Vladutiu AO, "Very High Values of Serum High-Density Lipoprotein Cholesterol," *Arch Pathol Lab Med*, 1992, 116(8):831-6.

Hill Plots *see* P-50 Blood Gas *on page 307*

Histalog™ Stimulation Test *replaced by* Gastric Analysis *on page 232*

Histamine

CPT 83088

Patient Care **PREPARATION:** Patient must be on a diet of microbially processed foods, such as cheeses or sauerkraut.

Specimen Blood, urine, or cerebrospinal fluid[1] **CONTAINER:** Special vial is required for blood **COLLECTION:** Collect 10 mL blood without preservative and transfer immediately to vial containing 20 mg potassium oxalate; 24-hour urine collection, send 50 mL aliquot **STORAGE INSTRUCTIONS:** Store blood or urine frozen. **SPECIAL INSTRUCTIONS:** Test is ordinarily available only from a few reference laboratories.

Interpretive **REFERENCE RANGE:** Blood: 3-9 μg/dL (SI: 98-293 nmol/L); urine: 17-68 μg/24 hours (SI: 553-2210 nmol/L); considerably method variable **USE:** Evaluate possible systemic mastocytosis **LIMITATIONS:** Test not very sensitive. There are false-positive results associated with urinary tract infections. Histamine level alone may not fully reflect the role of histamine in a disease process. Measurement of histamine and its metabolites may be necessary.[2] **METHODOLOGY:** Gas chromatography (GC),[1] fluorometry,[3] radioisotope enzymatic,[4,5] high performance liquid chromatography (HPLC),[6,7] chemical ionization mass spectrometry **ADDITIONAL INFORMATION:** Mast cells produce numerous biologically active materials, including histamine.[8] Histamine is often, but not consistently, elevated in cases of systemic mastocytosis,[9] and also in other myeloproliferative disorders such as chronic myelogenous leukemia and polycythemia vera. Some carcinoid tumors (particularly of gastric origin) produce excessive amounts of histamine. Measurement of urinary methylated and other histamine metabolites may be more sensitive and specific. In a study of 25 patients with urticaria pigmentosa, methylimidazoleacetic acid, the major histamine metabolite, was able to identify all cases of systemic mastocytosis (>4.1 mg/24 hours) while histamine was elevated in only half of cases.[10] In another study of systemic mast cell disease urinary histamine was elevated in only 1 of 26 cases.[11] Histamine release from basophils and mast cells in response to allergen and reagin complex is generally recognized. There is also evidence that histamine is synthesized by T cells/macrophages *de novo* through the action of histidine decarboxylase.[12,13] There is evidence suggesting that basophils have an interleukin 1 receptor that can modulate the response to IgE-related signals.[14]

Serum histamine levels are decreased with HIV infection, a finding of possible prognostic significance. Splenectomy results in a rise in histamine levels in AIDS patients with thrombocytopenic purpura. Histamine levels have been reported decreased in some 60% of patients with malignant disease.[15]

Footnotes

1. Khandelwal JK, Hough LB, Mornshow AM, et al, "Measurement of Tele-Methylhistamine and Histamine in Human Cerebrospinal Fluid, Urine, and Plasma," *Agents Actions*, 1982, 12:583-90.
2. Green JP, Prell GD, Khandelwal JK, et al, "Aspects of Histamine Metabolism," *Agents Actions*, 1987, 22:1-15.
3. Assem ESK and Chong EKS, "Simultaneous Fluorometric Assay of Histamine and Histidine in Biological Fluid Using an Automated Analyzer," *Agents Actions*, 1982, 12:26-9.
4. Horakova Z, Keiser HR, and Beaven MA, "Blood and Urine Histamine Levels in Normal and Pathological States as Measured by a Radiochemical Assay," *Clin Chim Acta*, 1977, 79:447-56.

5. Dyer J, Warren K, Merlin S, et al, "Measurement of Plasma Histamine: Description of an Improved Method and Normal Values," *J Allergy Clin Immunol*, 1982, 70:82-7.
6. Granerus G and Wass U, "Urinary Excretion of Histamine, Methylhistamine (1-MeHi), and Methylimidazoleacetic Acid (MelmAA) in Mastocytosis: Comparison of New HPLC Methods With Other Present Methods," *Agents Actions*, 1984, 14:341-5.
7. Liotet S, Meyohas MC, Batellier L, et al, "Blood Histamine Levels in Patients Infected With the Human Immunodeficiency Virus," *Presse Med*, 1988, 17:2240-2.
8. McBride P, Jacobs R, Bradley D, et al, "Use of Plasma Histamine Levels to Monitor Cutaneous Mast Cell Degranulation," *J Allergy Clin Immunol*, 1989, 83(2 Pt 1):374-80.
9. Friedman BS, Steinberg SC, Meggs WJ, et al, "Analysis of Plasma Histamine Levels in Patients With Mast Cell Disorders," *Am J Med*, 1989, 87(6):649-54.
10. Granerus G and Roupe G, "Increased Urinary Methylimidazoleacetic Acid (MelmAA) as an Indicator of Systemic Mastocytosis," *Agents Actions*, 1982, 12:29-31.
11. Webb TA, Li C-Y, and Yam LT, "Systemic Mast Cell Disease: A Clinical and Hematopathologic Study of 26 Cases," *Cancer*, 1982, 49:927-38.
12. Aoi R, Nakashima I, Kitamura Y, et al, "Histamine Synthesis by Mouse T Lymphocytes Through Induced Histidine Decarboxylase," *Immunology*, 1989, 66(2):219-23.
13. Oh C, Suzuki S, Nakashima I, et al, "Histamine Synthesis by Non-Mast Cells Through Mitogen-Dependent Induction of Histidine Decarboxylase," *Immunology*, 1988, 65:143-8.
14. Massey WA, Randall TC, Kagey-Sobotka A, et al, "Recombinant Human IL-1α and -1β Potentiate IgE-Mediated Histamine Release From Human Basophils," *J Immunol*, 1989, 143(6):1875-80.
15. Motoki T, Obara T, Ezoe H, et al, "Low Serum Histamine in Malignant Disease," *N Engl J Med*, 1984, 310, 391-2.

References

Jacobs R, Kaliner M, Shelhamer JH, et al, "Blood Histamine Concentrations Are Not Elevated in Humans With Septic Shock," *Crit Care Med*, 1989, 17(1):30-5.

Keyzer JJ, de Monchy JG, van Doormaal JJ, et al, "Improved Diagnosis of Mastocytosis by Measurement of Urinary Histamine Metabolites," *N Engl J Med*, 1983, 309:1603-5.

Hoesch Test *see* Porphobilinogen, Qualitative, Urine *on page 325*

Holmes Formula *see* Osmolality, Calculated *on page 299*

Homocysteine, Qualitative *see* Cystine, Qualitative *on page 205*

Homovanillic Acid, Urine

CPT *83150*

Related Information

Catecholamines, Fractionation, Plasma *on page 172*
Catecholamines, Fractionation, Urine *on page 174*
Metanephrines, Total, Urine *on page 289*
Vanillylmandelic Acid, Urine *on page 382*

Synonyms HVA

Test Commonly Includes Measurement of creatinine excretion as well as HVA

Patient Care PREPARATION: Patients should avoid aspirin, disulfiram, reserpine, and pyridoxine, if possible at least 48 hours prior to collection of the specimen. Levodopa should be avoided for 2 weeks before collection.

Specimen 24-hour urine CONTAINER: Plastic urine container COLLECTION: Urine specimen should not contact metal. Depending on laboratory, boric, acetic, or hydrochloric acid must initially be added to the container as a preservative. Check with your laboratory for volume and concentration. STORAGE INSTRUCTIONS: Measure 24-hour urine volume, adjust to pH 2-4 and aliquot 100 mL sample and refrigerate. Stable 7 days at 4°C. SPECIAL INSTRUCTIONS: For work-up for neuroblastoma, excretion of VMA should also be measured.

Homovanillic Acid, Urine

Age, y	μg HVA/mg creatinine	SI: mmol HVA/mol creatinine
0–1	1.2–35.0	0.7–21.7
1–2	4.0–23.0	2.5–14.3
2–5	0.5–20.0	0.3–12.4
5–10	0.5–15.0	0.3–9.3
10–15	0.25–12.0	0.2–7.4
Adults	0.25–7.0	0.2–4.4

Adults: <8 mg/24 h.

Interpretive REFERENCE RANGE: Adult normal range is usually <8 mg/24 hours (SI: <44 μmol/day). Pediatric values are up to 35 μg HVA/mg creatinine (SI: 22 mmol HVA/mol creatinine) in infancy. See table. USE: Diagnose neuroblastoma, ganglioneuroblastoma, and pheochromo-
(Continued)

Homovanillic Acid, Urine *(Continued)*

cytoma; follow course of tumor treatment **LIMITATIONS:** Almost all patients with neuroblastoma have elevations of HVA, while only about 80% have elevations of urinary catecholamines. Increased HVA levels, however, are not specific for neuroblastoma. **METHODOLOGY:** High performance liquid chromatography (HPLC), solvent extraction, and colorimetry[1,2] **ADDITIONAL INFORMATION:** HVA is the major terminal metabolite of the dopamine pathway. VMA is the major terminal metabolite of the norepinephrine pathway. HVA is often excreted in excess amounts by neuroblastomas, ganglioneuroblastomas, pheochromocytomas, and in Riley-Day syndrome. Excretion may be intermittent. Plasma HVA is increased in schizotypal personality disorders.[3] Approximately 20% of subjects with neuroblastoma do not have increased VMA.[1]

Footnotes

1. Rothstein A, "Determination of Urinary Homovanillic Acid Using the Nitrosonaphthol Reaction," *Am J Clin Pathol*, 1987, 87:644-8.
2. Davidson DF, "Simultaneous Assay for Urinary 4-Hydroxy-3-Methoxy-Mandelic Acid, 5-Hydroxyindoleacetic Acid and Homovanillic Acid by Isocractic HPLC With Electrochemical Detection," *Ann Clin Biochem*, 1989, 26(Pt 2):137-43.
3. Siever LJ, Amin F, Coccaro EF, et al, "Plasma Homovanillic Acid in Schizotypal Personality Disorder," *Am J Psychiatry*, 1991, 148(9):1246-8.

References

Javors MA, Bowden CL, and Maas LW, "3-Methoxy-4-Hydroxyphenylglycol, 5-Hydroxyindoleacetic Acid, and Homovanillic Acid in Human Cerebrospinal Fluid. Storage and Measurement by Reversed-Phase High Performance Liquid Chromatography and Coulometric Detection Using 3-Methoxy-4-Hydroxyphenylacetic Acid as an Internal Standard," *J Chromatogr*, 1984, 336:259-69.

Lavin N, "Neuroblastoma, Ganglioneuroblastoma, and Ganglioneuroma," Lavin N, ed, *Manual of Endocrinology and Metabolism*, Boston, MA: Little, Brown and Co, 1986, 141-2.

Leavelle DE, *Mayo Medical Laboratories Interpretive Handbook*, Rochester, MN: Mayo Medical Laboratories, 1990.

2-Hour PP Glucose *see* Glucose, 2-Hour Postprandial *on page 237*

HP *see* Haptoglobin, Serum *on page 247*

Hp *see* Haptoglobin, Serum *on page 247*

hPL *see* Placental Lactogen, Human *on page 324*

5-HT *see* Serotonin *on page 348*

Human Calcitonin *see* Calcitonin *on page 157*

Human Chorionic Gonadotropin, Serum

CPT *84702*

Related Information

Alpha$_1$-Fetoprotein, Serum *on page 115*
Placental Lactogen, Human *on page 324*
Pregnancy Test *on page 333*

Synonyms Beta Subunit, hCG; hCG; hCG, Beta Subunit

Applies to Pregnancy Testing; Tumor Detection

Patient Care **PREPARATION:** Patient must avoid having radioisotope scan prior to collection of specimen, if test is to be done by RIA.

Specimen Serum **CONTAINER:** Red top tube **STORAGE INSTRUCTIONS:** Serum stable 24 hours at 25°C and 4 days at 4°C. Freeze at -20°C for longer storage.[1,2] **CAUSES FOR REJECTION:** Recently administered radioisotopes **SPECIAL INSTRUCTIONS:** For females, state date of last menstrual period.

Interpretive **REFERENCE RANGE:** Depends on application and methodology. <3 mIU/mL (SI: <3 IU/L) usually normal (nonpregnant). **USE:** Work up and manage germ cell neoplasms. High levels may be found with choriocarcinoma, embryonal cell carcinoma, and gestational trophoblastic tumors. Islet cell tumors may make hCG, as may some carcinomas of lung, stomach, colon, pancreas, liver, and breast. hCG is used in prenatal screening for trisomy 21 (Down syndrome).[3] In combination with serum estriol and serum AFP, the detection of Down syndrome is greatly increased, from 25% to 65%. **LIMITATIONS:** Normal hCG levels do not rule out germinal tumor. The same test method may not be suitable for use as a tumor marker and for pregnancy testing. Several reference preparations may be used as standards, different methods calibrated against different materials, making interlaboratory comparisons difficult. **METHODOLOGY:** Two site immunoradiometric assay (IRMA), radioimmunoassay (RIA); two site enzyme-linked immunosorbent assay (ELISA) methods have been especially successful commercially to assist the diagnosis of early pregnancy.[4,5] Time resolved europium-chelate fluorescence procedures may exceed RIA in sensitivity.[6] Two site fluorescent immunoassay is capable of measurement to the 1 mIU/mL.[7] hCG by RIA measures the immunologic activities of both hCG and its free beta subunit (sometimes called total beta assays). **ADDITIONAL INFORMATION:** Human chorionic gonadotropin, a glycoprotein hormone, which is normally produced by the developing placenta, and aberrantly produced by some germ cell neoplasms, is composed of glycopeptide α- and β-subunits. The α-subunit, a 92-amino acid sequence, is identical with that of luteinizing hormone, follicle stimulating hormone, and thyroid stimulating hormone; and it is this shared structure which accounts for some false-positives in pregnancy tests not based on the β-subunit. The β-subunit, a 145 amino acid sequence, is unique to hCG and specific tests for it are not subject to hormonal cross reactivity. Tests specific for β-subunit are now available sensitive enough to detect a normal pregnancy 6-10 days after implantation, levels of hCG can be detected as low as 5 mIU/mL (SI: 5 IU/L).

Chorionic gonadotropin assays are sometimes used to support the diagnosis of ectopic pregnancy. Ectopic gestations do not develop or secrete hCG as do intrauterine pregnancies. Abnormally low hCG levels coupled with transvaginal ultrasound detect many ectopic pregnancies prior to rupture.[8] It is especially useful to measure hCG sequentially every other day to detect a lack of rise in the level.

hCG levels are extremely useful in following those germ cell neoplasms which produce hCG, particularly trophoblastic neoplasms. Following evacuation of a trophoblastic lesion, hCG β-subunit should fall to normal in 6-8 weeks and stay there. Oral contraceptive use may delay this fall. Any other delay in the fall, or subsequent rise, is an indication for other further evaluation.

In germ cell neoplasms in the male, β-hCG and α-fetoprotein are both useful tumor markers. They can be demonstrated histochemically in tissue to confirm diagnosis and can be followed in serum to evaluate recurrence.

hCG has high carbohydrate content, 30% of its molecular weight is due to sugars, 8% to 9% is the result of sialic acid. Removal of sialic acid residues from the β-subunit decreases biologic activity by 50%. A considerable understanding of the molecular structure and molecular biologic function has developed.

Footnotes

1. Hohnadel DC and Kaplan LA, "Hormones and Their Metabolites; β-hCG (β-Human Chorionic Gonadotropin)," *Clinical Chemistry: Theory, Analysis, and Correlation*, 2nd ed, Kaplan LA and Pesce AJ, eds, St Louis, MO: Mosby-Year Book Inc, 1989, 938-44.
2. Greene MF, Fencl MD, and Tulchinsky D, "Biochemical Aspects of Pregnancy," *Fundamentals of Clinical Chemistry*, 3rd ed, Tietz NW, ed, Philadelphia, PA: WB Saunders Co, 1987, 906-13.
3. Petrocik E, Wassman ER, and Kelly JC, "Prenatal Screening for Down Syndrome With Maternal Serum Human Chorionic Gonadotropin Levels," *Am J Obstet Gynecol*, 1989, 161(5):1168-73.
4. Bandi ZL, Schoen I, and DeLara M, "Enzyme-Linked Immunosorbent Urine Pregnancy Tests: Clinical Specificity Studies," *Am J Clin Pathol*, 1987, 87:236-42.
5. Braunstein GD, Kelley L, Farber S, et al, "Two Rapid, Sensitive, and Specific Immunoenzymatic Assays of Human Choriogonadotropin in Urine Evaluated," *Clin Chem*, 1986, 32:1413-4.
6. Lövgren T, Hemmilä I, Pettersson K, et al, "Time-Resolved Fluorometry in Immunoassays," *Alternative Immunoassays*, Collins WP, ed, New York, NY: John Wiley and Sons, 1985, 203-17.
7. Pettersson K, Siitari H, Hemmilä I, et al, "Time-Resolved Fluoroimmunoassay of Human Choriogonadotropin," *Clin Chem*, 1983, 29:60-4.
8. DiMarchi JM, Kosasa TS, and Hale RW, "What Is the Significance of the Human Chorionic Gonadotropin Value in Ectopic Pregnancy?" *Obstet Gynecol*, 1989, 74(6):851-5.

References

Khazaeli MB, Buchina ES, Pattillo RA, et al, "Radioimmunoassay of Free Beta-Subunit of Human Chorionic Gonadotropin in Diagnosis of High-Risk and Low-Risk Gestational Trophoblastic Disease," *Am J Obstet Gynecol*, 1989, 160(2):444-9.

Nomura F, Ohnishi K, and Tanabe Y, "Clinical Features and Prognosis of Hepatocellular Carcinoma With Reference to Serum Alpha-Fetoprotein Levels," *Cancer*, 1989, 64(8):1700-7.

Tyrey L, "Human Chorionic Gonadotropin Assays and Their Uses," *Obstet Gynecol Clin North Am*, 1988, 15:457-75.

Vaitukaitis JL, Braunstein GD, Ross GT, et al, "A Radioimmunoassay Which Specifically Measures Human Chorionic Gonadotropin in the Presence of Human Luteinizing Hormone," *Am J Obstet Gynecol*, 1972, 113:751-8.

Vaitukaitis JL, "Radioimmunoassay of Human Choriogonadotropin," *Clin Chem*, 1985, 31:1749-54.

Human Chorionic Gonadotropin, Urine *see* Pregnancy Test *on page 333*

Human Chorionic Somatomammotropin *see* Placental Lactogen, Human *on page 324*

Human Pancreatic Polypeptide *see* Pancreatic Polypeptide, Human *on page 310*

Human Placental Lactogen *see* Placental Lactogen, Human *on page 324*

HVA *see* Homovanillic Acid, Urine *on page 253*

Hydrocortisone, Serum *see* Cortisol, Blood *on page 191*

11-Hydroxyandrosterone *see* 17-Ketosteroids Fractionation, Urine *on page 267*

β-Hydroxybutyrate *see* Ketone Bodies, Blood *on page 265*

17-Hydroxycorticosteroids, Urine

CPT 83491

Related Information

Cortisol, Blood *on page 191*

17-Ketogenic Steroids, Urine *on page 265*

Synonyms 17-OHCS; Porter-Silber Chromogens, Urine

Patient Care PREPARATION: All drugs ideally should be withheld for several days prior to collection of urine, if possible, without doing harm to the patient. Avoid patient stress.

Specimen 24-hour urine CONTAINER: Plastic container with hydrochloric or acetic acid as preservative COLLECTION: Instruct the patient to void at 8 AM and discard the specimen. Then collect all urine including the final specimen voided at the end of the 24-hour collection specimen (ie, 8 AM the next morning). Container must be labeled with patient's name, date, and time. STORAGE INSTRUCTIONS: Refrigerate during collection, refrigerate or freeze after collection. Stable 45 days if refrigerated and acidified. CAUSES FOR REJECTION: Preservative not added

Interpretive REFERENCE RANGE: A modicum of variation exists between published ranges. See table. USE: Adrenal function test useful in evaluation of glucocorticoid production; increased in ectopic ACTH syndrome, Cushing's syndrome, and stress; decreased in Addison's disease, adrenogenital syndrome, pituitary insufficiency.[1] Urinary metabolites of glucocorticoids can be measured by 17-ketogenic steroids and 17-hydroxycorticosteroids. More metabolites are measured by the former.[2] LIMITATIONS: Subject to interferences and variability due to unreliable 24-hour urine collections. Now that they are available, serum or urine cortisol measurements are preferred. **Urinary free cortisol is a more sensitive and specific test for hypercortisolism.**[3] METHODOLOGY: Porter-Silber color reaction ADDITIONAL INFORMATION: The Porter-Silber color reaction detects steroids with a dihydroxyacetone group at carbon 17, including major glucocorticoid metabolites. By pretreating with a strong reducing agent one increases the number of metabolites detected (ie, 17-ketogenic steroids). Either 17-hydroxysteroid or 17-ketogenic steroid measurements can be used as an estimate of adrenal steroid production, either as baseline values or in stimulation or suppression tests.

17–Hydroxycorticosteroids, Urine

Age	Conventional Units	SI Units
<8 y	<1.5 mg/24 h	< 4.1 μmol/d
8–12 y	<4.5 mg/24 h	<12.4 μmol/d
Adults male female	 4.5–12.0 mg/24 h 2.5–10.0 mg/24 h	 12.4–33.1 μmol/d 6.9–27.6 μmol/d

Deoxycorticosterone (DOC), corticosterone (compound B) and aldosterone lack a 17-hydroxyl group and are not measured in 17-KG and 17-OHCS procedures.[2]

Footnotes

1. Zeiger MA, Nieman LK, Cutler GB, et al, "Primary Bilateral Adrenocortical Causes of Cushing's Syndrome," *Surgery*, 1991, 110(6):1106-15.
2. Speroff L, Glass RH, and Kase NG, *Clinical Gynecologic Endocrinology and Infertility*, 4th ed, Baltimore, MD: Williams & Wilkins, 1989.
3. Flack MR, Oldfield EH, Cutler GB Jr, et al, "Urine Free Cortisol in the High-Dose Dexamethasone Suppression Test for the Differential Diagnosis of the Cushing Syndrome," *Ann Intern Med*, 1992, 116(3):211-7.

References

Patel ST and Lott JA, "Cortisol," *Methods in Clinical Chemistry*, Pesce AJ and Kaplan LA, eds, St Louis, MO: Mosby-Year Book Inc, 1987, 224-31.

11-Hydroxyetiocholanolone *see* 17-Ketosteroids Fractionation, Urine *on page 267*

5-Hydroxyindoleacetic Acid, Quantitative, Urine

CPT *83497*

Related Information

Serotonin *on page 348*

Synonyms 5-HIAA, Quantitative, Urine

Applies to Serotonin, Metabolite

Abstract Derived from tryptophan, serotonin (5-hydroxytryptamine) (5-HT) is metabolized to 5-hydroxyindoleacetic acid. Increased excretions occur in the presence of carcinoid tumors. Carcinoid tumors are enterochromaffin neoplasms containing amine precursor uptake and decarboxylation cells (APUDomas). They occur in the multiple endocrine neoplasia syndrome (MEN) I or II but are often not a part of those entities. Occasional carcinoids secrete other substances, including ACTH, gastrin, insulin, VIP, and calcitonin.

Patient Care PREPARATION: Avoid bananas, avocados, chocolate, plums, eggplant, tomatoes, plantain, pineapples, walnuts, acetaminophen, salicylates, phenacetin, cough syrup containing glyceryl guaiacolate, naproxen (Naprosyn®, Anaprox®), mephenesin, methocarbamol, imipramine, isoniazid, MAO inhibitors, methenamine, methyldopa, phenothiazines, for a 48-hour period or more prior to and during the collection. Drug interference relates to method; check with laboratory.

Specimen 24-hour urine CONTAINER: Check with laboratory. Glacial acetic, hydrochloric, or boric acids are often recommended as preservative. COLLECTION: 24-hour urine STORAGE INSTRUCTIONS: Stable 7 days if acidified and refrigerated.

Interpretive REFERENCE RANGE: Approximately 1-9 mg/24 hours (SI: 5-48 μmol/day) CRITICAL VALUES: >25 mg/24 hours indicative of carcinoid syndrome USE: Diagnose carcinoid tumors and syndrome; values >25 mg/24 hours (higher if the patient has malabsorption) are strong evidence for carcinoid. LIMITATIONS: 5-HIAA may be normal with nonmetastatic carcinoid tumor and may be normal even with the carcinoid syndrome, particularly in subjects without diarrhea. Some patients with the carcinoid syndrome excrete nonhydroxylated indolic acids, not measured as 5-HIAA. Midgut carcinoids are most apt to produce the carcinoid syndrome with 5-HIAA elevation. Patients with renal disease may have falsely low 5-HIAA levels in the urine.[1] 5-HIAA is increased in untreated patients with malabsorption, who have increased urinary tryptophan metabolites. Such patients include those with celiac disease, tropical sprue, Whipple's disease, stasis syndrome, and cystic fibrosis. It is increased in those with chronic intestinal obstruction. Poor correlation exists between 5-HIAA level and the clinical severity of the carcinoid syndrome. Recent studies confirm its use as a prognostic factor in this disease.[2] CONTRAINDICATIONS: False elevated results if foods containing serotonin or drugs producing metabolites that react with nitrosonaphthol, a reagent used in this determination, are ingested within 2 days prior to collection. METHODOLOGY: Colorimetry after extraction, spectrophotometric, gas chromatography (GC), high performance liquid chromatography (HPLC),[3] fluorescence polarization immunoassay (FPIA) ADDITIONAL INFORMATION: 5-HIAA is the major urinary metabolite of serotonin, a ubiquitous bioactive amine. Serotonin, and consequently 5-HIAA, are produced in excess by most carcinoid tumors, especially those producing the carcinoid syndrome of flushing, hepatomegaly, diarrhea, bronchospasm, and heart disease. Quantitation of urinary 5-HIAA is the best test for carcinoid, but scrupulous care must be taken that specimen collection and patient preparation have been correct. Carcinoid tumors may cause increased excretion of tryptophan, 5-hydroxytryptophan and histamine as well as serotonin. Serum serotonin assay may detect some carcinoids missed by 5-HIAA assay. It may be done by HPLC, RIA, or radioenzymatic assay, but it is not offered by many laboratories, even prestigious reference laboratories. Of 75 patients with carcinoid tumors, 75% had above normal urinary 5-HIAA excretion and 64% had above normal serotonin excretion. Six patients with increased urinary serotonin had normal urinary 5-HIAA.

Footnotes

1. Schultz AL, "5-Hydroxyindoleacetic Acid," *Methods in Clinical Chemistry*, Pesce AJ and Kaplan LA, eds, St Louis, MO: Mosby-Year Book Inc, 1987, 714-20.
2. Agranovich AL, Anderson GH, Manji M, et al, "Carcinoid Tumour of the Gastrointestinal Tract: Prognostic Factors and Disease Outcome," *J Surg Oncol*, 1991, 47(1):45-52.
3. Stroomer AE, Overmars H, Abeling NG, et al, "Simultaneous Determination of Acidic 3,4-Dihydroxyphenylalanine Metabolites and 5-Hydroxyindole-3-Acetic Acid in Urine by High Performance Liquid Chromatography," *Clin Chem*, 1990, 36(10):1834-7.

(Continued)

5-Hydroxyindoleacetic Acid, Quantitative, Urine *(Continued)*

References

Lechago J, "Neuroendocrine Cells of the Gut and Their Disorders," *Gastrointestinal Pathology*, Goldman H, Appelman HD, and Kaufman N, eds, Baltimore, MD: Williams & Wilkins, 1990, 181-219.

Vinik AI, McLeod MK, Fig LM, et al, "Clinical Features, Diagnosis, and Localization of Carcinoid Tumors and Their Management," *Gastroenterol Clin North Am*, 1989, 18(4):865-96.

17-Hydroxyprogesterone, Blood or Amniotic Fluid

CPT 83498

Related Information

17-Ketogenic Steroids, Urine *on page 265*
17-Ketosteroids, Total, Urine *on page 267*
Pregnanetriol, Urine *on page 335*

Synonyms 17-OHP

Replaces Urine 17-Ketogenic Steroids; Urine Pregnanetriol Assay

Abstract A C-21 steroid, 17-hydroxyprogesterone is produced by adrenal cortices, ovaries, testes, and placenta. It is converted to pregnanetriol.

Patient Care PREPARATION: No radioactive isotopes

Specimen Serum or plasma, amniotic fluid[1] CONTAINER: Red top tube or lavender top (EDTA) tube; check with laboratory. STORAGE INSTRUCTIONS: Separate within 4 hours. Serum or plasma stable 7 days at 4°C to 25°C.

Interpretive REFERENCE RANGE: Ranges vary between laboratories. These are examples. Adults: male: 50-200 ng/dL (SI: 1.5-6.0 nmol/L), female follicular phase: 20-80 ng/dL (SI: 0.6-2.4 nmol/L), female luteal phase: 100-300 ng/dL (SI: 3.0-9.0 nmol/L), female postmenopausal: <50 ng/dL (SI: <1.5 nmol/L) CRITICAL VALUES: The lack of required levels of adrenocortical steroids in the adrenogenital syndrome can be life-threatening. Early diagnosis and therapy are indicated. USE: Markedly elevated in patients with congenital adrenal hyperplasia (adrenogenital syndrome) due to 21-hydroxylase deficiency. Evaluate hirsutism and/or infertility. Assess certain adrenal or ovarian tumors with endocrine activity. LIMITATIONS: Elevated, but less so, in 11-hydroxylase deficiency. Measurement of serum 11-desoxycortisol (substance S) can differentiate these abnormalities. METHODOLOGY: Radioimmunoassay (RIA), high performance liquid chromatography (HPLC) ADDITIONAL INFORMATION: 17-Hydroxyprogesterone is the substrate for subsequent 21- and 11-hydroxylation, to produce cortisol. The two critical enzymes, 21-hydroxylase and 11-beta-hydroxylase, participate in cortisol generation. If hydroxylation, at either position, cannot take place because of enzyme deficiency, cortisol synthesis decreases, accompanied by increased ACTH. Congenital adrenal hyperplasia and adrenogenital syndrome result from lack of normal glucocorticoids and build up of precursors (mostly virilizing). Lack of 21-hydroxylase is the most common cause of adrenogenital syndrome. Congenital adrenal hyperplasia caused by 21-hydroxylase deficiency is the most common cause of female hermaphroditism.[1] It is an autosomal recessive disease. Basal 17-hydroxyprogesterone levels can be normal in late-onset 21-hydroxylase deficiency presenting as hirsutism. Such patients are described as having a dramatically increased 17-hydroxyprogesterone response to ACTH. Patients with 21-hydroxylase deficiency have increased 17-ketosteroids, urine pregnanetriol, as well as, high 17-hydroxyprogesterone. 17-Hydroxyprogesterone can also be measured on heelstick blood collected on filter paper for infant screening. Prenatal diagnosis of congenital adrenal hyperplasia is possible by HLA typing, by DNA analysis, or by hormone measurements from amniotic fluid, including 17-hydroxyprogesterone.[1] Some nonspecificity is seen when amniotic fluid analysis is used.[2] Congenital adrenal hyperplasia with adult onset is among the causes of hirsutism and/or infertility.

Footnotes

1. Pang S, Pollack MS, Marshall RN, et al, "Prenatal Treatment of Congenital Adrenal Hyperplasia Due to 21-Hydroxylase Deficiency," *N Engl J Med*, 1990, 322(2):111-5.
2. Lee A and Ellis G, "Serum 17-Alpha-Hydroxyprogesterone in Infants and Children as Measured by a Direct Radioimmunoassay Kit," *Clin Biochem*, 1991, 24(6):505-11.

References

Check JH, Vaze MM, Epstein R, et al, "17-Hydroxyprogesterone Level as a Marker for Corpus Luteum Function in Aborters Versus Nonaborters," *Int J Fertil*, 1990, 35(2):112-5.

Robboy SJ, Lombardo JM, and Welch WR, "Disorders of Abnormal Sexual Development," *Blaustein's Pathology of the Female Genital Tract*, 3rd ed, Kurman RJ, ed, New York, NY: Springer-Verlag, 1987, 15-35.

Hydroxyproline, Total, Urine

CPT 83505

Abstract Collagen has a very high content of hydroxyproline (and proline). Urinary excretion of hydroxyproline reflects collagen catabolism and is high in periods of rapid bone turnover (eg, Paget's disease of bone).

Patient Care **PREPARATION:** Avoid foods containing gelatin and meat prior to and during urine collection. These include gelatin desserts (Jello®), ice creams, candies. Patient must avoid aspirin-containing drugs. Hormonal agents affect quantitation.

Specimen 24-hour urine **CONTAINER:** Plastic urine container **COLLECTION:** Add 10 mL toluene to container before the beginning of collection; will vary with the individual laboratory. Instruct the patient to void at 8 AM and discard the specimen. Then collect all urine including the final specimen voided at the end of the 24-hour collection period (ie, 8 AM the next morning). Refrigerate during collection. Container must be labeled with patient's name, date, and time. A 2-hour collection after overnight fast may also be used. **SPECIAL INSTRUCTIONS:** Requisition must state date and time collection started and date and time collection finished. Indicate patient's age and sex.

Interpretive **REFERENCE RANGE:** Adult male: 15-45 mg/24 hours (1-4 mg/2 hours) (7-20 μg/mg creatinine) (SI: 76-381 μmol/day). Adult female values are about one-half of the male ranges. Infants, children, and adolescents variably higher depending on growth spurts. Normal range is higher in infancy, childhood, and adolescence, especially during growth spurts. Care must be taken to note the type of diet employed in establishing the reference range of a given laboratory. Most reference values have been obtained on low-dose gelatin, not gelatin-free diets. **USE:** Evaluate collagen metabolism of bone. High in Paget's disease of bone, indicating increased bone resorption and formation. Congenital hydroxyprolinemias are extremely rare. Iminoglycinuria occurs with a frequency of about 1:16,000. A benign autosomal recessive disease, it represents a renal tubular defect. Excessive excretion of glycine, proline, and hydroxyproline occurs. Other hydroxyprolinurias also exist, also without established clinical entities. Measured in osteomalacia when serum alkaline phosphatase is normal, or with coexisting hepatic disease and secondary increase of alkaline phosphatase. Increased with healing fracture. Increased with elevated thyroid function probably because of increased bone turnover in this condition.[1] **METHODOLOGY:** Extraction/colorimetry; high performance liquid chromatography (HPLC) **ADDITIONAL INFORMATION:** Increases occur in osteoporosis, osteomalacia, rickets, primary and secondary hyperparathyroidism, with prolonged bedrest, pregnancy, and acromegaly. Hydroxyproline may be measured as a marker of metastasis of malignancy to bone.[2] Multiple myeloma may increase urinary hydroxyproline levels. Urinary hydroxyproline, like serum alkaline phosphatase, is useful in evaluation and response to treatment of Paget's disease of bone.[3]

Footnotes

1. Krakauer JC and Kleerekoper M, "Borderline-Low Serum Thyrotropin Level Is Correlated With Increased Fasting Urinary Hydroxyproline Excretion," *Arch Intern Med*, 1992, 152(2):360-4.
2. Kaplan LA, "Laboratory Approaches," *Methods in Clinical Chemistry*, Pesce AJ and Kaplan LA, eds, St Louis, MO: Mosby-Year Book Inc, 1987, 680-2.
3. Leavelle DE, *Mayo Medical Laboratories Interpretive Handbook*, Rochester, MN: Mayo Medical Laboratories, 1990.

References

Gilbertson TJ, Branden MN, Gruszczyk SB, et al, "Serum Total Hydroxyproline Assay Effects of Age, Sex, and Paget's Bone Disease," *J Clin Chem Clin Biochem*, 1983, 21:129-32.

Meites S, *Pediatric Clinical Chemistry: Reference (Normal) Values*, 3rd ed, Washington, DC: American Association of Clinical Chemistry Press, 1989, 162.

Phang JM and Scriver CR, "Disorders of Proline and Hydroxyproline Metabolism," *The Metabolic Basis of Inherited Disease*, 6th ed, Scriver CR, Beaudet AL, Sly WS, et al, eds, New York, NY: McGraw-Hill Inc, 1989, 577-97.

5-Hydroxytryptamine, Blood *see* Serotonin *on page 348*

25-Hydroxy Vitamin D_3 *see* Vitamin D_3, Serum *on page 387*

Hyperlipoproteinemias *see* Lipoprotein Electrophoresis *on page 281*

Hyperphenylalaninemia Screen *see* Phenylalanine, Blood *on page 317*

Hypothyroidism, Newborn Screen *see* Newborn Screen for Hypothyroidism and Phenylketonuria *on page 295*

ICSH *see* Luteinizing Hormone, Blood or Urine *on page 286*

IgE Allergen Specific *see* Allergen Specific IgE Antibody *on page 112*

IGF-I *see* Somatomedin-C *on page 354*

Immunoreactive Insulin *see* Insulin, Blood *on this page*

Immunoreactive PTH *see* Parathyroid Hormone *on page 311*

Inborn Errors of Metabolism Screen *see* Amino Acid Screen, Plasma *on page 118*

Inborn Errors of Metabolism Screen *see* Amino Acid Screen, Qualitative, Urine *on page 120*

Insulin Antibody, Serum

CPT 86337

Related Information

C-Peptide *on page 195*

Test Commonly Includes Antibodies to both beef and pork insulin

Abstract Development of IgG antibodies to insulin in diabetic subjects on exogenous insulin therapy may lead to need for larger insulin doses. IgE antibodies can also develop, leading to reactions such as urticaria.

Patient Care PREPARATION: Avoid radioisotopes prior to collection of specimen.

Specimen Serum CONTAINER: Red top tube STORAGE INSTRUCTIONS: Serum stable for 7 days at 4°C. CAUSES FOR REJECTION: Anticoagulated blood collected

Interpretive REFERENCE RANGE: Method dependent. Results may be reported as percent binding of patient's serum to labeled insulin or as greatest dilution that shows detectable binding. Reference ranges are <3% for the former, 0 for the latter. USE: Determine the presence of antibodies against heterologous insulins. The presence of insulin antibody points to exogenous insulin administration (eg, use of beef and pork insulins by diabetics) or to insulin autoimmune hypoglycemia. Insulin antibody may be found in factitious hypoglycemia. LIMITATIONS: Antibodies to insulin are frequently detected in diabetics, even those who use human insulin. These are usually of little significance; however, high levels may be associated with insulin resistance. There is no definite titer associated with insulin resistance, although 1:64 has been suggested. METHODOLOGY: Radioimmunoassay (RIA) or enzyme-linked immunosorbent assay (ELISA). Recent work suggests insulin autoantibodies measured by RIA are more related to IDDM than those measured by ELISA.[1] ADDITIONAL INFORMATION: Such antibodies develop from impurities in animal insulins. Beef insulin is more allergenic than either pork or human insulins. Antibodies to insulin develop in insulin autoimmune hypoglycemia, a rare entity. In management of autoimmune disorders such as systemic lupus erythematosus (SLE), steroids are used and can induce diabetes mellitus. Such steroid-induced diabetes is a widely recognized complication of therapy of SLE. When insulin is required, such diabetic patients may be subject to risk of immunologic complications, developing antibodies while on steroid therapy. A case is reported of insulin antibodies in a patient with SLE before treatment with steroids.[2]

Footnotes

1. Greenbaum CJ, Palmer JP, Kuglin B, et al, "Insulin Autoantibodies Measured by Radioimmunoassay Methodology Are More Related to Insulin-Dependent Diabetes Mellitus Than Those Measured by Enzyme-Linked Immunosorbent Assay: Results of the Fourth International Workshop on the Standardization of Insulin Autoantibody Measurement," *J Clin Endocrinol Metab*, 1992, 74(5):1040-4.
2. Varga J, Lopatin M, and Boden G, "Hypoglycemia Due to Anti-insulin Receptor Antibodies in Systemic Lupus Erythematosus," *J Rheumatol*, 1990, 17(9):1226-9.

References

Leavelle DE, *Mayo Medical Laboratories Interpretive Handbook*, Rochester, MN: Mayo Medical Laboratories, 1990.

Insulin, Blood

CPT 83525

Related Information

C-Peptide *on page 195*
C-Reactive Protein *on page 669*
Glucose, Fasting *on page 238*
Glucose, Random *on page 240*
Glucose Tolerance Test *on page 241*

Synonyms Immunoreactive Insulin

Test Commonly Includes Glucose must be drawn simultaneously. Glucose for hypoglycemia work-up should not be done by reflectance meter.

Abstract The earliest molecule is preproinsulin. The precursor of insulin is proinsulin. Proinsulin as well as insulin are secreted by islet beta cells in response to glucose ingestion. Causes of fasting hypoglycemia include islet cell tumor (insulinoma), exogenous insulin or oral hypoglycemic drugs, alcohol use, pituitary or adrenal insufficiency, bulky extrapancreatic tumor, and instances of very severe hepatic disease.

Patient Care PREPARATION: If insulin is requested, the patient ideally should be fasting for 7 hours. Avoid radioisotopes prior to collection of specimen.

Specimen Serum or plasma CONTAINER: Red top tube or green top (heparin) tube STORAGE INSTRUCTIONS: Stable 12 hours at room temperature and 1 week at 4°C.[1] CAUSES FOR REJECTION: Blood glucose >50 mg/dL

Interpretive REFERENCE RANGE: Fasting level: up to 20-25 µIU/mL (SI: 144-179 pmol/L), with slight differences in upper limit of normal between laboratories. POSSIBLE PANIC RANGE: Fasting insulin levels >35 µIU/mL (SI: >250 pmol/L) USE: Suspect islet cell tumor when fasting glucose is <50 mg/dL (SI: <2.8 mmol/L), especially if there is patient or family history of multiple endocrine neoplasia (MEN). Work-up for fasting hypoglycemia: evaluate for insulin-producing neoplasm (islet cell tumor, insulinoma) or pancreatic islet cell hyperplasia. The diagnosis of insulinoma is established when serum insulin and C-peptide levels are significantly increased, drawn when symptoms of hypoglycemia are present and plasma glucose is low. Serum insulin is high in factitious hypoglycemia from exogenous insulin. LIMITATIONS: The key finding in insulinoma is the presence of insulin levels >20-30 µIU/mL (SI: >144-215 pmol/L) with blood glucose <57 mg/dL (SI: <3.2 mmol/L) 2-3 hours after tolbutamide injection. Elevated insulin values are meaningless unless blood glucose is <50 mg/dL (SI: <2.8 mmol/L).

The assay fails to distinguish between endogenous and exogenous insulins. Insulin antibodies in diabetic subjects who have been treated with animal insulins may invalidate results of insulin assays. Many diabetics, particularly obese individuals, have been thought to have normal or high serum insulin, fasting and after glucose administration. However, a highly specific assay which does not cross react with proinsulin provides evidence that insulin falls in type II diabetics with glucose.[2] Proinsulin is increased in type II diabetics.

In work-up for insulinoma, factitious hypoglycemia must be considered, especially vis-a-vis the insulin/glucose ratio. C-peptide is useful for evaluation of insulinoma. Since C-peptide is the result of cleavage of proinsulin within the β-cell, it is not present in pharmaceutical insulin, and C-peptide level is low with surreptitious injection of insulin. It is increased in insulinoma when plasma glucose is <40 mg/dL (SI: <2.2 mmol/L). Insulin is taken up by the liver, but C-peptide is not; thus, C-peptide reflects beta-cell secretion.

Increased insulin levels are found in Cushing's syndrome, in women on oral contraceptives, in subjects on exogenous corticosteroids, and in acromegaly. Adrenocortical steroids and growth hormone are insulin antagonists. Levodopa causes increased levels.

Most insulin assays react immunologically with proinsulin related molecules, which exhibit little insulin-like activity.[2]

METHODOLOGY: Radioimmunoassay (RIA) ADDITIONAL INFORMATION: Relationship of fasting glucose to insulin is critical in work-up of insulinoma. Inappropriately elevated insulin is found in two conditions: insulinoma and exogenous administration of insulin. Criteria for insulinoma include hypoglycemia (plasma glucose <30 mg/dL; SI: <1.7 mmol/L) with hyperinsulinemia (>6 µIU/mL; SI: >43 pmol/L).[1] About 33% of insulinoma patients have a normal serum insulin level; it needs to be shown that insulin is high for the patient's glucose value. A diagnosis of islet cell tumor also includes a criterion of plasma glucose <57 mg/dL (SI: <3.2 mmol/L) and insulin >20 µIU/mL (SI: >144 pmol/L) 2-3 hours after tolbutamide. Fraker and Norton require, for preoperative evaluation of patients with islet cell tumors:

- 72-hour fasting hypoglycemia (blood glucose <40 mg/dL; SI: <2.2 mmol/L) and hyperinsulinism (serum insulin >6 µIU/mL; SI: >43 pmol/L)
- high or normal C-peptide and high proinsulin level (>25%)
- insulin/glucose ratio >0.3[3]

Since release of insulin from an insulinoma may be erratic, it may be necessary to have the patient fast for up to 72 hours, drawing a specimen every 4 hours for glucose and insulin assay. Occasionally, only a single specimen in such a long fasting period will show an insulin/glucose ratio diagnostic of insulinoma. Care must be taken in selecting a laboratory whose insulin results are sensitive and reliable.

(Continued)

Insulin, Blood *(Continued)*

The most common cause of hyperinsulinemia is obesity. Stimulation and inhibition tests are helpful in differentiating whether hyperinsulinism is due to obesity or to tumors.

Insulin secretory reserve distinguishes between two apparently different syndromes: induced serum insulin peak <60 μIU/mL (SI: <431 pmol/L), with complications of diabetes developing, and insulin peaks of ≥60 μIU/mL (SI: ≥431 pmol/L) without complications. If only one insulin is ordered, it should be a fasting specimen. Insulin levels can also be ordered with glucose tolerance tests, but in practice this is seldom necessary. Specimens so ordered are drawn each time a glucose specimen is drawn, unless otherwise specified. Obese patients may have insulin resistance and high fasting and postprandial insulin levels.

Boden provides a useful diagnostic summary.[4]

It has been shown that pancreatic secretion of insulin is pulsatile.[5]

Footnotes

1. Fody EP, Bennett BD, Richardson LD, et al, *Clinical Laboratory Handbook for Patient Preparation and Specimen Handling: Fascicle V, Endocrinology and Metabolism*, Skokie, IL: College of American Pathologists, 1989.
2. Gambino R, "Insulin and Proinsulin," *Lab Report for Physicians*, 1989, 11:77-9.
3. Fraker DL and Norton JA, "The Role of Surgery in the Management of Islet Cell Tumors," *Gastroenterol Clin North Am*, 1989, 18(4):805-30.
4. Boden G, "Glucagonomas and Insulinomas," *Gastroenterol Clin North Am*, 1989, 18(4):831-45.
5. Chou HF, Ipp E, Bowsher RR, et al, "Sustained Pulsatile Insulin Secretion From Adenomatous Human Beta-Cells. Synchronous Cycling of Insulin, C-Peptide, and Proinsulin," *Diabetes*, 1991, 40(11):1453-8.

References

Casali P, Nakamura M, Ginsberg-Fellner F, et al, "Frequency of B Cells Committed to the Production of Antibodies to Insulin in Newly Diagnosed Patients With Insulin-Dependent Diabetes Mellitus and Generation of High Affinity Human Monoclonal IgG to Insulin," *J Immunol*, 1990, 144(10):3741-7.

Leavelle DE, *Mayo Medical Laboratories Interpretive Handbook*, Rochester, MN: Mayo Medical Laboratories, 1990.

McMahon MM, O'Brien PC, and Service FJ, "Diagnostic Interpretation of the Intravenous Tolbutamide Test for Insulinoma," *Mayo Clin Proc*, 1989, 64(12):1481-8.

Ostlund RE Jr, Staten M, Kohrt WM, et al, "The Ratio of Waist-to-Hip Circumference, Plasma Insulin Level, and Glucose Intolerance as Independent Predictors of the HDL_2 Cholesterol Level in Older Adults," *N Engl J Med*, 1990, 322(4):229-34.

Samaan NA, Ouais S, Ordonez NG, et al, "Multiple Endocrine Syndrome Type I: Clinical, Laboratory Findings, and Management in Five Families," *Cancer*, 1989, 64(3):741-52.

Sheppard BC, Norton JA, Doppman JL, et al, "Management of Islet Cell Tumors in Patients With Multiple Endocrine Neoplasia: A Prospective Study," *Surgery*, 1989, 106(6):1108-17.

Shuster LT, Go VLW, Rizza RA, et al, "Potential Incretins," *Mayo Clin Proc*, 1988, 63:794-800.

Solcia E, Capella C, Fiocca R, et al, "The Gastroenteropancreatic Endocrine System and Related Tumors," *Gastroenterol Clin North Am*, 1989, 18(4):671-93.

Insulin C-Peptide *see* C-Peptide *on page 195*

Insulin-Like Growth Factor I *see* Somatomedin-C *on page 354*

Interstitial Cell Stimulating Hormone *see* Luteinizing Hormone, Blood or Urine *on page 286*

Ion Gap *see* Anion Gap *on page 132*

Ionized Calcium *see* Calcium, Ionized *on page 159*

Iontophoresis *see* Chloride, Sweat *on page 183*

Iron and Total Iron Binding Capacity/Transferrin

CPT *83540 (iron); 83550 (iron binding capacity); 84466 (transferrin)*

See Also Anemia Flowchart in the Hematology Appendix

Related Information

Complete Blood Count *on page 533*
Erythropoietin, Serum *on page 214*
Ferritin, Serum *on page 220*
Hemoglobin *on page 554*
Iron Stain, Bone Marrow *on page 562*
Protoporphyrin, Free Erythrocyte *on page 341*
Protoporphyrin, Zinc, Blood *on page 342*

Schilling Test *on page 598*
Transferrin *on page 369*

Synonyms Fe and TIBC; Iron Binding Capacity; Iron Profile; TIBC; Total Iron Binding Capacity

Test Commonly Includes Serum iron, total iron binding capacity and/or transferrin, percent of saturation

Patient Care PREPARATION: Specimen should be drawn fasting in the morning (circadian rhythm affects iron; levels are lower in the evening). Sample should be drawn before patient is given therapeutic iron or blood transfusion. Iron determinations on patients who have had blood transfusions should be delayed several days.

Specimen Serum CONTAINER: Red top tube SAMPLING TIME: Morning; marked daily variation occurs COLLECTION: Serum iron levels are 30% higher in the morning and blood levels should be determined on fasting AM samples. Blood should be drawn before other specimens which require anticoagulated tubes. Separate serum from cells as soon as possible. STORAGE INSTRUCTIONS: Stable 1 week at 4°C

Interpretive REFERENCE RANGE: A variety of approaches to the estimation of serum iron, TIBC, and transferrin are in use. Expect normal ranges to vary between laboratories as they are in part method dependent. Iron: 50-160 μg/dL (SI: 9.0-28.8 μmol/L) for adult males; slightly lower (5% to 10%) values for adult females. Iron binding capacity: 250-350 μg/dL (SI: 45-63 μmol/L). Percent saturation (transferrin saturation): 20% to 50%. TIBC is a chemical approximation of transferrin. Quantitative assays for transferrin are widely available. A mathematical relationship between TIBC and transferrin can be derived, depending on methodology, in which transferrin can be measured, then TIBC calculated. USE: Differential diagnosis of anemia, especially with hypochromia and/or low MCV. The **percent saturation** sometimes is more helpful than is the iron result to estimate iron stores and iron deficiency anemia. Evaluate thalassemia and possible sideroblastic anemia; work up hemochromatosis, in which iron is increased and iron saturation is high. Decrease in iron level after performance of a Schilling test supports the diagnosis of vitamin B_{12} deficiency, *vide infra*. Evaluate iron poisoning (toxicity) and overload in renal dialysis patients or patients with transfusion dependent anemias. Use of TIBC in iron toxicity may be less useful than previously believed.[1] TIBC or transferrin is a useful index of nutritional status.

Uncomplicated iron deficiency: Serum transferrin (and TIBC) high, serum iron low, saturation low. Usual causes of depleted iron stores include blood loss, inadequate dietary iron. RBCs in moderately severe iron deficiency are hypochromic and microcytic. The red cell distribution width increases and MCV decreases. Stainable marrow iron is absent. Serum ferritin decrease is the earliest indicator of iron deficiency if inflammation is absent.

Anemia of chronic disease: Serum transferrin (and TIBC) low to normal, serum iron low, saturation low or normal. Transferrin decreases with many inflammatory diseases. With chronic disease there is a block in movement to and utilization of iron by marrow. This leads to low serum iron and decreased erythropoiesis. Examples include acute and chronic infections, malignancy, and renal failure.

Sideroblastic anemia: Serum transferrin (and TIBC) normal to low, serum iron normal to high, saturation high.

Hemolytic anemias: Serum transferrin (and TIBC) normal to low, serum iron high, saturation high.

Hemochromatosis: Serum transferrin (and TIBC) slightly low, serum iron high, saturation very high.

Protein depletion: Serum transferrin (and TIBC) may be low, serum iron normal or low (if patient also is iron deficient). This may occur as a result of malnutrition, liver disease, renal disease (eg, nephrosis) or other entities.

Liver disease: Serum transferrin variable; with acute viral hepatitis, high along with serum iron and ferritin. With chronic liver disease (eg, cirrhosis), transferrin may be low. Patients who have cirrhosis and portacaval shunting have saturated TIBC/transferrin as well as high ferritin.

Chronic dialysis for renal failure: Monitor iron levels in patients undergoing dialysis. To follow treatment of iron overload with deferoxamine or with regimen of recombinant human erythropoietin and phlebotomy.[2]

LIMITATIONS: Except for iron poisoning, a serum iron without TIBC or transferrin is of limited value. Ferritin levels are also useful for iron deficiency. Low iron level may not indicate iron deficiency in acute infection with leukocytosis. Low iron levels may be misleading in chronic in-

(Continued)

Iron and Total Iron Binding Capacity/Transferrin *(Continued)*

fection, inflammation, and malignancy; high ferritin levels occur in many such states. TIBC and transferrin are increased in patients on oral contraceptives, with normal saturation. Gross hemolysis may interfere with serum iron. **CONTRAINDICATIONS:** Parenteral iron before sample is drawn will cause misleading high iron results. Recent blood transfusion may have only a small positive effect on iron. **METHODOLOGY:** Ferrozine, bathophenanthroline (iron); nephelometry (transferrin); $MgCO_3$ column, other methods (TIBC); atomic absorption (iron, TIBC), anodal stripping; inductively coupled plasma atomic emission spectroscopy **ADDITIONAL INFORMATION:** Serum iron is **increased** in hemosiderosis, hemolytic anemias especially thalassemia, sideroachrestic anemias, hepatitis, acute hepatic necrosis, hemochromatosis, and with inappropriate iron therapy. Iron may reach high levels with iron poisoning. Some patients who receive multiple transfusions (eg, some hemolytic anemias, thalassemia, renal dialysis patients) will have increased serum iron levels.

Serum iron is **decreased** with insufficient dietary iron, chronic blood loss (including the hemolytic anemias, paroxysmal nocturnal hemoglobinuria), inadequate absorption of iron and impaired release of iron stores as in inflammation, infection, and chronic diseases. The combination of low iron, high TIBC and/or transferrin, and low saturation indicates iron deficiency. Without all of these findings together, iron deficiency is unproven. Low ferritin supports the diagnosis of iron deficiency. **Detection of iron deficiency may lead to detection of adenocarcinoma of gastrointestinal tract, a point which cannot be overemphasized.** In recovery from pernicious anemia, especially just after B_{12} dose, iron levels are low. In fact, the drop in serum iron 1 to several days after the Schilling test flushing dose of vitamin B_{12} may be more useful in diagnosis than the radioactivity of the 24-hour urine collection. Serum iron is reported to drop with acute infarct of myocardium.

TIBC is increased in iron-deficiency, use of oral contraceptives, and in pregnancy.

TIBC decreased in hypoproteinemia from many causes, and in a number of inflammatory states.

Increased saturation occurs with HLA-related (classical) hemochromatosis before ferritin is greatly increased, and also with iron overload (eg, cirrhosis and portacaval shunt), in hemolytic anemias, and with iron therapy. Saturation >70% in females, >80% in males is described as prerequisite for parenchymal loading. However, sample contamination and the vagaries of fluctuation in serum iron levels can make such criteria misleading on occasion.

The serum ferritin is a more sensitive test than the serum iron or TIBC for iron deficiency and for iron overload. When all these tests are used together, as is often necessary, they usually can distinguish between iron deficiency anemia and the anemia of chronic disease. The best and most reliable evaluation of total body iron stores is by bone marrow aspiration and biopsy. The best evaluation of iron deficiency in childhood (unless lead toxicity is suspected) is free erythrocyte porphyrins.

With recombinant erythropoietin therapy serum iron, transferrin saturation, and ferritin levels decline due to rapid utilization by stimulated erythropoiesis with resultant decrease in storage iron.[2]

While iron is usually considered in relation to hematopoiesis and oxygen transport functions of red cells, it is also of prime import to the lymphomyeloid systems.[3]

Footnotes

1. Tenenbein M and Yatscoff RW, "The Total Iron-Binding Capacity in Iron Poisoning. Is It Useful?" *Am J Dis Child*, 1991, 145(4):437-9.
2. McCarthy JT, Johnson WJ, Nixon DE, et al, "Transfusional Iron Overload in Patients Undergoing Dialysis: Treatment With Erythropoietin and Phlebotomy," *J Lab Clin Med*, 1989, 114(2):193-9.
3. deSousa M and Brock JH, *Iron in Immunity, Cancer and Inflammation*, New York, NY: John Wiley and Sons, 1989.

References

Brown EB, "Iron Metabolism: A 40 Year Overview," *Am J Med*, 1989, 87(3N):35N-39N.

Burns ER, Goldberg SN, Lawrence C, et al, "Clinical Utility of Serum Test for Iron Deficiency in Hospitalized Patients," *Am J Clin Pathol*, 1990, 93(2):240-5.

Finch CA and Huebers H, "Perspectives in Iron Metabolism," *N Engl J Med*, 1982, 306:1520-8.

Oski FA, "Iron Deficiency in Infancy and Childhood," *N Engl J Med*, 1993, 329(3):190-3.

Iron Binding Capacity *see* Iron and Total Iron Binding Capacity/Transferrin *on page 262*

Iron Profile *see* Iron and Total Iron Binding Capacity/Transferrin *on page 262*

Isocitric Dehydrogenase *replaced by* Alanine Aminotransferase *on page 100*

Isoenzymes of Alkaline Phosphatase *see* Alkaline Phosphatase Isoenzymes *on page 107*

Isozymes of Alkaline Phosphatase *see* Alkaline Phosphatase Isoenzymes *on page 107*

11-Ketoandrosterone *see* 17-Ketosteroids Fractionation, Urine *on page 267*

11-Ketoetiocholanolone *see* 17-Ketosteroids Fractionation, Urine *on page 267*

17-Ketogenic Steroids, Urine

CPT *83582*

Related Information

Cortisol, Blood *on page 191*
Cortisol, Urine *on page 193*
17-Hydroxycorticosteroids, Urine *on page 256*
17-Hydroxyprogesterone, Blood or Amniotic Fluid *on page 258*

Synonyms 17-KGS

Abstract Derived from adrenal cortical steroids, 17-KGS determinations are now an obsolescent approach to laboratory investigation. It measures 17-ketosteroids (KS) after 17-OHCS, cortols, cortolones, and pregnanetriol are oxidized to 17-KS.[1]

Specimen 24-hour urine **CONTAINER:** Plastic urine container **COLLECTION:** Add preservative as required by the individual laboratory prior to collection. Acetic or hydrochloric acids are often used. **STORAGE INSTRUCTIONS:** Record total volume. Pour off proper aliquot and refrigerate. **CAUSES FOR REJECTION:** Incomplete collection

Interpretive **REFERENCE RANGE:** Adult levels vary among laboratories. Male: 5-24 mg/24 hours (SI: 17-83 μmol/day); female: 4-15 mg/24 hours (SI: 14-52 μmol/day). The levels are less in childhood. Somewhat different figures appear in current editions of *Cecil Textbook of Medicine* and *Williams Textbook of Endocrinology*. It is of interest that the index of the two volume Cecil set provides no other aspect of 17-ketogenic steroids.[2] **USE:** Adrenal function test; increased with stress, Cushing's syndrome, and some cases of adrenogenital syndrome; decreased with Addison's disease and hypopituitarism **LIMITATIONS:** Interference by drugs (including penicillin and meprobamate), glucose, and radiographic contrast material. Subject to all the vagaries of incorrect collection of 24-hour urine specimens. **Better tests are now available.** 17-KGS has no advantage over assays of 17-OHCS (17-hydroxycorticosteroids).[1] **METHODOLOGY:** Norymberski reaction (Zimmermann color reaction after treatment with a strong oxidizing agent such as periodate or bismuthate) **ADDITIONAL INFORMATION:** The Norymberski reaction measures most of the 17-hydroxysteroids and a few additional steroid metabolites, of which the most important is pregnanetriol, which is elevated in adrenogenital syndrome. 17-Ketogenic steroids may be measured as base line, or as part of stimulation or suppression tests. The assay requires the presence of a 17-alpha hydroxyl group, like that of 17-hydroxycorticosteroids (17-OHC). Deoxycorticosterone (DOC), corticosterone (compound B), and aldosterone lack a 17-hydroxyl group and are not measured as 17-KG or 17-OHC.[3] **The availability of immunoassays for serum and urine cortisol and 17-hydroxyprogesterone are among factors which make this test obsolescent**.

Footnotes

1. Orth DW, Kovacs WJ, and DeBold CR, "The Adrenal Cortex," *Williams Textbook of Endocrinology*, 8th ed, Wilson JD and Foster DW, ed, Philadelphia, PA: WB Saunders Co, 1992, 581.
2. Elin RJ, "Laboratory Reference Interval Values of Clinical Importance," *Cecil Textbook of Medicine*, 19th ed, Vol 2, Wyngaarden JB, Smith JH, and Bennett JC, eds, Philadelphia, PA: WB Saunders Co, 1992, 2370-80.
3. Speroff L, Glass RH, and Kase NG, *Clinical Gynecologic Endocrinology and Infertility*, 4th ed, Baltimore, MD: Williams & Wilkins, 1989.

Ketone Bodies, Blood

CPT *82009 (qualitative); 82010 (quantitative)*

Related Information

Alcohol, Blood or Urine *on page 936*
Anion Gap *on page 132*
Glucose, Fasting *on page 238*
(Continued)

Ketone Bodies, Blood *(Continued)*

Glucose, Quantitative, Urine *on page 1120*
Glucose, Random *on page 240*
Glucose, Semiquantitative, Urine *on page 1121*
HCO_3, Blood *on page 248*
Ketones, Urine *on page 1128*
Lactic Acid, Blood *on page 273*
Osmolality, Calculated *on page 299*
Osmolality, Serum *on page 300*
pH, Blood *on page 315*
Phosphorus, Serum *on page 319*
Red Blood Cell Indices *on page 592*
Reducing Substances, Urine *on page 1150*
Toxicology Drug Screen, Blood *on page 1005*
Volatile Screen *on page 1010*

Synonyms Ketones, Blood; Nitroprusside Reaction, Blood

Applies to Acetoacetate; Acetone; Beta-Hydroxybutyrate; β-Hydroxybutyrate

Abstract Carbohydrate deprivation and increased catabolism of fatty acids leads to increases in the ketone bodies (acetoacetate and acetone). β-hydroxybutyrate is also increased and is usually listed with the "ketone" bodies although it is not a ketone.

Specimen Serum **CONTAINER:** Red top tube **COLLECTION:** Capillary tubes should be filled as much as possible using technique to avoid air bubbles. Free flowing heelstick. Avoid hemolysis. **CAUSES FOR REJECTION:** Hemolysis **SPECIAL INSTRUCTIONS:** Placement of peripheral venous catheter on admission may be useful in selected cases, such as instances of ketoacidosis. Lactic acid, glucose, electrolytes, urea nitrogen, venous or arterial pH should also be measured in possible ketoacidosis, with alcohol level, CBC, and urinalysis if clinically indicated. Serum osmolality is often needed.

Interpretive **REFERENCE RANGE:** Negative in normal nutritional states by semiquantitative screening tests. **POSSIBLE PANIC RANGE:** Positivity in 1:32 dilution indicates severe ketosis. **USE:** Diagnose ketonemia, ketoacidosis resulting from diabetes mellitus, alcoholism, stress, starvation, intestinal disorders including emesis, glycogen storage disease (von Gierke's), infantile organic acidemias, and other metabolic disorders. Determination of the presence of ketone bodies is useful when isopropanol ingestion is suspected. **LIMITATIONS:** False-negatives or falsely weak reactions may occur. Up to 33% of cases of diabetic ketoacidosis also have lactic acidosis. Acidosis shifts ketone bodies to β-hydroxybutyrate. However, β-hydroxybutyrate is not measured by nitroprusside, which reacts with both acetoacetic acid and acetone. The reagent is 5 to 20 times more sensitive to acetoacetic acid than to acetone and does not react with β-hydroxybutyrate. Thus, as ketoacidosis is treated, an apparent positive Acetest® is found while there is an actual reduction of total plasma ketone body concentration. Acidosis shifts equilibrium toward β-hydroxybutyrate (unmeasured), but treatment of ketoacidosis results in increased acetoacetate (measured) and thus a more positive "acetone" reaction, before ketone bodies decrease. Ketostix® false-positives occur with large amounts of levodopa. Nonketotic coma in diabetes may be caused by hyperosmolarity. **METHODOLOGY:** Nitroprusside reaction (colorimetry). Gas chromatography (GC) and enzymatic methods are used in some institutions, but fast laboratory response is usually needed. **ADDITIONAL INFORMATION:** Strongly positive serum acetone without severe acidosis, with normal anion gap, bicarbonate, and plasma glucose suggests the possibility of rubbing alcohol intoxication. Look for dehydration with ketosis. Ketoacidosis in diabetes usually occurs with decreased plasma pH and bicarbonate, increased glucose and other abnormalities. As ketoacidosis and metabolic acidosis are treated, hypokalemia may become evident. A normal or low potassium on admission of a patient with ketoacidosis may indicate severe potassium depletion. Thus, potassium is especially important among the parameters to follow in treatment of ketoacidosis. Hypophosphatemia may evolve. Acetone may be elevated due to absolute or relative starvation, especially in children. A significant mortality rate exists; in children younger than 10 years of age, diabetic ketoacidosis is reported to account for 70% of diabetes related deaths.[1] A multipoint kinetic method allows determination of acetoacetate plus β-hydroxybutyrate and lactate plus pyruvate in a single cuvette.[2]

Footnotes

1. Bonadio WA, Gutzeit MF, Losek JD, et al, "Outpatient Management of Diabetic Ketoacidosis," *Am J Dis Child*, 1988, 142(4):448-50.

2. Nuwayhid NF, Johnson GF, and Feld RD, "Multipoint Kinetic Method for Simultaneously Measuring the Combined Concentrations of Acetoacetate-Beta-Hydroxybutyrate and Lactate-Pyruvate," *Clin Chem*, 1989, 35(7):1526-31.

References

Caraway WT and Watts NB, "Carbohydrates," *Fundamentals of Clinical Chemistry*, 3rd ed, Tietz NW, ed, Philadelphia, PA: WB Saunders Co, 1987, 438-40.

Kaplan LA, "Ketones," *Clinical Chemistry – Theory, Analysis, and Correlation*, 2nd ed, Kaplan LA and Pesce AJ, eds, St Louis, MO: Mosby-Year Book Inc, 1989, 856-8.

Shaffer PA, "Antiketogenesis: Its Mechanism and Significance. 1932 (Classical Article)," *Medicine (Baltimore)*, 1990, 69(5):317-23.

Ketones, Blood *see* Ketone Bodies, Blood *on page 265*

17-Ketosteroids Fractionation, Urine

CPT 83593

Related Information

17-Ketosteroids, Total, Urine *on this page*

Synonyms 17-KS Fractionation

Applies to Androsterone; Dehydroepiandrosterone; Etiocholanolone; 11-Hydroxyandrosterone; 11-Hydroxyetiocholanolone; 11-Ketoandrosterone; 11-Ketoetiocholanolone

Test Commonly Includes Quantitation of some or all of the following: androsterone, etiocholanolone, and dehydroepiandrosterone (DHEA); these are the three major metabolites of androgens in the urine. Such fractionation may also include 11-ketoandrosterone, 11-ketoetiocholanolone, 11-hydroxyandrosterone, 11-hydroxyetiocholanolone, pregnanediol, pregnanetriol, delta-5-pregnanetriol, and 11-ketopregnanetriol.

Abstract Metabolites of steroids from adrenal cortices (two-thirds) and from the testes (one-third).[1]

Specimen 24-hour urine **CONTAINER:** Plastic urine container with acetic acid or hydrochloric acid preservative, as requested by the laboratory. **COLLECTION:** Add preservative to the container prior to the start of collection. **STORAGE INSTRUCTIONS:** Adjust pH as required. Keep refrigerated. **CAUSES FOR REJECTION:** Incomplete collection

Interpretive **REFERENCE RANGE:** Normal ranges are usually provided by laboratories doing such fractionation. They are often stratified by age and sex. Typical values for adult males: androsterone: 2-5 mg/day; dehydroepiandrosterone: 0.1-2.0 mg/day; etiocholanolone: 2-5 mg/day; for adult females: androsterone: 0.5-2.5 mg/day; dehydroepiandrosterone: 0.1-1.5 mg/day; etiocholanolone: 1.0-3.5 mg/day. **USE:** Analysis useful in evaluation of adrenal and gonadal abnormalities including the adrenogenital syndrome, differential diagnosis of adrenocortical hyperplasia and carcinoma; arrhenoblastoma, Stein-Leventhal syndrome. **LIMITATIONS:** Generally, analysis of specific entities should be sought. **METHODOLOGY:** Column chromatography or gas-liquid chromatography (GLC)

Footnotes

1. Leavelle DE, *Mayo Medical Laboratories Interpretive Handbook*, Rochester, MN: Mayo Medical Laboratories, 1990.

References

Speroff L, Glass RH, and Kase NG, *Clinical Gynecologic Endocrinology and Infertility*, 4th ed, Baltimore, MD: Williams & Wilkins, 1989.

Weykamp CW, Penders TJ, Schmidt NA, et al, "Steroid Profile for Urine: Reference Values," *Clin Chem*, 1989, 35(12):2281-4.

17-Ketosteroids, Total, Urine

CPT 83586

Related Information

Dehydroepiandrosterone Sulfate *on page 206*
17-Hydroxyprogesterone, Blood or Amniotic Fluid *on page 258*
17-Ketosteroids Fractionation, Urine *on this page*
Testosterone, Free and Total *on page 358*

Synonyms 17-KS

Abstract A ketone on the steroid nucleus is at C-17. The major precursors of 17-KS are DHEA (dehydroepiandrosterone) and DHEA-S (dehydroepiandrosterone sulfate). DHEA-S is the only substance in blood which can replace 17-KS in the work-up for hirsutism. 17-KS are metabolites of androstenedione, testosterone, and other compounds.

(Continued)

17-Ketosteroids, Total, Urine *(Continued)*

Patient Care **PREPARATION:** ACTH will cause increases, as will stress.

Specimen 24-hour urine **CONTAINER:** Plastic urine container with hydrochloric acid or 33% acetic acid preservative, depending on laboratory. Some laboratories ask for pH adjustment following collection. **COLLECTION:** Add preservative to container prior to the start of collection. **STORAGE INSTRUCTIONS:** Record total volume. Pour off proper aliquot and refrigerate. **CAUSES FOR REJECTION:** Incomplete collection

Interpretive **REFERENCE RANGE:** Adults: male: 8-20 mg/24 hours (SI: 28-69 μmol/day), female: 6-15 mg/24 hours (SI: 21-52 μmol/day) with decrease in advancing years; exact ranges vary somewhat between laboratories. Prepubertal children are much lower. **USE:** Assess adrenal androgens. 17-Ketosteroids are elevated in Cushing's syndrome, adrenogenital syndrome, some adrenal and gonadal tumors, pregnancy, and female pseudohermaphrodism. This is a somewhat obsolete test that has been replaced by immunoassays for specific analytes. **LIMITATIONS:** Increased with obesity. Numerous drugs in common use cause spurious increase or decrease including carbamazepine, cephalothin, and tiaprofenic acid. Excretion of the 17-ketosteroids is variable over time. Although often used to evaluate androgenic status, this test essentially **does not detect the major androgens, testosterone and dihydrotestosterone**. If low androgens are anticipated, serum testosterone is the test of choice, not 17-KS. **METHODOLOGY:** Zimmermann reaction (colorimetry after extractions). Zimmermann reaction detects androsterone, dehydroepiandrosterone, etiocholanolone, 11-ketoetiocholanolone, dehydroepiandrosterone (DHEA), 11-ketoandrosterone, 11-beta-hydroxyandrosterone, and 11-beta-hydroxyetiocholanolone. **ADDITIONAL INFORMATION:** In men, about one-third of 17-KS is of gonadal origin; in women and children, the adrenal is the predominant source. Cortisol, estrogens, pregnanediol, pregnanetriol, testosterone, and dihydrotestosterone are not 17-KS. The adrenogenital syndromes, virilizing entities, include adrenal tumors and congenital hyperplasias. The latter include partial 21-hydroxylase deficiency, complete 21-hydroxylase deficiency (salt-losing), and 11-beta-hydroxylase deficiency (mostly hypertensive). Other types of congenital adrenal hyperplasia exist as well. **With the availability of specific hormone and hormone metabolite tests, this assay is obsolete**.

References

Leavelle DE, *Mayo Medical Laboratories Interpretive Handbook*, Rochester, MN: Mayo Medical Laboratories, 1990.

Salway JG, ed, *Drug-Test Interaction Handbook*, New York, NY: Raven Press, 1990, 938-41.

Weykamp CW, Penders TJ, Schmidt NA, et al, "Steroid Profile for Urine: Reference Values," *Clin Chem*, 1989, 35(12):2281-4.

17-KGS *see* 17-Ketogenic Steroids, Urine *on page 265*

Kidney Profile

CPT 80007

Related Information

Anti-DNA *on page 634*
Antinuclear Antibody *on page 638*
C3 Complement, Serum *on page 649*
C4 Complement, Serum *on page 650*
Complement, Total, Serum *on page 667*
Complete Blood Count *on page 533*
Cryoglobulin, Qualitative, Serum *on page 670*
Glomerular Basement Membrane Antibody *on page 681*
Immunoglobulin A *on page 709*
Kidney Biopsy *on page 68*
Osmolality, Serum *on page 300*
Osmolality, Urine *on page 302*
Platelet Count *on page 586*
Streptozyme *on page 749*
Urinalysis *on page 1162*

Synonyms Renal Panel; Renal Profile

Test Commonly Includes Urea nitrogen (BUN), creatinine, glucose, electrolytes

Abstract A test grouping ordered on a regular basis by nephrologists caring for patients with renal diseases.

Specimen Serum CONTAINER: Red top tube COLLECTION: See individual tests for specimen collection instructions.

Interpretive REFERENCE RANGE: See normals under individual test listings for tests in profile or panel. USE: Evaluate renal diseases ADDITIONAL INFORMATION: Electrolytes are needed to evaluate renal problems. The rationale for this test grouping is that patients who require frequent monitoring of renal function also require monitoring of serum electrolytes. Hyponatremia may indicate hyperglycemia. Many of these patients are diabetic and others are on intravenous glucose infusions, another reason to monitor glucose. Finally, interpretation and correction of potassium fluctuations are aided by current knowledge of glucose concentration.

For further possible work-up, see the following tests: Osmolality, Urine and Osmolality, Serum in this chapter and Complement Total, Serum; C3 Complement, Serum; and C4 Complement, Serum in the Immunology and Serology chapter. Patients with possible glomerulopathy, nephrotic syndrome, and/or glomerulonephritis may need some of the following tests, depending on the clinical picture: ANA; anti-DNA; streptozyme; cryoglobulins; platelet count (for nephrosis in anaphylactoid purpura, thrombotic thrombocytopenic purpura); IgA (for cases of IgA nephropathy); antiglomerular basement membrane antibody. Urinalyses are also needed.

References

Andreoli TE, "Approach to the Patient With Renal Disease," *Cecil Textbook of Medicine*, Wyngaarden JB, Smith LH, and Bennett JC, eds, 19th ed, Vol 1, Philadelphia, PA: WB Saunders Co, 1992, 477-82.

Dennis VW, "Investigations of Renal Function," *Cecil Textbook of Medicine*, Wyngaarden JB, Smith LH, and Bennett JC, eds, 19th ed, Vol 1, Philadelphia, PA: WB Saunders Co, 1992, 492-9.

Klahr S, "Structure and Function of the Kidneys," *Cecil Textbook of Medicine*, Wyngaarden JB, Smith LH, and Bennett JC, eds, 19th ed, Vol 1, Philadelphia, PA: WB Saunders Co, 1992, 482-92.

17-KS *see* 17-Ketosteroids, Total, Urine *on page 267*

K^+, Serum or Plasma *see* Potassium, Blood *on page 330*

17-KS Fractionation *see* 17-Ketosteroids Fractionation, Urine *on page 267*

K^+, Urine *see* Potassium, Urine *on page 332*

Lactate, Blood *see* Lactic Acid, Blood *on page 273*

Lactate Dehydrogenase

CPT 83615

Related Information

Alanine Aminotransferase *on page 100*
Aspartate Aminotransferase *on page 135*
Cardiac Enzymes/Isoenzymes *on page 170*
Creatine Kinase *on page 196*
Lactate Dehydrogenase Isoenzymes *on page 271*
Myoglobin, Blood *on page 293*
Troponin *on page 375*

Synonyms Lactic Acid Dehydrogenase; LD; LDH

Abstract This enzyme catalyzes the interconversion of lactate and pyruvate. It is found in all cells of the body and exists in five molecular forms (isoenzymes).

Specimen Serum CONTAINER: Red top tube, serum separator tube is acceptable. Green top (heparin) tube is also acceptable. STORAGE INSTRUCTIONS: Avoid hemolysis. Stable 2-3 days at room temperature.[1] CAUSES FOR REJECTION: Hemolysis in collection of sample

Interpretive REFERENCE RANGE: Normal ranges for serum LD (LDH) vary among methods. They are higher in childhood. For adults, in most laboratories, the range is up to approximately 200 units/L. See following table for approximate ranges. USE: Causes of **high LD:** Neoplastic states (especially with high alkaline phosphatase, very high total LD, and isomorphic pattern of LD isoenzymes); hypoxic cardiorespiratory diseases; hemolytic anemia; megaloblastic anemias, including pernicious anemia (levels may be >2000 units/L and LD isoenzymes reveal LD_1:LD_2 flip); infectious mononucleosis; inflammation; hypothyroidism (some cases); myocardial infarct: LD begins to rise about 12 hours after infarct and usually returns to normal after CK (CPK) and AST (SGOT) levels return to normal, isoenzymes usually most useful 48 hours from onset of infarct to reveal LD_1:LD_2 inversion; pulmonary infarct (rarely, triad of LD, bilirubin, AST increases occurs); other lung diseases.

Diseases of liver, including cirrhosis. Total LD in cirrhosis is usually not greatly increased. In acute viral hepatitis, LD is not greatly elevated and AST is usually three or more times higher (in relation to the upper limit of normal) than LD; chronic alcoholism is usually associated with

(Continued)

Lactate Dehydrogenase *(Continued)*

some combination of elevated MCV (mean corpuscular volume), triglyceride, alkaline phosphatase, AST (SGOT), ALT (SGPT), GGT, and bilirubin and low folate.

Renal infarct – high LD, out of proportion to AST and alkaline phosphatase; seizures, other CNS diseases; acute pancreatitis; collagen diseases; excessive destruction of cells; fracture, other trauma, including head trauma, muscle damage; muscular dystrophy; focal necrosis; shock, hypotension; intestinal obstruction.

LD isoenzymes may be useful in the diagnosis of a number of the disease states mentioned above including myocardial infarction, neoplastic states, hemolytic anemia, megaloblastic anemias including pernicious anemia, infectious mononucleosis, some cases of hypothyroidism, diseases of the liver, renal infarct, and excessive destruction of cells

Other causes of increased LD include specimen tube artifact, such as serum contact with clot or exposure to heat. Chemistry profile with very high LD and no glucose may relate to unseparated serum and cells in a tube at room temperature or higher. Since LD is found in virtually every tissue in the body, the diagnostic value of an elevated level is limited.

Lactate Dehydrogenase

Age	units/L
0–2 y	125–275
2–3 y	166–232
3–4 y	112–221
4–5 y	108–206
5–6 y	104–205
6–7 y	100–204
7–8 y	95–203
8–12 y	90–201
12–14 y	90–199
14–16 y	Up to 168
16–17 y	Up to 161
17–43 y	90–156
≥43 y	90–176

LIMITATIONS: Hemolysis elevates LD results, oxalate inhibits LD, ascorbic acid can decrease LD values. **METHODOLOGY:** Lactate to pyruvate monitored at 340 nm is predominant method but pyruvate to lactate is used. Pyruvate to lactate assay results in values about twice those of the lactate to pyruvate method. The temperature is usually 37°C but 30°C is also used. **ADDITIONAL INFORMATION:** In **infectious mononucleosis**, LD is usually more elevated than AST, and there is usually an isomorphic pattern of LD isoenzymes. In **viral hepatitis**, by contrast, AST and ALT (the transaminases) are much more increased than is LD, about three or more times higher than total LD, and LD_5 is high. The differential diagnosis of acute infarct of myocardium includes pericarditis and angina, entities in which enzymes are usually not substantially increased. LD is useful in selected settings as a tumor marker,[2,3,4,5,6] but LD is not helpful as a screening test for cancer. (Other applications as a tumor marker are included in the subsequent listing.) Bovine or porcine heparin therapy can cause increases of AST, ALT, and LD with elevated LD hepatic fractions.

Footnotes

1. Moss DW, Henderson AR, and Kachmar JF, "Enzymes," *Textbook of Clinical Chemistry*, Tietz NW, ed, Philadelphia, PA: WB Saunders Co, 1986, 379-83.
2. Barlogie B, Smallwood L, Smith T, et al, "High Serum Levels of Lactic Dehydrogenase Identify a High-Grade Lymphoma-Like Myeloma," *Ann Intern Med*, 1989, 110(7):521-5.
3. Farley FA, Healey JH, Caparros-Sison B, et al, "Lactase Dehydrogenase as a Tumor Marker for Recurrent Disease in Ewing's Sarcoma," *Cancer*, 1987, 59:1245-8.
4. Ganz PA, Yeung Ma P, Wang H-J, et al, "Evaluation of Three Biochemical Markers for Serially Monitoring the Therapy of Small-Cell Lung Cancer," *J Clin Oncol*, 1987, 5:472-9.
5. Hamrick RM III and Murgo AJ, "Lactate Dehydrogenase Values and Bone Scans as Predictors of Bone Marrow Involvement in Small-Cell Lung Cancer," *Arch Intern Med*, 1987, 147:1070-1.
6. Schwartz MK, "Lactic Dehydrogenase: An Old Enzyme Reborn as a Cancer Marker?" *Am J Clin Pathol*, 1991, 96(4):441-3.

References

Gulbis B, Unger P, Lenaers A, et al, "Mass Concentration of Creatine Kinase MB Isoenzyme and Lactate Dehydrogenase Isoenzyme 1 in Diagnosis of Perioperative Myocardial Infarction After Coronary Bypass Surgery," *Clin Chem*, 1990, 36(10):1784-8.

Kagawa FT, Kirsch CM, Yenokida GG, et al, "Serum Lactate Dehydrogenase Activity in Patients With AIDS and *Pneumocystis carinii* Pneumonia: An Adjunct to Diagnosis," *Chest*, 1988, 94:1031-3.

Reis GJ, Kaufman HW, Horowitz GL, et al, "Usefulness of Lactate Dehydrogenase and Lactate Dehydrogenase Isoenzymes for Diagnosis of Acute Myocardial Infarction," *Am J Cardiol*, 1988, 61:754-8.

Schiele F, "Lactate Dehydrogenase," *Drug Effects on Laboratory Test Results Analytical Interferences and Pharmacological Effects*, Siest G and Galteau MM, eds, Littleton, MA: PSG Publishing Co Inc, 1988, 269-306.

Lactate Dehydrogenase, Cerebrospinal Fluid *see* Cerebrospinal Fluid LD *on page 179*

Lactate Dehydrogenase Isoenzymes

CPT *83625*

See Also Anemia Flowchart in the Hematology Appendix

Related Information

Cardiac Enzymes/Isoenzymes *on page 170*
Creatine Kinase Isoenzymes *on page 197*
Lactate Dehydrogenase *on page 269*
Myoglobin, Blood *on page 293*
Troponin *on page 375*

Synonyms Lactic Acid Dehydrogenase Isoenzymes; LDH Isoenzymes; LD Isoenzymes

Replaces Alpha-Hydroxybutyric Dehydrogenase, Serum

Test Commonly Includes Total serum LD (LDH) and electrophoretic quantitation of isoenzymes

Abstract Changes of LD isoenzymes are periodically measured following onset of chest pain, to study the relationships of the anodic fractions and to provide important information for the differential diagnosis of acute infarct of myocardium ("LD_1/LD_2 flip"). The differential diagnosis of certain other diseases is enhanced as well with use of LD isoenzymes.

Specimen Serum **CONTAINER:** Red top tube **SAMPLING TIME:** Cardiac enzymes and isoenzymes are best interpreted as a sequential series. Typically, a series of three: one at admission (or initial event) and two more at 6- to 8-hour intervals. **COLLECTION:** Avoid hemolysis **CAUSES FOR REJECTION:** Hemolysis in collection of sample; specimen collected in oxalate, citrate, fluoride, or other anticoagulants **SPECIAL INSTRUCTIONS:** Normal total LD is not necessarily a complete contraindication to perform isoenzymes. LD_1:LD_2 flip occurs in some sera in which total LD is within normal range.

Interpretive **REFERENCE RANGE:** Method dependent. Normally LD separates electrophoretically into five bands, each an isoenzyme. One set of normal ranges, based on agarose: LD_1: 22% to 36%, LD_2: 35% to 46%, LD_3: 13% to 26%, LD_4: 3% to 10%, LD_5: 2% to 12%. LD_1 and LD_2 (anodal fractions) are associated with cardiac and RBC origin. LD_5 and LD_4 are associated with hepatic and skeletal muscle origin. LD_2 is greater than LD_1 normally. Thus, the LD_1:LD_2 ratio is normally 0.50-0.80. In myocardial damage, such as acute infarct of myocardium, there is flip or inversion of LD_1:LD_2 (LD_1 becoming greater than LD_2). LD_4 is normally less than LD_5, and the normal LD_5:LD_4 ratio is up to 0.8. **POSSIBLE PANIC RANGE:** LD_1:LD_2 flip in a patient not in a coronary unit, not known to have pernicious anemia or hemolytic anemia. **USE:** Useful in the differential diagnosis of acute myocardial infarction, megaloblastic anemia (folate deficiency, pernicious anemia), hemolytic anemia, and very occasionally renal infarct. These entities are characterized by LD_1 increases, often with LD_1:LD_2 inversion.

The isomorphic pattern (total LD significantly high with no increase in percentage, of any fraction) is seen with neoplasia, cardiorespiratory diseases, hypothyroidism, infectious mononucleosis, and other inflammatory states, uremia, and necrosis.[1]

LD_5 increases are seen with striated muscle lesions (eg, trauma) and with liver diseases (eg, hepatic congestion, congestive heart failure, hepatitis, cirrhosis, alcoholism). LD_5 increase is probably more significant when the LD_5:LD_4 ratio is increased.

Although a modicum of controversy exists regarding the most suitable criteria for LD isoenzymes for the diagnosis of acute myocardial infarction, **almost all laboratories recognize abnormality when LD_1** equals or is greater than LD_2. Alternatives to LD_1 greater than LD_2 have been proposed. Using an electrophoretic method (Helena), Rotenberg et al suggested the criterion of LD_1 >90 units/L.[2] Such expression of LD_1 in absolute units is helpful but, of course, may be misleading when total LD is substantially increased. Others have modified this suggested normal range. Application of LD_1:LD_4 ratio and other ratios found the LD_1:LD_4 ratio to be a powerful diagnostic ratio for acute myocardial infarction,[3,4] but others have not used the LD_1:LD_4 ratio successfully.

In many laboratories, a few percent of normal individuals may have LD_1:LD_2 ratios as high as 0.81. A ratio of 0.82-0.99 is suspicious of myocardial injury. A ratio >1.0 is diagnostic of myocardial injury, if other clinical criteria are met, especially in the absence of increased MCV (ie, without megaloblastic anemia). In unstable angina, an increase of the LD_1:LD_2 ratio is described with normal total LD. However, progressively increasing LD_1:LD_2 ratio without complete inversion may have diagnostic significance for acute myocardial infarct.

Persistent LD_1:LD_2 flip following acute myocardial infarct may represent a marker for reinfarction[5]. Especially when acute myocardial infarction is complicated by shock, the isomorphic pattern may be found.[6] LD_1:LD_2 inversion commonly appears subsequent to the isomorphic pattern in instances of acute myocardial infarction.[1]

(Continued)

Lactate Dehydrogenase Isoenzymes *(Continued)*

The appearance of an LD "flip" (when LD_1 is greater than LD_2) is extremely helpful in diagnosis of MI. The presence of a LD "flip" a day following or with the detection of CK-MB is essentially diagnostic of MI, if baseline cardiac enzymes/isoenzymes are normal and if rises and falls are as anticipated for the diagnosis of acute MI. While CK-MB peaks 12-24 hours after onset of infarction, LD isoenzymes usually become diagnostic at about 36-55 hours after onset and return to normal 3-14 days after onset. Each laboratory must define its own criteria for this important test.

LIMITATIONS: Timing is important in diagnosis of acute myocardial infarct (MI). In a small percentage of patients with acute myocardial infarction, the expected flip (reversal) of LD_1:LD_2 does not occur; in such patients there is often simply an increase in LD_1. **METHODOLOGY:** Electrophoresis; immunochemical methods have been introduced including immunoprecipitation **ADDITIONAL INFORMATION:** Patterns of LD isoenzymes in acute pulmonary edema include the isomorphic pattern and LD_5 increases.[7] Serum LD increases also in patients with bacterial pneumonia, in whom LD isoenzyme patterns are described.[8]

Macroenzymes, high molecular weight complexes, occur with LD as well as with CK and other enzymes. LD isoenzymes may complex to IgA or IgG. Such LD macroenzymes are characterized by abnormal position of isoenzyme bands, broadening or abnormal motility of a band, and otherwise unexplained increase of total serum LD. Some of these patients have abnormal ANA results and IgG complexes.[9] Some have abnormalities of light chains. Treatment with streptokinase was found to produce a LD-streptokinase complex which was seen as a band at the origin in electrophoresis.[10]

An isoenzyme band cathodal to LD_5 has been called **LD_6**. It is not an immunoglobulin complex. It has occurred in subjects with liver disease and is said to indicate a grave prognosis.[11]

The association between LD_1 and testicular seminoma has been widely recognized. Its relationship to nonseminomatous testicular tumors as well are described.[12] The ovarian equivalent of seminoma is dysgerminoma, which also may relate to LD_1 increases.[13,14] A variety of malignant tumors are characterized by total LD increases, sometimes with isomorphic patterns[1] or with LD_5 increases.[15] Increase LD_5:LD_1 ratio is suggestive of prostatic carcinoma or other cancers.[16]

In a series of 220 patients with carcinoma of breast, LD was the most common enzyme elevated. The nonspecificity of single enzyme elevation was discussed, but enzymes provide an inexpensive baseline for postoperative follow-up. Enzyme elevation defines a subgroup of patients deserving further evaluation.[17] In malignancy of various types, there is reported an abnormal isoenzyme of LD migrating between albumin and LD_1 on agarose gel electrophoresis.[18]

An inverted LD_5:LD_4 ratio is not to be confused with LD_1:LD_2 ratio, used to evaluate acute MI. There is evidence that when LD_5 sufficiently exceeds LD_4, liver disease might exist. Such liver disease might be primary or secondary (eg, congestive heart failure). Additional tests which may be useful, if clinically indicated, to work up such possible liver disease or injury might include ALT (SGPT), GGT, serum protein electrophoresis, and prothrombin time. LD_5 is the striated muscle as well as the liver fraction. Although striated muscle problems are usually clinically obvious, occasionally the physician does not get a clinical history of the postictal state or of various withdrawal syndromes. In such situations a CK may be helpful.

LD with LD isoenzymes is useful as a tumor marker. Schwartz has recently outlined applications in adenocarcinoma of lung, colorectal carcinoma, malignant germ cell tumors, and in lymph nodes.[19] LD_3 may be useful in chronic granulocytic leukemia.[20] High serum LDH is described as a marker for drug resistance with high tumor volume in multiple myeloma.[21]

Footnotes

1. Jacobs DS, Robinson RA, Clark GM, et al, "Clinical Significance of the Bisomorphic Pattern of the Isoenzymes of Serum Lactate Dehydrogenase," *Ann Clin Lab Sci*, 1977, 7:411-21.
2. Rotenberg Z, Davidson E, Weinberger I, et al, "The Efficiency of Lactate Dehydrogenase Isoenzyme Determination for the Diagnosis of Acute Myocardial Infarction," *Arch Pathol Lab Med*, 1988, 112(9):895-7.
3. Loughlin JF, Krijnen PM, Jablonsky G, et al, "Diagnostic Efficiency of Four Lactate Dehydrogenase Isoenzyme-1 Ratios in Serum After Myocardial Infarction," *Clin Chem*, 1988, 34(10):1960-5.
4. Galbraith LV, Leung FY, Jablonksy G, et al, "Time-Related Changes in the Diagnostic Utility of Total Lactate Dehydrogenase, Lactate Dehydrogenase Isoenzyme-1, and Two Lactate Dehydrogenase Isoenzyme-1 Ratios in Serum After Myocardial Infarction," *Clin Chem*, 1990, 36(7):1317-22.
5. Rotenberg Z, Weinberger I, Sagie A, et al, "Lactate Dehydrogenase Isoenzymes in Serum During Recent Acute Myocardial Infarction," *Clin Chem*, 1987, 33:1419-20.

6. Rotenberg Z, Weinberger I, Davidson E, et al, "Atypical Patterns of Lactate Dehydrogenase Isoenzymes in Acute Myocardial Infarction," *Clin Chem*, 1988, 34(6):1096-8.
7. Rotenberg Z, Weinberger I, Davidson E, et al, "Patterns of Lactate Dehydrogenase Isoenzymes in Serum of Patients With Acute Pulmonary Edema," *Clin Chem*, 1988, 34(9):1882-4.
8. Rotenberg Z, Weinberger I, Davidson E, et al, "Significance of Isolated Increases in Total Lactate Dehydrogenase and Its Isoenzymes in Serum of Patients With Bacterial Pneumonia," *Clin Chem*, 1988, 34(7):1503-5.
9. Gorus F, Aelbrecht W, and Van Camp B, "Circulating IgG-LD Complex, Dissociable by Addition of NAD^+," *Clin Chem*, 1982, 28:236-9.
10. Podlasek SJ, Dufour DR, and McPherson RA, "Alterations in Lactate Dehydrogenase Isoenzyme Patterns After Therapy With Streptokinase or Streptococcal Infection," *Clin Chem*, 1989, 35(8):1763-6.
11. Wolf PL, "Lactate Dehydrogenase-6: A Biochemical Sign of Serious Hepatic Circulatory Disturbance," *Arch Intern Med*, 1985, 145:1396-7.
12. Von Eyben FE, Blaabjerg O, Petersen PH, et al, "Serum Lactate Dehydrogenase Isoenzyme 1 as a Marker of Testicular Germ Cell Tumor," *J Urol*, 1988, 140(5):986-90.
13. Schwartz PE and Morris JM, "Serum Lactic Dehydrogenase: A Tumor Marker for Dysgerminoma," *Obstet Gynecol*, 1988, 72(3 Pt 2):511-5.
14. Yoshimura T, Takemori K, Okazaki T, et al, "Serum Lactic Dehydrogenase and Its Isoenzymes in Patients With Ovarian Dysgerminoma," *Int J Gynaecol Obstet*, 1988, 27:459-65.
15. Rotenberg Z, Weinberger I, Sagie A, et al, "Total Lactate Dehydrogenase and Its Isoenzymes in Serum of Patients With Non-Small-Cell Lung Cancer," *Clin Chem*, 1988, 34(4):668-70.
16. Manzo V, Sun T, and Lien YY, "Misdiagnosis of Acute Myocardial Infarction," *Ann Clin Lab Sci*, 1990, 20(5):324-8.
17. Clark CP 3d, Foreman ML, Peters GN, et al, "Efficacy of Preoperative Liver Function Tests and Ultrasound in Detecting Hepatic Metastasis in Carcinoma of the Breast," *Surg Gynecol Obstet*, 1988, 167(6):510-4.
18. Giannoulaki EE, Kalpaxis DL, Tentas C, et al, "Lactate Dehydrogenase Isoenzyme Pattern in Sera of Patients With Malignant Diseases," *Clin Chem*, 1989, 35(3):396-9.
19. Schwartz MK, "Lactic Dehydrogenase: An Old Enzyme Reborn as a Cancer Marker?" *Am J Clin Pathol*, 1991, 96(4):441-3.
20. Buchsbaum RM, Liu FJ, and Trujillo JM, "Serum Lactate Dehydrogenase-3 Isoenzyme in Chronic Granulocytic Leukemia," *Am J Clin Pathol*, 1991, 96(4):464-9.
21. Dimopoulos MA, Barlogie B, Smith TL, et al, "High Serum Lactate Dehydrogenase Level as a Marker for Drug Resistance and Short Survival in Multiple Myeloma," *Ann Intern Med*, 1991, 115(12):931-5.

References

Jacobs DS, Clark GM, Beers AL, et al, "Automation of Interpretive Clinical Laboratory Reports: Isoenzymes of Serum Lactate Dehydrogenase," *Lab Med*, 1979, 10:636-9.

Kagawa FT, Kirsch CM, Yenokida GG, et al, "Serum Lactate Dehydrogenase Activity in Patients With AIDS and *Pneumocystis carinii* Pneumonia: An Adjunct to Diagnosis," *Chest*, 1988, 94:1031-3.

Kippenberger DJ, "Electrophoretic Evidence of a Patient With Only Three Lactate Dehydrogenase Isoenzymes," *Lab Med*, 1979, 10:153.

Rotenberg Z, Selp R, Wolfe LA, et al, "Flipped Patterns of Lactate Dehydrogenase Isoenzymes in Serum of Elite College Basketball Players," *Clin Chem*, 1988, 34:2351-4.

Wolf PL, "Lactate Dehydrogenase Isoenzymes in Myocardial Disease," *Clin Lab Med*, 1989, 9(4):655-65.

Wukich DK, Callaghan JJ, Graeber GM, et al, "Operative Treatment of Acute Hip Fractures: Its Effect on Serum Creatine Kinase, Lactate Dehydrogenase and Their Isoenzymes," *J Trauma*, 1989, 29(3):375-9.

Lactate Dehydrogenase, Variable *see* Body Fluid Lactate Dehydrogenase *on page 149*

Lactic Acid, Blood

***CPT** 83605*

Related Information

Acetaminophen, Serum *on page 935*
Alcohol, Blood or Urine *on page 936*
Anion Gap *on page 132*
Creatinine, Serum *on page 202*
Ketone Bodies, Blood *on page 265*
Osmolality, Calculated *on page 299*
Osmolality, Serum *on page 300*
pH, Blood *on page 315*
Salicylate *on page 999*

Synonyms Blood Lactate; Lactate, Blood

Applies to Biotin; Phenformin

Abstract Hypoperfusion is the most common cause of lactic acidosis, and hyperlactacidemia may be the only marker of tissue hypoperfusion.[1]

(Continued)

Lactic Acid, Blood *(Continued)*

Specimen Whole blood, arterial or venous, or plasma **CONTAINER:** Gray top (sodium fluoride) tube **COLLECTION:** Avoid hand-clenching and use of a tourniquet. A tourniquet or a patient clenching and unclenching his/her hand will lead to build-up of potassium and lactic acid from the hand muscles. Commonly needed with or as stat follow-up to venous or arterial pH. Serial determinations are often valuable.[1] Send specimen on ice. **STORAGE INSTRUCTIONS:** Centrifuge immediately and take off plasma (unless laboratory uses a whole blood method). Keep plasma on ice or at 2°C to 8°C, analyze promptly. A recent study of blood handling techniques and their effect on lactate concentration has been published.[2] **CAUSES FOR REJECTION:** Specimen not received on ice **SPECIAL INSTRUCTIONS:** Keep tube on ice until delivered to the laboratory. Tube must be in laboratory within 15 minutes of being drawn.

Interpretive **REFERENCE RANGE:** Plasma values: venous: 4.5-19.8 mg/dL (SI: 0.5-2.2 mmol/L); arterial: 4.5-14.4 mg/dL (SI: 0.5-1.6 mmol/L) **POSSIBLE PANIC RANGE:** $\geq$45.0 mg/dL **USE:** Suspect lactic acidosis when unexplained anion gap metabolic acidosis is encountered, especially if azotemia or ketoacidosis are not present. Evaluate metabolic acidosis, regional or diffuse tissue hypoperfusion, hypoxia, shock, congestive heart failure, dehydration, complicated postoperative state, ketoacidosis or nonketotic acidosis in diabetes mellitus, patients with infections, inflammatory states, postictal state, certain myopathies, acute leukemia and other neoplasia, enzyme defects, glycogen storage disease (type I), thiamine deficiency, and hepatic failure. A spontaneous form of lactic acidosis occurs. It is a prognostic index in particular clinical settings, especially in critically ill patients in shock. A relationship to renal disease also exists. With skin rash, seizures, alopecia, ataxia, keratoconjunctivitis, and lactic acidosis in children, consider defective biotin metabolism. Phenformin, ethanol, methanol, and salicylate and ethylene glycol poisoning may cause lactic acidosis. Acetaminophen toxicity causes lactic acidosis, sometimes with hypoglycemia. Cyanide, isoniazid, and propylene glycol are among the causes of lactic acidosis.[1] Lactic acidosis may be due to inborn errors of metabolism. **LIMITATIONS:** Gross hemolysis depresses results. Intravenous injections or infusions which modify acid-base balance, may cause alterations in lactate levels. Epinephrine and exercise elevate lactate, as may I.V. sodium bicarbonate, glucose, and hyperventilation. False low values with a high LD (LDH) value. Normal L-lactate occurs with high D-lactate in D-lactic acidosis. Metabolic acidosis following bypass for obesity, related to altered gastrointestinal flora, is a feature of subjects who develop mental changes as well, in whom D-lactate is the causative anion.[1] **CONTRAINDICATIONS:** Lack of acidosis is **not** a contraindication for this test. **METHODOLOGY:** Enzymatic; other methods include gas chromatography (GC) **ADDITIONAL INFORMATION:** Phosphorus is sometimes significantly abnormal in lactic acidosis. Creatinine is higher in ketoacidosis than in lactic acidosis, by interference produced by acetoacetic acid on creatinine. Causes of lactic acidosis (usually $<$45 mg/dL (SI: $<$5.0 mmol/L)) include carbohydrate infusions, exercise, diabetic ketosis, alcohol. Causes of lactic acidosis ($>$45 mg/dL) include shock (in which lactic acidosis may occur early, before fall in blood pressure, decrease in urine output), hypoxia (including congestive failure, severe anemia, hypotension) and malignancies. Severe lactic acidosis can develop in minutes. Lactic acidosis can accompany dehydration. Blood lactate concentration correlates negatively with survival in patients with acute myocardial infarction, with persistent elevation, $>$36 mg/dL (SI: $>$4.0 mmol/L) for more than 12 hours, being associated with poor prognosis. At a given bicarbonate level, the average pCO_2 is lower in lactic acidosis than in diabetic ketoacidosis. Lactic acid determination is generally indicated if anion gap is $>$20 mmol/L and if pH is $<$7.25 and the pCO_2 is not elevated. (Mizock uses pH 7.35 as a diagnostic criterion.[1]) The measurement of lactate levels may be indicated in the clinical setting of metabolic acidosis. Serum salicylate, ethanol level, and osmolality may be helpful. Spontaneous lactic acidosis may be fatal. Protocols are available for measurement of lactate in cord blood.[3]

Footnotes

1. Mizock BA, "Lactic Acidosis," *Dis Mon*, 1989, 35(4):233-300.
2. Bishop PA, May M, Smith, JF, et al, "Influence of Blood Handling Techniques on Lactic Acid Concentrations," *Int J Sports Med*, 1992, 13(1):56-9.
3. Prentice A, Vadgama P, Appleton DR, et al, "A Protocol for the Routine Measurement of Lactate and Pyruvate in Cord Blood," *Br J Obstet Gynaecol*, 1989, 96(7):861-6.

References

Gau N, "Lactic Acid," *Methods in Clinical Chemistry*, Pesce AJ and Kaplan LA, eds, St Louis, MO: Mosby-Year Book Inc, 1987, 78-82.

Kreisberg RA, "Lactate Homeostasis and Lactic Acidosis," *Ann Intern Med*, 1980, 92:227-37.

Lactic Acid, Body Fluid *see* Body Fluid *on page 145*

Lactic Acid, Cerebrospinal Fluid *see* Cerebrospinal Fluid Lactic Acid *on page 178*

Lactic Acid Dehydrogenase *see* Lactate Dehydrogenase *on page 269*

Lactic Acid Dehydrogenase, Fluid *see* Cerebrospinal Fluid LD *on page 179*

Lactic Acid Dehydrogenase Isoenzymes *see* Lactate Dehydrogenase Isoenzymes *on page 271*

Lactose Tolerance Test

CPT *82951 (3 specimens); 82952 (more than 3 specimens)*

Related Information

Reducing Substances, Stool *on page 1149*

Synonyms Tolerance Test, Lactose

Test Commonly Includes Fasting, 30-, 60-, 120-, 180-, and 240-minute glucose measurements

Abstract Lactose intolerance provides an example of osmotic diarrhea from ingestion of solutes not absorbable by a given subject. The lactose tolerance test reflects lactase deficiency of enterocytes.

Patient Care PREPARATION: A trial of withdrawal from lactose-containing food is advocated before the lactose tolerance test. Such a trial may make the test unnecessary. Patient should fast for 8 hours before testing, usually overnight. No smoking or gum chewing allowed during test. Occurrence of any vomiting should be reported to the patient's physician. Patient is encouraged to drink a moderate amount of water during the test, one to two glasses. Patient should remain seated or in bed. AFTERCARE: Test may produce diarrhea and cramps.

Specimen Plasma or 24-hour urine CONTAINER: Gray top (sodium fluoride) tube, plastic 24-hour urine container COLLECTION: Draw specimens in gray top tubes fasting and at 30 minutes, 1, 2, 3, and 4 hours after lactose load to be analyzed for glucose. (Samples can be taken fasting, 15 minutes, 30 minutes, 45 minutes, 1 hour, and 2 hours.) Record patient symptoms (especially cramps, nausea, watery diarrhea). SPECIAL INSTRUCTIONS: Lactose load: Adults: 50 g/m^2 body surface or 1 g/kg body weight should be consumed in 5-10 minutes. If severe lactase deficiency is suspected, the dose should be lowered. **Since lactase deficiency can be inferred from effects of ingestion of milk, the lactose tolerance test is not often needed or done. If available, breath tests may be preferable.** Less than 10 ppm H_2 gas in the exhaled breath is normal. Lactase deficient subjects usually have ≥50 ppm H_2 in exhaled air.[1] In infants and young children suspected of severe intolerance, a lower lactose dose should be used to avoid extreme reaction.

Interpretive REFERENCE RANGE: An increase in plasma glucose of >20-30 mg/dL (SI: >1.1-1.7 mmol/L) is normal. An increase of plasma glucose of <20 mg/dL (SI: <1.1 mmol/L) over the fasting level, with symptoms, is considered abnormal and is evidence for lactase deficiency. A flat curve can be defined as an increase of <20 mg/dL (SI: <1.1 mmol/L) and is seen in most subjects with lactose deficiency who are not diabetic. Urine reference range: children: <1.5 mg/100 dL; adults: 12-40 mg/dL (SI: 0.7-2.2 mmol/L). USE: Work-up for distension, diarrhea and/or cramping after ingestion of milk. Diagnose idiopathic lactase deficiency, which is found in a majority of black and Oriental adults, as well as in 5% to 15% of adult Caucasians. It is also found in children. Evaluate lactose intolerance, malabsorption syndromes. May be abnormal with Crohn's disease, small bowel resections, jejunitis, sprue, *Giardia lamblia* infestation, Whipple's disease, and in cystic fibrosis of the pancreas. LIMITATIONS: Up to 20% incidence of false-positives and negatives is reported. Since lactase-deficient patients have had normal tolerance curves, this test is of questionable value. METHODOLOGY: Blood specimens are analyzed for glucose after an oral dose of lactose. ADDITIONAL INFORMATION: Lactose is a disaccharide digested by lactase. It yields glucose and galactose. The latter is converted to glucose by the liver after its absorption. Glucose is measured and it is the increase or lack of increase over the fasting specimen that is used for interpretation. Diabetic patients may have abnormal lactose tolerance curves due to abnormal carbohydrate metabolism and not necessarily due to lactose intolerance. Since 25% of normal individuals have flat glucose tolerance tests, it has been suggested that patients with flat lactose tolerance tests should also have a glucose tolerance test. Ethanol can prevent conversion of galactose to glucose by the liver; thus, blood or urine galactose can be measured. A test strip has been described which may replace the lactose tolerance test, at least for some purposes, such as mass screening. The H_2 lactose breath test can also establish the diagnosis of lactase deficiency.

(Continued)

Lactose Tolerance Test *(Continued)*

Footnotes

1. Kaplan LA and Pesce AJ, eds, *Clinical Chemistry - Theory, Analysis, and Correlation*, 2nd ed, St Louis, MO: Mosby-Year Book Inc, 1989, 409.

References

Ahnen DJ, "Disorders of Nutrient Assimilation," *Textbook of Internal Medicine*, Kelley WN, ed, Philadelphia, PA: JB Lippincott Co, 1989, 522-34.

Wright TL and Heyworth MF, "Maldigestion and Malabsorption," *Gastrointestinal Disease*, Sleisenger MH and Fordtran JS, eds, Philadelphia, PA: WB Saunders Co, 1989, 263-82.

LAP *see* Leucine Aminopeptidase *on this page*

L-Aspartate: 2-Oxoglutarate Aminotransferase *see* Aspartate Aminotransferase *on page 135*

LD *see* Lactate Dehydrogenase *on page 269*

LD, Body Fluid *see* Body Fluid *on page 145*

LD, Fluid *see* Body Fluid Lactate Dehydrogenase *on page 149*

LDH *see* Lactate Dehydrogenase *on page 269*

LDH Isoenzymes *see* Lactate Dehydrogenase Isoenzymes *on page 271*

LD Isoenzymes *see* Cardiac Enzymes/Isoenzymes *on page 170*

LD Isoenzymes *see* Lactate Dehydrogenase Isoenzymes *on page 271*

LDLC *see* Low Density Lipoprotein Cholesterol *on page 284*

LDLC/HDLC Ratio *see* Low Density Lipoprotein Cholesterol *on page 284*

LD Variable *see* Body Fluid Lactate Dehydrogenase *on page 149*

Lecithin/Sphingomyelin Ratio *see* Amniotic Fluid Lecithin/Sphingomyelin Ratio and Phosphatidylglycerol *on page 124*

Leucine Aminopeptidase

CPT *83670*

Related Information

Alkaline Phosphatase, Serum *on page 109*
Gamma Glutamyl Transferase *on page 230*
5' Nucleotidase *on page 297*

Synonyms Arylamidase; Arylamidase Naphthylamidase; LAP

Abstract A cellular peptidase used as a test of biliary excretory function. Not in widespread use.

Specimen Serum, ascitic fluid **CONTAINER:** Red top tube

Interpretive **REFERENCE RANGE:** Depends on method. 12-33 units/L; higher values in males. Little age-related change. **USE:** Like 5' nucleotidase and GGT, LAP is used to investigate the origin of increased serum alkaline phosphatase. LAP is not elevated in bone disease. Elevated levels are observed in biliary cirrhosis, other types of cirrhosis, obstructive jaundice, metastatic tumor and granulomas in liver, choledocholithiasis, other biliary and liver diseases. It is often increased in primary carcinomas of pancreas and in some patients with pancreatitis. LAP is found in high concentration in ascitic fluid in malignancy. **LIMITATIONS:** Increased in the last trimester of pregnancy. Seldom used at present. **METHODOLOGY:** Colorimetry, fluorometry, enzyme assay **ADDITIONAL INFORMATION:** Helpful in evaluation of the biliary tract. The tests of biliary function include total and direct bilirubin and alkaline phosphatase, as well as GGT, LAP, and 5' nucleotidase. LAP and 5' nucleotidase are comparable clinically. In the newborn, LAP activity is normal in hemolytic disease (Rh and ABO incompatibilities) and in physiological jaundice. LAP is normal in diseases of bone which cause increases of alkaline phosphatase.

L-Glyceric Acid, Urine *see* Oxalate, Urine *on page 303*

LH *see* Luteinizing Hormone, Blood or Urine *on page 286*

Liley Test *see* Amniotic Fluid Analysis for Erythroblastosis Fetalis *on page 122*

Lipase, Serum

***CPT** 83690*

Related Information

Amylase, Serum *on page 127*
Amylase, Urine *on page 129*
Body Fluid Amylase *on page 148*

Synonyms Triacylglycerol Acylhydrolase

Applies to Body Fluid Lipase

Abstract An enzyme produced by the pancreas which is elevated in pancreatitis. The new lipase methods are superior to total serum amylase in diagnosis of acute pancreatitis.[1]

Specimen Serum; lipase (unlike amylase) is not applicable to urine. Lipase may be run on pleural or peritoneal fluid. **CONTAINER:** Red top tube **STORAGE INSTRUCTIONS:** Stable 1 week at 25°C, 3 weeks at 4°C.

Interpretive **REFERENCE RANGE:** Method dependent but typically <200 units/L **USE:** Diagnose pancreatitis **LIMITATIONS:** EDTA anticoagulant may interfere. Hemoglobin at ≤250 mg/dL may interfere, depending on method. Fifty-five percent of patients with primary biliary cirrhosis had raised serum lipase activity.[2] Lipase is increased in about 50% of the patients with chronic renal failure. About 75% of such patients have increased serum amylase as well.[3] Serum lipase increases with hemodialysis.[4] This increase is apparently due to heparin-induced lipolytic activity. Therefore, predialysis blood samples are recommended for lipase measurement. Both serum amylase and lipase may be elevated in chronic alcoholics in the absence of acute pancreatitis.[5] **CONTRAINDICATIONS:** Urine specimens are inappropriate for lipase. Lipase activity is usually absent in urine, possibly from inactivation of the enzyme. **METHODOLOGY:** Turbidimetric (using triolein), other methods available **ADDITIONAL INFORMATION:** Serum lipase is usually normal in patients with elevated serum amylase, without pancreatitis, who have peptic ulcer, salivary adenitis, inflammatory bowel disease, intestinal obstruction, and macroamylasemia. Coexistence of increased serum amylase with normal lipase may be a helpful clue to the presence of macroamylasemia.[6] Lipase is elevated with amylase in acute pancreatitis, but the elevation of lipase is more prolonged.

In work-up of pancreatitis, in addition to serum lipase and amylase, the 2-hour urine amylase is of value. Pancreatic isoamylase may be useful in mild elevations of total serum amylase. Electrolytes, serum calcium, glucose, and acetone are also often needed. Immunoreactive trypsin is technically more difficult than lipase and probably no better. The serum lipase/amylase ratio may help distinguish alcoholic from nonalcoholic pancreatitis. Ratios >2 (expressed as multiples of the upper limits of normal) suggest an alcoholic etiology.[7] Higher lipase:amylase ratios in patients with alcoholic pancreatitis were described as well by others.[8] Lipase isoform or isoenzymes have been studied.[9]

Footnotes

1. Gambino R, "Pancreatitis: Acute and Nonacute," *Lab Report for Physicians*, 1987, 9:28-9.
2. Fonseca V, Epstein O, Katrak A, et al, "Serum Immunoreactive Trypsin and Pancreatic Lipase in Primary Biliary Cirrhosis," *J Clin Pathol*, 1986, 39:638-40.
3. Royse VL, Jensen DM, and Corwin HL, "Pancreatic Enzymes in Chronic Renal Failure," *Arch Intern Med*, 1987, 147:537-9.
4. Vaziri ND, Chang D, Malekpour A, et al, "Pancreatic Enzymes in Patients With End-Stage Renal Disease Maintained on Hemodialysis," *Am J Gastroenterol*, 1988, 83(4):410-2.
5. Gumaste VV, Sereny G, Dave P, et al, "Serum Lipase Levels in Chronic Alcoholics," *J Clin Gastroenterol*, 1991, 13(4):407-10.
6. Andrews PA and Thomas PA, "Macroamylasaemia as a Cause of Persistently Raised Serum Amylase," *Br J Surg*, 1988, 75(10):1035.
7. Gumaste VV, Dave PB, Weissman D, et al, "Lipase/Amylase Ratio. A New Index That Distinguishes Acute Episodes of Alcoholic From Nonalcoholic Acute Pancreatitis," *Gastroenterology*, 1991, 101(6):1361-6.
8. Tenner SM and Steinberg W, "The Admission Serum Lipase:Amylase Ratio Differentiates Alcoholic From Nonalcoholic Acute Pancreatitis," *Am J Gastroenterol*, 1992, 87(12):1755-8.
9. Lott JA and LU CJ, "Lipase Isoforms and Amylase Isoenzymes: Assays and Application in the Diagnosis of Acute Pancreatitis," *Clin Chem*, 1991, 37(3):361-8.

References

Thompson HJ, Obekpa PO, Smith AN, et al, "Diagnosis of Acute Pancreatitis: A Proposed Sequence of Biochemical Investigations," *Scand J Gastroenterol*, 1987, 22:719-24.

Lipid Profile

CPT *80061*

Related Information

Apolipoprotein A and B *on page 134*
Cholesterol *on page 185*
High Density Lipoprotein Cholesterol *on page 249*
Lipoprotein (a) *on page 280*
Lipoprotein Electrophoresis *on page 281*
Low Density Lipoprotein Cholesterol *on page 284*
Triglycerides *on page 370*

Synonyms Coronary Heart Disease Risk Index; Risk Index for Coronary Arterial Disease

Test Commonly Includes Triglycerides, total cholesterol, HDL cholesterol, LDL cholesterol, estimate (by calculation) of VLDL cholesterol (if triglycerides are <400 mg/dL)

Abstract A panel of tests involving serum lipids used to evaluate coronary heart disease risk.

Patient Care PREPARATION: Patient should be on stable diet ideally for 2-3 weeks prior to collection of blood and should fast for at least 12 hours before collection of the specimen. Inconclusive evidence for 72 hours of abstinence from alcohol exists before sampling for lipid profile. See Preparation in the Cholesterol listing.

Specimen Serum CONTAINER: Red top tube COLLECTION: Lipid profiles are best avoided following acute myocardial infarct, for up to 3 months, although cholesterol can be measured in the first 24 hours. STORAGE INSTRUCTIONS: Lipoproteins are labile. Even stored at 4°C, analysis should not be delayed more than a few days.

Interpretive REFERENCE RANGE: Reference values for blood lipids have been published as extensive tables, providing percentile distributions by age groups.[1] See tables 1-8. USE: Abbreviations used are as follows: HDLC, high density lipoprotein cholesterol; LDLC, low density lipoprotein cholesterol; VLDLC, very low density lipoprotein cholesterol. Evaluate hyperlipidemia as an index to coronary artery disease. Investigation of serum lipids is indicated in those with coronary and other arterial disease, especially when it is premature, and in those with family history of atherosclerosis or of hyperlipidemia. In this sense, the expression "premature" is mostly used to include those younger than 40 years of age. Patients with xanthomas should be worked up with lipid profiles, but not those with xanthelasmas or xanthofibromas in the sense of dermatofibromas. Those whose fasting serum is lipemic should have a lipid profile, but the serum of a subject with high cholesterol but normal triglyceride is not milky in appearance. The patient with high cholesterol (>240 mg/dL) should have a lipid profile. Patients with cholesterol levels between 200-240 mg/dL plus two other coronary heart disease risk factors should also have a lipid profile.[2] In addition to application in screening programs for evaluation of risk factors for coronary arterial disease, lipid profiling may lead to detection of some cases of hypothyroidism. If a patient has low LDLC, but very low HDLC, he/she may still be in jeopardy (Castelli of the Framingham study); therefore, LDLC/HDLC ratios are useful. **Primary hy-**

Table 1.—Selected Reference Values for Plasma Total Cholesterol (mg/dL) in White Male Subjects

Age (years)	No.	Mean	Percentiles			
			5	75	90	95
0–19	5749	155	115	170	185	200
20–24	882	165	125	185	205	220
25–29	2042	180	135	200	225	245
30–34	2444	190	140	215	240	255
35–39	2320	200	145	225	250	270
40–44	2428	205	150	230	250	270
45–69	7710	215	160	235	260	275
70+	850	205	150	230	250	270

Table 2.—Selected Reference Values for Plasma Low-Density Lipoprotein Cholesterol (mg/dL) in White Male Subjects

Age (years)	No.	Mean	Percentiles			
			5	75	90	95
5–19	713	95	65	105	120	130
20–24	118	105	65	120	140	145
25–29	253	115	70	140	155	165
30–34	403	125	80	145	165	185
35–39	371	135	80	155	175	190
40–44	385	135	85	155	175	185
45–69	1162	145	90	165	190	205
70+	119	145	90	165	180	185

Table 3.—Selected Reference Values for Plasma High-Density Lipoprotein Cholesterol (mg/dL) in White Male Subjects

Age (years)	No.	Mean	Percentiles		
			5	10	95
5-14	438	55	35	40	75
15-19	299	45	30	35	65
20-24	118	45	30	30	65
25-29	253	45	30	30	65
30-34	403	45	30	30	65
35-39	371	45	30	30	60
40-44	383	45	25	30	65
45-69	1162	50	30	30	70
70+	119	50	30	35	75

Table 4.—Selected Reference Values for Plasma Total Cholesterol (mg/dL) in White Female Subjects

Age (years)	No.	Mean	Percentiles			
			5	75	90	95
0-19	5470	160	120	175	190	200
20-24	1566	170	125	190	215	230
25-34	4340	175	130	195	220	235
35-39	2012	185	140	205	230	245
40-44	2050	195	145	215	235	255
45-49	2149	205	150	225	250	270
50-54	1992	220	165	240	265	285
55+	4478	230	170	250	275	295

Table 5.—Selected Reference Values for Plasma Low-Density Lipoprotein Cholesterol (mg/dL) in White Female Subjects

Age (years)	No.	Mean	Percentiles			
			5	75	90	95
5-19	652	100	65	110	125	140
20-24	199	105	55	120	140	160
25-34	646	110	70	125	145	160
35-39	299	120	75	140	160	170
40-44	318	125	75	145	165	175
45-49	326	130	80	150	175	185
50-54	256	140	90	160	185	200
55+	668	150	95	170	195	215

Table 6.—Selected Reference Values for Plasma High-Density Lipoprotein Cholesterol (mg/dL) in White Female Subjects

Age (years)	No.	Mean	Percentiles		
			5	10	95
5-19	666	55	35	40	70
20-24	199	55	35	35	80
25-34	649	55	35	40	80
35-39	298	55	35	40	80
40-44	318	60	35	40	90
45-49	328	60	35	40	85
50-54	256	60	35	40	90
55+	668	60	35	40	95

Table 7.—Selected Reference Values for Plasma Triglycerides (mg/dL) in White Male Subjects

Age (years)	No.	Mean	Percentiles		
			5	90	95
0-9	1491	55	30	85	100
10-14	2278	65	30	100	125
15-19	1980	80	35	120	150
20-24	882	100	45	165	200
25-29	2042	115	45	200	250
30-34	2444	130	50	215	265
35-39	2320	145	55	250	320
40-54	6862	150	55	250	320
55-64	2526	140	60	235	290
65+	1600	135	55	210	260

Table 8.—Selected Reference Values for Plasma Triglycerides (mg/dL) in White Female Subjects

Age (years)	No.	Mean	Percentiles		
			5	90	95
0-9	1304	60	35	95	110
10-19	4166	75	40	115	130
20-34	5906	90	40	145	170
35-39	2012	95	40	160	195
40-44	2050	105	45	170	210
45-49	2149	110	45	185	230
50-54	1992	120	55	190	240
55-64	2768	125	55	200	250
65+	1710	130	60	205	240

Rifkind BM and Segal P, "Lipid Research Clinics Program Reference Values for Hyperlipidemia and Hypolipidemia," *JAMA*, 1983, 250:1870-1, with permission.

(Continued)

Lipid Profile *(Continued)*

perlipoproteinemia includes hypercholesterolemia, a direct risk factor for coronary heart disease. **Secondary hyperlipoproteinemias** include increases of lipoproteins secondary to hypothyroidism, nephrosis, renal failure, obesity, diabetes mellitus, alcoholism, primary biliary cirrhosis, and other types of cholestasis. **Decreased** lipids are found with some cases of malabsorption, malnutrition, advanced liver disease. In abetalipoproteinemia, cholesterol is <70 mg/dL (SI: <1.81 mmol/L). **LIMITATIONS:** Patients with obstructive liver disease may develop lipoprotein abnormalities. Serum lipid factors have not been demonstrated to strongly influence recurrent stenosis following coronary angioplasty, the pathogenesis of which is presently not well understood. **CONTRAINDICATIONS:** Patient on antihyperlipidemic drugs, endocrine imbalance, unstable weight, abnormal diet. LDLC should not be calculated if triglyceride is >400 mg/dL (SI: >4.52 mmol/L). **METHODOLOGY:** See listings for cholesterol, triglycerides, and lipoproteins. LDLC is calculated as follows: LDLC = total cholesterol - (VLDLC + HDLC). VLDLC is estimated as follows: VLDLC = triglycerides/5. Lipoprotein electrophoresis has a very limited role. Ultracentrifugation is not available to many laboratories. **ADDITIONAL INFORMATION:** Several other factors are well-documented as risk factors in developing coronary heart disease and are known to be additive in effect to hyperlipidemia. These include "rich" diet – habitually high saturated fat, cholesterol, and calories in relation to energy expenditure; cigarette smoking; hypertension; obesity; glucose intolerance/diabetes mellitus; and left ventricular hypertrophy.

In contemporary medical practice, lipid analyses are presently very predominantly limited to cholesterol, triglyceride, HDL, and calculated LDL. **Apolipoproteins** can be measured but their major applications have so far been limited. Genetically determined, 13 lipoprotein apoproteins are presently recognized. Apoproteins AI and B are thought to have potential for atherosclerotic heart disease risk prediction. A ratio of apoprotein AI to apoprotein B may prove to be a useful predictor of cardiovascular risk – the lower the ratio, the higher the risk. However, lack of interlaboratory agreement and standardization, and the use of different methods are among the barriers to more widespread application of apoproteins. More work is needed.[3] Characteristics of apolipoproteins are outlined. Apolipoproteins act as acute phase reactants and should not be measured in ill subjects. **Lipoprotein (a)** has been demonstrated in atheromas. Its apolipoprotein component bears similarities to plasminogen. (See Plasminogen Activator Inhibitor in the Coagulation chapter.) It is measured by RIA or by rate nephelometry and ELISA. Increased levels are associated with coronary atherosclerosis. It presently is studied in research settings.[3]

Footnotes

1. Rifkind BM and Segal P, "Lipid Research Clinics Program Reference Values for Hyperlipidemia and Hypolipidemia," *JAMA*, 1983, 250:1869-72.
2. "Report of the National Cholesterol Treatment Program Expert Panel on Detection, Evaluation, and Treatment of High Blood Cholesterol in Adults," *Arch Intern Med*, 1988, 148(1):36-64.
3. Rosenfeld L, "Lipoprotein Analysis. Early Methods in the Diagnosis of Atherosclerosis," *Arch Pathol Lab Med*, 1989, 113(10):1101-10.

References

Austin GE, Hollman J, Lynn MJ, et al, "Serum Lipoprotein Levels Fail to Predict Postangioplasty Recurrent Coronary Artery Stenosis," *Cleve Clin J Med*, 1989, 56(5):509-14.

Mount JN, Kearney EM, Rosseneu M, et al, "Immunoturbidimetric Assays for Serum Apolipoproteins A1 and B Using Cobas Bio Centrifugal Analyzer," *J Clin Pathol*, 1988, 41:471-4.

Steiner G, "From an Excess of Fat, Diabetics Die," *JAMA*, 1989, 262(3):398-9, (editorial).

Stern MP, Patterson JK, Haffner SM, "Lack of Awareness and Treatment of Hyperlipidemia in Type II Diabetes in a Community Survey," *JAMA*, 1989, 262(3):360-4.

Tasaki H, Nakashima Y, Nandate H, et al, "Comparison of Serum Lipid Values in Variant Angina Pectoris and Fixed Coronary Artery Disease With Normal Subjects," *Am J Cardiol*, 1989, 63(20):1441-5.

Lipoprotein (a)

CPT 84999

Related Information

Apolipoprotein A and B *on page 134*

Lipid Profile *on previous page*

Synonyms Lp(a)

Abstract This is a plasma lipoprotein with a lipid composition very similar to low density lipoprotein (LDL). The apolipoprotein, however, is composed of two proteins linked by disulfide bonds. The plasma level of Lp(a) is positively correlated with the occurrence of coronary heart disease and cerebrovascular disease particularly in hypercholesterolemic subjects.

Specimen Plasma or serum **CONTAINER:** Lavender top (EDTA) tube, red top tube **STORAGE INSTRUCTIONS:** Spin at low temperature. Stable at 4°C for 1 week and frozen for months.

Interpretive REFERENCE RANGE: 10-20 mg/dL (ELISA).[1] Range is method dependent. Some other methods have higher expected ranges. CRITICAL VALUES: Plasma levels >30 mg/dL are associated with a two- to threefold increased risk of coronary artery disease (CAD). USE: Assess coronary artery disease (CAD) risk METHODOLOGY: Enzyme-linked immunosorbent assay (ELISA), rate and endpoint nephelometry, electroimmunodiffusion ADDITIONAL INFORMATION: The two proteins that make up the apoprotein are B-100 (a major apoprotein of LDL) and a second which has a very high homology with plasminogen. There is a significant variation in concentration of this lipoprotein among individuals, but within any individual it tends to remain relatively constant for long periods. At least six isoforms of apo Lp(a) exist and the molecular mass varies from 400,000-700,000. These isoforms react differently in most immunochemical tests which accounts for the wide range of expected values. High Lp(a) values in hyperlipidemic subjects are clearly an independent risk factor for CAD and possible cerebral infarction. The association is not as clear in normolipidemic subjects. There is evidence to suggest that Lp(a) may inhibit fibrinolysis by decreasing the activation of plasminogen to which it has high homology.[2]

Footnotes

1. Labeur C, Michiels G, Bury J, et al, "Lipoprotein (a) Quantified by an Enzyme-Linked Immunosorbent Assay With Monoclonal Antibodies," *Clin Chem*, 1989, 35(7):1380-4.
2. Albers JJ, Marcovina SM, and Lodge MS, "The Unique Lipoprotein (a): Properties and Immunochemical Measurement," *Clin Chem*, 1990, 36(12):2019-26.

References

Fless GM, Snyder ML, and Scanu AM, "Enzyme-Linked Immunoassay for Lp(a)," *J Lipid Res*, 1989, 30(5):651-2.

Labeur C, Shepherd J, and Rosseneu M, "Immunological Assays of Apolipoproteins in Plasma: Methods and Instrumentation," *Clin Chem*, 1990, 36(4):591-7.

Seed M, Hoppichler F, Reaveley D, et al, "Relation of Serum Lipoprotein (a) Concentration and Apolipoprotein (a) Phenotype to Coronary Heart Disease in Patients With Familial Hypercholesterolemia," *N Engl J Med*, 1990, 322(21):1494-9.

Utermann G, "The Mysteries of Lipoprotein (a)," *Science*, 1989, 246(4932):904-10.

Lipoprotein Electrophoresis

***CPT** 83715*

Related Information

Cholesterol *on page 185*

High Density Lipoprotein Cholesterol *on page 249*

Lipid Profile *on page 278*

Low Density Lipoprotein Cholesterol *on page 284*

Triglycerides *on page 370*

Synonyms Lipoprotein Phenotyping

Applies to Hyperlipoproteinemias; Lipoprotein X

Test Commonly Includes Separation of lipoprotein patterns and classification by electrophoresis. Serum triglyceride and cholesterol determination should also be ordered.

Abstract This procedure separates some of the lipid fractions based on electrophoretic mobility. It is outdated and not very useful.

Patient Care PREPARATION: Patient should be on a stable diet for 2-3 weeks and should be fasting for 12-14 hours.

Specimen Serum CONTAINER: Red top tube CAUSES FOR REJECTION: Patient not fasting for 12 hours

Interpretive REFERENCE RANGE: Quantitation not available from this procedure. Visual estimates of stain density in comparison to normal patterns are usually done. USE: Evaluate hyperlipidemia to determine abnormal lipoprotein distribution and concentration in the serum (eg, work up Tangier disease) LIMITATIONS: Does not directly provide cholesterol or HDL cholesterol quantitation. Patients with different Fredrickson phenotypes on lipoprotein electrophoresis were found within given families, and the same patient did not always fall within the same phenotype on repeat analyses. Examination of the fasting specimen following overnight refrigeration, with quantitation of cholesterol and triglyceride, often provides the same or better information than lipoprotein electrophoresis. Development of quantitative methods for HDLC further diminished the status of the lipoprotein electrophoresis. Few laboratories provide the assay. METHODOLOGY: **Electrophoresis** provides phenotypes as a classification of hyperlipoproteinemias. **Analytical ultracentrifugation** provides flotation rate, expressed as Svedberg units: smaller molecules are more dense and contain more protein and less lipid. ADDITIONAL INFORMATION: The lipid profile has generally replaced this test. Attempts to predict

(Continued)

Lipoprotein Electrophoresis *(Continued)*

high density lipoprotein cholesterol from lipoprotein electrophoretic patterns have been unsuccessful. Lipoprotein electrophoresis may still be used to establish the diagnosis of type III broad beta disease with cholesterol quantitation with subsequent ultracentrifugation to detect abnormal betalipoprotein. Familial dysbetalipoproteinemia occurs with palmar or tuberous xanthomas and with substantially elevated cholesterol levels. Phenotyping of Apo E (apolipoprotein work-up) supports this diagnosis. In hyperalphalipoproteinemia, cholesterol is increased as alphalipoprotein cholesterol as in familial hyperalphalipoproteinemia and also as a secondary entity. Lipoprotein electrophoresis provides a classification based on electrophoretic mobility as the designations in the left column as follows: See table. Lipoprotein-X measured following 2 weeks of cholestyramine may be helpful in work-up of extrahepatic obstruction. Its unique cathodal mobility on agar gel electrophoresis is noteworthy. It is absent from normal serum.

Lipoprotein Electrophoresis

Electrophoresis	Composition
Chylomicrons	About 90% triglyceride
Prebeta (very low density lipoprotein) (VLDL)	**Triglyceride,** phospholipid, cholesterol, protein
Beta (low density lipoprotein) (LDL)	**Cholesterol,** protein, phospholipid, triglyceride
Alpha (high density lipoprotein) (HDL)	**Protein, phospholipid,** cholesterol, triglyceride

Lipoprotein Phenotyping *see* Lipoprotein Electrophoresis *on previous page*

Lipoprotein X *see* Lipoprotein Electrophoresis *on previous page*

Liver Battery *see* Liver Profile *on this page*

Liver Panel *see* Liver Profile *on this page*

Liver Profile

CPT 80058

Related Information

Acetaminophen, Serum *on page 935*
Amiodarone *on page 939*
Bilirubin, Total *on page 139*

Synonyms Liver Battery; Liver Panel

Test Commonly Includes Liver profile most often includes total bilirubin, conjugated bilirubin, alkaline phosphatase, LD (LDH), AST (SGOT), with ALT (SGPT), GGT (GGTP). It may also include serum protein electrophoresis, prothrombin time, HB_sAg, perhaps LAP (leucine aminopeptidase) or 5' nucleotidase. $Alpha_1$-antitrypsin phenotype and quantitation on occasion explains cases otherwise difficult to classify but is rarely if ever included in liver profiles.

Abstract Characterization of liver disease requires intelligent correlation of the medical history, physical examination, and laboratory test results.[1]

Specimen Serum **CONTAINER:** Red top tube **STORAGE INSTRUCTIONS:** Protect bilirubin specimens from light. **CAUSES FOR REJECTION:** Hemolysis interferes with certain tests (see individual listings). **SPECIAL INSTRUCTIONS:** The specimen should be handled with extra precaution, especially if there is a greater than usual possibility of hepatitis. Prothrombin time tube should be spun down immediately, plasma separated from cells, placed in special plastic tube, kept refrigerated, and analyzed within 4 hours.

Interpretive **REFERENCE RANGE:** See individual test listings. **USE:** Evaluate liver disease, biliary disease, hepatoma, chronic active hepatitis, cirrhosis, including biliary cirrhosis; investigate otherwise unexplained increases in such tests as AST, ALT, alkaline phosphatase, or prolongation of the prothrombin time; work up possible alcoholism **LIMITATIONS:** A number of useful tests include those to work up pancreatitis, such as serum amylase and lipase and urine 2-hour amylase. Other tests helpful in evaluation of liver disease include 5' nucleotidase; immunoglobulins IgG, IgA, IgM; ANA; antimitochondrial antibody; smooth muscle antibody; LD isoenzymes; alpha-fetoprotein, and 2-hour urine urobilinogen. Ammonia is useful only in selected cases, (eg, Reye's syndrome).

Use of blood alcohol determinations for investigation of liver disease has been advocated, because the test is cheap and simple. Other tests useful in alcoholism include MCV and folate levels, triglycerides as well as GGT, AST, and bilirubin. Prothrombin time is often helpful. False-positive tests occur in asymptomatic patients. Repeat testing on initial abnormalities is important.[2] Viral hepatitis serological tests additional to HB_sAg may be indicated. Liver disease related to alpha$_1$-antitrypsin deficiency and to Wilson's disease must be considered.

CONTRAINDICATIONS: Many physicians prefer to order tests individually, as clinically indicated. Among the problems with such profiles, tests appropriate for specific clinical indications may not be included. Few physicians recall accurately the content of a liver profile offered by a specific clinical laboratory. **METHODOLOGY:** See individual test listings. **ADDITIONAL INFORMATION:** Liver profile interpretation can be considered as follows:

Cholestasis and biliary tract: alkaline phosphatase (very rarely, isoenzymes of alkaline phosphatase),[3] GGT, leucine aminopeptidase, 5' nucleotidase, total bilirubin, conjugated bilirubin, eosinophil count, urine bile (as part of urinalysis) are used. In extrahepatic biliary obstruction the serum alkaline phosphatase is increased two to three times or more while AST remains <300 units/L. Very high alkaline phosphatase levels may be found with intrahepatic cholestasis, such that alkaline phosphatase which is high out of proportion to the severity of jaundice, may indicate an intrahepatic disease.[1] Serum and urine amylase and lipase are often relevant. Viral, alcoholic, or drug-related cholestatic hepatitis may give rise to chemistry tests indistinguishable from those of extrahepatic obstruction.[1]

Liver excretory function: urine urobilinogen, total bilirubin, conjugated bilirubin.

Hepatoma and other tumors: alkaline phosphatase, GGT, total LD, CEA, HB_sAg (hepatitis B surface antigen). Alpha$_1$-fetoprotein may increase moderately in nonmalignant liver diseases; rising or high levels may indicate hepatoma.[1] Such clinical laboratory tests do not prove tumor without imaging and biopsy.

Hepatocellular disease: AST, ALT (more specific than AST), LD, LD_4, LD_5 (fractions related to liver in LD isoenzymes), liver biopsy, HB_sAg (hepatitis B surface antigen), anti-HB_s (antibody to hepatitis B surface antigen), anti-HB_c (antibody to hepatitis B core antigen), HB_eAg (hepatitis B "e" antigen), anti-HB_e (antibody to hepatitis B_e antigen), anti-HAV, IgM (antibody to hepatitis A virus, IgM).

Liver metabolic function: Serum ammonia may increase in liver necrosis and cirrhosis.[4]

Hemochromatosis: Mild abnormalities in liver profile tests (AST, ALT, ALP) may occur in hemochromatosis.[5]

Immunologic stimulation: Protein electrophoresis: features suggestive of cirrhosis but not always present in that disease include low albumin, low alpha$_2$, polyclonal or oligoclonal gammopathy, and beta/gamma bridging. Many but not all cases of conventional hepatic cirrhosis are accompanied by polyclonal gammopathy, sometimes with beta/gamma bridging. Oligoclonal gammopathy is found in <50% of cases of chronic active hepatitis (CAH).

Immunoglobulins: IgM: very helpful in primary biliary cirrhosis; high in acute and chronic hepatitis, cholangitis, and CAH. Alpha$_1$-globulin tends to fall with serum albumin. Both alpha and beta globulins may decrease in hepatocellular failure.[4]

Antibodies: ANA: A portion of cases of CAH have positive ANA and/or positive LE prep. **Antimitochondrial antibody**: Extremely useful in primary biliary cirrhosis; high more often in cholangitis than in cholecystitis. **Smooth muscle antibody:** Hepatitis and conventional as well as biliary cirrhosis; especially useful for CAH (chronic active hepatitis). Antibodies usually negative in drug jaundice and nonfebrile extrahepatic obstruction. In intrahepatic or extrahepatic biliary obstructive disease, the tests listed under Cholestasis and Biliary Tract are more abnormal than those listed under Hepatocellular Disease.

In **viral hepatitis**, AST is usually three to five times or more higher (as multiples of the upper limit of normal) than LD; in cases which clinically resemble hepatitis, but in which LD equals or exceeds AST, LD isoenzymes may be useful. LD_4 and LD_5 are the hepatic fractions. An isomorphic pattern, if detected, may suggest infectious mononucleosis, CMV infection, neoplasm, or cirrhosis/alcoholism, depending on clinical setting. Appropriate positive serological

(Continued)

Liver Profile *(Continued)*

tests support a diagnosis of viral hepatitis, while negative ones provide support for drug-induced hepatitis. Resolution of liver disease with removal of the offending agent enhances the latter diagnosis.

Hepatic functional reserve: Both albumin and prothrombin time are useful in evaluation of the liver, but they are nonspecific. Representing hepatic synthesis, albumin reflects also nutritional status and is lost in a variety of gastrointestinal and renal diseases.

Liver biopsy is not replaced by such testing. Liver biopsy remains a vital diagnostic modality. Its interpretation commonly requires and is supported by clinical laboratory investigation. Results of testing must be provided to the histopathologist who works up and holds responsibility for interpretation of the liver biopsy.

Footnotes

1. Frank BB and Members of the Patient Care Committee of the American Gastroenterological Association, "Clinical Evaluation of Jaundice – A Guideline of the Patient Care Committee of the American Gastroenterological Association," *JAMA*, 1989, 262(21):3031-4.
2. McKenna JP, Moskovitz M, and Cox JL, "Abnormal Liver Function Tests in Asymptomatic Patients," *Am Fam Physician*, 1989, 39(3):117-26.
3. Narayanan S, "Serum Alkaline Phosphate Isoenzymes as Markers of Liver Disease," *Ann Clin Lab Sci*, 1991, 21(1):12-8.
4. Friedman RB and Young DS, *Effects of Disease on Clinical Laboratory Tests*, Washington, DC: American Association of Clinical Chemistry Press, 1989.
5. Lin E and Adams PC, "Biochemical Liver Profile in Hemochromatosis. A Survey of 100 Patients," *J Clin Gastroenterol*, 1991, 13(3):316-20.

References

Sherwin JE, "Liver Function," *Clinical Chemistry Theory Analysis and Correlation*, Chapter 23, Kaplan LA and Pesce AJ, eds, St Louis, MO: Mosby-Year Book Inc, 1989, 359-72.

Low Density Lipoprotein Cholesterol

CPT 83721

Related Information

Apolipoprotein A and B *on page 134*
Cholesterol *on page 185*
Lipid Profile *on page 278*
Lipoprotein Electrophoresis *on page 281*
Triglycerides *on page 370*

Synonyms Beta Lipoproteins; LDLC

Applies to LDLC/HDLC Ratio

Abstract The concentration of cholesterol in this lipoprotein is positively correlated with coronary heart disease risk (see following table).

Patient Care PREPARATION: See Preparation in Cholesterol listing.

Specimen Serum CONTAINER: Red top tube SAMPLING TIME: 12- to 14-hour fast before drawing CAUSES FOR REJECTION: Patient not fasting

Interpretive REFERENCE RANGE: Up to approximately 130 mg/dL (SI: $\leq$3.36 mmol/L). CRITICAL VALUES: >160 mg/dL USE: An association exists between increased LDLC and total prediction of risk of coronary arterial atherosclerosis. High LDLC is a direct risk factor for coronary atherosclerosis. Screening early in life has been suggested.[1] LIMITATIONS: If triglyceride is >400 mg/dL, LDL cannot be calculated accurately by the Friedewald formula. See notes in methodology. For reliable LDLC levels, accurate HDLC, cholesterol, and triglyceride methods are necessary; *vide infra*. METHODOLOGY: Usually a calculation rather than a direct measurement. LDL can be separated in the analytical ultracentrifuge (*vide infra*), but that instrument is expensive, time consuming, and not very cost effective or practical for hospital laboratories. ADDITIONAL INFORMATION: LDL carries cholesterol in plasma. LDL is the major transport protein for cholesterol. LDL is derived using the Friedewald formula. The current formula when expressed in mg/dL: LDLC = total cholesterol – (HDLC + 0.20 x triglycerides [mg/dL]); or when concentrations are expressed in mmol/L: LDLC = total cholesterol – (HDLC + 0.46 x triglyceride).[2,3] This formula is not valid for specimens with chylomicrons present or triglyceride levels >400 mg/dL (SI: >4.52 mmol/L). LDLC/HDLC ratio provides a better signal for risk than either single result. Pseudocholinesterase/HDLC ratio has been studied. The National Cholesterol Education Program (NCEP) has defined a classification based on LDLC.[4] See table. However, Palumbo perceives some NCEP recommendations as only arbitrarily acceptable.[5] By analytical ultracentrifugation, LDL falls in the subgroup S_F 0-12, while VLDL are in S_F 12-400 (very low density lipoprotein). The major apoprotein of LDL is apoprotein B. Measurement of apoprotein B has been used to indicate possible elevations of LDLC.[6]

Classification Based on LDL Cholesterol

<130 mg/dL	(SI: <3.36 mmol/L)	Desirable LDL cholesterol
130-159 mg/dL	(SI: 3.36-4.11 mmol/L)	Borderline-high-risk LDL cholesterol
≥160 mg/dL	(SI: ≥4.14 mmol/L)	High-risk LDL cholesterol

- The LDL cholesterol level is the basis for decisions about initiating dietary or drug therapy.
- Patients with LDL cholesterol levels ≥160 mg/dL (SI: ≥4.14 mmol/L) are considered at high risk for CHD. These patients should be given cholesterol-lowering treatment.
- Patients with borderline-high-risk LDL cholesterol levels 130-159 mg/dL (SI: 3.36-4.11 mmol/L) should also be treated to lower their cholesterol if they have definite CHD or two other CHD risk factors (see Cholesterol listing for additional definition of risk factors).

"National Cholesterol Education Program, Adult Treatment Panel Report 1987," National Cholesterol Education Program, National Heart, Lung and Blood Institute, National Institutes of Health, C-200, Bethesda, MD 20892, 1987.

Footnotes

1. Webber LS, Srinivasan SR, Wattigney WA, et al, "Tracking of Serum Lipids and Lipoproteins From Childhood to Adulthood, The Bogalusa Heart Study," *Am J Epidemiol*, 1991, 133(9):884-99.
2. Warnick GR, Knopp RH, Fitzpatrick V, et al, "Estimating Low Density Lipoprotein Cholesterol by the Friedewald Equation Is Adequate for Classifying Patients on the Basis of Nationally Recommended Cutpoints," *Clin Chem*, 1990, 36(1):15-9.
3. Rifai N, Warnick GR, McNamara JR, et al, "Measurement of Low Density Lipoprotein Cholesterol in Serum: A Status Report," *Clin Chem*, 1992, 38(1):150-60.
4. "National Cholesterol Education Program, Adult Treatment Panel Report 1987," National Cholesterol Education Program, National Heart, Lung, and Blood Institute, National Institutes of Health, 1987, C-200, Bethesda, MD 20892.
5. Palumbo PJ, "National Cholesterol Education Program: Does the Emperor Have Any Clothes?" *Mayo Clin Proc*, 1988, 63(1):88-90.
6. Dennison BA, Kikuchi DA, Srinivasan SR, et al, "Measurement of Apolipoprotein B as a Screening Test for Identifying Children With Elevated Levels of Low Density Lipoprotein Cholesterol," *J Pediatr*, 1990, 117(3):358-63.

References

Dale JC, "Focus on Cholesterol, Low Density Lipoprotein (LDL), Serum," *Mayo Medical Laboratories Communique*, 1989, 14:3-4.

Garber AM, "Where to Draw the Line Against Cholesterol," *Ann Intern Med*, 1989, 111(8):625-7.

Goodman DS, Hulley SB, Clark LT, et al, "Report of the National Cholesterol Education Program Expert Panel on Detection, Evaluation, and Treatment of High Blood Cholesterol in Adults," *Arch Intern Med*, 1988, 148:36-69.

Grundy SM, Goodman DS, Rifkind BM, et al, "The Place of HDL in Cholesterol Management: A Perspective From the National Cholesterol Education Program," *Arch Intern Med*, 1989, 149(3):505-10.

Rifkind BM and Segal P, "Lipid Research Clinics Program Reference Values for Hyperlipidemia and Hypolipidemia," *JAMA*, 1983, 250:1869-72.

Steinberg D, Parthasarathy S, Carew TE, et al, "Beyond Cholesterol. Modifications of Low-Density Lipoprotein That Increase Its Atherogenicity," *N Engl J Med*, 1989, 320(14):915-24.

Stossel TP, Austin MA, Breslow JL, et al, "Clinical Investigation Low-Density Lipoprotein Subclass Patterns and Risk of Myocardial Infarction," *JAMA*, 1988, 260:1917-21.

Lp(a) *see* Lipoprotein (a) *on page 280*

L/S Ratio *see* Amniotic Fluid Lecithin/Sphingomyelin Ratio and Phosphatidylglycerol *on page 124*

Luteinizing Hormone, Blood or Urine

CPT 83002

Related Information

Clomiphene Test *on page 190*
Follicle Stimulating Hormone *on page 222*
Testosterone, Free and Total *on page 358*

Synonyms Follitropin; ICSH; Interstitial Cell Stimulating Hormone; LH; Pituitary Gonadotropins

Test Commonly Includes Usually measured with FSH

Abstract Levels of this hormone (along with FSH) are used to assess the level of anterior pituitary gonadotropic function.

Patient Care PREPARATION: Avoid radioisotope administration to patient prior to collection of specimen.

Specimen Serum or urine CONTAINER: Red top tube, plastic urine container STORAGE INSTRUCTIONS: Separate serum from cells. Stable 14 days at 4°C to 25°C. SPECIAL INSTRUCTIONS: In females, date of last menstrual period should be supplied. It is important to measure both FSH and LH.

Interpretive REFERENCE RANGE: Normal serum ranges vary among laboratories but these are typical: Adults: male: 7-24 mIU/mL (SI: 7-24 IU/L), female: 6-30 mIU/mL (SI: 6-30 IU/L) (baseline), midcycle peak for follicular or luteal phase: over four times baseline. Low levels are found in hypogonadotropic states. High values occur with castration, ovarian failure, and in the postmenopausal state (30-200 mIU/mL).[1] Lower values in children up to the midteens. USE: Excessive FSH and LH are found in hypogonadism, anorchia, gonadal failure, complete testicular feminization syndrome, menopause. FSH and LH are pituitary products, useful to distinguish primary gonadal failure from secondary (hypothalamic/pituitary) causes of gonadal failure, menstrual disturbances, and amenorrhea. Useful in defining menstrual cycle phases in infertility evaluation of women and testicular dysfunction in men. FSH is commonly used with LH, which also is a gonadotropin. Both are low with pituitary or hypothalamic failure. When one is high and the other low, a gonadotropin-producing pituitary tumor is likely.[1]

Elevated basal LH with high LH/FSH ratio, >2, with some increase of ovarian androgen, in an essentially nonovulatory adult female is presumptive evidence of Stein-Leventhal syndrome in the appropriate clinical setting.

LH acts upon and is used to assess Leydig cell function in males.

Urinary LH and FSH are used in children who have precocious puberty, in many of whom FSH and LH levels overlap the normal range. An advantage of 24-hour urine collections is that they overcome problems of pulsatile secretion spikes.

FSH, LH and testosterone are low in Kallmann's syndrome. Isolated LH deficiency is a variant of Kallmann's syndrome. Patients who have growth hormone deficiency have FSH and/or LH deficiency as well.

LIMITATIONS: Secretion of both LH and FSH are pulsatile, in response to the normal intermittent release of gonadotropin releasing hormone (GnRH). While both are pulsatile, LH exhibits a circadian rhythm while FSH does not.[2] In addition, in females both FSH and LH vary over the course of the menstrual cycle, with peaks at time of ovulation. Thus, interpretation of a single determination may be difficult. Only 75% of patients with polycystic ovary syndrome have increase of LH. Increased LH with normal or low FSH may occur with obesity, hyperthyroidism, and in liver disease. The extreme chemical similarity of LH and hCG can cause technical problems of cross reactivity. Use of multiple or pooled blood samples or urine (24-hour) is recommended. Monoclonal assays have provided improvement. Normal LH and FSH (RIA) levels can occur in hypoestrogenic patients. The glycoprotein hormones can be heterogeneous, inactive molecules which circulate but reagent antibodies in the radioimmunoassay can recognize sufficient material to generate a normal level response. FSH and LH within normal range can occur with CNS/pituitary failure.[1] METHODOLOGY: Radioimmunoassay (RIA), immunoradiometric assay (IRMA), radioreceptor assay[3] ADDITIONAL INFORMATION: FSH and LH are glycoprotein pituitary hormones which have unique β-subunits, and α-subunits in common with TSH and hCG. They are under complex regulation by hypothalamic GnRH and by gonadal sex hormones, estrogen and progesterone in females, and testosterone. On the simplest level, FSH and LH are high in conditions in which sex hormones cannot be elaborated, and low in conditions of primary pituitary dysfunction. High concentrations of LH (during the follicular phase) in patients with polycystic ovary syndrome interfere with conception and may contribute to early pregnancy loss in these patients.[4] In males, LH has been called interstitial cell stimulating hormone (ICSH) because of its effect on testosterone production by Leydig cells. This is necessary for normal maturation of spermatozoa.

Footnotes

1. Speroff L, Glass RH, and Kase NG, *Clinical Gynecologic Endocrinology and Infertility*, 4th ed, Baltimore, MD: Williams & Wilkins, 1989.
2. Dunkel L, Alfthan H, Stenman UH, et al, "Developmental Changes in 24-Hour Profiles of Luteinizing Hormone and Follicle-Stimulating Hormone From Prepuberty to Midstages of Puberty in Boys," *J Clin Endocrinol Metab*, 1992, 74(4):890-7.
3. Whitcomb RW and Schneyer AL, "Development and Validation of a Radioligand Receptor Assay for Measurement of Luteinizing Hormone in Human Serum," *J Clin Endocrinol Metab*, 1990, 71(3):591-5.
4. Homburg R, Armar NA, Eshel A, et al, "Influence of Serum Luteinizing Hormone Concentrations on Ovulation, Conception, and Early Pregnancy Loss in Polycystic Ovary Syndrome," *Br Med J [Clin Res]*, 1988, 297(6655):1024-6.

References

Apter D, Cacciatore B, Alfthan H, et al, "Serum Luteinizing Hormone Concentrations Increase 100-Fold in Females From 7 Years to Adulthood, as Measured by Time-Resolved Immunofluorometric Assay," *J Clin Endocrinol Metab*, 1989, 68(1):53-7.

Kossoy LR, Hill GA, Parker RA, et al, "Luteinizing Hormone and Ovulation Timing in a Therapeutic Donor Insemination Program Using Frozen Semen," *Am J Obstet Gynecol*, 1989, 160(5 Pt 1):1169-72.

Nippoldt TB, Reame NE, Kelch RP, et al, "The Roles of Estradiol and Progesterone in Decreasing Luteinizing Hormone Pulse Frequency in the Luteal Phase of the Menstrual Cycle," *J Clin Endocrinol Metab*, 1989, 69(1):67-76.

Magnesium, Serum

***CPT** 83735*

Related Information

Amikacin *on page 938*
Calcium, Serum *on page 160*
Cyclosporine *on page 957*
Digoxin *on page 959*
Gentamicin *on page 970*
Magnesium, Urine *on page 289*
Potassium, Blood *on page 330*
Tobramycin *on page 1004*

Synonyms Mg, Serum

Abstract Magnesium is one of the major inorganic cations; the others are sodium, potassium, and calcium. Intracellular magnesium concentrations are much higher than extracellular (serum) values. Most intracellular magnesium is complexed.

Specimen Serum **CONTAINER:** Red top tube **COLLECTION:** Draw without venous stasis, separate serum from red cells as soon as possible. **STORAGE INSTRUCTIONS:** Refrigerate. Serum separated from cells is stable at 2°C to 6°C for several days. **CAUSES FOR REJECTION:** Hemolysis

Interpretive **REFERENCE RANGE:** 1.5-2.3 mg/dL (SI: 0.60-0.95 mmol/L), not consistent among published papers, laboratories, and geographic areas. Four sets of units are in use to express concentration of magnesium: 1.0 mEq/L = 1.22 mg/dL = 0.5 mmol/L = 12.2 mg/L. Magnesium, like calcium, is partly protein bound. Slightly low values in the presence of hypoalbuminemia or hypoproteinemia should not, therefore, be of major concern. **CRITICAL VALUES:** In patients with acute myocardial infarct, serum magnesium $<$2.0 mg/dL (SI: $<$0.82 mmol/L) may increase the risk of ventricular arrhythmia in the presence of hypokalemia. **POSSIBLE PANIC RANGE:** Symptoms appear at $<$1.2 mg/dL (SI: $<$0.5 mmol/L); $<$1.2 mg/dL is severe depletion. Slightly low levels should be repeated on a new specimen. Hospital diet often improves magnesium levels, especially in those who have not been on a normal diet. Toxic symptoms appear $>$4.9 mg/dL (SI: $>$2.0 mmol/L). Possible death from respiratory failure $>$14.6 mg/dL (SI: $>$6.0 mmol/L). **USE:** **Magnesium deficiency** produces neuromuscular disorders. It may cause weakness, tremors, tetany, and convulsions. **Hypomagnesemia** is associated with hypocalcemia, hypokalemia, long-term hyperalimentation, intravenous therapy, diabetes mellitus, especially during treatment of ketoacidosis; alcoholism and other types of malnutrition; malabsorption; hyperparathyroidism; dialysis; pregnancy; and hyperaldosteronism. Renal loss of magnesium occurs with cis-platinum therapy. Alfrey also adds amphotericin toxicity to the causes of hypomagnesemia.

Magnesium deficiency is described with cardiac arrhythmias. The concept that magnesium deficiency may cause arrhythmias is repeatedly expressed.

Increased magnesium levels relate mostly to patients in renal failure. Marked increases may be found in such patients who take magnesium salts (eg, as antacids which contain magnesium). Increased serum magnesium is also found with Addison's disease and in pregnant pa-

(Continued)

Magnesium, Serum *(Continued)*

tients with severe pre-eclampsia or eclampsia who are receiving magnesium sulfate as an anticonvulsant. Hypermagnesemia may occur in patients using magnesium-containing cathartics.[1] High magnesium levels are manifested by decreased reflexes, somnolence, and heart block.

Indications for measurement of serum magnesium include the presence of unexplained hypocalcemia, instances in which hypokalemia is unresponsive to potassium supplementation, and in patients who have cardiac disorders in which hypomagnesemia may be especially hazardous such as congestive failure, ventricular ectopy, digitalis use, or left ventricular hypertrophy. Serum magnesium is indicated only selectively in patients on diuretics: those on high dose thiazides, loop diuretics or hydrochlorothiazide in doses $>$50 mg/day.

Because an association between aminoglycoside therapy and severe hypomagnesemia is described, a recommendation is published to measure serum magnesium in subjects receiving aminoglycosides. Recommendations also exist to measure it in patients on cyclosporine.[2]

LIMITATIONS: Hemolysis will yield elevated results as levels in erythrocytes are two to three times higher than serum. Bilirubin may cause falsely low values. **METHODOLOGY:** Spectrophotometry using calmagite dye, methylthymol blue; atomic absorption spectrophotometry. These methods were found to correlate, although a slight bias to higher values was reported with the Du Pont aca®, for levels $>$2.4 mg/dL (SI: $>$1.0 mmol/L). **ADDITIONAL INFORMATION:** Parathormone enhances tubular reabsorption of magnesium. Measure magnesium in patients with hypocalcemia, of whom 23%, without renal failure, were found in one study to have hypomagnesemia. Magnesium-containing drugs can cause toxic levels in patients with impaired renal function. A causal relation between decreased Mg^{2+} content of cardiac muscle/coronary arteries and nonocclusive sudden-death ischemic heart disease has been proposed. Serum magnesium constitutes only a small fraction of total body stores and may not predict magnesium status correctly.[3] Magnesium acts as a metallic cofactor in over 300 enzymatic reactions.[4] A positive correlation between normomagnesemia and successful resuscitation is reported. Serum magnesium has prognostic importance in congestive heart failure.[5]

Footnotes

1. Gerard SK, Hernandez C, and Khayam-Bashi H, "Extreme Hypermagnesemia Caused by an Overdose of Magnesium-Containing Cathartics," *Ann Emerg Med*, 1988, 17(7):728-31.
2. Chernow B, Bamberger S, Stoiko M, et al, "Hypomagnesemia in Patients in Postoperative Intensive Care," *Chest*, 1989, 95(2):391-7.
3. Elin RJ, "Assessment of Magnesium Status," *Clin Chem*, 1987, 33:1965-70.
4. Reinhart RA, "Clinical Correlates of the Molecular and Cellular Actions of Magnesium on the Cardiovascular System," *Am Heart J*, 1991, 121(5):1513-21.
5. Gottlieb SS, Baruch L, Kukin ML, et al, "Prognostic Importance of the Serum Magnesium Concentration in Patients With Congestive Heart Failure," *J Am Coll Cardiol*, 1990, 16(4):827-31.

References

Castelbaum AR, Donofrio PD, Walker FO, et al, "Laxative Abuse Causing Hypermagnesemia, Quadriparesis, and Neuromuscular Junction Defect," *Neurology*, 1989, 39(5):746-7.

Farrell EC Jr, "Magnesium," *Clinical Chemistry – Theory, Analysis, and Correlation*, 2nd ed, Kaplan LA and Pesce AJ, eds, St Louis, MO: Mosby-Year Book Inc, 1989, 875-9.

Gottlieb SS, "Importance of Magnesium in Congestive Heart Failure," *Am J Cardiol*, 1989, 63(14):39G-42G, (review).

Gren J and Woolf A, "Hypermagnesemia Associated With Catharsis in a Salicylate-Intoxicated Patient With Anorexia Nervosa," *Ann Emerg Med*, 1989, 18(2):200-3.

Lum G, "Hypomagnesemia in Acute and Chronic Care Patient Populations," *Am J Clin Pathol*, 1992, 97(6):827-30.

Quamme GA, "Laboratory Evaluation of Magnesium Status: Renal Function and Free Intracellular Magnesium Concentration," *Clin Lab Med*, 1993, 13(1):209-23.

Ryan MF, "The Role of Magnesium in Clinical Biochemistry: An Overview," *Ann Clin Biochem*, 1991, 28(Pt 1):19-26.

Sipes SL, Weiner CP, Gellhaus TM, et al, "The Plasma Renin-Angiotensin System in Pre-eclampsia: Effects of Magnesium Sulfate," *Obstet Gynecol*, 1989, 73(6):934-7.

Weber CA and Santiago RM, "Hypermagnesemia. A Potential Complication During Treatment of Theophylline Intoxication With Oral Activated Charcoal and Magnesium-Containing Cathartics," *Chest*, 1989, 95(1):56-9.

Magnesium, Urine

CPT 83735

Related Information

Calcium, Urine *on page 163*

Magnesium, Serum *on page 287*

Synonyms Mg, Urine

Patient Care PREPARATION: Patient should be instructed to use a plastic bedpan.

Specimen 24-hour urine CONTAINER: Plastic acid-washed urine container; addition of hydrochloric acid as preservative may be desirable; check with laboratory. COLLECTION: Instruct the patient to void at 8 AM and discard the specimen. Then collect all urine including the final specimen voided at the end of the 24-hour collection period (ie, 8 AM the next morning). Patient's name, date, and time collection started and date and time collection finished are needed. STORAGE INSTRUCTIONS: Refrigerate CAUSES FOR REJECTION: Specimen allowed to contact metal.

Interpretive REFERENCE RANGE: 7.3-12.2 mg/dL (SI: 3-5 mmol/day); a lack of uniformity exists among references regarding boundaries of reference range for urine magnesium. Lack of consistent normal ranges for serum magnesium between published papers, laboratories and geographic areas is also evident. Some laboratories report in mg/24 hours. See information regarding units in Magnesium, Serum listing. Values are slightly higher in males. USE: Magnesium excretion controls magnesium balance. Magnesium urinary excretion is enhanced by increasing blood alcohol levels, diuretics, Bartter's syndrome, corticosteroids, cis-platinum therapy and aldosterone. Renal magnesium wasting occurs in renal transplant recipients who are on cyclosporine and prednisone. Renal conservation of magnesium is diminished by hypercalciuria, salt-losing conditions, and the syndrome of inappropriate secretion of antidiuretic hormone. Magnesium deficiency is often inadequately documented by serum magnesium levels. Urinary magnesium analyses have been advocated before and after therapeutic magnesium administration to further investigate the significance of an apparent low serum magnesium.[1] METHODOLOGY: Atomic absorption (AA) ADDITIONAL INFORMATION: Hypercalcemia, hypophosphatemia, and acidosis are among inhibitors of tubular reabsorption of magnesium.

Footnotes

1. Chernow B, Bamberger S, Stoiko M, et al, "Hypomagnesemia in Patients in Postoperative Intensive Care," *Chest*, 1989, 95(2):391-7.

References

Nicoll GW, Struthers AD, and Fraser CG, "Biological Variation of Urinary Magnesium," *Clin Chem*, 1991, 37(10 Pt 1):1794-5.

Roelofsen JM, Berkel GM, Uttendorfsky OT, et al, "Urinary Excretion Rates of Calcium and Magnesium in Normal and Complicated Pregnancies," *Eur J Obstet Gynecol Reprod Biol*, 1988, 27:227-36.

Metabolic Screen for Amino Acids *see* Amino Acid Screen, Plasma *on page 118*

Metabolic Screen for Amino Acids *see* Amino Acid Screen, Qualitative, Urine *on page 120*

Metanephrines, Total, Urine

CPT 83835

Related Information

Catecholamines, Fractionation, Plasma *on page 172*

Catecholamines, Fractionation, Urine *on page 174*

Homovanillic Acid, Urine *on page 253*

Vanillylmandelic Acid, Urine *on page 382*

Synonyms Total Metanephrines

Applies to Catecholamines

Test Commonly Includes Metanephrine and normetanephrine

Abstract These compounds, the immediate metabolites of epinephrine and norepinephrine, are known collectively as catecholamines. Increases in catecholamine production by the adrenal medulla and, therefore, increased urinary excretion of metanephrines occur in the presence of a pheochromocytoma.

Patient Care PREPARATION: Consult the laboratory which will do the assay. Emotional and physical stress may interfere through stimulation of endogenous catecholamines.[1] Drugs may interfere including alpha$_2$-agonists, calcium channel blockers, converting enzyme inhibitors, (Continued)

Metanephrines, Total, Urine *(Continued)*

bromocriptine, phenothiazines, tricyclic antidepressants, and levodopa.[1] Endogenous and exogenous catecholamines and therapy with methyldopa, monoamine oxidase inhibitors increase metanephrine excretion.[1] See Limitations.

Specimen 24-hour urine **CONTAINER:** Plastic urine container **COLLECTION:** Specimens for catecholamines, VMA, and metanephrines should be obtained while the patient is resting, not on medications, and without recent exposure to imaging contrast materials.[1] The likelihood of detection of pheochromocytoma is enhanced if the collection period is initiated by or includes a crisis. If crises occur less often than once a day, the patient may bring in specimen initiated by a crisis. Acidify to pH 4 after collection is complete with hydrochloric acid. **STORAGE INSTRUCTIONS:** Keep collection cold

Interpretive **REFERENCE RANGE:** Mean 0.6 mg/24 hours (SI: 3.3 μmol/day), up to 1.3 mg/24 hours (SI: 7.1 μmol/day) or <1.2 μg/mg creatinine, with some variation between laboratories **CRITICAL VALUES:** >2.2 μg/mg creatinine indicative of pheochromocytoma **USE:** Evaluate the presence of abnormal catecholamine production. An established method, useful in the diagnosis of pheochromocytoma, secreting paraganglioma, neuroblastoma, and ganglioneuroblastoma. **LIMITATIONS:** False-negative results occur (eg, interference by methylglucamine in x-ray contrast medium).[1] False-positives occur; results should be confirmed by other means, such as urine catecholamines and VMA. False-positives can be caused by stress and drugs. Interfering substances partly depend on analytical methods. Drugs causing interference include phenacetin and antihypertensive drugs (eg, alpha-adrenergic receptor blocking agents). Propranolol interferes with a spectrophotometric assay. A valuable table of causes of interference with biochemical diagnosis of pheochromocytoma has been recently published.[1] **METHODOLOGY:** Colorimetry, fluorometry, gas chromatography (GC), and liquid chromatography (LC) techniques (particularly, HPLC) **ADDITIONAL INFORMATION:** Metanephrine and normetanephrine are metabolic products of epinephrine and norepinephrine, the adrenal medullary hormones secreted by pheochromocytomas. Because secretion is usually episodic, plasma catecholamine drawn during an asymptomatic period may be normal, while total metanephrines collected over 24 hours would be abnormal. On the other hand, a tumor could be intermittently active, but secrete over a full 24-hour period total metanephrines within normal limits. Analyses of 24-hour specimens are preferable to spot (random) samples for catecholamines, VMA, and metanephrines.

Assay of total metanephrines has provided the highest number of true positive results for pheochromocytoma. It has become the first choice as a screening test. Metanephrine has been positive in 98% to 99%, VMA in about 90% of patients with pheochromocytoma. A Mayo Clinic group advocates use of metanephrines as a screening test with confirmation by assay of urine catecholamine fractions.[1]

When only a spot urine sample is available or the 24-hour urine collection is incomplete, simultaneous measurement of urine creatinine permits expression of the metanephrine/creatinine ratio. Some clinicians use >2.2 μg metanephrines/mg creatinine to distinguish pheochromocytoma from normal with this ratio. Reference intervals for 24-hour urinary metanephrines in hypertensives have been published.[2] Pheochromocytomas cause hypertension that is classically paroxysmal. They may cause sudden headache, pallor, perspiration, and palpitation. Rarely hypotension presents as the initial manifestation.[1]

Footnotes

1. Sheps SG, Jiang N-S, Klee GG, et al, "Recent Developments in the Diagnosis and Treatment of Pheochromocytoma," *Mayo Clin Proc*, 1990, 65(1):88-95.
2. Kairisto V, Koskinen P, Mattila K, et al, "Reference Intervals for 24-Hour Urinary Normetanephrine, Metanephrine, and 3-Methoxy-4-Hydroxymandelic Acid in Hypertensive Patients," *Clin Chem*, 1992, 38(3):416-20.

References

Rosano TG, Swift TA, and Hayes LW, "Advances in Catecholamine and Metabolite Measurements for Diagnosis of Pheochromocytoma," *Clin Chem*, 1991, 37(10 Pt 2):1854-67.

MetHb *see* Methemoglobin *on this page*

Methemoglobin

CPT *83045 (qualitative); 83050 (quantitative)*

Related Information

Blood Gases, Arterial *on page 140*

Hemoglobin Electrophoresis *on page 556*

Synonyms MetHb; NADH-MetHb Reductase

Applies to Cytochrome b_5 Reductase

Abstract This pigment is hemoglobin in which the iron is in the trivalent state. It cannot act as an oxygen carrier.

Specimen Whole blood **CONTAINER:** Green top (heparin) tube **STORAGE INSTRUCTIONS:** Keep tube on ice. pH dependent. Should be run within 8 hours, or false-negatives may occur. Run as promptly as possible after draw. Studies have shown up to 10% drop in 4 hours, up to 16% drop in 8 hours, in samples kept on ice. Such studies have not been extensive. May be drawn into sodium fluoride-containing tubes and immediately frozen at 0°C to -4°C prior to analysis.

Interpretive **REFERENCE RANGE:** Up to 1.5% of total hemoglobin. Smokers have a slightly higher percent methemoglobin than do nonsmokers. **POSSIBLE PANIC RANGE:** Headache and other symptoms occur at levels >30%. Methemoglobinemia can be fatal, particularly >70% saturation levels. **USE:** Evaluate cyanosis, especially in the presence of normal arterial gases; evaluate polycythemia and hemoglobinopathies; work up dyspnea and headache; work up "poppers" and "sniffers"; evaluate drug or chemical toxicity, since most instances of methemoglobinemia are so acquired; monitor patients on high dose nitrate therapy; measurement in CSF may detect small cerebral and subdural hematomas.[1] **LIMITATIONS:** Sulfhemoglobin, methylene blue, and Evans blue dye may interfere. Methemoglobin exhibits pH sensitivity. **METHODOLOGY:** Spectrophotometry; Hb M variants are best detected by electrophoresis because spectrophotometry is unreliable due to their abnormal ferrihemoglobin spectra. **ADDITIONAL INFORMATION:** Methemoglobin is an inactive, oxidized form of hemoglobin resulting in decreased oxygen-carrying capacity of blood. Concentrations of methemoglobin of over 10% to 15% of hemoglobin will cause cyanosis. Sulfhemoglobin will interfere with methemoglobin determined by the above method. Methemoglobinemia may be hereditary or acquired. Polycythemia is occasionally present as a compensatory mechanism. Elevations of methemoglobin lead to dyspnea and headache, and can be lethal. Most instances of methemoglobinemia are acquired, from drugs and chemicals. Nitro and amino groups are especially involved, eg, aniline and derivatives, nitrites, nitroglycerin, nitrate salts in burn patients, dapsone (perhaps the most common cause of drug-induced methemoglobinemia), acetophenetidin, phenacetin and some sulfonamides, chlorates, quinones, large doses of ferrous sulfate, and many other drugs and some intestinal bacteria. Well water containing nitrate is the most common cause of methemoglobinemia in the newborn. Methemoglobinemia has been reported after exposure to automobile exhaust fumes.[2]

Hereditary methemoglobinemia is uncommon. It may be due to a deficiency of red cell NADH-methemoglobin reductase (diaphorase, also termed cytochrome b_5 reductase), which has an autosomal recessive mode of inheritance. It may also be the result of presence of certain hemoglobinopathies, members of the Hb M family including Hb M Saskatoon, Boston, Iwate, Hyde Park, and Milwaukee. These have autosomal dominant mode of inheritance and may be associated with clinical cyanosis. Hb Seattle and other hemoglobinopathies also show increase in the *in vitro* rate of methemoglobin formation.[3] A recently identified new hemoglobin variant, Hb Warsaw, is also characterized by elevated blood levels of methemoglobin.[4]

A study of postmortem methemoglobin levels showed a range of 0.8% to 57% in individuals who, clinically, should have had normal antemortem concentrations. There was no correlation with antemortem circumstances, autopsy findings, or interval of time from death to autopsy.[5]

Footnotes

1. Trbojevic-Cepe M, Vogrinc Z, and Brinar V, "Diagnostic Significance of Methemoglobin Determination in Colorless Cerebrospinal Fluid," *Clin Chem*, 1992, 38(8 Pt 1):1404-8.
2. Laney RF and Hoffman RS, "Methemoglobinemia Secondary to Automobile Exhaust Fumes," *Am J Emerg Med*, 1992, 10(5):426-8.
3. Beutler E, "Hemoglobinopathies Producing Cyanosis," *Hematology*, 4th ed, Chapter 78, Williams WJ, Beutler E, Ersler AJ, et al, eds, New York, NY: McGraw-Hill Inc, 1990, 746-51.
4. Honig GR, Telfer MC, Rosenblum BB, et al, "Hb Warsaw (β42 Phe → Val): An Unstable Hemoglobin With Decreased Oxygen Affinity. I. Hematologic and Clinical Expression," *Am J Hematol*, 1989, 32(1):36-41.
5. Reay DT, Insalaco SJ, and Eisele JW, "Postmortem Methemoglobin Concentrations and Their Significance," *J Forensic Sci*, 1984, 29:1160-3.

References

Beutler E and Gelbart T, "Carboxyhemoglobin, Methemoglobin, and Sulfhemoglobin Determinations," *Hematology*, 4th ed, Chapter A16, Williams WT, Beutler E, Erslev AJ, et al, eds, New York, NY: McGraw-Hill Inc, 1990, 1732-4.

Dean BS, Lopez G, and Krenzelok EP, "Environmentally-Induced Methemoglobinemia in an Infant," *J Toxicol Clin Toxicol*, 1992, 30(1):127-33.

(Continued)

Methemoglobin *(Continued)*

Fechner GG and Gee DJ, "Study on the Effects of Heat on Blood and on the Postmortem Estimation of Carboxyhemoglobin and Methaemoglobin," *Forensic Sci Int*, 1989, 40(1):63-7.

Jaffé ER and Hultquist DE, "Cytochrome b_5 Reductase Deficiency and Enzymopenic Hereditary Methemoglobinemia," Chapter 92, *The Metabolic Basis of Inherited Disease*, 6th ed, Scriver CR, Beaudet AL, Sly WS, et al, eds, New York, NY: McGraw-Hill Inc, 1989, 2267-80.

Johnson WS, Hall AH, and Rumack BH, "Cyanide Poisoning Successfully Treated Without Therapeutic Methemoglobin Levels," *Am J Emerg Med*, 1989, 7(4):437-40.

Weatherall DJ, Clegg JB, Higgs DR, et al, "The Hemoglobinopathies," Chapter 93, *The Metabolic Basis of Inherited Disease*, 6th ed, Scriver CR, Beaudet AL, Sly WS, et al, eds, New York, NY: McGraw-Hill Inc, 1989, 2304-5.

3-Methoxy-4-Hydroxymandelic Acid *see* Vanillylmandelic Acid, Urine *on page 382*

Metyrapone Test

CPT 82538

Related Information

Cortisol, Blood *on page 191*
Cortisol, Urine *on page 193*
Cosyntropin Test *on page 194*
Prolactin *on page 336*

Applies to 11-Deoxycortisol

Test Commonly Includes 8 AM serum 11-deoxycortisol and cortisol after oral metyrapone

Abstract Metyrapone is a 11-β-hydroxylase inhibitor and inhibits the conversion of 11-deoxycortisol to cortisol. Serum 11-deoxycortisol will increase and serum cortisol decrease if normal pituitary stimulation of the adrenal with ACTH occurs.

Patient Care PREPARATION: Other measures, possibly including the cosyntropin test, should be done first (ie, the patient's adrenals must be known to be able to respond to ACTH). If response to exogenous ACTH has not been demonstrated, then an attempt to measure response to release of endogenous ACTH may carry risk to the patient. No recent administration of radioisotopes. Metyrapone is given at 11 PM the night before the specimen is collected. Dose ranges (by patient weight) from 2-3 g.

Specimen Serum CONTAINER: Red top tube SAMPLING TIME: 8 AM, morning after oral metyrapone STORAGE INSTRUCTIONS: For 11-deoxycortisol, separate as soon as possible. Freeze serum if assay is not performed within 24 hours.

Interpretive REFERENCE RANGE: 11-deoxycortisol increased to >7 μg/dL (SI: >202 nmol/L); cortisol <10 μg/dL (SI: <276 nmol/L) USE: Differential diagnosis of Cushing's syndrome, pituitary adenoma (Cushing's disease), adrenal cortical tumor, and ectopic ACTH syndrome LIMITATIONS: Ectopic ACTH syndrome was not extensively studied in the key paper reporting this evaluation. The authors of this study did not encourage dexamethasone or metyrapone testing for this differential diagnosis. Later reports suggest that ectopic sources for ACTH versus pituitary sources in Cushing's syndrome can be differentiated by this test.[1] CONTRAINDICATIONS: Should not be used in patients with possible adrenal insufficiency. METHODOLOGY: Radioimmunoassay (RIA) ADDITIONAL INFORMATION: Metyrapone inhibits conversion of 11-deoxycortisol to cortisol. The decrease in cortisol levels causes increased secretion of ACTH. ACTH stimulates adrenocortical secretion of 11-deoxycortisol, precursor to cortisol. Thus, giving metyrapone tests pituitary ACTH reserve and the integrity of the adrenal cortical-pituitary feedback loop. Serum 11-deoxycortisol increases in patients with pituitary adenoma (Cushing's disease) and does not rise in patients with adrenal cortical tumor, in whom pituitary corticotrophe suppression is anticipated. In adrenogenital syndrome with 21-hydroxylase deficiency (the most common form) 11-deoxycortisol is low, but in 11-hydroxylase deficiency it is high. It may also be high in adrenal carcinoma. A 3-day metyrapone test protocol is also available.

Footnotes

1. Blunt SB, Sandler LM, Burrin JM, et al, "An Evaluation of the Distinction of Ectopic and Pituitary ACTH Dependent Cushing's Syndrome by Clinical Features, Biochemical Tests, and Radiological Findings," *Q J Med*, 1990, 77(283):1113-33.

References

von Bardeleben U, Stalla GK, Muller OA, et al, "Blunting of ACTH Response to Human CRH in Depressed Patients Is Avoided by Metyrapone Pretreatment," *Biol Psychiatry*, 1988, 24:782-6.

Watts NB and Keffer JH, "The Adrenal Cortex and Glucocorticoids," *Practical Endocrine Diagnosis*, 4th ed, Philadelphia, PA: Lea & Febiger, 1989.

Mg, Serum *see* Magnesium, Serum *on page 287*

Mg, Urine *see* Magnesium, Urine *on page 289*

Microbilirubin *see* Bilirubin, Neonatal *on page 138*

Murphy-Pattee *replaced by* Thyroxine *on page 364*

Myocardial Infarct Panel *see* Cardiac Enzymes/Isoenzymes *on page 170*

Myoglobin, Blood

CPT 83874

Related Information

Cardiac Enzymes/Isoenzymes *on page 170*
Creatine Kinase *on page 196*
Creatine Kinase Isoenzymes *on page 197*
Haptoglobin, Serum *on page 247*
Lactate Dehydrogenase *on page 269*
Lactate Dehydrogenase Isoenzymes *on page 271*
Muscle Biopsy *on page 75*
Myoglobin, Qualitative, Urine *on page 1135*
Troponin *on page 375*

Applies to Carbonic Anhydrase III

Abstract Myoglobin is a low molecular weight (17,900-d) cytoplasmic heme protein (oxygen-binding) which is found in cardiac and striated muscle. An increase in its concentration is a useful marker for early (30-60 minutes) detection of recent myocardial infarct, as a monitor for reinfarction, thrombolytic therapy, and myocardial injury during cardiac surgery.

Patient Care PREPARATION: No recent administration of radioactive substances if RIA method is used.

Specimen Serum CONTAINER: Red top tube STORAGE INSTRUCTIONS: Serum may be stored at 4°C for 2 years.

Interpretive REFERENCE RANGE: Approximate range: 5-70 μg/L (SI: 5-70 μg/L). Varies with method. Level is up to 25% higher in men. USE: Diagnose skeletal or myocardial muscle injury. Serum myoglobin is generally detectable earlier than is CK or CK-MB increase in patients with acute myocardial infarction.[1] Serum myoglobin was found also in 50% of patients with acute coronary insufficiency. It is thought to define a population of small infarcts of myocardium. Serum myoglobin concentrations correlate with size of infarct.[1] Diagnose rhabdomyolysis. Myoglobin appears with trauma, ischemia, malignant hyperthermia, exertion, dermatomyositis, polymyositis, muscular dystrophy. LIMITATIONS: Increased myoglobin levels occur after intramuscular injections. Increased serum myoglobin has been reported after a high voltage electrical accident. Many laboratories prefer CK isoenzymes (CK-MB does not rise after intramuscular injection) and do not provide plasma myoglobin levels. Recent technical improvements in the assay will allow more widespread use of the test. As an index of myocardial infarct, myoglobin returns rapidly to baseline levels.[1] It is not tightly bound to protein and is rapidly excreted.[2] CONTRAINDICATIONS: Administration of radioactive material before test if RIA method is used. METHODOLOGY: Radioimmunoassay (RIA), fluorometric immunoassay,[3] immunoturbidimetry,[4] dual-label time-resolved fluoroimmunoassay,[5] nephelometry[6] ADDITIONAL INFORMATION: Serum myoglobin is rapidly cleared by the kidneys.[2] Elevated levels may be associated with cocaine use.[7] It is increased in cardiac surgery, thrombolytic therapy,[8,9] myocardial infarction,[10] exercise, shock, renal failure, progressive muscular dystrophy, and rhabdomyolysis from any cause. Its **main advantage** is as a sensitive (99% to 100%) marker for **early myocardial injury** because it is released earlier from necrotic cells than CK, allowing for earlier detection of myocardial infarction.[10] Levels rise as early as 1 hour after infarct and peak within 4-12 hours.[11] Myoglobin is cleared rapidly, and therefore, its clinical sensitivity is reduced with time (after 18 hours it is not useful). Because myoglobin is not specific to myocardial muscle, the issue of specificity arises in cases of acute myocardial injury associated with muscle trauma, where a distinction cannot be made as to the origin of myoglobin. If one measures **carbonic anhydrase III**, an 18,000-d cytoplasmic protein present in skeletal muscle but **not** in cardiac muscle, the separation can be made.[5] Simultaneous assay of both proteins shows that in skeletal muscle injury the ratio of myoglobin to carbonic anhydrase III is constant; while in patients with AMI, the ratio shows a temporal pattern similar to myoglobin alone. Serum troponin concentrations may prove to be of benefit.

Footnotes

1. Isakov A, Shapira I, Burke M, et al, "Serum Myoglobin Levels in Patients With Ischemic Myocardial Insult," *Arch Intern Med*, 1988, 148(8):1762-5.

(Continued)

Myoglobin, Blood *(Continued)*

2. Faulkner MR, "Myoglobinuria and Hemoglobinuria," *Lab Report for Physicians*, 1989, 11:57-9.
3. Silva DP Jr, Landt Y, Porter SE, et al, "Development and Application of Monoclonal Antibodies to Human Cardiac Myoglobin in a Rapid Fluorescence Immunoassay," *Clin Chem*, 1991, 37(8):1356-64.
4. Mair J, Artner-Dworzak E, Lechleitner P, et al, "Early Diagnosis of Acute Myocardial Infarction by a Newly Developed Rapid Immunoturbidimetric Assay for Myoglobin," *Br Heart J*, 1992, 68(5):462-8.
5. Vuori J, Rasi S, Takala T, et al, "Dual-Label Time-Resolved Fluoroimmunoassay for Simultaneous Detection of Myoglobin and Carbonic Anhydrase III in Serum," *Clin Chem*, 1991, 37(12):2087-92.
6. Delanghe JR, Chapelle JP, and Vanderschueren SC, "Quantitative Nephelometric Assay for Determining Myoglobin Evaluated," *Clin Chem*, 1990, 36(9):1675-8.
7. Pogue VA and Nurse HM, "Cocaine-Associated Acute Myoglobinuric Renal Failure," *Am J Med*, 1989, 86(2):183-6.
8. McCullough DA, Harrison PG, Forshall JM, et al, "Serum Myoglobin and Creatine Kinase Enzymes in Acute Myocardial Infarction Treated With Anistreplase," *J Clin Pathol*, 1992, 45(5):405-7.
9. Laperche T, Steg PG, Benessiano J, et al, "Patterns of Myoglobin and MM Creatine Kinase Isoforms Release Early After Intravenous Thrombolysis of Direct Percutaneous Transluminal Coronary Angioplasty for Acute Myocardial Infarction, and Implications for the Early Noninvasive Diagnosis of Reperfusion," *Am J Cardiol*, 1992, 70(13):1129-34.
10. Apple FS, "Acute Myocardial Infarction and Coronary Reperfusion. Serum Cardiac Markers for the 1990's," *Am J Clin Pathol*, 1992, 97(2):217-26.
11. Van Blerk M, Maes V, Huyghens L, et al, "Analytical and Clinical Evaluation of Creatine Kinase MB Mass Assay by IMx: Comparison With MB Isoenzyme Activity and Serum Myoglobin for Early Diagnosis of Myocardial Infarction," *Clin Chem*, 1992, 38(12):2380-6.

References

Andersen PT, Miller-Petersen J, Henneberg EW, et al, "Hypermyoglobinemia After Successful Arterial Embolectomy," *Surgery*, 1987, 102:25-31.

Delanghe J, Chapelle JP, el Allaf M, et al, "Quantitative Turbidimetric Assay for Determining Myoglobin Evaluated," *Ann Clin Biochem*, 1991, 28(Pt 5):474-9.

Gibler WB, Gibler CD, Weinshenker E, et al, "Myoglobin as an Early Indicator of Acute Myocardial Infarction," *Ann Emerg Med*, 1987, 16:851-6.

Kasik JW, Leuschen MP, Bolam DL, et al, "Rhabdomyolysis and Myoglobinemia in Neonates," *Pediatrics*, 1985, 76:255-8.

Mair J, Smidt J, Artner-Dworzak E, et al, "Rapid Diagnosis of Myocardial Infarction by Immunoturbidimetric Myoglobin Measurement," *Lancet*, 1991, 337(8753):1343-4.

Seguin J, Saussine M, Ferriere M, et al, "Comparison of Myoglobin and Creatine Kinase MB Levels in the Evaluation of Myocardial Injury After Cardiac Operations," *J Thorac Cardiovasc Surg*, 1988, 95:294-7.

Serrano S, Chueca P, Carrasco E, et al, "Predictive Value of Myoglobin in Early Diagnosis of Acute Myocardial Infarction," *Ann Emerg Med*, 1990, 19(8):953.

Silva DP Jr, Landt Y, Porter SE, et al, "Development and Application of Monoclonal Antibodies to Human Cardiac Myoglobin in A Rapid Fluorescence Immunoassay," *Clin Chem*, 1991, 37(8):1356-64.

Vrenna L, Castaldo AM, Castaldo P, et al, "Comparison Between Nephelometric and RIA Methods for Serum Myoglobin, and Efficiency of Myoglobin Assay for Early Diagnosis of Myocardial Infarction," *Clin Chem*, 1992, 38(5):789-90.

Na^+ *see* Sodium, Blood *on page 349*

NADH-MetHb Reductase *see* Methemoglobin *on page 290*

Na, Urine *see* Sodium, Urine *on page 351*

Nephrogenous Cyclic AMP *see* Cyclic AMP, Plasma *on page 204*

Nephrogenous Cyclic AMP *see* Cyclic AMP, Urine *on page 204*

Neuron-Specific Enolase, Serum

CPT *83520*

Synonyms NSE; S-NSE

Abstract The gamma-gamma isoenzyme of enolase is found only in neuronal tissue (including cells of neuroendocrine origin). Serum levels may be elevated in processes characterized by nerve cell or neuroendocrine cell destruction, including neoplasms of neural or neuroendocrine origin. Serum levels may be useful as a marker for small cell carcinoma of lung, for staging of such tumors, and for monitoring for relapse after therapy.

Specimen Serum **CONTAINER:** Red top tube **COLLECTION:** Must avoid hemolysis. Place blood on ice immediately after collecting. **STORAGE INSTRUCTIONS:** Centrifuge within 30-45 minutes. Maintain at 4°C and analyze same day or freeze at -70°C until assayed. **CAUSES FOR REJECTION:** Specimen with hemolysis (RBCs contain $\gamma\gamma$-enolase) **TURNAROUND TIME:** Approximately 1 week, as this analysis will be performed by a reference laboratory in most situations

Interpretive REFERENCE RANGE: 9.6±0.7 (SE) ng/mL (RIA method);[1] 3.45±1.6 ng/mL (2SD) (EIA method);[2] 6±5 (SE) ng/mL (EIA method);[3] method and laboratory variable USE: Detect and identify neoplasms of neural or neuroectodermal derivation (eg, small cell carcinoma of lung, neuroblastoma, and others); useful in monitoring therapy and detection of relapse; not of use in screening for early stages of such neoplasms METHODOLOGY: Radioimmunoassay (RIA), enzyme immunoassay (EIA)[1], immunobioluminescence assay[2] ADDITIONAL INFORMATION: Enolase, one of the enzymes of the glycolytic pathway, exists in the serum as a number of isomeric variants. The enzyme exists as an intracytoplasmic dimer accounting for up to 3% of soluble protein in some tissues. There are three distinct subunits, α, β, and γ, five isoenzymes have been identified, $\alpha\alpha$, $\beta\beta$, $\gamma\gamma$, $\alpha\beta$, and $\alpha\gamma$. β-enolase ($\beta\beta$ isomer) is found in muscle, hybrid forms ($\alpha\alpha$, $\alpha\beta$) are found in megakaryocytes and platelets. The gamma-gamma isoenzyme appears to be found largely in neural tissue. This enzyme is released into the CSF when neural tissue is injured. Neoplasms derived from neural or neuroendocrine tissue may release NSE into the blood. The test may have value in predicting response to therapy. In a group of 13 patients with small cell carcinoma of lung, very high levels of NSE (≥100 ng/mL, mean of 490 ng/mL) were found in seven of eight responders. Levels <100 ng/mL (mean 28 ng/mL) were found in the remaining six patients, only two of whom were responders. These values are from samples obtained during the first 3-day course of chemotherapy. There is evidence that the level of serum neuron-specific enolase correlates with tumor burden.[1] Increase occurs more commonly and is at higher levels in advanced stage than in limited stage disease. The enzyme has been elevated in sera of all patients with three or more sites of metastases.

Serum NSE levels are increased in cases of neuroblastoma but also in other certain childhood tumors. Levels >100 ng/mL in children are, however, highly suggestive of advanced neuroblastoma. Use of NSE to monitor treated neuroblastoma patients has not been found to be a sensitive index of residual tumor. NSE levels may also be increased in some patients with seminoma[3] and some patients with uremia who have been on dialysis. The specificity of serum neuron-specific enolase may not yet be clearly established. In immunocytochemistry, its specificity leaves a great deal to be desired. Levels of this enzyme in spinal fluid seems to correlate with levels of S-100 protein and myelin basic protein in patients with neurological lesions.[4]

Footnotes

1. Anastasiades KD, Mullins RE, and Conn RB, "Neuron-Specific Enolase: Assessment by ELISA in Patients With Small Cell Carcinoma of the Lung," *Am J Clin Pathol*, 1987, 87:245-9.
2. Wevers RA, Theunisse AW, and Rijksen G, "An Immunobioluminescence Assay for Gamma-Gamma Enolase Activity in Human Serum and Cerebrospinal Fluid," *Clin Chim Acta*, 1988, 178:141-50.
3. Kuzmits R, Schernthaner G, and Krisch K, "Serum Neuron-Specific Enolase: A Marker for Response to Therapy in Seminoma," *Cancer*, 1987, 60:1017-21.
4. van Engelen BG, Lamers KJ, Gabreels FJ, et al, "Age-Related Changes of Neuron-Specific Enolase, S-100 Protein, and Myelin Basic Protein Concentrations in Cerebrospinal Fluid," *Clin Chem*, 1992, 38(6):813-6.

References

Kaiser E, Kuzmits R, Pregnant P, et al, "Clinical Biochemistry of Neuron Specific Enolase," *Clin Chim Acta*, 1989, 183(1):13-31, (review).

Virji MA, Mercer DW, and Herberman RB, "Tumor Markers in Cancer Diagnosis and Prognosis," *CA*, 1988, 38:105-26.

Newborn Screen for Hypothyroidism and Phenylketonuria

***CPT** 84030 (PKU); 84437 (neonatal T4)*

Related Information

Phenylalanine, Blood *on page 317*

T_4 Newborn Screen *on page 357*

Synonyms Hypothyroidism, Newborn Screen; Phenylketonuria, Newborn Screen; PKU, Neonatal; Thyroxine, Neonatal

Applies to Phenylalanine Hydroxylase Activity

Test Commonly Includes Phenylalanine and thyroxine by filter paper collection

Patient Care PREPARATION: Blood should be obtained 2-4 days after birth. For phenylalanine testing, 48 hours ideally should have elapsed after the first protein ingestion.

Specimen Whole blood CONTAINER: Filter paper specified for method SAMPLING TIME: Before infant is discharged from the nursery COLLECTION: Allow a large drop of blood to saturate filter paper, filling the printed circle. (More complete instructions appear in the listing Phenylalanine, Blood.) STORAGE INSTRUCTIONS: Allow blood spots to dry before sending to the labora-

(Continued)

Newborn Screen for Hypothyroidism and Phenylketonuria *(Continued)*

tory. **CAUSES FOR REJECTION:** Multiple applications of blood to the same spot, use of pipet or capillary device to soak filter paper, quantity not sufficient, application of blood to both sides of filter paper. Cord blood **cannot** be used for PKU.

Interpretive **REFERENCE RANGE:** Phenylalanine: <2 mg/dL (SI: <121 μmol/L); thyroxine: >7.5 μg/dL (SI: >97 nmol/L) **POSSIBLE PANIC RANGE:** Phenylalanine: >4 mg/dL (SI: >242 μmol/L); thyroxine (T_4): <7 μg/dL (SI: <90 nmol/L) **USE:** Used in screening for PKU and hypothyroidism in newborns, (mandatory in many areas); prevention of mental retardation by early diagnosis. Siblings of children with PKU, PHP (persistent hyperphenylalaninemias), and congenital hypothyroidism deserve special priority.[1] **LIMITATIONS:** When a baby is discharged early (before 72 hours of age), many states, hospitals, and physicians prefer to take a sample early, rather than risk no sample at all.[1] Early sampling for PKU risks some false-negative results. Recent work suggests that essentially all phenylketonurics will be positive within the first 24 hours if a cutoff of 2 mg/dL is used.[2] Subclassification of phenylalanine hydroxylase deficiency can be made based on blood phenylalanine levels.[3] If screening (PKU) occurs before 24 hours of life, rescreening should be done. Sick and/or premature infant should be screened (PKU) by age 7 days independent of feeding history or antibiotic therapy.[1]

Any inadequate specimen must be repeated.

When the infant is tested for PKU before 24 hours of age, there is a 16% chance of missing a positive case. When screened between 24 and 72 hours of age, there is a 4% chance of missing a positive. (See footnote 2.)

Normal T_4 (and in some cases including normal TSH) screening results do not ensure against failure of normal development due to presence of hypothyroidism. Even without technical error, 6% to 12% of cases of infantile hypothyroidism will have normal screening hormone levels.[4] Infants with plasma thyroxine levels <30 nmol/L were shown to have a significantly higher incidence of neonatal problems (prolonged jaundice, feeding difficulties, etc) in addition to hypothyroidism.[5] Recent studies clearly show the value of neonatal thyroid screening.[6]

Different geographic areas may be subject to relative iodine deficiency that effects thyroid function. Such effects may mask tertiary hypothyroidism in prematurity. Additional problems including delayed rise in TSH have been noted.

Screening must be integrated with follow-up, confirmation of diagnosis, and treatment. Problems have included failure to screen all neonates and imperfect compliance with follow-up screening.

METHODOLOGY: Guthrie method is widely used for neonatal PKU testing. Phenylalanine can also be quantitated by fluorometry. A T_4 radioimmunoassay (RIA) procedure is commonly done for thyroid screening. False-positive PKU tests due to antibiotic usage, in particular ampicillin, have been noted and methods for their avoidance (use of penicillinase in test agar or fixing with formic acid vapors) have been reported.[7,8,9] **ADDITIONAL INFORMATION:** Scriver and Clow indicate that an adequate sample is obtained from a term neonate at least 24 hours after milk feeding is started and as close to hospital discharge as possible. For the premature infant, they define an adequate sample as one obtained between the fifth and seventh days of life.

The Committee on Genetics of the American Academy of Pediatrics writes that **all** infants should be screened at discharge from the nursery, regardless of age.[1] The following is abbreviated from a Department of Health letter in one state.[10]

Some newborn infants are discharged from hospitals without receiving a test for PKU and congenital hypothyroidism. This increases the risk that some cases may be missed completely or that diagnosis and treatment of positive cases could be delayed beyond 1 month of age. There have been law suits filed against hospitals or physicians in some states. Obviously, both problems must be averted.

The original laws required testing for PKU only and earliest timing for this test was considered to be 72 hours of age. Recent information has found that most cases have abnormal laboratory results for this condition at an even earlier age. With changing patterns of maternity care an increasing number of mothers and babies are being discharged by 24-48 hours of age. Even though hospitals and physicians make arrangements for the patient to return for testing when early discharge occurs, there is a significant risk of missed appointments and missed cases or delayed diagnosis.

The standard is established that all infants be tested for PKU and congenital hypothyroidism prior to discharge.[10]

Footnotes

1. American Academy of Pediatrics, Committee on Genetics, "Newborn Screening Fact Sheets: Congenital Hypothyroidism," *Pediatrics*, 1989, 83:454-6 and 461-2.
2. Doherty LB, Rohr FJ, and Levy HL, "Detection of Phenylketonuria in the Very Early Newborn Blood Specimen," *Pediatrics*, 1991, 87(2):240-4.
3. Matalon R and Michals K, "Phenylketonuria: Screening, Treatment, and Maternal PKU," *Clin Biochem*, 1991, 24(4):337-42.
4. American Academy of Pediatrics, American Thyroid Association, "Newborn Screening for Congenital Hypothyroidism: Recommended Guidelines," *Pediatrics*, 1987, 80:745-9.
5. Grant DB, Smith I, Fuggle PW, et al, "Congenital Hypothyroidism Detected by Neonatal Screening: Relationship Between Biochemical Severity and Early Clinical Features," *Arch Dis Child*, 1992, 67(1):87-90.
6. Willi SM and Moshang T Jr, "Diagnostic Dilemmas. Results of Screening Tests for Congenital Hypothyroidism," *Pediatr Clin North Am*, 1991, 38(3):555-66.
7. Mabry CC, Reid MC, and Kuhn RJ, "A Source of Error in Phenylketonuria Screening," *Am J Clin Pathol*, 1988, 90(3):279-83.
8. Wilcken B, Brown AR, Liu A, et al, "Eliminating Some Possible Errors in Phenylketonuria Screening," *Am J Clin Pathol*, 1989, 92(3):396, (letter).
9. Kremensky I and Kalaydjieva L, "Avoiding Sources of Error in PKU Screening," *Am J Clin Pathol*, 1989, 92(3):396-7, (letter).
10. Schloesser PT and Hollowell JG, "State of Kansas, Department of Health and Environment," 1982, 10.

References

Allen DB, Sieger JE, Litsheim T, et al, "Age-Adjusted Thyrotropin Criteria for Neonatal Screening for Hypothyroidism," *J Pediatr*, 1990, 117(2 Pt 1):309-12.

Mabry CC, "Phenylketonuria: Contemporary Screening and Diagnosis," *Ann Clin Lab Sci*, 1990, 20(6):393-7.

Michals K, Azen C, Acosta P, et al, "Blood Phenylalanine Levels and Intelligence of 10-Year-Old Children With PKU in the National Collaborative Study," *J Am Diet Assoc*, 1988, 88:1226-9.

Scriver CR and Clow CL, "Phenylketonuria: Epitome of Human Biochemical Genetics," *N Engl J Med*, 1989, 303:1336-42, 1394-400.

Waisbren SE, Mahon BE, Schnell RR, et al, "Predictors of Intelligence Quotient and Intelligence Quotient Change in Persons Treated for Phenylketonuria Early in Life," *Pediatrics*, 1987, 79:351-5.

NH_3, Blood *see* Ammonia, Blood *on page 120*

Nitroprusside Reaction, Blood *see* Ketone Bodies, Blood *on page 265*

Norepinephrine, Urine *see* Catecholamines, Fractionation, Urine *on page 174*

NSE *see* Neuron-Specific Enolase, Serum *on page 294*

5'NT *see* 5' Nucleotidase *on this page*

5' Nucleotidase

***CPT** 83915*

Related Information

Alkaline Phosphatase, Serum *on page 109*
Gamma Glutamyl Transferase *on page 230*
Leucine Aminopeptidase *on page 276*

Synonyms Ecto-5'NT; 5'NT

Replaces BSP

Abstract A plasma membrane enzyme relevant to the biliary tract.

Patient Care **PREPARATION:** A fasting specimen is preferred.

Specimen Serum, synovial fluid **CONTAINER:** Red top tube **STORAGE INSTRUCTIONS:** Stable 4 days at 4°C or 3 months at -20°C. Unstable at room temperature.[1]

Interpretive **REFERENCE RANGE:** Varies with laboratory. Typically measured as units/dL activity. Henry lists normal range as 0-1.6 units/dL.[2] **USE:** Like GGT and LAP, 5' nucleotidase is used to investigate the origin of increased serum alkaline phosphatase. It is a liver-related enzyme used to work up cholestatic/biliary obstruction. It parallels the increases of alkaline phosphatase and leucine aminopeptidase in hepatobiliary diseases, but is not usually elevated in skeletal disorders such as Paget's disease of bone. It is increased with metastatic neoplasia in the liver, primary biliary cirrhosis, and biliary obstruction secondary to calculi or tumor. *Vide infra.* **LIMITATIONS:** Some feel that 5' nucleotidase and leucine aminopeptidase offer little which is not provided by GGT. **METHODOLOGY:** Varies widely. Activity is generally measured by hydrolyzing a particular nucleotide such as 5'-AMP, 5'-CMP, or 5'-IMP. Detection methods include detecting inorganic phosphate measured by a molybdate color reaction, detecting nucleoside reac-

(Continued)

5' Nucleotidase *(Continued)*

tion products after separation by high performance liquid chromatography, coupled reactions to detect ammonia, NADH, or urate, or radioligand release.[3] A method for measuring 5'NT cytosolic activity uses coupled reactions utilizing cytidine monophosphate as substrate, cytidine deaminase, and uridine nucleosidase, measuring ultraviolet differential absorption between CMP and uracil, the latter one of the end products of the coupled reactions.[4] **ADDITIONAL INFORMATION:** 5' Nucleotidase comprises a group of widely distributed enzymes that are found in both prokaryotic and eukaryotic organisms. It is located predominantly on plasma membranes in mammalian cells. In lymphocytes, hepatocytes, and placental cells, 5'NT is located on the external surface of the cell membrane and may be classified as an ectoenzyme "ecto-5'NT". 5'NT is probably a metalloprotein with zinc as the likely native constituent metal. Human erythrocytes contain at least two cytosolic 5'NT activities; several isoenzymes of erythrocyte pyrimidine 5'NT have been characterized. Primary function of ecto-5'NT is conversion of impermeable extracellular nucleotides to corresponding nucleosides which are permeable, and may be utilized as metabolic substrates or modulators (eg, adenosine).[3]

Isoforms of 5'NT with α_1-electrophoretic mobility vary inversely with serum bile acid concentrations. They increase in serum after surgical correction of biliary obstruction.[5] In rabbits myocardial activity of 5'NT is associated with improved postischemic recovery of ventricular functions.[6] Patients with multiple myeloma have increased numbers of plasma cells with cytoplasmic 5'NT activity when compared to control patients or patients with monoclonal gammopathy of undetermined significance.[7] Such determinations of plasma cell 5'NT activity are not currently used to study myeloma. 5'NT activity is increased in synovial fluid of patients with calcium pyrophosphate dehydrate deposition. Synovial fluid 5'NT activity is greater in patients with osteoarthritis compared to those with gout, pseudogout, or rheumatoid arthritis.[8] 5'NT activity has been shown to be increased in the myofiber interstitium in polymyositis.[9] Prostate epithelium in benign prostatic hyperplasia appears to express high levels of 5'NT activity compared with prostatic carcinomas.[10]

5' Nucleotidase did not change between the first and third trimesters of pregnancy in a study of 219 pregnant women.[11]

In patients receiving antiepileptic drugs, the frequency of enzyme elevation was similar to that of alkaline phosphatase but lower than that of GGT.[12]

Footnotes

1. Ellis G, "5' Nucleotidase," *Methods in Clinical Chemistry*, Pesce AJ and Kaplan LA, eds, St Louis, MO: Mosby-Year Book Inc, 1987, 1125-33.
2. Henry JB, *Clinical Diagnosis and Management by Laboratory Methods*, 18th ed, Philadelphia, PA: WB Saunders Co, 1991, 1371.
3. Sunderman FW Jr, "The Clinical Biochemistry of 5'-Nucleotidase," *Ann Clin Lab Sci*, 1990, 20(2):123-39.
4. Amici A, Natalini P, Ruggieri S, et al, "A Spectrophotometric Method for the Assay of Pyrimidine 5'-Nucleotidase in Human Erythrocytes," *Br J Haematol*, 1989, 73(3):392-5.
5. Novo FJ and Tutor JC, "Changes in Alkaline Phosphatase and 5'-Nucleotidase Multiple Forms After Surgical Management of Biliary Obstruction," *Clin Chem*, 1992, 38(7):1340-2.
6. Grosso MA, Banerjee A, St Cyr JA, et al, "Cardiac 5'-Nucleotidase Activity Increases With Age and Inversely Relates to Recovery from Ischemia," *J Thorac Cardiovasc Surg*, 1992, 103(2):206-9.
7. Majumdar G, Heard SE, and Singh AK, "Use of Cytoplasmic 5' Nucleotidase for Differentiating Malignant From Benign Monoclonal Gammopathies," *J Clin Pathol*, 1990, 43(11):891-2.
8. Wortmann RL, Veum JA, and Rachow JW, "Synovial Fluid 5'-Nucleotidase Activity – Relationship to Other Purine Catabolic Enzymes and to Arthropathies Associated With Calcium Crystal Deposition," *Arthritis Rheum*, 1991, 34(8):1014-20.
9. Hilton DA, Eagles ME, and Fletcher A, "Histochemical Demonstration of 5'-Nucleotidase Activity in Inflammatory Muscle Disease," *Arch Pathol Lab Med*, 1991, 115(4):362-4.
10. Rackley RR, Lewis TJ, Preston EM, et al, "5'-Nucleotidase Activity in Prostatic Carcinoma and Benign Prostatic Hyperplasia," *Cancer Res*, 1989, 49(13):3702-7.
11. Alvi MH, Amer NA, and Sumerin I, "Serum 5' Nucleotidase and Serum Sialic Acid in Pregnancy," *Obstet Gynecol*, 1988, 72(2):171-4.
12. Fortman CS and Witte DL, "Serum 5' Nucleotidase in Patients Receiving Antiepileptic Drugs," *Am J Clin Pathol*, 1985, 84:197-201.

Nutritional Status *see* Albumin, Serum *on page 102*

O_2 Capacity *see* Oxygen Saturation, Blood *on page 305*

O_2 Content *see* Oxygen Saturation, Blood *on page 305*

OD 450 Method *see* Amniotic Fluid Analysis for Erythroblastosis Fetalis *on page 122*

OGTT *see* Glucose Tolerance Test *on page 241*

1,25-$(OH)_2D_3$ *see* Vitamin D_3, Serum *on page 387*

1,25$(OH)_2$ D_3 *see* Vitamin D_3, Serum *on page 387*

17-OHCS *see* 17-Hydroxycorticosteroids, Urine *on page 256*

17-OHP *see* 17-Hydroxyprogesterone, Blood or Amniotic Fluid *on page 258*

***o*-Phosphoric-Monester Phosphohydrolase** *see* Acid Phosphatase *on page 96*

Oral Glucose Tolerance Test *see* Glucose Tolerance Test *on page 241*

Osmolal Gap *see* Osmolality, Calculated *on this page*

Osmolal Gap *see* Osmolality, Serum *on next page*

Osmolal Gap, Urine *see* Osmolality, Urine *on page 302*

Osmolality, Calculated

CPT 83930

Related Information

Alcohol, Blood or Urine *on page 936*
Anion Gap *on page 132*
Electrolytes, Blood *on page 212*
Ethylene Glycol *on page 965*
HCO_3, Blood *on page 248*
Ketone Bodies, Blood *on page 265*
Lactic Acid, Blood *on page 273*
Osmolality, Serum *on next page*
pH, Blood *on page 315*
Sodium, Blood *on page 349*

Applies to Holmes Formula; Osmolal Gap

Test Commonly Includes Sodium, urea nitrogen (BUN), glucose

Abstract The osmolal gap, the difference between measured serum osmolality and calculated serum osmolality, is useful for demonstration of the presence of osmotically active molecules within serum not attributable to electrolytes, glucose, or serum urea nitrogen. Use of osmolal gap may point to the presence of ethanol, other osmotically active alcohols,[1] or glycols. It is not very useful by itself.

Patient Care PREPARATION: Patient ideally should be fasting for 8 hours, a setting not usually possible when the need for investigation of osmolality arises.

Specimen Serum or plasma CONTAINER: Red top tube, green top (heparin) tube COLLECTION: Keep one green top tube on ice, should a pH be needed. CAUSES FOR REJECTION: Gross hemolysis

Interpretive REFERENCE RANGE: Calculated osmolality: 275-295 mOsm/kg (SI: 275-295 mmol/kg). The normal serum osmolal gap is about 9-15 mOsm/kg (SI: 9-15 mmol/kg). Measured osmolality is usually greater than the calculated value. Osmolality may be calculated by the Holmes formula: (1.86 x sodium) + (glucose/18) + (BUN/2.8), expressing sodium, glucose, and BUN in conventional units. It may be rounded off as: (2 x sodium) + (glucose/18) + (BUN/2.8). Dr Weisberg's formula: calculated osmolality = (2 x sodium) + (glucose/20) + (BUN/3). Still another formula in use is: (1.86 x sodium) + (glucose/18) + (BUN/2.8) + 9. POSSIBLE PANIC RANGE: >20 mOsm/kg (SI: >20 mmol/kg) USE: Screen, monitor electrolyte status, renal function. **Elevated osmolal gap** with decreased calculated value is found in shock, and in hyperglobulinemia and hyperlipidemia; in hyperproteinemia and hyperlipidemia water is being displaced, and serum sodium is decreased, but measured osmolality remains normal.[2] Increased osmolal gap occurs with chronic renal failure, as well as with methanol or ethanol ingestion, ketosis including diabetic ketoacidosis, mannitol therapy, and ethylene glycol toxicity. High anion gap metabolic acidosis with large osmolal gap is in keeping with ethylene glycol or methyl alcohol toxicity.[3] Writing in a surgical journal, Baker describes increased gaps in two settings, acute and chronic surgical illness, the latter accompanied by decreased serum water content. The former relates to the sick cell syndrome.[2] METHODOLOGY: The tests above can be done on a variety of instruments, that have in common the items necessary to calcu-

(Continued)

Osmolality, Calculated *(Continued)*

late osmolality and to follow many of the patients seen in hospital practice, with other tests ordered as clinically indicated. **ADDITIONAL INFORMATION:** Look for crystalluria in the urinary sediment to further investigate ethylene glycol toxicity. Calcium oxalate and/or hippurate crystals would support this impression, as would the documentation of severe high anion gap metabolic acidosis.[4] Elevated osmolal gap with normal blood pH and ketosis occurs with isopropyl alcohol intoxication.

Footnotes

1. Snyder H, Williams D, Zink B, et al, "Accuracy of Blood Ethanol Determination Using Serum Osmolality," *J Emerg Med*, 1992, 10(2):129-33.
2. Baker RJ, "Biochemical Gaps: Osmolal and Anion," *Curr Surg*, 1987, 44:378-81.
3. Light RT, Nelson KM, and Eckfeldt JH, "Ethylene Glycol Poisoning," *JAMA*, 1981, 246:1769, (letter).
4. Terlinsky AS, Grochowski J, Geoly KL, et al, "Identification of Atypical Calcium Oxalate Crystalluria Following Ethylene Glycol Ingestion," *Am J Clin Pathol*, 1981, 76:223-6.

References

Emmett M and Narins RG, "Clinical Use of the Anion Gap," *Medicine (Baltimore)*, 1977, 56:38-54.

Halperin ML, Margolis BL, Robinson LA, et al, "The Urine Osmolal Gap: A Clue to Estimate Urine Ammonium in "Hybrid" Types of Metabolic Acidosis," *Clin Invest Med*, 1988, 11:198-202.

Hertford JA, McKenna JP, and Chamovitz BN, "Metabolic Acidosis With an Elevated Anion Gap," *Am Fam Physician*, 1989, 39(4):159-68.

Hirasawa H, Odaka M, Sugai T, et al, "Prognostic Value of Serum Osmolality Gap in Patients With Multiple Organ Failure Treated With Hemopurification," *Artif Organs*, 1988, 12:382-7.

Norris SH, "Quiz of the Month. Severe Acidosis and an Osmolar Gap in an Alcoholic," *Am J Nephrol*, 1989, 9(2):144, 175-6.

Oster JR, Perez GO, and Materson BJ, "Use of the Anion Gap in Clinical Medicine," *South Med J*, 1988, 81:229-37.

Sklar AH and Linas SL, "The Osmolal Gap in Renal Failure," *Ann Intern Med*, 1983, 98:481-2.

Weisberg HF, "Unraveling the Laboratory Model of a Syndrome: The Osmolality Model," *Clinician and Chemist. The Relationship of the Laboratory to the Physician*, Young DS, Hicks J, Nipper H, et al, eds, Washington, DC: American Association of Clinical Chemistry, 1979, 200-43.

Osmolality, Serum

CPT 83930

Related Information

Alcohol, Blood or Urine *on page 936*
Electrolytes, Blood *on page 212*
Ethylene Glycol *on page 965*
Ketone Bodies, Blood *on page 265*
Ketones, Urine *on page 1128*
Kidney Profile *on page 268*
Lactic Acid, Blood *on page 273*
Osmolality, Calculated *on previous page*
Volatile Screen *on page 1010*

Synonyms Serum Osmolality

Applies to Osmolal Gap

Replaces Osmolarity

Abstract The osmolality of a solution is defined as the number of molecules or ions (particles) in a solution of water. Osmolality is independent of particle size or charge. Nonpolar solutions yield one molecule (eg, glucose) while polar solutions yield multiples of the number of ions solubilized (eg, sodium chloride yields two ions while magnesium chloride yields three ions).

Specimen Serum **CONTAINER:** Red top tube **COLLECTION:** Pediatrics: Blood drawn from heelstick **STORAGE INSTRUCTIONS:** Refrigerate or freeze serum if not run within 4 hours.

Interpretive **REFERENCE RANGE:** 275-295 mOsm/kg (SI: 275-295 mmol/kg) H_2O. Some consider normal to be 280-290 mOsm/kg (SI: 280-290 mmol/kg) H_2O and others within 270-310 mOsm/kg (SI: 270-310 mmol/kg) H_2O. **POSSIBLE PANIC RANGE:** <265 mOsm/kg (SI: <265 mmol/kg), >320 mOsm/kg (SI: >320 mmol/kg). Result of 385 mOsm/kg (SI: 385 mmol/kg) relates to stupor in hyperglycemia. Values 400-420 mOsm/kg (SI: 400-420 mmol/kg) can relate to grand mal seizures. Values >420 mOsm/kg (SI: >420 mmol/kg) may be lethal. **USE:** Evaluate electrolyte and water balance, hyperosmolar status and hydration status, dehydration, acid-base balance, seizures; evaluate antidiuretic hormone function, liver disease, hyperosmolar coma. Osmolality measures the concentration of particles in solution. Freezing point depression serum osmolality with calculated osmolal gap, is useful in screening for and approximating the serum concentrations of certain low molecular weight toxins, such as ethanol, ethylene glycol, isopropanol, and methanol,[1] especially as a rapid approximation for emergent situations. See Limitations.

High serum osmolality may result from hypernatremia, dehydration, hyperglycemia, mannitol therapy, azotemia, ingestion of ethanol, methanol, ethylene glycol. Thus, osmolality has a role in toxicology and in coma evaluation. Very low birth weight infants may have elevated serum osmolality for the first week of life.[2]

Low serum osmolality may be secondary to overhydration, hyponatremia, syndrome of inappropriate antidiuretic hormone secretion (SIADH) with carcinoma of lung and other entities.

Causes of hyperosmolality, hypo-osmolality, and of factors affecting ADH are published.[3] Serum osmolality measurements do not measure the fraction of serum that is water. Osmolality measurement by freezing point depression is also indifferent to permeability of solutes to cell membranes.[4]

LIMITATIONS: When vapor pressure osmometry is used, volatile solutes (eg, alcohols and glycols) may remain in the vapor phase and not be detected.[1] **METHODOLOGY:** Freezing point depression (more often used) or vapor pressure **ADDITIONAL INFORMATION:** Measured osmolality is usually more than calculated osmolality. If measured osmolality is more than 15 mOsm/kg (SI: >15 mmol/kg) greater than calculated, consider methanol, ethylene glycol, or ethanol ingestion or other toxicity; shock; or trauma. Elevated serum osmolality with normal sodium suggests possible hyperglycemia, uremia, or alcoholism.[3] Both serum and urine values and calculated osmolality (see prior listing) are sometimes needed. Although lactic acidosis theoretically should not contribute to the osmolal gap, increases in the osmolal gap in lactic acidosis have been reported.[5] Drugs including thiazide diuretics, steroids, cimetidine, and others have been implicated in the development of hyperosmolar hyperglycemic nonketotic coma.[6] Slight elevation of serum osmolality over expected values have been reported in the elderly.[7,8] After overnight dehydration, urine/serum ratio is usually ≥ 3.[3] Work-up of diabetes insipidus has been discussed by Bartter and Delea.[9]

Footnotes

1. Eisen TF, Lacouture PG, and Woolf A, "Serum Osmolality in Alcohol Ingestions: Differences in Availability Among Laboratories of Teaching Hospital, Nonteaching Hospital, and Commercial Facilities," *Am J Emerg Med*, 1989, 7(3):256-9.
2. Giacoia GP, Miranda R, and West KI, "Measured vs Calculated Plasma Osmolality in Infants With Very Low Birth Weights," *Am J Dis Child*, 1992, 146(6):712-7.
3. Weisberg HF, "Unraveling the Laboratory Model of a Syndrome: The Osmolality Model," *Clinician and Chemist. The Relationship of the Laboratory to the Physician*, Young DS, Hicks J, Nipper H, et al, eds, Washington, DC: American Association of Clinical Chemistry, 1979, 200-43.
4. Gennari FJ, "Current Concepts, Serum Osmolality, Uses and Limitations," *N Engl J Med*, 1984, 310:102-5.
5. Schelling JR, Howard RL, Winter SD, et al, "Increased Osmolal Gap in Alcoholic Ketoacidosis and Lactic Acidosis," *Ann Intern Med*, 1990, 113(8):580-2.
6. Pope DW and Dansky D, "Hyperosmolar Hyperglycemic Nonketotic Coma," *Emerg Med Clin North Am*, 1989, 7(4):849-57.
7. McLean KA, O'Neill PA, Davies I, et al, "Influence of Age on Plasma Osmolality: A Community Study," *Age Ageing*, 1992, 21(1):56-60.
8. O'Neill PA, Faragher EB, Davies I, et al, "Reduced Survival With Increasing Plasma Osmolality in Elderly Continuing-Care Patients," *Age Ageing*, 1990, 19(1):68-71.
9. Bartter FC and Delea CS, "Diabetes Insipidus: Its Nature and Diagnosis," *Lab Management*, Jan 1982, 23-8.

References

Baker RJ, "Biochemical Gaps: Osmolal and Anion," *Curr Surg*, 1987, 44:378-81.

Fraser CL and Arieff AI, "Fatal Central Diabetes Mellitus and Insipidus Resulting From Untreated Hyponatremia: A New Syndrome," *Ann Intern Med*, 1990, 112(2):113-9.

Leech S and Penney MD, "Correlation of Specific Gravity and Osmolality of Urine in Neonates and Adults," *Arch Dis Child*, 1987, 62:671-3.

Maffly RH, "Renal Function and Disorders of Water, Sodium, and Potassium Balance," *Scientific American Medicine*, Section 10, Chapter 1, Rubenstein E and Federman DD, eds, New York, NY: Scientific American Inc, 1990, 2-34.

Nose H, Mack GW, Shi XR, et al, "Role of Osmolality and Plasma Volume During Rehydration in Humans," *J Appl Physiol*, 1988, 65:325-31.

Penney MD and Walters G, "Are Osmolality Measurements Clinically Useful?" *Ann Clin Biochem*, 1987, 24:566-71.

Snyder H, Williams D, Zink B, et al, "Accuracy of Blood Ethanol Determination Using Serum Osmolality," *J Emerg Med*, 1992, 10(2):129-33.

Worthley LI, Guerin M, and Pain RW, "For Calculating Osmolality, the Simplest Formula Is the Best," *Anaesth Intensive Care*, 1987, 15:199-202.

Osmolality, Urine

CPT 83935

Related Information

Concentration Test, Urine *on page 1115*
Electrolytes, Urine *on page 213*
Kidney Profile *on page 268*
Sodium, Urine *on page 351*
Specific Gravity, Urine *on page 1152*
Urinalysis *on page 1162*

Synonyms Urine Osmolality

Applies to Osmolal Gap, Urine; U/P Ratio

Abstract Osmolality is a definitive measure of urine concentration.

Specimen Random urine or timed specimen **CONTAINER:** Clean urine container **STORAGE INSTRUCTIONS:** Refrigerate during collection and storage.

Interpretive **REFERENCE RANGE:** Random urine: neonates: 75-300 mOsm/kg (SI: 75-300 mmol/kg); children and adults: 250-900 mOsm/kg (SI: 250-900 mmol/kg). Normal range of serum sodium (mmol/L) to osmolality (mOsm/kg) ratio is 0.43-0.50.[1] Patients with normal renal function after 14-hour restriction of fluids should be able to concentrate to >800 mOsm/kg (SI: >800 mmol/kg); <400 mOsm/kg (SI: <400 mmol/kg) is interpreted by Weisberg as severe renal impairment.[2] Prolonged dehydration may be dangerous for some patients. **POSSIBLE PANIC RANGE:** <100 mOsm/kg (SI: <100 mmol/kg) in overhydration, >800 mOsm/kg (SI: >800 mmol/kg) in dehydration **USE:** Evaluate concentrating ability of the kidneys (eg, in acute and chronic renal failure); evaluate electrolyte and water balance; used in work-up for renal disease, syndrome of inappropriate antidiuretic hormone secretion (SIADH), and diabetes insipidus; may be used with urinalysis when patient has had radiopaque substances, has glycosuria or proteinuria;[2] evaluate dehydration, amyloidosis; estimate urinary ammonium concentrations using the urine osmolal gap and detect increased osmolality due to the presence of unusual molecules.[3] Osmolality is desirable in examination of neonatal urine when protein or glucose are present.[4] **LIMITATIONS:** Serum osmolality is often needed to interpret urine osmolality. **METHODOLOGY:** Freezing point depression **ADDITIONAL INFORMATION:** Osmolality is a better measurement of urine concentration than specific gravity. Osmolality is a measure of renal tubular concentration, depending on the state of hydration. Simultaneous determination of urine and serum osmolalities facilitates interpretation of results. High urinary/plasma ratio is seen in concentrated urine. Normal ranges for the U/P ratio are given by Weisberg as approximately 0.2-4.7, and >3.0 with overnight dehydration.[2] With poor concentrating ability the ratio is low but still ≥1.0. In SIADH urine sodium and urine osmolality are high for plasma osmolality.[5] Neonatal urine osmolality is discussed in a 1987 paper. Specifically derived regression equations are advocated to predict urine osmolality from specific gravity measurements.[4] Low birthweight infants have been reported to have increased serum osmolality with normal urine osmolality.[6]

The urine osmolal gap is described as the sum of urinary concentrations of sodium, potassium, bicarbonate, chloride, glucose, and urea compared to measured urine osmolality. The gap is normally 80-100 mOsm/kg (SI: 80-100 mmol/kg) H_2O. Determination of the urine osmolal gap is used to characterize metabolic acidosis. High urine osmolal gap can be used semiquantitatively.[7]

Footnotes

1. Preuss HG, Podlasek SJ, and Henry JB, "Evaluation of Renal Function and Water, Electrolyte, and Acid Base Balance," *Clinical Diagnosis and Management by Laboratory Methods*, 18th ed, Henry JB, ed, Philadelphia, PA: WB Saunders Co, 1991, 118-39.
2. Weisberg HF, "Unraveling the Laboratory Model of a Syndrome: The Osmolality Model," *Clinician and Chemist. The Relationship of the Laboratory to the Physician*, Young DS, Hicks J, Nipper H, et al, eds, Washington, DC: American Association of Clinical Chemistry, 1979, 200-43.
3. Kamel KS, Ethier JH, Richardson RM, et al, "Urine Electrolytes and Osmolality: When and How to Use Them," *Am J Nephrol*, 1990, 10(2):89-102.
4. Leech S and Penney MD, "Correlation of Specific Gravity and Osmolality of Urine in Neonates and Adults," *Arch Dis Child*, 1987, 62:671-3.
5. Goldstein CS, Braunstein S, and Goldfarb S, "Idiopathic Syndrome of Inappropriate Antidiuretic Hormone Secretion Possibly Related to Advanced Age," *Ann Intern Med*, 1983, 99:185-8.
6. Giacoia GP, Miranda R, and West KI, "Measured vs Calculated Plasma Osmolality in Infants With Very Low Birth Weights," *Am J Dis Child*, 1992, 146(6):712-7.
7. Halperin ML, Margolis BL, Robinson LA, et al, "The Urine Osmolal Gap: A Clue to Estimate Urine Ammonium in "Hybrid" Types of Metabolic Acidosis," *Clin Invest Med*, 1988, 11:198-202.

References

Fraser CL and Arieff AI, "Fatal Central Diabetes Mellitus and Insipidus Resulting From Untreated Hyponatremia: A New Syndrome," *Ann Intern Med*, 1990, 112(2):113-9.

Halperin ML and Skorecki KL, "Interpretation of the Urine Electrolytes and Osmolality in the Regulation of Body Fluid Tonicity," *Am J Nephrol*, 1986, 6:241-5, (editorial).

Osmolarity *replaced by* Osmolality, Serum *on page 300*

Oxalate, Urine

***CPT** 83945*

Related Information

Ethylene Glycol *on page 965*

Kidney Stone Analysis *on page 1129*

Synonyms Calcium Oxalate, Urine; Urine Oxalate

Applies to Glycolic Acid, Urine; Glyoxylic Acid, Urine; L-Glyceric Acid, Urine

Abstract Calcium oxalate stones are common in the urinary tract. Oxalate excretion is a predictor of oxalate nephrolithiasis.

Patient Care **PREPARATION:** Avoid vitamin C for 24 hours before collection. Pyridoxine is said to diminish oxaluria. The patient should be ambulatory, preferably at home, on usual fluid and food intake, to best interpret risk factors for nephrolithiasis.

Specimen 24-hour urine; first morning urine may give oxalate concentrations similar to 24-hour collections.[1] Total amount of oxalate excreted might be estimated using first morning urinary oxalate concentration and an estimate of daily urine output. **CONTAINER:** Acid-washed plastic container with 20 mL of 6N HCl added prior to collection (depending upon laboratory). No metal cap. **COLLECTION:** Instruct the patient to void at 8 AM and discard the specimen. Then collect all urine including the final specimen voided at the end of the 24-hour collection period (ie, 8 AM the next morning). Many laboratories request addition of acid to container before urine collection is started. Twenty-four hour urine volume must be recorded. **CAUSES FOR REJECTION:** Incomplete collection, no preservative or the wrong preservative, metal cap on container

Interpretive **REFERENCE RANGE:** 10-41 mg/24 hours (SI: 0.11-0.46 mmol/day).[2,3] Greater excretion of oxalic acid in men is recognized in healthy subjects as well as in stone formers. The differences were unexplained on the basis of body surface. A relationship with age was not found.[4] **USE:** Patients who form calcium oxalate kidney stones appear to absorb and excrete a higher fraction of dietary oxalate in urine than do normals. Hyperoxaluria is not uncommon in subjects with malabsorption. Twenty-four hour urine collections for oxalate are indicated in patients with surgical loss of distal small intestine, especially those with Crohn's disease. The incidence of nephrolithiasis in patients who have inflammatory bowel disease is 2.6% to 10%.[5] Hyperoxaluria is regularly present after jejunoileal bypass for morbid obesity; such patients may develop nephrolithiasis. **LIMITATIONS:** Interference by ascorbate is a major impediment in developing a simple assay. Urine specimens containing significant amounts of ascorbic acid (10-325 μg/dL) experience interference in two forms. First, ascorbic acid is converted nonenzymatically to oxalate at alkaline pH or if urine is not acidified after bicarbonate administration.[6] Second, ascorbate inhibits oxalate oxidase (enzymatic method) and markedly decreases recovery of oxalates.[7,8] Methods to eliminate ascorbate meet with varied success depending upon the urine ascorbate concentration.[8] **METHODOLOGY:** Colorimetry following anion exchange resin; atomic absorption (AA) after precipitation with calcium; enzymatic, oxalate oxidase; high performance liquid chromatography (HPLC). A method for routine clinical urinary oxalate has been reported.[9] **ADDITIONAL INFORMATION:** Oxaluria is characteristic of ethylene glycol intoxication. Oxalic acid excretion is increased with methoxyflurane. Serum calcium and urinary calcium excretion are also commonly needed; calcium oxalate renal stones are common.

Hyperoxaluria may occur with high intake of animal protein, purines, gelatin, calcium, strawberries, pepper, rhubarb, beans, beets, spinach, tomatoes, chocolate, cocoa, and tea. Hyperoxaluria is described with pyridoxine deficiency. Urinary oxalate derives from the metabolism of glycine and ascorbic acid more than from dietary ingestion. Oxalate excretion was increased in vegetarians, despite low animal protein ingestion.[10] Dietary intake of animal protein is also directly associated with the risk of stone formation. Limited calcium supplementation does not appear to increase the risk of nephrolithiasis in men. Calcium taken orally with oxalate loads decreases urinary oxalate excretion in patients with ileal disease. Calcium supplements taken with meals are less likely to lead to nephrolithiasis.[11]

Vitamin C increases oxalate excretion and may be a risk factor for calcium oxalate nephrolithiasis in individuals consuming "megadose" vitamin C. Such ingestion can usually be

(Continued)

Oxalate, Urine *(Continued)*

determined by history. If a vitamin C using stone former is found to have high urine oxalate excretion, the habit should be stopped. If oxalate excretion drops to normal, additional therapy to prevent stones may not be required.

Hyperoxaluria can result from intestinal hyperabsorption related to low calcium intake or high calcium enteric binding. Unabsorbed fat can bind calcium. Increased urinary uric acid excretion is frequently found in subjects who have calcium oxalate nephrolithiasis. Calcium nephrolithiasis in patients with hyperuricosuria has been related to urate-induced crystallization of calcium oxalate.[12] Urinary oxalate concentrations have been found to be increased in very low birth weight infants receiving parenteral amino acid solutions.[13]

Rare genetic disorders increase endogenous oxalate production; there are two types of primary hyperoxaluria. They are characterized by elevated urinary oxalate excretion and recurrent oxalate nephrocalcinosis. In type I, a defect in glyoxalate metabolism is found, leading to increased oxalate synthesis. Excessive quantities of urinary glyoxylic and glycolic acid excretion occur. Type II is rare; it is characterized by excessive urinary excretion of oxalic and L-glyceric acids with normal excretion of glycolic acid.[14]

Glycine irrigation during transurethral prostatic resections does not raise the urinary oxalate level during the postoperative period. This suggests that post-transurethral forced diuresis may not be indicated solely for bladder irrigation with glycine.[15]

Footnotes

1. Balchin ZEC, Moss PA, and Fraser CG, "Biological Variation of Urinary Oxalate in Different Specimens Types," *Ann Clin Biochem*, 1991, 28(Pt 6):622-3.
2. Leavelle DE, "Oxalate, Urine," *Mayo Medical Laboratories Interpretive Handbook*, Rochester MN: Mayo Medical Laboratories, 1990, 139.
3. Wilson DM and Liedtke RR, "Modified Enzyme-Based Colorimetric Assay of Urinary and Plasma Oxalate With Improved Sensitivity and No Ascorbate Interference: Reference Values and Sample Handling Procedures," *Clin Chem*, 1991, 37(7):1229-35.
4. Hesse A, Klocke K, Classen A, et al, "Age and Sex as Factors in Oxalic Acid Excretion in Healthy Persons and Calcium Oxalate Stone Patients," *Contrib Nephrol*, 1987, 58:16-20.
5. Earnest DL, "Enteric Hyperoxaluria," *Adv Intern Med*, 1979, 24:407-27.
6. Lemann J Jr, Hornick LJ, Pleuss JA, et al, "Oxalate Is Overestimated in Alkaline Urines Collected During Administration of Bicarbonate With No Specimen pH Adjustment," *Clin Chem*, 1989, 35(10):2107-10.
7. Li MG and Madappally MM, "Rapid Enzymatic Determination of Urinary Oxalate," *Clin Chem*, 1989, 35(12):2330-3.
8. Inamdar KV, Raghavan KG, and Pradhan DS, "Five Treatment Procedures Evaluated for the Elimination of Ascorbate Interference in the Enzymatic Determination of Urinary Oxalate," *Clin Chem*, 1991, 37(6):864-8.
9. Mazzuchin A, Michelutti L, and Falter H, "Modifications to Commercial Oxalate Oxidase Based Determination of Urinary Oxalate: A Method Suitable for Routine Clinical Analysis," *Clin Biochem*, 1990, 23(2):173-7.
10. Marangella M, Bianco I, Martini C, et al, "Effect of Animal and Vegetable Protein Intake on Oxalate Excretion in Idiopathic Calcium Stone Disease," *Br J Urol*, 1989, 63(4):348-51.
11. Curhan GC, Willett WC, Rimm EB, et al, "A Prospective Study of Dietary Calcium and Other Nutrients and the Risk of Symptomatic Kidney Stones," *N Engl J Med*, 1993, 328(12):833-8.
12. Pak CYC and Peterson R, "Successful Treatment of Hyperuricosuric Calcium Oxalate Nephrolithiasis With Potassium Citrate," *Arch Intern Med*, 1986, 146:863-7.
13. Campfield T and Braden G, "Urinary Oxalate Excretion by Very Low Birth Weight Infants Receiving Parenteral Nutrition," *Pediatrics*, 1989, 84(5):860-3.
14. Yendt ER and Cohanim M, "Response to Physiologic Dose of Pyridoxine in Type 1 Primary Hyperoxaluria," *N Engl J Med*, 1985, 312:953-7.
15. Hahn RG, "Glycine Irrigation and Urinary Oxalate Excretion," *Br J Urol*, 1989, 64(3):287-9.

References

Allen LC, Kadijevic L, and Romaschin AD, "An Enzymatic Method for Oxalate Automated With the Cobas Fara Centrifugal Analyzer," *Clin Chem*, 1989, 35(10):2098-100.

Barratt TM, Kasidas GP, Murdoch I, et al, "Urinary Oxalate and Glycolate Excretion and Plasma Oxalate Concentration," *Arch Dis Child*, 1991, 66(4):501-3.

Berckmans RJ and Boer P, "An Inexpensive Method for Sensitive Enzymatic Determination of Oxalate in Urine and Plasma," *Clin Chem*, 1988, 34:1451-5.

Brown JM, Stratmann G, Cowley DM, et al, "The Variability and Dietary Dependence of Urinary Oxalate Excretion in Recurrent Calcium Stone Formers," *Ann Clin Biochem*, 1987, 24:385-90.

Classen A and Hesse A, "Measurement of Urinary Oxalate: An Enzymatic and An Ion Chromatographic Method Compared," *J Clin Chem Clin Biochem*, 1987, 25:95-9.

Cowley DM, McWhinney BC, Brown JM, et al, "Effect of Citrate on the Urinary Excretion of Calcium and Oxalate: Relevance to Calcium Oxalate Nephrolithiasis," *Clin Chem*, 1989, 35(1):23-8.

Coyle P, Rofe AM, and Renfeng F, "Improved Urinary Oxalate Method for a Centrifugal Analyzer," *Clin Chem*, 1989, 35(8):1806, (letter).

Fry IDR and Starkey BJ, "The Determination of Oxalate in Urine and Plasma by High Performance Liquid Chromatography," *Ann Clin Biochem*, 1991, 28(Pt 6):581-7.

Knispel HH, Fitzner R, Kaiser M, et al, "Acute Acid Load in Recurrent Oxalate Stone Formers," *Urol Int*, 1988, 43:93-6.

Petrarulo M, Marangella M, Bianco O, et al, "Preventing Ascorbate Interference in Ion-Chromatographic Determinations of Urinary Oxalate: Four Methods Compared," *Clin Chem*, 1990, 36(9):1642-5.

Ryall RL, Harnett RM, Hibberd CM, et al, "Urinary Risk Factors in Calcium Oxalate Stone Disease: Comparison of Men and Women," *Br J Urol*, 1987, 60:480-8.

2-Oxoglutarate Aminotransferase *see* Alanine Aminotransferase *on page 100*

Oxygen Content *see* Blood Gases, Arterial *on page 140*

Oxygen-Hemoglobin Dissociation Curve (ODC) *see* Oxygen Saturation, Blood *on this page*

Oxygen-Hemoglobin Dissociation Curve (ODC) *see* P-50 Blood Gas *on page 307*

Oxygen Saturation *see* Blood Gases, Arterial *on page 140*

Oxygen Saturation, Blood

CPT *82792*

Related Information

Blood Gases, Arterial *on page 140*
Hemoglobin *on page 554*
P-50 Blood Gas *on page 307*
pH, Blood *on page 315*

Synonyms Hemoglobin Saturation, Percent; SaO_2; SO_2

Applies to 2,3-DPG; O_2 Capacity; O_2 Content; Oxygen-Hemoglobin Dissociation Curve (ODC); Transcutaneous Pulse Oximetry

Test Commonly Includes A part of blood gas determination in many laboratories.

Abstract The partial pressure of oxygen physically dissolved in plasma determines the amount of oxygen bound to hemoglobin = the oxygen saturation.

Specimen Whole blood, arterial **CONTAINER:** Heparinized syringe, capillary tubes, or green top (heparin) tube **COLLECTION:** Draw specimen into heparinized syringe, avoid air bubbles, and stopper tightly, knotting scalp vein infusion set tubing, fitting shank of syringe with a special closure or other means of insuring an airtight fit. Place heparinized specimen on ice. Take to the laboratory immediately. **CAUSES FOR REJECTION:** Specimen received with clots or air bubbles in the syringe, specimen not on ice, specimen not tightly stoppered **SPECIAL INSTRUCTIONS:** If capillaries are used to collect the specimen, warm skin 10-15 minutes prior to puncture, obtain free flow of blood with a sufficiently deep puncture ("arterialized capillary blood"), fill heparinized capillaries completely full (enough capillaries to provide at least 0.5 mL whole blood), cap and mix.

Interpretive **REFERENCE RANGE:** Children and adults: 95% to 99%. Arterial pO_2 of 80 mm Hg, SO_2 of 95% are normal for the aged. Arterial pO_2 of 100 mm Hg, SO_2 of 97% are normal for the young. **POSSIBLE PANIC RANGE:** Arterial pO_2 of 20 mm Hg, SO_2 of 35% are critically low, life-endangering levels; the same values from mixed venous blood indicate tissue hypoxia. Arterial pO_2 of 40 mm Hg, SO_2 of 75% are panic values that correlate with cyanosis, but these values are normal for mixed venous blood. **USE:** Evaluate the extent of oxygenation of hemoglobin and adequacy of tissue oxygenation, together with pO_2. Allows evaluation of oxygenation and oxyhemoglobin dissociation of blood with use of the oxygen dissociation curve (ODC). The dissociation curve expresses relationships between pO_2 and oxyhemoglobin saturation. Diagnose hypoxia; monitor respiratory function during mechanical ventilation.[1] Central venous oxygen saturation may also be used in detection of blood loss in cases of acute injury.[2] **LIMITATIONS:** Accuracy and precision may be affected by the presence of other pigments in the blood, including especially other heme derivatives (eg, carboxyhemoglobin), low hemoglobin concentrations, plasma turbidity (ie, as with lipemia), and presence of cell fragments. Interpretation is more meaningful if the nature of patient's inspired gas is recorded (ie, room air or mixture of gases with a controlled oxygen content). **CONTRAINDICATIONS:** Contraindications of arterial puncture **METHODOLOGY:** Spectrophotometric analysis of hemolysate with current automated analyzers directly measuring SO_2. Alternatively, a calculated SO_2 may be derived from the Hill equation using measured pH and pO_2. In the latter method, blood is analyzed at two

(Continued)

Oxygen Saturation, Blood *(Continued)*

wavelengths, one with a large difference in absorbance between oxygenated and deoxygenated hemoglobin, the other at the isobestic point (molar absorbance identical for the oxygenated and deoxygenated forms).[3] Transcutaneous pulse oximetry measures the absorption of different wavelengths of light passed through living tissue. See following discussion and footnotes. **ADDITIONAL INFORMATION:** The terms "O_2 content," "O_2 capacity," and "O_2 saturation" refer to various definitions of the amount of oxygen carried in the blood. **Oxygen content** is the total amount of oxygen present (bound to hemoglobin and dissolved in plasma) in the blood. Normally hemoglobin exists in blood in the oxygen-bound state (oxyhemoglobin) and in some unoxygenated forms (reduced hemoglobin, methemoglobin, carboxyhemoglobin, and sulfhemoglobin). Inactive forms account for about 4% of the total hemoglobin. **Oxygen capacity** is the amount of O_2 that would bind to hemoglobin if all the hemoglobin were oxygenated. **Oxygen saturation** is the ratio (in %) of oxyhemoglobin to the total amount of hemoglobin present.

The large pool of hemoglobin allows blood to transport 65 times the amount of oxygen dissolved in plasma. This relationship is dependent upon (primarily) pH (and thereby CO_2 parameters that contribute to the control of pH), temperature, the concentration of 2,3-diphosphoglycerate (2,3-DPG), and the molecular species of hemoglobin. When graphed, the relationship results in a sigmoid (S-shaped) oxygen-hemoglobin dissociation curve (ODC). The oxygen saturation (in %) is represented on the Y axis, the partial pressure of oxygen (in mm Hg) on the X axis with the curve shifted to the right or left (isobars) by changes in pH or other parameters. This is a physicochemically fixed relation such that if any two of the three determinants, pH, pO_2, or O_2 saturation are known, the other may be predicted. With the ODC in hand one can verify the accuracy of laboratory performance by assuring that the three reported values are consistent with each other as defined by the ODC (assuming normal molecular species of hemoglobin, concentration of 2,3-DPG, and constant temperature).

Red cell 2,3-DPG concentration plays an important role in regulation of hemoglobin's affinity for oxygen. 2,3-DPG binds to the β chains of deoxyhemoglobin and results in displacement of O_2 by the following equation:[4] $HgbO_2$ + 2,3-DPG = Hgb–2,3-DPG + O_2. An increase in 2,3-DPG will cause a shift of the reaction to the right. Greater affinity of fetal hemoglobin for oxygen has been ascribed to the poor binding of 2,3-DPG by the γ chains of fetal hemoglobin. Increased erythrocyte 2,3-DPG concentrations decrease intracellular pH resulting in a further reduction in oxygen affinity. 2,3-DPG is increased with hypoxia. Red cells of newborns contain approximately 80% hemoglobin F. Hemoglobin F has a slightly lower oxygen affinity compared to hemoglobin A (normal adult hemoglobin) and binds 2,3-DPG less strongly than hemoglobin A. Following birth, O_2 affinity decreases as red cell 2,3-DPG concentrations rise (20% during the first week of life). At 1-4 weeks, healthy prematures have P-50 values approaching those of normal adults.[5]

Decreased oxygen saturation relates to impaired cardiorespiratory function at the macro-organ level of heart and/or lungs (due to a variety of diseases) or at the intracellular chemical respiratory level (a number of pathologic mechanisms resulting in methemoglobinemia). The four mechanisms of abnormal gas exchange are hypoventilation, ventilation-perfusion disturbance, diffusion defect, and venous admixture. The hypoxemia accompanying right-to-left shunting in cardiac diseases (venous admixture) is preferentially evaluated with oxygen saturation. O_2 saturation provides a more direct indication of the size of the shunt than the pO_2 value.[6] Decreased central venous oxygen saturation was found to correlate better with estimated blood loss volumes in 26 trauma patients than vital signs including heart rate, blood pressure, central venous pressure, pulse pressure, and urine output. In this series of trauma patients, all had normal vital signs upon admission and a significant percentage of these patients had serious injuries and ongoing blood loss that required immediate attention.[2]

In some clinical situations, measurement of pO_2 alone may give misleading information as to sufficiency of the blood's oxygen-carrying ability. Partial pressure of oxygen may be normal or even increased while O_2 saturation may be decreased as the result of an abnormal heme compound (eg, carboxyhemoglobin as in cases of carbon monoxide poisoning).[7] Oxygen saturation is preferably measured directly (spectrophotometrically) and not derived from the pH and pO_2 values by use of the ODC relationships. Derived SO_2 values would give false normal results in the above example.

Arterial oxygen desaturation occurs after sedation for peritoneoscopy with resultant hypoxemia, hypercarbia, and acidosis.[8]

There is growing use of **transcutaneous pulse oximetry** to determine oxygen saturation, particularly in premature and in critically ill newborns and children. This noninvasive technique avoids the rigors of arterial puncture, necessity of subsequent proper sample handling, and can provide continual monitoring. This technique has generally been found reliable and useful in monitoring adequacy of oxygenation, effectiveness of resuscitative efforts, detection of development of prolonged periods of decreased SO_2 in neonates, and monitoring preterm infant's response to physical therapy.[1,9,10,11,12,13] Pulse oximetry has also been applied to detection of hyperoxemia in newborns but has low specificity.[14] Limitations of pulse oximetry have included overestimation of SO_2 at values 65% and less,[12,15] and variation from *in vitro* determined SO_2 in samples with >50% fetal hemoglobin as compared with samples having under 25% fetal hemoglobin.[11] A study of pulse oximeter determined oxygen saturation in pregnant patients and their newborns has found that SO_2 in neonates is commonly 90% or less within 10 minutes after birth and may not always be indicative of pathologic hypoxia.[16] Specialized devices (eg, balloon-tipped, thermodilution, fiberoptic, pulmonary arterial catheter) have been developed for the intraoperative monitoring of mixed venous oxygen saturation.[17]

Footnotes

1. Shannon DC, "Rational Monitoring of Respiratory Function During Mechanical Ventilation of Infants and Children," *Intensive Care Med*, 1989, 15(Suppl 1):S13-6.
2. Scalea TM, Hartnett RW, Duncan AO, et al, "Central Venous Oxygen Saturation: A Useful Clinical Tool in Trauma Patients," *J Trauma*, 1990, 30(12):1539-43.
3. Bruegger BB and Sherwin JE, "Blood Gas Analysis and Oxygen Saturation," *Methods in Clinical Chemistry*, Chapter 8, Pesce AJ and Kaplan LA, eds, St Louis, MO: Mosby-Year Book Inc, 1987, 54-66.
4. Ganong WF, *Review of Medical Physiology*, 15th ed, Norwalk, CT: Appleton & Lange, 1991, 616-22.
5. Bunn HF and Forget BG, "Oxygen and Carbon Dioxide Transport," *Hemoglobin: Molecular, Genetic and Clinical Aspects*, Chapter 5, Philadelphia, PA: WB Saunders Co, 1986, 91-125.
6. Siggaard-Andersen O, "Hydrogen Ions and Blood Gases," *Chemical Diagnosis of Disease*, Brown SS, Mitchell FL, and Young DS, eds, New York, NY: Elsevier/North Holland Biomedical Press, 1979, 219-38.
7. Browning RJ, "Pulmonary Disease: Putting Blood Gas Tests to Work," *Diagn Med*, 1982, 5:54-63.
8. Brady CE III, Harkleroad LE, and Pierson WP, "Alterations in Oxygen Saturation and Ventilation After Intravenous Sedation for Peritoneoscopy," *Arch Intern Med*, 1989, 149(5):1029-32.
9. Deckardt R, Schneider KT, and Graeff H, "Monitoring Arterial Oxygen Saturation in the Neonate," *J Perinat Med*, 1987, 15:357-60.
10. House JT, Schultetus RR, and Gravenstein N, "Continuous Neonatal Evaluation in the Delivery Room by Pulse Oximetry," *J Clin Monit*, 1987, 3:96-100.
11. Jennis MS and Peabody JL, "Pulse Oximetry: An Alternative Method for the Assessment of Oxygenation in Newborn Infants," *Pediatrics*, 1987, 79:524-8.
12. Lewallen PK, Mammel MC, Coleman JM, et al, "Neonatal Transcutaneous Arterial Oxygen Saturation Monitoring," *J Perinatol*, 1987, 7:8-10.
13. Kelly MK, Palisano RJ, and Wolfson MR, "Effects of a Developmental Physical Therapy Program on Oxygen Saturation and Heart Rate in Preterm Infants," *Phys Ther*, 1989, 69(6):467-74.
14. Bucher HU, Fanconi S, Baeckert P, et al, "Hyperoxemia in Newborn Infants: Detection by Pulse Oximetry," *Pediatrics*, 1989, 84(2):226-30.
15. Fanconi S, "Pulse Oximetry and Transcutaneous Oxygen Tension for Detection of Hypoxemia in Critically Ill Infants and Children," *Adv Exp Med Biol*, 1987, 220:159-64.
16. Porter KB, Goldhamer R, Mankad A, et al, "Evaluation of Arterial Oxygen Saturation in Pregnant Patients and Their Newborns," *Obstet Gynecol*, 1988, 71(3 Pt 1):354-7.
17. Thys DM, Cohen E, and Eisenkraft JB, "Mixed Venous Oxygen Saturation During Thoracic Anesthesia," *Anesthesiology*, 1988, 69(6):1005-9.

References

Chripko D, Bevan JC, Archer DP, et al, "Decreases in Arterial Oxygen Saturation in Paediatric Outpatients During Transfer to the Postanaesthetic Recovery Room," *Can J Anaesth*, 1989, 36(2):128-32.

Grebstad JA, Svendsen L, and Gulsvik A, "Precision of Arterial Blood Gases and Cutaneous Oxygen Saturation in Healthy Nonsmokers," *Scand J Clin Lab Invest*, 1989, 49(3):265-8.

Kwant B, Oeseburg B, and Zijistra WG, "Reliability of the Determination of Whole-Blood Oxygen Affinity by Means of Blood-Gas Analyzers and Multi-Wavelength Oximeters," *Clin Chem*, 1989, 35(5):773-7.

Porter KB, "Evaluation of Arterial Oxygen Saturation of the Newborn in the Labor and Delivery Suite," *J Perinatol*, 1987, 7:337-9.

Woolf CR, "Respiratory Disorders," *Applied Biochemistry of Clinical Disorders*, 2nd ed, Gornall AG, ed, Philadelphia, PA: J.B. Lippincott Co, 1986, 129-38.

P-50 Blood Gas

***CPT** 82820*

Related Information

Hemoglobin *on page 554*

Hemoglobin Electrophoresis *on page 556*

(Continued)

P-50 Blood Gas *(Continued)*

Oxygen Saturation, Blood *on page 305*

Synonyms Blood Gas P-50; pO_2 (0.5); pO_2 at Half Saturation

Applies to 2,3-DPG; Hill Plots; Oxygen-Hemoglobin Dissociation Curve (ODC)

Abstract P-50 is that pO_2 (partial pressure of oxygen) at which hemoglobin is 50% saturated. The oxygen-dissociation curve (ODC) is a graphical representation of the percent oxygen saturation versus pO_2. Hill plots are logarithmic curves representing an empirical expression for the equilibrium of hemoglobin or myoglobin with oxygen. Determination of P-50 value is an attempt to verify that a fairly tightly maintained physiologic relation between pO_2 and oxygen saturation exists in a particular patient and by implication that hemoglobin function (and thereby presumably structure as far as oxygen transport is concerned) is normal.

Specimen Whole blood **CONTAINER:** Heparinized syringe **COLLECTION:** Avoid contact with air, place on ice, and deliver to the laboratory immediately. **CAUSES FOR REJECTION:** Specimen clotted, air bubbles in syringe, needle not tightly capped (eg, needle not inserted into cork or hard rubber block)

Interpretive **REFERENCE RANGE:** pO_2 of approximately 27 mm Hg **METHODOLOGY:** The oxygen dissociation curve may be measured by discontinuous methods in which individual points of pO_2 are obtained with an oxygen electrode for a given saturation. Continuous methods utilize special cuvettes in which O_2 is generated at a constant rate. pO_2 is continuously measured as the oxygen content is increased. A review of instrumentation (including continuous technique) by Hedlund is informative.[1] Continuous oxygen saturation may be monitored *in vivo* by the use of pulse oximetry.[2] Single point methods have been described.[3,4] The reliability of such methods (using usually commonly available blood-gas analyzer/oximeter combinations) has been assessed.[5] The methods have been found suitable for detection of clinically significant abnormalities in O_2 affinity such as occur in patients with abnormal hemoglobins and CO poisoning. These procedures, however, did not provide truly accurate P_{50} and ^{n}Hill values. They were unable to discriminate between high and low values for P_{50} within the normal range.[5] Empirical equations and the use of a nomogram have been described that make possible calculation of P-50 from known values of pCO_2, pH, 2,3-DPG, and temperature present in physiological and pathological conditions.[6] **ADDITIONAL INFORMATION:** The **oxygen-hemoglobin dissociation curve (ODC)** is a graphical representation of the percent saturation of hemoglobin by exposure of blood to differing partial pressures of oxygen. The relation of oxygen saturation to pO_2 is dependent upon (primarily) pH (and thereby CO_2 parameters that contribute to the control of pH), temperature, 2,3-DPG (diphosphoglycerate) and the molecular species of hemoglobin. In the normal adult, the curve has a characteristic sigmoid configuration relating to the interaction of the components of the hemoglobin tetramer ("heme-heme interaction") and to the acceptance by the tetramer of DPG as oxygen is progressively bound or released. In effect, conformational changes occur on the molecular level (there is actually a physical change in the globin chain configuration and chain-to-chain positions with oxygenation/deoxygenation). The "normal" situation is taken at pH 7.4, temperature 37°C under which conditions a pO_2 of approximately 27 mm Hg results in 50% saturation of hemoglobin with oxygen. The P-50 value then is one point on the ODC (that pO_2 necessary to produce half saturation) reflecting the affinity of hemoglobin for oxygen. When the P-50 (and ODC curve) is shifted to the right, there will be less oxygen loaded on to hemoglobin at any given pO_2. This occurs with increased acidity (decreased pH) and with increased CO_2 content, ionic concentration, or temperature. With a "shift to the left" (as occurs with alkalosis or decrease in temperature), there is increased oxygen affinity (more oxygen loaded – higher oxygen saturation at any given pO_2). These characteristics have important implications to the availability of oxygen at the tissue level. The following is a summary:

$$\uparrow \begin{matrix}\text{RBC}\\ \text{2,3-DPG}\end{matrix} \rightarrow \uparrow \text{P-50} \begin{cases} \uparrow pO_2 \text{ necessary to } \rightarrow \text{50\% saturation Hgb with } O_2 \\ \downarrow O_2 \text{ affinity, } \uparrow \text{ tissue availability} \end{cases}$$

$$\downarrow \begin{matrix}\text{RBC}\\ \text{2,3-DPG}\end{matrix} \rightarrow \downarrow \text{P-50} \begin{cases} \downarrow pO_2 \text{ necessary to } \rightarrow \text{50\% saturation Hgb with } O_2 \\ \uparrow O_2 \text{ affinity, } \downarrow \text{ tissue availability} \end{cases}$$

Some hemoglobinopathies are characterized by an abnormal P-50 value, ODC right or left shifted, reflecting altered affinity for oxygen. A variety of molecular bases for 70 different hemoglobins with high oxygen affinities have been grouped by Perutz into eight classes.[7] Low oxygen affinity hemoglobins (28) fall into four classes based on molecular mechanism. Fairbanks lists 13 α-chain and 59 β-chain hemoglobin variants with increased oxygen affinity, not all of which have polycythemia or cyanosis.[8] Five α-chain and 22 β-chain variants have decreased O_2 affinity, some with cyanosis, and/or hemolysis and/or "anemia." The "anemia" may reflect a condition defined by a laboratory result rather than a physiologic deficiency, as the lowered affinity should allow a decreased mass of circulating hemoglobin to deliver a sufficient amount of oxygen. Hb Seattle, among many others, appears to be such an example.[9] A laboratory study of the ODC is important in cases of suspect hemoglobinopathy as some (eg, Hb Malmo[10]) have normal electrophoretic patterns using routine techniques.

Shifts in oxygen/hemoglobin relationships that favor survival appear to occur in ischemic heart disease,[11] but it is not clear if increased oxygen affinity is etiologic in occasional examples of myocardial ischemia and necrosis.[12] Interrelations between oxygen delivery, P-50, and oxygen consumption have been investigated in patients with acute myocardial infarct.[13] Oxygen consumption in nonsurvivors increased compared to survivors and was partially explained by an increased P-50. The authors noted that finding increased oxygen consumption in a patient with myocardial infarct should be interpreted with caution, as it may imply a precarious oxygen transport/requirement balance in peripheral tissue. Sodium bicarbonate, which is used to treat acidosis, has been found in one study[14] to decrease the P-50, decrease arterial pO_2 by 10 mm Hg, and increase blood lactate concentrations. P-50 has been found to decrease with use of some radiologic contrast agents.[15] Slight decrease in P-50 has also been reported in the critically ill.[16] Phosphates may increase the P-50.[17]

While normal pregnancy is associated with an increase in P-50, a significant decrease occurs in pre-eclampsia. This appears to be due in part to an increase in COHb present in pre-eclamptic pregnant women.[18]

Footnotes

1. Hedlund B, "Measurement of the Oxygen Dissociation Curve in the Clinical Laboratory," *Hemoglobinopathies and Thalassemias*, Fairbanks VF, ed, New York, NY: Thieme-Stratton Inc, 1980, 75-80.
2. Dodson SR, Hensley FA Jr, Martin DE, et al, "Continuous Oxygen Saturation Monitoring During Cardiac Catheterization in Adults," *Chest*, 1988, 94(1):28-31.
3. Pruden EL, Siggaard-Anderson O, and Tietz NW, "Blood Gases and pH," *Fundamentals of Clinical Chemistry*, 3rd ed, Chapter 19, Section 2, Philadelphia, PA: WB Saunders Co, 1987, 624-45.
4. Lichtman MA, Murphy MS, and Adamson JW, "Detection of Mutant Hemoglobins With Altered Affinity for Oxygen. A Simplified Technique," *Ann Intern Med*, 1976, 84:517-20.
5. Kwant G, Oeseburg B, and Zijistra WG, "Reliability of the Determination of Whole-Blood Oxygen Affinity by Means of Blood-Gas Analyzers and Multi-Wavelength Oximeters," *Clin Chem*, 1989, 35(5):773-7.
6. Samaja M, Melotti D, Rovida E, et al, "Effect of Temperature on the P-50 Value for Human Blood," *Clin Chem*, 1983, 29:110-4.
7. Perutz MF, "Molecular Anatomy, Physiology, and Pathology of Hemoglobin," *The Molecular Basis of Blood Diseases*, Chapter 5, Stamatoyannopoulos G, Nienhuis AW, Leder P, et al, eds, Philadelphia, PA: WB Saunders Co, 1987, 127-78.
8. Fairbanks VF, *Hemoglobinopathies and Thalassemias*, New York, NY: Thieme-Stratton Inc, 1980, 285-7.
9. Honig GR and Adams JG 3d, *Human Hemoglobin Genetics*, Chapter 6, New York, NY: Springer-Vehlay, Wien, 1986, 163-213, 292-349.
10. Fairbanks VF, Maldonado JE, Charache S, et al, "Familial Erythrocytosis Due to Electrophoretically Undetectable Hemoglobin With Impaired Oxygen Dissociation (Hemoglobin Malmo α_2 β_2^{97gln})," *Mayo Clin Proc*, 1971, 46:721-7.
11. Nevins MA, "Oxyhemoglobin Equilibrium in Ischemic Heart Disease," *JAMA*, 1974, 229:804-8.
12. Eliot RS and Bratt G, "The Paradox of Myocardial Ischemia and Necrosis in Young Women With Normal Coronary Arteriograms: Relation to Abnormal Hemoglobin-Oxygen Dissociation," *Am J Cardiol*, 1969, 23:633-8.
13. Sumimoto T, Takayama Y, Iwasaka T, et al, "Oxygen Delivery, Oxygen Consumption and Hemoglobin-Oxygen Affinity in Acute Myocardial Infarction," *Am J Cardiol*, 1989, 64(16):975-9.
14. Bersin RM, Chatterjee K, and Arieff AI, "Metabolic and Hemodynamic Consequences of Sodium Bicarbonate Administration in Patients With Heart Disease," *Am J Med*, 1989, 87(1):7-14.
15. Kim SJ, Salem MR, Joseph NJ, et al, "Contrast Media Adversely Affect Oxyhemoglobin Dissociation," *Anesth Analg*, 1990, 71(1):73-6.
16. Myburgh JA, Webb RK, and Worthley LIG, "The P50 Is Reduced in Critically Ill Patients," *Intensive Care Med*, 1991, 17(6):355-8.

(Continued)

P-50 Blood Gas *(Continued)*

17. Clerbaux T, Reynaert M, Willems E, et al, "Effect of Phosphate on Oxygen-Hemoglobin Affinity, Diphosphoglycerate and Blood Gases During Recovery From Diabetic Ketoacidosis," *Intensive Care Med*, 1989, 15(8):495-8.
18. Kambam JR, Entman S, Mouton S, et al, "Effect of Pre-eclampsia on Carboxyhemoglobin Levels: A Mechanism for a Decrease in P-50," *Anesthesiology*, 1988, 68(3):433-4.

References

Brown EG, Krouskop RW, McDonnell FE, et al, "A Technique to Continuously Measure Arteriovenous Oxygen Content Difference and P-50 *In Vivo*," *J Appl Physiol*, 1985, 58:1383-9.

Konzuki H, Enoki Y, Sakata S, et al, "A Simple Microtonometric Method for Whole Blood Oxygen Dissociation Curve and a Critical Evaluation of the "Single Point" Procedure for Blood P-50," *Jpn J Physiol*, 1983, 33:987-94.

Ostrander LE, Paloski WH, Barie PS, et al, "A Computer Algorithm to Calculate P-50 From a Single Blood Sample," *IEEE Trans Biomed Eng*, 1983, 30:250-4.

Paigen Test (*E. coli* Bacteriophage Resistance to Lysis Assay) *see* Galactose Screening Tests for Galactosemia *on page 228*

Pancreatic Polypeptide, Human

***CPT** 83520*

Synonyms Human Pancreatic Polypeptide; PP

Abstract Pancreatic polypeptide is a hormone of unknown physiologic function produced by pancreatic endocrine cells. Its release is stimulated by ingestion of food, and it is often, but not uniformly, increased in cases of neoplasms of the APUD system, for which it may serve as a marker. There is no evidence that it is pathogenetically associated with watery diarrhea-hypokalemia-achlorhydria (hypochlorhydria) syndrome.

Patient Care **PREPARATION:** Fasting, then sampled after food stimulation

Specimen Plasma **CONTAINER:** Lavender top (EDTA) tube; check with laboratory. Reference laboratories provide specific instructions. **CAUSES FOR REJECTION:** Recent radioactive scan

Interpretive **REFERENCE RANGE:** 50-200 or 250 pg/mL (SI: 50-200 or 250 mmol/L), fasting. Basal levels increase with age. **CRITICAL VALUES:** Fasting level >300 pg/mL (SI: >300 mmol/L) is suspicious of tumor-producing pancreatic polypeptide ("PPoma"). **USE:** Increased in some pancreatic APUD tumors. High levels may occur as a part of multiple endocrine adenomatosis type 1.[1] About half of the patients with endocrine pancreatic tumors have elevated levels. Assay of PP is useful for diagnosis of such tumors and to follow patients with them. It is described as an adjunctive marker for many pancreatic endocrine tumors.[2] **LIMITATIONS:** Levels of this polypeptide may be increased in a wide variety of settings other than PPoma, including renal failure, diabetes, hypoglycemia, and the postprandial state.[2] It has low sensitivity.[3,4] There usually are no characteristic clinical features of PPoma recognized. **METHODOLOGY:** Radioimmunoassay (RIA) **ADDITIONAL INFORMATION:** An atropine suppression test is used to distinguish tumor-related secretion of the peptide from normal. Release of the polypeptide from normal cells is under cholinergic control, inhibited by atropine, while autonomous secretion from a PPoma is anticipated.[2] Pancreatic endocrine tumors often secrete more than a single peptide. The peptides associated with such tumors include vasoactive intestinal polypeptide, gastrin, glucagon, somatostatin, and neurotensin.[2] Prediction of autonomic neuropathy in insulin-dependent diabetic patients; such patients, who are predisposed to the development of autonomic neuropathy may demonstrate a decreased pancreatic polypeptide (and epinephrine) response to insulin-induced hypoglycemia.[5] PP may be a glucoregulatory hormone.[6] Its release appears to be dependent upon intraluminal starch digestion.[7] The cholinergic system appears to be crucial and superimposed upon cholecystokinin in stimulating pancreatic polypeptide release.[8]

Footnotes

1. Gelston AL, Delisle MB, and Patel YC, "Multiple Endocrine Adenomatosis Type I. Occurrence in Octogenarian With High Levels of Circulating Pancreatic Polypeptide," *JAMA*, 1982, 247:665-6.
2. Adrian TE, Uttenthal LO, Williams SJ, et al, "Secretion of Pancreatic Polypeptide in Patients With Pancreatic Endocrine Tumors," *N Engl J Med*, 1986, 315:287-91.
3. Langstein HN, Norton JA, Chiang H-CV, et al, "The Utility of Circulating Levels of Human Pancreatic Polypeptide as a Marker for Islet Cell Tumors," *Surgery*, 1990, 108(6):1109-16.
4. Chiang H-CV, O'Dorisio TM, Huang SC, et al, "Multiple Hormone Elevations in Zollinger-Ellison Syndrome – Prospective Study of Clinical Significance and of the Development of a Second Symptomatic Pancreatic Endocrine Tumor Syndrome," *Gastroenterology*, 1990, 99(6):1565-75.
5. Kennedy FP, Go VL, Cryer PE, et al, "Subnormal Pancreatic Polypeptide and Epinephrine Responses to Insulin-Induced Hypoglycemia Identify Patients With Insulin-Dependent Diabetes Mellitus Predisposed to Develop Overt Autonomic Neuropathy," *Ann Intern Med*, 1988, 108(1):54-8.

6. Seymour NE, Brunicardi FC, Chaiken RL, et al, "Reversal of Abnormal Glucose Production After Pancreatic Resection by Pancreatic Polypeptide Administration in Man," *Surgery*, 1988, 104(2):119-29.
7. Layer P, Go VL, and DiMagno EP, "Carbohydrate Digestion and Release of Pancreatic Polypeptide in Health and Diabetes Mellitus," *Gut*, 1989, 30(9):1279-84.
8. Meier R, Hildebrand P, Thumshirn M, et al, "Effect of Loxiglumide, a Cholecystokinin Antagonist, on Pancreatic Polypeptide Release in Humans," *Gastroenterology*, 1990, 99(6):1757-62.

References

Brunicardi FC, Druck P, Sun YS, et al, "Regulation of Pancreatic Polypeptide Secretion in the Isolated Perfused Human Pancreas," *Am J Surg*, 1988, 155:63-9.

Feldman M, Samson WK, and O'Dorisio TM, "Apomorphine-Induced Nausea in Humans: Release of Vasopressin and Pancreatic Polypeptide," *Gastroenterology*, 1988, 95:721-6.

Green DW, Gomez G, and Greeley GH Jr, "Gastrointestinal Peptides," *Gastroenterol Clin North Am*, 1989, 18(4):695-733.

Inoue K, Tobe T, Suzuki T, et al, "Plasma Cholecystokinin and Pancreatic Polypeptide Response After Radical Pancreatoduodenectomy With Billroth I and Billroth II Type of Reconstruction," *Ann Surg*, 1987, 206:148-54.

PAP *see* Acid Phosphatase *on page 96*

Paracentesis Fluid Analysis *see* Body Fluid *on page 145*

Parathormone *see* Parathyroid Hormone *on this page*

Parathyroid Hormone

***CPT** 83970*

Related Information

Calcium, Serum *on page 160*
Calcium, Urine *on page 163*
Cyclic AMP, Plasma *on page 204*
Cyclic AMP, Urine *on page 204*
Kidney Stone Analysis *on page 1129*
Phosphorus, Serum *on page 319*
Phosphorus, Urine *on page 322*

Synonyms Immunoreactive PTH; Parathormone; PTH

Applies to Parathyroid Hormone, C-Terminal; Parathyroid Hormone, Intact; Parathyroid Hormone, N-Terminal; Parathyroid Hormone Related Protein; PRP; PTH-Related Protein

Test Commonly Includes Serum calcium is needed for interpretation. Serum phosphorus and creatinine are relevant.

Patient Care **PREPARATION:** Patient should be fasting. Recent injection of radioisotope may interfere, depending on assay system used.

Specimen Serum **CONTAINER:** Red top tube **SAMPLING TIME:** Diurnal rhythm exists. Nadir is in the morning. Morning draw is recommended. **COLLECTION:** Centrifuge promptly. Freeze immediately. Consult reference laboratory for specific instructions regarding exact PTH moiety being analyzed.

Interpretive **REFERENCE RANGE:** Typical reference range for PTH, intact: 10-50 pg/mL (SI: 1.1-5.3 pmol/L); N-terminal: 8-24 pg/mL (SI: 0.8-2.5 pmol/L); C-terminal: 0-340 pg/mL (SI: 0-35.8 pmol/L). Range for ICMA-PTH: 9-47 pg/mL (SI: 1-5 pmol/L); hypoparathyroid patients: $<$9 pg/mL (SI: $<$1.0 pmol/L); hyperparathyroidism patients: $>$47 pg/mL (SI: $>$5.0 pmol/L). **USE:** Evaluate hypercalcemia, differential diagnosis of primary hyperparathyroidism. In primary hyperparathyroidism serum PTH concentration is inappropriately high for the level of hypercalcemia. In hyperparathyroidism PTH correlates with bone disease.[1] May aid in distinction of hyperparathyroidism from nonparathyroid causes of hypercalcemia, such as neoplasia, vitamin D intoxication, and Graves' disease. Monitor therapy of secondary hyperparathyroidism in chronic renal failure; work up hypoparathyroidism, osteomalacia. **LIMITATIONS:** PTH is an 84-amino acid peptide that circulates in at least four molecular forms. Intact PTH possesses the greatest degree of activity and is present in the lowest plasma concentration. C-terminal peptide is inactive and is present in the highest concentration due to its long half-life. Older polyclonal assays measure more than one region of parathyroid hormone leading to substantial imprecision. Currently two-site assays are able to detect intact parathyroid hormone in the presence of excess amounts of inactive C-terminal fragments.[2] PTH measurements should always be interpreted in conjunction with a total calcium level. Ionized calcium, additionally, may be helpful. All PTH fragments accumulate in renal failure to a greater extent if hyperparathyroidism is present.

(Continued)

Parathyroid Hormone *(Continued)*

PTH may be increased with hypercalcemia of malignancy, but in the bulk of the cases a PTH-like factor, PTH-related protein (PRP), is involved.[2,3] PRP shows considerable homology with the N-terminus of parathyroid hormone, having eight of the first 13 amino acids identical.[4] Some patients with hyperparathyroidism have had normal serum PTH concentrations.

METHODOLOGY: Chemiluminescent immunoassay (CIA); bioassay of functional aminoterminal PTH; radioimmunoassay (RIA); immunoradiometric assay (IRMA). See footnote 2 for a good review of the state of detection of intact PTH. A rapid (modified immunoradiometric) parathyroid hormone assay has been described which may be utilized during surgery.[5,6] **ADDITIONAL INFORMATION:** No single assay previously has been suitable for evaluation of all suspected parathyroid disorders. Wood reports that utilization of two-site intact parathyroid hormone assays justifies the introduction of a national external quality assessment scheme in the UK.[2] This is a considerable improvement from the state of the art of parathyroid hormone detection just a few years ago.[7] Intact two-site PTH assays are direct measurements of parathyroid gland function, and are independent of renal disease. Such assays allow for excellent differentiation of hypoparathyroidism (low PTH, low calcium), primary hyperparathyroidism (high-normal to elevated PTH, high calcium), and nonparathyroid causes of hypercalcemia (Low or low-normal PTH, high calcium). In patients with chronic renal disease, these assays are also helpful for distinguishing patients with osteomalacia or aplasia (normal to slightly elevated PTH levels) from those with osteitis fibrosa (markedly elevated PTH levels). Consultation with reference laboratories regarding the specific performance of their assays in various clinical states is desirable. From November, 1989 to the present, ICMA-PTH is the conventional PTH assay at Mayo Medical Laboratories.[8]

In a series of 61 cases of primary hyperparathyroidism, calcium varied from 10.8-16.6 mg/dL (SI: 2.69-4.14 mmol/L) with poor correlation between calcium and PTH levels. Forty percent had increased alkaline phosphatase; 33% had hypercalciuria.[1] See chart.

Correlation of Clinical Diagnosis With Parathyroid Hormone and Calcium Levels

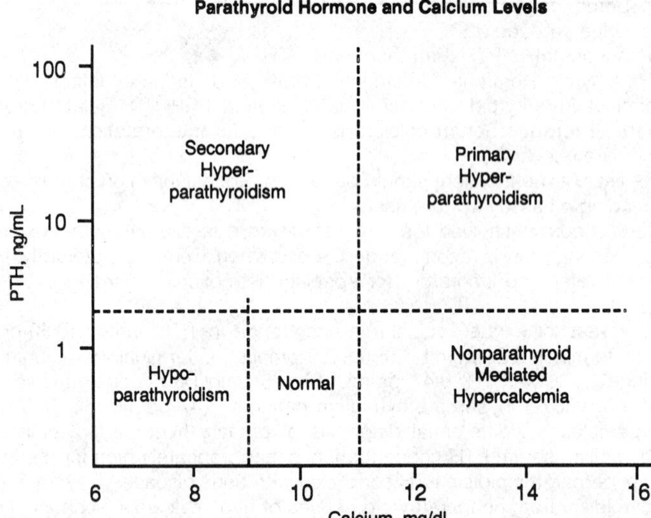

Consider parathyroid carcinoma when a patient presents with features of hyperparathyroidism, a palpable neck mass, both bone disease and nephrolithiasis, and marked increases of both serum calcium and PTH levels.[9]

When a nonparathyroid tumor is associated with hypercalcemia, decreased serum phosphorus and increased concentrations of parathyroid hormone related peptide, the neoplasm is most often squamous cell bronchogenic carcinoma, carcinoma of the breast, or renal cell carcinoma. The clinical syndrome is called **ectopic hyperparathyroidism**.

Familial benign hypercalcemia is a rare autosomal dominant entity which may be confused with primary hyperparathyroidism. Hypercalcemia begins in the first two decades. Although there is moderate hypercalcemia, hypercalciuria is not found. Serum calcium is elevated out of proportion to the concentration of PTH. Subtotal parathyroidectomy fails to eliminate hypercalcemia.

Footnotes

1. Nikkila MT, Saaristo JJ, and Koivula TA, "Clinical and Biochemical Features in Primary Hyperparathyroidism," *Surgery*, 1986, 105:148-53.
2. Wood PJ, "The Measurement of Parathyroid Hormone," *Ann Clin Biochem*, 1992, 29(Pt 1):11-21.
3. Pandian MR, Morgan CH, Carlton E, et al, "Modified Immunoradiometric Assay of Parathyroid Hormone-Related Protein: Clinical Application in the Differential Diagnosis of Hypercalcemia," *Clin Chem*, 1992, 38(2):282-8.
4. Lufkin EG, Kao PC, and Heath H, "Parathyroid Hormone Radioimmunoassays in the Differential Diagnosis of Hypercalcemia Due to Primary Hyperparathyroidism or Malignancy," *Ann Intern Med*, 1987, 106:559-60.
5. Ryan MF, Jones SR, and Barnes AD, "Clinical Evaluation of a Rapid Parathyroid Hormone Assay," *Ann Clin Biochem*, 1992, 29(Pt 1):48-51.
6. Ryan MF, Jones SR, and Barnes AD, "Modification to a Commercial Immunoradiometric Assay Permitting Intraoperative Monitoring of Parathyroid Hormone Levels," *Ann Clin Biochem*, 1990, 27(Pt 1):65-8.
7. Klee GG, Shikegawa J, and Trainer TD, "CAP Survey of Parathyroid Hormone Assays," *Arch Pathol Lab Med*, 1986, 110:588-91.
8. *Mayo Medical Laboratories 1993 Test Catalog*, Rochester, MN, 1993.
9. Wynne AG, van Heerden J, Carney JA, et al, "Parathyroid Carcinoma: Clinical and Pathologic Features in 43 Patients," *Medicine (Baltimore)*, 1992, 71(4):197-205.

References

Bourke E and Delaney V, "Assessment of Hypocalcemia and Hypercalcemia," *Clin Lab Med*, 1993, 13(1):157-81.

Budayr AA, Nissenson RA, Klein RF, et al, "Increased Serum Levels of a Parathyroid Hormone-Like Protein in Malignancy-Associated Hypercalcemia," *Ann Intern Med*, 1989, 111(10):807-12.

Firek AF, Kao PC, and Heath H 3d, "Plasma Intact Parathyroid Hormone (PTH) and PTH-Related Peptide in Familial Benign Hypercalcemia: Greater Responsiveness to Endogenous PTH Than in Primary Hyperparathyroidism," *J Clin Endocrinol Metab*, 1991, 72(3):541-6.

Flentje D, Schmidt-Gayk H, Fischer S, et al, "Intact Parathyroid Hormone in Primary Hyperparathyroidism," *Br J Surg*, 1990, 77(2):168-72.

Hage DS, Taylor B, and Kao PC, "Intact Parathyroid Hormone: Performance and Clinical Utility of an Automated Assay Based on High-Performance Immunoaffinity Chromatography and Chemiluminescence Detection," *Clin Chem*, 1992, 38(8 Pt 1):1494-1500.

Kao PC, van Heerden J, Grant CS, et al, "Clinical Performance of Parathyroid Hormone Immunometric Assays," *Mayo Clin Proc*, 1992, 67(7):637-45.

Lobaugh B, Neelon FA, Oyama H, et al, "Circadian Rhythms for Calcium, Inorganic Phosphorus, and Parathyroid Hormone in Primary Hyperparathyroidism: Functional and Practical Considerations," *Surgery*, 1989, 106(6):1009-16.

Mallette LE, Khouri K, Zengotita H, et al, "Lithium Treatment Increases Intact and Midregion Parathyroid Hormone and Parathyroid Volume," *J Clin Endocrinol Metab*, 1989, 68(3):654-60.

Quarles LD, Lobaugh B, and Murphy G, "Intact Parathyroid Hormone Overestimates the Presence and Severity of Parathyroid-Mediated Osseous Abnormalities in Uremia," *J Clin Endocrinol Metab*, 1992, 75(1):145-50.

Ross DS and Nussbaum SR, "Reciprocal Changes in Parathyroid Hormone and Thyroid Function After Radioiodine Treatment of Hyperthyroidism," *J Clin Endocrinol Metab*, 1989, 68(6):1216-9.

Rudnicki M, "Increasing Serum Parathormone in Progression of Primary Hyperparathyroidism," *J Intern Med*, 1992, 232:421-5.

Samaan NA, Ouais S, Ordonez NG, et al, "Multiple Endocrine Syndrome Type I: Clinical, Laboratory Findings, and Management in Five Families," *Cancer*, 1989, 64(3):741-52.

Silverberg SJ, Shane E, de la Cruz L, et al, "Abnormalities in Parathyroid Hormone Secretion and 1,25-Dihydroxyvitamin D_3 Formation in Women With Osteoporosis," *N Engl J Med*, 1989, 320(5):277-81.

Solal ME, Sebert JL, Boudailliez B, et al, "Comparison of Intact, Midregion, and Carboxy Terminal Assays of Parathyroid Hormone for the Diagnosis of Bone Disease in Hemodialyzed Patients," *J Clin Endocrinol Metab*, 1991, 73(3):516-24.

Watts NB and Keffer JH, "The Parathyroid Glands," *Practical Endocrine Diagnosis*, 4th ed, Philadelphia, PA: Lea & Febiger, 1989.

Woodhead JS, "The Measurement of Circulating Parathyroid Hormone," *Clin Biochem*, 1990, 23(1):17-21.

Young DS, *Effects of Drugs on Clinical Laboratory Tests*, 3rd ed, Washington, DC: AACC Press, 1990.

Parathyroid Hormone, C-Terminal *see* Parathyroid Hormone *on page 311*

Parathyroid Hormone, Intact *see* Parathyroid Hormone *on page 311*

Parathyroid Hormone, N-Terminal *see* Parathyroid Hormone *on page 311*

Parathyroid Hormone Related Protein *see* Parathyroid Hormone *on page 311*

PBI *replaced by* Thyroxine *on page 364*

PCE *see* Pseudocholinesterase, Serum *on page 343*

pCO_2 *see* Blood Gases, Arterial *on page 140*

pCO_2, Blood

CPT *82801*

Related Information

Blood Gases, Arterial *on page 140*
Blood Gases, Capillary *on page 143*
Carbon Dioxide, Blood *on page 165*
HCO_3, Blood *on page 248*
pH, Blood *on next page*

Applies to Acid-Base Status

Test Commonly Includes Test is part of blood gas panels and often, electrolyte panels

Abstract Disturbances of respiration primarily affect pCO_2, while metabolic disturbances are reflected more by bicarbonate levels.

Specimen Whole blood **COLLECTION:** See Blood Gases, Capillary listing. Deliver immediately to the laboratory. **STORAGE INSTRUCTIONS:** Must be analyzed within 1 hour. *In vitro* changes in blood gas parameters:[1] pO_2, 37°C: 33 mm Hg/10 minutes, 4°C: 3 mm Hg/10 minutes; pCO_2, 37°C: 1 mm Hg/10 minutes, 4°C: 0.1 mm Hg/10 minutes **CAUSES FOR REJECTION:** Specimen with clots, air bubbles, not received on ice, needle not tightly stoppered

Interpretive **REFERENCE RANGE:** Newborns, infants, and children up to approximately 2 years of age, with arterialized capillary blood (heel, fingertip, big toe) or arterial blood; 26.4-41.2 mm Hg; children older than 2 years of age and adults: arterial: 35-45 mm Hg, venous: 38-50 mm Hg **POSSIBLE PANIC RANGE:** $<$20 mm Hg, $>$70 mm Hg **USE:** Alveolar ventilation varies inversely as arterial pCO_2; therefore pCO_2 is an indication of adequacy of CO_2 elimination by the lungs. Diagnose respiratory alkalosis (pCO_2 low) with pH initially high (hyperventilation). pCO_2 is high with respiratory acidosis (hypoventilation). **LIMITATIONS:** Venous and arterial values are sensitive to sampling technique **METHODOLOGY:** pCO_2 electrode. This is a modified pH electrode which is present in a carbonate-bicarbonate buffer system. A plastic membrane (permeable to CO_2) is positioned between the blood sample and the electrode's surrounding buffer. CO_2 from the sample diffuses into the buffer; any pH change is detected by the electrode, and the resultant voltage change is read as pCO_2. **ADDITIONAL INFORMATION:** Respiratory compensation for metabolic acidosis and alkalosis involves adjustment of the pCO_2 level by hypoventilation (as in cases of metabolic alkalosis with resultant rise in pCO_2) or by hyperventilation (as in cases of metabolic acidosis with decreasing pCO_2). Helpful background is provided in the references listed. As CO_2 is highly soluble, there is a quickly attained equilibrium between arterial carbon dioxide tension ($PaCO_2$) and alveolar carbon dioxide tension. The arterial CO_2 measurement, then also determines the status of ventilation. $PaCO_2$ has a reverse relationship to alveolar ventilation.[1] The expression "**hypercapnia**" indicates the presence of excessive carbon dioxide in the blood. Disorders associated with hypercapnia include central depression, abnormal neuromuscular function, chest wall abnormality, upper or lower respiratory tract disease, or hypercapnia secondary to cardiac disease.[2] Arterial pCO_2 may be an indicator of systemic perfusion during cardiopulmonary resuscitation.[3] Increased venous-arterial pCO_2 gradients do not appear to be a reliable indicator of inadequate tissue perfusion during cardiopulmonary bypass.[4] Transcutaneous measurements of pCO_2 may be a convenient means of monitoring the neonate in intensive care units. Acidosis does affect the ability to correlate transcutaneous and arterial pCO_2 values.[5]

Footnotes

1. Bruegger BB and Sherwin JE, "Blood Gas Analysis and Oxygen Saturation," *Methods in Clinical Chemistry*, Chapter 8, Pesce AJ and Kaplan LA, eds, St Louis, MO: Mosby-Year Book Inc, 1987, 54-66.
2. Weinberger SE, Schwartzstein RM, and Weiss JW, "Hypercapnia," *N Engl J Med*, 1989, 321(18):1223-31.
3. Gazmuri RJ, von Planta M, Weil MH, et al, "Arterial PCO_2 as an Indicator of Systemic Perfusion During Cardiopulmonary Resuscitation," *Crit Care Med*, 1989, 17(3):237-40.
4. Ariza M, Gothard JW, Macnaughton P, et al, "Blood Lactate and Mixed Venous-Arterial pCO_2 Gradient as Indices of Poor Peripheral Perfusion Following Cardiopulmonary Bypass Surgery," *Intensive Care Med*, 1991, 17(6):320-4.
5. Hand IL, Shepard EK, Krauss AN, et al, "Discrepancies Between Transcutaneous and End-Tidal Carbon Dioxide Monitoring in the Critically Ill Neonate With Respiratory Distress Syndrome," *Crit Care Med*, 1989, 17(6):556-9.

References

Barrett CR Jr, "Pulmonary Physiologic Testing: Arterial Blood Gases," *The Laboratory in Clinical Medicine: Interpretation and Application*, Halsted JA and Halsted CH, eds, Philadelphia, PA: WB Saunders Co, 1981, 370-9.

Burnett RW and Itano M, "An Interlaboratory Study of Blood-Gas Analysis: Dependence of pO_2 and pCO_2 Results on Atmospheric Pressure," *Clin Chem*, 1989, 35(8):1779-81.

Hansen JE, Casaburi R, Crapo RO, et al, "Assessing Precision and Accuracy in Blood Gas Proficiency Testing," *Am Rev Respir Dis*, 1990, 141(5 Pt 1):1190-3.

Meyerhoff ME, "New *In Vitro* Analytical Approaches for Clinical Chemistry Measurements in Critical Care," *Clin Chem*, 1990, 36(8 Pt 2):1567-72.

Narins RG and Emmett M, "Simple and Mixed Acid-Base Disorders: A Practical Approach," *Medicine (Baltimore)*, 1980, 59:161-87.

Pentagastrin Stimulation Test *see* Gastric Analysis *on page 232*

Peptavlon® Stimulation Test *see* Gastric Analysis *on page 232*

Pericardial Fluid Analysis *see* Body Fluid *on page 145*

Peritoneal Fluid Analysis *see* Body Fluid *on page 145*

Peritoneal Fluid pH *see* Body Fluid pH *on page 150*

pH *see* Blood Gases, Arterial *on page 140*

pH, Blood

***CPT** 82800*

Related Information

Anion Gap *on page 132*
Blood Gases, Arterial *on page 140*
Blood Gases, Capillary *on page 143*
Blood Gases, Venous *on page 144*
Carbon Dioxide, Blood *on page 165*
Delta Base, Blood *on page 208*
Glucose, Fasting *on page 238*
Ketone Bodies, Blood *on page 265*
Lactic Acid, Blood *on page 273*
Osmolality, Calculated *on page 299*
Oxygen Saturation, Blood *on page 305*
pCO_2, Blood *on previous page*
pH, Urine *on page 1144*
Uric Acid, Serum *on page 378*

Synonyms Blood pH

Abstract Blood pH is an expression of acidity or acidemia.

Specimen Whole blood **CONTAINER:** Green top (heparin) tube or heparinized syringe **COLLECTION:** For venous sample, it is best to collect without tourniquet if possible. **Do not allow patient to clench/unclench his/her hand**. This builds up lactic acid. Draw specimen into air-free heparinized syringe with needle quickly stoppered, making sure that no air bubbles remain. Capillary tubes should be filled as much as possible, metal flea inserted, capped, and mixed well with magnet. All specimens should be on ice and brought to the laboratory immediately. For capillary collection, the skin area to be punctured should be warmed 10-15 minutes. The puncture should be deep enough to allow a free flow of blood. Place arterial or venous blood on ice and transport to the laboratory immediately. **STORAGE INSTRUCTIONS:** Keep on ice in a syringe. pH changes 0.01/10 minutes at 37°C and 0.001/10 minutes at 4°C.[1] **CAUSES FOR REJECTION:** Specimen with clots, air bubbles, not iced, needle not tightly stoppered **TURNAROUND TIME:** Stability of iced green top tube for pH is not in excess of 4 hours.

Interpretive **REFERENCE RANGE:** Pediatrics: newborns, with arterialized capillary blood (heel, fingertip, big toe) or arterial blood; 7.32-7.49; 2 months to 2 years, arterialized capillary or arterial blood: 7.34-7.46; children and adults: arterial: 7.35-7.45, venous: 7.32-7.43. Blood pH can be measured from either arterial or venous blood samples, usually with only very small differences in normal range. Such differences are partly addressed in the listing Blood Gases, Venous. **POSSIBLE PANIC RANGE:** <7.20, >7.60. Occasionally, patients with acidosis as severe as pH 6.80 survive. Many of these present with diabetic ketoacidosis, for which effective therapy is available. **USE:** Diagnose acidosis (eg, ketoacidosis), alkalosis (eg, emesis with loss of gas-
(Continued)

pH, Blood *(Continued)*

tric juice); evaluate acid-base balance, significance of serum or plasma potassium levels; work up hypokalemia; use of oxyhemoglobin dissociation curves. May be useful for assessment of birth asphyxia in the depressed newborn. **Increased** with uncompensated metabolic and respiratory alkalosis, **decreased** with uncompensated metabolic and respiratory acidosis. **LIMITATIONS:** pH values are sensitive to sampling technique. Concurrent metabolic acidosis and respiratory alkalosis may result in normal pH[1], pCO_2, HCO_3, and anion gap, but abnormality might be detected by potassium level and blood volume measurement. Organic acidemias of infancy are beyond the scope of this manual. **METHODOLOGY:** Glass pH electrode **ADDITIONAL INFORMATION:** pH should be judged in relation to other parameters such as pCO_2, HCO_3, Na^+, K^+, Cl^-, glucose, ketone bodies, phosphorus, and lactic acid, BUN, creatinine, and osmolality of serum and urine. A small amount of information about some acid base disorders is provided in the Anion Gap listing and the references which are included. The osmolal gap is addressed in the listing Osmolality, Calculated.

Causes of metabolic acidosis with normal and with increased anion gap are provided in Footnote 2. See Anion Gap listing as well.

Methanol, ethylene glycol, paraldehyde, and salicylate toxicity, diabetic ketoacidosis, alcoholic ketoacidosis, lactic acidosis, renal failure, and starvation are causes of **high anion gap metabolic acidosis**.

Additional to electrolytes and other tests listed above, relevant laboratory findings in acidemia may also include ketones, ethanol concentration, uric acid, albumin, CBC, urinalysis with examination for oxalate crystals, and salicylate concentration.

Hypoproteinemia causes a metabolic alkalosis.[3]

Umbilical artery pH may be useful in the assessment of birth asphyxia[4,5] of the depressed neonate. Others contend that infants must be severely depressed with Apgar scores ≤3 at 1 and 5 minutes to be reflected in a decreased serum pH.[6] Blood may be obtained from a clamped umbilical segment up to 1 hour after delivery.[7]

In hypotensive patients, tissue hypoxia may be assessed by measurements of arterial pH, mixed venous pH, and bicarbonate concentrations.[8] Such measurements do not appear to reliably assess tissue hypoxia in patients with fulminant hepatic failure.[9] For such patients, oxygen flux (the difference between arterial and venous oxygen) remains the best way to detect the presence of covert tissue hypoxia.

Footnotes

1. Bruegger BB and Sherwin JE, "Blood Gas Analysis and Oxygen Saturation," *Methods in Clinical Chemistry*, Chapter 8, Pesce AJ and Kaplan LA, eds, St Louis, MO: Mosby-Year Book Inc, 1987, 54-66.
2. Narins RG and Emmett M, "Simple and Mixed Acid-Base Disorders: A Practical Approach," *Medicine (Baltimore)*, 1980, 59:161-87.
3. McAuliffe JJ, Lind LJ, Leith DE, et al, "Hypoproteinemic Alkalosis," *Am J Med*, 1986, 81:86-90.
4. Nicolaides KH, Economides DL, and Soothill PW, "Blood Gases, pH, and Lactate in Appropriate- and Small-for-Gestational-Age Fetuses," *Am J Obstet Gynecol*, 1989, 161(4):996-1001.
5. Thorp JA, Sampson JE, Parisi VM, et al, "Routine Umbilical Cord Blood Gas Determinations?" *Am J Obstet Gynecol*, 1989, 161(3):600-5.
6. Gilstrap LC 3d, Leveno KJ, Burris J, et al, "Diagnosis of Birth Asphyxia on the Basis of Fetal pH, Apgar Score, and Newborn Cerebral Dysfunction," *Am J Obstet Gynecol*, 1989, 161(3):825-30.
7. Duerbeck NB, Chaffin DG, and Seeds JW, "A Practical Approach to Umbilical Artery pH and Blood Gas Determinations," *Obstet Gynecol*, 1992, 79(6):959-62.
8. Adrogué HJ, Rashad MN, Gorin AB, et al, "Assessing Acid-Base Status in Circulatory Failure: Differences Between Arterial and Central Venous Blood," *N Engl J Med*, 1989, 320(20):1312-6.
9. Wendon JA, Harrison PM, Keays R, et al, "Arterial-Venous pH Differences and Tissue Hypoxia in Patients With Fulminant Hepatic Failure," *Crit Care Med*, 1991, 19:(11)1362-4.

References

Adrogué HJ, Wilson H, Boyd AE III, et al, "Plasma Acid-Base Patterns in Diabetic Ketoacidosis," *N Engl J Med*, 1982, 307:1603-10.

Preuss HG, "Fundamentals of Clinical Acid-Base Evaluation," *Clin Lab Med*, 1993, 13:103-16.

Shapiro BA, "pH and Blood Gas Measurements: Discerning Innovation From Sophistication," *Crit Care Med*, 1989, 17(9):966.

Shapiro BA, Cane RD, Chomka CM, et al, "Preliminary Evaluation of an Intra-arterial Blood Gas System in Dogs and Humans," *Crit Care Med*, 1989, 17(5):455-60.

Wang F, Butler T, Rabbani GH, et al, "The Acidosis of Cholera: Contributions of Hyperproteinemia, Lactic Acidemia, and Hyperphosphatemia to an Increased Serum Anion Gap," *N Engl J Med*, 1986, 315:1591-5.

pH Body Fluid *see* Body Fluid pH *on page 150*

Phenformin *see* Lactic Acid, Blood *on page 273*

Phenylalanine, Blood

***CPT** 84030 (Guthrie)*

Related Information

Amino Acid Screen, Plasma *on page 118*
Amino Acid Screen, Qualitative, Urine *on page 120*
Newborn Screen for Hypothyroidism and Phenylketonuria *on page 295*
Phenylalanine Test, Urine *on page 1142*

Synonyms Guthrie Test; Hyperphenylalaninemia Screen; Phenylalanine Screening Test, Blood; Phenylketonuria Test; PKU Test

Abstract Autosomal recessive aminoacidopathy due to phenylalanine hydroxylase or biopterin (folic acid constituent) cofactor deficiencies. Detection by low cost dried blood spot screening can result in early treatment, sparing the afflicted individual from mental retardation.

Patient Care PREPARATION: Newborn should have milk (protein) feeding ideally for 48 hours before testing; sample as late as possible prior to discharge from hospital. Collection is recommended at 4-10 days for low birth weight infants.

Specimen Whole blood, serum or plasma CONTAINER: Newborns: PKU test card; screening: filter paper sheet. Pediatric: Small red top tube, gray top (sodium fluoride) tube or green top (heparin) tube; check with laboratory SAMPLING TIME: Just before infant is discharged from the nursery COLLECTION: Test card must be labeled with patient's name, date, time, date of birth and time of first milk feeding. In order to obtain accurate tests results for PKU, blood collection should preferably be made when the infant is 48-120 hours of age and has been on a protein feeding for at least 24 hours. Do not oversaturate filter paper. Do not fill circles on one side and then fill circles on reverse side. Do not collect blood with a capillary tube to apply to filter paper. Include information regarding blood transfusions and antibiotics or other medications administered to the infant, which may influence screening test results. STORAGE INSTRUCTIONS: Newborns: Air dry specimens at room temperature in a horizontal position for at least 2 hours. Do not use hermetically sealed envelopes. Pediatric: Separate serum and transfer to plastic vial containing 10 mg NaF. (Check with laboratory for other possible specimen requirements.) Separate within 4 hours of collection. Serum or plasma is stable 5 days at 4°C. Care in handling the filter paper specimens is essential, because exposure to extreme heat or light or touching the filter paper portion of the form can cause erroneous test results. Specimens containing contaminants, such as alcohol or other liquids, or antibiotics may not be satisfactory for testing. (See following discussion.) The phenylalanine in filter paper dried blood spots is stable for years when not exposed to environmental extremes. CAUSES FOR REJECTION: Filter paper not thoroughly saturated, inadequate specimen identification, specimens which are re-spotted (several drops of blood applied to the same circle), specimens which are QNS (quantity not sufficient). **Cord blood cannot be used. Phenylalanine is not significantly increased at birth.** Blood should not be drawn before milk diet of at least 24 hours prior to sampling, but need to sample before discharge from the nursery may take priority if outpatient sampling is not assured.

Interpretive REFERENCE RANGE: ≤2 mg/dL (SI: ≤121 μmol/L) by Guthrie bacterial-inhibition assay; <4 mg/dL (SI: <242 μmol/L) by fluorometry in some laboratories POSSIBLE PANIC RANGE: ≥4 mg/dL (SI: ≥242 μmol/L) by Guthrie bacterial-inhibition assay. Specific diagnosis after identification of a candidate case (by screening program) requires that plasma levels of phenylalanine be >2 mg/dL (SI: >121 μmol/L) on 2 consecutive days. USE: Evaluate patients for phenylketonuria, monitor therapy with phenylalanine restricted diet LIMITATIONS: Cases have been missed because blood phenylalanine was not increased, even after the third day of life.[1] Identification of non-PKU forms of hyperphenylalaninemia (see following information) requires additional testing for tetrahydrobiopterin pathway enzyme defects. **Not all individuals with increased blood phenylalanine have phenylketonuria.** When the infant is tested for PKU before 24 hours of age, there is a 16% chance of missing a positive case. When screened between 24 and 48 hours of birth, there is a 2.2% chance of missing a positive, between 48 and 72 hours, 0.3% chance. METHODOLOGY: Guthrie testing (microbiologic inhibition assay) (semiquantitative), chromatography, fluorometry ADDITIONAL INFORMATION: Successful detection of phenylketonuria by screening newborns for hyperphenylalaninemia has as its goal the identification of infants subject to central nervous system damage (in particular mental retardation) due to excessive levels of phenylalanine. Once identified, harmful CNS effects can be largely

(Continued)

Phenylalanine, Blood *(Continued)*

avoided by dietary measures, notably a semisynthetic diet low in phenylalanine. In young PKU patients, the tolerance for dietary phenylalanine (to maintain nontoxic plasma levels) is about 250-550 mg/day. Widespread institution of PKU screening programs, worldwide, is an outstanding public health triumph of the 20th century. Incidence is 1:10,000 to 1:25,000 in the United States. For blacks in Maryland the reported incidence is 1:50,000.[2]

State laws require PKU testing of infants within 28 days or less; in some states, prior to hospital discharge regardless of age. Disease caused by lack of phenylalanine hydroxylase leads to mental retardation if not treated. A second screening should be considered but is not universally mandated in infants whose first test occurred within the first 24 hours of life. Screening generally includes testing for hypothyroidism and in some areas for galactosemia and maple syrup disease as well as for phenylketonuria. Every effort must be made to assure that immediate diagnosis and treatment is provided for infants with abnormal results.

Presence of hyperphenylalaninemia implies a disorder of phenylalanine hydroxylation (to tyrosine). PKU due to phenylalanine hydroxylase (PAH) deficiency is the common example. However, in addition to PAH, hydroxylation requires oxygen and tetrahydrobiopterin (BH_4) as a cofactor. A defect in the metabolism of BH_4 that results in BH_4 deficiency will impair the hydroxylation and result in increased plasma phenylalanine concentrations. In the past 15 years three types of inborn errors of BH_4 metabolism ("atypical PKU") have been identified. Defects in BH_4 synthesis are guanosine triphosphate cyclohydrolase I deficiency and pyruvoyl tetrahydropterin synthase deficiency. The third type of defect involves the regeneration of BH_4 catalyzed by the enzyme dihydropteridine reductase. Experience with treatment of PKU over the past 25 years has shown that some 3% (variable between different populations) fail to respond.[3] These are largely cases of BH_4 cofactor deficiency. There are important differences in therapy between classical PKU and the various BH_4 cofactor deficiencies. "PKU positive" cases (identified as the result of phenylalanine screening tests) should be additionally tested for BH_4 deficiency. Clinical features; urine, blood, and enzyme analyses; prenatal diagnosis; and therapy of BH_4 deficiencies have been recently reviewed.[3]

Classical PKU is an autosomal recessive disorder. Relatives (eg, siblings) of a PKU homozygote or heterozygote have a 50% to 66.7% probability of being heterozygous for PKU. DNA hybridization techniques are undergoing evaluation for the identification of PKU heterozygotes.[4]

To maintain intellectual function, the importance of long-term (eg, beyond 10 years) dietary control of the blood phenylalanine level has been recently re-emphasized.[5,6] Significant phenylalanine hydroxylation *in vivo* in PKU homozygotes has been demonstrated.[7] Such findings suggest significant alternative pathway activity such as tyrosine hydroxylase. Promotion of such latent hydroxylating capabilities may eventually lead to therapies which will complement phenylalanine restriction.

Spuriously high blood phenylalanine levels (false-positives) may occur with Guthrie test screening due to uninterpretable "clear zone" effect, the result of antibiotics (usually ampicillin). Because of an increase in the number of cases and amounts of the awards in litigation involving PKU screening (usually false-negative cases), vagaries of PKU testing, while uncommon, are of considerable import and generate comment and innovation.[8,9,10]

A reference by Scriver et al provides a comprehensive review of the genetics and molecular biology of the hyperphenylalaninemias.

Intrauterine fetal injury results from exposure of the developing fetus to increased intrapartum maternal plasma phenylalanine levels. There is a high incidence of resultant fetal damage including microcephaly, intrauterine growth retardation, mental retardation, and congenital heart disease, as a result of maternal hyperphenylalaninemia.[11] Dietary management of mothers identified by newborn screening programs has as its goal the maintenance of near normal maternal phenylalaninemia throughout pregnancy.[12] In order to retain the achievements of over three decades of early detection and treatment of PKU, increasing attention is being turned to control of maternal hyperphenylalaninemia. The risk of maternal phenylketonuria and hyperphenylalaninemia syndrome is increasing. There is a nearly 100% risk of recurrence if treatment is not given. A number of suggestions have been made to deal with the growing problem of maternal PKU including use of genetic registers.[13] Polymerase chain reaction amplification of specific alleles, a modification of PCR technology, has been applied to screening for carriers of PKU.[14]

Footnotes

1. Committee on Genetics. American Academy of Pediatrics, "New Issues in Newborn Screening for Phenylketonuria and Congenital Hypothyroidism," *Pediatrics*, 1982, 69:104-6.
2. Hofman KJ, Steel G, Kazazian HH, et al, "Phenylketonuria in U.S. Blacks: Molecular Analysis of the Phenylalanine Hydroxylase Gene," *Am J Hum Genet*, 1991, 48(4):791-8.
3. Matalon R, Michals K, Blau N, et al, "Hyperphenylalaninemia Due to Inherited Deficiencies of Tetrahydrobiopterin," *Advanced Pediatrics*, eds, Barness LA, DeViro DC, Morrow G, et al, Chicago, IL: Year Book Medical Publishers, 1989, 36:67-89.
4. Lehmann WD, "Progress in the Identification of the Heterozygote in Phenylketonuria," *J Pediatr*, 1989, 114(6):915-24.
5. Waisbren SE, Mahon BE, Schnell RR, et al, "Predictors of Intelligence Quotient and Intelligence Quotient Change in Persons Treated for Phenylketonuria Early in Life," *Pediatrics*, 1987, 79:351-5.
6. Michals K, Azen C, Acosta P, et al, "Blood Phenylalanine Levels and Intelligence of 10-Year-Old Children With PKU in the National Collaborative Study," *J Am Diet Assoc*, 1988, 88(10):1226-9.
7. Thompson GN and Halliday D, "Significant Phenylalanine Hydroxylation *In Vivo* in Patients With Classical Phenylketonuria," *J Clin Invest*, 1990, 86(1):317-22.
8. Mabry CC, Reid MC, and Kuhn RJ, "A Source of Error in Phenylketonuria Screening," *Am J Clin Pathol*, 1988, 90(3):279-83.
9. Clemens PC and Plettner C, "Phenylketonuria Screening: Avoiding a Source of Error by Simplifying the Procedure," *Am J Clin Pathol*, 1989, 91(6):747, (letter).
10. Wilcken B, Brown AR, Liu A, et al, "Eliminating Some Possible Errors in Phenylketonuria Screening," *Am J Clin Pathol*, 1989, 92(3):396, (letter).
11. Brenton DP, "Cardiac Defects in the Children of Mothers With High Concentrations of Plasma Phenylalanine," *Br Heart J*, 1990, 63(3):143-4.
12. Thompson GN, Francis DEM, Kirby DM, et al, "Pregnancy in Phenylketonuria: Dietary Treatment Aimed at Normalising Maternal Plasma Phenylalanine Concentration," *Arch Dis Child*, 1991, 66(11):1346-9.
13. Luder AS and Greene CL, "Maternal Phenylketonuria and Hyperphenylalaninemia: Implications for Medical Practice in the United States," *Am J Obstet Gynecol*, 1989, 161(5):1102-5.
14. Sommer SS, Cassady JD, Sobell JL, et al, "A Novel Method for Detecting Point Mutations or Polymorphisms and Its Application to Population Screening for Carriers of Phenylketonuria," *Mayo Clin Proc*, 1989, 64(11):1361-72.

References

American Academy of Pediatrics Committee on Genetics, "Newborn Screening Fact Sheets: Phenylketonuria," *Pediatrics*, 1989, 83:461-2.

Atherton ND, "HPLC Measurement of Phenylalanine by Direct Injection of Plasma Onto an Internal-Surface Reverse-Phase Silica Support," *Clin Chem*, 1989, 35(6):975-8.

Gerasimova NS, Steklova IV, and Tuuminen T, "Fluorometric Method for Phenylalanine Microplate Assay Adapted for Phenylketonuria Screening," *Clin Chem*, 1989, 35(10):2112-5.

Scriver CR, Kaufman S, and Woo SLC, "The Hyperphenylalaninemias," *The Metabolic Basis of Inherited Disease*, 6th ed, Vol 1, Scriver CR, Beaudet AL, Sly WS, et al, eds, New York, NY: McGraw-Hill Inc, 1989, 495-546.

Tessari P, Inchiostro S, Vettore M, et al, "A Fast High-Performance Liquid Chromatographic Method for the Measurement of Plasma Concentration and Specific Activity of Phenylalanine," *Clin Biochem*, 1991, 24(5):425-8.

Phenylalanine Hydroxylase Activity *see* Newborn Screen for Hypothyroidism and Phenylketonuria *on page 295*

Phenylalanine Screening Test, Blood *see* Phenylalanine, Blood *on page 317*

Phenylketonuria, Newborn Screen *see* Newborn Screen for Hypothyroidism and Phenylketonuria *on page 295*

Phenylketonuria Test *see* Phenylalanine, Blood *on page 317*

Phosphatase, Acid *see* Acid Phosphatase *on page 96*

Phosphatase, Alkaline *see* Alkaline Phosphatase, Serum *on page 109*

Phosphatidylglycerol *see* Amniotic Fluid Lecithin/Sphingomyelin Ratio and Phosphatidylglycerol *on page 124*

Phosphatidylinositol *see* Amniotic Fluid Lecithin/Sphingomyelin Ratio and Phosphatidylglycerol *on page 124*

Phosphorus, Serum

CPT *84100*

Related Information

Alcohol, Blood or Urine *on page 936*

(Continued)

Phosphorus, Serum *(Continued)*

Calcium, Serum *on page 160*
Ketone Bodies, Blood *on page 265*
Kidney Stone Analysis *on page 1129*
Parathyroid Hormone *on page 311*

Synonyms PO_4, Blood

Abstract With exclusion of factitious types of hyperphosphatemia, causes of increased phosphate include diminished glomerular filtration, increased absorption in the renal tubules, and/or increased exogenous or endogenous phosphate loads. Hypophosphatemia and its complications are outlined.

Patient Care PREPARATION: Ideally, patient should be fasting. Phosphate levels are lower following meals.

Specimen Serum CONTAINER: Red top tube COLLECTION: Pediatric: Blood drawn from heelstick for capillary STORAGE INSTRUCTIONS: Serum should be promptly separated from the clot to avoid false elevations. CAUSES FOR REJECTION: Observable hemolysis

Interpretive REFERENCE RANGE: Both low and high ends of the normal range are higher in children than in adults. Children: approximately 4.0-6.0 mg/dL (SI: 1.29-1.94 mmol/L). Adults: 2.5-4.5 mg/dL (SI: 0.81-1.45 mmol/L). Some variation exists among authorities. POSSIBLE PANIC RANGE: <1.0 mg/dL is critical USE: Causes of **high phosphorus:** Youth; exercise; dehydration and hypovolemia; high phosphorus content enema; acromegaly; hypoparathyroidism; pseudohypoparathyroidism; bone metastases; hypervitaminosis D; sarcoidosis; milk-alkali syndrome; liver disease, such as portal cirrhosis; catastrophic events such as cardiac resuscitation, pulmonary embolism, renal failure; diabetes mellitus with ketosis; serum artifact – sample not refrigerated; overheated, hemolyzed sample, or serum allowed to remain too long on the clot.

Although phosphate accumulation occurs as renal disease progresses, hyperphosphatemia is not a feature of early renal failure;[1] it does not usually develop before renal function has diminished to about 25% of normal.[2] Osteitis fibrosa in uremic subjects, from excessive bone turnover, relates to hyperphosphatasia. The role of hyperphosphatemia in promotion of such secondary hyperparathyroidism is well established.[3] A relationship to osteomalacia in hemodialysis patients exists.[3]

Causes of **low phosphorus:** (Hypophosphatemia may occur with or without phosphate depletion. Serum levels vary as much as 2.0 mg/dL (SI: 0.65 mmol/L) during the day.)

Very severely malnourished subjects may have low phosphate levels, but even in starvation, phosphorus levels usually are normal. Antacids, diuretics, and long-term steroids are among the common agents bearing a relationship to severe hypophosphatemia.[4] Recent carbohydrate ingestion decreases phosphorus, as does intravenous glucose administration; cases of hypophosphatemia relate to I.V. carbohydrate,[4] dialysis, hyperalimentation, prolonged intravenous administration of phosphate-free fluids, metabolic states involving glucose, potassium, and pH. Depletion of phosphate occurs in diabetic ketoacidosis. Like potassium, phosphorus returns to the cell with therapy of diabetic ketoacidosis, and serum levels may diminish significantly during treatment. Osmotic diuresis induced by glycosuria in poorly controlled diabetes may lead to urinary phosphate losses with negative phosphorus balance. PO_4 levels may prove useful in initiation of insulin therapy, in diabetic ketoacidosis and other situations of insulin lack; with hyperglucagonemia, corticosteroid and epinephrine use, and in respiratory alkalosis. Association of hypophosphatemia with impaired glucose metabolism is thought to reflect decreased tissue sensitivity to insulin.[5] Alcoholism and other hepatic disorders are found very frequently among patients with low PO_4. Alcoholic ketosis and alcohol withdrawal are among causes of hypophosphatemia. There is a slight decrease in serum phosphorus in the last trimester of pregnancy.

Primary hyperparathyroidism and other causes of calcium elevation, including ectopic hyperparathyroidism (pseudohyperparathyroidism).

Patients with sepsis, including Legionnaires' disease and other respiratory infections. Twenty-two percent of instances of respiratory infections had serum phosphorous ≤ 2.4.[6] Halevy and Bulvik report gram-negative septicemia as a common cause of severe hypophosphatemia among 55,000 chemistry profiles of hospitalized patients they studied.[4] (Hypophosphatemia impairs bactericidal activity).

Vitamin D deficiency; osteomalacia, inherited and sporadic forms of hypophosphatemic rickets. In work-up for osteomalacia, look for decreased calcium and phosphorus and increased alkaline phosphatase. Biopsy, however, can be abnormal even when these biochemical parameters are within normal limits.

Renal tubular disorders (Fanconi syndrome, renal tubular acidosis); use of antacids that bind phosphorus (look for hypercalciuria, low urinary phosphorus, high alkaline phosphatase);[7] dialysis, vomiting; saline or lactate I.V.; steatorrhea, malabsorption, severe diarrhea, nasogastric suction; hypokalemia; negative nitrogen balance; decreased dietary PO_4 intake; recovery from severe burn injury; salicylate poisoning; acute gout; tumor-related: described as including hemangiopericytomas (uncommon pathologic entities) and neurofibromatosis; transfusion of blood; arteriography.

The signs and symptoms of phosphate depletion may include neuromuscular, neuropsychiatric, gastrointestinal, skeletal, and cardiopulmonary systems. Manifestations usually are accompanied by serum levels <1.0 mg/dL (SI: <0.32 mmol/L).

Severe hypophosphatemia is most common in elderly patients and is often found in postoperative subjects.[4]

Complications of hypophosphatemia: Effect on RBC 2,3-diphosphoglycerate and oxygen dissociation.[8] Depression of myocardial function (contractibility), decreased cardiac output; respiratory failure and respiratory muscle weakness; increased incidence of sepsis, impairment of bactericidal activities.[9] CNS consequences: polyradiculopathy, paresthesias, tremor, ataxia, weakness, slurred speech, stupor, coma, seizure; joint stiffness; myopathy; renal stones, hypercalciuria secondary to renal phosphate leak; insulin resistance, glucose intolerance. Rhabdomyolysis may complicate marked hypophosphatemia. A mortality rate of 20% is described in patients whose phosphorus concentration was 1.1-1.5 mg/dL (SI: 0.36-0.48 mmol/L).[4]

LIMITATIONS: Ninety-seven percent of hyperparathyroid subjects with normal renal function have <3.3 mg/dL serum phosphate, 80% <3.0 mg/dL and 40% <2.5 mg/dL.[10] Collection of multiple data points throughout the day may help to establish the diagnosis of primary hyperparathyroidism in patients with borderline serum biochemistries.[11] Thus, some hyperparathyroid patients have serum phosphorus levels within normal limits. Hemolysis, glassware contaminated with detergents, hyperbilirubinemia, or dysproteinemia may cause increased results. Spurious hyperphosphatemia may be due to increased serum triglycerides.[12] Phosphorus measurement on the Du Pont aca® was reported to be low with I.V. mannitol administration.[13,14,15] Falsely elevated serum phosphate concentrations have been reported in patients with multiple myeloma using a molybdate colorimetric assay on the Hitachi® 717.[16] Drug effects have been summarized.[17] **CONTRAINDICATIONS:** Sampling not long after a phosphorus-containing enema can provide startlingly high PO_4 levels. **METHODOLOGY:** Phosphomolybdate – colorimetric; modified molybdate – enzymatic, colorimetric[16] **ADDITIONAL INFORMATION:** Increasing dietary intake of potassium has been reported to increase serum phosphate concentrations apparently by decreasing renal excretion of phosphate.[18] During the last trimester of pregnancy, there is a sixfold increase in calcium and phosphorus accumulation as the fetus triples its weight. Plasma phosphorus concentrations may provide a useful means to assess response to phosphate supplements in the premature infant.[19]

Footnotes

1. Hakim RM and Lazarus JM, "Biochemical Parameters in Chronic Renal Failure," *Am J Kidney Dis*, 1988, 11(3):238-47.
2. Coburn JW and Salusky IB, "Control of Serum Phosphorus in Uremia," *N Engl J Med*, 1989, 320(17):1140-2, (editorial).
3. Delmez JA, Fallon MD, Harter HR, et al, "Does Strict Phosphorus Control Precipitate Renal Osteomalacia?" *J Clin Endocrinol Metab*, 1986, 62:747-52.
4. Halevy J and Bulvik S, "Severe Hypophosphatemia in Hospitalized Patients," *Arch Intern Med*, 1988, 148(1):153-5.
5. DeFronzo RA and Lang R, "Hypophosphatemia and Glucose Intolerance: Evidence for Tissue Insensitivity to Insulin," *N Engl J Med*, 1980, 303:1259-63.
6. Fisher J, Magid N, Kallman C, et al, "Respiratory Illness and Hypophosphatemia," *Chest*, 1983, 83: 504-8.
7. Insogna KL, Bordley DR, Caro JF, et al, "Osteomalacia and Weakness From Excessive Antacid Ingestion," *JAMA*, 1980, 244:2544-6.
8. Lichtman MA, Miller DR, Cohen J, et al, "Reduced Red Cell Glycolysis, 2,3-Diphosphoglycerate and Adenosine Triphosphate Concentration, and Increased Hemoglobin-Oxygen Affinity Caused by Hypophosphatemia," *Ann Intern Med*, 1971, 74:562-8.
9. Knochel JP, "The Pathophysiology and Clinical Characteristics of Severe Hypophosphatemia," *Arch Intern Med*, 1977, 137:203-20.

(Continued)

Phosphorus, Serum *(Continued)*

10. Kao PC, "Parathyroid Hormone Assay," *Mayo Clin Proc*, 1982, 57:596-7.
11. Lobaugh B, Neelon FA, Oyama H, et al, "Circadian Rhythms for Calcium, Inorganic Phosphorus, and Parathyroid Hormone in Primary Hyperparathyroidism: Functional and Practical Considerations," *Surgery*, 1989, 106(6):1009-16.
12. Leehey DJ, Daugirdas JT, and Ing TS, "Spurious Hyperphosphatemia Due to Hyperlipidemia," *Arch Intern Med*, 1985, 145:743-4.
13. Donhowe JM, Freier EF, Wong ET, et al, "Factitious Hypophosphatemia Related to Mannitol Therapy," *Clin Chem*, 1981, 27:1765-9.
14. Landesman PW, Lott JA, and Zager RA, "Mannitol Interferes With the Du Pont aca® Method for Inorganic Phosphorus," *Clin Chem*, 1982, 28:1994-5.
15. McCoy MT, Aguanno JJ, and Ritzmann SE, "Interferences of Mannitol With Phosphate Determination," *Am J Clin Pathol*, 1982, 77:468-70.
16. Bakker AJ, Bosma H, and Christen PJ, "Influence of Monoclonal Immunoglobulins in Three Different Methods for Inorganic Phosphorus," *Ann Clin Biochem*, 1990, 27(Pt 3):227-31.
17. Hitz J, Jaudon MC, and Galli A, "Phosphates," *Drug Effects on Laboratory Test Results Analytical Interferences and Pharmacological Effects*, Siest G and Galteau MM, eds, Littleton, MA: PSG Publishing Co Inc, 1988, 330-43.
18. Sebastian A, Hernandez RE, Portale AA, et al, "Dietary Potassium Influences Kidney Maintenance of Serum Phosphorus Concentration," *Kidney Int*, 1990, 37(5):1341-9.
19. Mayne PD and Kovar IZ, "Calcium and Phosphorus Metabolism in the Premature Infant," *Ann Clin Biochem*, 1991, 28(Pt 2):131-42.

References

Bourke E and Yanagawa M, "Assessment of Hyperphosphatemia and Hypophosphatemia," *Clin Lab Med*, 1993, 13(1):183-207.

Chan GM, Mileur L, and Hansen JW, "Calcium and Phosphorus Requirements in Bone Mineralization of Preterm Infants," *J Pediatr*, 1988, 113:225-9.

Gravelyn TR, Brophy N, Siegert C, et al, "Hypophosphatemia-Associated Respiratory Muscle Weakness in a General Inpatient Population," *Am J Med*, 1988, 84:870-6.

Hanukoglu A, Chalew SA, Sun CJ, et al, "Surgically Curable Hypophosphatemic Rickets. Diagnosis and Management," *Clin Pediatr (Phila)*, 1989, 28(7):321-5.

Laaban J-P, Waked M, Laromiguiere M, et al, "Hypophosphatemia Complicating Management of Acute Severe Asthma," *Ann Intern Med*, 1990, 112(1):68-9.

O'Connor LR, Klein KL, and Bethume JE, "Hyperphosphatemia in Lactic Acidosis," *N Engl J Med*, 1977, 297:707-9.

Peach H, Compston JE, Vedi S, et al, "Value of Plasma Calcium, Phosphate, and Alkaline Phosphatase Measurements in the Diagnosis of Histological Osteomalacia," *J Clin Pathol*, 1982, 35:625-30.

Tieder M, Modai D, Samuel R, et al, "Hereditary Hypophosphatemic Rickets With Hypercalciuria," *N Engl J Med*, 1985, 312:611-7.

Watchko J, Bifano EM, and Bergstrom WH, "Effect of Hyperventilation on Total Calcium, Ionized Calcium, and Serum Phosphorus in Neonates," *Crit Care Med*, 1984, 12:1055-6.

Weintraub Z, Iancu TC, Sheinfeld M, et al, "Urinary and Blood Levels of Adenosine 3', 5'-Monophosphate, Phosphorus, and Calcium in Infants," *Biol Neonate*, 1989, 55(4-5):233-7.

Phosphorus, Urine

CPT *84105*

Related Information

Calcitonin *on page 157*
Calcium, Serum *on page 160*
Calcium, Urine *on page 163*
Growth Hormone *on page 245*
Kidney Stone Analysis *on page 1129*
Parathyroid Hormone *on page 311*
Parietal Cell Antibody *on page 730*

Synonyms Urine Phosphorus

Test Commonly Includes Phosphorus on random or timed urine specimen

Specimen Timed or random urine. Diurnal variation exists. **CONTAINER:** Plastic urine container **COLLECTION:** For 24-hour urine collection: Instruct the patient to void at 8 AM and discard the specimen. Then collect all urine including the final specimen voided at the end of the 24-hour collection period (ie, 8 AM the next morning). Container must be labeled with patient's name, date and time collection started and date and time collection finished. **STORAGE INSTRUCTIONS:** Refrigerate. Laboratory adjusts final pH of urine aliquot to 6.

Interpretive **REFERENCE RANGE:** Adults: 0.9-1.3 g/24 hours (SI: 29-42 mmol/day), dependent on dietary intake **USE:** Evaluate calcium/phosphorus balance. **High** urinary phosphorus (ie, increased renal losses) occurs in primary hyperparathyroidism, vitamin D deficiency, renal tubular acidosis, diuretic use. Phosphates are among the substances which may be lost in the

Fanconi syndrome. Renal loss of phosphate may itself lead to rickets or osteomalacia. **Low** in hypoparathyroidism, pseudohypoparathyroidism, vitamin D intoxication

Evaluate nephrolithiasis. Hypophosphatemia with normal serum calcium, high alkaline phosphatase, hypercalciuria, low urinary phosphorus occurs with osteomalacia from excessive antacid ingestion. Observations of renal phosphate excretion have led to the classical theory of a maximal transport capacity (T_m). By this model, phosphate is reabsorbed to a maximum rate after which phosphate appears in the urine once the T_m is exceeded. Mechanisms and effectors of reabsorption are described.[1] The following table lists some important effectors of phosphate transport in the proximal nephron. Largely, however, urine phosphate simply reflects phosphate intake in patients not on phosphate-binding medications.

Effects on Phosphorus Transport

Atrial natriuretic peptide	↓
Calcitonin	↓
Glucocorticoid	↑
Growth hormone	↑
Insulin-like growth factor-I	↑
Metabolic acidosis (chronic)	↓
Metabolic alkalosis	↑
Parathyroid hormone	↓
Parathyroid hormone-related peptide (HHM factor)	↓
Phosphorus supply	↑ or ↓
Vasopressin	↓
Vitamin D	↑
Volume expansion	↓

From Hruska KA, "Phosphate Balance and Metabolism," *The Principles and Practice of Nephrology,* Chapter 19, Jacobson HR, Striker GE, and Klahr S, eds, Philadelphia, PA: Mosby-Year Book Inc, 1991, 122, with permission.

METHODOLOGY: Enzymatic, colorimetric[2] **ADDITIONAL INFORMATION:** Children with thalassemia may have normal phosphorus absorption but high renal phosphaturia, leading to a deficiency of phosphorus. Increasing dietary intake of potassium has been reported to increase serum phosphate concentrations apparently by decreasing renal excretion of phosphate.[3] During the last trimester of pregnancy, there is a sixfold increase in calcium and phosphorus accumulation as the fetus triples its weight. Plasma phosphorus concentrations and increased urinary phosphate may provide a useful means to assess response to phosphate supplements in the premature infant.[4]

Footnotes

1. Hruska KA, "Phosphate Balance and Metabolism," *The Principles and Practice of Nephrology*, Chapter 19, Jacobson HR, Striker GE, and Klahr S, eds, Philadelphia, PA: BC Decker Inc, 1991, 122.
2. Berti G, Fossati P, Tarenghi G, et al, "Enzymatic Colorimetric Method for the Determination of Inorganic Phosphorus in Serum and Urine," *J Clin Chem Clin Biochem*, 1988, 26:399-404.
3. Sebastian A, Hernandez RE, Portale AA, et al, "Dietary Potassium Influences Kidney Maintenance of Serum Phosphorus Concentration," *Kidney Int*, 1990, 37(5):1341-9.
4. Mayne PD and Kovar IZ, "Calcium and Phosphorus Metabolism in the Premature Infant," *Ann Clin Biochem*, 1991, 28(Pt 2):131-42.

References

Bakker AJ, Bosma H, and Christen PJ, "Influence of Monoclonal Immunoglobulins in Three Different Methods for Inorganic Phosphorus," *Ann Clin Biochem*, 1990, 27(Pt 3):227-31.

Juan D, "The Causes and Consequences of Hypophosphatemia," *Surg Gynecol Obstet*, 1981, 153:589-97.

Somell A and Alveryd A, "Diurnal Variations in the Urinary Excretion of Calcium and Phosphate in Hyperparathyroidism," *Acta Chir Scand*, 1976, 142:357-9.

Weintraub Z, Iancu TC, Sheinfeld M, et al, "Urinary and Blood Levels of Adenosine 3', 5'-Monophosphate, Phosphorus, and Calcium in Infants," *Biol Neonate*, 1989, 55(4-5):233-7.

PIIINP *see* CA 125 *on page 154*

Pituitary Gonadotropins *see* Luteinizing Hormone, Blood or Urine *on page 286*

PK Assay *see* Pyruvate Kinase Assay, Erythrocytes *on page 345*

PK Screen, Blood *see* Pyruvate Kinase Screen, Erythrocytes *on page 345*

PKU, Neonatal *see* Newborn Screen for Hypothyroidism and Phenylketonuria *on page 295*

PKU Test *see* Phenylalanine, Blood *on page 317*

Placental Lactogen, Human

CPT 83632

Related Information

Human Chorionic Gonadotropin, Serum *on page 254*

Synonyms Chorionic Somatomammotropin; hCS; hPL; Human Chorionic Somatomammotropin; Human Placental Lactogen

Abstract Related to the functional placental mass, hPL is an adjunctive rather than a definitive test.

Specimen Serum or plasma **CONTAINER:** Red top tube, lavender top (EDTA) tube, or green top (heparin) tube **STORAGE INSTRUCTIONS:** Freeze serum or plasma immediately. **CAUSES FOR REJECTION:** Recent radioactive scan

Interpretive **REFERENCE RANGE:** Varies with duration of gestation. Levels rise with advancing gestation to plateau at about 37 weeks. May reach 10 μg/mL (SI: 463 nmol/L). **CRITICAL VALUES:** Maternal serum hPL <4 μg/mL (SI: <185 nmol/L) after 30 weeks gestation; imperfect correlation exists with adverse outcome **USE:** Evaluate antepartum placental function: the maternal serum concentration correlates with placental weight; used as an index of fetal well-being, hPL tends to be low with intrauterine growth retardation **LIMITATIONS:** Single results are not as useful as a series over time. Test is not as useful as hCG in following course of trophoblastic neoplasia. Role of hPL in monitoring fetal well-being is controversial. Normal levels do not provide assurance of lack of complications. Low levels at term are especially difficult to interpret, since these have been reported in normal pregnancy. Intrauterine growth retardation is not always caused by placental disease. This test is seldom used. **METHODOLOGY:** Radioimmunoassay (RIA), turbidimetric latex immunoassay[1] **ADDITIONAL INFORMATION:** Human placental lactogen (chorionic somatomammotropin) is a growth-promoting hormone of placental origin, similar to chorionic gonadotropin. Placental lactogen appears to act through distinct PL receptors to regulate and coordinate growth and metabolism in the fetus and metabolism in the mother. Growth effects upon the fetus appear to be predominant in the first half of pregnancy. Metabolic effects appear to predominate in the last half of pregnancy.[2,3] It has been proposed that a major role of hPL is to provide optimum metabolic conditions for procurement of nutrients and use of these nutrients by the fetus, especially in the last half of pregnancy. A poor correlation of maternal serum concentrations with "fetal well-being" during the last half of pregnancy exists.

Immediately after its discovery, hPL was recommended to evaluate placental function and fetal well-being in pregnancies at risk, and prognosticate the inevitability of abortion (low levels or falling levels indicate poor prognosis). It was also recommended as a marker for trophoblastic neoplasia (elevated). These roles are controversial. Measurement of hPL has been suggested as a method for assessing gestational age.[4] hPL has been detected in some patients with nongerm cell neoplasms.[5]

High hPL may be found in instances of Rh isoimmunization and in multiple gestation, in each of which large placentas occur.[6] It is described as largely discarded in clinical practice of obstetrics.[7]

In twin pregnancy, hPL is described as an indicator of intrauterine growth retardation.[8]

Footnotes

1. Collet-Cassart D, Limet JN, Van Krieken L, et al, "Turbidimetric Latex Immunoassay of Placental Lactogen on Microtiter Plates," *Clin Chem*, 1989, 35(1):141-3.
2. Handwerger S, "Clinical Counterpoint: The Physiology of Placental Lactogen in Human Pregnancy," *Endocr Rev*, 1991, 12:329-36.
3. Parsons JA, Brelje TC, and Sorenson RL, "Adaptation of Islets of Langerhans to Pregnancy: Increased Islet Cell Proliferation and Insulin Secretion Correlates With the Onset of Placental Lactogen Secretion," *Endocrinology*, 1992, 130(3):1459-66.
4. Whittaker PG, Lind T, and Lawson JY, "A Prospective Study to Compare Serum Human Placental Lactogen and Menstrual Dates for Determining Gestational Age," *Am J Obstet Gynecol*, 1987, 156:178-82.
5. Heyderman E, Chapman DV, Richardson TC, et al, "Human Chorionic Gonadotropin and Human Placental Lactogen in Extragonadal Tumors, An Immunoperoxidase Study of Ten Nongerm Cell Neoplasms," *Cancer*, 1985, 56:2674-82.
6. Ray DA, "Biochemical Fetal Assessment," *Clin Obstet Gynecol*, 1987, 30:887-98.
7. Catanzarite VA, Perkins RP, and Pernoll ML, "Assessment of Fetal Well-Being," *Current Obstetric & Gynecologic Diagnosis & Treatment 1987*, Pernoll ML and Benson RC, eds, Norwalk, CT: Appleton & Lange, 1987, 279-302.
8. Trapp M, Kato K, Bohnet HG, et al, "Human Placental Lactogen and Unconjugated Estriol Concentrations in Twin Pregnancy: Monitoring of Fetal Development in Intrauterine Growth Retardation and Single Intrauterine Fetal Death," *Am J Obstet Gynecol*, 1986, 155:1027-31.

References

Halmesmaki E, Autti I, Granstrom ML, et al, "Alpha-Fetoprotein, Human Placental Lactogen, and Pregnancy-Specific Beta 1-Glycoprotein in Pregnant Women Who Drink: Relation to Fetal Alcohol Syndrome," *Am J Obstet Gynecol*, 1986, 155:598-602.

Hill DJ, Freemark M, Strain AJ, et al, "Placental Lactogen and Growth Hormone Receptors in Human Fetal Tissues: Relationship to Fetal Plasma Human Placental Lactogen Concentrations and Fetal Growth," *J Clin Endocrinol Metab*, 1988, 66:1283-90.

Southard JN and Talamantes F, "High Molecular Weight Forms of Placental Lactogen: Evidence for Lactogen-Macroglobulin Complexes in Rodents and Humans," *Endocrinology*, 1989, 125(2):791-800.

Stewart MO, Whittaker PG, Persson B, et al, "A Longitudinal Study of Circulating Progesterone, Oestradiol, hCG, and hPL During Pregnancy in Type I Diabetic Mothers," *Br J Obstet Gynaecol*, 1989, 96(4):415-23.

Walker WH, Fitzpatrick SL, Barrera-Saldana HA, et al, "The Human Placental Lactogen Genes: Structure, Function, Evolution, and Transcriptional Regulation," *Endocr Rev*, 1991, 12(4):316-28.

Plasma Cholinesterase *see* Pseudocholinesterase, Serum *on page 343*

Plasma Electrolytes *see* Electrolytes, Blood *on page 212*

Plasma Neuropeptide Y *see* Catecholamines, Fractionation, Plasma *on page 172*

Plasma Renin Activity *see* Renin, Plasma *on page 346*

Pleural Fluid Analysis *see* Body Fluid *on page 145*

Pleural Fluid pH *see* Body Fluid pH *on page 150*

pO_2 *see* Blood Gases, Arterial *on page 140*

pO_2 (0.5) *see* P-50 Blood Gas *on page 307*

pO_2 at Half Saturation *see* P-50 Blood Gas *on page 307*

PO_4, Blood *see* Phosphorus, Serum *on page 319*

Porphobilinogen *see* Porphyrins, Quantitative, Urine *on page 327*

Porphobilinogen *see* Uroporphyrinogen-I-Synthase *on page 381*

Porphobilinogen Deaminase Red Blood Cell *see* Uroporphyrinogen-I-Synthase *on page 381*

Porphobilinogen, Qualitative, Urine

CPT *84106*

Related Information

Delta Aminolevulinic Acid, Urine *on page 207*
Lead, Blood *on page 976*
Protoporphyrin, Free Erythrocyte *on page 341*
Urobilinogen, 2-Hour Urine *on page 1167*
Uroporphyrinogen-I-Synthase *on page 381*

Synonyms Watson-Schwartz Test

Applies to Hoesch Test

Test Commonly Includes Qualitative screen for urobilinogen and porphobilinogen

Abstract Porphobilinogen and delta aminolevulinic acid are porphyrin precursors, which are excreted.

Specimen Random urine **CONTAINER:** Any clean dark container, no preservative **COLLECTION:** Keep refrigerated during collection and thereafter. Prevent exposure to light. Some authorities suggest collecting in a dark bottle with 5 g sodium bicarbonate and keeping under refrigeration. **STORAGE INSTRUCTIONS:** Specimen may be stored for a brief period in refrigerator, but must be analyzed promptly. Adjust to pH 6-7 with sodium bicarbonate. Stabilized specimen is stable 12 hours at 25°C and 7 days at 4°C.

Interpretive **REFERENCE RANGE:** Negative **USE:** Porphobilinogen levels in the urine should be measured during acute attacks of abdominal pain, extremity pain or paresthesias, tachycardia, nausea and vomiting, neurologic abnormalities, and in the investigation of dark urine. It is a screen for **acute intermittent porphyria**, which is characterized by urinary excretion of porphobilinogen and delta aminolevulinic acid during acute attacks. The Watson-Schwartz test may detect some patients in latent periods who have acute intermittent porphyria. Increased urinary excretion of porphobilinogen may be caused also by acute attacks of **variegate porphyria** or of **hereditary coproporphyria**, and rarely in lead poisoning. In lead poisoning, uri-

(Continued)

Porphobilinogen, Qualitative, Urine *(Continued)*

nary aminolevulinic acid measurement is more useful. **LIMITATIONS:** False-negatives may occur. The major drawback of the Watson-Schwartz and Hoesch tests is the need for subjective interpretation of the visual endpoint.[1] Schreiber et al describe a new anion-exchange resin. Columns were prepared by packing polybenzimidazole resin.[1] Positive results must be confirmed by other methods, including quantitative tests for porphobilinogen and for aminolevulinic acid. A quantitative method using a condensation reaction with *p*-dimethylaminobenzaldehyde, with spectrophotometric analysis, is widely used. (Normal 0-2.0 mg/day or 0-8.8 mmol/day.)

May be negative in the patient with asymptomatic (latent) phase of acute intermittent porphyria, in whom uroporphyrinogen-I-synthase may detect the presence of acute intermittent porphyria; see listing for this assay.

The intoxication porphyrinurias (including lead poisoning) are better detected by delta aminolevulinic acid and other tests.

METHODOLOGY: Watson-Schwartz test, Ehrlich's reagent. A variant of the Watson-Schwartz test, the Hoesch test does not react with urobilinogen, an advantage. In both tests, there is a chemical interference (decrease in results) if indolic compounds (indole, indican, 5-HIAA) are present in large amounts.

Polybenzimidazole (PBI) resin columns:[1] A Dowex 2 resin is used to adsorb alkaline porphobilinogen, then acid elution of the porphobilinogen, followed by reaction with Ehrlich's reagent, and reading by spectrophotometry. The sensitivity is greatly increased.[2] Others have quantified the eluate by HPLC.[3]

ADDITIONAL INFORMATION: Acute attacks of acute intermittent porphyria are precipitated by drugs, including barbiturates, hydantoins, hormones, infection, and diet. The most common symptom of acute intermittent porphyria is abdominal pain. The most common sign is tachycardia.[4] Subjects with the porphyrias may pass urine the color of port wine. The term porphyria derives from the Greek "porphyria," an expression for the color purple.[4]

Quantitative porphobilinogen will pick up many but not all patients with acute intermittent porphyria in the latent period.

The Watson-Schwartz test is negative with cutanea tarda porphyria and in Günther's disease, congenital erythropoietic porphyria.

Footnotes

1. Schreiber WE, Jamani A, and Pudek MR, "Screening Tests for Porphobilinogen Are Insensitive. The Problem and Its Solution," *Am J Clin Pathol*, 1989, 92(5):644-9.
2. Buttery JE, Chamberlain BR, and Beng CG, "A Sensitive Method of Screening for Urinary Porphobilinogen," *Clin Chem*, 1989, 35(12):2311-2.
3. Jamani A, Pudek M, and Schreiber WE, "Liquid-Chromatographic Assay of Urinary Porphobilinogen," *Clin Chem*, 1989, 35(3):471-5.
4. Bloomer JR and Bonkovsky HL, "The Porphyrias," *Dis Mon*, 1989, 35(1):1-54.

References

Buttery JE, Carrera AM, and Pannall PR, "Analytical Sensitivity and Specificity of Two Screening Methods for Urinary Porphobilinogen," *Ann Clin Biochem*, 1990, 27(Pt 2):165-6.

Buttery JE, Chamberlain BR, and Beng CG, "Assessment of Two Anion-Exchange Resins for Direct Use in the Screening Method for Urinary Porphobilinogen," *Clin Chem*, 1990, 36(3):584.

Buttery JE and Stuart S, "Measurement of Porphobilinogen in Urine by a Simple Resin Method With Use of A Surrogate Standard," *Clin Chem*, 1991, 37(12):2133-6.

Galbraith RA, Sassa S, and Kappas A, "A Comparison of the Utility of Dowex Resin and Polybenzimidazole Aurorez Resin in the Determination of Urinary Porphobilinogen Concentrations," *Clin Chim Acta*, 1987, 164:235-9.

Holman JR and Green JB, "Acute Intermittent Porphyria. More Than Just Abdominal Pain," *Postgrad Med*, 1989, 86(5):295-8.

Porphyrins, Erythrocytes *see* Porphyrins, Quantitative, Urine *on next page*

Porphyrins, Feces *see* Porphyrins, Quantitative, Urine *on next page*

Porphyrins, Plasma *see* Porphyrins, Quantitative, Urine *on next page*

Porphyrins, Quantitative, Urine

CPT 84120

Related Information

Delta Aminolevulinic Acid, Urine *on page 207*
Protoporphyrin, Free Erythrocyte *on page 341*
Uroporphyrinogen-I-Synthase *on page 381*

Synonyms Coproporphyrins; Porphobilinogen; Uroporphyrins

Applies to Porphyrins, Erythrocytes; Porphyrins, Feces; Porphyrins, Plasma

Test Commonly Includes Uroporphyrins (octacarboxylporphyrins), heptacarboxylporphyrins, hexacarboxylporphyrins, pentacarboxylporphyrins, coproporphyrins (tetracarboxylporphrins)[1]

Abstract Porphyrins are byproducts of porphyrinogens. Accumulations of either cause porphyrias, which are characterized by increased excretion of porphyrins, porphyrinogens, or their precursors. Such precursors include delta aminolevulinic acid and porphobilinogen. The disease entities relate to specific enzyme defects.

Patient Care PREPARATION: Avoid alcohol and excessive fluid intake during collection. Phenothiazines may cause misleading porphobilinogen results.

Specimen 24-hour urine CONTAINER: Clean, dark container. Must be kept covered. COLLECTION: Check with laboratory; 5 g sodium bicarbonate is usually added to container before collection. Instruct the patient to void at 8 AM and discard the specimen. Then collect all urine including the final specimen voided at the end of the 24-hour collection period (ie, 8 AM the next morning). Specimen should be kept cool during collection. Container must be labeled with patient's name, date and time collection started, and date and time collection finished. Transport specimen immediately to the laboratory upon completion of collection. Adjust to pH 6-7 with sodium bicarbonate. STORAGE INSTRUCTIONS: Refrigerate during collection. Protect collection from light. SPECIAL INSTRUCTIONS: Do **not** expose to light.

Interpretive REFERENCE RANGE: See literature from individual laboratory. USE: Evaluate porphyrias, including those involving deficiencies of enzymes which are needed for heme synthesis and chemical porphyrias.

In **congenital erythropoietic porphyria**, elevations of urinary uroporphyrin and coproporphyrin occur, with the former exceeding the latter.

In **acute intermittent porphyria**, porphobilinogen and delta aminolevulinic acid are elevated in acute attacks, and mild increases of urinary uroporphyrin and coproporphyrin may be found. Porphobilinogen is increased in many but not all patients with acute intermittent porphyria in latent periods. Quantitative porphobilinogen is a better test than delta aminolevulinic acid overall for acute intermittent porphyria, but both are used (as well as the Watson-Schwartz test).[2]

Coproporphyrin and porphobilinogen excretion in urine are markedly increased during acute attacks of **hereditary coproporphyria**, increase of urinary uroporphyrin may be found, and increased fecal coproporphyrin III is described.

In **variegate porphyria** in acute attacks, results are similar to those of acute intermittent porphyria. Porphobilinogen and ALA are prone to become normal between attacks. Urine coproporphyrin exceeds uroporphyrin excretion during acute attacks.

Chemical porphyrias occur. Porphyrinogenic chemicals include certain halogenated hydrocarbons which cause the excretion of increased uroporphyrin.

In **lead poisoning** elevation of delta aminolevulinic acid greater than that of porphobilinogen occurs and porphobilinogen may be normal. Urinary coproporphyrin characteristically is increased. Free erythrocyte protoporphyrin is increased. Toxins such as lead interfere with heme synthesis and cause porphyrinuria.

Increased urine excretion of uroporphyrinogen, uroporphyrin, and coproporphyrin occurs in **porphyria cutanea tarda**. It is found in middle-aged men who like ethanol, young women on oral contraceptives, and in subjects on dialysis. These patients do not excrete increased porphobilinogen, but may have slight elevations of delta aminolevulinic acid.

LIMITATIONS: Increased porphobilinogen may occur in patients on oral contraceptives. This test and delta aminolevulinic acid will not detect protoporphyria. Coproporphyrinuria alone lacks specificity and sensitivity for lead screening. Erythrocyte uroporphyrinogen-I-synthase is decreased in latent acute intermittent porphyria, and is needed in patients with possible latent acute intermittent porphyria. Quantitative porphobilinogen is of value in active and in many cases of latent acute intermittent porphyria, but will miss some of the latter when compared to red cell uroporphyrinogen-I-synthase.

(Continued)

Porphyrins, Quantitative, Urine *(Continued)*

Porphyrias: Overview of Some Clinical Aspects and Chemical Findings

Disorder	Inheritance	Age of Clinical Onset	Primary Organ Involvement	Useful Tests	Primary Symptoms
Congenital erythropoietic porphyria Günther's disease	Autosomal recessive Rare	Birth — 5 y	Erythroid cells	Urinary porphyrins Fecal porphyrins Red cell porphyrins sometimes useful	Severe photosensitivity Red urine Stains diapers Hemolytic anemia
Acute intermittent porphyria Precipitating causes include barbiturates, hydantoins, sulfonamides	Autosomal dominant Most common acute hepatic porphyria in U.S.	Adults	Hepatic, probably erythroid cells	Urine porphobilinogen Urine porphyrins Urinary delta aminolevulinic acid Erythrocyte uroporphyrinogen-1-synthase Fecal porphyrins	Mild to severe neurologic/visceral symptoms Acute attacks
Hereditary coproporphyria	Autosomal dominant	Adults	Hepatic, possibly erythroid cells	Urine porphobilinogen Urine porphyrins including coproporphyrin Fecal porphyrins Erythrocyte uroporphyrinogen-1-synthase Plasma porphyrins	Similar to variegate porphyria Acute attacks
Variegate porphyria	Autosomal dominant	Adults	Hepatic, possibly erythroid cells	Urine porphobilinogen Urine porphyrins Fecal porphyrins Plasma porphyrins Erythrocyte uroporphyrinogen-1-synthase	Mild to severe photosensitivity and neurologic-visceral symptoms Acute attacks
Porphyria cutanea tarda	Unknown Most common porphyria in U.S.	Adults	Hepatic, possibly erythroid cells	Urine porphyrins Plasma porphyrins	Similar to variegate porphyria Photosensitization Liver damage
Protoporphyria	Autosomal dominant	Usually childhood	Erythroid cells, probably liver	Erythrocytic, plasma and fecal porphyrins	Photosensitization Liver damage
Acquired (intoxication) porphyria	Acquired	Children and adults	Hepatic, erythroid cells	Erythrocyte porphyrins Urinary delta aminolevulinic acid Urine porphobilinogen Urine porphyrins Fecal porphyrins	Mild photosensitivity

From Bauer JD, *Clinical Laboratory Methods*, 9th ed, St Louis, MO: Mosby-Year Book Inc, 1982, 707, with permission.

Increased urine porphyrin excretion may be secondary to other diseases (eg, hepatobiliary diseases), especially coproporphyrin excretion. These are secondary porphyrinurias. They lack increased urinary porphobilinogen or Δ-ALA, with the important exception of lead poisoning.[3]

METHODOLOGY: Chromatography, fluorometry, high performance liquid chromatography (HPLC) **ADDITIONAL INFORMATION:** The table provides an abbreviated overview of the porphyrias. Porphyrin fractionation of plasma can be done. Increases of urine porphyrins are found with congenital erythropoietic porphyria, acute intermittent porphyria, hereditary coproporphyria, variegate porphyria, and porphyria cutanea tarda.

Fecal porphyrin examination for hereditary coproporphyria, variegate porphyria, and protoporphyria can be used for adult patients. Stool examination for coproporphyrin and protoporphyrin is recommended for diagnosis of variegate porphyria.[4]

Neurologic dysfunction occurs in the **hepatic porphyrias**, the types of porphyria in which acute attacks develop: acute intermittent porphyria, variegate porphyria, hereditary coproporphyria, and ALA dehydrase deficiency. Abdominal pain, caused by autonomic neuropathy, occurs with acute attacks (eg, acute intermittent porphyria). It is the most common symptom of acute intermittent porphyria.[3]

Cutaneous aspects of the porphyrias are caused by photosensitization (eg, porphyria cutanea tarda, protoporphyria).

Hepatic complications are found with **porphyria cutanea tarda** and **protoporphyria**. Fluorescence is demonstrable in liver biopsies from patients with the former, as well as siderosis. Crystalline deposits may be found in protoporphyria.[3] The amount of porphobilinogen excreted in acute intermittent porphyria is usually greater than the excretion of delta aminolevulinic acid (Δ-ALA). When there is more Δ-ALA, another diagnosis should be considered, including lead poisoning, another type of porphyria, or hereditary tyrosinemia.[3] See also listing Protoporphyrin, Free Erythrocyte, which pertains to lead poisoning, and erythropoietic protoporphyria. The differential diagnosis of lead poisoning is relevant.[5]

Footnotes

1. Leavelle DE, *Mayo Medical Laboratories Interpretive Handbook*, Rochester, MN: Mayo Medical Laboratories, 1990.
2. Tschudy DP, "Porphyrins," *Chemical Diagnosis and Disease*, Brown SS, Mitchell FL, and Young DS, eds, Amsterdam, Holland: Elsevier/North Holland Biomedical Press, 1979, 1039-58.
3. Bloomer JR and Bonkovsky HL, "The Porphyrias," *Dis Mon*, 1989, 35(1):1-54.
4. Muhlbauer JE, Pathak MA, Tishler PV, et al, "Variegate Porphyria in New England," *JAMA*, 1982, 247:3095-102.
5. Bird TD, Wallace DM, and Labbe RF, "The Porphyria, Plumbism, Pottery Puzzle," *JAMA*, 1982, 247:813-4.

References

Billett HH, "Porphyrias: Inborn Errors in Heme Production," *Hosp Pract*, 1988, 41-60.

Deacon AC, "Performance of Screening Tests for Porphyria," *Ann Clin Biochem*, 1988, 25:392-7.

Edwards CQ, Griffen LM, Goldgar DE, et al, "HLA-Linked Hemochromatosis Alleles in Sporadic Porphyria Cutanea Tarda," *Gastroenterology*, 1989, 97(4):972-81.

Elder GH, "Recent Advances in the Identification of Enzyme Deficiencies in the Porphyrias," *Br J Dermatol*, 1983, 108:729-34, (review).

Elder GH, Urquhart AJ, De Salamanca RE, et al, "Immunoreactive Uroporphyrinogen Decarboxylase in the Liver in Porphyria Cutanea Tarda," *Lancet*, 1985, 2:229-33.

Ellefson RD, "Porphyrinogens, Porphyrins, and the Porphyrias," *Mayo Clin Proc*, 1982, 57:454-8.

Galbraith RA, Sassa S, and Kappas A, "A Comparison of the Utility of Dowex Resin and Polybenzimidazole Aurorez Resin in the Determination of Urinary Porphobilinogen Concentrations," *Clin Chim Acta*, 1987, 164:235-9.

Kimbrough RD, "Porphyrins and Hepatotoxicity," *Ann N Y Acad Sci*, 1987, 514:289-96.

Leahy DT and Brien TG, "A Simple Method for the Separation and Quantification of Urinary Porphyrins," *J Clin Pathol*, 1982, 35:1232-5.

Milo R, Neuman M, Klein C, et al, "Acute Intermittent Porphyria in Pregnancy," *Obstet Gynecol*, 1989, 73(3 Pt 2):450-2.

Ostrowski J, "Urinary Excretion of Porphyrins and Their Precursors in Chronic Liver Disease," *Mater Med Pol*, 1985, 17:240-5.

Pimstone NR, Gandhi SN, and Mukerji SK, "Therapeutic Efficacy of Oral Charcoal in Congenital Erythropoietic Porphyria," *N Engl J Med*, 1987, 316:390-3.

Rose IS, Young GP, St John DJ, et al, "Effect of Ingestion of Hemoproteins on Fecal Excretion of Hemes and Porphyrins," *Clin Chem*, 1989, 35(12):2290-6.

Scully RE, Mark EJ, and McNeely BU, "Case 39-1984: (Coproporphyria With Neuropathy), Presentation of Case," *Case Records of the Massachusetts General Hospital*, 1984, 839-47.

(Continued)

Porphyrins, Quantitative, Urine *(Continued)*

Stevens JF, "A Regional Quality Control Scheme for Urine Porphyrins," *Ann Clin Biochem*, 1989, 26(Pt 2):189-90.

Strik JJ, "Porphyrins in Urine as an Indication of Exposure to Chlorinated Hydrocarbons," *Ann N Y Acad Sci*, 1987, 514:219-21.

Toback AC, Sassa S, Poh-Fitzpatrick MB, et al, "Hepatoerythropoietic Porphyria: Clinical, Biochemical, and Enzymatic Studies in a Three-Generation Family Lineage," *N Engl J Med*, 1987, 316:645-50.

Vavra JD and Avioli LV, "Intermittent Acute Porphyria," *Arch Intern Med*, 1982, 142:1527.

Westerlund J, Pudek M, and Schreiber WE, "A Rapid and Accurate Spectrofluorometric Method for Quantification and Screening of Urinary Porphyrins," *Clin Chem*, 1988, 34:345-51.

Porter-Silber Chromogens, Urine *see* 17-Hydroxycorticosteroids, Urine *on page 256*

Postprandial Glucose *see* Glucose, 2-Hour Postprandial *on page 237*

Potassium, Arterial *see* Potassium, Blood *on this page*

Potassium, Blood

***CPT** 84132*

Related Information

Aldosterone, Blood *on page 104*
Aldosterone, Urine *on page 106*
Calcium, Serum *on page 160*
Chloride, Serum *on page 182*
Chloride, Urine *on page 184*
Concentration Test, Urine *on page 1115*
Electrolytes, Blood *on page 212*
Magnesium, Serum *on page 287*
Renin, Plasma *on page 346*

Synonyms K^+, Serum or Plasma

Applies to Electrolytes, Serum or Plasma; Potassium, Arterial

Abstract The major intracellular cation, potassium is very commonly measured as one of the serum or plasma electrolytes and as a urinary electrolyte as well.

Specimen Serum, plasma **CONTAINER:** Red top tube or green top (heparin) tube **COLLECTION:** Avoid very small needles if possible. Avoid stasis, use of tourniquet, and hand-clenching if possible. Avoid potassium-containing tubes such as potassium oxalate. Potassium can be reported from arterial as well as from venous blood. If arterial puncture is done for pO_2, plasma can be tested for Na^+, K^+, and Cl^- so long as lithium and not potassium heparinate anticoagulant is used. **STORAGE INSTRUCTIONS:** Remove plasma or serum from red cells within 4 hours before specimen is refrigerated. **CAUSES FOR REJECTION:** Hemolyzed specimen, serum specimen not removed from clot in patient with high platelet count. Such specimens may be analyzed but the likelihood of a falsely high potassium level must be recognized and stated in report. Preferably, sample should be rejected.

Interpretive **REFERENCE RANGE:** Plasma: 3.5-5.0 mmol/L (SI: 3.5-5.0 mmol/L). Add **approximately** 0.1 to normal ranges if serum is sampled rather than plasma. Pediatric ranges are sometimes reported as slightly higher than adult levels. Differences may well relate to the amount of hemolysis in specimens used to establish normal ranges. In daily practice some degree of hemolysis may occur in neonatal and pediatric specimens. Although grossly hemolyzed specimens are usually rejected, the acceptability of samples with slight hemolysis is debatable. Even slight hemolysis can increase potassium results; red cells have an intracellular concentration of 100-120 mmol/L or more potassium. **POSSIBLE PANIC RANGE:** Newborns: <2.5 mmol/L (SI: <2.5 mmol/L), >7.0 mmol/L (SI: >7.0 mmol/L); adults: <2.5 mmol/L (SI: <2.5 mmol/L), >6.5 mmol/L (SI: >6.5 mmol/L). With unanticipated high or low potassium, ECG may be indicated. If potassium is high and serum was used, examine peripheral blood smear for thrombocytosis and/or leukocytosis; obtain platelet and white count if indicated. **USE:** Evaluate electrolyte balance; potassium level should be followed especially in elderly patients, those on intravenous hyperalimentation, in patients on diuretic therapy and in cases of renal disease, particularly renal failure, patients on hemodialysis, and those with interstitial nephritis or nephropathy. Evaluate hypertension. Hyperkalemia may occur in and be caused by renal failure. Potassium should be monitored during treatment of acidosis, including ketoacidosis in diabetes mellitus. As one of the major electrolytes, potassium levels are a portion of regular assessment of acid-base balance and management of intravenous therapy.

Evaluate muscular weakness and irritability, mental confusion, weakness; manage leukemia, diseases of gastrointestinal tract including laxative abuse, large villous tumors, hepatic encephalopathy, emesis, fistulas and tube drainage; evaluate and prevent cardiac arrhythmias;[1,2] evaluate alcoholism with delirium tremens; detect, diagnose, and manage mineralocorticoid excess (primary aldosteronism, Cushing's syndrome, tumor with ectopic ACTH production, some cases of congenital adrenal hyperplasia), heat stroke, licorice ingestion mineralocorticoid effect.

LIMITATIONS: Inadequate sodium intake may mask the hypokalemia of aldosteronism; sodium loading in that setting may make hypokalemia recognizable. Heparinized plasma is probably the specimen of choice for potassium, because clotting causes cytolysis and may elevate serum values, usually but not always only slightly.

Since platelets release potassium during coagulation, samples from patients who have thrombocytosis (eg, some cases of polycythemia vera and other myeloproliferative diseases) will yield spuriously elevated potassium concentrations. Such "pseudohyperkalemia" may also occur in cases of leukemia with high WBC count (notably chronic myelogenous leukemia) as potassium is released from WBCs and platelets during clot formation. For such patients it is best to assay potassium on a heparinized sample. Pseudohyperkalemia in rheumatoid arthritis may be due to increased platelets.[3] Graber et al conclude that serum potassium increases with the platelet count in normal subjects and in those with thrombocytosis, and that the increment is an artifact.[4]

METHODOLOGY: Flame emission photometry or ion-selective electrode (ISE) **ADDITIONAL INFORMATION:** **Hypokalemia (low potassium)** has been found in >90% of hypertensive patients with primary aldosteronism (Conn's syndrome). This uncommon entity is a curable cause of hypertension. Low potassium occurs with endogenous or exogenous increase in other corticosteroids, including that in Cushing's syndrome as well as with dietary or parenteral deprivation of potassium (eg, parenteral therapy without adequate potassium replacement). Hypokalemia occurs with vomiting, diarrhea, fistulas, laxatives, diuretics, burns, excessive perspiration, Bartter's syndrome, some cases of alcoholism and folic acid deficiency, in alkalosis and in renal tubular acidosis, as well as in other entities.

Low potassium is much more significant with a low pH than with a high pH. When pH increases by 0.1, potassium decreases approximately 0.6 mmol/L. With low pH, as in ketoacidosis, as therapeutic adjustment towards normal is made, plasma/serum K^+ levels will decrease. Phosphorus levels tend to follow potassium levels downwards during therapy of diabetic ketoacidosis; both are largely intracellular. With insulin therapy (and increased utilization of carbohydrate), potassium moves into cells and serum/plasma level falls. Hyperalimentation may have a similar effect. Hypokalemia has been reported in slightly >50% of a series of 32 patients with acute myelogenous leukemia, but thrombocytosis can increase serum potassium levels, *vide supra*.

Thiazide/chlorthalidone therapy may cause hyperuricemia and hypercalcemia as well as hypokalemia.

The watery diarrhea-hypokalemia-achlorhydria (WDHA) syndrome most often is related to vasoactive intestinal polypeptide (VIP).

Consider magnesium status in patients who have hypokalemia.[5]

Hyperkalemia (high potassium) reflects generally inadequate renal excretion, mobilization of potassium from the tissues, or excessive intake or administration. Hyperkalemia occurs with hemolysis, trauma, with administration of potassium salts of some drugs, Addison's disease, acidosis, insulin lack, with increased osmolality (eg, glucose, mannitol), and in other entities as well as with renal diseases. Increased potassium can occur with potassium-sparing diuretics, nonsteroidal anti-inflammatory drugs, especially in the presence of renal disease. Systemic heparin therapy can suppress aldosterone release and increase potassium, especially in the presence of other factors.

A discussion of the relation between lactic acidosis and ketoacidosis and elevated serum potassium levels is provided in a paper by Fulop.[6]

Drug effects are summarized.[7]

Footnotes

1. Clausen TG, Brocks K, and Ibsen H, "Hypokalemia and Ventricular Arrhythmias in Acute Myocardial Infarction," *Acta Med Scand*, 1988, 224:531-7.
2. Borra S, Shaker R, and Kleinfeld M, "Hyperkalemia in an Adult Hospitalized Population," *Mt Sinai J Med*, 1988, 55:226-9.

(Continued)

Potassium, Blood *(Continued)*

3. Ralston SH, Lough M, and Sturrock RD, "Rheumatoid Arthritis: An Unrecognized Cause of Pseudohyperkalaemia," *Br Med J [Clin Res]*, 1988, 297(6647):523-4.
4. Graber M, Subramani K, Corish D, et al, "Thrombocytosis Elevates Serum Potassium," *Am J Kidney Dis*, 1988, 12(2):116-20.
5. Fulop M, "Serum Potassium in Lactic Acidosis and Ketoacidosis," *N Engl J Med*, 1979, 300:1087-9.
6. Fulop M, "Hyperkalemia in Diabetic Ketoacidosis," *Am J Med Sci*, 1990, 299(3):164-9.
7. Hitz J and Trivin F, "Potassium," *Drug Effects on Laboratory Test Results Analytical Interferences and Pharmacological Effects*, Siest G and Galteau MM, eds, Littleton, MA: PSG Publishing Co Inc, 1988, 362-74.

References

Alpern RJ and Toto RD, "Hypokalemic Nephropathy – A Clue to Cystogenesis?" *N Engl J Med*, 1990, 322(6):398-9.

Brem AS, "Disorders of Potassium Homeostasis," *Pediatr Clin North Am*, 1990, 37(2):419-27.

Corr LA, Grounds RM, Beacham JL, et al, "Effects of Circulating Endogenous Catecholamines on Plasma Glucose, Potassium, and Magnesium," *Clin Sci*, 1990, 78(2):185-91.

Jensen MD, Braun JS, Vetter RJ, et al, "Measurement of Body Potassium With a Whole-Body Counter: Relationship Between Lean Body Mass and Resting Energy Expenditure," *Mayo Clin Proc*, 1988, 63:864-8.

Kassirer JP and Harrington JT, "Fending Off the Potassium Pushers," *N Engl J Med*, 1985, 312:785-7.

Latta K, Hisano S, and Chan JC, "Perturbations in Potassium Balance," *Clin Lab Med*, 1993, 13(1):149-56.

Maffly RH, "Renal Function and Disorders of Water, Sodium, and Potassium Balance," *Scientific American Medicine*, Section 10, Chapter 1, Rubenstein E and Federman DD, eds, New York, NY: Scientific American Inc, 1990, 2-34.

Pierson RN Jr and Wang J, "Body Composition Denominators for Measurements of Metabolism: What Measurements Can Be Believed?" *Mayo Clin Proc*, 1988, 63:947-9, (editorial).

Quamme GA, "Laboratory Evaluation of Magnesium Status: Renal Function and Free Intracellular Magnesium Concentration," *Clin Lab Med*, 1993, 13:209-23.

Solomon R, Weinberg MS, and Dubey A, "The Diurnal Rhythm of Plasma Potassium: Relationship to Diuretic Therapy," *J Cardiovasc Pharmacol*, 1991, 17(5):854-9.

Tietz NW, Pruden EL, and Siggaard-Anderson O, "Electrolytes," *Fundamentals of Clinical Chemistry*, 3rd ed, Tietz NW, ed, Philadelphia, PA: WB Saunders Co, 1987, 616-20.

Torres VE, Young WF Jr, Offord KP, et al, "Association of Hypokalemia, Aldosteronism, and Renal Cysts," *N Engl J Med*, 1990, 322(6):345-51.

Young WF Jr, Hogan MJ, Klee GG, et al, "Primary Aldosteronism: Diagnosis and Treatment," *Mayo Clin Proc*, 1990, 65(1):96-110.

Potassium, Urine

***CPT** 84133*

Related Information

Chloride, Urine *on page 184*
Electrolytes, Urine *on page 213*
Kidney Stone Analysis *on page 1129*
Renin, Plasma *on page 346*

Synonyms K^+, Urine; Urine K^+

Specimen Random or timed urine (ie, 8-, 12-, or 24-hour) **CONTAINER:** Plastic urine container, no preservative **STORAGE INSTRUCTIONS:** Refrigerate

Interpretive **REFERENCE RANGE:** 26-123 mmol/24 hours (SI: 26-123 mmol/day), markedly intake dependent. If significantly decreased serum or plasma potassium has existed for days or more, urine K^+ excretion should be low: $\leq$15 mmol/L (SI: $\leq$15 mmol/L), or $\leq$30 mmol/24 hours (SI: $\leq$30 mmol/day). There is significant diurnal variation, output greater at night.[1] **USE:** Evaluate electrolyte balance, acid-base balance; evaluate hypokalemia; Carroll and Oh point out that urinary loss of 40 mmol/24 hours (SI: 40 mmol/day) in the presence of hypokalemia of <3 mmol/L is excessive.[2] In the presence of such hypokalemia, urine excretion is helpful to separate renal from nonrenal losses. Excretion <20 mmol/24 hours (SI: <20 mmol/day) is evidence that hypokalemia is not from renal loss.[1] Renal loss >50 mmol/L in a hypokalemic, hypertensive patient not on a diuretic may indicate primary or secondary aldosteronism. The kidneys do not respond quickly to potassium deprivation. There is renal wastage of potassium in secondary aldosteronism. Glucocorticoids, including endogenous steroids in Cushing's syndrome, are among the causes of kaliuresis. **METHODOLOGY:** Flame emission photometry, ion-selective electrode (ISE) **ADDITIONAL INFORMATION:** Urinary potassium may be elevated with dietary (food and/or medicinal) increase, hyperaldosteronism, renal tubular acidosis, onset of alkalosis, and with other disorders. Time relationships are important in interpretation. Potassium will decrease in Addison's disease and in renal disease with decreased urine flow (nephrosclerosis, pyelonephritis, glomerulonephritis).

Footnotes

1. Moore-Ede MC, Czeisler CA, and Richardson GS, "Circadian Timekeeping in Health and Disease, Part 2. Clinical Implications of Circadian Rhythmicity," *N Engl J Med*, 1983, 309:530-6.
2. Carroll HJ and Oh MS, *Water Electrolyte and Acid-Base Metabolism: Diagnosis and Management*, Philadelphia, PA: JB Lippincott Co, 1978.

References

Epstein M and Oster JR, "Disorders of Potassium Homeostasis," *The Laboratory in Clinical Medicine: Interpretation and Application*, 2nd ed, Halsted JA and Halsted CH, eds, Philadelphia, PA: WB Saunders Co, 1981, 296-303.

PP *see* Pancreatic Polypeptide, Human *on page 310*

PP, 2-Hour *see* Glucose, 2-Hour Postprandial *on page 237*

PRA *see* Renin, Plasma *on page 346*

Pregnancy Test

CPT *81025 (urine, qualitative); 84703*

Related Information

Human Chorionic Gonadotropin, Serum *on page 254*

Synonyms Beta-Subunit Human Chorionic Gonadotropin Urine or Serum; hCG, Slide Test, Stat; hCG, Urine; Human Chorionic Gonadotropin, Urine; β-Subunit of hCG

Specimen Urine or serum; first voided morning specimen is preferred if urine is tested (to obtain most concentrated specimen). **CONTAINER:** Plastic urine container or red top tube **STORAGE INSTRUCTIONS:** Urine stable 4 hours at 25°C and 3 days at 4°C. Serum should be frozen at -20°C if not run within 48 hours. **CAUSES FOR REJECTION:** Urine specimen grossly contaminated with blood or bacteria, inadequate labeling, low specific gravity, proteinuria, gross lipemia or turbidity **SPECIAL INSTRUCTIONS:** Centrifuge turbid urine specimens prior to testing.

Interpretive **REFERENCE RANGE:** Normal males and nonpregnant females: negative; normal pregnant females: positive. Sensitivity and specificity of β-subunit two point RIA or EIA tests may allow early diagnosis of pregnancy, within 6 days after conception. **USE:** Diagnose pregnancy; screen for women at risk of being pregnant prior to performance of x-ray, sterilization, menstrual regulation, and curettage procedures and/or prior to the initiation of gestation/embryo/fetal potentially injurious medication; detect and/or evaluate incomplete/complete abortions; detect ectopic gestation; screen for gestational trophoblastic neoplasia or ectopic hCG producing tumor. (A sensitive and quantitative test for the presence of hCG is preferable for these applications.) **LIMITATIONS:** Results may be negative in early pregnancy or whenever specific gravity is low. Large amounts of protein or phenothiazines may result in false-positive results with use of some earlier slide/tube tests, depending upon commercial supplier and technical characteristics of the test. In early pregnancy, incomplete abortion, recent complete abortion, ectopic pregnancy (in which hCG level is low), slide test end points may be difficult to interpret. Tube tests are generally more easily read than slide tests. Methods using covalent bonded latex particles and tests producing macroagglutination are more reliably interpreted. **METHODOLOGY:** Slide or tube agglutination-inhibition tests (urine), false-negative and false-positive results may occur. β-Subunit hCG by radioimmunoassay (serum or urine); immunoradiometric (IRMA) (eg, Tandem® hCG which incorporates two monoclonal antibodies, each with immunospecificity for different sites on the hCG molecule, one coated on a plastic bead on which the solid phase develops). Enzyme immunoassay, including sensitive (to 20-40 mIU/mL level of hCG, SI: 20-40 IU/L) two-point urine or serum qualitative/quantitative membrane based tests of which Tandem® ICON® is most well known. **ADDITIONAL INFORMATION:** Pregnancy testing is usually performed on urine. It is based on the the detection of human chorionic gonadotropin (hCG). Levels of hCG in the urine approach those seen in serum. In normal pregnancy, hCG levels rise at implantation and peak at 8-12 weeks. Although newer urine pregnancy tests are quite sensitive, false-negatives can occur early in gestation. In such cases, if ectopic pregnancy is suspected, serum hCG assays may be of value.

Early in the first trimester of pregnancy (1-2 weeks) serum hCG levels are from 50-500 mIU/mL (SI: 50-500 IU/L). Current generation sensitive tests can detect pregnancy shortly (2-3 days) after implantation of the ovum. By 3-4 weeks of gestation, hCG is at the 500-10,000 mIU/mL level (SI: 500-10,000 IU/L). Serum hCG level peaks during the second to third month of gestation (30,000-100,000 mIU/mL) (SI: 30,000-100,000 IU/L). Use of serum for pregnancy testing may provide greater sensitivity, of special value in cases of early pregnancy, and is of greater value in serial testing for follow-up of an abnormal gestation (eg, ectopic pregnancy or a ges-

(Continued)

Pregnancy Test *(Continued)*

tational trophoblastic neoplasm). If serum (or urine) hCG levels do not appear to correlate with the anticipated clinical situation, periodic repeat hCG determinations may be helpful. If there is demise of the developing embryo/fetus (eg, ectopic pregnancy), hCG levels will fall. Because of slow clearance from the serum, hCG may be detected in serum/urine for as long as 4 weeks following abortion.

Currently, the tests most commonly used to screen for pregnancy are two-point EIA "concentration" methods. A variety of different forms are commercially available. An antibody (frequently monoclonal) is immobilized on a membrane or other solid phase and the sample hCG is "concentrated" in a small central area of the surface (a membrane, bead, paddle, tube, or dipstick). Color development occurs within minutes of addition of enzyme tagged monoclonal anti-β-hCG. These tests are sensitive, specific, and fast. They have largely supplanted slide/tube screening procedures.

A study of specificity (six commercially available ELISA urine pregnancy tests) utilizing specimens from men and postmenopausal females found variable performance by the different methods, not explained by review of the medical records. Test systems with provision for a negative reference area gave fewer false-positive results (had greater specificity).[1] Correlation was found between mucous content of the postmenopausal female group's urine samples and the incidence of false-positive hCG results.

One year of routine use of Tandem® ICON® system for urine pregnancy testing (University of Texas) did not result in a report of known false-positive results. Stability of color development after addition of color reagents and presence or absence of a built in positive control could influence choice of a test system for routine use.

Serum progesterone levels used with beta-hCG levels may assist in differentiating normal intrauterine from abnormal intrauterine or ectopic pregnancy (cutoff point 15 ng/mL) (SI: 48 nmol/L). Beta-hCG and progesterone levels are lower in abnormal pregnancies. Less overlap occurs, however, between progesterone (as compared to beta-hCG) values in normal versus ectopic and abnormal pregnancies.[2] When a positive pregnancy test is obtained, differential considerations should include the possibility of simultaneous intrauterine and extrauterine gestations[3] (albeit unlikely) and the possibility of passively acquired hCG as in an individual recently transfused with fresh frozen plasma prepared from pregnant donors.[4]

A number of commercially successful home pregnancy tests have been introduced. They have been found to vary widely in performance (optimal accuracy, sensitivity, specificity, human factor useability).[5] A study of the use of such home pregnancy test kits has resulted in the suggestion that pharmacists have an opportunity in taking a more active role in promoting the appropriate use of such self-testing products.[6]

Footnotes

1. Bandi ZL, Schoen I, and DeLara M, "Enzyme-Linked Immunosorbent Urine Pregnancy Tests: Clinical Specificity Studies," *Am J Clin Pathol*, 1987, 87:236-42.
2. Riss PA, Radivojevic K, and Bieglmayer C, "Serum Progesterone and Human Chorionic Gonadotropin in Very Early Pregnancy: Implications for Clinical Management," *Eur J Obstet Gynecol Reprod Biol*, 1989, 32(2):71-7.
3. Boutiette LA and Anderson GV Jr, "Heterotopic Pregnancy," *J Emerg Med*, 1989, 7(1):33-5.
4. Kruskall MS, Owings DV, Donovan LM et al, "Passive Transfusion of Human Chorionic Gonadotropin from Plasma Donated During Pregnancy," *Vox Sang*, 1989, 56(2):71-4.
5. Latman NS and Bruot BC, "Evaluation of Home Pregnancy Test Kits," *Biomed Instrum Technol*, 1989, 23(2):144-9.
6. Coons SJ, "A Look at the Purchase and Use of Home Pregnancy Test Kits," *Am Pharm*, 1989, NS29(4):46-8.

References

Aziz K, "Sensitivity and Specificity of Pregnancy Tests," *Am Clin Lab*, 1989, 8:12, 5-6.

Christensen H, Thyssen HH, Schebye O, et al, "Three Highly Sensitive "Bedside" Serum and Urine Tests for Pregnancy Compared," *Clin Chem*, 1990, 36(9):1686-8.

Fields SA and Toffler WL, "Pregnancy Testing – Home and Office," *West J Med*, 1991, 154(3):327-8.

Hohnadel DC and Kaplan LA, "Hormones and Their Metabolites; β-hCG (β-Human Chorionic Gonadotropin)," *Clinical Chemistry – Theory, Analysis, and Correlation*, 2nd ed, Kaplan LA and Pesce AJ, eds, St Louis, MO: Mosby-Year Book Inc, 1989, 938-44.

Lee T, "Human Chorionic Gonadotropin Assays and Their Uses," *Obstet Gynecol Clin North Am*, 1988, 15:457-75.

Norman RJ, "Analytical and Clinical Sensitivity and Specificity in Pregnancy Testing," *Am J Obstet Gynecol*, 1989, 161(3):835-6.

Norman RJ, Gilmore TA, and McLoughlin JW, "Simple Quantitative Measurement of Serum Choriogonadotropin Compared With Immunoradiometric, Immunoenzymometric, and Chemiluminescent Assays," *Clin Chem*, 1992, 38(1):144-7.

Taylor CA Jr, Overstreet JW, Samuels SJ, et al, "Prospective Assessment of Early Fetal Loss Using An Immunoenzymometric Screening Assay for Detection of Urinary Human Chorionic Gonadotropin," *Fertil Steril*, 1992, 57(6):1220-4.

Pregnancy Testing *see* Human Chorionic Gonadotropin, Serum *on page 254*

Pregnanetriol, Urine

CPT 84138

Related Information

17-Hydroxyprogesterone, Blood or Amniotic Fluid *on page 258*

Test Commonly Includes May be included with 17-ketogenic steroids

Patient Care **PREPARATION:** Avoid muscular exercise before and during collection.

Specimen 24-hour urine **CONTAINER:** Plastic urine container **COLLECTION:** Preserve with boric acid.

Interpretive **REFERENCE RANGE:** Varies with age. Up to 2 mg/24 hours (SI: 5.9 μmol/day) for adults, less in children; it slightly increases in third trimester of pregnancy. **USE:** Increased in congenital adrenal hyperplasia, in the most common form of the adrenogenital syndrome, 21-hydroxylase deficiency. May be increased with certain tumors of ovary and adrenal cortices and in the Stein-Leventhal syndrome. **METHODOLOGY:** Extraction/gas-liquid chromatography (GLC), spectrophotometry **ADDITIONAL INFORMATION:** Muscular exercise may increase urinary pregnanetriol. Pregnanetriol is a major metabolite of 17-hydroxyprogesterone. Increased urinary 17-ketosteroids are usually found in 21-hydroxylase deficiency, with increased serum 17-hydroxyprogesterone. Pregnanetriol is not a ketosteroid; it is a ketogenic steroid.

References

Shackleton CH, Irias J, McDonald C, et al, "Late-Onset 21-Hydroxylase Deficiency: Reliable Diagnosis by Steroid Analysis of Random Urine Collections," *Steroids*, 1986, 48:239-50.

Weykamp CW, Penders TJ, Schmidt NA, et al, "Steroid Profile for Urine: Reference Values," *Clin Chem*, 1989, 35(12):2281-4.

Pressor Amines *see* Catecholamines, Fractionation, Plasma *on page 172*

Progesterone

CPT 84144

Abstract A C-21 steroid, progesterone is made by the corpus luteum. Its major source in pregnancy is the placenta.

Specimen Serum **CONTAINER:** Red top tube **STORAGE INSTRUCTIONS:** Serum stable 4 days at 4°C and 3 months at -20°C. **CAUSES FOR REJECTION:** Recently administered radioisotopes **SPECIAL INSTRUCTIONS:** Request should be completed with patient's sex, LMP (last menstrual period), and trimester of pregnancy.

Interpretive **REFERENCE RANGE:** Ovarian production of progesterone is low during the first (follicular) phase of the menstrual cycle. After the LH surge at the time of ovulation, progesterone levels rise for 4-5 days, and then fall. Progesterone levels are very high in early pregnancy and rise as pregnancy progresses. A rapid rise in the saliva estriol:progesterone ratio precedes the spontaneous onset of labor at term.[1] **USE:** A female sex hormone, serum progesterone is used to confirm the occurrence of ovulation and to assess corpus luteum function. A series of measurements can help define the day of ovulation.[2] Diagnose inadequate luteal phase;[3] investigate deficient progesterone production as a possible but unproven cause of habitual abortion.[4] The test is useful for monitoring patients having ovulation during induction with hCG, hMG, FSH/LHRH, or clomiphene. **METHODOLOGY:** Radioimmunoassay (RIA). A direct enzyme immunoassay for the measurement of salivary progesterone levels has been shown to be acceptable to patients and allows for a more comprehensive evaluation of ovarian function than can be obtained from a limited number of serum levels.[5] Direct time-resolved fluorescence immunoassay is available.[6] **ADDITIONAL INFORMATION:** Progesterone and 17-α-hydroxyprogesterone are weak androgens. Increased in congenital adrenal hyperplasia due to 21-hydroxylase, 17-hydroxylase, and 11-β-hydroxylase deficiency. It is decreased in threatened abortion, primary or secondary hypogonadism, and short luteal phase syndrome.

(Continued)

Progesterone *(Continued)*

Footnotes

1. Darne J, McGarrigle HH, and Lachelin GC, "Saliva Oestriol, Oestradiol, Oestrone and Progesterone Levels in Pregnancy: Spontaneous Labour at Term Is Preceded by a Rise in the Saliva Oestriol:Progesterone Ratio," *Br J Obstet Gynaecol*, 1987, 94:227-35.
2. Daya S, "Optimal Time in the Menstrual Cycle for Serum Progesterone Measurement to Diagnose Luteal Phase Defects," *Am J Obstet Gynecol*, 1989, 161(4):1009-11.
3. Soules MR, Clifton DK, Cohen NL, et al, "Luteal Phase Deficiency: Abnormal Gonadotropin and Progesterone Secretion Patterns," *J Clin Endocrinol Metab*, 1989, 69(4):813-20.
4. Glass RH and Golbus MS, "Habitual Abortion," *Maternal-Fetal Medicine: Principles and Practice*, 2nd ed, Creasy RK and Resnik R, eds, Philadelphia, PA: WB Saunders Co, 1989, 437-6.
5. Finn MM, Gosling JP, Tallon DF, et al, "Normal Salivary Progesterone Levels Throughout the Ovarian Cycle as Determined by a Direct Enzyme Immunoassay," *Fertil Steril*, 1988, 50(6):882-7.
6. Kakabakos SE and Khosravi MJ, "Direct Time-Resolved Fluorescence Immunoassay of Progesterone in Serum Involving the Biotin-Streptavidin System and the Immobilized-Antibody Approach," *Clin Chem*, 1992, 38(5):725-30.

References

Hilborn S and Krahn, "Effect of Time of Exposure of Serum to Gel-Barrier Tubes on Results for Progesterone and Some Other Endocrine Tests," *Clin Chem*, 1987, 33:203-4.

Nippoldt TB, Reame NE, Kelch RP, et al, "The Roles of Estradiol and Progesterone in Decreasing Luteinizing Hormone Pulse Frequency in the Luteal Phase of the Menstrual Cycle," *J Clin Endocrinol Metab*, 1989, 69(1):67-76.

Rebar RW, "The Ovaries," *Cecil Textbook of Medicine*, 18th ed, Vol 2, Wyngaarden JB and Smith LH Jr, eds, Philadelphia, PA: WB Saunders Co, 1988, 1425-46.

Romero R, Scoccia B, Mazor M, et al, "Evidence for a Local Change in the Progesterone/Estrogen Ratio in Human Parturition at Term," *Am J Obstet Gynecol*, 1988, 159:657-60.

Stewart MO, Whittaker PG, Persson B, et al, "A Longitudinal Study of Circulating Progesterone, Oestradiol, hCG and hPL During Pregnancy in Type 1 Diabetic Mothers," *Br J Obstet Gynaecol*, 1989, 96(4):415-23.

Proinsulin C-Peptide *see* C-Peptide *on page 195*

Prolactin

***CPT** 84146*

Related Information

Metyrapone Test *on page 292*

Patient Care PREPARATION: Patient should be fasting. No recently administered radioisotopes. Phenothiazines may cause hyperprolactinemia. Prolactin secretion is inhibited by levodopa, dopamine, bromocriptine, pergolide mesylate, and thyroid hormones. It is influenced by estrogens and antihypertensives.

Specimen Serum CONTAINER: Red top tube COLLECTION: Venipuncture itself can occasionally elevate prolactin level. Draw between 8 AM and 10 AM. Draw in chilled tube. Keep specimen on ice. STORAGE INSTRUCTIONS: Separate serum in refrigerated centrifuge and freeze. Stable 3 months at -20°C.

Interpretive REFERENCE RANGE: Normal range is given by one source as <20 ng/mL (SI: <20 μg/L) in nonlactating subjects. Normal ranges for prolactin are not interchangeable between all laboratories. Prolactin deficiency should be confirmed by lack of TRH response. CRITICAL VALUES: Although levels >200 ng/mL (SI: >200 μg/L) indicate prolactin-secreting tumor in a nonlactating woman, lower levels are found in instances of prolactinoma. USE: Prolactin level, for hyperprolactinemia, is the first test for work-up of galactorrhea (inappropriate lactation). About 75% of patients with galactorrhea and amenorrhea have hyperprolactinemia. A premenopausal female having amenorrhea and galactorrhea is suspect of pituitary prolactinoma and is considered a candidate for radiologic evaluation of the pituitary as well as serum prolactin levels. A pituitary function test, prolactin level is useful in the detection of prolactin-secreting pituitary tumors (microadenomas, macroadenomas) (Forbes-Albright syndrome) with or without galactorrhea, with or without evidence of sellar enlargement. Postpartum hyperprolactinemia is the Chiari-Frommel syndrome. Hirsutism occurs in occasional patients with prolactinomas, but there does not seem to be a relationship to virilization. Work up infertility, secondary amenorrhea, uncommonly primary amenorrhea, oligomenorrhea, and in males, impotence, gynecomastia, and hypogonadism. Of women with amenorrhea, 15% to 25% may have hyperprolactinemia. A transient increase of prolactin occurs often with generalized seizures. A sample can be drawn about 15-30 minutes after the episode and the baseline sampled after an hour.

Sequelae of hyperprolactinemia include amenorrhea, anovulation, and estrogen deficiency with secondarily decreased bone density. Both 17-KS and dehydroepiandrosterone sulfate are increased with hyperprolactinemia. Elevations are reported in some patients with renal cell carcinoma or with bronchogenic carcinoma.

Headache occurs in some patients with hyperprolactinemia and has been reported with lymphoid hypophysitis.

The only result of prolactin deficiency is the absence of postpartum lactation.

LIMITATIONS: Increased in patients on estrogens, antihypertensives, phenothiazines, tricyclic antidepressants, haloperidol, methyldopa, butyrophenones, cimetidine, metoclopramide, or reserpine, and in patients with hypothyroidism. Verapamil has been reported to have induced hyperprolactinemia and galactorrhea.[1] **Normal prolactin level does not rule out pituitary tumor.** Prolactin secretion is episodic and is influenced by stress and by low glucose levels.
METHODOLOGY: Immunoassay,[2] radioimmunoassay (RIA) **ADDITIONAL INFORMATION:** Levels rise during pregnancy and are elevated during lactation, in postpartum subjects, and following bilateral oophorectomy. Destructive pituitary diseases cause low levels. Hypothalamic lesions may be associated with increased values. Many pituitary tumors which previously were called chromophobe adenomas are now recognizable as prolactinomas.

Patients with hyperprolactinemia may have the multiple endocrine neoplasia syndrome, MEN-1.

Baseline work-up recommendations include FSH, LH, thyroxine, AM and PM cortisols, and testosterone.[1]

Provocative tests used in work-up of hyperprolactinemia include metyrapone stimulation of ACTH[1] and TRH provocative test.[3]

Antipsychotic drugs may elevate serum prolactin. Antipsychotics block dopamine, thereby elevating serum prolactin levels. Hyperprolactinemia is present in many patients receiving neuroleptics with an occasional patient developing amenorrhea, galactorrhea, and/or decreased libido. Amoxapine, a dibenzoxazepine type of tricyclic with antidepressant and antipsychotic characteristics, has been found to cause galactorrhea and oligomenorrhea with hyperprolactinemia. Amoxapine may have a dopamine blocking action. The prolactin level may rise significantly but only briefly. Point prolactin level determinations during therapy may be within normal range while total integrated 24-hour secretion is significantly increased. It has been recommended that patients who develop amenorrhea and/or galactorrhea during neuroleptic therapy should be observed regularly for possible emergence of a pituitary tumor.

Persistent elevations of plasma prolactin levels may be observed with, and after withdrawal from, chronic cocaine abuse, and may reflect a cocaine-induced derangement in the neural dopaminergic regulatory systems.[4]

Women with apparently normal ovarian function have been found with hyperprolactinemia. Many have been found to have big big prolactin, BBPRL. Presently it is thought to be a poorly understood scientific curiosity,[5] and a genetic basis is likely.[6] Prolactin has molecular heterogeneity.[7]

Footnotes

1. Gluskin LE, Strasberg B, and Shah JH, "Verapamil-Induced Hyperprolactinemia and Galactorrhea," *Ann Intern Med*, 1981, 95:66-7.
2. Babiel R, Willnow P, Baer M, et al, "A New Enzyme Immunoassay for Prolactin in Serum or Plasma," *Clin Chem*, 1990, 36(1):76-80.
3. Randall RV, Laws ER Jr, Abboud CF, et al, "Transsphenoidal Microsurgical Treatment of Prolactin-Producing Pituitary Adenomas. Results in 100 Patients," *Mayo Clin Proc*, 1983, 58:108-21.
4. Mendelson JH, Teoh SK, Lange U, et al, "Anterior Pituitary, Adrenal, and Gonadal Hormones During Cocaine Withdrawal," *Am J Psychiatry*, 1988, 145(9):1094-8.
5. Fraser IS, Lun ZG, Zhou JP, et al, "Detailed Assessment of Big Big Prolactin in Women With Hyperprolactinemia and Normal Ovarian Function," *J Clin Endocrinol Metab*, 1989, 69(3):585.
6. Larrea F, Escorza A, Valero A, et al, "Heterogeneity of Serum Prolactin Throughout the Menstrual Cycle and Pregnancy in Hyperprolactinemic Women With Normal Ovarian Function," *J Clin Endocrinol Metab*, 1989, 68(5):982.
7. Smith CR and Norman MR, "Prolactin and Growth Hormone: Molecular Heterogeneity and Measurement in Serum," *Ann Clin Biochem*, 1990, 27(Pt 6):542-50.

References

Baskin HJ, "Endocrinologic Evaluation of Impotence," *South Med J*, 1989, 82(4):446-9.
Berczi I, Cosby H, Hunter T, et al, "Decreased Bioactivity of Circulating Prolactin in Patients With Rheumatoid Arthritis," *Br J Rheumatol*, 1987, 26:433-6.

(Continued)

Prolactin *(Continued)*

Fujimoto VY, Clifton DK, Cohen NL, et al, "Variability of Serum Prolactin and Progesterone Levels in Normal Women: The Relevance of Single Hormone Measurements in the Clinical Setting," *Obstet Gynecol*, 1990, 76(1):71-8.

Kelly PA, Djiane J, Postel-Vinay MC, et al, "The Prolactin/Growth Hormone Receptor Family," *Endocr Rev*, 1991, 12(3):235-51.

Schlechte J, Dolan K, Sherman B, et al, "The Natural History of Untreated Hyperprolactinemia: A Prospective Analysis," *J Clin Endocrinol Metab*, 1989, 68(2):412-8.

Schulster D, Gaines-Das RE, and Jeffcoate SL, "International Standards for Human Prolactin: Calibration by International Collaborative Study," *J Endocrinol*, 1989, 121(1):157-66.

Smith CR, Butler J, Hashim I, et al, "Serum Prolactin Bioactivity and Immunoactivity in Hyperprolactinaemic States," *Ann Clin Biochem*, 1990, 27(Pt 1):3-8.

Tippet PD, Simon JA, Rifka SM, et al, "Luteal Phase Hyperprolactinemia During Ovulation Induction With Human Menopausal Gonadotropins: Incidence, Recurrence, and Effect on Pregnancy Rates," *Obstet Gynecol*, 1989, 73(4):613.

Veldhuis JD, Evans WS, and Stumpf PG, "Mechanisms That Subserve Estradiol's Induction of Increased Prolactin Concentrations: Evidence of Amplitude Modulation of Spontaneous Prolactin Secretory Bursts," *Am J Obstet Gynecol*, 1989, 161(5):1149-58.

Prostate Specific Antigen, Serum

CPT 84153

Related Information

Acid Phosphatase *on page 96*

Immunoperoxidase Procedures *on page 60*

Synonyms PSA

Abstract Marker for adenocarcinoma of prostate. PSA may also be increased in benign entities. Serially measured, PSA is extremely useful in monitoring presurgical as well as postsurgical patients and in anticipation of recurrence. PSA is proving to be an indispensable predictor of recurrent adenocarcinoma in postsurgical patients and an important aid in selection of adjunctive therapy.

Patient Care PREPARATION: Fasting specimen is preferred.

Specimen Serum CONTAINER: Red top tube SAMPLING TIME: PSA has little diurnal variation[1] but it is often sampled together with prostatic acid phosphatase (PAP), although PAP as a useful measurement has fallen into disrepute. COLLECTION: Rectal examination within 48 hours of specimen collection may cause elevation of results; mixed recommendations are published. STORAGE INSTRUCTIONS: PSA is stable in serum for 24 hours at room temperature. For longer periods, store at -20°C or colder.[1,2] No special treatment of serum is required. Ship to a reference laboratory in a plastic vial on dry ice. CAUSES FOR REJECTION: Recent prostatic manipulation should be avoided. SPECIAL INSTRUCTIONS: Individual patients should be followed with the same assay consistently; two major assays are available.

Interpretive REFERENCE RANGE: Male: <4 ng/mL; female <0.5 ng/mL (immunoassay method) USE: Prostate specific antigen (PSA) is a 34-kilodalton glycoprotein first detected in 1980.[3] It is a smaller molecule than PAP. It appears to be located only in the prostate,[4] where it is demonstrated in benign and malignant epithelium. Preoperative PSA serum levels correlate (but imperfectly) with extent of disease in patients with prostate cancer. PSA is useful in detecting residual tumor in postoperative stage of prostate cancer.[5] PSA has several advantages over prostatic acid phosphatase (PAP). It is more stable and does not have a significant diurnal variation.[1] It has been shown to be elevated in 95% of newly diagnosed cases of prostatic carcinoma (vs 60% for PAP) and in 97% of recurrent cases (PAP 66%).[6] PSA is reported to be directly proportional to increasing Gleason score.[7] (Unfortunately, Gleason scores are themselves problematical.) PSA has real utility as a screening test for prostatic cancer,[8] according to Labrie et al, although this point remains controversial. LIMITATIONS: Some cases of benign prostatic hypertrophy and prostatitis show elevation of PSA, but such increases are below those found with adenocarcinoma of prostate stages C and D. Neither PSA nor PAP has sufficient sensitivity or specificity to be used alone as a useful screen for asymptomatic men.[9] It is not acceptable used alone for staging,[10] and alone should not be used to select candidates for radical prostatectomy.[11] Elevations may also be associated with urethral instrumentation, TUR, prostatic needle biopsy, urinary retention, or prostatic infarct.[12] Used in preoperative patients, PSA does not sharply distinguish intracapsular from extracapsular carcinoma. No published paper claims diagnostic sensitivity early in prostate adenocarcinoma stage A. Digital rectal examination is claimed not to alter levels significantly.[13,14,15] METHODOLOGY: Radioimmunoassay, monoclonal two-site immunoradiometric assay.[16] An ultrasensitive RIA has been developed recently.[17] **ADDITIONAL INFORMATION:** Three to 6 months after radical prostatectomy, PSA is reported to provide a sensitive indicator of persistent disease.[10] Six months following introduction of antiandrogen therapy, PSA is reported as capable of distinguishing patients with favorable response from those in whom limited response is anticipated.[18]

Order of prognostic reliability for progression of adenocarcinoma of prostate is given as PSA, PAP, bone alkaline phosphatase, total acid phosphatase, and total alkaline phosphatase.[11] Transrectal ultrasound with PSA assay is a very effective screening procedure.[19,20]

Prostatic specific antigen has proven to be a reliable immunocytochemical marker for primary and metastatic adenocarcinoma of prostate, reacting with at least some cells in almost all adequate biopsies.

Footnotes

1. Schifman RB, Ahmann FR, Elvick A, et al, "Analytical and Physiological Characteristics of Prostate-Specific Antigen and Prostatic Acid Phosphatase in Serum Compared," *Clin Chem*, 1987, 33:2086-8.
2. Liedtke RJ and Batjer JD, "Measurement of Prostate-Specific Antigen by Radioimmunoassay," *Clin Chem*, 1984, 30:649-52.
3. Wang MC, Valenzuela LA, Murphy GP, et al, "Purification of a Human Prostate Specific Antigen," *Invest Urol*, 1980, 17:159-63.
4. Papsidero LD, Kuriyama M, Wang MC, et al, "Prostate Antigen: A Marker for Human Prostatic Epithelial Cells," *J Natl Cancer Inst*, 1981, 66:37-42.
5. Carter HB, Partin AW, Epstein JI, et al, "The Relationship of Prostate Specific Antigen Levels and Residual Tumor Volume in Stage A Prostate Cancer," *J Urol*, 1990, 144(5):1167-70.
6. Rainwater LM, Morgan WR, Klee GG, et al, "Prostate-Specific Antigen Testing in Untreated and Treated Prostatic Adenocarcinoma," *Mayo Clin Proc*, 1990, 65(8):1118-26.
7. Stamey TA and Kabalin JN, "Prostate Specific Antigen in the Diagnosis and Treatment of Adenocarcinoma of the Prostate. Untreated Patients," *J Urol*, 1989, 141(5):1070-5.
8. Labrie F, Dupont A, Suburu R, et al, "Serum Prostate Specific Antigen as Prescreening Test for Prostate Cancer," *J Urol*, 1992, 147(3 Pt 2):846-51.
9. Gambino R, "Prostatic Acid Phosphatase & Prostate-Specific Antigen: Immunoassays Should Replace Colorimetric Chemical Assays," *Lab Report for Physicians*, 1989, 11:9-13.
10. Lange PH, Ercole CJ, Lightner DJ, et al, "The Value of Serum Prostate Specific Antigen Determinations Before and After Radical Prostatectomy," *J Urol*, 1989, 141(4):873-9.
11. Chan DW and Oesterling JE, "Prostate-Specific Antigen (PSA) in the Diagnosis and Management of Prostatic Cancer," *ASCP Check Sample®*, Chicago, IL: The American Society of Clinical Pathologists, 1988, 28:1-5.
12. Brawer MK and Lange PH, "Prostate-Specific Antigen in Management of Prostatic Carcinoma," *Urology*, 1989, 33(5 Suppl):11-6.
13. Thomson RD and Clejan S, "Digital Rectal Examination-Associated Alterations in Serum Prostate-Specific Antigen," *Am J Clin Pathol*, 1992, 97(4):528-34.
14. Yuan JJ, Coplen DE, Petros JA, et al, "Effects of Rectal Examination, Prostatic Massage, Ultrasonography and Needle Biopsy on Serum Prostate Specific Antigen Levels," *J Urol*, 1992, 147(3 Pt 2):810-4.
15. Catalona WJ, Smith DS, Ratliff TL, et al, "Measurement of Prostate-Specific Antigen in Serum as a Screening Test for Prostate Cancer," *N Engl J Med*, 1991, 324(17):1156-61.
16. Lindstedt G, Jacobsson A, Lundberg PA, et al, "Determination of Prostate-Specific Antigen in Serum by Immunoradiometric Assay," *Clin Chem*, 1990, 36(1):53-8.
17. Graves HC, Wehner N, and Stamey TA, "Ultrasensitive Radioimmunoassay of Prostate-Specific Antigen," *Clin Chem*, 1992, 38(5):735-42.
18. Stamey TA, Kabalin JN, Ferrari M, et al, "Prostate Specific Antigen in the Diagnosis and Treatment of Adenocarcinoma of the Prostate. Antiandrogen Treated Patients," *J Urol*, 1989, 141(5):1088-90.
19. Babaian RJ and Camps JL, "The Role of Prostate-Specific Antigen as Part of the Diagnostic Triad and as a Guide When to Perform a Biopsy," *Cancer*, 1991, 68(9):2060-3.
20. Oesterling JE, "Prostate Specific Antigen: A Critical Assessment of the Most Useful Tumor Marker for Adenocarcinoma of the Prostate," *J Urol*, 1991, 145(5):907-23.

References

Babaian RJ, Mettlin C, Kane R, et al, "The Relationship of Prostate-Specific Antigen to Digital Rectal Examination and Transrectal Ultrasonography. Findings of the American Cancer Society National Prostate Cancer Detection Project," *Cancer*, 1992, 69(5):1195-200.

Barak M, Mecz Y, Lurie A, et al, "Evaluation of Prostate-Specific Antigen as a Marker for Adenocarcinoma of the Prostate," *J Lab Clin Med*, 1989, 113(1):598-603.

Benson MC, Whang IS, Olsson CA, et al, "The Use of Prostate Specific Antigen Density to Enhance the Predictive Value of Intermediate Levels of Serum Prostate Specific Antigen," *J Urol*, 1992, 147(3 Pt 2):817-21.

Brawer MK, Rennels MA, Nagle RB, et al, "Serum Prostate-Specific Antigen and Prostate Pathology in Men Having Simple Prostatectomy," *Am J Clin Pathol*, 1989, 92(6):760-4.

Brawer MK, Schifman RB, Ahmann FR, et al, "The Effect of Digital Rectal Examination on Serum Levels of Prostatic-Specific Antigen," *Arch Pathol Lab Med*, 1988, 112:1110-2.

Drago JR and York JP, "Prostate-Specific Antigen, Digital Rectal Examination, and Transrectal Ultrasound in Predicting the Probability of Cancer," *J Surg Oncol*, 1992, 49(3):172-5.

(Continued)

Prostate Specific Antigen, Serum *(Continued)*

Gillenwater JY, "Digital Rectal Examination-Associated Alterations in Serum Prostate-Specific Antigen," *Am J Clin Pathol*, 1992, 97(4):466-7, (editorial).

Glenski WJ, Malek RS, Myrtle JF, et al, "Sustained, Substantially Increased Concentration of Prostate-Specific Antigen in the Absence of Prostatic Malignant Disease: An Unusual Clinical Scenario," *Mayo Clin Proc*, 1992, 67(3):249-52.

Griffiths J, "Prostate Antigen – A New Perception of Use in Serum," *Am J Clin Pathol*, 1989, 92(6):845-6.

Grob BM, Haley C, Schellhammer PF, et al, "The Detection of Prostate Specific Antigen, MHS-5, and Other Markers in Invasive Prostate Cancer and Seminal Vesicle," *J Urol*, 1992, 147(5):1435-8.

Hortin GL, Bahnson RR, Daft M, et al, "Differences in Values Obtained With 2 Assays of Prostate Specific Antigen," *J Urol*, 1988, 139:762-5.

Killian CS, Emrich LJ, Vargas FP, et al, "Relative Reliability of Five Serially Measured Markers for Prognosis of Progression in Prostate Cancer," *J Natl Cancer Inst*, 1986, 76:179-85.

Lange PH, "Prostate-Specific Antigen for Staging Prior to Surgery and for Early Detection of Recurrence After Surgery," *Urol Clin North Am*, 1990, 17(4):813-7.

Littrup PJ, Kane RA, Williams CR, et al, "Determination of Prostate Volume With Transrectal US for Cancer Screening. Part I. Comparison With Prostate-Specific Antigen Assays," *Radiology*, 1991, 178(2):537-42.

Smith EM and Resnick MI, "Prostate Specific Antigen: Clinical Applications and New Developments," *The Kidney*, 1993, 25(5):1-6.

Prostatic Acid Phosphatase *see* Acid Phosphatase *on page 96*

Protein, Total, Serum

CPT *84155*

Related Information

Albumin, Serum *on page 102*
Cerebrospinal Fluid Protein Electrophoresis *on page 661*
Immunoelectrophoresis, Serum or Urine *on page 706*
Immunofixation Electrophoresis *on page 707*
Immunoglobulin A *on page 709*
Immunoglobulin G *on page 710*
Immunoglobulin G Subclasses *on page 711*
Immunoglobulin M *on page 712*
Protein Electrophoresis, Serum *on page 734*
Protein, Quantitative, Urine *on page 1145*

Synonyms Total Protein, Serum

Applies to Globulin

Test Commonly Includes Total protein, albumin, A/G ratio

Specimen Serum **CONTAINER:** Red top tube **COLLECTION:** Pediatric: Blood drawn from heelstick for capillary. **STORAGE INSTRUCTIONS:** Separate serum from cells. Refrigerate.

Interpretive **REFERENCE RANGE:** Adults: 6.0-8.0 g/dL (SI: 60-80 g/L) in later childhood and adults. Lower ranges occur in early childhood. Ambulatory values are slightly higher than are those found in recumbency. If normal ranges are set for inpatients, then many outpatients appear to be a little above the upper limit. **USE:** Evaluate nutritional status; investigate edema.

In the entities which follow, the diseases listed are sometimes increased or decreased as indicated, but are not always so.

Causes of **high total protein:** dehydration; some cases of chronic liver disease, including chronic active hepatitis and cirrhosis; neoplasms, especially myeloma; macroglobulinemia of Waldenström; tropical diseases (eg, kala-azar, leprosy, and others); granulomatous diseases, such as sarcoidosis; diseases in which total protein is sometimes high include collagen disease (eg, lupus erythematosus (SLE), and other instances of chronic infection/inflammation).

Causes of **low total protein:** pregnancy; intravenous fluids; cirrhosis or other liver disease, including chronic alcoholism; prolonged immobilization; heart failure; nephrotic syndromes; glomerulonephritis; neoplasia; protein losing enteropathies; Crohn's disease and chronic ulcerative colitis; starvation, malabsorption, or malnutrition; hyperthyroidism; burns; severe skin disease; and other chronic diseases.

Very low total protein (<4.0 g/dL (SI: <40 g/L)) and low albumin cause edema (eg, nephrotic syndromes).

LIMITATIONS: Venous stasis during venipuncture can lead to increased values. Hyperviscosity was reported to cause error in total protein through a discrete laboratory sampler-dilutor.[1] Hemolysis can falsely elevate total protein. Clinical interpretation is greatly enhanced by examination of the fractions composing total protein, when such separation is clinically indicated (ie, serum protein electrophoresis, quantitative immunodiffusion or other methods for IgG, IgA, IgM, immunofixation, immunoelectrophoresis). **METHODOLOGY:** Biuret for total protein, refractometry, BCG for albumin[2,3] **ADDITIONAL INFORMATION:** Total protein and albumin normally decrease by 5% to 10% upon recumbency, as in hospitalization. "Globulin" may be provided as a calculation, total protein - albumin = globulin. Such a result is a screening test much less definitive than otner methods. Total protein and albumin are commonly measured on chemistry profiling instruments. Drug effects are summarized.[4]

Footnotes

1. Chan KM and Ladenson JH, "Sample Viscosity Can Be a Source of Analytical Error When Discrete Sampler-Dilutors Are Used," *Clin Chem*, 1981, 27:1896-8.
2. Dawnay AB, Hirst AD, Perry DE, et al, "A Critical Assessment of Current Analytical Methods for the Routine Assay of Serum Total Protein and Recommendations for Their Improvement," *Ann Clin Biochem*, 1991, 28(Pt 6):556-67.
3. Camara PD, Wright C, Dextraze P, et al, "Comparison of a Commercial Method for Total Protein With a Candidate Reference Method," *Ann Clin Lab Sci*, 1991, 21(5):335-9.
4. Herbeth B, Diemert MC, and Galli A, "Total Proteins," *Drug Effects on Laboratory Test Results Analytical Interferences and Pharmacological Effects*, Siest G and Galteau MM, eds, Littleton, MA: PSG Publishing Co Inc, 1988, 375-90.

References

Koller A and Kaplan LA, "Total Serum Protein," *Methods in Clinical Chemistry*, Pesce AJ and Kaplan LA, eds, St Louis, MO: Mosby-Year Book Inc, 1987, 1134-8.

Protoporphyrin, Free Erythrocyte

CPT *84202 (quantitative); 84203 (screen)*

Related Information

Delta Aminolevulinic Acid, Urine *on page 207*
Hemoglobin *on page 554*
Iron and Total Iron Binding Capacity/Transferrin *on page 262*
Lead, Blood *on page 976*
Lead, Urine *on page 977*
Porphobilinogen, Qualitative, Urine *on page 325*
Porphyrins, Quantitative, Urine *on page 327*
Protoporphyrin, Zinc, Blood *on next page*

Synonyms FEP; Free Erythrocyte Protoporphyrin; Protoporphyrins, Fractionation, Erythrocytes; RBC Protoporphyrin

Abstract Free erythrocyte protoporphyrin expresses the amount of nonheme protoporphyrin in red cells.

Specimen Whole blood (test done on washed erythrocytes) **CONTAINER:** Lavender top (EDTA) tube or green top (heparin) tube **COLLECTION:** Pediatric: Blood drawn from heelstick for capillary. **STORAGE INSTRUCTIONS:** Stable 3 weeks at 4°C. Do not freeze. **SPECIAL INSTRUCTIONS:** Current hematocrit must be measured or specified.

Interpretive **REFERENCE RANGE:** Depends on method; ascertain ranges for individual testing laboratory. The FEP is considered unreliable in infants younger than 6 months of age.[1] Pediatric upper limit is 50 μg/dL (SI: 0.89 μmol/L) RBC. Adults: male: <30 μg/dL (SI: <0.53 μmol/L), female: <40 μg/dL (SI: <0.71 μmol/L) by hematofluorometer; 11-45 (SI: 0.20-0.80 μmol/L) for adult men and 19-52 (SI: 0.34-0.92 μmol/L) for adult women by Piomelli FEP expressed as μg/dL blood.[2] **POSSIBLE PANIC RANGE:** >190 μg/dL (SI: >3.38 μmol/L) **USE:** Differential diagnosis of disorders of heme production versus diseases of globin synthesis.[3] FEP is increased in lead poisoning, protoporphyria, in iron deficiency,[4,5,6,7] anemia of chronic disease and with some sideroblastic anemias.[3] FEP levels are also reported increased in entities characterized by marked increase in erythropoiesis, such as severe hemolytic anemias. Thus, FEP is useful in work-up of the microcytic anemias. FEP is increased with lead poisoning but not in acute intermittent porphyria.[8,9,10] FEP is reported normal with presumed alpha thalassemia trait, hemoglobin H, beta thalassemia trait, and hemoglobin E. **LIMITATIONS:** Fluorescent substances in plasma may interfere with hematofluorometer results. Elevated FEPs should be verified by retesting washed RBCs or by microextraction. Skin contamination may lead to false elevations. Both this test and blood lead are needed for full evaluation. **METHODOLOGY:** Hematofluorometer, extraction method, and high performance liquid chromatography (HPLC). The hematofluorometer measures porphyrins unbound in erythrocytes. With iron deficiency and diminished heme synthesis, free porphyrin accumulates in the red blood cell. **ADDITIONAL**

(Continued)

Protoporphyrin, Free Erythrocyte *(Continued)*

INFORMATION: "Free" protoporphyrin is not complexed, nonheme protoporphyrin. **Lead poisoning** is characterized by elevated plasma and urine delta aminolevulinic acid and increased urinary coproporphyrin. Urinary porphobilinogen and uroporphyrin are normal to slightly increased. Free erythrocyte protoporphyrin is a sensitive test for lead toxicity or chronic exposure,[10] **although, a careful study based on receiver operator curves showed that erythrocyte protoporphyrin levels should not be used as a screening test for lead poisoning in children**. The diagnosis of lead exposure or poisoning includes consideration of environmental exposure, as well as symptoms and abnormal erythrocyte protoporphyrin. FEP is given as 92-288 μg/dL (SI: 1.63-5.12 μmol/L) RBC in level II increased lead absorption, with higher FEP results in level III. Increased lead absorption is reported in the presence of iron deficiency.[11] Increased erythrocyte protoporphyrin exists as free protoporphyrin in protoporphyria, not as a zinc chelate, in contrast to lead poisoning and iron deficiency.[12] These two compounds, zinc protoporphyrin and metal free protoporphyrin, can be distinguished from each other by spectrophotofluorometry.[13]

Footnotes

1. Benjamin JT, Dickens MD, Ford RF, et al, "Normative Data of Hemoglobin Concentration and Free Erythrocyte Protoporphyrin in a Private Pediatric Practice," *Clin Pediatr (Phila)*, 1986, 25:206-8.
2. Marsh WL Jr, Nelson DP, and Koenig HM, "Free Erythrocyte Protoporphyrin (FEP) I. Normal Values for Adults and Evaluation of the Hematofluorometer," *Am J Clin Pathol*, 1983, 79:655-60.
3. Marsh WL Jr, Nelson DP, and Koenig HM, "Free Erythrocyte Protoporphyrin (FEP) II. The FEP Test Is Clinically Useful in Classifying Microcytic RBC Disorders in Adults," *Am J Clin Pathol*, 1983, 79:661-6.
4. Benjamin JT, Dickens MD, Ford RF, et al, "Normative Data of Hemoglobin Concentration and Free Erythrocyte Protoporphyrin in A Private Pediatric Practice: A 1990 Update," *Clin Pediatr (Phila)*, 1991, 30(2):74-6.
5. Parsons PJ, Stanton NV, Gunter EW, et al, "An Interlaboratory Comparison of Control Materials for Use With Hematofluorometers," *Clin Chem*, 1989, 35(10):2059-65.
6. Brown RG, "Determining the Cause of Anemia. General Approach, With Emphasis on Microcytic Hypochromic Anemias," *Postgrad Med*, 1991, 89(6):161-4, 167-70.
7. Beaton GH, Corey PN, and Steele C, "Conceptual and Methodological Issues Regarding the Epidemiology of Iron Deficiency and Their Implications for Studies of the Functional Consequences of Iron Deficiency," *Am J Clin Nutr*, 1989, 50(3 Suppl):575-88.
8. Turk DS, Schonfeld DJ, Cullen M, et al, "Sensitivity of Erythrocyte Protoporphyrin as a Screening Test for Lead Poisoning," *N Engl J Med*, 1992, 326(2):137-8.
9. McElvaine MD, Orbach HG, Binder S, et al, "Evaluation of the Erythrocyte Protoporphyrin Test as a Screen for Elevated Blood Lead Levels," *J Pediatr*, 1991, 119(4):548-50.
10. DeBaun MR and Sox HC Jr, "Setting the Optimal Erythrocyte Protoporphyrin Screening Decision Threshold for Lead Poisoning: A Decision Analytic Approach," *Pediatrics*, 1991, 88(1):121-31.
11. Carraccio CL, Bergman GE, and Daley BP, "Combined Iron Deficiency and Lead Poisoning in Children. Effect on FEP Levels," *Clin Pediatr (Phila)*, 1987, 26:644-7.
12. Bloomer JR and Bonkovsky HL, "The Porphyrias," *Dis Mon*, 1989, 35(1):1-54.
13. Gambino R, "Protoporphyrins," *Lab Report for Physicians*, 1986, 8:9.

References

Bird TD, Wallace DM, and Labbe RF, "The Porphyria, Plumbism, Pottery Puzzle," *JAMA*, 1982, 247:813-4.
Houk VN, "Protoporphyrins," *Lab Report for Physicians*, 1986, 8:60-1, (letter).
Schreiber WE, "Iron, Porphyrin, and Bilirubin Metabolism," *Clinical Chemistry – Theory, Analysis, and Correlation*, 2nd ed, Kaplan LA and Pesce AJ, eds, St Louis, MO: Mosby-Year Book Inc, 1989, 496-511.
Zanella A, Gridelli L, Berzuini A, et al, "Sensitivity and Predictive Value of Serum Ferritin and Free Erythrocyte Protoporphyrin for Iron Deficiency," *J Lab Clin Med*, 1989, 113(1):73-8.

Protoporphyrins, Fractionation, Erythrocytes *see* Protoporphyrin, Free Erythrocyte *on previous page*

Protoporphyrin, Zinc, Blood

CPT *84202*

Related Information

Delta Aminolevulinic Acid, Urine *on page 207*
Ferritin, Serum *on page 220*
Iron and Total Iron Binding Capacity/Transferrin *on page 262*
Lead, Blood *on page 976*
Protoporphyrin, Free Erythrocyte *on previous page*
Transferrin *on page 369*

Synonyms Zinc Protoporphyrin; ZPP

Abstract Zinc protoporphyrin measurement may be a useful adjunct in the diagnosis of nonanemic iron deficiency[1] but is not useful in screening programs for lead intoxication.[2]

Specimen Whole blood CONTAINER: Lavender top (EDTA) tube, green top (heparin) tube COLLECTION: Routine venipuncture STORAGE INSTRUCTIONS: Do not centrifuge. Refrigerate and protect from light. Stable 1 week at 4°C. CAUSES FOR REJECTION: Specimen not protected from light, specimen improperly collected, hemolysis, icterus

Interpretive REFERENCE RANGE: 17-77 μg/dL (SI: 0.27-1.23 μmol/L). Results may be obtained as ZPP/heme ratio; reference range: 30-80 μmol/mol heme CRITICAL VALUES: >100 μg/dL (SI: >1.6 μmol/L) USE: Evaluate iron deficiency, especially nonanemic iron deficiency. ZPP is superior to hemoglobin in identifying female blood donors with nonanemic iron deficiency.[1] LIMITATIONS: Zinc protoporphyrin may also be increased in lead poisoning, anemia of chronic disease, and erythropoietic protoporphyria. ZPP should **not** be used to screen or diagnose lead poisoning.[2,3] METHODOLOGY: Hematofluorometry (front-face); if washed erythrocytes are used, the assay becomes more specific and sensitive[4] ADDITIONAL INFORMATION: Zinc protoporphyrin levels increase as blood lead levels increase. Various authorities caution using ZPP as a screening test for lead poisoning. The Center for Disease Control has lowered the cutoff level for lead intoxication in children younger than 6 years of age to **10 μg/dL (SI: 0.48 μmol/L)**, and this level is so low that **ZPP is not useful** in this context because it is insensitive to such a lead level. Therefore, it is mandatory to measure lead levels in any screening program, rather than ZPP. ZPP appears only in new RBCs and remains for the life of the RBC; therefore, ZPP does not increase until several weeks after the onset of lead exposure and remains high long after exposure to lead. It is a reasonable indicator of total body burden of lead and remains a useful adjunct to the diagnosis of iron deficiency, particularly in nonanemic or questionably anemic patients. It reflects iron depletion in the bone marrow.

Footnotes

Baskin HJ, "Endocrinologic Evaluation of Impotence," *South M Portoporphyrin for Iron Deficiency in Nonanemic Female Blood Donors," Clin Chem*, 1990, 36(6):846-8.
2. Turk DS, Schonfeld DJ, Cullen M, et al, "Sensitivity of Erythrocyte Protoporphyrin as a Screening Test for Lead Poisoning," *N Engl J Med*, 1992, 326(2):137-8.
3. Rolfe PB, Marcinak JF, Nice AJ, et al, "Use of Zinc Protoporphyrin Measured by the Protofluor-Z Hematofluorometer in Screening Children for Elevated Blood Lead Levels," *Am J Dis Child*, 1993, 147(1):66-8.
4. Hastka J, Lasserre JJ, Schwarzbeck A, et al, "Washing Erythrocytes to Remove Interferents in Measurement of Zinc Protoporphyrin by Front-Face Hematofluorometry," *Clin Chem*, 1992, 38(11):2184-9.

References

Cone DC, "Lead Screening and Follow-Up in an Urban Pediatric Clinic," *N Y State J Med*, 1992, 92(8):338-42.
Labbe RF, "Clinical Utility of Zinc Protoporphyrin," *Clin Chem*, 1992, 38(11):2167-8.
Zwennis WC, Franssen AC, and Wijnans MJ, "Use of Zinc Protoporphyrin in Screening Individuals for Exposure to Lead," *Clin Chem*, 1990, 36(8 Pt 1):1456-9.

PRP *see* Parathyroid Hormone *on page 311*

PSA *see* Prostate Specific Antigen, Serum *on page 338*

Pseudocholinesterase Inhibition *see* Dibucaine Number *on page 209*

Pseudocholinesterase, Serum

CPT 82480

Related Information

Acetylcholinesterase, Red Blood Cell *on page 95*
Dibucaine Number *on page 209*

Synonyms Cholinesterase, Serum; PCE; Plasma Cholinesterase

Abstract Two types of cholinesterase are found in blood: "true" cholinesterase (acetylcholinesterase) in red cells and "pseudocholinesterase" (acylcholine acylhydrolase) in serum (plasma).

Specimen Serum CONTAINER: Red top tube STORAGE INSTRUCTIONS: Cholinesterase is stable in separated serum for 80 days at room temperature and 3 years at -20°C. However, specimens submitted to evaluate possible pesticide toxicity should be collected on ice, separated in a refrigerated centrifuge, and frozen until analyzed.[1]

Interpretive REFERENCE RANGE: Low in infancy, then increasing in early childhood. Ranges vary between methods and laboratories. POSSIBLE PANIC RANGE: Less than lower limit of normal USE: Screen preoperative patients for succinylcholine (suxamethonium) anesthetic sensitivity, genetic or secondary to insecticide exposure, in appropriate circumstances. Prevent or evaluate prolonged anesthetic effect, prolonged apnea, after surgery. Very small amounts (0.04-0.06 mg/kg) of succinylcholine are needed to obtain 90% of neuromuscular blockade in patients with low levels of plasma cholinesterase activity.[2]

(Continued)

Pseudocholinesterase, Serum *(Continued)*

Monitor organophosphorous or carbamate insecticide poisoning, in which level is decreased; establish patient's baseline value before exposure. Indications include such pesticide exposure, especially with miosis, blurred vision, muscle weakness, twitching, and fasciculation, bradycardia, nausea, diarrhea, vomiting, salivation, sweating, pulmonary edema, arrhythmias, and convulsions. The value of assessing risk status in persons exposed to organophosphate insecticides on the basis of plasma cholinesterase levels alone has been called into question.[3] Are normal levels indicative of no exposure or of a genetic variant with or without exposure? There are interpretive problems with low or high values.[3]

Family studies may be done when an individual with a genetically abnormal type is documented by serum pseudocholinesterase deficiency and, ideally, confirmed by phenotyping.

LIMITATIONS: Serum pseudocholinesterase may be decreased in patients on estrogens and oral contraceptives.[1] Fluoride interferes. Pseudocholinesterase is low also in some instances of liver disease, including decompensated cirrhosis, hepatitis, metastatic carcinoma, CHF, and in malnutrition, but not sufficiently consistently enough to be a useful clinical test for such disorders. Genetic atypical enzyme does not explain every instance of prolonged postsurgical apnea. Red cell cholinesterase is more useful for chronic insecticide exposure. Carbamate-poisoned persons can appear to have near normal or normal levels of pseudocholinesterase. **CONTRAINDICATIONS:** Not useful to screen for toxicity from chlorinated insecticides. **METHODOLOGY:** Colorimetry, kinetic enzyme utilizing different substrates, fluorometry[4] **ADDITIONAL INFORMATION:** Low serum cholinesterase activity may relate to exposure to insecticides or to one of a number of variant genotypes. Dibucaine and fluoride numbers are useful to phenotype such homozygous and heterozygous individuals, who are genetically sensitive to succinylcholine.

One patient in 1500 is susceptible to succinyldicholine anesthetic mishap.

Plasmapheresis has been noted to decrease the level of plasma cholinesterase. Patients with abnormally low cholinesterase activity after transfusion of blood or plasma will experience temporary augmentation of enzyme level. In estimating the duration of this enhanced activity, measures of plasma cholinesterase half-life have been utilized. The true half-life value has, however, been uncertain. A half-life value determined by measuring the rate of disappearance after intravenous injection of human cholinesterase has provided an average value of 11 days.[5]

A low level of activity of pseudocholinesterase has been demonstrated in cerebrospinal fluid, at about 1/20 to 1/100 the activity present in the corresponding plasma. With clinical conditions characterized by bleeding into the CSF, pseudocholinesterase activity increases 25% to 50% that of plasma.[6]

Patients with a variety of carcinomas have been reported to accumulate an embryonic type of cholinesterase activity in their sera. Such novel cholinesterase activity was found only in the sera of patients undergoing antitumor therapy (eg, chemotherapy or radiation therapy and/or hormone therapy).[7]

Increase in acetylcholinesterase activity, notably, in an acetylcholinesterase to butyrylcholine esterase ratio (histochemical study, not as measured in serum) has provided discriminatory diagnostic value in some cases of Hirschsprung's disease.[8]

Footnotes

1. Ladenson JH, "Nonanalytical Sources of Variation in Clinical Chemistry Results," *Gradwohl's Clinical Laboratory Methods and Diagnosis*, 8th ed, Sonnenwirth AC and Jarett L, eds, St Louis, MO: Mosby-Year Book Inc, 1980, 160.
2. Hickey DR, O'Connor JP, and Donati F, "Comparison of Atracurium and Succinylcholine for Electroconvulsive Therapy in a Patient With Atypical Plasma Cholinesterase," *Can J Anaesth*, 1987, 34:280-3.
3. Alexiou NG, Williams JF, Yeung HW, et al, "Paradoxical Elevation of Plasma Cholinesterase," *Am J Prev Med*, 1986, 2:235-81.
4. Kusu F, Tsuneta T, and Takamura K, "Fluorometric Determination of Pseudocholinesterase Activity in Postmortem Blood Samples," *J Forensic Sci*, 1990, 35(6):1330-4.
5. Ostergaard D, Viby-Mogensen J, Hanel HK, et al, "Half-Life of Plasma Cholinesterase," *Acta Anaesthesiol Scand*, 1988, 32:266-9.
6. Kambam JR, Horton B, Parris WC, et al, "Pseudocholinesterase Activity in Human Cerebrospinal Fluid," *Anesth Analg*, 1989, 68(4):486-8.
7. Zakut H, Even L, Birkenfeld S, et al, "Modified Properties of Serum Cholinesterases in Primary Carcinomas," *Cancer*, 1988, 61(4):727-37.
8. Causse E, Vaysse P, Fabre J, et al, "The Diagnostic Value of Acetylcholinesterase/Butyrylcholinesterase Ratio in Hirschsprung's Disease," *Am J Clin Pathol*, 1987, 88:477-80.

References

Hoffman RS, Henry GC, Howland MA, et al, "Association Between Life-Threatening Cocaine Toxicity and Plasma Cholinesterase Activity," *Ann Emerg Med*, 1992, 21(3):247-53.

Newman MA and Que Hee SS, "Interconversion and Comparison of Three Methods for Acetyl Cholinesterase in Serum," *Clin Chem*, 1984, 30:308-10.

PTH *see* Parathyroid Hormone *on page 311*

PTH-Related Protein *see* Parathyroid Hormone *on page 311*

Pulmonary Surfactant *see* Amniotic Fluid Pulmonary Surfactant *on page 126*

Pyridoxal Phosphate *see* Vitamin B_6 *on page 386*

Pyridoxine *see* Vitamin B_6 *on page 386*

Pyruvate Kinase Assay *see* Pyruvate Kinase Assay, Erythrocytes *on this page*

Pyruvate Kinase Assay, Erythrocytes

CPT *84220*

Related Information

Pyruvate Kinase Screen, Erythrocytes *on this page*

Synonyms PK Assay; Pyruvate Kinase Assay

Specimen Erythrocytes (washed) **CONTAINER:** Yellow top (ACD) tube, green top (heparin) tube, or lavender top (EDTA) tube **COLLECTION:** Mix tube three times by gentle inversion, place on ice. **CAUSES FOR REJECTION:** Specimen not fresh **SPECIAL INSTRUCTIONS:** Notify laboratory before specimen collection. Deliver specimen on ice. Specimen **must** be received in the laboratory within 30 minutes of collection.

Interpretive **REFERENCE RANGE:** Adults: 6-19 μmol $NAD(H)_2$/min/g Hgb (37°C) **USE:** Evaluate chronic hemolytic anemia **METHODOLOGY:** Spectrophotometric kinetic assay **ADDITIONAL INFORMATION:** Pyruvate kinase is the most common enzyme defect in anaerobic red cell glycolysis (Embden-Meyerhof glycolytic pathway) and the most common cause of congenital nonspherocytic hemolytic anemia.[1] The deficiency is inherited as an autosomal recessive trait. Current assay techniques preclude accurate distinction of all heterozygotes from normals. Specialized PK assays and the determination of red cell 2,3-DPG levels are often helpful in these cases. Most homozygous PK deficient children, younger than 2 years of age, have higher residual PK activities than those found in adult PK deficient homozygotes with comparable levels of reticulocytosis. Reductions of red cell pyruvate kinase activity to <20% of normal indicates hereditary PK deficiency. Slight to moderate decrease of red cell PK activity can be seen in some patients with leukemia and in aplasia. Further characterization may be necessary to diagnose hemolytic disease due to PK deficient variants, including doubly heterozygous individuals. A number of patients with hemolytic disease due to PK deficient variant will escape diagnosis if the enzyme is assayed only under conditions of substrate saturation.

Footnotes

1. Miwa S and Fujii H, "Pyruvate Kinase Deficiency," *Clin Biochem*, 1990, 23(2):155-7.

References

Zachee P, Staal GE, Rijksen G, et al, "Pyruvate Kinase Deficiency and Delayed Clinical Response to Recombinant Human Erythropoietin Treatment," *Lancet*, 1989, 1(8650):1327-8.

Pyruvate Kinase Deficiency Screen, RBCs *see* Pyruvate Kinase Screen, Erythrocytes *on this page*

Pyruvate Kinase Screen, Erythrocytes

CPT *84220*

Related Information

Pyruvate Kinase Assay, Erythrocytes *on this page*

Synonyms PK Screen, Blood; Pyruvate Kinase Deficiency Screen, RBCs

Specimen Erythrocytes (washed) **CONTAINER:** Lavender top (EDTA) tube **COLLECTION:** Routine venipuncture **STORAGE INSTRUCTIONS:** Refrigerate whole blood immediately.

Interpretive **REFERENCE RANGE:** Pyruvate kinase enzyme activity detected **USE:** Evaluate presence of pyruvate kinase enzyme deficiency; screen for inborn errors of erythrocyte metabolism associated with hemolytic anemia **LIMITATIONS:** This procedure can only differentiate between normal and grossly deficient samples and will not detect heterozygotes. **ADDITIONAL IN-**

(Continued)

Pyruvate Kinase Screen, Erythrocytes *(Continued)*

FORMATION: Pyruvate kinase (PK) deficiency in the red blood cell is a genetic disorder characterized by a lowered ATP level in the RBC and consequential membrane defect. The result is a nonspherocytic, chronic hemolytic anemia. PK deficiency is the most common and important form of hemolytic anemia due to a deficiency of glycolytic enzymes in the RBC.

Quantitative Fecal Fat, 72-Hour Collection *see* Fecal Fat, Quantitative, 72-Hour Collection *on page 219*

Radioallergosorbent Test *see* Allergen Specific IgE Antibody *on page 112*

Rapid ACTH Test *see* Cosyntropin Test *on page 194*

RAST® *see* Allergen Specific IgE Antibody *on page 112*

RBC Galactokinase *see* Galactokinase, Blood *on page 226*

RBC Protoporphyrin *see* Protoporphyrin, Free Erythrocyte *on page 341*

Red Cell Cholinesterase *see* Acetylcholinesterase, Red Blood Cell *on page 95*

Renal Panel *see* Kidney Profile *on page 268*

Renal Profile *see* Kidney Profile *on page 268*

Renin, Plasma

CPT 84244

Related Information

Aldosterone, Blood *on page 104*
Aldosterone, Urine *on page 106*
Electrolytes, Urine *on page 213*
Potassium, Blood *on page 330*
Potassium, Urine *on page 332*

Synonyms Plasma Renin Activity; PRA

Applies to Angiotensin

Test Commonly Includes Fasting supine or upright specimens, catheterization studies

Abstract The juxtaglomerular apparatus produces renin, an enzyme, which converts angiotensinogen to angiotensin I. Angiotensin I is in turn converted to angiotensin II, the biologically active metabolite. Angiotensin II stimulates the release of aldosterone from the adrenal cortex and has direct vasopressor effects.

Patient Care PREPARATION: Antihypertensive drugs, steroids, cyclic progestogens, estrogens, diuretics, licorice should be terminated at least 2 weeks and preferably, 4 weeks before a renin-aldosterone work-up is to begin. A special sodium diet may be ordered for 3 days only. A normal sodium diet is requested for 2-4 weeks unless renin activity is to be measured following salt depletion for aldosteronism. Upright posture, administration of diuretics, low-sodium diets stimulate renin release. Renins are commonly drawn at end of 24-hour collection of urine for sodium and creatinine and after several days of stable sodium intake controlled by the physician.

No recent administration of radioactivity; no recent radioactive tracers; no caffeine before or during collection. There are special instructions for preparation for sodium depletion renins, renal venous renin ratio, primary aldosteronism work-up. There are special diet instructions, sodium intake requirements. Check with laboratory for particular patient preparation instructions.

Specimen Plasma CONTAINER: Lavender top (EDTA) tube SAMPLING TIME: Normally, higher levels are found in upright subjects drawn in the morning. COLLECTION: Draw specimen into a prechilled syringe. Place in chilled lavender top tubes (with the rubber stopper off). Recap, mix, and immediately place on ice and deliver to the laboratory. STORAGE INSTRUCTIONS: Place in an ice-water bath. After the specimen is well cooled, centrifuge at 4°C. Separate plasma immediately and freeze in a plastic container. CAUSES FOR REJECTION: Clotted sample, patient preparation incorrect for the sample desired, recent radioisotope scan prior to collection of specimen SPECIAL INSTRUCTIONS: Request should state posture and dietary status.

Interpretive REFERENCE RANGE: 1-6 ng/mL/hour (SI: 0.77-4.6 nmol/L/hour). Depends upon sodium depletion, age, posture. Results depend on whether or not there has been stimulation (eg, furosemide). Values from right and left renal veins should normally be equal. In arterial constriction, a ratio >1.5 is considered abnormal. USE: Evaluate the role of renin in the differential diagnosis of hypertension. Renin is suppressed by high aldosterone levels in most patients with Conn's syndrome (primary aldosteronism). Evaluate hypokalemia; diagnose primary aldosteronism is made in the hypertensive patient with hypokalemia who excretes ≥50 mmol/L potassium in a 24-hour urine collection without diuretics. The patient with primary aldosteronism is characterized by low plasma renin and high serum and urine aldosterone.[1] The low renin which characterizes primary aldosteronism fails to increase appropriately with volume depletion (eg, upright posture, volume/sodium depletion). Such patients are not edematous.[2] Subjects with secondary aldosteronism may have elevated renin, in contrast to those with primary aldosteronism. Secondary aldosteronism occurs with accelerated hypertension and occurs in pregnancy.[2] Evaluate renovascular hypertension. Renin-producing tumors occur but are extremely rare (juxtaglomerular cell tumor).[2] Patients with them resemble subjects with renovascular hypertension chemically. Hyporeninemic hypoaldosteronism causes renal salt wasting, hyperkalemia, and metabolic acidosis. **LIMITATIONS:** Disease entities besides Conn's syndrome cause hypertension with low renin levels. Salt restricted diets increase supine renin levels by a factor of 2; upright renin levels by a factor of 6. Renin increases in pregnancy, patients on oral contraceptives and with salt loss, Addison's disease, diuretics, and certain types of renal diseases. Random samples may be difficult to interpret unless medications and state of sodium balance are defined. Specimen must be collected with scrupulous attention to technical detail. Drugs may alter results. **CONTRAINDICATIONS:** Random drawing of sample for renin activity rarely yields clinically meaningful information. **METHODOLOGY:** Radioimmunoassay (RIA). A kinetic assay in which renin's enzymatic activity is measured **indirectly** by the formation of angiotensin I from angiotensinogen.[3] **ADDITIONAL INFORMATION:** There exists a renin-aldosterone axis, involving angiotensin, which regulates sodium and potassium balance, blood volume and blood pressure. Renal reabsorption of sodium affects plasma volume. Low plasma volume, blood pressure, and low sodium induce renin release. Renin causes increased aldosterone through stimulation of angiotensin. Potassium loss suppresses renin release through aldosterone secretion. Aldosterone retains sodium, increasing plasma volume, elevating blood pressure and causing potassium loss. Adrenal vein sampling for aldosterone is useful; an increase on the side bearing the aldosteronoma supports diagnosis as well as location. Protocols for aldosterone/renin work-up are available,[2] and flow diagrams for hypertension are published.[1] The hypokalemia of Bartter's syndrome (a renal tubular nephropathy) is associated with edema, alkalosis, increased renin and aldosterone. Such patients are not edematous and have normal blood pressure.[2] Chapman et al have shown that the renin-angiotension-aldosterone system affects hypertension in polycystic kidney disease. They have also shown that use of angiotensin converting enzyme inhibitors can ameliorate the effect of increased renin levels.[4]

Footnotes

1. Beeler MF, "Hypertension," *Interpretations in Clinical Chemistry*, Chicago, IL: American Society of Clinical Pathologists, 1983, 72-5.
2. Williams GH and Dluhy RG, "Diseases of the Adrenal Cortex," *Harrison's Principles of Internal Medicine*, 12th ed, Vol 2, Wilson JD, Braunwald E, Isselbacher KJ, et al, eds, New York, NY: McGraw-Hill Inc, 1991, 1713-34.
3. Sealey JE, "Plasma Renin Activity and Plasma Prorenin Assays," *Clin Chem*, 1991, 37(10 Pt 2):1811-9.
4. Chapman AB, Johnson A, Gabow PA, et al, "The Renin-Angiotensin-Aldosterone System and Autosomal Dominant Polycystic Kidney Disease," *N Engl J Med*, 1990, 323(16):1091-6.

References

Andreoli TE, "Disorders of Fluid Volume, Electrolytes, and Acid-Base Balance," *Cecil Textbook of Medicine*, 19th ed, Vol 1, Wyngaarden JB, Smith LH Jr, and Bennett JC, eds, Philadelphia, PA: WB Saunders Co, 1992, 499-528.

Fievet P, Pleskov L, Desailly I, et al, "Plasma Renin Activity, Blood Uric Acid, and Plasma Volume in Pregnancy-Induced Hypertension," *Nephron*, 1985, 40:429-32.

Resnik LM, Laragh JH, Sealey JE, et al, "Divalent Cations in Essential Hypertension. Relations Between Serum Ionized Calcium, Magnesium, and Plasma Renin Activity," *N Engl J Med*, 1983, 309:888-91.

Scammell AM and Diver MJ, "Plasma Aldosterone and Renin Activity," *Arch Dis Child*, 1989, 64(1):139-41.

Torres VE, Young WF Jr, Offord KP, et al, "Association of Hypokalemia, Aldosteronism, and Renal Cysts," *N Engl J Med*, 1990, 322(6):345-51.

Trovati M, Massucco P, Anfossi G, et al, "Insulin Influences the Renin-Angiotensin-Aldosterone System in Humans," *Metabolism*, 1989, 38(6):501-3.

Resin Triiodothyronine Uptake *see* T_3 Uptake *on page 355*

Retinol, Serum *see* Vitamin A, Serum *on page 385*

Rheumatoid Factor, Body Fluid *see* Body Fluid *on page 145*

Risk Index for Coronary Arterial Disease *see* Lipid Profile *on page 278*

SaO_2 *see* Oxygen Saturation, Blood *on page 305*

Secretin *see* Vasoactive Intestinal Polypeptide *on page 384*

S-Epo *see* Erythropoietin, Serum *on page 214*

Serotonin

CPT 84260

Related Information

5-Hydroxyindoleacetic Acid, Quantitative, Urine *on page 257*

Synonyms 5-HT; 5-Hydroxytryptamine, Blood

Applies to Serotonin, Cerebrospinal Fluid

Abstract Serotonin is synthesized from tryptophan. Serotonin's major metabolite, 5-HIAA, is measured more commonly than 5-HT (parent compound).

Patient Care PREPARATION: Monoamine oxidase inhibitor drugs should be discontinued for at least 1 week prior to sampling, since they tend to increase the level of serotonin. Avoid application of radioisotopes (eg, scans) before sampling. Some methods require a low indole diet for several days. Avoid eggplant, avocado, bananas, tomatoes, pineapple, walnuts, and red plums.

Specimen Whole blood, cerebrospinal fluid CONTAINER: Tube with EDTA, sometimes with ascorbic acid. Check with laboratory. COLLECTION: Draw in chilled tubes. Keep on ice. STORAGE INSTRUCTIONS: Place whole blood in plastic bottle containing 10 mg EDTA and 75 mg ascorbic acid. Freeze within 4 hours of collection. Stable 7 days at -20°C. CAUSES FOR REJECTION: Stored specimen not frozen, specimen stored without preservatives

Interpretive REFERENCE RANGE: 10-30 μg/dL (SI: 570-1700 nmol/L). Values vary among laboratories and are method dependent. In serum, serotonin (5-hydroxytryptamine) levels in females were about 1.3-fold that of males. By RIA, a study provided ranges: male: 7-12 μg/dL (SI: 380-680 nmol/L), female: 9-16 μg/dL (SI: 520-900 nmol/L).[1] USE: Diagnose carcinoid syndrome. The classical syndrome includes flushing and vasomotor instability, diarrhea, hepatomegaly, and endocardial lesions. Ectopic production may occur from oat cell carcinomas of lung, islet cell tumors of pancreas, and medullary carcinoma of the thyroid. Carcinoid tumors occur in multiple endocrine neoplasia, types I or II. LIMITATIONS: Serotonin assays are not widely available and only rarely used. It may be useful to measure when normal or borderline increases of 5-HIAA are seen in a patient with clinical evidence of carcinoid syndrome. Urinary 5-HIAA is more sensitive and specific for diagnosis of carcinoid tumors. Engbaek and Voldby indicate that 5-methoxytryptamine and tryptamine cross react with their RIA method.[1] METHODOLOGY: Fluorometry, radioimmunoassay (RIA), gas chromatography (GC), liquid chromatography with electrochemical detection, radioenzymatic assay ADDITIONAL INFORMATION: Serotonin is produced by cells of the APUD system, including the enterochromaffin (Kulchitsky) cells distributed through the mucosa of the gastrointestinal tract. Most serotonin in blood is usually concentrated in platelets, which release it during platelet aggregation. Serotonin may be measured to confirm the diagnosis of carcinoid syndrome. The carcinoid syndrome is usually caused by primary carcinoids of the ileum, but the syndrome is occasionally caused by primary carcinoids of the stomach. Other organs give rise to carcinoids including pancreas, duodenum, bronchus, and ovary. Most patients with the carcinoid syndrome have hepatic metastases. The role of serotonin in psychiatric disorders is poorly established. A urinary serotonin assay is described but is not widely available.[2]

Footnotes

1. Engbaek F and Voldby B, "Radioimmunoassay of Serotonin (5-Hydroxytryptamine) in Cerebrospinal Fluid, Plasma, and Serum," *Clin Chem*, 1982, 624-8.
2. Feldman JM, "Urinary Serotonin in the Diagnosis of Carcinoid Tumors," *Clin Chem*, 1986, 32:840-4.

References

Anderson GM, Feibel FC, and Cohen DJ, "Determination of Serotonin in Whole Blood, Platelet-Rich Plasma, Platelet-Poor Plasma, and Plasma Ultrafiltrate," *Life Sci*, 1987, 40:1063-70.

Cryer PE, "The Carcinoid Syndrome," *Cecil Textbook of Medicine*, Wyngaarden JB, Smith LH Jr, and Bennett JC, eds, Philadelphia, PA: WB Saunders Co, 1992, 1394-7.

Schultz AL, "Serotonin," *Methods in Clinical Chemistry*, Pesce AJ and Kaplan LA, eds, 1987, 796-802.

Taqari PC, Boullin DJ, and Davies CL, "Simplified Determination of Serotonin in Plasma by Liquid Chromatography With Electrochemical Detection," *Clin Chem*, 1984, 30:131-5.

Tietz NW, ed, "5HIAA," *Textbook of Clinical Chemistry*, Philadelphia, PA: WB Saunders Co, 1986, 1160.

Wilson JD and Foster DW, eds, *Williams Textbook of Endocrinology*, 8th ed, Philadelphia, PA: WB Saunders Co, 1992, 1619-34.

Serotonin, Cerebrospinal Fluid *see* Serotonin *on previous page*

Serotonin, Metabolite *see* 5-Hydroxyindoleacetic Acid, Quantitative, Urine *on page 257*

Serum-Ascites Albumin Difference *see* Body Fluid *on page 145*

Serum Electrolytes *see* Electrolytes, Blood *on page 212*

Serum Osmolality *see* Osmolality, Serum *on page 300*

Sex Hormone Binding Globulin *see* Testosterone, Free and Total *on page 358*

SGOT *see* Aspartate Aminotransferase *on page 135*

SGPT *see* Alanine Aminotransferase *on page 100*

Shake Test *see* Amniotic Fluid Pulmonary Surfactant *on page 126*

SHBG *see* Testosterone, Free and Total *on page 358*

Siderophilin *see* Transferrin *on page 369*

Sm-C *see* Somatomedin-C *on page 354*

S-NSE *see* Neuron-Specific Enolase, Serum *on page 294*

SO_2 *see* Oxygen Saturation, Blood *on page 305*

Sodium, Arterial Blood *see* Sodium, Blood *on this page*

Sodium, Blood

CPT 84295

Related Information

Anion Gap *on page 132*
Chloride, Serum *on page 182*
Chloride, Urine *on page 184*
Electrolytes, Blood *on page 212*
Osmolality, Calculated *on page 299*
Sodium, Urine *on page 351*
Urea Nitrogen, Blood *on page 376*
Uric Acid, Serum *on page 378*

Synonyms Na^+

Applies to Sodium, Arterial Blood; Sodium, Corrected

Abstract Sodium with its accompanying anions is the most important extracellular osmotically active solute.[1]

Specimen Serum or plasma **CONTAINER:** Red top tube or green top (lithium heparin) tube **COLLECTION:** Pediatric: Blood drawn from heelstick for capillary sample. Na^+, with K^+ and Cl^-, can be reported from arterial or venous blood. If an arterial puncture is done for pO_2, lithium heparin anticoagulant must be used.

Interpretive **REFERENCE RANGE:** Adults: 135-145 mmol/L **POSSIBLE PANIC RANGE:** <120 mmol/L, >160 mmol/L **USE:** Evaluate electrolytes, acid-base balance, water balance, water intoxication, and diagnose dehydration.

Hypernatremia occurs in dehydration. For instance, nasogastric protein feeding with insufficient fluids may cause hypernatremia. Hypernatremia without obvious cause may relate to Cushing's syndrome, central or nephrogenic diabetes insipidus with insufficient fluids, primary aldosteronism, and other diseases. Severe hypernatremia may be associated with volume contraction, lactic acidosis, azotemia, weight loss, and increased hematocrit as evidence of dehydration. The corrected serum sodium is often high in nonketotic hyperosmolar coma. (A corrected Na^+ is calculated by increasing Na^+ by 1.3-1.6 mmol/L for each 100 mg/dL increment in serum or plasma glucose). 100 mg = 5.56 mmol/L. The corrected serum sodium level should be calculated in nonketotic hyperosmolar coma. Apparent mild hyponatremia with very high glucose may actually mean hypernatremia.[1]

Hyponatremia occurs with nephrotic syndrome, cachexia, hypoproteinemia, intravenous glucose infusion, congestive heart failure, and other clinical entities. Serum sodium is a predictor of cardiovascular mortality in patients with severe congestive heart failure.[2] **Hyponatremia** without congestive heart failure or dehydration may occur with hypothyroidism, the syndrome of inappropriate secretion of antidiuretic hormone (SIADH), renal failure, or renal sodium loss. (Continued)

Sodium, Blood *(Continued)*

The differential diagnosis of hyponatremia includes Addison's disease, hypopituitarism, liver disease including cirrhosis, hypertriglyceridemia, and psychogenic polydipsia. Diuretics and other drugs may cause hyponatremia. Sodium decreasing to levels <115 mmol/L can lead to significant neurological dysfunction with cerebral edema and increased intracranial pressure.

The differential diagnosis of hyponatremia includes determination of urine sodium and osmolality and serum urea nitrogen (BUN). BUN is often decreased in SIADH.

LIMITATIONS: Care should be taken that one is not dealing with "pseudohyponatremia." See the following comments. **METHODOLOGY:** Flame emission photometry, ion-selective electrode (ISE) **ADDITIONAL INFORMATION:** The ratio of serum sodium to osmolality is normally 0.43-0.50; a decreased ratio is found in uremia and other states in which there are increased substances with osmotic activity.

See Urea Nitrogen, Blood, regarding hyponatremia with sodium <128 mmol/L, hypoosmolality, low BUN, and the syndrome of inappropriate secretion of antidiuretic hormone.

A number of situations result in "pseudohyponatremia." In these circumstances, treatment may be undesirable. With pseudohyponatremia serum sodium is decreased but the serum is not hypotonic (serum osmolality is normal or even increased). This may occur as the result of other molecules replacing water in relation to sodium. The water content is effectively lowered – sodium is "diluted." In severe hypertriglyceridemia or paraprotein-related marked increase in protein, the concentration of sodium in relation to water is normal but the analytic result is determined as mmol/L of serum. Osmolality in this situation is determined as amount of particles per kg of water and will be normal. It has been shown that analyses by sodium electrode of the direct potentiometric type (requires no dilution) are not artifactually low in patients with hyperlipidemia.[3] If large amounts of solute, such as glucose or mannitol, are present, movement of intracellular water into the extracellular space may produce dilutional hyponatremia. In this case, sodium concentration in relation to water is actually low. "Osmolal gap" however exists between measured and calculated serum osmolality. Other substances capable of increasing serum osmolality (eg, ethanol) may also cause increase in the osmolal gap. Yet another cause of pseudohyponatremia is increased serum viscosity due to increased globulin proteins, occurring particularly in Waldenström's macroglobulinemia. The sodium analyzer may aspirate too little sample when viscosity is so high, leading to a factitious low sodium concentration. See discussion of "pseudohyponatremia" by Epstein and Osler.[4]

Hyponatremia may manifest lethal neurological complications (water intoxication with brain edema).

Drug effects are summarized.[5]

Footnotes

1. Daugirdas JT, Kronfol NO, Tzamaloukas AH, et al, "Hyperosmolar Coma: Cellular Dehydration and the Serum Sodium Concentration," *Ann Intern Med*, 1989, 110(11):855-7, (review).
2. Lee WH and Packer M, "Prognostic Importance of Serum Sodium Concentration and Its Modification by Converting Enzyme Inhibition in Patients With Severe Chronic Heart Failure," *Circulation*, 1986, 73:257-67.
3. Aw TC and Kiechle FL, "Pseudohyponatremia," *Am J Emerg Med*, 1985, 3:236-9.
4. Epstein M and Oster JR, "Disorders of Hyponatremia and Hypernatremia," *The Laboratory in Clinical Medicine. Interpretation and Application*, 2nd ed, Halsted JA and Halsted CH, eds, Philadelphia, PA: WB Saunders Co, 1981, 289-95.
5. Hitz J and Trivin F, "Sodium," *Drug Effects on Laboratory Test Results Analytical Interferences and Pharmacological Effects*, Siest G and Galteau MM, eds, Littleton, MA: PSG Publishing Co Inc, 1988, 391-404.

References

DeVita MV and Michelis MF, "Perturbations in Sodium Balance: Hyponatremia and Hypernatremia," *Clin Lab Med*, 1993, 13(1):135-48.

Fogh-Andersen N, Wimberly PD, Thade J, et al, "Determination of Sodium and Potassium With Ion Selective Electrodes," *Clin Chem*, 1984, 30:433-6.

Kaplan LA and Pesce AJ, eds, *Clinical Chemistry: Theory, Analysis, and Correlation*, St Louis, MO: Mosby-Year Book Inc, 1984.

Leehey DJ, Daugirdas JT, Manahan FJ, et al, "Prolonged Hypernatremia Associated With Azotemia and Hyponatruria," *Am J Med*, 1989, 86(4):494-6.

Maffly RH, "Renal Function and Disorders of Water, Sodium, and Potassium Balance," *Scientific American Medicine*, Section 10, Chapter 1, Rubenstein E and Federman DD, eds, New York, NY: Scientific American Inc, 1990, 2-34.

McCleane GJ, "Urea and Electrolyte Measurement in Preoperative Surgical Patients," *Anaesthesia*, 1988, 43:413-5. "With Severe Chronic Heart Failure," *Circulation*, 1986, 73:257-67.

Votey SR, Peters AL, and Hoffman JR, "Disorders of Water Metabolism: Hyponatremia and Hypernatremia," *Emerg Med Clin North Am*, 1989, 7(4):749-69.

Sodium, Corrected *see* Sodium, Blood *on page 349*
Sodium, Sweat *see* Chloride, Sweat *on page 183*

Sodium, Urine

***CPT** 84300*

Related Information

Chloride, Urine *on page 184*
Electrolytes, Urine *on page 213*
Kidney Stone Analysis *on page 1129*
Osmolality, Urine *on page 302*
Sodium, Blood *on page 349*

Synonyms Na, Urine; Urine Na

Specimen Timed or random urine **CONTAINER:** Plain urine container **CAUSES FOR REJECTION:** Improper labeling

Interpretive **REFERENCE RANGE:** 24-hour urine: 27-287 mmol/d, varies markedly with dietary intake of sodium. There is diurnal variation (output is lower at night). A European study provides average sodium excretion: male: 162 mmol/day, range: 143-208 mmol/day; female: 134 mmol/day, range: 119-165 mmol/day; within person CV: male: 30%, female: 34%.[1] **USE:** Work up volume depletion, acute renal failure, acute oliguria, and differential diagnosis of hyponatremia.[2] Division of hyponatremia into hypervolemia or not, edema or not, and urinary Na^+ less than or greater than 10 mmol/L provides a classification of hyponatremia.[3] History of diuretics, other drug intake, setting of osmotic diuresis or not, serum/plasma electrolytes, and other factors are needed. **LIMITATIONS:** It is often advantageous to request urine potassium and creatinine along with sodium measurement. High urine sodium does not necessarily indicate that total body sodium is increased (eg, salt-losing nephritis). This area is complex; the reader is referred to the footnotes and references. **METHODOLOGY:** Flame emission photometry or ion-selective electrode (ISE) **ADDITIONAL INFORMATION:** In cases of hyponatremia, random urine Na^+ <10 mmol/L may indicate extrarenal depletion: dehydration (gastrointestinal or sweat loss), congestive heart failure, liver disease or nephrotic syndromes.

Random urine Na^+ >10 mmol/L may indicate diuretics, emesis, intrinsic renal diseases, Addison's disease, hypothyroidism, or syndrome of inappropriate antidiuretic hormone (SIADH).[3] In hypothyroidism and in SIADH, Na^+ and Cl^- may be >40 mmol/L.[4] (Depending on intake, such results also can be found in normal individuals.) In SIADH, random urinary sodium usually is >20 mmol/L. Inappropriate secretion of antidiuretic hormone (SIADH) was found in 7% of 250 patients with small cell lung cancer.[5] Such patients have hyponatremia, often severe, with hypo-osmolar serum, high urinary sodium excretion with urine osmolality greater than that of serum. Acute and subacute diseases of the CNS, TB, and other chronic pulmonary diseases may also cause SIADH. SIADH may also be caused by acute intermittent porphyria, LE, occasional malignant neoplasms other than small cell carcinoma of the lung, and a number of drugs.[6]

The classification as presented here is overly abbreviated for clinical application. Pitfalls exist (eg, increase of Na^+ necessary to balance excretion of penicillin).[4]

Urine Na^+ >40 mmol/L in oliguria suggests acute tubular necrosis.[4,7] (However, spot urine sodiums without other data have been criticized for their applicability to this diagnosis.)

Low Na^+ excretion may be found with early obstructive uropathy and with the oliguria of acute glomerulonephritis[4] and in some patients with x-ray contrast acute renal failure.

Silver et al recommend measurement of urinary sodium excretion in patients with nephrolithiasis and hypercalciuria.[8]

It is important to know the urinary sodium level in patients with unexplained hyperchloremic metabolic acidosis when the diagnosis of distal renal tubular acidosis is being considered.[9]

Footnotes

1. Knuiman JT, Hautvast JG, van Der Heijden L, et al, "A Multi-Centre Study on Within-Person Variability in the Urinary Excretion of Sodium, Potassium, Calcium, Magnesium, and Creatinine in 8 European Centres," *Human Nutrition: Clinical Nutrition*, 1986, 40C:343-8.
2. Harrington JT and Cohen JJ, "Measurement of Urinary Electrolytes – Indications and Limitations," *N Engl J Med*, 1975, 293:1241-3.
3. DeVita MV and Michelis MF, "Perturbations in Sodium Balance: Hyponatremia and Hypernatremia," *Clin Lab Med*, 1993, 13(1):135-48.
4. Sherman RA and Eisinger RP, "The Use (and Misuse) of Urinary Sodium and Chloride Measurements," *JAMA*, 1982, 247:3121-4.

(Continued)

Evaluation and Treatment of the **Hypernatremic** Patient

CONDITION		ETIOLOGY	URINARY ELECTROLYTES	TREATMENT
Hypovolemic	Renal losses	Osmotic diuresis	Urinary sodium >30 mmol/L	Isotonic saline (0.9 NaCl) until hemodynamically stable, then hypotonic fluids
	Extrarenal losses	Sweating Diarrhea in children	Urinary sodium <30 mmol/L	
Euvolemic	Renal losses	Central diabetes insipidus Nephrogenic diabetes insipidus Partial diabetes insipidus Hypodipsia	Variable urinary sodium	Administer vasopressin and water replacement. If urine volume decreased, diagnosis is central diabetes insipidus or partial diabetes insipidus. If no response, diagnosis is nephrogenic diabetes insipidus. Give trial of hydrochlorothiazide.
	Extrarenal losses	Respiratory or skin losses		
Hypervolemic	Increased total body sodium	Primary or secondary aldosteronism, Cushing's syndrome, Hypertonic I.V. infusion, I.V. sodium bicarbonate administration, Sodium chloride tablets	Urinary sodium >30 mmol/L	Diuretics and water replacement

From Devita MV and Michelis MF, "Perturbations in Sodium Balance: Hyponatremia and Hypernatremia," *Clinics in Laboratory Medicine,* Vol 13, Preuss HG, ed, Philadelphia, PA: WB Saunders Co, 1993, 135-48, with permission.

Evaluation and Treatment of **Hyponatremic** Patient

CONDITION	CLINICAL PRESENTATION	URINARY ELECTROLYTES	ETIOLOGY	TREATMENT
Hypovolemic	Orthostatic hypotension Tachycardia Azotemia	Urinary sodium >30 mmol/L	Diuretics, RTA, mineralocorticoid deficiency, salt-wasting nephritis	0.9 NaCl I.V.
		Urinary sodium <30 mmol/L	Extrarenal losses; vomiting, diarrhea, burns, sequestration	0.9 NaCl I.V.
Euvolemic	No evidence of volume depletion or overload. Subclinical increase in TBW may be present.	Urinary sodium >20 mmol/L	Hypothyroidism	Thyroid replacement
			Glucocorticoid deficiency	I.V. glucocorticoids
			SIADH, drugs, acute water intoxication	Fluid restriction
Hypervolemic	Volume excess Edema	Urinary sodium >30 mmol/L	Acute and chronic renal failure	Fluid restriction; treat renal failure
		Urinary sodium <10 mmol/L	Cirrhosis Cardiac failure Nephrotic syndrome	Fluid restriction; sodium restriction; treat underlying disorders

From Devita MV and Michelis MF, "Perturbations in Sodium Balance: Hyponatremia and Hypernatremia," *Clinics in Laboratory Medicine*, Vol 13, Preuss HG, ed, Philadelphia, PA: WB Saunders Co, 1993, 135-48, with permission.

(Continued)

Sodium, Urine *(Continued)*

5. Hainsworth JD, Workman R, and Greco FA, "Management of the Syndrome of Inappropriate Antidiuretic Hormone Secretion in Small Cell Lung Cancer," *Cancer*, 1983, 51:161-5.
6. Streeten DHP and Moses AM, "Disorders of the Neurohypophysis," *Harrison's Principles of Internal Medicine*, Braunwald E, Isselbacher KJ, Petersdorf RG, et al, eds, New York, NY: McGraw-Hill Inc, 1991, 1682-91.
7. Schrier RW, "Acute Renal Failure," *JAMA*, 1982, 247:2518-22, 2524.
8. Silver J, Rubinger D, Friedlander MM, et al, "Sodium-Dependent Idiopathic Hypercalciuria in Renal-Stone Formers," *Lancet*, 1983, 2:484-6.
9. Batlle DC, von Riotte A, and Schlueter W, "Urinary Sodium in the Evaluation of Hyperchloremic Metabolic Acidosis," *N Engl J Med*, 1987, 316:140-4.

References

Brown MA, Gallery ED, Ross MR, et al, "Sodium Excretion in Normal and Hypertensive Pregnancy: A Prospective Study," *Am J Obstet Gynecol*, 1988, 159:297-307.

Intersalt Cooperative Research Group, "An International Study of Electrolyte Excretion and Blood Pressure, Results for 24-Hour Urinary Sodium and Potassium Excretion," *Br Med J [Clin Res]*, 1988, 297:319-28.

Kamel KS, Ethier JH, Richardson RM, et al, "Urine Electrolytes and Osmolality: When and How to Use Them," *Am J Nephrol*, 1990, 10(2):89-102.

Preuss HG, Podlasek SJ, and Henry JB, "Evaluation of Renal Function and Water, Electrolyte, and Acid-Base Balance," *Clinical Diagnosis and Management by Laboratory Methods*, 18th ed, Henry JB, ed, Philadelphia, PA: WB Saunders Co, 1991, 118-39.

Somatomedin-C

***CPT** 84305*

Related Information

Growth Hormone *on page 245*

Synonyms IGF-I; Insulin-Like Growth Factor I; Sm-C; Sulfation Factor

Abstract Secreted by the anterior pituitary, growth hormone (GH) stimulates growth through stimulation of synthesis of somatomedins. Somatomedins are GH-dependent peptides. Two peptides have a somatomedinic effect: IGF-I (Sm-C) and IGF II. The former is used in evaluation of growth disorders.[1] IGF-II increases in tumor-related hypoglycemia but not in acromegaly.

Patient Care **PREPARATION:** Overnight fast is preferable, no recent administration of radioactivity.

Specimen Plasma **CONTAINER:** Lavender top (EDTA) tube, check with laboratory **STORAGE INSTRUCTIONS:** Separate plasma immediately by centrifuging at 4°C. Freeze plasma in a plastic tube. **CAUSES FOR REJECTION:** Recent radioactive scan

Interpretive **REFERENCE RANGE:** GH and Sm-C are elevated during normal puberty. Values vary with age, sex, and among laboratories. Normal ranges are published in percentiles, stratified by age and sex.[2] **USE:** Diagnose acromegaly, in which Sm-C and GH are increased; evaluate hypopituitarism and hypothalamic lesions in children (diagnosis of dwarfism and response to therapy). IGF-I (Sm-C) is the assay of choice for the diagnoses of acromegaly since it has little variation in blood levels throughout the day, unlike GH. Normal somatomedin results are evidence against growth hormone deficiency. Low levels occur in Laron dwarfism, an entity in which GH is increased. **LIMITATIONS:** Malnutrition will cause low somatomedin-C levels in spite of normal amounts of circulating growth hormone. The Sm-C level does not distinguish pituitary dwarfism from constitutional delay of growth and development.[2] **METHODOLOGY:** Radioimmunoassay (RIA) following dissociation from binding protein and chromatography **ADDITIONAL INFORMATION:** Somatomedin-C is a polypeptide hormone produced by the liver and other tissues, with effect on growth promoting activity and glucose metabolism (insulin-like activity). Somatomedin-C is carried in blood bound to a carrier protein which prolongs its half-life. Its level is therefore more constant than that of growth hormones.

Low values are described with the extremes of age (first 5-6 years and advanced age), hypopituitarism, malnutrition, diabetes mellitus, Laron dwarfism, hypothyroidism, maternal deprivation syndrome, pubertal delay, cirrhosis, hepatoma, and some cases of short stature and normal GH response to pharmacologic tests.[1] Low values may be found with nonfunctioning pituitary tumors, with constitutional delay of growth and development and with anorexia nervosa.[2]

High values occur with adolescence, true precocious puberty, pregnancy, obesity, pituitary gigantism, **acromegaly**, and diabetic retinopathy.[1]

Since Sm-C is decreased with malnutrition, its concentration provides an index with which to monitor therapy for food deprivation.[3,4]

Provocative testing is done for assays of growth hormone; Sm-C provides another approach for evaluation of pituitary GH secretion.

Footnotes

1. Cacciari E and Cicognani A, "Somatomedin-C in Pediatric Pathophysiology," *Pediatrician*, 1987, 14:146-53.
2. Kao PC, Abboud CF, and Zimmerman D, "Somatomedin-C: An Index of Growth Hormone Activity," *Mayo Clin Proc*, 1986, 61:908-9.
3. Gambino R, "Update on Lab Tests for Nutritional Evaluation," *Lab Report for Physicians*,™ 1986, 8:81-4.
4. Isley WL, Newton G, Dev J, et al, "Somatomedin C in Rheumatoid Arthritis," *N Engl J Med*, 1985, 312:1197, (letter).

References

Daughaday WH, Salmon WD Jr, Van den Brande JL, et al, "On the Nomenclature of the Somatomedins and Insulin-Like Growth Factors," *J Clin Endocrinol Metab*, 1987, 65:1075-6, (letter).

Pintor C, Cella SG, and Baumann G, "Correction and Withdrawal of Conclusion – A Child With Phenotypic Laron Dwarfism and Normal Somatomedin Levels," *N Engl J Med*, 1992, 323(21):1485.

Pintor C, Loche S, Cella SG, et al, "A Child With Phenotypic Laron Dwarfism and Normal Somatomedin Levels," *N Engl J Med*, 1989, 320(6):376-9.

Rappaport R, Prevot C, and Brauner R, "Somatomedin-C and Growth in Children With Precocious Puberty: A Study of the Effect of the Level of Growth Hormone Secretion," *J Clin Endocrinol Metab*, 1987, 65:1112-7.

Underwood LE and D'Ercole AJ, "Anterior Pituitary Gland and Hypothalamus: Disorders Affecting Anterior Pituitary Function," *Pediatrics*, 18th ed, Rudolph AM and Hoffman JIE, eds, Norwalk, CT: Appleton & Lange, 1987, 1454-65.

Watts NB and Keffer JH, "Anterior Pituitary and Hypothalamus," *Practical Endocrinology*, 4th ed, Philadelphia, PA: Lea & Febiger, 1989, 11-36.

Williams JD and Foster DW, *Williams Textbook of Endocrinology*, 8th ed, Wilson JD and Foster DW, eds, Philadelphia, PA: WB Saunders Co, 1992, 268-80.

Somatomedins *see* Growth Hormone *on page 245*

Somatotropin *see* Growth Hormone *on page 245*

SPan-1 *see* CA 19-9 *on page 152*

Spectral Analysis, Amniotic Fluid *see* Amniotic Fluid Analysis for Erythroblastosis Fetalis *on page 122*

Stool Fat, Quantitative *see* Fecal Fat, Quantitative, 72-Hour Collection *on page 219*

S-TSH *see* Thyroid Stimulating Hormone *on page 361*

β-Subunit of hCG *see* Pregnancy Test *on page 333*

Sugar, Fasting *see* Glucose, Fasting *on page 238*

Sulfation Factor *see* Somatomedin-C *on previous page*

Sweat, Chloride *see* Chloride, Sweat *on page 183*

T_3 Resin Uptake *see* T_3 Uptake *on this page*

T_3 (RIA) *see* Triiodothyronine *on page 373*

T_3RU *see* T_3 Uptake *on this page*

T_3, Total *see* Triiodothyronine *on page 373*

T_3U *see* T_3 Uptake *on this page*

T_3 Uptake

CPT *84479*

Related Information

Free Thyroxine Index *on page 223*
Thyroid Antimicrosomal Antibody *on page 755*
Thyroid Antithyroglobulin Antibody *on page 756*
Thyrotropin-Receptor Antibody *on page 756*
Thyroxine *on page 364*
Thyroxine Binding Globulin *on page 366*

Synonyms Resin Triiodothyronine Uptake; T_3 Resin Uptake; T_3RU; T_3U

Test Commonly Includes T_3 uptake with T_4 or equivalent are part of the thyroid profile done very widely by most laboratories.

Abstract An indirect measure of thyroid binding globulin (measures unsaturated binding sites on the thyroid binding proteins). T_3 uptake does **not** measure serum T_3 levels. The first T_3 up-
(Continued)

T_3 Uptake *(Continued)*

take had been described by Hamolsky et al by 1957, using red blood cells. Radioactive T_3 was used in preference to T_4 because of lesser affinity of TBG for T_3 compared to T_4. Such red cells were subsequently replaced by resins.

Specimen Serum is preferred, plasma may also be used. **CONTAINER:** Red top tube; lavender top (EDTA) tube or green top (heparin) tube is also acceptable.[1] **STORAGE INSTRUCTIONS:** Separate within 48 hours. Store at 2°C to 8°C. **CAUSES FOR REJECTION:** Patient having a recent isotope scan before collection of specimen

Interpretive **REFERENCE RANGE:** Varies with different laboratories; the T_3 uptake can be expressed in several ways. It may be calculated to provide a normal value of unity. **USE:** Thyroid function test for the diagnosis of hypothyroidism or hyperthyroidism, used with T_4 or equivalent to provide free T_4 index, FT_4I. An indirect measure of binding protein, the T_3 uptake reflects available binding sites (ie, reflects TBG). T_3 uptake is **not** a measurement of serum T_3. It should never be used alone; rather, its usual application is in conjunction with total T_4 measurement. See table for typical examples of use.

Clinical Condition	T_4	T_3U	FT_4I
Normal	Normal	Normal	Normal
Hyperthyroid	Increased	Increased	Increased
Hypothyroid	Decreased	Decreased	Decreased
Increased TBG (eg, pregnancy)	Increased	Decreased	Normal
Decreased TBG (eg, nephrotic syndrome)	Decreased	Increased	Normal

LIMITATIONS: An **increase** in T_3U occurs in hyperthyroidism; in situations where drugs displace T_4 from TBG such as high doses of salicylates, phenytoin, phenylbutazone, etc; and in cases where the TBG concentration decreases such as in nephrotic syndrome, malnutrition, active acromegaly, etc. A **decrease** in T_3U occurs in hypothyroidism; and in cases where an increase in TBG occurs, such as estrogen administration (as contraceptive, during menopause, or treatment of osteoporosis), during pregnancy, and in conjunction with perphenazine.

Alterations in binding capacity of TBG are described with major illness and with high doses of salicylates and corticosteroids, and with use of heroin, methadone, phenytoin, and perphenazine. Alterations occur with malnutrition, such as in metastatic malignancy, and are found in patients with abnormal serum protein patterns (eg, nephrotic syndromes, cirrhosis). Other states in which changes in TBG occur include infancy, acromegaly, molar and ordinary pregnancy, oral contraceptives, and with exogenous hormones including androgens, anabolic steroids and estrogens. Hereditary increase and decrease of TBG occurs. Most authorities have abandoned this test in favor of more specific, sensitive tests such as FT_4, TSH, and FT_3.

CONTRAINDICATIONS: T_3 uptake cannot be run after administration of therapeutic or diagnostic radioactive material. This test should not be ordered alone; it is only useful with T_4 type tests. **METHODOLOGY:** Resin sponge uptake, charcoal bead uptake, related methods, based on *in vitro* competition for thyroid hormone between thyroid binding globulin and the added inert receptor. **ADDITIONAL INFORMATION:** When T_3 uptake is reported as a range, for example, such that 23% and less signifies low, and 34% and more indicates high, then the index may be calculated as follows:

$$FT_4I = \%\ T_3U\ (\text{patient}) / \%\ T_3U\ (\text{reference serum}) \times T_4\ (\mu g/dL)$$

The FT_4I range usually approximates the range for total T_4. In the presence of thyroid binding globulin abnormalities, the free thyroxine index is a useful laboratory parameter regarding clinical thyroid status.

Footnotes

1. Bhagavan NV, Caraway WT, Conn RB, et al, *Textbook of Clinical Chemistry*, Tietz NW, ed, Philadelphia, PA: WB Saunders Co, 1986, 1127.

References

Bakerman S, *A, B, C's of Interpretive Laboratory Data*, Greenville, NC: Interpretive Laboratory Data Inc, 1984.

Gruhn JG, Barsano CP, and Kumar Y, "The Development of Tests of Thyroid Function," *Arch Pathol Lab Med*, 1987, 111:84-100.

Helfand M and Crapo LM, "Screening for Thyroid Disease," *Ann Intern Med*, 1990, 112(11):840-9.
Larsen PR and Ingbar SH, "The Thyroid Gland," *Williams Textbook of Endocrinology*, 8th ed, Philadelphia, PA: WB Saunders Co, 1992, 357-458.
Surks MI, "Guidelines for Thyroid Testing," *Lab Med*, 1993, 24(5):270-4.

T_4 *see* Thyroxine *on page 364*

T_4-Binding Globulin *see* Thyroxine Binding Globulin *on page 366*

T_4 by EIA *see* Thyroxine *on page 364*

T_4 CPB *replaced by* Thyroxine *on page 364*

T_4, Free *see* Thyroxine, Free *on page 368*

T_4 Neonatal *see* T_4 Newborn Screen *on this page*

T_4 Newborn Screen

CPT 84437

Related Information

Galactose Screening Tests for Galactosemia *on page 228*
Newborn Screen for Hypothyroidism and Phenylketonuria *on page 295*
Thyroid Stimulating Hormone Screen, Filter Paper *on page 363*

Synonyms T_4 Neonatal; Thyroid Screen for Newborns

Abstract Screening for congenital hypothyroidism now occurs in all 50 states. The importance of newborn screening for hypothyroid case detection and early initiation of treatment has led to filter paper screening programs of T_4 and/or TSH in many countries of the world. If hypothyroidism is undetected, growth and mental retardation occurs, and in rare instances, death.

Specimen Whole blood. Unlike PKU testing, cord blood is satisfactory. Heel blood at discharge is also acceptable. **CONTAINER:** Special filter paper collection card **SAMPLING TIME:** T_4 peaks at 24 hours **COLLECTION:** Obtain heelstick whole blood sample and thoroughly saturate circles on the filter paper. Label the card with the patient's name, age, and physician. Prompt collection and processing of infants' blood samples is crucial to early detection of these disorders. Steps for collection: Warm the foot and/or massage the leg. Clean the puncture site with an alcohol swab, then dry with a sterile sponge to remove alcohol. Puncture the infant's heel with a sterile lancet of less than 2.5 mm. Wipe away the first drop of blood. Touch the filter paper to the drops and allow them to flow onto the filter paper and diffuse through the circles. Apply a sterile covering to the site. **STORAGE INSTRUCTIONS:** Exposure of card to extreme heat or light or touching the filter paper portion of the form can cause erroneous test results. **CAUSES FOR REJECTION:** Filter paper not thoroughly saturated, radioactive tracer given to baby before the sample is obtained, specimens which are QNS (quantity not sufficient), exposure of card to extreme heat or light or touching the filter paper portion of the form can cause erroneous test results **SPECIAL INSTRUCTIONS:** The T_4 specimen is usually collected at the same time the PKU specimen is obtained. Optimal collection time is 3-7 days after birth, when the baby has been on protein feeding for 24 hours (ie, usually just before discharge); 4-10 days after birth recommended for low birth weight infants.

Interpretive **REFERENCE RANGE:** T_4 results in infancy are higher than adult ranges. Thyroxine levels are lower in prematures. Peak occurs at about 24 hours; then T_4 decreases. Newborns that have a low T_4 are tested for TSH. **POSSIBLE PANIC RANGE:** Low result for T_4; high TSH. Abnormal value for infants 7 days old or younger: $T_4 \leq 6.5$ μg/dL (SI: ≤84 nmol/L); for infants 8 days old and older: $T_4 \leq 5.0$ μg/dL (SI: ≤64 nmol/L). See report of individual laboratory. **USE:** Screen for congenital hypothyroidism **LIMITATIONS:** Congenital thyroglobulin deficiency will result in low T_4 values even though the patient is euthyroid. TSH is low in TBG deficiency but T_3 uptake is high.[1] TSH is more sensitive for primary hypothyroidism. The risk of a false-negative result is increased when subjects with incomplete absence of thyroid parenchyma are screened only by T_4. **METHODOLOGY:** Radioimmunoassay (RIA). Thyroxine value may be determined from filter paper discs saturated with whole blood. Some laboratories do TSH to screen for congenital hypothyroidism, others do a T_4 as is done for adults, and most use the filter paper disc method. **ADDITIONAL INFORMATION:** There is evidence that growth becomes thyroid hormone dependent immediately after birth. Decreased growth rate, short stature, and abnormal epiphyseal maturation are clinical features of thyroid deficiency. While height may be normal at birth, growth velocity is decreased during the first weeks of life, increasing after the start of therapy.[2] Patients who are not detected and who do not receive early therapy will develop mental retardation, variable growth failure, metabolic changes of hypothyroidism, deaf-

(Continued)

T_4 Newborn Screen *(Continued)*

ness, and neurologic abnormalities. There is a higher incidence of detection from screening programs than from clinical surveillance since clinical signs in the great majority of cases are minimal at birth. Timing of sampling, retesting, and hazards of screening are important considerations.[3] Transient hypothyroxinemia and transient hyperthyroxinemia occur.[1]

If low values are obtained, the patient must have confirmatory tests run: T_4, TSH, sometimes T_3 uptake, and possibly TBG assessment. For rescreening, combined T_4 and TSH is recommended, when the initial T_4 is low.[3] Excessive quantities of TBG result in increased T_4, while deficiency in TBG has the opposite effect. Extrathyroidal conditions resulting in depressed T_4 levels include low birth weight (LBW). In normal as well as LBW infants, the T_4 will be lower between 5 and 9 days compared to 3-5 days after birth. The incidence of permanent abnormalities leading to hypothyroidism is approximately 1:3,600-5,000 live births (as determined by screening tests in the United States).[3] The incidence of congenital hypothyroidism in Bohemia/Moravia since 1985 is 1:5700 of live newborn infants.[4] In a Netherlands study the incidence of total organification defect (an autosomal process) was about 1 in 60,000 neonates.[5] Seven million newborns are screened annually for hypothyroidism. Three hundred and sixty are spared delayed growth and severe mental retardation while 1200 more babies avoid subnormal intelligence with early diagnosis.[6]

Footnotes

1. Howanitz JH, Howanitz PJ, and Henry JB, "Evaluation of Endocrine Function," *Clinical Diagnosis and Management by Laboratory Methods*, 18th ed, Henry JB, ed, Philadelphia, PA: WB Saunders Co, 1991, 308-20.
2. Leger J and Czernichow P, "Congenital Hypothyroidism: Decreased Growth Velocity in the First Week of Life," *Biol Neonate*, 1989, 55(4-5):218-23.
3. American Academy of Pediatrics, Committee on Genetics, "Newborn Screening Fact Sheets: Congenital Hypothyroidism," *Pediatrics*, 1989, 83:454-6.
4. Hnikova O, Kracmar P, Zelenka Z, et al, "Screening of Congenital Hypothyroidism in Newborns in Bohemia and Moravia," *Endocrinol Exp*, 1989, 23(2):117-23.
5. Vulsma T, Gons MH, and de Vijlder JJM, "Maternal-Fetal Transfer of Thyroxine in Congenital Hypothyroidism Due to a Total Organification Defect or Thyroid Agenesis," *N Engl J Med*, 1989, 321(1):13-6.
6. Willi SM and Moshang T Jr, "Diagnostic Dilemmas. Results of Screening Tests for Congenital Hypothyroidism," *Pediatr Clin North Am*, 1991, 38(3):555-66.

References

Fisher DA, "Euthyroid Low Thyroxine (T_4) and Triiodothyronine (T_3) States in Premature and Sick Neonates," *Pediatr Clin North Am*, 1990, 37(6):1297-312.

Gravdal JA, Meenan A, and Dyson AE, "Congenital Hypothyroidism," *J Fam Pract*, 1989, 29(1):47-50.

Gruters A, "Congenital Hypothyroidism," *Pediatr Ann*, 1992, 21(1):15, 18-21, 24-8.

LaFranchi SH, Hanna CE, Krainz PL, et al, "Screening for Congenital Hypothyroidism With Specimen Collection at Two Time Periods: Results of the Northwest Regional Screening Program," *Pediatrics*, 1985, 76:734-40.

Surks MI, "Guidelines for Thyroid Testing," *Lab Med*, 1993, 24(5):270-4.

T_4 (RIA) *see* Thyroxine *on page 364*

TAG 72 *see* CA 125 *on page 154*

TAG 72, Placental Alkaline Phosphatase *see* CA 15-3 *on page 152*

Tau Protein *see* Transferrin *on page 369*

TBG *see* Thyroxine Binding Globulin *on page 366*

tCO_2 *see* Carbon Dioxide, Blood *on page 165*

Testosterone, Free *see* Testosterone, Free and Total *on this page*

Testosterone, Free and Total

CPT *84402 (free); 84403 (total)*

Related Information

Androstenedione, Serum *on page 129*
Dehydroepiandrosterone Sulfate *on page 206*
Follicle Stimulating Hormone *on page 222*
17-Ketosteroids, Total, Urine *on page 267*
Luteinizing Hormone, Blood or Urine *on page 286*

Applies to Sex Hormone Binding Globulin; SHBG; Testosterone, Free

Abstract Testosterone is the major androgen responsible for sexual differentiations and male secondary sex characteristics. It is carried in the blood by the sex hormone binding globulin (SHBG). The major use of these assays is in the evaluation of hirsute women.

Specimen Serum or plasma **CONTAINER:** Red top tube, green top (heparin) tube, or lavender top (EDTA) tube **STORAGE INSTRUCTIONS:** Separate serum or plasma and freeze. **CAUSES FOR REJECTION:** Recent administration of radioactive isotope

Interpretive **REFERENCE RANGE:** **Free**: adults: male: 9-30 ng/dL (SI: 0.3-1.0 nmol/L), female: 0.3-1.9 ng/dL (SI: 0.01-0.06 nmol/L). **Total**: adults: male: 300-1200 ng/dL (SI: 10.4-41.6 nmol/L), female: 20-80 ng/dL (SI: 0.7-2.8 nmol/L). Values in children are lower. **USE:** An indicator of LH secretion and Leydig cell function. Evaluate gonadal and adrenal function. Helpful in the diagnosis of hypogonadism, hypopituitarism, Klinefelter's syndrome and impotence (low values), and hirsutism, anovulation, amenorrhea, and virilization in females due to Stein-Leventhal syndrome, masculinizing tumors of ovary such as Sertoli-Leydig cell tumor, tumors of the adrenal cortices, and congenital adrenal hyperplasia (high values). Hirsutism in females is most commonly caused by anovulation and excessive ovarian androgen production. Adrenal causes are uncommon. Contemporary investigation for female hirsutism includes testosterone, dehydroepiandrosterone sulfate, and 17-hydroxyprogesterone.[1] Testosterone is used in investigation of male precocious puberty. Male pseudohermaphroditism includes defective testosterone synthesis, androgen insensitivity syndromes, 5-α-reductase deficiency, and testicular dysgenesis. **LIMITATIONS:** Total serum testosterone may be normal in women with hirsutism, who may have abnormal free testosterone. Plasma testosterone level may be elevated in patients using cimetidine. In Klinefelter's syndrome, testosterone can be at the low end of the reference range or lower. Even when it is almost normal, LH levels are increased. **METHODOLOGY:** Radioimmunoassay (RIA), immunoassay (nonisotopic). Testosterone can be measured in saliva to provide an index of free testosterone.[2] Free testosterone generally done after ultrafiltration or equilibrium dialysis by RIA. **ADDITIONAL INFORMATION:** In males, testosterone may be normal or decreased in hypopituitarism, including selective gonadotropin deficiency (eg, Kallmann's syndrome). It may be decreased with hepatic cirrhosis, estrogen therapy, and with severe obesity. Low testosterone and high LH are encountered with renal failure and in malnutrition. It is decreased with excessive alcohol intake. Testosterone is usually increased in precocious puberty, related to idiopathic or CNS lesion, or to adrenal tumors or congenital adrenal hyperplasia.

Testosterone exists in serum both free (40%) and bound (60%) to albumin and to sex hormone binding globulin (SHBG) (testosterone binding globulin). Unbound (free) testosterone is the active moiety. Free and total testosterone can be measured. Usual testosterone assays measure both bound and unbound levels. In certain settings, total testosterone can be normal while free testosterone is increased, or the reverse. Free testosterone measured by analog RIA is reported to have greater diagnostic efficiency than total testosterone.[3]

The major androgens of normal females include dehydroepiandrosterone (DHEA) and androstenedione, both weak androgens. Each derives from adrenal glands as well as gonads, and can be converted to testosterone. About half of testosterone in the female derives from peripheral conversion of androstenedione.

LH stimulates androgen production. ACTH and TSH deficiencies are likelier causes of secondary testicular failure than is an LH decrease. Low LH with low testosterone is evidence of a pituitary lesion.

Footnotes

1. Speroff L, Glass RH, and Kase NG, *Clinical Gynecologic Endocrinology and Infertility*, 4th ed, Baltimore, MD: Williams & Wilkins, 1989.
2. Navarro MA, Juan L, Bonnin MR, et al, "Salivary Testosterone: Relationship to Total and Free Testosterone in Serum," *Clin Chem*, 1986, 32:231-2, (letter).
3. Wilke TJ and Utley DJ, "Total Testosterone, Free-Androgen Index, Calculated Free Testosterone, and Free Testosterone by Analog RIA Compared in Hirsute Women and in Otherwise Normal Women With Altered Binding of Sex-Hormone-Binding Globulin," *Clin Chem*, 1987, 33:1372-5.

References

Catrou PG and Beeler MF, "Disorders of Gonadal and Fetoplacental Function," *Interpretations in Clinical Chemistry*, 2nd ed, Chicago, IL: American Society of Clinical Pathologists, 1983, 76-82.

Henry JB, "Evaluation of Endocrine Function," Henry JB, ed, *Todd-Sanford-Davidsohn Clinical Diagnosis and Management by Laboratory Methods*, 18th ed, Henry JB, ed, Philadelphia, PA: WB Saunders Co, 1991, 343-5.

Leavelle DE, *Mayo Medical Laboratories Interpretive Handbook*, Rochester, MN: Mayo Medical Laboratories, 1990.

Ruutiainen K, Sannikka E, Santti R, et al, "Salivary Testosterone in Hirsutism: Correlations With Serum Testosterone and the Degree of Hair Growth," *J Clin Endocrinol Metab*, 1987, 64:1015-20.

Swinkels LM, van Hoof HJ, Ross HA, et al, "Low Ratio of Androstenedione to Testosterone in Plasma and Saliva of Hirsute Women," *Clin Chem*, 1992, 38(9):1819-23.

(Continued)

Testosterone, Free and Total *(Continued)*

Vittek J, Hommedieu DG, Gordon GG, et al, "Direct Radioimmunoassay (RIA) of Salivary Testosterone: Correlation With Free and Total Serum Testosterone," *Life Sci*, 1985, 37:711-6.

Wheeler JE and Rudy FR, "The Testis, Paratesticular Structures, and Male External Genitalia," *Principles and Practice of Surgical Pathology*, 2nd ed, Vol 2, Silverberg SG, ed, New York, NY: Churchill Livingstone, 1990, 1531-85.

Tetraiodothyronine *see* Thyroxine *on page 364*

Tg *see* Thyroglobulin, Serum *on this page*

Thermostable Alkaline Phosphatase *see* Alkaline Phosphatase, Heat Stable *on page 106*

Thoracentesis Fluid Analysis *see* Body Fluid *on page 145*

Thoracentesis Fluid pH *see* Body Fluid pH *on page 150*

Thymol Turbidity *replaced by* Alanine Aminotransferase *on page 100*

Thymol Turbidity *replaced by* Aspartate Aminotransferase *on page 135*

Thyrocalcitonin *see* Calcitonin *on page 157*

Thyroglobulin, Serum

CPT 84432

Synonyms Tg

Abstract Thyroglobulin is a secretory product of thyroid follicular epithelium, a high molecular weight iodinated glycoprotein. It is the storage form of the thyroid hormones. Its major clinical use is in the management of differentiated thyroid carcinomas.

Patient Care PREPARATION: Avoid scans and other recent prior administration of radioisotopes. Do not draw a specimen for this test soon after needle biopsy, thyroid surgery, or radioiodine therapy. Levels >15 ng/mL are more significant when patient has not been on thyroid hormone replacement therapy after thyroidectomy.

Specimen Serum CONTAINER: Red top tube SPECIAL INSTRUCTIONS: This is **not** thyroxine binding globulin (TBG).

Interpretive REFERENCE RANGE: Approximately 1.0-20.0 ng/mL. Detectable in most healthy adults; moderately elevated (several fold) in the last trimester of gestation and in neonates. CRITICAL VALUES: Thyroglobulin levels >50.0 ng/mL are associated with tumor recurrence in patients who lack thyroid tissue. USE: Thyroglobulin is elevated in three types of thyroid disorders: goiter and thyroid hyperfunction, inflammation or physical injury to the thyroid, and differentiated thyroid tumors.

Those thyroid cancer patients who have no remaining thyroid tissue, following surgery and/or irradiation, would not be expected to have a source of thyroglobulin. Thyroglobulin then is a tumor marker useful to assess the presence of residual papillary-follicular carcinoma of thyroid,[1] following resection, including tumors which fail to concentrate radioiodine. High values are found with many instances of tumor dissemination; thus, thyroglobulin assays are used to monitor postoperative thyroid carcinoma patients. Such assays are best used in concert with total body scans. Possibly it will be useful in patients with bone metastases in whom the primary site is unknown.

Low or undetectable levels in thyrotoxicosis are a clue to thyrotoxicosis factitia (surreptitious use of thyroid hormone). The assay may be useful to support a diagnosis of subacute thyroiditis. The absence of thyroglobulin from the serum of neonates suggests congenital athyreosis.[2] Thyroglobulin may prove useful as an indicator of T_4 therapy in patients with solitary nodules.[3]

LIMITATIONS: Thyroglobulin is useful in the management but not diagnosis of differentiated thyroid carcinomas. Thyroglobulin is not valid as a tumor marker for anaplastic or medullary carcinoma of thyroid. High values are reported with surgery or irradiation to the thyroid, with thyroiditis, T_4 binding globulin deficiency, with administration of TRH, TSH, iodine, and of anticancer drugs. High levels of thyroglobulin occur in goiter and in many types of hyperthyroidism. Normal levels are found in patients with small thyroid carcinomas. Low values occur with thyroid hormone administration. This is not a screening test for thyroid cancer. RIA methods are subject to interference in serums containing autoantibodies (eg, most patients with Hashimoto's thyroiditis). Newer methods, using IRMA technology can reliably measure thyroglobulin in the presence of antithyroglobulin autoantibodies,[4,5] an adjunct to ^{131}I

scanning in care of the thyroid cancer patient.[6] Thyroglobulin is decreased with fasting.[7] **METHODOLOGY:** Radioimmunoassay (RIA), immunoradiometric assay (IRMA) **ADDITIONAL INFORMATION:** Since functioning metastatic thyroid carcinoma causing hyperthyroidism is extremely uncommon, serial thyroglobulin assays provide a means of following such patients.[1] Serial thyroglobulin determinations may be helpful for detecting metastases which do not accumulate radioiodine.[8]

Footnotes

1. Black EG and Sheppard MC, "Serum Thyroglobulin Measurements in Thyroid Cancer: Evaluation of "False"-Positive Results," *Clin Endocrinol (Oxf)*, 1991, 35(6):519-20.
2. DiGeorge AM, "The Endocrine System," *Nelson Textbook of Pediatrics*, 14th ed, Behrman RE, Kliegman RM, and Nelson WE, eds, Philadelphia, PA: WB Saunders Co, 1992, 1414-28.
3. Morita T, Tamai H, Ohshima A, et al, "Changes in Serum Thyroid Hormone, Thyrotropin and Thyroglobulin Concentrations During Thyroxine Therapy in Patients With Solitary Thyroid Nodules," *J Clin Endocrinol Metab*, 1989, 69(2):227-30.
4. Piechaczyk M, Baldet L, Pau B, et al, "Novel Immunoradiometric Assay of Thyroglobulin in Serum With Use of Monoclonal Antibodies Selected for Lack of Cross-Reactivity With Autoantibodies," *Clin Chem*, 1989, 35(3):422-4.
5. Wilson R, McKillop JH, Jenkins C, et al, "Serum Thyroglobulin – Its Measurement and Clinical Use," *Ann Clin Biochem*, 1989, 26(Pt 5):401-6.
6. Aiello DP and Manni A, "Thyroglobulin Measurement vs Iodine-131 Total Body Scan for Follow-Up of Well-Differentiated Thyroid Cancer," *Arch Intern Med*, 1990, 150(2):437-9.
7. Unger J, "Fasting Induces a Decrease in Serum Thyroglobulin in Normal Subjects," *J Clin Endocrinol Metab*, 1988, 67(6):1309-11.
8. Botsch H, Glatz J, Shulz E, et al, "Long-Term Follow-Up Using Serial Serum Thyroglobulin Determinations in Patients With Differentiated Thyroid Carcinoma," *Cancer*, 1983, 52:1856-9.

References

Grant S, Luttrell B, Reeve T, et al, "Thyroglobulin May Be Undetectable in the Serum of Patients With Metastatic Disease Secondary to Differentiated Thyroid Carcinoma," *Cancer*, 1984, 54:1625-8.

Sheppard MC, "Serum Thyroglobulin and Thyroid Cancer," *Q J Med*, 1986, 59:429-33, (review).

Wilson JD and Foster DW, eds, *Williams Textbook of Endocrinology*, 8th ed, Philadelphia, PA: WB Saunders Co, 1992.

Thyroid Screen for Newborns *see* T_4 Newborn Screen *on page 357*

Thyroid Stimulating Hormone

***CPT** 84443*

Related Information

Amiodarone *on page 939*
Lithium *on page 979*
Thyroid Antimicrosomal Antibody *on page 755*
Thyroid Antithyroglobulin Antibody *on page 756*
Thyrotropin-Receptor Antibody *on page 756*

Synonyms S-TSH; Thyrotropin; Thyrotropin Stimulating Hormone; TSH; Ultrasensitive TSH

Abstract Produced by the anterior pituitary gland, thyroid stimulating hormone (TSH) stimulates secretion of T_4 (thyroxine) and T_3 (triiodothyronine). TSH secretion is physiologically regulated by T_3 and T_4 (feedback inhibition) and is stimulated by TRH (thyrotropin releasing hormone) from the hypothalamus. TSH assay is used to confirm hypothyroidism. The new sensitive assays permit recognition of hyperthyroidism.

Patient Care **PREPARATION:** Avoid radioisotope administration before collection of specimen.

Specimen Serum **CONTAINER:** Red top tube **SAMPLING TIME:** A diurnal rhythm exists. Peak levels occur at about 11 PM. TSH release is pulsatile.[1] **STORAGE INSTRUCTIONS:** Separate serum within 4 hours and refrigerate. Stable 4 days at 4°C.

Interpretive **REFERENCE RANGE:** Dependent on method. Pediatrics: neonates: <20 mIU/L by third day of life. Using one of the newer ultrasensitive assays (chemiluminometric two-site assay) Mayo Medical Laboratories has published age-stratified ranges, of which the lower limit is 0.4 mIU/L and the upper limit up to 10.0 mIU/L (for those 80 years of age and older). **USE:** Thyroid function test. Investigation of low T_4 result; the differential diagnosis of primary hypothyroidism from normal, and the differential diagnosis of primary hypothyroidism from pituitary/hypothalamic hypothyroidism. TSH is high in primary hypothyroidism. Low TSH occurs in hyperthyroidism. Evaluation of therapy in hypothyroid patients, receiving various thyroid hormone preparations: low values are found in states of excessive thyroid replacement. Normal result on a new sensitive TSH assay is acceptable evidence of adequate thyroid replacement.

(Continued)

Thyroid Stimulating Hormone *(Continued)*

Follow-up of patients who have had hyperthyroidism treated with radioiodine or surgery, and for low T_4 newborn screen results.

TSH had been used in the TRH stimulation test for borderline thyrotoxicosis. Such testing was not often needed[2] even before the introduction of sensitive immunoassays for serum thyrotropin, and is now mostly, but not completely, obviated.

The new highly sensitive TSH assays can be considered as a screening test for thyroid disease. A result within the accepted reference range provides strong evidence for euthyroidism.

LIMITATIONS: TSH may be affected by glucocorticoids, dopamine, and by severe illness,[3] and these remain limitations even for the new, sensitive TSH assays. TSH suppression in hypothyroidism with severe illness has been reported with TSH increase with recovery.[4] Normal TSH levels in the presence of hypothyroidism have been reported with head injury. TSH is not elevated in secondary (hypopituitarism) hypothyroidism nor in hypothalamic hypothyroidism.

The diagnosis of hyperthyroidism in pregnancy may require assay of free thyroid hormones and a TRH test.[5]

Probably no single test, even the sensitive immunoassays, can be expected to adequately reflect thyroid status under all circumstances. Among possible problems are the recovery phase of nonthyroidal illness, states of resistance to thyroid hormone, thyrotropin-producing tumors, thyroid status in acute psychiatric illness, early in thyrotoxicosis and in subacute thyroiditis.[6]

METHODOLOGY: Immunoassays including radioimmunoassay (RIA), immunochemiluminometric (ICMA) assays (chemiluminescent markers), sandwich immunoradiometric assays (IRMA), fluorometric enzyme immunoassay with use of monoclonal antibodies, microparticle enzyme immunoassay (MEIA) on IMx (Abbott Laboratories) **ADDITIONAL INFORMATION:** Unsuspected increase in the level of serum TSH is not uncommon in elderly subjects. TSH is the single most sensitive test for primary hypothyroidism. If there is clear evidence for hypothyroidism and the TSH is not elevated, hypopituitarism should be considered (secondary hypothyroidism).

TSH levels have been elevated or inappropriately detectable for high thyroid hormone levels in some patients with thyrotropin-secreting pituitary adenomas. Delay in diagnosis of these tumors may lead to visual compromise. The effects of such neoplasms can be misdiagnosed as those of primary hyperthyroidism.[7]

Until the late 1980s, TSH assays were not sufficiently sensitive to distinguish hyperthyroidism from euthyroid (normal) subjects. The new generation of ultrasensitive TSH immunoassays have provided a far more effective diagnostic separation of thyrotoxicosis from euthyroidism. They may well be the best possible screening test. Gambino is among those finding it difficult to accept a single screening test without a confirmatory test.[8]

Footnotes

1. Howanitz JH, Howanitz PJ, and Henry JB, "Evaluation of Endocrine Function," *Clinical Diagnosis and Management by Laboratory Methods*, 18th ed, Henry JB, ed, Philadelphia, PA: WB Saunders Co, 1991, 308-20.
2. Nicoloff JT and Spencer CA, "Clinical Review 12: The Use and Misuse of the Sensitive Thyrotropin Assays," *J Clin Endocrinol Metab*, 1990, 71(3):553-8.
3. Chopra IJ, Hershman JM, Pardridge MD, et al, "Thyroid Function in Nonthyroidal Illnesses," *Ann Intern Med*, 1983, 98:946-57.
4. Spencer CA, "Clinical Utility and Cost-Effectiveness of Sensitive Thyrotropin Assays in Ambulatory and Hospitalized Patients," *Mayo Clin Proc*, 1988, 63:1214-22.
5. Toft AD, "Use of Sensitive Immunoradiometric Assay for Thyrotropin in Clinical Practice," *Mayo Clin Proc*, 1988, 63(10):1035-42.
6. Ehrmann DA and Sarne DH, "Serum Thyrotropin and the Assessment of Thyroid Status," *Ann Intern Med*, 1989, 110(3):179-81.
7. Gesundheit N, Petrick PA, Nissim M, et al, "Thyrotropin-Secreting Pituitary Adenomas: Clinical and Biochemical Heterogeneity – Case Reports and Follow-Up of Nine Patients," *Ann Intern Med*, 1989, 111(10):827-35, (review).
8. Gambino R, "TSH and Thyroid Status," *Lab Report for Physicians*, 1989, 11:33-5.

References

Baskin HJ, "Endocrinologic Evaluation of Impotence," *South Med J*, 1989, 82(4):446-9.

Brennan MD, Klee GG, Preissner CM, et al, "Heterophilic Serum Antibodies: A Cause for Falsely Elevated Serum Thyrotropin Levels," *Mayo Clin Proc*, 1987, 62:894-98.

Clark PMS, Clark JDA, Holder R, et al, "Pulsatile Secretion of TSH in Healthy Subjects," *Ann Clin Biochem*, 1987, 24:470-6.

Cooper DS, "Thyroid Hormone Treatment: New Insights Into an Old Therapy," *JAMA*, 1989, 261(18):2694-5.

Ericsson UB, Fernlund P, and Thorell JI, "Evaluation of the Usefulness of a Sensitive Immunoradiometric Assay for Thyroid Stimulating Hormone as a First-Line Thyroid Function Test in an Unselected Patient Population," *Scand J Clin Lab Invest*, 1987, 47:215-21.

Gorman CA, "Symposium on Sensitivity TSH Assays - Introduction: Thyroid Function Testing: A New Era," *Mayo Clin Proc*, 1988, 63:1026-7.

Greenspan SL, Klibanski A, Schoenfeld D, et al, "Pulsatile Secretion of Thyrotropin in Man," *J Clin Endocrinol Metab*, 1986, 63:661-8.

Hamblin PS, Dyer SA, Mohr VS, et al, "Relationship Between Thyrotropin and Thyroxine Changes During Recovery From Severe Hypothyroxinemia of Critical Illness," *J Clin Endocrinol Metab*, 1986, 62:717-22.

Jackson JA, Verdonk CA, Spiekerman AM, et al, "Euthyroid Hyperthyroxinemia and Inappropriate Secretion of Thyrotropin: Recognition and Diagnosis," *Arch Intern Med*, 1987, 147:1311-3.

Klee GG, "Symposium on Sensitive TSH Assays - Part II: Sensitive Thyrotropin Assays: Analytic and Clinical Performance Criteria," *Mayo Clin Proc*, 1988, 63:1123-32.

Lawson N, Mike N, Wilson R, et al, "Assessment of a Time-Resolved Fluoroimmunoassay for Thyrotropin in Routine Clinical Practice," *Clin Chem*, 1986, 32:684-6.

Martinez M, Derksen D, and Kapsner P, "Making Sense of Hypothyroidism. An Approach to Testing and Treatment," *Postgrad Med*, 1993, 93(6):135-8, 141-5.

McDermott MT and Ridgway EC, "Thyroid Hormone Resistance Syndromes," *Am J Med*, 1993, 94(4):424-32.

Ridgway EC, "Symposium on Sensitive TSH Assay - Part I: Thyrotropin Radioimmunoassays: Birth, Life, and Demise," *Mayo Clin Proc*, 1988, 63:1028-34.

Rosenfeld L and Blum M, "Immunoradiometric Assay for Thyrotropin (TSH) Should Replace the RIA Method in the Clinical Laboratory," *Clin Chem*, 1986, 32:232-3, (letter).

Rosenthal MJ, Hunt WC, Garry PJ, et al, "Thyroid Failure in the Elderly: Microsomal Antibodies as Discriminant for Therapy," *JAMA*, 1987, 258:209-13.

Sawin CT, Geller A, Hershman JM, et al, "The Aging Thyroid: The Use of Thyroid Hormone in Older Persons," *JAMA*, 1989, 261(18):2653-5.

Spencer CA, "Symposium on Sensitive TSH Assays - Part III: Clinical Utility and Cost-Effectiveness of Sensitive Thyrotropin Assays in Ambulatory and Hospitalized Patients," *Mayo Clin Proc*, 1988, 63:1214-22.

Surks MI, "Guidelines for Thyroid Testing," *Lab Med*, 1993, 24(5):270-4.

Watts NB, "Use of a Sensitive Thyrotropin Assay for Monitoring Treatment With Levothyroxine," *Arch Intern Med*, 1989, 149(2):309-312.

Thyroid Stimulating Hormone Screen, Filter Paper

CPT 84443

Related Information

T_4 Newborn Screen *on page 357*

Synonyms TSH, Filter Paper

Patient Care **PREPARATION:** After cleansing infant's heel, puncture to obtain free-flowing blood for spotting on collection card. Spot blood directly on card, using no pipets or blood collection equipment. Avoid radioisotope administration before collection.

Specimen Whole blood, soaked through special collection paper **CONTAINER:** Special filter paper collection card **SAMPLING TIME:** Test newborn at 7-10 days. **COLLECTION:** Cord blood can be used, or sample can be collected at 3-5 days after birth. Using a large drop of blood, soak through the special collection paper at a minimum of one spot. **CAUSES FOR REJECTION:** Blood not soaked through collection card, recently administered radioisotope

Interpretive **REFERENCE RANGE:** TSH peaks just after birth to 2 to 3 times "normal", then declines.[1] "Normal" after immediate postpartum period is <7 μIU/mL (SI: <7 mIU/L). Adult levels reached by 10 days of age. **POSSIBLE PANIC RANGE:** Elevated TSH with low T_4, or high TSH with normal T_4 **USE:** Follow-up testing after, with, or instead of T_4 filter paper test for congenital hypothyroidism. **METHODOLOGY:** Radioimmunoassay (RIA) **ADDITIONAL INFORMATION:** The incidence of congenital hypothyroidism in the United States (on the basis of screening programs) is from 1:3600 to 1:5000. The incidence is significantly less in black populations. Without screening the diagnosis is likely to be missed because signs are usually minimal just after birth. Without detection and treatment mental and physical disability results including retardation, poor growth, low metabolic rate, constipation, bradycardia, and myxedema. Screening for congenital hypothyroidism is now performed by all states of the USA. Second screening at 2-6 weeks of age may be required to detect all cases. Combined screening for low T_4 and high TSH has greater specificity than the use of either test alone. Measurement of TSH is the best confirmatory test for primary hypothyroidism, in which it is elevated.

Footnotes

1. Howanitz JH, Howanitz PJ, and Henry JB, "Evaluation of Endocrine Function," *Clinical Diagnosis and Management by Laboratory Methods*, 18th ed, Henry JB, ed, Philadelphia, PA: WB Saunders Co, 1991, 308-20.

References

American Academy of Pediatrics Committee on Genetics, "Newborn Screening Fact Sheets: Congenital Hypothyroidism," *Pediatrics*, 1989, 83:454-6 and 461-2.

(Continued)

Thyroid Stimulating Hormone Screen, Filter Paper *(Continued)*

LaFranchi S, "Diagnosis and Treatment of Hypothyroidism in Children," *Compr Ther*, 1987, 13(10):20-30.

Meites S, *Pediatric Clinical Chemistry: Reference (Normal) Values*, 3rd ed, Washington, DC: American Association of Clinical Chemistry Press, 1989, 250-2.

Surks MI, "Guidelines for Thyroid Testing," *Lab Med*, 1993, 24(5):270-4.

Thorpe-Beeston JG, Nicolaides KH, and McGregor AM, "Fetal Thyroid Function," *Thyroid*, 1992, 2(3):207-17.

Thyrotropin *see* Thyroid Stimulating Hormone *on page 361*

Thyrotropin Stimulating Hormone *see* Thyroid Stimulating Hormone *on page 361*

Thyroxine

CPT *84436*

Related Information

Amiodarone *on page 939*
Kidney Stone Analysis *on page 1129*
Lithium *on page 979*
T_3 Uptake *on page 355*
Thyroid Antimicrosomal Antibody *on page 755*
Thyroid Antithyroglobulin Antibody *on page 756*
Thyrotropin-Receptor Antibody *on page 756*
Thyroxine Binding Globulin *on page 366*
Thyroxine, Free *on page 368*
Triiodothyronine *on page 373*

Synonyms T_4; T_4 by EIA; T_4 (RIA); Tetraiodothyronine; Thyroxine by RIA

Replaces T_4 CPB; Murphy-Pattee; PBI

Abstract Thyroxine (T_4) is the major secretory product of the thyroid gland. It is carried through the blood bound (in equilibrium) to thyroxine binding globulin (TBG), prealbumin, and albumin. T_4 secretion is stimulated by thyroid stimulating hormone (TSH).

Patient Care PREPARATION: Avoid radioisotope administration prior to collection of specimen.

Specimen Serum CONTAINER: Red top tube STORAGE INSTRUCTIONS: Separate serum within 48 hours and refrigerate. Separated serum stable 1 week at 25°C.

Interpretive REFERENCE RANGE: Pediatrics: Cord T_4 and values in the first few weeks are much higher, falling over the first months and years; 10 years and older: approximately 5.8-11.0 μg/dL (SI: 75-142 nmol/L), varying somewhat between laboratories. Borderline low is ≤4.5-5.7 μg/dL (SI: ≤58-73 nmol/L); low is ≤4.4 μg/dL (SI: ≤57 nmol/L); results <2.5 μg/dL (SI: <32 nmol/L) are strong evidence for hypothyroidism.[1]

Approximate adult normal range is given by Ingbar as 4.0-12.0 μg/dL (SI: 51-154 nmol/L)[2] and by Larsen as 5.0-11.0 μg/dL (SI: 64-142 nmol/L);[3] borderline high is 11.1-13.0 μg/dL (SI: 143-167 nmol/L); high is ≥13.1 μg/dL (SI: ≥169 nmol/L). High is sometimes given as ≥8-10 μg/dL (SI: ≥103-129 nmol/L). Normal range is increased in women on birth control pills, owing to increased TBG. Free thyroxine index will still be within the normal range. Normal range in pregnancy: approximately 5.5-16.0 μg/dL (SI: 71-206 nmol/L).

POSSIBLE PANIC RANGE: At values <2.0 μg/dL (SI: <26 nmol/L), myxedema coma is possible. At values >20 μg/dL (SI: >257 nmol/L), thyroid storm is possible. USE: Best general thyroid function screening test. **Decreased** in hypothyroidism, in genetically decreased TBG, and in the third stage of (painful) subacute thyroiditis; **increased** with hyperthyroidism, with subacute thyroiditis in its first stage, with thyrotoxicosis due to Graves' disease, with increased TBG (pregnancy, genetically increased TBG, acute intermittent porphyria, primary biliary cirrhosis), thyrotoxicosis factitia, and occasionally in euthyroid patients with familial dysalbuminemic hyperthyroxinemia. Used to diagnose T_4 thyrotoxicosis.

Primary hypothyroidism (hypometabolism) is caused by Hashimoto's thyroiditis, idiopathic myxedema, prior radioactive iodine therapy for hyperthyroidism, prior thyroid surgery, endemic goiter and other entities. Congenital causes include enzyme blocks and agenesis. Causes of **secondary hypothyroidism** include primary pituitary disease, eg, postpartum pituitary necrosis (Sheehan's syndrome) and pituitary tumors. The expression "myxedema" indicates advanced clinical hypothyroidism, with dermal mucopolysaccharide deposits. Comprehensive lists of causes of hypothyroidism are published.[2,3,4] A diagnosis of primary hypothyroidism should be confirmed by a TSH assay.

Graves' disease is classical thyrotoxicosis (hypermetabolism) caused by an immune or autoimmune disorder. Other causes of **hyperthyroidism** include toxic multinodular or uninodular goiter, phases of thyroiditis and a number of uncommon to rare entities, which cause increased T_4. Tabulations of causes of hyperthyroidism are widely available.[2,4]

T_4 and other tests are used to investigate goiter, an expression for thyroid enlargement, which may be found with hypothyroidism, euthyroidism, or hyperthyroidism.

LIMITATIONS: T_4 may be increased with excess intake of iodine or or with surreptitious use of thyroxine. T_4 levels may be abnormal in the presence of systemic nonthyroidal disease. Alterations in binding capacity or quantity of TBG may increase or decrease total thyroxine without causing symptoms. A common cause of elevated T_4 in nonthyroidal disease is said to be liver disease.

Serum thyroxine and free thyroxine (FT_4) are increased in familial dysalbuminemic hyperthyroxinemia, a euthyroid syndrome in which an abnormal binding site has affinity for thyroxine.[5] The T_3 is usually normal in this entity, as is T_3 uptake. Thus, T_3 uptake is commonly ordered with T_4.

T_4 is less sensitive than TSH in the diagnosis of hypothyroidism.

Euthyroid hyperthyroxinemia has been reviewed. It is an expression used as a collective term for nonthyroidal diseases and states which increase thyroxine levels with normal thyroid tissue and metabolism. In addition to thyroid hormone binding globulin changes and drug related phenomena, peripheral resistance to thyroid hormones and increases related to medical and acute psychiatric illness are described. Hyperemesis gravidarum and hyponatremia may cause euthyroid hyperthyroxinemia. Extensive tabulations of thyroid tests and some causes of changes in them have been published.[2,5]

Anti-T_4 antibodies may exist, interfering with T_4 and free T_4 determinations.

METHODOLOGY: Radioimmunoassay (RIA), enzyme-linked immunosorbent assay (ELISA), fluorescence polarization immunoassay (FPIA), chemiluminescence assay (CIA) **ADDITIONAL INFORMATION:** The combination of the serum T_4 and T_3 uptake as an assessment of TBG, helps to determine whether an abnormal T_4 value is due to alterations in serum thyroxine binding globulin or to changes of thyroid hormone levels. Deviations of both tests in the same direction usually indicate that an abnormal T_4 is due to abnormalities in thyroid hormone. Deviations of the two tests in opposite directions provide evidence that an abnormal T_4 may relate to alterations in TBG.

Thyroid Tests With Disease and Varying TBG

Diagnosis	T_4	FT_4 (or FT_4I)	TSH
Normal	Normal	Normal	Normal
Hyperthyroid	Increased	Increased	Decreased
Hypothyroid	Decreased	Decreased	Increased
Increased TBG	Increased	Normal	Normal
Decreased TBG	Decreased	Normal	Normal

Causes of increased TBG binding include neonatal state, molar and conventional pregnancy, estrogens, oral contraceptives, heroin, methadone, 5-fluorouracil, clofibrate, infectious hepatitis, chronic active hepatitis, and primary biliary cirrhosis, acute intermittent porphyria, lymphoma, and hereditary TBG increase.

Causes of decreased TBG binding include abnormal protein states. These include nephrotic syndrome, androgens, anabolic steroids, prednisone, acromegaly, liver or other systemic illness, severe stress, and hereditary TBG deficiency. Salicylates and diphenylhydantoin may lower T_4 significantly. Amiodarone may cause increased thyroxine levels and can cause hypothyroidism or hyperthyroidism.

Lithium carbonate may cause goiter with or without hypothyroidism.

Carbamazepine (Tegretol®) is reported to cause decreased values in thyroid function tests.

This brief review must point out that clinical interpretation of patients' signs and symptoms has primary significance. Definitive treatment based on insufficient laboratory tests is condemned.

The sensitive TSH assay has been advocated as a single screening test for thyroid disease. Such proposals are controversial; others find it difficult to accept one test as adequate for

(Continued)

Thyroxine *(Continued)*

screening[6] and warn that a single test cannot adequately, in all settings, reflect thyroid status.[7] An inverse relationship exists between thyroxine and TSH. While the former represents thyroid hormone concentration, the latter is a test of thyroid regulation.

Thyrotropin levels of treated hypothyroid subjects, triiodothyronine concentrations, and serum thyroxine levels are discussed with replacement doses of levothyroxine in a 1987 paper.[8]

Footnotes

1. Larsen RP and Ingbar SH, "The Thyroid," *Williams Textbook of Endocrinology*, 8th ed, Wilson J and Foster N, eds, Philadelphia, PA: WB Saunders Co, 1992, 357-488.
2. Wantofsky L and Ingbar SH, "Diseases of the Thyroid," *Harrison's Principles of Internal Medicine*, Braunwald E, Isselbacher KJ, Petersdorf RG, et al, eds, New York, NY: McGraw-Hill Inc, 1991, 1692-712.
3. Larsen PR, "The Thyroid," *Cecil Textbook of Medicine*, 18th ed, Vol 2, Wyngaarden JB, Smith LH Jr, and Bennett JC, eds, Philadelphia, PA: WB Saunders Co, 1992, 1248-71.
4. Fernandez-Ulloa M and Maxon HR III, "Thyroid," *Clinical Chemistry: Theory, Analysis, and Correlation*, Kaplan LA and Pesce AJ, eds, St Louis, MO: Mosby-Year Book Inc, 1989, 620-38.
5. Ruiz M, Rajatanavin R, Young RA, et al, "Familial Dysalbuminemic Hyperthyroxinemia: A Syndrome That Can Be Confused With Thyrotoxicosis," *N Engl J Med*, 1982, 306:635-9.
6. Gambino R, "TSH and Thyroid Status," *Lab Report for Physicians*, 1989, 11:33-5.
7. Ehrmann DA and Sarne DH, "Serum Thyrotropin and the Assessment of Thyroid Status," *Ann Intern Med*, 1989, 110(3):179-81.
8. Fish LH, Schwartz HL, Cavanaugh J, et al, "Replacement Dose, Metabolism, and Bioavailability of Levothyroxine in the Treatment of Hypothyroidism: Role of Triiodothyronine in Pituitary Feedback in Humans," *N Engl J Med*, 1987, 316:764-70.

References

de los Santos ET and Mazzaferri EL, "Thyroid Function Tests. Guidelines for Interpretation in Common Clinical Disorders," *Postgrad Med*, 1989, 85(5):333-40, 345-52, (review).

Franklyn JA, Davis JR, Ramsden DB, et al, "Phenytoin and Thyroid Hormone Action," *J Endocrinol*, 1985, 104:201-4.

Gharib H and Klee GG, "Familial Euthyroid Hyperthyroxinemia Secondary to Pituitary and Peripheral Resistance to Thyroid Hormones," *Mayo Clin Proc*, 1985, 60:9-15.

Griffin JE, "Hypothyroidism in the Elderly," *Am J Med Sci*, 1990, 299(5):334-45.

Gruhn JG, Barsano CP, and Kumar Y, "The Development of Tests of Thyroid Function," *Arch Pathol Lab Med*, 1987, 111:84-100.

Klee GG, Young WF, and Hay ID, "Biochemical Tests of Thyroid and Pituitary Function," *ASCP National Meeting*, Chicago, IL: American Society of Clinical Pathologists, 1990.

Larsen PR, Alexander NM, Chopra IJ, et al, "Revised Nomenclature for Tests of Thyroid Hormones and Thyroid-Related Proteins in Serum," *Arch Pathol Lab Med*, 1987, 111:1141-5.

Miller MJ, Pan C, and Barzel US, "The Prevalence of Subclinical Hypothyroidism in Adults With Low-Normal Blood Thyroxine Levels," *N Y State J Med*, 1990, 90(11):541-4.

Rallison ML, Dobyns BM, Meikle AW, et al, "Natural History of Thyroid Abnormalities: Prevalence, Incidence, and Regression of Thyroid Diseases in Adolescents and Young Adults," *Am J Med*, 1991, 91(4):363-70.

Schectman JM and Pawlson LG, "Screening for Thyroid Disease," *Ann Intern Med*, 1990, 113(11):896.

Schectman JM and Pawlson LG, "The Cost-Effectiveness of Three Thyroid Function Testing Strategies for Suspicion of Hypothyroidism in a Primary Care Setting," *J Gen Intern Med*, 1990, 5(1):9-15.

Staub JJ, Althaus BU, Engler H, et al, "Spectrum of Subclinical and Overt Hypothyroidism: Effect on Thyrotropin, Prolactin, and Thyroid Reserve, and Metabolic Impact on Peripheral Target Tissues," *Am J Med*, 1992, 92(6):631-42.

Surks MI, "Guidelines for Thyroid Testing," *Lab Med*, 1993, 24(5):270-4.

Wolf PG and Meek JC, "Practical Approach to the Treatment of Hypothyroidism," *Am Fam Physician*, 1992, 45(2):722-31.

Thyroxine Binding Globulin

CPT 84442

Related Information

Free Thyroxine Index *on page 223*
T_3 Uptake *on page 355*
Thyroxine *on page 364*
Thyroxine, Free *on page 368*

Synonyms T_4-Binding Globulin; TBG

Abstract Serum thyroid binding proteins include albumin, transthyretin (thyroid binding prealbumin), and, most important, thyroxine binding globulin. Familial TBG abnormalities may cause abnormalities in thyroid tests in essentially euthyroid subjects. TBG binds 70% to 80% of total T_4 normally; affected euthyroid persons have low T_4.[1] T_3 and T_4 circulate almost entirely bound to the three thyroid hormone binding proteins. TBG is a glycoprotein. Its abnormalities are not clinical diseases (ie, they do not themselves require treatment). This test is **not** for thyroglobulin.

Patient Care PREPARATION: No recent administration of radioactive isotopes or *in vivo* uptakes.

Specimen Serum CONTAINER: Red top tube

Interpretive REFERENCE RANGE: Adults: 21-52 μg/dL (SI: 270-669 nmol/L); 0-1 week: 21-90 μg/dL (SI: 270-1,158 nmol/L); 1-12 months: 21-76 μg/dL (SI: 270-978 nmol/L). Adult normals reached about age 14. USE: Determine binding capacity for T_4 to distinguish between hyperthyroidism causing high T_4, and euthyroid individuals with increased binding by TBG who have increased T_4 and normal levels of free hormones. Document cases of hereditary deficiency or increase of TBG. In work-up of thyroid disease, in patients with low T_4, high T_3 uptake or the reverse, who clinically seem eumetabolic and have normal FTI, measurement of TBG is only occasionally needed. Some such patients may have hereditary anomalies of TBG. TBG is increased by estrogens, tamoxifen, pregnancy, perphenazine, and in some cases of liver disease, including hepatitis. Decreased TBG is found with some instances of chronic liver disease, nephrosis and systemic disease and with large amounts of glucocorticoids, androgens/anabolic steroids, acromegaly; and increased TBG is found in certain genetically determined states. More information is provided in listing Thyroxine. Although alterations of TBG are usually resolved by the thyroid profile, TBG must occasionally be directly measured.

Kindreds are described with elevated TBG and hyperthyroxinemia as a harmless genetic abnormality. They have normal levels of TSH and free T_4 and decreased T_3 uptake. Structural variants of TBG are inherited as X-chromosome linked traits, most inherited structural abnormalities in TBG cause decreased affinity for thyroid hormone.[1] Six families have been described with complete TBG deficiency. Such kindreds appear to have no gross structural defects in the TBG gene.[2]

LIMITATIONS: TBG is normal in familial dysalbuminemic hyperthyroxinemia, an entity which can be incorrectly identified as thyrotoxicosis.[3] Low T_3 uptake and normal calculated free T_4 index often make measurement of TBG by RIA unnecessary. METHODOLOGY: Double antibody precipitation,[1] radioimmunoassay (RIA) ADDITIONAL INFORMATION: The usual thyroid function studies should be performed before considering this test. The major indication for TBG testing is in diagnosis of hereditary deficiency of TBG. A euthyroid subject with a structural abnormality such as TBG-San Diego can be expected to have low total T_4 and free T_4 (FT_4) index but normal TSH.[1] Serum TBG concentration is increased in adults with late-stage HIV infections[4] and in children with HIV infections.[5] It is unchanged in long-term fasting (protein sparing)[6] and decreased with nicotinic acid therapy.[7]

Footnotes

1. Sarne DH, Refetoff S, Nelson JC, et al, "A New Inherited Abnormality of Thyroxine-Binding Globulin (TBG-San Diego) With Decreased Affinity for Thyroxine and Triiodothyronine," *J Clin Endocrinol Metab*, 1989, 68(1):114-9.
2. Mori Y, Refetoff S, Flink IL, et al, "Detection of the Thyroxine-Binding Globulin (TBG) Gene in Six Unrelated Families With Complete TBG Deficiency," *J Clin Endocrinol Metab*, 1988, 67(4):727-33.
3. Ruiz M, Rajatanavin R, Young RA, et al, "Familial Dysalbuminemic Hyperthyroxinemia: A Syndrome That Can Be Confused With Thyrotoxicosis," *N Engl J Med*, 1982, 306:635-9.
4. Lambert M, Zech F, De Nayer P, et al, "Elevation of Serum Thyroxine-Binding Globulin (but Not of Cortisol-Binding Globulin and Sex Hormone-Binding Globulin) Associated With the Progression of Human Immunodeficiency Virus Infection," *Am J Med*, 1990, 89(6):748-51.
5. Laue L, Pizzo PA, Butler K, et al, "Growth and Neuroendocrine Dysfunction in Children With Acquired Immunodeficiency Syndrome," *J Pediatr*, 1990, 117(4):541-5.
6. Marine N, Hershman JM, Maxwell MH, et al, "Dietary Restriction on Serum Thyroid Hormone Levels," *Am J Med Sci*, 1991, 301(5):310-3.
7. O'Brien T, Silverberg JD, and Nguyen TT, "Nicotinic Acid-Induced Toxicity Associated With Cytopenia and Decreased Levels of Thyroxine-Binding Globulin," *Mayo Clin Proc*, 1992, 67(5):465-8.

References

Larsen PR, "The Thyroid," *Cecil Textbook of Medicine*, Wyngarden JB, Smith LH, and Bennett JC, eds, Philadelphia, PA: WB Saunders Co, 1992, 1248-71.

Nelson JC and Tomei RT, "Dependence of the Thyroxine/Thyroxine-Binding Globulin (TBG) Ratio and the Free Thyroxine Index on TBG Concentrations," *Clin Chem*, 1989, 35(4):541-4.

Refetoff S, "Inherited Thyroxine-Binding Globulin Abnormalities in Man," *Endocr Rev*, 1989, 10(3):275-93.

Surks MI, "Guidelines for Thyroid Testing," *Lab Med*, 1993, 24(5):270-4.

Thyroxine by RIA *see* Thyroxine *on page 364*

Thyroxine, Free

CPT 84439

Related Information

Free Thyroxine Index *on page 223*
Thyroid Antimicrosomal Antibody *on page 755*
Thyroid Antithyroglobulin Antibody *on page 756*
Thyrotropin-Receptor Antibody *on page 756*
Thyroxine *on page 364*
Thyroxine Binding Globulin *on page 366*
Triiodothyronine *on page 373*

Synonyms Free T_4; Free Thyroxine; FT_4; T_4, Free; Unbound T_4

Abstract Free T_4 is a very small fraction of total thyroxine (0.04%); it is the metabolically active fraction. Impetus for development of free T_4 emerged with recognition of euthyroid sick syndrome and euthyroid hyperthyroxinemia syndrome, settings in which conventional tests such as T_4 (total) and FTI fail to reliably reflect the patient's clinical thyroid status.[1]

Specimen Serum **CONTAINER:** Red top tube **STORAGE INSTRUCTIONS:** Separate serum within 48 hours. Stable 2 weeks at 4°C. **CAUSES FOR REJECTION:** Recent administration of radioisotopes

Interpretive **REFERENCE RANGE:** Approximately 0.7-1.8 ng/dL (SI: 9-23 pmol/L);[2] this example of a normal range is placed to permit comparison with the units in which conventional T_4 by RIA is expressed. Actual normal range varies somewhat between laboratories. Not increased in normal pregnancy. **USE:** A sensitive test for thyroid function, increased with hyperthyroidism.[2] Free T_4 is indicated when binding globulin (TBG) problems are perceived, or when conventional test results are borderline or seem inconsistent with clinical observations. It is normal in subjects with high thyroxine binding globulin hormone binding who are euthyroid (ie, free thyroxine should be normal in nonthyroidal diseases). It should be normal in familial dysalbuminemic hyperthyroxinemia. **LIMITATIONS:** FT_4 may be increased with radiologic contrast agents, propranolol, amiodarone, and heparin. It may be decreased with carbamazepine (Tegretol®). Free T_4 is a small part of total T_4 (0.04%). Free T_4 will not detect T_3 thyrotoxicosis. Increased free T_4 levels may occur in subjects with nonthyroid diseases. Such elevations are described as transient.[3] Low values were reported in patients with nonthyroidal illness. Discrepancies in free T_4 levels between methods are recognized.[1] Free T_4 is influenced by albumin concentration, requiring a number of follow up tests. Reliability problems continue to be discussed with the newer methods.[4] Results of kits intended to serve in place of equilibrium dialysis technique may differ from the reference method. **METHODOLOGY:** Equilibrium dialysis is the reference method; radioimmunoassay (RIA) **ADDITIONAL INFORMATION:** The free thyroxine index (FTI or FTI-2) is a calculation derived from T_3 uptake and T_4 RIA, which are tests which remain in widespread use. Generally, the FTI and the free T_4 provide comparable information, but this is a complex topic. Costs of each should be compared. FT_4 is increased with levothyroxine therapy. **A free T_3** test exists as well. It is briefly discussed in the listing Triiodothyronine.

Footnotes

1. Gruhn JG, Barsano CP, and Kumar Y, "The Development of Tests of Thyroid Function," *Arch Pathol Lab Med*, 1987, 111:84-100.
2. Gupta MK, Salazar R, and Schumacher OP, "A Solid Phase Radioimmunoassay for the Measurement of Free Thyroxine. A New Screening Test for Thyroid Function?" *Am J Clin Pathol*, 1983, 79:334-40.
3. Cooke RR and Pratt R, "Thyroid Function Tests in Acutely Ill Patients. Comparison of Analogue Based Free Thyroid Hormone Assays With Free Thyroxine Index," *Pathology*, 1986, 18:94-7.
4. Bethune JE, "Interpretation of Thyroid Function Tests," *Dis Mon*, 1989, 35(8):541-95.

References

Chattoraj SC and Watts NB, "Endocrinology," *Fundamentals of Clinical Chemistry*, 3rd ed, Tietz NW, ed, Philadelphia, PA: WB Saunders Co, 1987, 533-613.

Jansson R, Forberg R, and Levin K, "Free Thyroxine Index and Direct Measurements of Free Thyroxine Compared for Evaluating Postpartum Autoimmune Thyroid Dysfunction," *Clin Chem*, 1984, 30:903-5.

Martinez M, Derksen D, and Kapsner P, "Making Sense of Hypothyroidism. An Approach to Testing and Treatment," *Postgrad Med*, 1993, 93(6):135-8, 141-5.

Pearce CJ and Himsworth RL, "Total and Free Thyroid Hormone Concentrations in Patients Receiving Maintenance Replacement Treatment With Thyroxine," *Br Med J [Clin Res]*, 1984, 288:693-5.

Surks MI, "Guidelines for Thyroid Testing," *Lab Med*, 1993, 24(5):270-4.

Wantofsky L and Ingbar SH, "Diseases of the Thyroid," *Harrison's Principles of Internal Medicine*, Braunwald E, Isselbacher KJ, Petersdorf RG, et al, eds, New York, NY: McGraw-Hill Inc, 1991, 1692-712.

Wilkins TA, "Free Thyroxine Assays: Analogue Methods," *Lancet*, 1985, 2:884, (letter).

Thyroxine, Neonatal *see* Newborn Screen for Hypothyroidism and Phenylketonuria *on page 295*

TIBC *see* Iron and Total Iron Binding Capacity/Transferrin *on page 262*

Tissue Polypeptide Antigen *see* CA 19-9 *on page 152*

Tocopherol *see* Vitamin E, Serum *on page 389*

α-Tocopherol *see* Vitamin E, Serum *on page 389*

Tolbutamide Test *see* Glucose, Fasting *on page 238*

Tolerance Test, Lactose *see* Lactose Tolerance Test *on page 275*

Total Bilirubin *see* Bilirubin, Total *on page 139*

Total Bilirubin, Neonatal *see* Bilirubin, Neonatal *on page 138*

Total Calcium, Serum *see* Calcium, Serum *on page 160*

Total Iron Binding Capacity *see* Iron and Total Iron Binding Capacity/Transferrin *on page 262*

Total Metanephrines *see* Metanephrines, Total, Urine *on page 289*

Total Protein, Serum *see* Protein, Total, Serum *on page 340*

Total T_3 *see* Triiodothyronine *on page 373*

Total Urinary Catecholamines *replaced by* Catecholamines, Fractionation, Urine *on page 174*

Total Urinary Estrogens *see* Estrogens, Nonpregnant, Urine *on page 218*

TPA *see* CA 19-9 *on page 152*

Transaminase *see* Alanine Aminotransferase *on page 100*

Transaminase *see* Aspartate Aminotransferase *on page 135*

Transcutaneous Pulse Oximetry *see* Oxygen Saturation, Blood *on page 305*

Transferrin

CPT 84466

Related Information

Ferritin, Serum *on page 220*
Iron and Total Iron Binding Capacity/Transferrin *on page 262*
Protoporphyrin, Zinc, Blood *on page 342*

Synonyms Siderophilin; Tau Protein; TRF

Applies to Transferrin Index; Transferrin Receptors

Abstract Transferrin is an iron transport protein which binds iron released during hemoglobin catabolism as well as iron absorbed through the intestine, and transports it to the liver and reticuloendothelial system for storage.

Patient Care PREPARATION: Fasting specimen is preferred.

Specimen Serum CONTAINER: Red top tube SAMPLING TIME: Morning COLLECTION: See Iron and Total Iron Binding Capacity/Transferrin. CAUSES FOR REJECTION: Hemolysis

Interpretive REFERENCE RANGE: Approximately 200-360 mg/dL (SI: 2.0-3.6 g/L), with some variation between laboratories USE: Increased in iron deficiency anemia. It is decreased in chronic inflammatory states, hereditary atransferrinemia, some instances of acquired liver disease, neoplasia, and renal disease. Transferrin is an index of nutritional status. Transferrin (tau protein) can be used as a marker for the presence of CSF in patients presenting with a nasal discharge of clear fluid. LIMITATIONS: Increased in patients on oral contraceptives and in late pregnancy. May not be elevated in iron-deficient states in which there is severe protein malnutrition (eg, kwashiorkor) or chronic inflammation. METHODOLOGY: Radial immunodiffusion (RID), rate nephelometry, nephelometric scattering, immunoturbidity. The latter three immunochemical methods have shown good agreement in calibrator crossover and patient studies.[1] ADDITIONAL INFORMATION: Transferrin is responsible for 50% to 70% of the iron binding capacity of serum. Since other proteins may bind iron, transferrin is not the same as TIBC. Transferrin is an iron transport protein receiving and binding iron for delivery to receptors at recipient cells. The human transferrin gene, responsible for production of this single chain, 77,000 dalton polypeptide resides on chromosome 3, band q 21-25. Transferrin has two iron-binding sites and is largely but not exclusively synthesized by the liver. There are over 20 genetic variants, largely single amino acid substitutions. Transferrin levels rise with iron deficiency and fall in cases of iron overload. Transferrin is normally only about one-third saturated and is responsi-

(Continued)

Transferrin *(Continued)*

ble for circadian variation in serum iron (peak in AM) due to variable activity of the reticuloendothelial system. Transferrin saturation calculated as serum iron/TIBC may be used to screen for iron overload. **Transferrin index** calculated as serum iron/transferrin has been suggested as a better screen for iron overload.[2]

Recent studies have indicated that plasma **transferrin receptor concentrations** have a constant relationship to tissue receptors and reflect the rate of erythropoiesis except in iron deficiency.[3] Serum transferrin receptor concentrations appear to be independent of inflammation or liver disease,[4] unlike transferrin. Decreased binding of transferrin to erythroblasts[5] may lead to impaired iron uptake and may be a mechanism for the anemia of chronic disease. Decreased serum transferrin concentration may be associated with a poor progression-free survival in children with Hodgkin's disease.[6]

Footnotes

1. Christenson RH, Finley PR, and Silverman LM, "Immunochemical Assays for IgG, IgA, IgM and Transferrin Compared," *Clin Biochem*, 1989, 22(4):271-6.
2. Beilby J, Olynyk J, Ching S, et al, "Transferrin Index: An Alternative Method for Calculating the Iron Saturation of Transferrin," *Clin Chem*, 1992, 38(10):2078-81.
3. Huebers HA, Beguin Y, Pootrakul P, et al, "Intact Transferrin Receptors in Human Plasma and Their Relation to Erythropoiesis," *Blood*, 1990, 75(1):102-7.
4. Ferguson BJ, Skikne BS, Simpson KM, et al, "Serum Transferrin Receptor Distinguishes the Anemia of Chronic Disease From Iron Deficiency Anemia," *J Lab Clin Med*, 1992, 119(4):385-90.
5. Vreugdenhil G, Kroos MJ, van Eijk HG, et al, "Impaired Iron Uptake and Transferrin Binding by Erythroblasts in the Anaemia of Rheumatoid Arthritis," *Br J Rheumatol*, 1990, 29(5):335-9.
6. Hann HW, Lange B, Stahlhut MW, et al, "Prognostic Importance of Serum Transferrin and Ferritin in Childhood Hodgkin's Disease," *Cancer*, 1990, 66(2):313-6.

References

Bothwell TH, Charlton RW, and Motulsky AG, "Hemochromatosis," *The Metabolic Basis of Inherited Disease*, 6th ed, Scriver CE, Beaudet AL, Sly WS, et al, eds, New York, NY: McGraw-Hill Inc, 1989.

Keir G, Zeman A, Brookes G, et al, "Immunoblotting of Transferrin in the Identification of Cerebrospinal Fluid Otorrhoea and Rhinorrhoea," *Ann Clin Biochem*, 1992, 29(Pt 2):210-3.

Transferrin Index *see* Transferrin *on previous page*

Transferrin Receptors *see* Transferrin *on previous page*

TRF *see* Transferrin *on previous page*

Triacylglycerol Acylhydrolase *see* Lipase, Serum *on page 277*

Triacylglycerols *see* Triglycerides *on this page*

Triglycerides

CPT *84478*

Related Information

Apolipoprotein A and B *on page 134*
Cholesterol *on page 185*
High Density Lipoprotein Cholesterol *on page 249*
Lipid Profile *on page 278*
Lipoprotein Electrophoresis *on page 281*
Low Density Lipoprotein Cholesterol *on page 284*

Synonyms Triacylglycerols

Applies to Chylomicrons; VLDL

Test Commonly Includes Triglycerides are included in the lipid profiles of most laboratories.

Abstract Triglycerides are a family of complex lipids composed of glycerol esterified with three fatty acids (saturated or unsaturated) of the same or different lengths. Triglycerides are not soluble in blood and are therefore transported as chylomicrons (TG from exogenous source) or as VLDL (TG from endogenous source). Triglycerides constitute 95% of tissue storage fat.

Patient Care PREPARATION: The patient should be fasting for 12-14 hours and should be on a stable diet 3 weeks prior to collection of blood. Avoid alcohol for 3 days. See Preparation in Cholesterol listing.

Specimen Serum CONTAINER: Red top tube; lavender top (EDTA) tube is used by some outstanding laboratories CAUSES FOR REJECTION: Specimen collected in a glycerinated tube, nonfasting specimen

Interpretive REFERENCE RANGE: See tables. These tables are based on plasma triglycerides. Triglyceride values increase with aging. With cholesterol values within normal ranges, triglyce-

Reference Values for Plasma Triglycerides for White Males* (mg/L)

Age, y	Percentiles			
	5	50	90	95
0-9	300	550	850	1000
10-14	300	650	1000	1250
15-19	350	800	1200	1500
20-24	450	1000	1650	2000
25-29	450	1150	2000	2500
30-34	500	1300	2150	2650
35-39	550	1450	2500	3200
40-54	550	1500	2500	3200
55-64	600	1400	2350	2900
65+	550	1350	2100	2600

*From the LRC Prevalence Study (North America).

Reference Values for Plasma Triglycerides for White Females* (mg/L)

Age, y	Percentiles			
	5	50	90	95
0-9	350	600	950	1100
10-19	400	750	1150	1300
20-34	400	900	1450	1700
35-39	400	950	1600	1950
40-44	450	1050	1700	2100
45-49	450	1100	1850	2300
50-54	550	1200	1900	2400
55-64	550	1250	2000	2500
65+	600	1300	2050	2400

*From the LRC Prevalence Study (North America).

Reference Values for Plasma Triglycerides for Black Males* (mg/L)

Age, y	Percentiles†			
	5	50	90	95
0-9	310	470	750	880
10-19	310	530	880	1020
20-29	—	710	1250	—
30-39	420	910	1660	2240
40-49	520	970	2150	2940
50-59	—	1050	—	—
60+	—	960	—	—

*From the LRC Prevalence Study (North America).
†5th and 95th percentiles not given if $n < 100$; 90th percentile not given if $n < 75$.

Reference Values for Plasma Triglycerides for Black Females* (mg/L)

Age, y	Percentiles†			
	5	50	90	95
0-9	330	500	830	940
10-19	360	600	950	1100
20-29	380	680	1180	1370
30-39	380	740	1290	1500
40-49	430	840	1530	1880
50-59	—	940	1760	—
60+	—	1060	—	—

*From the LRC Prevalence Study (North America).
†5th and 95th percentiles not given if $n < 100$; 90th percentile not given if $n < 75$.

ride levels <250 mg/L (SI: <2.82 mmol/L) (90th percentile) are not thought to be related to risk; *vide infra*. **USE:** Evaluate turbid samples of blood, plasma, and serum; work up of chylomicronemia; evaluate hyperlipidemia; occasional cases of diabetes mellitus and/or pancreatitis are detected by hypertriglyceridemia. High levels may occur with hypothyroidism, nephrotic syndromes, carbohydrate-sensitive hypertriglyceridemia, glycogen storage disease, and in hyperlipoproteinemias type I, IIb, III, IV, and V. Some alcoholics have hypertriglyceridemia which disappears with abstinence. Extremely high triglyceride levels may occur with alcohol abuse. Triglyceride is needed for calculation of LDLC (low density lipoprotein cholesterol) concentration. Disturbances in triglyceride metabolism relate to diabetes and are an interactive risk factor for atherosclerotic disease.[1] Although the role of hypertriglyceridemia as a risk factor for coronary arterial disease has been controversial, men and women with low serum HDL cholesterol and high serum triglyceride concentrations have a higher relative risk of coronary artery disease (*vide infra*). In familial combined hyperlipidemia, hypertriglyceridemia may be found before hypercholesterolemia. Nevertheless, a strong case is not available for primary triglyceride screening of healthy persons without positive family history of coronary disease or other risk factors. Some knowledgeable authorities favor screening with lipid profiles, including triglycerides, for reasons discussed elsewhere in this listing and this chapter. In exogenous hypertriglyceridemia, chylomicrons float as a layer in the tube of refrigerated, stored serum. **LIMITATIONS:** If triglyceride is >400 mg/dL, LDL cannot be calculated accurately by the Friedewald formula.[2] Correction for free serum glycerol in critically ill patients or patients on hyperalimentation with glycerol-based solutions may be necessary in some enzymatic methods.[3] **METHODOLOGY:** Enzymatic, colorimetric. A method for direct measurement of LDLC is now available. In this procedure, HDL and VLDL are separated from LDL by a filter which traps antibody coated latex beads. **ADDITIONAL INFORMATION:** Classic research from the Framingham

(Continued)

Triglycerides *(Continued)*

studies in the 1970s identified major risk factors for coronary artery disease as hypertension, high serum cholesterol concentrations, and cigarette smoking. New analyses from the Framingham heart study demonstrate that men and women with high serum triglyceride concentrations (>151 mg/dL, SI: >1.7 mmol/L) and low serum HDL concentrations have a significantly higher rate of coronary artery disease. This high risk group (high serum triglycerides, low serum HDL) appears independent of the major risk factors including low serum HDL concentrations.[4] The Helsinki Heart Study reported a 5 year randomized coronary prevention trial among dyslipemic, middle-aged men.[5] This study found a relative risk of 3.8 for those men with an HDL cholesterol/LDL cholesterol ratio of 5 and serum triglycerides >203 mg/dL (>2.3 mmol/L). Men with HDL cholesterol/LDL cholesterol ratios >5 and serum triglyceride concentrations <2.3 mmol/L had a relative risk of 1.2. This high risk group also appeared to benefit the most from treatment with gemfibrozil. A similar type of study in Münster, Germany[6] reported similar findings. Clearly, serum triglyceride concentration is a powerful factor interacting with main effects of cholesterol and HDL cholesterol. Variations in apolipoprotein A-I and triglyceride concentrations account for two-thirds of the population variance in serum HDL cholesterol concentrations.[7] Fundamental relationships observed between HDL cholesterol, apolipoprotein A-I, and triglyceride were unaltered by levels of factors under personal volition such as obesity, physical activity, and smoking.[7] Triglycerides commonly increase with obesity and may increase with chronic renal or liver disease. A positive association exists between diabetes mellitus and hypertriglyceridemia. Extremely high triglyceride levels suggest the possibility of pancreatitis. **Chylomicronemia**, although associated with pancreatitis, is not accompanied by increased atherogenesis. Chylomicrons are not seen in normal fasting serum, but are found in the sera of normal subjects following a fatty meal as exogenous triglycerides. Left refrigerated, chylomicrons float to the surface of a sample overnight; VLDL remain in suspension. Triglyceride physiologically is carried mostly as very low density lipoproteins (VLDL). The triglyceride in VLDL is endogenous from hepatic synthesis.

When turbidity of blood, serum, or plasma is seen, triglyceride is often >350 mg/dL. **Fasting chylomicronemia** occurs with but is not limited to deficiency of apo-CII, (apolipoprotein work-up). It occurs also with deficiency of **lipoprotein lipase**.

A positive association exists between gout and hypertriglyceridemia.

Drug effects have been summarized.[8] Some women on estrogens and high estrogen oral contraceptives have an increase of triglyceride. Increases occur with pregnancy, similar to those with oral contraceptives. The most common cause of triglyceride increase is inadequate patient fasting which is a cause for rejection of the specimen. Hypertriglyceridemia is associated with use of thiazide diuretics and beta-adrenergic blocking agents.

Footnotes

1. Rifkind BM and Segal P, "Lipid Research Clinics Program Reference Values for Hyperlipidemia and Hypolipidemia," *JAMA*, 1983, 250:1869-72.
2. Friedewald WT, Levy RI, and Fredrickson DS, "Estimation of the Concentration of Low-Density Lipoprotein Cholesterol in Plasma, Without Use of the Preparative Ultracentrifuge," *Clin Chem*, 1972, 18:499-502.
3. Jessen RH, Dass CJ, and Eckfeldt JH, " Do Enzymatic Analyses of Serum Triglycerides Really Need Blanking for Free Glycerol?" *Clin Chem*, 1990, 36(7):1372-5.
4. Castelli WP, "Epidemiology of Triglycerides: A View from Framingham," *Am J Cardiol*, 1992, 70(19):3H-9H.
5. Manninen V, Tenkanen L, Koskinen P, et al, "Joint Effects of Serum Triglyceride and LDL Cholesterol and HDL Cholesterol Concentrations on Coronary Heart Disease Risk in the Helsinki Heart Study – Implications for Treatment," *Circulation*, 1992, 85(1):37-45.
6. Assmann G and Schulte H, "Role of Triglycerides in Coronary Artery Disease: Lessons From the Prospective Cardiovascular Münster Study," *Am J Cardiol*, 1992, 70(19):10H-13H.
7. Patsch W, Sharrett AR, Sorlie PD, et al, "The Relation of High Density Lipoprotein Cholesterol and Its Subfractions to Apolipoprotein A-I and Fasting Triglycerides: The Role of Environmental Factors – The Atherosclerosis Risk in Communities (ARIC) Study," *Am J Epidemiol*, 1992, 136(5):546-57.
8. Steinmetz J, Jouanel P, and Thuillier Y, "Triglycerides," *Drug Effects on Laboratory Test Results Analytical Interferences and Pharmacological Effects*, Siest G and Galteau MM, eds, Littleton, MA: PSG Publishing Co Inc, 1988, 405-22.

References

Criqui MH, Heiss G, Cohn R, et al, "Plasma Triglyceride Level and Mortality From Coronary Heart Disease," *N Engl J Med*, 1993, 328(17):1220-5.

Kihara S, Matsuzawa Y, Kubo M, et al, "Autoimmune Hyperchylomicronemia," *N Engl J Med*, 1989, 320(19):1255-9.

Maeda I, Hayashi S, Fushimi R, et al, "Error Detection of High Concentrations of Endogenous Free Glycerol in Determination of Serum Triglyceride With the TBA-80S Automated Discrete Analyzer," *Clin Chem*, 1992, 38(7):1376-7.

McQueen MJ, Henderson AR, Patten RL, et al, "Results of a Province-Wide Quality Assurance Program Assessing the Accuracy of Cholesterol, Triglycerides, and High-Density Lipoprotein Cholesterol Measurements and Calculated Low-Density Lipoprotein Cholesterol in Ontario, Using Fresh Human Serum," *Arch Pathol Lab Med*, 1991, 115(12):1217-22.

Naito HK, "Triglycerides," Pesce AJ and Kaplan LA, eds, *Methods in Clinical Chemistry*, St Louis, MO: Mosby-Year Book Inc, 1987, 1215-27.

O'Meara NM, Lewis GF, Cabana VG, et al, "Role of Basal Triglyceride and High Density Lipoprotein in Determination of Postprandial Lipid and Lipoprotein Responses," *J Clin Endocrinol Metab*, 1992, 75(2):465-71.

Peterson CM, Jovanovic-Peterson L, Mills JL, et al, "The Diabetes in Early Pregnancy Study: Changes in Cholesterol, Triglycerides, Body Weight, and Blood Pressure," *Am J Obstet Gynecol*, 1992, 166(2):513-8.

Sady SP, Thompson PD, Cullinane EM, et al, "Clinical Investigation: Prolonged Exercise Augments Plasma Triglyceride Clearance," *JAMA*, 1986, 256:2552-5.

Zimmerman BR, Palumbo PJ, O'Fallon WM, et al, "A Prospective Study of Peripheral Occlusive Arterial Disease in Diabetes. III. Initial Lipid and Lipoprotein Findings," *Mayo Clin Proc*, 1981, 56:233-42.

Triiodothyronine

***CPT** 84480*

Related Information

Free Thyroxine Index *on page 223*
Thyroxine *on page 364*
Thyroxine, Free *on page 368*

Synonyms T_3 (RIA); T_3, Total; Total T_3; Triiodothyronine, Total

Abstract T_3 is a thyroid hormone produced mainly from the peripheral conversion of T_4 (a prohormone). T_3 has a greater biological activity than T_4 and binds to TBG less tightly than T_4.

Patient Care PREPARATION: Avoid radioisotope administration prior to collection of specimen. T_3 may be decreased with radiologic contrast agents, propranolol, and amiodarone.

Specimen Serum CONTAINER: Red top tube STORAGE INSTRUCTIONS: Separate serum within 48 hours. Stable up to 2 weeks at 25°C.

Interpretive REFERENCE RANGE: Values in infancy and childhood are higher than in adults. Adults: Approximately 80-230 ng/dL (SI: 1.2-3.5 nmol/L) with some variation between laboratories. A computer-based method to validate reference ranges lists a normal range of 50-140 ng/dL (SI: 0.7-2.1 nmol/L).[1] Increase occurs in pregnancy. USE: Thyroid function test which measures T_3. It is particularly useful in the diagnosis of T_3 thyrotoxicosis, in which T_3 is increased and T_4 is within normal limits. T_3 toxicosis is occasionally found in Graves' disease. It occurs with a single toxic nodule, multinodular thyrotoxicosis, and following treatment with T_3 (Cytomel®).[2] It is increased in and helpful for confirmation of the diagnosis of conventional hyperthyroidism, in which commonly both serum T_3 and T_4 concentrations are increased. T_3 is needed in patients with clinical evidence for hyperthyroidism, in whom the usual thyroid profile is normal or borderline, and in particular, if the T_4 is normal and the patient is clinically hyperthyroid ("T_3 thyrotoxicosis"). It is normal to slightly increased with familial dysalbuminemic hyperthyroxinemia. Recommended for patients with supraventricular tachycardia, for patients with fatigue and weight loss not otherwise explained, or for those with proximal myopathy and in whom T_4 concentrations are not elevated. LIMITATIONS: T_3 is decreased with nonthyroidal chronic diseases and influenced by the state of nutrition. It is not helpful to work up hypothyroidism. It may be normal with thyrotoxicosis (thyroxine thyrotoxicosis).[3] Variations in TBG and other binding proteins can affect T_3. Such increases may be found with use of oral contraceptives, pregnancy, and other binding protein abnormalities outlined in the listing Thyroxine. Fasting causes T_3 and TSH to decrease.[4] METHODOLOGY: Radioimmunoassay (RIA), immunochemiluminometric assay, fluorescence polarization immunoassay (FPIA), fluorometric immunoassay ADDITIONAL INFORMATION: Thyroid hormones exist in human plasma as free and bound forms (ie, free T_3 and free T_4, as well as bound T_3 and bound T_4). Less than 1% of total serum T_3 is in the free form. Serum concentrations of the free forms of T_3 and T_4 are regulated by feedback systems and appear to parallel rates of cellular uptake. Thus, the free hormone fraction determines the thyroid status of the individual. Essentially, bound fractions are unavailable to exert metabolic effects. Proteins that bind T_3 include thyroxine binding globulin, transthyretin, and albumin. As the serum concentrations of the binding proteins rise so does the total T_3, while the free T_3 fraction may be unchanged. An example of when this occurs is in pregnancy. T_3 has a higher metabolic potency relative to T_4. As approximately one-third of T_4 is converted to T_3, T_4 appears to have little intrinsic metabolic activity in humans. See table on following page for comparison of T_3 with T_4.

(Continued)

Triiodothyronine *(Continued)*

Comparison of T_3 and T_4 in Humans

	T_3	T_4
Serum concentration total (μg/dL) free (ng/dL)	 0.14 0.4	 8 1.6
Fraction of total serum hormone that is in the free form (%)	0.3	0.02
Distribution volume (L)	35	10
Fraction intracellular (%)	64	10–20
Half-life (days)	1	7
Production rate (μg/day)	33	80
Fraction directly from thyroid (%)	20	100
Relative metabolic potency	1	0.3

From Larsen PR, "The Thyroid," *Cecil Textbook of Medicine,* Vol 2, Wyngarden JB, Smith LH, and Bennett JC, eds, Philadelphia, PA: WB Saunders Co, 1992, 1250, with permission.

Increased T_3 often occurs in hyperthyroidism, but in approximately 5% of cases only T_3 is elevated, "T_3 toxicosis." Do not confuse T_3 with T_3 uptake; these are two different tests. The latter is done very commonly as part of the usual thyroid profile. **Free T_3** may be assayed by an RIA procedure.

Decreased serum T_3 concentrations are reported in individuals with increased serum tumor necrosis factor.[5]

Footnotes

1. Luttrell B and Watters S, "Computerized Method for Validating Laboratory Reference Ranges for Triiodothyronine and Thyroxine Immunoassays," *Clin Chem*, 1991, 37(3):438-42.
2. Bethune JE, "Interpretation of Thyroid Function Tests," *Dis Mon*, 1989, 35(8):541-95.
3. Blank MS and Tucci JR, "A Case of Thyroxine Thyrotoxicosis," *Arch Intern Med*, 1987, 147:863-4.
4. Unger J, "Fasting Induces a Decrease in Serum Thyroglobulin in Normal Subjects," *J Clin Endocrinol Metab*, 1988, 67(6):1309-11.
5. Mooradian AD, Reed RL, Osterweil D, et al, "Decreased Serum Triiodothyronine Is Associated With Increased Concentrations of Tumor Necrosis Factor," *J Clin Endocrinol Metab*, 1990, 71(5):1239-42.

References

Austin D and Toivola B, "Laboratory Evaluation of an Immunochemiluminometric Assay of Triiodothyronine in Serum," *Clin Chem*, 1990, 36(2):334-7.

Camara PD, Velletri K, Krupski M, et al, "Evaluation of the Boehringer Mannheim ES 300 Immunoassay Analyzer and Comparison With Enzyme Immunoassay, Fluorescence Polarization Immunoassay, and Radioimmunoassay Methods," *Clin Biochem*, 1992, 25(4):251-4.

Larsen PR, "The Thyroid," *Cecil Textbook of Medicine*, 19th ed, Vol 2, Wyngarden JB, Smith LH, and Bennett JC, eds, Philadelphia, PA: WB Saunders Co, 1992, 1248-71.

Papanastasiou-Diamandi A, Shankaran P, and Khosravi MJ, "Immunoassay of Triiodothyronine in Serum by Time-Resolved Fluorometric Measurement of Europium-Chelate Complexes in Solution," *Clin Biochem*, 1992, 25(4):255-61.

Price A, Griffiths H, Kennedy L, et al, "Comparison of Methods for the Determination of Unbound Triiodothyronine in Pregnancy," *Clin Endocrinol (Oxf)*, 1992, 37(1):41-4.

Runnels BL, Garry PJ, Hunt WC, et al, "Thyroid Function in a Healthy Elderly Population: Implications for Clinical Evaluation," *J Gerontol*, 1991, 46(1):B39-44.

Surks MI, "Guidelines for Thyroid Testing," *Lab Med*, 1993, 24(5):270-4.

Takamatsu J, Kuma K, and Mozai T, "Serum Triiodothyronine to Thyroxine Ratio: A Newly Recognized Predictor of the Outcome of Hyperthyroidism Due to Graves' Disease," *J Clin Endocrinol Metab*, 1986, 62:980-3.

Watts NB and Keffer JH, *Practical Endocrine Diagnosis*, 4th ed, Philadelphia, PA: Lea & Febiger, 1989.

Triiodothyronine, Total *see* Triiodothyronine *on previous page*

Troponin

CPT *83520*

Related Information

Cardiac Enzymes/Isoenzymes *on page 170*
Creatine Kinase *on page 196*
Creatine Kinase Isoenzymes *on page 197*
Lactate Dehydrogenase *on page 269*
Lactate Dehydrogenase Isoenzymes *on page 271*
Myoglobin, Blood *on page 293*
Myoglobin, Qualitative, Urine *on page 1135*

Applies to Troponin C; Troponin I; Troponin T

Abstract Troponin I and troponin T are very useful in the diagnosis of acute myocardial injury because some of their isoforms show a high degree of cardiac specificity.[1]

Specimen Serum **CONTAINER:** Red top tube **STORAGE INSTRUCTIONS:** Serum stable 4 days at 4°C. **CAUSES FOR REJECTION:** Specimen hemolyzed

Interpretive **REFERENCE RANGE:** Depends on method. Troponin I: <3.1 μg/L (SI: <3.1 μg/L)[2]; troponin T: <0.2 μg/L (SI: <0.2 μg/L)[3] **USE:** Diagnose acute myocardial infarct (AMI) and minor myocardial cell damage from a few hours after onset of symptoms to as long as 120 hours. The sensitivity of troponin T for detecting AMI was 100% 10-190 hours after onset; sensitivity on the seventh day after admission was 84%.[4] In another study, CK-MB was more sensitive during the first 4 hours after onset of chest pain, but thereafter the sensitivities of troponin I and CK-MB were similar up to 48 hours.[2] However, troponin I remains increased longer than CK-MB and is more cardiac specific.[2] **METHODOLOGY:** Enzyme immunoassay (EIA), one-step[5]; double monoclonal sandwich enzyme immunoassay (EIA)[2] **ADDITIONAL INFORMATION:** Troponin T is more sensitive than CK-MB in the diagnosis of unstable angina with myocardial cell damage (30% vs <5%).[6] The contractile proteins of the myofibril include the regulatory protein, troponin. Troponin is a complex of three proteins, troponin C (the calcium-binding subunit, molecular weight 18 kd), troponin I (the actomyosin-adenosine triphosphatase-inhibiting subunit, molecular weight 26.5 kd), and troponin T (the tropomysin-binding subunit, molecular weight 39 kd).[1] The distribution of these isoforms varies between cardiac muscle and slow- and fast-twitch skeletal muscle. Their importance lies in the fact that some isoforms show a high degree of cardiac specificity. An enzyme immunoassay for cardiac troponin T showed a cross reactivity with troponin T extracted from mixed skeletal muscle fibers <2%.[7] The measurement of either troponin I or troponin T will become a very important addition to the clinical assessment of myocardial injury.

Footnotes

1. Apple FS, "Acute Myocardial Infarction and Coronary Reperfusion. Serum Cardiac Markers for the 1990s," *Clin Chem*, 1992, 97(2):217-26.
2. Bodor GS, Porter S, Landt Y, et al, "Development of Monoclonal Antibodies for An Assay of Cardiac Troponin I and Preliminary Results in Suspected Cases of Myocardial Infarction," *Clin Chem*, 1992, 38(11):2203-14.
3. Collinson PO, Moseley D, Stubbs PJ, et al, "Troponin T for the Differential Diagnosis of Ischaemic Myocardial Damage," *Ann Clin Biochem*, 1993, 30(Pt 1):11-6.
4. Mair J, Artner-Dworzak E, Lechleitner P, et al, "Cardiac Troponin T in Diagnosis of Acute Myocardial Infarction," *Clin Chem*, 1991, 37(6):845-52.
5. Katus HA, Looser S, Hallermayer K, et al, "Development and *in vitro* Characterization of A New Immunoassay of Cardiac Troponin T," *Clin Chem*, 1992, 38(3):386-93.
6. Hamm CW, Ravkilde J, Gerhardt W, et al, "The Prognostic Value of Serum Troponin T in Unstable Angina," *N Engl J Med*, 1992, 327(3):146-50.
7. Katus HA, Remppis A, Neumann FJ, et al, "Diagnostic Efficiency of Troponin T Measurements in Acute Myocardial Infarction," *Circulation*, 1991, 83(3):902-12.

References

Anderson PA, Malouf NN, Oakeley AE, et al, "Troponin T Isoform Expression in Humans. A Comparison Among Normal and Failing Adult Heart, Fetal Heart, and Adult and Fetal Skeletal Muscle," *Circ Res*, 1991, 69(5):1226-33.

Cummins B, Russell GJ, Chandler ST, et al, "Uptake of Radioiodinated Cardiac Specific Troponin I Antibodies in Myocardial Infarction," *Cardiovasc Res*, 1990, 24(4):317-27.

Donnelly R and Hillis WS, "Cardiac Troponin T," *Lancet*, 1993, 341(8842):410-1.

Gerhardt W, Katus H, Ravkilde J, et al, "S-Troponin T in Suspected Ischemic Myocardial Injury Compared With Mass and Catalytic Concentrations of S-Creatine Kinase Isoenzyme MB," *Clin Chem*, 1991, 37(8):1405-11.

Parmacek MS and Leiden JM, "Structure, Function, and Regulation of Troponin C," *Circulation*, 1991, 84(3):991-1003.

"Troponin T and Myocardial Damage," *Lancet*, 1991, 338(8758):23-4, (editorial).

(Continued)

Troponin *(Continued)*

Zabel M, Koster W, and Hohnloser SH, "Usefulness of CKMB and Troponin T Determinations in Patients With Acute Myocardial Infarction Complicated by Ventricular Fibrillation," *Clin Cardiol*, 1993, 16(1):23-5.

Troponin C *see* Troponin *on previous page*

Troponin I *see* Troponin *on previous page*

Troponin T *see* Troponin *on previous page*

True Cholinesterase *see* Acetylcholinesterase, Red Blood Cell *on page 95*

Trypsin, Immunoreactive *see* Amylase, Urine *on page 129*

TSH *see* Thyroid Stimulating Hormone *on page 361*

TSH, Filter Paper *see* Thyroid Stimulating Hormone Screen, Filter Paper *on page 363*

Tubeless Gastric Analysis *replaced by* Gastric Analysis *on page 232*

Tumor Detection *see* Human Chorionic Gonadotropin, Serum *on page 254*

UDP Galactose-4-Epimerase Deficiency *see* Galactose-1-Phosphate Uridyl Transferase, Erythrocyte *on page 227*

U-I-S *see* Uroporphyrinogen-I-Synthase *on page 381*

Ultrasensitive TSH *see* Thyroid Stimulating Hormone *on page 361*

Unbound T_4 *see* Thyroxine, Free *on page 368*

Unconjugated Estriol, Pregnancy *see* Estriol, Unconjugated, Pregnancy, Blood or Urine *on page 217*

U/P Ratio *see* Osmolality, Urine *on page 302*

Urate *see* Uric Acid, Serum *on page 378*

Urate, Urine *see* Uric Acid, Urine *on page 380*

Urea Clearance *replaced by* Creatinine Clearance *on page 201*

Urea Nitrogen, Blood

CPT *84520*

Related Information

BUN/Creatinine Ratio *on page 151*
Creatinine, Serum *on page 202*
Kidney Biopsy *on page 68*
Kidney Stone Analysis *on page 1129*
Sodium, Blood *on page 349*

Synonyms Blood Urea Nitrogen; BUN

Abstract Urea nitrogen reflects the ratio between urea **production** and **clearance**. Increased BUN may be due to increased production or decreased excretion. Although we commonly use the expression "BUN," most laboratories use serum, occasionally plasma but never whole blood.

Specimen Serum, plasma **CONTAINER:** Red top tube. Avoid fluoride and sodium citrate tubes if urease reaction is used and ammonium heparin tubes when conductimetric method is used. EDTA is suitable as well as lithium heparin for young children. **COLLECTION:** Pediatric: Blood drawn from heelstick for capillary (lithium heparin tube) **STORAGE INSTRUCTIONS:** Stable 1 day at room temperature, 3 days at 4°C to 8°C, and 3 months at -20°C.[1]

Interpretive **REFERENCE RANGE:** Birth to 1 year: 4-16 mg/dL (SI: 1.4-5.7 mmol/L); 1-40 years: 5-20 mg/dL (SI: 1.8-7.1 mmol/L); gradual slight increase subsequently occurs over 40 years of age. **POSSIBLE PANIC RANGE:** BUN >100 mg/dL (SI: >35.7 mmol/L) has been used in the definition of uremia.[2] **USE:** **High BUN** occurs in chronic glomerulonephritis, pyelonephritis, and other causes of chronic renal disease; with acute renal failure, decreased renal perfusion (prerenal azotemia) as in shock. With urinary tract obstruction BUN increases (postrenal azotemia), for example as caused by neoplastic infiltration of the ureters, hyperplasia, or carcinoma of the prostate. BUN is useful to follow hemodialysis and other therapy. "Uremia" was defined by Luke as an expression of a constellation of signs and symptoms in patients with severe azotemia secondary to acute or chronic renal failure.[2] Causes of increased BUN include severe congestive heart failure, increased protein catabolism, tetracyclines with diuretic use, hyperalimentation, ketoacidosis, and dehydration as in diabetes mellitus, but even moderate dehydration can cause BUN to increase. Corticosteroids tend to increase BUN by causing increased protein catabolism. Bleeding from the gastrointestinal tract is an important cause of high urea nitrogen, commonly accompanied by elevation of BUN/creatinine ratio. Nephrotoxic drugs must be considered.

Borderline high values may occur after recent ingestion of high protein meal and muscle wasting may cause an elevation as well.

With creatinine, BUN is used to monitor patients on dialysis.

Low BUN occurs in late normal pregnancy, decreased protein intake, with intravenous fluids, with some antibiotics, and in severe liver damage.

As described by DeCaux et al in 1980, in the syndrome of inappropriate secretion of antidiuretic hormone (SIADH), findings include hyponatremia with serum or plasma Na^+ $\leq$128 mmol/L, serum hypo-osmolality, <260 mOsm/kg, with urine osmolality >300 mOsm/kg (SI: >300 mmol/kg) with low BUN. Such findings occur in situations in which patients are overhydrated. Clinical findings included absence of edema or evidence of heart, liver, thyroid, renal or adrenal disease.[3] Hypouricemia, with uric acid levels in 16 of 17 patients <4 mg/dL (SI: <238 μmol/L), is reported with the syndrome of inappropriate secretion of antidiuretic hormone.[4] (SIADH can be seen with higher serum sodiums and higher osmolalities. Urine osmolality is greater than serum osmolality in SIADH. DeCaux in 1982 presented criteria modified from the 1980 paper.[5])

Osmolality (mOsm/kg H_2O) may be calculated as follows: Osmolality = [Na^+ (mmol/L) x 2] + urea N (mg/dL)/2.8 + glucose (mg/dL)/18.

LIMITATIONS: Uremia is best evaluated with creatinine as well as urea nitrogen. In both prerenal and postrenal azotemia, for instance, BUN is apt to be increased somewhat more than is creatinine. However, in a series of dehydrated children with gastroenteritis who had metabolic acidosis and increased anion gap, 88% had BUN concentration $\leq$18 mg/dL (SI: $\leq$6.4 mmol/L). The authors found bicarbonate and anion gap more sensitive indices in this setting.[6] In chronic progressive renal disease, about 75% of renal parenchyma must be damaged or destroyed before azotemia develops. BUN lacks sensitivity and specificity, but still remains a useful test. **METHODOLOGY:** Diacetyl monoxime; urease, Berthelot reaction; rate conductivity **ADDITIONAL INFORMATION:** Although creatinine is generally considered a more specific test to evaluate renal function, they are commonly used together. Luke points out that clinical renal failure is variable between individual patients.[2] Drug effects have been summarized.[7]

Footnotes

1. Rock RC, Walker WG, and Jennings CD, "Nitrogen Metabolites and Renal Function," *Textbook of Clinical Chemistry*, Tietz NW, ed, Philadelphia, PA: WB Saunders Co, 1986, 1254-1316.
2. Luke RG, "Uremia and the BUN," *N Engl J Med*, 1981, 305:1213-5, (editorial).
3. DeCaux G, Genette F, and Mockel J, "Hypouremia in the Syndrome of Inappropriate Secretion of Antidiuretic Hormone," *Ann Intern Med*, 1980, 93:716-7.
4. Beck LH, "Hypouricemia in the Syndrome of Inappropriate Secretion of Antidiuretic Hormone," *N Engl J Med*, 1979, 301:528-30.
5. DeCaux G, Unger J, Brimioulle S, et al, "Hyponatremia in the Syndrome of Inappropriate Secretion of Antidiuretic Hormone. Rapid Correction With Urea, Sodium Chloride, and Water Restriction Therapy," *JAMA*, 1982, 247:471-4.
6. Bonadio WA, Hennes HH, Machi J, et al, "Efficacy of Measuring BUN in Assessing Children With Dehydration Due to Gastroenteritis," *Ann Emerg Med*, 1989, 18(7):755-7.
7. Artur Y and Galimany R, "Urea," *Drug Effects on Laboratory Test Results Analytical Interferences and Pharmacological Effects*, Siest G and Galteau MM, eds, Littleton, MA: PSG Publishing Co Inc, 1988, 439-53.

References

Abuelo JG, "Benign Azotemia of Long-Term Hemodialysis: Increase in Blood Urea Nitrogen and Serum Creatinine Concentrations After the Initiation of Dialysis," *Am J Med*, 1989, 86(6 Pt 1):738-9.

Bidani A and Churchill PC, "Acute Renal Failure," *Dis Mon*, 1989, 35(2):57-132.

Comtois R, Bertrand S, Beauregard H, et al, "Low Serum Urea Level in Dehydrated Patients With Central Diabetes Insipidus," *Can Med Assoc J*, 1988, 139:965-8.

Urea Nitrogen Clearance *replaced by* Creatinine Clearance *on page 201*

Uric Acid, Serum

CPT 84550 (chemical); 84555 (uricase)

Related Information

Alcohol, Blood or Urine *on page 936*
Complete Blood Count *on page 533*
Creatinine, Serum *on page 202*
Kidney Stone Analysis *on page 1129*
Lead, Blood *on page 976*
pH, Blood *on page 315*
Sodium, Blood *on page 349*
Sputum Cytology *on page 510*
Uric Acid, Urine *on page 380*

Synonyms Urate

Abstract Uric acid, the end product of purine metabolism, is increased in a variety of clinicopathologic entities in addition to gout.

Patient Care PREPARATION: Ideally, patient should be fasting. Diurnal variations occur. Uric acid concentration is usually higher in the morning and lower in the evening.

Specimen Serum CONTAINER: Red top tube COLLECTION: Separate serum. Do not collect in lavender top (EDTA) tube or gray top (sodium fluoride) tube for urease method. STORAGE INSTRUCTIONS: Urate is stable in serum for 3 days at 25°C, 3-7 days at 4°C, and 6-12 months at -20°C.[1]

Interpretive REFERENCE RANGE: An increase occurs during childhood. Adults: male: 3.4-7.0 mg/dL (SI: 202-416 μmol/L), female: 2.4-6.0 mg/dL (SI: 143-357 μmol/L). Values >7.0 mg/dL (SI: >416 μmol/L) are sometimes arbitrarily regarded as hyperuricemia, but there is no sharp line between normals on the one hand, and the serum uric acid of those with clinical gout. Normal ranges cannot be adjusted for purine ingestion, but high purine diet increases uric acid. Uric acid may be increased with body size, exercise, and stress.[2] POSSIBLE PANIC RANGE: "Severe hyperuricemia" has been classified as uric acid >12 mg/dL (SI: >714 μmol/L) USE: An increased uric acid level does not necessarily translate to a diagnosis of gout; about 10% to 15% of instances of hyperuricemia are caused by gout.[2] The overlap between uric acid levels in those with and without gout is shown in a study in which the lowest level in a gouty subject was 6 mg/dL (SI: 357 μmol/L), while the highest uric acid in a nongouty person was 9.5 mg/dL (SI: 565 μmol/L).[3]

Elevations of uric acid occur in renal diseases with renal failure[4] and prerenal azotemia (eg, dehydration) as well as gout. Other drugs causing increased uric acid concentration include diuretics,[4] pyrazinamide, ethambutol, nicotinic acid, and aspirin in low doses.

Excessive cell destruction: neoplasia, even before as well as following chemotherapy and radiation therapy, especially lymphoma and leukemia; hemolytic anemia, resolving pneumonia and other inflammation; polycythemia, myeloma, pernicious anemia, infectious mononucleosis, congestive heart failure, large myocardial infarct.

Endocrine: hypothyroidism, hypoparathyroidism, hyperparathyroidism, pseudohypoparathyroidism; diabetes insipidus of nephrogenic type, Addison's disease.

Lead poisoning (saturnine gout) from paint, batteries, and moonshine. A causal relationship between plumbism and gout was recognized before 1876. Gout as a common complication of subclinical lead poisoning is described among the Roman aristocracy.[5]

Acidosis: lactic acidosis, diabetic ketoacidosis, recent alcohol ingestion, alcoholic ketosis. Shock and hypoxia relate to hyperuricemia. Attention has been directed at the cause of hyperuricemia in the intensive care unit; severely increased uric acid levels in acutely ill patients is explained by degradation of ATP with degradation of accumulated nucleotides to purine metabolites, uric acid among them. Such ATP degradation may occur with strenuous exercise and the adult respiratory distress syndrome. With metabolism of ethanol to acetyl CoA, the degradation of ATP explains the hyperuricemia of alcohol use. Hyperuricemia becomes then a marker for cell injury crisis.[6]

Toxemia of pregnancy, diet, weight loss, fasting, or starvation. Decreased urate clearance: cyclosporine-induced hyperuricemia.[7]

Triglyceride increase bears an association with hyperuricemia, as do diabetes mellitus and obesity. Hyperuricemia bears an association with obesity, hypertension and statistical association with myocardial infarct.

Hereditary gout: Lesch-Nyhan (X-linked) with deficiency of hypoxanthine-guanine phosphoribosyltransferase. Gout with partial absence HPRT. Increased 5-phosphoribosyl-1-pyrophosphate synthetase. Glycogen storage disease type I.[6]

Only a minority of individuals with hyperuricemia develop gout.

Three types of kidney disease are caused by precipitation: acute uric acid nephropathy, nephrolithiasis, and chronic urate nephropathy.[8]

Hyperuricemia in early essential hypertension correlates with renal vascular resistance and inversely with renal blood flow. Increased serum uric acid may indicate renal involvement.[9,10]

Low uric acid: Drugs: Drugs apparently bearing a relationship to low serum uric acid levels included aspirin (high doses), x-ray contrast agents, glyceryl guaiacolate or allopurinol. Corticosteroids and probenecid cause low uric. Massive doses of vitamin C are uricosuric.

Poor dietary intake of purines and protein; tea, coffee.

Renal tubular defects, Fanconi syndrome, late in Wilson's disease, outdated tetracycline, cystinosis, galactosemia, heavy metal poisoning, malignant neoplasms, hypereosinophilic syndrome.

Xanthinuria (deficiency of xanthine oxidase).

Hypouricemia is reported with acute intermittent porphyria, severe liver disease (especially obstructive biliary disease), and as an isolated defect in the tubular transport of uric acid.

With increased renal clearance of urate, hypercalciuria, and decreased bone density, diabetes,[11] and in SIADH.

With hyponatremia, serum hypo-osmolarity: Beck has described low uric acid with the syndrome of inappropriate secretion of antidiuretic hormone (SIADH): 16 of 17 patients with this syndrome were hypouricemic, with serum urate $\leq$4.0 mg/dL (SI: $\leq$238 μmol/L). All 13 patients with other causes of hyponatremia had serum urate $\geq$5.0 mg/dL (SI: $\geq$297 μmol/L).[12] Volume expansion, as with SIADH, causes decreased uric acid. The combination of low uric and low Na^+ may also be found in instances of liver disease and was anticipated with ticrynafen.

Azlocillin is reported to cause decrease of serum uric acid levels.[13] Drug effects on uric acid metabolism are published in tabular form.[14,15]

Idiopathic hypouricemia commonly is transient. Familial hypouricemia has been described.

LIMITATIONS: Positive interferences may be caused by ascorbic acid, caffeine, and theophylline. **METHODOLOGY:** Phosphotungstate, uricase, high performance liquid chromatography (HPLC) **ADDITIONAL INFORMATION:** Drug effects have been summarized.[16]

Footnotes

1. Tammes AR, "Uric Acid," *Quality Assurance Service*, CAP Computer Center, 1986.
2. Rock RC, Walker WG, and Jennings CD, "Nitrogen Metabolites and Renal Function," *Textbook of Clinical Chemistry*, Tietz NW, ed, Philadelphia, PA: WB Saunders Co, 1986, 1254-1316.
3. Seegmiller JE, Laster L, and Howell RR, "Biochemistry of Uric Acid and Its Relation to Gout," *N Engl J Med*, 1983, 268:712-6.
4. Langford HG, Blaufox MD, Borhani NO, et al, "Is Thiazide-Produced Uric Acid Elevation Harmful?" *Arch Intern Med*, 1987, 147:645-9.
5. Nriagu JO, "Saturnine Gout Among Roman Aristocrats," *N Engl J Med*, 1983, 308:660-3.
6. Fox IH, Palella TD, and Kelley WN, "Hyperuricemia: A Marker for Cell Energy Crisis," *N Engl J Med*, 1987, 317:111-2, (editorial).
7. Lin HY, Rocher LL, McQuillan MA, et al, "Cyclosporine-Induced Hyperuricemia and Gout," *N Engl J Med*, 1989, 321(5):287-92.
8. Dykman D and Simon EE, "Hyperuricemia and Uric Acid Nephropathy," *Arch Intern Med*, 1987, 147:1341-5.
9. Larson AW and Strong CG, "Initial Assessment of the Patient With Hypertension," *Mayo Clin Proc*, 1989, 64(12):1533-42.
10. Nunez BD, Frohlich ED, Garavaglia GE, et al, "Serum Uric Acid in Renovascular Hypertension: Reduction Following Surgical Correction," *Am J Med Sci*, 1987, 294:419-22.
11. Shichiri M, Iwamoto H, and Shiigai T, "Diabetic Renal Hypouricemia," *Arch Intern Med*, 1987, 147:225-8.
12. Beck LH, "Hypouricemia in the Syndrome of Inappropriate Secretion of Antidiuretic Hormone," *N Engl J Med*, 1979, 301:528-30.
13. Ernst JA and Sy ER, "Effect of Azlocillin on Uric Acid Levels in Serum," *Antimicrob Agents Chemother*, 1983, 24:609-10.
14. German DC and Holmes EW, "Gout and Hyperuricemia: Diagnosis and Management," *Hosp Pract [Off]*, 1986, 21:119-26, 131-2.
15. German DC and Holmes EW, "Hyperuricemia and Gout," *Med Clin North Am*, 1986, 70:419-36, (review).

(Continued)

Uric Acid, Serum *(Continued)*

16. Zhiri A and Jouanel P, "Urates," *Drug Effects on Laboratory Test Results Analytical Interferences and Pharmacological Effects*, Siest G and Galteau MM, eds, Littleton, MA: PSG Publishing Co Inc, 1988, 423-38.

References

Conger JD, "Acute Uric Acid Nephropathy," *Med Clin North Am*, 1990, 74(4):859-71.

Devgun MS and Dhillon HS, "Importance of Diurnal Variations on Clinical Value and Interpretation of Serum Urate Measurements," *J Clin Pathol*, 1992, 45(2):110-3.

Fievet P, Pleskov L, Desailly I, et al, "Plasma Renin Activity, Blood Uric Acid, and Plasma Volume in Pregnancy-Induced Hypertension," *Nephron*, 1985, 40:429-32.

Gores PF, Fryd DS, Sutherland DER, et al, "Hyperuricemia after Renal Transplantation," *Am J Surg*, 1988, 156:397-400.

Mejías E, Navas J, Lluberes R, et al, "Hyperuricemia, Gout, and Autosomal Dominant Polycystic Kidney Disease," *Am J Med Sci*, 1989, 297(3):145-8.

Menon RK, Mikhailidis DP, Bell JL, et al, "Warfarin Administration Increases Uric Acid Concentrations in Plasma," *Clin Chem*, 1986, 32:1557-9.

O'Connor JP and Emmerson BT, "The Treatment of Hyperuricaemia and Gout," *Aust Fam Physician*, 1985, 14:193-8.

Uric Acid, Urine

***CPT** 84560*

Related Information

Calcium, Urine *on page 163*
Creatinine, 12- or 24-Hour Urine *on page 200*
Kidney Stone Analysis *on page 1129*
Lead, Urine *on page 977*
Uric Acid, Serum *on page 378*

Synonyms Urate, Urine

Abstract Uric acid concentration is the product of *de novo* synthesis and dietary sources. Seventy-five percent of urate is eliminated through the kidney and 25% through the intestine. Renal excretion of urate involves reabsorption by the proximal tubules, secretion by the distal portion of the proximal tubules, and further reabsorption by the distal tubules.[1]

Patient Care PREPARATION: Twenty-four hour uric acid excretion is most often measured in patients with nephrolithiasis, in whom it is desirable to know the excretion of uric acid and other substances while the patient is on a **usual** diet. A number of drugs affect uric acid excretion including aspirin, other anti-inflammatory preparations, x-ray contrast agents, vitamin C, and warfarin. Diuretics decrease uric acid excretion.

Specimen 24-hour urine CONTAINER: To prevent precipitation in acid urine, add 10 mL of sodium hydroxide solution (12.5M) to specimen container prior to collection. COLLECTION: Instruct the patient to void at 8 AM and discard the specimen. Then collect all urine including the final specimen voided at the end of the 24-hour collection period (ie, 8 AM the next morning). Container must be labeled with patient's name, date and time collection started and finished. STORAGE INSTRUCTIONS: Do not refrigerate. Stable about 3 days.

Interpretive REFERENCE RANGE: Approximately 250-750 mg/24 hours (SI: 1.5-4.5 mmol/day) for women. Range for men may extend to 800 mg/24 hours (SI: 4.8 mmol/day). Increases on purine-rich diet. USE: Hyperuricosuria is associated with renal calculus formation. Identify overexcretors to determine risk of stone formation; identify genetic defects, influence of overexcretion on therapy of gout. Uric acid nephrolithiasis occurs in primary gout or in secondary hyperuricemia (eg, malignant diseases). Uric acid nephrolithiasis may complicate ulcerative colitis, Crohn's disease, and surgical jejunoileal bypass. Most subjects with uric acid stones do not have gout. Evaluate uric acid metabolism in gout. METHODOLOGY: Phosphotungstate, uricase, high performance liquid chromatography (HPLC) ADDITIONAL INFORMATION: Even mild renal failure decreases uric acid excretion. Uric acid excretion is decreased with hypertension.

A young patient with acute gouty arthritis, uric acid stones, and any patient who excretes >1000 mg uric acid/24 hours (SI: >5.9 mmol/day), should be screened for hypoxanthine-quanine phosphoribosyl-transferase (HPRT) deficiency.[2] The uric acid/creatinine ratio has been used as a screen for Lesch-Nyhan syndrome (HPRTase deficiency). Normal control patients 0.21-0.59; partial enzyme deficient group 0.62-2.00; complete enzyme deficiency 1.98-5.35.[3]

The ratio of uric acid to creatinine in morning samples of urine has been used as a screening test for detection of the Lesch-Nyhan syndrome, which is associated with virtually complete absence of activity of the enzyme hypoxanthine-guanine phosphoribosyltransferase. This ratio has also been applied to 24-hour urine samples from adult patients with gout for detection of partial deficiency of the same enzyme. Patients with gout exhibit uric acid:creatinine ratios of 0.15-0.73, whereas those patients with hyperuricemia associated with another disorder such as leukemia or glycogen storage disease have ratios of 0.25-1.77. The ratio is 0.27-0.58 for patients with nongouty arthritis. Patients with complete hypoxanthine-guanine phosphoribosyltransferase deficiency are reported to have urinary uric acid-to-creatinine ratios of 1.98-5.35, as compared to 0.62-2.00 for patients with gout accompanied by partial enzyme deficiency.

The ratio of uric acid to creatinine concentration on a random urine specimen has also been shown to be >1.0 in patients with acute renal failure secondary to acute uric acid nephropathy, but <1.0 in patients with acute renal failure resulting from other causes.

Footnotes

1. Bhagavan NV, Caraway WT, Conn RB, et al, *Textbook of Clinical Chemistry*, Tietz NW, ed, Philadelphia, PA: WB Saunders Co, 1986, 1283.
2. Wilson JM, Young AB, and Kelley WN, "Hypoxanthine-Guanine Phosphoribosyltransferase Deficiency. The Molecular Basis of the Clinical Syndromes," *N Engl J Med*, 1983, 309:900-10.
3. Pesce AJ and Kaplan LA, *Methods in Clinical Chemistry*, St Louis, MO: Mosby-Year Book Inc, 1987, 32.

References

Dykman D, Simon EE, and Avioli LV, "Hyperuricemia and Uric Acid Nephropathy," *Arch Intern Med*, 1987, 147:1341-5.

Schultz AL, "Uric Acid," *Clinical Chemistry – Theory, Analysis, and Correlation*, 2nd ed, Kaplan LA and Pesce AJ, eds, St Louis, MO: Mosby-Year Book Inc, 1989, 1024-8.

Urinary Anion Gap *see* Anion Gap *on page 132*

Urinary Free Cortisol *see* Cortisol, Urine *on page 193*

Urine 17-Ketogenic Steroids *replaced by* 17-Hydroxyprogesterone, Blood or Amniotic Fluid *on page 258*

Urine Cl *see* Chloride, Urine *on page 184*

Urine Cortisol *see* Cortisol, Urine *on page 193*

Urine Creatinine *see* Creatinine, 12- or 24-Hour Urine *on page 200*

Urine Electrolytes *see* Electrolytes, Urine *on page 213*

Urine K^+ *see* Potassium, Urine *on page 332*

Urine Na *see* Sodium, Urine *on page 351*

Urine Osmolality *see* Osmolality, Urine *on page 302*

Urine Oxalate *see* Oxalate, Urine *on page 303*

Urine Phosphorus *see* Phosphorus, Urine *on page 322*

Urine Pregnanetriol Assay *replaced by* 17-Hydroxyprogesterone, Blood or Amniotic Fluid *on page 258*

Uroporphyrinogen-Cosynthetase *see* Uroporphyrinogen-I-Synthase *on this page*

Uroporphyrinogen-I-Synthase

CPT 84999

Related Information

Porphobilinogen, Qualitative, Urine *on page 325*
Porphyrins, Quantitative, Urine *on page 327*

Synonyms Erythrocyte Porphobilinogen Deaminase; Erythrocyte Uroporphyrinogen-I-Synthase; U-I-S; Uroporphyrinogen-Cosynthetase

Applies to Porphobilinogen; Porphobilinogen Deaminase Red Blood Cell

Abstract The enzymatic defect of acute intermittent porphyria (AIP) is a deficiency of U-I-S in erythrocytes and other cells.[1]

Patient Care PREPARATION: Patient should fast for 12-14 hours, abstain from alcohol for 24 hours, and be off medications for 1 week ideally.

Specimen Whole blood (done on erythrocytes) CONTAINER: Green top (heparin) tube, lavender top (EDTA) tube STORAGE INSTRUCTIONS: If test can be done promptly, a red cell hemolysate (Continued)

Uroporphyrinogen-I-Synthase *(Continued)*

is prepared directly from whole blood. The whole blood sample can be stored for 1 week at 4°C. If there will be a delay of over a week, centrifuge heparinized specimen. After plasma and buffy layer are removed, wash red cells three times with cold isotonic saline. Pack by centrifugation. Freeze in dry ice-acetone.[1] Store at -20°C. There is loss of activity at 4°C, more at room temperature as red cells age. The test is done on a red cell hemolysate. **SPECIAL INSTRUCTIONS:** Hemoglobin and reticulocyte count should also be ordered.

Interpretive **REFERENCE RANGE:** 1.27-2.01 mU/g hemoglobin (SI: 81.9-129.6 U/mol Hgb). Varies among methods and among laboratories. Patients with acute intermittent porphyria have levels about half normal. Hemoglobin determination is done on the hemolysate for calculation of activity on a per gram of hemoglobin basis. **USE:** Evaluate subjects with episodes of abdominal pain, especially when such episodes are recurrent, and with tachycardia. U-I-S is low in the latent or carrier state of acute intermittent porphyria, normal in the other hereditary porphyrias. It is thought to provide support in the differential diagnosis of acute intermittent porphyria from other porphyrias.[1] **LIMITATIONS:** A small overlap with normals exists. Repeat assay at a later time is indicated to confirm carrier status. Qualitative and quantitative urinary porphobilinogen and family studies are also useful. Indeterminate or normal values for this enzyme may occur in some patients with acute intermittent porphyria. Red cell U-I-S activity varies with cell age. Younger red cells (newborn subjects) or other settings in which younger red cells are found, with reticulocytosis $\geq$5%, may lead to increased activity of this assay, which therefore may be high in various anemias, and may also mask the diagnosis of acute intermittent porphyria. **METHODOLOGY:** Fluorometric assay **ADDITIONAL INFORMATION:** This is the enzyme which converts porphobilinogen to uroporphyrinogen I. U-I-S is one of two methods of detection of asymptomatic carriers of acute intermittent porphyria. The other is quantitation of urine porphobilinogen. Both are recommended. U-I-S is normal or increased with lead poisoning, because of anemia in plumbism.[2] In acute intermittent porphyria excessive excretion of porphobilinogen and delta aminolevulinic acid occurs during acute attacks, but excretion may be normal between them. Red blood cell porphobilinogen deaminase activity, measured by a spectrofluorometric assay on erythrocytes, defines most patients with acute intermittent porphyria, while 55 of 56 subjects with other porphyrias were reported as having normal activity. This assay identified a number of latent carriers but not all patients with assumed acute intermittent porphyria.[3]

Footnotes

1. Forman DT, "Erythrocyte Uroporphyrinogen I Synthase Activity as an Indicator of Acute Porphyria," *Ann Clin Lab Sci*, 1989, 19(2):128-32.
2. Bird TD, Wallace DM, and Labbe RF, "The Porphyria, Plumbism, Pottery Puzzle," *JAMA*, 1982, 247:813-4.
3. Pierach CA, Weimer MK, Cardinal RA, et al, "Red Blood Cell Porphobilinogen Deaminase in the Evaluation of Acute Intermittent Porphyria," *JAMA*, 1987, 257:60-1.

References

Labbe RF and Lamon JW, "Porphyrins and Disorders of Porphyrin Metabolism," *Fundamentals of Clinical Chemistry*, 3rd ed, Tietz NW, ed, New York, NY: WB Saunders Co, 1987, 825-41.

Uroporphyrins *see* Porphyrins, Quantitative, Urine *on page 327*

Vanillylmandelic Acid, Urine

***CPT** 84585*

Related Information

Catecholamines, Fractionation, Plasma *on page 172*
Catecholamines, Fractionation, Urine *on page 174*
Homovanillic Acid, Urine *on page 253*
Metanephrines, Total, Urine *on page 289*

Synonyms 3-Methoxy-4-Hydroxymandelic Acid; VMA

Abstract Vanillylmandelic acid is a major metabolite of both epinephrine and norepinephrine, the result of the actions of both carboxy-o-methyl transferase and monoamine oxidase. As such it is significantly elevated in conditions with overproduction of catecholamines, notably pheochromocytoma. VMA, metanephrines and catecholamine assays are all useful screens for pheochromocytoma.

Patient Care **PREPARATION:** Interfering substances relate to methodology. Drug and diet recommendations from the laboratory used are desirable. Many laboratories restrict foods, such as coffee, tea, bananas, and other foods. Some ask for no drug use (except for digitalis) for

2 weeks before the test. Aspirin, pyridoxine, levodopa, amoxicillin, carbidopa, reserpine, and disulfiram commonly interfere. Monoamine oxidase inhibitors decrease VMA excretion. See Limitations.

Specimen 24-hour urine **CONTAINER:** Plastic container with hydrochloric or acetic acid preservative added before collection, according to the protocol of the laboratory which will perform the test. Adjust to pH 2-4 after collection, according to procedures of the laboratory doing the analysis. **COLLECTION:** Patient should be at rest during the collection, if possible taking no medication and without recent exposure to radiographic materials. **STORAGE INSTRUCTIONS:** Refrigerate. Stable up to 2 weeks. **CAUSES FOR REJECTION:** Preservative not added to container before collection **SPECIAL INSTRUCTIONS:** For neuroblastoma, both HVA (homovanillic acid) and VMA should be collected. Metanephrines are recommended as a first test for pheochromocytoma.[1]

Interpretive **REFERENCE RANGE:** Adult normal range is usually up to approximately 7-9 mg/24 hours (SI: 35-45 μmol/day). See table. **USE:** Diagnose pheochromocytoma; evaluate hypertension; diagnose and follow up neuroblastoma, ganglioneuroma, and ganglioneuroblastoma. Most neuroblastoma patients excrete excess HVA in 24-hour collections. If VMA and HVA are both used in work-up, up to 80% of all cases will be detected. **LIMITATIONS:** MAO inhibitors may produce false low value; coffee, vanilla, and chocolate should be omitted before testing; VMA in a random specimen may yield a false-negative; 24-hour collections are preferred.[2,3] Some neuroblastoma patients are positive for urinary homovanillic acid abnormality but do not excrete increased VMA.[4] Twenty percent to 32% of patients with neuroblastoma do **not** have elevation of VMA. Many will have other laboratory abnormalities such as increased metanephrines, homovanillic acid (HVA), or dopamine. **METHODOLOGY:** High performance liquid chromatography (HPLC), spectrophotometric following extraction **ADDITIONAL INFORMATION:** Virtually all pheochromocytomas (95%) may be diagnosed using VMA, metanephrine, and fractionated catecholamines in a 24-hour urine specimen. Creatinine is measured concomitantly to ensure adequate collection and to calculate the excretion ratio of VMA/creatinine and metanephrine/creatinine (see table). Ninety-five percent of patients with neuroblastoma have an increase in VMA or HVA, or both. Interpretation of all results should be tempered by knowledge of influences causing false-negatives and false-positives (eg, stress, drugs, compounds that interfere with the assays).[1]

Vanillylmandelic Acid, Urine

For 24–hour collection	mg/24 h	SI: μmol/d
0–1 y	Up to 1.8	Up to 9
1–4 y	Up to 3	Up to 15
4–15 y	Up to 4	Up to 20
15 y – adults	7–9	35–45
For 24– or 12–hour collection	**μg/mg of creatinine**	
<1 y	15–27	
1–5 y	11–13	
6–15 y	Up to 7	
15 y – adults	Up to 4.5	
Adults	Up to 7	
For 24–hour collection	**μg/g of body weight/24 h**	
<1 mo	Up to 180	
1 mo – 2 y	Up to 230	
>2 y	Up to 150	

Footnotes

1. Sheps SG, Jiang N-S, Klee GG, et al, "Recent Developments in the Diagnosis and Treatment of Pheochromocytoma," *Mayo Clin Proc*, 1990, 65(1):88-95.
2. Grumbach MM, "The Endocrine System," *Pediatrics*, 18th ed, Rudolph AM and Hoffman JIE, and Axelrod S, eds, Norwalk, CT: Appleton & Lange, 1987, 1447-57.
3. Bakken CL, "Mayo Medical Laboratories Test Catalog," Rochester, MN: Mayo Medical Laboratories, 1990.
4. Rothstein A, "Determination of Urinary Homovanillic Acid Using the Nitrosonaphthol Reaction," *Am J Clin Pathol*, 1987, 87:644-8.

References

Hanai J, Kawai T, Sato Y, et al, "Simple Liquid-Chromatographic Measurement of Vanillylmandelic Acid and Homovanillic Acid in Urine on Filter Paper for Mass Screening of Neuroblastoma in Infants," *Clin Chem*, 1987, 33:2043-6.

Knight JA and Wu JT, "Catecholamines and Their Metabolites: Clinical and Laboratory Aspects," *Lab Med*, 1987, 18:153-8.

(Continued)

Vanillylmandelic Acid, Urine *(Continued)*

Landsberg L and Young JB, "Catecholamines and the Adrenal Medulla," *Williams Textbook of Endocrinology*, 8th ed, Wilson JD and Foster DW, eds, Philadelphia, PA: WB Saunders Co, 1992, 621-705.

Meites S, *Pediatric Clinical Chemistry: Reference (Normal) Values*, 3rd ed, Washington, DC: American Association of Clinical Chemistry Press, 1989.

Melmon KL, "The Endocrinologic Function of Selected Antacoids: Catecholamines, Acetylcholine, Serotonin, and Histamine," *Williams Textbook of Endocrinology*, 8th ed, Wilson JD and Foster DW, eds, Philadelphia, PA: WB Saunders Co, 1992.

Scully RE, Mark EJ, and McNeely BU, "Weekly Clinicopathological Exercises," *Case Records of the Massachusetts General Hospital*, 1986, 314:431-9.

Tuchman M, Auray-Blais C, Ramnaraine ML, et al, "Determination of Urinary Homovanillic Acid and Vanillylmandelic Acids From Dried Filter Paper Samples: Assessment of Potential Methods for Neuroblastoma Screening," *Clin Biochem*, 1987, 20:173-7.

Vasoactive Intestinal Polypeptide

***CPT** 83519; 83520*

Related Information

Glucagon, Plasma *on page 236*

Synonyms VIP

Applies to Glucagon; Secretin

Abstract VIP is a 28 amino acid polypeptide produced by neuroendocrine cells in the gut and elsewhere. It has apparent paracrine activity on the gut, which relates to and is thought to be the major mediator of the symptoms of WDHA (watery diarrhea hypokalemia achlorhydria) syndrome or WDHH (watery diarrhea hypokalemia hypochlorhydria). The major entity which causes high VIP is a group of neural crest neoplasms (VIPomas). VIP mediates water transport, stimulates chloride secretion, and inhibits sodium absorption in the intestines.

Patient Care **PREPARATION:** Patient must be fasting for 10-12 hours. The fast must be complete (ie, not even water may be taken). No antacids for 24 hours prior to collection. All medications should be discontinued for 24-48 hours prior to collection.

Specimen Plasma **SAMPLING TIME:** 6 AM to 8 AM **COLLECTION:** Collect specimen in lavender top (EDTA) tube and transfer to red top tube containing 500 μL of 10,000 KIU/mL Trasylol®. **STORAGE INSTRUCTIONS:** Mix, centrifuge, and pour off plasma into transport tube supplied by reference laboratory. Transport frozen on dry ice. **CAUSES FOR REJECTION:** Recent administration of radioactive isotope

Interpretive **REFERENCE RANGE:** <76 ng/L.[1] Levels vary considerably between laboratories. **USE:** Hypersecretion of VIP is observed in "pancreatic cholera syndrome," also called Verner-Morrison syndrome, the watery diarrhea hypokalemia achlorhydria (WDHA) syndrome, or watery diarrhea hypokalemia hypochlorhydria (WDHH). It is characterized by hypermotility, watery diarrhea syndromes with hypokalemia and hypochlorhydria, dehydration and weakness; these symptoms can be reproduced by VIP. VIP can be secreted by pancreatic or ectopic islet cell tumors, and in islet-cell hyperplasia. **LIMITATIONS:** Not all patients with the syndrome have increased VIP. Increased VIP can be found in healthy controls and in laxative abusers.[2] **METHODOLOGY:** Radioimmunoassay (RIA), immunoassay **ADDITIONAL INFORMATION:** Other features of some cases of VIPoma have included hypercalcemia, flushing, and glucose intolerance.[2] A study of islet cell tumors in patients with multiple endocrine neoplasia (MEN) included vasoactive intestinal polypeptide tumor (VIPoma) as well as Zollinger-Ellison syndrome and insulinoma.[3] A VIP-producing tumor causing the pancreatic cholera syndrome was reported as a well differentiated mucinous adenocarcinoma which contained cells reactive for pancreatic peptide and VIP on immunocytochemistry.[4] Bronchial tumor, pheochromocytoma, ganglion-neuroma, ganglioneuroblastoma, and medullary thyroid carcinoma have been reported with the syndrome. The severe watery diarrhea is a secretory diarrhea. Peak output can exceed 3 L a day. The diarrhea is electrolyte rich; potassium loss can be 300 mmol/day. There is acidosis from bicarbonate loss.[5] Eighty percent of such patients have islet cell tumors, of which nearly 50% are malignant. Others have islet cell hyperplasia.[5] Normal levels of VIP have been reported in ulcerative colitis, Crohn's disease, cirrhosis, ascites, and diabetes.

Footnotes

1. Koch Tr, Michener SR, and Go VL, "Plasma Vasoactive Intestinal Polypeptide Concentration Determination in Patients With Diarrhea," *Gastroenterology*, 1991, 100(1):99-106.
2. Krejs GJ, "Noninsulin-Secreting Tumors of the Pancreatic Islets," *Williams Textbook of Endocrinology*, 8th ed, Wilson JD and Foster DW, eds, Philadelphia, PA: WB Saunders Co, 1992, 1567-76.
3. Sheppard BC, Norton JA, Doppman JL, et al, "Management of Islet Cell Tumors in Patients With Multiple Endocrine Neoplasia: A Prospective Study," *Surgery*, 1989, 106(6):1108-18.

4. Rood RP, DeLellis RA, Dayal Y, et al, "Pancreatic Cholera Syndrome Due to a Vasoactive Intestinal Polypeptide-Producing Tumor: Further Insights Into the Pathophysiology," *Gastroenterology*, 1988, 94(3):813-8.
5. Grunfeld C, "Pancreatic Islet Cell Tumors," *Cecil Textbook of Medicine*, 19th ed, Vol 2, Wyngaarden JB, Smith LH Jr, and Bennett JC, eds, Philadelphia, PA: WB Saunders Co, 1992, 1317-9.

References

Basson MD, Fielding LP, Bilchik AJ, et al, "Does Vasoactive Intestinal Polypeptide Mediate the Pathophysiology of Bowel Obstruction?" *Am J Surg*, 1989, 157(1):109-14.

Deveney CW and Way LW, "Regulatory Peptides of the Gut," *Basic and Clinical Endocrinology*, 3rd ed, Greenspan FS and Forsham PH, eds, Los Altos, CA: Lange Medical Publications, 1991, 569-91.

Fahrenkrug J and Emson PC, "Vasoactive Intestinal Polypeptide: Functional Aspects," *Br Med Bull*, 1982, 38:265-70, (review).

Fraker DL and Norton JA, "The Role of Surgery in the Management of Islet Cell Tumors," *Gastroenterol Clin North Am*, 1989, 18(4):805-30.

Green DW, Gomez G, and Greeley GH Jr, "Gastrointestinal Peptides," *Gastroenterol Clin North Am*, 1989, 18(4):695-733.

Venous Blood Gases *see* Blood Gases, Venous *on page 144*

VIP *see* Vasoactive Intestinal Polypeptide *on previous page*

Vitamin A, Serum

CPT 84590

Related Information

Carotene, Serum *on page 172*

Synonyms Retinol, Serum

Test Commonly Includes Vitamin A and beta-carotene determination

Patient Care **PREPARATION:** Patient must fast a minimum of 8 hours.

Specimen Serum **CONTAINER:** Red top tube **COLLECTION:** Draw in chilled tube. Protect from light. Keep specimen on ice. **STORAGE INSTRUCTIONS:** Separate serum in a 4°C centrifuge and freeze in a plastic vial immediately. Stable 2 years frozen. Stable 4 weeks at 4°C, although freezing is preferred. Protect from light. **CAUSES FOR REJECTION:** Specimen excessively exposed to light, patient not fasting, specimen not received on ice, hemolysis

Interpretive **REFERENCE RANGE:** Vitamin A: 30-95 μg/dL (SI: 1.05-3.32 μmol/L); beta-carotene: 50-200 μg/dL (SI: 0.93-3.72 μmol/L) **USE:** Differential diagnosis of hypervitaminosis A. A combination of a low serum carotene level and a low vitamin A suggests inadequate vitamin A nutrition. **LIMITATIONS:** Serum levels do not correlate well with liver stores because of homeostatic control exerted by the liver. Increased in patients on oral contraceptives. **METHODOLOGY:** Fluorescence or UV/VIS spectroscopy, high performance liquid chromatography (HPLC), electrochemical **ADDITIONAL INFORMATION:** Vitamin A is a fat-soluble vitamin which is necessary for the integrity of epithelial cells. It also plays an important role in the visual cycle, and is required for normal growth, development, and reproduction. Decreased levels of vitamin A are commonly due to dietary deficiency[1], or may occur in conditions of deficient pancreatic digestive enzymes, impaired intestinal absorption and zinc deficiency resulting in decreased retinol-binding protein (RBP) levels, or deficient bile. Hypovitaminosis A may lead to impaired skeletal growth, blindness, xerophthalmia, increased susceptibility to respiratory infections, and keratomalacia. Night blindness is the most usual result of this condition. Hypervitaminosis A may be due to increased intake, or conditions causing impaired disposal such as diabetes mellitus, chronic nephritis, or myxedema. The toxic effects of increased vitamin A include elevation of intracranial pressure, skin desquamation, hair loss, joint pain, headache, nausea, fever, vertigo, and visual disorientation. Chronic hypervitaminosis A may cause anorexia, dry skin, alopecia, hepatomegaly, and fatigue. Toxicity is best assessed by measuring retinyl esters which normally comprise 5% of total vitamin A, but in toxicity (taking >50,000 IU/day) may comprise >30% of total vitamin A. Toxicity appears when vitamin A levels exceed the capacity of RBP to bind to it. Vitamin A deficiency may occur when diseases or conditions impair the conversion of carotene to vitamin A or reduce the levels of RBP. Children with hypovitaminosis A have increased morbidity with measles.[2,3] Also there is a depressed immune response to tetanus in children with vitamin A deficiency.[4]

Footnotes

1. Usha N, Sankaranarayanan A, Walia BN, et al, "Early Detection of Vitamin A Deficiency in Children With Persistent Diarrhoea," *Lancet*, 1990, 335(8686):422.
2. Division fo Field Epidemiology, Centers for Disease Control, "Vitamin A Levels and Severity of Measles. New York City," *Am J Dis Child*, 1992, 146(2):182-6.

(Continued)

Vitamin A, Serum *(Continued)*

3. Hussey GD and Klein M, "A Randomized, Controlled Trial of Vitamin A in Children With Severe Measles," *N Engl J Med*, 1990, 323(3):160-4.
4. Semba RD, Muhilal S, Scott AL, et al, "Depressed Immune Response to Tetanus in Children With Vitamin A Deficiency," *J Nutr*, 1992, 122(1):101-7.

References

Bloem MW, Wedel M, Egger RJ, et al, "Mild Vitamin A Deficiency and Risk of Respiratory Tract Diseases and Diarrhea in Preschool and School Children in Northeastern Thailand," *Am J Epidemiol*, 1990, 131(2):332-9.

"Detecting Vitamin A Deficiency Early," *Lancet*, 1992, 339(8808):1514-5, (editorial).

Sommer A, "Vitamin A Deficiency and Childhood Mortality," *Lancet*, 1992, 340(8817):488-9.

Suan EP, Bedrossian EH Jr, Eagle RC Jr, et al, "Corneal Perforation in Patients Wtih Vitamin A Deficiency in the United States," *Arch Ophthalmol*, 1990, 108(3):350-3.

Vitamin B_6

***CPT** 84207*

Synonyms Pyridoxal Phosphate; Pyridoxine

Abstract Vitamin B_6 is a water soluble vitamin acts as a coenzyme (pyridoxal-5-phosphate) in protein, carbohydrate, and lipid metabolism, as well as in heme synthesis.

Specimen Plasma **CONTAINER:** Lavender top (EDTA) tube **COLLECTION:** Transport specimen **immediately** to the laboratory following collection. Avoid exposing specimen to light. **STORAGE INSTRUCTIONS:** Separate plasma or serum and freeze **immediately**. Avoid exposure to light. Stable 10 days at -80°C; 50% loss in 7 days at -20°C. **CAUSES FOR REJECTION:** Specimen more than 30 minutes in transit to the laboratory. Patient must avoid having radioisotope scan prior to collection of specimen (if RIA method used). **SPECIAL INSTRUCTIONS:** Communicate with laboratory before ordering this test; it is not routinely available. Scheduling and/or use of a reference laboratory may be required.

Interpretive **REFERENCE RANGE:** >50 ng/mL (SI: >243 nmol/L) (varies considerably with method). A broad range is approximately 25-80 ng/mL (SI: 122-389 nmol/L). HPLC method for pyridoxal phosphate has normal range of 3.5-18.0 ng/mL (SI: 17-88 nmol/L). **USE:** Detect vitamin B_6 deficiency **LIMITATIONS:** Evaluation is complicated by the knowledge that some individuals have an unusually high requirement for vitamin B_6. **METHODOLOGY:** Enzyme assay, high performance liquid chromatography (HPLC) with fluorometric detection, immunoradiometric assay (IRMA) **ADDITIONAL INFORMATION:** The family of "vitamin B_6" compounds includes pyridoxine as well as B_6 activity contributed by aldehyde (pyridoxal) and amine (pyridoxamine) derivatives, pyridoxine being the alcohol form of the 3-hydroxy-2-methylpyridine basic structure. In biologic material the B_6 compounds exist largely as phosphorylated derivatives. The vitamin is synthesized by plants and many microorganisms but not by the higher animals. It is widely available in natural diets, being present in fish, chicken, some fruits and vegetables, and wheat germ. It is partially destroyed by cooking and food processing. Vitamin B_6 is water soluble and is absorbed largely from the jejunum. A series of phosphorylase, oxidase, and kinase enzymes provide for extensive *in vivo* interconversion of pyridoxine and its derivatives. Most B_6-dependent enzymes utilize pyridoxal-5-phosphate (the aldehyde form) in a coenzyme role. Biologically critical amino acid/protein metabolic pathways (eg, transamination and decarboxylation reactions) are dependent upon B_6 enzymes, glycogen phosphorylase requires B_6 as does delta aminolevulinic acid synthetase, and pyridoxal phosphate is required for DNA synthesis. With dietary deficiency, conservation of pyridoxal phosphate-dependent enzymes occurs with redistribution of available coenzyme and maintenance of more essential functions, thus rendering some clinical deficiency states difficult to define.

Deficiency of this vitamin has been implicated in a wide variety of clinical conditions. Important in neonatology is the syndrome of jittery characteristics, colic, irritability, easy startling and seizures due to B_6 deficiency following ingestion of formula rendered B_6 depleted by excessive heating. B_6 may be decreased with malabsorption and inflammatory disease of the small bowel and in some cases of jejunoileal bypass.

Pyridoxine is required for heme synthesis. With deficiency, a hypochromic form of sideroblastic anemia may occur, characterized by the presence of ring sideroblasts (iron positive granules deposited about the nucleus of red cell precursors). Occasionally the anemia may have megaloblastic characteristics. It has been suggested that the underlying defect is a block in the conversion of pyridoxine to pyridoxal phosphate, which inhibits the production of delta aminolevulinic acid and thus the production of heme.[1] This form of sideroblastic anemia responds to large doses (over 2 g) of pyridoxal phosphate per day. Inherited abnormalities of apoenzymes that bind with pyridoxal phosphate are responsible for newborn conditions characterized by mental retardation, skeletal deformities, thrombotic conditions, osteoporosis, and visual defects. Some are associated with increased urinary amino acids (eg, homocystinuria, hypermethioninemia, cystathioninuria). Some can be controlled with large doses of vitamin B_6. In adults, elevated serum homocysteine levels due to vitamin B_6 deficiency may promote atherogenesis. With B_6 deficiency the activity of cystathionine β-synthase (which functions in amino acid metabolism) is inhibited. Pyridoxal-5'-phosphate is a cofactor for this enzyme. The influence of B_6 on serum cholesterol levels and platelet aggregation is controversial. Decreased plasma pyridoxal phosphate levels have been found in patients with acute MI.[2] There is evidence against increased need for vitamin B_6 by athletes.[3]

Penicillamine, levodopa, disulfiram, oral contraceptive agents, theophylline, and the antituberculous drugs isoniazid, cycloserine, and pyrazinoic acid may cause B_6 depletion in some cases with apparently associated sideroblastic anemia. B_6 supplements may be necessary.

B_6 may be decreased with pregnancy, lactation, alcoholism, diabetes mellitus, and in an uncommon B_6 dependency state, vitamin B_6 responsive neonatal convulsions. The effects of megadose vitamin B_6 consumption are controversial. There is evidence of significant neurotoxicity associated with pyridoxine megavitaminosis; tingling, numbness, clumsiness, gait disturbances, pseudoathetosis, with doses over 2 g per day.[4]

Vitamin B_6 deficiency impairs immune function by inhibiting interleukin-2 production and lymphocyte proliferation.[5]

Pais et al report that children with leukemia had lower pyridoxal-5 phosphate levels than age matched control children.[6]

Footnotes

1. Hines JD and Grasso JA, "The Sideroblastic Anemias," *Semin Hematol*, 1970, 7:86-106.
2. Kok FJ, Schrijver J, Hofman A, et al, "Low Vitamin B_6 Status in Patients With Acute Myocardial Infarction," *Am J Cardiol*, 1989, 63(9):513-6.
3. Dreon DM and Butterfield GE, "Vitamin B_6 Utilization in Active and Inactive Young Men," *Am J Clin Nutr*, 1986, 43:816-24.
4. Schaumburg H, Kaplan J, Windebank A, et al, "Sensory Neuropathy From Pyridoxine Abuse," *N Engl J Med*, 1983, 309:445-8.
5. Rosenburg, IH, "Vitamin B_6 and Immune Function in the Elderly and HIV-Seropositive Subjects," *Nutr Rev*, 1992, 50(5):145-7.
6. Pais RC, Vanous E, Hollins B, et al, "Abnormal Vitamin B_6 Status in Childhood Leukemia," *Cancer*, 1990, 66(11):2421-8.

References

Borschel MW, Kirksey A, and Hannemann RE, "Effects of Vitamin B_6 Intake on Nutriture and Growth of Young Infants," *Am J Clin Nutr*, 1986, 43:7-15.

Pesce AJ and Kaplan LA, *Methods in Clinical Chemistry*, Chapter 73, St Louis, MO: Mosby-Year Book Inc, 1987, 559.

Vitamin C *see* Ascorbic Acid, Blood *on page 135*

Vitamin D_1 *see* Vitamin D_3, Serum *on this page*

Vitamin D_3, Serum

***CPT** 82306 (calcifediol); 82307 (calciferol)*

Related Information

Calcium, Urine *on page 163*

Kidney Stone Analysis *on page 1129*

Synonyms Calcitriol; Cholecalciferol (25-OH D_3); 1,25-$(OH)_2D_3$

Applies to 1,25-Dihydroxy Vitamin D_3; 25-Hydroxy Vitamin D_3; 1,25$(OH)_2$ D_3; Vitamin D_1

Abstract With parathyroid hormone and calcitonin, 1,25-dihydroxy vitamin D_3 acts upon bone, parathyroid glands, kidneys and intestine, regulating calcium metabolism, osteoblast function, and parathormone release. It exerts effects or is involved in a wide range of tissues additional to its role in mineral homeostasis.

Patient Care PREPARATION: Fasting specimen is preferred.

Specimen Serum, plasma CONTAINER: Red top tube, green top (heparin) tube STORAGE INSTRUCTIONS: Stable 3 days at 4°C to 25°C. Processed serum stable for months at -20°C, tolerates freeze-thaw cycles.[1] CAUSES FOR REJECTION: Administration of radioisotopes

Interpretive REFERENCE RANGE: 25-hydroxy vitamin D_3: 10-60 ng/mL (SI: 25-150 nmol/L); 1,25-dihydroxy vitamin D_3: 20-76 pg/mL (SI: 48-182 pmol/L). The normal range is method depen-

(Continued)

Vitamin D_3, Serum *(Continued)*

dent and varies with diet, clothing, season, and UV light exposure. **USE:** Evaluate vitamin D deficiency as cause of osteopenia; both postmenopausal osteoporosis and senile osteoporosis are linked to vitamin D disturbances.[2] Its role includes investigation of the differential diagnosis of disorders of calcium metabolism; investigate diseases of bone including osteopenia, osteomalacia and rickets; work up malabsorption **LIMITATIONS:** Values of vitamin D vary with exposure to sunlight (in which increased levels of vitamin D_3 result from synthesis in the skin from 7-dehydrocholesterol, in a reaction catalyzed by UV light). Vitamin D_2, metabolically similar to vitamin D_3, derives only from diet.[2] There are also variations during the menstrual cycle, particularly at the time of ovulation. Reference ranges are not well established. Many assays detect inactive 24-hydroxy metabolites in addition to active metabolites. **METHODOLOGY:** Competitive binding assay, radioimmunoassay (RIA), high performance liquid chromatography (HPLC) **ADDITIONAL INFORMATION:** Vitamin D_3 (cholecalciferol) and vitamin D_2 (ergocalciferol) are hydroxylated in the liver to the 25-hydroxy form, and then to the active 1,25-dihydroxy form in the kidney. Functional abnormalities can result from failures of absorption or either hydroxylation step. In type II vitamin D-dependent rickets, there is end-organ unresponsiveness to 1,25-dihydroxy vitamin D. Long use of anticonvulsive drugs may lead to decreased levels of 25-hydroxy vitamin D, through induced increased hepatic metabolism, but this may not be clinically significant.

Vitamin D has a major action on intestinal absorption of calcium, bone calcium balance, and renal excretion of calcium. Thus, assessment of serum vitamin D levels are useful in the differential diagnosis of hypocalcemia, hypercalcemia, and hypophosphatemia. Specific measurement of both monohydroxy and dihydroxy forms can help pinpoint absorptive, hepatic, or renal abnormalities of vitamin D metabolism.

1,25-dihydroxy vitamin D is increased in sarcoidosis and hyperparathyroidism. It may be elevated in cases of hypercalcemia associated with malignant lymphoma. It is decreased in rickets, type I vitamin D-resistant rickets, hypoparathyroidism, pseudohypoparathyroidism, and renal osteodystrophy and psoriasis.[3]

Dietary intake of phosphorus is a determinant of 1,25-dihydroxy D_3 production. Increases of 1,25-dihydroxy D relating to hypocalcemia are thought to be mediated through increased output of parathyroid hormone. Vitamin D is also influenced by thyroid status, estrogens, calcitonin, growth hormone, prolactin, insulin, and glucocorticoids. The vitamin D endocrine system is linked to vitamin D-resistant rickets as well as classic vitamin D-deficient rickets and hypophosphatemic oncogenic rickets.

Because of the complex, multifactorial control of calcium balance, it is often useful to measure parathyroid hormone in conjunction with vitamin D.

D_2 is a commercially manufactured D vitamin derived from plants. It is used in vitamin preparations and therefore represents a fraction of the body's total vitamin D stores.[4] Vitamin D_1 (24,25-dihydroxy – also called calcidiol) is the major renal metabolite but has no physiological role.

Footnotes

1. Lissner D, Mason R, and Posen S, "Stability of Vitamin D Metabolites in Human Blood Serum and Plasma," *Clin Chem*, 1981, 27:773-4.
2. Reichel H, Koeffler HP, and Norman AW, "The Role of the Vitamin D Endocrine System in Health and Disease," *N Engl J Med*, 1989, 320(15):980-91.
3. Morimoto S and Yoshikawa K, "Psoriasis and Vitamin D_3. A Review of Our Experience," *Arch Dermatol*, 1989, 125(2):231-4.
4. Tietz NW, *Textbook of Clinical Chemistry*, Tietz NW, ed, Philadelphia, PA: WB Saunders Co, 1986, 1322.

References

Audran M and Kumar R, "The Physiology and Pathophysiology of Vitamin D," *Mayo Clin Proc*, 1985, 60:851-66.

Brommage R and DeLuca HF, "Evidence That 1,25-Dihydroxyvitamin D_3 Is the Physiologically Active Metabolite of Vitamin D_3," *Endocr Rev*, 1985, 6:491-511, (review).

Fournier A, Moriniere P, Boudaillez B, et al, "1,25 (OH) 2 Vitamin D_3 Deficiency and Renal Osteodystrophy: Should its Well-Accepted Pathogenetic Role in Secondary Hyperparathyroidism Lead to its Systematic Preventive Therapeutic Use?" *Nephrol Dial Transplant*, 1987, 2:498-503, (review).

Garabédian M, Jacqz E, Guillozo H, et al, "Elevated Plasma 1,25-Dihydroxyvitamin D Concentrations in Infants With Hypercalcemia and an Elfin Facies," *N Engl J Med*, 1985, 312:948-52.

Krall EA, Sahyoun N, Tannenbaum S, et al, "Effect of Vitamin D Intake on Seasonal Variations in Parathyroid Hormone Secretion in Postmenopausal Women," *N Engl J Med*, 1989, 321(26):1777-83.

Kumar R, "The Metabolism and Mechanism of Action of 1,25-Dihydroxyvitamin D_3," *Kidney Int*, 1986, 30:793-803, (review).

Lyles KW, Halsey DL, Friedman NE, et al, "Correlations of Serum Concentrations of 1,25-Dihydroxyvitamin D, Phosphorus, and Parathyroid Hormone in Tumoral Calcinosis," *J Clin Endocrinol Metab*, 1988, 67:88-92.

Silverberg SJ, Shane E, de la Cruz L, et al, "Abnormalities in Parathyroid Hormone Secretion and 1,25-Dihydroxyvitamin D_3 Formation in Women With Osteoporosis," *N Engl J Med*, 1989, 320(5):277-81.

Singer FR and Adams JS, "Abnormal Calcium Homeostasis in Sarcoidosis," *N Engl J Med*, 1986, 315:755-7, (editorial).

Vitamin E, Serum

CPT *84446*

Synonyms Alpha Tocopherol; Tocopherol; α-Tocopherol

Abstract Vitamin E is a lipid soluble vitamin that acts as antioxidant preventing damage to membranes by free radicals.

Specimen Serum, plasma **CONTAINER:** Red top tube, green top (heparin) tube **STORAGE INSTRUCTIONS:** Separate serum or plasma within 2 hours. Protect from light. Serum or plasma is stable 2 weeks at 25°C, 14 days at 4°C, and 1 year at -20°C.[1]

Interpretive **REFERENCE RANGE:** 0.8-1.5 mg/dL (SI: 19-35 μmol/L), varies with method **USE:** Evaluate vitamin E deficiency in hemolytic disease in premature infants and neuromuscular disease in infants (and adults) with chronic cholestasis; evaluate patients on long-term parenteral nutrition; patients with malignancy or malabsorption (eg, patients with cystic fibrosis, cases of intestinal bypass surgery); investigate brown-bowel syndrome **METHODOLOGY:** High performance liquid chromatography (HPLC), fluorometry after solvent extraction, colorimetry **ADDITIONAL INFORMATION:** Vitamin E (α-tocopherol) is an antioxidant so widely distributed in foodstuffs that deficiency rarely occurs from diet. However, vitamin E is fat soluble, and malabsorption and deficiency may develop in cases of chronic intraluminal intestinal bile deficiency. This has been particularly noted in premature infants and children with biliary atresia or cystic fibrosis (chronic intrahepatic cholestasis).[2] Clinically this may lead to a hemolytic anemia, due to increased erythrocyte fragility, or to a slowly progressive neurologic disorder characterized by ataxia, areflexia, gaze disturbances, and loss of proprioception and vibratory sensation. A similar syndrome has been reported in adults with malabsorption. The syndrome may respond to treatment with parenteral vitamin E.

Early treatment with vitamin E may delay or prevent the neuropathy with ataxia that develops during the course of abetalipoproteinuria. Vitamin E therapy, in some cases, may have a favorable effect on moderate and severe cases of the retinopathy of prematurity[3] and the retinopathy of abetalipoproteinemia. While lipid malabsorption syndrome (with steatorrhea and malabsorption of vitamin E) may be etiologically related to ataxic spinocerebellar neurologic degenerative disease, there are reports of familial and sporadic vitamin E deficiency with neurologic impairment in the absence of fat malabsorption or demonstrated plasma lipoprotein level abnormality.[4,5,6] An inherited defect in hepatocyte secretion of vitamin E into lipoprotein has been proposed.[3] The importance of not overlooking a treatable cause of neurologic degenerative disease has been emphasized.[6]

As an antioxidant, vitamin E assists the prevention of peroxidation of unsaturated fatty acids. Deficiency may result in accumulation of oxidized lipids which may polymerize with polysaccharides to form ceroid/lipofuscin pigment. This PAS positive material deposits in tissue as intracytoplasmic pigment granules. In three patients with "brown-bowel syndrome," vitamin E levels were found to be "extremely low" (0.1-0.2 mg/dL (SI: 2-5 μmol/L)).[7]

There continues to be interest in correlating plasma vitamin E levels with a variety of plasma constituents, with some positive and some negative results. Significance and/or validity of some associations is uncertain. Notably, abnormal serum levels of vitamin E have not been shown to relate significantly to clinical patency of ductus arteriosus,[8] sickle cell anemia,[9] moderate freshwater fish consumption,[10] insulin-dependent diabetics,[11] and risk of cancer (MRFIT study).[12] Plasma vitamin E level, in one study, showed a positive correlation with serum cholesterol, non-HDL cholesterol, triglycerides, and apolipoprotein B.[13] Vitamin E is reported to reduce the risk of coronary heart disease in men[14] and women.[15]

Footnotes

1. Tietz NW, *Clinical Guide to Laboratory Tests*, 2nd ed, Philadelphia, PA: WB Saunders Co, 1990, 588.
2. Issa S, Rotthauwe HW, and Burmeister W, "25-Hydroxyvitamin D and Vitamin E Absorption in Healthy Children and Children With Chronic Intrahepatic Cholestasis," *Eur J Pediatr*, 1989, 148(7):605-9.
3. Johnson L, Quinn GE, Abbasi S, et al, "Effect of Sustained Pharmacologic Vitamin E Levels on Incidence and Severity of Retinopathy of Prematurity: A Controlled Clinical Trial," *J Pediatr*, 1989, 114(5):827-38, (review).

(Continued)

Vitamin E, Serum *(Continued)*

4. Harding AE, Matthews S, Jones S, et al, "Spinocerebellar Degeneration Associated With a Selective Defect of Vitamin E Absorption," *N Engl J Med*, 1985, 313:32-5.
5. Sokol RJ, Kayden HJ, Bettis DB, et al, "Isolated Vitamin E Deficiency in the Absence of Fat Malabsorption - Familial and Sporadic Cases: Characterization and Investigation of Causes," *J Lab Clin Med*, 1988, 111(5):548-59.
6. Harding AE, Macevilly CJ, and Muller DPR, "Serum Vitamin E Concentrations in Degenerative Ataxias," *J Neurol Neurosurg Psychiatry*, 1989, 52(1):132, (letter).
7. Michowitz M, Noy S, Chayen D, et al, "Brown-Bowel Syndrome," *Am J Surg*, 1989, 55:566-9.
8. Rudolph N, Schiller MS, and Wong SL, "Vitamin E and Selenium in Preterm Infants: Lack of Effect on Clinical Patency of Ductus Arteriosus," *Int J Vitam Nutr Res*, 1989, 59(2):140-6.
9. Broxson EH Jr, Sokol RJ, and Githens JH, "Normal Vitamin E Status in Sickle Hemoglobinopathies in Colorado," *Am J Clin Nutr*, 1989, 50(3):497-503.
10. Hänninen OO, Agren JJ, Laitinen MV, et al, "Dose-Response Relationships in Blood Lipids During Moderate Freshwater Fish Diet," *Ann Med*, 1989, 21:203-7.
11. Basu TK, Tze WJ, and Leichter J, "Serum Vitamin A and Retinol-Binding Protein in Patients With Insulin-Dependent Diabetes Mellitus," *Am J Clin Nutr*, 1989, 50(2):329-31.
12. Connett JE, Kuller LH, Kjelsberg MO, et al, "Relationship Between Carotenoids and Cancer. The Multiple Risk Factor Intervention Trial (MRFIT) Study," *Cancer*, 1989, 64(1):126-34.
13. Rubba P, Mancini M, Fidanza F, et al, "Plasma Vitamin E, Apolipoprotein B and HDL Cholesterol in Middle-Aged Men From Southern Italy," *Atherosclerosis*, 1989, 77(1):25-9.
14. Rimm EB, Stampfer MJ, Ascherio A, et al, "Vitamin E Consumption and the Risk of Coronary Heart Disease in Men," *N Engl J Med*, 1993, 328(20):1450-6.
15. Stampfer MJ, Hennekens CH, Manson JE, et al, "Vitamin E Consumption and the Risk of Coronary Disease in Women," *N Engl J Med*, 1993, 328(20):1444-9.

References

Havel RJ and Kane JP, "Abetalipoproteinemia - Introduction: Structure and Metabolism of Plasma Lipoproteins," *The Metabolic Basis of Inherited Disease*, 6th ed, Chapter 44A, Scriver CR, Beaudet AL, Sly WS, et al, eds, New York, NY: McGraw-Hill Inc, 1989, 1145-51.

Kelleher J, Miller MG, Littlewood JM, et al, "The Clinical Effect of Correction of Vitamin E Depletion in Cystic Fibrosis," *Int J Vitam Nutr Res*, 1987, 57:253-9.

Munoz SJ, Heubi JE, Balistreri WF, et al, "Vitamin E Deficiency in Primary Biliary Cirrhosis: Gastrointestinal Malabsorption, Frequency and Relationship to Other Lipid-Soluble Vitamins," *Hepatology*, 1989, 9(4):525-31.

VLDL *see* Triglycerides *on page 370*

VMA *see* Vanillylmandelic Acid, Urine *on page 382*

Watson-Schwartz Test *see* Porphobilinogen, Qualitative, Urine *on page 325*

Wellness Programs *see* Chemistry Profile *on page 181*

Xylose Absorption Test *see* d-Xylose Absorption Test *on page 210*

Xylose Tolerance Test *see* d-Xylose Absorption Test *on page 210*

Zinc Protoporphyrin *see* Protoporphyrin, Zinc, Blood *on page 342*

ZPP *see* Protoporphyrin, Zinc, Blood *on page 342*

CHEMISTRY APPENDIX

International Unit (SI Unit) Conversion Tables

Analyte	Conventional Units	Conventional to SI (multiply by)	SI Units	SI to Conventional (multiply by)
Acetaminophen (Datril®, Tylenol®)	μg/mL	6.62	μmol/L	0.151
Acid phosphatase	units/L	NA	units/L	NA
Adrenocorticotropic hormone (ACTH)	pg/mL	1	ng/L	1
Albumin, serum	g/dL	10	g/L	0.10
Aldolase, serum	units/L	NA	units/L	NA
Aldosterone				
blood	ng/dL	0.0277	nmol/L	36.10
urine	μg/24 h	2.77	nmol/d	0.361
Alkaline phosphatase	units/L	NA	units/L	NA
$Alpha_1$-antitrypsin	mg/dL	0.01	g/L	100
$Alpha_1$-fetoprotein				
amniotic fluid	μg/mL	1	mg/L	1
serum	ng/mL	1	μg/L	1
Alanine aminotransferase (ALT)	units/L	NA	units/L	NA
Aluminum, serum	ng/mL	0.0371	μmol/L	26.95
Amikacin	μg/mL	1.71	μmol/L	0.585
Ammonia, blood	ng/dL	0.714	μmol/L	1.4
Amylase, serum	units/L	NA	units/L	NA
Androstenedione	ng/dL	0.0349	nmol/L	28.7
Angiotensin	ng/dL	10	ng/L	0.1
Angiotensin converting enzyme (ACE)	nmol/min/mL	1	units/L	1
Anion gap	mEq/L	1	mmol/L	1
Antidiuretic hormone (ADH) (vasopressin)	pg/mL	1	ng/L	1
Arsenic				
serum	μg/dL	0.133	μmol/L	7.52
urine	μg/L	0.0133	μmol/d	75.2
Ascorbic acid, blood	mg/dL	56.78	μmol/L	0.018
Aspartate aminotransferase (AST)	units/L	NA	units/L	NA
Base excess	mEq/L	1	mmol/L	1
Bicarbonate (HCO_3^-)	mEq/L	1	mmol/L	1
Bilirubin, serum				
direct	mg/dL	17.1	μmol/L	0.584
total	mg/dL	17.1	μmol/L	0.584
Bromide	mg/dL	0.125	mmol/L	79.9
Cadmium	μg/L	8.897	nmol/L	0.112
Caffeine	μg/mL	5.15	μmol/L	0.194

(continued)

Analyte	Conventional Units	Conventional to SI (multiply by)	SI Units	SI to Conventional (multiply by)
Calcitonin	pg/mL	1	ng/L	1
Calcium				
ionized	mg/dL	0.25	mmol/L	4
serum	mg/dL	0.25	mmol/L	4
urine	mg/24 h	0.025	mmol/d	40
Carbamazepine (Tegretol®)	µg/mL	4.23	µmol/L	0.236
Carbon dioxide	mEq/L	1	mmol/L	1
Carboxyhemoglobin	%	NA	%	NA
Carcinoembryonic antigen (CEA)	ng/mL	1	µg/L	1
Carotene, serum	µg/dL	0.0186	µmol/L	53.7
Catecholamines, fractionation, urine	µg/24 h	5.91	nmol/d	0.169
Ceruloplasmin	mg/dL	10	µmol/L	0.10
Chloramphenicol	µg/mL	3.09	µmol/L	0.323
Chlordiazepoxide (Librium®)	ng/mL	0.0033	µmol/L	303
Chloride				
serum	mEq/L	1	mmol/L	1
sweat	mEq/L	1	nmol/L	1
urine	mmol/24 h	1	mmol/d	1
Cholesterol	mg/dL	0.0259	mmol/L	38.61
HDL	mg/dL	0.0259	mmol/L	38.61
LDL	mg/dL	0.0259	mmol/L	38.61
Cholinesterase, serum	units/mL	1	kU/L	1
Chromium, serum	ng/mL	19.2	nmol/L	0.052
Clonazepam (Klonopin™)	ng/mL	3.17	nmol/L	0.316
Codeine	ng/mL	3.34	nmol/L	0.299
Compound S (11-deoxycortisol)	µg/dL	0.029	µmol/L	34.5
Copper				
serum	µg/dL	0.157	µmol/L	6.37
urine	µg/24 h	0.0157	µmol/d	63.69
Coproporphyrins (I and III)				
blood	µg/dL	15	nmol/L	0.067
fluid	µg/g	1.5	nmol/g	0.67
urine	µg/24 h	1.5	nmol/d	0.67
Cortisol				
blood	µg/dL	27.6	nmol/L	0.036
urine	µg/24 h	2.76	nmol/d	0.362
C-Peptide	ng/mL	0.33	nmol/L	3.03
Creatine kinase (CK)	units/L	NA	units/L	NA
Creatinine				
serum	mg/dL	88.4	µmol/L	0.0113
urine	mg/kg/24 h	8.84	µmol/kg/d	0.113
	mg/24 h	0.0088	µmol/d	113.1

(continued)

Analyte	Conventional Units	Conventional to SI (multiply by)	SI Units	SI to Conventional (multiply by)
Cyanide, blood	mg/L	38.4	μmol/L	0.026
Cyclic AMP				
plasma	ng/mL	3.04	nmol/L	0.329
urine	μg/L	3.04	μmol/L	0.329
Cystine, urine	mg/24 h	8.32	μmol/24 h	0.120
Delta aminolevulinic acid, urine	mg/24 h	7.626	μmol/d	0.131
DHEA	ng/mL	3.47	nmol/L	0.288
DHEA sulfate	μg/mL	2.6	μmol/L	0.38
Diazepam (Valium®)	ng/mL	0.0035	μmol/L	0.286
Digitoxin	ng/mL	1.31	nmol/L	0.765
Digoxin (Lanoxin®)	ng/mL	1.28	nmol/L	0.781
Diphenhydramine (Benadryl®)	μg/mL	3.92	μmol/L	0.255
Diphenylhydantoin (Dilantin®)	μg/mL	3.96	μmol/L	0.253
Disopyramide (Norpace®)	μg/mL	2.95	μmol/L	0.339
Doxepin (Sinequan®)	ng/mL	3.58	nmol/L	0.279
d-Xylose	mg/dL	0.066	mmol/L	15.01
Erythropoietin, serum	mIU/mL	1	IU/L	1
Estradiol (E_2), serum	pg/mL	3.67	pmol/L	0.272
Estriol (E_3), serum	μg/L	3.47	nmol/L	0.288
Estrone (E_1), serum	ng/dL	37	pmol/L	0.027
Ethanol	mg/dL	0.217	mmol/L	4.61
Ethchlorvynol (Placidyl®)	μg/mL	6.92	μmol/L	0.145
Ethosuximide (Zarontin®)	μg/mL	7.08	μmol/L	0.141
Ethylene glycol	mg/L	16.1	μmol/L	0.0621
Factor B (properdin)	mg/dL	10	mg/L	0.10
Fatty acids, free, serum	mg/dL	0.0354	mmol/L	28.25
Fecal fat	g/24 h	1	g/d	1
Ferritin, serum	ng/mL	1	μg/L	1
Fluoride	μg/mL	52.6	μmol/L	0.019
Folate				
red cell	ng/mL	2.265	nmol/L	0.442
serum	ng/mL	2.265	nmol/L	0.442
Follicle stimulating hormone (FSH)	mIU/mL	1	IU/L	1
Gamma glutamyl transferase (GGT)	units/L	NA	units/L	NA
Gastrin, serum	pg/mL	1	ng/L	1
Gentamicin	μg/mL	2.09	μmol/L	0.478
Glucose				
blood	mg/dL	0.0555	mmol/L	18.02
CSF	mg/dL	0.0555	mmol/L	18.02
urine	mg/dL	0.0555	mmol/L	18.02

(continued)

Analyte	Conventional Units	Conventional to SI (multiply by)	SI Units	SI to Conventional (multiply by)
Glutamine, CSF	mg/dL	68.5	μmol/L	0.0146
Glutethimide (Doriden®)	μg/mL	4.60	μmol/L	0.217
Glycated hemoglobin	% of total Hb	0.01	Fraction of total Hb	100
Gold	μg/dL	0.0508	μmol/L	19.68
Growth hormone (GH)	ng/mL	1	μg/L	1
Haloperidol (Haldol®)	ng/mL	2.66	nmol/L	0.376
Haptoglobin, serum	mg/dL	10	mg/L	0.10
Homovanillic acid (HVA), urine	mg/24 h μg/mg of creatinine	5.49 0.621	μmol/d mmol/mol of creatinine	0.182 1.61
Human chorionic gonadotropin (hCG), serum	mIU/mL	1	IU/L	1
17-Hydroxycorticosteroids (17-OHCS), urine	mg/24 h	2.76	μmol/d	0.362
5-Hydroxyindoleacetic acid (5-HIAA), urine	mg/24 h	5.2	μmol/d	0.19
17-Hydroxyprogesterone	ng/mL	3.03	nmol/L	0.330
Imipramine (Tofranil®)	ng/mL	3.57	nmol/L	0.280
Insulin, blood	μIU/mL	1	mIU/L	1
Iron	μg/dL	0.179	μmol/L	5.587
Iron binding capacity, total (TIBC)	μg/dL	0.179	μmol/L	5.587
Isopropanol	mg/L	0.0166	mmol/L	60.1
17-Ketogenic steroids, urine	mg/24 h	3.467	μmol/d	0.288
17-Ketosteroids	mg/24 h	3.467	μmol/d	0.288
Lactate dehydrogenase (LDH)	units/L	NA	units/L	NA
Lactic acid blood CSF	 mg/dL mg/dL	 0.111 0.111	 mmol/L mmol/L	 9.01 9.01
Lead serum urine	 μg/dL μg/24 h	 0.0483 0.00483	 μmol/L μmol/d	 20.70 207.04
Leucine aminopeptidase (LAP)	units/L	NA	units/L	NA
Lidocaine (Xylocaine®)	μg/mL	4.27	μmol/L	0.234
Lipase, serum	units/L	NA	units/L	NA
Lipids, total	mg/dL	0.01	g/L	100
Lithium	mEq/L	1	mmol/L	1
Lorazepam	ng/mL	3.11	nmol/L	0.321
Luteinizing hormone (LH)	mIU/mL	1	IU/L	1
Lysergic acid diethylamide (LSD)	μg/mL	3.09	μmol/L	0.323

(continued)

Analyte	Conventional Units	Conventional to SI (multiply by)	SI Units	SI to Conventional (multiply by)
Magnesium				
serum	mEq/L	0.50	mmol/L	2
urine	mEq/24 h	0.50	mmol/d	2
Manganese				
serum	μg/L	18.2	nmol/L	0.055
urine	μg/L	18.2	nmol/L	0.055
Mercury				
blood	μg/dL	0.0499	μmol/L	20.0
urine	μg/L	0.00499	μmol/d	200
Meperidine (Demerol®)	μg/mL	4.04	nmol/L	0.247
Meprobamate	μg/mL	4.58	μmol/L	0.218
Metanephrines, urine	mg/24 h	5.07	μmol/d	0.197
Methadone	ng/mL	0.00323	μmol/L	309
Methanol	mg/dL	0.312	mmol/L	3.2
Methsuximide (Celontin®)	μg/mL	5.29	μmol/L	0.189
Methyldopa (Aldomet®)	μg/mL	4.73	μmol/L	0.211
Methyprylon (Noludar®)	μg/mL	5.46	μmol/L	0.183
Myoglobin, blood	μg/L	NA	μg/L	NA
N-Acetylprocainamide (NAPA)	μg/mL	3.61	μmol/L	0.277
Nortriptyline (Aventyl®)	ng/mL	3.80	nmol/L	0.263
5' Nucleotidase	units/L	NA	units/L	NA
Osmolality				
serum	mOsm/kg	NA	mmol/kg	NA
urine	mOsm/kg	NA	mmol/kg	NA
Oxalate, urine	mg/24 h	11.4	μmol/d	0.088
Oxazepam (Serax®)	μg/mL	3.49	μmol/L	0.287
Parathyroid hormone	pg/mL	1	ng/L	1
Pentobarbital (Nembutal®)	μg/mL	4.42	μmol/L	0.266
Phencyclidine (PCP)	ng/mL	4.11	nmol/L	0.243
Phenobarbital	μg/mL	4.31	μmol/L	0.232
Phenylalanine, blood	mg/dL	0.0605	mmol/L	16.52
Phenytoin (Dilantin®)				
free	μg/mL	3.96	μmol/L	0.253
total	μg/mL	3.96	μmol/L	0.253
Phosphorus				
serum	mg/dL	0.323	mmol/L	3.10
urine	g/24 h	32.3	mmol/d	0.031
Porphobilinogen (PBG), urine	mg/24 h	4.42	μmol/d	0.226
Potassium				
blood	mEq/L	1	mmol/L	1
urine	mEq/24 h	1	mmol/d	1
Pregnanediol, urine	mg/24 h	3.12	μmol/24 h	0.321
Pregnanetriol, urine	mg/24 h	2.97	μmol/24 h	0.337
Primidone (Mysoline®)	μg/mL	4.58	μmol/L	0.218

(continued)

Analyte	Conventional Units	Conventional to SI (multiply by)	SI Units	SI to Conventional (multiply by)
Procainamide (Pronestyl®)	μg/mL	4.23	μmol/L	0.236
Progesterone	ng/dL	0.0318	nmol/L	0.314
Prolactin	ng/mL	1	μg/L	1
Propoxyphene (Darvon®)	μg/mL	2.95	μmol/L	0.339
Propranolol (Inderal®)	ng/mL	3.86	nmol/L	0.259
Protein				
CSF	mg/dL	10	mg/L	0.10
serum	g/dL	10	g/L	0.10
urine	mg/24 h	0.001	g/d	1000
Protoporphyrin, free erythrocyte	μg/dL	0.0178	μmol/L	56.18
Protoporphyrin, zinc (ZPP)	μg/dL	0.016	μmol/L	62.5
Quinidine	μg/mL	3.08	μmol/L	0.250
Salicylate	mg/dL	0.0724	mmol/L	13.81
Secobarbital (Seconal™)	μg/mL	4.20	μmol/L	0.238
Serotonin	ng/mL	0.00568	μmol/L	176
Sodium				
blood	mEq/L	1	mmol/L	1
urine	mEq/24 h	1	mmol/d	1
T_3 uptake (T_3U)	%	1	AU*	1
Testosterone	ng/dL	0.0347	nmol/L	28.8
Theophylline	μg/mL	5.55	μmol/L	0.18
Thiocyanate	μg/mL	17.2	μmol/L	0.058
Thyroglobulin	ng/mL	1	μg/L	1
Thyroid stimulating hormone (TSH)	μIU/mL	1	mIU/L	1
Thyrotropin-releasing hormone (TRH)	pg/mL	1	ng/L	1
Thyroxine binding globulin (TBG)	mg/dL	10	mg/L	0.10
Thyroxine (T_4)	μg/dL	12.9	nmol/L	0.0075
Thyroxine, free (FT_4)	ng/dL	12.9	pmol/L	0.0075
Tobramycin	μg/mL	2.14	μmol/L	0.467
Transferrin	mg/dL	0.01	g/L	100
Triglycerides	mg/dL	0.0113	mmol/L	88.5
Triiodothyronine (T_3)	ng/dL	0.0154	nmol/L	65.1
Troponin	μg/L	NA	μg/L	NA
Urea nitrogen, blood (BUN)	mg/dL	0.357	mmol/L	2.80
Uric acid				
serum	mg/dL	0.059	mmol/L	16.9
urine	mg/24 h	0.0059	mmol/d	169
Valproic acid (Depakene®)	μg/mL	6.93	μmol/L	0.144
Vancomycin	μg/mL	0.690	μmol/L	1.45

(continued)

Analyte	Conventional Units	Conventional to SI (multiply by)	SI Units	SI to Conventional (multiply by)
Vanillylmandelic acid (VMA), urine	mg/24 h	5.05	μmol/d	0.198
Vitamin				
A	μg/dL	0.0349	μmol/L	28.65
B_6	ng/mL	4.046	nmol/L	0.247
B_{12}	pg/mL	0.738	pmol/L	1.355
D_3 (calcitriol, 1,25-dihydroxy)	pg/mL	2.4	pmol/L	0.417
E	mg/dL	23.22	μmol/L	0.043
Warfarin (Coumadin®)	μg/mL	3.24	μmol/L	0.308
Zinc				
blood	μg/dL	0.153	μmol/L	6.54
urine	μg/24 h	0.0153	μmol/d	65.36

NA = not applicable.
AU = arbitrary unit.

COAGULATION

Wayne R. DeMott, MD

The prime functions of the coagulation mechanism are to protect the integrity of the blood vascular compartment, while reasonably maintaining its fluid state. Death may attend either the inability to stem the loss of blood or the conversion of blood to a solid. The illustrative comparable clinical problems are hemorrhage due to inability to form a normal clot on one hand versus intravascular thrombosis on the other. Thus, the modern medical environment focuses upon the results of panels of tests to assess hemorrhage (possibly due to consumptive coagulopathy) versus thrombosis (possibly the result of hypercoagulability). The exquisite and critically important equilibrium between these two states — irreversible sol vs irreversible gel — is inherent in the concept "disseminated intravascular coagulation" (consumptive coagulation). Excessive clotting occurs but mechanisms to maintain fluidity are activated resulting in coagulation failure-hemorrhage.

The following test listings describe clinical laboratory maneuvers that assist the clinician in the investigation and management of disorders of coagulation. Included importantly are the dichotomous states, intravascular coagulation, and hypercoagulation. Dichotomy of a different nature, a generation gap of sorts, must also be noted. Currently, the nature of many if not all coagulation abnormalities are biochemically highly defined. Earlier generations of tests, many of which persist (and are included amongst the entries which follow), suffer from lack of specificity. They are in reality crude screening procedures. On the other hand, they are not costly or difficult to perform and have some frequency of clinical applicability. Thus, they are readily maintained and are offered by many hospital clinical laboratories. Great strides in the understanding of diseases of coagulation at the molecular level have made possible analyses that are technically demanding and require a certain level of investment (in reagents, equipment, and personnel). Results of these more specific tests may have critical importance in defining a coagulation abnormality (eg, multimer analysis in von Willebrand's disease). The conditions defined by these "modern generation" procedures are usually clinically uncommon. In the "modern generation" fiscal environment in which most hospital clinical laboratories function, a high cost/low volume procedure equates to "refer" (to a reference laboratory). Thus, a certain "functional generation gap" has evolved which may not always have favorable implications to the welfare of particular patients.

The following listings attempt to include some of the "old" and some of the "new." There are hopefully sufficient footnote and reference citations to allow the user satisfactory access to additional detail.

Ac-Globulin *see* Factor V *on page 421*

ACT *see* Activated Coagulation Time *on this page*

Activated Clotting Time *see* Activated Coagulation Time *on this page*

Activated Coagulation Time

***CPT** 85347*

Related Information

Antithrombin III Test *on page 403*
Lee-White Clotting Time *on page 449*
Partial Thromboplastin Time *on page 450*

Synonyms ACT; Activated Clotting Time; Ground Glass Clotting Time

Applies to Heparin; Protamine Sulfate

Abstract Screening test for coagulation deficiencies, with special application to the monitoring of heparin effect. The test is utilized, in particular, to monitor heparin effect during cardiopulmonary bypass surgical procedures.

Patient Care **PREPARATION:** Tubes and syringes used to collect blood should be warmed to 37°C.

Specimen Whole blood **CONTAINER:** Blood sample is added or drawn into a tube containing an activator (silica, Celite, siliceous earth/diatomaceous earth or finely crushed ground glass). The Vacutainer® (Becton-Dickinson) line of evacuated glass tubes includes an appropriate tube Reorder #6522. This gray stoppered tube contains 12 mg of purified siliceous earth. **COLLECTION:** Test is done at bedside by the medical technologist. **TURNAROUND TIME:** Usually under 5 minutes **SPECIAL INSTRUCTIONS:** A two-syringe or two-tube collection method should be used. The initial 1 mL of blood collected into a plastic syringe or into a tube is discarded without removing needle from vein and the sample to be used for testing is then drawn into the tube containing siliceous earth.

Interpretive **REFERENCE RANGE:** Varies between laboratories as it is procedure, activator, and lot number of activator dependent. Normal result is generally 70-120 seconds. Hattersley originally found a normal range of 107 seconds (2SD ±26 seconds[1]) (5000 routine presurgical studies). Becton-Dickinson cautions that use of Vacutainer® tube #6522 will result in shorter ACT normal range than that reported by Hattersley. **CRITICAL VALUES:** A minimum ACT value for adequacy of heparinization has not yet been determined but there is evidence that it is under 400 seconds.[2] Gravlee et al suggest that during cardiopulmonary bypass the ACT range be kept within 300-500 seconds. **USE:** Screen for coagulation deficiencies using whole blood; establish baseline before heparin administration; monitor postheparin injection. ACT has been used to monitor the anticoagulant effect of heparin during percutaneous transluminal coronary angioplasty; use of an arterial blood sample may avoid a falsely low ACT level.[3] **LIMITATIONS:** Test is insensitive to factor VII deficiency and to some platelet abnormalities. Different activators and methods respond variably to heparinized blood so that heparin dose/response experience in one laboratory setting is not necessarily transferable to a different laboratory. Some authorities feel that the normal range is not sufficiently removed (different from) the heparin anticoagulated therapeutic desirable range.[4] Response to heparin anticoagulation may need to be considered with knowledge of other drugs being taken by the patient (see following information). Lysed platelets shortened the ACT of heparinized whole blood from 248 seconds (controls) to 127 seconds indicating the ACT can be artifactually low in the presence of heparin. There is evidence that platelet membrane fragments (rather than cytosol particles which contain platelet factor 4) are responsible for this effect.[5] This could present a problem in the use of the ACT for monitoring of heparin neutralization as platelet membrane fragmentation occurs during bypass open heart surgery.[6] See Additional Information for recommendation that baseline ACTs be determined after surgical incision. **METHODOLOGY:** Tubes of freshly drawn blood (usually 1 mL) are incubated at 37°C and tilted at 30-second intervals until flow of blood stops. The tilting, detection, and recording of clotting is performed manually or by relatively low cost and compact automated devices. **Manual and even machine results are dependent upon differences in test volume, intermachine variability, agitation speed and direction, and variation in individual technique.**[7] Quality control/assurance procedures must be in place and in practice. **ADDITIONAL INFORMATION:** While this test could readily replace the Lee and White and other older clotting time tests (which are considered obsolete by many and have not been offered in some laboratories for several years), it has found its greatest application in monitoring the results of heparin anticoagulation.

(Continued)

Activated Coagulation Time *(Continued)*

A voluminous and confusing literature has developed dealing with the pitfalls of heparin anticoagulation. It has been suggested that there is no advantage in laboratory monitoring to assist heparin anticoagulation (the insensitive and unwieldy whole blood clotting time was used in the initial prospective study, however).[8] At least 12 different (some closely related) tests have been proposed to measure heparin's anticoagulant effect.[9] These include clotting time, plasma recalcification time, partial thromboplastin time, thrombin time, polybrene titration, and synthetic substrate assay tests. That such diverse tests can be applied to this task reflects heparin's multisite inhibition of the coagulation mechanism. The APTT is most commonly used. This is in part because the APTT fits into laboratory routine of performance (it is fast, semiautomated, and, therefore, lends itself to batching and performance in the laboratory). The ACT, however, is justifiably preferred by some, including in particular, the cardiovascular surgeons.[10]

The following protocol of Hattersley et al was used in a study of 134 patients with thromboembolic disorders and resulted in no heparin failures and only two cases of dangerous bleeding.[11] Heparin used: porcine gut (Liquaemin®) made up 100 units/mL in 250 mL bag; I.V. bolus 50 units/kg body weight; subsequent infusion 15-25 units/kg/hour; modification of infusion rate to maintain ACT of 150-190 seconds; ACT obtained 4 hours after start of pump infusion, 4 hours after each change of rate, and at least once/24 hours. After 2-3 days of target range ACT, oral warfarin is given 5-10 mg/day according to body weight. After 3-5 days warfarin therapy and with PT at 2 to 2.5 times control, heparin is discontinued (warfarin continued).

The importance of laboratory monitoring of heparin anticoagulation is underscored by the known considerable individual variation in response. **Dose required for adequate anticoagulation is dependent on a variety of factors including severity of thrombotic process, potential risk for bleeding, variations in the heparin preparation (polymer length, degree of sulfonation), and medications that inactivate or inhibit heparin (antihistamines, digitalis, nicotine, penicillin, tetracyclines, streptomycin, erythromycin, gentamicin, ascorbic acid, chlorpromazine, and protamine).** The ACT, while favored by cardiovascular surgeons and recently considered operationally superior to the APTT for bedside monitoring of post-PTCA patients,[12] suffers a potential drawback. It assays overall coagulation activity. Prolonged values may not be exclusively the result of heparin. There is risk in giving protamine sulfate (heparin antagonist). When the protamine exceeds the amount of heparin, it begins to act as an anticoagulant; the ACT will lack specificity in this situation. It is likely that ACT is decreased as a result of a thromboplastic response induced with the surgical incision. Thus, in order to avoid false diagnosis of adequate protamine neutralization after cardiopulmonary bypass, baseline ACT should be determined after surgical incision.[13]

Footnotes

1. Hattersley PG, "Activated Coagulation of Whole Blood," *JAMA*, 1966, 196:436-40.
2. Metz S and Keats AS, "Low Activated Coagulation Time During Cardiopulmonary Bypass Does Not Increase Postoperative Bleeding," *Ann Thorac Surg*, 1990, 49(3):440-4.
3. Rath B and Bennett DH, "Monitoring the Effect of Heparin by Measurement of Activated Clotting Time During and After Percutaneous Transluminal Coronary Angioplasty," *Br Heart J*, 1990, 63(1):18-21.
4. Triplett DA, "Heparin: Clinical Use and Laboratory Monitoring," *Laboratory Evaluation of Coagulation*, Chicago, IL: ASCP Press, 1982, 292.
5. Bode AP and Eick L, "Lysed Platelets Shorten the Activated Coagulation Time (ACT) of Heparinized Blood," *Am J Clin Pathol*, 1989, 91(4):430-4.
6. George JN, Pickett EB, Saucerman S, et al, "Studies on Resting and Activated Platelets and Platelet Membrane Microparticles in Normal Subjects, and Observations in Patients During Adult Respiratory Distress Syndrome and Cardiac Surgery," *J Clin Invest*, 1986, 78:340-8.
7. Uden DL, Payne NR, Kriesmer P, et al, "Procedural Variables Which Affect Activated Clotting Time Test Results During Extracorporeal Membrane Oxygenation Therapy," *Crit Care Med*, 1989, 17(10):1048-51.
8. Salzman EW, Deykin D, Shapiro RM, et al, "Management of Heparin Therapy: Controlled Prospective Trial," *N Engl J Med*, 1975, 292:1046-50.
9. Triplett DA, "Heparin: Clinical Use and Laboratory Monitoring," *Laboratory Evaluation of Coagulation*, Chicago, IL: ASCP Press, 1982, 291.
10. Dauchot PJ, Berzina-Moettus L, Rabinovitch A, et al, "Activated Coagulation and Activated Partial Thromboplastin Times in Assessment and Reversal of Heparin-Induced Anticoagulation for Cardiopulmonary Bypass," *Anesth Analg*, 1983, 62:710-9.
11. Hattersley PG, Mitsuoka JC, and King JH, "Heparin Therapy for Thromboembolic Disorders. A Prospective Evaluation of 134 Cases Monitored by the Activated Coagulation Time," *JAMA*, 1983, 250:1413-6.
12. Varah N, Smith J, and Baugh RF, "Heparin Monitoring in the Coronary Care Unit After Percutaneous Transluminal Coronary Angioplasty," *Heart-Lung*, 1990, 19(3):265-70.
13. Gravlee GP, Whitaker CL, Mark LJ, et al, "Baseline Activated Coagulation Time Should Be Measured After Surgical Incision," *Anesth Analg*, 1990, 71(5):549-53.

References

Gravlee GP, Haddon WS, Rothberger HK, et al, "Heparin Dosing and Monitoring for Cardiopulmonary Bypass," *J Thorac Cardiovasc Surg*, 1990, 99(3):518-27.

Activated Partial Thromboplastin Substitution Test

CPT 85732

Related Information

Partial Thromboplastin Time *on page 450*

Synonyms APTT Correction Studies; Differential APTT Test; PTT Substitution

Test Commonly Includes Correction of patient's abnormal plasma with normal aged serum, normal absorbed plasma and normal plasma

Abstract Modification of the APTT to screen for specific coagulation factor deficiencies

Specimen Plasma **CONTAINER:** Blue top (sodium citrate) tube **COLLECTION:** Routine venipuncture. If multiple tests are being drawn, draw coagulation studies last. If only coagulation tests are being drawn, use two-syringe/tube technique, draw 1-2 mL into first syringe or Vacutainer®, discard, and then collect coagulation tests. This collection procedure avoids contamination of the specimen with tissue thromboplastins. **STORAGE INSTRUCTIONS:** Keep refrigerated **CAUSES FOR REJECTION:** Tube not full, specimen hemolyzed, specimen clotted, specimen received more than 2 hours after collection **SPECIAL INSTRUCTIONS:** These substitution correction studies are not offered routinely by all clinical laboratories. Schedule and arrange with laboratory before ordering.

Interpretive **REFERENCE RANGE:** The deficient factor is indicated by the results of APTT performed on mixtures of the patient's plasma and prepared correcting reagents (aged serum or absorbed normal plasma). Normal plasma contains factors VIII, IX, X, XI, and XII. The prepared reagents are deficient as indicated in the table. A factor V deficient plasma can be prepared by adsorption with a monoclonal antibody to factor V.[1] Tabulation and analysis will indicate the presumptive deficiency causing prolongation of patient's plasma APTT. **USE:** Presumptive identification of single coagulation factor deficiencies. Confirmation of the deficient factor requires specific factor assays/comparison with plasmas with known deficiencies. **LIMITATIONS:** Only useful with single coagulation factor deficiencies. Correction reactions may be difficult to interpret if patient's APTT is only modestly prolonged. **CONTRAINDICATIONS:** Current anticoagulant therapy

Activated Partial Thromboplastin Substitution Test

Plasma Deficient in:	APTT Corrected by:			
	Normal Plasma	Aged Normal Serum	$BaSO_4$ Plasma	Celite Plasma
V	+		+	+
VIII	+		+	+
IX	+	+		+
X	+	+		+
XI	+	+	+	
XII	+	+	+	+

Footnotes

1. Katzmann JA, Nesheim ME, Hibbard LS, et al, "Isolation of Functional Human Coagulation Factor V by Using a Hybridoma Antibody," *Proc Natl Acad Sci U S A*, 1981, 78:162-6.

References

Bowie EJW and Owen CA Jr, "Clinical and Laboratory Diagnosis of Hemorrhagic Disorders," Chapter 3, *Disorders of Hemostasis*, Ratnoff OD and Forbes CD, eds, Philadelphia, PA: WB Saunders Co, 1991, 55.

Activated Partial Thromboplastin Time *see* Partial Thromboplastin Time *on page 450*

Acute Phase Reactants *see* Fibrinogen *on page 435*

Aggregometer Test *see* Platelet Aggregation *on page 459*

AHF *see* Factor VIII *on page 424*

Antiaggregating Agents *see* Partial Thromboplastin Time *on page 450*

Anticoagulant, Circulating

***CPT** 85732*

Related Information

Anticardiolipin Antibody *on page 632*
Antinuclear Antibody *on page 638*
Cryoprecipitate *on page 1058*
Factor VIII Concentrate *on page 1064*
Factor IX Complex (Human) *on page 1065*
Inhibitor, Lupus, Phospholipid Type *on page 444*
Partial Thromboplastin Time *on page 450*
VDRL, Serum *on page 762*

Synonyms CAC; Lupus Anticoagulant

Patient Care PREPARATION: Coumadin® therapy should be discontinued for 2 weeks prior to test; heparin therapy should be discontinued 2 days prior to collection of the specimen.

Specimen Plasma CONTAINER: Blue top (3.2% or 3.8% sodium citrate) tube COLLECTION: Routine clean venipuncture. If multiple tests are being drawn, draw coagulation studies last. If only circulating anticoagulant is being drawn, use two-syringe (or Vacutainer® tube) technique. Avoid contamination of specimen with tissue thromboplastin. Draw first 1-2 mL in one syringe (or tube), discard, and (without moving needle) draw specimen into second tube (or with second syringe). Use only plastic syringes. STORAGE INSTRUCTIONS: Place specimen tube on ice and transport immediately to the laboratory. CAUSES FOR REJECTION: Patient receiving Coumadin® or heparin therapy; specimen hemolyzed, clotted, diluted or contaminated; specimen not on ice or received over 1 hour after collection

Interpretive REFERENCE RANGE: No circulating anticoagulant identified. Previous prothrombin and activated partial thromboplastin times are useful in interpretation of results. USE: Detection of circulating anticoagulants as may occur in multiple-transfused, factor-deficient patients, as associated with dysproteinemias (multiple myeloma), lupus erythematosus, rheumatoid arthritis, ulcerative colitis, postpartum complication and other conditions LIMITATIONS: Accurate quantitation of inhibitor may not be possible if patient is or has been receiving replacement or anticoagulant therapy or if test is done more than 2 hours after collection. Determination of presence of inhibitor may, however, be possible in some of these situations. METHODOLOGY: Serial dilutions of patient's plasma with fresh normal plasma incubated at room temperature and at 37°C for 2 hours followed by APTT. Factor specificity can be determined by measuring the specific factor activity remaining after incubation of normal plasma and dilutions of patient plasma. (For example, incubate equal parts of normal and test plasma for 30 minutes and compare factor levels before and after incubation). ADDITIONAL INFORMATION: Acquired circulating anticoagulants are of different types (usually immunoglobulins) and occur in a variety of disorders. In classic hemophilia, factor VIII antibody (usually of IgG class) can act as a circulating anticoagulant, negating the effect of exogenously administered factor VIII. These are the most common and important of the stage I inhibitors (against factors VIII, IX, XI, or XII) occurring in 5% to 20% of factor VIII deficient patients. They are more common in severe than mild cases of hemophilia A. They apparently arise as an immune response to that part of the factor VIII molecule (VIII:C or VIII:CAg) that is decreased or absent in these patients.[1] Less commonly, they may occur spontaneously (in patients without hemophilia) in some chronic inflammatory states, collagen diseases, postpartum, and in association with some drugs and some malignancies.[2] More common are the "lupus-like" or lupus anticoagulants, one of the most common causes of prolonged APTT (in absence of liver disease) and most often found during preoperative screening. These do not appear to be directed against a specific clotting factor and usually are not associated with clinically significant bleeding.

Detection of a circulating anticoagulant depends upon finding a prolonged clotting test result which is not corrected by adding normal plasma. Such inhibitors occur in some 5% to 10% of cases of systemic lupus erythematosus but are more often found in patients with other autoimmune processes or without demonstrable associated disease. A 32% incidence of this inhibitor has been reported in patients on long-term phenothiazine therapy.[3] Patients with lupus anticoagulant have a high incidence of positive ANA tests and may have a false-positive serology for syphilis. Lupus anticoagulant may appear as part of the procainamide-induced lupus syndrome. Patients with lupus anticoagulant often have prolonged prothrombin time, occasionally severe, due to associated deficiency of prothrombin activity. Of most importance clinically is that many patients (25% to 30%) with lupus "anticoagulant" have thromboembolism.[4] Cerebral ischemic episodes may be the result of cardioembolism occurring in patients who have a circulating lupus anticoagulant.[5] There is evidence that immunoadsorption (using extracorporeal staphylococcal protein A columns in hemophiliac patients) removes coagulation factor inhibitors and may allow successful factor replacement therapy.[6] Incubation with protein A bound to Sepharose (which removes IgG) has been used to show that a patient with acquired deficiency of both factor VII activity and antigen was likely the result of an IgG able to bind factor VII without neutralizing its activity. The bound immunoglobulin is hypothesized to have induced rapid plasma clearance of the factor VII molecule or to have modified its synthesis.[7]

Clinically significant inhibitors of factor XIII (eg, inhibitor New Haven) have been described.[8]

Footnotes

1. White GC II, McMillan CW, Blatt PM, et al, "Factor VIII Inhibitors: A Clinical Overview," *Am J Hematol*, 1982, 13:335-42.
2. Kessler CM, "An Introduction to Factor VIII Inhibitors: The Detection and Quantitation," *Am J Med*, 1991, 91(5A):1S-5S.
3. Canoso RT, Hutton RA, and Deykin D, "A Chlorpromazine-Induced Inhibitor of Blood Coagulation," *Am J Hematol*, 1977, 2:183-91.
4. Carreras LO, Defreyn G, Machin SJ, et al, "Arterial Thrombosis, Intrauterine Death, and "Lupus" Anticoagulant: Detection of Immunoglobulin Interfering With Prostacyclin Formation," *Lancet*, 1981, 1:244-6.
5. Young SM, Fisher M, Sigsbee A, et al, "Cardiogenic Brain Embolism and Lupus Anticoagulant," *Ann Neurol*, 1989, 26(3):390-2.
6. Uehlinger J, Button GR, McCarthy J, et al, "Immunoadsorption for Coagulation Factor Inhibitors," *Transfusion*, 1991, 31(3):265-9.
7. Weisdorf D, Hasegawa D, and Fair DS, "Acquired Factor VII Deficiency Associated With Aplastic Anemia: Correction with Bone Marrow Transplantation," *Br J Haematol*, 1989, 71(3):409-13.
8. Fukue H, Anderson K, McPhedran P, et al, "A Unique Factor XIII Inhibitor to a Fibrin-Binding Site on Factor XIIIA," *Blood*, 1992, 79(1):65-74.

References

Feinstein DI, "Acquired Inhibitors Against Factor VIII and Other Clotting Proteins," *Hemostasis and Thrombosis: Basic Principles and Clinical Practice*, Colman RW, Hirsh J, Marder VJ, et al, eds, Philadelphia, PA: JB Lippincott Co, 1982, 563-76.

Kaczor DA, Bickford NN, and Triplett DA, "Evaluation of Different Mixing Study Reagents and Dilution Effect in Lupus Anticoagulant Testing," *Am J Clin Pathol*, 1991, 95(3):408-11.

Kasper CK, "Treatment of Factor VIII Inhibitors," *Prog Hemost Thromb*, 1989, 9:57-86.

Antihemophilic Factor *see* Factor VIII *on page 424*

Antiphospholipid Antibody *see* Inhibitor, Lupus, Phospholipid Type *on page 444*

α_2-Antiplasmin *see* Plasminogen Assay *on page 457*

Antithrombin III Assay, Functional AT III *see* Antithrombin III Test *on this page*

Antithrombin III Test

***CPT** 85300 (activity); 85301 (antigen assay)*

Related Information

Activated Coagulation Time *on page 399*
Hypercoagulable State Coagulation Screen *on page 441*
Partial Thromboplastin Time *on page 450*
Platelet Aggregation, Hypercoagulable State *on page 461*
Prothrombin Fragment 1.2 *on page 467*

Synonyms Antithrombin III Assay, Functional AT III; Heparin Cofactor Activity; Immunologic Antithrombin III; Serine Protease Inhibitor

Abstract Test for antithrombin III level with applicability to testing for thromboembolic disease states.

Specimen Plasma **CONTAINER:** Two blue top (sodium citrate) tubes **COLLECTION:** Routine venipuncture. If multiple tests are being drawn, draw AT III with coagulation studies, last. If only antithrombin III is being drawn, draw 1-2 mL in another Vacutainer®, discard, and draw specimen into second tube (with citrate anticoagulant) avoiding contamination with tissue thromboplastin. Immediately invert gently at least five times, mixing thoroughly. Avoid excessively vigorous mixing. Tubes must be sufficiently full (eg, 4.5 mL blood added to 0.5 mL of liquid citrate anticoagulant). Place tubes on ice and deliver immediately to the laboratory. **STORAGE INSTRUCTIONS:** Separate plasma and keep refrigerated; deliver refrigerated specimen for testing within 2 hours. **CAUSES FOR REJECTION:** Specimen received more than 2 hours after collection,

(Continued)

Antithrombin III Test *(Continued)*

specimen not refrigerated, citrate tubes insufficiently filled, tubes not labeled, clotted specimens, specimen contaminated with heparin (as with heparin flush procedures) **TURNAROUND TIME:** 2-4 hours

Interpretive **REFERENCE RANGE:** 17-30 mg/dL (SI: 170-300 mg/L); 80% to 120% of normal activity, considerable method dependent variation. AT III is lower in serum than in plasma when using the thrombin neutralization test (some antithrombin is consumed when blood clots). Healthy premature infants at birth have decreased AT III, heparin cofactor II, protein C and protein S inhibitor levels, approximately 50% below normal adult values. With the exception of protein C and protein S, values have risen to those of normal adults by 6 months of age. Spontaneous hemorrhage or thromboses do not develop in healthy prematures, however, because of a balance that is maintained between procoagulants and inhibitors (see following references by Andrew et al). Potentially fatal hemorrhagic and thrombotic complications occur in sick (eg, respiratory distress, necrotizing enterocolitis, sepsis) prematures. There may be DIC, severe AT III deficiency, and/or dysfunctional AT III (see following references by Andrew et al and by Manco-Johnson). **USE:** Evaluate hypercoagulable state, fibrinogenolytic state, and response to heparin. Test for the hereditary deficiency of antithrombin III (autosomal dominant) which is characterized by predisposition to thrombosis. Acquired deficiency associated with severe cirrhosis, chronic liver failure, DIC, thrombolytic therapy, pulmonary embolism, nephrotic syndrome, or postsurgical state (especially liver transplant or partial hepatectomy). Also used to evaluate decreased synthesis or increased loss/consumption. Changes induced by drugs must be considered. Antithrombin III levels might also be of use in cases of suspected heparin failure, suspected DIC, or personal or familial history of thromboembolic disease. The test is indicated in the latter cases especially prior to heparinization, general or orthopedic surgery, prolonged bedrest, pregnancy, postpartum, or postoperative state or oral contraceptive use. AT III deficiency has been found **not** to be an inherent feature of SLE.[1] See table. **LIMITATIONS:** Test may measure functional or immunologic levels only. The functional anticoagulant effect may be variable. Presence of additional "antithrombins" (distinct from AT III, in particular heparin cofactor II) may contribute to functional "AT III" activity as determined variously by different clinical assays complicating their interpretation and comparability.[2] Antithrombin III activity may be decreased due to oral contraceptive use in women, in the third trimester of pregnancy, and in blood type O women taking high estrogen dose contraceptive preparations.[3] If specimen contains heparin (as with specimen drawn after heparin flush or patient receiving heparin), results may be erroneous. Patients receiving coumarin type anticoagulants may have increased AT III levels. **METHODOLOGY:** The numerous available methods (see references) fall into either functional (ie, thrombin neutralization, von Kaulla chromogenic/fluorogenic synthetic substrate) or immunologic based (ie, radial immunodiffusion (RID), electroimmunoassay, radioimmunoassay (RIA), enzyme-linked immunosorbent assay (ELISA)) groups. While RIA and ELISA methods are sensitive, they may give unreliable, misleading results in cases of inherited deficiency due to a functionally abnormal but antigenically nearly normal molecule. Increased heparin cofactor II in patients with type I diabetes and possibly in other clinical situations may lead to overestimation of functionally active AT III by the thrombin inhibition assay. Use of a factor Xa inhibition assay for functionally active AT III has been shown to give results similar to an immunoreactive method.[4] Synthetic chromogenic substrate-based methodology may now be considered the method of choice for determination of AT III activity.[5] **ADDITIONAL INFORMATION:** Antithrombin III has been shown to inhibit the activity of activated factors XII, XI, IX and X, as well as, II (thrombin). Antithrombin III is the main physiologic inhibitor of serine proteases generated during coagulation, in particular factor Xa, where it appears to exert its most critical effect. AT III is a "heparin cofactor." Heparin interacts with AT III and thrombin, increasing the rate of thrombin neutralization (inhibition) but decreasing the total quantity (of thrombin) inhibited. The understanding of "antithrombins" began in the early 1900s, is colorful as well as complex, and is still incomplete.[2] Two protein fractions were separated in 1974 and designated heparin cofactors A and B.[6] Heparin cofactor A (HC A) has an absolute requirement for heparin and did not inhibit activated factor X. AT III (heparin cofactor B) which neu-

Antithrombin III Levels

Increased With	Decreased With
Elevated ESR	Use of oral contraceptives
Elevated CRP	Pulmonary embolism
Hyperglobulinemia	Acute myocardial infarction
Coumarin type anticoagulation	Intravascular coagulation
	Thrombophlebitis
	Neoplastic disease of the liver

tralizes both thrombin and factor Xa was characterized and studied to the exclusion of HC A. An inhibitor (of thrombin) distinct from AT III has been purified,[7,8] partially sequenced, and designated heparin cofactor II (HC II). HC II has, essentially, the properties of HC A, is structurally similar to but different from AT III.[9] AT III and heparin, each alone or together, inhibit both the classical and alternative pathways of complement. AT III may act as a serine protease inhibitor of enzymatic stages of the complement system.[10]

Patients with low AT III levels usually exhibit some degree of resistance to heparin anticoagulation. AT III deficiency affects 1/2000 of the general population; 40% to 70% of these become symptomatic (experience thrombosis). Only some 2% to 3% of hospitalized patients with recurrent or extensive thrombosis have AT III deficiency.[5] In the more common forms of AT III deficiency, genetic molecular heterogeneity has been shown by the application of recombinant DNA techniques for molecular analysis.[11] Decrease in AT III may be associated with tendency to thrombosis with seemingly minor trauma in early adult years.

Thrombotic symptoms in cases of hereditary deficiency of antithrombin III have been reported with levels ranging from 40% to 60% of normal. Clinical picture of AT III deficiency may be similar to that of protein C deficiency.[12] Individuals with antithrombin III deficiency will show resistance to anticoagulation with heparin but can be anticoagulated with coumarin derivatives, in which case antithrombin III levels have been shown to rise. Antithrombin III levels may be decreased in women during hormonal contraceptive therapy. A significant number of patients with mesenteric venous thrombosis may have AT III deficiency. It has been recommended that patients with such thrombotic disease be screened for AT III levels to identify those patients that may benefit from coumarin anticoagulant prophylaxis.[13]

Synthetic nucleotides have been developed and applied to the analysis of AT III variants, AT III Northwick Park and AT III Glasgow. Inheritance of these variants is associated with thrombosis. Oligonucleotides, used as specific hybridization probes, have shown that these AT III variants result from a single base substitution that causes an amino acid substitution at Arg 393. Such nucleotide probe procedures could provide for early detection of AT III variants.[14]

Footnotes

1. Jarrett MP, Green D, and Ts'ao CH, "Relation Between Antithrombin III and Clinical and Serologic Parameters in Systemic Lupus Erythematosus," *J Clin Pathol*, 1983, 36:357-60.
2. Brandt JT, "The Role of Natural Coagulation Inhibitors in Hemostasis," *Clin Lab Med*, 1984, 4:247.
3. Burkman RT, Bell WR, Zacur HA, et al, "Oral Contraceptives and Antithrombin III: Variations by Dosage and ABO Blood Group," *Am J Obstet Gynecol*, 1991, 164(6 Pt 1):1453-8.
4. Gram J and Jespersen J, "Increased Concentrations of Heparin Cofactor II in Diabetic Patients, and Possible Effects on Thrombin Inhibition Assay of Antithrombin III," *Clin Chem*, 1989, 35(1):52-5.
5. Bick RL, *Disorders of Thrombosis and Hemostasis: Clinical and Laboratory Practice*, Chicago, IL, ASCP Press, 1992, 270.
6. Briginshaw GF and Shanberge JN, "Identification of Two Distinct Heparin Cofactors in Human Plasma: II. Inhibition of Thrombin and Activated Factor X." *Thromb Res*, 1974, 4:463-77.
7. Tollefsen DM and Blank MK, "Detection of a New Heparin-Dependent Inhibitor of Thrombin in Human Plasma," *J Clin Invest*, 1981, 68:589-96.
8. Tollefsen DM, Majerus DW, and Blank MK, "Heparin Cofactor II: Purification and Properties of a Heparin-Dependent Inhibitor of Thrombin in Human Plasma," *J Biol Chem*, 1982, 257:2162-9.
9. Griffith MJ, Noyes CM, and Church FC, "Reactive Site Peptide Structural Similarity Between Heparin Cofactor II and Antithrombin III," *J Biol Chem*, 1985, 260:2218-25.
10. Weiler JM and Linhardt RJ, "Antithrombin III Regulates Complement Activity *In Vitro*," *J Immunol*, 1991, 146(11):3889-94.
11. Prochownik EV, Antonarakis SE, Bauer KA, et al, "Molecular Heterogeneity of Inherited Antithrombin III Deficiency," *N Engl J Med*, 1983, 308:1549-52.
12. Broekmans AW, Veltkamp MD, and Bertina RM, "Congenital Protein C Deficiency and Venous Thromboembolism. A Study of Three Dutch Families," *N Engl J Med*, 1983, 309:340-4.
13. Wilson C, Walker ID, Davidson JF, et al, "Mesenteric Venous Thrombosis and Antithrombin III Deficiency," *J Clin Pathol*, 1987, 40:906-8.
14. Thein SL and Lane DA, "Use of Synthetic Oligonucleotides in the Characterization of Antithrombin III Northwick Park (393 CGT-TGT), and Antithrombin III Glasgow (393 CGT-CAT)," *Blood*, 1988, 72(5):1817-21.

References

Andrew M, Massicotte-Nolan P, Mitchell L, et al, "Dysfunctional Antithrombin III in Sick Premature Infants," *Pediatr Res*, 1985, 19:237-9.

Andrew M, Paes B, Milner R, et al, "Development of the Human Coagulation System in the Healthy Premature Infant," *Blood*, 1988, 72:1651-7.

Andrew M, Vegh P, Johnston M, et al, "Maturation of the Hemostatic System During Childhood," *Blood*, 1992, 80(8):1998-2005.

Bauer KA and Rosenberg RD, "Role of Antithrombin III as a Regulator of *In Vivo* Coagulation," *Semin Hematol*, 1991, 28(1):10-8.

(Continued)

Antithrombin III Test *(Continued)*

Blajchman MA, Austin RC, Fernandez-Rachubinski F, et al, "Molecular Basis of Inherited Human Antithrombin Deficiency," *Blood*, 1992, 80(9):2159-71.
Brandt JT and Ezenagu L, "Heparin Cofactor II, Thrombosis and Hemostasis," *ASCP Check Sample®*, Chicago, IL: American Society of Clinical Pathologists, 1987.
Buller HR and ten Cate JW, "Acquired Antithrombin III Deficiency: Laboratory Diagnosis, Incidence, Clinical Implications, and Treatment With Antithrombin III Concentrate," *Am J Med*, 1989, 87(3B):44S-48S.
Chuansumrit A, Manco-Johnson MJ, and Hathaway WE, "Heparin Cofactor II in Adults and Infants With Thrombosis and DIC," *Am J Hematol*, 1989, 31(2):109-13.
Conrad J, "Automation of Antithrombin III Methods on Routinely Available Instruments," *Semin Thromb Hemost*, 1983, 263-7.
Demers C, Ginsberg JS, Hirsh J, et al, "Thrombosis in Antithrombin-III-Deficient Persons: Report of a Large Kindred and Literature Review," *Ann Intern Med*, 1992, 116(9):754-61.
Edgar P, Jennings I, and Harper P, "Enzyme Linked Immunosorbent Assay for Measuring Antithrombin III," *J Clin Pathol*, 1989, 42(9):985-7.
Hathaway WE, "Clinical Aspects of Antithrombin III Deficiency," *Semin Hematol*, 1991, 28(1):19-23.
Manco-Johnson MJ, "Neonatal Antithrombin III Deficiency," *Am J Med*, 1989, 87(3B):49S-52S.
Menache D, "Antithrombin III: Biochemistry, Physiology, and Management of Patients With Hereditary Deficiency," *Semin Hematol*, 1991, 28:1-54.
Owen MC, Borg JY, and Carrell RW, "Antithrombin III Rouen-I (47 Arg to his) and (47 ser). Two New Variants With Decreased Heparin Affinity," *N Z Med J*, 1987, 100:566-7.
Rosenberg RD, "Role of Antithrombin III in Coagulation Disorders: State-of-the-Art Review," *Am J Med*, 1989, 87(3B):1S-67S.
Vinazzer H, "Therapeutic Use of Antithrombin III in Shock and Disseminated Intravascular Coagulation," *Semin Thromb Hemost*, 1989, 15(3):347-52.

APTT *see* Partial Thromboplastin Time *on page 450*

APTT Correction Studies *see* Activated Partial Thromboplastin Substitution Test *on page 401*

ASA Tolerance Test *see* Aspirin Tolerance Test *on this page*

Aspirin Tolerance Test

CPT 85999

Related Information

Bleeding Time, Duke *on page 408*
Bleeding Time, Ivy *on page 409*
von Willebrand Factor Antigen *on page 476*

Synonyms ASA Tolerance Test; Bleeding Time Aspirin Tolerance Test; Tolerance Test for Aspirin

Test Commonly Includes Bleeding time measurement before and after ingestion of aspirin

Patient Care PREPARATION: Patient must not have consumed aspirin (acetylsalicylic acid) or aspirin-containing preparations for the 10 days prior to testing. In adults, 10 grains (600 mg) of acetylsalicylic acid are given after the initial bleeding time has been performed. In children weighing less than 70 pounds, the dose of aspirin is 5 grains.

Specimen Blood; an *in vivo* test performed directly on the patient COLLECTION: Test is performed at patient's bedside by medical technologist. CAUSES FOR REJECTION: History of aspirin intake, presence of known abnormal bleeding time possibly due to abnormality of capillary vasculature

Interpretive REFERENCE RANGE: Test is to assess the degree of change that can be detected (using the bleeding time procedure) as a result of aspirin ingestion. The bleeding time will usually be prolonged by 2-3 minutes. If a vascular or platelet function defect is present or if the subject is a hyper-responder, there may be greater prolongation of the bleeding time after aspirin ingestion. USE: Assess the magnitude of aspirin effect on the bleeding time as an indirect reflection of the effect on platelet function; identify aspirin hyper-responders; may serve as a provocative test for von Willebrand's disease LIMITATIONS: Invalid if previous aspirin ingestion has occurred CONTRAINDICATIONS: Previous aspirin ingestion; markedly prolonged bleeding time before aspirin ingestion METHODOLOGY: A bleeding time test (preferably Mielke, template bleeding time) is performed before the patient ingests 600 mg of aspirin; 2 hours later the bleeding time is repeated using the opposite arm.[1] ADDITIONAL INFORMATION: There is evidence that some 15% of individuals may be aspirin "hyper-responders". These subjects are characterized by prolongation of over 5.9 minutes above normal baseline when the template bleeding time is determined 7 hours after a single 325 mg dose of aspirin is given.[2] An *in vitro* bleeding time test device and procedure have been described and applied to the detection of aspirin effect.[1] The device consists of a conical tube with a coated membrane covered window in which a slit has been placed. The nylon membrane is coated with collagen types I and III, factor VIII – von Willebrand's factor and fibronectin and then dried. A second square of nylon membrane is applied, dried, $CaCl_2$-$MgCl_2$ solution added and dried. This is the "subendothelial membrane." The conical-shaped tube is prepared from polyethylene tubing, a bulge produced, and a window cut into the tube. The membrane is then glued, coated side on the inside over the window. Within run precision had a coefficient of variation of 17%. Normal bleeding time by this method was less than 1 minute, postaspirin bleeding times were more than 7 minutes. The study group consisted, however, of only eight individuals.[3]

Footnotes

1. Bick RL, Adams T, and Schmalhorst WR, "Bleeding Times, Platelet Adhesion, and Aspirin," *Am J Clin Pathol*, 1976, 65:69-72.
2. Fiore LD, Brophy MT, Lopez A, et al, "The Bleeding Time Response to Aspirin. Identifying the Hyperresponder," *Am J Clin Pathol*, 1990, 94(3):292-6.
3. Brubaker DB, "An *In Vitro* Bleeding Time Test," *Am J Clin Pathol*, 1989, 91(4):422-9.

References

Mielke CH Jr, "Aspirin Prolongation of the Template Bleeding Time: Influence of Venostasis and Direction of Incision," *Blood*, 1982, 60:1134-42.

Autoprothrombin I *see* Factor VII *on page 422*

Autoprothrombin II *see* Factor IX *on page 426*

Beta-Thromboglobulin

CPT *85999*

Related Information

Fibrinopeptide A *on page 437*
Hypercoagulable State Coagulation Screen *on page 441*
Intravascular Coagulation Screen *on page 446*

Synonyms βTG; β-TG; β-Thromboglobulin

Abstract Beta-thromboglobulin (βTG) is a platelet α granule polypeptide protein formed of 81 amino acids. It is a marker of platelet activation applicable to the study of both prothrombotic states (hypercoagulability) and disseminated intravascular coagulation (DIC).

Specimen Blood or urine **CONTAINER:** Special siliconized tube containing EDTA, prostaglandin E_1, and theophylline must be used in order to stabilize platelets so that βTG will not be released during preparation of platelet-poor plasma.[1] **COLLECTION:** Blood should be harvested from a carefully performed clean venipuncture using a "two-tube" (or two-syringe) technique. The first 2-5 mL of blood (first tube) is discarded. The following 2.5 mL of blood is collected in special βTG assay tubes (see above under container), usually supplied by the manufacturer. Specimen must be transported on ice. **STORAGE INSTRUCTIONS:** Whole blood may be stored at 0°C to 4°C for up to 72 hours before processing. Platelet-poor plasma should be prepared from whole blood using a refrigerated centrifuge. **CAUSES FOR REJECTION:** Specimen improperly collected, specimen clotted, specimen not submitted in special βTG assay tubes or not submitted on ice **SPECIAL INSTRUCTIONS:** This test will most commonly be performed by a referral or research laboratory. Platelet-poor plasma should be prepared from whole blood using a refrigerated centrifuge (0°C to 4°C), centrifugation at 1900 g for 60 minutes. This will reduce the amount of βTG released from platelets during preparation to a minimum so that the plasma concentration will more closely reflect the true circulating level *in vivo*.[1]

Interpretive **REFERENCE RANGE:** 10-50 ng/mL **USE:** Differentiate DIC from primary lysis (βTG is elevated in the former); assess platelet hyperreactivity as in hypercoagulable states; studies of the prothrombotic state and of the effects of thrombolytic regimens in vascular occlusive disease,[2] heart failure,[3] coronary atherosclerosis,[4] inflammatory bowel disease,[5] and chronic uremia,[6] including diabetic nephropathy.[7] Urine, as well as plasma, levels of βTG were increased in patients with diabetic nephropathy. It was considered that the study of urine levels were less subject to methodological error.[7] **LIMITATIONS:** Dependent upon method of analysis, in particular specimen handling/processing, plasma levels of βTG may be artifactually increased due to platelet activation *in vitro*. Study of the ratio of plasma beta-thromboglobulin to plasma platelet factor 4 may allow distinction between *in vivo* and artifactual *in vitro* release.[8] **METHODOLOGY:** Radioimmunoassay (RIA), enzyme-linked immunosorbent assay (ELISA), procedure and reagents are commercially available **ADDITIONAL INFORMATION:** Beta-

(Continued)

Beta-Thromboglobulin *(Continued)*

thromboglobulin (βTG) is a platelet-secreted protein, with a molecular weight of 8800 daltons. It is present exclusively in megakaryocytes and in the α granules of platelets. βTG has a primary structure similar to platelet factor 4 (PF4). Platelet basic protein, another resident of α granules, is the apparent precursor for both βTG and PT4. βTG is a fibroblast chemoattractant and as such is involved in inflammatory reactions. Plasma βTG levels provide a specific marker of the *in vivo* platelet release reaction and are thus indicative of platelet activation.[2] Such activation may occur upon interaction of platelets with subendothelial collagen, or by the action of thrombin, ADP, or catecholamines. There is evidence that platelets from elderly individuals have increased levels of βTG.[9] Presence of a circadian rhythm of plasma βTG has been reported.[10]

Footnotes

1. Ludlam CA and Cash JD, "Studies on the Liberation of β-Thromboglobulin From Human Platelets *In Vitro*," *Br J Haematol*, 1976, 33:239-47.
2. Lonsdale RJ, Heptinstall S, Westby JC, et al, "A Study of the Use of the Thromboxane A_2 Antagonist, Sulotroban, in Combination With Streptokinase for Local Thrombolysis in Patients With Recent Peripheral Arterial Occlusions: Clinical Effects, Platelet Function, and Fibrinolytic Parameters," *Thromb Haemost*, 1993, 69(2):103-11.
3. Jafri SM, Ozawa T, Mammen E, et al, "Platelet Function, Thrombin and Fibrinolytic Activity in Patients With Heart Failure," *Eur Heart J*, 1993, 14:205-12.
4. Nilsson J, Volk-Jovinge S, Svensson J, et al, "Association Between High Levels of Growth Factors in Plasma and Progression of Coronary Atherosclerosis," *J Intern Med*, 1992, 232(5):397-404.
5. Webberley MJ, Hart MT, and Melikian V, "Thromboembolism in Inflammatory Bowel Disease: Role of Platelets," *Gut*, 1993, 34:247-51.
6. Sagripanti A, Cupisti A, Baicchi U, et al, "Plasma Parameters of the Prothrombotic State in Chronic Uremia," *Nephron*, 1993, 63(3):273-8.
7. Tóth L, Szénási P, Varsányi MN, et al, "Elevated Levels of Plasma and Urine Beta-Thromboglobulin or Thromboxane-B_2 as Markers of Real Platelet Hyperactivation in Diabetic Nephropathy," *Haemostasis*, 1992, 22(6):334-9.
8. Kaplan KL and Owen J, "Plasma Levels of β-Thromboglobulin and Platelet Factor 4 as Indices of Platelet Activation *In Vivo*," *Blood*, 1981, 57(2):199-202.
9. Abbate R, Prisco D, Rostagno C, et al, "Age-Related Changes in the Hemostatic System," *Int J Clin Lab Res*, 1993, 23(1):1-3, (editorial).
10. Stubbs F, "Circadian Rhythm of Plasma Beta-Thromboglobulin in Healthy Human Subjects," *Blood Coagul Fibrinolysis*, 1992, 3(4):497.

References

Brozović M and Mackie I, "Investigation of Thrombotic Tendency," *Practical Haematology*, 7th ed, Chapter 20, Dacie JV and Lewis SM, eds, New York, NY: Churchill Livingstone, 1991, 328-9.

Kerry PJ and Curtis AD, "Standardization of β-Thromboglobulin (β-TG) and Platelet Factor 4 (PF4): A Collaborative Study to Establish International Standards for β-TG and PF4," *Thromb Haemost*, 1985, 53:51-5.

Miller MD and Krangel MS, "Biology and Biochemistry of the Chemokines: A Family of Chemotactic and Inflammatory Cytokines," *Crit Rev Immunol*, 1992, 12(1-2):17-46.

Bleeding Time *see* Bleeding Time, Duke *on this page*

Bleeding Time Aspirin Tolerance Test *see* Aspirin Tolerance Test *on page 406*

Bleeding Time, Duke

CPT 85002

Related Information

Aspirin Tolerance Test *on page 406*
Bleeding Time, Ivy *on next page*
Bleeding Time, Mielke *on page 411*

Synonyms Bleeding Time

Abstract An *in vivo* screening test, largely of historic interest, for platelet and capillary function.

Specimen Blood; an *in vivo* test performed directly on the patient **CONTAINER:** Filter paper **CAUSES FOR REJECTION:** Low platelet count **TURNAROUND TIME:** Same day, usually within minutes or hours

Interpretive **REFERENCE RANGE:** 5 minutes; there is marked variation between laboratories in reported bleeding times performed on normal subjects.[1] As a corollary, each laboratory should have established its own normal range. **USE:** Evaluate platelet function **LIMITATIONS:** Not as sensitive as bleeding time, Ivy template **METHODOLOGY:** Ear lobe (after cleansing with 70% alcohol and allowing to dry) is punctured with a sterile lancet. Duration of flow of blood is timed (beginning with time of puncture and ending when flow stops). Filter paper is used to blot the drops of blood (must be done without touching skin or disturbing clot) at 15- to 30-second intervals. An *in vitro* bleeding time test device and procedure has been described. See Aspirin Tolerance Test. **ADDITIONAL INFORMATION:** Use is recommended only under special circumstances. Most laboratories no longer perform this test. The Ivy template bleeding time is a more standardized measure of the bleeding time. It is recommended in place of the Duke bleeding time except under unusual circumstances, such as bilateral arm casts. Test should be performed no sooner than 1 week after last dose of aspirin-containing medication.

Footnotes

1. Poller L, Thomson JM, and Tomenson JA, "The Bleeding Time: Current Practice in the UK," *Clin Lab Haematol*, 1984, 6:369-73.

References

Duke WW, "The Relation of Blood Platelets to Hemorrhagic Disease: Description of a Method for Determining the Bleeding Time and Coagulation Time and Report of Three Cases of Hemorrhagic Disease Relieved by Transfusion," *JAMA*, 1910, 55:1185-92.

Machin SJ, Preston E, and BSCH Haemostasis and Thrombosis Task Force of the British Society for Haematology, "Guidelines on Platelet Function Testing," *J Clin Pathol*, 1988, 41:1322-30.

Bleeding Time, Ivy

***CPT** 85002*

Related Information

Aspirin Tolerance Test *on page 406*
Bleeding Time, Duke *on previous page*
Bleeding Time, Mielke *on page 411*
Clot Retraction *on page 413*
Platelet Adhesion Test *on page 458*
Platelet Aggregation *on page 459*
von Willebrand Factor Antigen *on page 476*

Synonyms Ivy Bleeding Time

Abstract An *in vivo* functional test for platelet and capillary function

Patient Care **PREPARATION:** The skin of the volar surface of patient's forearm is prepared with alcohol wash and allowed to dry. **AFTERCARE:** If brisk bleeding has occurred (as with puncturing a vein) or if bleeding is prolonged, a pressure bandage should be placed over the puncture site.

Specimen Blood; an *in vivo* test performed directly on patient **CONTAINER:** Filter paper **COLLECTION:** Performed at bedside by a medical technologist. **CAUSES FOR REJECTION:** If the patient needs to be restrained, has excessively cold or edematous arms, or cannot have blood pressure cuff placed on either arm (as with casts, dressings, infection, or extensive rash). History of keloid formation. Some laboratories may require that patient or guardian signs informed consent. **TURNAROUND TIME:** Same day, usually within minutes or hours

Interpretive **REFERENCE RANGE:** 2-7 minutes, shorter in men than women, shorter in those over 50 years of age **POSSIBLE PANIC RANGE:** Greater than 12-15 minutes **USE:** A screening test used to assess capillary function, platelet number and function, and ability of platelets to adhere to vessel wall and form a plug. See reference by Burns and Lawrence for a comprehensive assessment of clinical utility. Useful in evaluation of ecchymosis, spontaneous bruising and bleeding, bleeding tendency. Prolonged in some patients after aspirin ingestion, in qualitative platelet disorders (eg, von Willebrand's disease, Bernard-Soulier syndrome, Glanzmann's thrombasthenia, and the "gray platelet syndrome"), with fibrinogen disorders, macroglobulinemia, some cases of myeloproliferative disease, renal failure, and with abnormalities of blood vessels. There is inconclusive evidence that the bleeding time is a good predictor of operative hemorrhage in patients with a negative history of bleeding diathesis. **LIMITATIONS:** Scarring of skin may occur. Patients with low platelet count ($<100,000/mm^3$) and some patients on aspirin therapy may have prolongation of the bleeding time. **CONTRAINDICATIONS:** Low platelet count ($<50,000/mm^3$); patient receiving medication containing aspirin; patient with established severe bleeding diathesis; patient with infectious disease of skin or taking any drug with acetyl groups; senile skin changes; prior history of keloid formation **METHODOLOGY:** A blood pressure cuff, placed on the arm above the elbow, is inflated and adjusted to 40 mm Hg. After the alcohol-cleansed puncture site has dried, the skin is held taut and two approximately 3 mm deep puncture wounds (test is performed in duplicate) are made in the volar skin of patient's forearm, immediately after which a stopwatch is started. Superficial veins should be avoided. At 30-second intervals the drops of blood are blotted using filter paper. When the flow of blood

(Continued)

Bleeding Time, Ivy *(Continued)*

ceases, the stop watch is triggered off. The classical Ivy bleeding time suffers from poor reproducibility. The test depends importantly on the ability to produce a uniform precise incision (freehand in the Ivy method). Characteristics of the incision may vary with the technologist, as well as, the site chosen for the test and the direction of the puncture wound. The use of template methods may not increase sensitivity or reproducibility (precision).[1] See listing, Bleeding Time, Mielke. Commercial versions with disposable equipment are available. A comparison of two such commercial adaptations have shown that the devices are fairly comparable, with some evidence that the horizontal incision may be more sensitive in detection of primary hemostasis.[2] There are compelling operational and practical reasons for preferring the Mielke (template) bleeding time over the nonstandardized Ivy bleeding time and for producing vertical (cephalocaudal, elbow to wrist) rather than horizontal cuts.[3] An *in vitro* bleeding time device and procedure has been described. See Aspirin Tolerance Test. **ADDITIONAL INFORMATION:** Test should be performed no sooner than 1 week after last dose of medication containing aspirin. Low platelet count or aspirin therapy will prolong the bleeding time. It may be prolonged in patients with senile skin changes in the presence of normal platelet function. Bleeding time is prolonged in both constitutional and acquired forms of von Willebrand's syndrome. The latter may relate to presence of dysproteinemia associated with lymphoproliferative disease.[4] There may be prolonged bleeding time in some patients with advanced renal failure who, however, have largely intact measurable parameters of platelet function.[5]

Either intravenous or subcutaneous administration of 1-deamino-8-D-arginine vasopressin (DDAVP®) has been shown to shorten the bleeding time in patients with uremia.[6]

The bleeding time may find application as a marker of thrombolytic activity in patients treated with streptokinase for deep vein thrombosis.[7] Oral administration of conjugated estrogens appears to decrease the bleeding time and improves clinical bleeding in patients with renal failure.[8]

Gray platelet syndrome is a rare autosomal recessive inherited isolated deficiency of platelet alpha granule content. It is associated with modest prolongation of the bleeding time, large degranulated (pale gray) platelets on the peripheral blood smear, increased plasma beta-thromboglobulin, decreased platelet factor 4, and decreased platelet aggregation with epinephrine, ADP, thrombin and collagen. Aggregation with ristocetin is normal.[9] Alpha granule depletion has also been reported with cardiopulmonary bypass[10] and as an *in vitro* artifact caused by EDTA-dependent platelet agglutinin.[11]

A current study found prolonged Ivy bleeding time in 33% of women with severe preeclampsia. Most of these subjects had an adequate number of platelets (>100,000/mm^3).Correlation of bleeding time with platelet count occurred only with platelet counts <100,000/mm^3.[12]

There is evidence that platelet storage pool deficiency may present with a prolonged bleeding time but without platelet aggregation abnormalities. Thus, storage pool deficiency enters into the differential consideration in all patients with unexplained prolongation of the bleeding time.[13]

Footnotes

1. Koster T, Caekebeke-Peerlinck KMJ, and Briet E, "A Randomized and Blinded Comparison of the Sensitivity and the Reproducibility of the Ivy and Simplate® II Bleeding Time Techniques," *Am J Clin Pathol*, 1989, 92(3):315-20.
2. Buchanan GR and Holtkamp CA, "A Comparative Study of Variables Affecting the Bleeding Time Using Two Disposable Devices," *Am J Clin Pathol*, 1989, 91(1):45-51.
3. Bick RL, *Disorders of Thrombosis and Hemostasis: Clinical and Laboratory Practice*, Chicago, IL: ASCP Press, 1992, 44.
4. Gan TE, Sawers RJ, and Koutts J, "Pathogenesis of Antibody-Induced Acquired von Willebrand Syndrome," *Am J Hematol*, 1980, 9:363-71.
5. Gordge MP, Faint RW, Rylance PB, et al, "Platelet Function and the Bleeding Time in Progressive Renal Failure," *Thromb Haemost*, 1988, 60:83-7.
6. Vigano GL, Mannucci M, Lattuada A, et al, "Subcutaneous Desmopressin (DDAVP®) Shortens the Bleeding Time in Uremia," *Am J Hematol*, 1989, 31(1):32-5.
7. Hirsch DR, Reis SE, Polak JF, et al, "Prolonged Bleeding Time as a Marker of Venous Clot Lysis During Streptokinase Therapy," *Am Heart J*, 1991, 122(4 Pt 1):965-71.
8. Shemin D, Elnour M, Amarantes B, et al, "Oral Estrogens Decrease Bleeding Time and Improve Clinical Bleeding in Patients With Renal Failure," *Am J Med*, 1990, 89(4):436-40.
9. Peerschke EIB, "The Gray Platelet Syndrome," *ASCP Check Sample®*, Chicago, IL: American Society of Clinical Pathologists, 1988.

10. Pumphrey CW and Dawes J, "Platelet Alpha Granule Depletion: Findings in Patients With Prosthetic Heart Valves and Following Cardiopulmonary Bypass Surgery," *Thromb Res*, 1983, 30:257-64.
11. Pegels JG, Bruynes ECE, Engelfriet CP, et al, "Pseudothrombocytopenia: An Immunologic Study on Platelet Antibodies Dependent on Ethylene Diamine Tetra-Acetate," *Blood*, 1982, 59:157-61.
12. Ramanathan J, Sibai BM, Vu T, et al, "Correlation Between Bleeding Times and Platelet Counts in Women With Pre-Eclampsia Undergoing Caesarean Section," *Anesthesiology*, 1989, 71(2):188-91.
13. Israels SJ, McNicole A, Robertson C, et al, "Platelet Storage Pool Deficiency: Diagnosis in Patients With Prolonged Bleeding Times and Normal Platelet Aggregation," *Br J Haematol*, 1990, 75(1):118-21.

References

Burns ER and Lawrence C, "Bleeding Time: A Guide to Its Diagnostic and Clinical Utility," *Arch Pathol Lab Med*, 1989, 113(11):1219-24.
Davis JM and Schwartz KA, "Bleeding Time," *Lab Med*, 1989, 20:759-62.
Lind SE, "The Bleeding Time Does Not Predict Surgical Bleeding," *Blood*, 1991, 77(12):2547-52.
Sirridge MS and Shannon R, *Laboratory Evaluation of Hemostasis and Thrombosis*, 3rd ed, Philadelphia, PA: Lea & Febiger, 1983, 72.

Bleeding Time, Mielke

***CPT** 85002*

Related Information

Bleeding Time, Duke *on page 408*
Bleeding Time, Ivy *on page 409*
Clot Retraction *on page 413*
Cryoprecipitate *on page 1058*
Platelet Concentrate, Donation and Transfusion *on page 1081*

Synonyms Bleeding Time, Simplate®; Bleeding Time, Template; Surgicutt®

Abstract An *in vivo* test for platelet function and capillary integrity

Patient Care **PREPARATION:** The advisability of informing patient as to the possibility of scar/keloid formation should be considered. **AFTERCARE:** Butterfly closure of puncture for 24 hours

Specimen Blood; an *in vivo* test performed directly on the patient **CONTAINER:** Filter paper **COLLECTION:** Performed at bedside by a laboratory technologist. **CAUSES FOR REJECTION:** If the patient needs to be restrained, has excessively cold or edematous arms, or cannot have blood pressure cuff placed on either arm (as with casts, dressings, infection, or extensive rash). History of keloid formation. Some laboratories may require that patient or guardian sign informed consent. **TURNAROUND TIME:** Same day, usually within minutes or hours

Interpretive **REFERENCE RANGE:** 2.5-10 minutes; using the Surgicutt® pediatric device the normal range in children 1-10 years of age is reported as 2.5-13 minutes; 11-16 years of age, 3-8 minutes; compared to an adult range of 1-7 minutes (using a Surgicutt® adult automated device). The children studied had no history of bleeding and did not have pathologic bleeding during their surgery. The difference between pediatric and adult bleeding time may relate to the length of the cut with the pediatric device.[1] **USE:** Screening for coagulation abnormality, in particular to assess capillary and platelet function. Useful in evaluation of ecchymosis, spontaneous bruising and bleeding, bleeding tendency. May be prolonged after aspirin ingestion, in cases of von Willebrand's disease, Bernard-Soulier syndrome, and Glanzmann's thrombasthenia (qualitative platelet disorders), macroglobulinemia, some case of myeloproliferative disease, fibrinogen disorders, and in renal failure.[2] **LIMITATIONS:** Low platelet count ($<100,000/mm^3$) or aspirin therapy may prolong the bleeding time. Scarring of skin may occur. If disease, injury, or I.V. therapy precludes access to the skin of the arm, test may be performed using medial aspect of the thigh. Results using normal controls and sensitivity to aspirin-induced prolongation are comparable at these two sites (arm compared to thigh).[3] **CONTRAINDICATIONS:** Low platelet count; patient receiving medication containing aspirin **METHODOLOGY:** This test is a modification of the Ivy bleeding time (see also that entry) and has replaced the classical Ivy bleeding time in most laboratories. The patient preparation (including use of a blood pressure cuff) is the same. Sensitivity and reproducibility of the test theoretically is increased by standardizing the method of production and length of the incision. This is achieved by use of a template or by use of the commercially available Simplate® or Surgicutt® devices, the latter two giving fairly comparable results.[4] A study comparing Ivy method and Simplate® II, however, did not find that the Simplate® II method was superior in sensitivity or reproducibility (precision) to the Ivy method.[5] There are significant practical reasons for producing vertical (elbow to wrist oriented) rather than horizontal cuts.[6] An *in vitro* bleeding time device and procedure have been described (see Aspirin Tolerance Test). **ADDITIONAL INFORMATION:** Test should be performed no sooner than 10 days after the last dose of medication

(Continued)

Bleeding Time, Mielke *(Continued)*

containing aspirin. There is no significant effect of therapeutic propranolol on template bleeding time.[7] In newborns, use of an automated bleeding time device resulted in bleeding times similar to or shorter than those of adults.[8]

Footnotes

1. Andrew M, Vegh P, Johnston M, et al, "Maturation of the Hemostatic System During Childhood," *Blood*, 1992, 80(8):1998-2005.
2. Gordge MP, Faint RW, Rylance PB, et al, "Platelet Function and the Bleeding Time in Progressive Renal Failure," *Thromb Haemost*, 1988, 60:83-7.
3. Hertzendorf LR, Stehling L, Kurec AS, et al, "Comparison of Bleeding Times Performed on the Arm and the Leg," *Am J Clin Pathol*, 1987, 87:393-6.
4. Buchanan GR and Holtkamp CA, "A Comparative Study of Variables Affecting the Bleeding Time Using Two Disposable Devices," *Am J Clin Pathol*, 1989, 91(1):45-51.
5. Koster T, Caekebeke-Peerlinck KMJ, and Briet E, "A Randomized and Blinded Comparison of the Sensitivity and the Reproducibility of the Ivy and Simplate® II Bleeding Time Techniques," *Am J Clin Pathol*, 1989, 92(3):315-20.
6. Bick RL, *Disorders of Thrombosis and Hemostasis: Clinical and Laboratory Practice*, Chicago, IL: ASCP Press, 1992, 44.
7. Pamphilon DH, Boon RJ, Prentice AG, et al, "Lack of Significant Effect of Therapeutic Propranolol on Measurable Platelet Function in Healthy Subjects," *J Clin Pathol*, 1989, 42(8):793-6.
8. Andrew M, Paes B, Bowker J, et al, "Evaluation of an Automated Bleeding Time Device in the Newborn," *Am J Hematol*, 1990, 35(4):275-7.

References

Braman AM and Schwartz KA, "Platelet Disorders," *Lab Med*, 1989, 20:831-5.

Machin SJ, Preston E, and BSCH Haemostasis and Thrombosis Task Force of the British Society for Haematology, "Guidelines on Platelet Function Testing," *J Clin Pathol*, 1988, 41:1322-30.

Montgomery RR and Scott JP, "Hemostasis: Diseases of the Fluid Phase," *Hematology of Infancy and Childhood*, 4th ed, Chapter 44, Nathan DG and Oski FA, eds, Philadelphia, PA: WB Saunders Co, 1993, 1609-10.

Sirridge MS and Shannon R, *Laboratory Evaluation of Hemostasis and Thrombosis*, 3rd ed, Philadelphia, PA: Lea & Febiger, 1983, 73-4.

Bleeding Time, Simplate® *see* Bleeding Time, Mielke *on previous page*

Bleeding Time, Template *see* Bleeding Time, Mielke *on previous page*

CAC *see* Anticoagulant, Circulating *on page 402*

Capillary Fragility Test

CPT 85999

Synonyms Negative Pressure Suction Cup Capillary Fragility; Rumpel-Leede Test; Rumpel-Leede Tourniquet Test; Tourniquet Test

Abstract Test for evaluation of capillary integrity

Specimen COLLECTION: Performed at bedside by medical technologist **CAUSES FOR REJECTION:** Presence of petechiae, ecchymoses, extensive infection, vesicle or bullae formation involving skin of patient's arms, casts on arms, or extensive intravenous attachments or wrappings impeding access to patient's upper extremities

Interpretive REFERENCE RANGE: Presence of 5 or less petechiae in men and 10 or less petechiae in women and children in an area of 2.5 cm radius. Normal range varies, dependent on technical differences in method. **USE:** Evaluate capillary endothelial integrity, ecchymosis, easy bruising, easy bleeding, spontaneous bruising, spontaneous bleeding **LIMITATIONS:** Results may be difficult to interpret if petechiae or other forms of hemorrhage in the skin are present before the test begins. Some normal individuals may show capillary fragility. Test may be normal in some patients with thrombocytopenia. **METHODOLOGY:** Negative- and/or positive-pressure methods may be employed.[1] Negative-pressure method uses a suction cup which is applied to the skin. Capillary resistance is the least negative pressure required for 1 minute to produce one or more petechiae. In the positive-pressure method, blood pressure cuff is maintained on the arm with pressure halfway between diastolic and systolic (maximum of 100 mm Hg) for 5 minutes. Cuff pressure is released and arm is observed for petechiae. The number of petechiae appearing in a given area is reported. **ADDITIONAL INFORMATION:** This test provides a relatively crude measure of capillary integrity. Positive reactions may occur with thrombocytopenia (platelet count $<10{,}000/mm^3$), toxic vascular reactions, and hereditary vascular abnormalities. Generally, large petechiae relate to thrombocytopenia while tiny pinpoint examples are more often associated with increase in vascular permeability. The results may vary with age and menstrual cycle. Positive results may occur prior to and immediately after menstruation and in the postmenopausal state. Hormones of the estrogen and cortisone type often improve capillary resistance. The prolonged use of steroids, however, eventually results in increased capillary fragility, possibly due to loss of subcutaneous tissue.

The tourniquet test lacks specificity and has been referred to as "abandoned by most laboratories." For use in children and the elderly, a standard petechiometer is commercially available.[2]

Footnotes

1. Bennington JL, "Saunders Dictionary & Encyclopedia of Laboratory Medicine and Technology," Philadelphia, PA: WB Saunders Co, 1984, 251.
2. Bick RL, *Disorders of Thrombosis and Hemostasis: Clinical and Laboratory Practice*, Chicago, IL: ASCP Press, 1992, 44, 51.

Christmas Disease Factor *see* Factor IX *on page 426*

Clot Lysis Time *see* Diluted Whole Blood Clot Lysis *on page 418*

Clot Retraction

***CPT** 85170*

Related Information

Bleeding Time, Ivy *on page 409*
Bleeding Time, Mielke *on page 411*
Factor XIII *on page 430*
Fibrinogen *on page 435*
Platelet Aggregation *on page 459*

Test Commonly Includes Description of clot retraction, size, firmness and RBC fallout. May include serum "drip-out" and serum and RBC escaping from clot.

Abstract Evaluation of clot formation, providing a window for possible platelet function (and/or number) abnormalities and/or fibrinogen level/function

Specimen Blood **CONTAINER:** Red top tube **COLLECTION:** Transport specimen to the laboratory within 1 hour of collection. May require special collection. **CAUSES FOR REJECTION:** Hemolyzed specimen, specimen received more than 1 hour after collection, tubes inadequately filled **SPECIAL INSTRUCTIONS:** Method may require collection directly into graduated centrifuge tube by laboratory technologist.

Interpretive **REFERENCE RANGE:** Amount of serum and RBC escaping from clot: ≥40%; RBC fallout: <5%; serum retained in clot: <20%; serum "drip-out": two drops or less in 2 minutes. Normally clot retraction starts in 1 hour and is complete within 24 hours. **USE:** Assess platelet function and fibrin structure in inducing clot retraction; a coagulation parameter used to investigate possibility of Glanzmann's disease **LIMITATIONS:** Concentration and functional ability of fibrinogen and hematocrit level should be within normal limits for valid interpretation and conclusions about platelet function. With low platelet count, aspirin therapy, increased fibrinolysis, altered fibrinogen/fibrin structure, or hypofibrinogenemia, abnormal clot retraction may occur and limit the ability to assess platelet function. In disseminated intravascular coagulation, afibrinogenemia, and severe hemophilic states, clot formation may not occur. **CONTRAINDICATIONS:** Patients with low platelet counts, hypofibrinogenemia, or those taking aspirin-containing medications **METHODOLOGY:** Whole blood without anticoagulant is placed in a clean, glass, graduated centrifuge tube. After 1 hour at 37°C a number of parameters can be measured (eg, amount of fluid remaining, RBC fallout, serum "dripout," others). The older literature describes a variety of quantitative methods using platelet-rich plasma.[1] **ADDITIONAL INFORMATION:** Clot retraction depends upon normal platelet function, a contractile protein present in the platelet membrane (thrombosthenin), and magnesium, ATP, and pyruvate kinase.[2] It is also influenced by the hematocrit level and fibrinogen structure and concentration. Thrombocytopenia and thrombasthenia are characterized by a soft friable clot with increased serum "drip-out" and decreased amount of serum expressed. With hypofibrinogenemia, the clot should be small, firm, and show increase in RBC fallout. With increased fibrinolysis, the clot should be soft and shaggy with increased RBC fallout. With disseminated intravascular coagulation, the clot is small and ragged with increased RBC fallout.[3] With congenital dysfibrinogenemia the clot should be of normal size but with increased RBC fallout. Coating of platelets with paraproteins (as in macroglobulinemia) may result in poor clot retraction. Thrombasthenia (Glanzmann's disease) is an inherited hemorrhagic condition with normal platelet count but with prolonged bleeding time, markedly decreased clot retraction, and abnormal platelet

(Continued)

Clot Retraction *(Continued)*

aggregation and adhesion. The defective clot retraction may reflect a failure of ADP activation of actin in the platelet membrane. A decrease in the amount of membrane glycoproteins II_b and III_a is accepted as the characteristic membrane abnormality in Glanzmann's thrombasthenia.[4] Clot retraction procedures have been largely replaced by platelet aggregation, platelet adhesion, and platelet release studies. An instrument has been developed, however, that measures force development during clot retraction. Force generated is transduced to a voltage change that is recorded. In this manner, the effect on clot retraction of change in platelet function and fibrin structure can be quantified. This device may extend the life of clot retraction studies by allowing quantification of retraction parameters in a more specific and reproducible manner. Qualitative platelet dysfunction may thus be characterized in part by measured functional abnormality of clot retraction. Practical clinical application must await results of patient studies. It has been shown that clot retraction parameters are temperature dependent with total inhibition at 15°C.[5]

Footnotes

1. Bang NU, Beller FK, Deutsch E, et al, *Thrombosis and Bleeding Disorders: Theory and Methods*, New York, NY: Academic Press, 1971, 441-5.
2. Corriveau DM and Fritsma GA, *Hemostasis and Thrombosis in the Clinical Laboratory*, Philadelphia, PA: JB Lippincott Co, 1988, 302.
3. Pittiglio DH and Sacher RA, *Clinical Hematology and Fundamentals of Hemostasis*, Philadelphia, PA: FA Davis Co, 1987, 451.
4. Forbes CD and Cuschieri A, *Management of Bleeding Disorders in Surgical Practice*, Oxford, UK: Blackwell Scientific Publications, 1993, 43.
5. Carr ME and Zekert SL, "Measurement of Platelet-Mediated Force During Plasma Clot Formation," *Am J Med Sci*, 1991, 302(1):13-8.

References

Owen CA Jr, "Historical Account of Tests of Hemostasis," *Am J Clin Pathol*, 1990, 93(4 Suppl 1):S3-8.

Sirridge MS and Shannon R, *Laboratory Evaluation of Hemostasis and Thrombosis*, 3rd ed, Philadelphia, PA: Lea & Febiger, 1983, 66, 83-5.

Clot Time *see* Lee-White Clotting Time *on page 449*

Coagulation Factor Assay

***CPT** 85611 (PT substitution); 85732 (PTT substitution)*

Related Information

Factor II *on page 420*
Factor V *on page 421*
Factor VII *on page 422*
Factor VIII *on page 424*
Factor IX *on page 426*
Factor X *on page 427*
Factor XI *on page 429*
Factor XII *on page 429*
Factor XIII *on page 430*
Factor, Fitzgerald *on page 431*
Factor, Fletcher *on page 432*
Partial Thromboplastin Time *on page 450*
Prothrombin Time *on page 468*

Synonyms Factor Assay

Applies to Coagulation Factor(s) II, V, VII, VIII, IX, X, XI, XII, and XIII (Screen)

Abstract Tests for specific clotting factors

Patient Care PREPARATION: Avoid Coumadin® therapy for 2 weeks and heparin therapy for 2 days prior to test

Specimen Plasma CONTAINER: Two blue top (sodium citrate) tubes COLLECTION: Routine venipuncture. If multiple tests are being drawn, draw coagulation studies last. If only factor assay is being drawn, draw 1-2 mL into another Vacutainer®, discard, and then collect the factor assay. This collection procedure avoids contamination of the specimen with tissue thromboplastins. Transport specimen to the laboratory immediately. STORAGE INSTRUCTIONS: Keep refrigerated. CAUSES FOR REJECTION: Tubes not full, tubes clotted, specimen hemolyzed, specimen received more than 2 hours after collection, specimen improperly labeled, specimen not refrigerated TURNAROUND TIME: Commonly sent to reference laboratories. SPECIAL INSTRUCTIONS: These assays are not usually routinely available. They may require referral to a specialized coagulation laboratory. Make arrangements with your local laboratory facility before drawing and submitting specimen.

Interpretive REFERENCE RANGE: Normal range varies with each factor and between laboratories but is generally broad, approximately 50% to 150% of normal activity. Factor XIII is usually estimated as present or absent on the basis of a urea solubility screening test. The normal finding is for the clot to be insoluble in 5M urea at 24 hours. Healthy premature infants have levels of vitamin K dependent factors (II, VII, IX, and X) and contact factors (XI, XII, PK, and HMWK) that are <50% of the level of normal adults (with the exception of VII which is somewhat higher). Healthy prematures, however, do not develop spontaneous hemorrhage because of a balance between procoagulant and inhibitors.[1] USE: Detect specific coagulation factor deficiency which may be present on a congenital basis or may be acquired secondary to a number of organ specific or generalized disease processes. Triplett[2] has provided a broad discussion of abnormalities that have been seen in association with liver, renal, immune, lymphoproliferative, and other disease processes. LIMITATIONS: Factors II, VII, IX, X may be increased in patients taking oral contraceptives. Interpretations of results may be limited if patient is receiving anticoagulant therapy or if test is done more than 2 hours after collection. CONTRAINDICATIONS: Patient on anticoagulant therapy METHODOLOGY: Results of mixing patient's plasma with naturally or treated deficient plasma and serum preparations are determined by using prothrombin time and activated partial thromboplastin time tests. Absorbed plasma and aged serum can be prepared and maintained locally. Storage and maintenance of a full set of known deficient plasmas, while commercially available (George King Biomedical, Olathe, Kansas), is usually only attempted by the specialized coagulation laboratory. ADDITIONAL INFORMATION: Stage II, intrinsic pathway coagulation deficiency states include the hemophilias, A (factor VIII deficiency), B (factor IX deficiency), and C (factor XI deficiency). Results of differential APTT testing using specially treated normal plasma and serum can be used to support these diagnoses. The reagents are commercially available or may be prepared in the laboratory. Consult the references for additional information. After absorption with $BaSO_4$ or Al $(OH)_3$ factors I, V, VIII, XI, and XII remain in the plasma (II, VII, IX, and X, the vitamin K dependent factors are removed). Adsorbed serum contains only factors XI and XII. Aged serum contains factor VII, IX, X, XI, and XII (lacks factors I, V, and VIII). Specific factor assay using known deficient plasma should be used to confirm results of differential (crossmixing) studies.

Use of Differential APTT in the Identification of Hemophilia

Hemophilia	PT	PTT	Adsorbed Plasma	Aged Normal Serum
A (VIII def)	Normal	↑	Corrects	No change
B (IX def)	Normal	↑	No change	Corrects
C (XI def)	Normal	↑	Corrects (partial)	Corrects (partial)
XII def	Normal	↑	Corrects	Corrects

Footnotes

1. Andrew M, Paes B, Milner R, et al, "Development of the Human Coagulation System in the Healthy Premature Infant," *Blood*, 1988, 72(5):1651-7.
2. Triplett DA, "Acquired Abnormalities of Hemostasis," *Laboratory Evaluation of Coagulation*, Chicago, IL: ASCP Press, 1982, 209-44.

References

Bloom AL and Thomas DP, eds, *Haemostasis and Thrombosis*, 2nd ed, New York, NY: Churchill Livingstone, 1987, 101-91.

Sirridge MS and Shannon R, *Laboratory Evaluation of Hemostasis and Thrombosis*, 3rd ed, Philadelphia, PA: Lea & Febiger, 1983, 115-33, 204-19.

Coagulation Factor(s) II, V, VII, VIII, IX, X, XI, XII, and XIII (Screen) *see* Coagulation Factor Assay *on previous page*

Coagulation Screen, Intravascular *see* Intravascular Coagulation Screen *on page 446*

Coagulation Time *see* Lee-White Clotting Time *on page 449*

Consumptive Coagulopathy Screen *see* Intravascular Coagulation Screen *on page 446*

Coumarins *see* Prothrombin Time *on page 468*

Cryocrit *see* Cryofibrinogen *on next page*

Cryofibrinogen

CPT 82585

Related Information

Cryoglobulin, Qualitative, Serum *on page 670*

Applies to Cryocrit

Abstract A test for one of the cold-precipitable plasma proteins in patients with cold intolerance.

Specimen Plasma **CONTAINER:** Blue top (sodium citrate) tube **CAUSES FOR REJECTION:** Improper tube, specimen more than 2 hours in transit to the laboratory **TURNAROUND TIME:** 24 hours **SPECIAL INSTRUCTIONS:** Transport to the laboratory immediately following collection. Must be allowed to clot at 37°C.

Interpretive **REFERENCE RANGE:** Negative: no cryofibrinogen detected **USE:** Detect cold precipitable fibrinogen. Cryofibrinogen has been reported in association with coagulation disorders, malignancies, phlebitis of pregnancy, inflammatory processes including neonatal infections, the use of oral contraceptives, and with scleroderma.[1] **CONTRAINDICATIONS:** Patients anticoagulated with heparin **METHODOLOGY:** Tube of plasma refrigerated overnight is compared to a control tube of patient's plasma kept covered at room temperature. Cryofibrinogen (precipitate from **plasma** on cooling) must be differentiated from cryoglobulin (precipitates or gels from **serum or plasma** when cooled at 4°C for 24 hours). Either of these may disappear on warming to 32°C. A "cold-precipitable protein study" to identify these cryoproteins is desirable. This involves keeping a sample of both patient's serum and plasma refrigerated for 24-72 hours. If samples are studied in Wintrobe tubes, any precipitating material can be measured by centrifuging (using a refrigerated centrifuge) and quantitated using the sedimentation scale (each mm of precipitate equates to 1% of **"cryocrit"**). **ADDITIONAL INFORMATION:** Cryofibrinogenemia can produce a clinical picture similar to that of cryoglobulinemia (cold sensitivity with purpura, vascular damage with bleeding, bullae, chronic ulcerations, and cold urticaria). Cryoprecipitable complexes between fibrinogen, globulins, and fibrinogen degradation products occur, such as fragments X and Y, forming complexes with fibrinogen and fibrin monomer and precipitating in the cold and in heparinized plasma.

Footnotes

1. Beightler E, Diven DG, Sanchez RL, et al, "Thrombotic Vasculopathy Associated With Cryofibrinogenemia," *J Am Acad Dermatol*, 1991, 24(2 Pt 2):342-5.

References

Gottlieb AJ, "Disorders of Hemostasis: Nonthrombocytopenic Purpuras," Section 12, *Hematology*, 4th ed, Williams WJ, Beutler E, Erslev AJ, et al, eds, New York, NY: McGraw-Hill Inc, 1990, 149:1437.

Klein AD and Kerdel FA, "Purpura and Recurrent Ulcers on the Lower Extremities. Essential Cryofibrinogenemia," *Arch Dermatol*, 1991, 127(1):113-8.

D-Dimer

CPT 85378 (semiquantitative); 85379 (quantitative)

Related Information

Fibrin Breakdown Products *on page 433*

Fibrin Split Products, Protamine Sulfate *on page 439*

Intravascular Coagulation Screen *on page 446*

Specimen Plasma **CONTAINER:** Collect whole blood in plastic tube that contains 0.11 mol/L sodium citrate and aprotinin (100 TIU/L (trypsin inhibiting units)) **STORAGE INSTRUCTIONS:** Test plasma may be stored at -80°C. The clinical situation in which these tests are employed, however, usually requires that samples be tested immediately. **TURNAROUND TIME:** Latex particle immunoassay, 30 minutes (applicable to clinical emergency situations); enzyme immunoassay (Dimertest EIA), 4-5 hours

Interpretive **USE:** Screening test for the detection of deep vein thrombosis (DVT); evaluation of acute myocardial infarction, unstable angina, and disseminated intravascular coagulation (DIC)[1] **LIMITATIONS:** Elevated D-dimer levels are not specific for the presence of deep vein thrombosis. **METHODOLOGY:** Enzyme-linked immunosorbent assay (ELISA), latex particle assay, immunoblotting[2] **ADDITIONAL INFORMATION:** The D-dimer is a fragment of fibrin that contains one intermolecular cross-link between the gamma chains of two fibrin monomers. This cross-linkage occurs in fibrin but not fibrinogen. It is thus specific for fibrin. Increased levels of D-dimer (cross-linked fibrin fragments) have been found in patients with deep vein thrombosis,[3] acute myocardial infarction,[4] acute pulmonary embolism,[5] unstable angina,[6] and disseminated intravascular coagulation.[1] D-dimer level <500 µg/L has been considered to exclude the diagnosis of acute pulmonary embolism.[5] In one study,[6] plasma from nearly 40% of pregnant women with pre-eclampsia was positive for D-dimer. Patients with D-dimer had more severe disease. The latex clumping tests have been found to have a low sensitivity, rendering them unsuitable for emergency screening.[7,8,9] While detection limits of 200 μg/L for one test and 500 μg/L for the other latex test are claimed, a low level of specificity (47%) does not allow a positive diagnosis of DVT when the level of D-dimer is >200 μg/L. On the other hand a level of D-dimer by ELISA <200 μg/L appears reliably to exclude presence of DVT. Results of D-dimer test by ELISA are 100% predictive for the absence of DVT (level <200 μg/L).[6,8] Results of this test (D-dimer by ELISA) may be considered to screen for those patients needing further evaluation to establish the presence of DVT.[8] Presence of increase in D-dimer supports the interpretation of presence of FDP, X, Y, D, and E fragments as indicative of acute DIC (eg, fibrin rather than fibrinogen fragments).[10] A lack of correlation has been found between thrombolysis (with resultant reperfusion) and increase in D-dimer levels (eg, D-dimer measurement does not distinguish between thrombolysis and fibrinolysis).[11,12]

On the other hand, presence of D-dimer confirms that both thrombin generation and plasmin generation have occurred. The in tandem use of fibrin degradation products (FDP) test and D-dimer measurement in the evaluation of DIC has been recommended. Sensitivity and specificity are thereby maximized. The FDP measurement, highly sensitive, is confirmed with the D-dimer test, very specific. Elevated FDP confirmed by D-dimer test result >0.5 mg/L is highly predictive of DIC in patients at risk.[1]

The use of plasma D-dimer levels in conjunction with other tests to follow clot lysis during thrombolytic therapy has been studied.[13,14] It is uncertain whether or not D-dimer originating from the degradation of soluble plasma fibrin should be subtracted from the total post-treatment level to obtain D-dimer resulting from lysis of thrombi.[15] D-dimer fragment in the plasma can then be considered a marker of solid-phase fibrin dissolution.[16] D-dimer analysis of cerebrospinal fluid has been found to accurately and rapidly differentiate cases of subarachnoid hemorrhage from traumatic lumbar puncture. D-dimer was superior to the use of xanthochromia or declining RBC count in sequential tubes for this distinction.[17]

Footnotes

1. Carr JM, McKinney M, and McDonagh J, "Diagnosis of Disseminated Intravascular Coagulation: Role of D-Dimer," *Am J Clin Pathol*, 1989, 91(3):280-7.
2. Francis CW, Connaghan DG, Scott WL, et al, "Increased Plasma Concentration of Cross-Linked Fibrin Polymers in Acute Myocardial Infarction," *Circulation*, 1987, 75:1170-7.
3. Kruskal JB, Commerford PJ, Franks JJ, et al, "Fibrin and Fibrinogen-Related Antigens in Patients With Stable and Unstable Coronary Artery Disease," *N Engl J Med*, 1987, 317:1361-5.
4. Bounameaux H, Cirafici P, de-Moerloose P, et al, "Measurement of D-dimer in Plasma as Diagnostic Aid in Suspected Pulmonary Embolism," *Lancet*, 1991, 337(8735):196-200.
5. Trofatter KF Jr, Howell ML, Greenberg CS, et al, "Use of the Fibrin D-Dimer in Screening for Coagulation Abnormalities in Pre-eclampsia," *Obstet Gynecol*, 1989, 73(3 Pt 1):435-40.
6. Rowbotham BJ, Carroll P, Whitaker AN, et al, "Measurement of Cross-Linked Fibrin Derivatives – Use in the Diagnosis of Venous Thrombosis," *Thromb Haemost*, 1987, 57:59-61.
7. Heaton DC, Billings JD, and Hickton CM, "Assessment of D-Dimer Assays for the Diagnosis of Deep Vein Thrombosis," *J Lab Clin Med*, 1987, 110:588-91.
8. Bounameaux H, Schneider P-A, Reber G, et al, "Measurement of Plasma D-Dimer for Diagnosis of Deep Venous Thrombosis," *Am J Clin Pathol*, 1989, 91(1):82-5.
9. Heaton DC, Billings JD, and Hickton CM, "Assessment of D-Dimer Assays for the Diagnosis of Deep Vein Thrombosis," *J Lab Clin Med*, 1987, 110:588-91.
10. Bick RL, "Disseminated Intravascular Coagulation and Related Syndromes: A Clinical Review," *Semin Thromb Hemost*, 1988, 14:299-338.
11. Brenner B, Francis CW, and Marder VJ, "The Role of Soluble Cross-Linked Fibrin in D-Dimer Immunoreactivity of Plasmic Digests," *J Lab Clin Med*, 1989, 113(6):682-8.
12. Mosesson MW, "D-Dimer, An Ambiguous Marker of Thrombolysis," *J Lab Clin Med*, 1989, 113(6):662.
13. Lawler CM, Bovill EG, Stump DC, et al, "Fibrin Fragment D-Dimer and Fibrinogen Bβ Peptides in Plasma as Markers of Clot Lysis During Thrombolytic Therapy in Acute Myocardial Infarction," *Blood*, 1990, 76(7):1341-8.
14. Boisclair MD, Lane DA, Wilde JT, et al, "A Comparative Evaluation of Assays for Markers of Activated Coagulation and/or Fibrinolysis: Thrombin-Antithrobmin Complex, D-Dimer and Fibrinogen/Fibrin Fragment E Antigen," *Br J Haematol*, 1990, 74(4):471-9.
15. Brenner B, Francis CW, Totterman S, et al, "Quantitation of Venous Clot Lysis With the D-Dimer Immunoassay During Fibrinolytic Therapy Requires Correction for Soluble Fibrin Degradation," *Circulation*, 1990, 81(6):1818-25.
16. Eisenberg PR, Jaffe AS, Stump DC, et al, "Validity of Enzyme-Linked Immunosorbent Assays of Cross-Linked Fibrin Degradation Products as a Measure of Clot Lysis," *Circulation*, 1990, 82(4):1159-68.
17. Lang DT, Berberian LB, Lee S, et al, "Rapid Differentiation of Subarachnoid Hemorrhage From Traumatic Lumbar Puncture Using the D-Dimer Assay," *Am J Clin Pathol*, 1990, 93(3):403-5.

DIC Screen *see* Intravascular Coagulation Screen *on page 446*

Differential APTT Test *see* Activated Partial Thromboplastin Substitution Test *on page 401*

Diluted Whole Blood Clot Lysis

CPT 85175

Related Information

Euglobulin Clot Lysis *on this page*
Plasminogen Activator Inhibitor *on page 455*
Plasminogen Assay *on page 457*

Synonyms Clot Lysis Time; Fibrinolysis Time

Specimen Laboratory personnel will usually collect specimen and initiate this test at the patient's bedside.

Interpretive REFERENCE RANGE: Rapid lysis implies excessive fibrinolytic activity. Clot still intact after 2 hours is "normal." Clot which lyses in less than 2 hours reflects lytic activity, time of dissolution is reported. A "control" tube with clot is kept in the refrigerator; lysis does not occur at that temperature. (Fibrinolytic activity of plasmin is inhibited.) POSSIBLE PANIC RANGE: 100% lysis in 1 hour or less USE: Monitor urokinase and streptokinase therapy, fibrinolytic activity; evaluate abnormal fibrinolysis; aids in differentiating primary pathologic fibrinolysis from secondary (physiologic) fibrinolysis with low levels of circulating plasmins LIMITATIONS: Testing must begin immediately upon drawing blood unless citrate-anticoagulated, chilled, platelet-poor plasma is tested.[1] Aspirin may influence fibrinolytic activity in addition to its antiplatelet activity. An inverse relationship has been shown between the degree of acetylation of fibrinogen and the clot lysis time.[2] METHODOLOGY: Whole blood is obtained and a 1:10 dilution in iced buffer solution is prepared. Test is started with the addition of 0.1 mL thrombin and is set up in triplicate. After 30 minutes refrigerator incubation (inactivates inhibitors), two of the tubes are heated at 37°C and the time to lysis noted. A clot in the refrigerated control tube assures that sufficient functional fibrinogen was present. ADDITIONAL INFORMATION: A tabular comparison of clot lysis tests is included in the listing, Euglobulin Clot Lysis.

Footnotes

1. Graeff H and Beller FK, "Fibrinolytic Activity in Whole Blood, Dilute Blood, and Euglobulin Clot Lysis Time Tests," Bang NU, Beller FK, Deutsch E, et al, eds, *Thrombosis and Bleeding Disorders: Theory and Methods*, New York, NY: Academic Press, 1971, 328-31.
2. Bjornsson TD, Schneider DE, and Berger H Jr, "Aspirin Acetylates Fibrinogen and Enhances Fibrinolysis. Fibrinolytic Effect Is Independent of Changes in Plasminogen Activator Levels," *J Pharmacol Exp Ther*, 1989, 250(1):154-61.

References

Sirridge MS and Shannon R, *Laboratory Evaluation of Hemostasis and Thrombosis*, 3rd ed, Philadelphia, PA: Lea & Febiger, 1983, 11-6, 169-74.

Disseminated Intravascular Coagulation Screen *see* Intravascular Coagulation Screen *on page 446*

Endothelial Cofactor *see* Thrombomodulin *on page 475*

Euglobulin Clot Lysis

CPT 85360

Related Information

Diluted Whole Blood Clot Lysis *on this page*
Fibrin Breakdown Products *on page 433*
Fibrinogen *on page 435*
Intravascular Coagulation Screen *on page 446*
Plasminogen Assay *on page 457*

Synonyms Euglobulin Clot Lysis Time; Euglobulin Lysis Time; Fibrinolysis Time

Abstract A measure of fibrinolytic activity, an older generation procedure

Patient Care PREPARATION: Prohibit exercise prior to drawing sample.

Specimen Plasma. Use of platelet-poor plasma is desirable, as platelets have antiplasmin activity and may prolong the lysis time. CONTAINER: Blue top (sodium citrate) tube COLLECTION: Use two-syringe or two-tube collection technique to avoid contamination by tissue proteins. A clean venipuncture is a necessity. To avoid release of plasminogen activator (which shortens the lysis time), do not massage vein vigorously, pump fist excessively, or leave tourniquet in place for a prolonged period. **STORAGE INSTRUCTIONS:** Deliver specimen immediately to the laboratory on ice. After centrifugation, the separated plasma should be kept on ice and tested within 30 minutes. **CAUSES FOR REJECTION:** Specimen not delivered promptly (within 15-20 minutes), hemolysis, clotted blood, dilution by I.V. fluids, specimen not iced, tubes not filled with correct amount of sample **SPECIAL INSTRUCTIONS:** It may be necessary to schedule this test with the laboratory.

Interpretive **REFERENCE RANGE:** Lysis time greater than 90 minutes. Shortened time to lysis indicates excessive fibrinolytic activity. Bleeding danger may exist if there is 100% lysis in 1 hour or less. **USE:** Detect and evaluate pathologic fibrinolytic activity; monitor urokinase or streptokinase fibrinolytic therapy. May be normal in cases of DIC. Useful in evaluation of lytic states during cardiovascular surgery, as the harvest of euglobulin fraction separates out inhibitors including heparin. **LIMITATIONS:** Decreased fibrinogen (<80 mg/dL) causes shortened (rapid) lysis time. Increased fibrinogen prolongs lysis time. Dysfibrinogen may be responsible for abnormal lysis time. If plasminogen is depleted (by *in vivo* fibrinolysis as in long-term cases of disseminated intravascular coagulation), a false normal lysis time may result. Clot dissolution will not occur because of the lack of plasminogen. See Methodology for use of control to detect this possibility. The euglobulin clot lysis test is nonspecific and is considered obsolete by some. **METHODOLOGY:** Plasma is acidified to form a "euglobulin clot" (antiplasmins are removed during treatment). Time required for lysis to occur is measured and reported. The lower the pH of plasma/acid, the longer the lysis time. (Maximal lysis results from precipitating euglobulins at pH 6.2.) With precipitation at pH 5.3, lysis may require 10-24 hours. Positive and negative plasma controls, as well as patient activated control (PAC), should be run concurrently with the test plasma. PAC consists of patient euglobulin fraction with streptokinase added. This should cause rapid clot dissolution. If plasminogen is depleted, the PAC will show no dissolution of clot, and the euglobulin lysis time will appear normal. A normal result in the PAC indicates that the actual test is unreliable.[1] **ADDITIONAL INFORMATION:** Lysis time of less than 60 minutes may be associated with presence of fibrin degradation products. Increased fibrinolysis may be associated with shock/circulatory collapse, epinephrine injection, pyrogen reactions, obstetric complication, and sudden death. See table. There is evidence that some (apparently most) patients with vascular ulcers have a prolonged euglobulin lysis time and an increased plasma fibrinogen level.[2] The exact role (primary or secondary) of the change in fibrinolytic activity has not been established.

Comparison of Clot Lysis Tests

Test	Measures	Sensitivity	Time Required (hours)
Whole blood clot lysis	Activator Plasminogen (plasmin) Fibrinogen Inhibitors	+/–	24
Diluted whole blood clot lysis	Activator Plasminogen (plasmin) Fibrinogen Inhibitors (decreased)	++	2–12
Euglobulin clot lysis	Activator Plasminogen (plasmin) Fibrinogen (decreased) Inhibitors (eliminated)	++ or +++	2

From Sirridge MS and Shannon R, *Laboratory Evaluation of Hemostasis and Thrombosis*, 3rd ed, Philadelphia, PA: Lea and Febiger, 1983, 171.

Footnotes

1. Fritsma GA, "Clot Based Assays of Coagulation," *Hemostasis and Thrombosis in the Clinical Laboratory*, eds, Corriveau DM and Fritsma GA, Philadelphia, PA: JB Lippincott Co, 1988, 4:124-5.
2. Falanga V, Moosa HH, Nemeth AJ, et al, "Dermal Pericapillary Fibrin in Venous Disease and Venous Ulceration," *Arch Dermatol*, 1987, 123:620-3.

References

Graeff H and Beller FK, "Fibrinolytic Activity in Whole Blood, Dilute Blood, and Euglobulin Clot Lysis Time Tests," Bang NU, Beller FK, Deutsch E, et al, eds, *Thrombosis and Bleeding Disorders: Theory and Methods*, New York, NY: Academic Press, 1971, 328-31.

Sirridge MS and Shannon R, *Laboratory Evaluation of Hemostasis and Thrombosis*, 3rd ed, Philadelphia, PA: Lea & Febiger, 1983, 69, 173-4.

Euglobulin Clot Lysis Time *see* Euglobulin Clot Lysis *on page 418*

Euglobulin Lysis Time *see* Euglobulin Clot Lysis *on page 418*

F 1.2 *see* Prothrombin Fragment 1.2 *on page 467*

F1+2 *see* Prothrombin Fragment 1.2 *on page 467*

Factor II

CPT *85210*

Related Information

Coagulation Factor Assay *on page 414*
Prothrombin Time *on page 468*

Synonyms Prothrombin

Abstract Factor II (prothrombin) is measured by functional or immunologic assays, results of which assist in identifying the presence of qualitative or quantitative deficiency. Such autosomal recessive defects are rare. If homozygous, they may be responsible for severe clinical bleeding and will be characterized by prolonged prothrombin time and partial thromboplastin time with normal thrombin time.

Patient Care PREPARATION: Avoid Coumadin® therapy for 2 weeks and heparin therapy for 2 days prior to test.

Specimen Plasma CONTAINER: Blue top (sodium citrate) tube COLLECTION: Routine venipuncture. If multiple tests are being drawn, draw coagulation studies last. If only coagulation tests are being drawn, draw 1-2 mL into another Vacutainer®, discard, and then collect coagulation tests. This collection procedure avoids contamination of the specimen with tissue thromboplastins. STORAGE INSTRUCTIONS: Keep refrigerated. CAUSES FOR REJECTION: Tube not full, specimen hemolyzed, specimen clotted, specimen received more than 2 hours after collection SPECIAL INSTRUCTIONS: Schedule or arrange for referral testing with laboratory, as prothrombin assay is not commonly available and is not the same test as a "prothrombin time" determination.

Interpretive REFERENCE RANGE: 83% to 117% of normal USE: Document specific factor deficiency LIMITATIONS: Interpretation of results may be limited if patient is receiving anticoagulant therapy or if test is done more than 2 hours after collection. CONTRAINDICATIONS: Patient on anticoagulant therapy METHODOLOGY: Test (patient's) plasma is diluted, mixed with factor II deficient substrate, clotting (prothrombin) time determined, and result obtained by comparison with dilution curve prepared by testing mixtures of factor II deficient plasma and dilutions of normal serum. Two-stage prothrombin assay may be used (does not require a factor II deficient preparation).[1] These are "functional" assays. Confirmation of prothrombin deficiency should include tests for both biologic (functional) and immunologically (or amidolytic-chromogenic substrate assay) defined prothrombin protein. Normal level determined by an immunologic- or chromogenic substrate-based method but decrease in function by biologic assay (eg, two-stage assay) indicates presence of dysprothrombinemia. One-stage assays for prothrombin using trypsin, tiger snake, taipan snake, and *Echis carinatus* snake venoms have been applied to the analysis of molecular defects of prothrombin. ADDITIONAL INFORMATION: Prothrombin, a vitamin K dependent, single polypeptide chain coagulation protein is synthesized in the liver. It achieves a plasma concentration of about 10 mg/dL and has a half-life of about 3 days.[2] It is formed of 581 amino acid residues organized into three domains and has a molecular weight of some 70,000. The enzyme factor Xa activates prothrombin (a zymogen) with the resultant formation of the enzyme thrombin. The prothrombin molecule is unique in that carboxylation of glutamic acid residues (by a vitamin K dependent carboxylase) occurs and is necessary for the binding of the protein to phospholipid surfaces and subsequent conversion to thrombin. Factor V, phospholipids, and calcium ions accelerate the rate of this conversion.

Two classes of autosomal recessive inherited abnormalities manifest, clinically; both are uncommon. Quantitative and qualitative (dysfunctional) defects occur. The latter are termed "dysprothrombinemias". The term "CRM-" (cross reacting material negative) is applied if factor II protein is absent while "CRM+" (cross reacting material positive) indicates presence of dysfunctional prothrombin. Inherited prothrombin deficiency is the rarest coagulopathy (incidence of 0.5/100,000 in most populations, 1/10,000 in the Italian population).[3] True hypoprothrombinemia is the most common form of congenital prothrombin deficiency.[4] Hypoprothrombinemia may be homozygous (prothrombin levels of 1% to 25%) or heterozygous (levels of 50% to 60%). Severe bleeding occurs in homozygous individuals with epistaxis, easy bruising, hematoma formation, menorrhagia, and post-trauma/postsurgical hemorrhage. Heterozygotes may have bleeding but usually very mild. Homozygotes have prolonged whole blood clotting times, APTT, and PT tests (prothrombin is required in the final common pathway of coagulation). A variety of genetic mechanisms underlie the dysprothrombinemias. Characteristics of Prothrombins Cardeza, Barcelona, San Juan I and II, Padua, Brussels, Quick, Molise, Metz, Madrid, Houston, Birmingham, Denver, Gainesville, Habana, Salakta, and Poissy have been summarized in a 1984 review by Maas and Triplett.[5] Bick, in his recent text (see reference), lists 19 examples of dysprothrombinemias described over the past two decades.

Transient acquired factor II deficiency has been briefly described, associated with *Mycoplasma pneumoniae* infection.[6]

Footnotes

1. Dacie JV and Lewis SM, *Practical Haematology*, 7th ed, New York, NY: Churchill Livingstone, 1991, 275-6.
2. Seegers WH, "Purification of Prothrombin and Thrombin," *Semin Thromb Hemost*, 1981, 7:199-212.
3. Shapiro SS and McCord S, "Prothrombin," *Prog Hemost Thromb*, 1978, 4:177-209.
4. Bithell TC, "Hereditary Coagulation Disorders," *Wintrobe's Clinical Hematology*, 9th ed, Vol 2, Chapter 56, Lee GR, Bithell TC, Foerster J, et al, eds, Philadelphia, PA: Lea and Febiger, 1993, 1442-3.
5. Maas R and Triplett DA, "Congenital Deficiency of Prothrombin," *ASCP Check Sample®*, Chicago, IL: American Society of Clinical Pathologists, 1984.
6. Collazos J, Egurbide MV, Atucha K, et al, "Transient Acquired Factor II Deficiency With *Mycoplasma pneumoniae* Infection," *J Infect Dis*, 1991, 164(2):434-5.

References

Bick RL, "Hereditary Coagulation Protein Defects," *Disorders of Thrombosis and Hemostasis: Clinical and Laboratory Practice*, Chapter 6, Chicago, IL: ASCP Press, 1992, 112-4.

Mammen EF, "Nature of Inherited Disorders," *Prothrombin and Other Vitamin K Proteins*, Vol 1, Seegers WA and Walz DA, eds, Boca Raton, FL: CRC Press, 1986, 115.

Factor V

***CPT** 85220*

Related Information

Coagulation Factor Assay *on page 414*
Plasma, Fresh Frozen *on page 1078*
Platelet Concentrate, Donation and Transfusion *on page 1081*

Synonyms Ac-Globulin; Labile Factor; Proaccelerin

Patient Care **PREPARATION:** Avoid Coumadin® therapy for 2 weeks and heparin therapy for 2 days prior to test.

Specimen Plasma **CONTAINER:** Blue top (sodium citrate) tube **COLLECTION:** Routine venipuncture. If multiple tests are being drawn, draw coagulation studies last. If only coagulation tests are being drawn, draw 1-2 mL into another Vacutainer®, discard, and then collect coagulation tests. This collection procedure avoids contamination of the specimen with tissue thromboplastins. **STORAGE INSTRUCTIONS:** Deliver specimen immediately to the laboratory on ice. Centrifuge (in refrigerated centrifuge at 4°C) and separate plasma. Keep refrigerated and test immediately, preferably within 1-2 hours. **CAUSES FOR REJECTION:** Tube not full, specimen hemolyzed, specimen clotted, specimen received more than 2 hours after collection **SPECIAL INSTRUCTIONS:** Not available in most general clinical laboratories. Communicate with laboratory for scheduling and referral as required.

Interpretive **REFERENCE RANGE:** 50% to 150% of normal. Homozygous factor V deficient patients have <10% (often <5%) activity. **USE:** Document specific factor deficiency **LIMITATIONS:** Interpretation of results may be limited if patient is receiving anticoagulant therapy or if test is done more than 2 hours after collection. **METHODOLOGY:** Modified one-stage prothrombin time using commercially available factor V deficient preparation, known factor V deficient patient plasma or artificially prepared factor V deficient plasma. Chromogenic substrate assay. **ADDITIONAL INFORMATION:** Factor V, a glycoprotein with molecular weight of 300,000, is synthesized in the liver. It is converted in the plasma from a single chain to a two chain molecule under the influence of thrombin activation. Activated V (Va) is a part of the prothrombin converting complex. Va is inactivated by protein Ca.[1] The molecular characterization of Va, in particular identification of the structural determinants responsible for acceleration of prothrombin activation and those that bind to phospholipid surfaces, have been described.[2] Factor V deficiency is inherited as an autosomal recessive, males and females are equally affected. Only homozygotes have bleeding symptoms; heterozygotes are largely asymptomatic. Symptoms include ecchymoses, epistaxis, menorrhagia, and bleeding following trauma and tooth extraction. GI hemorrhage and hemarthrosis may occur. Severity of bleeding does not correlate di-

(Continued)

Factor V *(Continued)*

rectly with factor V level, and symptoms are often mild, even in homozygotes. Cases of apparent combined factor V and factor VIII deficiency appear to be due to inherited deficiency of a plasma protein that inhibits activated protein C.[2] Protein C is yet another vitamin K dependent serine protease zymogen coagulation protein, an anticoagulant that when activated (by thrombin, trypsin, or plasmin) destroys activated factors V and VIII. Homozygous V deficient individuals usually have prolonged whole blood clotting time, prothrombin time, and APTT. Platelet factor V is present in α-granules of platelets and is necessary to the binding of Xa to the platelet surface. Factor V deficient patients have varying levels of platelet factor V (may not be fully deficient). Platelet transfusion may have a role in the treatment of factor V deficient patients.[3] It has been shown that commercial preparations of bovine thrombin may contain bovine factor V and patients exposed to topical thrombin (bovine) may develop antibodies to factor V.[4] Antithrombin antibodies may also develop and mask the factor V inhibitor of activity that is responsible in part for clinical bleeding.

Footnotes

1. Heeb MJ, España, and Griffin JH, "Inhibition and Complexation of Activated Protein C by Two Major Inhibitors in Plasma," *Blood*, 1989, 73(2):446-54.
2. Jackson CM, "The Biochemistry of Prothrombin Activation," *Haemostasis and Thrombosis*, Bloom AL and Thomas DP, eds, New York, NY: Churchill Livingstone, 1987, 173-80.
3. Triplett DA, *Laboratory Evaluation of Coagulation*, Chicago, IL: ASCP Press, 1982, 78.
4. Zehnder JL and Leung LL, "Development of Antibodies to Thrombin and Factor V With Recurrent Bleeding in a Patient Exposed to Topical Bovine Thrombin," *Blood*, 1990, 76(10):2011-6.

References

Mammen EF, "Factor V Deficiency; Congenital Coagulation Disorders," *Semin Thromb Hemost*, New York, NY: Thieme-Stratton Inc, 1983, 9:17-8.

Factor VII

***CPT** 85230*

Related Information

Coagulation Factor Assay *on page 414*
Hypercoagulable State Coagulation Screen *on page 441*
Plasma, Fresh Frozen *on page 1078*
Prothrombin Time *on page 468*

Synonyms Autoprothrombin I; Proconvertin; Stable Factor

Patient Care **PREPARATION:** Avoid coumarin-type anticoagulants for 2 weeks and heparin therapy for 2 days prior to test.

Specimen Plasma **CONTAINER:** Blue top (sodium citrate) tube **COLLECTION:** Routine venipuncture. If multiple tests are being drawn, draw coagulation studies last. If only coagulation tests are being drawn, draw 1-2 mL into another Vacutainer®, discard, and then collect coagulation tests. This collection procedure avoids contamination of the specimen with tissue thromboplastins. **STORAGE INSTRUCTIONS:** Keep refrigerated. **CAUSES FOR REJECTION:** Tube not full, specimen hemolyzed, specimen clotted, specimen received more than 2 hours after collection **SPECIAL INSTRUCTIONS:** Schedule with laboratory in advance as this test is not routinely available and usually requires transport to a specialized coagulation laboratory.

Interpretive **REFERENCE RANGE:** 50% to 150% of normal. Homozygous VII deficient patients have a less than 10% level of this factor. **USE:** Document specific factor deficiency **LIMITATIONS:** Interpretation of result may be limited if patient is receiving anticoagulant therapy or if test is done more than 2 hours after collection. **METHODOLOGY:** Modified one-stage prothrombin time utilizing commercially available factor VII deficient substrates or known factor VII deficient patient plasma (as condition is rare this is uncommonly available). A coupled amidolytic assay, tritiated peptide release assay, and an enzyme immunoassay (EIA) have been developed.[1] Use of a factor VII antigen assay (EIA) may be superior as it is not affected by the level of extrinsic pathway inhibitor. **ADDITIONAL INFORMATION:** Factor VII, a vitamin K dependent coagulation glycoprotein is synthesized in the liver. It is a single peptide chain of molecular weight 45,000-53,000 and is formed of 408 amino acids. Acute deficiencies may occur with severe hepatocellular disease. Glutamic acid residues are carboxylated (vitamin K dependent) as with prothrombin. At these γ-carboxyglutamic acid residues calcium binds factor VII to phospholipid surfaces. Factor VII is activated to VIIa by thrombin, Xa or XIIa fragments. The activated enzymic form of factor VII is a two chain molecule with the serine active site present on the heavy chain. Factor VII is unique in that it is the only factor in the extrinsic pathway of factor X activation. Deficiency of factor VII should be considered in patients with a prolonged prothrombin time but a normal APTT. Over 150 cases of hereditary deficiency have been described in the literature. About 20% of patients with functional hereditary factor VII defect are due to factor VII molecular variants (phenotypically abnormal proteins). While deficiency is rare, two forms exist. Both are autosomal recessive and affect both sexes. In one form the VII molecules are decreased while in the second group an abnormally formed molecule is produced. Bleeding symptoms may be severe in homozygotes and include epistaxis, ecchymoses, GI bleeding, hemarthroses, menorrhagia, and umbilical cord hemorrhage. Fatal cerebral hemorrhage may occur. Heterozygotes are usually asymptomatic. Homozygotes have prolonged prothrombin time (corrected by adding normal plasma) but normal APTT, cephalin activated clotting time, and thrombin time.

Phenotype expression in the form of hemorrhagic symptoms is quite variable; symptomatology does not always correlate with the degree of factor VII deficiency. There are some patients reported to have thrombotic episodes.[2] It is not clear if some of the clinical variation relates to molecular structural variants.

Homozygous homocystinuria is associated with thromboembolism. Factor VII, AT III, and protein C levels have been reported as decreased in two sisters with this disease.[3] Decreased synthesis of liver produced coagulation factors may occur in homocystinuria.

A growing body of evidence indicates greater risk of coronary artery disease with both higher plasma fibrinogen and factor VII coagulant activity relating to apparently associated lipid parameters.[4,5,6,7,8] Increase in dietary fat intake has been associated with increases in VIIC, serum lipids, and coronary heart disease.[9] Specifically, plasma VII level has been found higher in women than men and, in both sexes, increased relative to body size, triglyceride, LDL cholesterol, and HDL cholesterol.[10] Factor VII levels have been found inversely proportional to ethanol intake.[10] Postprandial triglyceridemia has been associated with an acute effect (increase) in VII activity.[11]

Footnotes

1. Hultin MB, "Fibrinogen and Factor VII as Risk Factors in Vascular Disease," *Prog Hemost Thromb*, 1991, 10:215-41.
2. Ogston D, *Venous Thrombosis: Causation and Prediction*, New York, NY: John Wiley and Sons, 1987.
3. Palareti G, Salardi S, Legnani C, et al, "Reduced Levels of Antithrombin III, Protein C and Factor VII in Homocystinuria. Long-Term Changes in Relation to Treatment," *Thromb Haemost*, 1985, 54:35, (abstract).
4. Meade TW, Mellow S, Brozovic M, et al, "Haemostatic Function and Ischaemic Heart Disease: Principal Results of the Northwick Park Heart Study," *Lancet*, 1986, ii:533-7.
5. Broadhurst P, Kelleher C, Hughes L, et al, "Fibrogen, Factor VII Clotting Activity and Coronary Artery Disease Severity," *Atherosclerosis*, 1990, 85(2-3):169-73.
6. Hubbard AR and Parr LJ, "The Effect of Phospholipase C on Plasma Factor VII," *Br J Haematol*, 1989, 73(3):360-4.
7. Hoffman CJ, Miller RH, Lawson WE, et al, "Elevation of Factor VII Activity and Mass in Young Adults at Risk of Ischemic Heart Disease," *J Am Coll Cardiol*, 1989, 14(4):941-6.
8. Mitropoulos KA, Miller GJ, Reeves BE, et al, "Factor VII Coagulant Activity Is Strongly Associated With the Plasma Concentration of Large Lipoprotein Particles in Middle-Aged Men," *Atherosclerosis*, 1989, 76(2-3):203-8.
9. Miller GJ, Cruickshank JK, Ellis LJ, et al, "Fat Consumption and Factor VII Coagulant Activity in Middle-Aged Men – An Association Between a Dietary and Thrombogenic Coronary Risk Factor," *Atherosclerosis*, 1989, 78(1):19-24.
10. Folsom AR, Wu KK, Davis CE, et al, "Population Correlates of Plasma Fibrinogen and Factor VII, Putative Cardiovascular Risk Factors," *Atherosclerosis*, 1991, 91(3):191-205.
11. Miller GJ, Martin JC, Mitropoulos KA, et al, "Plasma Factor VII Is Activated by Postprandial Triglyceridaemia, Irrespective of Dietary Fat Composition," *Atherosclerosis*, 1991, 86(2-3):163-71.

References

Fadel HE and Krauss JS, "Factor VII Deficiency and Pregnancy," *Obstet Gynecol*, 1989, 73(3 Pt 2):453-4.

Giddings JC, *Molecular Genetics and Immunoanalysis in Blood Coagulation*, Chichester, England: Ellis Horwood Ltd, 1988, 42-7.

Hayes TE, Pike J, and Tracy RP, "Factor VII Assays," *Arch Pathol Lab Med*, 1993, 117:52-7.

Mammen EF, "Factor VII Abnormalities," *Semin Thromb Hemost*, New York, NY: Thieme-Stratton Inc, 1983, 9:19-21.

Rao LV and Rapaport SI, "Factor VIIa-Catalyzed Activation of Factor X Independent of Tissue Factor: Its Possible Significance for Control of Hemophilic Bleeding by Infused Factor VIIa," *Blood*, 1990, 75(5):1069-73.

Factor VIII

CPT *85240*

Related Information

Coagulation Factor Assay *on page 414*
Cryoprecipitate *on page 1058*
Factor VIII Concentrate *on page 1064*
Factor IX *on page 426*
Factor IX Complex (Human) *on page 1065*
Partial Thromboplastin Time *on page 450*
Plasma, Fresh Frozen *on page 1078*
von Willebrand Factor Antigen *on page 476*
von Willebrand Factor Multimer Assay *on page 478*

Synonyms AHF; Antihemophilic Factor; F VIII; VIIIC:Ag

Applies to von Willebrand Protein; vWF

Specimen Plasma **CONTAINER:** Blue top (sodium citrate) tube **COLLECTION:** Routine venipuncture. If multiple tests are being drawn, draw coagulation studies last. If only coagulation tests are being drawn, draw 1-2 mL into another Vacutainer®, discard, and then collect coagulation tests. This collection procedure avoids contamination of the specimen with tissue thromboplastins. **STORAGE INSTRUCTIONS:** Deliver immediately on ice to the laboratory. Separate off platelet poor plasma. May store up to 2 hours at 2°C to 8°C or up to 2 weeks at -35°C. **CAUSES FOR REJECTION:** Clotted, hemolyzed or I.V. fluid diluted specimens, heparin contamination, improperly filled specimen tube, tube not iced, specimen received more than 1 hour after collection **SPECIAL INSTRUCTIONS:** Is not a routinely performed assay. May require scheduling or referral to a specialized or reference laboratory.

Interpretive **REFERENCE RANGE:** 50% to 150% of normal, plasma concentration is about 100 μg/L. See table in von Willebrand Factor Antigen listing. **USE:** Detect coagulant factor VIII deficiency **LIMITATIONS:** Increased in patients taking oral contraceptives. Does not measure antigenic reactivity. See listing, von Willebrand Factor Antigen. **METHODOLOGY:** Clotting times (one-stage or two-stage APTT) are performed on dilutions of patient plasma which have been mixed with APTT reagent and specific factor deficient plasma. The level of activity is determined by graphing results and comparing with those from pooled normal plasma similarly treated. Electroimmunoassay (Laurell rocket assay), two-dimensional crossed immunoelectrophoresis, immunoautoradiography, immunoblotting, radioimmunoassay (RIA), enzyme immunoassay (EIA) using monoclonal antibody. **ADDITIONAL INFORMATION:** Factor VIII deficiency (**hemophilia A**) is the most common of the hereditary bleeding disorders. Clinical features are the same as for factor IX deficiency. See listing, Factor IX. Deficiencies of factor VIII or IX are inherited as sex-linked recessive disorders.

Factor VIII is a molecular complex consisting of VIII:C, which corrects the abnormal clotting time, and VIII:R the "related protein" (the von Willebrand protein) which corrects the defect in von Willebrand's disease. VIII:C portion of the complex is a glycoprotein with molecular weight of about 285,000. There are both VIII:C deficient patients (cross reacting material negative (CRM$^-$) type also named hemophilia A$^-$, the common form) and VIII:C nonfunctional molecular variant patients (CRM$^+$ type also named hemophilia A$^+$).

Factor VIII circulates as a heterodimer bound to vWF through a C-terminal light chain.[1] The latter is metal ion-bridged to a N-terminal heavy chain. Proteolytic processing by thrombin produces expression of cofactor activity which correlates with cleavages at amino acid positions 372, 740, and 1689. Cleavages at positions 1689 and 372 are essential for cofactor activity in recombinant F VIII.[2] The factor VIII gene is large (186 kilobases). There is a high frequency of *de novo* mutations but in only about 50% of patients with severe hemophilia A are mutations in the gene itself detected.[3,4] It is hypothesized that mutations occur in locus-controlling regions or other sequences outside the gene that are important for its expression or in other genes necessary for factor VIII expression.[4] Use of factor VIII gene probes have confirmed the thesis that multiple different molecular abnormalities may result in clinical hemophilia A.[5] A case of severe hemophilia A, factor VIII 1689-Cys, a point mutation of a C to T transition in codon 1689 converting Arg to Cys at the light chain thrombin cleavage site has been shown to result in a failure to release the acidic peptide from the light chain on thrombin activation.[6]

Desmopressin (1-deamino-8-D-arginine vasopressin, DDAVP®), a synthetic analogue of ADH L-arginine vasopressin, can raise circulating levels of F VIII and vWF. As such, it has become established as a nontransfusional form for the therapy of mild and moderate forms of hemophilia A and von Willebrand's disease. In addition, there is evidence that DDAVP® reduces blood loss and transfusion requirements in cardiopulmonary bypass patients (who have defective hemostasis) and also in hemostatically normal individuals (eg, spinal fusion patients). DDAVP® may cause increase in factor VIII and vWF by increasing their release from storage sites. Mannucci has reviewed this important subject (see following reference).

Factor VIII concentrates, produced using recombinant technology, have been undergoing human clinical trials[7,8] and are available for clinical use (eg, Kogenate®, antihemophilic factor, recombinant). The manufacture of recombinant factor VIII, however, suffers from inefficiencies of production relating to the large size of this heterogeneous glycoprotein. To circumvent these difficulties, a B-domain-deleted form of FVIII has been developed. Residues 760-1639 are absent in this form (LA-VIII) of the molecule. It has been shown that the biochemical, immunologic, and *in vivo* functional characteristics are those of wild type rFVIII.[9] Potentially this source of factor VIII will allow large supply, low cost, and freedom from the threat of human virus infection. Molecular biologic techniques such as cloning of the VIII and IX genes and recombinant genetic technology may allow therapy to be directed at the underlying cause of the disease. On the near horizon is cure of factor VIII deficiency by "gene therapy."[10,11]

Family studies, combined with DNA (restriction fragment length polymorphism) and discriminant analyses, can determine if at-risk women are carriers for hemophilia A in most cases.[12]

Footnotes

1. Eaton DL and Vehar GA, "Factor VIII Structure and Proteolytic Processing," *Prog Hemost Thromb*, 1986, 8:47-70.
2. Pittman DD and Kaufman RJ, "Proteolytic Requirements for Thrombin Activation of Antihemophilic Factor (Factor VIII)," *Proc Natl Acad Sci U S A*, 1988, 85:2429-33.
3. Randall T, "Gene Scene: Factor VIII Gene Explains Just Half of Severe Cases of Hemophilia A," *JAMA* 1991, 226(12):1612-3.
4. Higuchi M, Kazazian HH Jr, Kasch L, et al, "Molecular Characterization of Severe Hemophilia A Suggests That About Half the Mutations Are Not Within the Coding Regions and Splice Junctions of the Factor VIII Gene," *Proc Natl Acad Sci U S A*, 1991, 88(16):7405-9.
5. Higuchi M, Kochhan L, Schwaab R, et al, "Molecular Defects in Hemophilia A: Identification and Characterization of Mutations in the Factor VIII Gene and Family Analysis," *Blood*, 1989, 74(3):1045-51.
6. O'Brien DP and Tuddenham EGD, "Purification and Characterization of Factor VIII 1,689-Cys: A Nonfunctional Cofactor Occurring in a Patient With Severe Hemophilia A," *Blood*, 1989, 73(8):2117-22.
7. Aronson DL, "The Current Status of Recombinant Human Factor VIII," *Semin Hematol*, 1991, 28(2 Suppl 1):55-6.
8. Schwartz RS and Rousell RH, "A Summary of the World-Wide Clinical Investigations of Recombinant Factor VIII," *Semin Hematol*, 1991, 28(2 Suppl 1):53-4.
9. Pittman DD, Alderman EM, Tomkinson KN, et al, "Biochemical, Immunological, and *In Vivo* Functional Characterization of B-Domain-Deleted Factor VIII," *Blood*, 1993, 81(11):2925-35.
10. Roberts HR, High VA, White GL, et al, "Ultra-Pure Factor VIII Products: The Impact for the Future of Hemophilia Care," Presented at the XVIII International Congress of the World Federation of Hemophilia, Madrid, May 26-31. 1988.
11. Israel DI and Kaufman RJ, "Retroviral-Mediated Transfer and Amplification of a Functional Human Factor VIII Gene," *Blood*, 1990, 75(5):1074-80.
12. Poon M-C, Hoar DI, Low S, et al, "Hemophilia A Carrier Detection by Restriction Fragment Length Polymorphism Analysis and Discriminant Analysis Based on ELISA of Factor VIII and vWf," *J Lab Clin Med*, 1992, 119(6):751-62.

References

Arkin CF, Bovill EG, Brandt JT, et al, "Factors Affecting the Performance of Factor VIII Coagulant Activity Assays," *Arch Pathol Lab Med*, 1992, 116(9):908-15.

Brandt JT, "Measurement of Factor VIII: A Potential Risk Factor for Vascular Disease," *Arch Pathol Lab Med*, 1993, 117(1):48-51.

Brettler DB and Levine PH, "Factor Concentrates for Treatment of Hemophilia: Which One to Choose?" *Blood*, 1989, 73(8):2067-73.

Mammen EF, "Factor VIII Abnormalities," *Semin Thromb Hemost*, New York, NY: Thieme-Stratton Inc, 1983, 9:22-7.

Mannucci PM, "Desmopressin: A Nontransfusional Form of Treatment for Congenital and Acquired Bleeding Disorders," *Blood*, 1988, 72:1449-55, (review).

Rao LV and Rapaport SI, "Factor VIIa-Catalyzed Activation of Factor X Independent of Tissue Factor: Its Possible Significance for Control of Hemophilic Bleeding by Infused Factor VIIa," *Blood*, 1990, 75(5):1069-73.

Schwaab R, Oldenburg J, Tuddenham EG, et al, "Mutations in Haemophilia A," *Br J Haematol*, 1993, 83(3):450-8.

Thompson AR, "Molecular Biology of the Hemophilias," *Prog Hemost Thromb*, 1991, 10:175-214.

White GC 2d and Shoemaker CB, "Factor VIII Gene and Hemophilia A," *Blood*, 1989, 73(1):1-12.

Zimmerman TS and Meyer D, "Structure and Function of Factor VIII and von Willebrand Factor," and Bloom AL, "Inherited Disorders of Blood Coagulation," *Hemostasis and Thrombosis*, Bloom AL and Thomas DP, eds, New York, NY: Churchill Livingstone, 1987, 131-47, 393-436.

Factor IX

CPT 85250

Related Information

Coagulation Factor Assay *on page 414*
Factor VIII *on page 424*
Factor IX Complex (Human) *on page 1065*
Partial Thromboplastin Time *on page 450*
Plasma, Fresh Frozen *on page 1078*

Synonyms Autoprothrombin II; Christmas Disease Factor; Hemophilia B; Plasma Thromboplastin Component

Patient Care PREPARATION: Avoid Coumadin® therapy for 2 weeks and heparin therapy for 2 days prior to test

Specimen Plasma CONTAINER: Blue top (sodium citrate) tube COLLECTION: Routine venipuncture. If multiple tests are being drawn, draw coagulation studies second. If only coagulation studies are being drawn, draw 1-2 mL into another Vacutainer®, discard, and then collect coagulation tests. This avoids contamination of the specimen with tissue thromboplastins. STORAGE INSTRUCTIONS: Keep refrigerated. CAUSES FOR REJECTION: Tube not full, specimen hemolyzed, specimen clotted, specimen received more than 2 hours after collection SPECIAL INSTRUCTIONS: Contact testing facility to schedule and possibly arrange for referral as this is an uncommonly available procedure unless you have access to a special coagulation laboratory.

Interpretive REFERENCE RANGE: 50% to 150% of normal. Patients with severe hemophilia will have levels of less than 1%, often undetectable. Moderate forms of the disease have levels of 1% to 10% while some mild cases may have 11% to 49% of normal factor IX. Plasma concentration is about 4 mg/L, biological half-life is 18-24 hours. Caution has been recommended in the interpretation of factor IX levels in prepubertal children and in particular, FIX functional to FIX antigen determined ratios, as there is evidence that values are lower in normal children than in adults.[1] USE: Document specific factor deficiency LIMITATIONS: Interpretation of results may be limited if patient is receiving anticoagulant therapy or if test is done more than 2 hours after collection. CONTRAINDICATIONS: Patient on anticoagulant therapy METHODOLOGY: One-stage and two-stage assays have been described. One-stage assay based on APTT involves testing mixtures of factor IX deficient plasma and dilutions of normal and test plasma. APTT results are obtained, and corrective effect of test plasma, as compared to normal plasma, is expressed as a percentage.[2] A 1988 College of American Pathologists Survey Program found that factor IX assay performance by participating laboratories showed improved assay precision as compared with performance in a 1980 survey.[3] There was significant difference, however, in the sensitivity of APTT reagents to factor IX deficiency. In addition, the least sensitive reagents included some that are in common use.[3] ADDITIONAL INFORMATION: Factor IX is a vitamin K dependent liver produced coagulation protein (a zymogen). It is a single chain glycoprotein with molecular weight of about 55,000 and plasma concentration of 4 μg/mL. It is about 18% carbohydrate; the complete amino acid sequence has been determined. As with factor II, glutamic acid residues are converted by a carboxylase (vitamin K dependent process) to γ-carboxyglutamic acid. Factor IX is activated to the enzyme IXa by XIa and calcium or, and perhaps predominantly by, VIIa, a tissue factor substance, and calcium.[4]

Factor IX deficiency (PTC, plasma thromboplastin component or **Christmas disease**) is commonly referred to as **hemophilia B**. It has a recessive sex-linked mode of inheritance, males are affected, females are carriers. It occurs in 1 of 25,000 males. There is genetic heterogeneity, not all cases are clinically severe; mild forms are more prevalent than severe, some may not be associated with spontaneous bleeding episodes. Carriers are asymptomatic, but some variants may have moderately prolonged prothrombin time (see following information). In some cases, the functional abnormality relates to production of an abnormal factor IX molecule. Over 20 variants have been described. Factor IX deficiency can be characterized and phenotypically classified on the basis of functional activity, level of antigenic-reacting material and reaction with bovine thromboplastin in relation to the presence of CRM (cross reacting material).[5] Clinical symptoms of hemophilia B include hematuria; GI hemorrhage; muscle and mucous membrane hemorrhage; intracranial, post-traumatic, and postsurgical bleeding; and joint hematomas (not significantly different from the features of hemophilia A – factor VIII deficiency). Low levels of factor IX may be present in patients with liver disease. Severity of the symptoms correlate directly with the degree of prolongation of APTT test (level of factor IX deficiency). Mildly affected patients may show excessive bleeding only with major trauma or surgery. The APTT may not be prolonged if the factor IX level is over 25%. In most cases of hemophilia B, the prothrombin time and thrombin times are normal. A subgroup of cross reacting material positive hemophilia B patients, however, is defined by its markedly prolonged ox-brain prothrombin time. The molecular defect of this "hemophilia B_m" (factor IX*Hilo*) has recently been described.[6]

A considerable body of knowledge concerning the molecular diversity of factor IX deficiency and the responsible genetic mechanisms has accumulated and is expanding. Application of oligonucleotide probes and endonuclease restriction enzymes has been applied to the study of factor IX polymorphisms. Recently a procedure based on DNA amplification using the polymerase chain reaction has been described.[7] It is described as rapid, avoids the use of radioisotopes, can be performed on small samples (under 1 mL) of whole blood, and has shown a high level of sensitivity. It is said to be applicable to any genetic polymorphism that overlaps a restriction enzyme recognition site.

A novel possibly curative therapy for factor IX deficiency has been described and could have application to other coagulation deficient states or abnormalities.[8] A retroviral vector encoding human clotting factor IX was introduced into normal human skin fibroblasts. More than 3 μg of factor IX per 1 million cultured cells was secreted over 24 hours. More than 70% of this protein was structurally and functionally indistinguishable from normal human factor IX. While this work was performed in rats and mice, it suggests that infected autologous fibroblasts might be capable of providing therapeutic levels of factor IX if transplanted into some hemophilia B patients.

Footnotes

1. Sweeney JD and Hoernig LA, "Age-Dependent Effect on the Level of Factor IX," *Am J Clin Pathol*, 1993, 99:687-8.
2. Dacie JV and Lewis SM, *Practical Haematology*, 7th ed, New York, NY: Churchill Livingstone, 1991, 275-6.
3. Brandt JT, Arkin CF, Bovill EG, et al, "Evaluation of APTT Reagent Sensitivity to Factor IX and Factor IX Assay Performance," *Arch Pathol Lab Med*, 1990, 114(2):135-41.
4. Bauer KA, Kass BL, ten Cate H, et al, "Factor IX Is Activated *In Vivo* by the Tissue Factor Mechanism," *Blood*, 1990, 76(4):731-6.
5. Giddings JC, *Molecular Genetics and Immunoanalysis in Blood Coagulation*, Chichester, England: Ellis Horwood Ltd, 1988, 51-71.
6. Huang M-N, Kasper CK, Roberts HR, et al, "Molecular Defect in Factor IX_{Hilo}, a Hemophilia B_m Variant: Arg → Gln at the Carboxyterminal Cleavage Site of the Activation Peptide," *Blood*, 1989, 73(3):718-21.
7. Graham JB, Kunkel GR, Tennyson GS, et al, "The Malmö Polymorphism of Factor IX: Establishing the Genotypes by Rapid Analysis of DNA," *Blood*, 1989, 73(8):2104-7.
8. Palmer TD, Thompson AR, and Miller AD, "Production of Human Factor IX in Animals by Genetically Modified Skin Fibroblasts: Potential Therapy for Hemophilia B," *Blood*, 1989, 73(2):438-45.

References

Goldsmith JC, Kasper CK, Blatt PM, et al, "Coagulation Factor IX: Successful Surgical Experience With a Purified Factor IX Concentrate," *Am J Hematol*, 1992, 40(3):210-5.

Mammen EF, "Congenital Coagulation Disorders," *Semin Thromb Hemost*, New York, NY: Thieme-Stratton Inc, 1983, 9:28-33.

Thompson AR, "Molecular Biology of the Hemophilias," *Prog Hemost Thromb*, 1991, 10:175-214.

Wilbers LL and Triplett DA, "Acquired Factor IX Inhibitors," *ASCP Check Sample®*, Chicago, IL: American Society of Clinical Pathologists, 1987.

Factor X

***CPT** 85260*

Related Information

Coagulation Factor Assay *on page 414*

Plasma, Fresh Frozen *on page 1078*

Synonyms Stuart Factor; Stuart-Prower Factor

Patient Care **PREPARATION:** Avoid Coumadin® therapy for 2 weeks and heparin therapy for 2 days prior to test.

Specimen Plasma **CONTAINER:** Blue top (sodium citrate) tube **COLLECTION:** Routine venipuncture. If multiple tests are being drawn, draw coagulation studies last. If only coagulation tests are being drawn, draw 1-2 mL into another Vacutainer®, discard, and then collect coagulation tests. This collection procedure avoids contamination of the specimen with tissue thromboplastins. **STORAGE INSTRUCTIONS:** Keep refrigerated. **CAUSES FOR REJECTION:** Tube not full, specimen hemolyzed, specimen clotted, specimen received more than 2 hours after collection **SPECIAL INSTRUCTIONS:** Test is not commonly available. Communicate with laboratory for scheduling and referral to a specialized coagulation laboratory.

Interpretive **REFERENCE RANGE:** 50% to 150%. Homozygotes have less than 2% activity, heterozygotes, 40% to 60%.[1] Plasma concentration is about 12 mg/L. **USE:** Document specific

(Continued)

Factor X *(Continued)*

factor deficiency **LIMITATIONS:** Interpretation of result may be limited if patient is receiving anticoagulant therapy or if test is done more than 2 hours after collection. **METHODOLOGY:** Modified one-stage prothrombin time utilizing commercially available factor X deficient substrate with test result read from normal plasma dilution curve; enzyme-linked immunosorbent assay (ELISA): chromogenic assay **ADDITIONAL INFORMATION:** Factor X is a vitamin K dependent glycoprotein coagulation factor (molecular weight of 59,000) produced by the liver. It circulates in plasma as a two chain molecule with a serine active center in the heavy chain. A 43,000 dalton heavy chain and a 16,000 dalton light chain are held together by a disulfide bond; the protein contains some 15% carbohydrate. Glutamic acid residues on the light chain are converted to γ-carboxyglutamic acid by carboxylase (vitamin K required). This process allows for binding (calcium dependent) to phospholipid surfaces during coagulation. Factor X activation occurs by the extrinsic path (thromboplastin) and by the intrinsic path (IXa, VIIa, Ca^{++}, and phospholipids). A protease in Russell's viper venom produces nonphysiological activation. All activation pathways cleave the same arginyl-isoleucyl heavy chain bond. Activated X (Xa) converts prothrombin to thrombin. The rare clinical condition (X deficiency) is inherited as autosomal, incompletely recessive, consanguinity present in less than 50% of affected families. About 50 families with hereditary factor X deficiency have been reported. Symptoms (homozygotes) include hematoma formation, hemorrhage, menorrhagia, hematuria, and umbilical cord hemorrhage. Hemarthrosis, petechiae, and cerebral hemorrhage occur only rarely. Acquired deficiencies occur with significant hepatic dysfunction and with oral anticoagulant (coumarin) therapy. Whole blood clotting time, prothrombin time (corrected by giving aged plasma), and APTT are prolonged while thrombin time, bleeding time, platelet count, platelet function, and other coagulation factor levels are normal. Factor X deficiency may be associated with primary systemic amyloidosis.[2] Successful treatment has been reported with the use of Autoplex® T (activated prothrombin complex).[3]

Coagulation profiles of known factor X variants indicate a number of molecular aberrations of factor X/Xa function. There are cases without detectable factor X antigen or function, cases with selective abnormalities involving one of the pathways of activation and a population (Friuli region of Italy) with moderate bleeding tendency, functional decrease in factor X (as defined by PT and APTT testing) but normal clotting times with Russell's viper venom and normal levels of factor X antigen. A structural defect in the heavy chain of factor X Friuli has been identified. The defect is probably produced by a point mutation affecting the activated heavy chain within the 195-424 segment of the amino acid sequences. The functional result is an approximately 33% decrease in the rate of activation of prothrombin to thrombin by activated factor X Friuli as compared to normal factor X.[4] Factor X Santo Domingo, a cause of severe bleeding, is caused by a homozygous transition in exon I which causes a substitution in the carboxy-terminus of the signal peptide, preventing cleavage by the signal peptidase resulting in impaired factor X secretion.[5] Major abnormalities of chromosome 13 and partial deletion of the factor X gene (resulting in severe deficiency of factor X activity and antigen) have also been reported.[6]

Footnotes

1. Mori K, Sakai H, Nakano N, et al, "Congenital Factor X Deficiency in Japan," *Tohoku J Exp Med*, 1981, 133:1-19.
2. McPherson RA, Onstad JW, Ugoretz RJ, et al, "Coagulopathy in Amyloidosis: Combined Deficiency of Factors IX and X," *Am J Hematol*, 1977, 3:225-35.
3. Henson K, Files JC, and Morrison FS, "Transient Acquired Factor X Deficiency: Report of the Use of Activated Clotting Concentrate to Control a Life-Threatening Hemorrhage," *Am J Med*, 1989, 87(5):583-5.
4. Fair DS, Revak DJ, Hubbard JG, et al, "Isolation and Characterization of the Factor X Friuli Variant," *Blood*, 1989, 73(8):2108-16.
5. Watzke HH, Wallmark A, Hamaguchi N, et al, "Factor X Santo Domingo. Evidence That the Severe Clinical Phenotype Arises From a Mutation Blocking Secretion," *J Clin Invest*, 1991, 88(5):1685-9.
6. Bernardi F, Marchetti G, Patracchini P, et al, "Partial Gene Deletion in a Family With Factor X Deficiency," *Blood*, 1989, 73(8):2123-7.

References

Jackson CM, "Factor X," *Prog Hemost Thromb*, 1984, 55-109.

Mammen EF, "Factor X Abnormalities," *Semin Thromb Hemost*, 1983, 9:31-3.

Factor XI

CPT 85270

Related Information

Coagulation Factor Assay *on page 414*
Plasma, Fresh Frozen *on page 1078*

Synonyms Plasma Thromboplastin Antecedent; PTA

Patient Care PREPARATION: Avoid Coumadin® therapy for 2 weeks and heparin therapy for 2 days prior to test.

Specimen Plasma CONTAINER: Blue top (sodium citrate) tube COLLECTION: Routine venipuncture. If multiple tests are being drawn, draw coagulation studies last. If only coagulation tests are being drawn, draw 1-2 mL into another Vacutainer®, discard, and then collect coagulation tests. This collection procedure avoids contamination of the specimen with tissue thromboplastins. STORAGE INSTRUCTIONS: Keep refrigerated. CAUSES FOR REJECTION: Tube not full, specimen hemolyzed, specimen clotted, specimen received more than 2 hours after collection SPECIAL INSTRUCTIONS: Schedule with laboratory in advance. Test is not routinely available, done by specialized coagulation laboratory.

Interpretive REFERENCE RANGE: 50% to 150% of normal. Homozygotes usually have levels of 1% to 10% while heterozygotes have about 50%. USE: Document specific factor deficiency LIMITATIONS: Interpretation of result may be limited if patient is receiving anticoagulant therapy or if test is done more than 2 hours after collection. METHODOLOGY: Modified APTT using commercially available factor XI deficient substrate with test result read from normal plasma dilution curve ADDITIONAL INFORMATION: Factor XI, a coagulation glycoprotein produced in the liver, circulates in the plasma as a dimer, the two chains held by disulfide bonds. Factor XI is activated (to XIa) by factor XIIa, and the dimer is broken into two chains. The serine active center is resident on the light chain. Activation of XI requires surfaces (usually phospholipid) and presence of prekallikrein and HMWK (high molecular weight kininogen). Structural organization of the complete factor XI gene has been described.[1] Inherited factor XI deficiency, while uncommon, is one of the more frequently encountered inherited defects of the coagulation mechanism. This condition is transmitted as an incomplete autosomal recessive, affecting males and females, and is seen especially in Ashkenazi Jews. Only homozygous patients have bleeding symptoms. They suffer post-trauma/postsurgical hemorrhage, epistaxis, hematuria, and menorrhagia. Excessive postpartum hemorrhage is especially common. Severity of bleeding does not always correlate with the plasma level of factor XI.[1] This may relate in part to the mechanism of activation of factor XI[2] and/or to use of aspirin. Heterozygotes are asymptomatic. Homozygotes have prolonged whole blood clotting time and APTT. Prothrombin time, thrombin time, bleeding time, platelet count, and platelet function tests are normal.

Footnotes

1. Giddings JC, *Molecular Genetics and Immunoanalysis in Blood Coagulation*, Chichester, England: Ellis Horwood Ltd, 1988, 35-7.
2. Gailani D and Broze GJ Jr, "Factor XI Activation in a Revised Model of Blood Coagulation," *Science*, 1991, 253(5022):909-12.

References

Kitchens CS, "Factor XI: A Review of Its Biochemistry and Deficiency," *Semin Thromb Hemost*, 1991, 17(1):55-72.
Mammen EF, "Factor XI Deficiency," *Semin Thromb Hemost*, 1983, 9:34-5.

Factor XII

CPT 85280

Related Information

Coagulation Factor Assay *on page 414*
Hypercoagulable State Coagulation Screen *on page 441*
Plasma, Fresh Frozen *on page 1078*

Synonyms Hageman Factor; XIIa

Patient Care PREPARATION: Avoid Coumadin® therapy for 2 weeks and heparin therapy for 2 days prior to test.

Specimen Plasma CONTAINER: Blue top (sodium citrate) tube COLLECTION: Routine venipuncture. If multiple tests are being drawn, draw coagulation studies last. If only coagulation tests are being drawn, draw 1-2 mL into another Vacutainer®, discard, and then collect coagulation tests. This collection procedure avoids contamination of the specimen with tissue thromboplastins. STORAGE INSTRUCTIONS: Keep refrigerated. CAUSES FOR REJECTION: Tube not full, specimen hemolyzed, specimen clotted, specimen received more than 2 hours after collection SPECIAL INSTRUCTIONS: Schedule with laboratory in advance as this is an uncommonly available test and is usually done only by specialized coagulation laboratories.

(Continued)

Factor XII *(Continued)*

Interpretive **REFERENCE RANGE:** 50% to 150% of normal; homozygotes have levels <1%; heterozygotes have levels of 15% to 80%. **USE:** Document specific coagulation deficiency **LIMITATIONS:** Interpretation of results may be limited if patient is receiving anticoagulant therapy or if test is done more than 2 hours after collection. **METHODOLOGY:** Modified APTT using a known factor XII deficient substrate, test result read from normal plasma dilution curve **ADDITIONAL INFORMATION:** Hageman factor (factor XII) is one of three proteins, XII, prekallikrein, and high molecular weight kininogen (HMWK), involved in the contact activation system. Factor XII is the first protein adsorbed onto negatively-charged surfaces (collagen fibers, platelet membranes, and other tissue surfaces) exposed after endothelial damage. With activation to XIIa, there is interaction with prekallikrein, HMWK, and XIIa fragments in a complex circular reinforcement loop in which activation of the fibrinolytic system (plasminogen), complement system (C1), and vasoactive system (HMWK to bradykinin) also occur. Factor XII is a single chain glycoprotein molecule synthesized and secreted by hepatocytes.[1] Upon activation by kallikrein, it is transformed to an enzyme with a light and heavy chain. The light chain contains the active enzymatic (serine) site, while the heavy chain is concerned with surface binding. Factor XII deficiency is usually inherited as an autosomal recessive condition, but a rare example appears to have autosomal dominant mode of inheritance. The condition affects both males and females. Patients, however, do not have bleeding symptoms as the clotting system can be activated by alternate paths that bypass the contact system. Occasionally, patients suffer thromboembolic episodes which can be fatal and apparently relate to impaired fibrinolytic activity (one of the functions of XIIa is to activate plasminogen to plasmin). Homozygous XII deficient patients have prolonged whole blood clotting times and APTT results. Euglobulin clot lysis time is usually significantly prolonged. Prothrombin time, thrombin time, and bleeding time are normal in the XII deficient patient.

A structurally abnormal F XII (F XII Bern) has been shown to have a defect in the light chain region (wherein the enzymatic active site is situated).[2]

While there are some apparent clinical associations between eosinophilia (marked) and thrombosis, a recent study indicates that eosinophils in suspension or eosinophil peroxidase, eosinophil major basic protein or eosinophil cationic protein, inhibit activation of Hageman factor.[3]

Footnotes

1. Gordon EM, Gallagher CA, Johnson TR, et al, "Hepatocytes Express Blood Coagulation Factor XII (Hageman Factor)," *J Lab Clin Med*, 1990, 115(4):463-9.
2. Wuillemin WA, Huber I, Furlan M, et al, "Functional Characterization of an Abnormal Factor XII Molecule (F XII Bern)," *Blood*, 1991, 78(4):997-1004.
3. Ratnoff OD, Gleich GJ, Shurin SB, et al, "Inhibition of the Activation of Hageman Factor (Factor XII) by Eosinophils and Eosinophilic Constituents," *Am J Hematol*, 1993, 42(1):138-45.

References

Braulke I, Pruggmayer M, Melloh P, et al, "Factor XII (Hageman) Deficiency in Women With Habitual Abortion: New Subpopulation of Recurrent Aborters?" *Fertil Steril*, 1993, 59(1):98-101.

Mammen EF, "Contact Factor Abnormalities," *Semin Thromb Hemost*, 1983, 9:36-41.

McDonough RJ and Nelson CL, "Clinical Implications of Factor XII Deficiency," *Oral Surg Oral Med Oral Pathol*, 1989, 68(3):264-6.

Factor XIII

CPT *85290; 85291 (screen)*

Related Information

Clot Retraction *on page 413*

Coagulation Factor Assay *on page 414*

Plasma, Fresh Frozen *on page 1078*

Synonyms Fibrin Stabilizing Factor; Fibrinoligase; Laki-Lorand Factor

Specimen Plasma **CONTAINER:** Blue top (sodium citrate) tube **COLLECTION:** Routine venipuncture **STORAGE INSTRUCTIONS:** Keep refrigerated. **CAUSES FOR REJECTION:** Tubes not full, blood clotted, hemolyzed specimen, specimen received more than 2 hours after collection, specimen not refrigerated

Interpretive **REFERENCE RANGE:** Clot stable in 5M urea for at least 24 hours. If factor XIII deficiency is present, clot will usually dissolve in 1-2 hours. **USE:** Evaluate bleeding disorders due to homozygous deficiency of factor XIII **METHODOLOGY:** Citrated plasma is recalcified, clotted at 37°C, and after 30 minutes placed in 5M urea at 37°C (screening test). A quantitative assay is based on the incorporation of monodansylcadaverine into casein (transaminase activity).[1]

ADDITIONAL INFORMATION: Factor XIII converts loose hydrogen bonded monomers into covalently bonded fibrin polymer. The resultant end product of fibrin formation has increased tensile strength and is resistant to fibrinolysis. Inactive factor XIII is present in plasma at a concentration of about 1 mg/dL. It is converted into its active transglutaminase enzymic form by thrombin. Then, in the presence of calcium, it causes covalent cross-linkage of fibrin molecules. Clinical symptoms and abnormal result in the factor XIII screening test do not occur unless only 1% to 2% or less of factor XIII activity remains (patients have near total deficiency) – there are no mild to moderate forms. The deficiency is inherited as an autosomal recessive condition, heterozygotes (with 50% of levels of XIII) are asymptomatic. Homozygotes have slow progressive bleeding, often hematomas-hemorrhagic cysts, bleeding after cuts, and poor wound healing. Death may be due to intracranial hemorrhage. An important early sign is persistent umbilical stump hemorrhage. Cases of liver disease, pregnancy, sickle cell disease, and Henoch-Schönlein purpura may have moderately decreased factor XIII levels (without resultant bleeding).

Activated factor XIII levels and cross-linked fibrin polymers are increased in patients with acute myocardial infarction.[2]

Intracranial hemorrhage, reported in infants with XIII deficiency, has lead to a recommendation that prophylactic life-long factor XIII concentrate (eg, Fibrogammin®) replacement therapy be considered in patients with severe deficiency.[3]

Hemorrhagic diarrhea in some patients with active Crohn's disease may be due (at least in part) to acquired factor XIII deficiency.[4,5] Clinically significant inhibitors of factor XIII have been described but are encountered only rarely, some 12 cases having been reported.[6]

Footnotes

1. Lorand L, Urayama T, de Kiewiet JWC, et al, "Diagnostic and Genetic Studies on Fibrin-Stabilizing Factor With a New Assay Based on Amine Incorporation," *J Clin Invest*, 1969, 48:1054-64.
2. Francis CW, Connaghan DG, Scott WL, et al, "Increased Plasma Concentration of Cross-Linked Fibrin Polymers in Acute Myocardial Infarction," *Circulation*, 1987, 75:1170-7.
3. Abbondanzo SL, Gootenberg JE, Lofts RS, et al, "Intracranial Hemorrhage in Congenital Deficiency of Factor XIII," *J Ped Hemat/Oncology*, 1988, 10:65-8.
4. Wisen O and Gardlund B, "Hemostasis in Crohn's Disease: Low Factor XIII Levels in Active Disease," *Scand J Gastroenterol*, 1988, 23:961-6.
5. Mamel JJ, "Gastrointestinal Bleeding in Crohn's Disease: The Role of Acquired Factor Deficiency," *Am J Gastroenterol*, 1990, 85(3):321-2.
6. Fukue H, Anderson K, McPhedran P, et al, "A Unique Factor XIII Inhibitor to a Fibrin-Binding Site on Factor XIIIA," *Blood*, 1992, 79(1):65-74.

References

Duckert F, Jung E, Shmerling DH, et al, "A Hitherto Undescribed Congenital Hemorrhagic Diathesis Probably Due to Fibrin Stabilizing Factor Deficiency," *Thromb Diath Hemorrh*, 1960, 5:179.

Loxand L, Losowsky MS, and Miloszewski KJM, "Human Factor XIII: Fibrin Stabilizing Factor," *Prog Hemost Thromb*, Spaet TH, ed, New York, NY: Grune and Stratton Inc, 1980, 5:245-90.

Factor Assay *see* Coagulation Factor Assay *on page 414*

Factor, Fitzgerald

***CPT** 85293*

Related Information

Coagulation Factor Assay *on page 414*
Factor, Fletcher *on next page*

Synonyms Fitzgerald Factor Assay; High Molecular Weight Kininogen; HMW Kininogen; Williams-Fitzgerald-Flaujeac Factor

Patient Care **PREPARATION:** Avoid Coumadin® therapy for 2 weeks and heparin therapy for 2 days prior to test.

Specimen Plasma **CONTAINER:** Blue top (sodium citrate) tube **COLLECTION:** Routine venipuncture. If multiple tests are being drawn, draw coagulation studies last. If only coagulation tests are being draw, draw 1-2 mL into another Vacutainer®, discard, and then collect coagulation tests. This collection procedure avoids contamination of the specimen with tissue thromboplastins. Place specimen in ice and transport immediately to the laboratory. **STORAGE INSTRUCTIONS:** Keep refrigerated (2°C to 8°C for up to 2 hours). May store frozen (at -35°C) for up to 2 weeks. **CAUSES FOR REJECTION:** Specimen hemolyzed, clotted, diluted, or contaminated with heparin; tubes not full, not iced, or received more than 1 hour after collection **SPECIAL INSTRUCTIONS:** Not a routine test. Contact laboratory to learn of availability and need for special arrangements.

(Continued)

Factor, Fitzgerald *(Continued)*

Interpretive REFERENCE RANGE: Patient's plasma is normal if upon mixing with known deficient plasma the combination has normal APTT, 90 mg/L (bioassay) USE: Investigate cause of prolonged APTT; confirmation of Fitzgerald factor deficiency LIMITATIONS: Interpretation of results may be limited if patient is receiving anticoagulant therapy. CONTRAINDICATIONS: Patient on anticoagulant therapy METHODOLOGY: Measurement of functional coagulant activity of a mixture of test (patient's) plasma with Fitzgerald factor deficient plasma, bioassay based on kinin formation, radioimmunoassay (RIA), enzyme-linked immunosorbent assay (ELISA), particle concentration fluorescence immunoassay[1] ADDITIONAL INFORMATION: Previous prothrombin time and partial thromboplastin time are useful for interpretation. Patients with deficiency of Fitzgerald factor deficiency do not have clinical bleeding disease. Some patients have been reported to have thromboembolic episodes. This rare condition is considered when an abnormal APTT is not explained by other significant factor deficiency. The prolonged APTT clotting time may be shortened or even normalized after incubation with contact activators. HMWK (high molecular weight kininogen), Hageman factor (factor XII), and prekallikrein are functionally and structurally closely related. The gene for human kininogen has been isolated and characterized.[2] HMWK augments the formation of activated Hageman factor. A functional domain for the binding of HMWK is present within the heavy chain region of factor XI.[3] HMWK has a binding site for prekallikrein (Fletcher factor).[4] These proteins are involved in the contact phase of coagulation and immune system mechanisms. As deficient states of these proteins lack bleeding manifestations, it could be considered that they are not true coagulation factors. The intrinsic pathway of coagulation is initiated when the four plasma proteins (Hageman factor, prekallikrein, HMWK, and factor XI) interact with particular negatively charged surfaces. Plasminogen activation, immune pathway activation (release of kinins and complement activation) may also be involved. HMWK is one of the proteins required for the generation of bradykinin (a vasoactive peptide).

Footnotes

1. Scott CF and Colman RW, "Sensitive Antigenic Determinations of High Molecular Weight Kininogen Performed by Covalent Coupling of Capture Antibody," *J Lab Clin Med*, 1992, 119(1):77-86.
2. Kitamura N, Kitagawa H, Fukushima D, et al, "Structural Organization of the Human Kininogen Gene and a Model for Its Evolution," *J Biol Chem*, 1985, 260:8610-7.
3. Baglia FA, Sinha D, and Walsh PN, "Functional Domains in the Heavy-Chain Region of Factor XI: A High Molecular Weight Kininogen-Binding Site and a Substrate-Binding Site for Factor IX," *Blood*, 1989, 74(1):244-51.
4. Reddigari SR and Kaplan AP, "Monoclonal Antibody to Human High-Molecular-Weight Kininogen Recognizes Its Prekallikrein Binding Site and Inhibits Its Coagulant Activity," *Blood*, 1989, 74(2):695-702.

References

Giddings JC, *Molecular Genetics and Immunoanalysis in Blood Coagulation*, Chichester, England: Ellis Horwood Ltd, 1988, 3:30-2.

Factor, Fletcher

***CPT** 85292*

Related Information

Coagulation Factor Assay *on page 414*
Factor, Fitzgerald *on previous page*

Synonyms Fletcher Factor Assay; Prekallikrein Assay

Patient Care PREPARATION: Avoid Coumadin® therapy for 2 weeks and heparin therapy for 2 days prior to test.

Specimen Plasma CONTAINER: Blue top (sodium citrate) tube COLLECTION: Routine venipuncture. If multiple tests are being drawn, draw coagulation studies last. If only coagulation tests are being drawn, draw 1-2 mL into another Vacutainer®, discard, and then collect coagulation tests. This collection procedure avoids contamination of the specimen with tissue thromboplastins. STORAGE INSTRUCTIONS: Keep refrigerated. Centrifuge at 2500 g for 15 minutes at 4°C and remove platelet-poor plasma with plastic pipette. Test immediately or freeze and store at -70°C. CAUSES FOR REJECTION: Tube not full, specimen hemolyzed, specimen clotted, specimen received more than 2 hours after collection SPECIAL INSTRUCTIONS: Not a routine test. Contact laboratory for special arrangements and scheduling.

Interpretive REFERENCE RANGE: Patient's plasma is normal if upon addition to known deficient plasma the mixture has normal APTT. A level of only 2% of prekallikrein provides complete correction. 50 mg/L (RIA), 100 mg/L (RID). USE: Investigate cause of prolonged APTT; identify prekallikrein deficiency (Fletcher factor deficit)[1] LIMITATIONS: Interpretation of results may be limited if patient is receiving anticoagulant therapy. Use of an ellagic acid-activated thromboplastin will usually not detect Fletcher factor deficiency. **CONTRAINDICATIONS:** Patient on anticoagulant therapy **METHODOLOGY:** Measurement of coagulant activity of a mixture of test (patient's) plasma with Fletcher factor deficient plasma; radioimmunoassay (RIA), radial immunodiffusion (RID) **ADDITIONAL INFORMATION:** Previous prothrombin time and partial thromboplastin time are useful for interpretation. Prekallikrein is one of the coagulation proteins involved in the generation of bradykinin (a vasoactive peptide), and one of the major factors required for contact activation (others are Hageman factor and high molecular weight kininogen (HMWK)). Prekallikrein is a single-chain glycoprotein with molecular weight of about 88,000. In plasma, complexes form between prekallikrein and HMWK (up to 70% of prekallikrein may be so bound); immune-based assays, therefore, may overestimate the actual value. Deficiency of any of the contact factors is associated with prolongation of APTT test. Prolonged APTT times may be shortened or even normal after incubation with contact activators. Deficiency is thought to be inherited as an autosomal recessive trait and does not result in bleeding tendency. Some patients may have thromboembolic episodes. Prekallikrein may be decreased in some newborns. Levels may be decreased in some patients with liver disease and in patients with uremia.[2]

Footnotes

1. LaDuca FM and Tourbaf KD, "Fletcher Factor Deficiency, Source of Variations of the Activated Partial Thromboplastin Time Test," *Am J Clin Pathol*, 1981, 75:626-8.
2. Saito H and Ratnoff OD, "Alteration of Factor VII Activity by Activated Fletcher Factor (A Plasma Kallikrein): A Potential Link Between the Intrinsic and Extrinsic Blood-Clotting Systems," *J Lab Clin Med*, 1975, 85:405-15.

References

Giddings JC, *Molecular Genetics and Immunoanalysis in Blood Coagulation*, Chichester, England: Ellis Horwood Ltd, 1988, 27-30.

Triplett DA, "Congenital Coagulation Factor Deficiencies (Excluding Abnormalities of Factor VIII)," *Laboratory Evaluation of Coagulation*, Chicago, IL: ASCP Press, 1982, 96-7.

Factor I *see* Fibrinogen *on page 435*

Factor VIIIR:Ag *see* von Willebrand Factor Antigen *on page 476*

Factor VIII-Related Antigen *see* von Willebrand Factor Antigen *on page 476*

FBP *see* Fibrin Breakdown Products *on this page*

FDP *see* Fibrin Breakdown Products *on this page*

Fibrin Breakdown Products

CPT 85362 (semiquantitative); 85370 (quantitative)

Related Information

Cryoprecipitate *on page 1058*
D-Dimer *on page 416*
Euglobulin Clot Lysis *on page 418*
Fibrinogen *on page 435*
Fibrinopeptide A *on page 437*
Fibrin Split Products, Protamine Sulfate *on page 439*
Intravascular Coagulation Screen *on page 446*
Partial Thromboplastin Time *on page 450*

Synonyms FBP; FDP; Fibrin Degradation Products; Fibrin Split Products; Staphylococcal Clumping Test; Thrombo-Wellcotest® for Fibrin Split Products

Abstract Test for disseminated intravascular coagulation (DIC). Test results, if positive, are indicative of clot formation and subsequent lysis or partial lysis by fibrinolytic activity.

Patient Care **PREPARATION:** Draw sample for fibrin breakdown products before instituting heparin therapy

Specimen Plasma **CONTAINER:** Special tube for fibrin split products, containing thrombin and an antifibrinolytic agent (protease inhibitor) **COLLECTION:** Routine venipuncture. Blood placed in special tube obtained from Coagulation Laboratory. Mix gently. The specimen will clot. **STORAGE INSTRUCTIONS:** Separate and refrigerate serum as soon as possible if test is not run immediately. **CAUSES FOR REJECTION:** Nonclotted blood, improper collection tube, tube overfilled, inadequate labeling, improper storage of serum

Interpretive **REFERENCE RANGE:** <10 μg/mL **POSSIBLE PANIC RANGE:** >40 μg/mL **USE:** Detect fibrin breakdown products (FBP) in serum. Helpful in establishing the diagnosis of dissemi-

(Continued)

Fibrin Breakdown Products *(Continued)*

nated intravascular coagulation. The presence of fibrin breakdown products at the higher titer level (>40 μg/mL – Thrombo-Wellcotest®) indicates that a fibrinolytic process has high likelihood of being associated with DIC. FBP are also elevated in primary fibrinolysis. May be of use in monitoring fibrinolytic therapy. Of use in study of pulmonary embolism, myocardial infarct, inflammation, and some liver diseases (in which clot formation and lysis occur or increased fibrinolytic activity is present).[1] **LIMITATIONS:** May be normal in fibrinolytic states if fragments have been degraded into portions too small to detect (method dependent). The presence of rheumatoid factor may rarely interfere and cause falsely high results. If rheumatoid arthritis (RA) is clinically suspect, it is advisable to perform RA testing. If the patient's RA is negative, the test is valid. However, if the RA is positive, the FBP should be interpreted with caution. The presence of fibrinogen in the test serum will cause a false-positive result. The collection tube must be fully clotted. **CONTRAINDICATIONS:** Patient on heparin therapy **METHODOLOGY:** Latex agglutination (LA) /clumping (Thrombo-Wellcotest®), tanned RBC hemagglutination inhibition, staphylococcal clumping test, radioimmunoassay (RIA), others, a variety of immunologic-based methods incorporating antisera to one or more of the fragments of fibrinogen (X, Y, D, and E). A comparative study of three different methods has found significant variation in sensitivity when dealing with normal and "suspicious" range samples but comparable results in the detection of abnormal levels of fibrin split products.[2] **ADDITIONAL INFORMATION:** Breakdown products of fibrinogen and fibrin (X, Y, D, and E) are released during the process of fibrinolysis. Fragment X (large) can polymerize slowly with thrombin but usually forms aggregates with fibrinogen, fibrin monomer, or other X and Y fragments. Fragment Y does not polymerize but interferes with the action of thrombin (acts as an antithrombin). Fragments D and E are small, D inhibits fibrin polymerization, while E is relatively inert. In addition, it has been shown (using B β-1-24 determinations) that FBP provide a surface for tissue plasminogen activator and plasminogen binding potentiating fibrinogen proteolysis by promoting plasmin generation.[3] Previous and recent red cell morphology, thrombin time, prothrombin time, partial thromboplastin time, fibrinogen, and platelet count are useful for interpretation.

Increased levels of fibrin degradation products may occur with a variety of pathologic processes in which clot formation and lysis are involved. In particular, application to the differentiation of pulmonary embolic lung disease from nonthromboembolic processes has been suggested. FBP and soluble fibrin complexes (measured using the serial dilution protamine sulfate test of Gurewich and Hutchinson) are positive in 55% of patients with pulmonary embolism but in only 4% of patients with nonthromboembolic disease. Eighty-three percent of 29 patients with pulmonary emboli were positive for FBP, but 50% of 80 patients with nonthromboembolic pulmonary disease were positive (indicative of poor specificity). Carcinoma was especially associated with presence of FBP. Use of the two tests together provides greater specificity, but this approach, generally, is not specific for the diagnosis of pulmonary embolism.[4,5] Reference must be made to the patient's clinical status (eg, results of lung scan studies) to establish presence of pulmonary embolus. Use of plasma FBP levels to exclude diagnosis of pulmonary embolism may be of value but is not firmly established.[4]

Presence of FBP in the urine does not correlate with serum FBP level. Over 2 mg/day of urinary FBP may indicate fibrin deposition and lysis in the kidney (if marked proteinuria is not present).[6]

Footnotes

1. Triplett DA, "Acquired Abnormalities of Hemostasis," *Laboratory Evaluation of Coagulation*, Chicago, IL: ASCP Press, 1982, 215-7.
2. Drewinko B, Surgeon J, Cobb P, et al, "Comparative Sensitivity of Different Methods to Detect and Quantify Circulating Fibrinogen/Fibrin Split Products," *Am J Clin Pathol*, 1985, 84:58-66.
3. Weitz JI, Leslie B, and Ginsberg J, "Soluble Fibrin Degradation Products Potentiate Tissue Plasminogen Activator-Induced Fibrinogen Proteolysis," *J Clin Invest*, 1991, 87(3):1082-90.
4. Bynum LJ, Crotty C, and Wilson JE III, "Use of Fibrinogen/Fibrin Degradation Products and Soluble Fibrin Complexes for Differentiating Pulmonary Embolism From Nonthromboembolic Lung Disease," *Am Rev Respir Dis*, 1976, 114:285-9.
5. Rowbotham BJ, Egerton-Vernon J, Whitaker AN, et al, "Plasma Cross Linked Fibrin Degradation Products in Pulmonary Embolism," *Thorax*, 1990, 45(9):684-7.
6. Stiehm ER, Kuplic LS, and Uehling DT, "Urinary Fibrin Split Products in Human Renal Disease," *J Lab Clin Med*, 1971, 77:843-52.

References

Bick RL, "Disseminated Intravascular Coagulation," *Disorders of Thrombosis and Hemostasis*, Chapter 7, Chicago, IL: ASCP Press, 1992, 137-73.

Graeff H and Hafter R, "Detection and Relevance of Cross-linked Fibrin Derivatives in Blood," *Semin Thromb Hemost*, 1982, 8:57-68.

Triplett DA, *Laboratory Evaluation of Coagulation*, Chicago, IL: ASCP Press, 1982, 42-5, 175-8, 185-8.

Fibrin Degradation Products *see* Fibrin Breakdown Products *on page 433*

Fibrindex™ *see* Thrombin Time *on page 474*

Fibrinogen

CPT 85384 (activity); 85385 (antigen)

Related Information

Clot Retraction *on page 413*
Cryoprecipitate *on page 1058*
Euglobulin Clot Lysis *on page 418*
Fibrin Breakdown Products *on page 433*
Fibrinopeptide A *on page 437*
Fibrin Split Products, Protamine Sulfate *on page 439*
Intravascular Coagulation Screen *on page 446*
Plasma, Fresh Frozen *on page 1078*
Plasma Protein Fraction (Human) *on page 1079*
Thrombin Time *on page 474*

Synonyms Factor I; Fibrinogen Level; Quantitative Fibrinogen

Applies to Acute Phase Reactants; Sedimentation Rate

Abstract Precursor of fibrin, major contributor to the meshwork of blood clots. Meaningful assay of fibrinogen is uniquely challenging. Fibrinogen is an acute phase reactant as well as the focal point in the coagulation process. Consumption of fibrinogen is a major and clinically threatening aspect of disseminated intravascular coagulation.

Specimen Plasma **CONTAINER:** Blue top (sodium citrate) tube **COLLECTION:** If multiple tests are being drawn, draw coagulation studies last. If only a fibrinogen is being drawn, draw 1-2 mL into another Vacutainer® or syringe (two-syringe technique), discard, and then collect the fibrinogen tube. This collection procedure avoids contamination of the specimen with tissue thromboplastin. **STORAGE INSTRUCTIONS:** Separate and freeze plasma as soon as possible if test is not run immediately. **CAUSES FOR REJECTION:** Tube not full, tube clotted, specimen improperly labeled, specimen hemolyzed, specimen more than 1 hour old, stored specimen not frozen

Interpretive **REFERENCE RANGE:** Quantitative: 200-400 mg/dL. The normal range in childhood (ages 1-16) is similar to that in adults (see reference by Andrew et al). **POSSIBLE PANIC RANGE:** <100 mg/dL **USE:** Identify congenital afibrinogenemia, disseminated intravascular coagulation, and fibrinolytic activity **LIMITATIONS:** Increased in patients on oral contraceptives. Interpretations of results may be limited if patient is receiving anticoagulant therapy depending upon method of analysis. In cases of dysfibrinogenemia, results of fibrinogen determination will vary widely (method dependent). Individual methods may very widely (see following information) and suffer specific, occasionally significant, limitation. **CONTRAINDICATIONS:** Patient receiving heparin less than 1 hour prior to specimen collection (depending upon method of analysis) **METHODOLOGY:** The many tests for fibrinogen proposed and in use over the past generation are a reflection of difficulties encountered in their clinical application. Generally, the most useful clinical information is obtained from "functional" based methods (ie, those that determine clottable plasma protein). These, however, are dependent upon fibrinogen activation with subsequent assessment of fibrin (which may or may not be contaminated with other protein). Functional methods are "blind" to the presence of nonclottable fibrinogen (molecular aberrant forms – dysfibrinogens). Most immunologic-based methods give misleading high results (from the vantage point of availability in the patient of useable-clottable fibrinogen). They will usually detect altered molecular forms but may include breakdown products (largely fragment X). Consideration should be given to employing two different methodologies depending on the clinical situation. Functional methods with different modes of activation and/or end point detection or one "functional" and one immunologic-based method, as available in the individual laboratory situation.

Earlier literature describes many methods based on harvesting the fibrin clot from plasma, washing, and determining the protein in the clot (by weight or chemically). These methods are generally time consuming, technically difficult, and suffer from inaccuracy due to inclusion of nonfibrinogen proteins in the clot, loss of clot fragments, and inaccuracies in measuring the clot protein. They will not measure the nonclottable fibrinogen derived protein.

(Continued)

Fibrinogen *(Continued)*

Modified thrombin time method, the Clauss assay (in which a high concentration of thrombin is added to diluted plasma, resultant clotting time then proportional to the fibrinogen concentration) has the advantage that the endpoint is measured as a rate reaction. It is a rapid and simple procedure. The Clauss assay, however, depends upon the reliable maintenance of an accurate reference dilution curve and may give falsely low results in patients with circulating FBPs or paraproteins.[1]

A method (Ellis and Stransky[2]) similar to the Clauss assay is growing in use due to its adaptation to several automated instruments. Thrombin and calcium are added to citrated plasma, and the change in resultant turbidity is measured. The extent of fibrin polymerization rather than the rate of fibrinogen conversion is the parameter utilized.

A variety of immunologic-based tests have been and continue to be developed. The FI™ test was a screening procedure utilizing antibody coated latex particles. When modified, it was used as a screen for FBP, a forerunner of the Thrombo-Wellcotest®. Radioimmunoassays have been developed for fibrinogen fragments, monomers, and fibrinopeptides A and B. Interest exists in RIA for released fibrinopeptide A as an indication of presence of thromboembolic process.[3] See also test listing, Fibrinopeptide A.

A number of less well established (and uncommonly available) approaches to the determination of fibrinogen have been proposed. As an example, the method of Frigola et al[4] combines electrophoresis and thrombin clotting of fibrinogen. Following protein electrophoresis of plasma, thrombin is applied to "fix" fibrinogen (it is converted to fibrin on the cellulose acetate electrophoretic membrane) and nonclotted proteins are washed away with saline. The membrane is then stained and quantitated by densitometry.

ADDITIONAL INFORMATION: Fibrinogen is a complex polypeptide which upon enzyme action (physiologically by thrombin but pathologically by other substances such as occur in snake venom, eg, Reptilase®-R) is converted to fibrin that forms along with platelets the meshwork of the common blood clot. Fibrinogen is formed of three different pairs of polypeptide chains (α, β, γ) linked by disulfide bonds and forming a dimer. With conversion to fibrin, two pairs of peptides are released from the N-terminals of the α- and β-chains (fibrinopeptides A are released from the α-chains, fibrinopeptides B from the β-chains). The detailed and intricate molecular biochemistry has been explored, and the primary structure completely established.[5] Fibrinogen levels are decreased with hereditary afibrinogenemia, intravascular coagulation, primary and secondary fibrinolysis, and liver disease. Increased levels may be seen with inflammation, pregnancy, and in women taking oral contraceptives. Very high levels of heparin or fibrin breakdown products may affect results of some assays. See Methodology for discussion of clinical implications of assay method. Some clinical problems may benefit from application of more than one test method (eg, in the assessment of cardiovascular risk).[6]

Fibrinogen, while of primary importance as a coagulation protein, is also an acute-phase protein reactant. As such, it is increased in disease processes involving tissue damage/inflammation. It is not often employed clinically as a measure of acute phase response as concurrent hemorrhage (fibrinogen concentration rises initially) and DIC (rise or fall in fibrinogen depending on method) renders interpretation problematic. Fibrinogen is one of the major determinants of the ESR/ZSR (sedimentation rate) phenomenon. Changes in fibrinogen may impair the reliability of erythrocyte sedimentation measurements.[7] There is evidence that increase in dietary fish oils results in decreased fibrinogen levels.[8]

Congenital hypofibrinogenemia may be responsible for mild hemorrhagic symptoms, fibrinogen levels are usually <100 mg/dL, and screening tests (eg, PT, APTT) may be normal or only slightly prolonged. There are a growing number of patients with fibrinogen variants. About 150 varieties of such dysfibrinogenemia have been recorded. These individuals are usually detected when prolonged clotting times are discovered as a result of routine laboratory testing. Over 50% of the cases are asymptomatic; only in about 33% of the cases has a mild bleeding tendency been noted. Some 20 cases have been associated with thrombocytopenia, recurrent thrombosis, or spontaneous abortion. Most cases show a pattern of autosomal dominant inheritance. Most are heterozygous, but in some there is a negative family history. Most cases of dysfibrinogenemia show discrepancy between the results of fibrinogen assays based on the thrombin clotting time (functional) and immune or chemical based methods.[9]

Footnotes

1. Timmis GC, Mammen EF, Ramos RG, et al, "Hemorrhage vs Rethrombosis After Thrombolysis for Acute Myocardial Infarction," *Arch Intern Med*, 1986, 146:667-72.

2. Ellis BC and Stransky A, "A Quick and Accurate Method for the Determination of Fibrinogen in Plasma," *J Lab Clin Med*, 1961, 58:477-88.
3. Joist JH, "Fibrinopeptide A in the Diagnosis and Treatment of Deep Venous Thrombosis and Pulmonary Embolism," *Clin Lab Med*, 1984, 4:363-80.
4. Frigola A, Angeloni S, and Cerqueti AR, "New Method for Determining Thrombin-Clottable Fibrinogen," *Clin Chem*, 1977, 23:2103-6.
5. Mosesson MW and Finlayson JS, "The Search for the Structure of Fibrinogen," *Prog Hemost Thromb*, 1976, 3:61-107.
6. Knapp ML, Feher MD, Carey H, et al, "Comparison of an Immunochemical Assay for Plasma Fibrinogen and a Turbidimetric Thrombin Clotting Technique to Discriminate Hyperlipidaemic Patients From Healthy Controls," *J Clin Pathol*, 1990, 43(6):508-10.
7. Fischer CL and Gill CW, "Acute Phase Proteins," *Serum Protein Abnormalities: Diagnostic and Clinical Aspects*, Ritzmann SE and Daniels JC, eds, New York, NY: Alan R Liss Inc, 1982, 336-7.
8. Radack K, Deck C, and Huster G, "Dietary Supplementation With Low-Dose Fish Oils Lowers Fibrinogen Levels: A Double-Blind Controlled Study," *Ann Intern Med*, 1989, 111(10):757-8.
9. Giddings JC, *Molecular Genetics and Immunoanalysis in Blood Coagulation*, Chichester, England: Ellis Horwood Ltd, 1988, 120-36.

References

Andrew M, Vegh P, Johnston M, et al, "Maturation of the Hemostatic System During Childhood," *Blood*, 1992, 80(8):1998-2005.

Bovill EG, McDonagh J, Triplett DA, et al, "Performance Characteristics of Fibrinogen Assays - Results of the College of American Pathologists Proficiency Testing Program 1988-1991," *Arch Pathol Lab Med*, 1993, 117(1):58-66.

Galanakis DK, "Dysfibrinogenemia: A Current Perspective," *Clin Lab Med*, 1984, 4:395-418.

Hermans J and McDonagh J, "Fibrin: Structure and Interactions," *Semin Thromb Hemost*, 1982, 8:11-24.

Hollensead SC and Triplett DA, "Review of Fibrinogen Methods: Clinical Considerations," *ASCP Check Sample®*, Chicago, IL: American Society of Clinical Pathologists, 1988.

Palareti G, Maccaferri M, Manotti C, et al, "Fibrinogen Assays: A Collaborative Study of Six Different Methods," *Clin Chem*, 1991, 37(5):714-9.

Fibrinogen Level *see* Fibrinogen *on page 435*

Fibrinogen Screen *see* Thrombin Time *on page 474*

Fibrinoligase *see* Factor XIII *on page 430*

Fibrinolysis Time *see* Diluted Whole Blood Clot Lysis *on page 418*

Fibrinolysis Time *see* Euglobulin Clot Lysis *on page 418*

Fibrinopeptide A

CPT 85999

Related Information

Beta-Thromboglobulin *on page 407*
Fibrin Breakdown Products *on page 433*
Fibrinogen *on page 435*
Hypercoagulable State Coagulation Screen *on page 441*
Inhibitor, Lupus, Phospholipid Type *on page 444*
Intravascular Coagulation Screen *on page 446*

Synonyms FpA; FPA

Abstract Fibrinopeptides A and B are removed proteolytically from fibrinogen by thrombin. Fibrinogen is a dimer formed of three polypeptide chains, alpha, beta, and gamma. Presence of FPA indicates that the enzyme thrombin is present and has acted on fibrinogen. FPA is elevated in patients with disseminated intravascular coagulation and is also increased in hypercoagulable states.[1]

Specimen Plasma, urine, cerebrospinal fluid, ascitic fluid **COLLECTION:** Specimen drawn into special anticoagulant (supplied by manufacturer) which contains EDTA, aprotinin, and a thrombin inhibitor. Special precautions are required during sample collection and handling to avoid exogenous conversion of fibrinogen. Clean venipuncture and gentle handling of the specimen is required. Double syringe technique should be used with the first 2-3 mL of blood being discarded. Draw sample into a prechilled collection tube and place immediately on ice. **STORAGE INSTRUCTIONS:** Centrifuge specimen at 4°C within 30 minutes of collection. Perform analysis immediately or freeze plasma specimen at -70°C. **CAUSES FOR REJECTION:** Specimen not collected in special anticoagulant, specimen not iced, specimen clotted, specimen improperly labeled **SPECIAL INSTRUCTIONS:** Special anticoagulant, handling, and processing as indicated above.

(Continued)

Fibrinopeptide A *(Continued)*

Interpretive **REFERENCE RANGE:** Male: 1.5 ± 1.1 ng/mL, female: 1.9 ± 1.2 ng/mL[2] **USE:** Results of FPA determinations are applicable to the study of hypercoagulable states, procoagulant conditions, and disseminated intravascular coagulation (DIC) in which FPA levels are increased. Levels are also elevated in a range of conditions in which there is activation of coagulation (eg, numerous malignancies, postoperative states, and disorders of fibrinolysis). FPA levels are decreased during therapeutic heparinization. **LIMITATIONS:** Careful attention must be given to proper specimen collection and handling to avoid artifactual elevation of FPA levels as the result of coagulation activation with exogenous conversion of fibrinogen. **METHODOLOGY:** Radioimmunoassay (RIA),[2] enzyme immunoassay (EIA),[3] established procedures are commercially available from a number of manufacturers **ADDITIONAL INFORMATION:** Fibrinopeptide A is a small peptide formed of 16 amino acids with a molecular weight of 1535 daltons. It is released from the N-terminus of the alpha chain of fibrinogen. Fibrinogen serves as a substrate for the enzymatic activity of thrombin which cleaves FPA from the amino terminal end of the Aα chain. FPA is a specific marker of the *in vivo* generation of thrombin and, as such, provides a measure of endogenous activation of coagulation. Assays of such peptides and of platelet-specific proteins (see also test listing Beta-Thromboglobulin) have been applied to the study of a variety of clinical problems involving the prethrombotic state and its control. A limited sampling of recent reports include applications of FPA levels in the fields of cardiology, hematology/oncology, nephrology, gastroenterology, and neurology. The threat of thromboembolism in patients with heart failure has been studied. Increased platelet and thrombin activation and fibrinolytic activity correlate with the severity of the cardiac failure.[4] FPA levels are elevated in cases of acute coronary thrombosis with transmural infarction within the first 10 hours after onset of symptoms.[5] While FPA levels are considered a sensitive marker for coronary artery thrombosis in acute ischemic coronary artery syndromes, results of single determinations did not provide prognostic information additional to that available on the basis of history, physical examination, or electrocardiogram.[6] FPA levels have been used to monitor fibrin formation in patients with acute myocardial infarction who have been heparinized. Findings suggested that higher than standard doses of heparin may be required to fully inhibit fibrin formation.[7] On the basis of FPA levels, there is evidence that the process of DIC does not contribute to the coagulopathy of chronic liver disease (cirrhosis).[8] In the field of dermatology, the condition livedo vasculitis is considered to represent a thrombogenic vasculopathy (rather than a small vessel vasculitis) on the basis of elevated FPA levels.[9] Hemostatic activation in patients with carcinoma of the prostate has been studied using measurements of FPA and D-dimer. In 40% of such patients, FPA levels were elevated. Higher levels were found in those patients with bone scan positive disease. Neither FPA nor D-dimer levels correlated with prostate specific antigen levels. These studies were interpreted as suggesting that changes of subclinical DIC occur in many patients on first presentation with prostate cancer.[10]

Footnotes

1. Bick RL, "Physiology of Hemostasis," *Disorders of Thrombosis and Hemostasis: Clinical and Laboratory Practice*, Chapter 1, Chicago, IL: ASCP Press, 1992, 12, 15.
2. Walenga JM, Hoppensteadt D, Emanuele RM, et al, "Performance Characteristics of a Simple Radioimmunoassay for Fibrinopeptide A," *Semin Thromb Hemost*, 1984, 10(4):219-27.
3. Amiral J, Walenga JM, and Fareed J, "Development and Performance Characteristics of a Competitive Enzyme Immunoassay for Fibrinopeptide A," *Semin Thromb Hemost*, 1984, 10(4):228-42.
4. Jafri SM, Ozawa T, Mammen E, et al, "Platelet Function, Thrombin and Fibrinolytic Activity in Patients With Heart Failure," *Eur Heart J*, 1993, 14(2):205-12.
5. Eisenberg PR, Sherman LA, Schectman K, et al, "Fibrinopeptide A: A Marker of Acute Coronary Thrombosis," *Circulation*, 1985, 71(5):912-8.
6. Alemán-Gómez JA, López-Candalez A, Freytes CO, et al, "Usefulness of Single Fibrinopeptide a Determination in Patients With Acute Ischemic Coronary Artery Syndromes," *Bol Asoc Med P R*, 1992, 84(4-5):134-8.
7. Mombelli G, Im Hof V, Haerberli A, et al, "Effect of Heparin on Plasma Fibrinopeptide A in Patients With Acute Myocardial Infarction," *Circulation*, 1984, 69(4):684-9.
8. Mombelli G, Fiori G, Monotti R, et al, "Fibrinopeptide A in Liver Cirrhosis: Evidence Against a Major Contribution of Disseminated Intravascular Coagulation to Coagulopathy of Chronic Liver Disease," *J Lab Clin Med*, 1993, 121(1):83-90.
9. McCalmont CS, McCalmont TH, Jorizzo JL, et al, "Livedo Vasculitis: Vasculitis or Thrombotic Vasculopathy?" *Clin Exp Dermatol*, 1992, 17(1):4-8.
10. Adamson AS, Francis JL, Witherow RO, et al, "Coagulopathy in the Prostate Cancer Patient: Prevalence and Clinical Relevance," *Ann R Coll Surg Engl*, 1993, 75(2):100-4.

References

Bick RL, "Disseminated Intravascular Coagulation," Chapter 7, and "Hypercoagulability and Thrombosis," Chapter 13, *Disorders of Thrombosis and Hemostasis: Clinical and Laboratory Practice*, Chicago, IL: ASCP Press, 1992, 137-73 and 261-89.

Fibrin Split Products *see* Fibrin Breakdown Products *on page 433*
Fibrin Split Products *see* Fibrin Split Products, Protamine Sulfate *on this page*

Fibrin Split Products, Protamine Sulfate

***CPT** 85366 (paracoagulation); 85370 (quantitative)*

Related Information

Cryoprecipitate *on page 1058*
D-Dimer *on page 416*
Fibrin Breakdown Products *on page 433*
Fibrinogen *on page 435*
Intravascular Coagulation Screen *on page 446*

Synonyms Fibrin Split Products; Plasma Protamine Paracoagulation; Protamine Sulfate Test for Fibrin Split Products; 3P Test; Triple P Test

Patient Care PREPARATION: Perform test prior to instituting heparin therapy for DIC.

Specimen Plasma CONTAINER: Blue top (sodium citrate) tube COLLECTION: Routine nontraumatic venipuncture. If multiple tests being drawn, draw coagulation studies last. If only a protamine sulfate test is being drawn, draw 1-2 mL into another Vacutainer® tube, discard, and then collect the blue top tube. This collection procedure avoids contamination of the specimen with tissue thromboplastin. CAUSES FOR REJECTION: Sample received more than 2 hours after collection, sample clotted, improperly labeled sample

Interpretive REFERENCE RANGE: Negative USE: Detection of fibrin monomers and early stage fibrin split products in plasma; useful in the diagnosis of disseminated intravascular coagulation, DIC LIMITATIONS: Thrombo-Wellcotest® is more specific. ADDITIONAL INFORMATION: Previous partial thromboplastin time, Thrombo-Wellcotest®, prothrombin time, and platelet count are often useful in interpretation of results. Protamine sulfate dissociates soluble fibrin monomer complexes, allowing fibrin monomers or early degradation products (fragment X) to polymerize, forming clot-like strands (precipitates) – the "paracoagulation" reaction. A positive test result reflects the presence of fibrin monomers, which is indicative of thrombin activity and is consistent with a diagnosis of intravascular coagulation (IVC). A negative result does not mean that IVC is not present. A positive result may also be seen in some cases of severe liver disease and inflammatory disorders due to accumulation of products of coagulation in the circulation. See table, Findings Indicative of DIC, in the listing, Intravascular Coagulation Screen.

Fibrin Stabilizing Factor *see* Factor XIII *on page 430*
Fibrin Time *see* Thrombin Time *on page 474*
Fitzgerald Factor Assay *see* Factor, Fitzgerald *on page 431*
Fletcher Factor Assay *see* Factor, Fletcher *on page 432*
FpA *see* Fibrinopeptide A *on page 437*
FPA *see* Fibrinopeptide A *on page 437*
F VIII *see* Factor VIII *on page 424*
Glass Bead Platelet Retention Test *see* Platelet Adhesion Test *on page 458*
Ground Glass Clotting Time *see* Activated Coagulation Time *on page 399*
Hageman Factor *see* Factor XII *on page 429*
Hemophilia B *see* Factor IX *on page 426*
Heparin *see* Activated Coagulation Time *on page 399*
Heparin *see* Lee-White Clotting Time *on page 449*
Heparin *see* Partial Thromboplastin Time *on page 450*
Heparin *see* Prothrombin Time *on page 468*
Heparin *see* Thrombin Time *on page 474*
Heparin Cofactor Activity *see* Antithrombin III Test *on page 403*
Heparin Inhibitors *see* Partial Thromboplastin Time *on page 450*
High Molecular Weight Kininogen *see* Factor, Fitzgerald *on page 431*

Hirudin Determination

CPT 85999

Related Information

Thrombin Time *on page 474*

Abstract Hirudin, an anticoagulant from medicinal leeches, was used in the late 1800s and is currently being produced by recombinant DNA techniques. Members of the hirudin family are potent inhibitors of thrombin. Clinical effects of this anticoagulant are preferentially monitored by results of the thrombin time in routine use.

Specimen Method dependent; citrate anticoagulated plasma (thrombin time assay); for chromogenic assay using plasma, heat-defibrinogenated, acid treated plasma must be used; ELISA method can measure hirudin in buffer or urine

Interpretive **USE:** Largely of use in nonclinical (in-laboratory) applications. Such uses include quantitation of thrombin or prothrombin, screening for abnormal plasma prothrombin activation, verification of the therapeutic range of oral anticoagulation, studies on fibrinopeptide release, studies on structure of fibrin and fibrinogen fragment/fibrin monomer interaction, research studies on thrombin binding to membrane receptors and applications in which removal of unwanted thrombin is of benefit. **LIMITATIONS:** The limits of sensitivity (ELISA) method are 8-7700 ng/mL. **METHODOLOGY:** Clotting methods (eg, thrombin titration[1]) based on the selective reaction between 1 mol of hirudin and 1 mol of thrombin (prolongation of thrombin time correlates linearly with the plasma concentration of hirudin); enzyme-linked immunosorbent assay (ELISA);[2] chromogenic substrate based procedures are the recommended method.[3] In the latter, patient's sample (containing hirudin) is mixed with standardized thrombin solution, chromogenic peptide substrate is added, and the residual thrombin activity determined by spectrophotometry. The residual thrombin activity is related to the amount of hirudin.[4] **ADDITIONAL INFORMATION:** Hirudin consists of a family of closely related small proteins, proteinase inhibitors with potent antithrombin effects. John Haycraft, in 1884, found that medicinal leeches (*Hirudo medicinalis*) containing a substance with anticoagulant properties. Markwardt et al isolated hirudin from leeches in the late 1950s.[5] It was characterized as a highly specific, very high affinity thrombin inhibitor, a polypeptide with 65 amino acids with a molecular weight of about 7000. The primary structures of members of the hirudin family are similar (eg, hirudins HV1 and PA, for which molecular sequences have been established and isoforms). In hirudins HV1 and PA, part of the active site of the inhibitor, a Lys residue flanked by two Pro residues, is thought to occupy the specificity pocket of thrombin.[6]

Methods for determining hirudin concentration are, in general, for in-laboratory/research applications. The most practical test for monitoring the clinical effects of hirudin anticoagulation is the thrombin time. The multiple nonclinical applications of hirudin have been reviewed by Stocker.[7] He considers three applications to be of special interest. These include use of hirudin as an inhibitor of meizothrombin, for discrimination between thrombin and other plasma proteinases, and use of hirudin as an anticoagulant to allow testing of blood and blood cell characteristics. The potential clinical applications of recombinant hirudin (r-hirudin) have been discussed.[8] These include postoperative prophylaxis against deep vein thrombosis and pulmonary embolus, prevention of reocclusion after percutaneous transluminal coronary angioplasty, anticoagulation during cardiovascular bypass surgery, and treatment of disseminated intravascular coagulation. Recombinant hirudin has been administered (on compassionate grounds and with benefit) to a patient with heparin-associated thrombocytopenia and deep vein thrombosis.[9] A specific antagonist for neutralization of hirudin is not available. This is seen as a significant current impediment to the clinical development and application of hirudin.[8]

Footnotes

1. Markwardt F, Nowak G, Stürzebecher J, et al, "Pharmacokinetics and Anticoagulant Effect of Hirudin in Man," *Thromb Hemost*, 1984, 52:160-3.
2. Spinner S, Stöffler G, and Fink E, "Quantitative Enzyme-Linked Immunosorbent Assay (ELISA) for Hirudin," *J Immunol Methods*, 1988, 87:79-83.
3. Stürzebecher J, "Methods for Determination of Hirudin," *Semin Thromb Hemost*, 1991, 17(2):99-112.
4. Griessbach U, Stürzebecher J, and Markwardt F, "Assay of Hirudin in Plasma Using a Chromogenic Thrombin Substrate," *Thromb Res*, 1985, 37:347-50.
5. Markwardt F, "The Comeback of Hirudin as an Antithrombotic Agent," *Semin Thromb Hemost*, 1991, 17(2):79-82.
6. Stürzebecher J and Walsmann P, "Structure-Activity Relationships of Recombinant Hirudins," *Semin Thromb Hemost*, 1991, 17(2):94-8
7. Stocker K, "Laboratory Use of Hirudin," *Semin Thromb Hemost*, 1991, 17(2):113-21.
8. Walenga JM, Markwardt F, Breddin K, et al, "Report on a Discussion Forum: Medical and Surgical Application of Recombinant Hirudin," *Semin Thromb Hemost*, 1991, 17(2):150-6.

9. Nand S, "Hirudin Therapy for Heparin-Associated Thrombocytopenia and Deep Venous Thrombosis," *Am J Hematol*, 1993, 43:310-1.

References

Dodt J, Müller H-P, Seemüller U, et al, "The Complete Amino Acid Sequence of Hirudin, a Thrombin Specific Inhibitor," *FEBS Lett*, 1983, 165(2):180-3.

Markwardt F, "Hirudin," *Semin Thromb Hemost*, 1991, 17(2):79-156.

HMW Kininogen *see* Factor, Fitzgerald *on page 431*

Hypercoagulable State Coagulation Screen

***CPT** 85230 (factor VII); 85280 (factor XII); 85300 (antithrombin III); 85303 (protein C); 85305 (protein S); 85575 (platelet aggregation)*

Related Information

Anticardiolipin Antibody *on page 632*
Antithrombin III Test *on page 403*
Beta-Thromboglobulin *on page 407*
Factor VII *on page 422*
Factor XII *on page 429*
Fibrinopeptide A *on page 437*
Inhibitor, Lupus, Phospholipid Type *on page 444*
Plasminogen Activator Inhibitor *on page 455*
Platelet Aggregation, Hypercoagulable State *on page 461*
Protein C *on page 464*
Protein S *on page 466*
Prothrombin Fragment 1.2 *on page 467*
Thrombomodulin *on page 475*

Synonyms Screen for Hypercoagulation; Thrombotic Disease Screen

Test Commonly Includes Availability and composition of screen may vary between laboratories. Commonly included are antithrombin III, protein C, protein S, factor VII, factor XII, platelet aggregation (spontaneous, second wave of aggregation with weak ADP, and response to dilutions of epinephrine). See the following listings, Platelet Aggregation, Hypercoagulable State; Plasminogen Activator Inhibitor; Plasminogen Assay; Euglobulin Clot Lysis; Diluted Whole Blood Clot Lysis; Fibrinogen; Platelet Count; Thrombin Time; and also tests for fibrin monomer and/or fibrin degradation products. Also applicable but less commonly available are plasma beta-thromboglobulin, fibrinopeptide A and B, tissue plasminogen activator, tissue plasminogen activator inhibitor, test for D-dimer fragment of fibrin, heparin cofactor II, and studies for dysfibrinogenemia/dysplasminogenemia.

Specimen Requires multiple specimens, approximately 30-50 mL of blood, dependent on the needs of constituent tests and whether some or all tests are performed "in-house" or by a reference laboratory **COLLECTION:** As for individual constituent tests. Sample for dilute clot lysis must be placed immediately into diluent after collection. **CAUSES FOR REJECTION:** Presence of anticoagulants (eg, heparin) may significantly alter the results of many tests in the screen, in particular, thrombin time, antithrombin III, and platelet aggregation studies **TURNAROUND TIME:** Dependent upon composition of screen and need to utilize reference laboratories. As some hypercoagulable clinical situations are of emergent nature an abbreviated screen ideally should have same day or even 2-4 hour turnaround time. **SPECIAL INSTRUCTIONS:** Initiate a dialogue with the Coagulation Laboratory concerning availability of, composition of, and special requirements for hypercoagulable screen.

Interpretive **REFERENCE RANGE:** See individual constituent tests. See also following table. Note that some tests employed in the study of the hypercoagulable state (eg, AT III, protein C, and protein S) may measure "functional" or "antigenic" (immunologic based) levels. Results may be incomplete or even misleading if both functional and antigenic based tests are not employed. **USE:** Screen for imbalance between procoagulants (factors that effect the conversion of prothrombin to thrombin) and anticoagulants (regulators of the formation of thrombin). Identify presence of hypercoagulable state. Dependent on the structure of the screen may be able to determine if the predisposition to clotting is due to a primary or secondary disorder. If primary, the screen may indicate or disclose the underlying etiology. **LIMITATIONS:** Test results must be considered in relation to the clinical situation. Test results may be misleading if obtained in close temporal proximity to an acute thrombotic disorder. Some apparent abnormalities may reflect physiologic as opposed to pathophysiologic thrombosis. **METHODOLOGY:** As per the individual test, many of the more specific tests may not be routinely available in most healthcare facilities. **ADDITIONAL INFORMATION:** Venous thromboembolic episodes result in approximately

(Continued)

Findings Indicative of Hypercoagulable State

Test Parameter	Finding
Antithrombin III antigenic functional	 ↓ or N ↓
APTT	↓ or N
Beta-thromboglobulin	↑
Clot lysis tests	
Fibrinogen	↓
Fibrinopeptide A	↑
Inhibitor, lupus, phospholipid type	present
Plasminogen	↓
Platelet aggregation spontaneous weak dilutions of epinephrine	↑
Platelet count	±
Protein C/S antigenic functional	 ↓ or N ↓↓
Prothrombin fragment 1.2	↑
Thrombin time	↓ or N

600,000 hospitalizations annually.[1] Screening tests for hypercoagulable states have as their goal the detection of abnormalities of the coagulation mechanism that predispose to thrombosis and thromboembolic disease.

Primary hypercoagulable states usually have their basis in an inherited quantitative or qualitative deficiency in one of the components of the coagulation system. Increased clotting occurs when there are significant deficiencies in the regulators AT III, heparin cofactor II, protein S or protein C, conditions usually inherited as autosomal dominant. Increased risk of thromboembolism may also occur with decrease in fibrinolysis, seen in patients with dysplasminogenemia, decreased plasminogen activator, or increased tissue plasminogen activator inhibitor plasma levels.

Acquired (secondary) hypercoagulable states are associated with clinical conditions that manifest wholly or in part by increased thromboembolism. Changes in platelet number and/or function, vessel wall and/or blood flow parameters may also predispose to thromboembolic episodes.

The primary thrombotic disorders include antithrombin III deficiency (present in 1 of 2000 individuals), protein C or S deficiency,[2,3] dysfibrinogenemia,[4] and dysplasminogenemia. A wide variety of disease processes are associated with secondary thrombotic states. See table. Any condition in which there is disruption of the endothelium of vessel wall or in which signifi-

Clinical Associations of Secondary Thrombotic States

Advanced age	Kawasaki disease
Collagen/vascular disorders	Neoplastic disease
Diabetes mellitus	Nephrotic syndrome
Hormone therapy	Myeloproliferative disease
estrogen	PNH
pregnancy	Severe serum protein abnormalities
birth control regimens	Postoperative status
Hyperlipidemia	Previous episode of thromboembolism
Hyperviscosity	Sepsis
Immobilization	Thrombotic thrombocytopenic purpura
Inflammatory bowel disease	

cant venous stasis occurs will increase the risk of thrombosis. Hereditary deficiency of heparin cofactor II (HC II) (see also Antithrombin III) is apparently very rare. The level of HC II in acquired disorders parallels activity of AT III and may not contribute to clinical evaluation of the hypercoagulable state. Measurement of HC II (in conjunction with AT III) may assist in differentiating acquired from hereditary changes in these inhibitors.[5]

Women with cerebrovascular accidents during oral contraceptive use were found to have persistent platelet coagulant hyperactivity (decreased plasma AT III, increased plasma β-thromboglobulin, normal platelet aggregation) even though use of contraceptives had been discontinued from 4 weeks to 14 years before the study.[6]

In patients younger than 51 years of age with lower limb ischemia, a high incidence of hypercoagulable states was found.[7] Presence of platelet aggregation showing increased activity, protein S or C deficiency, plasminogen deficiency, or lupus-like anticoagulant were common, only 24% of patients were normal. Arterial or graft thrombosis was common (20% incidence) in the early postoperative period.[8]

End-stage renal disease, while usually characterized by propensity to bleed, may also be predisposed to thrombo-embolic complications. Measures of fibrinolytic activity (euglobulin lysis activity, t-PA, urokinase), initially decreased, normalized after renal transplantation.[9] Thromboembolism (including renal vein thrombosis) is a serious complication of nephrotic syndrome, in particular with membranous nephropathy. Renal vein thrombosis complicating nephrotic syndrome has an overall incidence of some 35%. Thrombotic complications other than renal vein thrombosis occur in some 20% of nephrotic patients (pulmonary emboli account for 8%).[10] A variety of mechanisms may be involved.[11,12,13,14]

Homocystinuria has been associated with thromboembolism and decreased AT III and protein C levels.[15]

Patients who have thrombotic disease on the basis of an inherited abnormality of the coagulation mechanism should be considered for lifetime anticoagulation.[16] The apparent frequency (9.5%) of hypercoagulable states in some vascular surgery populations has been considered to support the practice of routine preoperative screening in such populations.[17]

Footnotes

1. Schafer, AI, "The Hypercoagulable States," *Ann Intern Med*, 1985, 102:814-28.
2. Hill RJ and Ens GE, "The Protein C Pathway," *Clin Hemost Rev*, 1987, 1:1-6, (review).
3. Camp PJ and Esmon CT, "Recurrent Venous Thromboembolism in Patients With a Partial Deficiency of Protein S," *N Engl J Med*, 1984, 311:1525-8.
4. Carrell N, Gabriel DA, Blatt PM, et al, "Hereditary Dysfibrinogenemia in a Patient With Thrombotic Disease," *Blood*, 1983, 62:439-47.
5. Brandt JT and Ezenagu L, "Heparin Cofactor II, Thrombosis and Hemostasis," *ASCP Check Sample*®, Chicago, IL: American Society of Clinical Pathologists, 1987.
6. Elam MB, Vicar MJ, Ratts TE, et al, "Mitral Valve Prolapse in Women With Oral Contraceptive-Related Cerebrovascular Insufficiency: Associated Persistent Hypercoagulable State," *Arch Intern Med*, 1986, 146:73-7.
7. Eldrup-Jorgensen J, Flanigan DP, Brace L, et al, "Hypercoagulable States and Lower Limb Ischemia in Young Adults," *J Vasc Surg*, 1989, 9(2):334-41.
8. Gomez MJ, Carroll RC, Hansard MR, et al, "Regulation or Fibrinolysis in Aortic Surgery," *J Vasc Surg*, 1988, 8(4):384-8.
9. Hong SY and Yang DH, "Fibrinolytic Activity in End-Stage Renal Disease," *Nephron*, 1993, 63(2):188-92.
10. Llach F, "Hypercoagulability, Renal Vein Thrombosis, and Other Thrombotic Complications of Nephrotic Syndrome," *Kidney Int*, 1985, 28:429-39.
11. Kanfer A, "Coagulation Factors in Nephrotic Syndrome," *Am J Nephrol*, 1990, 10(S1):63-8.
12. Ono T, Kanatsu K, Doi T, et al, "Relationship of Intraglomerular Coagulation and Platelet Aggregation to Glomerular Sclerosis," *Nephron*, 1991, 58:429-36.
13. Nakamura Y, Tomura S, Tachibana K, et al, "Enhanced Fibrinolytic Activity During the Course of Hemodialysis," *Clin Nephrol*, 1992, 38(2):90-6.
14. Du X-H, Glas-Greenwalt P, Kant KS, et al, "Nephrotic Syndrome With Renal Vein Thrombosis: Pathogenetic Importance of a Plasmin Inhibitor (α_2-Antiplasmin)," *Clin Nephrol*, 1985, 24(4):186-91.
15. Palareti G, Salardi S, Legnani C, et al, "Reduced Levels of Antithrombin III, Protein C and Factor VII in Homocystinuria. Long-Term Changes in Relation to Treatment," *Thromb Haemost*, 1985, 54:35, (abstract).
16. Bowen KJ and Vukelja SJ, "Hypercoagulable States. Their Causes and Management," *Postgrad Med*, 1992, 91(3):117-8, 123-5, 128.
17. Donaldson MC, Weinberg DS, Belkin M, et al, "Screening for Hypercoagulable States in Vascular Surgical Practice: A Preliminary Study," *J Vasc Surg*, 1990, 11(6):825-31.

References

Bick RL and Kunkel L, "Hypercoagulability and Thrombosis," *Lab Med*, 1992, 23(4):233-8.

Bolan CD and Alving BM, "Recurrent Venous Thrombosis and Hypercoagulable States," *Am Fam Physician*, 1991, 44(5):1741-51.

Büller HR and ten Cate JW, "Acquired Antithrombin III Deficiency: Laboratory Diagnosis, Incidence, Clinical Implications, and Treatment With Antithrombin III Concentrate," *Am J Med*, 1989, 87(3B):44S-48S.

Conard J and Samama MM, "Inhibitors of Coagulation, Atherosclerosis and Arterial Thrombosis," *Semin Thromb Hemost*, 1986, 12:87-103.

(Continued)

Hypercoagulable State Coagulation Screen *(Continued)*

Consensus Conference, "Prevention of Venous Thrombosis and Pulmonary Embolism," *JAMA*, 1986, 256:744-9.

Freed JA, "Hypercoagulability – Should Every Patient With Venous Thrombosis Be Tested?" *Postgrad Med*, 1991, 90(6):157-60, 165-6, 168.

Janssen HF, Schachner J, Hubbard J, et al, "The Risk of Deep Venous Thrombosis: A Computerized Epidemiologic Approach," *Surgery*, 1987, 101:205-12.

Lottenberg R, Dolly FR, and Kitchens CS, "Recurring Thromboembolic Disease and Pulmonary Hypertension Associated With Severe Hypoplasminogenemia," *Am J Hematol*, 1985, 19:181-93.

Mammen EF and Fujii Y, "Hypercoagulable States," *Lab Med*, 1989, 20:611-6.

Moake JL, "Hypercoagulable States," *Adv Intern Med*, Stollerman GH, Harrington WJ, LaMont JT, et al, eds, Chicago, IL: Year Book Medical Publishers Inc, 1990, 35:235-48.

Moake JL, "Hypercoagulable States: New Knowledge About Old Problems," *Hosp Pract Off Ed*, 1991, 26(3A):31-42.

Rosenberg RD and Bauer KA, "New Insights Into Hypercoagulable States," *Hosp Pract*, 1986, 21:131-47.

Schwarz HP, Fischer M, Hopmeier P, et al, "Plasma Protein S Deficiency in Familial Thrombotic Disease," *Blood*, 1984, 64:1297-1300.

Stead RB, "The Hypercoagulable State. Pulmonary Embolism and Deep Venous Thrombosis," Goldhaber SZ, ed, Philadelphia, PA: WB Saunders Co, 1985, 161-78.

Whitlock JA, Janco RL, and Phillips JA III, "Inherited Hypercoagulable States in Children," *Am J Pediatr Hematol Oncol*, 1989, 11(2):170-3.

Hypercoagulable State, Platelet Aggregation *see* Platelet Aggregation, Hypercoagulable State *on page 461*

Immunologic Antithrombin III *see* Antithrombin III Test *on page 403*

Inhibitor, Lupus, Phospholipid Type

***CPT** 85705*

Related Information

Anticardiolipin Antibody *on page 632*
Anticoagulant, Circulating *on page 402*
Fibrinopeptide A *on page 437*
Hypercoagulable State Coagulation Screen *on page 441*
Partial Thromboplastin Time *on page 450*
Plasminogen Activator Inhibitor *on page 455*
Protein S *on page 466*

Synonyms Lupus Anticoagulant; Phospholipid Type Anticoagulant

Applies to Antiphospholipid Antibody

Patient Care **PREPARATION:** Discontinue heparin therapy for 2 days and coumarin therapy for 2 weeks prior to collection of the specimen.

Specimen Plasma **CONTAINER:** Blue top (sodium citrate) tube **COLLECTION:** Obtain blood, using plastic syringe, from clean venipuncture without contamination by tissue thromboplastins. If blood is being drawn only for this test, use two-syringe technique. First draw 1-2 mL in one syringe (or tube if using Vacutainer® equipment), discard, and (without moving needle) draw specimen into second syringe (or tube). **STORAGE INSTRUCTIONS:** Centrifuge at 4°C for 20 minutes at 1500 g. Transfer plasma specimen using plastic pipettes.

Interpretive **REFERENCE RANGE:** Prolongation of APTT may result from presence of lupus anticoagulant[1] **USE:** Evaluate prolonged APTT, thrombotic states, fetal death **METHODOLOGY:** Dilute tissue thromboplastin time, platelet neutralization procedure,[2] APTT, enzyme immunoassay (EIA), enzyme-linked immunosorbent assay (ELISA) for anticardiolipin antibody. The more specific assays may not be routinely available. The dilute tissue thromboplastin inhibition test lacks specificity for lupus anticoagulant. Modifications have been described that assist in distinguishing lupus anticoagulant from other causes of a prolonged APTT.[3] Results of survey programs of the College of American Pathologists (1986 and 1987) have found significant variation in the sensitivity of APTT reagents to the presence of lupus-type anticoagulants. Use of the less responsive reagents could impair detection of such anticoagulants and in other cases the differentiation of a lupus anticoagulant from a specific factor inhibitor.[4] **ADDITIONAL INFORMATION:** Lupus anticoagulants (and also anticardiolipin antibodies) are immunoglobulins that cross react with phospholipids and interfere with phospholipid-dependent coagulation tests.[5] They are associated, therefore, with prolongation of the APTT, snake venom assays, plasma recalcification times and to a lesser extent, the prothrombin time. Presence of anticardiolipin antibody (by ELISA) may occur independent of demonstrable lupus anticoagulant activity. When the two occur together, adverse clinical events, thrombosis, or thrombocytopenia are of more common occurrence than if only anticardiolipin antibody is present.[6] The "lupus anticoagulant" while present in up to 10% of patients with systemic lupus erythematosus (SLE) is usually present in patients who do not have SLE. Patients with lupus anticoagulant are usually detected as the result of a prolonged APTT. While they usually do not manifest with abnormal bleeding, about 30% may have development of thromboses. Increased plasma levels of tissue plasminogen activator inhibitor, fibrinopeptide A, fibrinopeptide B beta 15-42 and thromboxane B_2 may have predictive value for occurrence of thrombotic events in cases of SLE who have lupus anticoagulant.[7,8] The lupus inhibitor may be present in otherwise normal individuals. It may occur as a complication of drug therapy, in particular, it is seen in association with the use of chlorpromazine. In some cases of valvular disease, the thrombotic tendency associated with lupus anticoagulant/phospholipid antibodies may be responsible for rheumatic-type deformities and severe **valvular heart disease**[9] (distortion of valve by layers of thrombus as in some patients with SLE, patients without a history of rheumatic fever).

There is evidence that lipoprotein-associated coagulation inhibitor contains three tandemly repeated serine protease inhibitory domains. When the inhibitory complex is generated, one domain binds to active site of Xa, two domains are required for the inhibition of VIIa/tissue factor (TF), and a third domain has no effect on the function of Xa or TF.[10] Some antiphospholipid antibodies decrease endothelial cell prostacyclin production apparently due to inhibition of phospholipase A_2 and thus predisposing to vascular thrombi.[11]

Pregnant women with high antiphospholipid antibody titers have an increased incidence of **midterm fetal death**. Steroid therapy does not improve (and may worsen) fetal outcome in asymptomatic pregnant women with antiphospholipid antibody and previous episode of fetal death.[12]

Lupus anticoagulants occurring in children have been reported only rarely. Nonhemophiliac examples of this condition have occurred in children 3-14 years of age, largely not associated with lupus erythematosus. Some have been associated with the use of antibiotics or antecedent viral infections. Presence of the inhibitor is usually transient and not associated with bleeding or thrombotic episodes.[13]

There is a high incidence (20% to 50%) of lupus anticoagulant in patients with **AIDS**. Rarely, associated inhibition of a specific coagulation factor has also been found.[14,15]

It has been recommended that patients undergoing evaluation for hypercoagulability be tested for the antiphospholipid syndrome even in the absence of a prolonged PTT.[16] This recommendation follows upon the results of a study of young patients with unusual thrombotic events (eg, cerebral thrombosis and coumarin associated skin necrosis), presence of "lupus anticoagulant," and binding of protein S by C4b-binding protein. Presumably, the decrease in free protein S is related to the hypercoagulable state in these patients.

Footnotes

1. Shapiro SS and Thiagarajan P, "Lupus Anticoagulants," *Prog Hemost Thromb*, 1982, 6:273-6, 263-85.
2. Triplett DA, Brandt JT, Kaczor D, et al, "Laboratory Diagnosis of Lupus Inhibitor. A Comparison of the Tissue Thromboplastin Inhibition Procedure With a New Platelet Neutralization Procedure," *Am J Clin Pathol*, 1983, 79:678-82.
3. Liu HW, Wong KL, Lin CK, et al, "The Reappraisal of Dilute Tissue Thromboplastin Inhibition Test in the Diagnosis of Lupus Anticoagulant," *Br J Haematol*, 1989, 72(2):229-34.
4. Brandt JT, Triplett DA, Rock WA, et al, "Effect of Lupus Anticoagulants on the Activated Partial Thromboplastin Time. Results of the College of American Pathologists Survey Program," *Arch Pathol Lab Med*, 1991, 115(2):109-14.
5. Kushner M and Simonian N, "Lupus Anticoagulants, Anticardiolipin Antibodies, and Cerebral Ischemia," *Stroke*, 1989, 20(2):225-9.
6. McHugh NJ, Moye DA, James IE, et al, "Lupus Anticoagulant: Clinical Significance in Anticardiolipin Positive Patients With Systemic Lupus Erythematosus," *Ann Rheum Dis*, 1991, 50(8):548-52.
7. Violi F, Ferro D, Valesini G, et al, "Tissue Plasminogen Activator Inhibitor in Patients With Systemic Lupus Erythematosus and Thrombosis," *Br Med J*, 1990, 300(6732):1099-102.
8. Mayumi T, Nagasawa K, Inoguchi T, et al, "Haemostatic Factors Associated With Vascular Thrombosis in Patients With Systemic Lupus Erythematosus and the Lupus Anticoagulant," *Ann Rheum Dis*, 1991, 50(8):543-7.
9. Ford SE, Lillicrap D, Brunet D, et al, "Thrombotic Endocarditis and Lupus Anticoagulant. A Pathogenetic Possibility for Idiopathic Type Valvular Heart Disease," *Arch Pathol Lab Med*, 1989, 113(4):350-3.
10. Girard TJ, Warren LA, Novotny WF, et al, "Functional Significance of the Kunitz-Type Inhibitory Domains of Lipoprotein-Associated Coagulation Inhibitor," *Nature*, 1989, 338(6215):518-20.
11. Schorer AE, Duane PG, Woods VL, et al, "Some Antiphospholipid Antibodies Inhibit Phospholipase A_2 Activity," *J Lab Clin Med*, 1992, 120(20):67-77.

(Continued)

Inhibitor, Lupus, Phospholipid Type *(Continued)*

12. Lockshin MD, Druzin ML, and Qamar T, "Prednisone Does Not Prevent Recurrent Fetal Death in Women With Antiphospholipid Antibody," *Am J Obstet Gynecol*, 1989, 160(2):439-43.
13. Singh AK, Rao KP, Kizer J, et al, "Lupus Anticoagulants in Children," *Ann Clin Lab Sci*, 1988, 18(5):384-7.
14. Ndimbie OK, Raman BKS, and Saeed SM, "Lupus Anticoagulant Associated With Specific Inhibition of Factor VII in a Patient With AIDS," *Am J Clin Pathol*, 1989, 91(4):491-3.
15. Taillan B, Roul C, Fuzibet JG, et al, "Circulating Anticoagulant in Patients Seropositive for Human Immunodeficiency Virus," *Am J Med*, 1989, 87(2):238.
16. Moreb J and Kitchens CS, "Acquired Functional Protein S Deficiency, Cerebral Venous Thrombosis, and Coumarin Skin Necrosis in Association With Antiphospholipid Syndrome: Report of Two Cases," *Am J Med*, 1989, 87(2):207-10.

References

Branch DW, "Antiphospholipid Antibodies and Pregnancy: Maternal Implications," *Semin Perinatol*, 1990, 14(2):139-46.

Branch DW, "Antiphospholipid Syndrome: Laboratory Concerns, Fetal Loss, and Pregnancy Management," *Semin Perinatol*, 1991, 15(3):230-7.

Eisenberg GM, "Antiphospholipid Syndrome: The Reality and Implications," *Hosp Pract (Off Ed)*, 1992, 27(6):119-22, 127-31.

Farrugia E, Torres VE, Gastineau D, et al, "Lupus Anticoagulant in Systemic Lupus Erythematosus: A Clinical and Renal Pathological Study," *Am J Kidney Dis*, 1992, 20(5): 463-71.

Feinstein DI, "Lupus Anticoagulant, Anticardiolipin Antibodies, Fetal Loss, and Systemic Lupus Erythematosus," *Blood*, 1992, 80(4):859-62.

Ferro D, Saliola M, Quintarelli C, et al, "Methods for Detecting Lupus Anticoagulants and Their Relation to Thrombosis and Miscarriage in Patients With Systemic Lupus Erythematosus," *J Clin Pathol*, 1992, 45(4):332-8.

Gastineau DA, Kazmier FJ, Nichols WL, et al, "Lupus Anticoagulant: An Analysis of the Clinical and Laboratory Features of 219 Cases," *Am J Hematol*, 1985, 19:265-75.

"Guidelines on Testing for the Lupus Anticoagulant. Lupus Anticoagulant Working Party on Behalf of the BCSH Haemostasis and Thrombosis Task Force," *J Clin Pathol*, 1991, 44(11):885-9.

Harris EN, "Syndrome of the Black Swan," *Br J Rheumatol*, 1987, 26:324-6.

Kaczor DA, Bickford NN, and Triplett DA, "Evaluation of Different Mixing Study Reagents and Dilution Effect in Lupus Anticoagulant Testing," *Am J Clin Pathol*, 1991, 95(3):408-11.

Levine SR and Welch KM, "Antiphospholipid Antibodies," *Ann Neurol*, 1989, 26(3):386-9.

Mackie IJ, Colaco CB, and Machin SJ, "Familial Lupus Anticoagulants," *Br J Haematol*, 1987, 67:359-63.

Mammen EF and Fujii Y, "Hypercoagulable States," *Lab Med*, 1989, 20:611-6.

Pope JM, Canny CL, and Bell DA, "Cerebral Ischemic Events Associated With Endocarditis, Retinal Vascular Disease, and Lupus Anticoagulant," *Am J Med*, 1991, 90(3):299-309.

Raz E, Michaeli J, Rosenmann E, et al, "Antinuclear Antibody-Negative Systemic Lupus Erythematosus (SLE) and Severe Renal Involvement: Close Correlation Between Disease Activity and Appearance of Circulating Anticoagulant," *Isr J Med Sci*, 1988, 24:105-8.

Rosner E, Pauzner R, Lusky A, et al, "Detection and Quantitative Evaluation of Lupus Circulating Anticoagulant Activity," *Thromb Haemost*, 1987, 57:144-7.

Saxena R, Saraya AK, Kotte VK, et al, "Inosithin Neutralization Test to Measure Lupus Anticoagulants," *Am J Clin Pathol*, 1993, 99(1):61-4.

Triplett DA, "Antiphospholipid Antibodies and Thrombosis: A Consequence, Coincidence, or Cause?" *Arch Pathol Lab Med*, 1993, 117(1):78-88.

Intravascular Coagulation Screen

CPT *85023 (CBC, platelet count, manual differential); 85362 (fibrin degradation products); 85384 (fibrinogen quantitative); 85610 (prothrombin time); 85730 (PTT)*

Related Information

Beta-Thromboglobulin *on page 407*
D-Dimer *on page 416*
Euglobulin Clot Lysis *on page 418*
Fibrin Breakdown Products *on page 433*
Fibrinogen *on page 435*
Fibrinopeptide A *on page 437*
Fibrin Split Products, Protamine Sulfate *on page 439*
Partial Thromboplastin Time *on page 450*
Plasminogen Assay *on page 457*
Platelet Count *on page 586*
Thrombin Time *on page 474*

Synonyms Coagulation Screen, Intravascular; Consumptive Coagulopathy Screen; DIC Screen; Disseminated Intravascular Coagulation Screen; Screen for Disseminated Intravascular Coagulation

Test Commonly Includes Availability and composition of screen varies between laboratories. Commonly included are platelet estimate or platelet count, PTT, dilute clot lysis or euglobulin clot lysis, fibrinogen, thrombin time, fibrin breakdown products, fibrin split products, and review of peripheral blood smear for microangiopathic changes in red blood cells. Work-up may also include tests for D-dimer, antithrombin III, heparin cofactor II, beta-thromboglobulin, and fibrinopeptide A.

Abstract Screens for DIC generally incorporate multiple tests which are individually sensitive but not specific. Individual test protocols must result in rapid turnaround time with limited expenditure of technologist resources. Correlation of the multiple test results usually allows specific conclusion as to the existence of a consumptive coagulopathy.

Specimen Approximately 15 mL of blood, see individual test listings for specific requirements. **COLLECTION:** As for individual constituent tests. Sample for dilute clot lysis must be collected at patient's side and placed directly into diluent. **TURNAROUND TIME:** It is possible and desirable that the DIC screen include largely tests that can be rapidly performed, so that a single experienced technologist can complete the tests in 60-90 minutes **SPECIAL INSTRUCTIONS:** Initiate a dialogue with the Coagulation Laboratory concerning availability of, composition of, and special requirements for the DIC screen.

Interpretive **REFERENCE RANGE:** See individual constituent tests and additional information. See table.

Findings Indicative of DIC

Test Parameter	Acute DIC	Chronic DIC
Antithrombin III	↓	
APTT (activated partial thromboplastin time)	↑ to ↑↑ to ↑↑↑	N
β-thromboglobulin	↑	
Clotting factor assays	↓	N or ↑
D-dimer, monoclonal Ab	↑	Usually ↑
Fibrin breakdown products present	++	+
Fibrinogen (clottable)	↓↓ or ↓↓↓	N or ↑
Fibrinolytic activity	N rarely ↑	N rarely ↑
Plasminogen	↓	N or ↓
Platelet count	↓↓ to ↓↓↓	N to ↑
Platelet factor IV	↑	
PT (prothrombin time)	↑	N
RBC microangiopathy	++	+
Reptilase time	↑	
Soluble fibrin/monomer complexes (protamine sulfate or ethanol gelation)	++	+
Thrombin time	↑↑	↑

USE: Identify the presence of or to follow course of the process of disseminated intravascular coagulation (DIC) including abnormalities in platelet count, fibrinogen, fibrin split products, fibrinolytic activity **LIMITATIONS:** One cannot distinguish physiologic from pathophysiologic clot formation and lysis in all cases. Results should be reviewed in relation to the clinical situation. **ADDITIONAL INFORMATION:** Platelet adhesion and aggregation with subsequent intravascular coagulation occur physiologically as early states in the reparative response to vascular injury, in which the nonthrombogenic endothelium has been torn or rubbed away. Naturally occurring inhibitors, including prostacyclin and antithrombin III, normally control the intravascular clotting process. With severe injury and/or entrance of thromboplastins into the circulation, the process may become pathologic and result in morbidity and/or mortality. The amount and rate of entry of thromboplastins into the circulation determine the severity and rapidity of the process. A corollary of primary importance in therapy is removal of the source of thromboplastic agents if possible.

The process of intravascular coagulation results in the partial to nearly complete conversion of plasma to serum. Clotting factors are variously converted with factors V and VIII completely destroyed, with small amounts of VII, IX, and X activated and lost due to the action of anti-

(Continued)

Intravascular Coagulation Screen *(Continued)*

thrombin. Platelets undergo changes in configuration and release reactions. Later and concurrently, fibrinogen is cleared and fibrin lysed to give rise to fibrin monomer aggregates and fibrin degradation products. Marked decrease in levels of heparin cofactor II have been reported in infants with DIC.[1]

Varying levels of complexity in interpretation are introduced by the multitest nature of the DIC screen and the need for clinical correlation. If all test results are normal, it is very unlikely that any significant degree of intravascular coagulation and lysis is in progress. With levels of fibrin breakdown products (FBP) <10 μg/mL, any significant level of DIC is unlikely. This is also a finding against physiologic clot formation and lysis of any significant degree. Intermediate levels of FBP (10-40 μg/mL) may be associated with mild or early DIC or with physiologic clot formation or lysis. Levels of FBP >40 μg/mL may still reflect only a physiologic process, but if associated with decreased (or decreasing) fibrinogen and/or platelet levels, possibility of DIC is likely. Process of DIC is frequently dynamic with changes occurring rapidly. Close monitoring of fibrinogen level and platelet count will reflect the rapidly changing picture and provide prognostic insight. With well developed, advanced DIC, PT and PTT become prolonged. Clot lysis may be active and shortened along with significantly decreased levels of fibrinogen and platelets and increased levels of FBP. The protamine sulfate paracoagulation test may be a useful adjunct for indication of increased levels of fibrin monomers.

Clinical states associated with intravascular coagulation (IVC) include gram-negative sepsis (endotoxin effect); gram-positive sepsis (some bacterial strains with a peptidoglycan that aggregates platelets in the presence of staphylococcal A protein);[2] pneumonia, severe (tissue destruction with thromboplastin generation); malaria (release of lipids from RBCs); malignancies involving pancreas, prostate, lung (necrosis and thromboplastin generation); Hodgkin's disease (necrosis and thromboplastin generation); some acute leukemias[3]; shock and trauma (stasis and thromboplastin); end state disease with tissue necrosis; placenta praevia and abruptio; toxemia of pregnancy; amniotic fluid embolus; dead fetus syndrome; ruptured uterus. Resulting from the observation that plasma D-dimer and serum FBP levels follow one another closely in cases of DIC, it has been considered that FBPs arise predominantly from plasmin's action on cross-linked fibrin rather than on fibrinogen.[4]

The rare association of severe thrombocytopenia and chronic consumptive coagulopathy with the Klippel-Trenaunay syndrome has been successfully treated with epsilon-aminocaproic acid (EACA).[5] The therapy was associated with a rise in platelet count to normal levels and technetium-99m-labeled autologous RBC imaging demonstration of regression of abnormal vascular channels. The Klippel-Trenaunay syndrome is an inherited abnormality which includes vascular malformations and varicose veins.

Therapy is based on removal of the inciting cause, replacement of deficient factors, and in only rare instances, heparin anticoagulant therapy. Replacement includes especially platelet infusion, whole blood, and fibrinogen rich cryoprecipitates. The risk of aggravation of bleeding must be carefully weighed in considering heparin therapy. In cases with evidence or threat of shock, renovascular thrombosis and necrosis, heparin (in the form of a constant I.V. infusion to maintain the APTT or activated coagulation time at 2.5 to 3 times control value) may be of protective value. Heparin should not be used until bleeding is controlled with replacement therapy and should never be used in patients with head injury or evidence of CNS bleeding.

Footnotes

1. Chuansumrit A, Manco-Johnson MJ, and Hathaway WE, "Heparin Cofactor II in Adults and Infants With Thrombosis and DIC," *AM J Hematol*, 1989, 31(2):109-13.
2. Kessler CM, Nussbaum E, and Tuazon CU, "Disseminated Intravascular Coagulation Associated With *Staphylococcus aureus* Septicemia Is Mediated by Peptidoglycan-Induced Platelet Aggregation," *J Infect Dis*, 1991, 164(1):101-7.
3. Lisiewicz J, "Disseminated Intravascular Coagulation in Acute Leukemia," *Semin Thromb Hemost*, 1988, 14:339-50.
4. Wilde JT, Kitchen S, Kinsey S, et al, "Plasma D-Dimer Levels and Their Relationship to Serum Fibrinogen/Fibrin Degradation Products in Hypercoagulable States," *Br J Haematol*, 1989, 71(1):65-70.
5. Poon M-C, Kloiber R, and Birdsell DC, "Epsilon-Aminocaproic Acid in the Reversal of Consumption Coagulopathy With Platelet Sequestration in a Vascular Malformation of Klippel-Trenaunay Syndrome," *Am J Med*, 1989, 87(2):211-13.

References

Baker WF Jr, "Clinical Aspects of Disseminated Intravascular Coagulation: A Clinician's Point of View," *Semin Thromb Hemost*, 1989, 15(1):1-57.

Bick RL, "Disseminated Intravascular Coagulation and Related Syndromes: A Clinical Review," *Semin Thromb Hemost*, 1988, 14:299-338.

Bick RL and Scates SM, "Disseminated Intravascular Coagulation," *Lab Med*, 1992, 23(3):161-5.

Büller HR and ten Cate JW, "Acquired Antithrombin III Deficiency: Laboratory Diagnosis, Incidence, Clinical Implications, and Treatment With Antithrombin III Concentrate," *Am J Med*, 1989, 87(3B):44S-48S.

Colman RW and Marder VJ, "Disseminated Intravascular Coagulation; (DIC): Pathogenesis, Pathophysiology, and Laboratory Abnormalities," *Hemostasis and Thrombosis: Basic Principles and Clinical Practice*, Colman W, Hirsh J, Marder VJ, et al, eds, Philadelphia, PA: JB Lippincott Co, 1982, 47:654-63.

Colman RW and Rubin RN, "Disseminated Intravascular Coagulation Due to Malignancy," *Semin Oncol*, 1990, 17(2):172-86.

Muller-Berghaus G, "Pathophysiologic and Biochemical Events in Disseminated Intravascular Coagulation: Dysregulation of Procoagulant and Anticoagulant Pathways," *Semin Thromb Hemost*, 1989, 15(1):58-87.

Ivy Bleeding Time *see* Bleeding Time, Ivy *on page 409*

Labile Factor *see* Factor V *on page 421*

Laki-Lorand Factor *see* Factor XIII *on page 430*

Lee-White *see* Lee-White Clotting Time *on this page*

Lee-White Clotting Time

CPT 85345

Related Information

Activated Coagulation Time *on page 399*

Partial Thromboplastin Time *on next page*

Synonyms Clot Time; Coagulation Time; Lee-White; Lee-White Coagulation Time; L-W

Applies to Heparin

Patient Care **PREPARATION:** No heparin therapy for a minimum of 3 hours prior to specimen collection.

Specimen Blood **CONTAINER:** Three 12 x 75 mm glass test tubes and syringe **COLLECTION:** Use two-syringe technique, draw blood into a plastic syringe. 1 mL of blood is placed into each of three tubes. Kept at 37°C. Start stopwatch upon filling of third tube. The test is complete when the last tube has clotted. **CAUSES FOR REJECTION:** Traumatic venipuncture, patient receiving heparin therapy within 3 hours of collection

Interpretive **REFERENCE RANGE:** 8-15 minutes **USE:** Evaluate whole blood clotting system; monitor therapy with heparin **LIMITATIONS:** Specimen obtained less than 3 hours after a dose of heparin will have markedly prolonged clotting time. The standard Lee-White clotting time lacks precision, as it is difficult to perform the test under truly standard conditions between individual technologists and individual laboratories. Prolonged CTs (as encountered when monitoring heparin use) are especially subject to inaccuracy. **A number of laboratories no longer offer this test.** **METHODOLOGY:** Time required for visual detection of clotting is determined after freshly drawn blood is subjected to standardized activation stimulus (timed periodic tube tilting) **ADDITIONAL INFORMATION:** Clotting time may be used to monitor effect of heparin therapy, but with occasional patients, no single test will allow unambiguous monitoring of such therapy. The addition of accelerators of coagulation (such as phospholipids or excessive contact activation as with some APTT reagents) will tend to overcome or mask the anticoagulant action of heparin. Heparin action is through the activation of antithrombin III. If AT III is greatly decreased, heparin will have little anticoagulant effect without the addition of plasma infusion. This may especially pertain to patients with disseminated intravascular coagulation. With severe lipemia, there will be a competitive attraction by lipase for heparin.

A table in the listing, Partial Thromboplastin Time, provides relationships of three coagulation tests which can be utilized to adjust heparin.

References

Sirridge MS and Shannon R, *Laboratory Evaluation of Hemostasis and Thrombosis*, 3rd ed, Philadelphia, PA: Lea & Febiger, 1983, 68, 112-5.

Lee-White Coagulation Time *see* Lee-White Clotting Time *on this page*

Low Molecular Weight *see* Partial Thromboplastin Time *on next page*

Lumi-Aggregometry *see* Platelet Aggregation *on page 459*

Lupus Anticoagulant *see* Anticoagulant, Circulating *on page 402*

Lupus Anticoagulant *see* Inhibitor, Lupus, Phospholipid Type *on page 444*

L-W *see* Lee-White Clotting Time *on this page*

Negative Pressure Suction Cup Capillary Fragility *see* Capillary Fragility Test *on page 412*

P62 *see* Platelet Aggregation *on page 459*

PAI *see* Plasminogen Activator Inhibitor *on page 455*

PAI Chromogenic Assay *see* Plasminogen Activator Inhibitor *on page 455*

Partial Thromboplastin Time

CPT *85730*

Related Information

Activated Coagulation Time *on page 399*
Activated Partial Thromboplastin Substitution Test *on page 401*
Anticoagulant, Circulating *on page 402*
Antithrombin III Test *on page 403*
Coagulation Factor Assay *on page 414*
Cryoprecipitate *on page 1058*
Factor VIII *on page 424*
Factor VIII Concentrate *on page 1064*
Factor IX *on page 426*
Factor IX Complex (Human) *on page 1065*
Fibrin Breakdown Products *on page 433*
Inhibitor, Lupus, Phospholipid Type *on page 444*
Intravascular Coagulation Screen *on page 446*
Lee-White Clotting Time *on previous page*
Plasma, Fresh Frozen *on page 1078*
Platelet Count *on page 586*
Thrombin Time *on page 474*

Synonyms Activated Partial Thromboplastin Time; APTT; PTT

Applies to Antiaggregating Agents; Heparin; Heparin Inhibitors; Low Molecular Weight; Protamine Sulfate; Thrombin Clotting Time Heparin Assay

Test Commonly Includes Patient time and control time

Abstract The activated partial thromboplastin time (APTT) is a readily available low cost screening test. The test procedure is usually automated, batch processing is efficient, and the turnaround time is reasonably rapid in the individual or stat mode. The test finds application in screening for intrinsic factor deficiencies and for monitoring of heparin anticoagulation.

Patient Care PREPARATION: Draw specimen 1 hour before next dose of heparin if heparin is being given by intermittent injection; not applicable to patients on continuous heparin infusion therapy. Do not draw from an arm with a heparin lock or heparinized catheter.

Specimen Plasma CONTAINER: Blue top (sodium citrate) tube COLLECTION: Routine venipuncture. If multiple tests are being drawn, draw coagulation studies last. If only a PTT is being drawn, draw 1-2 mL into another Vacutainer®, discard, and then collect the PTT (two-tube or two-syringe technique). This collection procedure avoids contamination of the specimen with tissue thromboplastins. Transport the specimen to the Hematology Laboratory as soon as possible. STORAGE INSTRUCTIONS: Keep refrigerated. CAUSES FOR REJECTION: Tube not full, specimen hemolyzed, specimen clotted, specimen received more than 2 hours after collection, specimen improperly labeled

Interpretive REFERENCE RANGE: 25-39 seconds, usually stated to be within 10 seconds of control. Healthy premature newborns have prolonged coagulation test screening results (eg, PT, PTT, TT) which return to normal adult values at about 6 months of age. Healthy prematures, however, do not develop spontaneous hemorrhage or thrombotic complications because of a balance between procoagulants and inhibitors. The normal range in childhood (ages 1-16) is similar to that in adults. (See reference by Andrew et al). POSSIBLE PANIC RANGE: Over 70 seconds USE: Evaluate intrinsic coagulation system; useful in monitoring heparin therapy; aid in screening for presence of classical hemophilia A and B; congenital deficiencies of factors II, V, VIII, IX, X, XI, and XII; dysfibrinogenemia; disseminated intravascular coagulation; liver failure; congenital hypofibrinogenemia; vitamin K deficiency; congenital deficiency of Fitzgerald factor; congenital deficiency of prekallikrein (Fletcher factor) CONTRAINDICATIONS: Specimen obtained less than 3 hours after dose of heparin METHODOLOGY: Methods involve addition of a contact activator (eg, Celite, kaolin, microsilicate, elagic acid). Plasma sample is added to activator and incubated at 37°C, usually for 5 minutes. Thromboplastin preparation is added, mixed, and with addition of $CaCl_2$, a timer is started. A variety of automated instruments have been designed to perform this test, often with the capability of also performing the prothrombin time test. A variety of instruments and reagents are used in the field resulting in many combinations, most monitored by the College of American Pathologists survey process. A handheld portable instrument that determines the APTT using a fingerstick sample of capillary whole blood has recently been developed.[1] **ADDITIONAL INFORMATION:** Hemolysis significantly shortens the activated partial thromboplastin time in normal but not in abnormal persons.[2] The APTT may be normal in persons with mild hereditary bleeding disorders. About 30% of normal concentration of factors V, VIII, IX, X, XI, and XII will maintain a rate of thrombin formation sufficient to produce a normal APTT. Prolongation of the APTT clotting time occurs if the concentration of any of the above single clotting factors falls below this level. Fibrinogen level, if <80 mg/dL, may result in an abnormal APTT. If Fletcher or Fitzgerald factors are <5% of normal the APTT may be abnormal. A prolonged APTT can be caused by inherited factor deficiency (I, II, V, VIII-XII), Fletcher or Fitzgerald, Coumadin® type therapy, liver disease, circulating anticoagulant (heparin, lupus anticoagulant, fibrin breakdown products), specific factor inhibitor (rheumatoid arthritis, penicillin reaction, occasional hemophiliacs), or intravascular coagulation.

The results of the College of American Pathologists surveys indicate that the source and type of heparinized specimen is important to consider when interpreting APTT test results.[3] Different reagent/instrument combinations effect the APTT response to heparin. Sensitivity is most influenced by the APTT reagent used while precision is most effected by the instrument utilized.

Control of heparin therapy: The control of heparin anticoagulant therapy is complex, controversial, and problematic. Recommendations for dosage and laboratory monitoring will be followed by a consideration of factors that may be responsible for "failures" (failure to achieve anticoagulated state, and/or excessive anticoagulation).

Heparin: Heparin is an acidic mucopolysaccharide found in mast cells and basophils, has a strong negative charge, a circulating half-life of only a few hours, and inhibits all of the active serine proteases (IIa, Xa, IXa, XIa, and XIIa). It is stable for 24 hours in a 5% dextrose solution. Low dose heparin activity relates to inactivation of Xa and possibly to cell surface repulsion effects. On the basis of minimum dose of heparin effective in producing comparable prolongations of clotting time, the whole blood PTT, APTT, whole blood clotting time, and PTT are about equivalent in measuring response to heparin. While some inactivation of heparin may occur in the liver (through action of heparinase), elimination is largely by the kidney so that heparin must be used cautiously in patients with impaired glomerular filtration.

Administration, dosage: Heparin is best administered intravenously, intermittently, or better as continuous infusion[4,5,6] in a dosage of 400-500 units/kg body weight/day divided into every 6-hour dosage (so that 100-125 units/kg body weight is given each 6 hours). Laboratory monitoring can be accomplished using the Lee-White clotting time, APTT, or activated clotting time (ACT). Dosage is adjusted to maintain the coagulation test result at about two times the control or "normal" level.

There are three levels of heparin therapy: low dose, moderate dose, and large dose. Before proceeding, one must decide on the level to be employed.[4] Low dose refers to small amounts of heparin (10,000-20,000 units/day) given subcutaneously and useful in the prophylaxis against venous thrombosis (selected patients). Measurable change in APTT does not usually occur. See review by Hirsh and Levine listed in references. Moderate dose implies full anticoagulation, requires 20,000-60,000 units/day, the APTT is adjusted to 1.5 to 2 times the control, and the regimen is applied to patients without active thromboembolic disease. Large dose heparin therapy utilizes dosage levels of 60,000-100,000 units/day during the first 24-48 hours and then reverting to 30,000-45,000 units/day. Large dose therapy is for patients with active thromboembolic disease.

Heparin should not be given intramuscularly. There is a trend to favor subcutaneous administration in the initial treatment of deep vein thrombosis. BIn support of this trend are studies claiming efficacy and safety, procedural simplification allowing outpatient or home therapy (see references by Hommes et al).

Complications: Not all individuals respond ideally or predictably to heparin. A voluminous literature deals with these exceptions and one must conclude that there is no shortcut to adequate and safe heparin anticoagulation. One must understand and investigate the causes and management of aberrant cases.

(Continued)

Partial Thromboplastin Time *(Continued)*

Drugs which antagonize the action of heparin include streptomycin, erythromycin, gentamicin, chlorpromazine, ascorbic acid, antihistamines, and digitalis.

Heparin should be given intravenously or subcutaneously but not intramuscularly due to the high risk of hematoma formation. Anaphylaxis and erythematous reactions may occur with the use of heparin in some individuals.

Untoward effects of heparin include development of osteoporosis with fractures (doses of 20,000 units/day over 6 months) for which a calcium intake of 1 g or more per day may be protective, anti-inflammatory effect, and inhibition of antidiuretic effect resulting in diuresis. Unusual reactions to heparin include anaphylaxis and erythematous reactions (species specific), alopecia, urticaria, headache, and bronchospasm.

An especially important complication of high dose heparin therapy is the development of thrombocytopenia which relates to heparin-induced aggregation. Because of the dangers attendant to a minority of heparin anticoagulated individuals, pretherapeutic laboratory evaluation has been recommended.[7] Abnormalities in platelet count, whole blood clotting time, activated PTT, or antithrombin III may indicate that the patient has a predisposition to an unusual heparin response. Hussey et al have emphasized the significant morbidity (including amputation of extremities) and mortality associated with heparin induced platelet aggregation resulting in new thrombosis and thrombocytopenia.[8] This phenomenon appears to have immune etiology and occurs in the presence of either an IgG or IgM heparin dependent platelet aggregating antibody.[9,10] These patients have a measurable abnormal response to ADP, heparin and ADP, and heparin alone in the platelet aggregation procedure when thrombocytopenia is present. See Platelet Aggregation listing.

The **progressive thromboembolic syndrome** appears to be always associated with thrombocytopenia. Monitoring of the heparinized patient has been recommended and includes daily physical examination for evidence of further thrombosis and periodic platelet counts, the need for which is determined clinically. Evidence of new thrombosis or decrease in platelet count to $<100,000/mm^3$ should be further investigated with aggregation studies to see if an abnormal response to platelet aggregation is present.

The platelet abnormality quickly reverses when heparin is discontinued. Added beneficial therapy includes antiaggregating agents such as dextran (Rheomacrodex®) I.V., 25 mL/hour; acetylsalicylic acid; dipyridamole; and Coumadin®. Iloprost® has been utilized to prevent heparin-induced thrombocytopenia during open heart surgery.[11,12]

The table summarizes the relation of three coagulation tests that have been and can be utilized to adjust the heparin anticoagulant effect.

Test	Usual Normal Control Results	Anticoagulant Range (Heparin Level 0.2–0.4 units/mL)
Lee-White clotting time	8–15 min	20–30 min
Activated clotting time	70–120 sec	180–240 sec
Activated PTT	25–39 sec	60–80 sec
(About twice the normal control value)		

Early studies[13,14] suggested that thrombi do not propagate when the heparin level is such as to prolong the Lee and White (L&W) clotting time to twice that of a normal control. The level of heparin required or desirable, however, varies on an individual basis depending on the severity of the thrombotic process, the potential bleeding risk, variations in the heparin preparation – varying polymer length, sulfonation of polymers, medications that inactivate or inhibit heparin (antihistamines, digitalis, nicotine, penicillin, tetracyclines, phenothiazines and protamine), poor coordination in timing the dose and collection of specimens, antithrombin III level, platelet factor IV level, and fibrinogen level.[15] If the latter factors are in normal range, heparin level of 0.3 units/mL of plasma is required to result in a Lee-White clotting time of twice the normal control. Heparin level of 0.6 units/mL (3 times normal Lee-White clotting time) may result in clinical bleeding. Therapeutic range is usually attained with heparin level of 0.2-0.4 units/mL. Heparin dose of 100-125 units/kg body weight given at six hourly intervals bolus I.V. or S.C. or 400-500 units/kg body weight/day as constant infusion will usually provide effective anticoagulation. Constant drip by pump infusion devices is probably most effective, while some have found the constant I.V. drip method to be cumbersome, difficult to control and to be without proven therapeutic superiority.[7,8] With intermittent pulse dosage, however, heparin effect must be monitored so as to provide high level anticoagulant action without accumulation with subsequent doses.

Monitoring: A bewildering number of coagulation tests and protocols have been recommended for monitoring heparin effect. The Lee and White clotting time, activated clotting time (ACT), and the activated plasma thromboplastin time (APTT) are currently used, as shown in the table.

The ACT has been favored during cardiovascular operations to monitor heparin dosage and neutralization. The ACT, however, assays overall coagulation activity such that prolonged values may not be exclusively the result of heparin. There is a risk, then, in giving protamine sulfate (heparin antagonist).[16] When the protamine sulfate concentration exceeds that of heparin, it begins to act as an anticoagulant with resultant at least potential lack of specificity. This can be identified by showing correction of the prolonged ACT by addition of protamine sulfate *in vitro* to the blood in question.[16] Some have held that laboratory control of heparin use is unnecessary.[17] They have found that the incidence of major bleeding complications during heparin anticoagulation is essentially the same when therapy is regulated with the whole blood clotting time (WBCT) as when heparin is given without clotting tests.[5]

A significantly larger amount of heparin is required for effective anticoagulation in the presence of active thromboembolic disease. It has been suggested that the heparin dosage required to maintain a target APTT of 1.5 to 2.5 times the control has diagnostic importance and can contribute to an understanding of whether or not thromboembolic disease is present.[4]

Simultaneous monitoring of APTT, WBCT, and the thrombin clotting time appears to have identified a population of patients in which a significant increase (more than double) in the level of factor VIII activity occurs.[18] This results in a misleading shortening of the APTT. To detect this situation, a combination of APTT and a **thrombin clotting time heparin assay (TCT)** has been recommended.[18] Discrepancy between a normal APTT and a prolonged TCT may indicate presence of antithrombin III deficiency. With dysfibrinogenemia, the TCT would be especially prolonged.

The APTT may be excessively sensitive, and while many studies show correlation with the whole blood clotting time, the series usually lack cases with prolonged APTT or the data show poor correlation with high levels of anticoagulation.

The Lee-White clotting time (WBCT) provides useable results but may require 30-40 minutes to achieve endpoint (clot formation) at high heparin levels. The microsilicate activated clotting time (ACT) obviates some of the difficulties with the WBCT, providing shorter clotting times.

Kurec AS et al have reported their experience comparing WBCT, ACT, and APTT in monitoring heparin anticoagulation.[19] They have found that the ACT correlates best with the APTT and is generally most useable.

Low molecular weight heparin (LMWH): Standard heparin is composed of sulfated mucopolysaccharides, heterogeneous fragments of different molecular weights. LMWH is less heterogeneous, consists of fragments with high and low affinity for AT III but LMWH use is associated with decreased antithrombin activity while anti-Xa activity is largely preserved. There is evidence that LMWH is able to protect against thromboembolic events while the risk of hemorrhage is reduced.[20] Conventional tests used in monitoring of standard heparin treatment (eg, APTT, TT, ACT) are not affected by LMWH at the doses usually employed. Laboratory control of the use of LMWH is, therefore, not applicable. Heparin-induced thrombocytopenia is usually seen, however, some 7-12 days after LMWH therapy begins so that periodic platelet counts are recommended.[20]

In recent years, increased emphasis has been placed on prevention of bleeding as a complication of anticoagulation, one of the goals of laboratory monitoring. To this end, use of a bleeding risk index for prospective evaluation has been developed and found to provide a valid estimate of the probability of major bleeding during anticoagulation.[21]

Patients with a prolonged APTT not corrected by mixing with normal plasma but with no family or clinical/surgical history of bleeding are (in screening situations) most commonly due to a phospholipid (lupus type) anticoagulant. College of American Pathologists surveys (1986 and

(Continued)

Partial Thromboplastin Time *(Continued)*

1987) found significant difference in the sensitivity of different APTT reagents to the presence of lupus anticoagulants. The difference in reagent responsiveness can affect the apparent factor activity and also the dilutional effect on mixing patient with normal plasma samples, thus impairing the ability to differentiate a lupus anticoagulant from a specific factor inhibitor.[22]

Appropriateness of prothrombin and partial thromboplastin time testing on the medical service of a teaching hospital (ordering patterns in relation to clinical indications) concludes that these tests are overutilized (at least 70% were not clinically indicated).[23,24]

Over 50% of cases of Noonan's syndrome (congenital heart disease, short stature, and dysmorphic facies) also have abnormal bleeding. Prolonged APTT was found in 40% of patients with the syndrome. A variety of specific individual and combined deficiencies were identified.[25]

Footnotes

1. Ansell J, Tiarks C, Hirsh J, et al, "Measurement of the Activated Partial Thromboplastin Time From a Capillary (Fingerstick) Sample of Whole Blood. A New Method for Monitoring Heparin Therapy," *Am J Clin Pathol*, 1991, 95(2):222-7.
2. Garton S and Larsen AE, "Effect of Hemolysis on the Partial Thromboplastin Time," *Am J Med Technol*, 1972, 38:408-10.
3. Gawoski JM, Arkin CF, Bovill T, et al, "The Effects of Heparin on the Activated Partial Thromboplastin Time of the College of American Pathologists Survey Specimens," *Arch Pathol Lab Med*, 1987, 111:785-90.
4. White TM, Bernene JL, and Marino AM, "Continuous Heparin Infusion Requirements. Diagnostic and Therapeutic Implications," *JAMA*, 1979, 241:2717-20.
5. Salzman EW, Deykin D, Shapiro RM, et al, "Management of Heparin Therapy: Controlled Prospective Trial," *N Engl J Med*, 1975, 292:1046-50.
6. Glazier RL and Crowell EB, "Randomized Prospective Trial of Continuous vs Intermittent Heparin Therapy," *JAMA*, 1976, 236:1365-7.
7. Forman WB, "The Risks of Heparin Therapy," *Hosp Formulary*, 1978, 779-84.
8. Hussey CU, Bernhard VM, McLean MR, et al, "Heparin Induced Platelet Aggregation: *In Vitro* Confirmation of Thrombotic Complications," *Ann Clin Lab Sci*, 1979, 9:487-93.
9. Trowbridge AA, Caraveo J, Green JB, et al, "Heparin-Related Immune Thrombocytopenia. Studies of Antibody-Heparin Specificity," *Am J Med*, 1978, 65:277-83.
10. Wahl TO, Lipschitz DA, and Stechschulte DJ, "Thrombocytopenia Associated With Antiheparin Antibody," *JAMA*, 1978, 240:2560-2.
11. Addonizio VP Jr, Fisher CA, Kappa JR, et al, "Prevention of Heparin-Induced Thrombocytopenia During Open Heart Surgery With Iloprost® (ZK36374)," *Surgery*, 1987, 102:796-807.
12. Sobel M, Adelman B, Szentpetery S, et al, "Surgical Management of Heparin-Associated Thrombocytopenia. Strategies in the Treatment of Venous and Arterial Thromboembolism," *J Vasc Surg*, 1988, 8(4):395-401.
13. Wessler S and Morris CE, "Studies in Intravascular Coagulation: IV. The Effect of Heparin and Dicumarol on Serum Induced Venous Thrombosis," *Circulation*, 1955, 12:553-6.
14. Carey LC and Williams RD, "Comparative Effects of Dicumarol, Tromexan, and Heparin on Thrombus Propagation," *Ann Surg*, 1960, 152:919-22.
15. Soloway HB, "Inappropriate Response to Heparin Therapy," *Diagnostic Medicine*, 1979, Sept/Oct, 2:31-3.
16. Roth JA, "Use of ACT to Monitor Heparin During Cardiac Surgery," *Ann Thorac Surg*, 1979, 28:69-72.
17. Bauer G, "Clinical Experiences of a Surgeon in the Use of Heparin," *Am J Cardiol*, 1964, 14:29-35.
18. Glynn MF, "Heparin Monitoring and Thrombosis," *Am J Clin Pathol*, 1979, 71:397-400.
19. Kurec AS, Morris MW, and Davey FR, "Clotting, Activated Partial Thromboplastin and Coagulation Times in Monitoring Heparin Therapy," *Ann Clin Lab Sci*, 1979, 9:494-500.
20. Samama M, "Low Molecular Weight Heparin," *ASCP Check Sample®*, Chicago, IL: American Society of Clinical Pathologists, 1987.
21. Landefeld CS, McGuire E 3d, and Rosenblatt MW, "A Bleeding Risk Index for Estimating the Probability of Major Bleeding in Hospitalized Patients Starting Anticoagulant Therapy," *Am J Med*, 1990, 89(5):569-78.
22. Brandt JT, Triplett DA, Rock WA, et al, "Effect of Lupus Anticoagulants on the Activated Partial Thromboplastin Time. Results of the College of American Pathologists Survey Program," *Arch Pathol Lab Med*, 1991, 115(2):109-14.
23. Erban SB, Kinman SL, and Schwartz JS, "Routine Use of the Prothrombin and Partial Thromboplastin Times," *JAMA*, 1989, 262(17):2428-32.
24. Janvier G, Winnock S, and Freyburger G, "Value of the Activated Partial Thromboplastin Time for Preoperative Detection of Coagulation Disorders Not Revealed by a Specific Questionnaire," *Anesthesiology*, 1991, 75(5):920-1.
25. Sharland M, Patton MA, Talbot S, et al, "Coagulation-Factor Deficiencies and Abnormal Bleeding in Noonan's Syndrome," *Lancet*, 1992, 339(8784):19-21.

References

Andrew M, Paes B, Milner R, et al, "Development of the Human Coagulation System in the Healthy Premature Infant," *Blood*, 1988, 72:1651-7.

Andrew M, Vegh P, Johnston M, et al, "Maturation of the Hemostatic System During Childhood," *Blood*, 1992, 80(8):1998-2005.

D'Angelo A, Seveso MP, D'Angelo SV, et al, "Effect of Clot-Detection Methods and Reagents on Activated Partial Thromboplastin Time (APTT). Implications in Heparin Monitoring by APTT," *Am J Clin Pathol*, 1990, 94(3):297-306.

Dhami MS and Bona RD, "Using Anticoagulants Safely. Guidelines for Therapeutic and Prophylactic Regimens," *Postgrad Med*, 1991, 90(1):121-2, 127-32.

Hirsh J and Levine MN, "Low Molecular Weight Heparin," *Blood*, 1992, 79(1):1-17.

Hommes DW, Bura A, Mazzolai L, et al, "Subcutaneous Heparin Compared With Continuous Intravenous Heparin Administration in the Initial Treatment of Deep Vein Thrombosis. A Meta-Analysis," *Ann Intern Med*, 1992, 116(4):279-84.

Middleton AL and Oakley E, "Activated Partial Thromboplastin Time (APTT): Review of Methods," *ASCP Check Sample®*, Chicago, IL: American Society of Clinical Pathologists, 1987.

Turpie AG, Robinson JG, and Doyle DJ, "Comparison of High-Dose With Low-Dose Subcutaneous Heparin to Prevent Left Ventricular Mural Thrombosis in Patients With Acute Transmural Anterior Myocardial Infarction," *N Engl J Med*, 1989, 320(6):352-7.

PC *see* Protein C *on page 464*

Phospholipid Type Anticoagulant *see* Inhibitor, Lupus, Phospholipid Type *on page 444*

Plasma Plasminogen Activator Inhibitor *see* Plasminogen Activator Inhibitor *on this page*

Plasma Protamine Paracoagulation *see* Fibrin Split Products, Protamine Sulfate *on page 439*

Plasma Thromboplastin Antecedent *see* Factor XI *on page 429*

Plasma Thromboplastin Component *see* Factor IX *on page 426*

Plasminogen Activator Inhibitor

CPT *85415*

Related Information

Diluted Whole Blood Clot Lysis *on page 418*
Hypercoagulable State Coagulation Screen *on page 441*
Inhibitor, Lupus, Phospholipid Type *on page 444*
Plasminogen Assay *on page 457*
Protein C *on page 464*
Protein S *on page 466*

Synonyms PAI; PAI Chromogenic Assay; Plasma Plasminogen Activator Inhibitor; Spectrolyse™/pL Procedure

Specimen Plasma **CONTAINER:** Blue top (sodium citrate) tube **SAMPLING TIME:** PAI-1 has a circadian rhythm, high in the early morning but falling in the afternoon and evening. This change should be considered when planning PAI-1 plasma studies. **COLLECTION:** Obtain **free flowing** venous blood sample using a two-syringe technique. If indwelling catheter is in place or Vacutainer® technique is utilized, use sample from second or third tube. Discard the first 3-5 mL of free flowing blood. Place gently mixed tube on ice and process (centrifuge) within 60 minutes. **STORAGE INSTRUCTIONS:** Plasma may be stored at -70°C (until analyzed). **CAUSES FOR REJECTION:** Correction procedure may be necessary if plasma sample is hemolyzed or has increase in bilirubin levels **SPECIAL INSTRUCTIONS:** Plasma must be absolutely platelet-free. Centrifugal force of at least 30,000 g/min used during centrifugation.[1]

Interpretive **REFERENCE RANGE:** 0-15 units/mL (average 4.5 units/mL).[2] Men generally have higher values than women. **USE:** Evaluate deep vein thrombosis, myocardial infarction (MI), and risk of postoperative thrombosis **LIMITATIONS:** Results may be affected by abnormally high levels of hemoglobin, bilirubin, or lipid levels present concurrently in the plasma test sample. There is evidence of significant intra-individual variation for 30 days following surgery or onset of deep vein thrombosis. Due to this acute phase reaction, it has been recommended that study of the fibrinolytic system should be postponed for at least 1 month after an acute episode.[3] **METHODOLOGY:** Two-stage indirect enzymatic assay (principle first developed by Chmielewska et al[4]), available commercially as Spectrolyse™/pL. In the first step a fixed

(Continued)

Plasminogen Activator Inhibitor *(Continued)*

amount of t-PA reacts with PAI in the test plasma, and sample is acidified to destroy other plasmin inhibitors. In the second step residual t-PA activity is measured by determining the color developed after any residual t-PA has generated plasmin that effects hydrolysis of the chromogen substrate. **ADDITIONAL INFORMATION:** There are two distinct plasminogen activator inhibitors, PAI-1 (present in normal plasma and platelet releasates) and PAI-2 (present in pregnancy plasma and leukocytes).[5] PAI-1 is a single chain glycoprotein, molecular weight of about 50,000. It is a serine protease inhibitor, a member of the "serpin" gene family. PAI-1 exists in latent (inactive), active, and complex (t-PA/PAI-1) forms in the blood. Increase in plasma PAI may be a cause of decreased fibrinolytic activity and may relate to clinical thrombotic disease. Patients with recurrent myocardial infarction, coronary artery disease, and deep vein thrombosis may have increased plasma PAI levels. There is increase in risk of recurrent MI in survivors of a first infarctive episode.[6] If plasma PAI is elevated prior to surgery, there is increase in risk of postoperative thrombosis. As PAI is an acute phase reactant of the inflammatory process, levels increase after surgery. Plasma PAI levels are increased with endotoxemia and with pregnancy. Perioperative (aortic surgery patients) increase in PAI may be due in part to release of inhibitor from platelets.[7]

There is evidence that human recombinant lymphotoxin, α and β interleukin-1, and recombinant tumor necrosis factor increase the production of plasminogen activator inhibitor. Increase in PAI activity might decrease fibrinolysis.[8]

Utilizing a radioimmunoassay to measure PAI-1 antigen levels before and after platelet aggregation, 85% of PAI-1 (in platelet-rich plasma) was found to be associated with platelets, about 4000 molecules per platelet.[4]

Plasminogen activation may play an important role in atherogenesis. Lipoprotein (a) (Lp(a)), a variant of low density lipoprotein, is a physiological inhibitor of plasminogen activation. Lp(a) competes with plasminogen for plasminogen binding sites, decreases binding of plasminogen by endothelial cells, thus suppressing fibrinolysis and contributing to a procoagulant state.[9]

Impaired fibrinolysis with elevated plasma plasminogen activator inhibitor levels was noted in a group of patients with malignant disease.[10] This finding may relate to the development of deep-vein thrombosis in some patients with malignant conditions.

Footnotes

1. Macy EM, Meilahn EN, Declerck PJ, et al, "Sample Preparation for Plasma Measurement of Plasminogen Activator Inhibitor-1 Antigen in Large Population Studies," *Arch Pathol Lab Med*, 1993, 117(1):67-70.
2. Wiman B, "The Role of the Fibrinolytic System in Thrombotic Disease," *Acta Med Scand Suppl*, 1987, 715:169-71.
3. Jansson J-H, Norberg B, and Nilsson TK, "Impact of Acute Phase on Concentrations of Tissue Plasminogen Activator and Plasminogen Activator Inhibitor in Plasma After Deep Vein Thrombosis or Open Heart Surgery," *Clin Chem*, 1989, 35(7):1544-5.
4. Chmielewska J and Wiman B, "Determination of Tissue Plasminogen Activator and Its Fast Inhibitor in Plasma," *Clin Chem*, 1986, 32:482-5.
5. Kruithof EK, Nicolosa G, and Bachmann F, "Plasminogen Activator Inhibitor 1: Development of a Radioimmunoassay and Observations on Its Plasma Concentration During Venous Occlusion and After Platelet Aggregation," *Blood*, 1987, 70:1645-53.
6. Hamsten A, De-Faire U, Walldius G, et al, "Plasminogen Activator Inhibitor in Plasma: Risk Factor for Recurrent Myocardial Infarction," *Lancet*, 1987, 2:3-9.
7. Gomez MJ, Carroll RC, Hansard MR, et al, "Regulation of Fibrinolysis in Aortic Surgery," *J Vasc Surg*, 1988, 8(4):384-8.
8. van Hinsbergh VW, Kooistra T, van den Berg EA, et al, "Tumor Necrosis Factor Increases the Production of Plasminogen Activator Inhibitor in Human Endothelial Cells *In Vitro* and Rats *In Vivo*," *Blood*, 1988, 72(5):1467-73.
9. Scott J, "Lipoprotein(a) Thrombogenesis Linked to Atherogenesis at Last?" *Nature*, 1989, 341(6237):22-3.
10. Newland JR and Haire WD, "Elevated Plasminogen Activator Inhibitor Levels Found in Patients With Malignant Conditions," *Am J Clin Pathol*, 1991, 96(5):602-4.

References

Chandler WL, Loo SC, Nguyen SV, et al, "Standardization of Methods for Measuring Plasminogen Activator Inhibitor Activity in Human Plasma," *Clin Chem*, 1989, 35(5):787-93.

Duncan A and Hunter RL, "Plasminogen Activator (PAI) in Plasma Samples," *Manual of Procedures for the Seminar on Diagnostic Hematology*, Sunderman FW, ed, Philadelphia, PA: Institute for Clinical Science, 1988, 29-37.

Krishnamurti C, Tang DB, Barr CF, et al, "Plasminogen Activator and Plasminogen Activator Inhibitor Activities in a Reference Population," *Am J Clin Pathol*, 1988, 89:747-52.

Loskutoff DJ, Sawdey M, and Mimuro J, "Type 1 Plasminogen Activator Inhibitor," *Prog Hemost Thromb*, 1989, 9:87-115.

Ranby M, Bergsdorf N, Nilsson T, et al, "Age Dependence of Tissue Plasminogen Activator Concentrations in Plasma, as Studied by an Improved Enzyme-Linked Immunosorbent Assay," *Clin Chem*, 1986, 32:2160-5.

Plasminogen Assay

***CPT** 85421*

Related Information

Diluted Whole Blood Clot Lysis *on page 418*
Euglobulin Clot Lysis *on page 418*
Intravascular Coagulation Screen *on page 446*
Plasminogen Activator Inhibitor *on page 455*

Synonyms Plasminogen, Quantitative

Applies to α_2-Antiplasmin

Specimen Plasma **CONTAINER:** Blue top (sodium citrate) tube **COLLECTION:** Routine venipuncture. If multiple tests are being drawn, draw coagulation studies last. If only coagulation tests are being drawn, draw 1-2 mL into another Vacutainer® tube, discard, and then collect coagulation tests (double syringe/tube technique). This collection procedure avoids contamination of the specimen with tissue thromboplastins. **STORAGE INSTRUCTIONS:** Keep refrigerated. **CAUSES FOR REJECTION:** Tube not full, specimen hemolyzed, specimen clotted, specimen received more than 2 hours after collection **SPECIAL INSTRUCTIONS:** Schedule with laboratory.

Interpretive **REFERENCE RANGE:** 3.8-8.4 CTA (Council on Thrombolytic Agents) units/mL (α-Caseinolytic method), may also be reported as percentage of normal for human plasma or in absolute concentration (immunologic assays). Levels are reduced in the newborn (in comparison with the mother).[1,2] **USE:** Determine plasminogen and plasmin activity in plasma, study dysplasminogens, monitor thrombolytic therapy, evaluate DIC **METHODOLOGY:** Caseinolytic method[3] and synthetic substrate based (amidolytic, chromogenic, fluorogenic)[4,5] **ADDITIONAL INFORMATION:** Plasminogen is a glycoprotein (molecular weight about 90,000 daltons) and is present in plasma as an inactive protein (zymogen) at a concentration of about 200 μg/mL and an *in vivo* half-life of 2.2 days. Molecular structure/function relationships are known and are nicely summarized in the following references. A series of five triple-loop structures (kringles) form a major part of the N-terminal region of the molecule and are binding sites for fibrin as well as for antifibrinolytic agents (eg, EACA). Activation of plasminogen (a single-chain protein) to the two-chain serine protease-plasmin, a potent enzyme, is accomplished by either an intrinsic pathway (factor XIIa is involved) or an extrinsic mechanism (serine proteases including urokinase are involved). Decreased plasminogen activity may be on an acquired or familial basis. Acquired decrease is seen in some cases of DIC, liver disease, L-asparaginase therapy (of acute leukemia), neonatal hyaline membrane disease, and following surgery.[6] Plasminogen assay has application to the monitoring of antifibrinolytic therapy.[7] After streptokinase therapy for acute myocardial infarction, the radial immunodiffusion assay did not show as great a decrease in plasma plasminogen as did a fluorogenic synthetic substrate assay.[8] This was shown to be the apparent result of a lack of specificity of the RID assay antibody to plasminogen. Decrease in plasminogen activity may be associated with tendency to thrombosis; altered molecular forms have been described.[9] Inhibitors of plasmin (eg, α_2-antiplasmin) are important in the regulation of fibrinolysis. There is evidence that regular vigorous physical exercise (participation in sporting activities) increases fibrinolytic activity of blood by decreasing plasminogen activator inhibitor capacity.[10]

Plasminogen polymorphism has been applied in the field of forensic hemogenetics.[11]

Footnotes

1. Biland L and Duckert F, "Coagulation Factors of the Newborn and His Mother," *Thromb Diath Haemorrh*, 1973, 29:644-51.
2. Corrigan JJ, Sleeth JJ, Jeter M, et al, "Newborn's Fibrinolytic Mechanism: Components and Plasmin Generation," *Am J Hematol*, 1989, 32(4):273-8.
3. Triplett DA and Harms CS, "Plasminogen Assay by α-Caseinolytic Method," *Procedures for the Coagulation Laboratory*, Chicago, IL: ASCP Press, 1981, 144-6.
4. Fareed J, Messmore HL, Walenga JM, et al, "Diagnostic Efficacy of Newer Synthetic-Substrates Methods for Assessing Coagulation Variables: A Critical Overview," *Clin Chem*, 1983, 29:225-36.
5. Friberger P, "Chromogenic Peptide Substrates. Their Use for the Assay of Factors in the Fibrinolytic and the Plasma Kallikrein-Kinin Systems," *Scand J Clin Lab Invest Suppl*, 1982, 162:1-298.
6. Pierson-Perry JF, Wehrly JA, and Siefring GE Jr, "Coagulation Testing With the Du Pont aca® Discrete Clinical Analyzer," *Semin Thromb Hemost*, 1983, 9:321-33.

(Continued)

Plasminogen Assay *(Continued)*

7. Marder VJ and Bell WR, "Fibrinolytic Therapy," *Hemostasis and Thrombosis*, Colman RW, Hirsch J, Marder VJ, et al, eds, Philadelphia, PA: JB Lippincott Co, 1982, 1037-57.
8. Hysell DC, Smith MR, Brewster PS, et al, "Discrepant Changes in Plasminogen by Two Different Assays in Patients Receiving Streptokinase," *Am J Clin Pathol*, 1988, 90(2):200-5.
9. Giddings JC, "Components of the Fibrinolytic Mechanism," *Molecular Genetics and Immunoanalysis in Blood Coagulation*, Chapter 7, Chichester, England: Ellis Horwood Ltd, 1988, 161-6.
10. Speiser W, Langer W, Pschaick A, et al, "Increased Blood Fibrinolytic Activity After Physical Exercise: Comparative Study in Individuals With Different Sporting Activities and in Patients After Myocardial Infarction Taking Part in a Rehabilitation Sports Program," *Thromb Res*, 1988, 51:543-55.
11. Skoda U, Klein A, Lübcke I, et al, "Application of Plasminogen Polymorphism to Forensic Hemogenetics," *Electrophoresis*, 1989, 9:422-6.

References

Benedict CR, Mueller S, Anderson HV, et al, "Thrombolytic Therapy: A State of the Art Review," *Hosp Pract*, 1992, 27(6):61-72.

Collen D and Lijnen HR, "Basic and Clinical Aspects of Fibrinolysis and Thrombolysis," *Blood*, 1991, 78(12):3114-24.

Müllertz S, "Fibrinolysis," *Semin Thromb Hemost*, 1984, 10:1, 1-103.

Rosenberg RD, "Physiology of Coagulation: The Fluid Phase," *Hematology of Infancy and Childhood*, 3rd ed, Nathan DG and Oski FA, eds, Philadelphia, PA: WB Saunders Co, 1987, 1248-70.

Plasminogen, Quantitative *see* Plasminogen Assay *on previous page*

Platelet Adhesion Test

CPT 85575

Related Information

Bleeding Time, Ivy *on page 409*
Platelet Aggregation *on next page*
Platelet Count *on page 586*

Synonyms Glass Bead Platelet Retention Test; Platelet Adhesiveness; Platelet Retention; Salzman Column Test

Patient Care PREPARATION: Avoid aspirin, phenylbutazone, antihistamines, phenothiazines for 10 days prior to test

Specimen Whole blood COLLECTION: Specimen will usually be collected by Hematology technologist. CAUSES FOR REJECTION: Specimen clotted SPECIAL INSTRUCTIONS: Schedule with laboratory in advance.

Interpretive REFERENCE RANGE: Method dependent. Normals usually have at least 75% platelet retention by glass bead column, commonly 90% to 95%; 35% to 75% may be considered borderline. USE: Evaluate platelet function; aid in the diagnosis of von Willebrand's disease, thrombasthenia (Glanzmann's disease), storage pool disease, and the Bernard-Soulier syndrome LIMITATIONS: This test is offered by very few laboratories because of difficulty in obtaining glass beads and columns of glass beads, in standardizing the technique and keeping glass beads (in the column) from settling. Procedure given in the reference by Zacharski and McIntyre provides for a low cost, reliable standardized test. Settling of beads is avoided by agitation with a vibrating hair management device just before use. A current authoritative reference indicates that *in vitro* platelet adhesion testing is **"unreliable"** and "has no clinical relevance" - thus, "should not be used".[1] CONTRAINDICATIONS: Thrombocytopenia or therapy with drugs listed above under patient preparation METHODOLOGY: Glass bead column. The relationship between the platelet count done on a presample (not exposed to glass beads) compared to a postsample (glass bead filtered) will give an indication of the adhesiveness of the platelets. ADDITIONAL INFORMATION: Useful in the evaluation of some thrombopathies. A defect in adhesion is present in **von Willebrand's disease**, **thrombasthenia**, **storage pool disease**, and the **Bernard-Soulier syndrome**. The Bernard-Soulier syndrome is a severe congenital hemorrhagic disorder characterized by large platelets, deficiency of platelet membrane glycoprotein I, and the inability of platelets to bind von Willebrand factor. Glass bead retention is decreased in vWD, the percent retention returns to normal, however, in columns that have been pretreated with normal plasma.[2] Platelet adhesion is defective in cases of complete afibrinogenemia. In a study designed to standardize platelet function tests there was wide variation between glass bead columns.[3] Some columns showed wide variation in normal subjects. It was felt columns would not detect abnormal platelet retention. These studies however, may not have controlled for glass bead settling in the column.

In normal individuals ingesting 200 IU of alpha-tocopherol (vitamin E) per day, platelet adhesion was decreased on average by 75%. A dose of 400 IU/day resulted in reduction of platelet adhesion by 82%. Scanning EM study showed decrease in pseudopodium formation in the alpha-tocopherol enriched platelets.[4]

There is evidence that some cases of mild bleeding disorders of von Willebrand disease type may be detected only by use of the McPherson and Zucker two-stage platelet retention assay.[5] In such cases platelets were defective in the second stage (platelet-platelet interaction) of the assay. The platelet retention defects normalized after treatment with desmopressin (d-DAVP). Thus, platelet adhesion studies may identify mild bleeding disorder patients who may improve after treatment with d-DAVP.[6]

Dietary supplementation with vitamin E (alpha-tocopherol) may result in significant decrease in platelet adhesion.[4]

Footnotes

1. Bick RL, "Qualitative (Functional) Platelet Disorders," Chapter 4, *Disorders of Thrombosis and Hemostasis: Clinical and Laboratory Practice*, Chicago, IL: ASCP Press, 1992, 49.
2. Davis GL and Fritsma GA, "Platelet Disorders," *Hemostasis and Thrombosis in the Clinical Laboratory*, Corriveau DM and Fritsma GA, eds, Philadelphia, PA: JB Lippincott Co, 1988, 334.
3. Roper-Drewinko PR, Drewinko B, Corrigan G, et al, "Standardization of Platelet Function Tests," *Am J Hematol*, 1981, 11:182-203.
4. Jandak J, Steiner M, and Richardson PD, "α-Tocopherol, an Effective Inhibitor of Platelet Adhesion," *Blood*, 1989, 73(1):141-9.
5. McPherson J and Zucker MB, "Platelet Retention in Glass Bead Columns: Adhesion to Glass and Subsequent Platelet-Platelet Interactions," *Blood*, 1976, 47:55-67.
6. Zeigler ZR, "Platelet Glass Bead Retention Is Useful in Monitoring Response to 1-Deamino-8-D-Arginine-Vasopressin (d-DAVP)," *Am J Hematol*, 1989, 31(4):248-52.

References

de Groot PG and Sixma JJ, "Platelet Adhesion," *Br J Haematol*, 1990, 75(3):308-12.
Packham MA and Mustard JF, "Platelet Adhesion," *Prog Hemost Thromb*, 1984, 7:211-88.
Zacharski LR and McIntyre OR, "A Standardized Test of Platelet Adhesiveness," *Am J Clin Pathol*, 1972, 58:422-7.

Platelet Adhesiveness *see* Platelet Adhesion Test *on previous page*

Platelet Aggregation

***CPT** 85575 (each agent)*

Related Information

Bleeding Time, Ivy *on page 409*
Clot Retraction *on page 413*
Platelet Adhesion Test *on previous page*
Platelet Aggregation, Hypercoagulable State *on page 461*
Platelet Count *on page 586*
von Willebrand Factor Assay *on page 478*

Synonyms Aggregometer Test; Platelet Function Studies

Applies to Lumi-Aggregometry; P62; Platelet Impedance Aggregation in Whole Blood

Test Commonly Includes Response to ADP, epinephrine, collagen, ristocetin, optionally arachidonic acid, thrombin

Patient Care PREPARATION: For 10 days prior to testing, drugs that inhibit platelet aggregation are contraindicated. See accompanying list. Any caffeine-containing products must not be consumed the day of test. Aspirin, ubiquitous in our society, will impair platelet aggregation.

Specimen Plasma CONTAINER: Plastic or siliconized glass syringe COLLECTION: Specimen may need to be specially drawn by laboratory. Keep at room temperature and transport to the laboratory immediately. STORAGE INSTRUCTIONS: Test should be run within 2 hours of obtaining the sample. Do not chill specimen, platelets are activated at low

Drugs That Inhibit Platelet Aggregation

Acetylsalicylic acid (ASA, Aspirin)	Indomethacin (Indocin)
Antihistamines	Marijuana
Chlordiazepoxide (Librium)	Phenothiazines
Clofibrate (Atromid)	Phenylbutazone (Butazolidin)
Cocaine	Propranolol (Inderal)
Corticosteroids	Pyrimidine compounds
Diazepam (Valium)	Sulfinpyrazone (Anturane)
Dipyridamole (Persantine)	Theophylline
Furosemide (Lasix)	Tricyclic antidepressants
Gentamicin	Others
Ibuprofen (Motrin)	

(Continued)

Platelet Aggregation *(Continued)*

temperatures. Blood should be processed at 20°C to 25°C and stored at 20°C to 37°C until tested. **CAUSES FOR REJECTION:** Platelet count <100,000/mm^3, clotted specimen, hemolysis, patient receiving therapy with drugs, particularly aspirin, antihistamines, anti-inflammatory drugs, psychotropic drugs, some antibiotics and others (unless one wishes to study effect of such medication upon platelet function) **SPECIAL INSTRUCTIONS:** Must usually be scheduled with laboratory.

Interpretive **REFERENCE RANGE:** ADP: 60% to 100%; epinephrine: 60% to 100%; collagen: 60% to 100%; ristocetin: 60% to 100%. Diagnostic information is present in the graphical representation of results. Response of normal platelets may vary with concentration of aggregating agent. **USE:** Evaluate platelet function; aid in diagnosis of von Willebrand's disease, Glanzmann's disease, storage pool disease, Bernard-Soulier syndrome, "gray platelet syndrome," and Raynaud's phenomenon **LIMITATIONS:** If drugs (as indicated above) are exerting an inhibitory effect, evaluation of pre-existing disease of platelet function may be impaired. Presence of lipemia or cryoglobulins may cause difficulty in interpretation. **METHODOLOGY:** Aggregating agent is added to platelet-rich plasma. Resultant change in optical density (if any) that occurs as the dispersed platelets form clumps is measured and recorded. Whole blood platelet aggregation methods have been developed and utilized (impedance aggregation).[1] Some aggregometers are fitted with a luminescence detector which monitors ATP release simultaneously with platelet aggregation (Lumi-aggregometers). Luciferase (firefly extract) acts on ATP as a substrate to emit light. **ADDITIONAL INFORMATION:** Ristocetin stimulated aggregation is of special value in study of von Willebrand's disease. Latter is characterized by decreased aggregation with ristocetin. It is suggested that about 50% of patients with chronic ITP have abnormal (decreased or absent) aggregation with ADP, collagen and epinephrine (using albumin density gradient concentrated platelets). These patients (with thrombopathy) also have demonstrable antiplatelet antibodies.[2] Abnormal platelet aggregation has been found in nearly one-half (44%) of beta-thalassemia major patients.[3] Enhanced platelet aggregation has been noted in insulin stress test induced by hypoglycemia, coinciding with the lowest blood glucose levels and with clinical signs of adrenaline release but without correlation with changes in cortisol, growth hormone, prolactin, or levodopa administration.[4] Platelets from diabetics are more sensitive to aggregating agents.[5] Aggregation responses with platelet concentration <100,000/mm^3, samples processed 90 minutes or longer at room temperature and ADP-induced responses in males as compared to females result in significantly lower values.[6]

Platelet aggregation and/or release is absent in a variety of conditions with qualitative platelet defects, generally termed thrombocytopathy. There are familial forms such as **Bernard-Soulier syndrome**, **Wiskott-Aldrich syndrome**, **storage pool disease**, **Hermansky-Pudlak syndrome**, and others.

Acquired disorders that affect platelet function are **uremia**, **macroglobulinemia**, **drug ingestion**, and others. Patients with **thrombasthenia** show no aggregation with ADP, epinephrine, or collagen.

Patients with **von Willebrand's disease** and **Bernard-Soulier syndrome** show defective aggregation with ristocetin. Whole blood platelet aggregation (along with RIA for platelet glycoprotein expression and monoclonal antibody immunochemical staining of whole blood smears) has been applied to establishing the diagnosis of Bernard-Soulier syndrome. Such patients have large platelets with decreased glycoprotein Ib expression. Platelet aggregation with ristocetin is absent.[7]

Patients with the **"gray platelet syndrome"** have large alpha granule content-depleted, pale staining platelets that aggregate with ristocetin but not with ADP, epinephrine, thrombin, or collagens[8]. See Bleeding Time, Ivy listing.

Patients with primary and secondary **Raynaud's phenomenon** have increased aggregation to the agonists serotonin and ADP but normal responses to adrenalin and collagen.[9] Aspirin effect is characterized by inhibition of collagen aggregation and absence of the secondary waves (release reaction) of ADP, epinephrine, and ristocetin. Aspirin and aspirin-containing drugs will inhibit platelet aggregation for about 7-10 days after ingestion.

Therapeutic propranolol levels have no significant influence on platelet function as determined by platelet aggregation studies with the possible exception of the agonists collagen and noradrenaline in which minor changes without likely biological import were noted.[10] On the other hand, a reversible effect of nitroglycerine (at therapeutic doses) has been shown on platelet function (platelet aggregation with ADP using an impedance aggregometer at bedside).[11]

A critical retrospective review of 188 patients with bleeding abnormalities resulted in the conclusion that results of aggregation and bleeding times were not highly correlated and that only rarely were previously undiagnosed platelet function diseases identified.[12] The authors find that 75% of patients with an abnormal bleeding time had normal aggregation while 26% of those with normal bleeding times had abnormal aggregation.

It has been shown that features of platelet storage pool deficiency may be present in some patients with prolonged bleeding times but no demonstrable abnormalities in platelet aggregation or von Willebrand factor.[13] Some patients with dense granule storage pool deficiency have decreased levels of granulophysin, a constituent of the platelet dense granule membrane.[14]

A patient with deficiency of P62 (a putative collagen receptor found in at least some patients with idiopathic thrombocytopenic purpura) has been shown to have defective collagen-induced platelet aggregation.[15]

Footnotes

1. Mackie IJ, Jones R, and Machin SJ, "Platelet Impedance Aggregation in Whole Blood and Its Inhibition by Antiplatelet Drugs," *J Clin Pathol*, 1984, 37:874-8.
2. Heyns AD, Fraser J, and Retief FP, "Platelet Aggregation in Chronic Idiopathic Thrombocytopenia Purpura," *J Clin Pathol*, 1978, 31:1239-43.
3. Hussain MA, Hutton RA, Pavlidou O, et al, "Platelet Function in Beta-Thalassemia Major," *J Clin Pathol*, 1979, 32:429-33.
4. Hutton RA, Mikhailidis D, Dormandy KM, et al, "Platelet Aggregation Studies During Transient Hypoglycemia: A Potential Method for Evaluating Platelet Function," *J Clin Pathol*, 1979, 32:434-8.
5. DiMinno G, Silver MJ, Cerbone AM, et al, "Increased Binding of Fibrinogen to Platelets in Diabetes: The Role of Prostaglandins and Thromboxane," *Blood*, 1985, 65:156-62.
6. Roper P, Drewinko B, Hasler D, et al, "Effects of Time, Platelet Concentrations, and Sex on the Human Platelet Aggregation Response," *Am J Clin Pathol*, 1979, 71:263-8.
7. Nichols WL, Kaese SE, Gastineau DA, et al, "Bernard-Soulier Syndrome: Whole Blood Diagnostic Assays of Platelets," *Mayo Clin Proc*, 1989, 64(5):522-30.
8. Peerschke EIB, "The Gray Platelet Syndrome," *ASCP Check Sample®*, Chicago, IL: American Society of Clinical Pathologists, 1988.
9. Biondi ML and Marasini B, "Abnormal Platelet Aggregation in Patients With Raynaud's Phenomenon," *J Clin Pathol*, 1989, 42(7):716-8.
10. Pomphilon DH, Boon RJ, Prentice AG, et al, "Lack of Significant Effect of Therapeutic Propranolol on Measurable Platelet Function in Healthy Subjects," *J Clin Pathol*, 1989, 42(8):793-6.
11. Diodati J, Théroux P, Latour J-G, et al, "Effects of Nitroglycerin at Therapeutic Doses on Platelet Aggregation in Unstable Angina Pectoris and Acute Myocardial Infarction," *Am J Cardiol*, 1990, 66(7):683-8.
12. Remaley AT, Kennedy JM, and Laposata M, "Evaluation of the Clinical Utility of Platelet Aggregation Studies," *Am J Hematol*, 1989, 31(3):188-93.
13. Israels SJ, McNicole A, Robertson C, et al, "Platelet Storage Pool Deficiency: Diagnosis in Patients With Prolonged Bleeding Times and Normal Platelet Aggregation," *Br J Haematol*, 1990, 75(1):118-21.
14. Shalev A, Michaud G, Israels SJ, et al, "Quantification of a Novel Dense Granule Protein (Granulophysin) in Platelets of Patients With Dense Granule Storage Pool Deficiency," *Blood*, 1992, 80(5):1231-7.
15. Ryo R, Yoshida A, Sugano W, et al, "Deficiency of P62, a Putative Collagen Receptor, in Platelets From a Patient With Defective Collagen-Induced Platelet Aggregation," *Am J Hematol*, 1992, 39(1):25-31.

References

Bick RL, "Acquired Platelet Function Defects," *Hematol Oncol Clin North Am*, 1992, 6(6):1203-28.

Braman AM and Schwartz KA, "Platelet Disorders," *Lab Med*, 1989, 20:831-5.

Fratantoni JC and Poindexter BJ, "Measuring Platelet Aggregation With Microplate Reader. A New Technical Approach to Platelet Aggregation Studies," *Am J Clin Pathol*, 1990, 94(5):613-7.

Hardisty RM, "Hereditary Disorders of Platelet Function," *Clin Lab Haematol*, 1983, 12:153-73.

Hutton RA and Ludlam CA, "ACP Broadsheet #122 Platelet Function Testing," *J Clin Pathol*, 1989, 42(8):858-64.

Machin SJ and Preston E, and BSCH Haemostasis and Thrombosis Task Force of the British Society for Haematology, "Guildlines on Platelet Function Testing," *J Clin Pathol*, 1988, 41:1322-30.

Platelet Aggregation, Hypercoagulable State

CPT *85575*

Related Information

Antithrombin III Test *on page 403*
Hypercoagulable State Coagulation Screen *on page 441*
Platelet Aggregation *on page 459*

Synonyms Hypercoagulable State, Platelet Aggregation; Platelet Autoaggregation

Test Commonly Includes Evaluation of spontaneous aggregation, second wave of aggregation with weak ADP, and platelet response to dilutions of epinephrine

(Continued)

Platelet Aggregation, Hypercoagulable State *(Continued)*

Patient Care PREPARATION: The patient should not receive aspirin, phenylbutazone, phenothiazines, antihistamines, or other drugs (see Platelet Aggregation) for 7-10 days prior to testing.

Specimen Plasma CONTAINER: Plastic tube or syringe with sodium citrate COLLECTION: Specimen is usually specially collected by Hematology technologist. SPECIAL INSTRUCTIONS: Consult laboratory as to availability of and need for scheduling this analysis. While a simple modification of standard platelet aggregation studies, in most laboratories such hypercoagulable aggregation tests are not routinely available.

Interpretive REFERENCE RANGE: Rapid spontaneous aggregation or aggregation with very dilute concentrations of epinephrine (as compared to control) may correlate with presence of hypercoagulable state. USE: Coagulation parameter used for evaluation of hypercoagulable states LIMITATIONS: Miale has noted that platelet autoaggregation should be a part of platelet aggregation studies but has not found hyperaggregability studies with dilute ADP or epinephrine reagents helpful.[1] CONTRAINDICATIONS: Thrombocytopenia, therapy with drugs as indicated under patient preparation METHODOLOGY: Platelet aggregation study techniques are used to evaluate platelet function for spontaneous aggregation and enhanced platelet response to standard aggregating agents, using platelet-rich plasma or whole blood (impedance method study of aggregation). ADDITIONAL INFORMATION: Spontaneous aggregation, second wave of aggregation with weak ADP, and enhanced platelet response with dilutions of epinephrine may be indications of platelet hyperactivity and may reflect presence of a hypercoagulable state. The results of whole blood aggregometry have been found significantly more sensitive than those of platelet-rich plasma optical aggregometry in the investigation of platelet hyperaggregability in patients with thromboembolic disease.[2] Hyperaggregation to ADP and to collagen, as well as, spontaneous aggregation has been reported in some but not all cases of myeloproliferative disease whose clinical characteristics included recurrent arterial and venous thromboses.[3]

Footnotes

1. Miale JB, *Laboratory Medicine: Hematology*, 6th ed, St Louis, MO: Mosby-Year Book Inc, 1982, 853-4.
2. Abbate R, Boddi M, Prisco D, et al, "Ability of Whole Blood Aggregometer to Detect Platelet Hyperaggregability," *Am J Clin Pathol*, 1989, 91(2):159-64.
3. Raman BKS, Van Slyck EJ, Riddle J, et al, "Platelet Function and Structure in Myeloproliferative Disease, Myelodysplastic Syndrome, and Secondary Thrombocytosis," *Am J Clin Pathol*, 1989, 91(6):647-55.

Platelet Antibody

CPT *86022*

Related Information

Platelet Antibody, Immunohematologic *on page 1080*
Platelet Count *on page 586*
Platelets, Apheresis, Donation *on page 1083*

Synonyms Serotonin Release

Specimen Plasma CONTAINER: Two blue top (sodium citrate) tubes COLLECTION: Routine venipuncture. If multiple tests are being drawn, draw coagulation test last. STORAGE INSTRUCTIONS: Separate plasma from red cells, transfer to plastic tube (12 x 75 mm) and freeze at -25°C. If the specimen is to be referred to a central laboratory (with resultant delay) for a test measuring platelet associated IgG, optimal collection is of whole blood into acid citrate dextrose, samples kept at 4°C.[1] This results in maximal yield of platelets without change in level of platelet associated IgG. A simplified test using preserved platelets has been described.[2] CAUSES FOR REJECTION: Specimen clotted, stored plasma not frozen, specimen hemolyzed SPECIAL INSTRUCTIONS: Communicate with laboratory before ordering. Platelet antibody tests are not commonly available.

Interpretive REFERENCE RANGE: Within control range that is determined with each test run USE: Detect the presence of an antibody that destroys platelets; diagnose and follow instances of immune thrombocytopenia LIMITATIONS: The serotonin release test may not reliably detect platelet antibodies in patients with idiopathic thrombocytopenia purpura[1] (ITP) METHODOLOGY: Serotonin release: Plasma from patient is mixed with a suspension of normal platelets labeled with ^{14}C-serotonin, and the amount of radioactivity (serotonin) released is measured.[2] More recently developed methods include direct and indirect antiplatelet antibody procedures utilizing fluorescein-conjugated antisera with immunofluorescence quantitated by flow cytometry;[3,4,5] direct and indirect immunoprecipitation utilizing polyacrylamide gel electrophoresis;[6] enzyme-linked immunosorbent assay (ELISA);[5] radiolabeled protein staph A assay;[7] direct chemiluminescence assay;[8] and immunoblot analysis.[9] Flow cytometry-based methods using platelets and lymphocytes can distinguish anti-HLA from platelet-specific antibodies.[10] **ADDITIONAL INFORMATION:** Determination of and significance of platelet antibodies presents an array of intriguing and complex issues. IgG is present on platelets of apparently normal nonthrombocytopenic individuals (about 4000 molecules per platelet).[1] Platelet-bound IgG is not necessarily pathogenic and might reflect immune complex binding or nonspecifically bound IgG, as well as, true antiplatelet antibody of probable more potential significance to immune platelet destruction. The many problems involved in developing an ideal test for platelet-associated IgG is reflected by the over 20 different tests available for platelet antibodies or complexes. The current status of this difficult area and its relation to the diagnosis of ITP has been the subject of informative reviews (see references). Platelet-associated autoantibodies against glycoprotein IIb/IIIa, as well as, against unidentified proteins have been reported in cases of ITP.[6] Radiolabeled allogeneic platelet kinetic (survival) studies indicate that platelet crossmatch tests, using radiolabeled protein staph A assay combined with the IgA ELISA test, provide the best indication of post-transfusion donor platelet survival.[7]

For additional information from the perspective of platelet transfusion see the listing Platelet Antibody, Immunohematologic in the Transfusion Service chapter.

Footnotes

1. Kelton JG and Gibbons S, "Autoimmune Platelet Destruction: Idiopathic Thrombocytopenic Purpura," *Semin Thromb Hemost*, 1982, 8:88-91.
2. Marmer DJ, Bowman RP, and Kennedy PS, "A Simplified (^{3}H) Serotonin Release Assay for the Detection of Platelet Antibodies," *Am J Hematol*, 1979, 6:45-50.
3. Lazarchick J and Jones T, "Antiplatelet Antibody Assay (Indirect Method)," *Manual of Procedures for the Seminar on Diagnostic Hematology*, Sunderman FW, Institute for Clinical Science, 1988, 101-8.
4. Lazarchick J and Hall S, "Platelet Associated Antibody Assay (Direct Method)," *Manual of Procedures for the Seminar on Diagnostic Hematology*, Sunderman FW, Institute for Clinical Science, 1988, 109-13.
5. Lin RY, Levin M, Nygren EN, et al, "Assessment of Platelet Antibody by Flow Cytometric and ELISA Techniques: A Comparison Study," *J Lab Clin Med*, 1990, 116:(4)479-86.
6. Tomiyama Y, Take H, Honda S, et al, "Demonstration of Platelet Antigens That Bind Platelet-Associated Autoantibodies in Chronic ITP by Direct Immunoprecipitation Procedure," *Br J Haematol*, 1990, 75(1):92-8.
7. Bensinger WI, Hadlock J, and Slichter SJ, "Identification of Alloimmunized Patients: Use of Radiolabeled Allogeneic Platelet Kinetic Measurements and Platelet Antibody Tests," *Blood*, 1991, 77(11):2372-8.
8. Kazemi A, Singh AK, and Slater NGP, "An *In Vitro* Direct Chemiluminescence Assay for Assessment of Platelet-Bound Antibody in Thrombocytopenic Patients," *Br J Haematol*, 1991, 79(4):624-7.
9. Lazarchick J, Russell R, and Horn B, "Maternal Platelet Antibody Levels in Neonatal Isoimmune Thrombocytopenia," *Ann Clin Lab Sci*, 1990, 20(3):200-4.
10. Freedman J and Hornstein A, "Simple Method for Differentiating Between HLA and Platelet-Specific Antibodies by Flow Cytometry," *Am J Hematol*, 1991, 38(4):314-20.

References

George JN, "Platelet IgG: Measurement, Interpretation, and Clinical Significance," *Prog Hemost Thromb*, 1991, 10:97-126.

Karpatkin S, "Autoimmune Thrombocytopenic Purpura," *Semin Hematol*, 1985, 22:260-88.

McMillan R, "Immune Thrombocytopenia," *Clin Lab Haematol*, 1983, 12:69-88.

Schwartz KA, "Platelet Antibody: Review of Detection Methods," *Am J Hematol*, 1988, 29:106-14.

Platelet Autoaggregation *see* Platelet Aggregation, Hypercoagulable State *on page 461*

Platelet Function Studies *see* Platelet Aggregation *on page 459*

Platelet Impedance Aggregation in Whole Blood *see* Platelet Aggregation *on page 459*

Platelet Retention *see* Platelet Adhesion Test *on page 458*

Prekallikrein Assay *see* Factor, Fletcher *on page 432*

Proaccelerin *see* Factor V *on page 421*

Proconvertin *see* Factor VII *on page 422*

Protamine Sulfate *see* Activated Coagulation Time *on page 399*

Protamine Sulfate *see* Partial Thromboplastin Time *on page 450*

Protamine Sulfate Test for Fibrin Split Products *see* Fibrin Split Products, Protamine Sulfate *on page 439*

Protein C

CPT 85302 (antigen); 85303 (activity)

Related Information

Hypercoagulable State Coagulation Screen *on page 441*
Plasminogen Activator Inhibitor *on page 455*
Protein S *on page 466*
Thrombomodulin *on page 475*

Synonyms PC; Protein C Antigen; Protein C, Functional

Applies to Protein Ca; Tissue Plasminogen Activator (t-PA)

Specimen Plasma **CONTAINER:** Blue top (sodium citrate) tube **COLLECTION:** Routine venipuncture. If multiple tests are being drawn, draw coagulation studies last. If only coagulation tests are being drawn, draw 1-2 mL into another Vacutainer® tube, discard, and then collect coagulation tests (double syringe/tube technique). This collection procedure avoids contamination of the specimen with tissue thromboplastins. **STORAGE INSTRUCTIONS:** May be stable for 1 month at -70°C. **CAUSES FOR REJECTION:** Patient receiving heparin (exception: chromogenic substrate based methods)[1] **TURNAROUND TIME:** 1 hour (automated synthetic substrate methods) **SPECIAL INSTRUCTIONS:** Determine if patient is on oral anticoagulants. Protein C (vitamin K dependent) levels may be decreased as a result of anticoagulation (as with coumarin derivatives). Snake venom activated chromogenic substrate based methods are not importantly affected by therapeutic levels of heparin.

Interpretive **REFERENCE RANGE:** 70% to 150% of normal pooled plasma, 0.60-1.13 units/mL (chromogenic assay and ELISA).[2] Quantitative antigen and activity are decreased (one-third adult normal) at birth, gradually increase but remain low during the first month of life.[3] Values are significantly decreased in children (ages 1-16 years) as compared to adults; 1-5 years of age: 0.40-0.92 units/mL; 6-10 years of age: 0.45-0.93 units/mL; 11-16 years of age: 0.55-1.11 units/mL.[2] **USE:** Investigate patients with thromboses, especially venous thromboses in young adults; study of patients with hypercoagulable state **LIMITATIONS:** Caution must be used in interpreting decreased protein C levels obtained from coumarin-anticoagulated patient samples (protein C level is decreased in patients taking Coumadin®). **METHODOLOGY:** Enzyme-linked immunosorbent assay (ELISA), radioimmunoassay (RIA), rocket immunoelectrophoresis (Laurell), particle concentration fluorescent immunoassay.[4] Functional assays include determination of activated protein C by chromogenic substrate after harvesting with immobilized antiprotein C antibody or determination of the effect of Ca on prolonging the APTT of normal plasma. Recently, automated chromogenic synthetic substrate methods suited to batch testing and screening have been developed utilizing a snake venom protein C activator derived from the Southern copperhead snake (Agkistrodon contortix).[1,5] The generation of *p*-nitroaniline measured at 405 nm is proportional to the level of protein Ca. **ADDITIONAL INFORMATION:** Protein C, a vitamin K dependent zymogen of a serine protease (activated protein C or Ca), has a molecular weight of 62,000 and neutralizes an inhibitor of tissue plasminogen activator (t-PA). It inactivates factors Va and VIIIa with prolongation of the conversion of prothrombin to thrombin by factor Xa. It thus has both profibrinolytic and anticoagulant properties. Protein C is synthesized in the liver and is activated to Ca rapidly by thrombin that has been bound by its endothelial cell receptor thrombomodulin. Protein Ca in the presence of protein S inhibits factor Va. By increasing the activity of t-PA, protein Ca enhances fibrinolysis. The protein C mechanism thus functions to prevent extension of intravascular thrombi.

Deficiency or functionally deficient forms of protein Ca are clinically, as would be expected, associated with thrombotic episodes. Griffin et al in 1981 described familial recurrent thrombophlebitis-associated with hereditary protein C deficiency.[6] Patients with partial protein C or with partial protein S deficiency (heterozygotes) may suffer venous thrombotic episodes, usually in early adult years. There may be deep vein thromboses, episodes of thrombophlebitis and/or pulmonary emboli, manifestations of an hypercoagulable state. Heterozygous protein C deficiency is an independent risk factor for the development of thrombotic episodes in some pedigrees.[7]

Homozygous protein C deficient patients have absent or near absent levels of C antigen and usually succumb in infancy with the picture of purpura fulminans neonatalis including lower extremity skin ecchymoses, anemia, fever, and shock. Heterozygous protein C deficient patients are of type I in which there is decreased C antigen or type II with normal C antigen levels but decreased functional activity. Protein C deficiency may be involved in some cases of Coumadin®-induced skin necrosis. Acquired deficiency may occur as with decreased protein C synthesis associated with liver disease. Patients may have combined deficiencies of protein C, antithrombin III, or protein S.[8]

The possible association of changes in protein C and/or protein S in patients having glomerular pathology with or without nephrosis has been studied (nephrotic patients are at risk for the development of thromboses). The mean levels of protein C, total protein S, and free protein S did not differ between patients with nephrosis and those without nephrosis. While mean free protein S levels were in the normal range for the four types of glomerular pathology studied, patients with diabetic glomerulopathy had significantly lower levels than those with membranous glomerulopathy. Hypercoagulability, however, is uncommon in patients with diabetic glomerulopathy but occurs with membranous glomerulonephritis. The presence of nephrosis, degree of proteinuria, or level of serum albumin did not correlate with changes in protein C or S.[9]

Decreased levels of protein C have been found during vaso-occlusive crises in children with sickle cell disease. With clinical improvement, protein C returned to preattack levels. In such cases, decreased levels of protein C may be due to increased consumption, as well as decreased production relating to changes in liver function.[10]

See tables, including Findings Indicative of Hypercoagulable State, in listing Hypercoagulable State Coagulation Screen.

Footnotes

1. Walker PA, Bauer KA, and McDonagh J, "A Simple, Automated Functional Assay for Protein C," *Am J Clin Pathol*, 1989, 92(2):210-3.
2. Andrew M, Vegh P, Johnston M, et al, "Maturation of the Hemostatic System During Childhood," *Blood*, 1992, 80(8):1998-2005.
3. Takamiya O, Kinoshita S, Niinomi K, et al, "Protein C in the Neonatal Period," *Haemostasis*, 1989, 19(1):45-50.
4. Miletech JP and Broze GJ, "Plasma Protein C Antigen in the Normal Population: What Is a Deficiency?" *Circulation*, 1986, 74(II):92.
5. Hales SC, "Measurement of Protein C Activity on the Multistat III Plus," *Lab Med*, 1989, 20:484-6.
6. Griffin JH, Evatt B, Zimmerman TS, et al, "Deficiency of Protein C in Congenital Thrombotic Disease," *J Clin Invest*, 1981, 68:1370-3.
7. Bovill EG, Bauer KA, Dickerman JD, et al, "The Clinical Spectrum of Heterozygous Protein C Deficiency in a Large New England Kindred," *Blood*, 1989, 73(3):712-7.
8. Bauer KA, Broekmans AW, Bertina RM, et al, "Hemostatic Enzyme Generation in the Blood of Patients With Hereditary Protein C Deficiency," *Blood*, 1988, 71(5):1418-26.
9. Allon M, Soffer O, Evatt BL, et al, "Protein S and C Antigen Levels in Proteinuric Patients: Dependence on Type of Glomerular Pathology," *Am J Hematol*, 1989, 31(2):96-101.
10. Karayalcin G and Lanzkowsky P, "Plasma Protein C Levels in Children With Sickle Cell Disease," *Am J Pediatr Hematol Oncol*, 1989, 11(3):320-3.

References

Berdeaux DH, Abshire TC, and Marlar RA, "Dysfunctional Protein C Deficiency (Type II) – A Report of 11 Cases in 3 American Families and Review of the Literature," *Am J Clin Pathol*, 1993, 99:677-86.

Brenner B, Shapira A, Bahari C, et al, "Hereditary Protein C Deficiency During Pregnancy," *Am J Obstet Gynecol*, 1987, 157:1160-1.

Civantos F, Kent J, and Pegelow CH, "Homozygous Protein C Deficiency," *ASCP Check Sample*®, Chicago, IL: American Society of Clinical Pathologists, 1987.

Clouse LH and Comp PC, "The Regulation of Hemostasis: The Protein C System," *N Engl J Med*, 1986, 314:1298-1300.

Esmon NL, "Thrombomodulin," *Prog Hemost Thromb*, 1989, 9:29-55.

Harrison RL and Alperin JB, "Concurrent Protein C Deficiency and Lupus Anticoagulants," *Am J Hematol*, 1992, 40(1):33-7.

Hill RT and Ens GE, "The Protein C Pathway," *Clin Hemost Rev*, 1987, 1:1-6, (review).

Manco-Johnson M and Nuss R, "Protein C Concentrate Prevents Peripartum Thrombosis," *Am J Hematol*, 1992, 40(1):69-70.

Marchetti G, Patracchini P, Gemmati D, et al, "Symptomatic Type II Protein C Deficiency Caused by a Missense Mutation (GLY 381 → Ser) in the Substrate-Binding Pocket," *Br J Haematol*, 1993, 84:285-9.

Melissari E and Kakkar VV, "Congenital Severe Protein C Deficiency in Adults," *Br J Haematol*, 1989, 72(2):222-8.

Rosenberg RD and Bauer KA, "New Insights Into Hypercoagulable States," *Hosp Pract*, 1986, 21:131-47.

Schofield KP, Thomson JM, and Poller L, "Protein C Response to Induction and Withdrawal of Oral Anticoagulant Treatment," *Clin Lab Haematol*, 1987, 9:255-62.

Tollefson DFJ, Friedman KD, Marlar RA, et al, "Protein C Deficiency: A Cause of Unusual or Unexplained Thrombosis," *Arch Surg*, 1988, 123:881-4.

Protein Ca *see* Protein C *on previous page*

Protein C Antigen *see* Protein C *on previous page*

Protein C, Functional *see* Protein C *on previous page*

Protein S

CPT 85305 (total); 85306 (free)

Related Information

Hypercoagulable State Coagulation Screen *on page 441*
Inhibitor, Lupus, Phospholipid Type *on page 444*
Plasminogen Activator Inhibitor *on page 455*
Protein C *on page 464*

Specimen Plasma **CONTAINER:** Blue top (sodium citrate) tube **STORAGE INSTRUCTIONS:** Sample may be stored up to 30 days at -20°C (preferably -70°C) prior to assay. **TURNAROUND TIME:** 48 hours

Interpretive **REFERENCE RANGE:** Total protein S, males: 78% to 103%; females: 70% to 122%; free protein S, males: 69% to 149%, females: 50% to 130%[1]; 0.60-1.13 units/mL using ELISA method, low end of ranges lower in children ages 1-16 (see reference by Andrew, et al). **LIMITATIONS:** There is evidence that functional deficiency of protein S may occur in patients who have demonstrable protein S antigen.[2] **METHODOLOGY:** Electroimmunodiffusion (Laurell rocket), enzyme immunoassay (EIA)[3] commercially available in kit form, (both involve measurement of antigen by immunologic means after precipitation of S complexed C4b-binding protein). Functional screening procedure has been developed. This test measures the contribution of patient's plasma to a mixture of purified protein C activated by a venom activator, protein S deficient plasma, cephalin, and $CaCl_2$. The clotting time is compared to results obtained with assayed standards using a standard curve.[4] **ADDITIONAL INFORMATION:** The activity of protein C is dependent upon a cofactor, protein S. Both protein C and protein S are vitamin K dependent coagulation proteins. Slightly over one-half of protein S is complexed with C 4b-binding protein and is inactive. The unbound fraction circulates in the plasma as the active form. Since protein S is required for the action of protein C, tendency to thrombosis would be expected (on a theoretic basis) in individuals with low levels of protein S. Recurrent thrombosis has been reported associated with congenital protein S deficiency.[5] Decrease in plasma protein S level has also been noted with use of oral contraceptives.[1] Before protein S deficiency can be excluded, both functional and antigenic levels should be studied.

Nonfamilial protein S deficiency has been reported in a 28-year old patient with inflammatory bowel disease and multiple episodes of deep vein thrombosis.[6] A possible role of congenital protein S deficiency in the development of intestinal arteriovenous malformations has been suggested.[7]

Presence of hypercoagulable state associated with decrease in free protein S levels has been reported with diabetic nephropathy, chronic renal failure due to hypertension, and antiphospholipid syndrome with cerebral venous thrombosis and coumarin-induced skin necrosis.[8,9]

See tables, including Findings Indicative of Hypercoagulable State, in listing Hypercoagulable State Coagulation Screen.

Footnotes

1. Boerger LM, Morris PC, Thurnau GR, et al, "Oral Contraceptives and Gender Affect Protein S Status," *Blood*, 1987, 69:692-4.
2. Comp PC, Doray D, Patton D, et al, "An Abnormal Plasma Distribution of Protein S Occurs in Functional Protein S Deficiency," *Blood*, 1986, 67:504-8.
3. Deutz-Terlouw P, Ballering L, van Wijngaarden A, et al, "Two ELISA's for Measurement of Protein S, and Their Use in the Laboratory Diagnosis of Protein S Deficiency," *Clin Chim Acta*, 1990, 186(3):321-34.
4. Kobayashi I, Amemiya N, Endo T, et al, "Functional Activity of Protein S Determined With Use of Protein C Activated by Venom Activator," *Clin Chem*, 1989, 35(8):1644-8.
5. Comp PC, Nixon RR, Cooper MR, et al, "Familial Protein S Deficiency Is Associated With Recurrent Thrombosis," *J Clin Invest*, 1984, 74:2082-8.
6. Wyshock E, Caldwell M, and Crowley JP, "Deep Venous Thrombosis, Inflammatory Bowel Disease, and Protein S Deficiency," *Am J Clin Pathol*, 1989, 90(5):633-5.
7. Guarner J, Grossman B, Judd R, et al, "Multiple Arteriovenous Malformations of the Small Intestine in a Patient With Protein S Deficiency," *Am J Clin Pathol*, 1989, 92(3):374-8.
8. Allon M, Soffer O, Evatt BL, et al, "Protein S and C Antigen Levels in Proteinuric Patients: Dependence on Type of Glomerular Pathology," *Am J Hematol*, 1989, 31(2):96-101.
9. Moreb J and Kitchens CS, "Acquired Functional Protein S Deficiency, Cerebral Venous Thrombosis, and Coumarin Skin Necrosis in Association With Antiphospholipid Syndrome: Report of Two Cases," *Am J Med*, 1989, 87(2):207-10.

References

Andrew M, Vegh P, Johnston M, et al, "Maturation of the Hemostatic System During Childhood," *Blood*, 1992, 80(8):1998-2005.

Graves-Hoagland RL and Walker FJ, "Laboratory Determination of Protein S," *Manual of Procedures for the Seminar on Diagnostic Hematology*, compiled by FW Sunderman, Institute for Clinical Science, Philadelphia, 1988.

Schwarz HP, Heeb MJ, Lottenberg R, et al, "Familial Protein S Deficiency With a Variant Protein S Molecule in Plasma and Platelets," *Blood*, 1989, 74(1):213-21.

Stahl CP, Wideman CS, Spira TJ, et al, "Protein S Deficiency in Men With Long-Term Human Immunodeficiency Virus Infection," *Blood*, 1993, 81(7):1801-7.

Prothrombin *see* Factor II *on page 420*

Prothrombin Fragment 1.2

CPT *85999*

Related Information

Antithrombin III Test *on page 403*
Hypercoagulable State Coagulation Screen *on page 441*
Prothrombin Time *on next page*

Synonyms F 1.2; F1+2; Prothrombin Fragment F1+2

Abstract Prothrombin fragment 1.2 is released from prothrombin during thrombin formation. Thus it is a prothrombin activation fragment. This test has clinical application as a marker of thrombin formation. F 1.2 levels may assist in study of the hypercoagulable state, assessment of thrombotic risk, and in monitoring anticoagulant therapy.

Specimen Plasma, lithium heparin anticoagulant. Some ELISA methods use plasma from 3.8% sodium citrate anticoagulated blood **STORAGE INSTRUCTIONS:** Dilute plasma 9:1 (by volume) with an EDTA-containing anticoagulant for use with heparinized plasma, assay immediately or store at -20°C (stable for at least 3 months).[1] **TURNAROUND TIME:** Currently, this test is not commonly available in most clinical environments and will be performed by a referral or reference laboratory. Some applications, however, would benefit from a rapid turnaround time.

Interpretive **REFERENCE RANGE:** 0.21-2.78 nmol/L in healthy individuals up to 44 years of age. F 1.2 levels rise slightly with age older than 44 years (ELISA, monoclonal antibody based) **USE:** Assessment of prethrombotic (hypercoagulable) state, risk of thrombosis, efficacy of anticoagulant therapy[1] **METHODOLOGY:** Enzyme-linked immunosorbent assay (ELISA), monoclonal antibody based,[1] polyclonal **ADDITIONAL INFORMATION:** With activation of prothrombin, factor Xa cleaves the bond Arg 273-Thr 274 resulting in liberation of prothrombin fragment F 1.2 and prethrombin 2. With cleavage of prethrombin, α-thrombin is formed. The latter enzyme converts fibrinogen to fibrin. Plasma F 1.2 is increased in clinical conditions in which there is increased risk of thrombosis. Such conditions have included patients with leukemia, severe liver disease, and postmyocardial infarction.[2] F 1.2 is decreased with oral anticoagulant therapy and in patients treated with antithrombin III.[1,3] Sample collection site, sex, and smoking status did not correlate significantly with the plasma concentration of F 1.2.[4] Venous occlusion for 2 minutes during sampling has not been noted to significantly alter plasma levels of F 1.2.[2]

Footnotes

1. Hursting MJ, Butman BT, Steiner JP, et al, "Monoclonal Antibodies Specific for Prothrombin Fragment 1.2 and Their Use in a Quantitative Enzyme-Linked Immunosorbent Assay," *Clin Chem*, 1993, 39(4):583-91.
2. Bruhn HD, Conard J, Mannucci M, et al, "Multicentric Evaluation of a New Assay for Prothrombin Fragment F 1+2 Determination," *Thromb Haemost*, 1992, 68(4):413-7.
3. Rodeghiero F, Castaman G, Gugliotta L, et al, "Supranormal Antithrombin III Levels Induced by Concentrate Administration Are Ineffective in Quenching Thrombin Generation in Acute Promyelocytic Leukemia," *Thromb Res*, 1993, 69:377-85.
4. Hursting MJ, Stead AG, Crout FV, et al, "Effects of Age, Race, Sex, and Smoking on Prothrombin Fragment 1.2 in a Healthy Population," *Clin Chem*, 1993, 39(4):683-6.

References

Bauer KA and Rosenberg RD, "Congenital Antithrombin III Deficiency: Insights into the Pathogenesis of the Hypercoagulable State and Its Management Using Markers of Hemostatic System Activation," *Am J Med*, 1989, 87(3B):39S-43S.

Bauer KA and Rosenberg RD, "The Pathophysiology of the Prethrombotic State in Humans: Insights Gained From Studies Using Markers of Hemostatic System Activation," *Blood*, 1987, 70(2):343-50.

Millenson MM, Bauer KA, Kistler JP, et al, "Monitoring 'Mini-Intensity' Anticoagulation With Warfarin: Comparison of the Prothrombin Time Using a Sensitive Thromboplastin With Prothrombin Fragment F 1+2 Levels," *Blood*, 1992, 79(8):2034-8.

Prothrombin Fragment F1+2 *see* Prothrombin Fragment 1.2 *on this page*

Prothrombin Time

CPT 85610

Related Information

Coagulation Factor Assay *on page 414*
Cryoprecipitate *on page 1058*
Factor II *on page 420*
Factor VII *on page 422*
Plasma, Fresh Frozen *on page 1078*
Plasma Protein Fraction (Human) *on page 1079*
Prothrombin Fragment 1.2 *on previous page*
Warfarin *on page 1011*

Synonyms Protime; PT

Applies to Coumarins; Heparin; PT Ratio

Test Commonly Includes Patient time and control time

Abstract A simple, low cost test useful for the evaluation of the extrinsic system of coagulation as it is sensitive to reduced levels of factors II, VII, and X. It is the time, in seconds, required for clot formation after addition of calcium and thromboplastin. A common application is monitoring the effect of warfarin type anticoagulation.

Specimen Plasma **CONTAINER:** Blue top (sodium citrate) tube **COLLECTION:** Routine venipuncture. If multiple tests are being drawn, draw coagulation studies last. If only a prothrombin time is being drawn, two-syringe collection technique is recommended to avoid contamination of the specimen with tissue thromboplastins. **STORAGE INSTRUCTIONS:** Plasma should be separated from cells as soon as possible and refrigerated if testing cannot be immediately performed. Testing should be performed within 4 hours. **CAUSES FOR REJECTION:** Tube not full; specimen clotted; specimen hemolyzed, lipemic, or icteric (possible interference with photo-optical clot detection); specimen received more than 3-4 hours after collection **SPECIAL INSTRUCTIONS:** Transport specimen to the hematology laboratory as soon as possible.

Interpretive **REFERENCE RANGE:** 10-13 seconds. Healthy premature newborns have prolonged coagulation test screening results (eg, PT, APTT, TT) which return to normal adult values at about 6 months of age. Healthy prematures, however, do not develop spontaneous hemorrhage or thrombotic complications because of a balance between procoagulants and inhibitors (see reference by Andrew et al). See table. The normal range in childhood (ages 1-16) is similar to that in adults.[1] **POSSIBLE PANIC RANGE:** Nonanticoagulated: >20 seconds; anticoagulated: more than three times control **USE:** Evaluate extrinsic coagulation system; aid in screening for congenital deficiencies of factors II, V, VII, X; deficiency of prothrombin; dysfibrinogenemia, afibrinogenemia (complete); heparin effect, coumarin or warfarin effect; liver failure; disseminated intravascular coagulation (DIC); and screen for vitamin K deficiency **LIMITATIONS:** Prothrombin times drawn less than 2 hours after heparin administration will be prolonged. The number of drugs which modify the hypoprothrombinemic action of the coumarins is remarkable.[2] Salicylates, phenylbutazone and clofibrate are mentioned by the St Paul Malpractice Digest.[3] Other references include barbiturates, chloral hydrate, chloramphenicol, ethchlorvynol, glutethimide, phenyramidol, quinidine, allopurinol, anabolic steroids, MAO-inhibitors, nortriptyline, phenytoin, propylthiouracil, antacids, sulfonamides, carbamazepine, estrogenic contraceptives, and griseofulvin.[2] Drugs lowering the PT include ethchlorvynol, glutethimide, anabolic steroids, antacids, estrogenic contraceptives, and griseofulvin. Nafcillin has been associated with warfarin resistance.[4] **METHODOLOGY:** The clotting time of citrate anticoagulated plasma is determined after the addition of an optimum concentration of calcium and an excess of thromboplastin. Clot detection is by manual (tilt tube visual) or, more commonly by an automated device for fibrin clot detection, electrode, electro-optical or other method. The result is always reported with that obtained on a commercial normal control plasma run at the same time. Coumatrak Protime Monitor® is a capillary whole blood (25 μL) method suitable for bedside testing.[5] A laser photometer detects cessation of flow by sensing change in light scatter from red blood cells. Time elapsed is converted to a plasma equivalent PT. Attempts in recent years to standardize prothrombin time results has led to growing interest in reporting of the "international normalized ratio" (INR).[6,7] See comments under Additional Information concerning INR and International Sensitivity Index (ISI). Chromogenic assays for determination of prothrombin have been developed. If the PT is prolonged repeat testing using half patient and half normal control plasma will identify presence of a circulating anticoagulant (prolonged PT will not correct). Further testing with aged serum (source of VII and X) and adsorbed plasma (source of V) may define the nature of the abnormality (see reference by Sirridge). **ADDITIONAL INFORMATION:** The prothrombin time determination is sensitive to the

Effect of Drugs on Anticoagulation and Monitoring Using the Prothrombin Time

Drug	PT	Increase in Coumarin*
Anabolic steroids	↑	
Antacids	↓	R
Barbiturates	↓	R
Carbamazepine	↓	R
Cephalosporins, 2nd, 3rd generation	↑	S
Cefamandole, 2nd, 3rd generation	↑	S
Chloral hydrate		None
Chloramphenicol		S
Cholestyramine	↓	R
Cimetidine (rarely)	↑	S
Clofibrate	↑	S
Corticosteroids		R
Disulfiram	↑	S
Erythromycin	↑	S
Estrogen contraceptives	↓	R
Ethchlorvynol	↓	R
Fluconazole	↑	
Glucagon		S
Glutethimide	↓	R
Griseofulvin	↓	R
Ibuprofen	↑	S
Ketoconazole	↑	
Meprobamate		R
Metronidazole	↑	S
Miconazole		S
Nafcillin	↓	R
Nonsteroidal AID, many		S
Oral hypoglycemic agents		S
Phenylbutazone	↑	S
Phenytoin sodium	↑	S
Primidone	↓	R
Rifampin	↓	R
Salicylates (aspirin)		S
Sulfamethoxazole trimethoprim		S
Sulfinpyrazone	↑	S
Tamoxifen	↑	
Tolbutamide		S
Tolmetin	↑	S
Vitamin E (large amount)	↑	S

*R = resistance, S = sensitivity.

(Continued)

Prothrombin Time *(Continued)*

ratio of plasma to citrate anticoagulant. That is, if enough blood is not added to the liquid citrate-containing tube when the specimen is drawn (tube usually contains 0.5 mL of 3.2% or 3.8% sodium citrate), a falsely elevated prothrombin time may result. The minimum amount of blood in the tube necessary to a reliable PT is therefore not readily predictable. **The citrate tube for PT/PTT must be completely filled.** An excellent discussion of important technical considerations in performance of the prothrombin time is given in the text by Sirridge and Shannon (reference following).

Antibiotic therapy and prolonged prothrombin time: Biochemical mechanisms have been defined that support results of clinical studies indicating that broad-spectrum antibiotics, in particular second- and third-generation cephalosporins exert an hypoprothrombinemic effect.[8,9] Destruction of menaquinone-producing GI bacteria and/or interference with prothrombin synthesis by N-methyl-thio-tetrazole side chains has resulted in recommendations that prophylactic vitamin K administration be considered.[10,11] A study controlled for condition and treatment variables by univariate and multivariate statistical analyses revealed, after multiple logistic regression analyses, increased risk of bleeding with the β-lactam antibiotics, moxalactam and possibly cefoxitin.[12]

Control of coumarin derivative therapy: Long-term anticoagulant therapy usually involves the use of a coumarin derivative (eg, Coumadin®). The prothrombin time (PT) provides for "control" of the dosage. The attempt is to impede thrombus formation without the threat of morbidity or mortality from hemorrhage. In the past this goal has been approached by administering a Coumadin® dosage that prolongs the PT to twice that of a normal control plasma. More recently it is considered that doses of warfarin derivatives (Coumadin®, dicumarol, Tromexan®) that result in prothrombin times of 1.25 times the control value (using rabbit brain thromboplastin) provide effective prophylaxis against thrombosis without excessive risk of hemorrhage.[13] Warfarin anticoagulant effect occurs gradually. Without a loading dose, 7.5 mg/day of warfarin anticoagulant will produce desired therapeutic effect in 5-7 days. With a loading dose of 10-15 mg the anticoagulant effect can be achieved in some 3 days but with greater risk of bleeding. When warfarin compounds are discontinued the PT will require 2-4 days to return to normal. If oral vitamin K is given PT returns to normal within about 24 hours. The over-anticoagulated state can be quickly reversed by giving vitamin K intramuscularly.

A joint committee of American College of Chest Physicians and National Heart, Lung, and Blood Institute (ACCP/NHLBI) has concluded that in North America patients may be unnecessarily at least slightly overanticoagulated when the use of warfarin preparations are monitored with rabbit brain reagent (as compared with human brain derived thromboplastins formerly used in the United Kingdom).[6] The ACCP/NHLBI task force recommends less intense oral anticoagulation with a PT ratio of 1.3 to 1.5 (prothrombin time of 15-18 seconds) when commercial rabbit brain thromboplastin is used for monitoring (exception – for patients with mechanical valves and/or with recurrent systemic embolism, PT ratio of 1.5 to 2.0 is recommended).

Two-step warfarin therapy has been found to decrease the incidence of postoperative deep vein thrombosis.[14]

Warfarin therapy can be started soon after the onset of heparin therapy in patients with venous thromboembolic disease with resultant savings in hospitalization costs.[15] A 1-year course of warfarin therapy may be needed for patients with prior deep vein thrombosis and indefinite treatment if there have been over two previous episodes.[16]

The characteristics of thromboplastins including results of human brain vs rabbit brain thromboplastin and the ISI (International Sensitivity Index) have been studied.[17] Consistency in the practice of warfarin type (coumarin) anticoagulation relating to its control by use of prothrombin time results has been elusive. This is due to variability in the sensitivity of thromboplastins. Historically, thromboplastins prepared locally by hospital laboratories and the human brain thromboplastin Manchester Comparative Reagent used as a reference plasma in the United Kingdom (UK) were more sensitive than rabbit brain or mixed commercial thromboplastin reagents introduced subsequently in North America.[18] Continued adherence to a 1948 American Heart Association recommendation that the therapeutic ranges for oral anticoagulation be kept at 2.0-2.5 that of a control PT (prothrombin time ratio of 2.0-2.5) led to a higher degree of anticoagulation. There was resultant increase in morbidity/mortality from bleeding. Nonhuman (largely rabbit) thromboplastins have also come into routine use throughout the UK (with advice to use the International Normalized Ratio) since withdrawal of Manchester Comparative Reagent in 1986.[19]

The variability in sensitivity of thromboplastins with resultant lack of between laboratory comparability in results of PT testing provided stimulus for standardization. In 1983, the International Normalized Ratio (INR) system was adopted by the International Committee for Standardization in Haematology, International Committee on Thrombosis and Haemostasis (ISCH/ICTH).[20] This system is based on the first World Health Organization (WHO) primary international reference preparation of thromboplastin. It has been considered to be an accepted international standard for clinical use.[18] The system is centered about the concept of an International Sensitivity Index (ISI). The ISI represents the responsiveness of a thromboplastin to the reduction in vitamin K-dependent factors. The ISI is derived by calibrating a thromboplastin reagent with a reference preparation. Use is made of a linear relation between the logarithm of the prothrombin time ratio of the reference material and that of the test thromboplastin. The goal of standardized reporting of the prothrombin time would be met with a reliable ISI in hand (provided by the manufacturer of the reagent thromboplastin) allowing conversion of the prothrombin time ratio measured with that reagent thromboplastin into an INR according to the formula: $INR = (PT\ ratio)^{ISI} = (patient\ PT/mean\ normal\ PT)^{ISI}$ where ISI is the International Sensitivity Index. Recent generation coagulation instruments, when provided with the ISI value, will calculate and report the INR value. Theoretically, the INR is the PT ratio that would result if the WHO reférence thromboplastin had been used in performing the test.

Acceptance (use) of the INR system by the North American medical community has been slow, leading to criticism and impassioned pleas for education and compliance.[18,21,22,23] Reliability of the INR system, however, which depends upon a valid ISI has recently come into question.[24,25,26,27,28,29] Ng et al could not obtain consistent reagent-independent INR values within three related laboratories and note reports that some automated coagulation analyzers produce inconsistent INR values.[24] They suggest that "further evaluation is necessary before universal implementation of the INR can be recommended". Swaim emphasizes the importance of ensuring that "ISI assignments permit accurate "normalization" of PT ratios". He has provided nine general recommendations to improve the INR system.[25] These include use of a single master International Reference Plasma, instrument-specific ISIs, commercial ISI assignments appropriate to specific instrument-thromboplastin combinations, ISI assignments based on three or more ISI determinations, and use of reagents with low ISI values. Recombinant human tissue factor, reputedly with very low ISI of 1.0 ± 0.1, has been developed. Commercial availability and use of such a thromboplastin reagent may allow for accurate and uniform reporting of PT results as an INR.

A statistical analysis program using Bayesian regression has been applied to the problem of early prediction of warfarin response. Study of this program has led to the conclusion that use of Bayesian regression analysis cannot be based exclusively on PT data from only the first 1-3 days of therapy.[30]

The prothrombin time has been shown to lack sensitivity (in its current form) as a monitor for the anticoagulant effect of recombinant hirudin (originally an anticoagulant from the medicinal leech *Hirudo medicinalis*).[31] See Hirudin Determination listing.

A study involving warfarin-derivative anticoagulated outpatients (562) found a 2% incidence of fatal bleeding, a 10% incidence of nonfatal major bleeding and a 12% incidence of minor bleeding. Important remedial lesions were present in 38% of cases with major bleeding. These lesions were unknown prior to bleeding, however, and represent a diagnostic yield from investigation of patients who bleed.[32,33]

A study of appropriateness of PT and APTT testing in a hospital setting (ordering patterns in relation to clinical indications) concludes that these tests are overutilized (at least 70% were not clinically indicated).[34]

Footnotes

1. Andrew M, Vegh P, Johnston M, et al, "Maturation of the Hemostatic System During Childhood," *Blood*, 1992, 80(8):1998-2005.
2. Bick RL, *Disorders of Thrombosis and Hemostasis: Clinical and Laboratory Practice*, Chicago, IL: ASCP Press, 1992, 297.
3. *Malpractice Digest*, St Paul Fire & Marine Insurance Co, July/Aug 1979, 3.
4. Fraser GL, Miller M, and Kane K, "Warfarin Resistance Associated With Nafcillin Therapy," *Am J Med*, 1989, 87(2):237-8.
5. Ansell JE, Hamke AK, Holden A, et al, "Cost-Effectiveness of Monitoring Warfarin Therapy Using Standard Versus Capillary Prothrombin Times," *Am J Clin Pathol*, 1989, 91(5):587-9.
6. Hirsh J, "Is the Dose of Warfarin Prescribed by American Physicians Unnecessarily High?" *Arch Intern Med*, 1987, 147:769-71.
7. Poller L, "A Simple Nomogram for the Derivation of International Normalized Ratios for the Standardization of Prothrombin Times," *Thromb Haemost*, 1988, 60:18-20.

(Continued)

Prothrombin Time *(Continued)*

8. Fainstein V, Bodey GP, McCredie KB, et al, "Coagulation Abnormalities Induced by Beta-Lactam Antibiotics in Cancer Patients," *J Infect Dis*, 1983, 148:745-50.
9. Bertino JS, Kozak AJ, Reese RE, et al, "Hypoprothrombinemia Associated With Cefamandole Use in a Rural Teaching Hospital," *Arch Intern Med*, 1986, 146:1125-8.
10. Lipsky JJ, "N-methyl-thio-tetrazole Inhibition of the Gamma Carboxylation of Glutamic Acid: Possible Mechanism for Antibiotic-Associated Hypoprothrombinemia," *Lancet*, 1983, 2:192-3.
11. Bechtold H, Andrassy K, Jahnchen E, et al, "Evidence for Impaired Hepatic Vitamin K_1 Metabolism in Patients Treated With N-methyl-thio-tetrazole Cephalosporin," *Thromb Haemost*, 1984, 51:358-61.
12. Brown RB, Klar J, Lemeshow S, et al, "Enhanced Bleeding With Cefoxitin or Moxalactam," *Arch Intern Med*, 1986, 146:2159-64.
13. Mohr DN, Ryu JH, Litin SC, et al, "Recent Advances in the Management of Venous Thromboembolism," *Mayo Clin Proc*, 1988, 63(3):281-90.
14. Francis CW, Marder VJ, Evarts M, et al, "Two-Step Warfarin Therapy: Prevention of Postoperative Venous Thrombosis Without Excessive Bleeding," *JAMA*, 1983, 249:374-8.
15. Rosiello RA, Chan CK, Tencza F, et al, "Timing of Oral Anticoagulation Therapy in the Treatment of Angiographically Proven Acute Pulmonary Embolism," *Arch Intern Med*, 1987, 147:1469-73.
16. Hirsh J and Hull RD, "Treatment of Venous Thromboembolism," *Chest*, 1986, 89(Suppl):4265-335.
17. Denson KW, "Thromboplastin – Sensitivity, Precision, and Other Characteristics," *Clin Lab Haematol*, 1988, 10:315-28.
18. Hirsh J, "Oral Anticoagulant Drugs," *N Engl J Med*, 1991, 324(26):1865-75.
19. Poller L, Taberner DA, Thomson JM, et al, "Survey of Prothrombin Time in National External Quality Assessment Scheme Exercises (1980-87)," *J Clin Pathol*, 1988, 41(4):361-4.
20. International Committee Communications, International Committee for Standardization in Haematology, International Committee on Thrombosis and Haemostasis, "ICSH/ICTH Recommendations for Reporting Prothrombin Time in Oral Anticoagulant Control," *Thromb Haemost*, 1985, 53:155-6.
21. Bussey HI, Force RW, Bianco TM, et al, "Reliance on Prothrombin Time Ratios Causes Significant Errors in Anticoagulation Therapy," *Arch Intern Med*, 1992, 152(2):278-82.
22. Hirsh J, "Substandard Monitoring of Warfarin in North America: Time for Change," *Arch Intern Med*, 1992, 152(2):257-8.
23. Ansell JE, "Imprecision of Prothrombin Time Monitoring of Oral Anticoagulation: A Survey of Hospital Laboratories," *Am J Clin Pathol*, 1992, 98(2):237-9.
24. Ng VL, Levin J, Corash L, et al, "Failure of the International Normalized Ratio to Generate Consistent Results Within a Local Medical Community," *Am J Clin Pathol*, 1993, 99:689-94.
25. Swain WR, "Prothrombin Time Reporting and the International Normalized Ratio System: Improvements Are Needed," *Am J Clin Pathol*, 1993, 99:653-5.
26. Poller L, Thomson JM, and Taberner DA, "Effect of Automation on Prothrombin Time Test in NEQAS Surveys," *J Clin Pathol*, 1989, 42(10):97-100.
27. Taberner DA, Poller L, Thomson JM, et al, "Effect of International Sensitivity Index (ISI) of Thromboplastins on Precision of International Normalised Ratios (INR)," *J Clin Pathol*, 1989, 42(10):92-6.
28. Poller L, Taberner DA, Thomson JM, et al, "Effect of the Choice of WHO International Reference Preparation for Thromboplastin on International Normalised Ratios," *J Clin Pathol*, 1993, 46(1):64-6.
29. Hirsh J, "Inadequate Monitoring of Warfarin Dosage," *Blood*, 1992, 80(2):562-3.
30. Boyle DA, Ludden TM, Carter BL, et al, "Evaluation of a Bayesian Regression Program for Predicting Warfarin Response," *Ther Drug Monit*, 1989, 11(3):276-84.
31. Walenga JM, Pifarre R, Hoppensteadt DA, et al, "Development of Recombinant Hirudin as a Therapeutic Anticoagulant and Antithrombotic Agent: Some Objective Considerations," *Semin Thromb Hemost*, 1989, 15(3):316-33.
32. Landefeld CS and Goldman L, "Major Bleeding in Outpatients Treated With Warfarin: Incidence and Prediction by Factors Known at the Start of Outpatient Therapy," *Am J Med*, 1989, 87(2):144-52.
33. Landefeld CS, Rosenblatt MW, and Goldman L, "Bleeding in Outpatients Treated With Warfarin: Relation to the Prothrombin Time and Important Remedial Lesions," *Am J Med*, 1989, 87(2):153-9.
34. Erban SB, Kinman JL, and Schwartz JS, "Routine Use of the Prothrombin and Partial Thromboplastin Times," *JAMA*, 1989, 262(17):2428-32.

References

Andrew M, Paes B, Milner R, et al, "Development of the Human Coagulation System in the Healthy Premature Infant," *Blood*, 1988, 72:1651-7.

D'Angelo A, Seveso MP, D'Angelo SV, et al, "Comparison of Two Automated Coagulometers and the Manual Tilt Tube Method for the Determination of Prothrombin Time," *Am J Clin Pathol*, 1989, 92(3):321-8.

James AH, Britt RP, Raskino CL, et al, "Factors Affecting the Maintenance Dose of Warfarin," *J Clin Pathol*, 1992, 45:704-6.

Millenson MM, Bauer KA, Kistler JP, et al, "Monitoring 'Mini-Intensity' Anticoagulation With Warfarin: Comparison of the Prothrombin Time Using a Sensitive Thromboplastin With Prothrombin Fragment F_{1+2} Levels," *Blood*, 1992, 79(8):2034-8.

Peterson CE and Kwaan HC, "Current Concepts of Warfarin Therapy," *Arch Intern Med*, 1986, 146:581-4.

Poller L and Hirsh J, "Special Report: A Simple System for the Derivation of International Normalized Ratios for the Reporting of Prothrombin Time Results With North American Thromboplastin Reagents," *Am J Clin Pathol*, 1989, 92(1):124-6.

Sirridge MS and Shannon R, *Laboratory Evaluation of Hemostasis and Thrombosis*, 3rd ed, Philadelphia, PA: Lea & Febiger, 1983, 151-5.
van den Besselaar AMHP, van Mansfeld H, and van der Meer FJM, "International Normalized Ratio (INR) for Monitoring Oral Anticoagulant Treatment," *ASCP Check Sample®*, Chicago, IL: American Society of Clinical Pathologists, 1987.

Protime *see* Prothrombin Time *on page 468*

PT *see* Prothrombin Time *on page 468*

PTA *see* Factor XI *on page 429*

3P Test *see* Fibrin Split Products, Protamine Sulfate *on page 439*

PT Ratio *see* Prothrombin Time *on page 468*

PTT *see* Partial Thromboplastin Time *on page 450*

PTT Substitution *see* Activated Partial Thromboplastin Substitution Test *on page 401*

Quantitative Fibrinogen *see* Fibrinogen *on page 435*

Reptilase®-R Time

CPT 85635

Related Information

Thrombin Time *on next page*

Abstract A clotting time procedure similar to the thrombin time but clotting is produced by action of the snake venom enzyme, Reptilase®.

Specimen Plasma **CONTAINER:** Plastic (preferred) coagulation tube with sodium citrate liquid anticoagulant. Invert tube gently 5-10 times to mix and prevent clotting. **COLLECTION:** By venipuncture only. Avoid contamination of specimen with tissue thromboplastin. Deliver immediately to the laboratory. **CAUSES FOR REJECTION:** Specimen clotted, hemolyzed, received in laboratory more than 2 hours after collection **TURNAROUND TIME:** Approximately 45 minutes

Interpretive **REFERENCE RANGE:** 18-22 seconds **USE:** Aids in distinguishing hypofibrinogenemias from heparin contamination and from effects of fibrin degradation products **METHODOLOGY:** A plasma clotting time is determined using Reptilase®-R reagent to activate and transform fibrinogen **ADDITIONAL INFORMATION:** Reptilase®-R has an action similar to that of thrombin, it clots fibrinogen. It is isolated from *Bothrops atrox* snake venom. It differs from thrombin's action on fibrinogen by releasing only fibrinopeptide A (thrombin hydrolyzes both fibrinopeptide A and B from fibrinogen). Reptilase®-R time is not inhibited by heparin and can be substituted for the thrombin time in fibrinogen evaluation in heparinized patients. In cases of afibrinogenemia and some cases of dysfibrinogenemia both the thrombin time and the Reptilase®-R time will be prolonged. In evaluation of a patient with hypercoagulability normal thrombin time or Reptilase® time essentially excludes presence of an abnormal fibrinogen.[1] Reptilase® time is infinitely prolonged in cases of congenital afibrinogenemia and cases of dysfibrinogenemias with the exception of fibrinogen Oklahoma and fibrinogen Oslow. If heparin effect is the only cause of a prolonged prothrombin time, the Reptilase®-R time will be normal.

Footnotes

1. Mammen EF and Fujii Y, "Hypercoagulable States," *Lab Med*, 1989, 20:611-2.

References

Wyrick-Glatzel J and Gwaltney-Krause S, "Laboratory Methods in Hematology and Hemostasis," *Clinical Hematology and Fundamentals of Hemostasis*, 1987, Chapter 31, Pittiglio DH and Sacher RA, eds, Philadelphia, PA: FA Davis Co, 1987, 462.

Ristocetin Cofactor *see* von Willebrand Factor Assay *on page 478*

Rumpel-Leede Test *see* Capillary Fragility Test *on page 412*

Rumpel-Leede Tourniquet Test *see* Capillary Fragility Test *on page 412*

Salzman Column Test *see* Platelet Adhesion Test *on page 458*

Screen for Disseminated Intravascular Coagulation *see* Intravascular Coagulation Screen *on page 446*

Screen for Hypercoagulation *see* Hypercoagulable State Coagulation Screen *on page 441*

Sedimentation Rate *see* Fibrinogen *on page 435*

Serine Protease Inhibitor *see* Antithrombin III Test *on page 403*

Serotonin Release *see* Platelet Antibody *on page 462*

Spectrolyse™/pL Procedure *see* Plasminogen Activator Inhibitor *on page 455*

Stable Factor *see* Factor VII *on page 422*

Staphylococcal Clumping Test *see* Fibrin Breakdown Products *on page 433*

Stuart Factor *see* Factor X *on page 427*

Stuart-Prower Factor *see* Factor X *on page 427*

Surgicutt® *see* Bleeding Time, Mielke *on page 411*

βTG *see* Beta-Thromboglobulin *on page 407*

β-TG *see* Beta-Thromboglobulin *on page 407*

Thrombin Clotting Time Heparin Assay *see* Partial Thromboplastin Time *on page 450*

Thrombin-Fibrindex *see* Thrombin Time *on this page*

Thrombin Time

CPT 85999

Related Information

Cryoprecipitate *on page 1058*
Fibrinogen *on page 435*
Hirudin Determination *on page 440*
Intravascular Coagulation Screen *on page 446*
Partial Thromboplastin Time *on page 450*
Reptilase®-R Time *on previous page*

Synonyms Fibrin Time; Fibrindex™; Fibrinogen Screen; Thrombin-Fibrindex

Applies to Heparin

Test Commonly Includes Patient time and control time

Specimen Plasma **CONTAINER:** Blue top (sodium citrate) tube **COLLECTION:** Routine venipuncture as for coagulation studies. If multiple tests are being drawn, draw coagulation studies last. If only a thrombin time is being drawn, draw 1-2 mL into another Vacutainer® or syringe (two-syringe technique), discard, and then collect the thrombin time. This collection procedure avoids contamination of the specimen with tissue thromboplastins. **STORAGE INSTRUCTIONS:** Keep refrigerated. Freeze plasma if test is not to be performed promptly. **CAUSES FOR REJECTION:** Tube not full, specimen clotted, hemolyzed specimen, specimen received more than 2 hours after collection **SPECIAL INSTRUCTIONS:** Transport the specimen to the hematology laboratory as soon as possible.

Interpretive **REFERENCE RANGE:** Less than $1\frac{1}{2}$ times control value **USE:** Determination of severe hypofibrinogenemia, dysfibrinogenemia, and presence of heparin-like anticoagulants; useful in diagnosis and monitoring of disseminated intravascular coagulation (DIC) and fibrinolysis; useful in monitoring fibrinolytic therapy.[1] The thrombin time test can be used to monitor therapy with heparin. See Limitations. **LIMITATIONS:** Affected by concentration and reactivity of fibrinogen, increased amounts of fibrin degradation products (FDP), and the presence of inhibitory substances, such as heparin and large amounts of fibrin degradation products. Use of this test to monitor heparin will be unreliable if hypofibrinogenemia is present or if fibrin breakdown products (FBP) have been generated by a process of DIC. See also previous test listing, Reptilase®-R Time. **CONTRAINDICATIONS:** Patient on heparin therapy **METHODOLOGY:** Clotting time is measured after exogenous thrombin is added. Reliable results and use depends upon the addition of a standard concentration of thrombin to test and control plasmas. Concentration of thrombin in commercial preparations varies. The amount of calcium chloride added in the test environment should be adjusted to give a "normal" plasma clotting time of 8-9 seconds. Loss of sensitivity (with resultant inability to detect some clinical abnormalities) will occur if the thrombin time control has risen into the 11-14 second range. **ADDITIONAL INFORMATION:** Thrombin time is a screening test for presence of sufficient amount of functional (clottable) fibrinogen. The thrombin time is often included as part of a panel of tests for detection and evaluation of DIC. Fibrinogen/FBP act as powerful antithrombins, prolong the thrombin time, and thereby indicate presence of DIC. If the thrombin time is prolonged, additional information can be obtained by repeating the analysis on a 1:1 mixture of patient's plasma and normal (control) plasma. If the clotting time of such a 1:1 mix approximates that of the control plasma, hypofibrinogenemia or a defective molecular form of fibrinogen (dysfibrinogenemia) may be present. If the clotting time after mixing does not correct (is closer to the patient's originally prolonged thrombin time) presence of a thrombin inhibitor in the patient's plasma is likely (eg, heparin, FBP). The thrombin time is nearly always prolonged with dysfibrinogenemia.[2]

See tables, including Findings Indicative of Hypercoagulable State in listing Hypercoagulable State Coagulation Screen, and the table, Findings Indicative of DIC in the listing, Intravascular Coagulation Screen.

Footnotes

1. Bick RL, "Thrombolytic Therapy," *Disorders of Thrombosis and Hemostasis*, Chapter 15, Chicago, IL: ASCP Press, 1992, 322.
2. Mammen EF and Fujii Y, "Hypercoagulable States," *Lab Med*, 1989, 20:611-2.

References

Brozović M, "Investigation of Acute Haemostatic Failure," *Practical Haematology*, Chapter 18, Dacie JV and Lewis SM, eds, New York, NY: Churchill Livingstone, 1991, 284.

Sirridge MS and Shannon R, *Laboratory Evaluation of Hemostasis and Thrombosis*, 3rd ed, Philadelphia, PA: Lea & Febiger, 1983, 161-3.

β-Thromboglobulin *see* Beta-Thromboglobulin *on page 407*

Thrombomodulin

***CPT** 85337*

Related Information

Hypercoagulable State Coagulation Screen *on page 441*
Protein C *on page 464*

Synonyms Endothelial Cofactor; TM

Abstract Thrombomodulin (TM) is the endothelial cell thrombin receptor. The thrombin-thrombomodulin complex activates protein C. TM is thus an anticoagulant protein cofactor modulating the specificity of thrombin for its receptor and activating the central enzyme (protein C) of a major anticoagulant pathway resulting in the inactivation of factors Va and VIIIa. Soluble TM is increased in the sera of patients with systemic lupus erythematosus (SLE), disseminating cancer, and a variety of conditions in which there is endothelial cell injury.

Specimen Plasma **CONTAINER:** Citrated blood drawn into siliconized tubes **STORAGE INSTRUCTIONS:** Centrifuge at 2000 g at 4°C for 20 minutes. May store plasma at -70°C. **SPECIAL INSTRUCTIONS:** This test will likely be available only from reference or research laboratories.

Interpretive **REFERENCE RANGE:** 44 ± 10.5 ng/mL[1] **USE:** TM fragments measured in plasma likely reflect endothelial cell injury occurring in diverse conditions including systemic lupus erythematosus,[2] cancer, in particular, disseminated forms,[1] disseminated intravascular coagulation (DIC),[3,4] pulmonary thromboembolism, adult respiratory distress syndrome, renal failure including diabetic nephropathy, acute hepatic failure,[4] and thrombotic thrombocytopenic purpura (TTP).[5] Plasma TM levels may have value in assessing prognosis in DIC and TTP.[5] **LIMITATIONS:** Results using tests based on different monoclonal antibodies may vary, dependent upon sensitivity of reagent antibody to fragments of TM.[5] **METHODOLOGY:** Enzyme-linked immunosorbent assay (ELISA), procedure and reagents available commercially **ADDITIONAL INFORMATION:** Thrombomodulin (TM) is an endothelial cell receptor with high affinity for thrombin. It exerts anticoagulant influence acting as a cofactor for thrombin-catalyzed activation of protein C. The latter is an important anticoagulant protease zymogen. TM is a single chain glycoprotein. It has six consecutive epidermal growth factor-like structural domains in an extracellular position. Monoclonal ELISA analytic systems have recently been developed.[1,2,4] Plasma thrombomodulin fragments reflect endothelial cell injury. They are reportedly increased in a variety of conditions with microvascular injury including SLE, DIC, acute hepatic failure, acute respiratory distress syndrome, and renal dysfunction.[1] A study of plasma TM levels in cancer patients found significant increase with the development of disseminated disease.[1] Marked variation in individual plasma TM levels were noted. Patients with colorectal cancer had normal levels at the time of diagnosis while some patients with pancreatic cancer had initial elevation of plasma TM.

(Continued)

Thrombomodulin *(Continued)*

Footnotes

1. Lindahl AK, Boffa MC, and Abildgaard U, "Increased Plasma Thrombomodulin in Cancer Patients," *Thromb Haemost*, 1993, 69(2):112-4.
2. Kodama S, Uchijima E, Nagai M, et al, "One-Step Sandwich Enzyme Immunoassay for Soluble Human Thrombomodulin Using Monoclonal Antibodies," *Clin Chim Acta*, 1990, 192(3):191-9.
3. Asakura H, Jokaji H, Saito M, et al, "Plasma Levels of Soluble Thrombomodulin Increase in Cases of Disseminated Intravascular Coagulation With Organ Failure," *Am J Hematol*, 1991, 38(4):281-7.
4. Takano S, Kimura S, Ohdama S, et al, "Plasma Thrombomodulin in Health and Diseases," *Blood*, 1990, 76(10):2024-9.
5. Wada H, Ohiwa M, Kaneko T, et al, "Plasma Thrombomodulin as a Marker of Vascular Disorders in Thrombotic Thrombocytopenic Purpura and Disseminated Intravascular Coagulation," *Am J Hematol*, 1992, 39(1):20-4.

References

Esmon NL, "Thrombomodulin," *Prog Hemost Thromb*, 1989, 9:29-55.

Sadler JE, Lentz SR, Sheehan JP, et al, "Structure-Function Relationships of the Thrombin-Thrombomodulin Interaction," *Haemostasis*, 1993, 23(Suppl 1):183-93.

Thrombotic Disease Screen *see* Hypercoagulable State Coagulation Screen *on page 441*

Thrombo-Wellcotest® for Fibrin Split Products *see* Fibrin Breakdown Products *on page 433*

Tissue Plasminogen Activator (t-PA) *see* Protein C *on page 464*

TM *see* Thrombomodulin *on previous page*

Tolerance Test for Aspirin *see* Aspirin Tolerance Test *on page 406*

Tourniquet Test *see* Capillary Fragility Test *on page 412*

Triple P Test *see* Fibrin Split Products, Protamine Sulfate *on page 439*

VIIIC:Ag *see* Factor VIII *on page 424*

VIIIR Antigen *see* von Willebrand Factor Antigen *on this page*

von Willebrand Factor Antigen

CPT 85246

Related Information

Aspirin Tolerance Test *on page 406*
Bleeding Time, Ivy *on page 409*
Cryoprecipitate *on page 1058*
Factor VIII *on page 424*
von Willebrand Factor Assay *on page 478*
von Willebrand Factor Multimer Assay *on page 478*

Synonyms Factor VIIIR:Ag; Factor VIII-Related Antigen; VIIIR Antigen

Specimen Plasma **CONTAINER:** Two blue top (sodium citrate) tubes **COLLECTION:** Routine venipuncture. If multiple tests are being drawn, draw coagulation studies last. If only a factor VIIIR antigen is being drawn, draw 1-2 mL into another Vacutainer®, discard, and then collect the factor VIIIR antigen. This collection procedure avoids contamination of the specimen with tissue thromboplastins. **STORAGE INSTRUCTIONS:** Keep refrigerated **CAUSES FOR REJECTION:** Specimen hemolyzed, specimen received more than 2 hours after collection, stored specimen not refrigerated **SPECIAL INSTRUCTIONS:** Transport the specimen to the laboratory as soon as possible. Usually not available as a routine test.

Interpretive **REFERENCE RANGE:** In classical hemophilia, factor VIII antigen levels are very low or undetectable; in von Willebrand's disease, the levels are normal or increased, however, in some type II variant cases levels of VIIIR:Ag may be normal. **USE:** A coagulation parameter useful in the differential diagnosis of hemophilia A and von Willebrand's disease (von Willebrand's syndrome) **LIMITATIONS:** Interpretation of results may be limited if specimen is received more than 2 hours after collection or if specimen is stored unrefrigerated **CONTRAINDICATIONS:** Current anticoagulant therapy **METHODOLOGY:** Crossed immunoelectrophoresis, Laurell one-dimensional "rocket" electrophoresis, radioimmunoassay (RIA), enzyme-linked immunosorbent assay (ELISA), or radiocrossed immunoelectrophoresis **ADDITIONAL INFORMATION:** Factor VIII assay results aid in interpretation of antigen level. The clinically diverse von Willebrand's disease is being related to underlying molecular diversity. The von Willebrand

Factor VIII/von Willebrand Factor Terminology

vWD	von Willebrand's disease
VIII:C	Factor VIII procoagulant activity, the AHF factor (protein which corrects abnormality in hemophilia A) Factor VIII-related protein
VIIIC:Ag	The immunologic determinant of VIIIC
VIIIR	von Willebrand factor, factor VIII carrier protein (corrects bleeding time abnormality in von Willebrand's disease)
VIIIR:Ag	Antigenic expression of von Willebrand factor
VIIIR:RCo VIIIR:RCF VIIIR:WF	Ristocetin cofactor (property of VIIIR which in presence of ristocetin, strongly aggregates platelets)

Factor VIII/von Willebrand Disease Terminologic Equivalents

Current (Intl Committee Thrombosis/Hemostasis)	Previous Terminology or Equivalents
Factor VIII (FVIII)	AHF VIIIC
Factor VIII antigen (FVIII Ag)	VIIIC Ag
von Willebrand factor (vWF)	RiCoF VIIIR:RCo VIIIR:RCF
von Willebrand factor antigen (vWF Ag)	VIIIR Ag FVIIIR Ag

factor is not a single discrete molecule but a series of multimers with molecular weight from 800,000 to some 20,000,000. Ratio of the mass of F VIII to VIII vWF complex is about 1:100. Smallest multimers are electrophoretically the most rapid (anodal) while the largest are slowest. The hemostatic efficacy of these multimers is proportional to their size. Types IA, IB, IC, IIA, IIB, IIC through IIH, and III vWD have been described. Types IIF, IIG, and IIH are defined on the basis of single case reports. In type I the multimeric structure of vW factor is normal – all forms present but reduced in amount. In type II the slow moving high molecular weight forms are missing. The remaining proteins are lacking in vWF activity. In type III, all multimers are markedly decreased or absent. See table. Coagulopathy may be an early sign of dysproteinemia, IgG bound factor VIII resulting in an acquired von Willebrand's syndrome with prolonged bleeding time and significantly decreased levels of vWF Ag (factor VIII related antigen), F VIII (factor VIII procoagulant activity) and vWF (VIII R:RCo, factor).[1]

von Willebrand's syndrome is characterized clinically by easy/spontaneous bruising, petechiae/purpura, mucosal (gastrointestinal, genitourinary, nasal, gingival) membrane bleeding, and hemorrhage, occasionally severe, with surgery or trauma. Bilateral epistaxis and easy bruising typically begin in early childhood. Type IA, IIA, and IIB have autosomal dominant mode of inheritance. Type III and IIC are inherited in autosomal recessive mode. Characteristically, bleeding time is prolonged while platelet count, clot retraction, and coagulation time are normal. Type III is characterized by severe hemorrhage, high incidence of consanguinity, and very long bleeding time consistent with absence or near absence of vWF multimer proteins.

Familiarity with the possible considerable variation (over time) in test results when dealing with mild vWD or when attempting to exclude the diagnosis has been re-emphasized.[2]

Footnotes

1. Gan TE, Sawers RJ, and Koutts J, "Pathogenesis of Antibody-Induced Acquired von Willebrand Syndrome," *Am J Hematol*, 1980, 9:363-71.
2. Blombäck M, Eneroth P, Andersson O, et al, "On Laboratory Problems in Diagnosing Mild von Willebrand's Disease," *Am J Hematol*, 1992, 40(2):117-20.

References

Bick RL, "Hereditary Coagulation Protein Defects – von Willebrand's Disease," *Disorders of Thrombosis and Hemostasis: Clinical and Laboratory Practice*, Chapter 6, Chicago, IL: ASCP Press, 1992, 123-6.

Bona RD, "von Willebrand Factor and von Willebrand's Disease: A Complex Protein and a Complex Disease," *Ann Clin Lab Sci*, 1989, 19(3):184-9.

Giddings JC, *Molecular Genetics and Immunoanalysis in Blood Coagulation*, Chichester, England: Ellis Horwood Ltd, 1988, 76-118.

(Continued)

von Willebrand Factor Antigen *(Continued)*

Ginsburg D, "The von Willebrand Factor Gene and Genetics of von Willebrand's Disease," *Mayo Clin Proc*, 1991, 66(5):506-15.

Hill RJ and Ens GE, "Thrombotic Thrombocytopenic Purpura," *Clin Hemost Rev*, 1989, 3:1-4.

Kirby EP and Mills CB, "Methods for Studying the von Willebrand Factor-Platelet Interaction – Method for Studying Platelets and Megakaryocytes," Colman RW and Smith JB, eds, *Modern Methods in Pharmacology*, New York, NY: Alan R. Liss Inc, 1987, 4:65-88.

Meyer D, Piétu G, Fressinaud E, et al, "von Willebrand Factor: Structure and Function," *Mayo Clin Proc*, 1991, 66(5):516-23.

Miller JL, "von Willebrand Disease," *Hematology/Oncology Clinics of North America: Platelets in Health and Disease*, Vol 4, Colman RW and Rao AK, eds, Philadelphia, PA: WB Saunders Co, 1990, 107-28.

Sadler JE, "von Willebrand Disease," *The Metabolic Basis of Inherited Disease*, Vol 2, 6th ed, Scriver CR, Beaudet AL, Sly WS, et al, eds, New York, NY: McGraw-Hill Inc, 1989, 2171-87.

Triplett DA, "Laboratory Diagnosis of von Willebrand's Disease," *Mayo Clin Proc*, 1991, 66(8):832-40.

Zimmerman TS and Meyer D, "Structure and Function of Factor VIII and von Willebrand Factor," and Bloom AL, "Inherited Disorders of Blood Coagulation," *Hemostasis and Thrombosis*, Bloom AL and Thomas DP, eds, New York, NY: Churchill Livingstone, 1987, 131-47 and 393-436.

von Willebrand Factor Assay

CPT *85245*

Related Information

Cryoprecipitate *on page 1058*
Platelet Aggregation *on page 459*
von Willebrand Factor Antigen *on page 476*
von Willebrand Factor Multimer Assay *on this page*

Synonyms Ristocetin Cofactor; vW Factor Assay

Specimen Plasma **CONTAINER:** Blue top (sodium citrate) tube **COLLECTION:** Specimen will be drawn by clinic or laboratory technologist. **STORAGE INSTRUCTIONS:** Separate into plastic vial, freeze immediately and send frozen. **CAUSES FOR REJECTION:** Tube not full, specimen hemolyzed, specimen clotted, specimen received more than 2 hours after collection **SPECIAL INSTRUCTIONS:** Must schedule with laboratory in advance.

Interpretive **REFERENCE RANGE:** Interpretation of platelet aggregation patterns, normal plasma/platelets aggregate when exposed to ristocetin **USE:** Aid with the differential diagnosis of hemophilia and von Willebrand's disease **METHODOLOGY:** Modified platelet aggregation (aggregation as stimulated by ristocetin – a measure of vWF binding to platelet glycoprotein Ib); measurement of agglutination of fresh washed or formalin-fixed platelets by patient's plasma as compared to agglutination produced by a "standard plasma" (donor pool or reference plasma) used to prepare a standard curve;[1] botrocetin snake venom based platelet agglutinating test[2] **ADDITIONAL INFORMATION:** Plasma from von Willebrand's disease patients lacks a factor causing platelet aggregation in response to ristocetin.

Footnotes

1. Brozović M and Mackie I, "Investigation of a Bleeding Tendency," *Practical Haematology*, 7th ed, Chapter 19, Dacie JV and Lewis SM, eds, New York, NY: Churchill Livingstone, 1991, 308-11.
2. Brinkhous KM and Read MS, "Use of Venom Coagglutinin and Lyophilized Platelets in Testing for Platelet-Aggregating von Willebrand Factor," *Blood*, 1980, 55(3):517-20.

References

Bloom AL, "von Willebrand Factor: Clinical Features of Inherited and Acquired Disorders," *Mayo Clin Proc*, 1991, 66(7):743-51.

Triplett DA, "Laboratory Diagnosis of von Willebrand's Disease," *Mayo Clin Proc*, 1991, 66(8):832-40.

von Willebrand Factor Multimer Assay

CPT *85247*

Related Information

Cryoprecipitate *on page 1058*
Factor VIII *on page 424*
von Willebrand Factor Antigen *on page 476*
von Willebrand Factor Assay *on this page*

Synonyms vWF Multimer Assays

Specimen Plasma **CONTAINER:** Blue top (sodium citrate) tube **COLLECTION:** Routine venipuncture. If multiple tests are being drawn, draw coagulation studies last. If only a prothrombin time is being drawn, two-syringe collection technique is recommended to avoid contamination of the specimen with tissue thromboplastins. **TURNAROUND TIME:** This is not a routine clinical laboratory procedure and will usually be performed at a reference laboratory. As such 5-7 days may be required before analytic results are available.

Interpretive **USE:** Classification of von Willebrand's disease variants **METHODOLOGY:** Immunoelectrophoresis using agarose gel and ^{125}I labeled anti-vWF followed by autoradiography for detection of vWF multimers. A Western blot nonradioactive chemiluminescence assay has been developed.[1] **ADDITIONAL INFORMATION:** The von Willebrand factor (vWF) is a family of protein multimers varying in molecular weight from 1-20 million daltons. There is evidence that a large, fully polymerized vWF multimer is released from vascular endothelial cells. vWF is found in plasma, α granules of platelets and subendothelial connective tissue. Plasma and basement membrane vWF are largely of endothelial cell origin. Extensive intracellular processing occurs before active vWF multimers are formed. A large precursor pro-vWF protein dimerizes, is transported to the Golgi apparatus after N-linked glycosylation and in subsequent acidic environment pro vWF dimers multimerize by formation of interchain disulfide bonds.[2] The protein accumulates in Weibel-Palade bodies of endothelial cells and is released from these compartments basolaterally.[3] The integrin $\alpha v\beta_3$ serves as an endothelial cell receptor for von Willebrand factor.[4] Plasma multimers are generated from the polymer after it is released into the circulation.[5] See table.

Subtypes of von Willebrand's Disease

Subtype	Multimer Composition	Multimer Level	Platelet Aggregation
I	Complete	↓	
II	Highest MW multimers absent		
III (clinically severe)	All multimers involved	Absent	
IIb	Highest MW multimers absent		↓ with ristocetin
Platelet type	Highest MW multimers absent		↓ with ristocetin

In von Willebrand's disease (vWD) there is abnormal vWF multimeric structure.[6] vWF bridges vascular subendothelium and a platelet membrane receptor on glycoprotein Ib. The spectrum of von Willebrand's disease may involve qualitative and/or quantitative abnormalities of plasma and/or platelet vWF.[7] Multimer analysis has formed the basis of subtype classification of vWD. See table. A platelet-type vWD (pseudo-vWD) is caused by an abnormal platelet receptor for vWF.[8,9]

Terminology: Factor VIII and von Willebrand Factor*

FVIII (FVIIIC)	Factor VIII	Procoagulant activity (deficient in hemophilia A)
FVIII Ag	Factor VIII antigen	Factor VIII, immunologic definition
vWD		von Willebrand disease
vWF (VIIIR)	von Willebrand factor	Activity of protein deficient in von Willebrand's disease measured using ristocetin cofactor assays (RiCoF)
vWF Ag	von Willebrand factor antigen	Immunologic determinants of von Willebrand factor previously termed factor VIII related antigen (VIIIR Ag)

* Recommendations of the International Committee for Thrombosis and Hemostasis, 1985

There is evidence that some, probably rare, cases of type I vWD are acquired and result from accelerated clearance of vWF from the circulation with or without involvement of inactivating antibodies against vWF:Ag.[10]

The increased platelet agglutinating activity occurring with thrombotic thrombocytopenic purpura (TTP) appears to result from release of platelet-agglutinating factor and unusually large

(Continued)

von Willebrand Factor Multimer Assay *(Continued)*

vWF multimers.[11] Platelet agglutination in patients with TTP can be inhibited by large dose infusion of human immunoglobulin G with resultant remission (in a majority of cases) of this once usually fatal disease.[12]

Footnotes

1. Wen LT, McPherson RA, and Smolec JM, "A Chemiluminographic Detection of von Willebrand's (Factor VIII-Related Antigen) Multimeric Composition," *Am J Clin Pathol*, 1993, 99(3):343.
2. Wagner DD and Bonfanti R, "Von Willebrand Factor and the Endothelium," *Mayo Clin Proc*, 1991, 66(6):621-7.
3. Wagner DD, Urban-Pickering M, and Marder VJ, "von Willebrand Protein Binds to Extracellular Matrices Independently of Collagen," *Proc Natl Acad Sci U S A*, 1984, 81:471-5.
4. Cheresh DA, "Human Endothelial Cells Synthesize and Express an Arg-Gly-Asp-Directed Adhesion Receptor Involved in Attachment to Fibrinogen and von Willebrand Factor," *Proc Natl Acad Sci U S A*, 1987, 84:6471-5.
5. Tsai H-M, Nagel RL, Hatcher VB, et al, "Multimeric Composition of Endothelial Cell-Derived von Willebrand Factor," *Blood*, 1989, 73(8):2074-6.
6. Ruggeri ZM and Zimmerman TS, "Variant von Willebrand's Disease. Characterization of Two Subtypes By Analysis of Multimeric Composition of Factor VIII/von Willebrand Factor in Plasma and Platelets," *J Clin Invest*, 1980, 65:1318-25.
7. Ruggeri ZM and Zimmerman TS, "von Willebrand Factor and von Willebrand Disease," *Blood*, 1987, 70:895-904.
8. Bloom AL, "Von Willebrand Factor: Clinical Features of Inherited and Acquired Disorders," *Mayo Clin Proc*, 1991, 66(7):743-51.
9. Scott JP and Montogmery RR, "The Rapid Differentiation of Type IIb von Willebrand's Disease From Platelet-Type (Pseudo-) von Willebrand's Disease by the 'Neutral' Monoclonal Antibody Binding Assay," *Am J Clin Pathol*, 1991, 96(6):723-8.
10. Igarashi N, Miura M, Kato E, et al, "Acquired von Willebrand's Syndrome With Lupus-Like Serology," *Am J Ped Hemat/Oncol*, 1989, 11(1):32-5.
11. Schmidt JL, "Thrombotic Thrombocytopenic Purpura: Successful Treatment Unlocks Etiologic Secrets," *Mayo Clin Proc*, 1989, 64(8):956-61.
12. Lian EC-Y, Mui PTK, Siddiqui FA, et al, "Inhibition of Platelet-Aggregating Activity in Thrombotic Thrombocytopenic Purpura Plasma by Normal Adult Immunoglobulin G," *J Clin Invest*, 1984, 73:548-55.

References

Bona RD and Carta CA, "von Willebrand Factor Multimer Assay," *Manual of Procedures for the Seminar on Diagnostic Hematology*, FW Sunderman, Philadelphia, PA: Institute for Clinical Science Inc, 1988, 193-8.

Cheresh DA, "Structural and Biologic Properties of Integrin-Mediated Cell Adhesion," *Clin Lab Med*, 1992, 12(2):217-36.

Gralnick HR, Williams SB, McKeown LP, et al, "Platelet von Willebrand Factor," *Mayo Clin Proc*, 1991, 66(6):634-40.

Handin RI and Wagner DD, "Molecular and Cellular Biology of von Willebrand Factor," *Prog Hemost Thromb*, 1989, 9:233-59.

Lian EC-Y, "Pathogenesis of Thrombotic Thrombocytopenic Purpura," *Semin Hematol*, 1987, 24:82-100.

Miller JL, "von Willebrand Disease," *Hematology/Oncology Clinics of North America: Platelets in Health and Disease*, Vol 4, Colman RW and Rao AK, eds, Philadelphia, PA: WB Saunders Co, 1990, 107-28.

Ruggeri ZM, "Structure and Function of von Willebrand Factor: Relationship to von Willebrand's Disease," *Mayo Clin Proc*, 1991, 66(8):847-61.

Sadler JE, "von Willebrand Disease," *The Metabolic Basis of Inherited Disease*, Vol 2, 6th ed, Scriver CR, Beaudet AL, Sly WS, et al, eds, New York, NY: McGraw-Hill Inc, 1989, 2171-87.

Triplett DA, "Laboratory Diagnosis of von Willebrand's Disease," *Mayo Clin Proc*, 1991, 66(8):832-40.

von Willebrand Protein *see* Factor VIII *on page 424*

vWF *see* Factor VIII *on page 424*

vW Factor Assay *see* von Willebrand Factor Assay *on page 478*

vWF Multimer Assays *see* von Willebrand Factor Multimer Assay *on page 478*

Williams-Fitzgerald-Flaujeac Factor *see* Factor, Fitzgerald *on page 431*

XIIa *see* Factor XII *on page 429*

CYTOPATHOLOGY

Melanie J. Castelli, MD
Paolo Gattuso, MD
Antimo Candel, MD
Eugene S. Olsowka, MD, PhD

Cytopathology is the study of pathologic alterations in individual cells that reflect changes in their environment and also in the spectrum from premalignant to neoplastic conditions. The accurate interpretation of cytologic changes cannot be separated from the clinical presentation. All pertinent clinical and radiologic information is of inestimable value to a good cytomorphologist. Other factors are of importance also, and these include an adequate specimen: good cellularity, correct site sampled, and proper fixation.

The most commonly performed cytologic examination is the familiar "Pap" smear, a cervicovaginal specimen, introduced in 1943[1] by Dr George Papanicolaou. This screening procedure has played a role in reducing morbidity and mortality in women from cervical carcinoma.

Cytologic screening of many body sites is now routine. Exfoliated cells in urine, spinal fluid, effusion fluids (ascites, pleural, pericardial, joint), and fiberoptic endoscopically obtained brushings of the oropharyngeal, gastrointestinal, and upper genitourinary tract are all obtained without difficulty and frequently will yield a diagnosis for the clinician.

In addition, the development of fine needle aspiration cytology of palpable masses as well as deep seated lesions (available with radiographic assistance) has greatly enlarged the scope of cytopathologic practice. The place for fine needle aspiration diagnosis is at the forefront of cytopathology; however, the decision as to indications for use must be made jointly by clinician and pathologist.

In addition, cytologic material can be studied at present with numerous special modalities, including flow cytometry, electron microscopy, immunoperoxidase staining, immunofluorescence, and standard tissue special stains. The studies may elucidate specific etiologies of neoplasms; however, the diagnosis of a neoplastic versus a non-neoplastic process remains a morphologic one.

In order for the Cytopathology Laboratory to maintain high standards of diagnostic accuracy, close communication with the clinical staff must be regarded as essential. In addition, the patients' welfare is of the utmost importance, and in no case in which a question exists, either on the part of clinician or cytopathologist, should the suggestion for tissue confirmation be withheld. A well trained, experienced cytopathology staff is an invaluable asset to clinicians and patients alike.

---

[1] Papanicolaou GN and Traut HF, *Diagnosis of Uterine Cancer by the Vaginal Smear*, The Commonwealth Fund, New York, NY: 1943.

Abdominal Mass Aspiration *see* Fine Needle Aspiration, Deep Seated Lesions *on page 498*

Amniotic Fluid Cytology

CPT *88104 (cytopathology, smear with interpretation)*

Related Information

Amniotic Fluid, Chromosome and Genetic Abnormality Analysis *on page 891*
Amniotic Fluid Lecithin/Sphingomyelin Ratio and Phosphatidylglycerol *on page 124*
Cytomegalic Inclusion Disease Cytology *on page 496*
Nile Blue Fat Stain *on page 505*

Synonyms Premature Rupture of Bag of Waters (BOW); Premature Rupture of Fetal Membranes

Test Commonly Includes Simple smear from external os in patients suspected of having prematurely ruptured the amniotic sac (bag of waters)

Specimen Amniotic fluid **SAMPLING TIME:** Less than 15 minutes **COLLECTION:** Obtain fluid with simple spatula or even wooden tongue depressor from the external os, fresh, smeared onto either a plain glass or frosted glass slide, and fixed in 95% ethyl alcohol. **CAUSES FOR REJECTION:** Unlabeled slide

Interpretive **REFERENCE RANGE:** In nonrupture, the fluid will show a smooth, even pattern when examined under the microscope. **USE:** Assess leakage of amniotic fluid from the cervical os in cases of rupture of the fetal membranes **CONTRAINDICATIONS:** Extensive bleeding precludes use of this method **METHODOLOGY:** Alcohol-fixed, Papanicolaou stained smear, examined for "ferning" of the fluid obtained. The smear will show branching in the pattern of fern leaves induced by the presence of sodium in high concentration leaking from the amniotic fluid. This is secondary to the high estrogen content of the fluid.[1] **ADDITIONAL INFORMATION:** One may sometimes be called upon to distinguish between maternal urine and amniotic fluid. Typically amniotic fluid contains more protein than urine and has concentrations of urea and creatinine similar to serum concentrations. Maternal urine typically contains higher urea and creatinine concentrations than amniotic fluid. Protein, urea, and creatinine concentrations may vary with the age of pregnancy.[2]

Footnotes

1. Gorodeski IG, Paz M, Insler V, et al, "Diagnosis of Rupture of Fetal Membranes by Glucose and Fructose Measurements," *Obstet Gynecol*, 1979, 53:611.
2. Schumann GB and Schweitzer SC, "Examination of Urine," *Clinical Diagnosis and Management by Laboratory Methods*, 18th ed, Henry JB, ed, Philadelphia, PA: WB Saunders Co, 1991, 388-9.

References

Cunningham FG, MacDonald PC, Leveno KJ, et al, *Williams Obstetrics*, 19th ed, Norwalk, CT: Appleton and Lange, 1993, 373.

Ascitic Fluid Cytology *see* Body Fluids Cytology *on this page*

BAL Cytology *see* Bronchoalveolar Lavage Cytology *on page 487*

Bladder, Ureteral, and Pelvicocalyceal Barbotage Specimens *see* Urine Cytology *on page 513*

Bladder Washings Cytology *see* Urine Cytology *on page 513*

Body Cavity Fluid Cytology *see* Body Fluids Cytology *on this page*

Body Fluids Cytology

CPT *88104*

Related Information

Biopsy or Body Fluid Aerobic Bacterial Culture *on page 778*
Biopsy or Body Fluid Anaerobic Bacterial Culture *on page 778*
Biopsy or Body Fluid Fungus Culture *on page 780*
Biopsy or Body Fluid Mycobacteria Culture *on page 782*
Body Fluid *on page 145*
Body Fluid Amylase *on page 148*
Body Fluid Glucose *on page 148*
Body Fluid Lactate Dehydrogenase *on page 149*
Body Fluid pH *on page 150*

Body Fluids Analysis, Cell Count *on page 523*
CA 125 *on page 154*
Carcinoembryonic Antigen *on page 167*
Cyst Fluid Cytology *on page 495*
Gene Rearrangement for Leukemia and Lymphoma *on page 911*
Gram Stain *on page 815*
Immunoperoxidase Procedures *on page 60*
Immunophenotypic Analysis of Tissues by Flow Cytometry *on page 65*
Polymerase Chain Reaction *on page 927*
Synovial Fluid Analysis *on page 1158*
Tumor Aneuploidy by Flow Cytometry *on page 88*
Viral Culture, Body Fluid *on page 1198*
Washing Cytology *on page 515*

Synonyms Body Cavity Fluid Cytology; Effusion Cytology; Fluids Cytology; Serous Effusion Cytology; Serous Fluid Cytology

Applies to Ascitic Fluid Cytology; Culdocentesis; Paracentesis Fluid Cytology; Pericardial Fluid Cytology; Peritoneal Fluid Cytology; Pleural Fluid Cytology; Synovial Fluid Cytology; Thoracentesis Fluid Cytology

Test Commonly Includes Cytologic evaluation of smears, cytocentrifuge preparations, filter preparations, and cell block preparations when indicated

Abstract Combined application of cytology with other laboratory studies enhances diagnosis.

Patient Care PREPARATION: Patient should sign informed consent prior to procedure. Puncture site should be carefully cleaned and prepared as for any tap. In cases of suspected malignancy, the smallest gauge needle (22 g) should be used, as tract seeding has been reported post-thoracentesis with large bore needles.

Specimen Fresh body fluid CONTAINER: 50 mL disposable (plastic) screw top container, heparinized. See Special Instructions. COLLECTION: Gently agitate the container as fluid is collected in order to mix the heparin with the fluid; fluid may also be collected fresh without anticoagulant and sent to the laboratory in the fresh state immediately. Other tests are usually needed as well. See Relation Information above. **Venous blood** drawn at the same time may be helpful; comparisons between serum and body fluid protein, LD, glucose, and other tests are often useful. See listing, Body Fluid in the Chemistry chapter. When pleural fluid is sampled, a **pleural biopsy** may provide diagnosis, especially of granulomatous diseases as well as carcinoma. STORAGE INSTRUCTIONS: Fluid with or without anticoagulant may be stored at 4°C; cells in the fluid can be preserved at this temperature for up to 1 week, without appreciable deterioration of cellular detail. With special techniques, specimens may be kept frozen at -70°C for 1 year without serious loss of cellular details.[1] CAUSES FOR REJECTION: Added fixation of any type, unless previously discussed with Cytology Laboratory personnel; improper labeling or requisition; gross contamination due to spillage; prolonged period (over 2 hours) at room temperature; improper container (thoracentesis and paracentesis drainage bags and large syringes are **not** acceptable containers) TURNAROUND TIME: Usually about 24 hours SPECIAL INSTRUCTIONS: Add 1 mL of heparin per 100 mL of fluid anticipated (each mL of heparin contains 1000 units). Include pertinent clinical information on requisition including previous malignancy, drugs, radiation therapy, or history of alcohol abuse.

Interpretive USE: Establish the presence of primary or metastatic neoplasms. Aid in the diagnosis of rheumatoid pleuritis; systemic lupus erythematosus; myeloproliferative and lymphoproliferative disorders; viral, fungal, and parasitic infestation of serous cavities, and fistulas involving serous cavities. Examination of effusion is more sensitive and specific than blind pleural biopsy in the diagnosis of malignant pleural disease. The presence of malignant neoplastic cells in the fluid usually indicates that the patient has widespread metastases, with the exception of patients with primary pulmonary lesions. Effusion fluid may be submitted for flow cytometric analysis in those cases suspected of myeloproliferative or lymphoproliferative disorder. Examination of synovial fluid from a joint effusion may aid in the diagnosis of metabolic arthritis (gout or pseudogout), rheumatoid arthritis, or traumatic arthritis as well as septic arthritis (gonococcal arthritis). LIMITATIONS: Allowing fluid to stand for prolonged period before processing may cause deterioration and artifacts. In these fluids, a second tap may be required after the reaccumulation of fluid for optimal cytologic interpretation. Clots may contain diagnostic cells which are available for recovery by preparation of a cell block; routine smears may fail to reveal such cells. Malignant cells cannot be recovered from all fluids from all subjects with malignant disease. Very well differentiated carcinomas may be difficult to distinguish from reactive states. CONTRAINDICATIONS: Documented bleeding diathesis and fully anticoagu-

(Continued)

Body Fluids Cytology *(Continued)*

lated patients are relative contraindications. **ADDITIONAL INFORMATION:** Fluids should be submitted **fresh, unfixed**, and **heparinized** to provide well-preserved, representative, diagnostic material. Exfoliated cells deteriorate rapidly in the effusion, both in and out of the body. The amount of heparin recommended is minimal but adequate to prevent clotting of body cavity fluids and act as a preservative; excess amounts will not alter cytologic detail. Cytologic evaluation may classify the type of neoplasm and suggest its site of origin. Fixatives, such as formalin and alcohol, or other types of fixatives must not be used since they prevent adherence of the cells to the slides, do not allow cells to flatten out for optimal presentation of cellular details, and hinder quality staining by the Papanicolaou method. Alcohol also causes precipitation of protein which may interfere with cell analysis. If feasible, cell blocks can be prepared from the fluid sediment. Immunocytochemical studies can be performed on the cytology slides and cell blocks as additional diagnostic methods.[2,3,4,5,6,7]

Tumor markers support discrimination between benign and malignant effusions. **Carcinoembryonic antigen** (CEA) is used both as an immunocytochemical marker and as a test available for serum and other body fluids. As a fluid marker, it is significantly increased with many carcinomas of lung,[8] especially adenocarcinomas,[9] while mesotheliomas do not cause significant elevations of fluid CEA. Other primary sites likely to cause CEA elevations include breast and gastrointestinal tract.

Fluid CA 125 elevation with negative CEA assay occurs with serous and endometrioid carcinomas of ovary and adenocarcinoma of endometrium and fallopian tube.[10,11] By contrast, increased fluid CEA with negative CA 125 results are found with mucinous adenocarcinomas of ovary, lungs, gastrointestinal tract (including pancreas), or breast.[11] Both antigens are within normal range with lymphoma, melanoma, and with benign effusions.

Ascitic fluid from patients with cirrhosis may contain markedly atypical cells which may be derived from mesothelial cells.[12]

Footnotes

1. McCorriston J, "New Method for Preserving Cytology Specimens," *J Clin Pathol*, 1989, 42(10):1101-3.
2. Bedrossian CW, Bonsib S, and Moran C, "Differential Diagnosis Between Mesothelioma and Adenocarcinoma: A Multimodal Approach Based on Ultrastructure and Immunocytochemistry," *Semin Diagn Pathol*, 1992, 9(2):124-40.
3. Nance KV and Silverman JF, "Immunocytochemical Panel for the Identification of Malignant Cells in Serous Effusions," *Am J Clin Pathol*, 1991, 95(6):887-94.
4. Kuhlmann L, Berghauser KH, and Schaffer R, "Distinction of Mesothelioma From Carcinoma in Pleural Effusions. An Immunocytochemical Study on Routinely Processed Cytoblock Preparations," *Pathol Res Pract*, 1991, 187(4):467-71.
5. Wirth PR, Legier J, and Wright GL Jr, "Immunohistochemical Evaluation of Seven Monoclonal Antibodies for Differentiation of Pleural Mesothelioma From Lung Adenocarcinoma," *Cancer*, 1991, 67(3):655-62.
6. Tickman RJ, Cohen C, Varma VA, et al, "Distinction Between Carcinoma Cells and Mesothelial Cells in Serous Effusions. Usefulness of Immunohistochemistry," *Acta Cytol*, 1990, 34(4):491-6.
7. Flens MJ, van der Valk P, Tadema TM, et al, "The Contribution of Immunocytochemistry in Diagnostic Cytology. Comparison and Evaluation With Immunohistology," *Cancer*, 1990, 65(12):2704-11.
8. Tamura S, Nishigaki T, Moriwaki Y, et al, "Tumor Markers in Pleural Effusion Diagnosis," *Cancer*, 1988, 61(2):298-302.
9. Kjeldsberg CR and Knight JA, *Body Fluids: Laboratory Examination of Amniotic, Cerebrospinal, Seminal, Serous, and Synovial Fluids*, 3rd ed, Chicago, IL: ASCP Press, 1993, 159-254.
10. Pinto MM, Bernstein LH, Brogan DA, et al, "Immunoradiometric Assay of CA 125 in Effusions," *Cancer*, 1987, 59:218-22.
11. Rudolph RA, Pinto MM, and Bernstein LH, "Measuring Decision Values for CEA and CA 125 in Effusions," *Lab Med*, 1990, 21(9):574-8.
12. Guzman J, Bross KJ, Schölmerich J, et al, "Immunocytochemical Analysis of Ascitic Fluid Due to Cirrhosis – A Contribution to Understanding the Origin of Markedly Atypical Cells," *Acta Cytol*, 1992, 36(2):236-40

References

Bedrossian CW, Mason MR, and Gupta PK, "Rapid Cytologic Diagnosis of *Pneumocystis*: A Comparison of Effective Techniques," *Semin Diagn Pathol*, 1989, 6(3):245-61.

Covell JL, Lowry EH, and Feldman PS, "Cytologic Diagnosis of Blastomycosis in Pleural Fluid," *Acta Cytol*, 1982, 26:833-6.

Drew PA and Krauss JS, "Identification of *Giardia lamblia* in Peritoneal Fluid of Trauma Patients," *Acta Cytol*, 1989, 33(2):283-4.

Ehya H, "The Cytologic Diagnosis of Mesothelioma," *Semin Diagn Pathol*, 1986, 3:196-203.

Fam AG, Voorneveld C, Robinson JB, et al, "Synovial Fluid Immunocytology in the Diagnosis of Leukemic Synovitis," *J Rheumatol*, 1991, 18(2):293-6.

Gerbes AL, Jüngst D, Xie Y, et al, "Ascitic Fluid Analysis for the Differentiation of Malignancy-Related and Nonmalignant Ascites: Proposal of a Diagnostic Sequence," *Cancer*, 1991, 68(8):1808-14.

Goodman ZD, Gupta PK, Frost JK, et al, "Cytodiagnosis of Viral Infections in Body Cavity Fluids," *Acta Cytol*, 1979, 23:204-8.
Hira PR, Lindberg LG, Ryd W, et al, "Cytologic Diagnosis of Bancroftian Filariasis in a Nonendemic Area," *Acta Cytol*, 1988, 32:267-9.
Mezger J, Stötzer O, Schilli G, et al, "Identification of Carcinoma Cells in Ascitic and Pleural Fluid – Comparison of Four Panepithelial Antigens With Carcinoembryonic Antigen," *Acta Cytol*, 1992, 36(1):75-81.
Naylor B, "Cytological Aspects of Pleural, Peritoneal, and Pericardial Fluids From in Patients With Systemic Lupus Erythematosus," *Cytopathology*, 1992, 3(1):1-8.
Naylor B, "The Pathognomonic Cytologic Picture of Rheumatoid Pleuritis," *Acta Cytol*, 1990, 34(4):465-73.
O'Hara MF, Cousar JB, Glick AD, et al, "Multiparameter Approach to the Diagnosis of Hematopoietic-Lymphoid Neoplasms in Body Fluids," *Diagn Cytopathol*, 1985, 1:33-8.
Okuyama T, Imai S, and Tsuburu Y, "Egg of *Schistosoma japonicum* in Ascitic Fluid," *Acta Cytol*, 1985, 29:651-2.
Reda MG and Baigelman W, "Pleural Effusion in Systemic Lupus Erythematosus," *Acta Cytol*, 1980, 24:553-7.
Spieler P and Gloor F, "Identification of Types and Primary Sites of Malignant Tumors by Examination of Exfoliated Tumor Cells in Serous Fluids," *Acta Cytol*, 1985, 29:753-67.
Stanley MW and Henry MJ, "The Significance of Leukemia and Lymphoma Cells in Cerebrospinal Fluid Contaminated by Blood Containing Malignant Cells: A Probabilistic Approach Based on the Poisson Frequency Distribution," *Diagn Cytopathol*, 1988, 4(3):193-5.
Stephenson RW, Britt DA, and Schumann GB, "Primary Cytodiagnosis of Peritoneal Extramedullary Hematopoiesis," *Diagn Cytopathol*, 1986, 2:241-3.
Wahl RW, "Curschmann's Spirals in Pleural and Peritoneal Fluids," *Acta Cytol*, 1986, 30:147-51.
Weaver KM, Novak PM, and Naylor B, "Vegetable Cell Contaminants in Cytologic Specimens. Their Resemblance to Cells Associated With Various Normal and Pathologic States," *Acta Cytol*, 1981, 25:210-4.
Yam LT, Lin DG, Janckila AJ, et al, "Immunocytochemical Diagnosis of Lymphoma in Serous Effusions," *Acta Cytol*, 1985, 29:833-41.

Bone Needle Aspiration Cytology *see* Fine Needle Aspiration, Deep Seated Lesions *on page 498*

Brain Cyst Fluid Cytology *see* Cyst Fluid Cytology *on page 495*

Brain Needle Aspiration *see* Fine Needle Aspiration, Deep Seated Lesions *on page 498*

Breast Cyst Aspiration Cytology *see* Fine Needle Aspiration, Superficial Palpable Masses *on page 499*

Breast Cyst Fluid Cytology *see* Cyst Fluid Cytology *on page 495*

Breast Discharge Cytology *see* Nipple Discharge Cytology *on page 505*

Bronchial Aspirate Cytology *see* Bronchial Washings Cytology *on this page*

Bronchial Aspiration for *Pneumocystis* *see Pneumocystis carinii* Preparation *on page 508*

Bronchial Brushings Cytology *see* Brushings Cytology *on page 489*

Bronchial Wash Cytology *see* Bronchial Washings Cytology *on this page*

Bronchial Washings Cytology

CPT *88104 (smears with interpretation); 88106 (filter method with interpretation); 88107 (smears and filter preparation with interpretation); 88108 (concentration technique, smears and interpretation)*

Related Information

Bronchial Aspirate Anaerobic Culture *on page 792*
Bronchoalveolar Lavage *on page 793*
Cytomegalic Inclusion Disease Cytology *on page 496*
Cytomegalovirus Antibody *on page 672*
Cytomegalovirus Culture *on page 1175*
Cytomegalovirus Isolation, Rapid *on page 1176*
Pneumocystis carinii Preparation *on page 508*
Pneumocystis Fluorescence *on page 732*
Sputum Culture *on page 849*
Sputum Cytology *on page 510*
Sputum Fungus Culture *on page 853*
Sputum Mycobacteria Culture *on page 855*
(Continued)

Bronchial Washings Cytology *(Continued)*

Viral Culture, Respiratory Symptoms *on page 1204*
Virus, Direct Detection by Fluorescent Antibody *on page 1208*

Synonyms Bronchial Aspirate Cytology; Bronchial Wash Cytology

Applies to Tracheal and Bronchial Washings; Tracheal Aspiration Cytology

Test Commonly Includes Cytologic evaluation of smears and cell block routinely; cytocentrifuge (cytospin) and filter preparations may be included. After the washings or aspirates have been centrifuged, direct smears and cell blocks can be prepared from the sediment or the fluid samples may be prepared using a membrane filtration technique. Use of both cytocentrifugation and membrane filtration techniques may be appropriate in some cases.[1,2]

Patient Care **PREPARATION:** Informed consent for bronchoscopy **AFTERCARE:** Postbronchoscopy sputum for cytology is advisable, as it may yield a more diagnostic specimen than that obtained during bronchoscopy.

Specimen Bronchial washings **CONTAINER:** 50 mL disposable centrifuge tube **COLLECTION:** Washings or aspirates are collected during endoscopic examination by instilling 3-5 mL of physiologic saline solution through the bronchoscope and reaspirating the fluid; the samples should be properly labeled and delivered to the laboratory immediately. **STORAGE INSTRUCTIONS:** After hours place in refrigerator. **CAUSES FOR REJECTION:** Improper labeling or fixation, prolonged period (more than 6 hours) at room temperature **SPECIAL INSTRUCTIONS:** Include type of specimen and pertinent clinical information on requisition (ie, age, clinical impression, past diagnoses, radiographic findings, and history of radiation or chemotherapy). Infectious diseases suspected, immunocompromised status of patient (ie, status postorgan or marrow transplant or AIDS), and special stains requested should be specified. Special handling of all cytologic specimens regarding infectious etiology is routine (universal precautions).

Interpretive **USE:** Establish the presence of primary or metastatic neoplasms; aid in the diagnosis of respiratory infections with herpesvirus, cytomegalovirus, measles virus, fungal diseases, *Pneumocystis carinii*, *Strongyloides*, *Echinococcus*, and *Paragonimus*; may be helpful in the diagnosis of lipoid pneumonitis, hemosiderosis (Goodpasture's syndrome), asbestosis, alveolar proteinosis, and allergic processes; diagnose opportunistic infection in immunocompromised patients **LIMITATIONS:** Specimen is considered unsatisfactory if respiratory epithelium is not present. **ADDITIONAL INFORMATION:** Special stains may be necessary for identification of organisms. The most commonly used are silver methenamine (Grocott), Diff-Quik™, or Giemsa for fungus and *Pneumocystis* and Ziehl-Neelsen for acid-fast bacteria. Immunoperoxidase staining for further diagnostic information can also be performed.[3] In addition, smears for immunofluorescence may be of use.

Footnotes

1. Taskinen E, Tukiainen P, and Renkonen R, "Bronchoalveolar Lavage – Influence of Cytologic Methods on the Cellular Picture," *Acta Cytol*, 1992, 36(5):680-6.
2. Thompson AB, Robbins RA, Ghafouri MA, et al, "Bronchoalveolar Lavage Fluid – Effect of Membrane Filtration Preparation on Neutrophil Recovery," *Acta Cytol*, 1989, 33(4):544-9.
3. Lyubsky S and Thorn R, "Application of Immunoperoxidase Staining to the Cell Blocks From Sputa and Bronchial Washings," *Arch Pathol Lab Med*, 1989, 113(1):94-5.

References

Broaddus C, Dake MD, Stulbarg MS, et al, "Bronchoalveolar Lavage and Transbronchial Biopsy for the Diagnosis of Pulmonary Infections in the Acquired Immunodeficiency Syndrome," *Ann Intern Med*, 1985, 102:747-52.

Chandler FW and Watts JC, "Fungal Infections," *Pulmonary Pathology*, Dail DH and Hammar SP, eds, New York, NY: Springer-Verlag, 1988.

Chandra P, Delaney MD, and Tuazon CU, "Role of Special Stains in the Diagnosis of *Pneumocystis carinii* Infection From Bronchial Washing Specimens in Patients With the Acquired Immune Deficiency Syndrome," *Acta Cytol*, 1988, 32:105-8.

Chaudhuri B, Nanos S, Soco JN, et al, "Disseminated *Strongyloides stercoralis* Infestation Detected by Sputum Cytology," *Acta Cytol*, 1980, 24:360-2.

Corwin RW and Irwin RS, "The Lipid-Laden Alveolar Macrophage as a Marker of Aspiration in Parenchymal Lung Disease," *Am Rev Respir Dis*, 1985, 132:576-81.

Marchevsky A, Rosen MJ, Chrystal G, et al, "Pulmonary Complications of the Acquired Immunodeficiency Syndrome," *Hum Pathol*, 1985, 16:659-70.

Riazmontazer N and Bedayat G, "Cytology of Plasma Cell Myeloma in Bronchial Washings," *Acta Cytol*, 1989, 33(4):519-22.

Strigle SM and Gal AA, "A Review of Pulmonary Cytopathology in the Acquired Immunodeficiency Syndrome," *Diagn Cytopathol*, 1989, 5(1):44-54.

Wheeler TM, Johnson ED, Coughlin D, et al, "The Sensitivity of Detection of Asbestos Bodies in Sputa and Bronchial Washings," *Acta Cytol*, 1988, 32:647-50.

Bronchoalveolar Lavage Cytology

CPT *88104*

Related Information

Bronchial Aspirate Anaerobic Culture *on page 792*
Bronchoalveolar Lavage *on page 793*
Brushings Cytology *on page 489*
Cytomegalic Inclusion Disease Cytology *on page 496*
Cytomegalovirus Antibody *on page 672*
Cytomegalovirus Culture *on page 1175*
Cytomegalovirus Isolation, Rapid *on page 1176*
Pneumocystis carinii Preparation *on page 508*
Pneumocystis Fluorescence *on page 732*
Sputum Culture *on page 849*
Sputum Cytology *on page 510*
Sputum Fungus Culture *on page 853*
Sputum Mycobacteria Culture *on page 855*
Transbronchial Fine Needle Aspiration *on page 512*
Viral Culture, Respiratory Symptoms *on page 1204*
Virus, Direct Detection by Fluorescent Antibody *on page 1208*

Synonyms BAL Cytology

Test Commonly Includes Cytologic evaluation of smears after processing. Special stains for microorganisms and/or cell count with differential; identification of hemosiderin-laden macrophages. Combined use of cytocentrifugation and membrane filtration techniques may be desirable in some circumstances.[1]

Patient Care PREPARATION: Informed consent for procedure. Topical anesthesia of the pharynx and upper respiratory tree is necessary. Sedation is useful but often precluded by patient's clinical status. AFTERCARE: Transient fever, chills, and myalgias have been reported to occur in up to 50% of cases. Antipyretic analgesics may be indicated.

Specimen Lavage fluid CONTAINER: Centrifuge tubes or other sterile, leakproof disposable containers SAMPLING TIME: 1-2 hours COLLECTION: More than 80% of pulmonologists use the right middle lobe as the sampling site. Both volume recovered and total cell count is higher from this area. The bronchoscope is wedged in a distal bronchial segment. 100-300 mL of warm, pyrogen-free, isotonic, sterile solution is infused with recovery of 40% to 60%. Fixative should not be used. STORAGE INSTRUCTIONS: Specimen should be forwarded to the Cytology Laboratory immediately. Cold storage is less than optimal but essential if processing is delayed. Detection of *Pneumocystis* is not compromised by delayed processing; however, it is more difficult to identify in patients who are already receiving treatment for this organism. CAUSES FOR REJECTION: Leaking container, insufficient clinical history SPECIAL INSTRUCTIONS: Requisition should specify need for special stains for microorganisms or cell count. Routine processing in many cytology laboratories includes only Papanicolaou stained smears.

Interpretive REFERENCE RANGE: 10-15 x 10^6 cells/100 mL, 80% to 90% macrophages, 10% lymphocytes USE: Useful in the diagnosis of infection of the lungs, bronchoalveolar lavage is now commonly used as the preliminary diagnostic procedure in severe diffuse lung infections in both normal and immunocompromised hosts, particularly opportunistic infectious organisms (CMV, *Pneumocystis*, herpes, and fungi).[2,3,4,5,6,7,8,9,10,11] BAL is also useful in the diagnosis and management of sarcoid and interstitial lung disease.[12,13,14,15] Neoplastic cells have also been identified by this method.[16,17,18,19] Atypical type II pneumocytes in the lavage fluid due to toxic injury may indicate progression of the damaged lung.[20,21] LIMITATIONS: Wide variability in cell type and numbers recovered, particularly in smokers. Standardized volumes and concentrations not yet established. CONTRAINDICATIONS: Severe hypoxemia with impending respiratory failure ADDITIONAL INFORMATION: Interstitial lung disease can be divided into BAL lymphocyte predominant groups (sarcoid, hypersensitivity pneumonitis) and neutrophil predominant (smoking, idiopathic pulmonary fibrosis, and histiocytosis-X). A Diff-Quik™ stained cytospin preparation of BAL is an excellent rapid screening procedure for pathogens, particularly in the immunocompromised patient. It can detect *Pneumocystis*, CMV, herpes, *Cryptococcus*, *Candida*, blastomycosis, and aspergillosis as well as *Nocardia* and *Actinomyces*. Detection of fat-laden macrophages in increased numbers (>40% of cells) correlates well with chronic aspiration pneumonia.

Footnotes

1. Thompson AB, Robbins RA, Ghafouri MA, et al, "Brochoalveolar Lavage Fluid Processing - Effect of Membrane Filtration Preparation on Neutrophil Recovery," *Acta Cytol*, 1989, 33(4):544-9.

(Continued)

Bronchoalveolar Lavage Cytology *(Continued)*

2. Broadus C, Drake MD, Stulbarg MS, et al, "Bronchoalveolar Lavage and Transbronchial Biopsy for the Diagnosis of Pulmonary Infections in the Acquired Immunodeficiency Syndrome," *Ann Intern Med*, 1985, 102:747-52.
3. Chandler FW and Watts JC, "Fungal Infections," *Pulmonary Pathology*, Dail DH and Hammar SP, eds, New York, NY: Springer-Verlag, 1988.
4. DeFine LA, Saleba KP, Gibson BB, et al, "Cytologic Evaluation of Bronchoalveolar Lavage Specimens in Immunosuppressed Patients With Suspected Opportunistic Infections," *Acta Cytol*, 1987, 31:235-42.
5. Emanuel D, Peppard J, Stover D, et al, "Rapid Immunodiagnosis of Cytomegalovirus Pneumonia by Bronchoalveolar Lavage Using Human and Murine Monoclonal Antibodies," *Ann Intern Med*, 1986, 104:476-81.
6. Ognibere FP, Shelhamer J, Gill V, et al, "The Diagnosis of *Pneumocystis carinii* Pneumonia in Patients With the Acquired Immunodeficiency Syndrome Using Segmental Bronchoalveolar Lavage," *Am Rev Respir Dis*, 1984, 129:929-32.
7. Orenstein M, Webber CA, and Heurich AE, "Cytologic Diagnosis of *Pneumocystis carinii* Infection by Bronchoalveolar Lavage in Acquired Immunodeficiency Syndrome," *Acta Cytol*, 1985, 29:727-31.
8. Rosenthal DL, "Cytology of Inflammatory Diseases of the Lung," *Compendium on Diagnostic Cytology*, 6th ed, Weid GL, Keebler CM, Koss LG, et al, eds, Chicago, IL: Tutorial of Cytology, 1988.
9. Stover DE, White DA, Romano PA, et al, "Diagnosis of Pulmonary Disease in Acquired Immunodeficiency Syndrome (AIDS): Role of Bronchoscopy and Bronchoalveolar Lavage," *Am Rev Respir Dis*, 1984, 130:659-62.
10. Strigle SM and Gal AA, "A Review of Pulmonary Cytopathology in the Acquired Immunodeficiency Syndrome," *Diagn Cytopathol*, 1989, 5(1):44-54.
11. Winn WC Jr and Walker DH, "Viral Infections," *Pulmonary Pathology*, Dail DH and Hammar SP, eds, New York, NY: Springer-Verlad, 1988.
12. Corwin RW and Irwin RS, "The Lipid-Laden Alveolar Macrophage as a Marker of Aspiration in Parenchymal Lung Disease," *Am Rev Respir Dis*, 1985, 132:576-81.
13. Daniele RP, Elias JA, Epstein PE, et al, "Bronchoalveolar Lavage: Role in the Pathogenesis, Diagnosis and Management of Interstitial Lung Disease," *Ann Intern Med*, 1985, 102:93-9.
14. Martin WJ, Williams DE, Dines DE, et al, "Interstitial Lung Disease Assessment by Bronchoalveolar Lavage," *Mayo Clin Proc*, 1983, 58:751-7.
15. Reynolds HY and Chuetien J, "Respiratory Tract Fluid Analysis of Content and Contemporary Use in Understanding of Lung Disease," *DM*, 1984, 30:1-91.
16. Linder J, Radio SJ, Robbins RA, et al, "Bronchoalveolar Lavage in the Cytologic Diagnosis of Carcinoma of the Lung," *Acta Cytol*, 1987, 31:796-801.
17. Sestin P, Rotto L, Gotti, et al, "Bronchoalveolar Lavage Diagnosis of Bronchoalveolar Carcinoma," *Eur J Respir Dis*, 1985, 66:55-8.
18. Springmeyer SC, Hackman R, Carlson JJ, et al, "Bronchoalveolar Cell Carcinoma Diagnosed by Bronchoalveolar Lavage," *Chest*, 1983, 83:278-9.
19. Wisecarver J, Ness MJ, Rennard SI, et al, "Bronchoalveolar Lavage in the Assessment of Pulmonary Hodgkin's Disease," *Acta Cytol*, 1989, 33(4):527-32.
20. Bedrossian CWM, "Iatrogenic and Toxic Injury," *Pulmonary Pathology*, Dail DH and Hammar SP, eds, New York, NY: Springer-Verlag, 1988.
21. Huang MS, Colby JR, and Martin WJ Jr, "Utility of Bronchoalveolar Lavage in the Diagnosis of Drug-Induced Pulmonary Toxicity," *Principles and Practice of Infectious Diseases*, Mandel GL, Douglas RA Jr, and Bennett JE, eds, New York, NY: John Wiley and Sons, 1979.

References

Allen JN, Davis WB, and Pacht ER, "Diagnostic Significance of Increased Bronchoalveolar Lavage Fluid Eosinophils," *Am Rev Respir Dis*, 1990, 142(3):642-7.

Baughman R, Strohofer S, and Kim K, "Variation of Differential Cell Counts of Bronchoalveolar Lavage Fluid," *Arch Pathol Lab Med*, 1986, 110:341-3.

Baughman RP, Dohn MN, Loudon RG, et al, "Bronchoscopy With Bronchoalveolar Lavage in Tuberculosis and Fungal Infections," *Chest*, 1991, 99(1):92-7.

Chamberlain DW, Braude AC, and Rebuck AS, "A Critical Evaluation of Bronchoalveolar Lavage; Criteria for Identifying Unsatisfactory Specimens," *Acta Cytol*, 1987, 31:599-605.

Fleury-Feith J, Escudier E, Pocholle MJ, et al, "The Effects of Cytocentrifugation on Differential Cell Counts in Samples Obtained by Bronchoalveolar Lavage," *Acta Cytol*, 1987, 31:606-10.

Krieger B, Blinder L, and Inchausti BC, "Clinical Utility of Bronchoalveolar Lavage in a General Hospital," *Arch Intern Med*, 1989, 149(7):1605-7.

Linder J and Rennard SI, *Bronchoalveolar Lavage*, Chicago, IL: American Society of Clinical Pathologists, 1988.

Martin WJ 2d, "Diagnostic Bronchoalveolar Lavage in Immunosuppressed Patients With New Pulmonary Infiltrates," *Mayo Clin Proc*, 1992, 67(3):296-8.

Meduri GU, Stover DE, Greeno RA, et al, "Bilateral Bronchoalveolar Lavage in the Diagnosis of Opportunistic Pulmonary Infections," *Chest*, 1991, 100(5):1272-6.

Murray N, *Respiratory Medicine*, New York, NY: WB Saunders Co, 1988.

Mylius EA and Gullvag B, "Alveolar Macrophage Count as an Indicator of Lung Reaction to Industrial Air Pollution," *Acta Cytol*, 1986, 30:157-62.

Pisani RJ, Witzig TE, Li CY, et al, "Confirmation of Lymphomatous Pulmonary Involvement by Immunophenotypic and Gene Rearrangement Analysis of Bronchoalveolar Lavage Fluid," *Mayo Clin Proc*, 1990, 65(5):651-6.

Popp W, Ritschka L, Scherak O, et al, "Bronchoalveolar Lavage in Rheumatoid Arthritis and Secondary Sjögren's Syndrome," *Lung*, 1990, 168(4):221-31.

Radio SJ, Rennard SI, Kessinger A, et al, "Breast Carcinoma in Bronchoalveolar Lavage. A Cytologic and Immunocytochemical Study," *Arch Pathol Lab Med*, 1989, 113(4):333-6.

Rennard SI, "Future Directions for Bronchoalveolar Lavage," *Lung*, 1990, 168(Suppl):1050-6.

Rennard SI, "Bronchoalveolar Lavage in the Diagnosis of Cancer," *Lung*, 1990, 168(Suppl):1035-40.

Roggli VL, Piantadosi CA, and Bell DY, "Asbestos Bodies in Bronchoalveolar Lavage Fluid: A Study of 20 Asbestos-Exposed Individuals and Comparison to Patients With Other Chronic Interstitial Lung Disease," *Acta Cytol*, 1986, 30:470-6.

Schumann GB and Swensen JJ, "Comparison of Papanicolaou's Stain With the Gomori Methenamine Silver (GMS) Stain for the Cytodiagnosis of *Pneumocystis carinii* in Bronchoalveolar Lavage (BAL) Fluid," *Am J Clin Pathol*, 1991, 95(4):583-6.

Silverman JF, Turner RC, West RL, et al, "Bronchoalveolar Lavage in the Diagnosis of Lipoid Pneumonia," *Diagn Cytopathol*, 1989, 5(1):3-8.

Stanley MW, Henry-Stanley MJ, and Iber C, "Bronchoalveolar Lavage," *Cytology and Clinical Application*, New York, NY: Igaku-Shoin, 1991.

Woods GL, Thompson AB, Rennard SL, et al, "Detection of Cytomegalovirus in Bronchoalveolar Lavage Specimens. Spin Amplification and Staining With a Monoclonal Antibody to the Early Nuclear Antigen for Diagnosis of Cytomegalovirus Pneumonia," *Chest*, 1990, 98(3):568-75.

Bronchopulmonary Lavage for *Pneumocystis* *see Pneumocystis carinii* Preparation *on page 508*

Brushings Cytology

CPT 88104

Related Information

Bronchoalveolar Lavage Cytology *on page 487*

Cytomegalic Inclusion Disease Cytology *on page 496*

Applies to Bronchial Brushings Cytology; Colonic Brushings Cytology; Esophageal Brushings Cytology; Gastric Brushings Cytology; Oropharyngeal Brushings Cytology; Small Bowel Brushings Cytology; Tracheal Brushings Cytology; Ureteral Brushings Cytology

Test Commonly Includes Examination of prepared smears; cytocentrifuge preparations may be prepared if the brush is submitted to the laboratory in physiologic saline solution.

Patient Care PREPARATION: Informed consent for procedure

Specimen Brush suspected lesions via a flexible fiberoptic bronchoscope or other endoscopic devices to examine and brush suspected lesions[1,2,3,4] CONTAINER: Coplin jar containing 95% ethanol COLLECTION: Roll brush gently over fully frosted glass slide and fix immediately in 95% ethanol. Label one end of glass slide as well as Coplin jar with patient's name and identification number. The exact site brushed should be indicated on the jar label and the requisition. For assistance in the diagnosis of infectious disease, a special double-sheathed brush should be sent sterile, separately, to the Microbiology Laboratory for cultures. CAUSES FOR REJECTION: Improper fixation, hypocellularity, unlabeled slides SPECIAL INSTRUCTIONS: Specify the site brushed and include all pertinent clinical data on requisition; indicate requests for special stains to identify unusual organisms (eg, ameba, fungus).

Interpretive USE: Establish the presence of primary or metastatic neoplasms; aid in the diagnosis of certain infections with herpesvirus, cytomegalovirus, measles virus, fungal diseases, *Pneumocystis carinii*, *Strongyloides*, *Echinococcus*, *Giardia lamblia*, *Entamoeba*, *Paragonimus*; aid in the diagnosis of Legionnaires' disease; aid in the diagnosis of anaerobic pulmonary infections; aid in the diagnosis of lipoid pneumonia, hemosiderosis (Goodpasture's syndrome), asbestosis, allergic processes, metaplastic glandular epithelium of esophagus (Barrett's esophagus). Brushing smears are suitable for immunocytochemical staining for bacterial or tumor antigens. LIMITATIONS: Allowing smears and brushes to dry before they are well fixed will introduce many artifacts and distortions hampering reliable interpretation. Such dried slides are reported as **unsatisfactory** for cytologic evaluation. If smears have not been air dried for longer than 30 minutes, a 30 second rehydration in normal saline prior to fixing in 95% alcohol may rehydrate cells sufficiently for smear to be interpretable.[5] Detailed clinical history is necessary as exemplified by a case report of marked post-tracheostomy atypia simulating squamous cell carcinoma.[6] ADDITIONAL INFORMATION: Special stains and culture may be indicated, especially in the diagnosis of infectious processes or inflammatory conditions.

(Continued)

Brushings Cytology *(Continued)*

Footnotes

1. Chen YL, "The Diagnosis of Colorectal Cancer With Cytologic Brushings Under Direct Vision at Fiberoptic Colonoscopy," *Dis Colon Rectum*, 1987, 30:342-4.
2. Dowlwatshahi K, Skinner DB, DeMeester TR, et al, "Evaluation of Brush Cytology as an Independent Technique for Detection of Esophageal Cancer," *J Thorac Cardiovasc Surg*, 1988, 89:849-51.
3. Festa VI, Hajdu SI, and Winawar SJ, "Colorectal Cytology in Chronic Ulcerative Colitis," *Acta Cytol*, 1985, 29:262-8.
4. Ryan ME, "Cytologic Brushing of Ductal Lesions During ERCP," *Gastrointest Endosc*, 1991, 37(2):139-42.
5. Chan JK and Kung IT, "Rehydration of Air-Dried Smears With Normal Saline - Application in Fine-Needle Aspiration Cytologic Examination," *Am J Clin Pathol*, 1988, 89(1):30-4.
6. Berman JJ, Murray RJ, and Lopez-Plaza IM, "Widespread Post-tracheostomy Atypia Simulating Squamous Cell Carcinoma - A Case Report," *Acta Cytol*, 1991, 35(6):713.

References

Chambers LA and Clark WE, "The Endoscopic Diagnosis of Gastroesophageal Malignancy: A Cytologic Review," *Acta Cytol*, 1986, 30:110-4.

Cook JJ, de Carlo DJ, and Haneman B, "The Role of Brush Cytology in the Diagnosis of Gastric Malignancy," *Acta Cytol*, 1988, 32:461-4.

Geisinger KR, Teot LA, and Richter JE, "A Comparative Cytopathologic and Histologic Study of Atypia, Dysplasia, and Adenocarcinoma in Barrett's Esophagus," *Cancer*, 1992, 69(1):8-16.

Jeevanandaur V, Treat MR, and Forde KA, "A Comparison of Direct Brush Cytology and Biopsy in the Diagnosis of Colorectal Cancer," *Gastrointest Endosc*, 1987, 33:370-1.

Melville DM, Richman PI, Shepherd NA, et al, "Brush Cytology of the Colon and Rectum in Ulcerative Colitis: An Aid to Cancer Diagnosis," *Am J Clin Pathol*, 1988, 41:1180-6.

Catheterized Urine Cytology *see* Urine Cytology *on page 513*

Cerebrospinal Fluid Cytology

***CPT** 88104*

Related Information

Beta$_2$-Microglobulin *on page 644*
Bone Marrow *on page 524*
Cerebrospinal Fluid Anaerobic Culture *on page 797*
Cerebrospinal Fluid Analysis *on page 527*
Cerebrospinal Fluid Culture *on page 798*
Cerebrospinal Fluid LD *on page 179*
Immunoperoxidase Procedures *on page 60*
Immunophenotypic Analysis of Tissues by Flow Cytometry *on page 65*
Polymerase Chain Reaction *on page 927*
Tumor Aneuploidy by Flow Cytometry *on page 88*

Synonyms Spinal Fluid Cytology

Applies to Cisternal Tap Cytology; Lumbar Tap Cytology; Ventricular Tap Cytology

Test Commonly Includes Smears, filter preparations, cytocentrifuge preparations, and immunocytochemistry when indicated[1]

Patient Care PREPARATION: Signed informed consent should be obtained. The patient is then prepped establishing a sterile field; 1% lidocaine is used for local anesthesia. AFTERCARE: A "fibrin patch" using the patient's own plasma may be necessary if severe headache and/or vertigo develops and persists.

Specimen Fresh cerebrospinal fluid CONTAINER: Use sterile tube from lumbar puncture tray or sterile, leakproof screw-top container SAMPLING TIME: 30-60 minutes COLLECTION: A 23-gauge spinal needle with stylet is inserted through the L1-L2 interspinous space, and dura mater into the cerebrospinal fluid space. In a three part collection, the third tube should be submitted in its entirety to the Cytology Laboratory immediately. Specimen must be labeled with patient's name, identification number, and date. STORAGE INSTRUCTIONS: Spinal taps for cytology should be done when the specimen can be processed immediately. If it is not possible to process the cellular sample immediately, it must be refrigerated or fixed 1:1 by volume with Carbowax® fixative. It is imperative to note that **without immediate processing, degeneration of cells within the spinal fluid begins within 20 minutes at room temperature.** CAUSES FOR REJECTION: Improper labeling, prolonged period (more than 3 hours) at room temperature, gross blood contamination SPECIAL INSTRUCTIONS: Specify specimen origin. Include pertinent clinical data on requisition (ie, admitting diagnosis, age, history, and prior diagnostic procedures). It is of utmost importance to alert the cytology laboratory if the fluid has been recovered from any type of ventricular shunt.[2]

Interpretive **REFERENCE RANGE:** Adults and children: acellular, or up to 3-5 mononuclear cells/μL; infants: 20-30 mononuclear cells/μL **USE:** Establish the presence of primary or metastatic neoplasm; aid in the diagnosis of fungal (particularly cryptococcal), bacterial, viral, and aseptic meningitis; may be of assistance in patients with demyelinating disease (ie, multiple sclerosis). Of patients with untreated acute lymphoblastic leukemia (ALL), approximately 80% will have leukemic cells in CSF at some time. Of patients with acute myeloblastic leukemia, about 60% will be shown to have such cells in the CSF. Other malignant neoplasms metastatic to the CNS include primaries of the lung, breast, kidney, gastrointestinal tract, melanomas, and choriocarcinomas. Of the primary tumors from the lung, small cell undifferentiated carcinoma is the most common source of CNS metastases.[3] Cytologic studies may provide evidence of cytomegalovirus infection of the CNS (eg, in subjects with AIDS). Examination of CSF in AIDS patients is also helpful in detection of cryptococcal meningitis and lymphoma but less helpful in diagnosis of *Toxoplasma*.[4] **LIMITATIONS:** Malignant cells are shed into cerebrospinal fluid only from tumors which extend the subarachnoid space or into the ventricles. Metastatic tumors and leukemias have better detection rates than primary CNS tumors. Meningeal carcinomatosis or lymphoma may be diagnosed in this fluid, however they shed fewer cells at intermittent periods. Herpes meningitis **cannot** be diagnosed by CSF cytology: brain biopsy is required. **CONTRAINDICATIONS:** Elevated intracranial pressure; abnormal coagulation profile **ADDITIONAL INFORMATION:** Myelography, radiation, and especially intrathecal therapy can all produce striking cytologic changes.

Footnotes

1. Vick WW, Wikstrand CJ, Bullard DE, et al, "The Use of a Panel of Monoclonal Antibodies in the Evaluation of Cytologic Specimens From the Central Nervous System," *Acta Cytol*, 1987, 31:815-24.
2. Bigner SH, Elmore PD, Dee AL, et al, "The Cytopathology of Reactions to Ventricular Shunts," *Acta Cytol*, 1985, 29(3):391.
3. Kjeldsberg CR and Knight JA, "Cerebrospinal Fluid," *Body Fluids: Laboratory Examination of Amniotic, Cerebrospinal, Seminal, Serous, and Synovial Fluids*, 3rd ed, Chapter 2, Chicago, IL: ASCP Press, 1993, 65-157.
4. Katz RL, Alappattu C, Glass JP, et al, "Cerebrospinal Fluid Manifestations of the Neurologic Complications of Human Immunodeficiency Virus Infection," *Acta Cytol*, 1989, 33(2):233-44.

References

Bigner SH, Elmore PD, Dee AL, et al, "Unusual Presentations of Inflammatory Conditions in Cerebrospinal Fluid," *Acta Cytol*, 1985, 29(3):291.

Bigner SH and Johnston WW, *Cytopathology of the Central Nervous System*, New York, NY: Masson Publishing USA Inc, 1983.

Wertlake PT, Markovits BA, and Stellar S, "Cytologic Evaluation of Cerebrospinal Fluid With Clinical and Histologic Correlation," *Acta Cytol*, 1972, 16:224-39.

Cervical Smear *see* Cervical/Vaginal Cytology *on this page*

Cervical/Vaginal Cytology

***CPT** 88150; 88156 (Bethesda system)*

Related Information

Chlamydia trachomatis Culture *on page 1171*
Chlamydia trachomatis Direct FA Test *on page 1173*
Cytomegalovirus Culture *on page 1175*
Cytomegalovirus Isolation, Rapid *on page 1176*
Endometrial Cytology *on page 497*
Hormonal Evaluation, Cytologic *on page 503*
Human Papillomavirus DNA Probe Test *on page 916*
Neisseria gonorrhoeae Culture *on page 831*
Trichomonas Preparation *on page 879*
Viral Culture, Urogenital *on page 1207*

Synonyms Cervical Smear; Pap Smear; Vaginal Cytology

Applies to Herpes Smear; The Bethesda System; Vira Pap®; Vira Type®; Vulvar Cytology

Test Commonly Includes Fast smear, cervical scraping smear, vaginal pool smear, lateral vaginal wall smear, direct scraping smear

Patient Care **PREPARATION:** Patients are advised to avoid douches 48-72 hours prior to examination; however, this should not preclude taking of the smear. Provide relevant information including age and last menstrual period (LMP).

Specimen Endocervical and cervical scrape or brush are recommended in all cases. Aspiration of posterior vaginal fornix fluid (vaginal pool) may also be used and is actually the smear of

(Continued)

Cervical/Vaginal Cytology *(Continued)*

choice for hormonal evaluation and is particularly useful if endometrial cancer is being sought; however it is not a substitute for cervical specimens. Endometrial aspirations are not advised for routine use. For lesions of the vagina or vulva, scrapings made directly from the lesion are most diagnostic. Cellular samples obtained by scraping the upper lateral vaginal wall may be used for hormonal evaluation; however, due to variation in site chosen and technique in obtaining the smear, a true reflection of hormonal status may not result. **CONTAINER:** Glass slides with frosted ends; spray fixative containing 95% ethanol and water or liquid fixative such as PRO-FIXX™ (Lerner Laboratories, Stanford, CT), also containing ethanol and water. **Hair spray should never be used to fix Pap smear slides.** The slides may be sent to the laboratory in cardboard slide containers; if the smears are wet-fixed in 95% alcohol in a Coplin jar, this may be sent to the laboratory. **COLLECTION:** Preferred fixatives: Spray or liquid fixatives as mentioned above or 95% ethanol. Patient identification of specimen: Each slide must be labeled with patient's name and site sampled, written with graphite pencil on the frosted end of the slide. It is possible to label nonfrosted slides only with a diamond point pen. The speculum must be introduced **without** lubricant; in certain cases, running the speculum through warm saline will prove helpful prior to insertion into atrophic, stenotic, or small introitus.

Sampling:

Endocervix: Gentle scrape or brush of endocervical canal

- Scrape – Rotate narrow end of spatula in the cervical os and gently smear onto labeled glass slide and fix immediately.
- Brush – Use a tapered synthetic fiber brush to sample endocervical cells and mucous. Do not scrub onto the slide; rather, lightly roll brush over the slide.

Ectocervical scrape: With spatula thoroughly scrape the entire ectocervix with emphasis on the squamocolumnar junction. Spread material evenly onto labeled glass slide and fix immediately.

Vaginal pool smear: Use pipette, tongue blade, spatula, or lip of speculum to obtain material (fluid) from the posterior fornix. Place drop of fluid directly on glass slide and spread fluid evenly over the slide with glove. This material may contain cells from the vagina, cervix, endometrium, fallopian tubes, and ovaries. Immediate fixation is imperative. The vaginal pool smear is valuable for cytohormonal as well as radiation effect evaluation. This smear will detect approximately 90% of endometrial carcinomas when the cellular and hormonal patterns are interpreted in combination. Although this is not the smear of choice for cancer detection, up to 90% of cervical carcinomas may be detected in this smear. A vaginal pool smear may be obtained in children with a nasal speculum.

Cervical scraping smear: Made by introducing cervical spatula through the external os endocervical canal, rotating 360°, sampling the entire squamocolumnar junction, and spreading onto slide with immediate fixation. Although not the smear of choice for cancer detection, it will detect approximately 97% of early cervical lesions. Perhaps 25% of endometrial lesions will be detected by this method.

Fast smear: Combines vaginal pool and cervical scraping smear material on one slide and detects 90% of endometrial carcinomas and 97% of cervical carcinomas; it is therefore considered the smear of choice for cancer detection. First, the vaginal pool material is obtained, and one drop placed 1 inch from the end of the glass slide. Do **not** smear. Obtain cervical scraping as described above, remove quickly, and mix with lower part of vaginal pool material. Over open fixative container, quickly draw gloved fifth finger from combined drop to opposite end of slide **twice**. Immediately drop into fixative.

Lateral vaginal wall smear: Scraping from upper lateral one-third of vaginal mucosa. Used in cytohormonal evaluations.

Direct scraping smear: Direct scrape of grossly visible lesion, smeared and fixed as previously described.

CAUSES FOR REJECTION: Improper fixation, lack of identification **SPECIAL INSTRUCTIONS:** Include pertinent clinical history such as age, LMP, parity, postmenopausal status, surgery, exogenous hormones, history of carcinoma, radiation, chemotherapy, abnormal vaginal bleeding, and history of previous abnormal Pap smears.

Interpretive **POSSIBLE PANIC RANGE:** Any smear with definitely malignant cells should ideally be verbally relayed directly to the clinician in addition to forwarding the formal report. **USE:** Diagnose primary or metastatic neoplasms; diagnose cervical dysplasia (cervical intraepithelial

Cervical/Vaginal Cytology

Traditional Class	Bethesda System
	ADEQUACY OF THE SPECIMEN
	Satisfactory for evaluation
	Satisfactory for evaluation but limited by...(specify reason)
	Unsatisfactory for evaluation...(specify reason)
	GENERAL CATEGORIZATION (optional)
1	Within normal limits
2	Benign cellular changes: see Descriptive Diagnoses.
3, 4, 5	Epithelial cell abnormality: see Descriptive Diagnoses.
	DESCRIPTIVE DIAGNOSES
	Benign Cellular Changes
2	Infection
	Trichomonas vaginalis
	Fungal organisms morphologically consistent with *Candida* spp
	Predominance of coccobacilli consistent with shift in vaginal flora
	Bacteria morphologically consistent with Actinomyces spp
	Cellular changes associated with herpes simplex virus
	Other*
2	Reactive Changes
	Reactive cellular changes associated with:
	Inflammation (includes typical repair)
	Atrophy with inflammation ("atrophic vaginitis")
	Radiation
	Intrauterine contraceptive device (IUD)
	Other
3, 4, 5	**Epithelia Cell Abnormalities**
	Squamous Cell
2 or 3†	Atypical squamous cells of undetermined significance: qualify†
3	Low grade squamous intraepithelial lesion (LSIL) encompassing: HPV* mild dysplasia/CIN 1
3 or 4	High grade squamous intraepithelial lesion (HSIL) encompassing: moderate and severe dysplasia, CIS/CIN 2, and CIN 3
5	Squamous cell carcinoma
	Glandular Cell
2	Endometrial cells, cytologically benign in a postmenopausal woman
2 or 3†	Atypical glandular cells of undetermined significance: qualify†
5	Endocervical adenocarcinoma
5	Endometrial adenocarcinoma
5	Extrauterine adenocarcinoma
5	Adenocarcinoma, NOS
5	**Other Malignant Neoplasms:** Specify
	Hormonal Evaluation (applies to vaginal smears only)
	Hormonal pattern compatible with age and history
	Hormonal pattern incompatible with age and history: specify
	Hormonal evaluation not possible due to: specify

*Cellular changes of human papillomavirus (HPV) — previously termed **koilocytosis, koilocytotic atypia,** and **condylomatous atypia** — are included in the category of LSIL.

†Atypical squamous or glandular cells of undetermined significance should be further qualified, if possible, as to whether a reactive or premalignant/malignant process is favored.

(Continued)

Cervical/Vaginal Cytology *(Continued)*

neoplasia (CIN)); diagnose genital infections with herpes, *Candida* sp, *Trichomonas vaginalis*, cytomegalovirus and *Actinomyces*; aid in the diagnosis of vaginal adenosis, cervicovaginal endometriosis, condyloma, human papillomavirus infection, lymphogranuloma venereum; aid in evaluating hormonal function (formerly referred to as MI, maturation index); useful in suggesting chlamydial infection **LIMITATIONS:** Failure to obtain adequate ectocervical, endocervical, or vaginal cell population is considered to indicate an unsatisfactory smear. Use of lubricating jelly on the speculum will interfere with the cytologic assessment and cause a suboptimal specimen. Inflammatory smears should not be assessed for hormonal status, as the inflammation will itself alter the maturation of the mucosa. Because the smears are only a screening method, a lesion may be completely missed due to sampling error. Chlamydial infection must be documented with associated culture. **ADDITIONAL INFORMATION:** Suggested criteria for follow-up:

- No atypical cells – annual cytologic follow-up in women of reproductive age
- Inflammation with associated change – annual follow-up
- Inflammation with possible underlying dysplasia – clear inflammation and repeat smear
- Low grade dysplasia (mild CIN I) (LSIL) – follow-up smear 3-6 months, if abnormality persists, colposcopic exam suggested
- High grade dysplasia (CIN II-CIN III) (HSIL) – colposcopy with biopsy

In postmenopausal women, an atypia of atrophy may appear to mimic a high grade dysplasia. Frequently an estrogen proliferation test, in which topical vaginal estrogen is applied and a subsequent smear taken, is advised. In a true dysplasia, such estrogen will cause the cells to mature, however, dysplasia will persist; in atrophic atypia, maturation will occur, but no dysplasia will be identified.

In patients of childbearing years who have had three consecutive annual normal smears, a smear biannually is acceptable. Patients on oral contraceptives should have smears every 6 months. When a colposcopic biopsy fails to reveal a high grade lesion seen on the smear, a cone biopsy should be considered.

If the smear is repeated too soon (less than 6 weeks), a lesser degree of atypia or dysplasia may be noted. This does not negate the original findings and the abnormality should be pursued. A strong association between HPV DNA and cervical dysplasia and neoplasia has been found. Specific subtypes are considered more causal of neogenesis. Because of the increased frequency of finding this lesion in young adults, the importance of Pap screening should not be underestimated.[1] There are some proponents of detecting the HPV in cervical swab specimens and/or biopsies by ViraPap® and *in situ* hybridization to identify high-risk patients. This remains controversial at present.[2] The listing, Human Papillomavirus DNA Probe Test in the Molecular Pathology chapter, is intended to provide a modicum of discussion relevant to papillomavirus and cervical/vaginal cytopathology.

The practitioner and patients should insist on smear review by licensed cytotechnologists and board certified pathologists and should be cautious about simply seeking the lowest price.

Conferences of leading cytopathologists and gynecologists, held at Bethesda in 1988 and 1991, formulated recommendations for uniform diagnostic terminology for cervical/vaginal cytology. Such recommendations eliminated reporting by classes. These conferences, sponsored by the National Cancer Institute, led to a new classification, the Bethesda System (TBS). See table.[3,4,5,6]

Footnotes

1. Levine AJ, Harper J, Hillborne L, et al, "HPV DNA and Risk of Intraepithelial Lesions of the Uterine Cervix in Young Women," *Am J Clin Pathol*, 1993, 100:6-11.
2. Meyer M, Carbonell R, Mauser N, et al, "Detection of Human Papillomavirus in Cervical Swab Samples by ViraPap® and in Cervical Biopsy Specimens by *in situ* Hybridization," *Am J Clin Pathol*, 1993, 100:12-7.
3. "The 1988 Bethesda System for Reporting Cervical/Vaginal Cytological Diagnoses: National Cancer Institute Workshop", *JAMA*, 1989, 262(7):931-4.
4. "The Revised Bethesda System for Reporting Cervical/Vaginal Cytological Diagnoses: National Cancer Institute Workshop," *Acta Cytol*, 1992, 36(3):273-6.
5. Luff RD, "The Bethesda System for Reporting Cervical/Vaginal Cytologic Diagnoses: Report of the 1991 Bethesda Workshop," *Hum Pathol*, 1992, 23(7):719-21.
6. Sherman ME, Schiffman MH, Erozan YS, et al, "The Bethesda System. A Proposal Reporting Abnormal Cervical Smears Based on the Reproducibility of Cytopathologic Diagnosis," *Arch Pathol Lab Med*, 1992, 116(11):1155-8.

References

Atkinson B, *Atlas of Diagnostic Cytopathology*, Philadelphia, PA: WB Saunders Co, 1992.

Betsill WL and Clark AH, "Early Endocervical Glandular Neoplasia," *Acta Cytol*, 1986, 30:115-26.

Bibbo M and Wied GL, "Inflammation Reaction and Microbiology of the Female Productive Tract," *Compendium on Diagnostic Cytology*, Wied GL, Keebler CM, Koss LG, et al, eds, Chicago, IL: Tutorials of Cytology, 1992, 63-8.

Erozan Y, *Manual for the Thirty-Third Postgraduate Institute for Pathologists in Cytopathology*, Baltimore, MD: John Hopkins University School of Medicine and John Hopkins Hospital, 1992.

Gay JD, Donaldson LD, and Goellner JR, "False-Negative Results in Cervical Cytologic Studies," *Acta Cytol*, 1985, 29:1043-6.

Genest DR, Stein L, Cibas E, et al, "A Binary (Bethesda) System for Classifying Cervical Cancer Precursors: Criteria, Reproducibility, and Viral Correlates," *Hum Pathol*, 1993, 24:730-6.

Gupta PK, "Microbiology, Inflammation, and Viral Infection," *Comprehensive Cytopathology*, 1st ed, Bibbo M, ed, Philadelphia, PA: WB Saunders Co, 1991, 115-52.

Hudson EA, Coleman DV, and Brown CL, "The 1988 Bethesda System for Reporting Cervical/Vaginal Cytologic Diagnoses," *Acta Cytol*, 1990, 34(6):902-3.

Koss LG, "The New Bethesda System for Reporting Results of Smears of the Uterine Cervix," *J Natl Cancer Inst*, 1990, 82(12):988-91.

Luff RD, "The Bethesda System for Reporting Cervical/Vaginal Cytologic Diagnoses: Report of the 1991 Bethesda Workshop," *Am J Clin Pathol*, 1992, 98(2):152-4.

Luff RD, "The Bethesda System for Reporting Cervical/Vaginal Diagnoses," *Acta Cytol*, 1993, 37(2):115-24.

Maguire NC, "Current Use of the Papanicolaou Class System in Gynecologic Cytology," *Diagn Cytopathol*, 1988, 4:169-76.

Paris AL, "Conference on the State of the Art in Quality Control Measures for Diagnostic Cytology Laboratories," *Acta Cytol*, 1989, 33(4):423-90.

Sherman ME, Schiffman MH, Kurman RJ, et al, "The Bethesda System: Interobserver Reproducibility of Cytopathologic Diagnoses," The Bethesda System Second Conference, April 1991.

Wied G, Bonfiglio TA, Cardin V, et al, "Questions on Quality Assurance Measures in Cytopathology," *Acta Cytol*, 1988, 32:913-39.

***Chlamydia* Smears Cytology** *see* Ocular Cytology *on page 506*

Cisternal Tap Cytology *see* Cerebrospinal Fluid Cytology *on page 490*

CMV Smear *see* Cytomegalic Inclusion Disease Cytology *on next page*

Colonic Brushings Cytology *see* Brushings Cytology *on page 489*

Colon Washings Cytology *see* Washing Cytology *on page 515*

Conjunctival Smear Cytology *see* Ocular Cytology *on page 506*

Corneal Cytology *see* Ocular Cytology *on page 506*

Cornification Count *replaced by* Hormonal Evaluation, Cytologic *on page 503*

CT-Guided FNA *see* Fine Needle Aspiration, Deep Seated Lesions *on page 498*

Cul-de-sac Fluid Cytology *see* Cyst Fluid Cytology *on this page*

Culdocentesis *see* Body Fluids Cytology *on page 482*

Cyst Fluid Cytology

***CPT** 88104*

Related Information

Alpha$_1$-Fetoprotein, Serum *on page 115*
Body Fluids Cytology *on page 482*
Breast Biopsy *on page 40*
CA 125 *on page 154*
Carcinoembryonic Antigen *on page 167*
Fine Needle Aspiration, Deep Seated Lesions *on page 498*
Fine Needle Aspiration, Superficial Palpable Masses *on page 499*
Nipple Discharge Cytology *on page 505*

Applies to Brain Cyst Fluid Cytology; Breast Cyst Fluid Cytology; Cul-de-sac Fluid Cytology; Hydrocele Fluid Cytology; Ovarian Cyst Fluid Cytology; Pancreatic Cyst Fluid Cytology; Renal Cyst Fluid Cytology

Test Commonly Includes Filter preparation, smears, cytocentrifuge preparations

Specimen Freshly aspirated fluid **CONTAINER:** Sterile, leakproof, screw-top tube **COLLECTION:** Label with patient's name, identification number, date, and anatomic site. **STORAGE INSTRUCTIONS:** Specimen should be processed as soon as possible; specimens must be kept refrigerated, but not frozen, if processing is delayed. **SPECIAL INSTRUCTIONS:** Specify anatomic site and provide relevant clinical data. If culture is also required, this should be forwarded as a separate specimen directly to the Microbiology Laboratory.

(Continued)

Cyst Fluid Cytology *(Continued)*

Interpretive USE: Establish nature of cystic process (ie, malignancy, inflammatory, retention, infection) ADDITIONAL INFORMATION: After aspiration of a palpable cyst, the area should be reexamined for evidence of a residual mass. If the lesion has not entirely disappeared after fluid aspiration, aspiration biopsy of the residual mass is required in order to exclude cystic malignant lesion.

Breast cyst fluid is usually sparsely cellular and may contain a few apocrine cells. Bloody, cellular fluids may indicate papilloma or intracystic papillary carcinoma (older age groups).

Benign **thyroid cysts** often reveal dark green to brown fluid containing numerous hemosiderin-laden macrophages, a result of intracystic hemorrhage. However, cystic variants of papillary thyroid carcinoma do exist, and a remaining mass should also be aspirated to exclude this possibility.

During laparoscopy, **ovarian cysts** are encountered for which aspiration may be indicated.[1,2] Tumor-associated antigens CEA, CA 125, and alpha-fetoprotein (AFP) are low in follicular and lutein cysts. Both benign and malignant serous cystadenomas contain fluid low in CEA and AFP but marked by high CA 125. High CEA and CA 125 are reported in primary mucinous cystadenomas and cystadenocarcinomas. High CEA with normal CA 125 is described in adenocarcinoma of colon metastatic to ovary,[3] an entity easily mistaken in histopathology for primary ovarian carcinoma. Elevated AFP was reported with a malignant teratoma.

Footnotes

1. Patel KR and Boon AP, "Metastatic Breast Cancer Presenting as an Ovarian Cyst: Diagnosis by Fine Needle Aspiration Cytology," *Cytopathology*, 1992, 3(3):191-5.
2. Stanley MW, Horwitz CA, and Frable WJ, "Cellular Follicular Cyst of the Ovary: Fluid Cytology Mimicking Malignancy," *Diagn Cytopathol*, 1991, 7(1):48-52.
3. Pinto MM, Bernstein LH, Brogan DA, et al, "Measurement of CA 125, Carcinoembryonic Antigen, and Alpha-Fetoprotein in Ovarian Cyst Fluid: Diagnostic Adjunct to Cytology," *Diagn Cytopathol*, 1990, 6(3):160-3.

References

Ingram EA and Helikson MA, "Echinococcosis (Hydatid Disease) in Missouri: Diagnosis by Fine Needle Aspiration of a Lung Cyst," *Diagn Cytopathol*, 1991, 7(5):527-31.

Katz LB and Ehya H, "Aspiration Cytology of Papillary Cystic Neoplasm of the Pancreas," *Am J Clin Pathol*, 1990, 94(3):328-33.

Lewandrowski KB, Southern JF, Pins MR, et al, "Cyst Fluid Analysis in the Differential Diagnosis of Pancreatic Cysts. A Comparison of Pseudocysts, Serous Cystadenoma, Mucinous Cystic Neoplasm, and Mucinous Cystadenocarcinoma," *Ann Surg*, 1993, 217(1):41-7.

Orell SR, Sterrett GF, Walters MN, et al, *Manual and Atlas of Fine Needle Aspiration Cytology*, New York, NY: Churchill Livingstone, 1992.

Rogers LR and Barnett G, "Percutaneous Aspiration of Brain Tumor Cysts Via the Ommaya Reservoir System," *Neurology*, 1991, 41(2 Pt 1):279-82.

Cytology, Sputum *see* Sputum Cytology *on page 510*

Cytomegalic Inclusion Bodies *see* Cytomegalic Inclusion Disease Cytology *on this page*

Cytomegalic Inclusion Disease Cytology

CPT 87207

Related Information

Amniotic Fluid Cytology *on page 482*
Bronchial Washings Cytology *on page 485*
Bronchoalveolar Lavage *on page 793*
Bronchoalveolar Lavage Cytology *on page 487*
Brushings Cytology *on page 489*
Cytomegalovirus Antibody *on page 672*
Cytomegalovirus Culture *on page 1175*
Cytomegalovirus Isolation, Rapid *on page 1176*
Urine Cytology *on page 513*

Synonyms CMV Smear; Cytomegalic Inclusion Bodies; Cytomegalovirus Cytology; Viral Study

Test Commonly Includes Filter or cytocentrifuge preparations for identification of nuclear and/or cytoplasmic viral inclusion bodies

Abstract Bronchoalveolar lavage is reported to be a superb means for detection of CMV infection of the lower respiratory tract.[1]

Specimen Fresh urine, lavage fluid, washing fluid, or alcohol-fixed brushing specimen COLLECTION: All specimens should be labeled with patient's name, identification number, and date. Pertinent history should be provided. CAUSES FOR REJECTION: Specimen not processed within 6 hours SPECIAL INSTRUCTIONS: History of immunosuppression, radiation, and/or chemotherapy especially is needed.

Interpretive USE: Establish the presence of cytomegalovirus infection, especially in immunosuppressed patients, including those with bone marrow and other transplantation procedures and AIDS. LIMITATIONS: Viral culture is the method of choice for definitive diagnosis of CMV, but cytology can provide more rapid information. Cytology is less sensitive than culture for CMV even when immunohistochemical staining is employed. Therefore, a negative cytologic examination for CMV does not exclude the possibility of this etiology, and culture results are needed. The differentiation of whether CMV is a cause of clinical disease or present as an incidental finding in a given patient remains a problem.[1] METHODOLOGY: Conventional cytologic methods, immunofluorescence microscopy

Footnotes

1. Martin WJ II, "Diagnostic Bronchoalveolar Lavage in Immunosuppressed Patients With New Pulmonary Infiltrates," *Mayo Clin Proc*, 1992, 67(3):296-8.

References

Bibbo M, *Comprehensive Cytopathology*, Philadelphia, PA: WB Saunders Co, 1991, 340-1.
Crawford SW, Bowden RA, Hackson RC, et al, "Rapid Detection of Cytomegalovirus Pulmonary Infection by Bronchoalveolar Lavage and Centrifugation Culture," *Ann Intern Med*, 1988, 108:180-5.
Emanuel D, Peppard J, Stover D, et al, "Rapid Immunodiagnosis of Cytomegalovirus Pneumonia by Bronchoalveolar Lavage Using Human and Murine Monoclonal Antibodies," *Ann Intern Med*, 1986, 104:476-81.
Linder J and Rennard S, *Bronchoalveolar Lavage*, Chicago, IL: ASCP Press, 1988, 89-90.
Traystman MD, Gupta PK, Shah KV, et al, "Identification of Viruses in the Urine of Renal Transplant Recipients by Cytomorphology," *Acta Cytol*, 1980, 24:501-10.

Cytomegalovirus Cytology *see* Cytomegalic Inclusion Disease Cytology *on previous page*

Effusion Cytology *see* Body Fluids Cytology *on page 482*

Endometrial Cytology

CPT 88160 (screening and interpretation); 88162 (extended study, 5 or more slides)

Related Information

Cervical/Vaginal Cytology *on page 491*

Synonyms Endo-Pap®; Gravlee Jet® Wash; Isaac's Aspirator®; Medhosa Cannula®; Mi-Mark® Procedure; Vakutage®

Test Commonly Includes Smears, filter, cytocentrifuge, and cell block preparations

Specimen Endometrial scrape, wash, or aspiration COLLECTION: Smear cellular material from collecting instrument thinly and evenly on a clean glass slide. Immediately spray or wet fix. Any remaining cellular material is deposited in a formalin bottle for cell block preparation. Slides and specimen bottle are labeled with patient's name and identification number. Aspirated fluid must be brought to the laboratory at once. Fluid specimens may be processed either by cytocentrifuge or cell block method. CAUSES FOR REJECTION: Unlabeled slides or specimens SPECIAL INSTRUCTIONS: Include all relevant clinical data on requisition including LMP, age, prior diagnoses, history of bleeding, hypertension, diabetes, parity, as well as hormone use.

Interpretive USE: Evaluate possible endometrial carcinoma or hyperplasia LIMITATIONS: Hypocellular specimen, poorly fixed specimen limits interpretation CONTRAINDICATIONS: Cervical or vaginal infections, cervical stenosis METHODOLOGY: Smears and cytocentrifuged specimens are examined microscopically; cell blocks and tissue fragments are processed as surgical tissue specimens for histopathologic examination. ADDITIONAL INFORMATION: This procedure may be useful in women who are at high risk of developing endometrial carcinoma or in women on whose routine cervical Pap smear endometrial cells were identified. Evidence supporting screening for endometrial carcinoma is scanty. Moreover, patients may be screened with a well performed combined Fast smear. See Cervical Vaginal Cytology. The presence of noncyclic endometrial cells in a routine PAP smear may be abnormal depending upon clinical history and cellular appearance.[1]

Footnotes

1. Means M, "The Significance of Noncyclic Endometrial Cells," *Cytopathology II*, The American Society of Clinical Pathologists Continuing Education Program, 1991, 2(8).

(Continued)

Endometrial Cytology *(Continued)*

References

Bibbo M, *Comprehensive Cytopathology*, Philadelphia, PA: WB Saunders Co, 1991.

Coscia-Porrazzi LO, Maiello FM, and de Falco ML, "The Cytology of the Normal Cyclic Endometrium," *Diagn Cytopathol*, 1986, 2:198-203.

Koss LG, Schreiber K, Oberlander SG, et al, "Detection of Endometrial Carcinoma and Hyperplasia in Asymptomatic Women," *Obstet Gynecol*, 1984, 64:1-11.

Meisels A and Jolicoeur C, "Criteria for the Cytologic Assessment of Hyperplasias in Endometrial Samples Obtained by the Endopap Endometrial Sampler," *Acta Cytol*, 1985, 29:297-302.

Meucaglia L, "Endometrial Cytology: Six Years of Experience," *Diagn Cytopathol*, 1987, 3:185-90.

Palermo VG, "Interpretation of Endometrium Obtained by the Endo-Pap Sampler and a Clinical Study of Its Use," *Diagn Cytopathol*, 1985, 1:5-12.

Pritchard KI, "Screening for Endometrial Cancer: Is It Effective?" *Ann Intern Med*, 1989, 110(3):177-9.

Endo-Pap® *see* Endometrial Cytology *on previous page*

Esophageal Brushings Cytology *see* Brushings Cytology *on page 489*

Esophageal Washings Cytology *see* Washing Cytology *on page 515*

Estrogen Effect, Cytologic *see* Hormonal Evaluation, Cytologic *on page 503*

Eye Smear for Cytology *see* Ocular Cytology *on page 506*

Fat Cells *see* Nile Blue Fat Stain *on page 505*

Fetal Maturity Determination *see* Nile Blue Fat Stain *on page 505*

Fine Needle Aspiration Biopsy Cytology *see* Fine Needle Aspiration, Superficial Palpable Masses *on next page*

Fine Needle Aspiration, Deep Seated Lesions

***CPT** 88170*

Related Information

Abscess, Aerobic and Anaerobic Bacterial Culture *on page 768*
Biopsy or Body Fluid Aerobic Bacterial Culture *on page 778*
Biopsy or Body Fluid Anaerobic Bacterial Culture *on page 778*
Biopsy or Body Fluid Fungus Culture *on page 780*
Biopsy or Body Fluid Mycobacteria Culture *on page 782*
Cyst Fluid Cytology *on page 495*
Electron Microscopy *on page 45*
Fine Needle Aspiration, Superficial Palpable Masses *on next page*
Immunoperoxidase Procedures *on page 60*
Immunophenotypic Analysis of Tissues by Flow Cytometry *on page 65*
Transbronchial Fine Needle Aspiration *on page 512*

Synonyms CT-Guided FNA; FNA; FNAB; Ultrasound Guided FNA

Applies to Abdominal Mass Aspiration; Bone Needle Aspiration Cytology; Brain Needle Aspiration; Liver Needle Aspiration Cytology; Lung Needle Aspiration Cytology; Lymph Node Aspiration Cytology; Mediastinal Mass Aspiration; Neck Mass Aspiration; Needle Biopsy Cytology; Pancreas Needle Aspiration Cytology; Retroperitoneal Mass Aspiration; Thyroid Needle Aspiration Cytology

Test Commonly Includes Examination of air-dried, Diff-Quik™ stained, and/or ethanol-fixed, Papanicolaou stained direct smears, cytospin or cell block preparations. Useful adjuncts include microbiological cultures, special stains, flow cytometry, and immunohistochemistry.

Patient Care PREPARATION: Signed informed consent from the patient is required. The patient is prepped surgically to produce a sterile field. One percent lidocaine is used for local anesthesia of skin and overlying subcutaneous tissue. Sedation and/or analgesics may be needed. The suite in which the biopsies are done should be equipped for the handling of complications, such as pneumothorax (chest tube trays, etc). AFTERCARE: Patient should be advised of possible discomfort, local pain, and bleeding. A postpulmonary biopsy routine chest x-ray is obtained, as are routine cuts of liver, etc; post-CT biopsy to exclude hematoma. Occasionally, antibiotics may be required, dependent upon clinical circumstances.[1]

Specimen Needle aspirated material, needle rinse CONTAINER: Plain glass slides with frosted end; Coplin jar containing 95% ethanol; 50 mL plastic capped centrifuge tube containing 25 mL balanced salt solution SAMPLING TIME: 45 minutes to 2 hours COLLECTION: Aspiration equipment needed includes a 15 cm graduated 22-gauge sterile Chiba needle with stylet and attached 10-20 mL plastic syringe. The aspiration is usually performed by the radiologist in the CT or ultrasound suites. Most important is the localization of the needle tip within the mass. Smears and needle rinse are usually prepared by a cytotechnologist or cytopathologist present at the procedure. Immediate evaluation of air-dried Diff-Quik™ stained smears is possible, and rapidly determines the adequacy of the specimen, and need for more material or ending of the procedure. Appropriate material for culture may be obtained by this method. **STORAGE INSTRUCTIONS:** All material should be immediately brought to the Cytology Laboratory. All slides must be labeled with the patient's name, and a requisition with all required information must accompany the material. The needle rinse, if immediate delivery to the laboratory is not possible, should be refrigerated at 4°C. **CAUSES FOR REJECTION:** Unlabeled specimens. Insufficient material can result in an "unsatisfactory" reading. **TURNAROUND TIME:** Often 24 hours; longer if special studies are required. Immediate evaluation can be given within 30 minutes. **SPECIAL INSTRUCTIONS:** Requisition should include all pertinent clinical data including age, sex, primary diagnosis, and any history of malignancy or infectious disease.

Interpretive **USE:** Diagnosis of deep-seated lesions not accessible to superficial aspiration but visible and approachable with radiologic assistance **LIMITATIONS:** Sampling error, particularly with small (1 cm or less) pulmonary nodules; lesions completely surrounded by bone; or when the procedure must be terminated due to complications or patient discomfort **CONTRAINDICATIONS:** Severe chronic obstructive pulmonary disease is a contraindication to pulmonary aspiration, which has a 15% to 30% risk of pneumothorax; abnormal coagulation profile; adrenal or extra-adrenal mass in which the diagnosis of pheochromocytoma is being considered. **ADDITIONAL INFORMATION:** The smallest gauge needle should be used, routinely a 22-gauge needle is used. Needle tracking of malignancy has been reported in the literature. Although the majority of these cases were 18-gauge or greater needles, incidents of tracking with 22- and 23-gauge needles, especially of high grade pancreatic carcinoma, have been reported. Other significant complications include pneumothorax, empyema, hemorrhage, nerve damage, and sudden death due to aspiration or to pheochromocytoma. Most deep seated FNA biopsies proceed uneventfully. Good communication among radiologist, cytopathologist, and clinician maximizes the usefulness of this procedure.

Footnotes

1. Ulich TR and Layfield LJ, "Fatal Septic Shock After Fine Needle Aspiration of a Pancreatic Pseudocyst," *Acta Cytol*, 1985, 29(5):879.

References

Frias-Hidvegi D, *Guides to Clinical Aspiration Biopsy: Liver and Pancreas*, New York, NY: Igaku-Shoin, 1988.

Koss LG, Wayke S, and Olsewski W, *Aspiration Biopsy: Cytologic Interpretation and Histologic Bases*, New York, NY: Igaku-Shoin, 1984.

Orell SR, Sterrett GF, Walters MN, et al, *Manual and Atlas of Fine Needle Aspiration Cytology*, New York, NY: Churchill Livingstone, 1992.

Salzman AJ, "Imaging Techniques in Aspiration Biopsy," *Clinical Aspiration Cytology*, 2nd ed, Linsk JA and Franzen S, eds, 1989.

Tao L, *Guides to Clinical Aspiration Biopsy: Pleura and Mediastinum*, New York, NY: Igaku-Shoin, 1988.

Tao L, *Transabdominal Fine Needle Aspiration Biopsy*, New York, NY: Igaku-Shoin, 1990.

Fine Needle Aspiration of Lung *see* Transbronchial Fine Needle Aspiration *on page 512*

Fine Needle Aspiration, Superficial Palpable Masses

***CPT** 88170*

Related Information

Abscess, Aerobic and Anaerobic Bacterial Culture *on page 768*
Biopsy or Body Fluid Aerobic Bacterial Culture *on page 778*
Biopsy or Body Fluid Anaerobic Bacterial Culture *on page 778*
Biopsy or Body Fluid Fungus Culture *on page 780*
Biopsy or Body Fluid Mycobacteria Culture *on page 782*
Breast Biopsy *on page 40*
Cyst Fluid Cytology *on page 495*
Electron Microscopy *on page 45*
Estrogen Receptor Immunocytochemical Assay *on page 51*
Fine Needle Aspiration, Deep Seated Lesions *on previous page*
Histopathology *on page 57*
Image Analysis *on page 58*
(Continued)

Fine Needle Aspiration, Superficial Palpable Masses *(Continued)*

Immunoperoxidase Procedures *on page 60*
Immunophenotypic Analysis of Tissues by Flow Cytometry *on page 65*
Progestogen Receptor Immunocytochemical Assay *on page 79*
Transbronchial Fine Needle Aspiration *on page 512*
Tumor Aneuploidy by Flow Cytometry *on page 88*

Synonyms Fine Needle Aspiration Biopsy Cytology; FNA; FNAB; "Skinny" or "Thin" Needle Aspiration

Applies to Breast Cyst Aspiration Cytology; Intraoral Needle Aspiration; Lymph Node Needle Aspiration; Neck Mass Needle Aspiration; Needle Biopsy Cytology; Prostate Needle Aspiration; Subcutaneous Fat Pad Aspiration; Subcutaneous Mass Needle Aspiration; Thyroid Needle Aspiration

Test Commonly Includes Examination of both air-dried Diff-Quik™ and 95% ethanol-fixed Papanicolaou stained smears, with needle rinsed material submitted for cytospins or cell block preparation. Useful adjuncts include microbiological cultures, special stains for organisms (ethanol-fixed smears); direct fluorescent antibody (DFA) staining (air-dried smears): flow cytometric immunophenotyping for cell surface markers (RPMI media used for needle rinse); DNA ploidy analysis (Hank's balanced salt solution used in needle rinse); estrogen receptor immunohistochemical analysis (ethanol-fixed smears); and special stains for amyloid, copper, or iron (ethanol-fixed smears)

Patient Care PREPARATION: A signed informed consent should be obtained. The patient should be comfortably seated or supine in a position which maximizes exposure of and access to the area to be biopsied. The overlying skin should be cleansed with an alcohol or Betadine® wipe and allowed to dry. Local anesthesia with 1% lidocaine is used only in rare cases (ie, possible traumatic neuroma). Intraoral lesions should be sprayed with topical anesthetic spray. Assistance of an otolaryngologist is recommended for biopsies of the posterior mouth and pharynx. AFTERCARE: Adequate pressure of at least 5 minutes is essential to prevent significant deep hematoma, especially in hyperplastic lymph nodes, thyroid gland, and salivary gland aspirates. If the patient regularly takes aspirin, longer pressure with ice pack may be required, as in patients on Coumadin®. Mild analgesics may be needed by the patients for 24-48 hours postbiopsy if the area is painful.

Specimen Aspirated cellular material from nodule with needle rinse material saved in a balanced salt solution CONTAINER: Plain glass slides with frosted end for labeling with patient information; Coplin jar containing 95% ethanol; 50 mL plastic centrifuge tube containing 25 mL of a balanced salt solution SAMPLING TIME: 15 minutes COLLECTION: Aspiration equipment needed includes a 1" to 1.5" long 22- to 25-gauge sterile needle with a **clear hub** and an attached 10 or 20 mL syringe. The clear-hubbed needle allows the aspirated material to be seen easily. Commercially available syringe holders ("guns") are available. Fine needle aspiration technique requires extensive familiarization and experience. (See figures.) Steps include the following:

1. Palpation and immobilization of mass with nondominant hand; the mass may either be fixed between the index finger and the thumb or between the index and third finger (see figures 1A and 1B). Gloves must be worn throughout the entire procedure.
2. Insertion of needle into the mass in a single motion (figure 2).
3. Application of suction (5 mL) with subsequent rapid back and forth movement of the needle within the mass (figures 3A and 3B); the needle should also be rotated simultaneously in a 360° fashion in order to sample the entire lesion.
4. Release of suction when material can be seen in the hub of the needle (figure 4). **It is not necessary to see material in the barrel of the syringe.**
5. Removal of the needle from the mass (figure 5).
6. Expression of the material onto glass slide for smears by first removing the needle, aspirating 3 mL air into the syringe, replacing the syringe onto the needle and forcing the material out onto a slide.

Alternate slides are air-dried and alcohol fixed. Normally, the procedure is performed twice to ensure adequate material for diagnosis. As noted in Cyst Fluid Cytology, if a cystic lesion is drained, the area should be re-examined for residual mass, and if present this mass should be aspirated. If an infectious process is suspected, appropriate culture apparatus should be inoculated and immediately sent to the Microbiology Laboratory. The needle should be rinsed with balanced salt solution, and this residue placed in the 50 mL container for cytospin or cell block preparation.

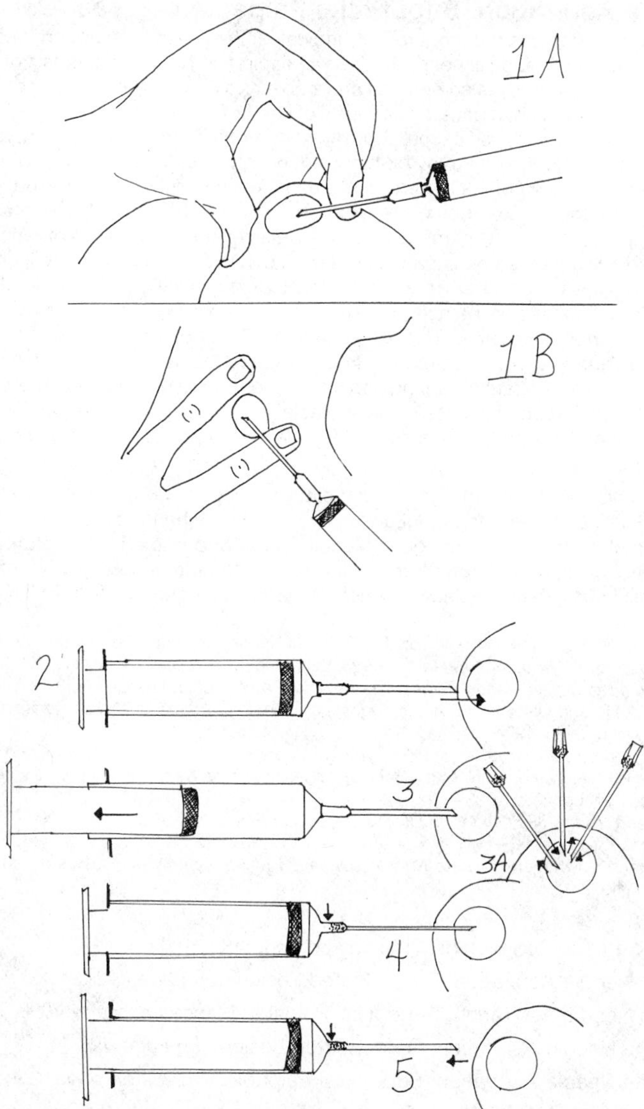

STORAGE INSTRUCTIONS: All materials should be forwarded immediately to the Cytology Laboratory. If the needle rinse cannot be immediately brought to the laboratory, it should be kept refrigerated at 4°C. **CAUSES FOR REJECTION:** Unlabeled specimen, improper fixation, insufficient material **TURNAROUND TIME:** 1 hour for immediate evaluation of air-dried slides; routine: 24-48 hours; longer if special studies are necessary **SPECIAL INSTRUCTIONS:** The clinician should consider discussing the case and biopsy with the cytopathologist before it is performed, as this sometimes improves handling of the specimen especially when special studies are needed. All pertinent clinical history must be provided.

Interpretive **USE:** Screen and diagnose superficial palpable masses including both primary benign and malignant lesions as well as metastatic lesions; particularly useful in situations where a rapid diagnosis is important to the clinician and patient. FNA can assist in the diagnosis of bacterial and fungal infections, and amyloidosis (abdominal fat pad aspiration). Aspirated material may be used for immunophenotyping, DNA ploidy analysis, estrogen receptor immunohistochemistry, and electron microscopy. **LIMITATIONS:** Needle aspiration is subject to sampling error (1% to 10%). Intraepidermal lesions, small, mobile subcutaneous lesions, extensively necrotic lesions, and diffuse plaque-like lesions may cause the most difficulty. Thy-

(Continued)

Fine Needle Aspiration, Superficial Palpable Masses *(Continued)*

roid aspirations of neoplasm cannot reliably indicate if the lesion is an adenoma or carcinoma; histopathologic examination is needed. When an aspiration primary diagnosis of lymphoma is made, an excisional biopsy is sometimes preferable and usually definitive for classification of the lymphoma. In addition, a primary diagnosis of soft tissue sarcoma requires histopathologic evaluation for definitive classification. **CONTRAINDICATIONS:** Significantly abnormal coagulation profile. Patients on Coumadin® may be biopsied, however, extensive and lengthy postbiopsy pressure and application of ice are advised. Such a case should be discussed with the cytopathologist beforehand. **ADDITIONAL INFORMATION:** Routinely, FNA of palpable masses is a procedure causing only minor discomfort with local bruising and 24-58 hours of tenderness in the area biopsied. However, some situations **must** be considered if doing FNA, including the following. A neck mass in an elderly patient may represent a calcified atherosclerotic carotid; ultrasound prior to biopsy may be needed to exclude this possibility, as FNA may induce embolization of atheromatous plaque. Thyroid laceration with extensive bleeding may occur if the patient moves during thyroid aspiration. Rarely, tracheal laceration can complicate aspiration if the needle enters the trachea during aspiration and the patient coughs. Pneumothorax can be induced by aspiration of a mass in the supraclavicular fossa, most frequently in a markedly cachectic patient. Infarction of nodule due to FNA and, rarely, infection of aspiration site or nerve damage may occur.

Good communication between clinician and cytopathologist maximizes the usefulness of this procedure. FNA has a high degree of accuracy when in the hands of experienced physicians and cytopathologists. Its use has been steadily increasing in the United States as a consequence of its low morbidity, rapid turnaround time, and high accuracy. FNA of the prostate gland has essentially been replaced by use of the "biopsy" gun method.

References

Abele JS and Miller TR, "Implementation of an Outpatient Needle Aspiration Biopsy Service and Clinic," *Personal Perspective Cytopathology Annual 1993*, Baltimore, MD: Williams & Wilkins, 1993, 113-7.

Frable WJ, *Thin Needle Aspiration Biopsy*, Philadelphia, PA: WB Saunders Co, 1983.

Koss LG, Wayke S, and Olsewski W, *Aspiration Biopsy: Cytologic Interpretation and Histologic Bases*, New York, NY: Igaku-Shoin, 1984.

Linsk JA and Franzen S, *Clinical Aspiration Cytology*, 2nd ed, New York, NY: JB Lippincott Co, 1989, 1-15.

Orell SR, Sterrett GF, Walters MN, et al, *Manual and Atlas of Fine Needle Aspiration Cytology*, New York, NY: Churchill Livingstone, 1992.

Qizilbash A and Young JE, *Guides to Clinical Aspiration Biopsy: Head and Neck*, New York, NY: Iguku-Shorn, 1988.

Stanley MW and Lowhagent T, *Fine Needle Aspiration of Palpable Masses*, Boston, MA: Butterworth-Heinemann, 1993.

Fluids Cytology *see* Body Fluids Cytology *on page 482*

FNA *see* Fine Needle Aspiration, Deep Seated Lesions *on page 498*

FNA *see* Fine Needle Aspiration, Superficial Palpable Masses *on page 499*

FNAB *see* Fine Needle Aspiration, Deep Seated Lesions *on page 498*

FNAB *see* Fine Needle Aspiration, Superficial Palpable Masses *on page 499*

Gastric Brushings Cytology *see* Brushings Cytology *on page 489*

Gastric Washings Cytology *see* Washing Cytology *on page 515*

Gravlee Jet® Wash *see* Endometrial Cytology *on page 497*

Herpes Cytology

CPT 87207

Related Information

Herpes Simplex Antibody *on page 692*
Herpes Simplex Virus Antigen Detection *on page 1181*
Herpes Simplex Virus Culture *on page 1182*
Herpes Simplex Virus Isolation, Rapid *on page 1184*
Herpesvirus Antigen *on page 693*
Skin Biopsies *on page 84*
Varicella-Zoster Virus Serology *on page 761*

Synonyms Herpetic Inclusion Bodies; Inclusion Body Cytology; Tzanck Smear

Applies to Polymerase Chain Reaction Detection of HSV, VZV

Test Commonly Includes Preparation of cytological smears, both air-dried and Diff-Quik™ stained, as well as alcohol-fixed Papanicolaou stained, with microscopic examination for cellular features of herpes virus infection

Abstract Tzanck smears may be difficult to interpret. They are positive in approximately 50% of herpes simplex virus (HSV) infections and 80% of varicella-zoster virus (VZV) infections. Herpes may cause aseptic meningitis. Genital herpes simplex virus may be transmitted to neonates; such transmission may be catastrophic.

Specimen Scrape of lesion. If a blister is present, the smear should be taken at the edge of the lesion after the blister has been "deroofed". A direct scrape of the area under the blister will be useless, and will reveal only neutrophils. COLLECTION: Firmly scrape the edge of the lesion, preferably a bullous lesion after removal of the bulla. The edge of normal skin and ulcer is to be scraped. In sites other than skin, a direct scrape is done. The scrape may be done with a wooden spatula or tongue blade. Use of cotton swab or Culturette® will recover fewer cells. If a nonblistering lesion is to be scraped, it may be moistened first with sterile saline before scraping. Label slides with patient's name. CAUSES FOR REJECTION: Hypocellular smears or smears composed only of neutrophilic exudate TURNAROUND TIME: A stat smear can usually be ready within an hour if required.

Interpretive USE: Establish the presence of herpes virus infection LIMITATIONS: Tzanck smears cannot provide distinction between HSV 1 and HSV 2, and treatment is not the same for each. Herpes inclusions may not be seen in 50% of active lesions, however, peripheral margination of nuclear chromatin, multinucleated giant cells, and other cellular changes suggestive of herpes infection may point to the correct diagnosis. Interpretation can be difficult. **Viral culture is the definitive diagnostic method.** METHODOLOGY: Air-dried, Diff-Quik™ stained or alcohol-fixed, Pap stained smear. Both types of smears may be submitted for immunoperoxidase stain for herpes viral antigen. Giemsa or Wright's stain may also be used. ADDITIONAL INFORMATION: Diagnostic yield is increased by immunoperoxidase or immunofluorescent procedures, which become positive before characteristic viral cytopathic changes develop. Smears with a heavy inflammatory exudate may be especially difficult to interpret because of nonspecific staining. Smears must be done with and without the primary antibody, and positive and negative controls must be run concurrently. Polymerase chain reaction has been utilized successfully in detection of HSV and VZV DNA sequences and has been reported as equivalent or superior to viral culture. Biopsy is also useful.

References

Corey L and Spear PG, "Infections With Herpes Simplex Viruses," *N Engl J Med*, 1986, 314:686-91, 749-56.

Drew WL, "Diagnostic Virology," *Clin Lab Med*, 1987, 7:721-40.

Koelle DM, Benedetti J, Langenberg A, et al, "Asymptomatic Reactivation of Herpes Simplex Virus in Women After the First Episode of Genital Herpes," *Ann Intern Med*, 1992, 116(6):433-7.

Mertz GJ, Benedetti J, Ashley R, et al, "Risk Factors for the Sexual Transmission of Genital Herpes," *Ann Intern Med*, 1992, 116(3):197-202.

Nahass GT, Goldstein BA, Zhu WY, et al, "Comparison of Tzanck Smear, Viral Culture, and DNA Diagnostic Methods in Detection of Herpes Simplex and Varicella-Zoster Infection," *JAMA*, 1992, 268(18):2541-4.

Herpes Smear *see* Cervical/Vaginal Cytology *on page 491*

Herpetic Inclusion Bodies *see* Herpes Cytology *on previous page*

Hormonal Evaluation, Cytologic

CPT *88155*

Related Information

Cervical/Vaginal Cytology *on page 491*

Synonyms Estrogen Effect, Cytologic; Maturation Index

Replaces Cornification Count

Test Commonly Includes Count of at least 200 squamous cells, with assessment of maturation as to parabasal, intermediate, or superficial (mature)

Patient Care PREPARATION: Douches should be avoided for 24 hours prior to obtaining the smear.

Specimen Scrape of lateral vaginal wall; distal third is preferred CONTAINER: Smear on plain glass slide COLLECTION: Prelabel frosted end of plain glass slide with graphite pencil with patient's name and LVW (lateral vaginal wall). The scrape, with a wooden spatula or tongue blade, is smeared across a glass slide and immediately fixed in 95% ethanol. CAUSES FOR REJECTION: Improper labeling, improper fixative, air drying, specimen taken from site other than

(Continued)

Hormonal Evaluation, Cytologic *(Continued)*

lateral vaginal wall, presence of inflammatory changes due to trichomonads, *Candida* sp, severe bacterial cytolysis **TURNAROUND TIME:** 24 hours **SPECIAL INSTRUCTIONS:** Slide should be labeled LVW (lateral vaginal wall). Include age, last menstrual period (LMP), pertinent history (ie, drugs, history of radiation therapy hormone use, previous gynecological surgery).

Interpretive **REFERENCE RANGE:** The hormonal evaluation will be reported in general terms, such as "normal for age and menstrual status", or "hormonal pattern incompatible with patient's age and menstrual status". When specifically requested, a count or maturation index can be given and is reported in in percentages of cell types, parabasal:intermediate:superficial (ie, 10/60/20 indicating 10% parabasal, 60% intermediate, and 20% superficial). The interpretation of this test is dependent upon the clinical situation. **USE:** Evaluate the maturation status of the vaginal squamous epithelium, which reflects the balance of estrogen and progesterone effects upon this target tissue; also useful in the diagnosis of conditions producing abnormal cytohormonal balance (ie, pituitary dysfunction, ovarian dysfunction, feminizing tumor, and virilizing tumor). **Note**: Any dysplastic or malignant changes noted are treated as they would be on a routine smear, and must be reported to the clinician. **LIMITATIONS:** This test cannot be performed in the presence of inflammation of the vaginal or cervical mucosa. Maturation index is of extremely limited value when applied to a given individual as an isolated procedure because of the great overlap of normal indices and because of great interobserver variability in counts. A series of smears for MI is more useful, but seldom warranted now that sensitive hormonal assays are available. **CONTRAINDICATIONS:** Cervicitis, vaginitis **ADDITIONAL INFORMATION:** A few agents affecting cytohormonal pattern are estrogen, cortisone, digitalis, and tetracycline suppositories (causing misleading massive desquamation).

References

Bibbo M, *Comprehensive Cytopathology*, Philadelphia, PA: WB Saunders Co, 1991.

Erozan Y, *Manual for the Thirty-Third Postgraduate Institute for Pathologists in Cytopathology*, Baltimore, MD: John Hopkins University School of Medicine and John Hopkins Hospital, 1992.

Wied GL and Bibbo M, "Hormonal Cytology," *Comprehensive Cytopathology*, 1st ed, Bibbo M, ed, Philadelphia, PA: WB Saunders Co, 1991, 85-114.

Hydrocele Fluid Cytology *see* Cyst Fluid Cytology *on page 495*

Inclusion Body Cytology *see* Herpes Cytology *on page 502*

Inclusion Conjunctivitis *see* Ocular Cytology *on page 506*

Induced Sputum Technique *see Pneumocystis carinii* Preparation *on page 508*

Intraoral Needle Aspiration *see* Fine Needle Aspiration, Superficial Palpable Masses *on page 499*

Isaac's Aspirator® *see* Endometrial Cytology *on page 497*

Lavage Cytology *see* Washing Cytology *on page 515*

Lipid, Cytology *see* Nile Blue Fat Stain *on next page*

Liver Needle Aspiration Cytology *see* Fine Needle Aspiration, Deep Seated Lesions *on page 498*

Lumbar Tap Cytology *see* Cerebrospinal Fluid Cytology *on page 490*

Lung Needle Aspiration Cytology *see* Fine Needle Aspiration, Deep Seated Lesions *on page 498*

Lymph Node Aspiration Cytology *see* Fine Needle Aspiration, Deep Seated Lesions *on page 498*

Lymph Node Needle Aspiration *see* Fine Needle Aspiration, Superficial Palpable Masses *on page 499*

Maturation Index *see* Hormonal Evaluation, Cytologic *on previous page*

Medhosa Cannula® *see* Endometrial Cytology *on page 497*

Mediastinal Mass Aspiration *see* Fine Needle Aspiration, Deep Seated Lesions *on page 498*

Mi-Mark® Procedure *see* Endometrial Cytology *on page 497*

Neck Mass Aspiration *see* Fine Needle Aspiration, Deep Seated Lesions *on page 498*

Neck Mass Needle Aspiration *see* Fine Needle Aspiration, Superficial Palpable Masses *on page 499*

Needle Biopsy Cytology *see* Fine Needle Aspiration, Deep Seated Lesions *on page 498*

Needle Biopsy Cytology *see* Fine Needle Aspiration, Superficial Palpable Masses *on page 499*

Nile Blue Fat Stain

CPT *88313*

Related Information

Amniotic Fluid Cytology *on page 482*
Amniotic Fluid Lecithin/Sphingomyelin Ratio and Phosphatidylglycerol *on page 124*

Applies to Fat Cells; Fetal Maturity Determination; Lipid, Cytology

Test Commonly Includes Special stain and count of cells positive for intracellular fat

Abstract This test was an early study to try to assess fetal maturity. This is essentially an obsolescent test.

Specimen Amniotic fluid **CONTAINER:** Sealed test tube **STORAGE INSTRUCTIONS:** If immediate processing is not possible, place in refrigerator. **CAUSES FOR REJECTION:** Improper fixation, lack of cellular material **TURNAROUND TIME:** 72 hours

Interpretive **REFERENCE RANGE:** Negative for fat to positive for fat. Amniotic fluid: less than 34 weeks maturity: <1% of cells positive for intracellular fat; 34-38 weeks maturity: 1% to 10% of cells positive; 38-40 weeks maturity: 10% to 50% or more of cells positive; more than 40 weeks maturity: >50% of cells positive. **USE:** Determine the presence of intracellular fat; amniotic fluid test for fetal maturity **LIMITATIONS:** Not as specific as more recent tests including the lecithin/sphingomyelin ratio measured on amniotic fluid; additional spectrophotometric determinations on amniotic fluid are more precise than the Nile Blue fat stain. **METHODOLOGY:** Test based on the staining of neutral lipid in fetal cells obtained by amniocentesis. The neutral lipid is stained by oxazone present in commercial Nile blue sulfate. A smear of the amniotic fluid is made on a clean slide. No fixative is required. The stain solution is a 0.1% aqueous solution of Nile Blue sulfate, which is a differential stain for neutral fat. The preparation is examined under low power (10x) for the presence of fetal cells. Notation is made between the anucleate fetal cells with the orange lipid droplets and the blue nucleated, lipid-free cells. The test is based on staining characteristics and detailed knowledge of cellular morphology is not required by the examiner.

References

Kjeldsberg CR and Knight JA, "Amniotic Fluid," *Body Fluids: Laboratory Examination of Amniotic, Cerebrospinal, Seminal, Serous, and Synovial Fluids*, 3rd ed, Chapter 1, Chicago, IL: ASCP Press, 1993, 1-63.

Nipple Discharge Cytology

CPT *88104*

Related Information

Breast Biopsy *on page 40*
Cyst Fluid Cytology *on page 495*

Synonyms Breast Discharge Cytology

Test Commonly Includes Examination of smeared stained slides

Abstract Examination of nipple discharge may aid in the evaluation of inflammatory or neoplastic lesions of the breast.

Specimen Nipple discharge **COLLECTION:** Clean nipple and areola with warm saline; then gently grip subareolar area and nipple with thumb and forefinger. Using a milking action, when liquid appears, allow a pea sized drop to accumulate on the nipple apex. Place a plain glass slide (with one frosted end for labeling) upon the nipple and slide across quickly. Place slide immediately in 95% ethanol. See diagram. Prepare four to six smears, as the amount of specimen allows. If clinician has difficulty expressing liquid, allow the patient to do it herself. If an eczematous areolar lesion exists, a separate scraping should be made with a wooden spatula or tongue blade for examination to exclude Paget's disease of the breast.

CAUSES FOR REJECTION: Improper fixative, drying artifact, unlabeled slides, hypocellularity **TURNAROUND TIME:** 24 hours **SPECIAL INSTRUCTIONS:** Specify nipple discharge. Include pertinent clinical data on requisition, specifically indicating presence of subareolar mass, other dominant breast masses, or fibrocystic disease.

(Continued)

Nipple Discharge Cytology *(Continued)*

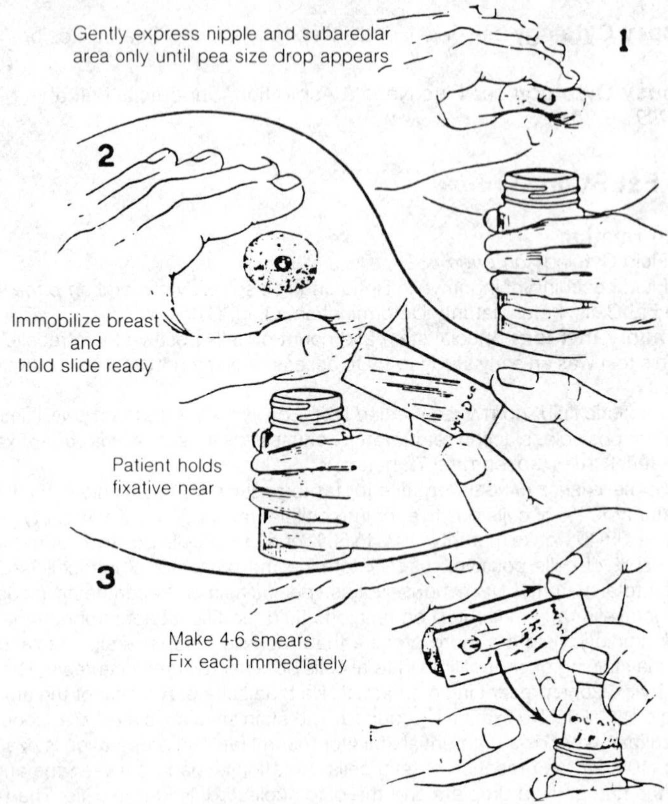
Gently express nipple and subareolar area only until pea size drop appears
1
2
Immobilize breast and hold slide ready
Patient holds fixative near
3
Make 4-6 smears
Fix each immediately

Interpretive USE: Assist in the diagnosis of neoplastic and inflammatory disease LIMITATIONS: Drying of smear before fixation will render it unsatisfactory for evaluation. Hypocellular smears with poor cytologic detail are not uncommon. ADDITIONAL INFORMATION: If material obtained is scanty and quickly air dries, submit the air-dried smear for Diff-Quik™ or Giemsa stains.

References

Fung A, Rayter Z, Fisher C, et al, "Preoperative Cytology and Mammography in Patients With Single-Duct Nipple Discharge Treated by Surgery," *Br J Surg*, 1990, 77(11):1211-2.

Johnson TL and Kini SR, "Cytologic and Clinicopathologic Features of Abnormal Nipple Secretions: 225 Cases," *Diagn Cytopathol*, 1991, 7(1):17-22.

Takada T, Matsui A, Sato Y, et al, "Nipple Discharge Cytology in Mass Screening for Breast Cancer," *Acta Cytol*, 1990, 31:161-4.

Uei Y, Watanabe Y, Hirota T, et al, "Cytologic Diagnosis of Breast Carcinoma With Nipple Discharge. Special Significance of the Spherical Cell Cluster," *Acta Cytol*, 1980, 24:522-8.

Ocular Cytology

***CPT** 88104*

Related Information

Chlamydia trachomatis Direct FA Test *on page 1173*

Conjunctival Culture *on page 803*

Viral Culture, Eye or Ocular Symptoms *on page 1202*

Synonyms *Chlamydia* Smears Cytology; Conjunctival Smear Cytology; Corneal Cytology; Eye Smear for Cytology

Applies to Inclusion Conjunctivitis

Test Commonly Includes Smears fixed in 95% ethanol and stained with Papanicolaou stain; or air-dried smears stained with Giemsa or Diff-Quik™ stain

Specimen Direct smear of ocular lesion or fine needle aspiration specimen[1,2,3] COLLECTION: Swab lesion with cotton-tipped applicator or scrape with sterile ophthalmic spatula and smear on two clean, glass slides, **immediately** spray-fix one slide, let other air dry. Label frosted end of slide with patient's name and identification number. FNA performed in standard manner (see FNA). **CAUSES FOR REJECTION:** Inadequate fixation, hypocellularity **TURNAROUND TIME:** 24 hours; 24-48 hours if fluorescent or immunohistochemical stains used

Interpretive **USE:** Diagnose trachoma-inclusion conjunctivitis and evaluate possible dysplastic or malignant conjunctival lesions; diagnose intraocular and/or orbital tumors **ADDITIONAL INFORMATION:** Diagnosis of viral and chlamydial infections is considerably improved by immunofluorescent and immunoperoxidase stains for organisms. A study of 292 palpable orbital and eyelid tumors reported a false-positive rate for malignancy of 1.6% and a false-negative rate of 1.8%.[4] Experience with intraocular fine needle aspirations is limited, but published reports exist.[3]

Footnotes

1. Scroggs MW, Johnston WW, and Klintworth GK, "Intraocular Tumors: A Cytopathologic Study," *Acta Cytol*, 1990, 34(3):401-8.
2. Arora R, Rewari R, and Betharia SM, "Fine Needle Aspiration Cytology of Orbital and Adnexal Masses," *Acta Cytol*, 1992, 36(4):483-91.
3. O'Hara BJ, Ehya H, Shields JA, et al, "Fine Needle Aspiration Biopsy in Pediatric Ophthalmic Tumors and Pseudotumors," *Acta Cytol*, 1993, 37(2):125-30.
4. Zajdela A, Vielh P, Schlienger P, et al, "Fine Needle Cytology of 292 Palpable Orbital and Eyelid Tumors," *Am J Clin Pathol*, 1990, 93:100-4.

References

Arora R, Rewari R, and Betheria SM, "Fine Needle Aspiration Cytology of Eyelid Tumors," *Acta Cytol*, 1990, 34(2):227-32.

Cristallini EG, Bolis GB, and Ottaviano P, "Fine Needle Aspiration Biopsy of Orbital Meningioma – Report of a Case," *Acta Cytol*, 1990, 34(2):236-8.

Gadkari SS, Adrianwala SD, Prayag AS, et al, "Conjunctival Impression Cytology – A Study of Normal Conjunctiva," *J Postgrad Med*, 1992, 38(1):21-3.

Paridaens AD, McCartney AC, Curling OM, et al, "Impression Cytology of Conjunctival Melanosis and Melanoma," *Br J Ophthalmol*, 1992, 76(4):198-201.

Sanderson TL, Pustai W, Shelley L, et al, "Cytologic Evaluation of Ocular Lesions," *Acta Cytol*, 1980, 24:391-400.

Tsubota K, Kajiwara K, Ugajin S, et al, "Conjunctival Brush Cytology," *Acta Cytol*, 1990, 34(2):233-5.

Oral Cavity Cytology

***CPT** 88104*

Related Information

Buccal Smear for Sex Chromatin Evaluation *on page 896*
Chromosome Analysis, Blood or Bone Marrow *on page 898*
Herpes Simplex Virus Antigen Detection *on page 1181*
Herpes Simplex Virus Culture *on page 1182*
Herpes Simplex Virus Isolation, Rapid *on page 1184*
Immunofluorescence, Skin Biopsy *on page 708*
Morphine, Urine *on page 987*
Skin Biopsies *on page 84*

Synonyms Oral Scraping Cytology; Pemphigus Smear

Test Commonly Includes Evaluation of 95% ethanol-fixed, Papanicolaou-stained smears or 95% ethanol-fixed, Aceto-Orcein-stained smears; smears may also be used for immunofluorescent studies screening for monosomies or trisomies.

Abstract Used to diagnose various conditions of the oral cavity including, but not limited to, dysplastic and neoplastic lesions.

Patient Care **PREPARATION:** Patient should rinse mouth vigorously several times before scrape is done.

Specimen For grossly visible lesion, a direct scrape of the area with a tongue blade or wooden spatula is done. **CONTAINER:** Glass slides, with one frosted end; Coplin jar filled with 95% ethanol **SAMPLING TIME:** 10-15 minutes **COLLECTION:** Scrape grossly visible lesion with spatula or tongue blade. Smear gently on labeled glass slide and fix **immediately** in 95% ethanol or with spray or liquid fixative (described in Cervical/Vaginal Cytology). For genetic assessments, a scraping is taken from the lateral buccal mucosa just above the dentate line along the anterior two-thirds of the buccal mucosa. All materials should be submitted to the laboratory with a completed requisition containing full history. **CAUSES FOR REJECTION:** Unlabeled slides, incomplete requisition, hypocellular smears **TURNAROUND TIME:** Routine: 24 hours, immunofluorescence: 48 hours **SPECIAL INSTRUCTIONS:** Requisition should include age, physical findings, his-

(Continued)

Oral Cavity Cytology *(Continued)*

tory of smoking, presence of dentures, skin lesions, reverse smoking, radiation or chemotherapy, and clinical findings suggestive of chromosomal abnormality. If pemphigus is suspected, the lesion should be scraped at the edge, where normal mucosa and affected mucosa are identified.

Interpretive USE: Diagnose dysplastic and malignant disease of the oral cavity, oral pemphigus, oral herpes or *Candida* sp, and rarely, neoplasm of minor palatal salivary glands; screen for Turner's syndrome, Klinefelter's syndrome, multiple X syndrome, and trisomy 21, 13, and 18 LIMITATIONS: Poorly fixed or hypocellular specimens METHODOLOGY: Tissue biopsy may be more rewarding in cases of neoplasm, as many oral cancers show extensive overlying hyperkeratosis (leukoplakia) which reveals only anucleate squames on smear. Buccal smears for Barr body analysis have been almost replaced by karyotyping studies. With the advent of monoclonal anticentromeric antibodies for specific chromosomes, rapid screening for Turner's syndrome, trisomy 21, 13, and 18 is becoming increasingly efficacious.

References

Bibbo M, *Comprehensive Cytopathology*, Philadelphia, PA: WB Saunders Co, 1991, 399.

Das DK, Gulati A, Bhatt NC, et al, "Fine Needle Aspiration Cytology of Oral and Pharyngeal Lesions – A Study of 45 Cases," *Acta Cytol*, 1993, 37(3):333-42.

Günhan O, Doğan N, Celasun B, et al, "Fine Needle Aspiration Cytology of Oral Cavity and Jaw Bone Lesions – A Report of 102 Cases," *Acta Cytol*, 1993, 37(2):135-41.

Medak H and Burlakow P, "Cytology of Pemphigus Vulgaris," *ASCP Check Sample®*, Chicago, IL: American Society of Clinical Pathologists, 1981.

Oral Scraping Cytology *see* Oral Cavity Cytology *on previous page*

Oropharyngeal Brushings Cytology *see* Brushings Cytology *on page 489*

Ovarian Cyst Fluid Cytology *see* Cyst Fluid Cytology *on page 495*

Pancreas Needle Aspiration Cytology *see* Fine Needle Aspiration, Deep Seated Lesions *on page 498*

Pancreatic Cyst Fluid Cytology *see* Cyst Fluid Cytology *on page 495*

Pap Smear *see* Cervical/Vaginal Cytology *on page 491*

Paracentesis Fluid Cytology *see* Body Fluids Cytology *on page 482*

Pemphigus Smear *see* Oral Cavity Cytology *on previous page*

Pericardial Fluid Cytology *see* Body Fluids Cytology *on page 482*

Peritoneal Fluid Cytology *see* Body Fluids Cytology *on page 482*

Peritoneal Washings Cytology *see* Washing Cytology *on page 515*

Pleural Fluid Cytology *see* Body Fluids Cytology *on page 482*

Pneumocystis carinii Preparation

CPT *88312*

Related Information

Bronchial Washings Cytology *on page 485*
Bronchoalveolar Lavage *on page 793*
Bronchoalveolar Lavage Cytology *on page 487*
Pneumocystis Fluorescence *on page 732*
Sputum Cytology *on page 510*
Viral Culture, Respiratory Symptoms *on page 1204*

Applies to Bronchial Aspiration for *Pneumocystis*; Bronchopulmonary Lavage for *Pneumocystis*; Induced Sputum Technique; Transbronchial Aspiration Biopsy for *Pneumocystis*; Transthoracic Needle Aspiration for *Pneumocystis*

Test Commonly Includes Papanicolaou, Diff-Quik™, Giemsa, methenamine silver stains, or monoclonal antibodies to *Pneumocystis*

Abstract Diagnosis of *Pneumocystis* pneumonia in any immunocompromised patient including AIDS patients, postorgan transplant patients, and patients receiving chemotherapeutic regimens.

Patient Care PREPARATION: Induced sputum technique: A common method used consists of using a heated (37°C) solution of 15% NaCl and 20% propylene glycol, the vapors of which the patient inhales for 15-20 minutes. Subsequent to this inhalation, the patient usually will produce a large amount of satisfactory sputum.

Specimen Lung biopsy, transthoracic needle aspirate, bronchoalveolar lavage fluid, or induced sputum. **Routine sputum is not acceptable** for identification of *Pneumocystis*. **CONTAINER:** Sterile jar, clean glass slides **COLLECTION:** For bronchoalveolar lavage, see Bronchoalveolar Lavage Cytology. For tissue lung biopsy, touch preparations made from the fresh surgical specimen are made by lightly touching the fresh tissue in rapid succession along the length of three to four slides. Induced sputum is sent to the laboratory fresh, and prepared in the laboratory. **CAUSES FOR REJECTION:** Inadequate material, unlabeled specimen, inadequate history **TURNAROUND TIME:** Routine: 24 hours; stat: 1 hour

Interpretive **USE:** Identify *Pneumocystis carinii* organisms, predominantly in immunocompromised patients **LIMITATIONS:** *Pneumocystis* preparations applied to spontaneously expectorated sputum have an extremely low yield. In about 40% of individuals with AIDS and symptomatic pneumonia caused by other agents, one may anticipate *P. carinii* in bronchoalveolar lavage fluid, unless the patient is receiving treatment for this organism prophylactically. *P. carinii* was correctly identified in 94% of adequate transbronchial biopsies, 95% of bronchoalveolar lavage cell block specimens, 88% of bronchoalveolar smears, and 79% of brushings in a series of 36 autopsy-proven cases.[1] Although a paper from the city of New York indicates that *Pneumocystis* can be reliably identified in smears of bronchial washes,[2] others recommend lavage cytologic procedures.[3,4] Martin explains that although sputum analysis remains useful for the diagnosis of *P. carinii* pneumonia in subjects who have AIDS, its utility for diagnosis of *P. carinii* in immunosuppressed patients who do not have AIDS is limited.[4] An NIH paper recommends the induced sputum technique and provides details of methods.[5] **METHODOLOGY:** In the hands of an experienced cytopathologist, *P. carinii* can be identified with Pap, Giemsa, Diff-Quik™, and methenamine silver stains. **ADDITIONAL INFORMATION:** Impaired cellular immunity is the major predisposing background for *Pneumocystis carinii* infection: AIDS, malnutrition, prematurity, immunodeficiency disease entities, and use of immunosuppressive drugs and/or corticosteroids. In subjects with AIDS, the risk of *P. carinii* correlates with the number of CD4 lymphocytes.[6]

This entity is found in patients with clinical diffuse interstitial pneumonitis. Immunocompromised patients have a high incidence of *Pneumocystis carinii* infection (as high as 44% in some series). *Pneumocystis carinii* pneumonia may be, but is not always, rapidly progressive. It may be life-threatening, so that rapid diagnosis is important to allow prompt institution of therapy. *Pneumocystis carinii* is the most frequent cause of death in children with ALL in remission, such that some institutions routinely give prophylactic trimethoprim-sulfamethoxazole to their leukemic children undergoing antineoplastic therapy. *P. carinii* is also the most common infection and most common cause of death in patients with AIDS. If a patient has been receiving prophylactic therapy for *P. carinii* and presents with pneumonitis, the cytopathologist must be notified, because if organisms are present, they will have destroyed or partially destroyed cyst walls, and examination must be extremely meticulous to identify the organisms. Under circumstances of prophylactic therapy for *Pneumocystis*, such organisms are best identified through use of an immunohistochemical or immunofluorescent method.

Serum carcinoembryonic antigen has been proposed but not proven prognostic in HIV-related *P. carinii* pneumonia.[7]

Footnotes

1. Gal AA, Klatt EC, Koss MN, et al, "The Effectiveness of Bronchoscopy in the Diagnosis of *Pneumocystis carinii* and Cytomegalovirus Pulmonary Infections in Acquired Immunodeficiency Syndrome," *Arch Pathol Lab Med*, 1987, 111:238-41.
2. Rorat E, Garcia RL, and Skolom J, "Diagnosis of *Pneumocystis carinii* Pneumonia by Cytologic Examination of Bronchial Washings," *JAMA*, 1985, 254:1950-1.
3. DeFine LA, Saleba KP, Gibson BB, et al, "Cytologic Evaluation of Bronchoalveolar Lavage Specimens in Immunosuppressed Patients With Suspected Opportunistic Infections," *Acta Cytol*, 1987, 31:235-42.
4. Martin WJ II, "Diagnostic Bronchoalveolar Lavage in Immunosuppressed Patients With New Pulmonary Infiltrates," *Mayo Clin Proc*, 1992, 67(3):296-8.
5. Masur H, Gill VJ, Ognibene FP, et al, "Diagnosis of *Pneumocystis* Pneumonia by Induced Sputum Technique in Patients Without the Acquired Immunodeficiency Syndrome," *Ann Intern Med*, 1988, 109(9):755-6.
6. Walzer PD, "*Pneumocystis carinii* – New Clinical Spectrum?" *N Engl J Med*, 1991, 324(4):263-5.
7. Bedos JP, Hignette C, Lucet JC, et al, "Serum Carcinoembryonic Antigen: A Prognostic Marker in HIV-Related *Pneumocystis carinii* Pneumonia," *Scand J Infect Dis*, 1992, 24(3):309-15.

References

Bibbo M, *Comprehensive Cytopathology*, Philadelphia, PA: WB Saunders Co, 1991.

Koss LG, *Diagnostic Cytology and Its Histopathologic Bases*, 4th ed, Philadelphia, PA: JB Lippincott Co, 1992, 741-2.

(Continued)

Pneumocystis carinii Preparation *(Continued)*

Linder J and Rennard S, *Bronchoalveolar Lavage*, Chicago, IL: ASCP Press, 1988, 94-6.
Scully RE, ed, "Case Records of the Massachusetts General Hospital," *N Engl J Med*, 1987, 316:466-75.

Polymerase Chain Reaction Detection of HSV, VZV *see* Herpes Cytology *on page 502*

Premature Rupture of Bag of Waters (BOW) *see* Amniotic Fluid Cytology *on page 482*

Premature Rupture of Fetal Membranes *see* Amniotic Fluid Cytology *on page 482*

Prostate Needle Aspiration *see* Fine Needle Aspiration, Superficial Palpable Masses *on page 499*

Pulmonary Cytology Series *see* Sputum Cytology *on this page*

Renal Cyst Fluid Cytology *see* Cyst Fluid Cytology *on page 495*

Renal Pelvic Washings Cytology *see* Urine Cytology *on page 513*

Retroperitoneal Mass Aspiration *see* Fine Needle Aspiration, Deep Seated Lesions *on page 498*

Serous Effusion Cytology *see* Body Fluids Cytology *on page 482*

Serous Fluid Cytology *see* Body Fluids Cytology *on page 482*

"Skinny" or "Thin" Needle Aspiration *see* Fine Needle Aspiration, Superficial Palpable Masses *on page 499*

Small Bowel Brushings Cytology *see* Brushings Cytology *on page 489*

Spinal Fluid Cytology *see* Cerebrospinal Fluid Cytology *on page 490*

Sputum Cytology

CPT 88104

Related Information

Bronchial Aspirate Anaerobic Culture *on page 792*
Bronchial Washings Cytology *on page 485*
Bronchoalveolar Lavage Cytology *on page 487*
Coccidioidomycosis Antibodies *on page 664*
Cytomegalovirus Antibody *on page 672*
Cytomegalovirus Culture *on page 1175*
Cytomegalovirus Isolation, Rapid *on page 1176*
Pneumocystis carinii Preparation *on page 508*
Pneumocystis Fluorescence *on page 732*
Sputum Culture *on page 849*
Sputum Fungus Culture *on page 853*
Sputum Mycobacteria Culture *on page 855*
Uric Acid, Serum *on page 378*
Viral Culture, Respiratory Symptoms *on page 1204*
Virus, Direct Detection by Fluorescent Antibody *on page 1208*

Synonyms Cytology, Sputum; Pulmonary Cytology Series

Test Commonly Includes Three to five consecutive first morning deep cough specimens

Abstract Cytopathological examination of sputum may aid in the evaluation of respiratory infections or neoplasms.

Patient Care PREPARATION: It should be explained to the patient that the contents of the collection container (fixative material) should not be consumed by the patient.

Specimen Expectorated sputum, **not saliva or nasal aspirates** CONTAINER: 50 mL screw-top plastic container; for sputum series it will contain cytologic fixative (Carbowax®) and antibiotic to prevent bacterial overgrowth COLLECTION: Upon arising the patient rinses his mouth with water and expectorates a deep cough into the container. The **first** cough specimen is the most rewarding. STORAGE INSTRUCTIONS: Specimens not delivered during laboratory hours should be placed in a refrigerator (but not allowed to freeze) and delivered as soon as possible. If it is not possible to bring unfixed material to the laboratory, a prefixed specimen (using Carbowax® or 70% ethanol) may be substituted. The best preparations are from **fresh** sputum. **CAUSES FOR REJECTION:** Specimen consists of saliva or nasal secretions **TURNAROUND TIME:** 24 hours **SPECIAL INSTRUCTIONS:** Include admitting diagnosis and pertinent clinical history on requisition (ie, age, clinical diagnosis, exposure to carcinogens, radiographic findings, and history of radiation or chemotherapy).

Interpretive **USE:** Establish the presence of neoplasm; aid in the diagnosis of respiratory infections with herpesvirus, cytomegalovirus,[1] fungal diseases, *Strongyloides*, *Echinococcus*, and *Paragonimus*; aid in the diagnosis of lipoid pneumonitis, allergic processes, hemosiderosis, Goodpasture's syndrome, asbestosis, and alveolar proteinosis **LIMITATIONS:** If no carbon bearing histiocytes are identified in the specimen, it is considered to be an unsatisfactory specimen (not a deep cough specimen). **METHODOLOGY:** Sputa may be collected fresh, without fixative; make direct smears from white flecks and blood-tinged areas;[2,3] fix smears immediately in 95% ethanol. Sputa may be collected in Carbowax® if Saccomanno's technique is used.[4] Saccomanno's technique involves the collection of sputum material in a mixture of 50% ethanol and 2% polyethylene glycol. If the patient cannot produce sputum spontaneously by deep coughing, it should be induced as described under *Pneumocystis carinii* Preparation listing. **ADDITIONAL INFORMATION:** Special stains are sometimes needed. When a pulmonary lesion is suspected, a complete sputum series should be examined. The complete sputum series consists of a fresh, early morning, deep cough specimen each day for 3-5 days. A postbronchoscopy sputum should be included in the series. The complete sputum series increases the detection of primary bronchogenic carcinoma from 45% (one specimen) to 86% (three specimens). A 12- to 24-hour specimen is collected in Carbowax® in patients with scanty sputum, when previous single sputum contains rare malignant cells, or cells highly suspicious for malignancy are present. Sputum cytology can distinguish between undifferentiated carcinoma, small cell type and other (nonsmall cell) bronchogenic carcinomas In cases where infectious agents are identified by cytology, culture confirmation is advised. Although some institutions report high accuracy of diagnosis of *P. carinii* with induced sputa, our laboratory has not been able to duplicate these results.

Footnotes

1. Lyubski S and Thorn R, "Application of Immunoperoxidase Staining to the Cell Blocks From Sputa and Bronchial Washings," *Arch Pathol Lab Med*, 1989, 113(1):94-5.
2. Risse EKJ, Van't Hof MA, and Vooijs GP, "Relationship Between Patient Characteristics and the Sputum Cytologic Diagnosis of Lung Cancer," *Acta Cytol*, 1987, 31:159-65.
3. Risse EKJ, Vooijs GP, and Van't Hof MA, "Relationship Between the Cellular Composition of Sputum and the Cytologic Diagnosis of Lung Cancer," *Acta Cytol*, 1987, 31:170-6.
4. Saccomanno G, Saunders RP, Ellis H, et al, "Concentration of Carcinoma or Atypical Cells in Sputum," *Acta Cytol*, 1963, 7:305-10.

References

Bibbo M, *Comprehensive Cytopathology*, Philadelphia, PA: WB Saunders Co, 1991, 320-98.

Bleumenfeld W and Griffiss JM, "*Pneumocystis carinii* in Sputum," *Arch Pathol Lab Med*, 1988, 112:816-20.

Dao AH, "*Entamoeba gingivalis* in Sputum Smears," *Acta Cytol*, 1985, 29:632-3.

Fontana RS, Sanderson DR, Woolner LB, et al, "Screening for Lung Cancer. A Critique of the Mayo Lung Project," *Cancer*, 1991, 67(4 Suppl):1155-64.

Gupta RK, "Diagnosis of Unsuspected Pulmonary Cryptococcosis With Sputum Cytology," *Acta Cytol*, 1985, 39:154-6.

Koss LG, *Diagnostic Cytology and Its Histopathologic Bases*, 4th ed, Philadelphia, PA: JB Lippincott Co, 1992, 687-768.

Midgley J, Parsons PA, Shanson DC, et al, "Monoclonal Immunofluorescence Compared With Silver Stain for Investigating *Pneumocystis carinii* Pneumonia," *J Clin Pathol*, 1991, 44(1):75-6.

O'Brien RF, Quinn JL, Miyahara BT, et al, "Diagnosis of *Pneumocystis carinii* Pneumonia by Induced Sputum in a City With Moderate Incidence of AIDS," *Chest*, 1989, 95(1):136-8.

Subcutaneous Fat Pad Aspiration *see* Fine Needle Aspiration, Superficial Palpable Masses *on page 499*

Subcutaneous Mass Needle Aspiration *see* Fine Needle Aspiration, Superficial Palpable Masses *on page 499*

Synovial Fluid Cytology *see* Body Fluids Cytology *on page 482*

The Bethesda System *see* Cervical/Vaginal Cytology *on page 491*

Thoracentesis Fluid Cytology *see* Body Fluids Cytology *on page 482*

Thyroid Needle Aspiration *see* Fine Needle Aspiration, Superficial Palpable Masses *on page 499*

Thyroid Needle Aspiration Cytology *see* Fine Needle Aspiration, Deep Seated Lesions *on page 498*

Tracheal and Bronchial Washings *see* Bronchial Washings Cytology *on page 485*

Tracheal Aspiration Cytology *see* Bronchial Washings Cytology *on page 485*

Tracheal Brushings Cytology *see* Brushings Cytology *on page 489*

Transbronchial Aspiration Biopsy for *Pneumocystis* *see Pneumocystis carinii* Preparation *on page 508*

Transbronchial Fine Needle Aspiration

***CPT** 88170*

Related Information

Bronchoalveolar Lavage Cytology *on page 487*
Fine Needle Aspiration, Deep Seated Lesions *on page 498*
Fine Needle Aspiration, Superficial Palpable Masses *on page 499*

Synonyms Fine Needle Aspiration of Lung; Wang Needle Biopsy of Lung

Test Commonly Includes Examination of direct air-dried, Diff-Quik™ stained or 95% ethanol-fixed, Papanicolaou stained smears; cytospin or cell block preparations may be included.

Abstract Cytopathological examination of transbronchial aspirates may aid in the evaluation of infections or neoplastic central pulmonary lesions.

Patient Care PREPARATION: Radiographic studies (ie, CT scan) for exact location of lesion. Informed consent from patient. Topical anesthesia of the pharynx and upper respiratory tree is necessary. Sedation may be used.

Specimen Needle aspirate smears; needle rinse in balanced salt solution CONTAINER: Plain glass slides with frosted end for labeling; Coplin jar containing 95% ethanol; 50 mL plastic centrifuge tube containing 25 mL balanced salt solution SAMPLING TIME: 1-2 hours COLLECTION: Fiberoptic bronchoscopic placement of a long flexible tube with attached fine needle and subsequent placement of needle into mass through the bronchial wall;[1,2] subsequent aspiration with preparation of aspirated material as described under Fine Needle Aspiration, Superficial Palpable Masses. STORAGE INSTRUCTIONS: All material should be forwarded to the Cytology Laboratory as soon as possible. The needle rinse material should be refrigerated if immediate delivery to the laboratory is not possible. This technique may also be applied to submucosal gastrointestinal lesions with an endoscope.[3] CAUSES FOR REJECTION: Improper labeling, insufficient material, insufficient clinical information TURNAROUND TIME: Routine: 24 hours SPECIAL INSTRUCTIONS: The diagnoses of this type of biopsy depends greatly on the skill of the pulmonologist who is obtaining the specimen. Bloody specimens should be smeared as soon as possible to avoid clotting. If the specimen appears to consist almost entirely of blood, it may be entirely placed in the salt solution for cell block preparation. Requisition should contain all pertinent clinical information, particularly if infection is suspected, and culture to exclude tuberculosis and histoplasmosis might be indicated in selected cases.

Interpretive USE: Diagnose neoplastic or infectious central pulmonary lesions LIMITATIONS: Sampling error may be as high as 10% to 25%. Lack of lymphocytes in transbronchial aspirates should be regarded as tantamount to an inadequate specimen.[4] CONTRAINDICATIONS: Abnormal coagulation profile; severe hypoxemia with impending respiratory failure ADDITIONAL INFORMATION: Bronchoalveolar lavage and/or bronchial brushings are usually performed in association with the FNA. At times, a simultaneous transbronchial biopsy may also be obtained. Lesions which ulcerate the bronchial mucosa may be more accessible to direct forceps tissue biopsy or bronchial brushing. An alternative approach to deep seated thoracic lesions is a percutaneous CT-guided fine needle aspiration. Although transbronchial FNA specimens tend to be scanty, specimens provided by experienced pulmonologists often include sufficient and adequate material to permit cytologic diagnosis. A recent review at the Mayo Clinic found transbronchial fine needle aspiration of benefit when a submucosal mass was present, extrinsic compression of bronchi was present, or when an extrabronchial mass was found radiographically.[5]

Footnotes

1. Horsley JR, Miller RE, and Amy RW, "Bronchial Submucosal Needle Aspiration Performed Through the Fiberoptic Bronchoscope," *Acta Cytol*, 1984, 28:211-7.
2. Rosenthal DL and Wallace JM, "Fine Needle Aspiration of Pulmonary Lesions in Fiberoptic Bronchoscopy," *Acta Cytol*, 1984, 28:203-10.

3. Ingoldby CJH, Mason MK, and Hall RI, "Endoscopic Needle Aspiration Cytology: A New Method for the Diagnosis of Upper Gastrointestinal Cancer," *Gut*, 1987, 28:1142-4.
4. Baker JJ, Solanki PH, Schenk DA, et al, "Transbronchial Fine Needle Aspiration of the Mediastinum – Importance of Lymphocytes as an Indicator of Specimen Adequacy," *Acta Cytol*, 1990, 34(4):517-23.
5. Gay PC and Brutinel WM, "Transbronchial Needle Aspiration in the Practice of Bronchoscopy," *Mayo Clin Proc*, 1989, 64(2):158-62.

References

Murray N, *Respiratory Medicine*, New York, NY: WB Saunders Co, 1988.
Wagner ED, Ramzy I, Greenberg SD, et al, "Transbronchial Fine Needle Aspiration, Reliability and Limitations" *Am J Clin Pathol*, 1989, 92(1):36-50.

Transthoracic Needle Aspiration for *Pneumocystis* *see* Pneumocystis carinii Preparation *on page 508*

Tzanck Smear *see* Herpes Cytology *on page 502*

Ultrasound Guided FNA *see* Fine Needle Aspiration, Deep Seated Lesions *on page 498*

Ureteral Brushings Cytology *see* Brushings Cytology *on page 489*

Ureteral Washings Cytology *see* Urine Cytology *on this page*

Urine Cytology

CPT *88104*

Related Information

Cytomegalic Inclusion Disease Cytology *on page 496*
Cytomegalovirus Culture *on page 1175*
Cytomegalovirus Isolation, Rapid *on page 1176*
Herpes Simplex Virus Antigen Detection *on page 1181*
Ova and Parasites, Urine *on page 839*
Tumor Aneuploidy by Flow Cytometry *on page 88*
Urine Fungus Culture *on page 883*
Viral Culture, Urine *on page 1207*

Applies to Bladder, Ureteral, and Pelvicocalyceal Barbotage Specimens; Bladder Washings Cytology; Catheterized Urine Cytology; Renal Pelvic Washings Cytology; Ureteral Washings Cytology; Voided Urine Cytology

Test Commonly Includes Smears, cytocentrifuge preparations, millipore filter preparations, flow cytometry, immunocytochemistry

Abstract Urine cytology may be useful in the evaluation of inflammatory and neoplastic conditions in the urinary system.

Patient Care PREPARATION: Hydrate patient (give several glasses of water) 30 minutes to 1 hour prior to collection. Patient should **not** have had mineral oil cathartics. Inform patient to discard first early morning voided urine. Taking 1 g vitamin C at bedtime the night before the examination can help to improve cell preservation.

Specimen Voided or catheterized urine; intraoperative washings of urinary bladder, ureters, or renal pelvis; ileal conduit urine CONTAINER: 100 mL plastic, leakproof, screw-top container; specimen should be submitted in the fresh state as soon as possible to the Cytology Laboratory. SAMPLING TIME: Ideally, the specimen should be as fresh as possible. Urine which has been in the bladder for prolonged periods shows extensive cellular degeneration. Specimens sitting out fresh at room temperature demonstrate cellular degeneration within 1 hour. COLLECTION: For detection of upper urinary tract lesions: Catheterize ureters to pelvis for suspected renal or pelvic lesions. Repeat procedure using either ureter for control. For ureteral lesion, catheterize ureter to a point just below the level of the suspected lesion. Catheterize other ureter for control. Collect urine for 30 minutes. Label appropriately, right and left ureteral or right and left pelvic specimen. Bring specimen immediately to the Cytology Laboratory. STORAGE INSTRUCTIONS: If the specimen cannot be brought immediately to the Cytology Laboratory, it must be refrigerated at 4°C. CAUSES FOR REJECTION: 24-hour collection, prolonged period at room temperature with extensive degeneration of cellular detail, unlabeled specimen, leaking container, contaminated specimen SPECIAL INSTRUCTIONS: First morning voided specimen is unsatisfactory, due to cellular degeneration. Bladder washings should not be collected in a hypotonic solution. Voided urine is the specimen of choice for male patients, and catheterized urine is the specimen of choice for female patients (to avoid vaginal-vulvar squamous contamination). If cytomegalovirus infection is suspected, this concern should be noted on the requisition.

(Continued)

Urine Cytology *(Continued)*

Interpretive USE: Indicate presence of primary benign or malignant as well as metastatic disease; routine surveillance for recurrent transitional cell carcinoma; follow-up patients receiving intravesicular therapy for transitional cell carcinoma; aid in diagnoses of infections with herpesvirus, polymovirus, cytomegalovirus, fungal diseases, and *Schistosoma*; detect malacoplakia, renal hemosiderosis, hemolytic anemia, cerebral metachromatic leukodystrophy, and endometriosis of the urinary tract LIMITATIONS: Low grade (grade 1) papillary transitional cell carcinoma cannot be diagnosed reliably by cytology alone. Polyoma virus infections may sometimes be confused with high grade transitional cell carcinoma.[1] Recent instrumentation and calculi may produce atypical changes in urothelial cells simulating malignancy. History of instrumentation of the bladder must be provided. Numerous chemotherapeutic agents (Cytoxan®, thiotepa, BCG) may produce cell changes almost indistinguishable from true dysplasia or neoplasia. For these reasons, complete clinical history is of utmost importance. Urine cytology has a very low sensitivity for detection of primary renal and prostate neoplasms. Diagnostic accuracy of urine cytology appears closely related to the grade of bladder tumors, pretreatment and post-treatment status, and minimally to the type of therapy (radiation, chemotherapy, surgery).[2] METHODOLOGY: Two preparatory methods to evaluate urine cytology have been compared.[3] ADDITIONAL INFORMATION: Voided urine is much preferred over a catheterized sample due to atypical cell changes induced by trauma of the catheter itself. Barbotage (instilled saline insufflated with air in tiny bubbles to gently exfoliate the urothelium) cytology has the highest sensitivity for the detection of transitional cell carcinoma. Although poorly-differentiated carcinomas are diagnosed with relative ease, well-differentiated (low grade) carcinomas may not be diagnosed by routine cytologic methods. DNA flow cytometry (DNA analysis) may detect the presence of an aneuploid population of cells with or without an increased S-phase. It is a sensitive indicator for recurrent transitional neoplasia but is of no use in cases in which the primary transitional cell carcinoma is diploid. Maximum sensitivity is obtained using both cell morphology and DNA analysis. Renal tubular cells may be found in the urine secondary to acute tubular injury.[4] Lymphomas may rarely be diagnosed in urine cytology.[5]

Footnotes

1. Boon ME, van Keep J-PM, and Kok LP, "Polyomavirus Infection Versus High-Grade Bladder Carcinoma - The Importance of Cytologic and Comparative Morphometric Studies of Plastic-Embedded Voided Urine Sediments," *Acta Cytol*, 1989, 33(6):887-93.
2. Wiener HG, Vooijs GP, van't Hof-Grootenboer B, "Accuracy of Urinary Cytology in the Diagnosis of Primary and Recurrent Bladder Cancer," *Acta Cytol*, 1993, 37(2):163-9.
3. Dhundee J and Rigby HS, "Comparison of Two Preparatory Techniques for Urine Cytology," *J Clin Pathol*, 1990, 43(12):1034-5.
4. Tanaka T, Yoshimi N, Sawada K, et al, "Ki-1-Positive Large Cell Anaplastic Lymphoma Diagnosed by Urinary Cytology - A Case Report," *Acta Cytol*, 1993, 37(4):520.
5. Racusen LC and Solez K, "Exfoliation of Renal Tubular Cells," *Mod Pathol*, 1991, 4(3):368.

References

Betz SA, See WA, and Cohen MB, "Granulomatous Inflammation in Bladder Wash Specimens After Intravesical Bacillus Calmette-Guérin Therapy for Transitional Cell Carcinoma of the Bladder," *Am J Clin Pathol*, 1993, 99(3):244-8.

Crosby JH, Allsbrook WC Jr, Koss LG, et al, "Cytologic Detection of Urothelial Cancer and Other Abnormalities in a Cohort of Workers Exposed to Aromatic Amines," *Acta Cytol*, 1991, 35(3):263.

Eldidi MM and Patten SF, "New Cytologic Classification of Normal Urothelial Cells: An Analytical and Morphometric Study," *Acta Cytol*, 1982, 26:725.

Kern W, "The Diagnostic Accuracy of Sputum and Urine Cytology," *Acta Cytol*, 1988, 32:651-4.

Koss LG, Czerniak B, Herz F, et al, "Flow Cytometric Measurements of DNA and Other Cell Components in Human Tumors: A Critical Appraisal," *Hum Pathol*, 1989, 20(6):528-48.

Murphy WM, "Current Status of Urinary Cytology in the Evaluation of Bladder Neoplasms," *Acta Cytol*, 1990, 21(9):886.

Murphy WM, "Urinary Cytology in Diagnostic Pathology," *Diagn Cytopathol*, 1985, 1:173-5.

Vaginal Cytology *see* Cervical/Vaginal Cytology *on page 491*

Vakutage® *see* Endometrial Cytology *on page 497*

Ventricular Tap Cytology *see* Cerebrospinal Fluid Cytology *on page 490*

Viral Study *see* Cytomegalic Inclusion Disease Cytology *on page 496*

Vira Pap® *see* Cervical/Vaginal Cytology *on page 491*

Vira Type® *see* Cervical/Vaginal Cytology *on page 491*

Voided Urine Cytology *see* Urine Cytology *on page 513*

Vulvar Cytology *see* Cervical/Vaginal Cytology *on page 491*

Wang Needle Biopsy of Lung *see* Transbronchial Fine Needle Aspiration *on page 512*

Washing Cytology

CPT *88104*

Related Information

Body Fluid *on page 145*
Body Fluids Cytology *on page 482*

Synonyms Lavage Cytology

Applies to Colon Washings Cytology; Esophageal Washings Cytology; Gastric Washings Cytology; Peritoneal Washings Cytology

Test Commonly Includes Smears, cytocentrifuge preparations, filter preparations, cell block

Abstract Used to establish the presence of inflammatory or neoplastic lesions in various body sites.

Patient Care PREPARATION: For gastric or esophageal washings, patient must be fasting at least 12 hours prior to procedure. Soft supper the night before, water ad lib 1 hour before. For intubation patient should be sitting upright. Dentures, if worn, should be removed. Colon washings specimens should be collected prior to barium examination. If this is not possible, wait at least 24 hours after the barium exam before attempting a cytologic study.

Specimen Gastric washings, colon washings, esophageal washings, peritoneal washings CONTAINER: Sterile, plastic, screw-top container, 50 mL; may contain 50% ethanol; **packed in ice** COLLECTION: Gastric washing: Evaluation for neoplasm: Collect resting gastric contents and discard. Then instill 300 mL of a balanced salt solution through the gastric tube. Have patient then sit, lie on back, lie on stomach, lie on right side, and lie on left side. Aspirate as much of injected saline as possible and place in container packed in ice. Label with patient name, identification number, and date. Deliver immediately on ice to the Cytology Laboratory.

Peritoneal washings: Wash peritoneal site vigorously with several hundred mL of a balanced salt solution. Retrieve as much as possible and submit as above, labeled by anatomic site (ie, "subdiaphragm", "cul-de-sac", "left gutter wash", "right gutter wash").

STORAGE INSTRUCTIONS: Due to rapid degeneration of cellular material, storage, even at 4°C for any extended length of time, is not recommended. SPECIAL INSTRUCTIONS: Include pertinent clinical history on requisition (eg, suspicion for neoplasm, history of peptic ulcer, endoscopic findings).

Interpretive USE: Establish the presence of primary or metastatic neoplasms, reactive processes, or infectious disease. Aid in staging of gynecologic and gastrointestinal neoplasms. LIMITATIONS: Nondiagnostic if epithelium is not present or poorly preserved; if specimen is grossly contaminated with food or barium sulfate; if no mesothelial cells are identified in peritoneal washings, the specimen is unsatisfactory; may be of limited value in intestinal cases where the lesion is submucosal; a Wang transmucosal needle aspirate may be helpful (see Transbronchial Needle Aspirate Cytology). CONTRAINDICATIONS: Collection of specimen at a time when it cannot be immediately processed. ADDITIONAL INFORMATION: Lavage is not as sensitive or specific as endoscopically directed brushings or biopsy (aspiration biopsy or tissue forceps biopsy). However, a complete set of peritoneal, pelvic, and diaphragmatic washings are an essential part of the staging of gynecologic, particularly ovarian carcinomas.

References

Drake M, "Esophageal and Gastric Cytology," *Compendium on Diagnostic Cytology*, 6th ed, Wied GL, Keebler CM, Koss LG, et al, eds, Chicago, IL: Tutorials of Cytology, 1988, 364-78.

Gupta RK and Rogers KE, "Endoscopic Cytology and Biopsy in the Diagnosis of Gastroesophageal Malignancy," *Acta Cytol*, 1983, 27:17-22.

Ingoldby CJH, Mason MK, and Hall RI, "Endoscopic Needle Aspiration Cytology: A New Method for the Diagnosis of Upper Gastrointestinal Cancer," *Gut*, 1987, 28:1142-4.

Ishi H, Yamamoto R, Tatsuta M, et al, "Evaluation of Fine Needle Aspiration Biopsy Under Direct Vision Gastrofiberoscopy in Diagnosis of Diffusely Infiltrative Carcinoma of the Stomach," *Cancer*, 1986, 57:1365-9.

Layfield LJ, Reichman A, and Weinstein WM, "Endoscopically Directed Fine Needle Aspiration Biopsy of Gastric and Esophageal Lesions," *Acta Cytol*, 1992, 36(1):69-74.

Martin JK and Goether JR, "Abdominal Fluid Cytology in Patients With Gastrointestinal Malignant Lesions," *Acta Cytol*, 1986, 61:467-71.

Ravinsky E, "Cytology of Peritoneal Washings in Gynecologic Patients," *Acta Cytol*, 1986, 30:8-16.

(Continued)

Washing Cytology *(Continued)*

Shida S and Ishioka K, "Gastric Cytology: Its Evaluation for the Diagnosis of Early Gastric Cancer," *Compendium on Diagnostic Cytology*, 6th ed, Wied GL, Keebler CM, Koss LG, et al, eds, Chicago, IL: Tutorials of Cytology, 1988, 382-7.

Wang HH, Jonasson JG, and Ducatman BS, "Brushing Cytology of the Upper Gastrointestinal Tract: Obsolete or Not?" *Acta Cytol*, 1991, 35(2):195-8.

HEMATOLOGY

Wayne R. DeMott, MD
Lowell L. Tilzer, MD, PhD

Hematology is the study of blood and bone marrow, and the physiologic and biochemical processes that affect the quantity and function of the cellular components of blood: red cells, white cells, and platelets. It has deep roots in morphology and recently has witnessed great advances in the understanding of the biochemical basis of such disorders as thalassemia, the hemoglobinopathies, and the enzyme deficiency anemias.

Table of Unit Equivalency

Procedure	Conventional Unit	SI Equivalent
Red blood cell count	$10^6/mm^3$	$10^{12}/L$
White blood cell count	$10^3/mm^3$	$10^9/L$
Platelet count	$10^3/mm^3$	$10^9/L$
Reticulocyte count	% (or .../mm^3)	% (or ... x $10^9/L$)
Hemoglobin	g/100 mL	g/dL
Mean cell volume		fL
Mean cell hemoglobin		pg
Mean cell hemoglobin concentration	%	g/dL
Mean cell diameter		μm
Plasma hemoglobin	mg/100 mL	mg/L
Vitamin B_{12}, Serum	ng/L	pmol/L
Folate, serum	μg/L	nmol/L

Absolute Eosinophil Count *see* Eosinophil Count *on page 539*

Acid β-Galactosidase *see* Tests for Uncommon Inherited Diseases of Metabolism and Cell Structure *on page 605*

Acid Elution for Fetal Hemoglobin *see* Kleihauer-Betke *on page 563*

Acid-Fast, Ziehl-Neelsen, Stain for Intracellular Pigment *see* Leukocyte Cytochemistry *on page 567*

Acidified Serum Test *see* Ham Test *on page 549*

Acid Phosphatase Stain With and Without Tartrate *see* Leukocyte Cytochemistry *on page 567*

Acid Phosphatase, Tartrate Resistant, Leukocytes *see* Tartrate Resistant Leukocyte Acid Phosphatase *on page 603*

Acid Serum Test *see* Ham Test *on page 549*

Acid Serum Test for PNH *see* Ham Test *on page 549*

Adrenal Function Eosinophil Count *see* Thorn Test *on page 609*

Alpha-Naphthyl Esterase Stain With and Without Fluoride *see* Leukocyte Cytochemistry *on page 567*

Amyloid *see* Leukocyte Cytochemistry *on page 567*

Antipernicious Anemia Factor *see* Vitamin B_{12} *on page 612*

APT Test

CPT 83033

Synonyms Apt Test for Swallowed Blood Syndrome; Fetal Hemoglobin Test in Newborn

Abstract This test uses alkali denaturation of fetal hemoglobin to determine if blood present in the stool of a newborn is the result of swallowing maternal blood or is due to perinatal/neonatal GI hemorrhage.

Specimen Blood stained diaper, grossly bloody (red) stool, or bloody vomitus or mucus **CONTAINER:** Use clean uncontaminated glass or plastic container for specimen or send blood stained diaper. **CAUSES FOR REJECTION:** Reject if specimen received is not grossly bloody or if there is evidence of melena/coffee ground aspirate.

Interpretive **REFERENCE RANGE:** Report will provide indication if blood is of maternal or infant origin (adult or fetal hemoglobin). **USE:** Diagnose swallowed blood syndrome and differentiate this condition from gastrointestinal hemorrhage in the newborn. The test is performed infrequently. **LIMITATIONS:** The specimen must be grossly bloody, red, not tarry. Test performed in cases of melena or with coffee ground material (denatured blood) may produce a false-positive as oxyhemoglobin has been converted to hematin.[1] **METHODOLOGY:** Dissolved blood (one volume of bloody stool or vomitus mixed with five volumes of water) is treated with 1% NaOH, 1-4 mL of hemolysate (alkali denaturation test). The mixture is then centrifuged at 2000 rpm for 1-2 minutes. Fetal hemoglobin is alkali resistant, and the solution will remain pink. Maternal blood will be converted to alkaline hematin in 1-2 minutes, and the solution becomes yellow brown. Thus, if the supernatant remains pink (indicative of fetal blood), additional clinical investigation must be pursued.[2] The newborn's blood should be tested concurrently as a control to exclude the possibility of adult Hgb in the test infant. **ADDITIONAL INFORMATION:** In the swallowed blood syndrome, blood or bloody stools are passed usually on the second or third day of life. The blood may be swallowed during delivery or may be from a fissure of the mother's nipple. This condition must be differentiated from gastrointestinal hemorrhage of the newborn. The test is based on the fact that the infant's blood contains >60% fetal hemoglobin that is alkali resistant. Swallowed blood of maternal origin contains adult hemoglobin which is converted to brownish alkaline hematin on the addition of alkali. In a study of 94 infants younger than 30 days of age with gastrointestinal bleeding, 49 had no obvious source of bleeding, in 19 definite evidence of a bleeding diathesis was found, and in 12 hematemesis or melena resulted from previously swallowed maternal blood as demonstrated by the Apt Test.[3]

Footnotes

1. Apt L and Downey WS, "Melena Neonatorum: The Swallowed Blood Syndrome. A Simple Test for the Differentiation of Adult and Fetal Hemoglobin in Bloody Stools," *J Pediatr*, 1955, 47:6-12.
2. Glader BE, "Recognition of Anemia and Red Blood Cell Disorders During Infancy," *Perinatal Hematology*, Vol 21, Chapter 6, *Methods in Hematology*, Alter BD, ed, New York, NY: Churchill Livingstone, 1989, 158-9.

3. Sherman NJ and Clatworthy HW Jr, "Gastrointestinal Bleeding in Neonates: A Study of 94 Cases," *Surgery*, 1967, 62:614-9.

References

Apt L, "Melena Neonatorum: An Experimental Study of the Effect of the Oral Administration of Blood on the Stools," *J Pediatr*, 1955, 47:1-5.

Berry R and Perrault J, "Gastrointestinal Bleeding," *Pediatric Gastrointestinal Disease: Pathophysiology-Diagnosis-Management*, Vol 1, Chapter 10, Walker WA, Durie PR, Hamilton JR, et al, eds, Philadelphia, PA: BC Decker Inc, 1991, 111-31.

Mougenot JF, "Gastrointestinal Haemorrhage," *Paediatric Gastroenterology*, Chapter 38, New York, NY: Oxford University Press, 1992, 446-57.

Apt Test for Swallowed Blood Syndrome *see* APT Test *on previous page*

Ascitic Fluid Analysis *see* Body Fluids Analysis, Cell Count *on page 523*

ASD Chloroacetate Esterase Stain *see* Leukocyte Cytochemistry *on page 567*

Autohemolysis Test

***CPT** 86940 (screen); 86941 (incubated)*

Related Information

Glucose-6-Phosphate Dehydrogenase, Quantitative, Blood *on page 547*
Glucose-6-Phosphate Dehydrogenase Screen, Blood *on page 548*
Osmotic Fragility *on page 573*
Osmotic Fragility, Incubated *on page 575*
Peripheral Blood: Red Blood Cell Morphology *on page 584*
Red Blood Cell Enzyme Deficiency, Quantitative *on page 591*

Abstract Autohemolysis test measures the degree to which patient's red cells lyse without additives, with glucose, and with ATP. Sterile conditions are required. Test has some application to diagnosis of hereditary spherocytosis and RBC enzyme deficiencies but is tedious to perform and is of limited value.

Specimen Defibrinated sterile blood **CONTAINER:** Sterile syringe **COLLECTION:** Using sterile technique, 25 mL of blood is drawn and immediately defibrinated by swirling in a bottle which contains glass beads. **STORAGE INSTRUCTIONS:** Specimen is immediately taken to the laboratory, blood defibrinated, and tubes prepared for incubation. **CAUSES FOR REJECTION:** Specimen hemolyzed, specimen clotted, specimen more than 5 minutes in transit, specimen with bacteria (as from a patient with septicemia) **SPECIAL INSTRUCTIONS:** Defibrinated blood must usually be obtained by laboratory personnel.

Interpretive **REFERENCE RANGE:** Percent of red cell lysis at 48 hours: blood alone: 0.2-2.0; blood and 10% glucose: 0-0.9; blood and 0.4M ATP: 0.5-2.5 **USE:** Diagnose hereditary spherocytosis; detect conditions producing spontaneous hemolysis, particularly hereditary spherocytosis; categorize RBC enzyme deficiencies; work up hemolytic anemia **LIMITATIONS:** Large sample of blood required and obtained by a trauma-free venipuncture. Test lacks sensitivity and specificity. While this test finds application in the diagnosis of hereditary spherocytosis, it has largely been supplanted by specific enzyme spot assays for the diagnosis of nonspherocytic congenital hemolytic anemia.[1,2] **CONTRAINDICATIONS:** Bacteremic patients **METHODOLOGY:** Defibrinated blood from patient and from a control are incubated without additives, with glucose, and with ATP. Subsequently absorbance determinations are used to calculate the percent hemolysis. Procedure is technically laborious. Sterile glassware must be used. **ADDITIONAL INFORMATION:** The test must always be run with and compared to a control. Test should be run in duplicate. This may allow detection of reagent inactivity or bacterial contamination of specimen or reagent. It is difficult to maintain sterility but also full activity of ATP. Normal red cells hemolyze minimally when incubated. G-6-PD deficient RBCs (Dacie type I hemolytic anemia) have increased autohemolysis which corrects significantly with glucose or ATP. Pyruvate kinase deficiency (Dacie type II hemolytic anemia) has increased autohemolysis which does not correct and may be aggravated with glucose but does correct toward normal with ATP. Triosephosphate isomerase deficiency corrects completely with glucose or ATP. Hereditary spherocytosis is a type I hemolytic anemia; the addition of glucose usually, but not always, decreases the rate of autohemolysis to about the same proportion as normal blood.

Glucose by itself can induce hemolysis in the autohemolysis test in patients with hereditary spherocytosis.[3] Streichman et al suggest this was the result of a direct effect of glucose on already swollen red cells. They found that the problem could be ameliorated by adding NaCl to isotonic conditions. With autoimmune hemolytic anemia, autohemolysis may be increased,

(Continued)

Autohemolysis Test *(Continued)*

but the effect of adding glucose is unpredictable. Autohemolysis is usually normal in cases of paroxysmal nocturnal hemoglobinuria. Hemolytic anemia due to oxidant drugs is usually associated with increased autohemolysis. Generally, failure of glucose to decrease autohemolysis indicates presence of a glycolytic block. Schröter et al have found the autohemolysis test, along with the fresh osmotic fragility test, to be highly diagnostic for hereditary spherocytosis in the newborn.[4] This is especially important since the MCHC may not be elevated in hereditary spherocytosis in the newborn and because spherocytes are not uncommon in newborns without hereditary spherocytosis. See table.

Autohemolysis Test

Condition	Incubation 37°C 48 Hours	Incubation + 10% Glucose	Incubation + ATP
Normal	0.2%–2.0%	0.0%–0.9%	0.5%–2.5%
G-6-PD deficiency	3.0%–5.0%	Normal	Normal
Pyruvate kinase deficiency	12%–16%	12%–16%	Normal
Hereditary spherocytosis	12.0%–15.0%	3.0%–5.0%	3.0%–5.0%

Footnotes

1. Beutler E, "Why Has the Autohemolysis Test Not Gone the Way of the Cephalin Flocculation Test?" *Blood*, 1978, 51:109-10.
2. Fukagawa N, Friedman S, Gill FM, et al, "Hereditary Spherocytosis With Normal Osmotic Fragility After Incubation: Is the Autohemolysis Test Really Obsolete?" *JAMA*, 1979, 242:63-4.
3. Streichman S, Cohen S, and Tatarsky J, "Glucose-Induced Hemolysis of Spheric Red Blood Cells in Hereditary Spherocytosis: New Aspects of the Autohemolysis Test," *Am J Clin Pathol*, 1984, 81:122-7.
4. Schröter W and Kahsnitz E, "Diagnosis of Hereditary Spherocytosis in Newborn Infants," *J Pediatr*, 1983, 103:460-3.

References

Dacie J, "Haemolytic Anaemia in Man: Clinical Findings, Blood Picture and Other Pathological Changes, Methods of Investigation, Diagnosis and Treatment," *The Haemolytic Anaemias: The Hereditary Haemolytic Anaemias*, Vol 1, Part 1, Chapter 3, New York, NY: Churchill Livingstone, 1985, 101-5.

Dacie JV and Lewis SM, *Practical Haematology*, 7th ed, New York, NY: Churchill Livingstone, 1991, 202-4.

Grimes AJ, Leets I, and Dacie JV, "The Autohemolysis Test: Appraisal of the Method for the Diagnosis of Pyruvate Kinase Deficiency and the Effect of pH and Additives," *Br J Haematol*, 1968, 14:309-22.

Lee GR, "The Hemolytic Disorders: General Considerations," *Wintrobe's Clinical Hematology*, Chapter 32, Lee RG, Bithell TC, Foerster J, et al, eds, Philadelphia, PA: Lea & Febiger, 1993, 958-9.

Selwyn J and Dacie J, "Autohemolysis and Other Changes Resulting From the Incubation *In Vitro* of Red Cells From Patients With Congenital Hemolytic Anemia," *Blood*, 1954, 9:414.

Automated Differential *see* Peripheral Blood: Differential Leukocyte Count *on page 576*

B_{12} *see* Vitamin B_{12} *on page 612*

Bacteremia Detection, Buffy Coat Micromethod

CPT 85009

Related Information

Bacterial Antigens, Rapid Detection Methods *on page 775*
Blood Culture, Aerobic and Anaerobic *on page 784*
Buffy Coat Smear Study of Peripheral Blood *on page 526*
Microfilariae, Peripheral Blood Preparation *on page 571*
Peripheral Blood: Differential Leukocyte Count *on page 576*

Synonyms Buffy Coat Method for Detection of Bacteremia; Microbuffy Coat Method for Detection of Bacteremia; Septicemia Detection, Buffy Coat Micromethod

Abstract Glass slide smears of buffy coat of blood (relatively concentrated white cells) are stained for pathogenic microorganisms. The procedure is a simple, quick, cost efficient method that can assist in establishing the presence of bacteremia but lacks sensitivity and to some extent, specificity.

Specimen Blood **CONTAINER:** Heparinized capillary tubes **COLLECTION:** Transport immediately to the laboratory for processing. Blood should be cultured concurrently. **TURNAROUND TIME:** 1-2 hours

Interpretive **REFERENCE RANGE:** Negative **POSSIBLE PANIC RANGE:** Positive **USE:** Aid in the diagnosis of acute bacterial blood infection, bacteremia **LIMITATIONS:** There have been conflicting reports on the usefulness of this technique. A high incidence of false-positives and negatives has been reported.[1] **METHODOLOGY:** Gram stain is applied to smear of buffy coat; Wright stain of buffy coat can show histoplasmosis; Ziehl-Neelsen stain can show mycobacteria **ADDITIONAL INFORMATION:** A variety of unusual organisms, sites of infection and clinical circumstances may produce septicemia. Attempts to stain buffy coat of blood samples obtained from children with suspected bacteremia using acridine orange (a DNA intercalating agent) has proven to be of low diagnostic efficiency.[2] The QBC® tube (quantitative buffy coat, utilizing tubes precoated with acridine orange) has been considered to have value in the rapid detection of *Wuchereria bancrofti* microfilarial organisms[3] but had low sensitivity and was frequently (40% of specimens) unable to provide species identification when utilized for malaria case identification in the field.[4] The ability to detect and diagnose *Mycobacterium avium-intracellulare* and *Cryptococcus neoformans* using both a stain of the buffy coat and culture of the buffy coat from AIDS patients has been studied. The results showed that culture of buffy coat was much more effective in early diagnosis of those organisms than examining the stained buffy coat smear microscopically.[5] Another group found that use of the buffy coat smear was rapid and specific for detection of *Mycobacterium avium* complex infection in AIDS patients although lacking in sensitivity (positive predictive value of 100%, negative predictive value of 22%).[6] Buffy coat smears have been employed in the diagnosis of histoplasmosis in AIDS patients[7] and in the detection of *Malassezia* sp deep-line catheter-associated sepsis.[8]

Footnotes

1. Coppen MJ, Noble CJ, and Aubrey C, "Evaluation of Buffy Coat Microscopy for the Early Diagnosis of Bacteremia," *J Clin Pathol*, 1981, 34:1375-7.
2. Henrickson KJ, Powell KR, and Ryan DH, "Evaluation of Acridine Orange Stained Buffy Coat Smears for Identification of Bacteremia in Children," *J Pediatr*, 1988, 112(1):65-6.
3. Freedman DO and Berry RS, "Rapid Diagnosis of Bancroftian Filariasis by Acridine Orange Staining of Centrifuged Parasites," *Am J Trop Med Hyg*, 1992, 47(6):787-93.
4. Mak JW, Normaznah Y, and Chiang GL, "Comparison of the Quantitative Buffy Coat Technique With the Conventional Thick Blood Film Technique for Malaria Case Detection in the Field," *Singapore Med J*, 1992, 33(5):452-4.
5. Danseker B and Boltone EJ, "Mycobacteria and Cryptococci Cultured From the Buffy Coat of AIDS Patients Prior to Symptomatology: A Rationale for Early Therapy," *AIDS Res Hum Retroviruses*, 1986, 2:343-8.
6. Nussbaum JM, Dealist C, Lewis W, et al, "Rapid Diagnosis by Buffy Coat Smear of Disseminated *Mycobacterium avium* Complex Infection in Patients With Acquired Immunodeficiency Syndrome," *J Clin Microbiol*, 1990, 28(3):631-2.
7. Kurtin PJ, McKinsey DS, Gupta MR, et al, "Histoplasmosis in Patients With Acquired Immunodeficiency Syndrome," *Am J Clin Pathol*, 1990, 93(3):367-72.
8. Marcon MJ and Powell DA, "Human Infections Due to *Malassezia* spp," *Clin Microbiol Rev*, 1992, 5(2):101-19.

References

Kleiman MB, Reynolds JK, Schreiner RL, et al, "Rapid Diagnosis of Neonatal Bacteremia With Acridine Orange Stained Buffy Coat," *J Pediatr*, 1984, 105:419-21.

Kostiala AA, Jormalainen S, and Kosunen TU, "Detection of Experimental Bacteremia and Fungemia by Examination of Buffy Coat Prepared by a Micromethod," *Am J Clin Pathol*, 1979, 72:437-43.

Studer JP, Glauser MP, and Schapira M, "Value of Examining Buffy Coats for Intragranulocytic Microorganisms in Patients With Fever," *Br Med J*, 1979, 1:85-6.

Beta-Glucuronidase Stain *see* Leukocyte Cytochemistry *on page 567*

Blood Cell Profile *see* Complete Blood Count *on page 533*

Blood Count *see* Complete Blood Count *on page 533*

Blood Smear for Malarial Parasites *see* Malaria Smear *on page 569*

Blood Smear for Trypanosomal/Filarial Parasites *see* Microfilariae, Peripheral Blood Preparation *on page 571*

Blood Smear Morphology *see* Peripheral Blood: Red Blood Cell Morphology *on page 584*

Blood Viscosity *see* Viscosity, Blood *on page 610*

Blood Volume

***CPT** 78120 (red cell volume single sample); 78121 (multiple samples)*

Related Information

Erythropoietin, Serum *on page 214*
Hematocrit *on page 552*
Peripheral Blood: Red Blood Cell Morphology *on page 584*
Phlebotomy, Therapeutic *on page 1075*
Red Blood Cell Indices *on page 592*
Red Cell Mass *on page 595*

Synonyms Plasma/Blood Volume; Total Blood Volume

Applies to Plasma Volume Measurement; Red Cell Volume

Test Commonly Includes Total blood volume, red cell mass, and plasma volume, measured and predicted

Abstract This procedure measures the patient's total circulating volume of blood and/or fractions (eg, red cell mass) of the blood volume. A component of the blood (eg, albumin) is labeled, usually with a radioisotope. The dilution of the label is inversely proportional to the size (volume) of the compartment in which it has been diluted. Blood volume study may be an invaluable contribution to some clinical situations (eg, polycythemia, acute blood loss) in which determination of Hgb, a concentration, or Hct, a fraction, could be misleading.

Patient Care PREPARATION: Patient should have all RIA blood work performed, at least drawn, prior to injection of any radioactive material. Technologist will administer injected dose to patient and withdraw blood samples after the appropriate interval (usually 10 minutes). Patient must be available since timing is important.

Specimen Whole blood CONTAINER: Method dependent. For ^{51}Cr-labeled red cell methods, ACD-NIH or Strumia's ACD solution, ratio of one part ACD to five parts blood. EDTA anticoagulated blood may be used, but excess EDTA must be avoided. EDTA causes shrinkage of red cells, the resultant red cell volume is too low unless used in a concentration of 1.5 ± 0.25 mg/mL of blood. Samples of blood for ^{125}I or ^{131}I labeled albumin plasma volume methods may be collected in heparinized syringe.

Interpretive REFERENCE RANGE: Normal values are method dependent. Blood volume varies with body habitus, age, sex, weight, and height. There is special correlation with body surface area. As the amount of blood in fat is about 2/35 that of lean tissue, the normal value for an obese individual is less than that for a lean person of same weight. Careful clinical assessment as to degree of obesity, edema, etc, must be a part of the determination of normal. See table. USE: Differentiate relative from absolute polycythemia. Polycythemia may be defined as increased red cells and, in a sense, is the opposite of anemia. Polycythemia is usually considered when hemoglobin is 18 g/dL, hematocrit is 52%, and RBC count is 6 million/mm^3. These values do not tell whether the red cell mass is increased or the plasma volume is decreased. Relative polycythemias are caused by decreased plasma volumes such as in burns, severe sweating, shock, dehydration, or any other cause of hemoconcentration. Absolute polycythemia occurs when red cell mass is increased. This can be because of increased erythropoietin in secondary polycythemia (appropriate or inappropriate[1]) or occurs spontaneously as in the myeloproliferative syndrome, polycythemia vera (splenomegaly usually present). LIMITATIONS: Any *in vivo* isotope test will affect blood volume (eg, bone scans, liver scans, brain scans). Check with the laboratory to see if blood volume determination would be valid. Cost of radioisotope label has increased substantially in recent years. A decline in orders for blood volume determination has occurred over the past two decades relating to technical variations, accuracy concerns, and in part to FDA related-withdrawal of some partially automated analytic systems. A dependable, accurate, "double tag" method (simultaneous use of ^{125}I albumin and ^{51}Cr-labeled RBCs) is technically rigorous and time consuming compared to other clinical laboratory procedures. CONTRAINDICATIONS: Patient actively bleeding, edema METHODOLOGY: General concept of dilution technique using ^{125}I-tagged albumin and/or ^{51}Cr-tagged red blood cells. Technetium (Tc-99m) or indium (^{113m}In or ^{111}In) labeled red cells have also been used for red cell volume measurements. ADDITIONAL INFORMATION: Hgb, Hct, or RBC count determinations are concentration expressed parameters and may be

Blood Volume Parameters
Normal Adult Males and Females
^{51}Cr RBC Label Method

Measurement	Men (mL/kg)	Women (mL/kg)
Blood volume	61.54±8.59	58.95±4.94
Erythrocyte volume	28.27±4.11	24.24±2.59
Plasma volume	33.45±5.18	34.77±3.24

misleading when the clinical situation requires assessment of the absolute volume of blood or one of its components. Acute shift in body fluids between the intravascular and extravascular spaces as may occur with heart failure, shock, and third space pooling are examples of such misleading circumstances. There is increase in plasma volume in the last trimester of pregnancy, toxemia of pregnancy, and in uremia. Blood volume may be as much as 16% higher in the evening than in the morning.[2] See references for further information and comprehensive table of predicted normal blood volumes.

Footnotes

1. Shouval D, Anton M, Galun E, et al, "Erythropoietin-Induced Polycythemia in Athymic Mice Following Transplantation of Human Renal Carcinoma Cell Line," *Cancer Res*, 1988, 48(12):3430-4.
2. Finlayson DC, "Diurnal Variation in Blood Volume of Man," *J Surg Res*, 1964, 4:286.

References

Dacie JV and Lewis SM, "Blood Volume," *Practical Haematology*, 7th ed, New York, NY: Churchill Livingstone, 1991, 361-9.

Langan JK, Scheffel U, and McIntyre PA, "The Hematopoietic System," *Nuclear Medicine Technology and Techniques*, Chapter 18, Bernier DR, Christian PE, Langan JK, et al, eds, St Louis, MO: Mosby-Year Book Inc, 1989, 485.

Pollycove M and Tono M, "Blood Volume," *Diagnostic Nuclear Medicine*, 2nd ed, Vol 2, Chapter 42, Gottschalk A, Hoffer PB, Potchen EJ, et al, eds, Baltimore, MD: Williams & Wilkins, 1988, 690-7.

"Recommended Methods for Measurement of Red-Cell and Plasma Volume: International Committee for Standardization in Haematology," *J Nucl Med*, 1980, 21:793-800.

Williams WJ, Beutler E, Erslev AJ, et al, *Hematology*, 4th ed, New York, NY: McGraw-Hill Inc, 1990, 414-6.

Body Fluids Analysis, Cell Count

***CPT** 89050 (cell count); 89051 (with differential)*

Related Information

Biopsy or Body Fluid Aerobic Bacterial Culture *on page 778*
Biopsy or Body Fluid Anaerobic Bacterial Culture *on page 778*
Biopsy or Body Fluid Fungus Culture *on page 780*
Biopsy or Body Fluid Mycobacteria Culture *on page 782*
Body Fluid *on page 145*
Body Fluid Amylase *on page 148*
Body Fluid Glucose *on page 148*
Body Fluid Lactate Dehydrogenase *on page 149*
Body Fluid pH *on page 150*
Body Fluids Cytology *on page 482*
CA 125 *on page 154*
Carcinoembryonic Antigen *on page 167*
Cerebrospinal Fluid Analysis *on page 527*
Synovial Fluid Analysis *on page 1158*

Applies to Ascitic Fluid Analysis; Cyst Fluid Analysis; Joint Fluid Analysis; Paracentesis Fluid Analysis; Pericardial Fluid Analysis; Peritoneal Fluid Analysis; Pleural Fluid Analysis; Thoracentesis Fluid Analysis

Test Commonly Includes Total WBC count and differential, total RBC count, (protein, sugar, LD (LDH), amylase, and multiple additional tests are commonly done on body fluids)

Patient Care **PREPARATION:** Aseptic preparation for aspiration

Specimen Body fluid, (ie, pleural fluid, synovial fluid, cyst fluid, paracentesis fluid, pericardial fluid, etc) **CONTAINER:** Glass test tube or large glass container **COLLECTION:** Add heparin to specimen. **STORAGE INSTRUCTIONS:** Specimen should be brought directly to the laboratory after collection. Do **not** store. **CAUSES FOR REJECTION:** Clotted specimen, inadequate volume of specimen for the procedures requested **SPECIAL INSTRUCTIONS:** Requisition must state site of origin. Commonly cytologic, microbiologic and chemical examinations are also helpful.

Interpretive **REFERENCE RANGE:** See following table. Glucose and amylase levels in fluids approximate whole blood levels. A pleural fluid LD to serum LD ratio >0.6 suggests exudate. In pleural fluids, total protein >3.0 g/dL indicates exudate, protein <3.0 g/dL indicates transudate. For peritoneal fluid, the cutoff point is lower, 2.0-2.5. Pericardial fluids have no established cutoff point in differentiating transudates from exudates. **USE:** Evaluate body fluids; differential diagnosis of exudate, transudate **ADDITIONAL INFORMATION:** Cultures, cytology, and chemical studies usually must be requested separately and should have a separate specimen if possible. See listings for Body Fluid, Body Fluid Glucose, Body Fluid Amylase, and Body Fluid pH in the Chemistry chapter and Body Fluids Cytology in the Cytopathology chapter. Elevated lymphocytes can be associated with congestive heart failure (pleural fluid), tuberculosis,

(Continued)

Body Fluids Analysis, Cell Count *(Continued)*

Expected Normal Findings — Body Fluids

Type of Fluid	Appearance	Amount	Cells	Glucose	Total Protein
Pleural	Clear, colorless to pale yellow	1-10 mL	<1000/mm^3 <25% polys 0 RBC	Approximates WB glucose	
Peritoneal	Clear, colorless to pale yellow	<100 mL	<500/mm^3 <25% polys <100,000 RBC/mm^3		
Pericardial	Clear, colorless to pale yellow	20-25 mL	<500 WBC/mm^3 <25% polys 0 RBC		
Synovial	No crystals	<4 mL	<200 WBC/mm^3 <25% polys	Blood/synovial difference <10 mg/dL	1.0-3.0 g/dL

tumors, lymphomas, lymphatic leukemia, rheumatoid arthritis, and postpneumonia effusions. Elevated polymorphonuclear leukocytes are associated with acute infectious processes, (ie, bacterial inflammation, eg, bacterial peritonitis). The difference between uninfected ascitic fluid and that of bacterial peritonitis is reported as WBC count of 122/mm^3 vs 2686/mm^3. PMN count provides the highest sensitivity; its reliability is enhanced with pH (low with peritonitis, <7.35).[1] Elevated eosinophils are associated with tumors, infarcts, SLE, rheumatoid arthritis, rheumatic fever, parasites, postpneumonic effusions, pneumothorax, or may have no clinical significance. Elevated plasma cells can be associated with lymphoma, especially Hodgkin's disease or with chronic inflammation. Sometimes atypical plasma cells are seen in the presence of multiple myeloma. A low glucose level supports diagnosis of rheumatoid effusion. Creatinine level distinguishes ascitic collection from tap of an overdistended bladder.

A cost efficient management of body fluid clinical laboratory testing is recommended by Albright et al with the description of "transport and rapid accessioning for additional procedures," a two-tiered analytic system.[2] Physician understanding and logistic considerations for standardized handling are involved. Storage of and access to body fluid samples for subsequent testing after limited initial study are the cornerstone of this concept. Cell count, however, must be performed as soon as possible to avoid distortions produced by storage. Microbiologic study and cytology must also receive timely consideration.

Footnotes

1. Garcia-Tsao G, Conn HO, and Lerner E, "The Diagnosis of Bacterial Peritonitis: Comparison of pH, Lactate Concentration and Leukocyte Count," *Hepatology*, 1985, 5:91-6.
2. Albright RE Jr, Christenson RH, Habig RL, et al, "Cerebrospinal Fluid (CSF) TRAP: A Method to Improve CSF Laboratory Efficiency," *Am J Clin Pathol*, 1988, 90:707-10.

References

Albright RE Jr, "Management of Cerebrospinal Fluid and Other Body Fluids," *Practical Laboratory Hematology*, Chapter 13, Koepke JA, ed, New York, NY: Churchill Livingstone, 1991, 295-310.

Kjeldsberg CR and Knight JA, *Body Fluids: Laboratory Examination of Amniotic, Cerebrospinal, Seminal, Serous, and Synovial Fluids*, 3rd ed, Chicago, IL: ASCP Press, 1993, 159-253, 265-301.

Strasinger SK, *Urinalysis and Body Fluids: A Self-Instructional Test*, Philadelphia, PA: FA Davis Co, 1985, 169-74.

Bone Marrow

CPT *85095 (aspiration); 85097 (smear interpretation)*

Related Information

Biopsy or Body Fluid Aerobic Bacterial Culture *on page 778*
Biopsy or Body Fluid Anaerobic Bacterial Culture *on page 778*
Biopsy or Body Fluid Fungus Culture *on page 780*
Biopsy or Body Fluid Mycobacteria Culture *on page 782*
Breakpoint Cluster Region Rearrangement in CML *on page 895*
Buffy Coat Smear Study of Peripheral Blood *on page 526*
Cerebrospinal Fluid Cytology *on page 490*
Chromosome Analysis, Blood or Bone Marrow *on page 898*
Chromosome *In Situ* Hybridization *on page 901*

Complete Blood Count *on page 533*
Gene Rearrangement for Leukemia and Lymphoma *on page 911*
Iron Stain, Bone Marrow *on page 562*
Leishmaniasis Serological Test *on page 717*
Leukocyte Cytochemistry *on page 567*
Lymph Node Biopsy *on page 72*
Peripheral Blood: Differential Leukocyte Count *on page 576*
Schilling Test *on page 598*
Terminal Deoxynucleotidyl Transferase *on page 604*
Viral Culture *on page 1195*
Viral Culture, Body Fluid *on page 1198*
Vitamin B_{12} *on page 612*
White Blood Count *on page 616*

Synonyms Bone Marrow Aspirate; Bone Marrow Biopsy

Test Commonly Includes H & E stain, Wright's stain, and iron stain; special histochemistry in certain indicated circumstances

Abstract A glass or plastic syringe is used to suck marrow (the "aspirate") from cancellous bone and/or a "core" biopsy is obtained by using special needles (eg, Jamshidi needle). The specimens can be studied microscopically using a variety of routine and special stains, tested for the presence of microorganisms, and/or studied using molecular biologic techniques. Marrow study has broad application to disease processes.

Patient Care PREPARATION: Physician explains procedure to patient. Hopefully, patient apprehension is allayed. Aseptic aspiration under local anesthetic is performed. AFTERCARE: Keep site dry for 24 hours.

Specimen Bone marrow aspirate and/or biopsy CONTAINER: Coverslips are prepared at bedside, and biopsy and clot are placed in fixative (formalin or Zenker's solution). SPECIAL INSTRUCTIONS: Marrow procedures must generally be planned in advance with coordination and scheduling allowing for indicated cultures, biopsy, or other special studies (eg, electron microscopy, flow cytometry, gene rearrangement, or chromosome analysis).

Interpretive REFERENCE RANGE: Results interpreted by pathologist/hematologist/oncologist USE: Evaluate bone marrow morphology, erythropoiesis, myelopoiesis, myeloid/erythroid ratio, megakaryocytes, cellularity, and marrow iron stores; evaluate platelet dependent clotting dysfunction; evaluate anemia; marrow culture can make a valuable contribution to the study of fever of undetermined origin and possible systemic infection, in particular, histoplasmosis and tuberculosis; establish the presence of, classify, or follow up neoplasia (myeloma, macroglobulinemia of Waldenström, carcinomatosis, lymphoproliferative diseases, myeloproliferative diseases, ie, myelofibrosis, leukemias). In general, serum ferritin level with the CBC, serum iron, TIBC, and peripheral smear evaluation can supplant bone marrow exam when the **only** indication for marrow exam is evaluation of iron stores. LIMITATIONS: Presence of normal or nondiagnostic marrow at one site may not exclude the possibility of disease elsewhere in the marrow. Aspiration prior to biopsy does not disturb the estimation of cellularity of the biopsy at that same site (provided an adequate sized biopsy is obtained).[1] CONTRAINDICATIONS: Sternal site – aneurysm of thoracic aorta; very severe bleeding diathesis METHODOLOGY: A variety of sites and needles are available. Jamshidi needle for marrow biopsy is effective and currently enjoys widespread use. Sternum or posterosuperior iliac spine are common sites for marrow aspirate. Posterosuperior iliac spine is the most common site for biopsy and is usually favored over the anterior iliac crest.[2] Anterior iliac crest and vertebral spinous process may also be used in adults; anterior tibia is the desirable site in infants and young children. ADDITIONAL INFORMATION: A bone marrow biopsy may not be part of the routine marrow study but is desirable in most cases. Biopsy may be necessary in cases of "packed marrow" as with some forms of malignancy, myeloproliferative disease, and with granulomatous entities. Information obtained from the study of different types of marrow specimens is complementary.[3] An unusual cause of depleted iron stores may be iron storage preferentially by tumor cells.[4] The marrow is said to be always involved in cases of hairy cell leukemia (leukemic reticuloendotheliosis).[5] Marrow study is important in the classification of a number of diseases involving the reticuloendothelial system, including the uncommon entity hairy cell leukemia. In recent years the French, American, British (FAB) classifications have achieved increasing acceptance.[6,7,8] Bone marrow culture is sometimes helpful, for instance, in diagnoses of miliary tuberculosis and histoplasmosis. Orders for appropriate cultures must accompany such samples, which require sterile containers. Serial bone marrow biopsy samples have been utilized to follow the course of *in vivo* differentiation of myeloid cells in cases of acute leukemia that are receiving

(Continued)

Bone Marrow *(Continued)*

chemotherapy. The method uses monoclonal antibody to a purine analogue with subsequent identification by immunofluorescence. *In vivo* differentiation as detected in this manner has been found to indicate favorable long-term prognosis and may assist in the choice of effective therapeutic regimens.[9]

Footnotes

1. Wolff SN, Katzenstein AL, Phillips GL, et al, "Aspiration Does Not Influence Interpretation of Bone Marrow Biopsy Cellularity," *Am J Clin Pathol*, 1983, 80:60-2.
2. Hernández-García MT, Hernández-Nieto L, Pérez-González E, et al, "Bone Marrow Trephine Biopsy: Anterior Superior Iliac Spine *Versus* Posterior Superior Iliac Spine," *Clin Lab Haematol*, 1993, 15(1):15-9.
3. Brynes RK, McKenna RW, and Sundberg RD, "Bone Marrow Aspiration and Trephine Biopsy. An Approach to a Thorough Study," *Am J Clin Pathol*, 1978, 70:753-9.
4. Udoji WC and Husain I, "Microcytic Normochromic Anemia Associated With Iron Storage by Hypernephroma," *Am J Clin Pathol*, 1978, 70:944-6.
5. Bartl R, Frisch B, Hill W, et al, "Bone Marrow Histology in Hairy Cell Leukemia. Identification of Subtypes and Their Prognostic Significance," *Am J Clin Pathol*, 1983, 79:531-45.
6. Bennett JM, Catovsky D, Daniel M-T, et al, "Proposals for the Classification of the Myelodysplastic Syndromes," *Br J Haematol*, 1982, 51:189-99.
7. Bennett JM, Catovsky D, Daniel M-T, et al, "Proposed Revised Criteria for the Classification of Acute Myeloid Leukemia," *Ann Intern Med*, 1985, 103:626-9.
8. Bennett JM, Catovsky D, Daniel M-T, et al, "Criteria for the Diagnosis of Acute Leukemia of Megakaryocyte Lineage (M7): A Report of the French-American-British Cooperative Group," *Ann Intern Med*, 1985, 103:460-2.
9. Raza A, Preisler H, Lampkin B, et al, "Clinical and Prognostic Significance of *In Vivo* Differentiation in Acute Myeloid Leukemia," *Am J Hematol*, 1993, 42(2):147-57.

References

Bartl R, Frisch B, and Wilmanns W, "Potential of Bone Marrow Biopsy in Chronic Myeloproliferative Disorders (MPD)," *Eur J Haematol*, 1993, 50(1):41-52.

Bloomfield CD and Brunning RD, "The Revised French-American-British Classification of Acute Myeloid Leukemia: Is New Better?" *Ann Intern Med*, 1985, 103:614-5.

Hyun BH, Gulati GL, and Ashton JK, *Color Atlas of Clinical Hematology*, New York, NY: Igaku-Shoin, 1986.

Karcher DS and Frost AR, "The Bone Marrow in Human Immunodeficiency Virus (HIV)-Related Disease: Morphology and Clinical Correlation," *Am J Clin Pathol*, 1991, 95(1):63-71.

Kass L, *Bone Marrow Interpretation*, 2nd ed, Philadelphia, PA: JB Lippincott Co, 1985.

Paulman PM, "Bone Marrow Sampling," *Am Fam Physician*, 1989, 40(6):85-9.

Rothstein G, "Origin and Development of the Blood and Blood Forming Tissues," *Wintrobe's Clinical Hematology*, Chapter 3, Lee GR, Bithell TC, Foerster J, et al, eds, Philadelphia, PA: Lea and Febiger, 1993, 41-78.

Wittels B, *Surgical Pathology of Bone Marrow: Core Biopsy Diagnosis*, Philadelphia, PA: WB Saunders Co, 1985.

Bone Marrow Aspirate *see* Bone Marrow *on page 524*

Bone Marrow Biopsy *see* Bone Marrow *on page 524*

Bone Marrow Iron Stain *see* Iron Stain, Bone Marrow *on page 562*

Buffy Coat Method for Detection of Bacteremia *see* Bacteremia Detection, Buffy Coat Micromethod *on page 520*

Buffy Coat Smear Study of Peripheral Blood

CPT 85009

Related Information

Bacteremia Detection, Buffy Coat Micromethod *on page 520*
Blood Culture, Aerobic and Anaerobic *on page 784*
Bone Marrow *on page 524*
Lymph Node Biopsy *on page 72*

Abstract The detection of some pathologic elements potentially present in peripheral blood can be enhanced by preparing and staining the concentrated white cell fraction ("buffy coat") of blood

Specimen Blood **CONTAINER:** Lavender top (EDTA) tube

Interpretive **USE:** Low cost maneuver to detect uncommon cells or organisms in blood, largely for detection of abnormal, immature, blast, or malignant white blood cell or other nucleated cell forms; usually used to detect leukemic cells, circulating malignant cells, or immature blood cells in cases of myelofibrosis or other marrow myelophthisic processes; may be used in histocytochemical evaluation of leukemias when a "dry tap" of the marrow occurs **LIMITATIONS:** Preparation of buffy coat smears may distort cells; artifact affects especially fragile cells **METHODOLOGY:** Wright's stained smear of buffy coat developing in centrifuged tube or capillary of anticoagulated whole blood **ADDITIONAL INFORMATION:** Utility of buffy coat study has been questioned. In a series of 96 children with ALL, buffy coat study found no cases of relapse not detected by WBC count or usual peripheral blood smear.[1] On the other hand, it has been suggested that erroneous results from buffy coat study are the result of an uneven distribution of WBCs in the buffy coat layer. Removal and mixing of the entire buffy coat layer prior to making smears prevents uneven distribution of the leukocytes and avoids artifactual distortion of WBC morphology.[2] Unusual organisms (eg, *Strongyloides stercoralis* present as overwhelming hyperinfection in an immune suppressed individual,[3] microfilaremia[4]) may be detected by buffy coat study.

Footnotes

1. Franklin IM, "A Comparison of Peripheral Blood and Buffy Coat Smear Examination for the Prediction of Bone Marrow Relapse of Acute Lymphoblastic Leukemia in Childhood," *J Clin Pathol*, 1983, 36:192-4.
2. Pereira TT, Hargrove GH, and Cornbleet PJ, "Preparation of Buffy Coat Smears in Leukopenic Patients," *Lab Med*, 1981, 12:2, 96-8.
3. Gambino R, "Examination of the Buffy Coat in Patients With FUO," *Lab Report for Physicians*, 1983, 5:43-4.
4. Freedman DO and Berry RS, "Rapid Diagnosis of Bancroftian Filariasis by Acridine Orange Staining of Centrifuged Parasites," *Am J Trop Med Hyg*, 1992, 47(6):787-93.

References

Brown BA, "Routine Hematology Procedures," *Hematology: Principles and Procedures*, 6th ed, Philadelphia, PA: Lea & Febiger, 1993, 99.

CBC *see* Complete Blood Count *on page 533*

Cell Count, CSF *see* Cerebrospinal Fluid Analysis *on this page*

Ceramidase *see* Tests for Uncommon Inherited Diseases of Metabolism and Cell Structure *on page 605*

Ceramidetrihexoside α-Galactosidase *see* Tests for Uncommon Inherited Diseases of Metabolism and Cell Structure *on page 605*

Cerebrospinal Fluid Analysis

***CPT** 82947 (glucose); 84155 (protein quantitative); 89050 (cell count); 89051 (with differential count)*

Related Information

Bacterial Antigens, Rapid Detection Methods *on page 775*
Body Fluids Analysis, Cell Count *on page 523*
Cerebrospinal Fluid Culture *on page 798*
Cerebrospinal Fluid Cytology *on page 490*
Cerebrospinal Fluid Fungus Culture *on page 800*
Cerebrospinal Fluid Glucose *on page 176*
Cerebrospinal Fluid IgG Ratios and IgG Index *on page 653*
Cerebrospinal Fluid Lactic Acid *on page 178*
Cerebrospinal Fluid LD *on page 179*
Cerebrospinal Fluid Mycobacteria Culture *on page 801*
Cerebrospinal Fluid Protein *on page 659*
FTA-ABS, Cerebrospinal Fluid *on page 679*
Gram Stain *on page 815*
Viral Culture, Central Nervous System Symptoms *on page 1199*

Synonyms Cell Count, CSF; CSF Analysis

Test Commonly Includes Color of supernatant, volume, turbidity, WBC/mm^3, polys/mm^3, lymphs/mm^3, RBC/mm^3, percent of crenated RBC, protein, sugar, sometimes VDRL, sometimes FTA-ABS, and protein electrophoresis in selected cases may be helpful additional analyses.

Abstract Cerebrospinal fluid (CSF) exists in the cerebral ventricles and subarachnoid spaces. Examination of CSF contributes to diagnosis and sometimes management of various disease entities of the central nervous system including meningitis, encephalitis, instances of vasculitis, demyelinating diseases, tumors, paraneoplastic entities, polyneuritis, instances of cerebrovascular disease, cases of seizure disorders and confusional states.[1] For diagnosis of

(Continued)

Initial Cerebrospinal Fluid Findings in Suppurative Diseases of the Central Nervous System and Meninges

Condition	Pressure (mm H_2O)	Leukocytes/mm^3	Protein (mg/dL)	Sugar (mg/dL)	Specific Findings
Acute bacterial meningitis	Usually elevated; average, 300	Several hundred to more than 60,000; usually a few thousand; occasionally fewer than 100 (especially meningococcal or early in disease); PMNs* predominate	Usually 100-500, occasionally >1000	<40 in >50% of cases	Organism usually seen on smear or culture in >90% of cases
Subdural empyema	Usually elevated; average, 300	Fewer than 100 to a few thousand; PMNs predominate	Usually 100-500	Normal	No organisms seen on smear or culture unless concurrent meningitis
Brain abscess	Usually elevated	Usually 10-200; fluid is rarely acellular; lymphocytes predominate	Usually 75-400	Normal	No organisms seen on smear or culture
Ventricular empyema (rupture of brain abscess)	Considerably elevated	Several thousand to 100,000; usually >90% PMNs	Usually several hundred	Usually <40	Organism may be seen on smear or culture
Cerebral epidural abscess	Slightly to modestly elevated	Few to several hundred or more cells; lymphocytes predominate	Usually 50-200	Normal	No organisms seen on smear or culture
Spinal epidural abscess	Usually reduced with spinal block	Usually 10-100; lymphocytes predominate	Usually several hundred	Normal	No organisms seen on smear or culture
Thrombophlebitis (often associated with subdural empyema)	Often elevated	Few to several hundred; PMNs and lymphocytes	Slightly to moderately elevated	Normal	No organisms seen on smear or culture
Bacterial endocarditis (with embolism)	Normal or slightly elevated	Few to fewer than 100; lymphocytes and PMNs	Slightly elevated	Normal	No organisms seen on smear or culture
Acute hemorrhagic encephalitis	Usually elevated	Few to more than 1000; PMNs predominate	Moderately elevated	Normal	No organisms seen on smear or culture

(continued)

Condition	Pressure (mm H_2O)	Leukocytes/mm^3	Protein (mg/dL)	Sugar (mg/dL)	Specific Findings
Tuberculous infection	Usually elevated; may be low with dynamic block in advanced stages	Usually 25-100, rarely more than 500; lymphocytes predominate, except in early stages when PMNs may account for 80% of the cells	Nearly always elevated, usually 100-200; may be much higher if dynamic block	Usually reduced; <50 in 75% of cases	Acid-fast organisms may be seen on smear of protein coagulum (pellicle) or recovered from inoculated guinea pig or by culture
Cryptococcal infection	Usually elevated; average, 225	Average, 50 (0-800); lymphocytes predominate	Average, 100; usually 20-500	Reduced in $>50\%$ the cases; average 30; often higher in patients with concomitant diabetes mellitus	Organisms may be seen in India ink preparation and on culture (Sabouraud's medium); will usually grow on blood agar; may produce alcohol in cerebrospinal fluid from fermentation of glucose
Syphilis (acute)	Usually elevated	Average, 500; usually lymphocytes; rare PMNs	Average, 100; γ-globulin often high, with abnormal colloidal gold curve	Normal (rarely reduced)	Positive results of reagin test for syphilis; spirochetes not demonstrable by usual techniques of smear or culture
Sarcoidosis	Normal to considerably elevated	0 to <100 mononuclear cells	Slight to moderate elevation	Normal	No specific findings

*Polymorphonuclear leukocytes
From Feigin RD and Cherry JD, eds, *Textbook of Pediatric Infectious Diseases*, Vol 1, Philadelphia, PA: WB Saunders, 1992, 410, with permission.

(Continued)

Cerebrospinal Fluid Analysis *(Continued)*

meningitis, culture, and then Gram staining have priority over all other testing, when only a small quantity of cerebrospinal fluid (CSF) is available. Cell count with differential deserve the next priority, followed by glucose and protein.

Patient Care PREPARATION: Aseptic preparation for aspiration

Specimen Cerebrospinal fluid. A sample of peripheral blood for serum should be obtained concurrently if CSF is being studied for presence of oligoclonal bands (eg, as in demyelinating diseases, in particular multiple sclerosis) or when glucose and protein levels are needed as in cases of possible infection (eg, meningitis or encephalitis). Blood culture and plasma glucose should be drawn in cases of possible meningitis as well as CBC and differential. CONTAINER: Sterile test tubes from lumbar puncture tray COLLECTION: Specimens of spinal fluid and blood for culture should be obtained prior to initiation of antibiotic treatment of meningitis. Tubes must be labeled with patient's name, date, and labeled with number indicating sequence in which tubes were obtained. Specimen should be delivered to the laboratory **promptly**. STORAGE INSTRUCTIONS: Do **not** store; place in the hands of a laboratory technologist. CAUSES FOR REJECTION: Unlabeled tubes, insufficient or clotted specimen SPECIAL INSTRUCTIONS: When a diagnosis of meningitis is considered, culture of other materials as well as culture of CSF may be helpful. Most children with bacterial meningitis are initially bacteremic, and blood cultures are of value. In neonates and small children, urine culture may be positive. Cultures and Gram stains of petechiae may provide immediate diagnosis.

Interpretive REFERENCE RANGE: Adults: 0-5 cells/mm^3, all lymphocytes and monocytes; 0 red blood cells; protein: lumbar 15-50 mg/dL, cisternal 15-25 mg/dL, ventricular 6-15 mg/dL; glucose 50-80 mg/dL. Younger than 1 month: <32 cells/mm^3, 1 month to 1 year: <10 cells/mm^3, 1-4 years: <8 cells/mm^3, 5 years to puberty: <5 cells/mm^3; in the premature neonate: <29 cells/mm^3 POSSIBLE PANIC RANGE: Increased number of cells USE: Evaluate bacterial or viral encephalitis, meningitis, meningoencephalitis, mycobacterial or fungal infection, parasitic infestations, primary or secondary malignancy, leukemia/malignant lymphoma of CNS, trauma, vascular occlusive disease, vasculitis, heredofamilial and/or degenerative processes. The table outlines findings, including those with subdural empyema, brain abscess, ventricular empyema, cerebral epidural abscess, spinal epidural abscess, tuberculosis, syphilis, sarcoidosis, and other entities.[1]

The nucleated blood cell count in the cerebrospinal fluid is described as superior to any combination of the other CSF tests for bacterial meningitis. In patients who have not received antimicrobial agents the ultimate diagnosis of bacterial meningitis is based on results of culture.[2] The cell count and differential count are mandatory, and a Gram stain must be examined promptly in work-up of possible meningitis. Glucose and protein are necessary, as well, in the work-up for possible meningitis.[3] In a study of aseptic versus bacterial meningitis, the mean CSF cell counts in aseptic and bacterial meningitis were respectively 228 cells/mm^3 (range 6-2650) and 4035 cells/mm^3 (range 16-17,650).[4] **Early viral infection** as well as **bacterial meningitis** can elicit neutrophil leukocytosis in blood and CSF. In viral meningitis, a shift to mononuclear predominance often occurs subsequently.[5,6,7] In 205 cases of acute **viral** meningitis, the 25th percentile, median, and 75th percentile leukocyte counts (10^6/L) were 37/100/250, with 3%, 33%, and 75%, respectively PMNs. In 217 cases of acute **bacterial** meningitis, leukocyte counts (10^6/L) were 330/1195/4400 with 70%, 86%, and 97% PMNs, respectively.[8] Seasonal curves for viral and bacterial infection go in opposite directions; viral meningitis is a disease of midsummer, while bacterial meningitis is relatively more common in the winter.[8]

Signals of possible meningeal infection in the newborn: Leukocyte count >30 cells/mm^3 with more than 60% PMNs, CSF protein >100 mg/dL, CSF glucose lower than 40% of the level in blood are findings in bacterial meningitis.[9] CSF WBC >10 cells/mm^3 in very young infants, and 5 cells/mm^3 in older infants and children with >1 PMN/mm^3 is abnormal.

LIMITATIONS: A traumatic (bloody) tap may make interpretation difficult. Normal CSF may be found early in meningitis. METHODOLOGY: Manual cell count using hemacytometer. Electronic cell counters lack precision and validity when used to analyze most CSF specimens (background is high relative to total white cell count). Differential cell study using manually prepared smears or cytocentrifuge methods. Bovine albumin, 22%, mixed with spinal fluid specimen is helpful in maintaining the morphologic integrity of smeared cells. For chemical, microbiologic, and other analyses, see appropriate entries in other chapters. ADDITIONAL INFORMATION: **More extensive testing:** Cytology, conventional cultures and cultures for mycobacteria, fungi, and viruses, additional chemistry and serologic determinations must usually be ordered separately.

Correction for traumatic tap: If cell counts and protein determinations are performed on CSF and blood obtained at the same time, correction for "bloody tap" can be calculated. All CSF measurements should be made from the same tube. The ratio of RBC count CSF to RBC count blood provides a factor which when multiplied by the blood WBC count or blood protein level indicates the expected level of contribution of these parameters from the blood to the spinal fluid. These contributed WBC or protein values can then be subtracted from the respective values measured in the spinal fluid. For example:

1. RBCs (CSF)/RBCs (blood) x WBCs (blood) or x protein (blood).
2. WBCs (CSF) or protein (CSF) – product calculated in 1 = true CSF WBC or true CSF protein.

If the peripheral blood is normal and traumatic tap had occurred, about 1 WBC is added to the CSF for each 700 RBCs that have been transferred into the CSF.[10] RBC contamination from a traumatic tap does not adversely affect the laboratory diagnosis of bacterial meningitis.

When only a small amount of CSF can be obtained, Gram stain and culture must always have priority over antigen detection testing.[11] Antigen detection methods cannot replace culture and Gram stain. A bacterial culture is the first test to be performed on cerebrospinal fluid for meningitis. It is the "gold standard" for diagnosis.[12] A requirement for 50 or more leukocytes per μL of CSF has been proposed as justification for bacterial antigen testing.[11] Another group found a CSF nucleated blood cell count $<6/mm^3$ provided a criterion for an abbreviated CSF evaluation.[2] Correlation exists between bacterial concentration in CSF and the numbers of PMNs found.[13]

There is substantial mortality and morbidity in subjects with bacterial meningitis. Neurologic sequelae are found in as many as 33% of all survivors in one study.[14] Sequelae occur especially in newborns and children.[11] Particularly when bacterial meningitis follows an insidious pattern, diagnostic delay may be unavoidable.[15] Eight of 21 survivors of neonatal meningitis were normal, eight had mild sequelae, and five had moderate to severe sequelae in a culture-proven series.[16] Despite early diagnosis and the use of appropriate therapy, both complications of meningitis and deaths may occur. As many as 50% of survivors of meningitis have some sequelae, as summarized by the Task Force on Diagnosis and Management of Meningitis.[17]

White cell pleocytosis is found in only 33% of patients with multiple sclerosis (MS). The white count rarely exceeds 20 cells/mm^3. Most patients with MS (66%) have normal total protein. In contrast, patients with Guillain-Barré syndrome usually have no excess white cells but show elevated CSF protein of 100-500 mg/dL.[18]

Footnotes

1. Felgin RD and Cherry JD, *Textbook of Pediatric Infectious Diseases*, Philadelphia, PA: WB Saunders Co, 1987, 488.
2. Rodewald LE, Woodin KA, Szilagyi PG, et al, "Relevance of Common Tests of Cerebrospinal Fluid in Screening for Bacterial Meningitis," *J Pediatr*, 1991, 119(3):363-9.
3. Fishman RA, *Cerebrospinal Fluid in Diseases of the Nervous System*, 2nd ed, Philadelphia, PA: WB Saunders Co, l992, 157-351.
4. Walsh-Kelly C, Nelson DB, Smith DS, et al, "Clinical Predictors of Bacterial Versus Aseptic Meningitis in Childhood," *Ann Emerg Med*, 1992, 21(8):910-4.
5. Connolly KJ and Hammer SM, "The Acute Aseptic Meningitis Syndrome," *Infect Dis Clin North Am*, 1990, 4(4):599-622.
6. Hammer SM and Connolly KJ, "Viral Aseptic Meningitis in the United States: Clinical Features, Viral Etiologies, and Differential Diagnosis," *Curr Clin Top Infect Dis*, 1992, 12:1-25.
7. Amir J, Harel L, Frydman M, et al, "Shift of Cerebrospinal Polymorphonuclear Cell Percentage in the Early Stage of Aseptic Meningitis," *J Pediatr*, 1991, 119(6):938-41.
8. Spanos A, Harrell FE Jr, and Durack DT, "Differential Diagnosis of Acute Meningitis: An Analysis of the Predictive Value of Initial Observations," *JAMA*, 1989, 262(19):2700-7.
9. McCracken GH Jr, "Current Management of Bacterial Meningitis in Infants and Children," *Pediatr Infect Dis J*, 1992, 11(2):169-74.
10. Bauer JD, *Clinical Laboratory Methods*, 9th ed, St Louis, MO: Mosby-Year Book Inc, 1982, 759.
11. Gray LD and Fedorko DP, "Laboratory Diagnosis of Bacterial Meningitis," *Clin Microbiol Rev*, 1992, 5(2):130-45.
12. Smith AL, "Bacterial Meningitis," *Pediatr Rev*, 1993, 14(1):11-8.
13. La Scolea LJ Jr and Dryja D, "Quantitation of Bacteria in Cerebrospinal Fluid and Blood of Children With Meningitis and Its Diagnostic Significance," *J Clin Microbiol*, 1984, 19:187-90.
14. Sáez-Llorens X, Ramilo O, Mustafa MM, et al, "Molecular Pathophysiology of Bacterial Meningitis: Current Concepts and Therapeutic Implications," *J Pediatr*, 1990, 116(5):671-84.
15. Kilpi T, Anttila M, Kallio MJ, et al, "Severity of Childhood Bacterial Meningitis and Duration of Illness Before Diagnosis," *Lancet*, 1991, 338(8764):406-9.

(Continued)

Cerebrospinal Fluid Analysis *(Continued)*

16. Franco SM, Cornelius VE, and Andrews BF, "Long-Term Outcome of Neonatal Meningitis," *Am J Dis Child*, 1992, 146(6):567-71.
17. Klein JO, Feigin RD, and McCracken GH Jr, "Report of the Task Force on Diagnosis and Management of Meningitis," *Pediatrics*, 1986, 78(5):959-82.
18. Harrington MG and Kennedy PG, "The Clinical Use of Cerebrospinal Fluid Studies in Demyelinating Neurological Diseases," *Postgrad Med J*, 1987, 63:735-40.

References

Bonadio WA, Smith DS, Goddard S, et al, "Distinguishing Cerebrospinal Fluid Abnormalities in Children With Bacterial Meningitis and Traumatic Lumbar Puncture," *J Infect Dis*, 1990, 162(1):251-4.

Feigin RD, McCracken GH Jr, and Klein JO, "Diagnosis and Management of Meningitis," *Pediatr Infect Dis J*, 1992, 11:785-814.

Levy M, Wong E, and Fried D, "Diseases That Mimic Meningitis. Analysis of 650 Lumbar Punctures," *Clin Pediatr (Phila)*, 1990, 29(5):258-61.

CHBHA *see* Heinz Body Stain *on page 551*

Chromium-51 Tagged RBC Survival Test *see* ^{51}Cr Red Cell Survival *on page 536*

Cold Hemolysin Test

CPT 86941

See Also Anemia Flowchart in the Hematology Appendix

Synonyms Donath-Landsteiner Test; PCH Test; Test for D-L Antibody; Test for Paroxysmal Cold Hemoglobinuria

Abstract Test for paroxysmal cold hemoglobinuria (PCH), a condition caused by sensitization of red blood cells (at temperatures less than 30°C) by a complement binding IgG biphasic hemolysin. Warming to 37°C causes hemolysis of patient's RBCs.

Specimen Blood **CONTAINER:** Red top tube **COLLECTION:** Obtain 7 mL of blood by routine venipuncture from patient in previously warmed (37°C) red top tube and another 7 mL of blood in previously cooled (3°C to 4°C) red top tube in an ice water bath. Collect similar samples from a normal individual for a negative control. Deliver to hematology laboratory immediately. **SPECIAL INSTRUCTIONS:** Consult laboratory as test may need to be arranged in advance.

Interpretive **REFERENCE RANGE:** Negative **USE:** Diagnosis of the uncommon disorder, paroxysmal cold hemoglobinuria. PCH may occur with syphilis, infectious mononucleosis, influenza, measles, mumps, chickenpox, and other viral illnesses. **METHODOLOGY:** Observation of red cell lysis by patient's cold activated serum **ADDITIONAL INFORMATION:** There are two types of cold autoantibodies, the cold autoagglutinins/hemolysins (as found in cold-antibody autoimmune hemolytic anemia) and the biphasic hemolysins. These antibodies are characterized by optimal reaction at temperatures less than 30°C. The cold autoagglutinins are usually monoclonal or polyclonal IgM antibodies with anti-H, anti-IH, or anti-i immunospecificity. Anti-Pr is the second most commonly associated antibody. Classic paroxysmal cold hemoglobinuria is caused by an IgG complement binding biphasic hemolysin,[1] an autoantibody that attaches to the RBC membrane at 4°C to 20°C. The antibody causes only weak agglutination of red cells in saline. When the temperature rises to 37°C, hemolysis occurs. The immunohematologic specificity of the Donath-Landsteiner type PCH antibody is usually anti-P.[2] While PCH was the first hemolytic anemia to be recognized, it has become the least common type of autoimmune hemolytic anemia. Previously associated with syphilis, it is now more commonly seen in viral-like illness, largely in children.[3] The re-emergence of syphilis associated with AIDS may cause a comeback of PCH.

Footnotes

1. Engelfriet CP, Overbeeke MA, and von dem Borne AE, "Autoimmune Hemolytic Anemia," *Semin Hematol*, 1992, 29(1):3-12.
2. Judd WJ, Wilkinson SL, Issitt PD, et al, "Donath-Landsteiner Hemolytic Anemia Due to an Anti-Pr-Like Biphasic Hemolysin," *Transfusion*, 1986, 26:423-5.
3. Nordhagen R, Stensvold A, Winses A, et al, "Paroxysmal Cold Hemoglobinuria," *Acta Paediatr Scand*, 1984, 73:258-62.

References

Dacie JV and Lewis SM, *Practical Haematology*, 7th ed, New York, NY: Churchill Livingstone, 1991, 500-2.

Petz LD and Garratty G, *Acquired Immune Hemolytic Anemias*, New York, NY: Churchill Livingstone, 1980, 50-7, 175-8.

Sherry C Sr, "Acquired Immune Anemia of Increased Destruction," *Clinical Hematology: Principles, Procedures, Correlations*, Chapter 19, Lotspeich-Steininger CA, Stiene-Martin EA, and Koepke JA, eds, Philadelphia, PA: JB Lippincott Co, 1992, 274.

Williams WJ, Beutler E, Erslev AJ, et al, *Hematology*, 4th ed, New York, NY: McGraw-Hill Inc, 1990, 678-9.

Complete Blood Count

CPT *85021 (hemogram, automated [RBC, WBC, Hgb, Hct, and indices only]); 85022 (hemogram, automated and manual differential WBC count [CBC]); 85023 (hemogram and platelet count, automated and manual differential WBC count [CBC]); 85024 (hemogram and platelet count, automated and automated partial differential WBC count [CBC]); 85025 (hemogram and platelet count, automated and automated complete, differential WBC count [CBC])*

See Also Anemia Flowchart in the Hematology Appendix

Related Information

Bone Marrow *on page 524*
Eosinophil Count *on page 539*
Ferritin, Serum *on page 220*
Folic Acid, RBC *on page 544*
Folic Acid, Serum *on page 545*
Hematocrit *on page 552*
Hemoglobin *on page 554*
Iron and Total Iron Binding Capacity/Transferrin *on page 262*
Kidney Profile *on page 268*
Lymph Node Biopsy *on page 72*
Lymphocyte Subset Enumeration *on page 720*
Peripheral Blood: Differential Leukocyte Count *on page 576*
Peripheral Blood: Red Blood Cell Morphology *on page 584*
Platelet Count *on page 586*
Platelet Sizing *on page 588*
Red Blood Cell Indices *on page 592*
Red Cell Count *on page 594*
Uric Acid, Serum *on page 378*
Vitamin B_{12} *on page 612*
White Blood Count *on page 616*

Synonyms Blood Cell Profile; Blood Count; CBC; Hemogram

Test Commonly Includes WBC, Hct, Hgb, differential count, RBC, WBC and RBC morphology, RBC indices, platelet estimate, platelet count, RDW, and histograms. Although RBC, WBC, and platelet histograms are not usually available on patient charts, they are helpful to the technologist in detecting problems with patients and quality control. Even though the histograms are not on the chart, they can be viewed in the laboratory along with the blood smear. New analyzers also provide automated 5-part white cell differentials: granulocytes, monocytes, lymphocytes, eosinophils, and basophils.

Abstract The standard broadly inclusive automated test for evaluation of RBC, WBC, and platelets. The majority of CBC results are generated by highly automated electronic and pneumatic multichannel analyzers based on aperture-impedance and/or laser beam cell sizing and counting (see reference by Koepke).

Red Cell Values on First Postnatal Day*

Gestational Age (wk)	24–25	26–27	28–29	30–31	32–33	34–35	36–37	Term
RBC (x 10^6/mm^3)	4.65 ±0.43	4.73 ±0.45	4.62 ±0.75	4.79 ±0.74	5.0 ±0.76	5.09 ±0.5	5.27 ±0.68	5.14 ±0.7
Hgb (g/dL)	19.4 ±1.5	19.0 ±2.5	19.3 ±1.8	19.1 ±2.2	18.5 ±2.0	19.6 ±2.1	19.2 ±1.7	19.3 ±2.2
Hct (%)	63 ±4	62 ±8	60 ±7	60 ±8	60 ±8	61 ±7	64 ±7	61 ±7.4
MCV (fL)	135 ±0.2	132 ±14.4	131 ±13.5	127 ±12.7	123 ±15.7	122 ±10.0	121 ±12.5	119 ±9.4
Retic (%)	6.0 ±0.5	9.6 ±3.2	7.5 ±2.5	5.8 ±2.0	5.0 ±1.9	3.9 ±1.6	4.2 ±1.8	3.2 ±1.4

From Zaizov R and Matoth Y,[1] "Red Cell Values on the First Postnatal Day During the Last 16 Weeks of Gestation," *Amer J Hematol,* 1976, 1:2, 275–8, with permission.
*Mean values ± SD.

(Continued)

Mean Hematologic Values for Full-Term Infants, Children, and Adults*

Age	Hemoglobin (g/dL)	Hematocrit (%)	RBC (10^6/mm^3)	MCV (fL)	MCH (pg)	MCHC (g/dL)
Birth (cord blood)	17.1 ± 1.8	52.0 ± 5	4.64 ± 0.5	113 ± 6	37 ± 2	33 ± 1
1 d	19.4 ± 2.1	58.0 ± 7	5.30 ± 0.5	110 ± 6	37 ± 2	33 ± 1
2-6 d	19.8 ± 2.4	66.0 ± 8	5.40 ± 0.7	122 ± 14	37 ± 4	30 ± 3
14-23 d	15.7 ± 1.5	52.0 ± 5	4.92 ± 0.6	106 ± 11	32 ± 3	30 ± 2
24-37 d	14.1 ± 1.9	45.0 ± 7	4.35 ± 0.6	104 ± 11	32 ± 3	31 ± 3
40-50 d	12.8 ± 1.9	42.0 ± 6	4.10 ± 0.5	103 ± 11	31 ± 3	30 ± 2
2-2.5 mo	11.4 ± 1.1	38.0 ± 4	3.75 ± 0.5	101 ± 10	30 ± 3	30 ± 2
3-3.5 mo	11.2 ± 0.8	37.0 ± 3	3.88 ± 0.4	95 ± 9	29 ± 3	30 ± 2
5-7 mo	11.5 ± 0.7	38.0 ± 3	4.21 ± 0.5	91 ± 9	27 ± 3	30 ± 2
8-10 mo	11.7 ± 0.6	39.0 ± 2	4.35 ± 0.4	90 ± 8	27 ± 3	30 ± 1
11-13.5 mo	11.9 ± 0.6	39.0 ± 2	4.44 ± 0.4	88 ± 7	27 ± 2	30 ± 1
1.5-3 y	11.8 ± 0.5	39.0 ± 2	4.45 ± 0.4	87 ± 7	27 ± 2	30 ± 2
5 y	12.7 ± 1.0	37.0 ± 3	4.65 ± 0.5	80 ± 4	27 ± 2	34 ± 1
10 y	13.2 ± 1.2	39.0 ± 3	4.80 ± 0.5	81 ± 6	28 ± 3	34 ± 1
Men	15.5 ± 1.1	46.0 ± 3.1	5.11 ± 0.38	—	—	—
Women	13.7 ± 1.0	40.9 ± 3	4.51 ± 0.36	—	—	—
Men and women	—	—	—	90.1 ± 4.8	30.2 ± 1.8	33.7 ± 1.1

From Johnson TR, "How Growing Up Can Alter Lab Values in Pediatric Laboratory Medicine," *Diag Med* (special issue), 1982, 5:13-8, with permission.
*Mean ± 1 SD.

Mean Hematologic Values for Low-Birth-Weight Infants*

Weight and Gestational Age at Birth	Age at Testing	Hemoglobin (g/dL)	Hematocrit (%)	Reticulocytes (%)
<1500 g 28–32 wk	3 d	17.5 ± 1.5	54 ± 5	8.0 ± 3.5
	1 wk	15.5 ± 1.5	48 ± 5	3.0 ± 1.0
	2 wk	13.5 ± 1.1	42 ± 4	3.0 ± 1.0
	3 wk	11.5 ± 1.0	35 ± 4	—
	4 wk	10.0 ± 0.9	30 ± 3	6.0 ± 2.0
	6 wk	8.5 ± 0.5	25 ± 2	11.0 ± 3.5
	8 wk	8.5 ± 0.5	25 ± 2	8.5 ± 3.5
	10 wk	9.0 ± 0.5	28 ± 3	7.0 ± 3.0
1500–2000 g 32–36 wk	3 d	19.0 ± 2.0	59 ± 6	6.0 ± 2.0
	1 wk	16.5 ± 1.5	51 ± 5	3.0 ± 1.0
	2 wk	14.5 ± 1.1	44 ± 5	2.5 ± 1.0
	3 wk	13.0 ± 1.1	39 ± 4	—
	4 wk	12.0 ± 1.0	36 ± 4	3.0 ± 1.0
	6 wk	9.5 ± 0.8	28 ± 3	6.0 ± 2.0
	8 wk	9.5 ± 0.5	28 ± 3	5.0 ± 1.5
	10 wk	9.5 ± 0.5	29 ± 3	4.5 ± 1.5
2000–2500 g 36–40 wk	3 d	19.0 ± 2.0	59 ± 6	4.0 ± 1.0
	1 wk	16.5 ± 1.5	51 ± 5	3.0 ± 1.0
	2 wk	15.0 ± 1.5	45 ± 5	2.5 ± 1.0
	3 wk	14.0 ± 1.1	43 ± 4	—
	4 wk	12.5 ± 1.0	37 ± 4	2.0 ± 1.0
	6 wk	10.5 ± 0.9	31 ± 3	3.0 ± 1.0
	8 wk	10.5 ± 0.9	31 ± 3	3.0 ± 1.0
	10 wk	11.0 ± 1.0	33 ± 3	3.0 ± 1.0

From Johnson TR, "How Growing Up Can Alter Lab Values in Pediatric Laboratory Medicine," *Diag Med* (special issue), 1982, 5:13-8, with permission.
*Mean ± 1 SD.

Proposed Classification of Anemic Disorders Based on Red Cell Mean (MCV) and Heterogeneity (RDW)

MCV Low RDW Normal (microcytic homogeneous)	MCV Low RDW High (microcytic heterogeneous)	MCV Normal RDW Normal (normocytic homogeneous)	MCV Normal RDW High (normocytic heterogeneous)	MCV High RDW Normal (macrocytic homogeneous)	MCV High RDW High (macrocytic heterogeneous)
Heterozygous thalassemia*	Iron deficiency*	Normal	Mixed deficiency*	Aplastic anemia	Folate deficiency*
Chronic disease*	S/β–thalassemia	Chronic disease* chronic liver disease*†	Early iron or folate deficiency*	Preleukemia†	Vitamin B_{12} deficiency
	Hemoglobin H	Nonanemic hemoglobinopathy (eg, AS, AC)	Anemic hemoglobinopathy (eg, SS, SC)*		Immune hemolytic anemia
	Red cell fragmentation	Transfusion†	Myelofibrosis		Cold agglutinins
		Chemotherapy	Sideroblastic*		Chronic lymphocytic leukemia, high count
		Chronic lymphocytic leukemia			
		Chronic myelocytic leukemia†			
		Hemorrhage			
		Hereditary spherocytosis			

From Bessman JD Jr, Gilmer PR, and Gardner FH, "Improved Classification of Anemias by MCV and RDW," *Am J Clin Pathol,* 1983, 80:324, with permission. The data for sensitivity of RDW and MCV in each disease category can be obtained from the authors.
*MCV alone <90% sensitive.
†RDW alone <90% sensitive.

(Continued)

Complete Blood Count *(Continued)*

Specimen Whole blood **CONTAINER:** Lavender top (EDTA) tube **COLLECTION:** Mix specimen 10 times by gentle inversion. If specimen is not brought to the laboratory immediately refrigeration is required. If the anticipated delay in arrival is more than 4 hours, two blood smears should be prepared immediately after the venipuncture and submitted with the blood specimen. **CAUSES FOR REJECTION:** Improper tube, clotted specimen, hemolyzed specimen, dilution of blood with I.V. fluid

Interpretive **REFERENCE RANGE:** Accompanying tables summarize differences in red cell parameter normal ranges, note especially important age and sex variances. Refer to tables. **CRITICAL VALUES:** **Critical values**: Hematocrit: <18% or >54%; hemoglobin: <6.0 g/dL or >18.0 g/dL; WBC on admission: <2500/mm^3 or >30,000/mm^3; platelets: <20,000/mm^3 or >1,000,000/mm^3 **USE:** Evaluate anemia, leukemia, reaction to inflammation and infections, peripheral blood cellular characteristics, state of hydration and dehydration, polycythemia, hemolytic disease of the newborn; manage chemotherapy decisions **LIMITATIONS:** Hemoglobin may be falsely high if the plasma is lipemic or if the white count is >50,000 cells/mm^3. "Spun" (manual centrifuged) microhematocrits are approximately 3% higher (due to plasma trapping) compared to automated hematocrit levels. The increase is especially pronounced in cases of polycythemia (increased Hct levels) and when the cells are hypochromic and microcytic. The spun Hct level (as compared to Coulter S) may be 12% higher at Hct levels of 70% and MCV of 48 fL with decrease in change to 3% higher at Hct levels of 70% with MCV of 100 fL.[1] Cold agglutinins (high titer) may cause spurious macrocytosis and low RBC count. This results when RBC couplets are "seen" and processed as single cells by the detection circuitry. Keeping the blood warm and warming the diluent prior to and during counting can correct this problem.[2] See also discussion under Hematocrit. **METHODOLOGY:** Varies considerably between institutions. Most laboratories have high capacity multichannel instruments in place (available from multiple commercial sources). The majority measure RBC and WBC parameters on the basis of changes in electrical impedance as cells and platelets are pulled through a tiny aperture. These are highly automated devices with extensive computer processing of the electrical signals after analog/digital conversion. Accuracy (with proper standardization) and precision (usually in the 0.5% to 2% range) is significantly improved over older manual and semiautomated methods. Some instruments count light impulses that are generated as cells flow across a laser beam. Proper calibration is a prime requisite (see references by Koepke, Lewis et al, and Rowan et al). **ADDITIONAL INFORMATION:** Presence of one or more of the following may be indications for further investigation: hemoglobin <10 g/dL, hemoglobin >18 g/dL, MCV >100 fL, MCV <80 fL, MCHC >37%, WBC >20,000/mm^3, WBC <2000/mm^3, presence of sickle cells, significant spherocytosis, basophilic stippling, stomatocytes,significant schistocytosis, oval macrocytes, tear drop red blood cells, eosinophilia (>10%) monocytosis (>15%), nucleated red blood cells in other than the newborn, malarial organisms or the possibility of malarial organisms, hypersegmented (five or more nuclear segments) PMNs, agranular PMNs, Pelger-Huët anomaly, Auer rods, Döhle bodies, marked toxic granulation, mononuclears in which apparent nucleoli are prominent (blast type cells), presence of metamyelocytes, myelocytes, promyelocytes, neutropenia, presence of plasma cells, peculiar atypical lymphocytes, significant increase or decrease in platelets. Some quantitative elements of the CBC are related to each other, normally, such that examination of the results of any individual analysis allow for the application of a simple but effective case individualized quality control maneuver. The RBC count, hemoglobin, and hematocrit may be analyzed by applying a "rule of three." If red cells are normochromic/normocytic, the RBC count times 3 should approximately equal the hemoglobin and the hemoglobin multiplied by 3 should approximate the hematocrit.[3] If there is significant deviation from this relation, one should check for supporting abnormalities in RBC indices and peripheral smear. The indices themselves offer a quick quality control check of the CBC. If patient transfusion can be excluded, then RBC indices should vary little consecutively from day to day.

Anemias have been classified on the basis of their MCV and RDW (RBC heterogeneity). This classification has been especially helpful in the separation of iron deficiency from thalassemia. Heterozygous thalassemia (thalassemia minor) when associated with normal hemoglobin has a normal RDW (13.4 ±1.2%) while RDW is high with iron deficiency (16.3 ±1.8%).[4] RDW will be increased slightly in cases of thalassemia with slight anemia.[4] Some studies have found that the RDW does not reliably separate iron deficiency from thalassemia minor unless, possibly, a higher cutoff value of 17.0% is utilized.[5] See also the entry, Ferritin, Serum in the Chemistry chapter.

In patients who do not have disorders known to result in anisocytosis (eg, liver disease, alcoholism, combined nutritional deficiency) and who have not received a recent blood transfusion, it has been claimed RDW may be helpful in separating the anemia of chronic disease (RDW in normal range) from iron deficiency (RDW increased) thereby reducing the need for marrow study to determine iron stores.[6] It has also been reported, however, on the basis of serum ferritin levels in relatively undefined patient populations that RDW is not clinically useful in distinguishing the anemia of chronic disease from iron deficiency.[7]

Bessman claims that the RDW is increased before the MCV decreases in iron deficiency.[8] Although this is somewhat controversial,[9] perhaps even a simple marketing tool copied by all hematology instrument manufacturers, it serves as an inexpensive screen for the common iron deficiency anemia. See tables.

As might be anticipated, the RDW is an insensitive parameter for the diagnosis of vitamin B_{12} deficiency, as well as for the diagnosis of folate deficiency, and the RDW has no value in separating alcohol-related macrocytosis from B_{12}/folate deficiency.[10] It has been found that in a hospitalized urban patient population, zidovudine treatment of AIDS is the most common cause of macrocytosis (44%) and B_{12}/folate deficiency are relatively decreased (3% and 4%, respectively).[11]

Footnotes

1. Dosik H and Prasad B, "Coulter S Hematocrit and Microhematocrit in Polycythemic Patients," *Am J Hematol*, 1978, 5:51-4.
2. Hattersley PG, Gerard PW, Caggiano V, et al, "Erroneous Values on the Model S Coulter Due to High Titer Cold Agglutinins," *Am J Clin Pathol*, 1971, 55:442-6.
3. Lofsness KG, "Correlation of Hematologic Data From the Individual Patient as a Quality Control Tool," *Am J Med Technol*, 1983, 49:655-9.
4. Bessman JD Jr, Gilmer PR, and Gardner FH, "Improved Classification of Anemias by MCV and RDW," *Am J Clin Pathol*, 1983, 80:322-6.
5. van Zeben D, Bieger R, van Wermeskerken RK, et al, "Evaluation of Microcytosis Using Serum Ferritin and Red Blood Cell Distribution Width," *Eur J Haematol*, 1990, 44(2):106-9.
6. Kaye FJ and Alter BP, "Red-Cell Size Distribution Analysis: An Evaluation of Microcytic Anemia in Chronically Ill Patients," *Mt Sinai J Med*, 1985, 52:319-23.
7. Rice LE, Saleem A, Dunn K, et al, "RDW Fails to Distinguish Iron-Deficiency from Anemia of Chronic Disease," *Blood*, 1987, 70:55a.
8. McClure S, Custer E, and Bessman JD, "Improved Detection of Early Iron Deficiency in Nonanemic Subjects," *JAMA*, 1985, 253:1021-3.
9. Flynn MM, Reppun TS, and Bhagavan NV, "Limitation of Red Cell Distribution Width (RDW) in Evaluation of Microcytosis," *Am J Clin Pathol*, 1986, 85:445-9.
10. Zuiable A and Wickramasinghe SN, "RDW in Vitamin B_{12} and Folate Deficiency and in Patients With Alcohol-Related Macrocytosis," *Clin Lab Haematol*, 1992, 14(2):164-6.
11. Snower DP and Weil SC, "Changing Etiology of Macrocytosis: Zidovudine as a Frequent Causative Factor," *Am J Clin Pathol*, 1993, 99(1):57-60.

References

Beautyman W and Bills T, "Osmotic Error in Erythrocyte Volume Determinations," *Am J Hematol*, 1982, 12:383-9.

Burgess PR, Kershaw GW, Coleman RH, et al, "A Computerized Expert System for Handling the Output of the Technicon H1 Haematology Analyser," *Clin Lab Haematol*, 1993, 15(1):21-32.

Fraser CG, Wilkinson SP, Neville RG, et al, "Biologic Variation of Common Hematologic Laboratory Quantities in the Elderly," *Am J Clin Pathol*, 1989, 92(4):465-70.

Koepke J, "Quantitative Blood Cell Counting," *Practical Laboratory Hematology*, Chapter 3, Koepke J, ed, New York, NY: Churchill Livingstone, 1991, 43-60.

Lee GR, "Microcytosis and the Anemias Associated With Impaired Hemoglobin Synthesis," *Wintrobe's Clinical Hematology*, 9th ed, Vol 1, Chapter 25, Lee GR, Bithell TC, Foerster J, et al, eds, Philadelphia, PA: Lea & Febiger, 1993, 791-807.

Lewis SM, England JM, and Rowan RM, "Current Concerns in Haematology 3: Blood Count Calibration," *J Clin Pathol*, 1991, 44(11):881-4.

Penn D, Williams PR, Dutcher TF, et al, "Comparison of Hematocrit Determinations by Microhematocrit and Electronic Particle Counter," *Am J Clin Pathol*, 1979, 72:71-4.

Rowan RM and England JM, "Special Aspects in Haematology," *Evaluation Methods in Laboratory Medicine*, Chapter 7, Haeckel R, ed, New York, NY: VCH Publishers, 1993, 141-51.

Second National Health and Nutrition Examination Survey, "Hematological and Nutritional Biochemistry Reference Data for Persons 6 Months-74 Years of Age: United States, 1976-80," *Vital and Health Statistics*, DHHS Publication No (PHS) 83-1682, 1982.

^{51}Cr Labeled Red Cell Volume *see* Red Cell Mass *on page 595*

^{51}Cr Red Cell Survival

CPT 78130; 78135 (with splenic and/or hepatic sequestration)

Related Information

Occult Blood, Stool *on page 1138*

Reticulocyte Count *on page 597*

Synonyms Chromium-51 Tagged RBC Survival Test; Erythrocyte Survival; Red Cell Survival; Survival of Red Blood Cells

Patient Care PREPARATION: Obtain signed procedure permit for "^{51}Cr red cell survival." Patient's own ^{51}Cr labeled red cells are infused. Patient should be provided a schedule for serial blood samples to be drawn.

Specimen Whole blood is drawn, processed (tagged with ^{51}Cr), and reinfused into the patient. CONTAINER: Lavender top (EDTA) tube COLLECTION: Scheduled periodic blood samples are drawn for determination of residual radioactivity. CAUSES FOR REJECTION: Previous isotope procedure with significant radioactivity remaining in patient's blood, significant transfused blood, intermittent bleeding episodes TURNAROUND TIME: Time required for procedure depends on half-time of disappearance of labeled cells and averages 3 weeks. SPECIAL INSTRUCTIONS: At least 21 days should be allowed for this study. When selective splenic sequestration as cause of hemolysis is suspected, liver and spleen readings may be performed in conjunction with ^{51}Cr RBC Survival Test.

Interpretive REFERENCE RANGE: Presence of half of ^{51}Cr label remaining at 25-35 days (red cell survival half-life of 25-35 days).[1] Given an isotope label that would act as a "perfect" tracer (no loss through elution), one would expect half of the label to disappear at about 55-60 days, half of the average red cell life span of 110-120 days (see discussion that follows). The ratio of spleen to liver counts is usually 1:1 in normal individuals. USE: Provide proof of hemolytic process, (ie, determine if patient's RBCs have decreased survival); determine red cell survival in cases of increased red cell destruction, (ie, immunohemolytic anemia;[2] spherocytosis, red cell enzyme deficiency, and hemoglobinopathies); evaluate occult blood loss, especially subdural hematomas,[3] and splenic sequestration. In the spleen/liver (S/L) ratio, the average patient with splenomegaly ratio is 1:1; hemolytic anemias show 3:1 or 4:1. LIMITATIONS: This test cannot discriminate between red cell loss due to intravascular hemolysis and red cell loss due to bleeding that results in blood loss from the intravascular compartment. Test is expensive. METHODOLOGY: Patient's own RBCs incubated with ^{51}Cr under sterile conditions are injected back into the patient's vascular system and periodic blood samples are obtained for measurement of residual radioactivity over a 2- to 3-week period. Activity (counts/minute/mL of RBCs) obtained at 24 hours is usually taken at the starting point (is given a value of 100%). A plot is constructed (should include hematocrit correction)[4] and the ^{51}Cr half-life is determined. ADDITIONAL INFORMATION: The ^{51}Cr red cell survival does not equate numerically with one-half of the physiologic RBC lifespan (110-120 days). This is due to elution of the ^{51}Cr label from red cells during the procedure. As a result, the ^{51}Cr survival time does not relate in a simple or direct manner to the red cell lifespan and is best viewed as a semiquantitative index of survival. Given a "perfect" label, half of the activity would be lost at 55-60 days. Diisopropylfluorophosphate (DFP) ^{14}C, ^{32}P, or tritium labels act, essentially, as a perfect label but are not in common routine clinical use as, lacking gamma emission, imaging or organ uptake studies cannot be performed. In patients with hemolysis, the RBC survival curve results from the rate of elution of the label combined with the rate of random hemolysis. In addition to DFP, red cells may be labeled for survival studies with ^{14}C cyanate, ^{75}Se selenomethionine, ^{14}C or ^{15}N glycine or ^{55}Fe or ^{59}Fe iron. Because of the penetrance capability of gamma emitting ^{51}Cr, patients with ^{51}Cr-labeled RBCs can undergo *in vivo* count rate measurements over the spleen and liver during red cell survival study. See reference by Landaw for clinical significance of spleen/liver ratio, RBC sequestration index, and RBC survival.

Footnotes

1. International Committee for Standardization in Haematology, "Recommended Method for Radioisotope Red-Cell Survival Studies," *Br J Haematol*, 1980, 45:659-66.
2. Levy GJ, Selset G, McQuiston D, et al, "Clinical Significance of Anti-Yt^{b}. Report of a Case Using ^{51}Chromium Red Cell Survival Study," *Transfusion*, 1988, 28(3):265-7.
3. Ito H, Yamamoto S, Saito K, et al, "Quantitative Estimation of Hemorrhage in Chronic Subdural Hematoma Using the ^{51}Cr Erythrocyte Labeling Method," *J Neurosurg*, 1987, 66:862-4.
4. Milam JD, Samuels MS, Hidalgo JU, et al, "Use of Hematocrit Values in Evaluation of Red Cell Survival With Chromium-51," *Am J Clin Pathol*, 1966, 45:56-60.

References

Brucer M, "How Long Will Red Cells Last?" "Development of the Red Cell Survival Test," *Vignettes in Nuclear Medicine*, St Louis, MO: Mallinckrodt Chemical Works, 1973, 55.

Henry JB, Nelson DA, Tomar RH, et al, *Clinical Diagnosis and Management by Laboratory Methods*, 18th ed, Philadelphia, PA: WB Saunders Co, 1991, 642-3.

Langan JK, Scheffel U, and McIntyre PA, "The Hematopoietic System," *Nuclear Medicine Technology and Techniques*, Chapter 18, Bernier DR, Christian PE, Langan JK, et al, eds, St Louis, MO: Mosby-Year Book Inc, 1989, 493-5.

Landaw SA, "Hemostasis, Survival, and Red Cell Kinetics: Measurement and Imaging of Red Cell Production," *Hematology Basic Principles and Practice*, Chapter 24, Hoffman R, Benz EJ Jr, Shattil SJ, et al, eds, New York, NY: Churchill Livingstone, 1991, 274-90.

CSF Analysis *see* Cerebrospinal Fluid Analysis *on page 527*

Cyanocobalamin, True *see* Vitamin B_{12} *on page 612*

Cyst Fluid Analysis *see* Body Fluids Analysis, Cell Count *on page 523*

Cytochemistry, Leukocyte *see* Leukocyte Cytochemistry *on page 567*

Cytokines *see* Eosinophil Count *on this page*

Differential *see* Peripheral Blood: Differential Leukocyte Count *on page 576*

Differential Smear *see* Peripheral Blood: Differential Leukocyte Count *on page 576*

Dithionite Test *see* Sickle Cell Tests *on page 600*

Donath-Landsteiner Test *see* Cold Hemolysin Test *on page 532*

Eos Count *see* Eosinophil Count *on this page*

Eosinophil Count

CPT 85999

Related Information

Complete Blood Count *on page 533*
Eosinophil Smear *on page 541*
Muramidase, Blood and Urine *on page 571*
Ova and Parasites, Stool *on page 836*
Ova and Parasites, Urine *on page 839*
Parasite Antibodies *on page 729*
Peripheral Blood: Differential Leukocyte Count *on page 576*
Thorn Test *on page 609*

Synonyms Absolute Eosinophil Count; Eos Count; Total Eosinophil Count

Applies to Cytokines; Granulocyte/Macrophage Colony Stimulating Factor; Interleukin-3; Interleukin-5

Abstract Manual (using phloxine stain) or automated absolute eosinophil count is requested in certain clinical situations because of expected greater precision/accuracy than is usually obtained using the relative number of eosinophils from the manual differential count. Eosinophil count is increased in a wide variety of conditions including especially, allergy, drug reaction, parasitism, collagen vascular disease, and some malignant states. Eosinophils are decreased with hyperadrenalism.

Specimen Whole blood **CONTAINER:** Lavender top (EDTA) tube **CAUSES FOR REJECTION:** Clotted specimen, specimen more than 4 hours old

Interpretive **REFERENCE RANGE:** 50-350/mm^3 **USE:** Aid in the diagnosis of allergy, drug reaction, parasitic infestations, collagen disease, Hodgkin's disease, and myeloproliferative diseases. Increased also in a broad range of less common conditions including the acute hypereosinophilic syndrome,[1] angioneurotic edema, acute renal allograft rejection,[2] eosinophilic nonallergic rhinitis,[3] anisakiasis,[4] eosinophilic gastroenteritis,[5] eosinophilia myalgia syndrome,[6] and others. Decrease in eosinophils occurs in Cushing's disease (hyperadrenalism). **LIMITATIONS:** Manual method is subject to an inherent error of 20% to 30%.[7] **METHODOLOGY:** Manual, using Fuchs-Rosenthal or Speirs-Levy special large volume hemocytometer and eosinophil stain diluent (eg, Pilot's solution or phloxine B solution as used in the Unopette™ Brand System, Becton Dickinson, Rutherford, NJ). Automated method (eg, Technicon®, Coulter, Sysmex) should provide greater precision/accuracy and is recommended for obtaining an absolute eosinophil count.[7] **ADDITIONAL INFORMATION:** Toxocaral disease (visceral larva migrans) is a typical parasitic disease in which eosinophil counts (eosinophils >30% on differential) are usually elevated. Taylor et al[8] point out, however, that up to 27% of children with toxocariasis have normal eosinophil counts. Thus, normal eosinophil counts do not rule out toxocaral disease or other par-

(Continued)

Eosinophil Count *(Continued)*

asitic infestations. The T-cell produced cytokines interleukin-3, granulocyte/macrophage colony stimulating factor, and interleukin-5 (IL-5) stimulate eosinophil production *in vitro*. Murine eosinophil differentiation factor (IL-5) has its most specific effect on eosinophil growth in culture with no significant effect on growth/development of other myeloid cell lines.[9] IL-5 appears to be the prime mediator of eosinophilia in patients with certain parasitic diseases.[10,11]

An important although rare cause of increased eosinophils in the peripheral blood is the acute hypereosinophilic syndrome (HES). Reported mortalities range from 81% to 95% in 1-3 years. The HES syndrome includes high peripheral WBC count, circulating early eosinophil forms without blast cells, mental confusion, delusions, near coma, and severe cardiac symptoms. Consistently associated with a poor prognosis are WBC count $\geq$90,000/mm^3, blast forms in blood, heart failure, and severe CNS symptoms (confusion, organic psychosis and coma). This condition may not be a true leukemic myeloproliferative disease, although concepts of HES are controversial.

Infiltrative lung diseases, in which peripheral blood eosinophils may be increased, include eosinophilic pneumonia, Löffler's syndrome (often related to *Ascaris* infestation), and tropical eosinophilia (usually related to filariasis).[12]

Eosinophilic gastroenteritis may occur with blood eosinophilia.[5]

Eosinophilia myalgia syndrome (EMS) characterized by an eosinophil count of 1000 cells/mm^3 or more and severe often incapacitating myalgia is possibly associated with the use of L-tryptophan-containing products (LTCPs). Further definition of this syndrome, causal association between LTCPs and EMS, and modifying etiologic factors/cofactors has been recommended and is being pursued by CDC.[6,13] An EMS-like syndrome has been considered to result from several factors including ingestion of tryptophan, inactivation of indoleamine-2,3-dioxygenase, and possible impairment of the hypothalamic-pituitary-adrenal axis.[14] The differential diagnosis of EMS (causes other than L-tryptophan) is discussed by Dicker et al (see References). Sarcoidosis, granulomatous myositis, collagen vascular diseases, neoplastic myositis, and other entities should be considered. EMS is potentially fatal (Guillain-Barré like ascending polyneuropathy) with a clinical course resembling the toxic oil syndrome that was epidemic in Spain in 1981.[15]

Footnotes

1. Chusid MJ, Dale DC, West BC, et al, "The Hypereosinophilic Syndrome: Analysis of Fourteen Cases With Review of the Literature," *Medicine (Baltimore)*, 1975, 54:1-27.
2. Weir MR, Hall-Craggs M, Shen SY, et al, "The Prognostic Value of the Eosinophil in Acute Renal Allograft Rejection," *Transplantation*, 1986, 41:709-12.
3. Rupp GH and Friedman RA, "Eosinophilic Nonallergic Rhinitis in Children," *Pediatrics*, 1983, 70:437-9.
4. Valdiserri, RO, "Intestinal Anisakiasis. Report of a Case and Recovery of Larvae From Market Fish," *Am J Clin Pathol*, 1981, 76:329-33.
5. Pavli P and Doe WF, "The Alimentary Tract in Disorders of the Immune System," *Gastrointestinal and Oesophageal Pathology*, Whitehead R, ed, Edinburgh, England: Churchill Livingstone, 1989, 187.
6. Center for Disease Control, "Eosinophilia-Myalgia Syndrome – New Mexico," *MMWR Morb Mortal Wkly Rep*, 1989, 38(45):765-7.
7. McNeely JC and Brown D, "Laboratory Evaluation of Leukocytes: Absolute Eosinophil Counting Procedure," *Clinical Hematology: Principles, Procedures, Correlations*, Chapter 25, Lotspeich-Steininger CA, Stiene-Martin EA, and Koepke JA, eds, Philadelphia, PA: JB Lippincott Co, 1992, 329-31.
8. Taylor MR, Keane CT, O'Connor P, et al, "The Expanded Spectrum of Toxocaral Disease," *Lancet*, 1988, 1(8587):692-5.
9. Clutterbuck EJ, Hirst EM, and Sanderson CJ, "Human Interleukin-5 (IL-5) Regulates the Production of Eosinophils in Human Bone Marrow Cultures: Comparison and Interaction With IL-1, IL-3, IL-6, and GMCSF," *Blood*, 1989, 73(6):1504-12.
10. Limaye AP, Abrams JS, Silver JE, et al, "Regulation of Parasitic Induced Eosinophilia: Selectively Increased Interleukin-5 Production in Helminth-Infected Patients," *J Exp Med*, 1990, 172(1):399-402.
11. Limaye AP, Abrams JS, Silver JE, et al, "Interleukin-5 and the Post-treatment Eosinophilia in Patients With Onchocerciasis," *J Clin Invest*, 1991, 88(4):1418-21.
12. Colby TV and Carrington CB, "Infiltrative Lung Disease," Chapter 20, *Pathology of the Lung*, Thurlbeck WM, ed, New York, NY: Thieme Medical Publishers Inc, 1988, 425-517.
13. Center for Disease Control, "Eosinophilia-Myalgia Syndrome and L-Tryptophan-Containing Products – New Mexico, Minnesota, Oregon and New York," *MMWR Morb Mortal Wkly Rep*, 1989, 38(46):785-8.
14. Silver RM, Heyes MP, Maize JC, et al, "Scleroderma, Fasciitis, and Eosinophilia Associated With the Ingestion of Tryptophan," *N Engl J Med*, 1990, 322(13):874-81.
15. Kilbourne EM, Rigau-Perez JG, Heath CW Jr, et al, "Clinical Epidemiology of Toxic-Oil Syndrome: Manifestations of a New Illness," *N Engl J Med*, 1983, 309:1408-14.

References

Dicker RM, James N, and Cunha BA, "The Eosinophilia-Myalgia Syndrome With Neuritis Associated With L-Tryptophan Use," *Ann Intern Med*, 1990, 112(12):957-8.

Duffy J, "Eosinophilia-Myalgia Syndrome," *Mayo Clin Proc*, 1992, 67:1201-2.
Mahmond, AAF, Austen, KF, and Simon, AS, *The Eosinophil in Health and Disease*, New York, NY: Grune and Stratton Inc, 1980.
Martin RW, Duffy J, Engel AG, et al, "The Clinical Spectrum of the Eosinophilia-Myalgia Syndrome Associated With L-Tryptophan Ingestion. Clinical Features in 20 Patients and Aspects of Pathophysiology," *Ann Intern Med*, 1990, 113(9):124-34.
Mayeno AN, Belongia EA, Lin F, et al, "3-(Phenylamino)alanine, a Novel Aniline-Derived Amino Acid Associated With the Eosinophilia-Myalgia Syndrome: A Link to the Toxic Oil Syndrome?," *Mayo Clin Proc*, 1992, 67(12):1134-9.
Randolph TG, "Differentiation and Enumeration of Eosinophils in the Counting Chamber With a Glycol Stain; A Valuable Technique in Appraising ACTH Dosage," *J Lab Clin Med*, 1949, 34:1696-1701.
Shurin SB, "Eosinophil and Basophil Structure and Function," *Hematology Basic Principles and Practice*, Chapter 41, Hoffman R, Benz EJ Jr, Shattil SJ, et al, eds, New York, NY: Churchill Livingstone, 1991, 538-42.
Van Slyck EJ and Adamson TC III, "Acute Hypereosinophilic Syndrome. Successful Treatment With Vincristine, Cytarabine, and Prednisone," *JAMA*, 1979, 242:175-6.
Smith H and Cook RM, *Immunopharmacology of Eosinophils, The Handbook of Immunopharmacology*, Page C, ed, San Diego, CA: Academic Press, 1993, 1-250.

Eosinophil Smear

***CPT** 89190*

Related Information

Eosinophil Count *on page 539*

Synonyms Fecal Smear for Eosinophils; Nasal Smear for Eosinophils; Sputum Smear for Eosinophils

Specimen Two slides of nasal secretion, smear or swab of feces or sputum. No fixation is required for slides. Nasal secretions may be submitted on wax paper or plastic wrap. **CONTAINER:** Slides or nasal secretions on wax paper **CAUSES FOR REJECTION:** Slides received in cytology fixative, no specimen on slide, smear, or swab **SPECIAL INSTRUCTIONS:** Requisition must state site of specimen.

Interpretive **REFERENCE RANGE:** No eosinophils identified **USE:** Investigate allergy, asthmatic disorders, and parasitic infestations **METHODOLOGY:** Wright's stain and microscopic examination of smear **ADDITIONAL INFORMATION:** Eosinophils are often increased in the blood and sputum of patients with asthma, usually in relation to the severity of the process.[1] There is no percentage of eosinophils in sputum diagnostic of asthma, but levels >80% (related to proportion of neutrophils) are very suggestive of asthma or of chronic bronchitis with wheezing. There is evidence of an inverse correlation between the numbers of eosinophils in the circulation and/or sputum and pulmonary function (eg, airway flow rates).[2,3,4] Gram stained smears of microbiology specimens will not stain eosinophils.

Footnotes

1. Busse WW and Sedgwick JB, "Eosinophils in Asthma," *Ann Allergy*, 1992, 68(3):286-90.
2. Griffin E, Håkansson L, Formgren H, et al, "Blood Eosinophil Number and Activity in Relation to Lung Function in Patients With Asthma and With Eosinophilia," *J Allergy Clin Immunol*, 1991, 87(2):548-57.
3. O'Connor GT, Sparrow D, and Weiss ST, "The Role of Allergy and Nonspecific Airway Hyperresponsiveness in the Pathogenesis of Chronic Obstructive Pulmonary Disease," *Am Rev Respir Dis*, 1989, 140(1):225-52.
4. Alfaro C, Sharma OP, Navarro L, et al, "Inverse Correlation of Expiratory Lung Flows and Sputum Eosinophils in Status Asthmaticus," *Ann Allergy*, 1989, 63(3):251-4.

References

Middleton E, "Chronic Rhinitis in Adults," *J Allergy Clin Immunol*, 1988, 81:971-5.
Viera VG and Prolla JC, "Clinical Evaluation of Eosinophils in the Sputum," *J Clin Pathol*, 1979, 32:1054-7.

Erythrocyte Count *see* Red Cell Count *on page 594*

Erythrocyte Enzyme Deficiency, Quantitative *see* Red Blood Cell Enzyme Deficiency, Quantitative *on page 591*

Erythrocyte Enzyme Deficiency Screen *see* Red Blood Cell Enzyme Deficiency Screen *on page 592*

Erythrocyte Indices *see* Red Blood Cell Indices *on page 592*

Erythrocyte Sedimentation Rate *see* Zeta Sedimentation Ratio *on page 617*

Erythrocyte Survival *see* ^{51}Cr Red Cell Survival *on page 536*

Extrinsic Factor of Castle *see* Vitamin B_{12} *on page 612*

Fecal Smear for Eosinophils *see* Eosinophil Smear *on previous page*

Fetal Hemoglobin

CPT 83030

Related Information

Hemoglobin Electrophoresis *on page 556*
Hemolytic Disease of the Newborn, Antibody Identification *on page 1070*
Kleihauer-Betke *on page 563*
Sickle Cell Tests *on page 600*

Synonyms Hb F; Hemoglobin, Fetal

Specimen Whole blood **CONTAINER:** Lavender top (EDTA) tube for venipuncture specimen; lavender top Microtainer™ tube for capillary specimen

Interpretive REFERENCE RANGE: 6 months to adult: up to 2% of the total hemoglobin; 0-6 months: up to 75% **USE:** Evaluate hemoglobinopathies, hemolytic anemia; diagnose hereditary persistence of fetal hemoglobin, thalassemia; evaluate sickling hemoglobins **LIMITATIONS:** Carboxyhemoglobin A is also resistant to alkali denaturation. Assay for Hb F should initially convert carboxyhemoglobin to cyanmethemoglobin or false-positive elevations of Hb F may be obtained.[1] **METHODOLOGY:** Alkali denaturation, high resolution hemoglobin electrophoresis (some methods), acid elution (Kleihauer-Betke), radial immunodiffusion (RID), isoelectric focusing, high performance liquid chromatography (HPLC), enzyme immunoassay (EIA)[2] **ADDITIONAL INFORMATION:** Fetal hemoglobin is formed of two α-chains and two γ-chains. It is the major hemoglobin during fetal life. Hb F levels decrease after birth by about 3% to 4% per week. In 2-3 weeks fetal hemoglobin is about 65%. By 6 months of age fetal hemoglobin is <2% of the total hemoglobin. See graph. The oxygen dissociation curve of Hb F is shifted to the left as compared with normal Hb A. This may be due to decreased binding of 2,3-DPG by Hb F (γ-chains). This facilitates placental oxygen transfer. With erythroblastosis fetalis and anoxic states of the newborn, however, Hb F is proportionally lower than in a normal newborn. Some 15 inherited abnormalities of γ-chain structure have been described[3], but most are without clinical significance (fetal Hgb normally forms <2% of total hemoglobin). An exception is Hb F Poole which has been reported as a cause of hemolytic disease of the newborn.[4]

In the adult, hereditary persistence of fetal hemoglobin (HPFH) of multiple varieties, is associated with varying elevations of Hb F. The homozygous form of HPFH is found only in blacks. In the heterozygous state, the Hb F level is 15% to 35% in the black type, and 5% to 20% in the Greek type. Homozygous β-thalassemia is associated with Hb F levels of >10% to <90%. About 50% of heterozygotes for β-thalassemia have elevated levels around 2%, rarely >5%. The remainder have normal Hb F. Heterozygous S/β thalassemia may have Hb F in the 5% to 20% range. With homozygous Hb S disease the level of Hb F varies from 0% to 20%.[5] Other conditions associated with elevated Hb F include various anemias, spherocytosis, Fanconi's, acquired aplastic, hemolytic, hypoplastic, megaloblastic, myelophthisic, and untreated pernicious anemia; all types of leukemia (especially erythroleukemia and juvenile chronic myelogenous leukemia), multiple myeloma and lymphomas, metastatic disease of the bone marrow; pregnancy; miscellaneous disorders reported include infants small for gestational age, infants with chronic intrauterine anoxia with developmental anomalies; during anticonvulsant drug therapy; diabetes; hyper and hypothyroidism; and macroglobulin. Elevation of Hb F should, then, raise the question of possible underlying disease.

Footnotes

1. Hoagland HC, "Interpretation of Increased Concentration of Hemoglobin F," *Hemoglobinopathies and Thalassemias: Laboratory Methods and Case Studies*, Fairbanks VF, ed, New York, NY: Thieme-Stratton Inc, 1980, 69.
2. Moscoso H, Shyamala M, Kiefer CR, et al, "Monoclonal Antibody to the γ-Chain of Human Fetal Hemoglobin Used to Develop an Enzyme Immunoassay," *Clin Chem*, 1989, 35(10):2066-9.
3. Weatherall DJ, Clegg JB, Higgs DR, et al, "The Hemoglobinopathies," *The Metabolic Basis of Inherited Disease*, 6th ed, Scriver CR, Beaudet AL, Sly WS, et al, eds, New York, NY: McGraw-Hill Inc, 1989, 2323-4.
4. Lee-Potter JP, Deacon-Smith RA, Simpkiss MJ, et al, "A New Cause of Hemolytic Anemia in the Newborn. A Description of an Unstable Fetal Hemoglobin: F. Poole, $\alpha_2\gamma_2$ 130 Tryptophan Yields Glycine," *J Clin Pathol*, 1975, 28:317-20.
5. Warth JA and Rucknagal DL, "The Increasing Complexity of Sickle Cell Anemia," *Prog Hematol*, 1983, 13:25-47.

References

Bunn HF and Forget BG, *Hemoglobin: Molecular, Genetic and Clinical Aspects*, Philadelphia, PA: WB Saunders Co, 1986, 68-75.

Nonmalignant Conditions Associated With Increased Proportions of Hb F

Condition	Hb F Value (%)
Anemias	
Aplastic anemia (both congenital and acquired)	5–25
Pernicious anemia	2–6
Hereditary spherocytosis	2–5
Hereditary elliptocytosis	2–5
Congenital nonspherocytic hemolytic anemia	3–4
Anemia of chronic infection	2–3
Anemia of blood loss	2–8
Erythropoietic porphyria	2–10
Paroxysmal nocturnal hemoglobinuria	2–25
Hemoglobinopathies	
Unstable hemoglobins	<10
Homozygous Hb S disease	<20
Hb Lepore trait	<5
Hb Kenya trait	6–13
Thalassemias	
β-thalassemia minor	<5
$\delta\beta$-thalassemia minor	5–20
β-thalassemia major	30–95
α-thalassemia minor	~1
Hb H disease	5–15
Hemoglobinopathy–thalassemia interactions	
S/β-thalassemia	10–30
E/β-thalassemia	10–50
C/β-thalassemia	10–30
Hereditary persistence of fetal hemoglobin (HPFH)	
African-type	
heterozygous	15–40
homozygous	100
Greek-type	
heterozygous	10–20
Swiss-type	
heterozygous	1–3

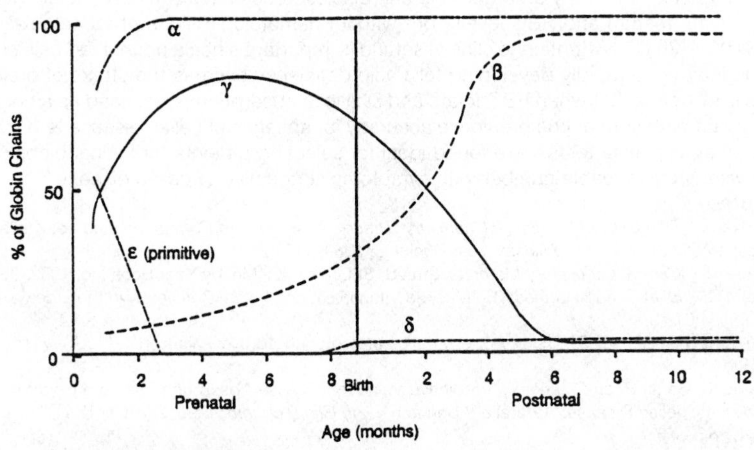

Relative amounts of the several globin chains (ε, α, γ, β, and δ) present during fetal development and the first year of life.

(Continued)

Fetal Hemoglobin *(Continued)*

Castro O, Winter WP, Lee TC, et al, "Prevalence of α-Chain Variants at Birth," *Am J Clin Pathol*, 1981, 75:56-9.

Embury SH and Mentzer WC, "The Thalassemia Syndromes," *The Hereditary Hemolytic Anemias*, Chapter 3, Mentzer WC and Wagner GM, New York, NY: Churchill Livingstone, 1989, 93-144.

Fucharoen S, Rowley PT, Paul NW, et al, *Thalassemia: Pathophysiology and Management*, March of Dimes Birth Defects Foundation Original Article Series, Vol 23, No 5A, New York, NY: Alan R Liss Inc, 1987.

Kaufman RE, "Analysis of Abnormal Hemoglobins," *Practical Laboratory Hematology*, Koepke JA, ed, New York, NY: Churchill Livingstone, 1991, 251-94.

Fetal Hemoglobin Test in Newborn *see* APT Test *on page 518*

Filarial Infestation *see* Microfilariae, Peripheral Blood Preparation *on page 571*

Filariasis Peripheral Blood Preparation *see* Microfilariae, Peripheral Blood Preparation *on page 571*

Folate Level *see* Folic Acid, Serum *on next page*

Folic Acid, RBC

CPT *82747*

See Also Anemia Flowchart in the Hematology Appendix

Related Information

Complete Blood Count *on page 533*
d-Xylose Absorption Test *on page 210*
Folic Acid, Serum *on next page*
Hemoglobin *on page 554*
Schilling Test *on page 598*
Vitamin B_{12} *on page 612*
Vitamin B_{12} Unsaturated Binding Capacity *on page 615*

Synonyms RBC Folate; Red Cell Folate

Patient Care **PREPARATION:** Avoid radioisotope scan prior to collection of specimen.

Specimen Erythrocytes **CONTAINER:** Lavender top (EDTA) tube. Green top (heparin) tube may also be used for folate assay, but heparin interferes with vitamin B_{12} determinations, which are often performed simultaneously. **SAMPLING TIME:** Fasting specimen is preferred. **STORAGE INSTRUCTIONS:** Red cells (or hemolysate) can be stored at 4°C or frozen until assay.

Interpretive **REFERENCE RANGE:** 125-600 ng/mL (SI: 283-1360 nmol/L). The megaloblastic anemia of folate deficiency is usually associated with red cell folate levels <100 ng/mL (SI<227 nmol/L) RBCs.[1,2] **USE:** Detect folate deficiency **METHODOLOGY:** Radioimmunoassay (RIA), competitive protein binding **ADDITIONAL INFORMATION:** Since serum folate values fluctuate significantly with diet, measurement of red cell folate is a better measure of tissue folate stores. It is widespread practice to measure serum and red cell folate with vitamin B_{12} levels. A study of patients in an inner city area geriatric unit disclosed 50 cases with decreased vitamin B_{12} and/or folate (serum and RBC levels) but without hematologic signs of megaloblastosis (all had MCV <100 fL).[3] Attention to clinical setting is important since a normal red cell folate level can be found in a rapidly developing folic acid deficiency such as the stress of pregnancy.[4] There is evidence that when RBC folate and D-xylose absorption tests, used as a noninvasive screen, are both normal, the predictive accuracy for absence of celiac disease is 100%. When used together, these tests were found ideal for selecting patients for jejunal biopsy from an otherwise unmanageable number with symptoms suggestive of celiac disease.[5]

Footnotes

1. McNeely MD, "Folic Acid," *Clinical Chemistry: Theory, Analysis, and Correlation*, 2nd ed, Kaplan LA and Pesce AJP, St Louis, MO: Mosby-Year Book Inc, 1989, 1131-2.
2. Bauer JD, *Clinical Laboratory Methods*, 9th ed, St Louis, MO: Mosby-Year Book Inc, 1982, 95-6.
3. Craig GM, Elliot C, and Hughes KR, "Masked Vitamin B_{12} and Folate Deficiency in the Elderly," *Br J Nutr*, 1985, 54:613-9.
4. Williams WJ, Beutler E, Erslev AJ, et al, *Hematology*, 4th ed, New York, NY: McGraw-Hill Inc, 1990, 456-9.
5. Labib M, Gama R, and Marks V, "Predictive Value of D-Xylose Absorption Test and Erythrocyte Folate in Adult Coeliac Disease: A Parallel Approach," *Ann Clin Biochem*, 1990, 27(Pt 1):75-7.

References

Chanarin I, "Megaloblastic Anaemia, Cobalamin, and Folate," *J Clin Pathol*, 1987, 40:978-84.

Davis RE and Nicol DJ, "Folic Acid," *Int J Biochem*, 1988, 20:133-9, (minireview).

Folic Acid, Serum

CPT 82746

See Also Anemia Flowchart in the Hematology Appendix

Related Information

Complete Blood Count *on page 533*
Folic Acid, RBC *on previous page*
Hemoglobin *on page 554*
Intrinsic Factor Antibody *on page 714*
Parietal Cell Antibody *on page 730*
Schilling Test *on page 598*
Vitamin B_{12} *on page 612*
Vitamin B_{12} Unsaturated Binding Capacity *on page 615*

Synonyms Folate Level; Serum Folate

Patient Care PREPARATION: Patient should be fasting overnight. Collect prior to transfusion or initiation of folate therapy.

Specimen Serum CONTAINER: Red top tube COLLECTION: Avoid hemolysis. Transport specimen to the laboratory promptly after collection. Avoid exposure to light. STORAGE INSTRUCTIONS: Stable 24 hours at 4°C or store frozen early in hospital stay (feeding malnourished patient may rapidly elevate folate level to normal). Protect from light. CAUSES FOR REJECTION: Hemolyzed specimen, stored specimen not frozen or protected from light, patient having had isotope scan or Schilling's test prior to collection of specimen

Interpretive REFERENCE RANGE: >2 ng/mL (SI>5 nmol/L). See table for pediatric reference ranges.

Pediatric Serum Folate Reference Chart

Age, y	Male (nmol/L)		Female (nmol/L)	
	Low	High	Low	High
0–1	16.3	50.8	14.3	51.5
2–3	5.7	34.0	3.9	35.6
4–6	1.1	29.4	6.1	31.9
7–9	5.2	27.0	5.4	30.4
10–12	3.4	24.5	2.3	23.1
13–18	2.7	19.9	2.7	16.3

From Hicks JM, Cook J, Godwin ID, et al, "Vitamin B_{12} and Folate — Pediatric Reference Ranges," *Arch Pathol Lab Med,* 1993, 117:705, with permission.

USE: Detect folate deficiency; monitor therapy with folate; evaluate megaloblastic and macrocytic anemia; evaluate alcoholic patients and those with prior jejunoileal bypass for morbid obesity or those with intestinal blind-loop syndrome LIMITATIONS: May be decreased in patients on oral contraceptives. Folate will deteriorate on exposure to light. Usually measured with red cell folate and vitamin B_{12} levels. METHODOLOGY: Competitive protein binding radioimmunoassay. Patient's endogenous unlabeled serum folate competes with radiolabeled folate for specific sites on a binding protein (eg, as derived from milk) and is compared to a standard curve. A chemiluminescence receptor assay has been developed. It employs an acridinium-ester-coupled folate molecule as tracer and folate binding protein on magnetic particles as the solid phase.[1] ADDITIONAL INFORMATION: Naturally occurring folates are present widely in plant and animal foods taken in the diet and absorbed in the small intestine. Folic acid (pteroylglutamic acid) has a number of biologically active forms (largely conjugates of glutamic acid, eg, N-5-methyltetrahydrofolic acid and N-5-formyltetrahydrofolic acid – folinic acid) that function as coenzymes. Lack of folic acid inhibits DNA synthesis in rapidly dividing cells, thus producing megaloblastic anemia. While a specific folate-binding protein is present in the serum, some 90% of folate is unbound. The binding protein increases with folate deficiency and returns to normal with treatment.

Serum levels are affected by present dietary intake. Drugs that are folate antagonists, such as methotrexate and pentamidine, may induce a deficiency state. Some drugs, such as oral contraceptives, phenytoin, and ethanol impair absorption of folate. In the pH range of physiologic significance, folate binds to aluminum hydroxide. Chronic use of antacids or H_2-receptor

(Continued)

Folic Acid, Serum *(Continued)*

antagonists by patients with diets marginal in folate has been considered as a cause of folic acid deficiency.[2] Levels are commonly high in patients with B_{12} deficiency since this vitamin is needed to allow incorporation of folate into tissue cells. Folate (folic acid) deficiency is present in some 33% of pregnant women, many alcoholics, patients with a wide variety of malabsorption syndromes including celiac disease, sprue, Crohn's disease, and jejunal/ileal bypass procedure.

Measurement of both serum and red cell folate levels constitutes a reliable means of determining the existence of folate deficiency. These tests are recommended for all patients who have megaloblastic anemia, as well as for patients who have anemia, hypersegmentation of the granulocytic nuclei, and coincident evidence of iron deficiency. The finding of a low serum folate means that the patient's recent diet has been subnormal in folate content and/or that recent absorption of folate has been subnormal, but does not prove that the patient either has or will develop tissue folate depletion requiring folate therapy. Therefore, serum folate assays have a very poor predictive value in diagnosis and should be interpreted with caution. A low red cell folate can mean either that there is tissue folate depletion due to folate deficiency requiring folate therapy, or alternatively, that the patient has primary vitamin B_{12} deficiency blocking the ability of cells to take up folate. In the latter case, the proper therapy would be with vitamin B_{12} rather than with folic acid. It is for these reasons that it is advisable to determine red cell folate in addition to serum folate, and thereby definitively determine that the diagnosis is folate deficiency for which the proper treatment is folic acid. For thoroughness, the serum vitamin B_{12} level should also be determined. In the past it was considered that over 50% of all patients with significant megaloblastic anemia have primary deficiency of vitamin B_{12}.[3] Currently however, in some geographic areas (hospitalized urban patient populations), zidovudine, used in the treatment of acquired immune deficiency syndrome, has been the most common cause of macrocytosis.[4]

Folate deficient diets have been proposed for methotrexate responsive malignancy. It has also been suggested that plasma folate concentrations in patients who do and do not respond to folate deprivation/antagonism be compared and ratioed to methotrexate levels as part of tumor therapy regimes.[5] The levels of serum and RBC folate may be significantly increased in hyperthyroidism.[6] The biochemical events underlying the phenomenon of megaloblastosis and the pathways of thymidylate synthesis has recently been reviewed.[7]

Footnotes

1. Klukas C, Comerci C, Campbell J, et al, "A Chemiluminescence Receptor Assay for Folate," *Clin Chem*, 1989, 35:1194.
2. Russell RM, Golner BB, Krasinski SD, et al, "Effect of Antacid and H_2 Receptor Antagonists on the Intestinal Absorption of Folic Acid," *J Lab Clin Med*, 1988, 112(4):458-63.
3. Bauer JD, *Clinical Laboratory Methods*, 9th ed, St Louis, MO: Mosby-Year Book Inc, 1982, 95-6.
4. Snower DP and Weil SC, "Changing Etiology of Macrocytosis: Zidovudine as a Frequent Causative Factor," *Am J Clin Pathol*, 1993, 99(1):57-60.
5. Cohen P and Dix D, "On the Role of Folate Deficiency in Cancer Therapy," *Clin Chem*, 1988, 34(9):1945-6 (letter).
6. Ford HC, Carter JM, and Rendle MA, "Serum and Red Cell Folate and Serum Vitamin B_{12} Levels in Hyperthyroidism," *Am J Hematol*, 1989, 31(4):233-6.
7. Das KC and Herbert V, "*In Vitro* DNA Synthesis by Megaloblastic Bone Marrow: Effect of Folates and Cobalamins on Thymidine Incorporation and De Novo Thymidylate Synthesis," *Am J Hematol*, 1989, 31(1):11-20.

References

Chanarin I, "Megaloblastic Anaemia, Cobalamin, and Folate," *J Clin Pathol*, 1987, 40:978-84.

Craig GM, Elliot C, and Hughes KR, "Masked Vitamin B_{12} and Folate Deficiency in the Elderly," *Br J Nutr*, 1985, 54:613-9.

Davis RE and Nicol DJ, "Folic Acid," *Int J Biochem*, 1988, 20:133-9, (minireview).

Hicks JM, Cook J, Godwin ID, et al, "Vitamin B_{12} and Folate: Pediatric Reference Ranges," *Arch Pathol Lab Med*, 1993, 117:704-6.

Free Hemoglobin *see* Hemoglobin, Plasma *on page 559*

α-Fucosidase *see* Tests for Uncommon Inherited Diseases of Metabolism and Cell Structure *on page 605*

G-6-PD, Qualitative *see* Glucose-6-Phosphate Dehydrogenase Screen, Blood *on page 548*

G-6-PD, Quantitative, Blood *see* Glucose-6-Phosphate Dehydrogenase, Quantitative, Blood *on this page*

G-6-PD Screen, Blood *see* Glucose-6-Phosphate Dehydrogenase Screen, Blood *on next page*

Galactocerebroside *see* Tests for Uncommon Inherited Diseases of Metabolism and Cell Structure *on page 605*

β-Galactosidase *see* Tests for Uncommon Inherited Diseases of Metabolism and Cell Structure *on page 605*

Glucocerebroside *see* Tests for Uncommon Inherited Diseases of Metabolism and Cell Structure *on page 605*

Glucose-6-Phosphate Dehydrogenase, Quantitative, Blood

CPT *82955*

See Also Anemia Flowchart in the Hematology Appendix

Related Information

Autohemolysis Test *on page 519*
Glucose-6-Phosphate Dehydrogenase Screen, Blood *on next page*
Heinz Body Stain *on page 551*
Red Blood Cell Enzyme Deficiency, Quantitative *on page 591*
Red Blood Cell Enzyme Deficiency Screen *on page 592*

Synonyms G-6-PD, Quantitative, Blood

Applies to Heinz Bodies

Specimen Erythrocytes **CONTAINER:** Lavender top (EDTA) tube, green top (heparin) tube, or acid-citrate-dextrose (ACD) solution **STORAGE INSTRUCTIONS:** In above anticoagulants, RBC enzymes stable at 4°C for at least 6 days and stable at 25°C for at least 24 hours. If sample must be sent to a referral laboratory, ship on wet ice, do not freeze.[1]

Interpretive **REFERENCE RANGE:** 8.34 ± 1.59 IU/g hemoglobin **USE:** Evaluate G-6-PD deficiency; determine the cause of drug-induced hemolysis or hemolysis secondary to acute bacterial or viral infection or metabolic disorder such as acidosis **LIMITATIONS:** False normal results after hemolysis may occur; *vide infra.* **CONTRAINDICATIONS:** Normal G-6-PD screen, marked reticulocytosis **METHODOLOGY:** Using hemolysate, measurement of formation of NADPH by following change in absorbance at 340 nm at 37°C **ADDITIONAL INFORMATION:** A G-6-PD screen is recommended before G-6-PD quantitative is requested (see Glucose-6-Phosphate Dehydrogenase Screen, Blood). G-6-PD hemolysis is associated with formation of Heinz bodies in peripheral red blood cells. It is the older erythrocytes which are most G-6-PD deficient in affected individuals. These cells are first eliminated in a hemolytic crisis. The younger cells and reticulocytes contain more G-6-PD. For these reasons after a hemolytic crisis, when only younger erythrocytes and reticulocytes are present, the G-6-PD values may be spuriously normal. Quantitative assay of G-6-PD may be helpful in establishing the diagnosis in female patients (who have two RBC populations) or in males with mild G-6-PD deficiency who have had recent hemolysis. In such cases, assay of the reticulocyte-poor bottom fraction of a centrifuged blood sample may be useful.[2] Mutations responsible for the G-6-PD deficient state can be identified by use of molecular biologic techniques.[3]

Footnotes

1. Beutler E, Blume KG, Kaplan JC, et al, "International Committee for Standardization in Haematology: Recommended Methods for Red-Cell Enzyme Analysis," *Br J Haematol*, 1977, 35:331-40.
2. Beutler E, "Glucose-6-Phosphate Dehydrogenase Deficiency," *N Engl J Med*, 1991, 324(3):169-74.
3. Huang CS, Tang CJ, Huang MJ, et al, "Diagnosis of Glucose-6-Phosphate Dehydrogenase (G6PD) Mutations by DNA Amplification and Allele-Specific Oligonucleotide Probes," *Acta Haematol*, 1992, 88(2-3):92-5.

References

Beutler E, "Study of Glucose-6-Phosphate Dehydrogenase: History and Molecular Biology," *Am J Hematol*, 1993, 42(1):53-8.

Dacie J, "The Haemolytic Anaemias," *The Hereditary Haemolytic Anaemias*, 3rd ed, Vol 1, Part 1, Chapter 9, Edinburgh, Scotland: Churchill Livingstone, 1985, 364-418.

Mentzer WC and Wagner GM, *The Hereditary Haemolytic Anaemias*, Chapter 6, New York, NY: Churchill Livingstone, 1989, 289-92.

Williams WJ, Beutler E, Erslev AJ, et al, *Hematology*, 4th ed, New York, NY: McGraw-Hill Inc, 1990, 1723-6.

Glucose-6-Phosphate Dehydrogenase Screen, Blood

CPT 82960

See Also Anemia Flowchart in the Hematology Appendix

Related Information

Autohemolysis Test *on page 519*
Glucose-6-Phosphate Dehydrogenase, Quantitative, Blood *on previous page*
Red Blood Cell Enzyme Deficiency, Quantitative *on page 591*
Red Blood Cell Enzyme Deficiency Screen *on page 592*

Synonyms G-6-PD, Qualitative; G-6-PD Screen, Blood

Abstract G-6-PD is a red cell enzyme with an X-linked mode of inheritance that is important in maintaining RBC proteins in the reduced state. There are over 400 different mutations recorded,[1] resulting in premature hemolysis of red cells when the mutant enzyme is stressed.

Specimen Erythrocytes **CONTAINER:** Lavender top (EDTA) tube

Interpretive **REFERENCE RANGE:** G-6-PD enzyme activity detected **USE:** Detect drug sensitive populations of red cells due to G-6-PD deficiency; determine the cause of hemolysis. G-6-PD deficient hemolysis may also be secondary to acute bacterial or viral infection and metabolic disorder such as acidosis. **LIMITATIONS:** A blood enzyme screen, performed after a hemolytic episode often will not detect G-6-PD deficiency even if present because the most deficient cells have been destroyed. This procedure can only differentiate between normal and grossly deficient samples. **Test may need to be repeated (if initial result is normal) after the patient recovers from an undiagnosed episode of anemia.** **CONTRAINDICATIONS:** Marked reticulocytosis **METHODOLOGY:** Fluorescent NADPH spot test **ADDITIONAL INFORMATION:** G-6-PD quantitation may be useful if a deficiency is detected in the screening test. In a large group of American black males the incidence of G-6-PD deficiency was found to be 11% (methemoglobin reduction test and fluorescent spot test). Approximately 20% of female blacks are heterozygous. G-6-PD deficiency had no adverse effect on the course and fatality rates of a spectrum of diseases (including those with thrombotic associations).[2] While usually mild in black children G-6-PD deficiency may be severe and life-threatening with oxidative stress, especially that relating to infection (viral in particular), fava bean ingestion, and less often relating to naphthalene exposure. A number of commonly used drugs/chemicals can induce hemolysis in individuals with G-6-PD deficiency (see table), while evidence has accumulated that some occasionally suspect drugs can be given in therapeutic doses without inducing hemolysis.[3] Distinctive abnormal RBC "eccentrocytes" may occur. While G-6-PD screens may be normal after hemolytic episodes significant reticulocytosis (usually >7%) will reflect presence of the deficiency.[4] Infection rather than use of ASA appears to precipitate hemolytic episodes in cases of G-6-PD deficiency.[5] If deficiency is severe, impaired granulocyte function occurs with increased susceptibility to infection.[6] Occasionally, a few of this group can be symptomatic. There are many genetic variants of G-6-PD, some causing marked clinical manifestations, others none. The nonblack variant found in high frequency in such areas as India, Japan, Southeast Asia, and certain Mediterranean countries tends to present as a more severe form of the disease. Molecular heterogeneity, as reflected by the numerous mutant isoenzymes, is accompanied by biochemical functional diversity including decreased catalytic effectiveness, impaired substrate and cofactor kinetics, variable reactivity with substrate analogues, and variations in electrophoretic migration rates and pH optima. Cloning of the G-6-PD gene has been accomplished, and there is ongoing activity in cDNA sequencing of G-6-PD variants.[3,7,8]

Drugs/Chemicals Capable of Inducing Hemolytic Episode in G–6–PD Deficient Individuals

Acetanilid	Niridazole
Doxorubicin	Nitrofurantoin
Furazolidone	Phenazopyridine
Methylene blue	Primaquine
Nalidixic acid	Sulfamethoxazole

From Beutler E, "Glucose–6–Phosphate Dehydrogenase Deficiency," *N Engl J Med,* 1991, 324:171, with permission.

Footnotes

1. Beutler E, "The Genetics of Glucose-6-Phosphate Dehydrogenase Deficiency," *Semin Hematol*, 1990, 27(2):137-64.
2. Heller P, Best WR, Nelson RB, et al, "Clinical Implications of Sickle Cell Trait and Glucose-6-Phosphate Dehydrogenase Deficiency in Hospitalized Black Male Patients," *N Engl J Med*, 1979, 300:1001-5.
3. Beutler E, "Glucose-6-Phosphate Dehydrogenase Deficiency," *N Engl J Med*, 1991, 324(3):169-74.

4. Shannon K and Buchanan GR, "Severe Hemolytic Anemia in Black Children With Glucose-6-Phosphate Dehydrogenase Deficiency," *Pediatrics*, 1982, 70:3, 364-9.
5. Glader BE, "Evaluation of the Hemolytic Role of Aspirin in Glucose- 6-Phosphate Dehydrogenase Deficiency," *J Pediatr*, 1976, 89:1027-8.
6. Vives Corrons JL, Feliu E, Pujades MA, et al, "Severe Glucose- 6-Phosphate Dehydrogenase Deficiency (G-6-PD) Associated With Chronic Hemolytic Anemia, Granulocyte Dysfunction and Increased Susceptibility to Infections: Description of a New Molecular Variant (G-6-PD Barcelona)," *Blood*, 1982, 59:428-34.
7. Martini G, Toniolo D, Vulliamy T, et al, "Structural Analysis of the X-Linked Gene Encoding Human Glucose-6-Phosphate Dehydrogenase," *EMBO J*, 1986, 5:1849-55.
8. Chiu DT, Zuo L, Chao L, et al, "Molecular Characterization of Glucose-6-Phosphate Dehydrogenase (G6PD) Deficiency in Patients of Chinese Descent and Identification of New Base Substitutions in the Human G6PD Gene," *Blood*, 1993, 81(8):2150-4.

References

Beutler E, "Study of Glucose-6-Phosphate Dehydrogenase: History and Molecular Biology," *Am J Hematol*, 1993, 42(1):53-8.

Paglia DE, "Enzymopathies," *Hematology Basic Principles and Practice*, Chapter 37, Hoffman R, Benz EJ Jr, Shattil SJ, et al, eds, New York, NY: Churchill Livingstone, 1991, 504-13.

Williams WJ, Beutler E, Erslev AJ, et al, *Hematology*, 4th ed, New York, NY: McGraw-Hill Inc, 1990, 591-606.

β-Glucosidase *see* Tests for Uncommon Inherited Diseases of Metabolism and Cell Structure *on page 605*

Glutathione Reductase Deficiency, RBC *see* Red Blood Cell Enzyme Deficiency, Quantitative *on page 591*

Glycogen Storage Diseases *see* Tests for Uncommon Inherited Diseases of Metabolism and Cell Structure *on page 605*

Granulocyte/Macrophage Colony Stimulating Factor *see* Eosinophil Count *on page 539*

Hairy Cell Leukemia Test *see* Tartrate Resistant Leukocyte Acid Phosphatase *on page 603*

Ham Test

CPT 85475

Related Information

Peripheral Blood: Red Blood Cell Morphology *on page 584*

Sugar Water Test Screen *on page 603*

Synonyms Acid Serum Test; Acid Serum Test for PNH; Acidified Serum Test; Paroxysmal Nocturnal Hemoglobinuria Test; PNH Test; Serum Lysis

Specimen Erythrocytes **CONTAINER:** Lavender top (EDTA) tube **CAUSES FOR REJECTION:** Improper tube, specimen clotted, specimen hemolyzed

Interpretive **REFERENCE RANGE:** A positive result shows lysis of red cells in acidified serum samples with patient's cells (not with normal cells). **USE:** Evaluate patients with suspected PNH (paroxysmal nocturnal hemoglobinuria) or suspected congenital dyserythropoietic anemia, type II (HEMPAS); evaluate hemolytic anemia, especially with hemosiderinuria, pancytopenia, decreased RBC acetylcholinesterase, decreased leukocyte alkaline phosphatase, negative direct Coombs' test, and/or apparent marrow failure. Positive in PNH: 10% to 50% lysis in acidified noninactivated serum. Can be as low as 5% or as much as 80%. Low or negative after transfusion. Diagnosis of PNH rests upon showing that the suspected patient's red cells have a high sensitivity to complement mediated hemolysis.[1] **LIMITATIONS:** False-positive results may occur in other hematologic diseases: hereditary and acquired spherocytosis, hereditary dyserythropoietic anemia (CDA type II, HEMPAS, *vide infra*), aged red cells (as with old transfused blood), aplastic anemia, leukemia, and myeloproliferative syndromes.[1] In these conditions hemolysis will also occur in the acidified inactivated serum. The latter is negative in PNH since hemolysis is complement dependent. **CONTRAINDICATIONS:** Transfusion **METHODOLOGY:** Acidified serum test of Ham. PNH suspect RBCs will lyse in acidified normal and acidified patient's serum. The normal serum used must be fresh and ABO blood group compatible with test RBCs. Alternatives to acidification of the testing serum are the addition of bovine thrombin, cobra venom factor, insulin, heating, or use of specific antibodies to activate complement. Probably these tests do not offer advantages over the Ham test. False-negative results may occur with any of these tests in which the PNH patient's serum (which may have low serum complement activity) is used.[2] **ADDITIONAL INFORMATION:** PNH red cells are unusually

(Continued)

Ham Test *(Continued)*

susceptible to lysis by complement. The Ham (acidified serum) and sucrose hemolysis test can demonstrate this lysis *in vitro*. A positive acidified-serum test (performed with careful attention to proper controls) defines the PNH condition. A positive test is necessary for the diagnosis. In PNH, 10% to 50% of lysis (measured as liberated hemoglobin) is usually obtained but lysis may be as great as 80% or as little as 5%.

In some cases, three populations of cells exist in patients with PNH. One is markedly hypersensitive to complement (type III cells), one has a midlevel of sensitivity (type II cells), and the third population has normal sensitivity (type I cells). Type III cells are variably present, are the population which undergoes lysis in the Ham test and relate to the severity of illness.[3] The young PNH cells (reticulocyte-rich) are more susceptible to lysis than the older red cells. PNH RBCs will undergo lysis in acidified normal serum and in the patient's acidified serum.[3]

The only other disorder which may give a positive Ham test is one of the congenital dyserythropoietic anemias. In CDA type II (HEMPAS - hereditary erythroblastic multinuclearity with positive acidified serum test) the red cells undergo lysis in only a proportion (about 30%) of normal sera, and these RBCs do not undergo lysis in the patient's own acidified serum. The sucrose lysis test is negative in cases of HEMPAS. Lysis occurring in HEMPAS probably occurs due to the presence on the red cells of an unusual antigen which reacts with a complement-fixing IgM antibody ("anti-HEMPAS") which is present in some normal sera.[4] Heating at 56°C, which destroys the complement in serum, inactivates the lytic system so that if lysis occurs with inactivated serum this cannot be considered positive.

Another type of cell that may lyse in inactivated serum is the spherocyte. Spherocytes may lyse in acidified serum possibly due to the lowered pH.[3]

PNH has been considered a "candidate" myeloproliferative disease.[5] A 55% to 65% incidence of PNH occurs in primary myelofibrosis and myeloid metaplasia.

PNH is a disease not only of increased complement sensitivity of red cell membranes, but also granulocytes and platelet membranes. A new diagnostic test using flow cytometry and monoclonal antibodies has been developed.[6] This technique reveals and detects missing proteins from granulocytes in patients with PNH. The method correlates well with the Ham test for abnormal red cells.

The membrane defect is due to a deficiency of DAF (decay accelerating factor) and HRF (homologous restriction factor)/MIRL (membrane inhibitor of reactive lysis). These are complement regulating proteins. DAF, a membrane protein, accelerates the spontaneous decay of C3 convertase enzyme of the complement activation pathways. This membrane protein deficiency affects granulocytes, monocytes, red cells, and platelets.[7,8] HRF/MIRL inhibits complement mediated lysis by C5b-9.[9,10]

Footnotes

1. Conrad ME and Barton JC, "The Aplastic Anemia-Paroxysmal Nocturnal Hemoglobinuria Syndrome," *Am J Hematol*, 1979, 7:61-7.
2. Harruff RC and Rohn RJ, "Potential Errors in the Laboratory Diagnosis of Paroxysmal Nocturnal Hemoglobinuria," *Am J Clin Pathol*, 1983, 80:152-8.
3. Dacie JV and Lewis SM, "Laboratory Methods Used in the Investigation of Paroxysmal Nocturnal Hemoglobinuria (PNH)," *Practical Haematology*, 7th ed, Chapter 16, New York, NY: Churchill Livingstone, 1991, 260-2.
4. Verwilghen RL, Lewis SM, Dacie JV, et al, "HEMPAS: Congenital Dyserythropoietic Anemia (Type II)," *Q J Med*, 1973, 42:257-78.
5. Dameshek W, "Foreword and a Proposal for Considering Paroxysmal Nocturnal Hemoglobinuria (PNH) as a "Candidate" Myeloproliferative Disorder," *Blood*, 1969, 33:263-4.
6. van der Schoot CE, Huizinga TW, van't Veer Korthof ET, et al, "Deficiency of Glycosyl-Phosphatidylinositol-Linked Membrane Glycoproteins of Leukocytes in Paroxysmal Nocturnal Hemoglobinuria, Description of a New Diagnostic Cytofluorometric Assay," *Blood*, 1990, 76(7):1853-9.
7. Nicholson-Weller A, Spicer DB, and Austen KF, "Deficiency of the Complement Regulatory Protein, 'Decay-Accelerating Factor,' on Membranes of Granulocytes, Monocytes, and Platelets in Paroxysmal Nocturnal Hemoglobinuria," *N Engl J Med*, 1985, 312:1091-7.
8. Rosse WF, "Paroxysmal Nocturnal Hemoglobinuria and Decay-Accelerating Factor," *Annu Rev Med*, 1990, 41:431-6.
9. Zalman LS, Wood LM, Frank MM, et al, "Deficiency of the Homologous Restriction Factor in Paroxysmal Nocturnal Hemoglobinuria," *J Exp Med*, 1987, 165:572-7.
10. Wilcox LA, Ezzell JL, Bernshaw NJ, et al, "Molecular Basis of the Enhanced Susceptibility of the Erythrocytes of Paroxysmal Nocturnal Hemoglobinuria to Hemolysis in Acidified Serum," *Blood*, 1991, 78(3):820-9.

References

Desforges JF, "Paroxysmal Nocturnal Hemoglobinuria," *Hematology Basic Principles and Practice*, Chapter 16, Hoffman R, Benz EJ Jr, Shattil SJ, et al, eds, New York, NY: Churchill Livingstone, 1991, 210-20.

Grenier KA, "Hemolytic Anemias: Intracorpuscular Defects: V. Paroxysmal Nocturnal Hemoglobinuria," *Clinical Hematology and Fundamentals of Hemostasis*, 2nd ed, Chapter 13, Harmening DM, ed, Philadelphia, PA: FA Davis Co, 1992, 183-92.

Williams WJ, Beutler E, Erslev AJ, et al, *Hematology*, 4th ed, New York, NY: McGraw-Hill Inc, 1990, 1730.

H and H *see* Hematocrit *on next page*

H and H *see* Hemoglobin *on page 554*

Hb *see* Hemoglobin *on page 554*

Hb A_2 *see* Hemoglobin A_2 *on page 555*

Hb F *see* Fetal Hemoglobin *on page 542*

Hct *see* Hematocrit *on next page*

Heat Denaturation *see* Hemoglobin, Unstable, Heat Labile Test *on page 560*

Heinz Bodies *see* Glucose-6-Phosphate Dehydrogenase, Quantitative, Blood *on page 547*

Heinz Bodies *see* Hemoglobin, Unstable, Heat Labile Test *on page 560*

Heinz Bodies *see* Hemoglobin, Unstable - Isopropanol Precipitation Test *on page 561*

Heinz Bodies *see* Red Blood Cell Enzyme Deficiency, Quantitative *on page 591*

Heinz Bodies *see* Red Blood Cell Enzyme Deficiency Screen *on page 592*

Heinz Body Stain

CPT *85441*

See Also Anemia Flowchart in the Hematology Appendix

Related Information

Glucose-6-Phosphate Dehydrogenase, Quantitative, Blood *on page 547*
Hemoglobin, Unstable, Heat Labile Test *on page 560*
Hemoglobin, Unstable - Isopropanol Precipitation Test *on page 561*
Peripheral Blood: Red Blood Cell Morphology *on page 584*
Red Blood Cell Enzyme Deficiency, Quantitative *on page 591*
Red Blood Cell Enzyme Deficiency Screen *on page 592*
Reticulocyte Count *on page 597*

Synonyms Methyl Violet Stain for Heinz Bodies

Applies to CHBHA

Abstract Heinz bodies are intraerythrocyte insoluble inclusions of oxidatively denatured hemoglobin. They reflect the presence of a metabolic derangement of or abnormality in the secondary structure of hemoglobin.

Specimen Whole blood **CONTAINER:** Lavender top (EDTA) tube, green top (heparin) tube **COLLECTION:** Obtain a tube of normal control blood at the time patient sample is drawn. **STORAGE INSTRUCTIONS:** Refrigerate **CAUSES FOR REJECTION:** Clotted specimen, hemolyzed specimen

Interpretive **REFERENCE RANGE:** No Heinz bodies identified. Using blood incubated with acetylphenylhydrazine, normal control may have one to a few (under five) Heinz bodies in about one-third of the RBCs. A positive result (indicative of a defective reducing system) will find five or more Heinz bodies in about one-third or more of the RBCs. The definition of "abnormal" may vary somewhat between different laboratories. **USE:** Test for hemolytic disorders associated with Heinz body formation (eg, G-6-PD deficiency, thalassemia, unstable hemoglobin) **METHODOLOGY:** Supravital stain (methyl violet, new methylene blue, crystal violet, or brilliant cresyl blue) using blood incubated (60 minutes or more) at room temperature with acetylphenylhydrazine or sterile blood incubated 24 and 48 hours at 37°C. Heinz bodies are intraerythrocytic, purple, vary in shape (round, oval, serrated), 1-3 μm across, single or multiple, and close to the cell membrane. **ADDITIONAL INFORMATION:** Heinz bodies are uncommon except with G-6-PD deficiency immediately following hemolysis and in patients with unstable hemoglobin variants. They are present characteristically in the congenital Heinz body hemolytic anemias (CHBHA). There are over 30 different molecular variants of hemoglobin underlying CHBHA. The three major causes for Heinz body formation and increased hemolysis are exposure to certain

(Continued)

Heinz Body Stain *(Continued)*

chemicals and drugs, deficiency of one of the reducing systems of blood, and presence of an unstable hemoglobin. Oxidative denaturation of the hemoglobin molecule leads to Heinz body formation with the first two situations and is probably the mechanism for the precipitation of unstable hemoglobin. A variety of detailed molecular mechanisms have been proposed and defined to underlie the actual production of the Heinz body phenomenon.[1] Heinz bodies are usually removed by the spleen; postsplenectomy they increase in the peripheral blood. It has also been proposed that they may be actively extruded in cases of drug-induced hemolytic anemia.[2] While absent in the blood of normal individuals presplenectomy, they occur in sulfonamide-induced hemolytic crisis in cases of Hb Zurich and in cases of Hb Shepherd's Bush, Hb Gun Hill, and Hb Philly. Postsplenectomy, Heinz bodies occur in >50% of cells in blood stained supravitally, especially with methyl violet. They can be generated in red cells of unsplenectomized patients by 60 minutes or more incubation with acetylphenylhydrazine or by incubation of sterile blood for 24-48 hours at 37°C. Ability to demonstrate the bodies relates to the degree of instability of the hemoglobin. Cells of Hb Koln require up to 48 hours incubation and the Heinz bodies are small. With Hb Seattle and Hb Shepherd's Bush the bodies are seen readily after 24 hours incubation.[3] Heinz bodies may be found after the administration of sulfonamides, nitrofurans, Dilantin®, streptomycin, fava beans, chlorates, phenylhydrazine, primaquine (in sensitive individuals), and likely, other compounds.

Footnotes

1. Dacie J, "The Haemolytic Anaemias," *The Hereditary Haemolytic Anaemias*, 3rd ed, Vol 1, Part 1, Chapter 3, Edinburgh, Scotland: Churchill Livingstone, 1985, 84-6.
2. Amare M, Lawson B, and Larsen WE, "Active Extrusion of Heinz Bodies in Drug-Induced Hemolytic Anemia," *Br J Haematol*, 1972, 23:215-9.
3. White JM and Dacie JV, "The Unstable Hemoglobins - Molecular and Clinical Features," *Prog Hematol*, 1971, 7:85-9.

References

Brown BA, *Hematology: Principles and Procedures*, 6th ed, Philadelphia, PA: Lea & Febiger, 1993, 143-5.
Jaffe ER, "Oxidative Hemolysis or What Made the Red Cell Break?" *N Engl J Med*, 1972, 286:156-7.
Jandl JH, "Heinz Body Hemolytic Anemia," *Blood*, 1st ed, Boston, MA: Little, Brown and Co, 1987, 335-9.
Wyrick-Glatzel J and Gwaltney-Krause S, "Laboratory Methods in Hematology and Hemostasis," *Clinical Hematology and Fundamentals of Hemostasis*, 2nd ed, Chapter 30, Section 1, Harmening DM, ed, Philadelphia, PA: FA Davis Co, 1992, 540.

Helminths, Blood *see* Microfilariae, Peripheral Blood Preparation *on page 571*

Hematocrit

***CPT** 85013 (spun hematocrit); 85014 (other than spun hematocrit)*

See Also Anemia Flowchart in the Hematology Appendix

Related Information

Blood Volume *on page 522*
Complete Blood Count *on page 533*
Hemoglobin *on page 554*
Peripheral Blood: Red Blood Cell Morphology *on page 584*
Red Blood Cell Indices *on page 592*
Red Blood Cells *on page 1087*
Red Cell Count *on page 594*
Red Cell Mass *on page 595*
Reticulocyte Count *on page 597*

Synonyms Hct; Microhematocrit; Packed Cell Volume; PCV

Applies to H and H

Abstract Percent of whole blood that is red blood cells. A determination that is of importance in the detection and follow-up of anemia and polycythemia. The hematocrit value is used in the calculation of the MCV and MCHC.

Specimen Whole blood **CONTAINER:** Lavender top (EDTA) tube **COLLECTION:** Routine venipuncture. Invert tube gently to mix. For capillary puncture, establish free flow of blood to minimize dilution with tissue fluid. **STORAGE INSTRUCTIONS:** If specimen is not brought to the laboratory within 4 hours, refrigeration should be provided. **CAUSES FOR REJECTION:** Clotted or hemolyzed specimen

Interpretive **REFERENCE RANGE:** Males: 2 years: 35% to 44%, 6 years: 31% to 43%, adult: 42% to 52%; females: 2 years: 35% to 44%, 6 years: 31% to 43%, adult: 35% to 47%. In general, spun hematocrits are 2% to 3% higher than automated hematocrits, due to plasma trapping.

See tables. **USE:** Evaluate anemia, blood loss, hemolytic anemia, polycythemia, and other conditions **LIMITATIONS:** When dealing with results of automated instruments falsely high results may occur with cryoproteins, significant leukocytosis, giant platelets; false low results may be seen with microcytosis, *in vitro* hemolysis or in presence of autoagglutinins. **METHODOLOGY:** Manual microhematocrit centrifugation; automated - electronic cell counters such as Coulter S, Coulter S Plus, subsequent Coulter S models including STKR® and JT series, H-1, Sysmex, others; derived by electronic calculation considering that Hct = RBC x MCV / 10 (latter two are directly measured). Data ReCap, a summary compilation of data of College of American Pathologists indicates that for the year 1980, hematocrit had a SD of 2.2 and CV of 5.3%.[1] Reference to the results of current CAP surveys indicate a trend toward a further decrease in SD and CV of the hematocrit. **ADDITIONAL INFORMATION:** The degree of plasma trapping is increased in disease with less deformable RBCs (eg, sickle cell disease, hereditary spherocytosis, and iron deficiency). A study[2] using ^{125}I labeled human serum albumin found trapped plasma volume to be 1.53% (25 normals), somewhat less than earlier work[3] which found a level of 3% and the work of Miale, who reported the calculated hematocrit (Coulter S and Coulter S Plus derived) to be 2% lower than the microhematocrit at the 40% level.[4]

Hematocrit Values — First Postnatal Day[5]

Gestational Age (wk)	Hct (%)	Gestational Age (wk)	Hct (%)
24-25	63	32-33	60
26-27	62	34-35	61
28-29	60	36-37	64
30-31	60	Term	61

Normal Hematocrit Values — Newborn

Age	Hct (%)	Age	Hct (%)
Birth - 2 d	54-68	6-7 d	47-61
2-3 d	54-66	7-8 d	47-64
3-4 d	52-71	1-2 wk	50-62
4-5 d	39-55	2-3 wk	39-53
5-6 d	50-64	3-4 wk	37-49

A large study (17,274 children in apparent good health and residing in the Washington, DC, metropolitan area) found that the lower mean Hct and Hgb value in African-American children (as compared to white children) was the result not only of α and β thalassemia but also of the presence of Hb AS and Hb AC. The mean Hct of children with Hb AC and Hb AS was 1.5 and 1.0 point lower, respectively, than that of subjects with Hb AA.[5]

The red cell indices, MCV and MCHC, depend on the Hct for their derivation and are of use in the evaluation of anemia. See also discussion under the entry, Complete Blood Count.

Footnotes

1. Elevitch FR and Noce PS, eds, *Data ReCap: 1970-1980. A Compilation of Data From the College of American Pathologists Clinical Laboratory Improvement Programs*, Skokie, IL: College of American Pathologists, 1981, 208-10.
2. Pearson TC and Guthrie DL, "Trapped Plasma in the Microhematocrit," *Am J Clin Pathol*, 1982, 78:770-2.
3. England JM, Walford DM, Waters DA, et al, "Reassessment of the Reliability of the Hematocrit," *Br J Haematol*, 1972, 23:247-56.
4. Miale JB, *Laboratory Medicine: Hematology*, 6th ed, St Louis, MO: Mosby-Year Book Inc, 1982, 360.
5. Rana SR, Sekhsaria S, and Castro OL, "Hemoglobin S and C Traits: Contributing Causes for Decreased Mean Hematocrit in African-American Children," *Pediatrics*, 1993, 91(4):800-2.

References

Brown BA, *Hematology: Principles and Procedures*, 6th ed, Philadelphia, PA: Lea & Febiger, 1993, 85-7, 345-79.

Henry JB, Nelson DA, Tomar RH, et al, *Clinical Diagnosis and Management by Laboratory Methods*, 18th ed, Philadelphia, PA: WB Saunders Co, 1991, 560-1, 582, 597-8.

Second National Health and Nutrition Examination Survey, "Hematological and Nutritional Biochemistry Reference Data for Persons 6 Months-74 Years of Age: United States, 1976-80," *Vital and Health Statistics*, DHHS Publication No (PHS), 83-1682, 1982.

Wyrick-Glatzel J and Gwaltney-Krause S, "Laboratory Methods in Hematology and Hemostasis," *Clinical Hematology and Fundamentals of Hemostasis*, 2nd ed, Chapter 30, Section 1, Harmening DM, ed, Philadelphia, PA: FA Davis Co, 1992, 523-53.

Zaizov R and Matoth Y, "Red Cell Values on the First Postnatal Day During the Last 16 Weeks of Gestation," *Am J Hematol*, 1976, 1:275-8.

Hemoflagellates *see* Microfilariae, Peripheral Blood Preparation *on page 571*

Hemoglobin

CPT 85018

See Also Anemia Flowchart in the Hematology Appendix

Related Information

Complete Blood Count *on page 533*
Cyanide, Blood *on page 956*
Erythropoietin, Serum *on page 214*
Ferritin, Serum *on page 220*
Folic Acid, RBC *on page 544*
Folic Acid, Serum *on page 545*
Hematocrit *on page 552*
Iron and Total Iron Binding Capacity/Transferrin *on page 262*
Oxygen Saturation, Blood *on page 305*
P-50 Blood Gas *on page 307*
Protoporphyrin, Free Erythrocyte *on page 341*
Red Blood Cell Indices *on page 592*
Red Blood Cells *on page 1087*
Red Cell Count *on page 594*
Red Cell Mass *on page 595*
Reticulocyte Count *on page 597*
Sickle Cell Tests *on page 600*
Vitamin B_{12} *on page 612*

Synonyms Hb; Hgb

Applies to H and H

Abstract This procedure determines the concentration of hemoglobin (Hgb) in whole blood. Hemoglobin is the major component of the red cell and functions to transport oxygen. It also acts to buffer carbon dioxide formed during metabolic activity. The Hgb level is important in the detection and follow up of anemia and polycythemia. The Hgb value is used in the calculation of the MCH and MCHC.

Specimen Whole blood **CONTAINER:** Lavender top (EDTA) tube **COLLECTION:** Routine venipuncture. Invert tube gently to mix. **CAUSES FOR REJECTION:** Clotted or hemolyzed specimen

Interpretive **REFERENCE RANGE:** See table in the listing, Complete Blood Count. **USE:** Evaluate anemia, blood loss, hemolysis, polycythemia, and other conditions **LIMITATIONS:** Hyperlipemic plasma (especially Fredrickson and Lees type I and V in which chylomicronemia is present) or white count >50,000/mm^3 may falsely elevate the hemoglobin result with corresponding increase in the MCH. A method correcting for lipemia has been suggested.[1] **METHODOLOGY:** While oxyhemoglobin and other chemical approaches to hemoglobinometry exist, nearly all current procedures involve a one or two step procedure in which RBC lysis/dilution occurs with the formation of a cyanmethemoglobin compound. Dilutions are read by spectrophotometer at 540 nm. The majority of routine hematology laboratories obtain the hemoglobin level as one of a number of parameters from an automated multichannel instrument. **ADDITIONAL INFORMATION:** The hemoglobin determination is one of the best standardized and accurate of available clinical laboratory analyses. Data ReCap, a summary compilation of data of College of American Pathologists, indicates that for the year 1980, the hemoglobin determination had a SD of 0.3 and a CV of 2.2%.[2] The results of current CAP surveys continue to show good interlaboratory performance for the Hgb procedure with low SD and CV values. The clinical utility of subject-specific reference values has been delineated and emphasized.[3]

In cyanide poisoned individuals treated with methemoglobin-forming agents (to protect cytochrome oxidase) oxygen carrying capacity is decreased in direct proportion to the amount of methemoglobin (nonoxygen carrying) that is formed. A multiwavelength spectrophotometric method has been developed which allows monitoring of hemoglobin derivatives present in the blood of treated cyanide poisoned patients.[4]

The red cell indices, MCH and MCHC, depend on the Hgb for their derivation and are of use in the evaluation of anemia. See also the discussion under Complete Blood Count.

Footnotes

1. Williams GJ, *Coulter Currents*, 1980, 3:2, (letters to the editor).
2. Elevitch FR and Noce PS, eds, *Data ReCap: 1970-1980. A Complication of Data From the College of American Pathologists Clinical Laboratory Improvement Programs*, Skokie, IL: College of American Pathologists, 1981, 211-3.
3. Fraser CG, Wilkinson SP, Neville RG, et al, "Biologic Variation of Common Hematologic Laboratory Quantities in the Elderly," *Am J Clin Pathol*, 1989, 92(4):465-70.

4. Zijlstra WG and Buursma A, "Rapid Multicomponent Analysis of Hemoglobin Derivatives for Controlled Antidotal Use of Methemoglobin-Forming Agents in Cyanide Poisoning," *Clin Chem*, 1993, 39(8):1685-9.

References

Brown BA, *Hematology: Principles and Procedures*, 6th ed, Philadelphia, PA: Lea & Febiger, 1993, 83-5, 345-79.

Henry JB, Nelson DA, Tomar RH, et al, *Clinical Diagnosis and Management by Laboratory Methods*, 18th ed, Philadelphia, PA: WB Saunders Co, 1991, 555-60, 608-13, 627-76.

Second National Health and Nutrition Examination Survey, "Hematological and Nutritional Biochemistry Reference Data for Persons 6 Months-74 Years of Age: United States, 1976-80," *Vital and Health Statistics*, DHHS Publication No (PHS) 83-1682, 1982.

Wyrick-Glatzel J and Gwaltney-Krause S, "Laboratory Methods in Hematology and Hemostasis," *Clinical Hematology and Fundamentals of Hemostasis*, 2nd ed, Chapter 30, Section 1, Harmening DM, ed, Philadelphia, PA: FA Davis Co, 1992, 523-53.

Zwart A, "Spectrophotometry of Hemoglobin: Various Perspectives," *Clin Chem*, 1993, 39:1570-2.

Hemoglobin A_2

***CPT** 83020 (electrophoresis)*

See Also Anemia Flowchart in the Hematology Appendix

Related Information

Hemoglobin Electrophoresis *on next page*

Peripheral Blood: Red Blood Cell Morphology *on page 584*

Red Blood Cell Indices *on page 592*

Synonyms Hb A_2

Abstract Hemoglobin A_2 (Hb A_2) is a tetramer of α- and δ-globulin chains ($\alpha_2\,\delta_2$). Concentration fluctuates in the thalassemia syndromes and some acquired diseases.

Specimen Whole blood **CONTAINER:** Lavender top (EDTA) tube **CAUSES FOR REJECTION:** Specimen clotted

Interpretive **REFERENCE RANGE:** The stable adult Hb A_2 level is 2.5% to 3.5% of total hemoglobin. See table.

Alterations in Hb A_2 in Various Disorders

	Elevated	Reduced
Congenital	β–thalassemia trait Unstable hemoglobin variants Sickle trait (AS) SS with α–thalassemia	α–thalassemia $\delta\beta$–thalassemia δ–thalassemia HPFH
Acquired	Megaloblastic anemias Hyperthyroidism	Iron deficiency Sideroblastic anemias

From Bunn HF and Forget BG, *Hemoglobin: Molecular, Genetic, and Clinical Aspects,* Philadelphia, PA: WB Saunders Co, 1986, 61–7, with permission.

USE: Investigate microcytic anemia, for hemoglobinopathies, especially thalassemia, particularly beta-thalassemia trait **LIMITATIONS:** Blood transfusion prior to hemoglobin electrophoresis may make interpretation inconsistent. High levels of hemoglobin F usually are accompanied by lower levels of A_2. Sickle cell trait range is from 1.7% to 4.5% hemoglobin A_2. Presence of Hb S or Hb C will interfere with column chromatographic method. Presence of Hb C interferes with routine electrophoretic method. Quantitation of Hb A_2 by densitometric scanning of electrophoretic pattern may result in misleading (high) results as this method is not uniformly reliable. **CONTRAINDICATIONS:** Recent blood transfusion **METHODOLOGY:** Electrophoresis, DEAE cellulose chromatography is preferred; radial immunodiffusion (RID) is also available. **ADDITIONAL INFORMATION:** This test is done in many laboratories as part of the hemoglobin electrophoresis. Hemoglobin A_2 levels have special application to the diagnosis of beta-thalassemia trait, which may be present even though peripheral blood smear is normal. (This reflects the underlying genetic spectrum of beta-thalassemia which in reality is a complex of 20-30 distinct conditions and over 50 different mutations.) The microcytosis and other morphologic changes of beta-thalassemia trait must be differentiated from iron deficiency. Low MCV may include the majority of beta-thalassemia trait patients but does not differentiate iron deficient individuals. Low Hb A_2 levels occur in untreated iron deficiency. If the beta-thalassemia is associated with iron deficiency, the Hb A_2 level falls, making the differentiation even more difficult (corrected after iron therapy).[1]

(Continued)

Hemoglobin A_2 *(Continued)*

The most definitive evidence for presence of beta-thalassemia trait is genetic (family study). A well documented report, however, indicates the occurrence of beta-thalassemia minor as a result of a spontaneous initiation codon mutation.[2] Offspring of a person with thalassemia major will have beta-thalassemia trait. Apart from such genetic studies (which are subject to practical difficulties) gene probes are the most definitive method for identifying beta-thalassemia trait. This method identifies "silent" carriers but is a research level procedure. Elevated percent Hb A_2 is the next best evidence for the diagnosis of beta-thalassemia trait. Sufficient criteria for the diagnosis of thalassemia trait are an elevated Hb A_2 percentage by a reliable method (Hgb electrophoresis with elution and quantitation by spectrophotometry) or column chromatography (assuming Hb S, C, or an unstable hemoglobin are not present).

Hb A_2 may be increased in megaloblastic anemia and may be decreased in sideroblastic anemia, Hb H disease, and erythroleukemia. Approximately one-third of zidovudine (AZT) treated human immunodeficiency virus-1 positive individuals have elevated Hb A_2 levels.[3]

Footnotes

1. Wasi P, Disthasongchan P, and Na-Nakorn S, "The Effect of Iron Deficiency on the Levels of Hemoglobins A_2 and E," *J Lab Clin Med*, 1968, 71:85-91.
2. Beris P, Darbellay R, Speiser D, et al, "De Novo Initiation Codon Mutation (ATG → ACG) of the β-Globin Gene Causing β-Thalassemia in a Swiss Family," *Am J Hematol*, 1993, 42(3):248-53.
3. Routy JP, Monte M, Beaulieu R, et al, "Increase of Hemoglobin A_2 in Human Immunodeficiency Virus-1-Infected Patients Treated With Zidovudine," *Am J Hematol*, 1993, 43:86-90.

References

Adams JG 3d and Coleman MB, "Structural Hemoglobin Variants That Produce the Phenotype of Thalassemia," *Semin Hematol*, 1990, 27(3):229-38.

Bunn HF and Forget BG, *Hemoglobin: Molecular, Genetic, and Clinical Aspects*, Philadelphia, PA: WB Saunders Co, 1986, 61-7.

Erdem S and Aksoy M, "The Increase of Hemoglobin A_2 to its Adult Level," *Isr J Med Sci*, 1969, 5:427-8.

Kazazian HH Jr, "The Thalassemia Syndromes: Molecular Basis and Prenatal Diagnosis in 1990," *Semin Hematol*, 1990, 27(3):209-28.

Lukens JN, "The Thalassemias and Related Disorders: Quantitative Disorders of Hemoglobin Synthesis," *Wintrobe's Clinical Hematology*, 9th ed, Vol 1, Chapter 39, Lee GR, Bithell TC, Foerster J, et al, eds, Philadelphia, PA: Lea & Febiger, 1993, 1102-45.

Steinberg MH and Adams JG 3d, "Hemoglobin A_2: Origin, Evolution, and Aftermath," *Blood*, 1991, 78(9):2165-77.

Thonglairoam V, Winichagoon P, Fucharoen S, et al, "Hemoglobin Constant Spring in Bangkok: Molecular Screening by Selective Enzymatic Amplification of the α_2-Globin Gene," *Am J Hematol*, 1991, 38(4):277-80.

Hemoglobin Electrophoresis

CPT 83020

See Also Anemia Flowchart in the Hematology Appendix

Related Information

Fetal Hemoglobin *on page 542*
Hemoglobin A_2 *on previous page*
Methemoglobin *on page 290*
P-50 Blood Gas *on page 307*
Peripheral Blood: Red Blood Cell Morphology *on page 584*
Reticulocyte Count *on page 597*
Sickle Cell Tests *on page 600*

Test Commonly Includes Electrophoresis for separation and distribution of hemoglobins

Abstract In this procedure, hemoglobins are caused to separate and migrate. A variety of techniques are utilized. Most commonly bands are developed on a substrate in a buffer solution across an electric field with subsequent visualization after fixation and staining. Clinical applications include detection and identification of hemoglobin variants and the investigation of some hemolytic anemias resulting from red cell intracorpuscular defects.

Specimen Whole blood **CONTAINER:** Lavender top (EDTA) tube for venipuncture specimen; lavender top Microtainer™ tube for capillary specimen **CAUSES FOR REJECTION:** Specimen clotted **TURNAROUND TIME:** Method dependent, usually 1-2 days

Interpretive **REFERENCE RANGE:** Hemoglobin A: 95% to 98%; hemoglobin A_2: 1.5% to 3.5%; hemoglobin F: 0% to 2%; hemoglobin C: absent; hemoglobin S: absent **USE:** Diagnose hemoglobinopathies; evaluate hemolytic anemia; diagnose thalassemia; evaluate sickling hemoglobins, hemoglobin C; with other and specialized techniques, evaluate unstable, low and high oxygen affinity hemoglobinopathies (eg, one cause of polycythemia) **LIMITATIONS:** Blood transfusion prior to hemoglobin electrophoresis may make interpretations inconsistent. Many abnormal hemoglobins will not separate from normal adult Hb A during application of routine electrophoretic techniques. Rarely, there may be lack of specificity for Hgb (eg, monoclonal immunoglobulin).[1] **METHODOLOGY:** Electrophoresis using cellulose acetate, agarose gel, citrate agar gel, or starch gel substrates; isoelectric focusing using polyacrylamide or agarose gel substrates; alkali denaturation for fetal hemoglobin; anion exchange resin chromatography for hemoglobin A_2 quantitation **ADDITIONAL INFORMATION:** In this procedure, hemoglobin (Hgb), released from lysed red blood cells, is caused to migrate through a substrate in a buffer by application of an electric current. Different types of hemoglobin are separated into specific bands that are subsequently visualized by application of one of a variety of staining procedures. Migration of hemoglobin is defined by interaction of a specific hemoglobin molecule with substrate structure, buffer pH, ionic strength, and other characteristics. The test is of central importance in establishing the presence of common hemoglobinopathies (Hb S, C, D, and E) and in the evaluation of some cases of hemolytic anemia. Study of peripheral blood smear RBC morphology can assist in the decision to order hemoglobin electrophoresis. Hemoglobin electrophoresis (including determination of Hb F) is indicated if a positive sickle screening test has been obtained. Hb F and Hb A_2 quantitation (often included as part of an "Hb electrophoresis" package) are important in establishing the presence of thalassemia. In some cases additional study will be needed. Depending upon the abnormality encountered this might include reticulocyte count, haptoglobin level, citrate agar gel electrophoresis at acidic pH and family studies. Complete characterization of abnormal hemoglobin states may require sophisticated laboratory studies usually available only in a research setting (eg, some of the thalassemia syndromes).[2] Ultimately, amino acid globin chain sequencing may be necessary to establish the presence of a hemoglobinopathy. Hemoglobin electrophoresis of umbilical cord blood can detect α-chain variants Hb F/G and Hb G as well as S and C gene products. Results have been reported as consistent with the predicted frequency (1 in 625) of sickle anemia at birth.[3] Newer techniques of analysis, globin chain electrophoresis,[4,5] isoelectric focusing,[6,7] restriction endonuclease studies,[8] and polymerase chain reaction[9] are powerful additions to the laboratory's ability to detect and identify hemoglobin variants. Interest and capability in these areas is growing, but the procedures are still not routinely available in most clinical laboratories. Some alkaline gel electrophoretic systems may offer advantages in glycohemoglobin quantitation because of their ability to discriminate Hb F and to simultaneously detect common hemoglobinopathies.[10] It has been shown that capillary electrophoresis can separate hemoglobin variants within 10 minutes.[11]

Screening of the general population for sickle cell and other hemoglobinopathies had vocal proponents in the late 1960s and early 1970s. Interest waned, largely the result of possible socioeconomic implications of case detection. During the past decade, however, there has been growing activity in (and state support of) newborn screening for sickle cell and other hemoglobinopathies. Problem areas include false-negative results (associated with the use of dried blood filter paper samples) and the detection of maternal contamination of cord blood.[12,13,14]

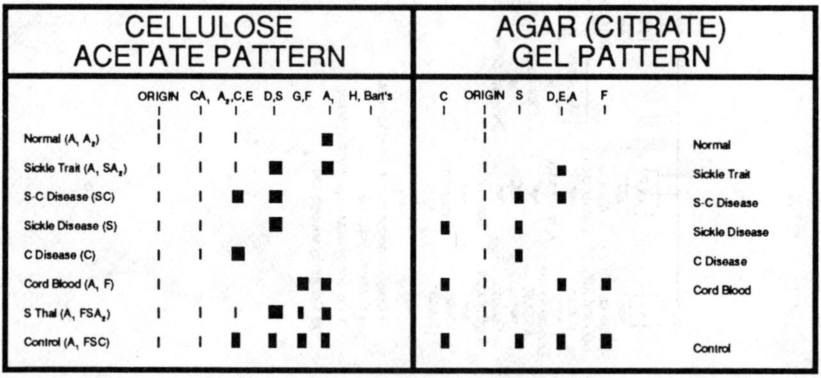

CELLULOSE ACETATE PATTERN

ORIGIN CA, A_2,C,E D,S G,F A_1 H, Bart's

Normal (A_1 A_2)
Sickle Trait (A_1 SA_2)
S-C Disease (SC)
Sickle Disease (S)
C Disease (C)
Cord Blood (A_1 F)
S Thal (A_1 FSA_2)
Control (A_1 FSC)

AGAR (CITRATE) GEL PATTERN

C ORIGIN S D,E,A F

Normal
Sickle Trait
S-C Disease
Sickle Disease
C Disease
Cord Blood
Control

(Continued)

Hemoglobin Electrophoresis *(Continued)*

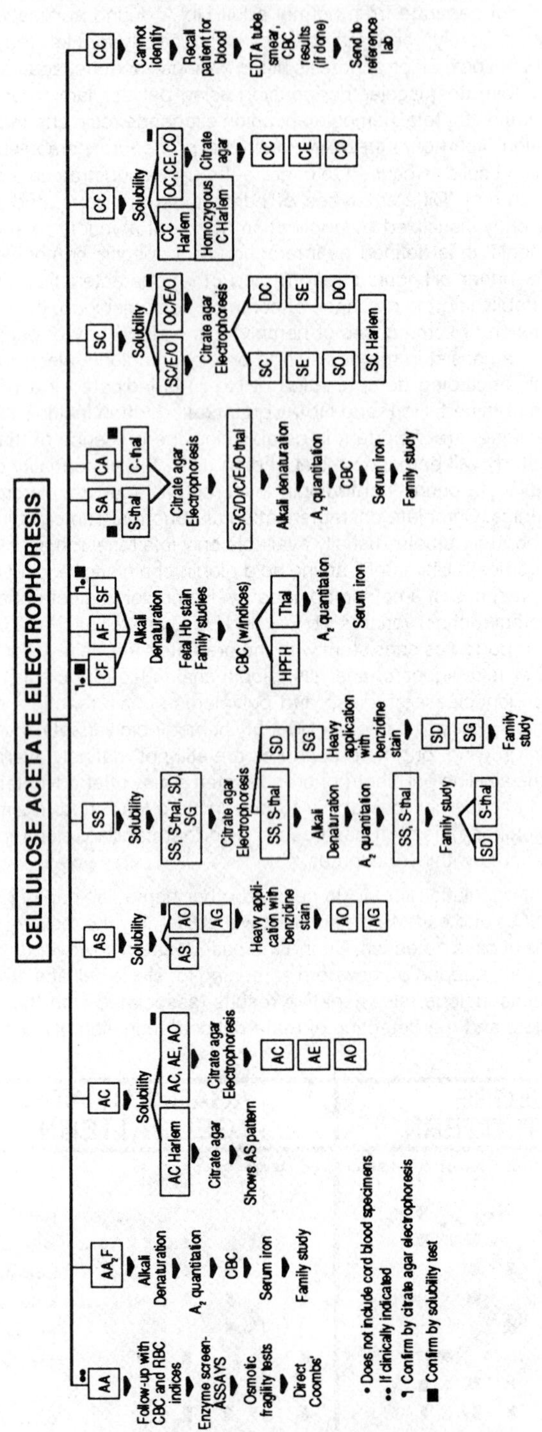

Footnotes

1. Sughayer MA and Arkin CF, "Unusual Band on Hemoglobin Electrophoresis Produced by a Monoclonal Immunoglobulin in Serum," *Clin Chem*, 1989, 35(8):1794.
2. Huisman TH, "Sickle Cell Anemia as a Syndrome: A Review of Diagnostic Features," *Am J Hematol*, 1979, 6:173-84.
3. Castro O, Winter WP, Lee TC, et al, "Prevalence of α-Chain Variants at Birth," *Am J Clin Pathol*, 1981, 75:56-9.
4. Alter BP, "Gel Electrophoretic Separation of Globin Chains," *Prog Clin Biol Res*, 1981, 60:157-75.
5. Alter BP, Coupal E, and Forget BG, "Globin Chain Electrophoresis for Prenatal Diagnosis of Beta Thalassemia," *Hemoglobin*, 1981, 5:357-70.
6. Basset P, Beuzard Y, Garel MC, et al, "Isoelectric Focusing of Human Hemoglobin: Its Application to Screening, to the Characterization of 70 Variants, and to the Study of Modified Fractions of Normal Hemoglobins," *Blood*, 1978, 51:971-82.
7. Cossu G, Manca M, Pirastu G, et al, "Neonatal Screening of β-Thalassemias by Thin Layer Isoelectric Focusing," *Am J Hematol*, 1982, 13:149-57.
8. Gutmann DH, "The Use of Restriction Endonucleases in the Prenatal Diagnosis of Hemoglobinopathies," *Am J Med Technol*, 1982, 48:361-6.
9. Skogerboe KJ, West SF, Murillo MD, et al, "Genetic Screening of Newborns for Sickle Cell Disease: Correlation of DNA Analysis With Hemoglobin Electrophoresis," *Clin Chem*, 1991, 37(3):454-8.
10. Bayliss KM, Kopinski WS, and Kueck BD, "Glycohemoglobin Quantitation by Alkaline Gel Electrophoresis. A Reliable Technique with Practical Clinical Advantages," *Am J Clin Pathol*, 1989, 91(5):570-4.
11. Chen FT, Liu CM, Hsieh YZ, et al, "Capillary Electrophoresis - A New Clinical Tool," *Clin Chem*, 1991, 37(1):14-9.
12. Kutlar A, Ozcan O, Brisco JT, et al, "The Detection of Hemoglobin Variants by Isoelectrofocusing Using EDTA-Collected and Filter Paper-Dried Cord Blood Specimens," *Am J Clin Pathol*, 1990, 94(2):199-202.
13. Githens JH, Lane PA, McCurdy RS, et al, "Newborn Screening for Hemoglobinopathies in Colorado. The First 10 Years," *Am J Dis Child*, 1990, 144(4):466-70.
14. Scott RB, "Newborn Screening for Sickle Cell Disease and Other Hemoglobinopathies," *Pediatrics*, 1989, 83(5 Pt 2):908-9.

References

Alter BP, "Prenatal Diagnosis of Hemoglobinopathies and Other Hematologic Diseases," *J Pediatr*, 1979, 95:501-3.

Bunn HF and Forget BG, *Hemoglobin: Molecular, Genetic and Clinical Aspects*, Philadelphia, PA: WB Saunders Co, 1986.

Dickerson RE and Geis I, *Hemoglobin: Structure, Function, Evolution and Pathology*, Menlo Park, CA: The Benjamin/Cummings Publishing Co Inc, 1983.

Fairbanks VF, *Hemoglobinopathies and Thalassemias: Laboratory Methods and Case Studies*, Chapter 6, New York, NY: Thieme-Stratton Inc, 1980.

Harrison CR, "Hemolytic Anemias: Intracorpuscular Defects, IV. Thalassemia," *Clinical Hematology and Fundamentals of Hemostasis* 2nd ed, Chapter 12, Harmening DM, ed, Philadelphia, PA: FA Davis Co, 1992.

Stamatoyannopoulos G, Nienhuis AW, Leder P, et al, eds, *The Molecular Basis of Blood Diseases*, Chapter 2-6, Philadelphia, PA: WB Saunders Co, 1987, 28-206.

Thonglairoam V, Winichagoon P, Fucharoen S, et al, "Hemoglobin Constant Spring in Bangkok: Molecular Screening by Selective Enzymatic Amplification of the α_2-Globin Gene," *Am J Hematol*, 1991, 38(4):277-80.

Zeringer H and Harmening DM, "Hemolytic Anemias: Intracorpuscular Defects, III. The Hemoglobinopathies," *Clinical Hematology and Fundamentals of Hemostasis* 2nd ed, Chapters 11, Harmening DM, ed, Philadelphia, PA: FA Davis Co, 1992.

Hemoglobin, Fetal *see* Fetal Hemoglobin *on page 542*

Hemoglobin, Free *see* Hemoglobin, Plasma *on this page*

Hemoglobin, Plasma

CPT 83051

Related Information

Haptoglobin, Serum *on page 247*

Hemoglobin, Qualitative, Urine *on page 1122*

Synonyms Free Hemoglobin; Hemoglobin, Free; Plasma Free Hemoglobin

Abstract Test used to detect intravascular hemolysis

Patient Care PREPARATION: Special precautions and patient preparation are usually required to draw the specimen. Laboratory should be contacted directly. AFTERCARE: A pressure bandage should be applied to the site of 18-gauge needle puncture (following the puncture) to stop residual bleeding.

Specimen Plasma CONTAINER: Lavender top (EDTA) tube COLLECTION: Recommended procedure for collecting sample without inducing hemolysis: Use 18-gauge needle with attached in-

(Continued)

Hemoglobin, Plasma *(Continued)*

fusion tubing. Place tourniquet lightly around the upper arm. Puncture antecubital vein with as little trauma as possible. Release tourniquet and clamp tubing off as soon as blood return is seen. Collect 3 mL of blood first in a red top tube with the rubber stopper off. Follow by a 5 mL collection in a green top (heparin) tube with the stopper off. Clamp tubing, withdraw needle, and apply pressure to the site until residual bleeding is stopped. Cap green top tube and gently mix three to five times. Use this specimen for the plasma hemoglobin determination. **STORAGE INSTRUCTIONS:** Separate and freeze plasma as soon as possible if test is not run immediately. **CAUSES FOR REJECTION:** Traumatic venipuncture causing hemolysis

Interpretive **REFERENCE RANGE:** <10 mg/dL,[1] optimally (with absence of artifactual hemolysis during collection of blood) <1 mg/dL **USE:** Evaluate hemolytic anemia, especially intravascular hemolysis **LIMITATIONS:** Plasma hemoglobin is increased with intravascular hemolysis, ABO incompatible transfusion, traumatic hemolysis, falciparum malaria, burns, and march hemoglobinuria. Increase may occur in some cases of extravascular hemolysis, delayed transfusion reaction, slight increase in sickle cell anemia, and β-thalassemia. High bilirubin, turbidity, methemalbuminemia, lipemic plasma, and hemolysis during or after venipuncture may cause falsely elevated values in the plasma hemoglobin test (method based on peroxide oxidation of benzidine). Method based on the fractional absorbance of oxyhemoglobin at 578 nm is proportional even in the presence of those interfering substances.[2] Use of benzidine has been restricted because of reports that it is carcinogenic. **METHODOLOGY:** An established method utilizes fractional absorbance of oxyhemoglobin at 578 nm. A method utilizing first-derivative spectroscopy (procedure of Soloni et al) has undergone evaluation. It is rapid and not affected by bilirubin, myoglobin, lipemia, or turbidity. It is sensitive down to a level of 1 mg/dL.[3] **ADDITIONAL INFORMATION:** High bilirubin (up to 36 mg/dL), turbidity of the specimen, or a fair amount of methemalbumin will not affect the method based on fractional absorbance of oxyhemoglobin at 578 nm or the method of Soloni et al.[4] Hemoglobinemia can be easily detected by gross examination of centrifuged blood when plasma hemoglobin is >50 mg/dL.

Footnotes

1. Copeland BE, Dyer PJ, and Pesce AJ, "Hemoglobin by First Derivative Spectrophotometry: Extent of Hemolysis in Plasma and Serum Collected in Vacuum Container Devices," *Ann Clin Lab Sci*, 1989, 19(5):383-8.
2. Watkins BF and Bermes EJ, "Measurement of Plasma Hemoglobin," *Seminar on Biochemical Hematology*, FW Sunderman, ed, Philadelphia, PA: Institute for Clinical Science Inc, 1979, 57-62.
3. Soloni FG, Cunningham MT, and Amazon K, "Plasma Hemoglobin Determination by Recording Derivative Spectrophotometry," *Am J Clin Pathol*, 1986, 85:342-7.
4. Copeland BE, Dyer PJ, and Pesce AJ, "Hemoglobin Determination in Plasma or Serum by First-Derivative Recording Spectrophotometry," *Am J Clin Pathol*, 1989, 92(5):619-24.

References

Fairbanks VF, Ziesmer SC, and O'Brien PC, "Methods for Measuring Plasma Hemoglobin in Micromolar Concentration Compared," *Clin Chem*, 1992, 38(1):132-40.

Lee GR, "The Hemolytic Disorders: General Considerations," *Wintrobe's Clinical Hematology*, 9th ed, Vol 1, Chapter 32, Lee GR, Bithell TC, Foerster J, et al, eds, Philadelphia, PA: Lea & Febiger, 1993, 944-64.

Hemoglobin, Unstable, Heat Labile Test

***CPT** 83065*

Related Information

Heinz Body Stain *on page 551*

Hemoglobin, Unstable - Isopropanol Precipitation Test *on next page*

Synonyms Heat Denaturation; Test for Congenital Heinz Body Hemolytic Anemia; Unstable Hemoglobins

Applies to Heinz Bodies

Abstract A simple, low cost test for the detection of unstable hemoglobin. Most of such variant hemoglobins will not separate from Hb A on routine electrophoresis.

Specimen Whole blood **CONTAINER:** Lavender top (EDTA) tube **CAUSES FOR REJECTION:** Specimen more than 4 hours old

Interpretive **REFERENCE RANGE:** Less than 1% unstable hemoglobin (quantitation by hemoglobinometry of centrifuged lysate). Normally, test should result in little or no precipitate. A positive result (denatured hemoglobin present) is the presence of turbidity and/or fine flocculation, a readily visible precipitate. **USE:** Determine the presence of unstable hemoglobins, most of which will not be identified by routine hemoglobin electrophoresis **LIMITATIONS:** The visual end point in this test may be difficult to interpret. Test should be run along with a normal control. Some degree of slight precipitation may occur in an erratic manner in normals. Quantitation of

% unstable hemoglobin (by hemoglobinometry) is desirable. Result can be compared to the isopropanol precipitation test for unstable hemoglobin (see following listing). **METHODOLOGY:** Washed cells lysed, acidified, lysate heated at 50°C for 1 hour and examined for turbidity/flocculation (compared to control). Percent unstable hemoglobin may be reported. **ADDITIONAL INFORMATION:** Another approach to detection of unstable hemoglobins is to search for Heinz bodies. Heinz body test is less specific than heat instability study. Hemolysates containing unstable hemoglobin may precipitate spontaneously on standing a few days in the refrigerator. Some unstable hemoglobins are associated with hemolytic anemia and an appropriate clinical picture including intermittent jaundice and usually splenomegaly. If hypersplenism is present there may be thrombocytopenia. There have been many different unstable hemoglobins reported after the early study of Hb Köln.[1] Lukens and Lee in the 9th edition (1993) of *Wintrobe's Clinical Hematology* indicate that over 125 unstable hemoglobins have been identified. On the basis of clinical severity, these authors have divided the unstable hemoglobin variants into five groups. Eleven are classified as "severe hemolytic disease, no response to splenectomy"; 15 are associated with "moderately severe hemolytic disease improved by splenectomy"; 52 are classified as "moderate to mild hemolytic disease with hemolytic crises"; 33 have "no clinical or hematologic abnormality"; and 28 are considered to have "insufficient data to classify". The most common unstable Hb variant is Hb Köln which has wide geographic distribution. Most unstable hemoglobins have been demonstrated only in single individuals or families. Most unstable hemoglobin diseases have an autosomal dominant mode of inheritance, however, in over 40 some cases the disease has occurred as a result of a spontaneous mutation.[2] Some of these unstable hemoglobins also have abnormal affinity for oxygen.

Footnotes

1. White JM and Dacie JV, "The Unstable Hemoglobins – Molecular and Clinical Features," *Prog Hematol*, 1971, 7:69-109.
2. Lukens JN and Lee GR, "Unstable Hemoglobin Disease," *Wintrobe's Clinical Hematology*, 9th ed, Vol 1, Chapter 37, Lee GR, Bithell TC, Foerster J, et al, eds, Philadelphia, PA: Lea & Febiger, 1993, 1054-60.

References

Bunn HF and Forget BG, *Hemoglobin: Molecular, Genetic and Clinical Aspects*, Philadelphia, PA: WB Saunders Co, 1986, 565-94.

Williams WJ, Beutler E, Erslev AJ, et al, *Hematology*, 4th ed, New York, NY: McGraw-Hill Inc, 1990, 644-52.

Zinkham WH and Winslow RM, "Unstable Hemoglobins: Influence of Environment on Phenotypic Expression of a Genetic Disorder," *Medicine (Baltimore)*, 1989, 68(5):309-20.

Hemoglobin, Unstable – Isopropanol Precipitation Test

CPT 83068

Related Information

Heinz Body Stain *on page 551*

Hemoglobin, Unstable, Heat Labile Test *on previous page*

Synonyms Unstable Hemoglobins

Applies to Heinz Bodies

Abstract A simple, low cost test for unstable hemoglobins. Most of such variant hemoglobins will not be detected by routine hemoglobin electrophoresis as they migrate with Hb A.

Specimen Whole blood **CONTAINER:** Lavender top (EDTA) tube

Interpretive **REFERENCE RANGE:** Absence of a precipitate in buffered isopropanol. Solution should remain clear for 30-40 minutes. **USE:** Differential diagnosis of hemolytic anemias; detect unstable hemoglobins many of which will not be identified (separated from Hb A) by standard electrophoretic techniques **LIMITATIONS:** Hemoglobin F begins to precipitate about halfway through the incubation period – about the time that one expects unstable Hgb to appear. If the patient's Hb F is increased, a false-positive result for unstable Hgb may result.[1] **METHODOLOGY:** Mix 2 mL of 17% (unit/unit) isopropanol with 0.2 mL of hemolysate. Incubate at 37°C; check for precipitate at 20 minutes. **ADDITIONAL INFORMATION:** Heat lability and Heinz body tests are also applicable to the detection and study of unstable hemoglobins. While simple to perform, interpretation may be difficult. A multitest approach has been suggested.[2]

Footnotes

1. Dacie JV and Lewis SM, *Practical Haematology*, 7th ed, New York, NY: Churchill Livingstone, 1991, 252.
2. Carrell RW, "Hemoglobin Stability Tests," *The Detection of Hemoglobinopathies*, Schmidt RM, et al, eds, Cleveland, OH: CRC Press, 1974.

References

Bunn HF and Forget BG, *Hemoglobin: Molecular, Genetic and Clinical Aspects*, Philadelphia, PA: WB Saunders Co, 1986, 565-94.

Carrell RW and Kay R, "A Simple Method for the Detection of Unstable Hemoglobins," *Br J Haematol*, 1972, 23:615-9.

(Continued)

Hemoglobin, Unstable – Isopropanol Precipitation Test *(Continued)*

Williams WJ, Beutler E, Erslev AJ, et al, *Hematology*, 4th ed, New York, NY: McGraw-Hill Inc, 1990, 644-52.
Zinkham WH and Winslow RM, "Unstable Hemoglobins: Influence of Environment on Phenotypic Expression of a Genetic Disorder," *Medicine (Baltimore)*, 1989, 68(5):309-20.

Hemogram *see* Complete Blood Count *on page 533*
Hemosiderin Stain *see* Iron Stain, Bone Marrow *on this page*
Hemosiderin Stain *see* Siderocyte Stain *on page 602*
Hexosaminidase A *see* Tests for Uncommon Inherited Diseases of Metabolism and Cell Structure *on page 605*
Hexosaminidase A and B *see* Tests for Uncommon Inherited Diseases of Metabolism and Cell Structure *on page 605*
Hgb *see* Hemoglobin *on page 554*
Inborn Errors of Metabolism *see* Tests for Uncommon Inherited Diseases of Metabolism and Cell Structure *on page 605*
Incubated Osmotic Fragility *see* Osmotic Fragility *on page 573*
Indices *see* Red Blood Cell Indices *on page 592*
Interleukin-3 *see* Eosinophil Count *on page 539*
Interleukin-5 *see* Eosinophil Count *on page 539*
Iron Stain *see* Siderocyte Stain *on page 602*

Iron Stain, Bone Marrow

CPT 85535

Related Information

Bone Marrow *on page 524*
Ferritin, Serum *on page 220*
Iron and Total Iron Binding Capacity/Transferrin *on page 262*
Siderocyte Stain *on page 602*

Synonyms Bone Marrow Iron Stain; Hemosiderin Stain; Marrow Iron Stores; Perls' Test; Prussian Blue Stain; Sideroblast Stain

Test Commonly Includes Iron stain on sections of marrow aspirate clot and/or bone marrow biopsy and iron stain marrow cover slip smears

Specimen Bone marrow glass coverslip or slide smears, marrow aspirate, or biopsy **CONTAINER:** Coverslips or glass microslides are prepared at the bedside. Biopsy and clot fixed in formalin or other fixative (eg, B-5 or Zenker's solution). **COLLECTION:** Physician obtains bone marrow aspirate specimen by aseptic aspiration technique. Phlebotomist simultaneously obtains blood specimen for the preparation of peripheral blood smears. **CAUSES FOR REJECTION:** No marrow obtained ("dry tap") or no bone marrow particles on smears **SPECIAL INSTRUCTIONS:** Requisition should include a brief clinical history.

Interpretive **REFERENCE RANGE:** Results should be interpreted in light of clinical background. Peripheral blood: no stainable iron is usually present (ie, no siderocytes are normally found). Bone marrow: stainable iron present as extracellular granules/globules and/or intracellular in cytoplasm of histiocytes – cells of the RE system. About one-third of the rubricytes in the marrow may be iron-positive sideroblasts (but not "ringed sideroblasts"). **USE:** Semiquantitation of bone marrow iron stores; sensitive test for the evaluation of iron reserve; aid in the diagnosis of iron deficiency; aid in the diagnosis of hemosiderosis/hemochromatosis; aid in the diagnosis of sideroblastic anemia including refractory anemia with ringed sideroblasts **LIMITATIONS:** Specimen should include sufficiently large spicules of marrow. **METHODOLOGY:** Ferrocyanide ion reacts in acid with ferric ion to form a dark blue precipitate called Prussian blue. A silver stain has been proposed as a sensitive alternative for the demonstration of ringed sideroblasts.[1] **ADDITIONAL INFORMATION:** It would appear that when a bone biopsy specimen is decalcified for over 2 hours, "leaching" of iron may occur so that a bone biopsy may be negative for iron while aspirate smear is positive. Krause et al, however, found that in only 35% of 270 cases with iron negative aspirate smears were there also iron negative biopsies (65% iron positive biopsies with iron negative smears).[2] Therefore, without evaluation of both types of specimens a significant overdiagnosis of iron deficiency may occur. Hemochromatosis, hemolytic anemias, and those with ineffective erythropoiesis (eg, thalassemia, megaloblastic and sideroblastic anemias) and anemias of chronic disease (especially inflammation) are characterized by increase in iron stores. The usual sideroblast has small iron positive granules without pattern in the cytoplasm. Ringed sideroblasts are rubricytes with tiny particles of iron located in mitochondria forming a ring around at least two-thirds of the nucleus. These pathologic sideroblasts occur in cases of normoblastic refractory anemia, B_6 responsive anemia, thalassemia, a variety of sideroblastic anemias, in some cases of B_{12}/folic acid deficiency, and in chloramphenicol toxicity. See table.

Siderocytes in Peripheral Blood Normal vs Hemolytic States

	Average (%)	Range (%)
Normal	0	0
Normal, postsplenectomy	4	0–14
Hereditary spherocytosis	0–2	0–2
HS, postsplenectomy	10	2–45
Acquired hemolytic anemia	2.3	0–21
Acquired hemolytic anemia postsplenectomy	20	1–67
Thalassemia	0	0
Sickle cell anemia	0.2	0.2
Hemolytic disease newborn	3.7	0–35

From Miale JB, *Laboratory Medicine: Hematology*, 6th ed, St Louis, MO: Mosby–Year Book Inc, 1982, 582, with permission.

A proposed silver stain for ringed sideroblasts may have as its chemical basis the demonstration of insoluble phosphates and/or carbonates of iron or other metals. Thus, when marrow iron is decreased (eg, sideroblastic anemia with iron deficiency due to GI bleeding), silver staining may be used to demonstrate ringed sideroblasts that would not be seen with Perls' reaction. Decalcified bone biopsy specimens, however, cannot be used to demonstrate sideroblasts (reaction is negative) by this method.[1] Silver staining is not considered to substitute for the Prussian blue reaction in identification of ringed sideroblasts.[1]

A cost efficient and noninvasive alternative to bone marrow iron study is the proposed combined determination of zinc protoporphyrin/heme ratio and serum ferritin.[3,4] In a study of the anemia of chronic disease (rheumatoid arthritis) it was concluded that a combination of peripheral blood parameters (MCV, ferritin, and transferrin) could detect iron deficiency without resorting to marrow aspiration.[5]

Footnotes

1. Tham KT, Cousar JB, and Macon WR, "Silver Stain for Ringed Sideroblasts. A Sensitive Method That Differs From Perls' Reaction in Mechanism and Clinical Application," *Am J Clin Pathol*, 1990, 94(1):73-6.
2. Krause JR, Brubaker D, and Kaplan S, "Comparison of Stainable Iron in Aspirated and Needle Biopsy Specimens of Bone Marrow," *Am J Clin Pathol*, 1979, 72:68-70.
3. Labbe RF, "Zinc Protoporphyrin/Heme Ratio as an Indicator of Marrow Iron Stores," *Am J Clin Pathol*, 1991, 95(5):758.
4. Labbe RF and Rettmer RL, "Zinc Protoporphyrin: A Product of Iron-Deficient Erythropoiesis," *Semin Hematol*, 1989, 26(1):40-6.
5. Vreugdenhil G, Baltus CA, Van Eijk HG, et al, "Anaemia of Chronic Disease: Diagnostic Significance of Erythrocyte and Serological Parameters in Iron Deficient Rheumatoid Arthritis Patients," *Br J Rheumatol*, 1990, 29(2):105-10.

Itano Solubility Test *see* Sickle Cell Tests *on page 600*

Joint Fluid Analysis *see* Body Fluids Analysis, Cell Count *on page 523*

K-B *see* Kleihauer-Betke *on this page*

Kleihauer-Betke

CPT 85460

Related Information

D[u] *on page 1063*
Fetal Hemoglobin *on page 542*
Rh_o(D) Immune Globulin (Human) *on page 1091*
Rosette Test for Fetomaternal Hemorrhage *on page 1097*

Synonyms Acid Elution for Fetal Hemoglobin; K-B

Abstract Staining of a postpartum maternal blood specimen for identification of percentage of fetal cells present

(Continued)

Kleihauer-Betke *(Continued)*

Specimen Whole blood **CONTAINER:** Lavender top (EDTA) tube **STORAGE INSTRUCTIONS:** Blood must be less than 6 hours old. Smears must be fixed within 1 hour after preparation. **CAUSES FOR REJECTION:** Clotted specimen, improper labeling, inadequate specimen, gross hemolysis **SPECIAL INSTRUCTIONS:** A cord blood specimen should also be sent as a source of fetal blood (for use as a positive control).

Interpretive **REFERENCE RANGE:** Full-term newborns: Hb F cells are >90%; normal adults: Hb F cells are <0.01% **USE:** Determine possible fetal-maternal hemorrhage in the newborn; aid in diagnosis of certain types of anemia in adults; assess the magnitude of fetal-maternal hemorrhage; calculate dosage of Rh immune globulin (eg, RhoGAM™) to be given **LIMITATIONS:** Possibility of presence of an hemoglobinopathy with increase in Hb F must be considered when this test is used to assess fetal-maternal hemorrhage. Specimens must be obtained prior to transfusion. **CONTRAINDICATIONS:** Known pre-existing elevation of maternal Hb F (eg, mothers with hereditary persistence of fetal hemoglobin)[1,2] **METHODOLOGY:** Acid elution. After fixation with alcohol Hb F remains as a precipitate within the cell while Hb A is soluble in citric acid phosphate buffer. The adult RBCs containing little or no Hb F appear as ghosts under microscope. **ADDITIONAL INFORMATION:** The Kleihauer-Betke test is helpful in distinguishing some forms of thalassemia from hereditary persistence of fetal hemoglobin (HPFH). The hereditary persistence of fetal hemoglobin reveals a uniform distribution of fetal hemoglobin in each red cell. Δ-β-thalassemia, in contrast, demonstrates a heterogeneous distribution of fetal hemoglobin, (ie, some cells are stained and others are ghost RBCs).

Some RhoGAM™ failures are due to a failure to suspect and diagnose fetal- maternal hemorrhage that may require more than one dose of RhoGAM™. Ultimate purpose is to prevent evolution of anti-D antibodies in the postpartum woman and subsequent hemolytic disease of the newborn (erythroblastosis fetalis). The amount of fetal blood contamination can be calculated. Each vial of Rh immune globulin contains 300 μg of anti-D. This is enough to prevent maternal immunization when the fetal bleed is up to 30 mL of whole blood (15 mL packed cells). One vial of Rh immune globulin is given to the Rh-negative mother for every 30 mL of fetal blood contamination from an Rh-positive fetus.

In cases of maternal hereditary persistence of fetal hemoglobin, an alternative method for detection and quantification of fetal Rh (D)-positive hemorrhage has been developed.[1] In this method, a flow cytometer is used to quantitate an indirect immunofluorescent reaction in which IgG anti-D is used as the primary antibody.

A study designed to determine the incidence of fetomaternal hemorrhage following cesarean section utilizing Kleihauer-Betke testing found some degree of hemorrhage in 18.5% of the study patients. In 2.5%, there was evidence of more than 30 mL of fetal blood lost into the maternal circulation. This finding led to the recommendation that all Rh-negative patients having a C-section be screened (Kleihauer-Betke test) for fetomaternal hemorrhage.[3]

Footnotes

1. Patton WN, Nicholson GS, Sawers AH, et al, "Assessment of Fetal-Maternal Haemorrhage in Mothers With Hereditary Persistence of Fetal Haemoglobin," *J Clin Pathol*, 1990, 43(9):728-31.
2. Holcomb WL, Gunderson E, and Petrie RH, "Clinical Use of the Kleihauer-Betke Test," *J Perinat Med*, 1990, 18(5):331-7.
3. Feldman N, Skoll A, and Sibai B, "The Incidence of Significant Fetomaternal Hemorrhage in Patients Undergoing Cesarean Section," *Am J Obstet Gynecol*, 1990, 163(3):855-8.

References

Henry JB, Nelson DA, Tomar RH, et al, *Clinical Diagnosis and Management by Laboratory Methods*, 18th ed, Philadelphia, PA: WB Saunders Co, 1991, 493-4.

Kleihauer E, "Determination of Fetal Hemoglobin: Elution Technique," *The Detection of Hemoglobinopathies*, Schmidt RM, et al, eds, Cleveland, OH: CRC Press, 1974.

Von Stein GA, Munsick RA, Stiver K, et al, "Fetomaternal Hemorrhage in Threatened Abortion," *Obstet Gynecol*, 1992, 79(3):383-6.

LAP *see* Leukocyte Alkaline Phosphatase *on page 566*

LAP Score *see* Leukocyte Alkaline Phosphatase *on page 566*

LAP Smear *see* Leukocyte Alkaline Phosphatase *on page 566*

Large Molecule Diseases *see* Tests for Uncommon Inherited Diseases of Metabolism and Cell Structure *on page 605*

LE Cell Test

CPT 87205

Related Information

Anti-DNA *on page 634*
Antinuclear Antibody *on page 638*
Scleroderma Antibody *on page 745*
Sjögren's Antibodies *on page 746*
Smooth Muscle Antibody *on page 747*

Synonyms LE Prep; LE Preparation; LE Slide Cell Test; Lupus Test

Abstract Historically, an important test for systemic lupus erythematosus (SLE), it is currently outmoded.

Patient Care PREPARATION: Avoid heparin therapy for 2 days prior to collection. Large doses of heparin may increase the incidence of false-negative results.

Specimen Whole blood CONTAINER: Green top (heparin) tube; EDTA anticoagulated blood may cause false-negative results COLLECTION: Routine venipuncture. Invert gently to mix. Transport to the laboratory within 30 minutes. CAUSES FOR REJECTION: Insufficient volume, clotted specimen, patient on heparin

Interpretive REFERENCE RANGE: Negative USE: Evaluate autoimmune diseases, specifically SLE (systemic lupus erythematosus); aid in the diagnosis of "lupoid" hepatitis (chronic active hepatitis). The discovery of the LE cell more than 40 years ago has been important in understanding autoimmune disease. As stated by Tan and associates, however, "It has been superseded by modern ANA tests with greater sensitivity and rapidity, but its fundamental contribution to understanding of ANAs cannot be overlooked."[1] A few authors[2] still advocate the use of this test. LIMITATIONS: This test is an indirect method for detecting one of the antinuclear antibodies. It is less sensitive than fluorescent antibody techniques for ANA and not specific for lupus erythematosus. Positive tests have been reported in a variety of drug induced lupus syndromes, in rheumatoid arthritis, chronic and active hepatitis, drug hypersensitivity, and other collagen diseases. One negative result, therefore, should not be considered to rule out the possibility of LE. EDTA anticoagulated blood may cause a false-negative reaction. CONTRAINDICATIONS: Patients receiving large doses of heparin or with severe leukopenia/neutropenia METHODOLOGY: Blood cells are ruptured by a variety of methods – glass beads are commonly used. Nuclear material is thereby released to interact with any antibody that may be present. One hour incubation at 37°C allows time for interaction of nuclear material and antibody and for the altered nuclear material to be phagocytosed (a complement dependent process). Buffy coat smears are prepared, stained, and studied for presence of phagocytosed homogenous lavender staining material. Presence of extracellular LE material or formation of rosettes does not add specific diagnostic information. ADDITIONAL INFORMATION: SLE is a disease of protean clinical manifestations commonly with rash, arthralgia, fever, anemia, leukopenia, thrombocytopenia, and hypocomplementemia, occurring especially in women. The LE slide cell test is relatively insensitive. It is positive in only 60% to 80% of acutely ill cases of LE. A negative LE slide cell test does not exclude the diagnosis of lupus erythematosus. The patient's serum should be studied for antinuclear antibody (ANA). The antibody may be of IgG, A, or M specificity but is most commonly of IgG class. A negative ANA test nearly excludes the diagnosis of LE (>95% sensitivity) if the patient is not being treated with corticosteroid or immunosuppressive drugs. Some drugs (in particular Dilantin®) may relate to lupus erythematosus and cause positive LE slide cell tests. Up to 25% of individuals taking Dilantin® (diphenylhydantoin) develop antinuclear antibodies. See table.

Drugs Capable of Inducing Lupus Syndromes Positive LE Slide Tests

Dilantin	Phenelzine sulfate
Ethosuximide	Phenylbutazone
Griseofulvin	Primidone
Hydralazine	Procainamide
Isoniazid	Propylthiouracil
Mesantoin	Reserpine
Methyldopa	Streptomycin
Methylthiouracil	Sulfonamides
Oral contraceptives	Tetracycline
Penicillin	Tridione

Footnotes

1. Tan EM, Robinson CA, and Nakamura RM, "ANAs in Systemic Rheumatic Disease: Diagnostic Significance," *Postgrad Med*, 1985, 78:141-2, 145-8.
2. Hidalgo C and Vladutin AO, "Lupus Erythematosus Cells in Serum and Pleural Fluid of a Patient With Negative Fluorescent Antinuclear Antibody Test," *Am J Clin Pathol*, 1987, 87:660-2.

References

Dacie JV and Lewis SM, "Demonstration of LE Cells," *Practical Haematology*, 7th ed, New York, NY: Churchill Livingstone, 1991, 530-2.

(Continued)

LE Cell Test *(Continued)*

Hargraves MM, "Discovery of the LE Cell and Its Morphology," *Mayo Clin Proc*, 1969, 44:579.

Hargraves MM, Richmond H, and Morton R, "Presentation of Two Bone Marrow Elements: The "Tart" Cell and the "LE" Cell," *Proc Staff Meet Mayo Clin*, 1948, 23:25.

Nakamura RM, Peebles CL, Rubin RL, et al, "Autoantibodies to Nuclear Antigens (ANA): Advances in Laboratory Tests and Significance in Systemic Rheumatic Disease" 1st ed, Chicago, IL: ASCP Press, 1985, 7-33.

Steinberg AD, Gourley MF, Klinman DM, et al, "NIH Conference. Systemic Lupus Erythematosus," *Ann Intern Med*, 1991, 115(7):548-59.

LE Prep *see* LE Cell Test *on previous page*

LE Preparation *see* LE Cell Test *on previous page*

LE Slide Cell Test *see* LE Cell Test *on previous page*

Leukemic Reticuloendotheliosis Test *see* Tartrate Resistant Leukocyte Acid Phosphatase *on page 603*

Leukocyte Acid Phosphatase *see* Tartrate Resistant Leukocyte Acid Phosphatase *on page 603*

Leukocyte Alkaline Phosphatase

CPT 85540

Related Information

Breakpoint Cluster Region Rearrangement in CML *on page 895*
Leukocyte Cytochemistry *on next page*
White Blood Count *on page 616*

Synonyms LAP; LAP Score; LAP Smear

Abstract A cytochemical reaction useful in differential diagnosis of myeloproliferative diseases, in particular, distinguishing leukemoid reaction from leukemia.

Specimen Whole blood **CONTAINER:** Slides with smears of blood **COLLECTION:** Make six smears on long slides from fingerstick blood. Air dry the slides. Transport to Hematology immediately, (ie, within 30 minutes). **STORAGE INSTRUCTIONS:** Slides must be fixed with cold 10% formalin methanol or citrated buffered acetone, rinsed, air dried, and frozen within 8 hours (preferably within 30 minutes) after obtaining the blood. After fixation, smears can be stored for up to 8 weeks before staining. **CAUSES FOR REJECTION:** Blood collected in EDTA anticoagulant, transit time to the laboratory in excess of 30 minutes, neutrophil count $<1000/mm^3$ in peripheral blood

Interpretive **REFERENCE RANGE:** 11-95 **USE:** Aid in the differential diagnosis of chronic granulocytic leukemia versus leukemoid reaction; aid in the evaluation of polycythemia and myelofibrosis **LIMITATIONS:** Pregnancy, increased number of immature forms of neutrophils, and postoperative or "stressful" states are associated with increased scores. The differential must have adequate numbers of mature neutrophilic granulocytes to perform the LAP. **METHODOLOGY:** Enzyme reaction with leukocyte alkaline phosphatase liberating naphthol or a substituted naphthol compound which then couples with fast blue RR or other chromogen to form an insoluble precipitate. Color of the precipitate relates to the type of substituted naphthol substrate and diazonium dye used (color is reagent dependent). Cells are scored as to the degree of phosphatase activity present, 0 to 4+. One hundred cells are counted and the score totaled. **ADDITIONAL INFORMATION:** Low scores have been associated with CML, PNH, thrombocytopenic purpura, and hereditary hypophosphatasia. In CML regardless of the total white count, the score remains low. In CML, it has been demonstrated that the mRNA for leukocyte alkaline phosphatase by Northern blotting is undetectable.[1] This suggests either rapid degradation of the message or no transcription of the LAP gene. In nonleukemic neutrophilia, the LAP rises as the WBC rises. High scores have been seen in polycythemia vera, myelofibrosis, aplastic anemia, mongolism, hairy cell leukemia, leukemoid reactions, and neutrophilia either physiological or secondary to infection. It is also increased in Hodgkin's disease. Serial LAP activity can be a useful adjunct in evaluating the activity of Hodgkin's disease as well as its response to therapy. Increase in LAP does not occur in cases of sickle cell crisis, possibly due to zinc deficiency (leukocyte alkaline phosphatase is a zinc metalloenzyme) but more likely relating to a mild defect in the hypothalamic-pituitary-adrenal axis with decreased plasma cortisol response in patients in sickle cell crisis.[2]

Footnotes

1. Rambaldi A, Terao M, Bettoni S, et al, "Differences in the Expression of Alkaline Phosphatase mRNA in Chronic Myelogenous Leukemia and Paroxysmal Nocturnal Hemoglobinuria Polymorphonuclear Leukocytes," *Blood*, 1989, 73(5):1113-5.
2. Rosenbloom BE, Odell WD, and Tanaka KR, "Pituitary-Adrenal Axis Function in Sickle Cell Anemia and Its Relationship to Leukocyte Alkaline Phosphatase," *Am J Hematol*, 1980, 9:373-9.

References

Catovsky D, "Leukocyte Cytochemical and Immunological Techniques," *Practical Haematology*, 7th ed, Chapter 10, Dacie JV and Lewis SM, eds, New York, NY: Churchill Livingstone, 1991, 125-55.

Cline MJ, "Laboratory Evaluation of Benign Quantitative Granulocyte and Monocyte Disorders," *Hematology: Clinical and Laboratory Practice*, Vol 2, Chapter 75, Bick RL, ed, St Louis, MO: Mosby-Year Book Inc, 1993, 1155-60.

Kaplow LS, "Cytochemistry of Leukocyte Alkaline Phosphatase: Use of Complex Naphthol AS Phosphates in Azo Dye-Coupling Technics," *Am J Clin Pathol*, 1963, 39:439-49.

Leukocyte Count *see* White Blood Count *on page 616*

Leukocyte Cytochemistry

***CPT** 88313 (each stain)*

Related Information

Bone Marrow *on page 524*
Breakpoint Cluster Region Rearrangement in CML *on page 895*
Leukocyte Alkaline Phosphatase *on previous page*
Muramidase, Blood and Urine *on page 571*
Peripheral Blood: Differential Leukocyte Count *on page 576*
Tartrate Resistant Leukocyte Acid Phosphatase *on page 603*
White Blood Count *on page 616*

Synonyms Cytochemistry, Leukocyte

Applies to Acid-Fast, Ziehl-Neelsen, Stain for Intracellular Pigment; Acid Phosphatase Stain With and Without Tartrate; Alpha-Naphthyl Esterase Stain With and Without Fluoride; Amyloid; ASD Chloroacetate Esterase Stain; Beta-Glucuronidase Stain; Methenamine Silver; Methyl Green-Pyronine; Nonspecific Esterase; Oil Red O Stain; PAS Stain; Peroxidase Stain; Sudan Black Stain

Test Commonly Includes Any of the above stains indicated by examination of routinely stained preparations or specific request

Abstract Cytochemical reactions useful in differential diagnosis, in particular, in the study and characterization of acute leukemia.

Specimen Blood or bone marrow smears, imprints or smears of cell suspensions **CONTAINER:** Green top (heparin) tube **COLLECTION:** Smears are prepared at the patient's bedside. **STORAGE INSTRUCTIONS:** Transport specimen to the laboratory immediately.

Interpretive **REFERENCE RANGE:** Interpretation and significance usually requires correlation with other cytologic and cytochemical aspects of the specific case. **USE:** Cytochemically evaluate neoplasms and abnormal cells in bone marrow, peripheral blood, or other specimens such as imprints; detect amyloidosis; classify leukemias and plasma cell dyscrasias; evaluate myeloproliferative/lymphoproliferative disorders **ADDITIONAL INFORMATION:** See also test listing Tartrate Resistant Leukocyte Acid Phosphatase, for hairy cell leukemia. In the technique of Yam et al for esterase reactions, a single slide preparation is consecutively stained for two different enzyme activities.[1] The nonspecific esterase (α-naphthyl acetate substrate – black granulation) is monocyte specific, while the chloroacetate esterase (naphthol ASD chloroacetate – red granulation) is granulocyte specific.[1] These reactions should be helpful in some cases in distinguishing acute granulocytic from acute monocytic leukemia and are of value in distinguishing acute myelomonocytic leukemia from acute granulocytic leukemia and acute monocytic leukemia (Schilling type). In acute myelomonocytic leukemia, both granulocytic and monocytic markers are present simultaneously in the leukemic cells. Nonspecific esterase activity inhibited by fluoride has been described in red cell precursors – including megaloblasts in cases of untreated pernicious anemia, megaloblastoid rubricytes in cases of DiGuglielmo syndrome, and rubricytes in cases of severe untreated iron deficiency. Rubricytes from normal marrow lack nonspecific esterase activity.[2] By use of high resolution isoelectric focusing in polyacrylamide gel, isoenzymes of nonspecific esterases extracted from leukemic blasts can be visualized. For each type of leukemic blast (ie, lymphoblast, myeloblast, and monoblast), a consistent and distinctive pattern of nonspecific esterase ac-

(Continued)

Leukocyte Cytochemistry *(Continued)*

tivity has been reported.[3] Isoenzyme fractions of acid phosphatases and nonspecific esterases appear to be unique for lymphoblasts, myeloblasts, and immature or leukemic monocytes. The fluoride inhibited nonspecific esterase reaction indicates monocytic origin and is unusual in T- lymphocyte cell malignancy. The laboratory may be unable to perform the peroxidase reaction as this test utilizes a chemical, benzidine, which has been shown to be carcinogenic. Alternate methods are available.[4] The following table lists cytochemical reactions for leukemias. A current study was designed to assess the value of PAS (periodic acid-Schiff) stain in delineating lymphoblastic and myeloblastic leukemia. It was concluded that a positive PAS reaction combined with negative myeloperoxidase, Sudan black B, and alpha-naphthyl butyrate esterase results continues to have a diagnostic role in differentiating lymphoblastic and myeloblastic leukemia.[5] Another study showed that PAS and iron stain together or PAS and double esterase together was helpful in excluding a diagnosis of myelodysplastic syndrome.[6] Flow cytochemistry study has been applied to the differentiation of acute leukemias.[7]

Cytochemical Reactions in Normal Blood Cells and Blast Cells of Acute Leukemias

	Peroxidase Sudan Black B	α-Naphthyl Acetate	α-Naphthyl Butyrate	Naphthol-AS-D Chloroacetate	PAS	Acid Phosphatase
Promyelocyte	+/++	—/±	—	+/++	± /+	+/++
Neutrophil	++	—/±	—	+/++	+++	+
Monocyte	—/±	+++	++/+++	—/±	±	++
Lymphocyte	—	—/±[a]	—/±[a]	—	—/+	—/++
Erythroblast	—	—/±[b]	—	—	—	±/—
Megakaryocyte	—	+++	±	—	++	++
ALL	—	—/+[c]	—	—	+/++[d]	—/+[c]
AML(M1)	+	—	—	+	+	—
AML(M2)	++	—/+	—/+	++	+	+
APL(M3)	+++	—/++	—	+++	± /++	++
AMML(M4)	++	++/+++	++	++	—/++	++
AMoL(M5)	—/±	+++	+++	—/±	++	+
EL(M6)	—	++	+	—	++	—
MegL(M7)	—	+	—/±	—	++	+
AUL	—	—	—	—	—	—

From Williams WJ, Beutler E, Erslev AJ, et al, eds, *Hematology,* 4th ed, New York, NY: McGraw-Hill Inc, 1990, 1745-53, with permission.
— = negative
± = weak or few positive cells
\+ = moderate
++ = moderately strong
+++ = strongly positive (most cells)
ALL = acute lymphocytic leukemia
AML(M1) = acute myeloblastic leukemia
AML(M2) = acute myeloblastic leukemia with maturation
APL(M3) = acute promyelocytic leukemia
AMML(M4) = acute myelomonocytic leukemia
AMoL(M5) = acute monocytic leukemia
EL(M6) = acute erythroleukemia
MegL(M7) = acute megakaryocytic leukemia
AUL = acute undifferentiated leukemia
[a]Positivity is focal, not diffuse.
[b]In erythroleukemia and in some erythroid maturation defects, positivity is strong.
[c]Focal cytoplasmic positivity in a small proportion of ALL.
[d]Coarse blocks are typical.

Note: In M1 through M5, the cytochemical reactions for the esterases apply to all the mononuclear nonerythroid, nonlymphocytic cells. In M6, the cytochemical reactions in the table apply to the erythroblasts. Myeloblasts are also present and are likely to be Sudan black B- or peroxidase-positive.

Footnotes

1. Yam LT, Li CY, Crosby WH, et al, "Cytochemical Identification of Monocytes and Granulocytes," *Am J Clin Pathol*, 1971, 55:283-90.
2. Kass L and Peters CL, "Nonspecific Esterase Activity in Pernicious Anemia and Chronic Erythremic Myelosis: A Cytochemical and Electrophoretic Study," *Am J Clin Pathol*, 1977, 68:273-5.

3. Tavassoli M, Shaklai M, and Crosby WH, "Cytochemical Diagnosis of Acute Myelomonocytic Leukemia," *Am J Clin Pathol*, 1979, 72:59-62.
4. Hanker JS, Yates PE, Metz CB, et al, "A New Specific, Sensitive and Noncarcinogenic Reagent for the Demonstration of Horseradish Peroxidase," *Histochem J*, 1977, 9:789-92, (letter).
5. Snower DP, Smith BR, Munz UJ, et al, "Re-Evaluation of the Periodic Acid-Schiff Stain in Acute Leukemia With Immunophenotypic Analyses," *Arch Pathol Lab Med*, 1991, 115(4):346-50.
6. Seo IS, Li CY, and Yam LT, "Myelodysplastic Syndrome: Diagnostic Implications of Cytochemical and Immunocytochemical Studies," *Mayo Clin Proc*, 1993, 68(1):47-53.
7. Tsakona CP, Kinsey SE, and Goldstone AH, "Use of Flow Cytochemistry Via the H*1 in FAB Identification of Acute Leukaemias," *Acta Haematol*, 1992, 88(2-3):72-7.

References

Goasguen J and Bennett JM, "The Acute Myeloid Leukemias: Morphology and Cytochemistry," (including Appendix of Methods), *Hematology: Clinical and Laboratory Practice*, Vol 2, Chapter 77, Bick RL, ed, St Louis, MO: Mosby-Year Book Inc, 1993, 1195-216.

Kass L and Elias JM, "Cytochemical and Immunocytochemistry in Bone Marrow Examination: Contemporary Techniques for the Diagnosis of Acute Leukemia and Myelodysplastic Syndrome," *Hematology/Oncology Clinics of N America*, Philadelphia, PA: WB Saunders Co, 1988.

Li CY and Yam LT, "Cytochemical Characterization of Leukemic Cells With Numerous Cytoplasmic Granules," *Mayo Clin Proc*, 1987, 62:978-85.

Williams WJ, Beutler E, Erslev AJ, et al, *Hematology*, 4th ed, New York, NY: McGraw-Hill Inc, 1990, 1745-53.

Lupus Test *see* LE Cell Test *on page 565*

Lysosomal Storage Diseases *see* Tests for Uncommon Inherited Diseases of Metabolism and Cell Structure *on page 605*

Lysozyme, Blood *see* Muramidase, Blood and Urine *on page 571*

Lysozyme, Urine *see* Muramidase, Blood and Urine *on page 571*

Malarial Parasites *see* Malaria Smear *on this page*

Malaria Smear

***CPT** 87207*

See Also Anemia Flowchart in the Hematology Appendix

Related Information

Parasite Antibodies *on page 729*

Peripheral Blood: Red Blood Cell Morphology *on page 584*

Synonyms Blood Smear for Malarial Parasites; Malarial Parasites

Test Commonly Includes Examination of thick and thin smears

Abstract Malaria is still the most common infectious disease in the world. Its rapid diagnosis in the laboratory is extremely important. Although there are not many cases in the United States, with more world travel, it can be expected to increase.

Specimen Fresh blood – fresh fingerstick smears (two or three of each thick and thin film type) made at bedside preferred, EDTA anticoagulated blood for saponin lysis.[1] To make a thick film smear, spread a drop of blood centrally placed on a slide into a square about four times area of original drop. Spreading is conveniently achieved with the corner of another slide. Ideally, blood should be thinned until small newsprint is just visible.[2] **CONTAINER:** Slides and lavender top (EDTA) tube **COLLECTION:** Specimen should be drawn immediately before a fever spike is anticipated. **CAUSES FOR REJECTION:** Specimen clotted **SPECIAL INSTRUCTIONS:** If the patient has traveled to a malaria endemic area the date and area traveled should be specified on the requisition. Most cases of malaria seen in the U.S. are found in foreign nationals traveling in the United States.[3]

Malaria Species Infecting Human Red Cells

Plasmodium Species	Malaria	Length of Cycle (hours)
P. vivax	Tertian	45
P. falciparum	Malignant tertian	48
P. ovale	Ovale	48
P. malariae	Quartan	72

Interpretive **REFERENCE RANGE:** No organisms identified **USE:** Diagnose malaria, parasitic infestation of blood; evaluate febrile disease of unknown origin **LIMITATIONS:** One negative result does not rule out the possibility of parasitic infestation. If protozoal, filarial, or trypanosomal infection is strongly suspected, test should be performed at least three times with samples obtained at different times in the fever cycle. **METHODOLOGY:** Microscopic exam-

(Continued)

Malaria Smear *(Continued)*

Changes in Infected RBCs Useful in Identification of Malaria Species

Plasmodium Species	Infected RBC Enlarged	Presence of Schffner Dots	Presence of Maurer Dots	Multiple Parasites per RBC	Parasite With Double Chromatin Dots	Parasite With Sausage-Shaped Gametocytes
P. vivax	+	+	—	Rare	Rare	—
P. falciparum	—	—	+	+	+	+
P. ovale	±	+	—	—	—	—
P. malariae	—	—	+	—	—	—

ination of thick and thin peripheral blood Romanovsky dye (in particular Giemsa) stained smears. Thick films are more difficult to interpret but greatly increase sensitivity (by concentrating cells and organisms). Thick smears require considerable experience with malaria. They increase the number of cells examined in a given time period by a factor of about 12.[2] Screening for malaria can also be accomplished by fluorescent microscopy using acridine orange or benzothiocarboxypurine.[4,5,6,7] These methods are sensitive and can provide consistent results without the need for highly experienced observers. DNA hybridization probes for detection of malaria have been described,[8,9] but in one study, sensitivity was not comparable to that obtained with use of thick films.[9] Thin smears, although not as sensitive, are far superior for determining the species of *Plasmodium* on morphological grounds.[10] **ADDITIONAL INFORMATION:** Proper therapy depends upon identification of the specific variety of malaria parasite. Release of trophozoites and RBC debris results in a febrile response. Periodicity of fever correlates with type of malaria (see table). Organisms are most likely to be detected just before onset of fever which is predictable in many cases. Sampling immediately upon onset of fever is the most desirable time to obtain blood. Alternatively in cases negative by these means but with a strong clinical history, multiple sampling at different times in the fever cycle may prove successful. Malarial parasites are destroyed in AS and SS patients. The cause of parasite death in AS cells is potassium loss, in SS cells Hb S aggregates destroy the parasites by physical penetration.[11]

Footnotes

1. Keffer JH, "Malarial Parasites. Concentration by Saponin Hemolysis," *Tech Bull Regist Med Technol*, 1966, 36:153-5.
2. Dacie JV and Lewis SM, *Practical Haematology*, 7th ed, New York, NY: Churchill Livingstone, 1991, 80-1.
3. Gordon S, Brennessel DJ, Goldstein JA, et al, "Malaria: A City Hospital Experience," *Arch Intern Med*, 1988, 148(7):1569-71.
4. Jahanmehr SAH, Hyde K, Geary CG, et al, "Simple Technique for Fluorescence Staining of Blood Cells With Acridine Orange," *J Clin Pathol*, 1987, 40:926-9.
5. Rickman LS, Long GW, Oberst R, et al, "Rapid Diagnosis of Malaria by Acridine Orange Staining of Centrifuged Parasites," *Lancet*, 1989, 1(8629):68-71.
6. Long GW, Jones TR, Rickman LS, et al, "Acridine Orange Detection of *Plasmodium falciparum* Malaria: Relationship Between Sensitivity and Optical Configuration," *Am J Trop Med Hyg*, 1991, 44(4):402-5.
7. Makler MT, Ries LK, Ries J, et al, "Detection of *Plasmodium falciparum* Infection With the Fluorescent Dye, Benzothiocarboxypurine," *Am J Trop Med Hyg*, 1991, 44(1):11-6.
8. Barker RH Jr, Suebsaeng L, Rooney W, et al, "Detection of *Plasmodium falciparum* Infection in Human Patients: A Comparison of the DNA Probe Method to Microscopic Diagnosis," *Am J Trop Med Hyg*, 1989, 41(3):266-72.
9. Lanar DE, McLaughlin GL, Wirth DF, et al, "Comparison of Thick Films, *In Vitro* Culture and DNA Hybridization Probes for Detecting *Plasmodium falciparum* Malaria," *Am J Trop Med Hyg*, 1989, 40(1):3-6.
10. Pammenter MD, "Techniques for the Diagnosis of Malaria," *S Afr Med J*, 1988, 74:55-7.
11. Friedman MJ and Trager W, "The Biochemistry of Resistance to Malaria," *Sci Am*, 1981, 244:154-5, 158-64.

References

Henry JB, Nelson DA, Tomar RH, et al, *Clinical Diagnosis and Management by Laboratory Methods*, 18th ed, Philadelphia, PA: WB Saunders Co, 1991, 1168-72.

Makler MT and Gibbins B, "Laboratory Diagnosis of Malaria," *Clin Lab Med*, 1991, 11(4):941-56.

Marrow Iron Stores *see* Iron Stain, Bone Marrow *on page 562*

MCHC (Mean Corpuscular Hemoglobin Concentration) MCH (Mean Corpuscular Hemoglobin) *see* Red Blood Cell Indices *on page 592*

MCV (Mean Corpuscular Volume) *see* Red Blood Cell Indices *on page 592*

Methenamine Silver *see* Leukocyte Cytochemistry *on page 567*

Methyl Green-Pyronine *see* Leukocyte Cytochemistry *on page 567*

Methylmalonic Acid *see* Vitamin B_{12} *on page 612*

Methyl Violet Stain for Heinz Bodies *see* Heinz Body Stain *on page 551*

Microbuffy Coat Method for Detection of Bacteremia *see* Bacteremia Detection, Buffy Coat Micromethod *on page 520*

Microfilariae, Peripheral Blood Preparation

CPT *87207*

Related Information

Bacteremia Detection, Buffy Coat Micromethod *on page 520*
Filariasis Serological Test *on page 679*
Peripheral Blood: Red Blood Cell Morphology *on page 584*

Synonyms Blood Smear for Trypanosomal/Filarial Parasites; Filariasis Peripheral Blood Preparation; Helminths, Blood; Trypanosomiasis, Peripheral Blood Preparation

Applies to Filarial Infestation; Hemoflagellates

Test Commonly Includes Examination of both thick and thin smears, wet preparation

Specimen Fresh blood from fingerstick **CONTAINER:** Slides **COLLECTION:** Recommended procedure is for specimen to be obtained when patient spikes a fever. Optimal yield results from examination of a daytime specimen (ie, noon), and a night time specimen (ie, midnight). Timing of sampling relates to geographic place of exposure. **CAUSES FOR REJECTION:** Specimen clotted **SPECIAL INSTRUCTIONS:** If patient has traveled to an endemic area, the date of travel, the area, and the parasite suspected should be specified.

Interpretive **REFERENCE RANGE:** No parasites identified **USE:** Diagnose trypanosomiasis or microfilariasis; work up of elephantiasis, parasitic infestation of blood **LIMITATIONS:** One negative result does not rule out the possibility of parasitic infestation. Since some species of blood parasites can be found during the day and others are nocturnal, both day and night specimens enhance identification. Most filariae generate microfilariae which can be found in peripheral blood, but *Onchocerca volvulus* and *Dipetalonema streptocerca* give rise to microfilariae which do not circulate. **METHODOLOGY:** Fresh wet blood film, with a coverslip, in which motile microfilariae cause agitation of adjacent red cells. Stained films are used as well. **ADDITIONAL INFORMATION:** Biopsy of skin and subcutaneous mass is used in diagnosis of *D. streptocerca* and *O. volvulus.* Differential diagnosis of species of circulating microfilariae requires distinction between the presence or absence of a sheath, the pattern of nuclei in the tail and sometimes the history of geographic exposure and time of sampling.

References

Garcia LS, "Laboratory Methods for Diagnosis of Parasitic Infections," *Bailey and Scott's Diagnostic Microbiology*, Chapter 44, Finegold SM and Baron EJ, eds, St Louis, MO: Mosby-Year Book Inc, 1986, 838-42, 854-6.

Microhematocrit *see* Hematocrit *on page 552*

Morphology *see* Peripheral Blood: Red Blood Cell Morphology *on page 584*

MPV *see* Platelet Sizing *on page 588*

Mucopolysaccharidoses *see* Tests for Uncommon Inherited Diseases of Metabolism and Cell Structure *on page 605*

Muramidase, Blood and Urine

CPT *85549*

Related Information

Eosinophil Count *on page 539*
Leukocyte Cytochemistry *on page 567*
Lymph Node Biopsy *on page 72*

Synonyms Lysozyme, Blood; Lysozyme, Urine

Specimen Serum, 24-hour urine **CONTAINER:** Red top tube; EDTA plasma (lavender top tube)

(Continued)

Muramidase, Blood and Urine *(Continued)*

may also be used; 24-hour urine container **COLLECTION:** Collect urine for 24-hour period on ice, no preservative. **STORAGE INSTRUCTIONS:** Separate serum and freeze **immediately** in plastic vial on dry ice. Upon receipt of urine specimen, freeze on dry ice **immediately** in plastic vial.

Interpretive **REFERENCE RANGE:** Serum: 4.0-15.6 μg/mL (0.28-1.10 μmol/L); urine: 0-1.4 μg/mL (0-0.097 μmol/L)[1] **USE:** Differential diagnosis of leukemia; present in association with some cases of myelogenous and most cases of monocytic leukemia **METHODOLOGY:** Turbidimetric, immunochemical (nephelometry), enzymatic - colorimetric, radioimmunoassay (RIA), agarose gel diffusion (recommended method)[1] **ADDITIONAL INFORMATION:** Lysozyme when present in large amounts, may appear as a far cathodal migrating ("cationic") band occasionally on serum or urine protein electrophoresis. It is elevated in some cases of myelogenous, and most cases of myelomonocytic and monocytic leukemia. Lysozyme has been found within the granules of normal and leukemic eosinophils by immunoelectron microscopic study. Elevated serum lysozyme may not establish presence of monocytic differentiation in cases of acute myelogenous leukemia with eosinophilia.[3] The level of serum lysozyme has been used as a predictor of CNS involvement in these leukemias.[2] Serum lysozyme has been shown to be elevated in a number of conditions, including tuberculosis and sarcoidosis as well as leukemia, and it is markedly elevated in sarcoid lymph nodes.[4]

Footnotes

1. Schultz AL, "Lysozyme," *Methods in Clinical Chemistry*, Chapter 95, Pesce AJ and Kaplan LA, eds, St Louis, MO: Mosby-Year Bood Inc, 1987, 742-6.
2. Peterson BA, Brunning RD, Bloomfield CD, et al, "Central Nervous System Involvement in Acute Nonlymphocytic Leukemia," *Am J Med*, 1987, 83:464-70.
3. Moscinski LC, Kasnic G Jr, and Saker A Jr, "The Significance of an Elevated Serum Lysozyme Value in Acute Myelogenous Leukemia With Eosinophilia," *Am J Clin Pathol*, 1992, 97(2):195-201.
4. Silverstein E, Friedland J, and Ackerman T, "Elevation of Granulomatous Lymph-Node and Serum Lysozyme in Sarcoidosis and Correlation With Angiotensin-Converting Enzyme," *Am J Clin Pathol*, 1977, 68:219-24.

References

Williams WJ, Beutler E, Erslev AJ, et al, *Hematology*, 4th ed, New York, NY: McGraw-Hill Inc, 1990, 1761-2.

Zucker S, Hanes DJ, Vogler WR, et al, "Plasma Muramidase: A Study of Methods and Clinical Applications," *J Lab Clin Med*, 1970, 75:83-92.

Murayama Test *see* Sickle Cell Tests *on page 600*

Nasal Smear for Eosinophils *see* Eosinophil Smear *on page 541*

NBT Test *see* Nitroblue Tetrazolium Test *on this page*

Neutral β-Galactosidase *see* Tests for Uncommon Inherited Diseases of Metabolism and Cell Structure *on page 605*

Nitroblue Tetrazolium Test

CPT 86384

Synonyms NBT Test; Tetrazolium Reduction Test

Abstract NBT test is used mainly for the diagnosis of chronic granulomatous disease (CGD), an X-linked inherited disease, characterized by disabled phagocyte NADPH oxidase with inability to efficiently kill phagocytized bacteria.

Specimen Whole blood **CONTAINER:** Green top (heparin) tube **STORAGE INSTRUCTIONS:** Specimen cannot be stored (test utilizes live granulocytes). **CAUSES FOR REJECTION:** Transit to the laboratory of more than 1 hour, specimen clotted **SPECIAL INSTRUCTIONS:** Advance scheduling with the laboratory may be required as the specimen must be tested while the neutrophils are still viable. Transport to the laboratory **immediately** following collection.

Interpretive **REFERENCE RANGE:** 2% to 8% segmented neutrophils reduce dye **USE:** Diagnose chronic granulomatous disease (CGD) of childhood **LIMITATIONS:** Requires fresh blood for live white blood cells. **METHODOLOGY:** Assessment of reduction of a tetrazolium dye by stimulated and unstimulated neutrophils. Neutrophils reduce the dye to a dark blue-black formazan pigment upon phagocytosis. **ADDITIONAL INFORMATION:** Usually a reliable aid in the diagnosis of CGD in which neutrophils are unable to reduce the dye (which correlates with their inability to kill bacteria). In patients with CGD, the NADPH oxidase system fails to generate superoxide and related oxygen intermediates with resultant susceptibility to recurrent bacterial and fungal infections. The NBT test is unreliable in the differentiation of bacterial from viral and other infections, producing unacceptable false-negative and false-positive results. Forty-three nonbacterial infections and other clinical states have been associated with false-positive NBT tests.[1] There are also reports of bacterial infections accompanied by false-negative results. One study suggests that peripheral segmented neutrophils from patients with solid cancer (nonlymphomatous tumors) have decreased capacity to reduce NBT dye to formazan when maximally stimulated with endotoxin.[2] NBT reduction in lymphoma patients was comparable to that of controls. It was also found that stimulated NBT reduction apparently declines with age.[2] Chronic granulomatous disease can now be diagnosed using restriction fragment length polymorphism with labeled gene probes.[3] The abnormal gene located on the short arm of the X chromosome codes for cytochrome b558.[4] The CGD may result from genetic defects in at least four different components of the multicomponent NADPH oxidase system.[5]

Treatment of CGD patients with recombinant interferon-γ has been shown to result in a near-normal level of superoxide production and return of granulocyte bactericidal capacity to normal control levels. Interferon-γ stimulates progenitor cells and their mature progeny. Colonies of such cells regain the ability to generate superoxide.[5]

Footnotes

1. Lace JV, Tan JS, and Watanakunakorn C, "An Appraisal of the Nitroblue Tetrazolium Reduction Test," *Am J Med*, 1975, 58:685-94.
2. Haim N, Obedeanu N, Meshulam T, et al, "Comparative Study of the Endotoxin-Stimulated Nitroblue Tetrazolium Test in Disease and Health," *J Clin Pathol*, 1978, 31:1249-52.
3. Antonarakis SE, "Diagnosis of Genetic Disorders at the DNA Level," *N Engl J Med*, 1989, 320(3):153-63.
4. Francke U, Ochs HD, Darras BT, et al, "Origin of Mutations in Two Families With X-Linked Chronic Granulomatous Disease," *Blood*, 1990, 76(3):602-6.
5. Ezekowitz RAB, "Chronic Granulomatous Disease: An Update and a Paradigm for the Use of Interferon-γ as Adjunct Immunotherapy in Infectious Diseases," *Curr Top Microbiol Immunol*, 1992, 181:283-92.

References

Babior BM and Woodman RC, "Chronic Granulomatous Disease," *Semin Hematol*, 1990, 27(3):247-59.

Forrest CB, Forehand JR, Axtell RA, et al, "Clinical Features and Current Management of Chronic Granulomatous Disease," *Hematol Oncol Clin North Am*, 1988, 2:253-63.

Quie PG, "Chronic Granulomatous Disease of Childhood: A Saga of Discovery and Understanding," *Pediatr Infect Dis J*, 1993, 12(5):395-8.

Smith RM and Curnutte JT, "Molecular Basis of Chronic Granulomatous Disease," *Blood*, 1991, 77(4):673-86.

Van der Valk P and Herman CJ, "Biology of Disease: Leukocyte Function," *Lab Invest*, 1987, 57:127-37.

Nonspecific Esterase *see* Leukocyte Cytochemistry *on page 567*

Oil Red O Stain *see* Leukocyte Cytochemistry *on page 567*

Osmotic Fragility

***CPT** 85555*

Related Information

Autohemolysis Test *on page 519*
Osmotic Fragility, Incubated *on page 575*
Peripheral Blood: Red Blood Cell Morphology *on page 584*
Reticulocyte Count *on page 597*

Synonyms Incubated Osmotic Fragility; RBC Fragility; Red Cell Fragility

Specimen Whole blood **CONTAINER:** Lavender top (EDTA) tube or green top (heparin) tube **STORAGE INSTRUCTIONS:** Store refrigerated (4°C) if test performance must be delayed. **CAUSES FOR REJECTION:** Hemolysis, clotted specimen, blood more than 6 hours old, oxalate or citrate anticoagulated blood collected **SPECIAL INSTRUCTIONS:** May need to schedule this test in advance.

Interpretive **REFERENCE RANGE:** Hemolysis begins 0.45%, hemolysis complete 0.35% **USE:** Evaluate hemolytic anemia, especially hereditary spherocytosis; evaluate immune hemolytic states **LIMITATIONS:** Any severe anemia including iron deficiency will yield an abnormal curve. Test measures presence of spherocytes and "spheroidal" cells. Test is **not** specific for hereditary spherocytosis. Trauma-free venipuncture is needed. **METHODOLOGY:** Erythrocytes are placed in graded dilutions of sodium chloride solution; swelling and hemolysis in the lower dilutions provide an index of the resistance of the cells to hypotonic saline. Percent hemolysis is determined using optical density measurements. A modification of osmotic fragility using glycerol and Bis-Tris, is purportedly more sensitive for the diagnosis of hereditary spherocytosis.[1] **ADDITIONAL INFORMATION:** Hereditary spherocytosis may be the result of an autosomal dominant transmitted defect in red cell structural proteins.[2] It is associated with a compensated or uncompensated hemolytic state which is relieved by splenectomy. Uncompensated

(Continued)

Osmotic Fragility *(Continued)*

Osmotic Fragility of Erythrocytes in Various Diseases

Disease	Initial Hemolysis (% saline ±1 SD)	Complete Hemolysis (% saline ±1 SD)	Remarks
Normal	0.44 ± 0.02	0.32 ± 0.02	
Hereditary spherocytosis	0.68 ± 0.14	0.46 ± 0.10	Abnormal in all cases; initial hemolysis may occur in 0.85% saline solution
Acquired hemolytic anemia	0.52 ± 0.04	0.42 ± 0.04	Abnormal in most cases; degree varies with severity
Hemolytic disease caused by ABO incompatibility	0.50 ± 0.02	0.40 ± 0.02	Abnormal in many cases; degree varies with severity
Hemolytic disease caused by Rh incompatibility	0.60 ± 0.06	0.40 ± 0.04	Abnormal in many cases; degree varies with severity
Hemolytic anemia caused by drugs	0.50 ± 0.04	0.40 ± 0.04	Abnormal in most cases during onset; may be normal in later stages
Hemolytic anemia caused by burns	0.50 ± 0.04	0.40 ± 0.04	Abnormal in about 50% of cases during first few days; usually normal after a few days
Pernicious anemia	0.48 ± 0.04	0.36 ± 0.02	Occasionally very abnormal; normal in most cases
Congenital nonspherocytic hemolytic anemia	0.44 ± 0.02	0.32 ± 0.02	Fragility may be increased after blood is incubated
Elliptocytosis, asymptomatic	0.44	0.32	
Elliptocytosis with hemolytic anemia	0.50	0.32	
Thalassemia	0.38 ± 0.04	0.20 ± 0.06	Complete hemolysis may not be achieved until salt concentration of 0.1% is reached
Sickle cell anemia	0.36 ± 0.02	0.20 ± 0.04	Abnormal in all cases
Sickle cell trait (S/A)	0.44 ± 0.04	0.32 ± 0.04	Always normal
Hb C disease	0.34	0.22	Abnormal in almost all cases
Erythremia	0.40 ± 0.02	0.28 ± 0.02	Not a constant finding
Iron deficiency anemia	0.38 ± 0.02	0.28 ± 0.02	Typical in severe anemia; not common otherwise
Obstructive jaundice (severe)	0.36 ± 0.02	0.28 ± 0.04	Decreased fragility usually noted in severely jaundiced patients

From Miale JB, *Laboratory Medicine: Hematology,* 6th ed, St Louis, MO: Mosby–Year Book Inc, 1982, 584, with permission.

forms of the disease (ie, with anemia) may be associated with reticulocytosis (usually mild to moderate) and mild elevation of serum indirect bilirubin. Patients are susceptible to pigment stones of the gallbladder and to aplastic marrow crises. Spherocytes are more susceptible than are normal red cells to hemolysis in dilute (hypotonic) saline. They show increased osmotic fragility. Spherocytes of any origin (including conditions other than hereditary spherocytosis, eg, autoimmune hemolytic anemia) will cause increased osmotic fragility. Generally, fully expanded cells (eg, spheroidal cells or spherocytes) have increased osmotic fragility while cells with higher surface area to volume ratios (eg, thin cells, hypochromic, target) have decreased osmotic fragility, including some cases of stomatocytosis.[3] The molecular pathology of spherocytosis and other red cell membrane structural protein defects has been partially established and described (see references). Most hereditary hemolytic anemias (including spherocytosis and elliptocytosis) involve mutations of membrane structural proteins, the majority code for abnormal spectrin molecules. Red cell protein 4.2 deficiency has been described. It has been reported recently in Japanese individuals who have related anemia and whose red cells show osmotic fragility.[4] Decreased osmotic fragility (resistance to lysis) may be seen with iron deficiency (hypochromic cell population), other hemoglobinopathies (especially hemoglobin C disease)[5] likely due to the target cell population, and is characteristic of thalassemia. Osmotic fragility is increased in cases of malaria infestation. Both infected and uninfected cells show the increased osmotic fragility. Both osmotic and mechanical fragility of RBCs in patients with multiple sclerosis has been reported as increased.[6] See table.

Footnotes

1. VeHore L, Zanella A, Molaro GL, et al, "A New Test for the Laboratory Diagnosis of Spherocytosis," *Acta Haematol*, 1984, 72:258-63.
2. Boivin P and Galand C, "Isoelectric Focusing of Spectrin Components in Hereditary Spherocytosis," *Clin Chim Acta*, 1976, 71:165-71.
3. McGrath KM, Collecutt MF, Gordon A, et al, "Dehydrated Hereditary Stomatocytosis – A Report of Two Families and A Review of the Literature," *Pathology*, 1984, 16:146-50.
4. Rybicki AC, Qiu JJ, Musto S, et al, "Human Erythrocyte Protein 4.2 Deficiency Associated With Hemolytic Anemia and a Homozygous ^{40}Glutamic Acid → Lysine Substitution in the Cytoplasmic Domain of Band 3 (Band $3^{\text{Montefiore}}$)," *Blood*, 1993, 81(8):2155-65.
5. Booth F and Mead SV, "Resistance to Lysis of Erythrocytes Containing Hemoglobin C – Detected in a Differential White Cell Counting System," *J Clin Pathol*, 1983, 36:816-8.
6. Schauf CL, Frischer H, and Davis FA, "Mechanical Fragility of Erythrocytes in Multiple Sclerosis," *Neurology*, 1980, 30:323-5.

References

Dacie JV and Lewis SM, *Practical Haematology*, 7th ed, New York, NY: Churchill Livingstone, 1991, 196-200.

DiPaolo BR, Speicher KD, and Speicher DW, "Identification of the Amino Acid Mutations Associated With Human Erythrocyte Spectrin αII Domain Polymorphisms," *Blood*, 1993, 82(1):284-91.

Henry JB, Nelson DA, Tomar RH, et al, *Clinical Diagnosis and Management by Laboratory Methods*, 18th ed, Philadelphia, PA: WB Saunders Co, 1991, 644-5.

Palek J, "Introduction: Red Blood Cell Membrane Proteins, Their Genes and Mutations," *Semin Hematol*, 1993, 30(1):1-3.

Peters LL and Lux SE, "Ankyrins: Structure and Function in Normal Cells and Hereditary Spherocytes," *Semin Hematol*, 1993, 30:85-118.

Winkelmann JC and Forget BG, "Erythroid and Nonerythroid Spectrins," *Blood*, 1993, 81(12):3173-85.

Osmotic Fragility, Incubated

***CPT** 85557*

Related Information

Autohemolysis Test *on page 519*

Osmotic Fragility *on previous page*

Synonyms RBC Fragility; Red Cell Fragility

Abstract The same as the previous test (osmotic fragility) except blood is incubated at 37°C for 24 hours. The test is mainly for diagnosis of hereditary spherocytosis.

Specimen Whole blood **CONTAINER:** Lavender top (EDTA) tube or green top (heparin) tube **COLLECTION:** Sterile technique must be used. **CAUSES FOR REJECTION:** Specimen hemolyzed, specimen clotted, improper anticoagulant (oxalate or citrate), improper venipuncture technique

Interpretive **USE:** Evaluate hemolytic anemia, particularly hereditary spherocytosis, congenital nonspherocytic hemolytic anemia, thalassemia **ADDITIONAL INFORMATION:** Incubation accentuates increased osmotic fragility. In cases of nonspherocytic hemolytic anemia, fragility may be normal in the unincubated osmotic fragility test but increased after incubation. See graph.

(Continued)

Osmotic Fragility, Incubated *(Continued)*

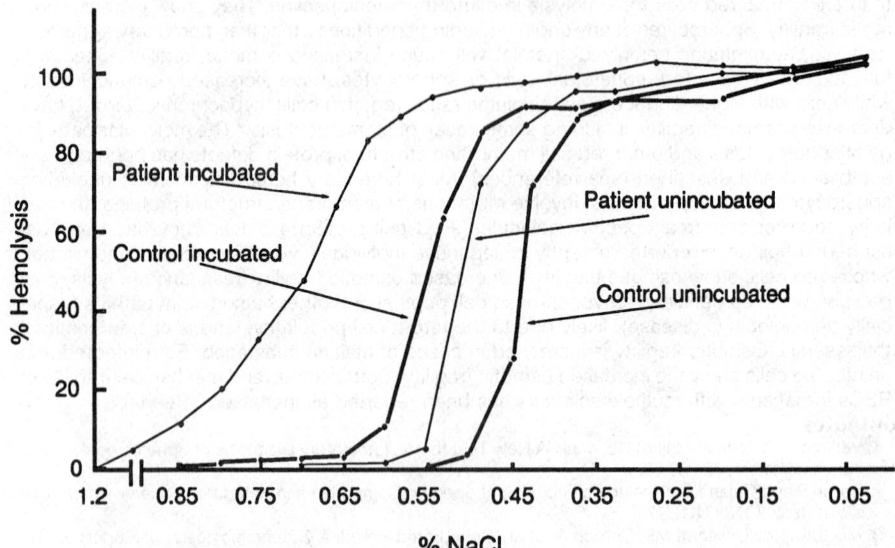

Osmotic fragility of unincubated and incubated RBCs from a normal individual and from a patient with hereditary sphercytosis. Note the increase in fragility produced by incubation of hereditary spherocytosis RBCs.

From Rapaport SI, *Introduction to Hematology*, 2nd ed, Philadelphia, PA: J.B. Lippincott Co., 1987, with permission.

References

Dacie JV and Lewis SM, *Practical Haematology*, 7th ed, New York, NY: Churchill Livingstone, 1991, 196-200.

Ovalocytes Smear *see* Peripheral Blood: Red Blood Cell Morphology *on page 584*

Packed Cell Volume *see* Hematocrit *on page 552*

Pappenheimer Body Stain *see* Siderocyte Stain *on page 602*

Paracentesis Fluid Analysis *see* Body Fluids Analysis, Cell Count *on page 523*

Paroxysmal Nocturnal Hemoglobinuria Test *see* Ham Test *on page 549*

PAS Stain *see* Leukocyte Cytochemistry *on page 567*

PCH Test *see* Cold Hemolysin Test *on page 532*

PCV *see* Hematocrit *on page 552*

PDW *see* Platelet Sizing *on page 588*

Pericardial Fluid Analysis *see* Body Fluids Analysis, Cell Count *on page 523*

Peripheral Blood: Differential Leukocyte Count

CPT 85007

Related Information

Bacteremia Detection, Buffy Coat Micromethod *on page 520*
Bone Marrow *on page 524*
Complete Blood Count *on page 533*
Eosinophil Count *on page 539*
Infectious Mononucleosis Screening Test *on page 713*

Leukocyte Cytochemistry *on page 567*
Lymph Node Biopsy *on page 72*
Lymphocyte Subset Enumeration *on page 720*
Peripheral Blood: Red Blood Cell Morphology *on page 584*
Platelet Count *on page 586*
White Blood Count *on page 616*

Synonyms Automated Differential; Differential; Differential Smear; Peripheral Differential; White Blood Cell Morphology

Test Commonly Includes Relative frequency (%) of the white blood cells, RBC morphology, platelet evaluation

Specimen Whole blood, fresh, anticoagulated (EDTA preferred). Heparin or oxalate may induce morphologic artifact in WBC. **CONTAINER:** Lavender top (EDTA) tube or smears prepared directly from fingerstick or heelstick blood. Heparin or oxalate may produce artifactual distortion especially of white blood cells.

Interpretive **REFERENCE RANGE:** See tables on following pages. **USE:** Determine qualitative and quantitative variations in white cell numbers and morphology, morphology of red cells and platelet evaluation; evaluate anemia, leukemia, infections, inflammatory states, and inherited disorders of red cells, white cells, and platelets **LIMITATIONS:** Because of sampling, large statistical variation exists, particularly with 100 cell count manual method and with low incidence cells. Day-to-day changes should be interpreted in relation to known method-related variation. **METHODOLOGY:** One or a combination of methods: manual enumeration of white cells on Wright's stained peripheral blood smear; computer image analysis (automated); continuous flow system (automated) using cytochemical/light scattering measurements; cell volume (impedance related/conductivity/light scattering) measurements; resultant electronic signals of combined methods are further manipulated with computer-assisted synthesis and derivations. See in particular, second and third references for details of how white blood cells (including eosinophils and basophils) are differentiated by different commercially available automated systems. **ADDITIONAL INFORMATION:** Significantly abnormal findings (automated or manual method) should be the subject of further study and review. Changes in leukocyte fractions are a window to a spectrum of minor to serious physiologic and pathologic changes. Some of these are tabulated in the following table and in tables in the Hematology Appendix.

The past decade has seen significant contributions to the definition of WBC differential reference values. The considerable increase in available data (as compared to that of the 1940-1970 period) cannot be summarized comprehensively in a simple manner. Variations, often not clinically significant, relate to differences in sex, race, physiologic state, and method of analysis. More significant variation is seen with age. A continuous flow cytochemical based automated analytic system determines immaturity of the neutrophilic granulocytic series on the basis of a peroxidase reaction. This is not directly comparable to identification of band (stab) population using morphologic criteria. Enumeration of band population is definition dependent. Automated differential determinations may vary between instruments and manual techniques but clinical significance of such differences may be minimal. Black individuals have lower neutrophil values than whites.[1] The greatest variation, both in relative and absolute terms occurs as the result of age. High WBC levels are present in the newborn and lymphocytes are increased in childhood (as compared to adult values). Both relative (%) and absolute (actual number of cells/mm^3) values need to be considered in relation to the clinical situation.

The overuse of the manual differential has become an important issue in times of cost containment[2] and technologist shortages. Current hematology instruments can produce automated differentials by cytochemistry/light scattering or cell volume/conductivity/light scattering ("VCS") techniques. Conductivity measurements utilize a high frequency electromagnetic probe. Leukocytes are separated into granulocytes, lymphocytes, monocytes, eosinophils, and basophil categories and an immaturity index (not exactly bands) of the granulocytes. With modern hematology instruments, manual differentials are probably overordered. High white counts[3,4] and fever are better indicators of clinical infection than the percentage of bands. This is because of the high variability of manual differential band counts from technologist to technologist. In the words of Shapiro et al, "The leukocyte differential is overused, only occasionally useful, and amenable to real cost reduction."[2] On the other hand, any particular patient (albeit uncommonly encountered) may present with very few but very significantly abnormal peripheral leukocytes (eg, blast cells of acute leukemia) allowing timely diagnosis not possible by other initial methods of evaluation. See also comments under Additional Information of Peripheral Blood: Red Blood Cell Morphology listing.

(Continued)

Differential Leukocyte Count

Age	Segmented Neutrophils (%)	Band Neutrophils (%)	Eosinophils (%)	Basophils (%)	Lymphocytes (%)	Monocytes (%)
Birth	47 ± 15	14.1 ± 4	2.2	0.6	31 ± 5	5.8
12 h	53	15.2	2.0	0.4	24	5.3
24 h	47	14.2	2.4	0.5	31	5.8
1 wk	34	11.8	4.1	0.4	41	9.1
2 wk	29	10.5	3.1	0.4	48	8.8
2 mo	25	8.4	2.7	0.5	57	5.9
6 mo	23	8.8	2.5	0.4	61	4.8
10 mo	22	8.3	2.5	0.4	63	4.6
2 y	25	8.0	2.6	0.5	59	5.0
6 y	43	8.0	2.7	0.6	42	4.7
10 y	46 ± 15	8.0 ± 3	2.4	0.5	38 ± 10	4.3
14 y	48	8.0	2.5	0.5	37	4.7
21 y	51 ± 15	8.0 ± 3	2.7	0.5	34 ± 10	4.0

From Miale JB, *Laboratory Medicine: Hematology,* 6th ed, St Louis, MO: Mosby-Year Book Inc, 1982, with permission.

Review of Peripheral Blood Smear

Red Cell Variant*†	Clinical Associations
Crenated cell (Echinocyte)	Variant form of normal RBC
Burr cell Schizocyte Helmet cell (Schizocyte)	DIC, I.V. fibrin deposition Microangiopathic hemolytic anemia Hypertension Cardiac valve disease Uremia, burns Metastatic malignancy Severe iron deficiency/bleeding lesion Normal newborn
Elliptocyte Ovalocyte (Elliptocyte)	Few seen normally Many may mean primary elliptocytosis Iron deficiency Thalassemia Hb S or C Other hemolytic anemias
Target cell (Codocyte)	Hemoglobinopathies (S, C, D, thalassemia, esp) Iron deficiency Liver disease LCAT deficiency
Oval macrocyte (Megalocyte)	Megaloblastic anemia B_{12}/folate deficiency Myeloproliferative disease Chemotherapy patients
Spherocyte (Spherocyte)	Hereditary spherocytosis Immune and other hemolytic states
Tear drop cell (Dacryocyte)	Myeloproliferative diseases Myelophthisic processes Pernicious anemia Thalassemia
Sickle cell (Drepanocyte)	Sickle cell disease and variants (ie, sickle/thalassemia, SD disease, SC disease
Acanthocyte (Acanthocyte)	Abetalipoproteinemia Alcoholic cirrhosis with hemolysis Pyruvate kinase deficiency Postheparin in some individuals[1]
Stomatocyte (Stomatocyte)	Hereditary stomatocytosis Alcoholism Rh *null* disease
Schistocyte Helmet cell Spurr cell (Schizocyte) (Keratocyte)	Microangiopathic hemolysis Cardiac valve disease DIC Severe burns Uremia
Triangulocytes[2]	Alcoholism Rarely, Hb C disease Thalassemia Nonalcohol liver disease TTP Antimitotic chemotherapy
Eccentrocytes[3] (Asymmetric distribution of Hgb)	G-6-PD deficiency

(Continued)

(continued)

Red Cell Variant*†	Clinical Associations
Bite cells[4,5] (Degmacyte)	Heinz body hemolytic anemia Oxidative hemolysis Methemoglobinemia due to phenazopyridine sulfanilamide Unstable hemoglobin (eg, Hb Koln) Thalassemia
Hemighosts[6]	Severe oxidative injury Heinz body hemolytic anemia Oxidative hemolysis
Polychromatophil Reticulocyte Nucleated RBC	Increased erythropoiesis Myelophthisic states Hemolytic states Postsplenectomy
Basophilic stippling (Punctate basophilis)	Lead poisoning Hemolytic states, other anemias Thalassemia Pyrimidine-5'-nucleotidase deficiency
Pappenheimer bodies (Siderocytes)	Some hemolytic anemias Postsplenectomy Some megaloblastic anemias Some sideroblastic states
Parasites	*Plasmodium* (malaria) *Bartonella* Microfilaria (not intracellular)
Rouleaux of RBCs	Reflects increased protein concentration May be associated with multiple myeloma Waldenstrom's macroglobulinemia blue staining background
Howell-Jolly bodies (Nuclear fragments)	Hemolytic anemia Hyposplenism/Asplenism (splenectomy) Megaloblastic anemia
Cabot Ring (Nuclear remnants)	Megaloblastic anemia
Heinz bodies (Denatured Hb)	Some drug sensitive oxidative hemolytic anemias Unstable hemoglobinopathies
WBC Abnormalities	**Clinical Associations**
Leukocytosis Increase % bands (left shift) Toxic granulation Toxic vacuolation	Acute reactive state metabolic basis infections (esp bacterial) basis
Döhle bodies	Acute infection, esp pneumonia scarlet fever measles septicemia May-Hegglin anomaly
Hypersegmented neutrophils	Megaloblastic states as pernicious anemia
Hypogranular neutrophils	Some cases of chronic myelogenous leukemia

(continued)

WBC Abnormalities	Clinical Associations
Auer rods (present in blast cells)	Acute myelogenous leukemia
Chediak/Higashi inclusions	Congenital deficiency Lysosomal membrane Phospholipid
Alder-Rielly anomaly	Mucopolysaccharidosis
Pelger-Huët anomaly (mono and bilobed neutrophils with clumped nuclear chromatin)	Congenital form Acquired form - associated with myelogenous leukemia
Platelet Abnormalities	**Clinical Associations**
Platelet satellitosis	No definite causal clinical association
Platelet clumping	May cause spurious leukocytosis and thrombocytopenia[7]

From Bessis M, *Blood Smears Reinterpreted,* New York, NY: Springer International, 1977, with permission.
From Bessis M, Weed RI, and Leblond PF, *Red Cell Shape: Physiology, Pathology, Ultrastructure,* New York, NY: Springer Verlag, 1973, with permission.

[1]Silber R, "Of Acanthocytes, Spurs, Burrs, and Membranes," *Blood,* 1969, 34:111.
[2]Schumacher HR, Khanna S, and Moyer B, "Letter: Triangulocytes in Alcoholism," *JAMA,* 1976, 235:2285-6.
[3]Ham TH, Grauel JA, Dunn RF, et al, "Physical Properties of Red Cells as Related to Effects *in Vivo.* IV. Oxidant Drugs Producing Abnormal Intracellular Concentration of Hemoglobin (Eccentrocytes) With a Rigid Red-Cell Hemolytic Syndrome," *J Lab Clin Med,* 1973, 82:898-910.
[4]Ward PC, Schwartz BS, and White JG, "Heinz Body Anemia: "Bite Cell" Variant — A Light and Electron Microscopic Study," *Am J Hematol,* 1983, 15:135-46.
[5]Greenberg MS, "Heinz Body Hemolytic Anemia: "Bite Cells" — A Clue to Diagnosis," *Arch Intern Med,* 1976, 136:153-5.
[6]Chan TK, Chan WC, and Weed RI, "Erythrocyte Hemighosts: A Hallmark of Severe Oxidative Injury *in Vivo," Br J Haematol,* 1982, 50:575.
[7]Solanki DL and Blackburn BC, "Spurious Leukocytosis and Thrombocytopenia. A Dual Phenomenon Caused by Clumping of Platelets *in Vitro," JAMA,* 1983, 250:2514-5.

*Established terminology is followed (parentheses) by that of Bessis M, et al, introduced on the basis of ultrastructural analyses.
†Some abnormal red cell forms may represent artifact introduced during preparation of the blood smear (esp stomatocytes and elliptocytes, occasionally target like cells).

(Continued)

Leukocyte Values From Birth to Maturity*

Age	Leukocyte count (x 10^3/mm^3)	Neutrophils			Eosinophils	Basophils	Lymphocytes	Monocytes
		Total	Band	Segmented				
At birth	18.1 (0.0–30.0)	11.0 (6.0–26.0) 61%	1.65 9.1%	9.4 52%	0.40 (0.02–0.85) 2.2%	0.10 (0–0.64) 0.6%	5.5 (2.0–11.0) 31%	1.05 (0.40–3.1) 5.8%
12 h	22.8 (13.0–38.0)	15.5 (6.0–28.0) 68%	2.33 10.2%	13.2 58%	0.45 (0.02–0.95) 2.0%	0.10 (0–0.50) 0.4%	5.5 (2.0–11.0) 24%	1.20 (0.40–3.6) 5.3%
24 h	18.9 (9.4–34.0)	11.5 (5.0–21.0) 61%	1.75 9.2%	9.8 52%	0.45 (0.05–1.00) 2.4%	0.10 (0–0.30) 0.5%	5.8 (2.0–11.5) 31%	1.10 (0.20–3.1) 5.8%
1 wk	12.2 (5.0–21.0)	5.5 (1.5–10.0) 45%	0.83 6.8%	4.7 39%	0.50 (0.07–1.10) 4.1%	0.05 (0–0.25) 0.4%	5.0 (2.0–17.0) 41%	1.10 (0.30–2.7) 9.1%
2 wk	11.4 (5.0–20.0)	4.5 (1.0–9.5) 40%	0.63 5.5%	3.9 34%	0.35 (0.07–1.00) 3.1%	0.05 (0–0.23) 0.4%	5.5 (2.0–17.0) 48%	1.00 (0.20–2.4) 8.8%
4 wk	10.8 (5.0–19.5)	3.8 (1.0–9.0) 35%	0.49 4.5%	3.3 30%	0.30 (0.07–0.90) 2.8%	0.05 (0–0.20) 0.5%	6.0 (2.5–16.5) 56%	0.70 (0.15–2.0) 6.5%
2 mo	11.0 (5.5–18.0)	3.8 (1.0–9.0) 34%	0.49 4.4%	3.3 30%	0.30 (0.07–0.85) 2.7%	0.05 (0–0.20) 0.5%	6.3 (3.0–16.0) 57%	0.65 (0.13–1.8) 5.9%
4 mo	11.5 (6.0–17.5)	3.8 (1.0–9.0) 33%	0.45 3.9%	3.3 29%	0.30 (0.07–0.80) 2.6%	0.05 (0–0.20) 0.4%	6.8 (3.5–14.5) 59%	0.60 (0.10–1.5) 5.2%
6 mo	11.9 (6.0–17.5)	3.8 (1.0–8.5) 32%	0.45 3.8%	3.3 28%	0.30 (0.07–0.75) 2.5%	0.05 (0–0.20) 0.4%	7.3 (4.0–13.5) 61%	0.58 (0.10–1.3) 4.8%
8 mo	12.2 (6.0–17.5)	3.7 (1.0–8.5) 30%	0.41 3.3%	3.3 27%	0.30 (0.07–0.70) 2.5%	0.05 (0–0.20) 0.4%	7.6 (4.5–12.5) 62%	0.58 (0.08–1.2) 4.7%
10 mo	12.0 (6.0–17.5)	3.6 (1.0–8.5) 30%	0.40 3.3%	3.2 27%	0.30 (0.06–0.70) 2.5%	0.05 (0–0.20) 0.4%	7.5 (4.5–11.5) 63%	0.55 (0.05–1.2) 4.6%
12 mo	11.4 (6.0–17.5)	3.5 (1.5–8.5) 31%	0.35 3.1%	3.2 28%	0.30 (0.05–0.70) 2.6%	0.05 (0–0.20) 0.4%	7.0 (4.0–10.5) 61%	0.55 (0.05–1.1) 4.8%

*From Altman PL and Dittmer DS, eds, *Blood and Other Body Fluids,* Bethesda, MD: Federation of American Societies for Experimental Biology, 1961, with permission.

(continued)

Age	Leukocyte count (x $10^3/mm^3$)	Neutrophils			Eosinophils	Basophils	Lymphocytes	Monocytes
		Total	Band	Segmented				
2 y	10.6 (6.0–17.0)	3.5 (1.5–8.5) 33%	0.32 3.0%	3.2 30%	0.28 (0.04–0.65) 2.6%	0.05 (0–0.20) 0.5%	6.3 (3.0–9.5) 59%	0.53 (0.05–1.0) 5.0%
4 y	9.1 (5.5–15.5)	3.8 (1.5–8.5) 42%	0.27 (0–1.0) 3.0%	3.5 (1.5–7.5) 39%	0.25 (0.02–0.65) 2.8%	0.05 (0–0.20) 0.6%	4.5 (2.0–8.0) 50%	0.45 (0–0.8) 5.0%
6 y	8.5 (5.0–14.5)	4.3 (1.5–8.0) 51%	0.25 (0–1.0) 3.0%	4.0 (1.5–7.0) 48%	0.23 (0–0.65) 2.7%	0.05 (0–0.20) 0.6%	3.5 (1.5–7.0) 42%	0.40 (0–0.8) 4.7%
8 y	8.3 (4.5–13.5)	4.4 (1.5–8.0) 53%	0.25 (0–1.0) 3.0%	4.1 (1.5–7.0) 50%	0.20 (0–0.50) 2.4%	0.05 (0–0.20) 0.6%	3.3 (1.5–6.8) 39%	0.35 (0–0.8) 4.2%
10 y	8.1 (4.5–13.5)	4.4 (1.8–8.0) 54%	0.24 (0–1.0) 3.0%	4.2 (1.8–7.0) 51%	0.20 (0–0.60) 2.4%	0.04 (0–0.20) 0.5%	3.1 (1.5–6.5) 38%	0.35 (0–0.8) 4.3%
12 y	8.0 (4.5–13.5)	4.4 (1.8–8.0) 55%	0.25 (0–1.0) 3.0%	4.2 (1.8–7.0) 52%	0.20 (0–0.55) 2.5%	0.04 (0–0.20) 0.5%	3.0 (1.2–6.0) 38%	0.35 (0–0.8) 4.4%
14 y	7.9 (4.5–13.0)	4.4 (1.8–8.0) 56%	0.24 (0–1.0) 3.0%	4.2 (1.8–7.0) 53%	0.20 (0–0.50) 2.5%	0.04 (0–0.20) 0.5%	2.9 (1.2–5.8) 37%	0.38 (0–0.8) 4.7%
16 y	7.8 (4.5–13.0)	4.4 (1.8–8.0) 57%	0.23 3.0%	4.2 54%	0.20 (0–0.50) 2.6%	0.04 (0–0.20) 0.5%	2.8 (1.2–5.2) 35%	0.40 (0–0.8) 5.1%
18 y	7.7 (4.5–12.5)	4.4 (1.8–7.7) 57%	0.23 3.0%	4.2 54%	0.20 (0–0.45) 2.6%	0.04 (0–0.20) 0.5%	2.7 (1.0–5.0) 35%	0.40 (0–0.8) 5.2%
20 y	7.5 (4.5–11.5)	4.4 (1.8–7.7) 59%	0.23 (0–0.7) 3.0%	4.2 (1.8–7.0) 56%	0.20 (0–0.45) 2.7%	0.04 (0–0.20) 0.5%	2.5 (1.0–4.8) 33%	0.38 (0–0.8) 5.2%
21 y	7.4 (4.5–11.0)	4.4 (1.8–7.7) 59%	0.22 (0–0.7) 3.0%	4.2 (1.8–7.0) 56%	0.20 (0–0.45) 2.7%	0.04 (0–0.20) 0.5%	2.5 (1.0–4.8) 34%	0.30 (0–0.8) 4.0%

(Continued)

Footnotes

1. Karayalcin G, Rosner F, and Sawitsky A, "Pseudoneutropenia in Blacks: A Normal Phenomenon," *N Y State J Med*, 1972, 72:1815-7.
2. Shapiro MF, Hatch RL, and Greenfield S, "Cost Containment and Labor-Intensive Tests: The Case of the Leukocyte Differential Count," *JAMA*, 1984, 252:231-4.
3. Banez EI and Bacaling JH, "An Evaluation of the Technicon® HI Automated Hematology Analyzer in Detecting Peripheral Blood Changes in Acute Inflammation," *Arch Pathol Lab Med*, 1988, 112(9):885-8.
4. Bentley SA, "Alternatives to the Neutrophil Band Count," *Arch Pathol Lab Med*, 1988, 112(9):883-4.

References

Cornbleet J, "Spurious Results From Automated Hematology Cell Counters," *Lab Med*, 1983, 14:509-14.

Hope E and Peerschke EIB, "Principles of Automated Differential Analysis," *Clinical Hematology and Fundamentals of Hemostasis*, 2nd ed, Chapter 30, Section II, Harmening DM, ed, Philadelphia, PA: FA Davis Co, 1992, 554-67.

Pierre RV, "Leukocyte Differential Counting," *Practical Laboratory Hematology*, Chapter 7, Koepke JA, ed, New York, NY: Churchill Livingstone, 1991, 131-56.

Rich EC, Crowson TW, and Connelly DP, "Effectiveness of Differential Leukocyte Count in Case Finding in the Ambulatory Care Setting," *JAMA*, 1983, 249:633-6.

Robertson EP, Lai HW, and Wei DC, "An Evaluation of Leukocyte Analysis on the Coulter STKS," *Clin Lab Haematol*, 1992, 14(1):53-68.

Swaim WR, "Laboratory and Clinical Evaluation of White Blood Cell Differential Counts: Comparison of the Coulter VCS, Technicon H-1, and 800-Cell Manual Method," *Am J Clin Pathol*, 1991, 95(3):381-8.

Wardlaw SC and Levine RA, "Quantitative Buffy Coat Analysis. A New Laboratory Tool Functioning as a Screening Complete Blood Cell Count," *JAMA*, 1983, 249:617-20.

Peripheral Blood: Red Blood Cell Morphology

***CPT** 85008*

See Also Anemia Flowchart in the Hematology Appendix

Related Information

Autohemolysis Test *on page 519*
Blood Volume *on page 522*
Complete Blood Count *on page 533*
Ham Test *on page 549*
Heinz Body Stain *on page 551*
Hematocrit *on page 552*
Hemoglobin A_2 *on page 555*
Hemoglobin Electrophoresis *on page 556*
Malaria Smear *on page 569*
Microfilariae, Peripheral Blood Preparation *on page 571*
Osmotic Fragility *on page 573*
Peripheral Blood: Differential Leukocyte Count *on page 576*
Red Blood Cell Indices *on page 592*
Red Cell Count *on page 594*
Schilling Test *on page 598*

Synonyms Blood Smear Morphology; Morphology; Peripheral Smear, Blood; RBC Morphology; RBC Smear; Red Blood Cell Morphology

Applies to Ovalocytes Smear; Schistocytes Smear; Sickle Cells Smear; Spherocytes Smear; Stippled RBCs Smear

Specimen Whole blood **CONTAINER:** Lavender top (EDTA) tube or smears prepared directly from fingerstick or heelstick blood. Heparin or oxalate may produce artifactual distortion especially of white blood cells. **COLLECTION:** Routine venipuncture. Invert tube gently to mix. **STORAGE INSTRUCTIONS:** Refrigerate **CAUSES FOR REJECTION:** Clotted or hemolyzed specimen

Interpretive **REFERENCE RANGE:** Normal morphology. It may not be possible to correlate minor changes in RBC morphology (eg, 5% to 10% elliptocytosis) with identifiable disease. **USE:** Evaluate red cell disorders, white cell disorders, platelet disorders, and correlation of findings to CBC parameters as quality control function **METHODOLOGY:** Study of red blood cell morphology as it presents on Wright's stained peripheral blood. Red blood cell indices as determined by automated cell counters (eg, MCV, MCH, MCHC, RDW) also give insight into morphologic red cell abnormalities. **ADDITIONAL INFORMATION:** Diverse trends at all levels of the medical care system have combined to focus attention on the utility/cost-effectiveness of manual review of the peripheral blood smear (PBS), in particular, as a routine incorporated in the CBC. The CBC has evolved from highly labor intensive to highly capital intensive, while the PBS has remained highly labor intensive. Automated devices continue to expand their repertoire, adding new parameters that digitize and in some cases improve upon information formerly gleaned from study of the PBS (eg, red cell distribution width which quantitates the morphologic observation anisocytosis). Radical changes in reimbursement, some in effect, others yet to occur, provide economic incentive to retain only laboratory procedures that have very strongly favorable cost/benefit ratios. Studies have suggested that physician criteria for ordering WBC differential on patients in the hospital are inconsistent (demand vs need is not clear)[1] and that differential leukocyte counting has no value in case finding in the "ambulatory care setting."[2] There appears to be a growing trend to perform WBC differential only in cases of abnormal WBC count or only upon specific order. That is, the trend is to delete the differential (blood smear review) from the "complete blood count" routine however the latter is defined. Differential counts have been found unproductive in a specialized clinical environment (healthy midshipmen being considered for nuclear submarine duty).[3] Patients requiring hospitalization, however, should present with greater hematologic abnormality (variable with type of patient and institution). The review of PBS is a part of the quality control cross check system built into each CBC and available to the medical technologist performing the test and to physicians and others who may subsequently question the integrity of the results. Each CBC (when truly complete with review of PBS, WBC differential count, and RBC indices) is a self-contained case individualized quality control unit.[4] Spurious results from automated counters may arise from a surprisingly large number of different sources, many requiring review of the PBS for detection and/or analysis.[5]

Cost and utilization considerations briefly reviewed above seem to indicate that review of PBS and differential study of WBCs should be relegated to the occasional special situation (ie, on physician order or to assist with evaluation of an abnormal result from an automated cell counter). This role in itself would necessitate review of some 10% to 30% of CBC studies depending on the type of institution. Computer assisted automated differential analyzers flag and require some 10% to 20% of cases for manual review, also institution variable. While labor intensive, the study of PBS is nearly devoid of capital costs. On the other hand, automated counters are not free of labor costs and are highly capital intensive. These expensive units are not centralized, due in part to the perceived need for "stat" capability. They are, therefore, not efficiently utilized; they are idle for part of the day. In effect a costly instrument is used to screen (CBC without differential) for performance of a low cost but in some respects more definitive test. A "variable effort" approach to the WBC differential utilizing a computer and "linkage patterns" of linked abnormalities has been proposed.[6] Here, the number of cells examined per slide varies with the apparent abnormality of the slide. Another alternative, quantitative buffy coat analysis (QBCA), has been proposed and may find acceptance. It is based on lower cost technology in which WBCs are differentially stained with a fluorescent dye in a specialized hematocrit tube having a float that expands the buffy coat layer.[7] In a critique, QBCA has been challenged, somewhat unrealistically, as not cost-competitive with manual methods.[8] The clinician will likely find a variable and changing approach to these problems.

Efforts expended on technical and economic aspects of delivering a CBC for patient/physician use unfortunately may becloud the fact that a wealth of information may be hidden from the sensory mechanisms and microcomputers of automated counters. This data, beneficial to the patient, may be lost without the manual study of the PBS. Examples of blood cell morphologic abnormalities (not comprehensive) are given in tabular form in listing, Peripheral Blood: Differential Leukocyte Count.

Footnotes

1. Rock WA Jr and Grogan JE, "Demand vs Need vs Physician Prerogatives in the Use of the WBC Differential," *JAMA*, 1983, 249:613-6.
2. Rich EC, Crowson TW, and Connelly DP, "Effectiveness of Differential Leukocyte Count in Case Finding in the Ambulatory Care Setting," *JAMA*, 1983, 249:633-6.
3. Wesson SK, Mercado T, Austin M, et al, "Differential Counts and Overuse of the Laboratory," *Lancet*, 1980, 1:552, (letter).
4. Lafsness KG, "Correlation of Hematologic Data From the Individual Patient as a Quality Control Tool," *Am J Med Technol*, 1983, 49:655-9.
5. Cornbleet J, "Spurious Results From Automated Hematology Cell Counters," *Lab Med*, 1983, 14:509-14.
6. Korpman RA and Bull B, "Whither the WBC Differential? – Some Alternatives," *Blood Cells*, 1980, 6:421-9.
7. Wardlaw SC and Levine RA, "Quantitative Buffy Coat Analysis. A New Laboratory Tool Functioning as a Screening Complete Blood Cell Count," *JAMA*, 1983, 249:617-20.
8. Fischer P and Addison L, "Quantitative Buffy Coat Analysis," *JAMA*, 1983, 250:1272, (letter).

References

Van Assendelft OW, "Interpretation of the Quantitative Blood Cell Count," *Practical Laboratory Hematology*, Chapter 4, Koepke JA, ed, New York, NY: Churchill Livingstone, 1991, 78-98.

(Continued)

Peripheral Blood: Red Blood Cell Morphology *(Continued)*

Williams WJ, "Polychrome Staining," *Hematology*, 4th ed, Appendix, Chapter A2, Williams WJ, Beutler E, Ersler AJ, et al, eds, New York, NY: McGraw-Hill Publishing Co, 1990, 1699-700.

Peripheral Differential *see* Peripheral Blood: Differential Leukocyte Count *on page 576*

Peripheral Smear, Blood *see* Peripheral Blood: Red Blood Cell Morphology *on page 584*

Peritoneal Fluid Analysis *see* Body Fluids Analysis, Cell Count *on page 523*

Perls' Test *see* Iron Stain, Bone Marrow *on page 562*

Peroxidase Stain *see* Leukocyte Cytochemistry *on page 567*

Plasma/Blood Volume *see* Blood Volume *on page 522*

Plasma Free Hemoglobin *see* Hemoglobin, Plasma *on page 559*

Plasma Volume Measurement *see* Blood Volume *on page 522*

Platelet Count

CPT *85590 (manual); 85595 (automated)*

Related Information

Complete Blood Count *on page 533*
Intravascular Coagulation Screen *on page 446*
Kidney Profile *on page 268*
Partial Thromboplastin Time *on page 450*
Peripheral Blood: Differential Leukocyte Count *on page 576*
Platelet Adhesion Test *on page 458*
Platelet Aggregation *on page 459*
Platelet Antibody *on page 462*
Platelet Antibody, Immunohematologic *on page 1080*
Platelet Concentrate, Donation and Transfusion *on page 1081*
Platelets, Apheresis, Donation *on page 1083*
Platelet Sizing *on page 588*

Synonyms Thrombocyte Count

Specimen Whole blood **CONTAINER:** Lavender top (EDTA) tube **CAUSES FOR REJECTION:** Clotted specimen, platelet clumping

Interpretive **REFERENCE RANGE:** 150,000-450,000/mm^3 (150-450 x 10^9/L or 150,000-450,000/μL).[1] Considerable interlaboratory variation exists, manual vs electronic automated procedures. Count is method dependent; results of manual count have high coefficient of variation as compared to automated methods.[2] Occasionally, apparently normal children, in particular those under 24 months of age, may have platelet counts in the 500,000-750,000 range.[3] **POSSIBLE PANIC RANGE:** <50,000/mm^3 or >1,000,000/mm^3 **USE:** Evaluate, diagnose, and follow up bleeding disorders, purpura/petechiae, drug-induced thrombocytopenia, idiopathic thrombocytopenia purpura, disseminated intravascular coagulation, leukemia, and chemotherapeutic management of malignant disease **LIMITATIONS:** Clumping may cause false low count.[4] Platelet satellitism around neutrophils may cause pseudothrombocytopenia. RBC (eg, microspherocytes) or WBC fragments including fragmented fragile leukemic cells and neutrophil pseudoplatelets[5] may cause falsely elevated counts. EDTA-induced platelet clumping has been considered the most frequent cause of spuriously low platelet counts[6] and appears to result from a variety of platelet antigen/antibody reactions occurring *in vitro* (eg, IgM autoantibody against 78-KD platelet glycoprotein).[7] **METHODOLOGY:** Variety of automated/semiautomated devices are in use. Counts are performed on platelet-rich plasma or whole blood by optical or impedance matching counting techniques. Carefully controlled phase microscopy manual count is usually considered the reference method but suffers from a wide coefficient of variation (Brecher-Cronkite phase contrast method has CV of 7% to 17%). **ADDITIONAL INFORMATION:** The platelet, of growing practical clinical importance in hemostatic considerations and a variety of medical/surgical processes, is also fundamental to etiologic considerations of arteriosclerotic and malignant disease.[8] Platelets are generally 2-3 microns in diameter but large forms (megathrombocytes) appear when production is increased. The production of platelets is controlled by thrombopoietin. Platelets survive for 8-10 days and are subject to circadian periodicity, highest platelet counts occurring during midday.[9] Some drugs may increase the platelet count by stimulating thrombopoietin production. Deaths from cardiovascular disease may relate temporally to the circadian rhythm of platelet production.[9]

Careful estimate of platelet number from stained peripheral blood smear can provide useful information. A variety of factors affect the distribution of platelets on a peripheral blood smear, and thus platelet estimates lack precision. Capillary blood platelet counts (c.f. to venous blood counts) may be significantly underestimated. Platelets are often clumped on smears obtained from capillary blood, contributing to imprecision. A small whole blood clot or very small fibrin clots in the EDTA anticoagulated specimen will usually be associated with clumping of platelets on the slide and with a false low platelet count.

Quantitative platelet disorders have varied etiology. Thrombocytopenia may have an immunologic basis, the result of production deficiency due to the effect of drugs or physical agents, abnormal platelet pooling or increased destruction (eg, sequestration by large vascular tumor), or result from a variety of probably nonimmunologic mechanisms (eg, hypersplenism). Decreases may occur after bleeding, transfusion, infections, or relating to defective production of or regulation by thrombopoietin.

Drugs and chemicals associated with thrombocytopenia often on an immune mediated basis[10] or as the result of marrow suppression include quinidine, quinine, heparin, gold salts, sulfas, rifampicin, ASA, digitoxin, apronal, chlorothiazides, chlorpropamide, meprobamate, antihistamines, chloramphenicol, penicillin, DDT, benzol, a variety of other industrial organic chemicals, diphenylhydantoin, PAS, hydrochlorothiazide, phenylbutazone, and a variety of antineoplastic chemotherapeutic agents. ASA acts by acetylating cyclo-oxygenase.

Thrombocytosis is less common, but likewise varied in etiology: physiologic (eg, postpartum or after exercise); myeloproliferative syndromes, (eg, thrombocythemia, some cases of chronic myelogenous leukemia, myelofibrosis with myeloid metaplasia); rebound following thrombocytopenia, marrow regenerative activity after bleeding episode, hemophilia, iron deficiency; asplenism, infections, inflammatory or malignant disease, especially carcinomatosis. Oral contraceptives may cause slight increase in platelet count. Slight to moderate decrease in platelet count has been noted during pregnancy in most women who have essential thrombocythemia.[11]

Inherited Abnormalities of Platelet Production (Characterized by Thrombocytopenia)

Condition	Inheritance	Abnormality	Therapy
May-Hegglin	Autosomal Dominant	Severe thrombocytopenia	Platelet replacement
Wiskott-Aldrich	Sex-linked	Severe thrombocytopenia with small platelets	Possibly splenectomy
Congenital thrombopoietin deficiency	? Autorecessive	Severe thrombocytopenia	Plasma transfusion
Thrombocytopenia with absent radius	Autorecessive	Moderate thrombocytopenia	Platelet replacement
Abnormalities of Platelet Function, Familial Transmission, Autorecessive			
Thrombasthenia		Absent clot retraction, absent aggregation, mild thrombocytopenia	Platelet replacement, steroids
Bernard-Soulier syndrome		Giant platelets, absent Ristocetin® aggregation	Platelet replacement
Platelet storage pool disease		Absent aggregation with collagen, mild thrombocytopenia, absent dense granules with decreased platelet serotonin	Splenectomy, platelet replacement
Hermansky-Pudlak syndrome		Aggregation abnormal with epinephrine and collagen, decreased dense granules and absent ADP stores	Platelet replacement
Release reaction abnormalities		Absent second wave aggregation with epinephrine and collagen, absent PF-3 release, varied inheritance	Platelet replacement

From Penner J, *Blood Coagulation Laboratory Manual,* University of Michigan Medical School, Sept, 1979, with permission.

(Continued)

Platelet Count *(Continued)*

Congenital causes of thrombocytopenia include Wiskott-Aldrich syndrome, May-Hegglin anomaly, thrombocytopenia with absent radius, and Bernard-Soulier syndrome. See table on previous page.

Footnotes

1. Rowan RM, "Platelet Counting and the Assessment of Platelet Function," *Practical Laboratory Hematology*, Chapter 8, Koepke JA, ed, New York, NY: Churchill Livingstone, 1991, 164.
2. Lohmann RC, Crawford LN, and Wood DE, "Proficiency Testing of Platelet Counting in Ontario," *Am J Clin Pathol*, 1992, 98(2):231-6.
3. Novak RW, Tschantz JA, and Krill CE Jr, "Normal Platelet and Mean Platelet Volumes in Pediatric Patients," *Lab Med*, 1987, 18:613-4.
4. Solanki DL and Blackburn BC, "Spurious Leukocytosis and Thrombocytopenia. A Dual Phenomenon Caused by Clumping of Platelets *In Vitro*," *JAMA*, 1983, 250:2514-5.
5. Merz B, "Newly Identified Particle May Explain Spurious Platelet Count," *JAMA*, 1983, 249:3146-7.
6. Payne BA and Pierre RV, "Pseudothrombocytopenia: A Laboratory Artifact With Potentially Serious Consequences," *Mayo Clin Proc*, 1984, 59:123-5.
7. De Caterina M, Fratellanza G, Grimaldi E, et al, "Evidence of a Cold Immunoglobulin M Autoantibody Against 78-kD Platelet Glycoprotein in a Case of EDTA-Dependent Pseudothrombocytopenia," *Am J Clin Pathol*, 1993, 99(2):163-7.
8. Doolittle RF, Hunkapillar MW, Hood LE, et al, "Simian Sarcoma Virus onc Gene, v-sis, Is Derived From the Gene (or Genes) Encoding a Platelet-Derived Growth Factor," *Science*, 1983, 221:275-7.
9. de Nicola P and Casale G, "Platelets," *Blood Diseases in the Aged*, Stuttgart, West Germany: Schwer Verlag, 1988, 71-6.
10. Moss RA, "Drug-Induced Immune Thrombocytopenia," *Am J Hematol*, 1980, 9:439-46.
11. Chow EY, Haley LP, and Vickars LM, "Essential Thrombocythemia in Pregnancy: Platelet Count and Pregnancy Outcome," *Am J Hematol*, 1992, 41(4):249-51.

References

Cornbleet PJ and Kessinger S, "Accuracy of Low Platelet Counts on the Coulter S-Plus IV®," *Am J Clin Pathol*, 1985, 83:78-80.

Feusner JH, Behrens JA, Detter JC, et al, "Platelet Counts in Capillary Blood," *Am J Clin Pathol*, 1979, 72:410-4.

Rowan RM, "Platelet Counting and the Assessment of Platelet Function," *Practical Laboratory Hematology*, Chapter 8, Koepke JA, ed, New York, NY: Churchill Livingstone, 1991, 157-70.

Thompson CE, Damon LE, Ries CA, et al, "Thrombotic Microangiopathies in the 1980s: Clinical Features, Response to Treatment, and the Impact of the Human Immunodeficiency Virus Epidemic," *Blood*, 1992, 80(8):1890-5.

Vora AJ and Lilleyman JS, "Secondary Thrombocytosis," *Arch Dis Child*, 1993, 68:88-90.

Platelet Sizing

***CPT** 85029*

Related Information

Complete Blood Count *on page 533*
Platelet Count *on page 586*

Synonyms MPV; PDW; Platelet Indices

Test Commonly Includes MPV (mean platelet volume), platelet count, PDW (platelet distribution width)

Abstract Modern automated cell counters may generate platelet sizing parameters (eg, MPV and PDW) which may be abnormal in some clinical situations. Platelet indices are analogous to red blood cell indices (eg, MCV and RDW) but have only modest clinical application. MPV and PDW are increased in patients with idiopathic thrombocytopenic purpura (ITP).

Specimen Whole blood **CONTAINER:** Lavender top (EDTA) tube; green top (heparin) tube may cause platelet clumping

Interpretive REFERENCE RANGE: See tables for mean platelet volume and platelet "crit" reference values. **USE:** Differential diagnosis of hematologic disease, assess platelet function, and guide need for platelet transfusion in thrombocytopenic patients **LIMITATIONS:** May be unreliable if platelet count is $<10,000/mm^3$ **METHODOLOGY:** Flow cytometry (FC) with measurement of platelet volume and size parameters by changes in electrical impedance (resistance of an individual cell is proportional to its volume) and microprocessor assisted mathematical analysis. Electrical signals (proportional to particle size) are sorted according to magnitude. Upper and lower thresholds define the central platelet volume distribution (2-20 fL).[1] **ADDITIONAL INFORMATION:** The clinical significance of variation in platelet size has only recently begun to be explored. Generally, large platelets are young platelets and have better hemostatic function than average age or old platelets.[2] MPV (in normal subjects) bears an inverse relation to plate-

Platelet Parameters in Males (mean ± SD)*

Age (y)	n	Platelet Count (x 10^9 mm^3) (x 10^9/L)	MPV (fL)	PCT (%)
1-5	24	357 ± 70	8.6 ± 0.7	0.304 ± 0.059
6-10	24	351 ± 85	8.6 ± 0.8	0.300 ± 0.058
11-15	16	282 ± 63	9.8 ± 1.0	0.274 ± 0.053
16-20	16	266 ± 63	10.2 ± 1.1	0.266 ± 0.049
21-30	24	238 ± 49	9.6 ± 0.6	0.277 ± 0.045
31-40	12	244 ± 56	9.8 ± 1.2	0.237 ± 0.044
41-50	17	271 ± 66	9.4 ± 1.0	0.250 ± 0.045
51-60	22	258 ± 61	9.8 ± 1.2	0.248 ± 0.045
61-70	29	256 ± 53	9.4 ± 1.1	0.238 ± 0.047
71-86	23	237 ± 49	9.6 ± 1.0	0.226 ± 0.048

From Graham SS, Traub B, and Minic IB, "Automated Platelet-Sizing Parameters on a Normal Population," *Am J Clin Pathol,* 1987, 87:365-9, with permission.
*SI conversion units for platelet count x 10^3 mm^3 is platelet count x 10^9/L.

Platelet Parameters in Females (mean ± SD)

Age (y)	n	Platelet Count (x 10^3 mm^3) (x 10^9/L)	MPV (fL)	PCT (%)
1-5	25	381 ± 76	8.9 ± 0.8	0.337 ± 0.069
6-10	18	336 ± 76	9.7 ± 1.1	0.326 ± 0.080
11-15	31	298 ± 72	9.8 ± 1.2	0.288 ± 0.058
16-20	22	270 ± 58	9.7 ± 0.7	0.262 ± 0.058
21-30	43	270 ± 58	9.8 ± 1.0	0.261 ± 0.046
31-40	30	282 ± 56	9.8 ± 1.2	0.271 ± 0.046
41-50	26	279 ± 65	9.8 ± 0.9	0.274 ± 0.072
51-60	21	285 ± 54	9.7 ± 0.7	0.276 ± 0.045
61-70	30	274 ± 61	9.6 ± 0.9	0.262 ± 0.052
71-83	24	279 ± 65	9.5 ± 1.0	0.261 ± 0.054

From Graham SS, Traub B, and Minic IB, "Automated Platelet-Sizing Parameters on a Normal Population," *Am J Clin Pathol,* 1987, 87:365-9, with permission.

let count. MPV rises with increased platelet turnover due to production of megathrombocytes. Platelet size parameters may be an example of a "test in search of a disease". Platelet sizing does find application in the evaluation of acute thrombocytopenia, in cases of suspected idiopathic thrombocytopenic purpura (ITP). MPV and PDW are increased with ITP. Use of increased platelet volume as an indicator of ITP versus acute leukemia will not likely replace bone marrow study for evaluation of megakaryocytes in cases of thrombocytopenia. Large platelets are present in the recovery stage of alcohol-induced thrombocytopenia.[3] Platelet size, while often a marker for platelet age, may in some cases reflect altered platelet production (eg, dyspoietic states such as the May-Hegglin anomaly in which increased platelet volume occurs).[1] Small platelets are seen in the Wiskott-Aldrich syndrome. Autoimmune thrombocytopenia and leukemia may be associated with presence of platelet fragments and decreased platelet volume. Hypersplenetic patients have smaller platelet size. Low MPV may be seen in patients with septic thrombocytopenia and in some cases of myeloproliferative disease after treatment with cytotoxic drugs. In the Bernard-Soulier syndrome, there is thrombocytopenia with large platelets.[4] Large platelets, occasionally with abnormal morphology, occur in the myeloproliferative syndromes. Increased MPV may also be seen in hyperthyroidism.[5] Mediterranean macrothrombocytopenia is characterized by low platelet count, large platelets, and a generally normal platelet "crit".[6] There is evidence that mean platelet volume correlates

(Continued)

Platelet Sizing *(Continued)*

with bleeding tendency in thrombocytopenic patients.[7] A significantly lower frequency of bleeding occurs with mean platelet volumes >6.4 fL. This measure, then, may be of use in assessing the need for platelet transfusion.

MPV and platelet count are normal and constant between the first trimester and the end of normal pregnancy, but MPV is increased in patients with pre-eclampsia. Platelet count is decreased in cases of pre-eclampsia but was also found to be decreased in 10% of normal pregnancies.[8] Platelet count is decreased in pre-eclamptic women with the HELLP syndrome (hemolysis, elevated liver tests, and low platelet count). Platelets have also been found to decrease in pre-eclamptic women with platelet count in the normal range.[9] Increase in MPV has been noted in neonates with coagulase-negative staphylococcal septicemia.[10] Platelet volume has been noted to decrease during cardiopulmonary bypass and to increase in atherosclerotic smokers.[11,12] Increase in MPV due to smoking has been proposed as a risk factor for atherosclerotic disease.[12]

Footnotes

1. Paulus JM, "Platelet Size in Man," *Blood*, 1975, 46:321-36.
2. Haver VM and Gear AR, "Functional Fractionation of Platelets," *J Lab Clin Med*, 1981, 97:187-204.
3. Sahud MA, "Platelet Size and Number in Alcoholic Thrombocytopenia," *N Engl J Med*, 1973, 286:355-6.
4. Howard MA, Hutton RA, and Hardisty RM, "Hereditary Giant Platelet Syndrome: A Disorder of a New Aspect of Platelet Function," *Br Med J [Clin Res]*, 1983, 2:586-8.
5. Henry JB, Nelson DA, Tomar RH, et al, *Clinical Diagnosis and Management by Laboratory Methods*, 18th ed, Philadelphia, PA: WB Saunders Co, 1991, 567-8.
6. England JM, "Blood Cell Sizing," *Practical Laboratory Hematology*, Chapter 6, Koepke JA, ed, New York, NY: Churchill Livingstone, 1991, 127-8.
7. Eldor A, Avitzour M, Or R, et al, "Prediction of Hemorrhagic Diathesis in Thrombocytopenia by Mean Platelet Volume," *Br Med J [Clin Res]*, 1982, 285:397-400.
8. Ahmed Y, van Iddekinge B, Paul C, et al, "Retrospective Analysis of Platelet Numbers and Volumes in Normal Pregnancy and in Pre-eclampsia," *Br J Obstet Gynaecol*, 1993, 100(3):216-20.
9. Neiger R, Contag SA, and Coustan DR, "Pre-eclampsia Effect on Platelet Count," *Am J Perinatol*, 1992, 9(5-6):378-80.
10. O'Connor TA, Ringer KM, and Gaddis ML, "Mean Platelet Volume During Coagulase-Negative Staphylococcal Sepsis in Neonates," *Am J Clin Pathol*, 1993, 99(1):69-71.
11. Boldt J, Zickmann B, Benson M, et al, "Does Platelet Size Correlate With Function in Patients Undergoing Cardiac Surgery?" *Intensive Care Med*, 1993, 19(1):44-7.
12. Kario K, Matsuo T, and Nakao K, "Cigarette Smoking Increases the Mean Platelet Volume in Elderly Patients With Risk Factors for Atherosclerosis," *Clin Lab Haematol*, 1992, 14(4):281-7.

References

Bithell TC, "Thrombocytopenia Caused by Immunologic Platelet Destruction," *Wintrobe's Clinical Hematology*, 9th ed, Vol 2, Chapter 50, Philadelphia, PA: Lea & Febiger, 1993, 1335.

Corash L, "Platelet Sizing: Techniques, Biological Significance, and Clinical Applications," *Current Topics in Hematology*, Piomelli S and Yachnin S, eds, New York, NY: Alan R Liss Inc, 1983, 4:99-122.

Graham SS, Traub B, and Mink IB, "Automated Platelet-Sizing Parameters on a Normal Population," *Am J Clin Pathol*, 1987, 87:365-9.

Jackson SR and Carter JM, "Platelet Volume: Laboratory Measurement and Clinical Application," *Blood Rev*, 1993, 7:104-13.

Thompson CB, Diaz DD, Quinn PG, et al, "The Role of Anticoagulation in the Measurement of Platelet Volumes," *Am J Clin Pathol*, 1983, 80:327-32.

Pleural Fluid Analysis *see* Body Fluids Analysis, Cell Count *on page 523*

PNH Test *see* Ham Test *on page 549*

PNH Test Screen *see* Sugar Water Test Screen *on page 603*

Prussian Blue Stain *see* Iron Stain, Bone Marrow *on page 562*

Radioactive Vitamin B_{12} Absorption Test With or Without Intrinsic Factor *see* Schilling Test *on page 598*

RBC *see* Red Cell Count *on page 594*

RBC Enzyme Screen *see* Red Blood Cell Enzyme Deficiency Screen *on page 592*

RBC Enzymes, Quantitative *see* Red Blood Cell Enzyme Deficiency, Quantitative *on next page*

RBC Folate *see* Folic Acid, RBC *on page 544*

RBC Fragility *see* Osmotic Fragility *on page 573*

RBC Fragility *see* Osmotic Fragility, Incubated *on page 575*

RBC Indices *see* Red Blood Cell Indices *on next page*

RBC Morphology *see* Peripheral Blood: Red Blood Cell Morphology *on page 584*

RBC Smear *see* Peripheral Blood: Red Blood Cell Morphology *on page 584*

RDW (Red Cell Distribution Width) *see* Red Blood Cell Indices *on next page*

Red Blood Cell Count *see* Red Cell Count *on page 594*

Red Blood Cell Enzyme Deficiency, Quantitative

CPT 82955 (G-6-PD)

See Also Anemia Flowchart in the Hematology Appendix

Related Information

Autohemolysis Test *on page 519*
Glucose-6-Phosphate Dehydrogenase, Quantitative, Blood *on page 547*
Glucose-6-Phosphate Dehydrogenase Screen, Blood *on page 548*
Heinz Body Stain *on page 551*
Red Blood Cell Enzyme Deficiency Screen *on next page*

Synonyms Erythrocyte Enzyme Deficiency, Quantitative; RBC Enzymes, Quantitative

Applies to Glutathione Reductase Deficiency, RBC; Heinz Bodies

Test Commonly Includes Glucose-6-phosphate dehydrogenase, pyruvate kinase, and any of over 20 RBC enzymes included in the following reference by E. Beutler

Specimen Erythrocytes **CONTAINER:** Lavender top (EDTA) tube **CAUSES FOR REJECTION:** Clotted or hemolyzed specimen

Interpretive **REFERENCE RANGE:** G-6-PD: 8.6-18.6 IU/g hemoglobin; phosphohexoisomerase: 14.7-42.2 IU/g hemoglobin; pyruvate kinase: 2.0-8.8 IU/g hemoglobin **USE:** Investigation of hemolytic anemia **LIMITATIONS:** False normal results may occur if testing is performed on a sample obtained just after a hemolytic episode (deficiency may be obscured by the presence of a young, enzyme-rich population of RBCs, the older enzyme-deficient red cells having been destroyed). **ADDITIONAL INFORMATION:** Individuals with low levels of RBC G-6-PD are susceptible to hemolytic episodes after exposure to certain chemicals, drugs, and fava beans. Drugs that may precipitate hemolysis in patients with G-6-PD deficiency include: analgesics/antipyretics: aspirin; sulfa drugs: sulfapyridine, sulfisoxazole; antimalarias: primaquine, pentaquine, quinine; nitrofurantoin; Chloromycetin®, quinidine, para-aminosalicylic acid; others. Deficient or absent RBC enzyme activity may relate to absence of or decreased level of the enzyme, presence of an inactive molecular form or of an isoenzyme with altered activity.[1] In some hematologic diseases (eg, PNH, aplastic anemia and acute leukemia), acquired red cell enzyme deficiency is not infrequently seen.[2] RBC glutathione reductase deficiency bears an association with a variety of chemotherapeutically treated malignant states (up to 43% in a study of hospitalized patients).[3] Glutathione reductase deficiency also occurred in some cases of malnutrition, liver disease, and sepsis.

Footnotes

1. Paglia DE, Valentine WN, Williams KD, et al, "An Isozyme of Erythrocyte Pyruvate Kinase (Pk-Los Angeles) With Impaired Kinetics Corrected by Fructose-1, 6-Diphosphate," *Am J Clin Pathol*, 1977, 68:229-34.
2. Miwa S, "Significance of the Determination of Red Cell Enzyme Activities," *Am J Hematol*, 1979, 6:163-72.
3. Frischer H, "Erythrocytic Glutathione Reductase Deficiency in a Hospital Population in the United States," *Am J Hematol*, 1977, 2:327-34.

References

Beutler E, *Red Cell Metabolism: A Manual of Biochemical Methods*, 3rd ed, New York, NY: Grune and Stratton Inc, 1984.

Beutler E, "Study of Glucose-6-Phosphate Dehydrogenase: History and Molecular Biology," *Am J Hematol*, 1993, 42(1):53-8.

Feng CS, Tsang SS, and Mak YT, "Prevalence of Pyruvate Kinase Deficiency Among the Chinese: Determination by the Quantitative Assay," *Am J Hematol*, 1993, 43:271-3.

Miwa S, Kanno H, and Fujii H, "Concise Review: Pyruvate Kinase Deficiency: Historical Perspective and Recent Progress of Molecular Genetics," *Am J Hematol*, 1993, 42(1):31-5.

Williams WJ, Beutler E, Erslev AJ, et al, *Hematology*, 4th ed, New York, NY: McGraw-Hill Inc, 1990, 591-612.

Red Blood Cell Enzyme Deficiency Screen

CPT 82960 (G-6-PD)

Related Information

Glucose-6-Phosphate Dehydrogenase, Quantitative, Blood *on page 547*
Glucose-6-Phosphate Dehydrogenase Screen, Blood *on page 548*
Heinz Body Stain *on page 551*
Red Blood Cell Enzyme Deficiency, Quantitative *on previous page*
Reticulocyte Count *on page 597*

Synonyms Erythrocyte Enzyme Deficiency Screen; RBC Enzyme Screen

Applies to Heinz Bodies

Test Commonly Includes G-6-PD qualitative, pyruvate kinase, triosephosphate isomerase, NADH diaphorase (NADH methemoglobin reductase), glutathione reductase. Completeness varies between laboratories.

Specimen Erythrocytes **CONTAINER:** Lavender top (EDTA) tube **CAUSES FOR REJECTION:** Clotted or hemolyzed specimen

Interpretive **REFERENCE RANGE:** Enzyme present, reported as normal **USE:** Detect etiology of hemolytic state **LIMITATIONS:** Does not detect heterozygotes. False normal results may occur if testing is performed on a sample obtained just after a hemolytic episode. **ADDITIONAL INFORMATION:** Phenotyping of RBC enzymes has been applied to paternity testing.[1]

Footnotes

1. Lee CL and Ying RL, "Phenotyping of Eight Erythrocytic Enzymes in One Acrylamide Gel," *Am J Clin Pathol*, 1979, 71:672-6.

References

Dacie JV, Lewis SM, and Luzzatto L, "Investigation of the Hereditary Haemolytic Anaemias: Membrane and Enzyme Abnormalities," *Practical Haematology*, 7th ed, Chapter 14, New York, NY: Churchill Livingstone, 1991, 195-225.

Luzzatto L and Mehta A, "Glucose-6-Phosphate Dehydrogenase Deficiency," *The Metabolic Basis of Inherited Disease*, 6th ed, Chapter 91, Scriver CR, Beaudet AL, Sly WS, et al, eds, New York, NY: McGraw-Hill Information Services Co, 1989, 2237-65.

Meloon JR, "Introduction to Hemolytic Anemias: Intracorpuscular Defects, II. Hereditary Enzyme Deficiencies," *Clinical Hematology and Fundamentals of Hemostasis*, 2nd ed, Chapter 10, Harmening DM, ed, Philadelphia, PA: FA Davis Co, 1992, 134-41.

Valentine WN, Tanaka KR, and Paglia DE, "Pyruvate Kinase and Other Enzyme Deficiency Disorders of the Erythrocyte," *The Metabolic Basis of Inherited Disease*, 6th ed, Chapter 94, Scriver CR, Beaudet AL, Sly WS, et al, eds, New York, NY: McGraw-Hill Information Services Co, 1989, 2341-65.

Red Blood Cell Indices

CPT 85029 (1-3 indices); 85030 (4 or more indices)

See Also Anemia Flowchart in the Hematology Appendix

Related Information

Aluminum, Serum *on page 1019*
Blood Volume *on page 522*
Complete Blood Count *on page 533*
Hematocrit *on page 552*
Hemoglobin *on page 554*
Hemoglobin A_2 *on page 555*
Ketone Bodies, Blood *on page 265*
Peripheral Blood: Red Blood Cell Morphology *on page 584*
Red Cell Count *on page 594*
Schilling Test *on page 598*
Vitamin B_{12} *on page 612*

Synonyms Erythrocyte Indices; Indices

Applies to MCHC (Mean Corpuscular Hemoglobin Concentration) MCH (Mean Corpuscular Hemoglobin); MCV (Mean Corpuscular Volume); RBC Indices; RDW (Red Cell Distribution Width)

Test Commonly Includes MCV, MCH, MCHC, RBC, RDW, Hct, Hgb

Abstract The RBC indices are measured or mathematically derived from Hgb, Hct, and red blood cell count. The values can be used for quick assessment of anemia.

Specimen Whole blood **CONTAINER:** Lavender top (EDTA) tube for venipuncture specimen; lavender top Microtainer™ tube for capillary specimen **COLLECTION:** Routine venipuncture. Invert the tube 5 to 10 times gently to mix. There must be no clots. **STORAGE INSTRUCTIONS:** Specimen cannot be used if stored over 10 hours at room temperature or 18 hours at 4°C refrigerated temperature. Specimen must not be frozen. **CAUSES FOR REJECTION:** Hemolyzed or clotted specimen

Interpretive **REFERENCE RANGE:** Normal values: RBC indices, healthy white and black subjects data from Coulter S, Sysmex, or H-1 Counters as of Miale.[1] See table. Values represent the mean and 95% range. **USE:** Evaluate red cell parameters; differential diagnosis of anemia, iron deficiency, hereditary spherocytosis, immune spherocytosis, thalassemia, chronic lead poisoning, folate deficiency, vitamin B_{12} deficiency, vitamin B_6 deficiency, pernicious anemia, and anemia of pregnancy **LIMITATIONS:** Patients showing both macrocytosis and microcytosis of the red cells may have indices within the reference range because of the averaging method used in determining indices. Patients with autoagglutination will show spurious results. Although MCV is commonly elevated early in pernicious anemia, it may be normal, especially later when micropoikilocytosis develops. **METHODOLOGY:** The great majority of RBC indices are obtained by the use of microcomputerized, highly automated electronic and pneumatic multichannel analyzers based on aperture-impedance cell sizing and counting (see reference by Koepke). **ADDITIONAL INFORMATION:** The group of three red cell indices are a productive and economically efficient approach to screening for hematologic abnormality, in particular the compensated and uncompensated anemias. The MCV (mean corpuscular volume) is the size (volume) of the average red cell. The MCH (mean corpuscular hemoglobin) is the weight of hemoglobin in the average red cell. The MCHC (mean corpuscular hemoglobin concentration) is the amount of hemoglobin present in the average red cell as compared to its size. The RBC indices are a valuable guide to the choice of more specific measurements such as serum iron, ferritin, folic acid, and/or vitamin B_{12} levels. The MCV decreases before MCHC in evolving iron deficiency anemia[1] while the MCHC decreases before the MCV in evolving anemia of chronic disease.[2] In hemolytic anemias, particularly the hemoglobinopathies, the RBC indices are less helpful. Decreased MCV levels may be due to thalassemia minor although they are not specific for this condition; A_2 hemoglobin levels should be studied to follow-up low MCV levels in appropriate clinical settings. Screening for high A_2 hemoglobin levels will discriminate a population of beta-thalassemics with normal MCV levels. Hemoglobin A_2 levels are most useful using the column chromatography method.

Blood Indices

	MCV (fL)	MCH (pg)	MCHC (%)	RDW
Adult male	90 (80–100)	30 (25.4–34.6)	34 (31–37)	13.0 (11.5–14.5)
Adult female	88 (79–98)	30 (25.4–34.6)	33 (30–36)	13.0 (11.5–14.5)

Changes in RBC Indices With Disease

Condition	MCV	MCH	MCHC	RDW
Iron deficiency anemia	↓	↓	↓	↑
Chronic inflammation	↓	N±	N±	N±
Pernicious anemia	↑	N or high N	high N	↑
B_{12}/folate deficiency	↑	N or high N	high N	↑
Hereditary spherocytosis	N or ↓	↑	↑	N±
Hemolytic/aplastic anemia	N±	N±	N±	N±
Anemia 2° acute blood loss	N±	N±	N±	N±
Polycythemia	N±	N±	N±	N±

A number of conditions (usually characterized by the generation of numerous RBC fragments) may show "relative microcytosis" as reflected by slightly decreased to low normal MCV. This has been described with sickle cell anemia. In children, low MCV for age suggests iron deficiency, lead poisoning, thalassemia syndrome, or very rarely, a pyridoxine-responsive anemia. Examination of the peripheral smear, family history, dietary history, and stool guaiac are helpful in this setting. MCV may be significantly increased in diabetic ketoacidosis[3] (this is due to plasma hyperosmolarity). The high molar concentration of glucose is the main contributing factor to the increased plasma osmolarity, producing an hypertonic intracellular state of

(Continued)

Red Blood Cell Indices *(Continued)*

RBCs. When such cells are put into a relatively hypotonic diluent (eg, Coulter cell counting), water enters the cell, it swells and may produce erroneously high MCV. Recognition of increase in MCV may alert the clinician to presence of the hyperosmolar state.[3]

Aluminum toxicity, occurring in uremic patients on chronic hemodialysis, is associated in some cases with decreased MCV, microcytic anemia.[4,5]

RDW is an electronic measurement of anisocytosis (red cell size variability). RDW is typically elevated in iron deficiency anemia while usually normal in beta thalassemia minor (heterozygous thalassemia). RDW is elevated in beta thalassemia major.

A recent study suggests that zidovudine (AZT) treatment of AIDS has become the most common cause of macrocytosis (increase in MCV) in the hospitalized urban patient population.[6]

Footnotes

1. Miale JB, *Laboratory Medicine: Hematology*, 6th ed, St Louis, MO: Mosby-Year Book Inc, 1982, 378.
2. England JM, Ward SM, and Down MC, "Microcytosis, Anisocytosis and the Red Cell Indices in Iron Deficiency," *Br J Haematol*, 1976, 34:589-97.
3. Evan-Wong LA and Davidson RJ, "Raised Coulter Mean Corpuscular Volume in Diabetic Ketoacidosis and Its Underlying Association With Marked Plasma Hyperosmolarity," *J Clin Pathol*, 1983, 36:334-6.
4. Touam M, Martinez F, Lacour B, et al, "Aluminum-Induced, Reversible Microcytic Anemia in Chronic Renal Failure: Clinical and Experimental Studies," *Clin Nephrol*, 1983, 19:295-8.
5. Mladenovic J, "Aluminum Inhibits Erythropoiesis *In Vitro*," *J Clin Invest*, 1988, 81(6):1661-5.
6. Snower DP and Weil SC, "Changing Etiology of Macrocytosis: Zidovudine as a Frequent Causative Factor," *Am J Clin Pathol*, 1993, 99(1):57-60.

References

Brown RG, "Normocytic and Macrocytic Anemias," *Postgrad Med*, 1991, 89(8):125-32, 135-6.

Fraser CG, Wilkinson SP, Neville RG, et al, "Biologic Variation of Common Hematologic Laboratory Quantities in the Elderly," *Am J Clin Pathol*, 1989, 92(4):465-70.

Kjeldsberg CR, "Principles of Hematologic Examination," *Wintrobe's Clinical Hematology*, Chapter 2, Lee GR, Bithell TC, Foerster J, et al, eds, Philadelphia, PA: Lea & Febiger, 1993, 7-37.

Koepke JA, "Quantitative Blood Cell Counting," *Practical Laboratory Hematology*, Chapter 3, Koepke JA, ed, New York, NY: Churchill Livingstone, 1991, 43-60.

Van Assendelft OW, "Interpretation of the Quantitative Blood Cell Count," *Practical Laboratory Hematology*, Chapter 4, Koepke J, ed, New York, NY: Churchill Livingstone, 1991, 61-98.

Williams WJ, Beutler E, Erslev AJ, et al, *Hematology*, 4th ed, New York, NY: McGraw-Hill Inc, 1990, 10-5.

Red Blood Cell Morphology *see* Peripheral Blood: Red Blood Cell Morphology *on page 584*

Red Cell Count

***CPT** 85041*

See Also Anemia Flowchart in the Hematology Appendix

Related Information

Complete Blood Count *on page 533*
Erythropoietin, Serum *on page 214*
Ferritin, Serum *on page 220*
Hematocrit *on page 552*
Hemoglobin *on page 554*
Peripheral Blood: Red Blood Cell Morphology *on page 584*
Red Blood Cell Indices *on page 592*
Vitamin B_{12} *on page 612*

Synonyms Erythrocyte Count; RBC; Red Blood Cell Count

Specimen Whole blood **CONTAINER:** Lavender top (EDTA) tube for venipuncture specimen; properly filled lavender top Microtainer™ tubes for capillary specimen **CAUSES FOR REJECTION:** Hemolyzed or clotted specimen

Interpretive **REFERENCE RANGE:** Male: 4.6-6.0 x $10^6/mm^3$; female: 3.9-5.5 x $10^6/mm^3$. See Complete Blood Count for age related normals. **USE:** Evaluate anemia, polycythemia **LIMITATIONS:** Presence of cold agglutinins may result in falsely low RBC counts. Modern electronic cell counters have a level of precision and accuracy greatly improved over manual counting techniques. With correct threshold setting, properly controlled and functioning instrumentation, reliability, and reproducibility of the RBC count is equivalent to or better than most laboratory tests. Surveys (College of American Pathologists) indicate a coefficient of variation (CV) of 1% to 2%. Some instruments commonly perform with CVs <1%. Between laboratory precision has been reported as 2.8%.[1] **METHODOLOGY:** Manual hemocytometer chamber count of diluted blood sample or electronic counting and sizing of red cells made to flow through a fine aperture or capillary, microcomputer control and analysis of data developed from changes in impedance or flow past a laser beam **ADDITIONAL INFORMATION:** Decrease in RBC count may be the result of red cell loss by bleeding or hemolysis, (intravascular or extravascular), failure of marrow production (due to a broad variety of causes), or may be secondary to dilutional factors (eg, intravenous fluids). Increase in RBC count may be the result of primary polycythemia (polycythemia vera) or secondary polycythemia (hypoxemia of lung or cardiovascular disease, increased erythropoietin production associated with renal cyst, renal cell carcinoma, cerebellar hemangioblastoma, or high O_2 affinity hemoglobinopathy) including stress polycythemia (hemoconcentration associated with exercise, exertion, fright, etc). RBC count is normally higher in individuals residing at high altitudes.

Footnotes

1. Elevitch FR and Noce PS, eds, *Data ReCap: 1970-1980. A Compilation of Data From College of American Pathologists Clinical Laboratory Improvement Programs*, Skokie, IL: College of American Pathologists, 1981, 216-7.

References

Henry JB, Nelson DA, Tomar RH, et al, *Clinical Diagnosis and Management by Laboratory Methods*, 18th ed, Philadelphia, PA: WB Saunders Co, 1991, 562-3.

Red Cell Folate *see* Folic Acid, RBC *on page 544*

Red Cell Fragility *see* Osmotic Fragility *on page 573*

Red Cell Fragility *see* Osmotic Fragility, Incubated *on page 575*

Red Cell Mass

CPT *78120 (single sample); 78121 (multiple samples)*

Related Information

Blood Volume *on page 522*
Erythropoietin, Serum *on page 214*
Hematocrit *on page 552*
Hemoglobin *on page 554*

Synonyms ^{51}Cr Labeled Red Cell Volume; Red Cell Volume

Test Commonly Includes Red cell mass, plasma volume, and total blood volume

Specimen Laboratory will usually manage sampling and reinjecting. **SPECIAL INSTRUCTIONS:** May require scheduling with laboratory in order to procure radioisotope. Patient's weight and height must be made available to the laboratory.

Interpretive **REFERENCE RANGE:** Male: 28.2 ± 4 mL/kg; female: 24.2 ± 2.6 mL/kg.[1] See table for reference values relating to body surface area. **USE:** Determine red cell mass; support the diagnosis of polycythemia vera; monitor therapy with antineoplastic drugs **LIMITATIONS:** Radiation from isotopes used in bone scans, liver scans, brain scans, and other isotope procedures may interfere with red cell mass determination. Application of "normal range" tables based on weight and height must be made cautiously. An individual patient may not be comparable to the normal (eg, severely edematous individuals). Dilutional relationship will be unrepresentative and RBC mass overestimated. Severe edema might also be associated with isotope loss but is especially problematic due to unrepresentative normal range comparisons. Test is expensive and time consuming. **CONTRAINDICATIONS:** Severe active bleeding **METHODOLOGY:** Patient blood sample is drawn, red cells are labeled with ^{51}Cr and then reinjected into patient. Separate blood samples are obtained prior to injection and at a timed interval after injection. RBC mass is calculated on the basis of dilution principle. While other isotope labels are used, ^{51}Cr is the most convenient and widely used. Technetium-99m can be used for red cell mass determination after treatment of patient's red blood cells with stannous ion ($SnCl_2$) before incubation with pertechnetate. This results in the binding of nearly all of the added technetium to pa-

Formulas for Calculating RBC Volume Reference Values From Body Surface Area (S)

Men	RCV = (1100) (S) RCV = (1486) (S^2) – (4106) (S) + 4514 RCV = (1550) (S) – 890
Women	RCV = (840) (S) RCV = (1167) (S) – 479

From International Committee for Standardization in Hematology," "Recommended Methods for Measurement of Red Cell and Plasma Volume: *J Nucl Med,* 1980, 21:793–800, with permission.

(Continued)

Red Cell Mass *(Continued)*

tient's red cells. **ADDITIONAL INFORMATION:** The assessment of anemia and polycythemia (assessment of whether or not one of these conditions truly exists) depends foremost upon a reliable and direct determination of red cell volume. RBC count, Hgb level, and Hct provide only concentration parameters, the measured number or amount relative to the solution in which it exists. In a number of clinical situations (eg, acute blood loss) the RBC count, Hgb, and Hct will not indicate the actual decrease or increase in circulating red cell mass. Components (RBC count, etc) do correlate with RBC volume. Due to technical complexity (resulting in high cost and prolonged turnaround time) CBC is usually used, especially for follow-up or monitoring situations, even though RBC mass study would provide a more meaningful result. Nevertheless, some clinical situations (eg, polycythemia, complicated fluid and electrolyte management problems) will benefit from at least initial red cell volume determination.

Causes of decreased red cell volume include anemia, nutritional (iron, B_{12}, folate deficit, etc), hemolytic (intravascular or extravascular hemolysis), production deficit (marrow failure, drug or chemical related), acute and/or chronic blood loss; acute blood loss (decreased RBC volume may be present with normal or increased Hgb/Hct/RBC count); chronic disease (inflammation/infection); radiation, starvation, or severe edema.

Causes of increased red cell volume include: a) polycythemia vera ("primary" polycythemia); b) secondary polycythemia, hypoxia may be due to **lung disease** (eg, emphysema, Pickwickian syndrome); **CV disease** with right to left shunt or due to high altitude; **Hemoglobin variants** eg, high O_2 affinity hemoglobinopathies such as Hb $M_{Saskatoon}$ and Hb $M_{Hyde\ Park}$, methemoglobinemia, carboxyhemoglobinemia (increased CO due to smoking), **erythropoietin producing tumors/cysts**, rarely (eg, renal cyst, renal cell adenocarcinoma, hepatoma, large uterine myomas, cerebellar hemangioblastoma) or, **hereditary overproduction of erythropoietin**;[2] and c) stress (relative, spurious, pseudo, benign) polycythemia; due to decreased plasma volume, as in cases of severe dehydration, burns, fluid and electrolyte abnormalities with Addison's or Cushing's diseases. Also relative polycythemia is seen in a population of "stressed" hypertensive middle aged males. The table shows relationship between increased and decreased red cell and plasma volumes.

Clinical Effect of Variable Relationship Between Red Cell Volume and Plasma Volume

Red Cell Volume	Plasma Volume	Cause	Effect
Normal	High	Pregnancy Cirrhosis Nephritis Congestive cardiac failure	Pseudoanemia
Normal	Low	Stress Peripheral circulatory failure Dehydration Edema Prolonged bed rest	Pseudopolycythemia
Low	Normal	Anemia	Accurate reflection of degree of anemia
Low	High	Anemia	Anemia less severe than indicated by blood count
Low	Low	Hemorrhage Severe anemia (when hematocrit <0.2)	Anemia more severe than indicated by blood count
High	Normal to low	Polycythemia	Accurate reflection of polycythemia or polycythemia less severe than apparent
High	High	Polycythemia (when hematocrit >0.5)	Polycythemia more severe than apparent
Normal or even high	High	Marked splenomegaly	Pseudoanemia

From Dacie JV and Lewis SM, *Practical Haematology*, 7th ed, New York, NY: Churchill Livingstone, 1991, 362, with permission.

Footnotes

1. Henry JB, *Todd-Sanford-Davidsohn Clinical Diagnosis and Management by Laboratory Methods*, 18th ed, Philadelphia, PA: WB Saunders Co, 1991, 1015-6.
2. Yonemitsu H, Yamaguchi K, Shigeta H, et al, "Two Cases of Familial Erythrocytosis With Increased Erythropoietin Activity in Plasma and Urine," *Blood*, 1973, 42:793-7.

References

Dacie JV and Lewis SM, *Practical Haematology*, 7th ed, New York, NY: Churchill Livingstone, 1991, 361-9.

"Recommended Methods for Measurement of Red Cell and Plasma Volume: International Committee for Standardization in Hematology," *J Nucl Med*, 1980, 21:793-800.

Red Cell Survival *see* ^{51}Cr Red Cell Survival *on page 536*

Red Cell Volume *see* Blood Volume *on page 522*

Red Cell Volume *see* Red Cell Mass *on page 595*

Retic Count *see* Reticulocyte Count *on this page*

Reticulocyte Count

CPT *85044 (manual); 85045 (flow cytometry)*

See Also Anemia Flowchart in the Hematology Appendix

Related Information

^{51}Cr Red Cell Survival *on page 536*
Heinz Body Stain *on page 551*
Hematocrit *on page 552*
Hemoglobin *on page 554*
Hemoglobin Electrophoresis *on page 556*
Osmotic Fragility *on page 573*
Red Blood Cell Enzyme Deficiency Screen *on page 592*
Sickle Cell Tests *on page 600*

Synonyms Retic Count

Specimen Whole blood **CONTAINER:** Lavender top (EDTA) tube or green top (heparin) tube for venipuncture specimen; heparinized capillary tube for capillary specimen **STORAGE INSTRUCTIONS:** Store EDTA anticoagulated blood at room temperature for up to 48 hours. **CAUSES FOR REJECTION:** Clotted or hemolyzed specimen

Interpretive **REFERENCE RANGE:** Adults: 0.5% to 1.5%; newborns: ≤7%, expressed as a percentage of 1000 RBCs. Normal values at birth: 2.5% to 6.5%, falling to normal adult level by the end of the second week. The elderly (older than 70 years of age) have a slightly higher percent of reticulocytes than young individuals but still fall within the normal range.[1] **USE:** Evaluate erythropoietic activity. Increased in acute and chronic hemorrhage, hemolytic anemias. Evaluate erythropoietic response to therapy of various anemias. **The test is underutilized, especially when one considers it is at a pivotal decision-making conjuncture.** The reticulocyte production index will decide if one is working with a hyperproliferative or nonproliferative anemia, and thus, which tests should be subsequently ordered. **LIMITATIONS:** In recently transfused patients reticulocytes may decrease on a dilutional basis due to transfusion. **CONTRAINDICATIONS:** Patients receiving a large number of blood transfusions **METHODOLOGY:** Vital stains, new methylene blue is commonly used; brilliant cresyl blue may be used. Recently, flow cytometric methods have been developed that have the advantage of reproducibility.[2] The disadvantage is that not every laboratory has a flow cytometer. The assay may be adapted to standard hematology instruments in the future. **ADDITIONAL INFORMATION:** Demonstration of an increase in the number of circulating reticulocytes provides reliable and inexpensive evidence of increased red cell production. Care should be exercised during interpretation of results that an apparent increase in reticulocytes is not the result of decrease in the number of nonreticulated RBCs (ie, anemia with fewer mature red cells). A variety of corrections have been proposed and are in use. Absolute reticulocyte count = reticulocytes (%) x RBC count. This gives the number of reticulocytes per mm^3 of blood. Reticulocyte index (RI) = reticulocytes (%) x patient Hct/normal Hct or patient RBC/normal RBC or patient Hgb/normal Hgb. This corrects the reticulocyte count for anemia. Reticulocyte production index (RPI) = RI x (1/maturation time), or RPI = patient's absolute reticulocyte count/normal absolute reticulocyte count x (1/maturation time). Maturation time is usually taken as 2. RPI corrects for the premature release of reticulocytes from the marrow as might occur in cases of brisk hemolysis or significant bleeding. RPI gives a reticulocyte percent value that reliably estimates RBC production. Failure of marrow production would be reflected by anemia with absence of the expected

(Continued)

Reticulocyte Count *(Continued)*

increase in RPI.[3] Reticulocyte count should be performed prior to transfusion. Image recognition and flow cytometry methods of reticulocyte determination appear to provide greater precision and comparable accuracy compared to the manual method for reticulocyte counting.[4,5,6]

Footnotes

1. Kosower NS, "Altered Properties of Erythrocytes in the Aged," *Am J Hematol*, 1993, 42(3):241-7.
2. Metzger DK and Charache S, "Flow Cytometric Reticulocyte Counting With Thioflavin T in a Clinical Hematology Laboratory," *Arch Pathol Lab Med*, 1987, 111:540-4.
3. Prouty HW, "Correcting the Reticulocyte Count," *Lab Med*, 1979, 10:161-3.
4. Hackney JR, Cembrowksi GS, Prystowsky MB, et al, "Automated Reticulocyte Counting by Image Analysis and Flow Cytometry," *Lab Med*, 1989, 20:551-5.
5. Pappas AA, Owens RB, and Flick JT, "Reticulocyte Counting by Flow Cytometry. A Comparison With Manual Methods," *Ann Clin Lab Sci*, 1992, 22(2):125-32.
6. Serke S and Huhn D, "Improved Specificity of Determination of Immature Erythrocytes (Reticulocytes) by Multiparameter Flow-Cytometry and Thiazole Orange Using Combined Staining With Monoclonal Antibody ($_{anti}$-Glycophorin-A)," *Clin Lab Haematol*, 1993, 15(1):33-44.

References

Brecher G, "New Methylene Blue as a Reticulocyte Stain," *Am J Pathol*, 1949, 19:895.

Brown BA, *Hematology: Principles and Procedures*, 6th ed, Philadelphia, PA: Lea & Febiger, 1993, 111-6, 279-80, 386-90.

Davis BH and Bigelow NC, "Flow Cytometric Reticulocyte Analysis and the Reticulocyte Maturity Index," *Ann N Y Acad Sci*, 1993, 677:281-92.

Houwen B, "Reticulocyte Maturation," *Blood Cells*, 1992, 18(2):167-86.

Lee GR, "The Hemolytic Disorders: General Considerations," *Wintrobe's Clinical Hematology*, 9th ed, Chapter 32, Lee GR, Bithell TC, Foerster J, et al, eds, Philadelphia, PA: Lea and Febiger, 1993, 944-64.

Schilling Test

***CPT** 78270 (without intrinsic factor); 78271 (with intrinsic factor)*

See Also Anemia Flowchart in the Hematology Appendix

Related Information

Bone Marrow *on page 524*
Folic Acid, RBC *on page 544*
Folic Acid, Serum *on page 545*
Gastrin, Serum *on page 234*
Intrinsic Factor Antibody *on page 714*
Iron and Total Iron Binding Capacity/Transferrin *on page 262*
Parietal Cell Antibody *on page 730*
Peripheral Blood: Red Blood Cell Morphology *on page 584*
Red Blood Cell Indices *on page 592*
Vitamin B_{12} *on page 612*
Vitamin B_{12} Unsaturated Binding Capacity *on page 615*

Synonyms Radioactive Vitamin B_{12} Absorption Test With or Without Intrinsic Factor; Vitamin B_{12} Absorption Test

Test Commonly Includes Measure of B_{12} absorption before and after administration of intrinsic factor (two stage procedure)

Abstract *In vivo* test for pernicious anemia, vitamin B_{12} malabsorption, and integrity of distal small intestine

Patient Care PREPARATION: Patient must be fasting from midnight the day of the test. Patient should have received no B vitamins for a period of 3 days before the test.

Specimen CAUSES FOR REJECTION: Patient having radioisotope scan prior to test, patient receiving vitamin B_{12} prior to the test, patient not fasting, incomplete collection of urine, failure to administer the parenteral B_{12}, contamination of urine with stool (which will contain some unabsorbed B_{12})

Interpretive REFERENCE RANGE: Normal values vary with the laboratory and procedure used. Generally, >10% excretion in the urine of radioactive B_{12} indicates intact intrinsic factor (IF) function. When only a few percent of B_{12} absorption occurs without IF, with improvement into normal range with exogenous IF, the presence of pernicious anemia is essentially established. Poor absorption (<6% or 7%) with, as well as without, IF suggests intestinal malabsorption. USE: Assess vitamin B_{12} absorption in the diagnosis of malabsorption due to the lack of intrinsic factor, [eg, Addisonian (pernicious) anemia], a diagnostic adjunct in other defects of small intestinal absorption; evaluate extent of Crohn's disease in terminal ileum. Part I of the Schilling test is ^{57}Co by itself. If abnormal, 5 days later it is repeated with intrinsic factor administered orally at the same time (Part II). If this part of the test is still abnormal, it suggests that the cause is not gastric in origin (PA) but lower in the GI tract. Dual tracer assays have been available to perform both assays at once but caution should be exercised, as described by Zuckler et al[1]. **LIMITATIONS:** If other isotope tests are to be performed, Schilling test should be completed first. The presence of renal dysfunction, pancreatic insufficiency, bacterial overgrowth of intestinal content, antibodies against IF in gastric secretions, myxedema, liver disease, or any other condition resulting in the decreased absorption of B_{12} from the GI tract, its concentration in the liver, or its excretion in the urine may result in abnormal values. Incomplete urine collection may invalidate results. **METHODOLOGY:** Patient swallows radiolabeled B_{12} dose and receives a B_{12} intramuscular injection. The patient's urine is collected for 24 hours. The total activity from the B_{12} label is measured and calculated. The percent excretion of vitamin B_{12} is then determined. **ADDITIONAL INFORMATION:** B_{12} tagged with ^{57}Co without (and on a repeat test, as indicated, with) intrinsic factor is given orally. A large parenteral dose of unlabeled B_{12} is given 1 hour later to load the cyanocobalamin serum binding sites. All orally absorbed (radioactively-tagged) B_{12} will be excreted in the urine. The 24-hour urine is analyzed, radioactive ^{57}Co is counted. This radiopharmaceutical should not be administered to patients who are pregnant or during lactation unless the information to be gained outweighs the potential hazards. The test should not be started within 2-3 days of a therapeutic dose (1000 μg) of B_{12} or previous Schilling test. Bone marrow examinations and B_{12} and folate levels must be obtained before the Schilling test is performed.

Fairbanks et al[2] have found that better separation of normal individuals from those with pernicious anemia occurs with oral B_{12} dose of <1 μg (eg, 0.5 μg). They further confirmed earlier reports that some patients with pernicious anemia do not absorb B_{12} adequately, even when given with IF. Such malabsorption is reversible so that after B_{12} therapy, the vitamin then is normally absorbed with IF (reversible malabsorption). These findings complicate the diagnosis of pernicious anemia using the Schilling test. The importance of establishing the diagnosis and commencing life-long B_{12} maintenance therapy (so as to reverse the severe effects of the megaloblastic anemia and nervous system degenerative process - combined systems disease) dictates that a combination of clinical and laboratory findings be considered. The laboratory picture should include appropriate abnormalities of RBC indices (in particular high MCV), presence of anemia, peripheral blood smear findings of oval macrocytes, tear drop shaped RBCs, leukopenia, thrombocytopenia, hypersegmented PMNs, megaloblastic marrow picture, decreased serum B_{12} level, usually increased serum LD, all to be correlated with Schilling test result and the clinical presentation.

Footnotes

1. Zuckler LS and Cherun LR, "Schilling Evaluation of Pernicious Anemia: Current Status," *J Nucl Med*, 1984, 25:1032-9.
2. Fairbanks VF, Wahner HW, and Phyliky RL, "Tests for Pernicious Anemia: The Schilling Test," *Mayo Clin Proc*, 1983, 58:541-4.

References

Carethers M, "Diagnosing Vitamin B_{12} Deficiency, A Common Geriatric Disorder," *Geriatrics*, 1988, 43:89-112.

Lindenbaum J, "Status of Laboratory Testing in the Diagnosis of Megaloblastic Anemia," *Blood*, 1983, 61:624-7.

Williams WJ, Beutler E, Erslev AJ, et al, *Hematology*, 4th ed, New York, NY: McGraw-Hill Inc, 1990, 462-4.

Schistocytes Smear *see* Peripheral Blood: Red Blood Cell Morphology *on page 584*

Sedimentation Rate *see* Sedimentation Rate, Erythrocyte *on this page*

Sedimentation Rate, Erythrocyte

CPT 85651

Related Information

C-Reactive Protein *on page 669*
Zeta Sedimentation Ratio *on page 617*

Synonyms Sedimentation Rate; Westergren Sed Rate

Abstract This test is not a very specific measure of inflammation and infection. It is used mainly to follow management of rheumatology patients.

Specimen Whole blood **CONTAINER:** Lavender top (EDTA) tube or citrated plasma in 4:1 dilution (9:1 dilution is **not** acceptable) **COLLECTION:** Specimen must be received within 12 hours of collection. **CAUSES FOR REJECTION:** Insufficient blood, clotted, hemolyzed specimen

(Continued)

Sedimentation Rate, Erythrocyte *(Continued)*

Interpretive REFERENCE RANGE: Male: younger than age 50: 0-15 mm/hour, older than age 50: 0-20 mm/hour; female: younger than age 50: 0-25 mm/hour, older than age 50: 0-30 mm/hour by Westergren method USE: Evaluate the nonspecific activity of infections, inflammatory states, autoimmune disorders, and plasma cell dyscrasias LIMITATIONS: Anemia and paraproteinemia invalidate results; some procedural methods may be associated with hazardous exposure of medical technologists to fresh whole blood. METHODOLOGY: Red cell sedimentation rate expressed in mm/hour, utilizing Westergren type sedimentation tubes. A validation procedure and method for the in laboratory production of a sedimentation rate reference material has been developed for and can be used for quality assurance programs.[1] ADDITIONAL INFORMATION: Elevations in fibrinogen, alpha- and beta-globulins (acute phase reactants), and immunoglobulins increase the sedimentation rate of red cells through plasma. The test is important in the diagnosis of temporal arteritis, as well as its management.[2] Use of the ESR, ZSR, and/or CRP may aid in the differential diagnosis of the anemia of chronic disease from iron deficiency anemia.[3]

Footnotes

1. Thomas RD, Westengard JC, Hay KL, et al, "Calibration and Validation for Erythrocyte Sedimentation Tests: Role of the International Committee on Standardization in Hematology Reference Procedure," *Arch Pathol Lab Med*, 1993, 117:719-23.
2. Wong RL and Kern JH, "Temporal Arteritis Without an Elevated Erythrocyte Sedimentation Rate," *Am J Med*, 1986, 80:959-64.
3. Johnson MA, "Iron: Nutrition Monitoring and Nutrition Status Assessment," *J Nutr*, 1990, 120(Suppl 11):1486-91.

References

Gambino R, DiRe JJ, Monteleone M, et al, "The Westergren Sedimentation Rate, Using K_3 EDTA," *Am J Clin Pathol*, 1965, 43:173-80.

Henry JB, Nelson DA, Tomar RH, et al, *Clinical Diagnosis and Management by Laboratory Methods*, 18th ed, Philadelphia, PA: WB Saunders Co, 1991, 599-601.

Singer JI and Buchino JJ, "Selected Laboratory in Pediatric Emergency Care," *Emerg Med Clin North Am*, 1986, 4:377-96.

Stuart J and Nash GB, "Technological Advances in Blood Rheology," *Crit Rev Clin Lab Sci*, 1990, 28(1):61-93.

Sed Rate *see* Zeta Sedimentation Ratio *on page 617*

Septicemia Detection, Buffy Coat Micromethod *see* Bacteremia Detection, Buffy Coat Micromethod *on page 520*

Serum Folate *see* Folic Acid, Serum *on page 545*

Serum Lysis *see* Ham Test *on page 549*

Serum Viscosity *see* Viscosity, Serum/Plasma *on page 611*

Sickle Cell Preparation, Metabisulfite Test *see* Sickle Cell Tests *on this page*

Sickle Cell Solubility Test *see* Sickle Cell Tests *on this page*

Sickle Cells Smear *see* Peripheral Blood: Red Blood Cell Morphology *on page 584*

Sickle Cell Tests

CPT *83020 (electrophoresis); 85660 (reduction slide method)*

See Also Anemia Flowchart in the Hematology Appendix

Related Information

Cytapheresis, Therapeutic *on page 1060*
Fetal Hemoglobin *on page 542*
Hemoglobin *on page 554*
Hemoglobin Electrophoresis *on page 556*
Reticulocyte Count *on page 597*

Synonyms Dithionite Test; Itano Solubility Test; Murayama Test; Sickle Cell Preparation, Metabisulfite Test; Sickle Cell Solubility Test; Sickledex™

Test Commonly Includes A variety of similar but usually slightly modified tests have been developed, described, and achieved varying degrees of acceptance. In some institutions a positive is confirmed by performing an alternate confirmatory sickle cell test and/or hemoglobin electrophoresis (the preferred procedure).

Abstract Screening tests for sickle cell anemia and related entities which include hemoglobin S.

Specimen Whole blood **CONTAINER:** Lavender top (EDTA) tube for venipuncture specimen; lavender top Microtainer™ for capillary specimen **COLLECTION:** Routine venipuncture. Invert tube gently to mix. **CAUSES FOR REJECTION:** Clotted specimen, hemolyzed specimen

Interpretive **REFERENCE RANGE:** Negative **USE:** Detect sickling hemoglobins; evaluate hemolytic anemia, undiagnosed hereditary anemia with morphologic (sickle-like) abnormalities on peripheral blood smear **LIMITATIONS:** False-positive solubility test for sickling may be due to polycythemic blood; excess blood in relationship to the quantity of reagent; interference by some forms of hyperglobulinemia (if suspect, test should be repeated using patient's washed red cells); and a variety of abnormal hemoglobins including I, Bart's, $C_{Georgetown}$, Alexandra, C_{Harlem}, Porto Alegre, Memphis/S, $C_{Ziguinchor}$ and S_{Travis}. False-negative solubility test reaction may occur with inadequate quantities of blood from anemic patients (hemoglobin levels <8.0 g/dL); deterioration of reducing agents (detected by negative result on positive control); deterioration of the lytic agent (detected by negativity of positive control); improper illumination and visualization of the line-reader scale and high concentration of Hb F or of phenothiazines may inhibit the sickle reaction; quantities of hemoglobin S too small to detect, as at birth or with transfusions of nonhemoglobin S into patients with hemoglobin S. The appearance of hemoglobin S is genetically delayed and is not usually present in sufficient quantity for a positive screening test result until after 3 months of age. Maximum levels are not reached until about 6 months of age. Solubility tests and sodium metabisulfite test are unlikely to be reliably positive until after 6 months of age. **METHODOLOGY:** Hgb high salt solubility – Sickledex™ and a number of other commercially available products; alternate: slide test with 2% sodium metabisulfite **ADDITIONAL INFORMATION:** Hb S is the result of a single amino acid substitution (valine for the normally present glutamic acid) at the 6th position of the β-globin chain of the hemoglobin molecule. The homozygous state results in sickle cell disease, a condition with significant morbidity and mortality. The heterozygous state causes sickle trait, a condition ordinarily characterized by little or no morbidity. Sickle disease presents a spectrum of clinical severity. Amelioration results from coincidental occurrence of other hemoglobinopathies, notably those with increased levels of Hb F (eg, thalassemia and different types of hereditary persistence of fetal hemoglobin). Variation in clinical expression is also the result of DNA polymorphism in the β-globin gene cluster.[1,2]

The incidence of sickle cell trait amongst African Americans in the U.S. is 8.5%. Because of possible anterior segment ischemia (a significant complication of retinal detachment surgery) that may occur in otherwise asymptomatic sickle trait individuals, it has been recommended that blacks undergo preoperative sickle tests prior to such procedures.[3]

Distinction between Hb S beta-thalassemia and sickle cell anemia is not always possible on clinical, hematologic, or electrophoretic grounds. Thalassemia heterozygotes have hypochromia and microcytosis, but overlap values exist. Differentiation can best be made by family or molecular pathology methods. Regional prevalence in the midwest area of Hb S beta-thalassemia is estimated to be 1:23,000 of the black population. It is recommended that positive sickle cell screen patients be further evaluated with cellulose acetate or agarose gel hemoglobin electrophoresis at pH 8.6, citrate agar gel electrophoresis at pH 6.0, Hb F studies and family studies. Complete characterization may require sophisticated laboratory studies with DNA amplification.[4] Erythrocyte ecdysis (long free filamentous processes stripping away from the surface of red cells) has been described in sickle cell anemia associated with elevated cold agglutinin titer.[5]

Survey testing to determine the incidence and significance of hereditary anemias (including the sickle hemoglobinopathies) continues on a worldwide basis.[6,7,8] The application of molecular biologic (DNA) based techniques for population screening is currently cost prohibitive but in future years is likely to be the preferred method for detection of sickle hemoglobinopathies, in particular for detection of the heterozygous states.[9,10]

A survey of laboratory results, methods and problems in screening for sickle cell disease with emphasis on laboratory responsibilities has recently been published by the US Department of Health and Human Services.[11]

The rare condition, "hemoglobin Munchausen" has been reviewed.[12]

Footnotes

1. El-Hazmi MA, Bahakim HM, and Warsy AS, "DNA Polymorphism in the Beta-Globin Gene Cluster in Saudi Arabs: Relation to Severity of Sickle Cell Anaemia," *Acta Haematol*, 1992, 88(2-3):61-6.
2. El-Hazmi MA, "Heterogeneity and Variation of Clinical and Haematological Expression of Haemoglobin S in Saudi Arabs," *Acta Haematol*, 1992, 88(2-3):67-71.

(Continued)

Sickle Cell Tests *(Continued)*

3. Cartwright MJ, Blair CJ, Combs JL, et al, "Anterior Segment Ischemia: A Complication of Retinal Detachment Repair in a Patient With Sickle Cell Trait," *Ann Ophthalmol*, 1990, 22(9):333-4.
4. Chehab FF and Kan YW, "Detection of Sickle Cell Anaemia Mutation by Colour DNA Amplification," *Lancet*, 1990, 335(8680):15-7.
5. Ward PC, Smith CM, and White JG, "Erythrocytic Ecdysis: An Unusual Morphologic Finding in a Case of Sickle Cell Anemia With Intercurrent Cold Agglutinin Syndrome," *Am J Clin Pathol*, 1979, 72:479-85.
6. Aluoch JR and Aluoch LH, "Survey of Sickle Disease in Kenya," *Trop Geogr Med*, 1993, 45:18-21.
7. Ali M and Lafferty J, "The Clinical Significance of Hemoglobinopathies in the Hamilton Region: A Twenty Year Review," *Clin Invest Med*, 1992, 15(5):401-5.
8. Martins MC, Olim G, Melo J, et al, "Hereditary Anaemias in Portugal: Epidemiology, Public Health Significance, and Control," *J Med Genet*, 1993, 30(3):235-9.
9. Steinberg MH, "DNA Diagnosis for the Detection of Sickle Hemoglobinopathies," *Am J Hematol*, 1993, 43:110-5.
10. McCabe ER, "Genetic Screening for the Next Decade: Application of Present and New Technologies," *Yale J Biol Med*, 1991, 64(1):9-14.
11. Guideline: Laboratory Screening for Sickle Cell Disease, U.S. Department of Health and Human Services, *Lab Med*, 1993, 24(8):515-22.
12. Ballas SK, "Munchausen Sickle Cell Painful Crisis," *Ann Clin Lab Med*, 1992, 22(4):226-8.

References

Huisman TH, "Sickle Cell Anemia as a Syndrome: A Review of Diagnostic Features," *Am J Hematol*, 1979, 6:173-84.

Serjeant GR, *Sickle Cell Disease*, 2nd ed, Oxford, England: Oxford U Pr, 1992.

Steinberg MH and Dreiling BJ, "Clinical, Hematologic and Biosynthetic Studies in Sickle Cell Beta-Thalassemia: A Comparison With Sickle Cell Anemia," *Am J Hematol*, 1976, 1:35-44.

Sickledex™ *see* Sickle Cell Tests *on page 600*

Sideroblast Stain *see* Iron Stain, Bone Marrow *on page 562*

Siderocyte Stain

CPT 85535

Related Information

Iron Stain, Bone Marrow *on page 562*

Synonyms Hemosiderin Stain; Iron Stain; Pappenheimer Body Stain

Specimen Blood: coverslip or slide smears; bone marrow: coverslip smears preferred

Interpretive **REFERENCE RANGE:** Peripheral blood: no siderocytes identified; bone marrow: stainable iron present **USE:** Detect sideroblastic anemias and hemolytic anemia; semiquantitation of marrow iron stores evaluation of iron reserve; assist in the diagnosis of iron deficiency and hemosiderosis/hemochromatosis **LIMITATIONS:** Siderocytes may be present in asplenic patients. **METHODOLOGY:** Prussian blue (potassium ferrocyanide) reaction **ADDITIONAL INFORMATION:** Siderotic granules represent iron not yet incorporated into hemoglobin and occur primarily when there is impaired hemoglobin synthesis (eg, sideroblastic anemia, lead poisoning). Savage et al[1] have shown that 36% of alcoholic patients with bone marrow proven sideroblastic anemia have siderocytes in the peripheral blood. Otherwise, siderocytes are uncommon in the peripheral blood unless a splenectomy has been performed on the patient. Iron staining of bone marrow is more important in terms of deciding on questionable causes of anemia. Numerous siderocytes are noted postsplenectomy and in some hemoglobinopathies. They are absent with iron deficiency.

Footnotes

1. Savage D and Lindenbaum J, "Anemia in Alcoholics," *Medicine (Baltimore)*, 1986, 65:322-38.

References

Douglas AS and Dacie JV, "The Incidence and Significance of Iron Containing Granules in Human Erythrocytes and Their Precursors," *J Clin Pathol*, 1953, 6:307.

Williams WJ, Beutler E, Erslev AJ, et al, *Hematology*, 4th ed, New York, NY: McGraw-Hill Inc, 1990, 1703-8.

Small Molecule Diseases *see* Tests for Uncommon Inherited Diseases of Metabolism and Cell Structure *on page 605*

Spherocytes Smear *see* Peripheral Blood: Red Blood Cell Morphology *on page 584*

Sphingolipidoses *see* Tests for Uncommon Inherited Diseases of Metabolism and Cell Structure *on page 605*

Sphingomyelinase *see* Tests for Uncommon Inherited Diseases of Metabolism and Cell Structure *on page 605*

Sputum Smear for Eosinophils *see* Eosinophil Smear *on page 541*

Stippled RBCs Smear *see* Peripheral Blood: Red Blood Cell Morphology *on page 584*

Sucrose Hemolysis Test *see* Sugar Water Test Screen *on this page*

Sudan Black Stain *see* Leukocyte Cytochemistry *on page 567*

Sugar Water Test Screen

CPT *86941*

Related Information

Ham Test *on page 549*

Synonyms PNH Test Screen; Sucrose Hemolysis Test

Test Commonly Includes Sucrose hemolysis if hemolysis is found in the sugar water screen test

Abstract The screening test for suspected paroxysmal nocturnal hemoglobinuria (PNH). Confirm with the Ham test.

Specimen Blood **CONTAINER:** Blue top (sodium citrate) tube **CAUSES FOR REJECTION:** Specimen clotted, hemolyzed specimens

Interpretive **REFERENCE RANGE:** Absence of hemolysis is the normal condition. If no hemolysis is present, the patient probably does not have PNH provided multiple recent transfusions have not reduced the proportion of abnormal cells. The screening test is not definitive. **USE:** Screen for PNH **LIMITATIONS:** False-positives may be seen in cases of megaloblastic anemias and autoimmune hemolytic anemias. False-negative results may occur if heparin or EDTA is used as an anticoagulant. **METHODOLOGY:** Erythrocytes exposed to a solution of low ionic strength (sucrose in water) will fix complement to the cell surface. PNH red cells have unusual susceptibility to complement and will hemolyze under these conditions. **ADDITIONAL INFORMATION:** If the sugar water test is positive, a subsequent Ham test is strongly recommended. A negative sugar water test rules out PNH in most instances, provided the proportion of patient cells has not been reduced by previous transfusion. It has been demonstrated that the most complement sensitive cells in PNH are younger RBCs and reticulocytes. Increased sensitivity can be obtained for the assays by separating young RBCs from old by centrifugation.[1]

Footnotes

1. Shimoda M and Yawata Y, "An Increased Calcium Accumulation in ATP-Dependent Red Cells of the Patients With Paroxysmal Nocturnal Hemoglobinuria," *Am J Hematol*, 1985, 20:325-35.

References

Hartmann RC and Jenkins DE, "The "Sugar Water" Test for Paroxysmal Nocturnal Hemoglobinuria," *N Engl J Med*, 1966, 275:155-7.

Williams WJ, Beutler E, Erslev AJ, et al, *Hematology*, 4th ed, New York, NY: McGraw-Hill Inc, 1990, 1729-30.

Sulfatidase *see* Tests for Uncommon Inherited Diseases of Metabolism and Cell Structure *on page 605*

Survival of Red Blood Cells *see* ^{51}Cr Red Cell Survival *on page 536*

Tartrate Resistant Leukocyte Acid Phosphatase

CPT *88313*

Related Information

Leukocyte Cytochemistry *on page 567*

Lymph Node Biopsy *on page 72*

Synonyms Acid Phosphatase, Tartrate Resistant, Leukocytes; Hairy Cell Leukemia Test; Leukemic Reticuloendotheliosis Test; Leukocyte Acid Phosphatase; TRAP Test

Test Commonly Includes Leukocyte acid phosphatase reaction with and without tartrate inhibition

Specimen Glass microscope slide smears prepared from fresh capillary or heparinized whole blood, fixed immediately (glutaraldehyde-acetone) after preparation **CONTAINER:** Green top (heparin) tube **STORAGE INSTRUCTIONS:** Smeared glass slides may be stored at least 1 week prior to assay if fixed immediately after preparation. **CAUSES FOR REJECTION:** Smears unfixed, blood not fresh

(Continued)

Tartrate Resistant Leukocyte Acid Phosphatase *(Continued)*

Interpretive REFERENCE RANGE: Most white cells of peripheral blood as well as platelets are acid phosphatase positive. Most white cells of blood have the acid phosphatase reaction inhibited by L(+) tartrate. USE: Diagnose "hairy cell leukemia" ("leukemic reticuloendotheliosis") METHODOLOGY: Naphthol AS-BI, fast garnet GBC, with and without L(+) tartaric acid ADDITIONAL INFORMATION: There are some six isoenzymes of leukocyte acid phosphatase. Of the six, isoenzyme V is not inhibited by L(+) tartrate acid. It has been found that the malignant mononuclear cells of leukemic reticuloendotheliosis ("hairy cell leukemia") contain isoenzyme V and are resistant to inhibition by L(+) tartaric acid. There is evidence the reaction is not entirely specific as tartrate resistant acid phosphatase reactions have been reported in cases of prolymphocytic leukemia and malignant lymphoma as well as some cases of infectious mononucleosis.[1] There have also been reports of rare false-negative results (patients with leukemic reticuloendotheliosis having negative tartrate resistant acid phosphatase reactions). Recently, a new assay based on antibody against band V acid phosphatase has been described. The immunoassay has greater specificity[2] than the standard cytochemical procedure.

Footnotes

1. Brown BA, *Hematology: Principles and Practice*, 6th ed, Philadelphia, PA: Lea & Febiger, 1993, 137-8.
2. Whitaker KB, Cox TM, and Moss DW, "An Immunoassay of Human Band-5 (Tartrate Resistant) Acid Phosphatase That Involves the Use of Antiporcine Uteroferrin Antibodies," *Clin Chem* 1989, 35(1):86-9.

References

Williams WJ, Beutler E, Erslev AJ, et al, *Hematology*, 4th ed, New York, NY: McGraw-Hill Inc, 1990, 1750-1.

Yam LT, Phyliky RL, and Li CY, "Benign and Neoplastic Disorders Simulating Hairy Cell Leukemia," *Semin Oncol*, 1984, 11:353-61.

TdT *see* Terminal Deoxynucleotidyl Transferase *on this page*

Terminal Deoxynucleotidyl Transferase

CPT 85999

Related Information

Bone Marrow *on page 524*
Immunophenotypic Analysis of Tissues by Flow Cytometry *on page 65*
Lymph Node Biopsy *on page 72*

Synonyms TdT; Terminal Deoxyribonucleotidyl Transferase; Terminal Transferase

Specimen Blood or bone marrow (avoid heparin) for leukocyte separation, pelletization, and storage at -20°C. Glass slide smears, air dried, of blood or marrow COLLECTION: Store dried smears at room temperature for up to 5 days.

Interpretive REFERENCE RANGE: Peripheral blood: negative for TdT-positive cells; bone marrow: <1.8% TdT-positive cells USE: Classify certain leukemias and lymphomas, normally used to distinguish lymphoblastic from nonlymphoblastic leukemia; diagnose acute lymphoblastic leukemia, lymphoid blast crisis of chronic myelogenous leukemia, and lymphoblastic lymphomas METHODOLOGY: Enzyme-linked immunosorbent assay (ELISA), indirect fluorescent antibody (IFA), peroxidase-antiperoxidase, avidin-biotin, immunoperoxidase, and incorporation of radiolabeled thymidine. A variety of methods for the enzyme assay of Ficoll/Hypaque® separated cell extracts have been described.[1] The radiometric assays are technically difficult and are usually available only in a research setting. Avidin-biotin immunoperoxidase[2] and flow cytometric[3] methods have been developed. ADDITIONAL INFORMATION: TdT acts to catalyze the polymerization of deoxynucleoside triphosphates (by addition to the 3' hydroxyl ends of oligodeoxynucleotides or polydeoxynucleotides without DNA template instructions). Thymus is the primary site of TdT positive cells and TdT is found in the nucleus of the more primitive T cells. A thymus related population of TdT positive cells resides in the bone marrow (normally a minor population - 1% to 2%). TdT is increased in more than 90% of the cases of ALL of childhood.[1] This is true for even pre-B cell as well as B-

Terminal Deoxynucleotidyl Transferase (TdT) in Hematologic Disease

Disease	Percent Positive
Acute lymphoblastic leukemia	80–90
Lymphoblastic lymphoma	90
Chronic granulocytic leukemia in blast crisis	30
Acute undifferentiated leukemia	60
Acute nonlymphocytic leukemia	2–5

From Rubin E, MD and Farber JL, MD, *Pathology*, Philadelphia, PA: JB Lippincott Co, 1077, with permission.

cell ALL.[4] A minor (5% to 10%) population of patients with acute nonlymphoblastic leukemia have TdT positive blasts. TdT positive blasts are prominent in some cases of chronic myelogenous leukemia relating to the development of an acute blast phase. TdT has been reported to assist in establishing the diagnosis of acute lymphoblastic leukemia.[5] TdT positive cases of blast phase CML correlate with a positive response to chemotherapy (vincristine and prednisone).[6,7] Combined assessment of nuclear TdT and cell surface antigens may assist in the detection of minimal residual disease after therapy of acute leukemia.[8,9] A 1991 study found that frequency of response to chemotherapy, response duration, and overall survival did not correlate with TdT expression.[10]

Footnotes

1. Beutler E and Blume KG, "Terminal Deoxynucleotidyl Transferase: Biochemical Properties, Cellular Distribution, and Hematologic Significance," *Prog Hematol*, 1979, 11:47-63.
2. Miller RT and Groothuis CL, "Improved Avidin-Biotin Immunoperoxidase Method for Terminal Deoxyribonucleotidyl Transferase and Immunophenotypic Characterization of Blood Cells," *Am J Clin Pathol*, 1990, 93(5):670-4.
3. Almasri NM, Iturraspe JA, Benson NA, et al, "Flow Cytometric Analysis of Terminal Deoxynucleotidyl Transferase," *Am J Clin Pathol*, 1991, 95(3):376-80.
4. Michiels JJ, Adriaansen HJ, Hagemeijer A, et al, "TdT Positive B-Cell Acute Lymphoblastic Leukemia (B-ALL) Without Burkitt Characteristics," *Br J Haematol*, 1988, 68(4):423-6.
5. Braziel RM, Keneklis T, and Donlon JA, "Terminal Deoxynucleotidyl Transferase in Non-Hodgkin's Lymphoma," *Am J Clin Pathol*, 1983, 80:655-9.
6. Tanaka M, Kaneda T, Hirota Y, et al, "Terminal Deoxynucleotidyl Transferase in the Blastic Phase of Chronic Myelogenous Leukemia: An Indicator of Response to Vincristine and Prednisone Therapy," *Am J Hematol*, 1980, 9:287-93.
7. Paciucci PA, Keaveney Y, Cuttner J, et al, "Mitoxantrone Vincristine, and Prednisone in Adults With Relapsed or Primarily Refractory Acute Lymphocytic Leukemia and Terminal Deoxynucleotidyl Transferase Positive Blastic Phase Chronic Myelocytic Leukemia," *Cancer Res*, 1987, 47:5234-7.
8. Drach J, Gattringer C, and Huber H, "Combined Flow Cytometric Assessment of Cell Surface Antigens and Nuclear TdT for the Detection of Minimal Residual Disease in Acute Leukaemia," *Br J Haematol*, 1991, 77(1):37-42.
9. Smith RG and Kitchens RL, "Phenotypic Heterogeneity of TDT+ Cells in the Blood and Bone Marrow: Implications for Surveillance of Residual Leukemia," *Blood*, 1989, 74(1):312-9.
10. Gucalp R, Paietta E, Weinberg V, et al, "Terminal Transferase Expression in Acute Myeloid Leukaemia: Biology and Prognosis," *Br J Haematol*, 1991, 78(1):48-54.

Terminal Deoxyribonucleotidyl Transferase *see* Terminal Deoxynucleotidyl Transferase *on previous page*

Terminal Transferase *see* Terminal Deoxynucleotidyl Transferase *on previous page*

Test for Congenital Heinz Body Hemolytic Anemia *see* Hemoglobin, Unstable, Heat Labile Test *on page 560*

Test for D-L Antibody *see* Cold Hemolysin Test *on page 532*

Test for Paroxysmal Cold Hemoglobinuria *see* Cold Hemolysin Test *on page 532*

Tests for Uncommon Inherited Diseases of Metabolism and Cell Structure

CPT 85999

Related Information

Amniotic Fluid, Chromosome and Genetic Abnormality Analysis *on page 891*
Muscle Biopsy *on page 75*
Urinalysis *on page 1162*

Synonyms Glycogen Storage Diseases; Inborn Errors of Metabolism; Large Molecule Diseases; Lysosomal Storage Diseases; Mucopolysaccharidoses; Small Molecule Diseases; Sphingolipidoses

Applies to Acid β-Galactosidase; Ceramidase; Ceramidetrihexoside α-Galactosidase; α-Fucosidase; Galactocerebroside; β-Galactosidase; Glucocerebroside; β-Glucosidase; Hexosaminidase A; Hexosaminidase A and B; Neutral β-Galactosidase; Sphingomyelinase; Sulfatidase

Test Commonly Includes Under this heading recognition is given to an ever growing number of genetically determined disorders having a biochemical/metabolic defect (usually an enzyme deficiency or abnormality). The limitations of space allow only brief mention. Most of

(Continued)

Tests for Uncommon Inherited Diseases of Metabolism and Cell Structure *(Continued)*

these disorders can be categorized as to biochemical type (eg, sphingolipidoses, mucopolysaccharidoses, lysosomal storage diseases) with overlap between these concepts and with some independent entities.

Of some 250 diseases with a defined biochemical basis, a majority involve abnormalities in enzymes. The 6th (1989) edition of the monumental text, *The Metabolic Basis of Inherited Disease*, has descriptions of inborn errors of metabolism that include over 180 entities tabulated over 1020 pages. They are grouped by biochemical type (eg, carbohydrate, amino acid, lipoprotein/lipid, purine/pyrimidine, acid lipase), tissue/function type (eg, blood and blood forming organs, transport, peroxisome, immune, etc) and include a broad category, **disorders of lysosomal enzymes**, with which this listing will be largely concerned. The 8th edition of McKusik's *Mendelian Inheritance in Man* describes over 4500 inherited diseases at the beginning of 1989. This book is being constantly updated as a computerized database through John Hopkins University.

Patient Care PREPARATION: Appropriate preliminary studies may be critically important to allow narrowing the range of diagnostic testing possibilities. Such investigation might include eye examination (cherry red macula occurs in some gangliosidoses; corneal opacities in Fabry disease; optic atrophy in metachromatic leukodystrophy and Krabbe disease), blood/urine screening tests (Berry spot test positive in G_{M1} gangliosidosis, cetylpyridinium chloride citrate, or thin-layer chromatography for mucopolysaccharidoses (see reference by Pennock); anemia; vacuolated lymphocytes in fucosidosis), x-ray studies (for developmental changes in bone as with mucopolysaccharidoses, EEG, nerve conduction time, and bone marrow in search of inclusion bearing or foamy histocytes, eg, as with Gaucher cells).

Specimen The majority of tests in this area involve lysosomal enzymes, present in body tissues and fluids. Blood (serum, plasma, or white cells), urine, and tears are the most easily obtained samples for analysis. Solid tissue may be biopsied (eg, skin, liver, muscle). Most commonly used are serum, leukocytes, and culture fibroblasts (from tissue biopsy). Heparin anticoagulated whole blood, usually at least 5 mL is needed, along with the serum. Specimen preference may be disease dependent (eg, the α-glucosidase deficiency of Pompe disease is best detected by using cultured skin fibroblasts or skeletal muscle).[1] Leukocytes provide a favorable substrate for sphingolipidosis testing but for detection of heterozygotes of Niemann-Pick or Krabbe disease cultured fibroblasts are preferred.[1] Referral of a leukocyte pellet or biopsy in culture media or even a growing culture of fibroblasts may be required. SPECIAL INSTRUCTIONS: For a number of reasons (a sampling follows), the reference laboratory should be contacted before specimens are sent. Details of the preliminary findings can be reviewed, appropriate tests recommended, the preferred samples obtained, need for a clinical photograph established, mode of transport decided, and any other special requirement arranged.

Interpretive USE: Assist in the diagnosis of sphingolipid and mucopolysaccharide lysosomal storage diseases by demonstrating presence of a partial or complete enzyme deficiency. Major symptoms, lipids accumulating, and enzymes involved in the sphingolipidoses are given in the following table. METHODOLOGY: Tests for enzyme deficiency utilizing synthetic substrates (eg, monosaccharide derivatives of 4-methylumbelliferone) have found recent and growing application in this group of diseases.[2] In addition to serum or plasma assays, recent years have seen the fruitful application of tests utilizing pelleted leukocytes and fibroblast cultures. ADDITIONAL INFORMATION: One group of lysosomal storage diseases, the mucopolysaccharidoses are due to genetic defects in enzymes that degrade connective tissue glycosaminoglycan. The following table relates the type of mucopolysaccharidosis to the enzyme defect. Urine screening tests are available for initial diagnosis of these diseases.

A table of glycogen storage diseases follows. Most of these disorders of carbohydrate metabolism are not lysosomal storage diseases. They are all autosomal recessive except one form of liver phosphorylase kinase deficiency in which only males are affected and the inheritance is X-linked.[3]

Disease severity and symptoms vary widely with type and organ site of the defective enzyme activity.

The recognized spectrum of inherited abnormalities of metabolism and structure is continually enlarging. The majority are uncommon to rare, so that resources of equipment and experienced personnel for testing are justifiably limited to the specialized laboratory. Even so there are a sufficient number of laboratories performing these assays so as to raise the question if

Mucopolysaccharidoses

Type	Eponymic Designation	Lysosomal Enzyme Defect
I	Three allelic disorders Hurler-Scheie	α-L-iduronidase
II	Hunter severe, mild	iduronate sulfatase
III A-D	Four nonallelic disorders Sanfilippo syndromes A-D	IIIA heparan N-sulfatase
		IIIB N-acetyl-α-D-glucosaminidase
		IIIC acetyl-CoA: α-glucosaminide N-acetyl transferase
		IIID N-acetyl-α-D-glucosaminide 6-sulfate sulfatase
IV A,B	Two nonallelic disorders Morquio syndromes A,B	IVA galactosamine 6-sulfate sulfatase
		IVB β-galactosidase
VI	Several allelic types Maroteaux-Lamy syndrome	arylsulfatase B
VII	Sly syndrome	β-glucuronidase

Glycogen Storage Diseases

I	Von Gierke's Ia, Ib	Glucose-6-phosphatase
II	Pompe's infantile, adult form	Lysosomal α-1,4-glucosidase
III	Cori's Forbe's	Amylo-1,6-glucosidase (debrancher enzyme)
IV	Andersen's	Amylo-(1,4:1,6)-transglucosidase (brancher enzyme)
V	McArdle's	Muscle phosphorylase
VI	Hers', glycogenoses	Hepatic phosphorylase X-linked phosphorylase-b-kinase Autosomal phosphorylase-b-kinase
VII	Tarui's	Muscle phosphofructokinase

any one can develop necessary case experience. Dialogue between the referring physician and the specialty laboratory is essential (discussed above in relation to technical considerations) in particular because of the biochemical heterogeneity frequently seen with these conditions. Clinical expression may be variable and unpredictable.

Each of the sphingolipidoses represents not one but several diseases differing in clinical signs and/or enzyme activity. They are characterized by differing age of onset, site of pathology, and amount of residual enzyme activity (total or partial deficiency). As in Tay-Sachs disease more than one form of the involved enzyme may be present. Two lysosomal glycoproteins (hexosaminidase A and G_{M2} activator protein) account for the enzymatic hydrolysis of glycolipids (largely ganglioside G_{M2}). With defective lysosomal degradation, glycolipid accumulates in neurones. Hexosaminidase A is formed of subunits α and β, each under different chromosome control. Hexosaminidase, the enzyme involved exists as two isoenzymes, A and B. In Tay-Sachs disease, hexosaminidase A is decreased or absent while hexosaminidase B is increased. In Sandhoff's disease, a variant form of Tay-Sachs, there is deficiency of both hexosaminidase A and B due to hexosaminidase β-subunit defect (encoded on chromosome 5).[4]

(Continued)

Tests for Uncommon Inherited Diseases of Metabolism and Cell Structure *(Continued)*

In addition, the usual sources of variance may affect enzyme deficiency testing. The activity of β-N-acetyl hexosaminidases in Tay-Sachs is affected by pregnancy, chronic diseases of liver, heart, joints, endocrine system, skin and medications including oral contraceptives, some steroids, thyroid, and Butazolidin®. These factors do not affect the result of hexosaminidase assays performed on leukocytes, fibroblasts, or tears.

Sphingolipid storage diseases involve most cells of the body and thus are expressed as multisystem diseases. Gaucher's disease is the most common and may show hepatosplenomegaly, thrombocytopenia, erosion of bone with tendency to pathologic fracture and in a few cases, CNS involvement. All of the lipid storage diseases show autosomal recessive inheritance with the exception of Fabry's disease (which is transmitted as X-linked).

The advent of treatment strategies (eg, enzyme infusion[5,6]) and enzyme targeting may add further impetus to establishing the diagnosis, detection of carriers, and monitoring of pregnancies at risk (through amniocentesis and culturing of epithelial cells in the amniotic fluid).[7]

Steroid sulfatase deficiency, characterized clinically by low maternal estrogen excretion with normal fetal growth/development, is important to recognize by antenatal diagnosis so that it can be differentiated from more serious fetal defects that are associated with low estrogen levels.[8]

Peroxisomes, cellular organelles involved in oxidative functions are deficient in cases of Zellweger syndrome. There is accumulation of long chain fatty acids, phytanic acid, pipecolic acid, bile acid intermediates, and lack of plasmalogen biosynthesis. Other diseases in this group include adrenoleukodystrophy and a form of chondrodysplasia punctata.[9]

See the references by Applegarth et al and the text by Scriver et al for investigation of small molecule diseases; organic acid, urea cycle, and peroxisomal disorders.

The rapidly expanding field of molecular genetics as it applies to the diagnosis of inherited disease has been succinctly discussed with emphasis on the nature of available tests in a recent review by Ostrer and Hejtmancik (see references).

Sphingolipid Storage Diseases (Sphingolipidoses)

Disease	Signs and Symptoms	Enzyme Defect
Fabry's disease	Reddish-purple skin rash, kidney failure, pain in lower extremities	Ceramidetrihexoside α-galactosidase
Farber's disease	Hoarseness, dermatitis, skeletal deformation, mental retardation	Ceramidase
Fucosidosis	Cerebral degeneration, muscle spasticity, thick skin	α-fucosidase
Gaucher's disease	Spleen and liver enlargement, erosion of long bones and pelvis, mental retardation only in infantile form	Glucocerebroside β-glucosidase
Generalized gangliosidosis	Mental retardation, liver enlargement, skeletal deformities, about 50% with red spot in retina	β-galactosidase
Krabbe's disease (globoid leukodystrophy)	Mental retardation, almost total absence of myelin, globoid bodies in white matter of brain	Galactocerebroside β-galactosidase
Niemann-Pick disease type I, II and subtypes	Liver and spleen enlargement, mental retardation, about 30% with red spot in retina	Sphingomyelinase
Metachromatic leukodystrophy	Mental retardation, psychological disturbances in adult form, nerves stain yellow-brown with cresyl violet dye	Sulfatidase
Sandhoff's disease	Same as Tay-Sachs disease but progressing more rapidly	Hexosaminidase A and B
Shindler disease	Neurodegeneration, psychomotor retardation, cortical blindness, myoclonic seizures	α-N-acetyl-galactosaminidase
Tay-Sachs disease	Mental retardation, red spot in retina, blindness, muscular weakness	Hexosaminidase A

From Brady RO and Kolodny EH, "The Sphingolipid Storage Disorders: Diagnosis and Detection," *Lab Management,* 1982, 20:28, with permission.

Footnotes

1. Kolodny EH, "General Principles and Techniques of Case Identification, Carrier Testing, and Prenatal Diagnosis," *Practical Enzymology of the Sphingolipidoses, Laboratory and Research Methods in Biology and Medicine*, Glew RH and Peters SP, eds, New York, NY: Alan R Liss Inc, 1977, 1:35-7, 17.
2. Brady RO and Kolodny EH, "The Sphingolipid Storage Disorders: Diagnosis and Detection," *Lab Management*, 1982, 20:7, 30-2.
3. Hers H-G, Van Hoof F, and de Barsy T, "Glycogen Storage Diseases," *The Metabolic Basis of Inherited Disease*, 6th ed, Chapter 12, Scriver CR, Beaudet AL, Sly WS, et al, eds, New York, NY: McGraw-Hill Information Services Co, 1989, 425-52.
4. Sandhoff K, Conzelmann E, Neufeld EF, et al, "The G_{M2} Gangliosidoses," *The Metabolic Basis of Inherited Disease*, 6th ed, Scriver CR, Beaudet AL, Sly WS, et al, eds, New York, NY: McGraw-Hill Information Services Co, 1989, 1807.
5. Brady RO, Barranger JA, Gal AE, et al, "Treatment of Lipidoses by Enzyme Infusion," *Lysosomes and Lysosomal Storage Diseases*, Callahan JW and Lowden JA, eds, New York, NY: Raven Press, 1981, 373-9.
6. Neuwelt EA, Barranger JA, Brady RO, et al, "Delivery of Hexosaminidase A to the Cerebrum After Osmotic Modification of the Blood-Brain Barrier," *Proc Natl Acad Sci U S A*, 1981, 78:5838-41.
7. Kudoh T, Kikuchi K, Nakamura F, et al, "Prenatal Diagnosis of G_{M1}-gangliosidosis: Biochemical Manifestations in Fetal Tissues," *Hum Genet*, 1978, 44:287-93.
8. Sherwood RA and Rocks BF, "Antenatal Diagnosis of Steroid Sulfatase Deficiency: Case Report and Literature Survey," *J Clin Pathol*, 1982, 35:1236-9.
9. Moser HW, "Peroxisomal Disorders," *Clin Biochem*, 1991, 24(4):343-51.

References

Applegarth DA, Dimmick JE, and Toone JR, "Laboratory Detection of Metabolic Disease," *Pediatr Clin North Am*, 1989, 36(1):49-65.

McKusik VA, *Mendelian Inheritance in Man*, 8th ed, Baltimore, MD: John Hopkins Press, 1988.

Ostrer H and Hejtmancik JF, "Prenatal Diagnosis and Carrier Detection of Genetic Diseases by Analysis of Deoxyribonucleic Acid," *J Pediatr*, 1988, 112:679-87.

Pennock CA, "A Review and Selection of Simple Laboratory Methods Used for the Study of Glycosaminoglycan Excretion and the Diagnosis of the Mucopolysaccharidoses," *J Clin Pathol*, 1976, 29:111-23.

Peters TJ, "Investigation of Tissue Organelles by a Combination of Analytical Subcellular Fractionation and Enzymic Microanalysis: A New Approach to Pathology," *J Clin Pathol*, 1981, 34:1-12.

Rhead WJ, "Inborn Errors of Fatty Acid Oxidation in Man," *Clin Biochem*, 1991, 24(4):319-29.

Roth KS, "Inborn Errors of Metabolism: The Essentials of Clinical Diagnosis," *Clin Pediatr (Phila)*, 1991, 30(3):183-90.

Scriver CR, Beaudet AI, Sly WS, et al, eds, "Lysosomal Enzymes," Part II, *The Metabolic Basis of Inherited Disease*, 6th ed, New York, NY: McGraw-Hill Inc, 1989, 1563-1839.

Shih VE, "Detection of Hereditary Metabolic Disorders Involving Amino Acids and Organic Acids," *Clin Biochem*, 1991, 24(4):301-9.

Tetrazolium Reduction Test *see* Nitroblue Tetrazolium Test *on page 572*

Thoracentesis Fluid Analysis *see* Body Fluids Analysis, Cell Count *on page 523*

Thorn Test

CPT 85999

Related Information

Adrenocorticotropic Hormone *on page 98*
Cortisol, Blood *on page 191*
Cortisol, Urine *on page 193*
Cosyntropin Test *on page 194*
Eosinophil Count *on page 539*

Synonyms Adrenal Function Eosinophil Count

Abstract Eosinophil count is performed before and 4 hours following an injection of ACTH as a test of adrenal cortical function.

Patient Care PREPARATION: Hold breakfast. Draw blood for initial eosinophil count. Give 25 units ACTH intramuscularly. May eat breakfast. Hold lunch. Repeat eosinophil count 4 hours after ACTH is given. May have lunch after second count is taken.

Specimen Whole blood CONTAINER: Lavender top (EDTA) tube CAUSES FOR REJECTION: Patient not fasting

Interpretive USE: This test is of largely historical interest. LIMITATIONS: The test is rather antiquated and nonspecific. Addison's disease is most appropriately diagnosed using modern ACTH and cortisol levels. Borderline values are further investigated by stimulation tests of the pituitary and adrenals. ADDITIONAL INFORMATION: If adrenal cortical function is normal, the eosinophil count will act as follows: The eosinophil count before the injection will be about twice

(Continued)

Thorn Test *(Continued)*

the value of the eosinophil count after the injection (eg, eosinophil count of 200 before injection vs 100 after injection). If the adrenal cortical function is decreased, eosinophil count before the injection will be approximately the same as the eosinophil count after the injection (eg, eosinophil count before the injection of 200, after the injection, 195). When adrenal cortical function is decreased, it indicates hypoadrenalism (Addison's disease).

References

McNeely JC and Brown D, "Laboratory Evaluation of Leukocytes," *Clinical Hematology: Principles, Procedures, Correlations*, Chapter 25, Lotspeich-Steininger CA, Stiene-Martin EA, and Koepke JA, eds, Philadelphia, PA: JB Lippincott Co, 1992, 331.

Thrombocyte Count *see* Platelet Count *on page 586*

Total Blood Volume *see* Blood Volume *on page 522*

Total Eosinophil Count *see* Eosinophil Count *on page 539*

Total WBC *see* White Blood Count *on page 616*

TRAP Test *see* Tartrate Resistant Leukocyte Acid Phosphatase *on page 603*

Trypanosomiasis, Peripheral Blood Preparation *see* Microfilariae, Peripheral Blood Preparation *on page 571*

UBBC *see* Vitamin B_{12} Unsaturated Binding Capacity *on page 615*

Unsaturated Vitamin B_{12} Binding Capacity *see* Vitamin B_{12} Unsaturated Binding Capacity *on page 615*

Unstable Hemoglobins *see* Hemoglobin, Unstable, Heat Labile Test *on page 560*

Unstable Hemoglobins *see* Hemoglobin, Unstable - Isopropanol Precipitation Test *on page 561*

Viscosity, Blood

CPT 85810

Related Information

Erythropoietin, Serum *on page 214*
Viscosity, Serum/Plasma *on next page*

Synonyms Blood Viscosity

Specimen Whole blood **CONTAINER:** Green top (heparin) tube **CAUSES FOR REJECTION:** Specimen clotted or hemolyzed **SPECIAL INSTRUCTIONS:** While this is an infrequently performed test and may not be routinely available, there is evidence that neonatal hyperviscosity is common,[1] suggesting that the test should be more frequently utilized. Consult the laboratory to determine if the requisite microviscometer can be obtained.

Interpretive **REFERENCE RANGE:** See references for normal range data. Viscosity normally rises with increase in hematocrit and is lower with lower shear rates. Study has shown that umbilical cord and venous hematocrits (not capillary) correlate with microviscometer readings in newborns.[2] **USE:** Detect hyperviscosity states including especially hyperviscosity in the neonatal period. **METHODOLOGY:** Wells-Brookfield microviscometer.[3] Viscosity is measured at low and high shear rates at 37°C. **ADDITIONAL INFORMATION:** The relatively new fields of haemorheology and clinical haemorheology focus upon the characteristics and resultant clinical effects of the flow behavior of blood. Somer and Meiselman have classified the haematological hyperviscosity syndromes as of polycythemic, sclerocythaemic, or plasma type.[4] The polycythemic category includes syndromes the result of erythrocytosis (primary or secondary) or of hyperleukocytic leukemia. Sclerocythaemic cases are the result of decreased deformability of red cells (as occur with sickle hemoglobinopathies, other hemolytic anemias, some forms of malaria, and with rigid leukemic cells). In the plasma category are paraproteinemias (eg, multiple myeloma and Waldenström's macroglobulinemia) and reactive polyclonal dysproteinemias.

Neonatal hyperviscosity, usually but not always associated with polycythemia, may be accompanied by a fairly typical clinical picture. Plethora, hypoglycemia, lethargy, and jitteriness/seizures (CNS symptoms) occur. There may be symptoms and findings suggesting congenital heart disease (CHD) (ie, respiratory distress, cardiac enlargement, and cyanosis). False diagnoses of CHD have been made in such cases. About 50% of such infants have modest hyperbilirubinemia (bilirubin >12 mg/dL). Blood viscosity of small or large-for-gestational age infants does not differ from average-for-gestational age infants. About 50% of the cases have schistocytes and increased nucleated RBC on peripheral blood smear. The whole blood viscosity test can be used to follow the result of exchange transfusion therapy of neonatal hyperviscosity syndrome. Whole blood viscosity is increased after splenectomy (adults).[5]

Footnotes

1. Hathaway WE, "Neonatal Viscosity," *Pediatrics*, 1983, 72:567-9.
2. Ramamurthy RS and Berlanga M, "Postnatal Alteration in Hematocrit and Viscosity in Normal and Polycythemic Infants," *J Pediatr*, 1987, 110:929-34.
3. Wells RE, Denton R, and Merrill EW, "Measurement of Viscosity of Biologic Fluids by Cone Plate Viscometer," *J Lab Clin Med*, 1961, 57:646-56.
4. Somer T and Meiselman HJ, "Disorders of Blood Viscosity," *Ann Med*, 1993, 25(1):31-9.
5. Robertson DA, Simpson FG, and Losowsky MS, "Blood Viscosity After Splenectomy," *Br Med J [Clin Res]*, 1981, 283:573-5.

References

Black VD and Lubchenko LO, "Neonatal Polycythemia and Hyperviscosity," *Pediatr Clin North Am*, 1982, 29:1137-48.

Crowley JP, Metzger JB, Merrill EW, et al, "Whole Blood Viscosity in Beta Thalassemia Minor," *Ann Clin Lab Sci*, 1992, 22(4):229-35.

Williams WJ, Beutler E, Erslev AJ, et al, *Hematology*, 4th ed, New York, NY: McGraw-Hill Inc, 1990, 427-9.

Viscosity, Serum/Plasma

***CPT** 85820*

Related Information

Immunofixation Electrophoresis *on page 707*
Protein Electrophoresis, Serum *on page 734*
Protein Electrophoresis, Urine *on page 737*
Viral Culture, Respiratory Symptoms *on page 1204*
Viscosity, Blood *on previous page*

Synonyms Serum Viscosity

Specimen Serum or plasma **CONTAINER:** Red top tube or lavender top (EDTA) tube

Interpretive **REFERENCE RANGE:** 1.4-1.8 relative to water **USE:** Evaluate hyperviscosity syndromes associated with monoclonal gammopathy states (myeloma, macroglobulinemia of Waldenström and other dysproteinemias), including occasional cases of rheumatoid arthritis, systemic lupus erythematosus, hyperfibrinogenemia **LIMITATIONS:** Does not measure whole blood viscosity, which increases with high hemoglobin/hematocrit. Subjective endpoint, temperature dependent, large technical error, less than ideal correlation exists between measured viscosity levels and clinical symptoms. **METHODOLOGY:** Viscometer (Viscosimeter), Cannon-Feuske, Ostwald. Water and plasma "flow times" are determined with the use of a viscometer RBC or WBC pipette and stopwatch.[1] Test may be performed at room temperature or 37°C. The relative viscosity is expressed as a ratio of plasma "flow time" to water "flow time." A viscometer is commercially available which gives an automated measurement of plasma viscosity.[2] **ADDITIONAL INFORMATION:** Hyperviscosity is most frequent (33% of cases)[3] with IgM monoclonal gammopathy (Waldenström's macroglobulinemia); next with IgA myeloma. When IgG myeloma leads to hyperviscosity IgG levels are usually very significantly elevated. Kappa light chain myeloma may (rarely) be responsible for hyperviscosity syndrome apparently as a result of true polymer formation.[4] A relative viscosity of 6-7 usually results in symptoms of the hyperviscosity syndrome, they have however been described with lower levels of relative viscosity (ie, 4).[5] Results of plasma viscosity obtained with an automated capillary viscometer show good precision and close correlation with the Harkness manual method (standard method selected by the International Committee for Standardization in Hematology).[2]

Footnotes

1. Wright DJ and Jenkins DE Jr, "Simplified Method for Estimation of Serum and Plasma Viscosity in Multiple Myeloma and Related Disorders," *Blood*, 1970, 36:516-22.
2. Cooke BM and Stuart J, "Automated Measurement of Plasma Viscosity by Capillary Viscometer," *J Clin Pathol*, 1988, 41(11):1213-6.
3. Gandara DR and Mackenzie MR, "Differential Diagnosis of Monoclonal Gammopathy," *Med Clin North Am*, 1988, 72(5):1155-67, (review).
4. Carter PW, Cohen HJ, and Crawford J, "Hyperviscosity Syndrome in Association with Kappa Light Chain Myeloma," *Am J Med*, 1989, 86(5):591-5.
5. Fahey JL, Barth WF, and Solomon A, "Serum Hyperviscosity Syndrome," *JAMA*, 1965, 192:464-7.

References

Foerster J, "Plasma Cell Dyscrasias: General Considerations," *Wintrobe's Clinical Hematology*, 9th ed, Chapter 83, Section 4, Lee RG, Bithell TC, Foerster J, et al, eds, Philadelphia, PA: Lea & Febiger, 1993, 2202-10.

(Continued)

Viscosity, Serum/Plasma *(Continued)*

Henry JB, Nelson DA, Tomar RH, et al, *Clinical Diagnosis and Management by Laboratory Methods*, 18th ed, Philadelphia, PA: WB Saunders Co, 1991, 709.
Somer T and Meiselman HJ, "Disorders of Blood Viscosity," *Ann Med*, 1993, 25(1):31-9.

Vitamin B_{12}

CPT 82607

See Also Anemia Flowchart in the Hematology Appendix

Related Information

Bone Marrow *on page 524*
Complete Blood Count *on page 533*
Folic Acid, RBC *on page 544*
Folic Acid, Serum *on page 545*
Gastrin, Serum *on page 234*
Hemoglobin *on page 554*
Intrinsic Factor Antibody *on page 714*
Parietal Cell Antibody *on page 730*
Red Blood Cell Indices *on page 592*
Red Cell Count *on page 594*
Schilling Test *on page 598*
Vitamin B_{12} Unsaturated Binding Capacity *on page 615*

Synonyms Antipernicious Anemia Factor; B_{12}; Cyanocobalamin, True; Extrinsic Factor of Castle

Applies to Methylmalonic Acid

Abstract Radioisotopic method replaces *Euglena* microbiological assay for detection of cobalamin deficiency

Patient Care PREPARATION: A fasting specimen is preferred; draw before transfusions or B_{12} therapy is started.

Specimen Serum CONTAINER: Red top tube STORAGE INSTRUCTIONS: Separate serum and freeze; protect from light. Obtain hematocrit from EDTA tube before freezing the whole blood specimen. CAUSES FOR REJECTION: Stored specimen not frozen

Interpretive REFERENCE RANGE: The lower reference limit, which is critical to the diagnosis of B_{12} deficiency/pernicious anemia, is not clearly established. It is likely in the range of 100-250 pg/mL (SI: 74-185 pmol/L).[1,2,3] Most commercial methods have in the past undergone modification, in particular after the report by Kolhouse et al.[1] (See following information.) Clinical correlation and multiple test documentation of the etiology of macrocytic anemia is advised. Occasionally, patients with significant neuropsychiatric abnormalities may have no hematologic abnormalities (absence of anemia or macrocytosis), but vitamin B_{12} level >200 pg/mL (SI: >150 pmol/L), or more commonly between 100 and 200 pg/mL (SI: 75-150 pmol/L).[4] See table for pediatric reference ranges. USE: Detect B_{12} deficiency as in pernicious anemia in those patients who have hematologic (weakness, anemia, oval macrocytosis, hypersegmented neutrophils, leukopenia/thrombocytopenia) or neurologic (numbness, tingling, loss of vibratory sensation in extremities) findings suggestive of such deficiency state. Because of problems associated with verifying the lower limits of "normal," this assay should not be employed as a screening test for functional cobalamin deficiency.[2,3,4] Diagnose folic acid deficiency[5]; evaluate hypersegmentation of granulocyte nuclei; investigate MCV >100 fL; diagnose macrocytic and megaloblastic anemia; work up alcoholism; prenatal care; evaluate malabsorption, including jejunoileal bypass patients operated for massive obesity; work up certain neurological disorders

Pediatric Serum B_{12} Reference Ranges

Age, y	Male (pg/mL)		Female (pg/mL)	
	Low	High	Low	High
0–1	216	891	168	1117
2–3	195	897	307	892
4–6	181	795	231	1038
7–9	200	863	182	866
10–12	135	803	145	752
13–18	158	638	134	605

From Hicks JM, Cook J, Godwin ID, et al, "Vitamin B_{12} and Folate — Pediatric Reference Ranges," *Arch Pathol Lab Med*, 1993, 117:705, with permission.

LIMITATIONS: Drugs capable of interference with absorption of B_{12} and/or folic acid include chemotherapeutic (methotrexate), antimalarial (pyrimethamine), diuretics (triamterene), protozoacides (pentamidine, isethionate), antibacterials (trimethoprim), anticonvulsants (phenytoin), sedatives (barbiturates), oral contraceptives, antituberculosis agents (cycloserine, para-aminosalicylic acid), antigout (colchicine), oral hypoglycemic, biguanide group (metformin, phenformin). Establishing functional cobalamin (B_{12}) sufficiency in any individual patient may require consideration of intra-individual variation, functional status of the gastric mucosa (in particular in elderly individuals) and transcobalamin II binding.[3,6] See following discussion of application of serum methylmalonic acid. **CONTRAINDICATIONS:** B_{12}/folate levels should be drawn before performance of Schilling test and before administration of any other radioactivity. **METHODOLOGY:** Radioimmunoassay (RIA) based on competitive protein binding has largely replaced earlier microbiologic assays. Patient's unlabeled endogenous serum B_{12} competes with radiolabeled B_{12} for specific sites on a binding protein (intrinsic factor) and is compared to the behavior of a standard. Some commercially available procedures combine B_{12} and folate testing in a single simultaneous method using two different isotopes (generally, with B_{12}, ^{57}Co and folate, ^{125}I labels). A chemiluminescence receptor assay utilizing intrinsic factor immobilized on magnetic particles (solid phase) has been developed.[7] **ADDITIONAL INFORMATION:** Vitamin B_{12} (cyanocobalamin) analogues form the base compound in coenzymes having important biologic functions. The vitamin has an intriguing ring structure, a planar tetrapyrrole corrin ring around an asymmetric cobalt atom. The structure is reminiscent of the relation of iron to heme. The corrin system, like porphyrin (heme), is synthesized from delta aminolevulinic acid. The basic compound is named cobalamin, the form with attached cyanide group (cyanocobalamin) is vitamin B_{12}. Two metabolically important cobamides (vitamin B_{12} containing coenzymes) are adenosyl cobamide and methyl cobamide. Cobamides are required for DNA synthesis, methylation, and citric acid cycle reactions.[4]

Vitamin B_{12} is not synthesized by humans. It is a requisite dietary component widely available in animal products (meat, fish, eggs, butter, milk, and cheese). The minimum daily requirement (MDR) is 1-5 μg/day, body stores are 2000-5000 μg, and daily loss is only about 0.1%. B_{12} is absorbed by mucosal epithelial cells (microvilli) of the terminal ileum, a pH and divalent cation dependent process. The vitamin is ingested in food sources bound to protein. Its absorption is dependent upon a gastric glycoprotein, intrinsic factor (IF). Gastric acid splits the B_{12} protein linkage. IF binding is by a benzimidazole nucleotide, which is independent of the analogue chemical form and which protects the enzyme from digestive enzymes. After the B_{12} intrinsic factor complex is absorbed by the ileal mucosa, the vitamin enters the portal circulation where it is bound by a system of carrier proteins, the transcobalamins I, II, and III. See the following listing, Vitamin B_{12} Unsaturated Binding Capacity. Transcobalamins I and III are of leukocyte origin, transcobalamin II is synthesized by the liver.

Competitive protein binding methods measure total or "true" cobalamin levels. Kolhouse et al[1] have shown that cobalamin analogues are present in some human plasmas. These may have higher affinity for "R proteins" (B_{12} binding proteins without intrinsic factor activity that have rapid electrophoretic mobility) than for intrinsic factor. Such analogues may result in falsely high levels of B_{12} with some radioisotope dilution assays (cobalamin deficiency would be masked[1]). In order to avoid failure to detect cobalamin deficiency (including pernicious anemia) Kolhouse et al have cautioned that only "true" cobalamin be measured (requires use of a purified, R factor free or blocked, intrinsic factor assay procedure). Spurious high B_{12} results have been reported in the past relating to anti-intrinsic factor-blocking antibodies and high or low results relating to endogenous B_{12} binding proteins; a variety of interferences have been reported.[8,9,10]

Conditions associated with decreased vitamin B_{12} include hypochlorhydria; pernicious anemia (PA) in which cobalamin levels may vary from 0 to overlapping lower limits of patients without PA; dietary deficiency (uncommon); disorders of intestinal absorption; inflammatory bowel disease; bacterial overgrowth, small intestine; *Diphyllobothrium* fish tapeworm, small intestine; prior gastric surgery; intestinal surgery (diminished B_{12} or folate or both are found in 88% of patients with jejunoileal bypass operated for morbid obesity);[11] resection of terminal ileum as for Crohn's disease prevents absorption of B_{12}; oral contraceptives; abnormalities of cobalamin transport or metabolism;[6] Imerslund's syndrome.[12,13] **A significant rise in red blood cell mean corpuscular volume (MCV) may be an important early indicator of B_{12} deficiency.**[14] Conditions associated with increased vitamin B_{12} include chronic granulocytic leukemia (and to a lesser degree leukemoid states); chronic renal failure; severe congestive heart failure; diabetes; obesity; COPD; and cases of liver cell damage.

(Continued)

Vitamin B_{12} *(Continued)*

There is growing evidence that elevated serum or urine methylmalonic acid (MMA) levels may be a more definitive indication of early cobalamin (B_{12}) deficiency. MMA serum level, when increased, reflects decreased tissue cobalamin and is an early indicator of B_{12} deficiency. Cobalamin dependent neurologic disease with normal hematologic parameters and serum B_{12} levels may be associated with significant elevations of serum methylmalonic acid.[4,15] GC/MS methodology for MMA determinations is preferred, is not currently in widespread use, but there have been important recent advances in sample preparation (simplification).[16] To avoid dietary influence serum MMA levels have preference over urine studies in nonfasting patients.[17]

Footnotes

1. Kolhouse JF, Kondo H, Allen NC, et al, "Cobalamin Analogues Are Present in Human Plasma and Can Mask Cobalamin Deficiency Because Current Radioisotope Dilution Assays Are Not Specific for True Cobalamin," *N Engl J Med*, 1978, 299:785-92.
2. Schilling RF, Fairbanks VF, Miller R, et al, "Improved Vitamin B_{12} Assays: A Report on Two Commercial Kits," *Clin Chem*, 1983, 29:582-3.
3. Lindstedt G, Lundberg P-A, Johansson P-M, et al, "High Prevalence of Atrophic Gastritis in the Elderly: Implications for Health-Associated Reference Limits for Cobalamin in Serum," *Clin Chem*, 1989, 35(7):1557-9.
4. Lindenbaum J, Healton EB, Savage DG, et al, "Neuropsychiatric Disorders Caused by Cobalamin Deficiency in the Absence of Anemia or Macrocytosis," *N Engl J Med*, 1988, 318(26):1720-8.
5. Tisman G and Herbert V, "B_{12} Dependence of Cell Uptake of Serum Folate: An Explanation for High Serum Folate and Cell Folate Depletion in B_{12} Deficiency," *Blood*, 1973, 41:465-9.
6. Herzlich B and Herbert V, "Depletion of Serum Holotranscobalamin II. An Early Sign of Negative Vitamin B_{12} Balance," *Lab Invest*, 1988, 58(3):332-7.
7. Leonard H, Klukas C, Williams M, et al, "A Chemiluminescence Receptor Assay for Vitamin B_{12}," *Clin Chem*, 1989, 35:1194.
8. Zucker RM, Podell ER, and Allen RH, "Multiple Problems With Current No-Boil Assays for Serum Cobalamin," *Ligand Q*, 1981, 4:52-8, 60-3; 1982, 5:48-9.
9. LeFebvre RJ, Virji AS, and Mertens BF, "Erroneously Low Results Due to High Nonspecific Binding Encountered With a Radioassay Kit That Measures "True" Serum Vitamin B_{12}," *Am J Clin Pathol*, 1980, 74:209-13.
10. El Shami AS and Durham AP, "More on Vitamin B_{12} Results as Measured With "Boil" and "No-Boil" Kits," *Clin Chem*, 1983, 29:2115-6.
11. Hocking MP, Duerson MC, O'Leary JP, et al, "Jejunoileal Bypass for Morbid Obesity. Late Follow-up in 100 Cases," *N Engl J Med*, 1983, 308:995-9.
12. Abdelaal MA and Ahmed AF, "Imerslund-Gräsbeck Syndrome in a Saudi Family," *Acta Paediatr Scand*, 1991, 80(11):1109-12.
13. Russo CL, Hyman PE, and Oseas RS, "Megaloblastic Anemia Characterized by Microcytosis: Imerslund-Gräsbeck Syndrome With Coexistent Alpha-Thalassemia," *Pediatrics*, 1988, 81(6):875-6.
14. Hall CA, "Vitamin B_{12} Deficiency and Early Rise in Mean Corpuscular Volume," *JAMA*, 1981, 245:1144-6.
15. Rasmussen K, Moelby L, and Jensen MK, "Studies on Methylmalonic Acid in Humans. II. Relationship Between Concentrations in Serum and Urinary Excretion, and the Correlation Between Serum Cobalamin and Accumulation of Methylmalonic Acid," *Clin Chem*, 1989, 35(12):2277-80.
16. Rasmussen K, "Solid Phase Sample Extraction for Rapid Determinations of Methylmalonic Acid in Serum and Urine by a Stable-Isotope-Dilution Method," *Clin Chem*, 1989, 35(2):260-4.
17. Rasmussen K, "Studies on Methylmalonic Acid in Humans. I. Concentrations in Serum and Urinary Excretion in Normal Subjects After Feeding and During Fasting and After Loading With Protein, Fat, Sugar, Isoleucine, and Valine," *Clin Chem*, 1989, 38(12):2271-6.

References

Carethers M, "Diagnosing Vitamin B_{12} Deficiency, A Common Geriatric Disorder," *Geriatrics*, 1988, 43:89-94, 105-7, 111-2.

Chanarin I, "Megaloblastic Anaemia, Cobalamin, and Folate," *J Clin Pathol*, 1987, 40:978-84.

Gimsing P and Nexo E, "Cobalamin-Binding Capacity of Haptocorrin and Transcobalamin: Age-Correlated Reference Intervals and Values From Patients," *Clin Chem*, 1989, 35(7):1447-51.

Herbert V, "Don't Ignore Low Serum Cobalamin (Vitamin B_{12}) Levels," *Arch Intern Med*, 1988, 148:1705-7, (editorial).

Herbert V, "The 1986 Herman Award Lecture. Nutrition Science as a Continually Unfolding Story: The Folate and Vitamin B_{12} Paradigm," *Am J Clin Nutr*, 1987, 46:387-402.

Hicks JM, Cook J, Godwin ID, et al, "Vitamin B_{12} and Folate: Pediatric Reference Ranges," *Arch Pathol Lab Med*, 1993, 117:704-6.

Lee GR, "Megaloblastic and Nonmegaloblastic Macrocytic Anemias," *Wintrobe's Clinical Hematology*, 9th ed, Chapter 24, Lee GR, Bithell TC, Foerster J, et al, eds, Philadelphia, PA: Lea & Febiger, 1993, 745-90.

Lindenbaum J, et al, "Neuropsychiatric Disorders Caused by Cobalamin Deficiency in the Absence of Anemia or Macrocytosis," *N Engl J Med*, 1988, 318:1720-8.

Steiner, et al, "Sensory Peripheral Neuropathy of Vitamin B_{12} Deficiency: A Primary Demyelinating Disease?" *J Neurol*, 1988, 235:163-4.

Thompson WG, Babitz L, Cassino C, et al, "Evaluation of Current Criteria Used to Measure Vitamin B_{12} Levels," *Am J Med*, 1987, 82:291-4.

Vitamin B_{12} Absorption Test *see* Schilling Test *on page 598*

Vitamin B_{12} UBC *see* Vitamin B_{12} Unsaturated Binding Capacity *on this page*

Vitamin B_{12} Unsaturated Binding Capacity

***CPT** 82608*

Related Information

Erythropoietin, Serum *on page 214*
Folic Acid, RBC *on page 544*
Folic Acid, Serum *on page 545*
Intrinsic Factor Antibody *on page 714*
Parietal Cell Antibody *on page 730*
Schilling Test *on page 598*
Vitamin B_{12} *on page 612*

Synonyms UBBC; Unsaturated Vitamin B_{12} Binding Capacity; Vitamin B_{12} UBC

Specimen Serum is most commonly used by most reference laboratories but use of EDTA plasma avoids increase in binding protein released from granulocytes (see following information). **CONTAINER:** Red top tube **STORAGE INSTRUCTIONS:** Refrigerate serum if not delivered to the laboratory immediately. Stable for days. Very stable when stored at -20°C.

Interpretive **REFERENCE RANGE:** 1000-2000 pg/mL binding capacity **USE:** Differential diagnosis of polycythemia vera from secondary/relative polycythemias; evaluate macrocytic/megaloblastic anemia; diagnose congenital absence of transcobalamin II or cobalophilin (transcobalamin I and III) **LIMITATIONS:** Increased with pregnancy and use of contraceptive hormones. Unrepresentative increase may occur during clotting of blood samples by release of unsaturated binding protein (cobalophilin) from granulocytes.[1] May give low values in samples with low protein content. Usually available only at reference or research laboratories. **METHODOLOGY:** Binding proteins are determined by their B_{12} binding capacity. Uptake of radiolabeled B_{12} is quantitated after saturation of serum transport systems and removal of excess vitamin with albumin or hemoglobin-coated charcoal. DEAE cellulose ion-exchange chromatography and isoelectric focusing are also used (in research environments). **ADDITIONAL INFORMATION:** Serum transport of vitamin B_{12} is accomplished by normally occurring proteins termed transcobalamins including I (an α-globulin), II (a β-globulin), and III (a group of transport factors – "R-type" binders or binder III – found also in some tissues, saliva, milk, and tears). The term "R-type" refers to binding protein with "rapid" mobility on electrophoresis. A family of immunologically identical proteins is known, not all of which have the initially described rapid mobility. They are known also as cobalophilins. Transcobalamin I is the major B_{12} transport protein and bears immunologic identity to granulocyte cobalophilin. Isoelectric focusing has shown that the cobalophilins are a microheterogenous group of plasma binding proteins. Stenman has reviewed this subject in detail.[1] Cobalophilin is increased in diseases characterized by excess granulocyte production, reactive leukocytosis, chronic myelogenous leukemia, and other myeloproliferative states, in particular polycythemia vera. UBBC levels are increased in over two-thirds of cases of polycythemia vera. Most cases of secondary/relative polycythemia patients have normal levels of UBBC. High levels occur in some patients with hepatoma.[2] The transcobalamins are normally about 25% saturated with vitamin B_{12}.

Footnotes

1. Stenman U-H, "Intrinsic Factor and the Vitamin B_{12} Binding Proteins," *Megaloblastic Anemia, Clinics in Haematology*, Hoffbrand AV, ed, Philadelphia, PA: WB Saunders Co, 1976, 5:473-95.
2. Waxman S and Gilbert HS, "A Tumor-Related Vitamin B_{12} Binding Protein in Adolescent Hepatoma," *N Engl J Med*, 1973, 289:1053-6.

References

Hall CA, Horch C, and Begley JA, "The Forms and Transport of Plasma Cobalamins in Normal Man and in Myeloproliferative States," *J Lab Clin Med*, 1979, 94:772-83.

Lee GR, "Nutritional Factors in the Production and Function of Erythrocytes," *Wintrobe's Clinical Hematology*, 9th ed, Chapter 7, Lee GR, Bithell TC, Foerster J, et al, eds, Philadelphia, PA: Lea & Febiger, 1993, 158-94.

Zittoun J, Farcet JP, Marquet J, et al, "Cobalamin (Vitamin B_{12}) and B_{12} Binding Proteins in Hypereosinophilic Syndromes and Secondary Eosinophilia," *Blood*, 1984, 63:779-83.

WBC *see* White Blood Count *on this page*

Westergren Sed Rate *see* Sedimentation Rate, Erythrocyte *on page 599*

White Blood Cell Morphology *see* Peripheral Blood: Differential Leukocyte Count *on page 576*

White Blood Count

CPT 85048

Related Information

Antineutrophil Antibody *on page 636*
Bone Marrow *on page 524*
Chromosome Analysis, Blood or Bone Marrow *on page 898*
Complete Blood Count *on page 533*
HIV-1/HIV-2 Serology *on page 696*
Leukocyte Alkaline Phosphatase *on page 566*
Leukocyte Cytochemistry *on page 567*
Lymph Node Biopsy *on page 72*
Lymphocyte Subset Enumeration *on page 720*
Peripheral Blood: Differential Leukocyte Count *on page 576*

Synonyms Leukocyte Count; Total WBC; WBC; White Count

Abstract This procedure determines the white blood cell concentration in a body fluid, usually blood. The count is most commonly generated by an automated analyzer using aperture-impedance and/or laser beam technology. Different types of white blood cells (eg, granulocytes, monocytes, lymphocytes, etc) are included in the total count. The results have widespread application to the diagnosis and monitoring of a variety of clinical conditions including infectious, neoplastic, and immunologic disease states.

Specimen Whole blood or other body fluid **CONTAINER:** Lavender top (EDTA) tube **CAUSES FOR REJECTION:** Clotted specimen, hemolyzed specimen

Interpretive **REFERENCE RANGE:** Peripheral blood: 4500-11,000/mm^3 (SI: 4.5-11.0 x 10^9/L) **POSSIBLE PANIC RANGE:** On admission <2500/mm^3 (SI: 2.5 x 10^9/L) or >30,000/mm^3 (SI: >30.0 x 10^9/L) **USE:** White cell enumeration; evaluate myelopoiesis, bacterial and viral infections, toxic metabolic processes; diagnose/evaluate leukemic states **LIMITATIONS:** If nucleated RBCs are found in differential count, the white blood count should be corrected. Electronic counters are subject to spurious high WBC counts in cases where clumped platelet aggregates are "seen" as white cells.[1] **METHODOLOGY:** Manual – hemocytometer counting chambers. Most WBC count determinations are obtained from one channel of a highly automated multichannel electronic and pneumatic analyzer using aperture-impedance and/or aperture conductance and/or laser light scattering technologies. WBC differential determination is provided by recent generations of analyzers. Excellent performance (precision, linearity, and lack of carryover) has been found on field evaluation of a commonly utilized multichannel device.[2] **ADDITIONAL INFORMATION:** In newborn infants WBC counts from different vascular sources (ie, capillary vs venous vs arterial blood) should not necessarily be considered equivalent. WBC counts from actively crying babies may show leukocytosis with left shift, possibly erroneously suggesting bacterial infections. Any stressful situation in newborns, children, or adults which leads to increase in endogenous epinephrine production may cause a rapid (15-30 minutes) increase in WBC count. In the evaluation of infection in newborns and young children, it is recommended that several counts be obtained from a consistent vascular source in resting individuals. A study of within subject and between subject variation has reaffirmed that hematologic parameters have significant individuality. Screening using conventional reference limits may be misleading. Subject specific reference values are likely to have greater clinical utility.[3] There is modest progressive leukocytosis (due to neutrophils) throughout pregnancy into the third trimester with subsequent decline in white count after about 34 weeks gestation.[4] Included in the broad differential consideration for the cause of neutropenia is collagen-vascular disease, notably lupus erythematosus and other autoimmune neutropenias (see References). Many drugs result in leukopenia including bezafibrate, an antihyperlipidemic fibric acid.[5]

Footnotes

1. Solanki DL and Blackburn BC, "Spurious Leukocytosis and Thrombocytopenia. A Dual Phenomenon Caused by Clumping of Platelets *In Vitro*," *JAMA*, 1983, 250:2514-5.
2. Warner BA and Reardon DM, "A Field Evaluation of the Coulter STKS®," *Am J Clin Pathol*, 1991, 95(2):207-17.
3. Fraser CG, Wilkinson SP, Neville RG, et al, "Biologic Variation of Common Hematologic Laboratory Quantities in the Elderly," *Am J Clin Pathol*, 1989, 92(4):465-70.

4. Balloch AJ and Cauchi MN, "Reference Ranges for Haematology Parameters in Pregnancy Derived From Patient Populations," *Clin Lab Haematol*, 1993, 15(1):7-14.
5. Ariad S and Hechtlinger V, "Bezafibrate-Induced Neutropenia," *Eur J Haematol*, 1993, 50(3):179, (letter).

References

Christensen RD and Rothstein G, "Pitfalls in the Interpretation of Leukocyte Counts of Newborn Infants," *Am J Clin Pathol*, 1979, 72:608-11.

Second National Health and Nutrition Examination Survey, "Hematological and Nutritional Biochemistry Reference Data for Persons 6 Months to 74 Years of Age: United States, 1976-80," *Vital and Health Statistics*, DHHS Publication No (PHS) 83-1682, 1982.

Shastri KA and Logue GL, "Autoimmune Neutropenia," *Blood*, 1993, 81(8):1984-95.

White Count *see* White Blood Count *on previous page*

Zeta Sedimentation Rate, ESR *see* Zeta Sedimentation Ratio *on this page*

Zeta Sedimentation Ratio

***CPT** 85651*

Related Information

Burn Culture, Quantitative *on page 794*
C-Reactive Protein *on page 669*
Sedimentation Rate, Erythrocyte *on page 599*

Synonyms Erythrocyte Sedimentation Rate; Sed Rate; Zeta Sedimentation Rate, ESR; ZSR

Test Commonly Includes Sedimentation rate expressed in percent

Abstract An automated sedimentation rate method, which however is not entirely analogous to other ESR methods. The ZSR requires a special centrifuge (which is no longer under manufacture) for its performance.

Patient Care **AFTERCARE:** If results are equivocal or inconsistent with clinical impression, the C-reactive protein (CRP) is a useful test which is comparable and which also is an acute phase reactant.

Specimen Whole blood **CONTAINER:** Lavender top (EDTA) tube **COLLECTION:** Specimen must be received within 4 hours of collection. **CAUSES FOR REJECTION:** Insufficient blood, clotted specimen, hemolyzed specimen

Interpretive **REFERENCE RANGE:** Younger than 50 years: <55%; 50-80 years: 40% to 60% **USE:** Nonspecific indicator of infectious disease and inflammatory states, reflects acute phase reactant levels; screen for collagen diseases; screen for and follow activity of rheumatic diseases, especially rheumatoid arthritis **LIMITATIONS:** The ZSR centrifuge is no longer produced. There are, however, many instruments still in use in the country. The majority of laboratories use the manual Westergren sed rate method (see Sedimentation Rate, Erythrocyte). **METHODOLOGY:** Standardized stress is applied to a column of red cells and the extent of red cell packing is determined. **ADDITIONAL INFORMATION:** The ZSR is rapidly performed, reproducible, and independent of the hematocrit, requiring no hematocrit correction. Sedimentation rate is increased, generally, in cases of infection/inflammation/tissue necrosis, especially where fibrinogen and inflammatory or macroglobulins are increased. May be increased with pregnancy, malignancy, and dysproteinemias (eg, especially macroglobulinemia and myeloma). Sedimentation rate may be decreased in sickle cell disease and spherocytosis. Poikilocytosis acts to inhibit red cell sedimentation. Use of the ESR, ZSR, and/or CRP may aid in the differentiation of the anemia of chronic disease from iron deficiency.[1] In a series of 981 measurements, Bucher et al found the ZSR a useful monitor of disease activity and found good correlation with the Wintrobe or Westergren ESR.[2] Comparison of ZSR with modified Westergren ESR and with clinical assessment of disease activity in rheumatoid arthritis has shown good correlation.[3] The erythrocyte sedimentation rate (including the ZSR) is usually markedly elevated in temporal (giant cell) arteritis.[4]

Footnotes

1. Johnson MA, "Iron: Nutrition Monitoring and Nutrition Status Assessment," *J Nutr*, 1990, 120(Suppl 11):1486-91.
2. Bucher WC, Gall EP, and Becker PT, "The Zeta Sedimentation Ratio (ZSR) as the Routine Monitor of Disease Activity in a General Hospital," *Am J Clin Pathol*, 1979, 72:65-7.
3. Morris MW, Pinals RS, and Nelson DA, "The Zeta Sedimentation Ratio (ZSR) and Activity of Disease in Rheumatoid Arthritis," *Am J Clin Pathol*, 1977, 68:760-2.
4. Molloy DW, Brooymans MA, and Borrie MJ, "Acute Chest Pain in An Elderly Woman," *Can J Cardiol*, 1988, 4:144-5.

References

Stuart J and Nash GB, "Technological Advances in Blood Rheology," *Crit Rev Clin Lab Sci*, 1990, 28(1):61-93.

ZSR *see* Zeta Sedimentation Ratio *on previous page*

HEMATOLOGY APPENDIX

Anemia Flowchart

The flowchart that follows is intended as an aid in diagnosis of anemia and is a supplement to this chapter to demonstrate how the entries might be placed in a logical order. The flowchart is not meant to replace a standard history and physical for diagnosis. Instead, it is intended as a teaching tool to develop patterns for test ordering in the work-up of anemia. Cost-effectiveness is made a prime concern. Thus, the beginning is based on the initial screen by the CBC, including the RDW. (See Complete Blood Count and the tables in that listing.) The method of Bessman[1] has been adapted for this beginning classification. In real life, some diagnoses may not fit the flowchart exactly, but the majority of cases do. The bulk of the flowchart centers around the reticulocyte count (section C) and the reticulocyte production index (RPI). See Reticulocyte Count entry for more information.

It will soon become apparent that the flowchart often ends with the diagnosis of iron deficiency anemia. This should not be surprising since iron deficiency anemia is the most common cause of decreased hemoglobin, especially in the outpatient setting. Normal values for many tests will vary between laboratories. Use reference ranges (normal values) from your own laboratory when appropriate. This flowchart is not intended to cover every hematologic possibility.

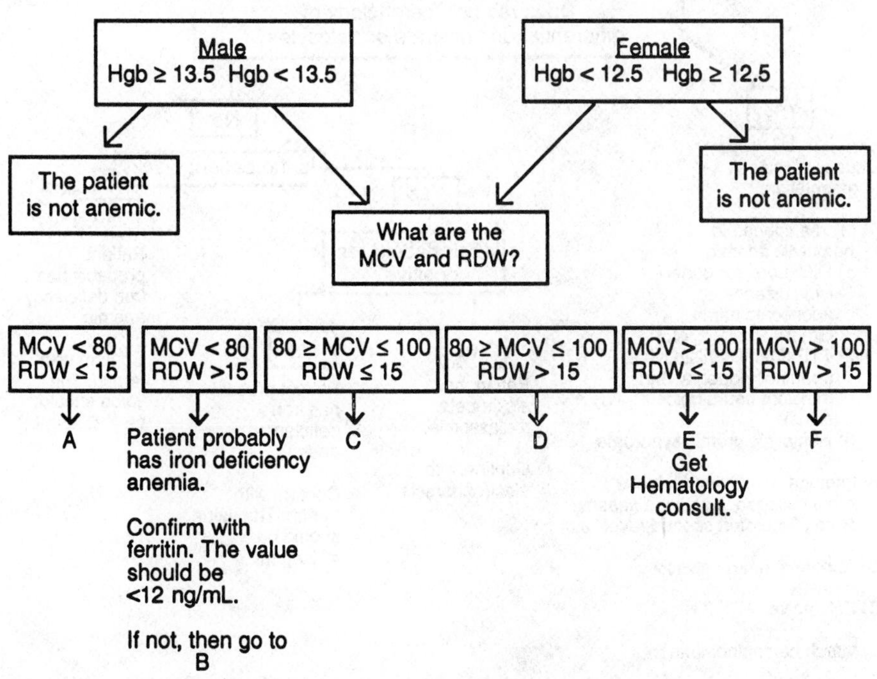

[1] JD Bessman, "Improved Classification of Anemias by MCV and RDW," *Am J Clin Pathol,* 1983, 80:322-6.

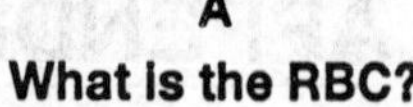

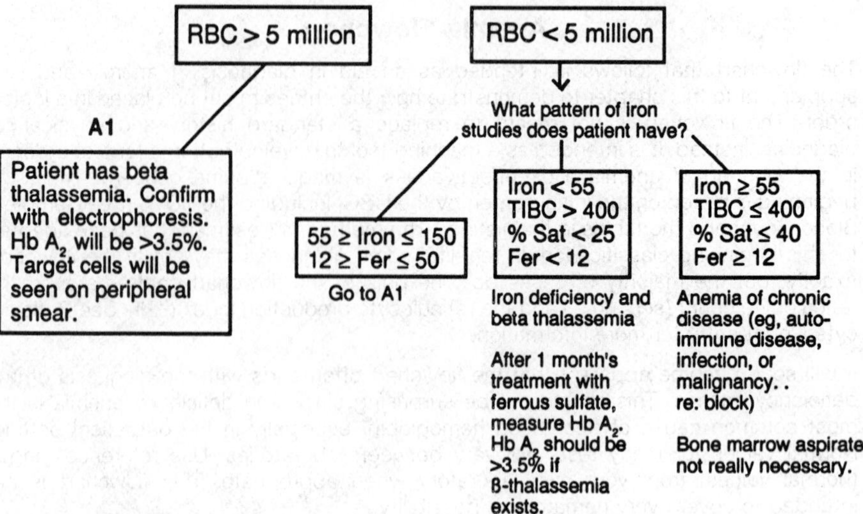
A
What is the RBC?
RBC > 5 million
RBC < 5 million
A1
Patient has beta thalassemia. Confirm with electrophoresis. Hb A2 will be >3.5%. Target cells will be seen on peripheral smear.
What pattern of iron studies does patient have?
55 ≥ Iron ≤ 150
12 ≥ Fer ≤ 50
Go to A1
Iron < 55
TIBC > 400
% Sat < 25
Fer < 12
Iron deficiency and beta thalassemia
After 1 month's treatment with ferrous sulfate, measure Hb A2. Hb A2 should be >3.5% if ß-thalassemia exists.
Iron ≥ 55
TIBC ≤ 400
% Sat ≤ 40
Fer ≥ 12
Anemia of chronic disease (eg, autoimmune disease, infection, or malignancy. . re: block)
Bone marrow aspirate not really necessary.

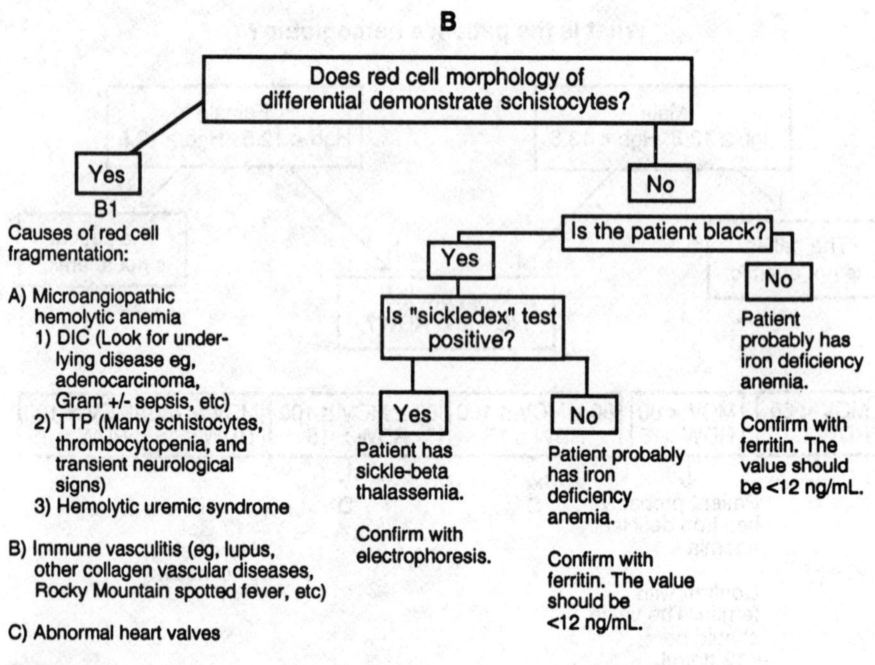
B
Does red cell morphology of differential demonstrate schistocytes?
Yes
B1
Causes of red cell fragmentation:
A) Microangiopathic hemolytic anemia
1) DIC (Look for underlying disease eg, adenocarcinoma, Gram +/- sepsis, etc)
2) TTP (Many schistocytes, thrombocytopenia, and transient neurological signs)
3) Hemolytic uremic syndrome
B) Immune vasculitis (eg, lupus, other collagen vascular diseases, Rocky Mountain spotted fever, etc)
C) Abnormal heart valves
D) Eclampsia
E) March hemoglobinuria
F) Severe burns
G) Others
No
Is the patient black?
Yes
Is "sickledex" test positive?
Yes
Patient has sickle-beta thalassemia.
Confirm with electrophoresis.
No
Patient probably has iron deficiency anemia.
Confirm with ferritin. The value should be <12 ng/mL.
No
Patient probably has iron deficiency anemia.
Confirm with ferritin. The value should be <12 ng/mL.

C

What is the uncorrected reticulocyte count?

S = Single correction reticulocyte count

S = Ret Count x (.xx/.45), where .xx is patient's hematocrit

Double correction reticulocyte count or reticulocyte production index (RPI) is calculated by dividing the single correction reticulocyte count by the maturation index (T).

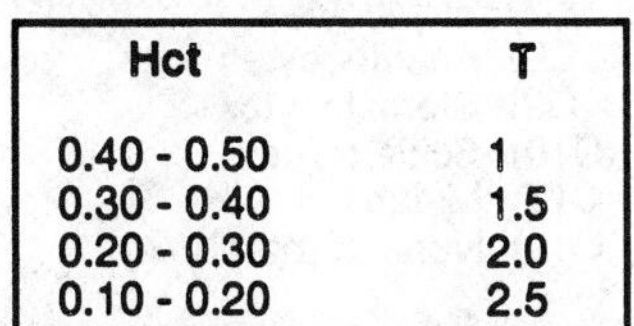

Hct	T
0.40 - 0.50	1
0.30 - 0.40	1.5
0.20 - 0.30	2.0
0.10 - 0.20	2.5

Reticulocyte Production Index = U

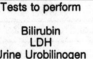

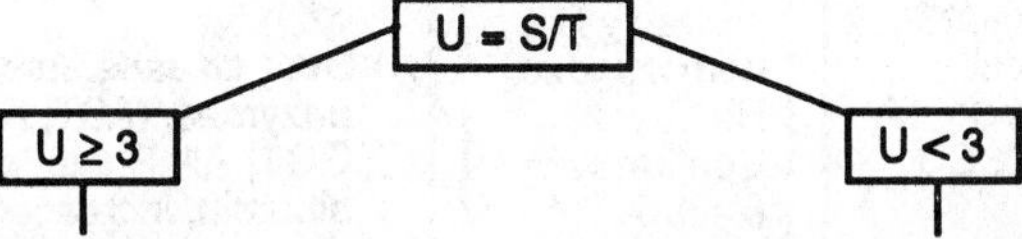

RPIs >3 are consistent with the hyperproliferative anemias (acute hemorrhage or hemolysis).

Go to C1

RPIs <3 are consistent with ineffective erythropoiesis or hypoproliferative anemias.

Go to C100

C1

Tests to perform

Bilirubin
LDH
Urine Urobilinogen
Hemoglobinemia
Hemoglobinuria
Hemosiderinuria

and

Haptoglobin

Haptoglobin >25 mg/dL; Bleeding

Patient probably has an acute hemorrhage.

Of course, you are most likely aware of this because you are covered with the patient's blood.

However, patients can lose large volumes of blood internally and either have obvious sources (eg, esophageal varices or duodenal ulcer) or not so obvious sources (eg, retroperitoneal blood or quadriceps bleed).

Haptoglobin <25 mg/dL; Hemolysis

The patient probably has a hemolytic anemia. Just a quick comment about the above tests. Bilirubin in hemolytic anemia is usually between 1.0 and 5.0 mg/dL. The majority (about 85%) should be indirect bilirubin. Urine urobilinogen may not be elevated unless the hemolysis is moderate to severe. The serum LDH isozymes will show a flipped 1:2 pattern similar to that of an acute infarction of myocardium.

If the patient has intravascular hemolysis, hemoglobinemia, hemoglobinuria, and hemosiderinuria should be present. A bone marrow aspirate (usually not needed) will reveal erythroid hyperplasia with fairly normal maturation.

The next easiest and most cost-effective part of the work-up is to look at the differential.

Go to C2

C2

Does the patient have any of the following abnormal morphology?

- C3) Sickle cells
- C4) Hb C crystals
- C5) Target cells
- C6) Spherocytes
- C7) Elliptocytes
- C8) Acanthocytes
- C9) Stomatocytes
- C10) Schistocytes
- C11) Malaria
- C12) None of the above

C3

Do hemoglobin electrophoresis. The patient either has sickle cell disease (SS) or is doubly heterozygous (SC, SD, SO, S-thal, etc).

C4

The patient probably is homozygous Hb C. Confirm with electrophoresis.

C5

Three possibilities:

A) Liver disease...elevated enzymes, (AST, ALT, LDH, GGT, Alk Phos), decreased albumin, increased PT, etc.

B) Hemoglobin C trait or disease, confirm by electrophoresis.

C) Thalassemia, confirm with elevated A2 (>3.5%) by electrophoresis.

C6

Are the results of direct Coombs' test positive?

<u>Yes</u>

C13

Is IgG type positive?

Yes

1) Primary idiopathic warm reactive
2) Secondary warm reactive (eg, lymphoreticular malignancy, SLE, infectious mononucleosis)
3) Drug dependent warm reactive (eg, penicillin, quinidine, Aldomet®..take careful history)

No

Is complement only positive?

Yes

1) Idiopathic cold agglutinin disease
2) Secondary to *Mycoplasma*, infectious mononucleosis, lymphoma
3) PCH

No

Lab error IgG and/or complement are likely to be positive; repeat Coombs'.

Go to C2

<u>No</u>

What is MCHC?

Patient probably has hereditary spherocytosis.

The MCHC is usually >34 but can drop below during reticulocytosis, confirm diagnosis with osmotic fragility test.

The patient should have splenomegaly and a history of jaundice. The disease is inherited as an autosomal dominant.

C7

Have test repeated to assure that the result is not an artifact.

If results are repeatable then the diagnosis is hereditary elliptocytosis (very rarely of clinical significance).

C8

Due to:

1) Severe (end-stage) liver disease...do Liver Chem Profile.

2) Congenital abetalipoproteinemia Publish it!

C9

Patient has hereditary stomatocytosis, or smear may be an artifact.

C10

Causes of red cell fragmentation:

A) Microangiopathic hemolytic anemia

1) DIC (look for underlying disease eg, adenocarcinoma, Gram +/- sepsis, etc)

2) TTP (many schistocytes, thrombocytopenia, and transient neurological signs)

3) Hemolytic uremic syndrome

B) Immune vasculitis (eg, lupus, other collagen vascular diseases, Rocky Mountain spotted fever, etc)

C) Abnormal heart valves

D) Eclampsia

E) March hemoglobinuria

F) Severe burns

C11

The patient has malaria. Confirm with thick smear.

C12

Do a direct Coombs'. Are the results of direct Coombs' positive?

Yes — Go to C13

No — Possible hemoglobinopathy. Do hemoglobin electrophoresis

Are results positive?

Yes — 8% of American blacks have sickle trait (AS). 0.15% of American blacks have sickle cell disease (SS). Hemoglobin C is 10 times less likely than hemoglobin S. Hundreds of rare hemoglobin variants exist, most of them quite rare.

No — Go to C14

C14

Do PK and G-6-PD enzyme screens.

Is PK present?

Is G-6-PD present?

PK (Yes) G-6-PD (No)

The patient has G-6-PD deficiency. Be careful. False-negatives can occur if measured at time of hemolytic crisis.

PK (No) G-6-PD (Yes)

Patient has PK deficiency

PK (Yes) G-6-PD (Yes)

Other enzyme deficiencies could be the cause of the hemolysis. A reference lab screens the other red cell enzymes, but the price is exceedingly high. The chance of such deficiency is 1 in 300,000. Shall we send the studies?

- Yes → C15
- No → C16

PK (No) G-6-PD (No)

Publish it!

C15

Are the results positive?

- Yes: Publish it!
- No: Sorry, your health insurance payment has gone up $10.00 per month.

C16

Sorry, but we are fresh out of lab tests to work up this patient's anemia.

Go back to the patient and repeat history and physical.

Look for splenomegaly.

If still no clues, get hematology consultation.

C25

What values does patient have? B_{12}, Folate and RBC Folate

300 > B_{12} < 1000, Folate < 2, RBC Folate < 200

Patient has folate deficiency.

The bone marrow aspirate will show hyperplastic, megaloblastic changes.

B_{12} < 300, Folate > 2, RBC Folate > 200

The patient has B_{12} deficiency.

Do Schilling test, parts 1 & 2, to distinguish gastric from ileal problem.

The bone marrow aspirate will show hyperplastic, megaloblastic changes.

B_{12} < 300, Folate < 2, RBC Folate < 200

The patient has both B_{12} and folate deficiencies.

The bone marrow aspirate will show hyperplastic, megaloblastic changes.

Any other combination?

Do bone marrow aspirate and biopsy and evaluate microscopically.

A) Myelophthisic state - this will show crowding out of the normal hematopoietic elements of the bone marrow by leukemia, metastic carcinoma, TB, etc.

B) Hypoplasia/aplasia - bone marrow will show decrease in erythrocytic precursors only (pure red cell aplasia) or panhypoplasia of marrow elements.

C) Endocrinopathy - slight hypoplasia due to Hashimoto's thyroiditis, Addison's disease, etc. Do appropriate endocrine tests.

D) Normal marrow - get home consult.

C100

What pattern of iron studies does patient have?

- **Iron < 55, TIBC > 400, % Sat < 25, Fer < 12**
  The patient has iron deficiency.
  A bone marrow is not necessary, but would show absence of stainable iron.
- **Iron < 55, TIBC ≤ 400, % Sat ≤ 40, Fer > 12**
  Anemia of chronic disease, (autoimmune disease, infection, or malignancy...re: iron block)
- **Iron > 150, TIBC < 250, % Sat > 25, Fer > 50**
  The patient has sideroblastic anemia, either congenital, or acquired (lead poisoning, alcohol, isoniazid, etc).
- **55 ≥ Iron ≤ 150, 12 ≥ Fer ≤ 50**
  A1
  Patient has beta thalassemia.
  Confirm with electrophoresis.
  Hb A_2 will be >3.5%.
  Target cells will be seen on peripheral smear.
- **Any other combination**
  What is patient's BUN?
  - **BUN ≤ 50**: Go to C25
  - **BUN > 50**: Chronic renal failure
    Bone marrow will show hypoplasia due to lack of erythropoietin and toxicity of urea.

D

The patient has a normocytic, heterogeneous anemia.

Probable early iron, sideroblastic, or folate deficiency (or mixed deficiency)

What values does patient have for ferritin and RBC folate?

- **Fer < 12, RBC Folate < 200**
  The patient has mixed iron and folate deficiency.
- **Fer > 12, RBC Folate < 200**
  The patient has early folate deficiency.
- **Fer > 50, RBC Folate < 200**
  The patient has a mixed sideroblastic anemia and folate deficiency... Publish it!
- **Fer < 12, RBC Folate > 200**
  The patient has early iron deficiency anemia.
- **12 < Fer < 50, RBC Folate > 200**
  Is the patient black?
  - **Yes**: Do hemoglobin electrophoresis.
    Results positive?
    - **Yes**: The patient has an "anemic" hemoglobinopathy, probably hemoglobin SS or SC.
    - **No**: (D2)
  - **No**: Go to D2
- **Fer > 50, RBC Folate > 200**
  The patient has sideroblastic anemia, confirm with oberservation of ringed sideroblasts in the bone marrow.

D2

The patient may have myelofibrosis. The differential should show a leukoerythroblastic reaction (nucleated RBCs and young WBCs).

Do bone marrow aspirate and biopsy to confirm.

If not myelofibrosis, repeat CBC and let's see what else might have caused the anemia.

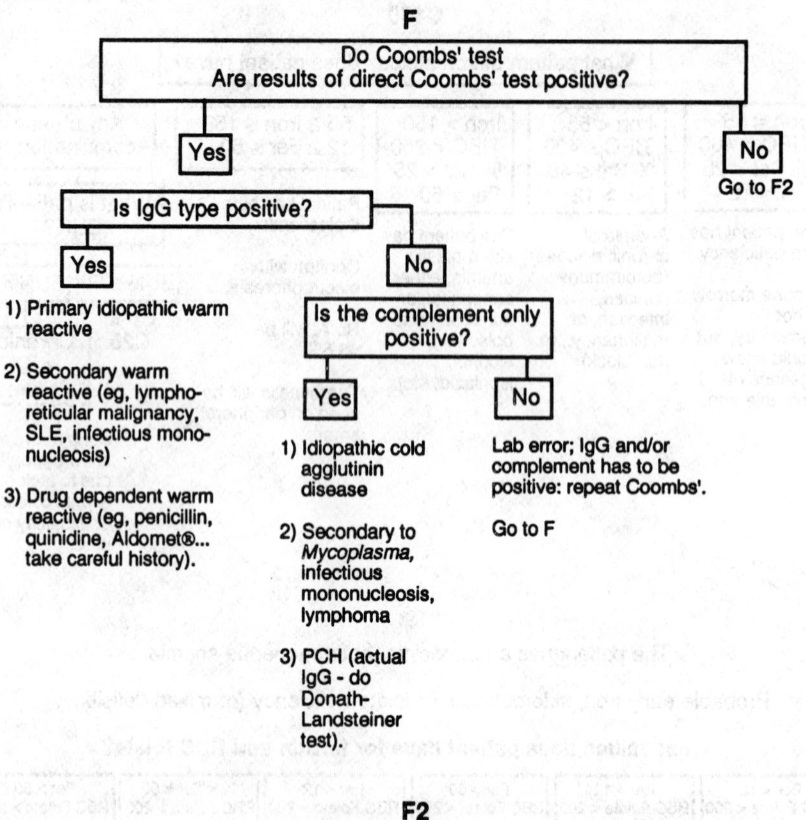
F
Do Coombs' test
Are results of direct Coombs' test positive?
Yes
No
Go to F2
Is IgG type positive?
Yes
1) Primary idiopathic warm reactive
2) Secondary warm reactive (eg, lympho-reticular malignancy, SLE, infectious mono-nucleosis)
3) Drug dependent warm reactive (eg, penicillin, quinidine, Aldomet®... take careful history).
No
Is the complement only positive?
Yes
1) Idiopathic cold agglutinin disease
2) Secondary to Mycoplasma, infectious mononucleosis, lymphoma
3) PCH (actual IgG - do Donath-Landsteiner test).
No
Lab error; IgG and/or complement has to be positive: repeat Coombs'.
Go to F

F2

Macrocytic, heterogeneous anemia

What pattern of iron studies does patient have?

$300 > B_{12} < 1000$ Folate < 2 RBC Folate < 200	$B_{12} < 300$ Folate > 2 RBC Folate > 200	$B_{12} < 300$ RBC Folate < 200	Any other combination?
The patient has folate deficiency. Go to F3	The patient has B_{12} deficiency. Do Schilling test, Part 1 & 2 to distinguish gastric from ileal problems. Go to F3	The patient has both B_{12} and folate deficiencies. Go to F3	Do bone marrow aspirate and biopsy and evaluate microscopically. If the diagnosis is not apparent then repeat CBC and begin work-up again.

F3

The bone marrow aspirate will show hyperplastic, megaloblastic changes.

IMMUNOLOGY AND SEROLOGY

David F. Keren, MD

Automation of serologic tests, broad availability of monoclonal antibody reagents, and dramatic improvements in flow cytometry instrumentation and software have combined to expand the readily available immunologic evaluation of many clinical laboratories. With this expanded capability, however, comes the problem of interpreting the occasional unusual result, handling the unusual specimen, being responsible to only offer in-house tests which are cost-effective, and educating laboratory staff and the clinical personnel as to their proper use and misuse to avoid needless expense to the patient.

For instance, we have recently learned that antibodies against antigens present in neutrophil cytoplasm have significance for diagnosing and following patients with Wegener's granulomatosis and many forms of systemic vasculitis. In addition, however, we now recognize that serum from the majority of patients with ulcerative colitis will also give positive reactions with neutrophils which resembles the perinuclear staining pattern seen with many forms of vasculitis. These are useful new assays that improve our diagnosis and prognosis for specific patients. However, the actual reading of some of these patterns can be tricky and subjective. Therefore, individuals must be trained by experienced workers before some of the newer assays are incorporated into the laboratory.

Patients with acquired immunodeficiency syndrome often have a profound polyclonal expansion of their immunoglobulins, often with readily detectable clones (oligoclonal). It may create problems in interpretation of serum protein electrophoresis and produce false-positives in some serologic studies.

Many new assays and markers are available for subtyping lymphoproliferative disorders, following patients with immunodeficiency diseases, and detecting unusual infections. Whereas many of these provide diagnostically useful information, we need to be cautious in our enthusiasm about new technologies to eliminate unnecessary costs. Some clinicians and laboratorians are tempted to perform an assay because the information the test would provide may be "interesting" though the information is not needed for diagnosis or prognosis. This type of thinking can no longer be afforded. Certainly there is a place for performing assays of interest. That place is when using an approved, carefully thought out, research protocol or at the expense of the individual who wants the information. The old adage which I learned during my training from Dr Rex B. Conn is still correct, "Ask yourself what you will change about the patient's care or prognosis if the test is positive or negative. If there is no difference in what you will do, don't do the test."

A_1AT *see* Alpha$_1$-Antitrypsin, Serum *on page 631*

A_1AT Phenotype *see* Alpha$_1$-Antitrypsin Phenotyping *on page 630*

AAT *see* Alpha$_1$-Antitrypsin, Serum *on page 631*

AAT Phenotype *see* Alpha$_1$-Antitrypsin Phenotyping *on page 630*

AAT-Pi *see* Alpha$_1$-Antitrypsin Phenotyping *on page 630*

ACA *see* Anticardiolipin Antibody *on page 632*

ACA *see* Centromere/Kinetochore Antibody *on page 653*

***Acanthocheilonema perstans* Serology** *see* Filariasis Serological Test *on page 679*

Acetylcholine Modulating Antibody *see* Acetylcholine Receptor Antibody *on this page*

Acetylcholine Receptor Antibody

CPT 84238

Synonyms Acetylcholine Modulating Antibody; Receptor Blocking Antibody; Receptor Modulating Antibody

Abstract Myasthenia gravis is an acquired autoimmune disease in which weakness and easy fatigability occur. Involvement of extraocular or general voluntary muscles is found.

Specimen Serum **CONTAINER:** Red top tube **STORAGE INSTRUCTIONS:** Separate serum and freeze in plastic vial **CAUSES FOR REJECTION:** Recent radioactive scan

Interpretive **REFERENCE RANGE:** Normal: <0.03 nmol/L; 1-20 nmol/L in 50% of patients; 20-400 nmol/L in 50% of patients **USE:** Contribute to diagnosis of myasthenia gravis **LIMITATIONS:** Poor concordance between antibody titer and clinical activity. Use of nonhuman substrates may produce false-negative results. Antibodies are not found in congenital myasthenia. **CONTRAINDICATIONS:** Recent radioactive scan **METHODOLOGY:** Radioimmunoassay (RIA), enzyme-linked immunosorbent assay (ELISA) **ADDITIONAL INFORMATION:** Antibodies to acetylcholine receptors are present in 90% of patients with generalized myasthenia gravis and in 75% to 80% of patients with ocular disease. These antibodies bind to a site different from that which binds acetylcholine or α-bungarotoxin, and receptor injury may be mediated by complement. The specificity of the antibodies vary from patient to patient. Those patients with antibody that inhibits the binding of α-bungarotoxin pursue an aggressive course. Antibodies to the neurotransmitter binding site (receptor blocking antibodies) can be detected in 30% of patients with myasthenia. Receptor modulating antibodies are present in 90% of myasthenic patients, and may be useful in patients with recent onset of disease. Myasthenia gravis is often associated with other autoantibodies (striational antibody 50%, thyroglobulin antibodies 40%) and with HLA-B8 and DR3. Sixty-six percent have thymic hyperplasia and up to 15% develop thymoma.

References

Biesecker G and Koffler D, "Immunology of Myasthenia Gravis," *Hum Pathol*, 1983, 14:419-23.

Bigazzi PE, Burek CL, and Rose NR, "Antibodies to Tissue-Specific Endocrine, Gastrointestinal, and Surface-Receptor Antigens," *Manual of Clinical Laboratory Immunology*, 4th ed, Vol 2, Rose NR, Conway de Macario E, Fahey JL, et al, eds, Washington, DC: American Society for Microbiology, 1992, 765-74.

Colvin RB, Bhan AK, and McCluskey RT, eds, *Diagnostic Immunopathology*, New York, NY: Raven Press, 1988, 112.

Engel AG, "Disorders of Neuromuscular Transmission," *Cecil Textbook of Medicine*, Vol 2, Wyngaarden JB, Smith LH Jr, and Bennett JC, eds, Philadelphia, PA: WB Saunders Co, 1992, 2265-7.

Lennon VA and Howard FM, "Serological Diagnosis of Myasthenia Gravis" *Clinical Lab Molecular Analyses*, Nakamura RM and O'Sullivan MB, eds, New York, NY: Grune and Stratton Inc, 1985, 29-44.

Pachner AR, "Antiacetylcholine Receptor Antibodies Block Bungarotoxin Binding to Native Human Acetylcholine Receptor on the Surface of TE671 Cells," *Neurology*, 1989, 39(8):1057-61.

ACL *see* Anticardiolipin Antibody *on page 632*

ACPA *see* Antineutrophil Cytoplasmic Antibody *on page 636*

Acquired Immune Deficiency Syndrome Serology *see* HIV-1/HIV-2 Serology *on page 696*

Acute Phase Proteins *see* Alpha$_1$-Antitrypsin, Serum *on page 631*

Acute Phase Reactant *see* Alpha$_1$-Antitrypsin, Serum *on page 631*

Acute Phase Reactant *see* C-Reactive Protein *on page 669*

Adenovirus Antibody Titer

***CPT** 86603*

Related Information

Adenovirus Culture *on page 1169*
Adenovirus Culture, Rapid *on page 1170*
Conjunctival Culture *on page 803*
Viral Culture, Respiratory Symptoms *on page 1204*
Virus, Direct Detection by Fluorescent Antibody *on page 1208*

Synonyms Adenovirus Serology

Test Commonly Includes Detection of increased antibody response to adenovirus

Specimen Serum **CONTAINER:** Red top tube **COLLECTION:** Acute and convalescent sera drawn 2-3 weeks apart are required **SPECIAL INSTRUCTIONS:** Acute and convalescent sera must be tested simultaneously. Tests will, therefore, not be performed unless both specimens are received.

Interpretive **REFERENCE RANGE:** A fourfold increase in titer in paired sera is indicative of a virus infection. Expected value single specimen: ≤1:16. **USE:** Establish the diagnosis of adenovirus infection; useful in differential diagnosis of respiratory ailments, hemorrhagic cystitis, and keratoconjunctivitis **LIMITATIONS:** The specific adenovirus serotype responsible for infection cannot be determined by complement fixation test. Complement fixation tests are of low sensitivity, particularly in children. Thus, not all adenovirus infections are accompanied by a predictable increase in detectable antibody response. **METHODOLOGY:** Complement fixation (CF), hemagglutination inhibition (HAI), enzyme-linked immunosorbent assay (ELISA), serum neutralization **ADDITIONAL INFORMATION:** There are 41 different types of adenovirus, and many infections are both asymptomatic and persistent. Thus, serologic evidence of adenovirus, and even isolation of an adenovirus from a patient, may be coincidental rather than the cause of the patient's present complaints.

References

Abzug MJ and Levin MJ, "Neonatal Adenovirus Infection: Four Patients and Review of the Literature," *Pediatrics*, 1991, 87(6):890-6.

Bryan JA, "The Serologic Diagnosis of Viral Infections," *Arch Pathol Lab Med*, 1987, 111:1015-23.

Hierholzer JC, "Adenoviruses," *Manual of Clinical Laboratory Immunology*, 4th ed, Vol 2, Rose NR, Conway de Macario E, Fahey JL, et al, eds, Washington, DC: American Society for Microbiology, 1992, 590-5.

Adenovirus Serology *see* Adenovirus Antibody Titer *on this page*

ADNase-B *see* Antideoxyribonuclease-B Titer, Serum *on page 633*

Adrenal Antibody, Serum

***CPT** 86255 (screen); 86256 (titer)*

Synonyms Antiadrenal Cortex Antibodies

Specimen Serum **CONTAINER:** Red top tube

Interpretive **REFERENCE RANGE:** Negative **USE:** Evaluate adrenal insufficiency **METHODOLOGY:** Indirect fluorescent antibody (IFA) **ADDITIONAL INFORMATION:** Serum antibodies to adrenal cortical cells, usually of all three zones, are seen in 60% of patients with **idiopathic Addison's disease**. They are present in only 5% to 17% of patients with tuberculous, fungal or metastatic destruction of the adrenals, and in 38% of unclassified cases. Antiadrenal antibodies are also present in such apparently unrelated processes as idiopathic hypoparathyroidism (28% of cases) and Hashimoto's disease (7%).

References

Bigazzi PE, Burek CL, and Rose NR, "Antibodies to Tissue-Specific Endocrine, Gastrointestinal, and Surface-Receptor Antigens," *Manual of Clinical Laboratory Immunology*, Vol 2, 4th ed, Rose NR, Conway de Macario E, Fahey JL, et al, eds, Washington, DC: American Society for Microbiology, 1992, 765-74.

Colvin RB, Bhan AK, and McCluskey RT, eds, *Diagnostic Immunopathology*, New York, NY: Raven Press, 1988, 107.

Agglutinins, Febrile *see* Febrile Agglutinins, Serum *on page 678*

AHBC *see* Hepatitis B Core Antibody *on page 684*

AH Titer *see* Antihyaluronidase Titer *on page 635*

AIDS Screen *see* HIV-1/HIV-2 Serology *on page 696*

Air Conditioner Lung *see* Hypersensitivity Pneumonitis Serology *on page 704*

Allergic Lung Serology *see* Hypersensitivity Pneumonitis Serology *on page 704*

Alpha$_1$-Antitrypsin Phenotyping

CPT 82104

Related Information

Alpha$_1$-Antitrypsin, Serum *on next page*

Protein Electrophoresis, Serum *on page 734*

Synonyms A_1AT Phenotype; AAT Phenotype; AAT-Pi; Alpha$_1$-Protease Inhibitor; Pi Phenotype; Protease Inhibitors

Test Commonly Includes Serum trypsin inhibitory capacity

Abstract Alpha$_1$-antitrypsin deficiency (alpha$_1$-protease inhibitor deficiency) is a genetic disease characterized by varying levels of severity. Alpha$_1$-antitrypsin is a glycoprotein which is the largest fraction (65%) in the alpha$_1$ globulins. Patients are detected by lack or diminution of the alpha$_1$ band on serum protein electrophoresis, abnormal migration of the alpha$_1$ band or by decreased levels determined immunochemically.

Cases of emphysema which are caused by hereditary alpha$_1$-antitrypsin deficiency make up about 2% of the incidence of emphysema.

Patient Care PREPARATION: Fasting preferred

Specimen Serum CONTAINER: Red top tube COLLECTION: Routine venipuncture STORAGE INSTRUCTIONS: Separate serum and refrigerate or freeze. CAUSES FOR REJECTION: Hemolyzed serum, serum stored at room temperature

Interpretive REFERENCE RANGE: Interpretation usually accompanies report; phenotypes are designated. PiMM phenotype is normal; PiMZ is heterozygous, intermediate deficient; and PiZZ is homozygous, severely deficient. Over 75 alleles are described; biosynthesis of A_1AT is controlled at the Pi locus by a pair of genes. There is codominant expression. The phenotype is "Pi" for protease inhibitor. Z and S are mutant proteins. A null-null state occurs as well. In the dysfunctional type, A_1AT is found in normal amounts but does not function normally. USE: Definitive analysis of hereditary alpha$_1$-antitrypsin deficiency which is associated with chronic obstructive pulmonary disease (COPD) (panacinar or panlobular emphysema), hepatic cirrhosis, and hepatoma. Cholestasis with neonatal hepatitis is found in a minority of neonates with A_1AT deficiency. METHODOLOGY: Crossed immunoelectrophoresis, isoelectric focusing; ***vide infra*** ADDITIONAL INFORMATION: Most pathologic is homozygous ZZ. An M null genotype will have phenotype as MM but low serum level of A_1AT. Alpha$_1$-antitrypsin deficiency may eventuate in or be associated with cholestatic hepatopathy in infants, a chronic hepatitis, familial infantile cirrhosis, or familial emphysema. The risks of cirrhosis and development of hepatoma are greater in males.

Alpha$_1$-antitrypsin (A_1AT) is a glycoprotein synthesized in the liver. It is the main component of the alpha$_1$ globulins. A_1AT serves to counter the effects of several serine proteases including elastase and trypsin. When A_1AT is deficient, unopposed activity of these enzymes results in emphysema. The age of occurrence of emphysema varies with the type of deficiency, ZZ being most severe, ZS less severe, and SS least severe. It often varies with the personal habits of the individual, especially regarding smoking.

In individuals with A_1AT deficiency, PAS-positive diastase-negative globules accumulate in periportal hepatocytes. Eventually, damage occurs which may result in cirrhosis.

It is especially important to detect A_1AT deficiency early, as an experimental replacement therapy is now available which has received favorable review in a recent NIH study. Although the long-term effects of this therapy are still unknown, it does have great potential to decrease the severity of emphysema.

A_1AT is a positive acute phase protein because it rises whenever there is tissue injury, necrosis, inflammation, or infection. Therefore, patients with A_1AT deficiency who suffer from bronchitis, pneumonia, or similar respiratory inflammation may have falsely normal levels during acute illness. After the acute phase of illness has passed, repeat determinations often reveal the "true" or "resting" A_1AT level which is indicative of the heterozygous phenotypic deficiency.

Therefore, use of high-resolution electrophoresis which would detect the slower electrophoretic migration of the Z and S variants is preferred over quantification of A_1AT by nephelometry as a screen for this deficiency. Further, a high-resolution electrophoretic system will detect heterozygotes which could lead to important family studies of potentially deficient first-degree relatives who may benefit from therapy.

Serum A_1AT may be increased in patients during normal pregnancy, chronic pulmonary diseases, hereditary angioneurotic edema, gastric diseases, liver diseases, pancreatitis, diabetes, carcinomas, renal diseases, and rheumatic diseases and may be decreased in patients with severe protein loss or in improper storage of specimen.

More than 95% of subjects who are severely deficient are homozygous for the Z allele (PiZZ). PiZZ subjects who smoke have a shorter life expectancy than do nonsmoking PiZZ persons. Variation in severity of clinical manifestations is recognized; some subjects with deficiency do not have significant impairment, but development of airway disease is partly a function of age.

References

Buist AS, "Alpha 1-Antitrypsin Deficiency – Diagnosing Treatment and Control: Identification of Patients," *Lung*, 1990, 168(Suppl):543-51.

Buist AS, "Alpha 1-Antitrypsin Deficiency in Lung and Liver Disease," *Hosp Pract Off Ed*, 1989, 24(5):51-9.

Cohen AB, "Unraveling the Mysteries of $Alpha_1$-Antitrypsin Deficiency," *N Engl J Med*, 1986, 314:778-9.

Crystal RG, "Alpha-1-Antitrypsin Deficiency: Pathogenesis and Treatment," *Hosp Pract Off Ed*, 1991, 26(2):81-4, 88-9, 93-4.

Eriksson S, Carlson J, and Velez R, "Risk of Cirrhosis and Primary Liver Cancer in $Alpha_1$-Antitrypsin Deficiency," *N Engl J Med*, 1986, 314:736-9.

Garver RI Jr, Mornex J-F, Nukiwa T, et al, "$Alpha_1$-Antitrypsin Deficiency and Emphysema Caused by Homozygous Inheritance of Nonexpressing $Alpha_1$-Antitrypsin Genes," *N Engl J Med*, 1986, 314:762-66.

Hutchison DC, "Natural History of Alpha-1-Protease Inhibitor Deficiency," *Am J Med*, 1988, 84:3-12.

Ishak KG and Sharp HL, "Metabolic Errors and Liver Disease," *Pathology of the Liver*, Chapter 4, MacSween RNM, Anthony PP, and Scheuer PJ, eds, New York, NY: Churchill Livingstone, 1987, 118-23.

Keren DF, *High-Resolution Electrophoresis and Immunofixation: Techniques and Interpretation*, Boston, MA: Butterworth's Publishers, 1987, 31-5.

Pierce JA, "Antitrypsin and Emphysema. Perspective and Prospects," *JAMA*, 1988, 259:2890-5.

Schmidt EW, Rasche B, Ulmer WT, et al, "Replacement Therapy for Alpha-1-Protease Inhibitor Deficiency in PiZ Subjects With Chronic Obstructive Lung Disease," *Am J Med*, 1988, 84:63-9.

Silverman EK, Pierce JA, Province MA, et al, "Variability of Pulmonary Function in $Alpha_1$-Antitrypsin Deficiency: Clinical Correlates," *Ann Intern Med*, 1989, 111(12):982-91.

Snider GL, "Pulmonary Disease in $Alpha_1$-Antitrypsin Deficiency," *Ann Intern Med*, 1989, 111(12):957-9.

Weinberger SE, "Recent Advances in Pulmonary Medicine," *N Engl J Med*, 1993, 328(19):1389-97.

$Alpha_1$-Antitrypsin, Serum

***CPT** 82103*

Related Information

$Alpha_1$-Antitrypsin Phenotyping *on previous page*
C-Reactive Protein *on page 669*
Protein Electrophoresis, Serum *on page 734*

Synonyms A_1AT; AAT; Acute Phase Proteins; α-1-Antitrypsin

Applies to Acute Phase Reactant; Specific Protein Analysis

Specimen Serum **CONTAINER:** Red top tube **CAUSES FOR REJECTION:** Lipemic serum

Interpretive **REFERENCE RANGE:** 78-200 mg/dL (SI: 0.78-2.00 g/L) **USE:** Detect hereditary decreases in the production of $alpha_1$-antitrypsin (A_1AT). Decreased or nearly absent levels of AAT can be a factor in chronic obstructive lung disease and liver disease. An increased prevalence of non-MM phenotypes is found with cryptogenic cirrhosis and with CAH. Cirrhosis in a child should raise consideration of AAT deficiency or Wilson's disease. Diagnosis of inflammatory states, if AAT is elevated (eg, rheumatoid arthritis, bacterial infection, vasculitis, neoplasia). **LIMITATIONS:** AAT may be elevated into normal range in heterozygous deficient patients during concurrent infection, pregnancy, estrogen therapy, steroid therapy, cancer, and during postoperative periods. Homozygous deficient patients will not show such elevation. Normal AAT levels may occur in patients with liver disease who are heterozygotes. In normals, pregnancy and contraceptive medication may elevate levels. Levels are normally low at birth but rise soon thereafter. **CONTRAINDICATIONS:** If CRP positive, retest AAT in 10-14 days. **METHODOLOGY:** Radial immunodiffusion (RID), nephelometry **ADDITIONAL INFORMATION:** Should be run when $alpha_1$ globulin in serum protein electrophoresis is low, when two bands are seen in the $alpha_1$ region, or when the $alpha_1$ region is obscured by $alpha_1$ lipoprotein. Heterozygous patients exhibit AAT levels which are commonly about 60% of normal. Homozygous recessive AAT patients exhibit levels at about 10% of normal. Phenotyping is desirable on patients with low values and on all patients being worked up for AAT-deficient liver disease. Most patholog-

(Continued)

Alpha$_1$-Antitrypsin, Serum *(Continued)*

ic is homozygous state ZZ. An M null genotype will have phenotype as MM but low serum level. AAT is one of the alpha globulins which together are called "acute phase reactants." These rise rapidly, but nonspecifically, in response to inflammatory insults.

References

Brantly ML, Wittes JT, Vogelmeier CF, et al, "Use of a Highly Purified Alpha$_1$-Antitrypsin Standard to Establish Ranges for the Common Normal and Deficient Alpha$_1$-Antitrypsin Phenotypes," *Chest*, 1991, 100(3):703-8.

Hodges JR, Millward-Sadler GH, Barbatis C, et al, "Heterozygous MZ Alpha$_1$ Antitrypsin Deficiency in Adults With Chronic Active Hepatitis and Cryptogenic Cirrhosis," *N Engl J Med*, 1981, 304:557-68.

Alpha$_1$-Protease Inhibitor *see* Alpha$_1$-Antitrypsin Phenotyping *on page 630*

Alternate Complement Pathway *see* Factor B *on page 678*

AMA *see* Antimitochondrial Antibody *on page 635*

Amebiasis Serological Test *see* *Entamoeba histolytica* Serological Test *on page 675*

ANA *see* Antinuclear Antibody *on page 638*

ANCA *see* Antineutrophil Cytoplasmic Antibody *on page 636*

ANF *see* Antinuclear Antibody *on page 638*

Antiadrenal Cortex Antibodies *see* Adrenal Antibody, Serum *on page 629*

Anti-B19 IgG Antibodies *see* Parvovirus B19 Serology *on page 731*

Anti-B19 IgM Antibodies *see* Parvovirus B19 Serology *on page 731*

Antibody to *Coccidioides immitis* *see* Coccidioidomycosis Antibodies *on page 664*

Antibody to Double-Stranded DNA *see* Anti-DNA *on page 634*

Antibody to HAV, IgM *see* Hepatitis A Antibody, IgM *on page 683*

Antibody to Hepatitis B Core Antigen *see* Hepatitis B Core Antibody *on page 684*

Antibody to Hepatitis B Surface Antigen *see* Hepatitis B Surface Antibody *on page 687*

Antibody to Native DNA *see* Anti-DNA *on page 634*

Anticardiolipin Antibody

CPT *86147*

Related Information

Anticoagulant, Circulating *on page 402*
Antinuclear Antibody *on page 638*
Automated Reagin Test *on page 642*
Hypercoagulable State Coagulation Screen *on page 441*
Inhibitor, Lupus, Phospholipid Type *on page 444*
RPR *on page 742*
Sjögren's Antibodies *on page 746*
VDRL, Serum *on page 762*

Synonyms ACA; ACL

Applies to Antiphospholipid Antibody; Lupus Anticoagulant (LA)

Test Commonly Includes Detection of antibody to the phospholipid, cardiolipin

Abstract Anticardiolipin and lupus anticoagulant are acquired antiphospholipid antibodies. They are autoantibodies found in subjects with systemic lupus erythematosus and related entities.[1]

Specimen Serum **CONTAINER:** Red top tube

Interpretive **REFERENCE RANGE:** Negative **USE:** Differential diagnosis of recurrent thromboses, lupus-like syndromes, false-positive VDRL or RPR, recurrent fetal loss, and rarely, severe hemorrhage **LIMITATIONS:** Anticardiolipin levels by enzyme-linked immunosorbent assay (ELISA) are associated with poor reproducibility. **METHODOLOGY:** Enzyme immunoassay (EIA) **ADDITIONAL INFORMATION:** Antibody to a cardiolipin, the diphosphatidyl glycerol component of many phospholipid membranes, is at least partially cross reactive with the reagin antibody of syphilis and the lupus anticoagulant. ACA is associated with a host of clinical and laboratory abnormalities. Abnormal tests include thrombocytopenia, reactive VDRL or RPR, SS-A/Ro antibodies, and prolonged activated partial thromboplastin time (APTT) (lupus anticoagulant). Clinically, patients have lupus-like symptoms, often "ANA negative," recurrent venous and arterial thromboses, recurrent fetal loss (usually more than two episodes for a strong association), mitral valve endocarditis, chorea, and epilepsy. The entire constellation is sometimes called the antiphospholipid antibody syndrome. The association between thrombosis and recurrent fetal loss and ACA in patients with a prolonged APTT is especially strong in patients in whom ACA is not induced by infection or medication. IgG anticardiolipin is more influenced by disease activity than is IgM anticardiolipin. Plasmapheresis along with anticoagulant therapy is often used in symptomatic cases. Lupus anticoagulant and anticardiolipin antibodies are found together in about 70% of patients with antiphospholipid antibody syndrome. LA is found in about 34% and ACA is found in 44% of subjects with SLE.[2]

Footnotes

1. Love PE and Santoro SA, "Antiphospholipid Antibodies: Anticardiolipin and the Lupus Anticoagulant in Systemic Lupus Erythematosus (SLE) and in Non-SLE Disorders," *Ann Intern Med*, 1990, 112(9):682-98.
2. Arnold WJ and Ike RW, "Specialized Procedures in the Management of Patients With Rheumatic Diseases," *Cecil Textbook of Medicine*, Vol 2, Wyngaarden JB, Smith LH Jr, and Bennett JC, eds, Philadelphia, PA: WB Saunders Co, 1992, 1505.

References

Alving BM, Barr CF, and Tang DB, "Correlation Between Lupus Anticoagulants and Anticardiolipin Antibodies in Patients With Prolonged Activated Partial Thromboplastin Times," *Am J Med*, 1990, 88(2):112-6.

Creagh MD, Malia RG, Cooper SM, et al, "Screening for Lupus Anticoagulant and Anticardiolipin Antibodies in Women With Fetal Loss," *J Clin Pathol*, 1991, 44(1):45-7.

Deegan MJ, "Anti-Phospholipid Antibodies," *Am J Clin Pathol*, 1992, 98(4):390-1.

Greisman SG, Thayaparan RS, Godwin TA, et al, "Occlusive Vasculopathy in Systemic Lupus Erythematosus. Association With Anticardiolipin Antibody," *Arch Intern Med*, 1991, 151(2):389-92.

Levine SR and Welch KMA, "The Spectrum of Neurologic Disease Associated With Antiphospholipid Antibodies: Lupus Anticoagulants and Anticardiolipin Antibodies," *Arch Neurol*, 1987, 44:876-83.

Lockshin MD, "Anticardiolipin Antibody," *Arthritis Rheum*, 1987, 30:471-2.

Lopez LR, Santos ME, Espinoza LR, et al, "Clinical Significance of Immunoglobulin A *Versus* Immunoglobulins G and M Anti-Cardiolipin Antibodies in Patients With Systemic Lupus Erythematosus – Correlation with Thrombosis, Thrombocytopenia, and Recurrent Abortion," *Am J Clin Pathol*, 1992, 98(4):449-54.

Meyer O, Piette J-C, Bourgeois P, et al, "Antiphospholipid Antibodies: A Disease Marker in 25 Patients With Antinuclear Antibody Negative Systemic Lupus Erythematosus (SLE)," *J Rheumatol*, 1987, 14:502-6.

Out HJ, de Groot PG, Hasselaar P, et al, "Fluctuations of Anticardiolipin Antibody Levels in Patients With Systemic Lupus Erythematosus: A Prospective Study," *Ann Rheum Dis*, 1989, 48(12):1023-8.

Scully RE, ed, "Case Records of the Massachusetts General Hospital," *N Engl J Med*, 1988, 319:699-712.

Antideoxyribonuclease-B Titer, Serum

CPT *86215*

Related Information

Antihyaluronidase Titer *on page 635*
Antistreptolysin O Titer, Serum *on page 640*
Streptozyme *on page 749*
Throat Culture *on page 876*

Synonyms ADNase-B; Anti-DNase-B Titer; Antistreptococcal DNase-B Titer; Streptodornase

Abstract Of four DNases produced by streptococci, DNase B is antigenically the most conserved.[1]

Specimen Serum **CONTAINER:** Red top tube **CAUSES FOR REJECTION:** Excessive hemolysis, lipemic serum

Interpretive **REFERENCE RANGE:** Children: preschool: ≤60 units; school: ≤170 units; adults: ≤85 units; a rise in titer of two or more dilution increments between acute and convalescent sera is significant. **USE:** Document recent streptococcal infection **LIMITATIONS:** Normal ranges may vary in different populations. **CONTRAINDICATIONS:** Not valid in patients with hemorrhagic pancreatitis **METHODOLOGY:** Colorimetry based on hydrolysis of DNA **ADDITIONAL INFORMATION:** Presence of antibodies to streptococcal DNase is an indicator of recent infection, especially if a rise in titer can be documented. This test has both theoretical and technical advantages over the ASO test: it is more sensitive to streptococcal pyoderma, it is not so subject to false-positives due to liver disease, and one need not worry about test invalidation due to oxidation of reagents. It is positive, like ASO, in about 80% to 85% of patients with streptococcal infections. Application of both tests detects about 95%.[1]

(Continued)

Antideoxyribonuclease-B Titer, Serum *(Continued)*

Footnotes

1. Leavelle DE, *Mayo Medical Laboratories Interpretive Handbook*, Mayo Medical Laboratories, 1990, 169-70.

References

Weinstein AJ and Farkas S, "Serologic Tests in Infectious Diseases: Clinical Utility and Interpretation," *Med Clin North Am*, 1978, 62:1099-1118.

Anti-DNA

***CPT** 86225 (double-stranded); 86226 (single-stranded)*

Related Information

Antinuclear Antibody *on page 638*
Kidney Profile *on page 268*
LE Cell Test *on page 565*

Synonyms Antibody to Double-Stranded DNA; Antibody to Native DNA; Anti-Double-Stranded DNA; Anti-ds-DNA; DNA Antibody; n-DNA; ss-DNA

Test Commonly Includes Titers on positive specimens

Specimen Serum **CONTAINER:** Red top tube **STORAGE INSTRUCTIONS:** Refrigerate immediately.

Interpretive **REFERENCE RANGE:** Normal: low levels of antibody or none (units and reference range will depend on laboratory and methodology) **USE:** Confirmatory test for systemic lupus erythematosus (SLE); monitor clinical course and response to treatments **METHODOLOGY:** Indirect fluorescent antibody (IFA) using *Crithidia luciliae* substrate, radioimmunoassay (RIA), enzyme immunoassay (EIA) **ADDITIONAL INFORMATION:** Antibodies to DNA, either single or double-stranded, are found primarily in systemic lupus erythematosus and are important, but not necessary or sufficient, for diagnosing that condition. Such antibodies are present in 80% to 90% of SLE cases. They are also present in smaller fractions of patients with other rheumatic disorders and in chronic active hepatitis, infectious mononucleosis, and biliary cirrhosis. In part, sensitivity for the different diseases is methodology dependent, and correlation with local laboratory experience is necessary.

In the past it was a rule of thumb that it was unnecessary to test for anti-DNA in patients with a negative test for antinuclear antibodies. A group of "ANA-negative lupus" patients has been described with anti-ss-DNA and anti-SS-A/Ro and anti-SS-B/La. However, HEp-2 substrate is much more sensitive than frozen section substrates; and it is uncommon for anti-SS-A/Ro to be negative with these newer substrates.

False-positive tests due to antibodies against histones have been reported with use of the *Crithidia luciliae* substrate assay.

Following titers of anti-DNA antibody may be of use in evaluating response to therapy, but should be regarded as a guide rather than a rigid dictator of treatment. Titers correlate particularly well with activity of lupus nephritis.

Procainamide and hydralazine may induce anti-ss-DNA antibodies and antihistone antibodies.

Antibodies to ss-DNA are not as diagnostically useful as those against ds-DNA which are associated with renal disease and clinical activity.

References

Carson DA, "The Specificity of Anti-DNA Antibodies in Systemic Lupus Erythematosus," *J Immunol*, 1991, 146(1):1-2.

Christian CL, "Prognostic and Therapeutic Implications of Immunologic Test Results in Rheumatic Disease," *Hum Pathol*, 1983, 14:446-8.

Colvin RB, Bhan AK, and McCluskey RT, eds, *Diagnostic Immunopathology*, New York, NY: Raven Press, 1988, 97-8.

Harmon CE, "Antinuclear Antibodies in Autoimmune Disease," *Med Clin North Am*, 1985, 69:547-63.

James K and Meek G, "Evaluation of Commercial Enzyme Immunoassays Compared to Immunofluorescence and Double Diffusion for Autoantibodies Associated With Autoimmune Diseases," *Am J Clin Pathol*, 1992, 97(4):559-65.

Suenaga R, Evans M, and Abdou NI, "Idiotypic and Immunochemical Differences of Anti-DNA Antibodies of a Lupus Patient During Active and Inactive Disease," *Clin Immunol Immunopathol*, 1991, 61(3):320-1.

Anti-DNase-B Titer *see* Antideoxyribonuclease-B Titer, Serum *on previous page*

Anti-Double-Stranded DNA *see* Anti-DNA *on this page*

Anti-ds-DNA *see* Anti-DNA *on this page*

Anti-GBM *see* Glomerular Basement Membrane Antibody *on page 681*

Antiglomerular Basement Membrane Antibody *see* Glomerular Basement Membrane Antibody *on page 681*

Anti-HAV, IgM *see* Hepatitis A Antibody, IgM *on page 683*

Anti-HB$_c$ *see* Hepatitis B Core Antibody *on page 684*

Anti-HB$_e$ *see* Hepatitis B$_e$ Antibody *on page 685*

Anti-HB$_s$ *see* Hepatitis B Surface Antibody *on page 687*

Anti-HCV (IgM) *see* Hepatitis C Serology *on page 690*

Antihepatitis B Core *see* Hepatitis B Core Antibody *on page 684*

Antihyaluronidase Titer

CPT *86060 (ASO titer); 86215 (antideoxyribonuclease-B titer)*

Related Information

Antideoxyribonuclease-B Titer, Serum *on page 633*
Antistreptolysin O Titer, Serum *on page 640*
Kidney Biopsy *on page 68*
Throat Culture *on page 876*

Synonyms AH Titer; Antistreptococcal Hyaluronidase Titer

Test Commonly Includes Antideoxyribonuclease-B, antihyaluronidase titer, ASO titer

Patient Care PREPARATION: A fasting specimen is preferred.

Specimen Serum CONTAINER: Red top tube

Interpretive REFERENCE RANGE: A fourfold rise in titer between acute and convalescent specimens is considered to be significant, regardless of the magnitude of the titer. For a single specimen, AH titers ≤1:250 are considered normal. USE: Document recent streptococcal infection LIMITATIONS: Test is less reproducible than ASO or anti-DNase-B. METHODOLOGY: Tube enzyme neutralization test ADDITIONAL INFORMATION: In addition to ASO, antihyaluronidase is used to aid in the diagnosis of streptococcal infections. The AHT test is a better test than the ASO test for the detection of antibodies in acute glomerulonephritis which follows a streptococcal pyoderma.

Anti-immunoglobulin A *see* IgA Antibodies *on page 705*

Antimitochondrial Antibody

CPT *86255 (IFA)*

Related Information

Smooth Muscle Antibody *on page 747*

Synonyms AMA; Mitochondrial Antibody

Abstract Primary biliary cirrhosis is a progressive cholestatic disease in which intrahepatic bile ducts undergo damage, leading ultimately to cirrhosis and hepatic failure. Mitochondrial antibodies are found in up to 95% of patients with primary biliary cirrhosis, but may be found in other circumstances as well.[1]

Specimen Serum CONTAINER: Red top tube

Interpretive REFERENCE RANGE: ≤1:20 considered nondiagnostic USE: Tests for mitochondrial antibody are recommended in differential diagnosis of chronic liver disease and to provide confirmatory evidence for a diagnosis of primary biliary cirrhosis LIMITATIONS: Titers <1:16 seen in 10% of cases of primary biliary cirrhosis. Level of antibody does not correlate with severity or duration of disease. Low, transient titers are sometimes seen with chlorpromazine or halothane sensitivity. METHODOLOGY: Indirect fluorescent antibody (IFA), enzyme-linked immunosorbent assay (ELISA) ADDITIONAL INFORMATION: Antimitochondrial antibody is present in 85% to 95% of cases of primary biliary cirrhosis. AMA is also found in 25% to 30% of cases of chronic active hepatitis and in cryptogenic cirrhosis. AMA is rarely found in patients with extrahepatic biliary obstruction, drug-induced hepatitis, viral hepatitis, alcoholic and other forms of cirrhosis, hepatic malignancy and other collagen diseases. There is an incidence of 1% positives in a general hospital population, mostly people with autoimmune disease. Primary biliary cirrhosis (PBC) is a chronic intrahepatic cholestatic disease found more frequently in women than in men with an incidence which is highest in the 30- to 60-year age group. The diagnosis of PBC is based upon clinical observations, histologic findings on liver biopsy, increased alka-

(Continued)

Antimitochondrial Antibody *(Continued)*

line phosphatase activity, elevated IgM levels, and presence of mitochondrial antibodies. Increases of 5'-nucleotidase and gamma-glutamyl transferase parallel those of alkaline phosphatase. In >90% of patients, the key M2 antigen has been identified as the E_2 component of the pyruvate dehydrogenase complex. Enzyme-linked immunosorbent assays developed using pyruvate, branched-chain ketoacid, and alpha-ketoglutarate dehydrogenase promise to add objectivity to analysis of these antibodies.

Footnotes

1. Kaplan MM, "Primary Biliary Cirrhosis," *N Engl J Med*, 1987, 316:521-8.

References

Berg PA and Klein R, "Antimitochondrial Antibodies in Primary Biliary Cirrhosis and Other Disorders: Definition and Clinical Relevance," *Dig Dis*, 1992, 10(2):85-101.

Brenard R and Geubel AP, "Antimitochondrial and Antinuclear Antibodies in Primary Biliary Cirrhosis: An Update in Relation to Their Biochemical Characterization and Clinical Significance," *Acta Clin Belg*, 1991, 46(5):305-12.

Butler P, Valle F, and Burroughs AK, "Mitochondrial Antigens and Antibodies in Primary Biliary Cirrhosis," *Postgrad Med J*, 1991, 67(791):790-7.

Colvin RB, Bhan AK, and McCluskey RT, eds, *Diagnostic Immunopathology*, New York, NY: Raven Press, 1988, 101.

Fussey SP, West SM, Lindsay JG, et al, "Clarifiation of the Identity of the Major M2 Autoantigen in Primary Biliary Cirrhosis," *Clin Sci*, 1991, 80(5):451-5.

Heseltine L, Turner IB, Fussey SP, et al, "Primary Biliary Cirrhosis. Quantitation of Autoantibodies to Purified Mitochondrial Enzymes and Correlation With Disease Progression," *Gastroenterology*, 1990, 99(6):1786-92.

James SP, Hoofnagle JH, Strober W, et al, "NIH Conference: Primary Biliary Cirrhosis: A Model Autoimmune Disease," (Clinical Conference) *Ann Intern Med*, 1983, 99:500-12.

Klion FM, Fabry TL, Palmer M, et al, "Prediction of Survival of Patients With Primary Biliary Cirrhosis," *Gastroenterology*, 1992, 102(1):310-3.

Manns MP and Nakamura RM, "Autoimmune Liver Diseases," *Clin Lab Med*, 1988, 8:281-301.

Neuberger J, Lombard M, and Galbraith R, "Primary Biliary Cirrhosis," *Gut*, 1991, S73-8.

Van de Water J, Cooper A, Surh CD, et al, "Detection of Autoantibodies to Recombinant Mitochondrial Proteins in Patients With Primary Biliary Cirrhosis," *N Engl J Med*, 1989, 320(21):1377-80.

Yeaman SJ, Danner DJ, Mutimer DJ, et al, "Primary Biliary Cirrhosis: Identification of Two Major M2 Mitochondrial Autoantigens," *Lancet*, 1988, 1:1067-9.

Yoshida T, Bonkovsky H, Ansari A, et al, "Antibodies Against Mitochondrial Dehydrogenase Complexes in Primary Biliary Cirrhosis," *Gastroenterology*, 1990, 99(1):187-94.

Antineutrophil Antibody

***CPT** 86255 (screen); 86256 (titer)*

Related Information

White Blood Count *on page 616*

Synonyms Granulocyte Antibody; Neutrophil Antibody

Specimen Serum **CONTAINER:** Red top tube **COLLECTION:** Routine venipuncture **STORAGE INSTRUCTIONS:** Remove serum from clot as soon as possible. Freeze serum. **CAUSES FOR REJECTION:** Specimen collected in the incorrect tube, gross hemolysis, quantity not sufficient, serum not frozen

Interpretive **REFERENCE RANGE:** Negative **USE:** Investigate for possible immune origin of neutropenia; detect antibodies against granulocyte-specific antigens to evaluate neonatal alloimmune neutropenia, autoimmune neutropenia, and transfusion reactions **METHODOLOGY:** Immunoassay **ADDITIONAL INFORMATION:** Recent advances in antibody detection have made possible the detection of autoantibodies specific for neutrophils. Autoantibodies to the two antigen sites, NA_2 and ND_1, are detected providing compelling evidence of the existence of autoimmune neutropenia. In some patients with autoimmune neutropenia, autoantibodies have specificity to action. This condition is associated with idiopathic thrombocytopenia purpura and responds to steroids. Resulting neutropenia may be moderate to severe.

References

Hartman KR, Mallet MK, Nath J, et al, "Antibodies to Actin in Autoimmune Neutropenia," *Blood*, 1990, 75(3):736-43.

Antineutrophil Cytoplasmic Antibody

***CPT** 86255 (screen); 86256 (titer)*

Related Information

Glomerular Basement Membrane Antibody *on page 681*

Kidney Biopsy *on page 68*

Synonyms ACPA; ANCA

Applies to Proteinase 3 (PR3)

Abstract The pathologic triad of Wegener's granulomatosis (WG) includes granulomatous inflammation of the upper and lower respiratory tract, vasculitis, and glomerulonephritis. ANCA represents the most useful marker available for WG.

Specimen Serum **CONTAINER:** Red top tube; do **not** use serum separator tube.

Interpretive **REFERENCE RANGE:** Negative; titer falls with remission **USE:** Diagnose Wegener's granulomatosis; assess disease activity. Microscopic polyarteritis, Churg-Strauss syndrome, idiopathic necrotizing and crescentic glomerulonephritis may also be detected.[1] A relationship between P-ANCA and inflammatory bowel disease is described.[2,3] ANCA may be found with drug-induced lupus syndrome, SLE, Felty's syndrome, and rheumatoid arthritis.[3] **LIMITATIONS:** Technically demanding; requires expert interpretation of fluorescent patterns. A negative result does not exclude the diagnosis of Wegener's granulomatosis.[4] **METHODOLOGY:** Indirect fluorescent antibody (IFA) **ADDITIONAL INFORMATION:** Serum antibodies against components of neutrophil cytoplasm can be demonstrated in patients with Wegener's granulomatosis (WG) and other forms of vasculitis. Two major patterns of reactivity are seen when the indirect fluorescent antibody technique is used – diffuse cytoplasmic staining (C-ANCA) and perinuclear staining (P-ANCA). The C-ANCA pattern has been attributed to reaction with proteinase 3 (PR3) in neutrophil granules, whereas the P-ANCA has several reactivities including myeloperoxidase, cathepsin G, and neutrophil elastase. The C-ANCA pattern is most typically seen in Wegener's granulomatosis. The P-ANCA pattern can also be seen in that condition. However, it is described as not a useful diagnostic method for WG.[5] Other forms of vasculitis most typically display the P-ANCA pattern. A P-ANCA pattern has also been seen in patients with ulcerative colitis, primary sclerosing cholangitis, and in some with rheumatoid arthritis. The antigenic specificity of the latter two has not been defined and has been referred to as granulocyte specific-ANA (GS-ANA). Although ANCA testing is a very useful test for vasculitis and Wegener's, false-positive and false-negatives do occur. C-ANCA is reported in 88% of patients with active WG and 43% of those in remission.[5] Unless the procedure is done with utmost critical evaluation of the patterns of immunofluorescence, there will be unacceptable nonspecificity.

Footnotes

1. Fienberg R, Mark EJ, Goodman M, et al, "Correlation of Antineutrophil Cytoplasmic Antibodies With the Extrarenal Histopathology of Wegener's (Pathergic) Granulomatosis and Related Forms of Vasculitis," *Hum Pathol*, 1993, 24(2):160-8.
2. Hardarson S, LaBrecque DR, Mitros FA, et al, "Antineutrophil Cytoplasmic Antibody in Inflammatory Bowel and Hepatobiliary Diseases. High Prevalence in Ulcerative Colitis, Primary Sclerosing Cholangitis, and Autoimmune Hepatitis," *Am J Clin Pathol*, 1993, 99(3):277-81.
3. Jennette JC and Falk RJ, "Antineutrophil Cytoplasmic Autoantibodies in Inflammatory Bowel Disease," *Am J Clin Pathol*, 1993, 99(3):221-3, (editorial).
4. Colby TV, Tazelaar HD, Specks U, et al, "Nasal Biopsy in Wegener's Granulomatosis," *Hum Pathol*, 1991, 22(2):101-4.
5. Hoffman GS, Kerr GS, Leavitt RY, et al, "Wegener Granulomatosis: An Analysis of 158 Patients," *Ann Intern Med*, 1992, 116(6):488-98.

References

Braun MG, Csernok E, Gross WL, et al, "Proteinase 3, the Target Antigen of Anticytoplasmic Antibodies Circulating in Wegener's Granulomatosis. Immunolocalization in Normal and Pathologic Tissues," *Am J Pathol*, 1991, 139(4):831-8.

Cohen-Tervaert JW, van der Woude FJ, Fauci AS, et al, "Association Between Active Wegener's Granulomatosis and Anticytoplasmic Antibodies," *Arch Intern Med*, 1989, 149(11):2461-5.

Kalina PH, Garrity JA, Herman DC, et al, "Role of Testing for Anticytoplasmic Autoantibodies in the Differential Diagnosis of Scleritis and Orbital Pseudotumor," *Mayo Clin Proc*, 1990, 65(8):1110-7.

Lesavre P, "Antineutrophil Cytoplasmic Autoantibodies Antigen Specificity," *Am J Kidney Dis*, 1991, 18(2):159-63.

Nölle B, Specks U, Lüdemann J, et al, "Anticytoplasmic Autoantibodies: Their Immunodiagnostic Value in Wegener's Granulomatosis," *Ann Intern Med*, 1989, 111(1):28-40.

Specks U, Rohrbach MS, and DeRemee RA, "Antineutrophil Cytoplasmic Autoantibodies," *N Engl J Med*, 1988, 318:1416-7.

Specks U, Wheatley CL, McDonald TJ, et al, "Anticytoplasmic Autoantibodies in the Diagnosis and Follow-Up of Wegener's Granulomatosis," *Mayo Clin Proc*, 1989, 64(1):28-36.

Ulmer M, Rautmann A, and Gross WL, "Immunodiagnostic Aspects of Autoantibodies Against Myeloperoxidase," *Clin Nephrol*, 1992, 37(4):161-8.

Wieslander J, "How Are Antineutrophil Cytoplasmic Autoantibodies Detected?" *Am J Kidney Dis*, 1991, 18(2):154-8.

Antinuclear Antibody

CPT *86038; 86039 (titer); 86255 (fluorescent screen); 86256 (fluorescent titer)*

Related Information

Anticardiolipin Antibody *on page 632*
Anticoagulant, Circulating *on page 402*
Anti-DNA *on page 634*
Kidney Biopsy *on page 68*
Kidney Profile *on page 268*
LE Cell Test *on page 565*
RPR *on page 742*
Sjögren's Antibodies *on page 746*
Skin Biopsies *on page 84*
VDRL, Cerebrospinal Fluid *on page 761*
VDRL, Serum *on page 762*

Synonyms ANA; ANF; FANA

Applies to Extractable Nuclear Antigens; MA Antibody; Nucleolar Antibody; RNP Antibody; Scl-70; Sm Antibody; SS-A/Ro; SS-B/La

Test Commonly Includes Titers and pattern of nuclear fluorescence on all positive samples

Abstract The antinuclear antibody (ANA) test detects autoantibodies which are directed against a wide variety of antigens which reside mainly in the nucleus. Such autoantibodies are found in a wide variety of rheumatic diseases; especially systemic lupus erythematosus, progressive systemic sclerosis, Sjögren's syndrome, and mixed connective tissue disease. The specific autoantibody detected can be helpful in distinguishing between these and other alternatives.

Specimen Serum **CONTAINER:** Red top tube **CAUSES FOR REJECTION:** Hemolysis

Interpretive **REFERENCE RANGE:** Negative. If the fluorescent ANA test is positive, follow-up antibody testing can quantitate and specify the type of antibody as an aid to diagnosis and management. If the fluorescent ANA test is negative and the clinical picture suggests a "collagen-vascular" disease, testing for antibody to nonhistone antigens may be done. Reference ranges vary from one laboratory to another. **USE:** Screening test for autoimmune diseases, systemic lupus erythematosus, and chronic active hepatitis; ANA is a hallmark of SLE and related disorders. **LIMITATIONS:** This test is not specific for any one collagen vascular disease. For specific tests for SLE see listings for Anti-DNA. Specimen is screened at a dilution which should be determined by each laboratory. Typically, dilutions of 1:20, 1:40, or 1:80 have been used. A small percent of SLE patients may have a titer of less than the screening dilution. Men and women older than 80 years of age have a 50% incidence of low titer ANA. Various medications can induce a "lupoid" condition and elevated ANA titers. Usually the titer decreases following removal of the drug. Drugs significantly associated with positive ANA tests include, among others: para-aminosalicylic acid (PAS, Parasol®), carbamazepine (Tegretol®), chlorpromazine (Thorazine®), Dilantin®, ethosuximide (Zarontin®), griseofulvin (Fulvicin®, Grifulvin® V), hydralazine (Apresoline®), isoniazid (INH, Nydrazid®), mephenytoin (Mesantoin®), methyldopa (Aldomet®), penicillin, phenylbutazone (Butazolidin®, Azolid®), phenytoin (Dilantin®) – hydantoin group, primidone (Mysoline®), procainamide (Pronestyl®), propylthiouracil, trimethadione (Tridione®).

ANA-negative lupus patients are known; ***vide infra***.

METHODOLOGY: Indirect fluorescent antibody (IFA) on tissue slices or cell monolayers. Results may vary with test substrate (ie, SS-A/Ro may be detected on a HEp-2 cell line) but not mouse kidney. **ADDITIONAL INFORMATION:** The indirect fluorescent antibody test has three elements to consider in the result: 1. Positive or negative fluorescence. A negative test is strong evidence against a diagnosis of SLE but not conclusive. 2. The titer (dilution) to which fluorescence remains positive provides a reflection of the concentration or avidity of the antibody. Many individuals, particularly the elderly, may have low titer ANA without significant disease substantiated after work-up. 3. The pattern of nuclear fluorescence reflects specificity for various diseases. Nuclear rim (peripheral) pattern correlates with antibody to native DNA and deoxynucleoprotein and bears correlation with SLE, SLE activity, and lupus nephritis. Homogenous (diffuse) pattern suggests SLE or other connective tissue diseases. Speckled pattern correlates with antibody to nuclear antigens extractable by saline; it is found in many disease states, including SLE and scleroderma. When antibodies to DNA and deoxyribonucleoprotein are present (rim and homogenous pattern), there may be interference with the detection of speckled pattern. Nucleolar pattern is seen in sera of patients with progressive systemic sclerosis and Sjögren's syndrome. Centromere pattern is seen in CREST syndrome.

Antinuclear Antibody

ANA Pattern	Corresponding Antibody	Found In
Rim and/or homogeneous	Double-stranded DNA Double and single-stranded DNA "LE cell antibody"	SLE SLE and other rheumatic diseases SLE, drug induced LE
Homogeneous	Histones	Drug induced LE
Speckled	Sm ("Smith") MA RNP	SLE SLE (severe) Mixed connective tissue disease
Atypical speckled	Scl-70 (Scl-1)	Scleroderma
Speckled	SS-B/La, SS-A/Ro	Sjogren's syndrome
Nucleolar	Nucleolar	Progressive systemic sclerosis

Five percent of the apparently "normal population" demonstrate serum ANA. Low titers of ANA reactivity may be seen in patients with rheumatoid arthritis (40% to 60% of patients), scleroderma (60% to 90%), discoid lupus, necrotizing vasculitis, Sjögren's syndrome (80%), chronic active hepatitis, pulmonary interstitial fibrosis, pneumoconiosis, tuberculosis, malignancy, age older than 60 years (18%), as well as in SLE, especially if the disease is inactive or under treatment. Titers ≥1:160 usually indicate the presence of active SLE, although occasionally other autoimmune disease may induce these high titers. ANA cannot be regarded as a foolproof screening test for either SLE or other rheumatic disorders, since it detects some significant nuclear antibodies poorly or not at all. Some of these failures may be related to the substrate used (rat kidney, mouse kidney, liver, tissue culture), while others may be intrinsic failures of the test. There are now known groups of "ANA-negative" lupus patients. Such patients often have antibodies to SS-A/Ro antigen (usually when a frozen section substrate is used) and subacute cutaneous lupus. Ten percent of patients with SLE manifest biologic false-positive tests for syphilis; this may even be the initial manifestation. Some other tests used in differentiation of autoimmune states include antibody to double-stranded DNA, rheumatoid factor, antibody to extractable nuclear antigens, total hemolytic complement, (C3, C4, etc). Although ANA tests are occasionally ordered on cerebrospinal fluid or synovial fluid, the current assays are not standardized for these fluids and such assays do not add to the diagnostic process.

American Rheumatism Association preliminary criteria for SLE: Facial erythema, discoid lupus, Raynaud's phenomenon, alopecia, photosensitivity, oral or nasopharyngeal ulceration, arthritis without deformity, LE cells, chronic false-positive syphilis serology, profuse proteinuria >3.5 g/day, cellular casts, pleuritis and/or pericarditis, psychosis and/or convulsions; hemolytic anemia/leukopenia/thrombocytopenia.

References

Aho K, Koskela P, Makitalo R, et al, "Antinuclear Antibodies Heralding the Onset of Systemic Lupus Erythematosus," *J Rheumatol*, 1992, 19(9):1377-9.

Astion ML, Orkand AR, Olsen GB, et al, "ANA-Tutor: A Computer Program That Teaches the Antinuclear Antibody Test," *Lab Med*, 1993, 24(6):341-4.

Bridges AJ, Anderson JD, McKay J et al, "Antinuclear Antibody Testing in a Referral Laboratory," *Lab Med*, 1993, 24(6):345-9.

Clegg DO, Williams HJ, Singer JZ, et al, "Early Undifferentiated Connective Tissue Disease. II. The Frequency of Circulating Antinuclear Antibodies in Patients With Early Rheumatic Diseases," *J Rheumatol*, 1991, 18(9):1340-3.

Colvin RB, Bhan AK, and McCluskey RT, eds, *Diagnostic Immunopathology*, New York, NY: Raven Press, 1988, 89-92.

Harmon CE, "Antinuclear Antibodies in Autoimmune Disease," *Med Clin North Am*, 1985, 69:547-63.

Nakamura RM and Binder WL, "Current Concepts and Diagnostic Evaluation of Autoimmune Disease," *Arch Pathol Lab Med*, 1988, 112:869-77.

Nakamura RM and Tan EM, "Autoantibodies to Nonhistone Nuclear Antigens and Their Clinical Significance," *Hum Pathol*, 1983, 14:392-400.

Nakamura RM and Tan EM, "Recent Progress in the Study of Autoantibodies to Nuclear Antigens," *Hum Pathol*, 1978, 9:85-91.

(Continued)

Antinuclear Antibody *(Continued)*

Senecal JL and Raymond Y, "Autoantibodies to DNA, Lamins, and Pore Complex Proteins Produce Distinct Peripheral Fluorescent Antinuclear Antibody Patterns on the HEp-2 Substrate," *Arthritis Rheum*, 1991, 34(2):249-51.

Antiparietal Cell Antibody *see* Parietal Cell Antibody *on page 730*

Antiphospholipid Antibody *see* Anticardiolipin Antibody *on page 632*

Antiskeletal Muscle Antibody *see* Skeletal Muscle Antibody *on page 747*

Antismooth Muscle Antibody *see* Smooth Muscle Antibody *on page 747*

Antistreptococcal DNase-B Titer *see* Antideoxyribonuclease-B Titer, Serum *on page 633*

Antistreptococcal Hyaluronidase Titer *see* Antihyaluronidase Titer *on page 635*

Antistreptolysin O Titer, Serum

CPT 86060 (titer); 86063 (screen)

Related Information

Antideoxyribonuclease-B Titer, Serum *on page 633*
Antihyaluronidase Titer *on page 635*
Group A *Streptococcus* Screen *on page 818*
Streptozyme *on page 749*
Throat Culture *on page 876*

Synonyms ASO

Test Commonly Includes Detection of antibody to streptolysin O

Abstract Detection of elevated ASO titer is useful to detect patients with acute rheumatic fever and other sequelae of poststreptococcal infections.

Specimen Serum **CONTAINER:** Red top tube **CAUSES FOR REJECTION:** Excessive hemolysis

Interpretive **REFERENCE RANGE:** Younger than 2 years of age: usually <50 Todd units; 2-5 years: <100 Todd units; 5-19 years: <166 Todd units; adults: <125 Todd units. A rise in titer of four or more dilution increments between acute and convalescent specimens is considered to be significant regardless of the magnitude of the titer. For a single specimen, ASO titers ≤166 Todd units are considered normal; but higher titers may be "normal" in demographic groups or may be associated with chronic pharyngeal carriage. **USE:** Document exposure to streptococcal infection. A marked rise in titer or a persistently elevated titer indicates that a *Streptococcus* infection or poststreptococcal sequelae are present. Elevated titers are seen in 80% to 85% of patients with acute rheumatic fever and in 95% of patients with acute glomerulonephritis. **LIMITATIONS:** False-positive ASO titers can be caused by increased levels of serum beta-lipoprotein produced in liver disease and by contamination of the serum with *Bacillus cereus* and *Pseudomonas* sp. ASO is not sensitive to sequelae of streptococcal pyoderma. Test is subject to technical false-positives due to oxidation of reagents. **METHODOLOGY:** Hemolysis inhibition, latex agglutination (LA) **ADDITIONAL INFORMATION:** Streptolysin is a hemolysin produced by group A streptococci. In an infected individual streptolysin O acts as a protein antigen, and the patient mounts an antibody response. A rise in titer begins about 1 week after infection and peaks 2-4 weeks later. In the absence of complications or reinfection, the ASO titer will usually fall to preinfection levels within 6-12 months. Both clinical and laboratory findings should be correlated in reaching a diagnosis.

References

Escobar MR, "Hemolytic Assays: Complement Fixation and Antistreptolysin O," *Manual of Clinical Microbiology*, 5th ed, Chapter 10, Balows A, Hausler WJ, Herrmann K, et al, eds, Washington DC: American Society for Microbiology, 1991, 73-8.

Keren DF and Warren JS, *Diagnostic Immunology*, Baltimore, MD: Williams & Wilkins, 1992, 168-70.

Antithyroglobulin Antibody *see* Thyroid Antithyroglobulin Antibody *on page 756*

Antithyroid Microsomal Antibody *see* Thyroid Antimicrosomal Antibody *on page 755*

α-1-Antitrypsin *see* $Alpha_1$-Antitrypsin, Serum *on page 631*

ART *see* Automated Reagin Test *on page 642*

ART Test *replaced by* RPR *on page 742*

Ascariasis Serological Test

CPT *86317 (quantitative); 86318 (qualitative or semiqualitative)*

Related Information

Ova and Parasites, Stool *on page 836*
Parasite Antibodies *on page 729*

Synonyms *Ascaris lumbricoides* Serological Test; *Toxocara canis* Serological Test; VLM (Visceral Larva Migrans) Serological Test

Abstract *Ascaris lumbricoides* is a nematode which inhabits the human small intestine. *Ascaris pneumonitis* or Loeffler's syndrome is the entity associated with larval migration.

Patient Care PREPARATION: Fasting blood sample required.

Specimen Serum CONTAINER: Red top tube STORAGE INSTRUCTIONS: Refrigerate at 4°C. CAUSES FOR REJECTION: Inadequate labeling, excessive hemolysis, lipemic serum, gross contamination of the specimen SPECIAL INSTRUCTIONS: Physician requesting the test must supply the laboratory with patient's age, sex, occupation, address, clinical symptoms, and date of onset of illness.

Interpretive REFERENCE RANGE: ELISA: <1:32; IHA: <1:128 USE: Support the clinical diagnosis of visceral larva migrans LIMITATIONS: False-negative results and false-positive results due to cross reactivity of related antigens occur. IHA tests for VLM due to *Toxocara* have shown almost 100% cross reaction with *Ascaris lumbricoides*. ELISA tests done with *Ascaris* absorbed antigen are more specific. METHODOLOGY: Indirect hemagglutination (IHA) or enzyme-linked immunosorbent assay (ELISA) The diagnosis of *Ascaris lumbricoides* intestinal infestation is established by demonstration of eggs in feces. ADDITIONAL INFORMATION: Visceral larva migrans and systemic ascariasis are usually associated with significant tissue and blood eosinophilia.

References

Ash LR and Orihel TC, *Atlas of Human Parasitology*, 3rd ed, Chicago, IL: ASCP Press, 1990, 134-7.

Ascaris lumbricoides **Serological Test** *see* Ascariasis Serological Test *on this page*

ASO *see* Antistreptolysin O Titer, Serum *on previous page*

Aspergillosis Complement Fixation Test *see Aspergillus* Serology *on this page*

Aspergillosis ID Test *see Aspergillus* Serology *on this page*

Aspergillus fumigatus **Precipitating Antibodies** *see* Hypersensitivity Pneumonitis Serology *on page 704*

Aspergillus niger **Precipitating Antibodies** *see* Hypersensitivity Pneumonitis Serology *on page 704*

Aspergillus Serology

CPT *86606*

Related Information

Biopsy or Body Fluid Fungus Culture *on page 780*
Blood Fungus Culture *on page 789*
Sputum Fungus Culture *on page 853*

Synonyms Aspergillosis Complement Fixation Test; Aspergillosis ID Test

Test Commonly Includes Detection of precipitating antibodies to *Aspergillus* sp in patients' serum

Specimen Serum CONTAINER: Red top tube CAUSES FOR REJECTION: Inadequate labeling, excessive hemolysis, lipemic serum, gross contamination of the specimen SPECIAL INSTRUCTIONS: Acute and convalescent serum specimens are desirable.

Interpretive REFERENCE RANGE: Immunodiffusion: negative; positive: titer >1:64 or fourfold increase in titer over 3 weeks. Three or more precipitin bands indicate fungus ball or invasive disease. Precipitin bands of nonidentity and reactions with C-reactive protein are seen. Complement fixation: titer <1:8 or less than fourfold increase. USE: Confirm the presence of precipitating antibodies to *Aspergillus* sp LIMITATIONS: A negative test does not rule out aspergillosis. METHODOLOGY: Immunodiffusion (ID), complement fixation (CF), enzyme-linked immuno-

(Continued)

Aspergillus Serology *(Continued)*

sorbent assay (ELISA) **ADDITIONAL INFORMATION:** *Aspergillus* precipitins are seen in 90% of patients with fungus balls, 70% of patients with allergic bronchopulmonary aspergillosis, and less often in patients with invasive aspergillosis. The value of complement fixing antibodies in the diagnosis of pulmonary aspergillosis is not established. Both sensitivity and specificity are poor. A battery of different *Aspergillus* sp antigens may be necessary.

The demonstration of *Aspergillus* antigen in serum is extremely sensitive and specific for the diagnosis of aspergillosis, but is not yet widely available.

Aspergillosis immunodiffusion: Sera can be tested against a polyvalent antigen mixture, or a series of species preparations. The greater the number of bands, the greater the likelihood of either a fungus ball or invasive aspergillosis. A negative test does not rule out aspergillosis. Nonidentity bands could be due to presence of CRP. Cross reactions occur in cases of histoplasmosis, coccidioidomycosis and blastomycosis, or may indicate antibody to an *Aspergillus* species other than *Aspergillus fumigatus*. Bands due to reaction with C-reactive protein can be removed by sodium citrate.

References

Brummund W, Resnick A, Fink JN, et al, "*Aspergillus fumigatus* Specific Antibodies in Allergic Bronchopulmonary Aspergillosis and Aspergilloma: Evidence for a Polyclonal Antibody Response," *J Clin Microbiol*, 1987, 25:5-9.

Chandler FW and Watts JC, "Fungal Infections," *Pulmonary Pathology*, Dail DH and Hammar SP, eds, New York, NY: Springer-Verlag, 1988, 222-8.

Knutsen AP, Hutcheson PS, Mueller KR, et al, "Serum Immunoglobulins E and G Anti-*Aspergillus fumigatus* Antibody in Patients With Cystic Fibrosis Who Have Allergic Bronchopulmonary Aspergillosis," *J Lab Clin Med*, 1990, 116(5):724-7.

Weiner MH, Talbot GH, Gerson SL, et al, "Antigen Detection in the Diagnosis of Invasive Aspergillosis," *Ann Intern Med*, 1983, 99:777-82.

Australian Antigen *replaced by* Hepatitis B Surface Antigen *on page 688*

Australian Antigen Antibody *replaced by* Hepatitis B Surface Antibody *on page 687*

Automated Reagin Test

***CPT** 86592*

Related Information

Anticardiolipin Antibody *on page 632*
Darkfield Examination, Syphilis *on page 808*
FTA-ABS, Serum *on page 680*
MHA-TP *on page 724*
Risks of Transfusion *on page 1093*
RPR *on page 742*
VDRL, Cerebrospinal Fluid *on page 761*
VDRL, Serum *on page 762*

Synonyms ART

Applies to Serologic Test for Syphilis; Syphilis Screening Test

Test Commonly Includes Reactive specimens often titered, and/or FTA-ABS test performed if the patient is not a known positive.

Specimen Serum **CONTAINER:** Red top tube **CAUSES FOR REJECTION:** Excessive hemolysis, lipemic serum, or gross contamination of the specimen

Interpretive **REFERENCE RANGE:** Negative **USE:** Screening test for syphilis **LIMITATIONS:** Biological false-positives have been reported in diseases such as infectious mononucleosis, leprosy, malaria, lupus erythematosus, vaccinia, and virus pneumonia. Pregnancy, narcotic addiction, and autoimmune diseases may also give false-positive reactions (of course, the coexistence of one of these processes does not exclude true syphilis as well!). The test will be positive in the antiphospholipid antibody syndrome (see Anticardiolipin Antibody). Pinta, yaws, bejel, and other related treponemal diseases produce positive reactions in this test and should not be considered false. Gross lipemia and hemolysis also interfere. False-negatives due to the prozone phenomenon have been reported. Additional dilutions may be needed when a suspicious patient tests negative with the routine screen. **CONTRAINDICATIONS:** Cannot be performed on spinal fluid or cord serum **METHODOLOGY:** Autoanalyzer modification of reagin agglutination test **ADDITIONAL INFORMATION:** The number of cases of syphilis has been increasing since 1987. The increase seems to be associated with HIV infection and prostitution associated with drug abuse. Because most infants with congenital syphilis lack signs of infection, serology for both nontreponemal and treponemal antibodies is needed for diagnosis. ART is a nontreponemal test for "reagin," an antibody which cross reacts with extracts of cardiac muscle and treponemal cell wall components. All such nontreponemal tests (including RPR and VDRL) are subject to the false-positives listed above. Such tests start becoming positive 2 weeks after exposure, and 100% of patients will be positive by 12 weeks. With adequate treatment, titers will return to normal (unlike treponemal tests).

References

Berkowitz J, Baxi L, and Fox HE, "False-Negative Syphilis Screening: The Prozone Phenomenon, Nonimmune Hydrops, and Diagnosis of Syphilis During Pregnancy," *Am J Obstet Gynecol*, 1990, 163(3):975-7.

Giansiracusa DF, "Case Records of the Massachusetts General Hospital," *N Engl J Med*, 1988, 319:699-712.

Huber TW, Storms S, Young P, et al, "Reactivity of Microhemagglutination, Fluorescent Treponemal Antibody Absorption, Venereal Disease Research Laboratory, and Rapid Plasma Reagin Tests in Primary Syphilis," *J Clin Microbiol*, 1983, 17:405-9.

Kirchner JT, "Syphilis - An STD on the Increase," *Am Fam Physician*, 1991, 44(3):843-54.

McGrew BE and Lantz MA, "Quantitative Automated Reagin Test for Syphilis," *Am J Med Technol*, 1970, 36.

Stevens RW and Stroebel E, "The Automated Reagin Test: Results Compared With VDRL and FTA-ABS Tests," *Am J Clin Pathol*, 1970, 53:32-4.

Young H, Moyes A, McMillan A, et al, "Enzyme Immunoassay for Anti-Treponemal IgG: Screening or Confirmatory Test?" *J Clin Pathol*, 1992, 45(1):37-41.

B27 *see* HLA-B27 *on page 701*

***Babesia* Species Serological Test** *see* Babesiosis Serological Test *on this page*

Babesiosis Serological Test

***CPT** 86317*

Related Information

Arthropod Identification *on page 774*
Lyme Disease Serology *on page 719*
Risks of Transfusion *on page 1093*

Synonyms *Babesia* Species Serological Test; Nantucket Fever Serological Test

Abstract This is an intraerythrocytic parasite which can cause symptoms which resemble those of *Plasmodium falciparum*. Like malaria, it causes hemolytic anemia. Asplenic, immunocompromised, and elderly subjects are especially at risk, but immunocompetent persons can develop the disease. These organisms are known to cause disease in cattle, including Texas fever.

Specimen Serum **CONTAINER:** Red top tube **STORAGE INSTRUCTIONS:** Refrigerate at 4°C.

Interpretive REFERENCE RANGE: Negative **CRITICAL VALUES:** A single value of 1:1024 is strongly suggestive or diagnostic. A fourfold increase in titer establishes diagnosis.[1] **USE:** Aid in the diagnosis of babesiosis **LIMITATIONS:** Sensitivity and specificity not fully determined. **METHODOLOGY:** Indirect immunofluorescent antibody. Intraerythrocytic ring forms and tetrads are found in the peripheral blood film. The former resemble those of *P. falciparum* malaria, but the rare tetrad forms are diagnostic. Organisms can resemble Pappenheimer bodies, which are found in asplenic persons. An acridine orange technique is available.[1] **ADDITIONAL INFORMATION:** *Babesia* is an intraerythrocytic parasite endemic in the Northeastern U.S. It can be transmitted by tick bite or blood transfusion. It is particularly severe in patients who have undergone splenectomy (and who lack the RBC "pitting" function of the spleen). In a series of six patients with babesiosis, all had high titers of antibody while acutely ill. Titers declined with clinical improvement but remained elevated for 4-16 weeks. A tick, *Ixodes dammini*, which transmits one of the *Babesia* species (*B. microti*, a rodent parasite) also transmits Lyme disease. Subjects with either disease should be considered for the other.

Footnotes

1. Scully RE, Mark EJ, McNeely WF, et al, "Case Records of the Massachusetts General Hospital," *N Engl J Med*, 1993, 329(3):194-9.

References

Ash LR and Orihel TC, *Atlas of Human Parasitology*, 3rd ed, Chicago, IL: ASCP Press, 1990, 115-7.

Bove JR, "Transfusion-Transmitted Diseases Other Than AIDS and Hepatitis," *Yale J Biol Med*, 1990, 63(5):347-51.

Dammin GJ, Spielman A, Benach JL, et al, "The Rising Incidence of Clinical *Babesia microti* Infection," *Hum Pathol*, 1981, 12:398-400.

(Continued)

Babesiosis Serological Test *(Continued)*

Gombert ME, "Human Babesiosis: Clinical and Therapeutic Considerations," *JAMA*, 1982, 248:3005-7.

Quick RE, Herwaldt BL, Thomford JW, "Babesiosis in Washington State: A New Species of *Babesia*?" *Ann Intern Med*, 1993, 119(4):284-90.

Wittner M, Rowin KS, Tanowitz HB, et al, "Successful Chemotherapy of Transfusion Babesiosis," *Ann Intern Med*, 1982, 96:601-4.

Bacterial Serology

CPT *86171 (complement fixation); 86403 (agglutination)*

Related Information

Bordetella pertussis Nasopharyngeal Culture *on page 790*
Brucellosis Agglutinins *on page 647*
Throat Culture *on page 876*
Throat Culture for *Corynebacterium diphtheriae on page 878*
Tularemia Agglutinins *on page 760*
Yersinia enterocolitica Antibody *on page 765*

Applies to *Bordetella pertussis* Titer; Diphtheria Neutralizing Antibody; *Leptospira* Agglutination; Leptospirosis Antibody Titers; Pertussis Titers; Rickettsial Antibody Titer; Whooping Cough Titers; *Yersinia pestis* Antibody Titer

Test Commonly Includes Detection of antibody titers to specific bacterial pathogens in patients' serum

Specimen Serum or cerebrospinal fluid **CONTAINER:** Red top tube; clean, sterile CSF tube **SPECIAL INSTRUCTIONS:** A single specimen is not usually diagnostic of acute infection. A second convalescent specimen drawn 2-3 weeks after acute onset is strongly recommended. The physician should arrange for the convalescent serum to be collected 2-3 weeks after the acute serum is collected.

Interpretive **REFERENCE RANGE:** Less than a fourfold difference between acute and convalescent samples **USE:** Serological support of suspected bacterial infection **LIMITATIONS:** Cross reactions between antibodies **METHODOLOGY:** Complement fixation (CF), agglutination, counterimmunoelectrophoresis (CIE) **ADDITIONAL INFORMATION:** A single determination of antibodies to bacterial antigens should not be depended upon to support a diagnosis, since cross reactions and persistent low-level titers are common phenomena. A rising titer over 2-3 weeks is more specific and more diagnostic of acute infection. Antibody titers to some organisms may rise as a side effect of other immune stimulation (ie, an infection with some other organism). Detection of bacterial antigens by counter immunoelectrophoresis can be extremely useful, especially in partially treated infections. Differentiation of IgG and IgM classes of antibody may help distinguish acute from previous infection. Methodologies differ in their ability to detect immunity or infection. For more information refer to the sections on specific bacteria.

Basement Membrane Antibodies *see* Immunofluorescence, Skin Biopsy *on page 708*

Bence Jones Protein *see* Immunofixation Electrophoresis *on page 707*

Bence Jones Protein *replaced by* Protein Electrophoresis, Urine *on page 737*

Bence Jones Protein Test *replaced by* Immunoelectrophoresis, Serum or Urine *on page 706*

Beta$_2$-Microglobulin

CPT *82232*

Related Information

Cerebrospinal Fluid Cytology *on page 490*
Gentamicin *on page 970*
HIV-1/HIV-2 Serology *on page 696*
Zidovudine *on page 1012*

Specimen Serum or 24-hour urine **CONTAINER:** Red top tube, plastic urine container **CAUSES FOR REJECTION:** Recent radioactive scan

Interpretive **REFERENCE RANGE:** Serum: <2 μg/mL (SI: <170 nmol/L); urine: <120 μg/24 hours (SI: <10 nmol/day) **USE:** Evaluate renal disease, activity of chronic lymphocytic leukemia, activity of AIDS **LIMITATIONS:** Increased synthesis of β_2-microglobulin in Crohn's disease, hepatitis, sarcoidosis, vasculitis, hyperthyroidism, viral infections, and some malignancies decreases the usefulness of serum levels. **CONTRAINDICATIONS:** Recent radioactive scan **METHODOLOGY:** Radioimmunoassay (RIA) **ADDITIONAL INFORMATION:** β_2-microglobulin is a cell membrane-associated 100 amino acid peptide, a component of the class I HLA complex. It is increased nonspecifically in inflammatory reactions and in active chronic lymphocytic leukemia in which there is increased lymphocyte turnover. Serum β_2-microglobulin predicts response in subjects with low grade lymphoma: at 42 months no patient with a level of $\geq$3.0 mg/L was projected to be in remission.[1] It is also a prognostic marker in multiple myeloma. It may be a useful differentiator of glomerular and tubular dysfunction: in glomerular disease β_2-microglobulin is increased in serum and decreased in urine, while in tubular disorders the opposite changes occur. Urinary retinol-binding protein and β_2-microglobulin levels may delineate those nephrotic subjects likelier to respond to steroids.[2] Urinary β_2-microglobulin becomes abnormal before serum creatinine in aminoglycoside nephrotoxicity. β_2-microglobulin is increased in AIDS patients with progressive disease, particularly those with opportunistic infection. The serum β_2-microglobulin level has been a useful marker for *in vivo* antiretroviral drug activity. It decreases in response to therapy with AZT. Its use has been combined with CD4 lymphocyte counts to calculate the probability of an HIV-infected person developing AIDS within the next 3 years.

Although some studies point to elevated β_2-microglobulin level in the CSF of patients with neurologic involvement by HIV, this is unlikely to provide significant information to guide therapy.

It is reported to delineate a subset of subjects who have primary amyloidosis whose outcomes are unfavorable, but it is not useful in such patients as an index of response to therapy.[3]

Footnotes

1. Litam P, Swan F, Cabanillas F, et al, "Prognostic Value of Serum β-2 Microglobulin in Low-Grade Lymphoma," *Ann Intern Med*, 1991, 114(10):855-60.
2. Sesso R, Santos AP, Nishida SK, et al, "Prediction of Steroid Responsiveness in the Idiopathic Nephrotic Syndrome Using Urinary Retinol-Binding Protein and Beta-2-Microglobulin," *Ann Intern Med*, 1992, 116(11):905-9.
3. Gertz MA, Kyle RA, Greipp PR, et al, "Beta 2-Microglobulin Predicts Survival in Primary Amyloidosis," *Am J Med*, 1990, 89(5):609-14.

References

Anderson RE, Lang W, Shiboski S, et al, "Use of β_2-Microglobulin Level and CD4 Lymphocyte Count to Predict Development of Acquired Immunodeficiency Syndrome in Persons With Human Immunodeficiency Virus Infection," *Arch Intern Med*, 1990, 150(1):73-7.

Calabrese LH, "Autoimmune Manifestations of Human Immunodeficiency Virus (HIV) Infection," *Clin Lab Med*, 1988, 8:269-79.

Gambino R, "Tests for AIDS," *Lab Report for Physicians,*™ 1987, 9:17-22.

Jacobson MA, Abrams DI, Volberding PA, et al, "Serum β_2-Microglobulin Decreases in Patients With AIDS or ARC Treated With Azidothymidine," *J Infect Dis*, 1989, 159(6):1029-36.

Lucey PR, McGuire SA, Clerici M, et al, "Comparison of Spinal Fluid β_2-Microglobulin Levels With CD4+ T-Cell Count, *In Vitro* T Helper Cell Function, and Spinal Fluid IgG Parameters in 163 Neurologically Normal Adults Infected With the Human Immunodeficiency Virus Type 1," *J Infect Dis*, 1991, 163(5):971-5.

Roiter I, Da Rin G, De Menis E, et al, "Increased Serum β_2-Microglobulin Concentrations in Hyperthyroid States," *J Clin Pathol*, 1991, 44(1):73-4.

Tolkoff-Rubin NE, Rubin RH, and Bonventre JV, "Noninvasive Renal Diagnostic Studies," *Clin Lab Med*, 1988, 8:510-3.

Beta-Gamma Bridging *see* Protein Electrophoresis, Serum *on page 734*

Bilharziasis *see* Schistosomiasis Serological Test *on page 745*

Blastomycosis Serology

***CPT** 86612*

Related Information

Biopsy or Body Fluid Fungus Culture *on page 780*
Fungus Smear, Stain *on page 813*
Sputum Fungus Culture *on page 853*
Urine Fungus Culture *on page 883*

Test Commonly Includes Detection of antibodies specific for *Blastomyces* in patient's serum

Abstract Blastomycosis is caused by the dimorphic mold *Blastomyces dermatitidis*. This mold is a natural inhabitant of the soil, and most cases in the United States occur around the Great Lakes and Upper Mississippi River. The disease almost always begins as a pulmonary infection. However, it can progress to a disseminated infection in immunocompromised individuals.

(Continued)

Blastomycosis Serology *(Continued)*

Specimen Serum **CONTAINER:** Red top tube **CAUSES FOR REJECTION:** Failure to collect a convalescent serum, inadequate labeling, excessive hemolysis, lipemic serum, gross contamination of the specimen

Interpretive **REFERENCE RANGE:** Complement fixation: titers <1:8; immunodiffusion: no precipitin band **USE:** Establish the diagnosis of infection due to *Blastomyces dermatitidis* **LIMITATIONS:** Failure to demonstrate precipitin antibodies does not rule out blastomycosis. Cross reactions are seen in patients with histoplasmosis and coccidioidomycosis. Skin testing prior to the test may elevate the complement fixation titer. The complement fixation test lacks sensitivity and specificity and gives positive results in <50% of culture proven cases. Newer EIA tests for blastomycosis have shown greater sensitivity with no compromise in specificity compared to 10 other tests. **METHODOLOGY:** Complement fixation (CF), immunodiffusion (ID), enzyme immunoassay (EIA) **ADDITIONAL INFORMATION:** **Blastomycosis immunodiffusion:** A band of identity with the "A" reference antibody from an infected human indicates active infection or recent past infection. This detects about 80% of cases. A negative test has little value and in no way excludes the existence of blastomycosis. Cross reactions producing lines of partial identity are seen in patients with histoplasmosis and coccidioidomycosis. Repeated testing at 3-week intervals may be needed to secure a diagnosis. EIA for antibody to purified A antigen is 90% sensitive, with some cross reaction with cases of histoplasmosis. After diagnosis is established, falling titers are a good prognostic sign.

References

Kaufman L and Reiss E, "Serodiagnosis of Fungal Diseases," *Manual of Clinical Laboratory Immunology*, 4th ed, Vol 2, Chapter 78, Rose NR, Conway de Macario E, Fahey JL, et al, eds, Washington, DC: American Society for Microbiology, 1992, 506-28.

Lo CY and Notenboom RH, "A New Enzyme Immunoassay Specific for Blastomycosis," *Am Rev Respir Dis*, 1990, 141(1):84:8.

Turner S and Kaufman L, "Immunodiagnosis of Blastomycosis," *Semin Respir Infect*, 1986, 1:22-8.

Blood Mononuclear Cells *see* Mixed Lymphocyte Culture *on page 725*

***Bordetella pertussis* Antibodies** *see Bordetella pertussis* Serology *on next page*

Bordetella pertussis Direct Fluorescent Antibody

CPT *87206*

Related Information

Bordetella pertussis Nasopharyngeal Culture *on page 790*
Bordetella pertussis Serology *on next page*

Synonyms *Bordetella pertussis* Smear; Nasopharyngeal Smear for *Bordetella pertussis*

Replaces Cough Plate Culture for Pertussis

Test Commonly Includes Fluorescent antibody stain to detect *Bordetella pertussis* on smear

Patient Care **PREPARATION:** Patient must not be on antimicrobial therapy.

Specimen Nasopharyngeal swab **CONTAINER:** Nasopharyngeal swab, sterile saline **COLLECTION:** Swab is passed through nose gently and into nasopharynx. Stay near septum and floor of nose. Rotate and remove. Specimen must be hand transported to the laboratory immediately following collection. **STORAGE INSTRUCTIONS:** Do not refrigerate. Transport to the laboratory immediately. **CAUSES FOR REJECTION:** Specimen not received in appropriate sterile container or on appropriate isolation medium, specimen more than 2 hours old. Cough plates are unacceptable. **SPECIAL INSTRUCTIONS:** Laboratory supervisor should be notified 24 hours before collection of specimen so that a special isolation medium can be prepared.

Interpretive **REFERENCE RANGE:** No *B. pertussis* detected **USE:** Detect and identify *B. pertussis* and *B. parapertussis*, establish diagnosis of whooping cough **LIMITATIONS:** Direct detection assays are always limited by the adequacy of the sample. Bacteria may be difficult to detect if there are few bacteria present in the specimen or too much mucoid material. **CONTRAINDICATIONS:** Lack of clinical symptoms of pertussis; previous antibiotic therapy **METHODOLOGY:** Direct fluorescent antibody (DFA) **ADDITIONAL INFORMATION:** The procedure enables early presumptive identification of *Bordetella pertussis*, the agent of whooping cough. Definitive cultural identification should be completed. There is also available a test for serum agglutinating antibodies, which if present may be titered over time to indicate exposure.

Bordetella pertussis Serology

CPT 86615

Related Information

Bordetella pertussis Direct Fluorescent Antibody *on previous page*
Bordetella pertussis Nasopharyngeal Culture *on page 790*
Sputum Culture *on page 849*

Synonyms *Bordetella pertussis* Antibodies; *Bordetella pertussis* Titer; Pertussis Serology

Test Commonly Includes Enzyme-linked immunosorbent assay to detect antibodies to *Bordetella pertussis* and/or pertussis toxin

Specimen Serum **CONTAINER:** Red top tube **STORAGE INSTRUCTIONS:** Refrigerate serum at 4°C.

Interpretive **REFERENCE RANGE:** Absent IgM antibody; less than fourfold rise in titer in paired sera **USE:** Evaluate acute infection with or immunity following vaccination for *Bordetella pertussis* **METHODOLOGY:** Microhemagglutination, enzyme-linked immunosorbent assay (ELISA) **ADDITIONAL INFORMATION:** Patients with acute infection develop IgG, IgM, and IgA antibodies to febrile agglutinogens; and IgM and IgA antibodies are probably diagnostic. Following vaccination, IgG and IgM antibodies can be demonstrated, except in infants. IgA antibodies do not develop.

References

Manclark CR, Meade BD, and Burstyn DG, "Serologic Response to *Bordetella pertussis*," *Manual of Clinical Laboratory Immunology*, 4th ed, Vol 2, Rose NR, Conway de Macario E, Fahey JL, et al, eds, Washington, DC: American Society for Microbiology, 1986, 388-94.

Mertsola J, Ruuskanen O, Kuronen T, et al, "Serologic Diagnosis of Pertussis: Evaluation of Pertussis Toxin and Other Antigens in Enzyme-Linked Immunosorbent Assay," *J Infect Dis*, 1990, 161(5):966-71.

Tomoda T, Ogura H, and Kurashige T, "Immune Responses to *Bordetella pertussis* Infection and Vaccination," *J Infect Dis*, 1991, 163(3):559-63.

***Bordetella pertussis* Smear** *see Bordetella pertussis* Direct Fluorescent Antibody *on previous page*

***Bordetella pertussis* Titer** *see* Bacterial Serology *on page 644*

***Bordetella pertussis* Titer** *see Bordetella pertussis* Serology *on this page*

Brucella abortus *see* Brucellosis Agglutinins *on this page*

Brucella melitensis *see* Brucellosis Agglutinins *on this page*

Brucella suis *see* Brucellosis Agglutinins *on this page*

Brucellosis Agglutinins

CPT 86000

Related Information

Bacterial Serology *on page 644*
Blood Culture, *Brucella on page 788*
Febrile Agglutinins, Serum *on page 678*

Applies to *Brucella abortus*; *Brucella melitensis*; *Brucella suis*

Test Commonly Includes Detection of antibody titers to *Brucella* antigens

Specimen Serum **CONTAINER:** Red top tube **CAUSES FOR REJECTION:** Excessive hemolysis, lipemic serum, gross contamination of the specimen

Interpretive **REFERENCE RANGE:** Negative. The most meaningful reference is less than a fourfold titer rise on paired sera drawn 10-14 days apart. Titers of 1:160 are suggestive of active disease. Ninety percent of patients with titers ≥1:320 have bacteremia. **USE:** Support the clinical diagnosis of brucellosis **LIMITATIONS:** Previous vaccination may have an effect on the titer. Test must be done utilizing a standard antigen prepared from *B. abortus* strain 1119. This will not detect antibodies to *B. canis*. Blocking antibodies may interfere at low titers. There are cross reactions with *Proteus* OX-19, *Yersinia enterocolitica*, *Francisella tularensis*, and *Vibrio cholerae*. **METHODOLOGY:** Tube agglutination, complement fixation, enzyme linked immunosorbent assay (ELISA) **ADDITIONAL INFORMATION:** *Brucella* agglutinins appear during the second week in acute cases and peak in 3-6 weeks. The *B. abortus* antigen used in the *Brucella* agglutination test is group specific and not species specific. If infection with *B. canis* is possible, a specific test for those antibodies must be done. Although cross reactions occur with several other organisms, usually homologous titers will be much higher than the cross reactants. With newer ELISA assays, IgG and IgM antibodies to *Brucella* are used both for initial diagnosis and for follow-up of patient.

(Continued)

Brucellosis Agglutinins *(Continued)*

References

Gazapo E, Gonzalez-Lahoz J, Subiza JL, et al, "Changes in IgM and IgG Antibody Concentrations in Brucellosis Over Time, Importance for Diagnosis and Follow-Up," *J Infect Dis*, 1989, 159(6):219-25.

Bunya Virus Titer *see* California Encephalitis Virus Titer *on page 651*

C1 Esterase Inhibitor, Serum

CPT 85335

Related Information

Complement Components *on page 665*

Synonyms C1 Inactivator; C1 Inhibitor; Esterase Inhibitor; HANE Assay; Hereditary Angioneurotic Edema Test

Applies to Esterase, Subunit of C1

Test Commonly Includes Functional (activity) analysis by complement decay and total immunoreactive level by immunodiffusion and CH_{50}

Abstract C1 esterase inhibitor is decreased in both genetic and acquired angioedema.

Specimen Serum **CONTAINER:** Red top tube **COLLECTION:** Collect sample on ice. Specimen must be chilled (in ice bath) during clotting. Separate from clot with minimum centrifugation. Freeze serum immediately. **STORAGE INSTRUCTIONS:** Specimen must be chilled (in ice bath) during clotting. Separate from clot with minimum centrifugation. Freeze serum immediately. **CAUSES FOR REJECTION:** Stored specimen not frozen, specimen more than 30 minutes in transit to the laboratory, hemolysis

Interpretive **REFERENCE RANGE:** Total: 8-24 mg/dL; functional: "present" **USE:** C1 esterase inhibitor is decreased in hereditary angioneurotic edema; decrease may be functional or quantitative **METHODOLOGY:** Radial immunodiffusion (RID) or nephelometry for measurement of antigenic material; functional assay of C1's activity on acetyl-L-tyrosine ethyl ester or by antigenic masking **ADDITIONAL INFORMATION:** The more common form (85% of patients) of hereditary angioneurotic edema is due to an absolute decrease in the amount of C1 esterase inhibitor. A less common form (15% of patients) is due to a functional defect. Both abnormalities must be tested for due to the potential life-threatening nature of the illness.

In addition to decreased C1 esterase inhibitor in the serum of patients with hereditary angioneurotic edema, a unique polypeptide kinin is increased in plasma from C1 esterase inhibitor deficient patient during attacks of swelling. Danazol, a synthetic androgenic inhibitor of gonadotropin release with little virilizing potential, decreases the number of clinical attacks in cases of hereditary angioneurotic edema. Patients with attacks of hereditary angioneurotic edema also have low total complement, C4 and C2. Consequently, measurement of serum C4 titer is an often used screening test. Hereditary angioneurotic edema is transmitted as an autosomal dominant trait. Heterozygotes also show decreased levels of C1 esterase inhibitor. During acute attacks of the disease, complement factors C4 and C2 can be markedly reduced, but C1 and C3 are normal. The initiating stimulus of clinical attacks is often unknown.

Angioedema may also be an acquired illness. The acquired form includes nonhereditary C1 esterase deficiency; drug-induced, allergic, and idiopathic forms; angioedema associated with autoimmune disease, especially with systemic lupus erythematosus and hypereosinophilia; angioedema occasionally associated with malignancy; and angioedema caused by physical stimuli. Angioedema has occasionally been known to precede development of lymphoproliferative disorders.

References

Alsenz J, Bork K, and Loos M, "Autoantibody-Mediated Acquired Deficiency of C1 Inhibitor," *N Engl J Med*, 1987, 316:1360-6.

Baldwin J, Pence HL, Karibo JM, et al, "C1-Esterase Inhibitor Deficiency: Three Presentations," *Ann Allergy*, 1991, 67(2 Pt 1):107-13.

Colten HR, "Hereditary Angioneurotic Edema, 1887-1987," *N Engl J Med*, 1987, 317:43-4.

Donaldson VH, "Hereditary Angioneurotic Edema," *DM*, 1979, 26:1-37.

Greaves M and Lawlor F, "Angioedema: Manifestations and Management," *J Am Acad Dermatol*, 1991, 25(1 Pt 2):155-61.

Markowitz H, "Hereditary Angioneurotic Edema and Functional C1 Esterase Inhibitor," *Mayo Clin Proc*, 1982, 57:326.

Nusinow SR, Zuraw BL, and Curd JG, "The Hereditary and Acquired Deficiencies of Complement," *Med Clin North Am*, 1985, 69:487-504.

C1 Inactivator *see* C1 Esterase Inhibitor, Serum *on previous page*

C1 Inhibitor *see* C1 Esterase Inhibitor, Serum *on previous page*

C1q Binding Test *see* C1q Immune Complex Detection *on this page*

C1q Immune Complex Detection

***CPT** 86332*

Related Information

C3 Complement, Serum *on this page*
Complement Components *on page 665*
Complement, Total, Serum *on page 667*

Synonyms C1q Binding Test; Circulating Immune Complexes; Immune Complex Detection by C1q

Applies to Synovial Fluid C1q Immune Complexes Detection

Specimen Serum **CONTAINER:** Red top tube

Interpretive **REFERENCE RANGE:** None detected **USE:** Assays for circulating immune complexes have little practical use for following autoimmune diseases. Although they have been proposed to follow conditions such as systemic lupus erythematosus, glomerulonephritis, and even Lyme disease, they are not superior to tests such as CH_{50} or CH_{100} which are better standardized between laboratories and less expensive. Further, assays like C1q do not correlate well with other assays such as Raji cell or immune conglutinins. Therefore, these assays are considered to be of research use only. **LIMITATIONS:** Correlates poorly with other immune complex assays **METHODOLOGY:** Radioimmunoassay (RIA), protein precipitation, coagglutination **ADDITIONAL INFORMATION:** The C1q assay is based on the binding of this component of complement to the Fc portion of immunoglobulins in antigen-antibody complexes. The entire complex can be precipitated with polyethylene glycol, and if the C1q is properly labeled, the complexes can be quantitated. Circulating immune complexes can be demonstrated in rheumatic, infectious, and neoplastic diseases, as well as most immunologically mediated illnesses (inflammatory bowel disease, thrombotic thrombocytopenic purpura). The 1981 WHO/IUIS survey of laboratory tests in clinical immunology concluded that the detection of circulating immune complexes is not essential to any specific diagnosis.

References

Agnello V, "Immune Complex Assays in Rheumatic Diseases," *Hum Pathol*, 1983, 14:343-9.

Endo L, Corman LC, and Panush RS, "Clinical Utility of Assays for Circulating Immune Complexes," *Med Clin North Am*, 1985, 69:623-36.

Keren DF, "Assays for Circulating Immune Complexes," *Clinical Laboratory Annual*, Batsakis JG and Homburger HA, eds, New York, Appleton-Century-Crofts, 1985, 105.

Kilpatrick DC and Weston J, "Immune Complex Assays and Their Limitations," *Med Lab Sci*, 1985, 42:178-85.

McDougal JS and McDuffie FC, "Immune Complexes in Man: Detection and Clinical Significance," *Adv Clin Chem*, 1985, 24:1-60.

C3 *see* C3 Complement, Serum *on this page*

C3 Activator *see* Factor B *on page 678*

C3 Complement, Serum

***CPT** 86160 (antigen); 86161 (functional activity)*

Related Information

C1q Immune Complex Detection *on this page*
C4 Complement, Serum *on next page*
Complement Components *on page 665*
Complement, Total, Serum *on page 667*
Factor B *on page 678*
Kidney Profile *on page 268*
Phagocytic Cell Immunocompetence Profile *on page 732*

Synonyms C3; Complement C3

Test Commonly Includes Quantitation of C3 component of complement

Abstract Complement levels can be a useful index for following autoimmune disease activity. Genetic deficiencies may be associated with pyogenic infections.

Specimen Serum **CONTAINER:** Red top tube **STORAGE INSTRUCTIONS:** Allow sample to clot 15-30 minutes at room temperature, then 30-60 minutes at 4°C. Refrigerate serum at 4°C if assay cannot be run at once.

(Continued)

C3 Complement, Serum *(Continued)*

Interpretive REFERENCE RANGE: Fresh serum: 900-2000 μg/mL (SI: 0.90-2.00 g/L) USE: Quantitation of C3 is used to detect individuals with inborn deficiency of this factor or those with immunologic disease in whom complement is consumed at an increased rate. These include lupus erythematosus, chronic active hepatitis, certain chronic infections, poststreptococcal and membranoproliferative glomerulonephritis, and others. LIMITATIONS: Detects both biologically active and inactive C3 METHODOLOGY: Radial immunodiffusion (RID), rate nephelometry ADDITIONAL INFORMATION: C3 comprises about 70% of the total protein in the complement system and is central to activation of both the classical and alternate pathways. Increased levels are found in numerous inflammatory states as an acute phase response. CH_{50} (total complement hemolytic activity), C3 and/or C4 may be decreased in cases of systemic lupus erythematosus, especially in cases with lupus nephritis, acute and chronic hypocomplementemic nephritis, subacute bacterial endocarditis, DIC, and partial lipodystrophy (with associated nephritis-like activity in serum.) However, C3 level is a poor indicator of diagnosis or prognosis. The "nongamma" (C3) Coombs' test may detect C3 on red cell membranes in some cases of autoimmune hemolytic anemias, but C3 levels are seldom decreased. In cases of disseminated intravascular coagulation, plasmin attacks C3 directly, and C3 levels have been found low in the hemolytic uremic syndrome form of disseminated intravascular coagulation (DIC). Cases of hereditary C3 deficiency, while rare, have been reported and are characterized clinically by recurrent infections (eg, pneumonia, meningitis, paronychia, impetigo). Pathogenic bacteria causing infections in these cases have included both gram-positive and gram-negative organisms. C3 levels have also been found deficient in cases of uremia, chronic liver diseases, anorexia nervosa, and celiac disease. See table.

General Guide to Evaluation of C4 and C3 Protein Levels in Presence of Decreased Hemolytic Complement Activity

	Normal C4	Decreased C4
Normal C3	Alterations *in vitro* (eg, improper specimen handling) Coagulation-associated complement consumption Inborn errors (other than C4 or C3)	Immune complex disease Hypergammaglobulinemic states Cryoglobulinemia Hereditary angioedema Inborn C4 deficiency
Decreased C3	Acute glomerulonephritis Membranoproliferative glomerulonephritis Immune complex disease Active SLE Inborn C3 deficiency	Active SLE Serum sickness Chronic active hepatitis Subacute bacterial endocarditis Immune complex disease

From *Gradwohl's Clinical Laboratory Methods and Diagnosis,* 8th ed, Sonnenwirth AC and Jarett L, eds, St Louis, MO: Mosby-Year Book Inc, 1980, 1233, with permission.

References

Colvin RB, Bhan AK, and McCluskey RT, eds, *Diagnostic Immunopathology*, New York, NY: Raven Press, 1988.

Frank MM, "Complement in the Pathophysiology of Human Disease," *N Engl J Med*, 1987, 316:1525-30.

Nusinow SR, Zuraw BL, and Curd JG, "The Hereditary and Acquired Deficiencies of Complement," *Med Clin North Am*, 1985, 69:487-504.

C3 Proactivator *see* Factor B *on page 678*

C4 *see* C4 Complement, Serum *on this page*

C4 Complement, Serum

CPT *86160 (antigen); 86161 (functional activity)*

Related Information

C3 Complement, Serum *on previous page*
Complement Components *on page 665*
Complement, Total, Serum *on page 667*
Factor B *on page 678*
Kidney Profile *on page 268*
Phagocytic Cell Immunocompetence Profile *on page 732*

Synonyms C4; Complement C4

Test Commonly Includes Quantitation of C4 component of complement

Specimen Serum **CONTAINER:** Red top tube **STORAGE INSTRUCTIONS:** Allow sample to clot 15-30 minutes at room temperature, then 30-60 minutes at 4°C. Refrigerate serum at 4°C if assay cannot be run at once.

Interpretive **REFERENCE RANGE:** 200-800 μg/mL (SI: 0.20-0.80 g/L) **USE:** Quantitation of C4 is used to detect individuals with inborn deficiency of this factor or those with immunologic disease in whom hypercatabolism of complement causes reduced levels. These diseases include lupus erythematosus, serum sickness, certain glomerulonephritides, chronic active hepatitis, hereditary angioedema, and others. **LIMITATIONS:** Complement proteins are acute phase reactants and have short half-lives. Serum level is a balance of synthesis and catabolism. Serial measurements are more useful than single values. **METHODOLOGY:** Radial immunodiffusion (RID), rate nephelometry **ADDITIONAL INFORMATION:** C4 is utilized only by the classical pathway, so that it is decreased only when this arm is activated. In diseases activating the alternate pathway alone, C4 levels will be normal. Total hemolytic activity (CH_{50}), C3, and C4 are frequently decreased in a variety of conditions producing immune complexes. C4 levels are sensitive indicators of lupus disease activity. In hereditary angioedema, the lack of C1 esterase inhibitor allows unopposed lysis of C2 and C4 by C1 esterase, so C4 levels will be low. C4 deficiency has been described in association with a clinical SLE-like disease but with absence of LE cells and variable immunoglobulin or C3 deposits in the skin biopsy, and with Henoch-Schönlein purpura or glomerulonephritis. The condition is inherited as an autosomal recessive trait with close HLA linkage. Hereditary C4 deficiency has been associated with an increased incidence of pyogenic bacterial infections. See table in C3 Complement, Serum.

References

Bishof NA, Welch TR, and Beischel LS, "C4B Deficiency: A Risk Factor for Bacteremia With Encapsulated Organisms," *J Infect Dis*, 1990, 162(1):248-50.

Colvin RB, Bhan AK, and McCluskey RT, eds, *Diagnostic Immunopathology*, New York, NY: Raven Press, 1988.

Frank MM, "Complement in the Pathophysiology of Human Disease," *N Engl J Med*, 1987, 316:1525-30.

Jackson CG, Ochs HD, and Wedgwood RU, "Immune Response of a Patient With Deficiency of the Fourth Component of Complement and Systemic Lupus Erythematosus," *N Engl J Med*, 1979, 300:1124-9.

Nusinow SR, Zuraw BL, and Curd JG, "The Hereditary and Acquired Deficiencies of Complement," *Med Clin North Am*, 1985, 69:487-504.

Ruddy S, "Complement," *Manual of Clinical Laboratory Immunology*, 4th ed, Vol 2, Chapter 18, Rose NR, Conway de Macario E, Fahey JL, et al, eds, Washington, DC: American Society for Microbiology, 1992, 114-23.

c100-3 *see* Hepatitis C Serology *on page 690*

CA2 *see* Thyroid Antithyroglobulin Antibody *on page 756*

California Encephalitis Virus Titer

CPT 86651

Related Information

Eastern Equine Encephalitis Virus Serology *on page 673*
St Louis Encephalitis Virus Serology *on page 749*
Viral Culture, Central Nervous System Symptoms *on page 1199*
Western Equine Encephalitis Virus Serology *on page 765*

Synonyms Bunya Virus Titer; Encephalitis Virus Titer, California; LaCrosse Virus Titer

Test Commonly Includes Complement fixation and hemagglutination inhibition

Abstract The California encephalitis virus is a member of the Bunyaviridae family. It is often referred to as the LaCrosse virus. This virus commonly causes aseptic meningitis, especially during the summer. Other members of the California serogroup are the Jamestown Canyon virus and snowshoe hare virus.

Specimen Serum **CONTAINER:** Red top tube **COLLECTION:** Acute and convalescent sera drawn 10-14 days apart are required. **CAUSES FOR REJECTION:** Failure to collect a convalescent serum

Interpretive **REFERENCE RANGE:** Less than a fourfold increase in titer in paired sera **USE:** Support diagnosis of California encephalitis virus infection **LIMITATIONS:** Complement fixing antibodies appear slowly **METHODOLOGY:** Counterimmunoelectrophoresis (CIE), complement fixation (CF), hemagglutination **ADDITIONAL INFORMATION:** Despite its name, California virus is rare in western states. It is more commonly the cause of an encephalitis occurring in children (5-9 years of age) in the North Central states during the summer. The organism, a bunyavirus, is harbored in small field animals and rodents and is transmitted by mosquitoes.

(Continued)

California Encephalitis Virus Titer *(Continued)*

References

Campbell GL, Eldridge BF, Reeves WC, et al, "Isolation of Jamestown Canyon Virus From Boreal Aedes Mosquitoes From the Sierra Nevada of California," *Am J Trop Med Hyg*, 1991, 44(3):244-9.

Tsai TF, "Arboviruses," *Manual of Clinical Laboratory Immunology*, 4th ed, Vol 2, Chapter 91, Rose NR, Conway de Macario E, Fahey JL, et al, eds, Washington, DC: American Society for Microbiology, 1992, 606-18.

***Campylobacter pylori* Serology** *see Helicobacter pylori* Serology *on page 682*

Candida Antigen

CPT 86403

Related Information

Biopsy or Body Fluid Fungus Culture *on page 780*
Blood Fungus Culture *on page 789*
Candidiasis Serologic Test *on this page*
Fungus Smear, Stain *on page 813*
Stool Fungus Culture *on page 861*

Test Commonly Includes Detection of *Candida* antigens in serum specimen

Specimen Serum **CONTAINER:** Red top tube **STORAGE INSTRUCTIONS:** Separate and refrigerate serum at 4°C.

Interpretive **REFERENCE RANGE:** Negative **USE:** Detect candidiasis in immunocompromised patients **LIMITATIONS:** Latex test is relatively insensitive. **METHODOLOGY:** Latex agglutination (LA), enzyme-linked immunosorbent assay (ELISA) **ADDITIONAL INFORMATION:** Detection of specific *Candida* sepsis is particularly important in immunocompromised patients due to the life-threatening nature of the illness. Unfortunately, the sensitivity of *Candida* antigen tests are too low to rule out candidemia despite a negative test result. Consequently, a negative result does not preclude the use of empiric antifungal therapy. A positive test, however, provides useful information.

References

Escuro RS, Jacobs M, Gerson SL, et al, "Prospective Evaluation of a *Candida* Antigen Detection for Invasive Candidiasis in Immunocompromised Adult Patients With Cancer," *Am J Med*, 1989, 87(6):621-7.

Hayette MP, Strecker G, Faille C, et al, "Presence of Human Antibodies Reacting With *Candida albicans* O-Linked Oligomannosides Revealed by Using an Enzyme-Linked Immunosorbent Assay and Neoglycolipids," *J Clin Microbiol*, 1992, 30(2):411-7.

Walsh TJ, Hathorn JW, Sobel JD, et al, "Detection of Circulating *Candida* Enolase by Immunoassay in Patients With Cancer and Invasive Candidiasis," *N Engl J Med*, 1991, 324(15):1026-31.

Candidiasis Serologic Test

CPT 86628

Related Information

Biopsy or Body Fluid Fungus Culture *on page 780*
Blood Fungus Culture *on page 789*
Candida Antigen *on this page*
Fungus Smear, Stain *on page 813*
Sputum Fungus Culture *on page 853*
Stool Fungus Culture *on page 861*
Urine Fungus Culture *on page 883*

Test Commonly Includes Precipitin test by agar gel diffusion

Specimen Serum **CONTAINER:** Red top tube **STORAGE INSTRUCTIONS:** Store serum at 4°C. **SPECIAL INSTRUCTIONS:** Paired sera drawn 10-14 days apart are strongly recommended in cases of suspected acute infection.

Interpretive **REFERENCE RANGE:** Negative. A fourfold increase in titer in paired sera drawn 10-14 days apart is usually indicative of acute infection. Titer >1:8 in the latex agglutination test is presumptive for systemic disease. **USE:** Evaluate suspected systemic candidiasis **LIMITATIONS:** Cross reactions occur in cases of cryptococcosis and tuberculosis with the latex agglutination test. Negative results do not rule out candidiasis. **CONTRAINDICATIONS:** Very severe cases of vaginitis or mucocutaneous candidiasis can produce positive results. **METHODOLOGY:** Latex agglutination (LA), crossed electrophoresis, immunodiffusion (ID), enzyme-linked immunosorbent assay (ELISA) **ADDITIONAL INFORMATION:** This test is difficult to interpret because precipitins are found in 20% to 30% of the normal population. Clinical correlation must exist for the test to be useful. Rising titers of agglutinins are believed to be reliable indicators of the presence of visceral candidiasis. Quantitative tests on sera taken at biweekly intervals are of value in monitoring the progress of infection before and after therapy.

References

Fujita S, Matsubara F, and Matsuda T, "Enzyme-Linked Immunosorbent Assay Measurement of Fluctuations in Antibody Titer and Antigenemia in Cancer Patients With and Without Candidiasis," *J Clin Microbiol*, 1986, 23:568-75.

Hayette MP, Strecker G, Faille C, et al, "Presence of Human Antibodies Reacting With *Candida albicans* O-Linked Oligomannosides Revealed by Using an Enzyme-Linked Immunosorbent Assay and Neoglycolipids," *J Clin Microbiol*, 1992, 30(2):411-7.

Centromere/Kinetochore Antibody

CPT *86235*

Related Information

Scleroderma Antibody *on page 745*

Synonyms ACA

Specimen Serum **CONTAINER:** Red top tube

Interpretive **REFERENCE RANGE:** Negative **USE:** Aid in diagnosis of CREST syndrome **METHODOLOGY:** Indirect fluorescent antibody (IFA) **ADDITIONAL INFORMATION:** CREST syndrome (calcinosis, Raynaud's phenomenon, esophageal dysfunction, sclerodactyly, telangiectasia) is a variant of systemic sclerosis. Patients have changes largely confined to the skin and digits. Patients' sera demonstrate speckled fluorescent antinuclear antibody patterns. When indirect immunofluorescence is applied to substrates with mitotic cells, the serum antibody is associated with chromosome centromeres. Seventy percent to 90% of patients with CREST and 10% to 20% of patients with diffuse scleroderma will be positive. The presence of ACA in patients without scleroderma or CREST often indicates the presence of another sometimes serious underlying connective tissue disease.

References

Goldman JA, "Anticentromere Antibody in Patients Without CREST and Scleroderma: Association With Active Digital Vasculitis, Rheumatic and Connective Tissue Disease," *Ann Rheum Dis*, 1989, 48(9):771-5.

Harmon CE, "Antinuclear Antibodies in Autoimmune Disease," *Med Clin North Am*, 1985, 69:547-63.

Tan EM and Nakamura RM, "Biology and Significance of Autoantibodies to Nuclear Antigens in Systemic Rheumatic Diseases," *Clinical Laboratory Molecular Analyses*, Nakamura RM and O'Sullivan MB, eds, New York, NY: Grune and Stratton Inc, 1985, 3-15.

Cerebrospinal Fluid IgG *see* Cerebrospinal Fluid Immunoglobulin G *on page 656*

Cerebrospinal Fluid IgG Ratios and IgG Index

CPT *82784*

Related Information

Cerebrospinal Fluid Analysis *on page 527*
Cerebrospinal Fluid Immunoglobulin G *on page 656*
Cerebrospinal Fluid Myelin Basic Protein *on page 657*
Cerebrospinal Fluid Oligoclonal Bands *on page 658*

Synonyms CSF IgG/CSF α_2-Macroglobulin; CSF IgG/CSF Albumin Ratio; CSF IgG/CSF Total Protein Ratio; IgG Ratios and IgG Index, Cerebrospinal Fluid

Test Commonly Includes Protein measurements, frequently immunochemical, on CSF and/or serum with determination of ratio or ratios of one protein to another.

Abstract The IgG index can be calculated with use of serum and CSF albumin and IgG.

Specimen Cerebrospinal fluid and serum **CONTAINER:** Clean, sterile CSF tube; red top tube **COLLECTION:** Tube should be labeled with the number indicating the sequence in which tubes were obtained. **STORAGE INSTRUCTIONS:** Store CSF in refrigerator at 4°C. **SPECIAL INSTRUCTIONS:** Before performing lumbar puncture, communicate with laboratory to determine which measurements and ratios are offered or can be obtained on a referral basis. The third tube of routinely obtained three tube set of CSF should be used for these studies.

Interpretive **REFERENCE RANGE:** CSF IgG index: 0.3-0.85.[1] Published information is relevant only to lumbar CSF. Ventricular, cisternal, or cervical CSF will have different reference ranges. **USE:** Detect and measure the level of IgG production by the central nervous system; has been applied to the diagnosis of multiple sclerosis (CSF IgG index, CSF immunoglobulin synthesis

(Continued)

Cerebrospinal Fluid IgG Ratios and IgG Index *(Continued)*

rate and CSF immunoglobulin "oligoclonal" bands) **LIMITATIONS:** Conditions in which lymphoreticular elements of the CNS produce immunoglobulins will result in false-positive (in relation to multiple sclerosis) elevations. Such conditions include but are not limited to aseptic meningitis, lymphoma, neurosyphilis, Guillain-Barré syndrome, and cerebral lupus erythematosus. These conditions, however, are either uncommon or are not frequently associated with an increased IgG index. It has recently been asserted that without presence of CSF oligoclonal bands the IgG index has no diagnostic value for multiple sclerosis (MS). The index has been noted to have limitations even as a screening test. Even a small amount of bloody contamination elevates the IgG index and IgG synthesis rate.[1] **METHODOLOGY:** Wide variety of generally immunochemical based methods (eg, nephelometry). See also listing Cerebrospinal Fluid Immunoglobulin G. **ADDITIONAL INFORMATION:** The finding that patients with multiple sclerosis frequently have increased CSF IgG has led to a quest for a test that would provide sensitive and specific support for the diagnosis. The three contenders, IgG index, synthesis rate, and oligoclonal bands, have shown sensitivity at the 80% to 90% level but are not uniformly specific. CSF IgG may be increased, generally with inflammatory disorders of the CNS (eg, idiopathic polyneuropathy, neurosyphilis). Rents in the interface between blood and CSF will allow increase in CSF IgG. The three contending methods attempt to differentiate between increased barrier permeability and increased CNS immunoglobulin synthesis, each in a different manner. The ratio technique relates CSF IgG level to another protein that hopefully reflects protein present on the basis of increased blood/CSF permeability. CSF IgG/CSF total protein is such a measure. CSF IgG/CSF albumin has been proposed by Tourtellotte et al as equally discriminative for MS as the CSF IgG/CSF total protein ratio. Both methods as originally described utilize electroimmunodiffusion described by Tourtellotte as "easy, rapid, sensitive, and reliable." The method requires only 5 μL of CSF (no concentration needed). This procedure, however, is being supplanted by less technically demanding automated immunochemical analyses. These ratios and a third, CSF IgG/CSF α_2-macroglobulin, are being supplanted by the IgG index, a ratio of ratios (CSF/Serum IgG / CSF/Serum albumin), which compares CSF with serum parameters. The index provides good separation of increased CNS IgG production from protein increases, the result of altered permeability of blood/CNS interface.

Hershey and Trotter have compared sensitivity/specificity (weighted equally) of four tests (not including IgG synthetic rate) and found the CSF IgG index superior with sensitivity of 91% and specificity of 96.5%.[2] Gambino, however, has emphasized that these results are with cerebral infections and immunologic diseases eliminated so that considerable clinical judgment must be exercised.[3] Currently studies comparing results of the three (or more) contenders continue. Results of IgG index testing appear to correlate with those of oligoclonal banding determinations, but the IgG index may have no specific value independent of the presence of oligoclonal bands.

Recommendations continue for careful clinical neurologic evaluation in cases of suspected multiple sclerosis as all of the laboratory testing procedures produce nonspecific results. Free kappa light chains in the CSF may represent a relatively specific laboratory abnormality to support a clinical diagnosis of multiple sclerosis.

Footnotes

1. Fishman RA, *Cerebrospinal Fluid in Diseases of the Nervous System*, 2nd ed, Philadelphia, PA: WB Saunders Co, 1992, 207-8.
2. Hershey LA and Trotter JL, "The Use and Abuse of the Cerebrospinal Fluid IgG Profile in the Adult: A Practical Evaluation," *Ann Neurol*, 1980, 8:426-34.
3. Gambino R, "CSF Immunoglobulins," *Lab Report for Physicians*, 1981, 3:42-4.

References

Barna BP, Valenzuela R, and Gupta MK, "Laboratory Analyses of Cerebrospinal Fluid," *Laboratory Handbook of Neuroimmunologic Disease*, Chapter 5, Barna BP, ed, Chicago, IL: ASCP Press, 1987, 65-104.

Christenson RH, Behlmer P, Howard JF Jr, et al, "Interpretation of Cerebrospinal Fluid Protein Assays in Various Neurologic Diseases," *Clin Chem*, 1983, 29:1028-30.

Giles PD, Heath JP, and Wroe SJ, "Oligoclonal Bands and the IgG Index in Multiple Sclerosis: Uses and Limitations," *Ann Clin Biochem*, 1989, 26(Pt 4):317-23.

Hische EA, van der Helm HJ, and van Walbeek HK, "The Cerebrospinal Fluid Immunoglobulin G Index as a Diagnostic Aid in Multiple Sclerosis: A Bayesian Approach," *Clin Chem*, 1982, 28:354-5.

Keren DF, "Multiple Sclerosis and Oligoclonal Bands," *High-Resolution Electrophoresis: Techniques and Interpretation*, Chapter 3, Boston, MA: Butterworth's Publishers, 1987, 86-93.

Rudick RA, French CA, Breton D, et al, "Relative Diagnostic Value of Cerebrospinal Fluid Kappa Chains in MS: Comparison With Other Immunoglobulin Tests," *Neurology*, 1989, 39(7):964-8.

Thompson EJ, Riches PG, and Kohn J, "Antibody Synthesis Within the Central Nervous System: Comparisons of CSF IgG Indices and Electrophoresis," *J Clin Pathol*, 1983, 36:312-5.

Tourtellotte WW, Tavolato B, Parker JA, et al, "Cerebrospinal Fluid Electroimmunodiffusion. An Easy, Rapid, Sensitive, Reliable, and Valid Method for the Simultaneous Determination of Immunoglobulin G and Albumin," *Arch Neurol*, 1971, 25:345-50.

Cerebrospinal Fluid IgG Synthesis Rate

***CPT** 82784*

Related Information

Cerebrospinal Fluid Immunoglobulin G *on next page*
Cerebrospinal Fluid Oligoclonal Bands *on page 658*
Cerebrospinal Fluid Protein Electrophoresis *on page 661*

Synonyms IgG Synthesis Rate, Cerebrospinal Fluid

Test Commonly Includes Serum and CSF IgG and albumin levels, calculation of IgG synthesis rate

Abstract Estimation of amount of IgG synthesized daily in the CNS, with the intention to correct for the amount of IgG entering from serum. Used to help confirm diagnosis of multiple sclerosis.

Specimen Cerebrospinal fluid and serum obtained concurrently **CONTAINER:** Clean, sterile CSF tube; red top tube **STORAGE INSTRUCTIONS:** Refrigerate CSF at 4°C. **SPECIAL INSTRUCTIONS:** Before performing lumbar puncture, communicate with laboratory to determine availability and specimen requirements. As a number of possibly helpful tests and ratios (applicable to the diagnosis of multiple sclerosis) based on protein immunochemical determinations have become available, individual laboratories may perform only a select few. Commercial (referral) laboratories may also be selective.

Interpretive **REFERENCE RANGE:** 0.14 ± 1.8 mg IgG synthesized/day, dependent upon the individual laboratories; normal values for CSF albumin and immunoglobulin G **USE:** Evaluate the *de novo* rate of synthesis of IgG in the CNS. Useful in diagnosis of inflammatory and autoimmune diseases involving the CNS, in particular, multiple sclerosis. Determination of IgG synthesis rate is based on the quotient of average normal serum IgG/average normal CSF IgG. As such it is dependent upon the validity of each individual laboratories' IgG method and normal range. As indicated previously, there are a variety of different testing approaches in use. Good laboratory practice requires establishing one's own normal range, especially important in this area. A sufficiently large sample of "normal" CSF, however, is not easily obtained. **LIMITATIONS:** The following formula involves a constant described as "a ratio constant that quantitatively determines the proportion of CSF IgG that normally passes by filtration from the serum into the CSF across an intact BBB" (blood brain barrier). Even a small amount of bloody contamination elevates IgG index and IgG synthesis rate. Fishman notes a lack of unanimity of opinion regarding the virtues of the various calculations which have been advocated, and concludes that he prefers the IgG-albumin index.[1] **METHODOLOGY:** A variety of usually immunochemical based methods are available. Nephelometry, rate immunonephelometry and electroimmunodiffusion have been used. See Cerebrospinal Fluid Immunoglobulin G listing. **ADDITIONAL INFORMATION:** Tourtellotte's IgG synthesis rate is theoretically the most definitive approach to determining IgG production by the central nervous system. It is based upon an empirically derived formula, the validity of which, however, has been verified by radiolabeled IgG experiments. The formula is given as: *de novo* CNS $IgG_{syn} = ((IgG_{CSF} - IgG_s/369) - (Alb_{CSF} - Alb_s/230)(IgG_s/Alb_s)\ 0.43) \times 5$. The constants (eg, 369 and 230) are method dependent and may vary from laboratory to laboratory. Controversy concerning the accuracy of the IgG synthesis formula has been expressed. A study by Tourtellotte and associates has shown that about 90% of multiple sclerosis patients show evidence of enhanced IgG synthesis. A study from the Cleveland Clinic indicates a sensitivity and specificity comparable to that for the IgG index (see Cerebrospinal Fluid IgG Ratios and IgG Index listing) in predictive value for MS. Sensitivity (96%) and specificity (98%) applied to a group considered as definite multiple sclerosis. A group of "possible multiple sclerosis" patients included a number of cases in which CNS IgG synthesis was normal – just 55% had an elevated rate. In the group with "neurologic diseases other than MS," 96% of patients had normal CNS IgG synthesis. The study suggests that determination of CSF IgG synthesis rate contributes importantly to the diagnosis of MS. The study also emphasizes that correlations between test results and diagnoses are dependent upon the validity of what must remain a clinical neurologic diagnosis.

Footnotes

1. Fishman RA, *Cerebrospinal Fluid in Diseases of the Nervous System*, 2nd ed, Philadelphia, PA: WB Saunders Co, 1992, 207-8.

(Continued)

Cerebrospinal Fluid IgG Synthesis Rate *(Continued)*

References

Barna BP, Valenzuela R, and Gupta MK, "Laboratory Analyses of Cerebrospinal Fluid," *Laboratory Handbook of Neuroimmunologic Disease*, Chapter 5, Barna BP, ed, Chicago, IL: ASCP Press, 1987, 65-104.

Mandler R, Goven H, and Valenzuela R, "Value of Central Nervous System IgG Daily Synthesis Determination in the Diagnosis of Multiple Sclerosis," *Neurology*, 1982, 32:296-8.

Thompson EJ and Keir G, "Laboratory Investigation of Cerebrospinal Fluid Proteins," *Ann Clin Biochem*, 1990, 27(Pt 5):425-35.

Tourtellotte WW, Potvin AR, Fleming JO, et al, "Multiple Sclerosis: Measurement and Validation of Central Nervous System IgG Synthesis Rate," *Neurology*, 1980, 30:240-4.

Tourtellotte WW, Staugaitis SM, Walsh MJ, et al, "The Basis of Intra-Blood-Brain-Barrier IgG Synthesis," *Ann Neurol*, 1985, 17:21-7.

Valenzuela R, Mandler R, and Goren H, "Immunonephelometric Quantitation of Central Nervous System IgG Daily Synthesis in Multiple Sclerosis. Clinical Evaluation Using Predictive Value Theory," *Am J Clin Pathol*, 1982, 78:22-8.

Cerebrospinal Fluid Immunoglobulin G

CPT *82784*

Related Information

Cerebrospinal Fluid IgG Ratios and IgG Index *on page 653*
Cerebrospinal Fluid IgG Synthesis Rate *on previous page*
Cerebrospinal Fluid Oligoclonal Bands *on page 658*

Synonyms Cerebrospinal Fluid IgG; CSF Gamma G; CSF IgG; CSF Immunoglobulin; Gamma G, CSF; IgG, CSF; Immunoglobulin G, Cerebrospinal Fluid; Spinal Fluid Globulin; Spinal Fluid Immunoglobulin

Replaces Colloidal Gold Curve

Specimen Cerebrospinal fluid **CONTAINER:** Clean, sterile CSF tube **COLLECTION:** Tube should be labeled with the sequence in which tubes were obtained. **STORAGE INSTRUCTIONS:** Store in refrigerator. **SPECIAL INSTRUCTIONS:** The third tube of a routinely obtained three tube set of CSF should be used for CSF IgG study.

Interpretive **REFERENCE RANGE:** Normal CSF IgG: 5% to 12% of total CSF protein.[1] There is no evidence of intraday variation, diurnal variation. **USE:** Evaluate central nervous system involvement by infection, neoplasm, or primary neurologic disease (in particular, multiple sclerosis) **LIMITATIONS:** Normal levels do not exclude disease; clinical correlation must be applied **METHODOLOGY:** Radial immunodiffusion (RID), electroimmunodiffusion, immunofluorometry, immunoprecipitation, immunonephelometry, rate immunonephelometry. A comparison of immunochemical methods (RID, rate nephelometry, and nephelometric light scattering at quasi-equilibrium) showed that calibrator crossover studies agreed well although precipitating diameters were difficult to read below IgG levels <3 mg/dL (SI: <0.03 g/L). **ADDITIONAL INFORMATION:** Cerebrospinal fluid protein is elevated in many conditions which affect the central nervous system primarily or secondarily. In inflammatory or destructive processes in which serum leaks into CSF, both IgG and albumin will be present in the CSF in increased amounts. Since albumin is not, but immunoglobulins are, synthesized in the central nervous system, a relative increase in CSF IgG indicates presence of a process involving the central nervous system primarily, in particular multiple sclerosis.

The study by Berner et al utilized the radial immunodiffusion technique. While this method suffers from a high and variable CV (about 10% to 20%), it is advantageous compared to electrophoretic techniques because of technical simplicity; there is no need to concentrate the spinal fluid. IgG showed marked elevation (>16 mg/dL) (SI: >0.16 g/L) in 36% of MS patients with only 1% of non-MS controls having this degree of increase. In the slightly elevated category (11% to 16%), there was considerable overlap with 38% of MS patients and 27% of non-MS patients falling into this category. While MS patients are maintained on ACTH and/or steroid therapy or during remission, CSF IgG levels decrease but generally remain significantly elevated.

Electrophoresis of CSF may also be enlightening if oligoclonal gamma globulin bands are demonstrated, which also suggest multiple sclerosis. See also Cerebrospinal Fluid Oligoclonal Bands test listing.

Footnotes

1. Fishman RA, *Cerebrospinal Fluid in Diseases of the Nervous System*, 2nd ed, Philadelphia, PA: WB Saunders Co, 1992, 206-14.

References

Barna BP, Valenzuela R, and Gupta MK, "Laboratory Analyses of Cerebrospinal Fluid," *Laboratory Handbook of Neuroimmunologic Disease*, Chapter 5, Barna BP, ed, Chicago, IL: ASCP Press, 1987, 65-104.

Ben-Menachem E, Persson L, Schechter PJ, et al, "Cerebrospinal Fluid Parameters in Healthy Volunteers During Serial Lumbar Punctures," *J Neurochem*, 1989, 52(2):632-5.
Berner JJ, Ciemins VA, and Schroeder EF Jr, "Radial Immunodiffusion of Spinal Fluid: Diagnostic Value in Multiple Sclerosis," *Am J Clin Pathol*, 1972, 58:145-52.
Christenson RH, Russell ME, and Hassett BJ, "Cerebrospinal Fluid: Electrophoresis and Methods for Determining Immunoglobulin G Compared," *Clin Biochem*, 1989, 22(6):429-32.
Marshall DW, Brey RL, Cahill WT, et al, "Spectrum of Cerebrospinal Fluid Findings in Various Stages of Human Immunodeficiency Virus Infection," *Arch Neurol*, 1988, 45:954-8.

Cerebrospinal Fluid Myelin Basic Protein

CPT 83873

Related Information

Cerebrospinal Fluid IgG Ratios and IgG Index *on page 653*
Cerebrospinal Fluid Oligoclonal Bands *on next page*

Synonyms CSF Myelin Basic Protein; MBP Assay; Myelin Basic Protein, Cerebrospinal Fluid

Abstract Myelin basic protein, a component of the myelin nerve sheath, is a product of oligodendroglia. Assay for MBP is more of an assessment of disease activity than a diagnostic test for any particular disease.

Specimen Cerebrospinal fluid **CONTAINER:** Clean, sterile CSF tube **STORAGE INSTRUCTIONS:** Freeze immediately after obtaining specimen. **SPECIAL INSTRUCTIONS:** Communicate with laboratory to obtain details of specimen collection. Sample is usually referred to reference laboratory. CSF sample should preferably be obtained when patient is symptomatic (ie, not between acute episodes).

Interpretive **REFERENCE RANGE:** (Immunoassay) no active demyelination: <4 ng/mL (or 4 μg/L);[1] weakly positive result: 5.1-6.0 μg/L; consistent with active demyelinating process: >6.0 μg/L **USE:** Estimate activity of demyelinating diseases of the central nervous system, in particular multiple sclerosis (MS) **LIMITATIONS:** Multiple sclerosis is often episodic. The MBP level may be low to undetectable between attacks. Patients in remission usually have no detectable MBP in their spinal fluid. MBP is optimally detected in CSF within 5-15 days of the onset of an acute exacerbation. The MBP molecule fragments readily undergo conformational changes in relation to solid surfaces versus liquid environment, and exhibit multiple immunologic determinants with different binding affinities. These and other considerations have led to disparate results of MBP RIA analyses from laboratory to laboratory. The variable expression of antigenic sites in relation to conformational changes occurring in the parent MBP molecule and its fragments also provide an explanation for the observation that MBP antigen and antibody to MBP antigen sometimes exist together in the same CSF or serum. Possibly, utilization of a radioligand of human MBP synthetic peptide 69-89 or human MBP peptide 43-88 as antigen for radioimmunoassay may improve sensitivity, but the nature of specificity for MBP would remain to be established. The level is increased in a number of entities which cause breakdown of myelin, including stroke, hypoxia, trauma, neoplasms, leukodystrophies, Wernicke's disease, Guillain-Barré syndrome, and CNS LE.[2,3] **METHODOLOGY:** Radioimmunoassay (RIA), enzyme immunoassay (EIA) **ADDITIONAL INFORMATION:** This test provides a measure of myelin fragments released into the spinal fluid as a result of the breakdown of myelin during acute phases in the course of demyelinating disease of the CNS (most common example of which is multiple sclerosis). MBP is a 169 amino acid peptide which comprises 30% of the protein of the myelin sheath. While MBP is a useful test in the diagnosis of active MS, some patients with this disorder will have normal levels, especially during remissions, and elevations may be seen in other disorders as well. Therefore, tests such as CSF oligoclonal bands and IgG index, which are positive in 90% of MS patients during active disease **or** revision, are preferred for the initial diagnosis. However, MBP is useful for providing objective evidence of disease activity.

CSF MBP levels were found to decrease to the level of controls in a group of 11 cases of chronic progressive multiple sclerosis receiving immunosuppressive therapy (cyclophosphamide and prednisone). These findings suggest that RIA for MBP might be used to monitor the hoped for beneficial effect of such therapy in some cases of MS.

It has been suggested that MBP levels in the CSF might be used in the assessment of radiation-induced myelopathy. MS patients in relapse have been shown to have increased interleukin 1 and interleukin 2 production as the result of MBP-stimulated peripheral blood mononuclear cells.

Initial evaluation of 130 HIV-infected patients for the presence of CSF myelin basic protein found none with MBP. Subsequent development of CNS symptoms with abnormal IgG parameters was not associated with abnormal MBP levels.

(Continued)

Cerebrospinal Fluid Myelin Basic Protein *(Continued)*

Footnotes

1. Mukherjee A, Vogt RF, and Linthicum DS, "Measurement of Myelin Basic Protein by Radioimmunoassay in Closed Head Trauma, Multiple Sclerosis, and Other Neurological Diseases," *Clin Biochem*, 1985, 18:304-7.
2. Fishman RA, *Cerebrospinal Fluid in Diseases of the Nervous System*, 2nd ed, Philadelphia, PA: WB Saunders Co, 1992, 210.
3. Kjeldsberg CR and Knight JA, *Body Fluids: Laboratory Examination of Amniotic, Cerebrospinal, Seminal, Serous and Synovial Fluids*, 3rd ed, Chicago, IL: ASCP Press, 1993, 93-4.

References

Barna BP, Valenzuela R, and Gupta MK, "Laboratory Analyses of Cerebrospinal Fluid," *Laboratory Handbook of Neuroimmunologic Disease*, Chapter 5, Barna BP, ed, Chicago, IL: ASCP Press, 1987, 65-104.

Day ED, "Radioimmunoassay for Myelin Basic Protein," *Clin Immunol Newslet*, 1982, 3:53-9.

Lamers KJ, Uitdehaag BM, Hommes OR, et al, "The Short-Term Effect of an Immunosuppressive Treatment on CSF Myelin Basic Protein in Chronic Progressive Multiple Sclerosis," *J Neurol Neurosurg Psychiatry*, 1988, 51:1334-7.

Marshall DW, Brey RL, and Butzin CA, "Lack of Cerebrospinal Fluid Myelin Basic Protein in HIV-Infected Asymptomatic Individuals With Intrathecal Synthesis of IgG," *Neurology*, 1989, 39(8):1127-9.

Rubin P, Whitaker JN, Ceckler TL, et al, "Myelin Basic Protein and Magnetic Resonance Imaging for Diagnosing Radiation Myelopathy," *Int J Radiat Oncol Biol Phys*, 1988, 15:1371-81.

Selmaj K, Nowak Z, and Tchorzewski H, "Multiple Sclerosis: Effect of Myelin Basic Protein on Interleukin 1, Interleukin 2 Production and Interleukin 2 Receptor Expression *In Vitro*," *Clin Exp Immunol*, 1988, 72:428-33.

Whitaker JN and Herman PK, "Human Myelin Basic Protein Peptide 69-89: Immunochemical Features and Use in Immunoassays of Cerebrospinal Fluid," *J Neuroimmunol*, 1988, 19:47-57.

Whitaker JN, Gupta M, and Smith OF, "Epitopes of Immunoreactive Myelin Basic Protein in Human Cerebrospinal Fluid," *Ann Neurol*, 1986, 20:329-36.

Cerebrospinal Fluid Oligoclonal Bands

***CPT** 83916*

Related Information

Cerebrospinal Fluid IgG Ratios and IgG Index *on page 653*
Cerebrospinal Fluid IgG Synthesis Rate *on page 655*
Cerebrospinal Fluid Immunoglobulin G *on page 656*
Cerebrospinal Fluid Myelin Basic Protein *on previous page*
Cerebrospinal Fluid Protein Electrophoresis *on page 661*

Synonyms Oligoclonal Bands, Cerebrospinal Fluid

Test Commonly Includes High-resolution electrophoresis of cerebrospinal fluid and serum obtained concurrently

Abstract Oligoclonal bands on CSF electrophoresis are typical of but not pathognomonic for multiple sclerosis. Quantitative and qualitative tests for multiple sclerosis and other inflammatory and immunological disorders of the CNS are complementary.[1]

Specimen Cerebrospinal fluid and serum obtained concurrently **CONTAINER:** Clean, sterile CSF tube; red top tube **STORAGE INSTRUCTIONS:** Refrigerate at 4°C.

Interpretive **REFERENCE RANGE:** Normal CSF has no demonstrable oligoclonal bands. **USE:** Oligoclonal CSF bands contribute to the diagnosis of inflammatory and autoimmune disease of the CNS. In particular, they are found in 83% to 94% of subjects with definite multiple sclerosis and in 100% of patients with subacute sclerosing panencephalitis,[1] and in other degenerative states as well (eg, presenile dementia). **LIMITATIONS:** Test has a satisfactorily high level of sensitivity (90%, approximately) for association with multiple sclerosis, but it is not specific. Serum protein electrophoresis must be run concurrently to assure that any CSF bands detected do not have origin in the serum. **METHODOLOGY:** Thin gel agarose high-resolution electrophoresis. Requires 80 times concentration of CSF. Cellulose acetate and agarose systems generally may detect "oligoclonal" bands but at a much lower level of sensitivity. Isoelectric focusing is preferred by some but results in decreased specificity. **ADDITIONAL INFORMATION:** Important to the diagnosis of multiple sclerosis is the demonstration of "oligoclonal" bands either by high-resolution agarose electrophoresis or by isoelectric focusing. For practical technical/interpretive reasons, high-resolution agarose techniques are preferred over isoelectric focusing. See also listings Cerebrospinal Fluid IgG Synthesis Rate and Cerebrospinal Fluid IgG Ratios and IgG Index. The oligoclonal band test is a specialized CSF electrophoresis test using unique "high resolution" gels and particular equipment. It is not sufficient to order routine CSF electrophoresis and assume that oligoclonal banding will be detected. Many studies indicate a high frequency of oligoclonal bands occurring in CNS of patients with MS. Some have found isoelectric focusing to be more sensitive. IEF, however, is technically more demanding and is not routinely available in the majority of routine clinical laboratories. A combination of oligoclonal bands in CSF and an elevated CSF IgG index may provide the best biochemical indication of the presence of multiple sclerosis. It has also been considered, however, that in patients without oligoclonal bands the IgG index has no diagnostic value relative to multiple sclerosis. Oligoclonal bands are not specific for MS but have been described in many other disorders, including subacute sclerosing panencephalitis, Jakob-Creutzfeldt disease, encephalitis, Guillain-Barré syndrome, neurosyphilis, stroke, cerebral vasculitis, and neoplasms. However, in most of these diseases, oligoclonal bands are uncommon, whereas they are present in about 90% or more of patients with MS.

Evidence that multiple sclerosis is mediated by the immune system is persuasive but circumstantial. The initial target in multiple sclerosis may well be the oligodendrocyte, with degeneration of myelin processes secondary to damage to the myelin-forming function of those cells.[2,3]

Footnotes

1. Fishman RA, *Cerebrospinal Fluid in Diseases of the Nervous System*, 2nd ed, Philadelphia, PA: WB Saunders Co, 1992, 208-10.
2. Ebers GC, "Multiple Sclerosis: New Insights From Old Tools," *Mayo Clin Proc*, 1993, 68:711-2.
3. Rodriguez M, Scheithauer BW, Forbes G, et al, "Oligodendrocyte Injury Is an Early Event in Lesions of Multiple Sclerosis," *Mayo Clin Proc*, 1993, 68:627-36.

References

Davenport RD and Keren DF, "Oligoclonal Bands in Cerebrospinal Fluid: Significance of Corresponding Bands in Serum for Diagnosis of Multiple Sclerosis," *Clin Chem*, 1988, 34:764.

Gerson B, Krolikowski J, and Gerson IM, "Two Agarose Electrophoretic Systems for Demonstration of Oligoclonal Bands in Cerebrospinal Fluid Compared," *Clin Chem*, 1980, 26:343-5.

Giles PD, Heath JP, and Wroe SJ, "Oligoclonal Bands and the IgG Index in Multiple Sclerosis: Uses and Limitations," *Ann Clin Biochem*, 1989, 26(Pt 4):317-23.

Hosein ZZ and Johnson KP, "Isoelectric Focusing of Cerebrospinal Fluid Proteins in the Diagnosis of Multiple Sclerosis," *Neurology*, 1981, 31:70-6.

Keren DF, "Multiple Sclerosis and Oligoclonal Bands," *High Resolution Electrophoresis: Techniques and Interpretation*, Chapter 3, Boston, MA: Butterworth's Publishers, 1987, 86-93.

Keren DF and Warren JS, *Diagnostic Immunology*, Baltimore, MD: Williams & Wilkins, 1992, 263-6.

Lasne Y, Benzerara O, Chazot G, et al, "A Sensitive Method for Characterization of Oligoclonal Immunoglobulins in Unconcentrated Cerebrospinal Fluid," *J Neurochem*, 1981, 36:1872-4.

Mehta PD and Patrick BA, "Oligoclonal IgG Bands in CSF: A Diagnostic Tool," *Clin Immunol Newslet*, 1982, 3:101-6.

Wybo I, Van Blerk M, Malfoit R, et al, "Oligoclonal Bands in Cerebrospinal Fluid Detected by Phastsystem Isoelectric Focusing," *Clin Chem*, 1990, 36(1):123-5.

Cerebrospinal Fluid Protein

***CPT** 84155*

Related Information

Bacterial Antigens, Rapid Detection Methods *on page 775*
Cerebrospinal Fluid Analysis *on page 527*
Cerebrospinal Fluid Culture *on page 798*
Cerebrospinal Fluid Fungus Culture *on page 800*
Cerebrospinal Fluid Glucose *on page 176*
Cerebrospinal Fluid Lactic Acid *on page 178*
Cerebrospinal Fluid LD *on page 179*
Cerebrospinal Fluid Mycobacteria Culture *on page 801*
Cerebrospinal Fluid Protein Electrophoresis *on page 661*
FTA-ABS, Cerebrospinal Fluid *on page 679*
Gram Stain *on page 815*
VDRL, Cerebrospinal Fluid *on page 761*
Viral Culture, Central Nervous System Symptoms *on page 1199*

Synonyms Protein, Cerebrospinal Fluid

Test Commonly Includes Culture, Gram stain, glucose, and protein are usually ordered together.

Abstract For diagnosis of meningitis, culture and then Gram staining have priority over all other testing, when only a small quantity of cerebrospinal fluid (CSF) is available. Cell count with differential deserve the next priority, followed by glucose and protein.

Specimen Cerebrospinal fluid **CONTAINER:** Clean, sterile CSF tube **COLLECTION:** Tubes should be labeled with patient's name, hospital number, and date and time of collection. **STORAGE IN-**

(Continued)

Cerebrospinal Fluid Protein *(Continued)*

STRUCTIONS: **Do not store. Must be delivered to clinical laboratory immediately.** SPECIAL INSTRUCTIONS: Usually three tubes of CSF are collected for count and culture in addition to protein and glucose with collection of 1 mL in each tube labeled #1, #2, #3 in order of collection.

Interpretive REFERENCE RANGE: Lumbar CSF: 0-1 month: <150 mg/dL (SI: <1.5 g/L); 1-6 months: approximately 30-100 mg/dL (SI: 0.30-1.00 g/L); 6 months and up: approximately 15-50 mg/dL (SI: 0.15-0.50 g/L). Ventricular CSF protein is generally lower. A recent study found a reference interval (biuret method) of 14-62 mg/dL (SI: 0.14-0.62 g/L).[1] POSSIBLE PANIC RANGE: Results above upper limits, especially with additional abnormalities (increased cells and/or decreased glucose) USE: **Increased** with bacterial meningitis, tuberculous meningitis, brain abscess, meningovascular syphilis, diabetes mellitus, CVA (including cases in which no hemorrhage has occurred), arachnoiditis, dehydration, drug effects, and subarachnoid hemorrhage. Used for differential diagnosis of multiple sclerosis; encephalomyelitis; other degenerative processes causing neurologic disease, some neoplastic diseases, some cases of myxedema and other instances of endocrine disorders, traumatic tap, and in CSF recovered from below the level of an obstruction of the spinal cord.

Decreased CSF protein may be seen in normal children 6-24 months of age, with dilution from water intoxication, CSF leak (CSF rhinorrhea or otorrhea, leaks following lumbar puncture, other fistulae), with removal of large volumes of CSF, in some patients with benign intracranial hypertension, in some leukemic subjects, and with hyperthyroidism. Low CSF protein is 10-20 mg/dL.[2]

LIMITATIONS: Fresh blood in the specimen (traumatic tap) will invalidate the protein result; turbid samples may exhibit a positive interference; hemolyzed or xanthochromic specimens may falsely depress results; ampicillin, gentamicin, and vancomycin increase the apparent CSF protein in at least some cases when measured with Ektachem® slides.[1] Problems in the differential diagnosis of multiple sclerosis, meningitis, and other entities are discussed in following paragraphs. METHODOLOGY: Quantitative turbidimetric (sulfosalicylic acid, trichloroacetic acid, TCA); colorimetric (Biuret, Folin-Lowry phenol); dye binding (bromocresol green); Kjeldahl technique (reference method) and a number of other methods including UV spectrophotometry of diluted serum at wavelength 210-220 nm. Sulfosalicylic acid gives greater turbidity with albumin than with globulin. TCA method is less subject to inaccuracy from this source.[3] Colorimetric methods may also suffer from the albumin/globulin specificity problem but in addition the reagents may react with nonprotein nitrogenous compounds. The use of gel filtration prior to direct UV spectrophotometry may eliminate chemical and drug interference. A micromethod utilizing benzethonium chloride and microtiter plates has been described with similar reactivity to IgG and albumin.[4] ADDITIONAL INFORMATION: Because of a less than sharply defined upper limit of normal,[2] a "borderline increased" range of 45-60 mg/dL (SI: 0.45-0.60 g/L) may be useful. The significance of elevated CSF protein should be carefully considered, in relation to the clinical findings, in particular if blood found its way into the CSF. This could occur at the time of needling the subarachnoid space ("bloody tap") and be clinically misleading, or reflect clinically significant CNS hemorrhage, trauma, vascular anomaly or tumor, and have prime clinical significance. The three tube collection procedure allows for helpful clinical differentiation; bloody CSF clearing between the first and third tubes usually indicates "traumatic tap." If such is the case, centrifuging the specimen should yield a supernatant fluid that is crystal clear. Pigmented (xanthochromic) supernatant indicates subarachnoid hemorrhage with lysis of RBCs as may occur if red cells reside more than a few hours in CSF. The fluid may be clear, however, up to 12 hours after subarachnoid hemorrhage in some cases while traumatic tap itself may be responsible for xanthochromia for as long as 2-5 days after lumbar puncture. If traumatic tap is reasonably certain clinically, the RBC count of patient's blood can be ratioed against the RBC count of CSF to obtain a factor that can be compared against total protein of blood vs CSF protein. This is not a particularly exacting or reliable procedure but may provide an indication that the CSF protein is higher than would be expected on the basis of contamination by peripheral blood. Patients with elevated CSF protein should have additional analyses (eg, IgG/albumin index, IgG synthetic rate, and high resolution agarose protein electrophoresis for demonstration of "oligoclonal" bands), in particular if there are clinical findings of multiple sclerosis. Total protein in CSF is within normal limits in of 66% of subjects with MS. Protein levels >100 mg/dL are very atypical, and bring a diagnosis of MS into question.[2]

Protein may be normal or increased in viral meningitis but is usually slightly increased, 50-80 mg/dL. Protein in most cases of viral meningitis is <100 mg/dL.[5] It is usually 100-500 mg/dL in acute bacterial meningitis and is occasionally >1000 mg/dL. Protein was <45 mg/dL in fewer than 2% of a series of 157 patients with acute bacterial meningitis. It is almost always high in tuberculous meningitis.[2] Smith and Haas caution that for a premature or term newborn, CSF protein >100 mg/dL (among other criteria) places the baby at risk for bacterial meningitis.[6] **The gold standard for the diagnosis of bacterial meningitis is the culture, isolation of a bacterium from the CNS.**[7] For subjects who have not been given antimicrobial drugs, the ultimate diagnosis of bacterial meningitis is based on cultures.[8]

CSF cellular and protein abnormalities occur with 10% to 20% of subjects who have primary syphilis and with 30% to 70% of those with secondary lues.[9]

Footnotes

1. Lott JA and Warren P, "Estimation of Reference Intervals for Total Protein in Cerebrospinal Fluid," *Clin Chem*, 1989, 35(8):1766-70.
2. Fishman RA, *Cerebrospinal Fluid in Diseases of the Nervous System*, 2nd ed, Philadelphia, PA: WB Saunders Co, 1992, 197-214.
3. Schriever H and Gambino S, "Protein Turbidity Produced by Trichloroacetic Acid and Sulfosalicylic Acid at Varying Temperatures and Varying Ratios of Albumin and Globulin," *Am J Clin Pathol*, 1975, 44:667-72.
4. Luxton RW, Patel P, Keir G, et al, "A Micro-Method for Measuring Total Protein in Cerebrospinal Fluid by Using Benzethonium Chloride in Microtiter Plate Wells," *Clin Chem*, 1989, 35(8):1731-4.
5. Hammer SM and Connolly KJ, "Viral Aseptic Meningitis in the United States: Clinical Features, Viral Etiologies, and Differential Diagnosis," *Curr Clin Top Infect Dis*, 1992, 12:1-25.
6. Smith AL and Haas J, "Neonatal Bacterial Meningitis," *Infections of the Central Nervous System*, Scheld WM, Whitley RJ, and Durack DT, eds, New York, NY: Raven Press, 1991, 313-33.
7. Smith AL, "Bacterial Meningitis," *Pediatr Rev*, 1993, 14(1):11-8.
8. Rodewald LE, Woodin KA, Szilágyi PG, et al, "Relevance of Common Tests of Cerebrospinal Fluid in Screening for Bacterial Meningitis," *J Pediatr*, 1991, 119(3):363-9.
9. Hook EW 3d and Marra CM, "Acquired Syphilis in Adults," *N Engl J Med*, 1992, 326:1060-9, (review).

References

Behrman RE, Kliegman RM, Nelson WE, et al, *Nelson Textbook of Pediatrics*, 14th ed, Philadelphia, PA: WB Saunders Co, 1992, 664-6, 683-91.

Kjeldsberg CR and Knight JA, *Body Fluids: Laboratory Examination of Amniotic, Cerebrospinal, Seminal, Serous and Synovial Fluids*, 3rd ed, Chicago, IL: ASCP Press, 1993, 89-102.

Roos KL, Tunkel AR, and Scheld WM, "Acute Bacterial Meningitis in Children and Adults," *Infections of the Central Nervous System*, Scheld WM, Whitley RJ, and Durack DT, eds, New York, NY: Raven Press, 1991, 335-409.

Cerebrospinal Fluid Protein Electrophoresis

***CPT** 84175*

Related Information

Cerebrospinal Fluid IgG Synthesis Rate *on page 655*
Cerebrospinal Fluid Oligoclonal Bands *on page 658*
Cerebrospinal Fluid Protein *on page 659*
Protein Electrophoresis, Serum *on page 734*
Protein, Total, Serum *on page 340*

Synonyms CSF Electrophoresis; Protein Electrophoresis, Spinal Fluid; Spinal Fluid Electrophoresis

Applies to Tau Fraction; Transthyretin

Test Commonly Includes Total protein

Abstract On electrophoresis, CSF normally includes a prealbumin fraction and a tau fraction. Its gamma globulin proportionally is less in CSF than in serum.

Specimen Cerebrospinal fluid, serum obtained at the same time that lumbar puncture is performed **CONTAINER:** Clean, sterile CSF tube **COLLECTION:** Tube should be labeled with the number indicating the sequence in which tubes were obtained. **STORAGE INSTRUCTIONS:** Store refrigerated. **SPECIAL INSTRUCTIONS:** The third tube of routinely obtained three tube set of CSF should be used for protein electrophoretic study.

Interpretive **REFERENCE RANGE:** Depends on methodology. Gamma: 3% to 11%, beta: 7.3% to 17.9%, $alpha_2$: 3.0% to 12.6%, $alpha_1$: 1.1% to 6.6%, albumin: 56.8% to 76.9%, prealbumin: 2.2% to 7.1%, total protein: 15-50 mg/dL, CSF albumin: 13.4-23.7 mg/dL, beta-gamma ratio: 1.67-2.3, oligoclonal bands: absent. A recent study, using preconcentration of samples and agarose (high resolution) gels, found lower albumin and higher beta and gamma globulin fractions. **USE:** Quantitate CSF protein fractions, aid in diagnosis of inflammatory, demyelinating disease of CNS, although routine CSF protein electrophoresis is highly insensitive and nonspecific for presence of multiple sclerosis (MS). Routine CSF protein electrophoresis has no role in screening for demyelinating diseases (eg, MS). For this either high-resolution electro-

(Continued)

Cerebrospinal Fluid Protein Electrophoresis *(Continued)*

phoresis or isoelectric focusing is required. For tests with greater sensitivity/specificity for MS, see Cerebrospinal Fluid Oligoclonal Bands and Cerebrospinal Fluid IgG Synthesis Rate. **LIMITATIONS:** Not specific, large volume of specimen needed (must be concentrated) **METHODOLOGY:** Cellulose acetate, agarose electrophoresis, "high resolution" agarose gel systems **ADDITIONAL INFORMATION:** Most CSF proteins reflect their counterparts in the serum (from which they are derived). CSF protein is only approximately 1/200 as concentrated as serum protein, necessitating concentration (usually 100 times) and therefore a minimal sample volume of 1 mL or greater is required. Serum protein electrophoresis should be performed simultaneously with CSF protein electrophoresis in order to determine if unique bands are of CNS origin or have been transferred in from the serum. Two protein populations usually not seen on serum protein electrophoretic studies (although possibly present in low concentration) are demonstrable routinely in CSF. These are **prealbumin**, now called **transthyretin**, (just anodal to albumin) and the **tau fraction** (just cathodal to the β-fraction near the origin). The tau fraction is not present on serum protein electrophoretic patterns and represents asialated transferrin. Indeed, the detection of asialated transferrin in drawing from nasal or auditory canals is strong evidence of CSF leakage due to skull fracture. CSF protein includes only small amounts of glycoproteins as compared to serum. As is the case with serum, they migrate as α_1-, α_2-, and β-globulins. Similarly there is very little lipoprotein (an α_1-globulin) in CSF as compared to serum. Severe craniocerebral trauma is characterized by a three- to fourfold increase in α_2 globulins over the first week post-trauma. Elevation of gamma globulin, increase in IgG to albumin ratio, IgG indices, increase in IgG synthetic rate and/or the presence of "oligoclonal" bands on thin gel agarose high resolution electrophoresis has special significance to the diagnosis of multiple sclerosis (see also discussion under these entries.) Earlier studies indicated that a significant number (75%, even 89%) of patients with clinically documented multiple sclerosis had elevated gamma globulin (some studies using paper electrophoresis). Most of the increase in gamma globulin is due to an increase in IgG. IgA and IgM is present largely in cases with >80-100 mg/dL (SI: >0.8-1.0 g/L) total protein and appears to be without diagnostic significance.

References

Auer L and Petek W, "Serum Globulin Changes in Patients With Craniocerebral Trauma," *J Neurol Neurosurg Psychiatry*, 1976, 39:1076-80.

Christenson RH, Russell ME, and Hassett BJ, "Cerebrospinal Fluid: Electrophoresis and Methods for Determining Immunoglobulin G Compared," *Clin Biochem*, 1989, 22(6):429-32.

Fishman RA, *Cerebrospinal Fluid in Diseases of the Nervous System*, 2nd ed, Philadelphia, PA: WB Saunders Co, 1992, 201-3.

Keren DF, "Interpretation of High-Resolution Electrophoresis Patterns in Serum, Urine, and Cerebrospinal Fluid," *High Resolution Electrophoresis and Immunofixation: Techniques and Interpretation*, Boston, MA: Butterworth's Publishers, 1987, 86-93.

Kjeldsberg CR and Knight JA, *Body Fluids: Laboratory Examination of Amniotic, Cerebrospinal, Seminal, Serous and Synovial Fluids*, 3rd ed, Chicago, IL: ASCP Press, 1993, 89-102.

Zaret D, Morrison N, Gulbranson R, et al, "Immunofixation to Quantify β 2-Transferrin in Cerebrospinal Fluid to Detect Leakage of CSF From Skull Injury," *Clin Chem*, 1992, 38(9):1909-12.

Cerebrospinal Fluid VDRL *see* VDRL, Cerebrospinal Fluid *on page 761*

CH_{50} *see* Complement, Total, Serum *on page 667*

CH_{100} *see* Complement, Total, Serum *on page 667*

Chagas' Disease Serological Test

CPT 86317

Related Information

Ova and Parasites, Stool *on page 836*
Parasite Antibodies *on page 729*
Risks of Transfusion *on page 1093*

Abstract American trypanosomiasis (Chagas' disease) is caused by a protozoan, *Trypanosoma cruzi*. The chronic disease includes myocarditis, cardiomyopathy, and megadisease of esophagus and colon. It can cause placentitis, and maternal transmission to the fetus leads to congenital Chagas' disease or abortion. Laboratory workers may be accidentally infected. Found only in the Western hemisphere, Chagas' disease is thought to cause the deaths of 50,000 people annually. Severe recrudescence may occur with immunosuppression (eg, organ transplantation, AIDS).

Specimen Serum **CONTAINER:** Red top tube

Interpretive **REFERENCE RANGE:** Indirect hemagglutination titer: <1:128; complement fixation titer: <1:8; immunoelectrophoresis titer: <1:64 **USE:** Support the clinical diagnosis of chronic Chagas' disease. In endemic areas, serologic testing is needed in blood banks, since transfusion from donors with chronic infection results in transmission of *T. cruzi* to the recipient in 13% to 23% of cases per contaminated unit. **LIMITATIONS:** Distinction between infection with positive serological findings and clinical disease must be kept in mind. False-positives occur in persons with leishmaniasis, malaria, syphilis, and collagen diseases. **METHODOLOGY:** Indirect hemagglutination (IHA), complement fixation (CF), indirect fluorescent antibody (IFA), direct agglutination, enzyme-linked immunosorbent assay (ELISA), immunoelectrophoresis (IEP) Acute disease can be diagnosed by microscopic demonstration of organisms on smears of blood or buffy coat. **ADDITIONAL INFORMATION:** IHA is more sensitive but less specific than the CF. CF shows a high degree of sensitivity in the acute stages of the disease. Because of the chronicity of Chagas' disease, stable low to moderate titers by IHA or CF are difficult to interpret. Serum from patients with Chagas' heart disease contain antibodies which bind to endocardial, vascular, and interstitial elements of heart tissue. Such an "EVI" factor may be predictive of cardiac Chagas' disease. Serologic tests return to normal in a large majority of patients 12-24 months after treatment. Chagas' disease, usually transmitted as a zoonosis by reduviids, is a life-long infection. Its highest incidence is found in Brazil, Argentina, Chile, Bolivia, and Venezuela.[1]

Footnotes

1. Neva FA, "American Trypanosomiasis (Chagas' Disease)," *Cecil Textbook of Medicine*, 19th ed, Chapter 426, Wyngaarden JB, Smith LH Jr, and Bennett JC, eds, Philadelphia, PA: WB Saunders Co, 1992, 1978-82.

References

Araujo FG, "Serological Diagnosis – Perspectives for Confirmatory Tests," *Chagas' Disease (American Trypanosomiasis): Its Impact on Transfusion and Clinical Medicine*, Wendel S, Brener Z, Camargo ME, et al, eds, São Paulo, Brazil: Cartgraf Editoru Ltd, 1992, 219-23.

Kerndt PR, Waskin HA, Kirchhoff LV, et al, "Prevalence of Antibody to *Trypanosoma cruzi* Among Blood Donors in Los Angeles, California," *Transfusion*, 1991, 31:814-8.

Kirchhoff LV, "American Trypanosomiasis (Chagas' Disease) – A Tropical Disease Now in the United States," *N Engl J Med*, 1993, 329(9):639-44.

Chickenpox Titer *see* Varicella-Zoster Virus Serology *on page 761*

Chlamydia Group Titer

***CPT** 86631; 86632 (IgM)*

Related Information

Chlamydia trachomatis Culture *on page 1171*
Chlamydia trachomatis Direct FA Test *on page 1173*
Chlamydia trachomatis DNA Probe *on page 897*
Lymphogranuloma Venereum Titer *on page 722*
Psittacosis Titer *on page 737*

Test Commonly Includes Detection of antibody titer to *Chlamydia* species

Specimen Serum **CONTAINER:** Red top tube **COLLECTION:** Collect acute phase blood as soon as possible after onset (no later than 1 week). Convalescent blood should be drawn 1-2 weeks after acute (no less than 2 weeks after onset).

Interpretive **REFERENCE RANGE:** Negative. A fourfold increase in titer in paired sera is usually indicative of chlamydial infection. Determination of IgM antibody may be helpful in differentiating acute infection from prior exposure. **USE:** Evaluate possible chlamydial infection **LIMITATIONS:** The antigen used in the test is group specific and not species specific. In cases of conjunctivitis, nongonococcal urethritis, and pneumonia of the newborn, there is usually **not** an antibody response detectable by complement fixation. A very high "background" of immunity in the general population makes interpretation of levels difficult. **METHODOLOGY:** Complement fixation (CF), indirect fluorescence antibody (IFA), enzyme immunoassay (EIA) **ADDITIONAL INFORMATION:** Because of the high prevalence of antibodies to *Chlamydia*, especially in patients being evaluated for urethritis or possible venereal disease, serologic diagnosis must be interpreted with caution. Very high titers, rising titers, or IgM specific antibody should be sought. In a patient being evaluated for chlamydial disease of the genitourinary tract, culture as well as serology should be obtained, as well as a serologic test for syphilis and a culture for *Neisseria gonorrhoeae*.

References

Ehret JM and Judson FN, "Genital *Chlamydia* Infections," *Clin Lab Med*, 1989, 9(3):481-500.

(Continued)

Chlamydia Group Titer *(Continued)*

Miettinen A, Heinonen PK, Teisala K, et al, "Antigen-Specific Serum Antibody Response to *Chlamydia trachomatis* in Patients With Pelvic Inflammatory Disease," *J Clin Pathol*, 1990, 43(9):758-61.

***Chlamydia psittaci* Antibodies** *see* Psittacosis Titer *on page 737*

***Chlamydia psittaci* Titer** *see* Psittacosis Titer *on page 737*

Circulating Immune Complexes *see* C1q Immune Complex Detection *on page 649*

CMV-IFA *see* Cytomegalovirus Antibody *on page 672*

CMV-IFA, IgG *see* Cytomegalovirus Antibody *on page 672*

CMV-IFA, IgM *see* Cytomegalovirus Antibody *on page 672*

CMV Titer *see* Cytomegalovirus Antibody *on page 672*

Coccidioidomycosis Antibodies

***CPT** 86635*

Related Information

Fungus Smear, Stain *on page 813*
Myoglobin, Qualitative, Urine *on page 1135*
Sputum Cytology *on page 510*
Sputum Fungus Culture *on page 853*

Applies to Antibody to *Coccidioides immitis*; Spherulin®

Test Commonly Includes Complement fixing or precipitating antibodies

Specimen Serum, cerebrospinal fluid **CONTAINER:** Red top tube; clean, sterile CSF tube

Interpretive **REFERENCE RANGE:** Negative 1:8 **USE:** Diagnose and evaluate the prognosis of coccidioidomycosis **LIMITATIONS:** When low titers are obtained, a diagnosis of coccidioidomycosis must be based on subsequent serological tests and on clinical and mycological studies. Cross reactions may occur in sera from patients with active histoplasmosis. False-negative results often occur in patients with solitary pulmonary lesions. **METHODOLOGY:** Complement fixation (CF), tube precipitation, enzyme-linked immunosorbent assay (ELISA), immunodiffusion (ID) **ADDITIONAL INFORMATION:** Low titers are usually associated with mild and localized disease. Patients with CF titers ≥1:16 should be observed for evidence of pulmonary or extrapulmonary dissemination. The higher the CF titer, the poorer the prognosis in assessing the extent and severity of both acute and chronic coccidioidomycosis. Falling CF titers indicate an improved clinical status. Specific IgM antibodies may be detected early in the course of the disease.

The tube precipitin test is effective in detection of early disease, 1-3 weeks after infection. These antibody levels are not prognostic. There are complement fixing antibodies to either coccidioidin (a culture filtrate) or Spherulin® (an extract of spherules). These become positive later and parallel the course of infection.

In immunodiffusion testing, a band of identity with coccidioidin indicates infection but may be negative early. Some individuals continue to produce detectable antibodies up to 1 year after clinical recovery from active disease. A negative test does not exclude coccidioidomycosis.

Finding CF antibody in CSF makes the diagnosis of coccidioidal meningitis (if fungal osteomyelitis of the base of the skull can be excluded).

References

Galgiani JN, Grace GM, and Lundergan LL, "New Serologic Tests for Early Detection of Coccidioidomycosis," *J Infect Dis*, 1991, 163(3):671-4.

Hedges E and Miller S, "Coccidioidomycosis: Office Diagnosis and Treatment," *Am Fam Physician*, 1990, 41(5):1499-506.

Kaufman L and Reiss E, "Serodiagnosis of Fungal Diseases," *Manual of Clinical Laboratory Immunology*, 4th ed, Vol 2, Chapter 78, Rose NR, Conway de Macario E, Fahey JL, et al, eds, Washington, DC: American Society for Microbiology, 1992, 506-28.

Cold Agglutinin Titer

***CPT** 86156 (screen); 86157 (titer)*

Related Information

Mycoplasma Serology *on page 727*

Applies to I Antigen; i Antigen

Test Commonly Includes Titer of patient's serum against type O blood cells at 2°C to 8°C

Specimen Serum **CONTAINER:** Red top tube **STORAGE INSTRUCTIONS:** After clotting at 37°C, separate serum from cells if specimen is to be stored overnight in refrigerator. **CAUSES FOR REJECTION:** Refrigeration of the specimen before separating serum from cells, specimen not allowed to clot at 37°C **SPECIAL INSTRUCTIONS:** Transport blood immediately to the laboratory.

Interpretive **REFERENCE RANGE:** Screen: negative; titer: <1:32 **USE:** Useful in supporting the diagnosis of primary atypical pneumonia (infection with *Mycoplasma pneumoniae*) **LIMITATIONS:** False-negatives may occur if serum is refrigerated on the clot; only half of patients with *M. pneumoniae* infection will have positive test; there are many positive results associated with a wide and nonspecific variety of other conditions **ADDITIONAL INFORMATION:** *M. pneumoniae* has I-like antigen specificity. The i and I RBC antigens appear to be ceramide heptasaccharides and decasaccharides. The fetal i RBCs change after birth so that by 18 months red cells carry largely I. The i substance has been found in saliva, milk, amniotic fluid, ovarian cyst fluid, and serum.

The most common cause of elevated cold agglutinin in high titers is an infection with *Mycoplasma pneumoniae*. Fifty-five percent of patients with disease have rising titers. In primary atypical *Mycoplasma pneumoniae*, cold agglutinins are demonstrated 1 week after onset; the titer increases in 8-10 days, peaks at 12-25 days, and rapidly falls after day 30. Antibiotic therapy may interfere with antibody formation. Ninety percent of these are severely affected or have prolonged illness.

Cold agglutinins are usually IgM autoantibodies directed against the Ii antigens of human RBCs. These antibodies may be found in patients with cold agglutinin disease or may occur transiently following a number of acute infectious illnesses. Cold agglutinins of cold agglutinin disease are usually monoclonal IgM kappa. Cold antibodies of IgG, IgA, or IgM type directed against Ii antigens may be found in infectious mononucleosis. Antibodies reacting near physiologic temperatures are more likely to be clinically important. Detection of cold agglutinins may be particularly important in patients where cold blood is to be used such as in a blood cardioplegia unit.

References

Branch DR, "Rapid, Reliable Cold Agglutinin Method," *Lab Med*, 1979, 10:481.

Boughton BJ, "Anti-i Cold Agglutinins in Choriocarcinomatosis: Trophoblastic i Antigen," *J Clin Pathol*, 1979, 32:523-7.

Dake SB, Johnston MF, Brueggeman P, et al, "Detection of Cold Hemagglutination in a Blood Cardioplegia Unit Before Systemic Cooling of a Patient With Suspected Cold Agglutinin Disease," *Ann Thorac Surg*, 1989, 47(6):914-5.

Colloidal Gold Curve *replaced by* Cerebrospinal Fluid Immunoglobulin G *on page 656*

Complement C3 *see* C3 Complement, Serum *on page 649*

Complement C4 *see* C4 Complement, Serum *on page 650*

Complement Components

***CPT** 86160 (antigen, each component); 86161 (activity, each component)*

Related Information

C1 Esterase Inhibitor, Serum *on page 648*
C1q Immune Complex Detection *on page 649*
C3 Complement, Serum *on page 649*
C4 Complement, Serum *on page 650*
Complement, Total, Serum *on page 667*
Factor B *on page 678*
Phagocytic Cell Immunocompetence Profile *on page 732*

Test Commonly Includes Quantitation of antigenic (immunologic) and/or functional complement components – C1, C1q, C1r, C1s, C2, C3, C4, C5, C6, C7, C8, C9; Factor B; Factor D

Specimen Serum **CONTAINER:** Red top tube **COLLECTION:** Samples for complement analysis should be allowed to clot 15-30 minutes at room temperature and then 30-60 minutes at 4°C. If the assay cannot be run at once, the specimen should be stored at -70°C.

Interpretive **REFERENCE RANGE:** C1q: 70 μg/mL; C1r: 34 μg/mL; C1s: 31 μg/mL; C2: 25 μg/mL; C3: 1600 μg/mL; C4: 600 μg/mL; C5: 85 μg/mL; C6: 75 μg/mL; C7: 55 μg/mL; C8: 55 μg/mL; C9:

(Continued)

Complement Components *(Continued)*

60 μg/mL; factor B: 200 μg/mL; factor D: 1 μg/mL **USE:** Assess patients with hereditary deficiency of complement components or acquired decrease in levels which may be seen due to hypercatabolism in hereditary angioneurotic edema, or consumption or loss as in vasculitides, glomerulonephritides, immune complex diseases **METHODOLOGY:** Radial immunodiffusion (RID), nephelometry, functional analysis in hemolytic system **ADDITIONAL INFORMATION:** Complement is an array of almost 25 proteins which can interact sequentially to produce a number of biologically active products which are implicated in the pathophysiology of numerous diseases with an immunologic basis. Complement is most often "activated" through either the "classical" pathway, beginning with antigen-antibody complexes (usually on some biologic surface) or the "alternate" pathway which is less clearly understood but may be independent of antigen and antibody. Calcium is also necessary. See figure.

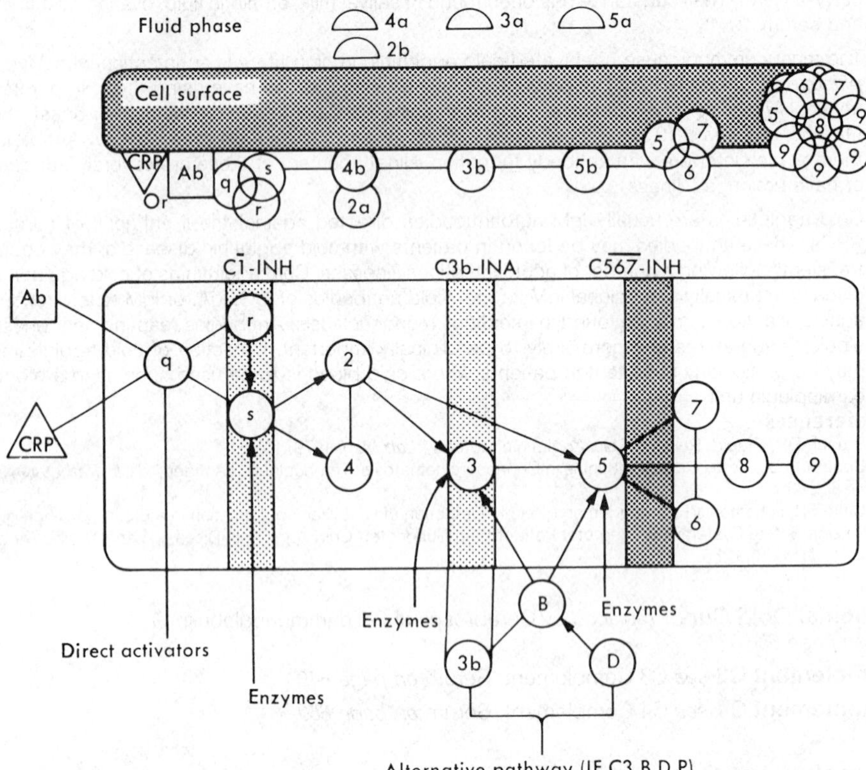

Diagram of primary complement pathway *(enclosed in rectangle)* showing alternative (properdin) pathway and additional modes of complement activation. Enzymatic cleavages are represented by **arrows,** and inhibitory activities are shown by **shading.** Interactions of complement components at cell surface **(stipple)** and cleavage products released into fluid phase are shown at top. From *Gradwohl's Clinical Laboratory Methods and Diagnosis,* 8th ed, Sonnenwirth AC and Jarett L, eds, St Louis, MO: Mosby–Year Book Inc, 1980, 1230, with permission.

In the course of activation several byproducts are produced which are active mediators of inflammation. C3a, C3b, C5a, and C5,6,7 are particularly important chemotactic factors and opsonins. The last three complement components are sometimes called the "membrane attack complex."

Measurement of total complement activity or components, particularly C3 and C4 which can reflect both complement pathways, may be useful in evaluating the activity of rheumatic disorders in which complement may be involved in pathogenesis. These include lupus, arteritis, and arthritis in particular.

There are also congenital deficiencies of complement components associated with distinct clinical syndromes (see table).

Summary of Complement Deficiencies in Man and Their Association With Repeated Infection and/or Collagen Disease

Deficient Component	No. of Patients	Disease/Symptoms
C1r	4	SLE (1), renal disease (1), repeated infections (1)
C1s	2	SLE (2)
C4	3	SLE (3)
C2	23	LE (7), vasculitis (3), MPGN (1), dermatomyositis (1)
C3	4	Repeated infections (3), fever/rash/arthralgias (1)
C5	3	SLE (1), gonococcal disease
C6	5	Relapsing meningococcal meningitis (4), gonococcal disease (1)
C7	5	Raynaud's disease (1), chronic renal disease (1), gonococcal disease (2), SLE (1)
C8	3	SLE (1), gonococcal disease (1)

From *Gradwohl's Clinical Laboratory Methods and Diagnosis,* 8th ed, Sonnenwirth AC and Jarett L, eds, St Louis, MO: Mosby-Year Book Inc, 1980, 1233, with permission.

Deficiency of C3 is associated with severe recurrent infections, usually with encapsulated microorganisms. Infections with *Neisseria* are associated with deficiencies of C5, C6, C7, and C8. Deficiencies of C1 components, C2 and C4 are associated with rheumatic diseases, including lupus, vasculitis, and dermatomyositis. Some individuals with deficiency may have no evidence of disease.

The most common complement deficiency is C2, which is a homozygous abnormality in 1 in 10,000 to 40,000 individuals, and is heterozygous in 1% to 2% of the general population. Patients with C2 deficiency and lupus often have negative or low titer ANA.

Complement components may drop in patients with active rheumatic diseases, particularly lupus nephritis, sometimes decreasing prior to the clinical attack.

References

Colvin RB, Bhan AK, and McCluskey RT, eds, *Diagnostic Immunopathology*, New York, NY: Raven Press, 1988.

Frank MM, "Complement in the Pathophysiology of Human Disease," *N Engl J Med*, 1987, 316:1525-30.

Nusinow SR, Zuraw BL, and Curd JG, "The Hereditary and Acquired Deficiencies of Complement," *Med Clin North Am*, 1985, 69:487-504.

Complement, Total, Serum

CPT 86162

Related Information

C1q Immune Complex Detection *on page 649*
C3 Complement, Serum *on page 649*
C4 Complement, Serum *on page 650*
Complement Components *on page 665*
Factor B *on page 678*
Kidney Profile *on page 268*
Phagocytic Cell Immunocompetence Profile *on page 732*

Synonyms CH_{50}; CH_{100}; Total Hemolytic Complement

Test Commonly Includes Quantitation of total functional serum complement

Specimen Serum **CONTAINER:** Red top tube **STORAGE INSTRUCTIONS:** Allow sample to clot 15-30 minutes at room temperature, then 30-60 minutes at 4°C. Store serum at -70°C if assay cannot be run at once.

Interpretive **REFERENCE RANGE:** 40-100 CH_{50} units. Synovial fluid levels are 33% to 50% of serum levels in patients with nonimmune processes. **USE:** Evaluate and follow-up SLE (systemic lupus erythematosus) patient's response to therapy. May predict disease flare in SLE. Screen for complement component deficiency; evaluate complement activity in cases of immune complex disease, glomerulonephritis, rheumatoid arthritis, SBE, cryoglobulinemia. The CH_{50} assay mainly evaluates the classical pathway. **LIMITATIONS:** Levels are affected by patient's age, stage and activity of disease, treatment, and genetic factors. A single normal re-

(Continued)

Complement, Total, Serum *(Continued)*

sult may be misleading; longitudinal studies are clinically more helpful. **METHODOLOGY:** Quantitative hemolysis, radial immunodiffusion (RID) **ADDITIONAL INFORMATION:** Complement is a system of 25 cell membrane associated and plasma proteins, which when activated produce multiple inflammatory mediators, opsonins, lysins, and down regulators vital to the normal function of the immune system. Complement components belong to a "classical" and "alternative" pathway whose activation steps differ. Complement proteins can be increased as part of the acute phase response to inflammation or infection, and they can be decreased or absent due to hypercatabolism, expenditure in immune complexes, or hereditary deficiency.

Patients with hereditary absence of a complement protein may have decreased total complement and recurrent bacterial infections or a rheumatic illness. Conversely, patients with rheumatic diseases, particularly with active illness and activation of complement and formation of immune complexes, may have low total complement. Falling complement levels may presage clinical flares, particularly of lupus nephritis.

References

Buyon JP, Tamerius J, Ordorica S, et al, "Activation of the Alternative Complement Pathway Accompanies Disease Flares in Systemic Lupus Erythematosus During Pregnancy," *Arthritis Rheum*, 1992, 35(1):55-61.

Colvin RB, Bhan AK, and McCluskey RT, eds, *Diagnostic Immunopathology*, New York, NY: Raven Press, 1988, 32.

Frank MM, "Complement in the Pathophysiology of Human Disease," *N Engl J Med*, 1987, 316:1525-30.

Katz P, "Clinical and Laboratory Evaluation of the Immune System," *Med Clin North Am*, 1985, 69:453-64.

Schur PH, "Complement Studies of Sera and Other Biologic Fluids," *Hum Pathol*, 1983, 14:338-42.

Conglutinin Solid-Phase Assay *see* Immune Complex Assay *on page 705*

Core Antibody *see* Hepatitis B Core Antibody *on page 684*

Cough Plate Culture for Pertussis *replaced by Bordetella pertussis* Direct Fluorescent Antibody *on page 646*

***Coxiella burnetii* Titer** *see* Q Fever Titer *on page 738*

Coxsackie A Virus Titer

CPT 86658

Related Information

Enterovirus Culture *on page 1178*
Viral Culture, Blood *on page 1197*
Viral Culture, Central Nervous System Symptoms *on page 1199*
Viral Culture, Respiratory Symptoms *on page 1204*

Test Commonly Includes Detection of antibody titer to Coxsackie A virus

Specimen Serum **CONTAINER:** Red top tube **SAMPLING TIME:** Acute and convalescent sera drawn at least 14 days apart are required.

Interpretive **REFERENCE RANGE:** Less than a fourfold increase in titer in paired sera **USE:** Establish the diagnosis of Coxsackie A virus infection **LIMITATIONS:** Neutralizing antibodies develop quickly and persist for many years after infection, making demonstration of a rise in titer difficult. Complement fixation test is not sensitive. **METHODOLOGY:** Viral neutralization, complement fixation (CF) **ADDITIONAL INFORMATION:** Coxsackie A virus produces a wide spectrum of disease including meningitis, myositis, pericarditis, respiratory illnesses, rash, and generalized systemic infection. Documentation of infection by serology is difficult, and diagnosis may depend on culture.

References

Melnick JL, "Enteroviruses," *Manual of Clinical Laboratory Immunology*, 4th ed, Vol 2, Chapter 93, Rose NR, Conway de Macario E, Fahey JL, et al, eds, Washington, DC: American Society for Microbiology, 1992, 631-3.

Coxsackie B Virus Titer

CPT 86658

Related Information

Enterovirus Culture *on page 1178*
Viral Culture, Blood *on page 1197*
Viral Culture, Central Nervous System Symptoms *on page 1199*
Viral Culture, Respiratory Symptoms *on page 1204*

Test Commonly Includes Coxsackie B_1, B_2, B_3, B_4, B_5, B_6 virus titers

Specimen Serum CONTAINER: Red top tube SAMPLING TIME: Acute and convalescent sera drawn 10-14 days apart are required.

Interpretive REFERENCE RANGE: Less than a fourfold increase in titer in paired sera USE: Establish the diagnosis of Coxsackie B virus infection LIMITATIONS: Neutralizing antibodies arise quickly and last for years and may make the demonstration of a rising titer difficult. Complement fixing antibodies are insensitive and nonspecific. METHODOLOGY: Complement fixation (CF), viral neutralization ADDITIONAL INFORMATION: Coxsackie B virus causes a wide variety of clinical illness, including pleurodynia (Bornholm's disease), meningitis, rash, pulmonary infection, pericarditis, and a generalized systemic infection. Approximately 50% of clinical myocarditis and pericarditis is caused by Coxsackie B. Since culture is frequently unrewarding, diagnosis may hinge on serologic studies. Recently there has been interest in various viral assays for postviral fatigue syndrome. Antibody to Coxsackie B virus is not helpful in this assessment.

References

Drew WL, "Diagnostic Virology," *Clin Lab Med*, 1987, 7:721-40.

Miller NA, Carmichael HA, Calder BD, et al, "Antibody to Coxsackie B Virus in Diagnosing Postviral Fatigue Syndrome," *BMJ*, 1991, 302(6769):140-3.

See DM and Tilles JG, "Viral Myocarditis," *Rev Infect Dis*, 1991, 13(5):951-6.

C-Reactive Protein

***CPT** 86140*

Related Information

Alpha$_1$-Antitrypsin, Serum *on page 631*
Insulin, Blood *on page 260*
Sedimentation Rate, Erythrocyte *on page 599*
Zeta Sedimentation Ratio *on page 617*

Synonyms Acute Phase Reactant; CRP

Abstract Produced by hepatocytes, C-reactive protein is a useful but nonspecific indicator of acute injury, infection, or inflammation. It is used to try to distinguish bacterial from viral infection. The former cause higher concentrations.

Specimen Serum CONTAINER: Red top tube CAUSES FOR REJECTION: Excessive hemolysis, lipemic serum

Interpretive REFERENCE RANGE: $<8\ \mu g/mL$ USE: Used similarly to erythrocyte sedimentation rate. CRP is nonspecific acute phase reactant used as an indicator of infectious disease and inflammatory states, including active rheumatic fever and rheumatoid arthritis. Progressive increases correlate with increases of inflammation/injury. CRP is a more sensitive, rapidly responding indicator than ESR. CRP may be used to detect early postoperative wound infection and to follow therapeutic response to anti-inflammatory agents. LIMITATIONS: Frozen specimens may give false-positive results; oral contraceptives may affect results. METHODOLOGY: Agglutination, nephelometry, radioimmunoassay (RIA) ADDITIONAL INFORMATION: CRP is a pentameric globulin with mobility near the gamma zone. It is an acute phase reactant which rises rapidly, but nonspecifically in response to tissue injury and inflammation. It is particularly useful in detection of occult infections, acute appendicitis, particularly in leukemia and in postoperative patients. In uncomplicated postoperative recovery, CRP peaks on the 3rd postop day and returns to preop levels by day 7. It may also be helpful in evaluation of extension or reinfarction after myocardial infarction and in following response to therapy in rheumatic disorders. It may help to differentiate Crohn's disease (high CRP) from ulcerative colitis (low CRP) and rheumatoid arthritis (high CRP) from uncomplicated lupus (low CRP). When used to evaluate patients with arthritis, serum is the preferred specimen. There is no advantage to examining synovial fluid for CRP.

References

Delpuech P, Desch G, Magnan F, et al, "C-Reactive Protein in Inflammatory Articular Diseases: Comparison of Concentrations in Blood and Synovial Fluid," *Clin Biochem*, 1989, 22(4):305-8.

Downton SR and Colten HR, "Acute Phase Reactants in Inflammation and Infection," *Semin Hematol*, 1988, 25:84-90.

Schofield KP, Voulgari F, Gozzard DI, et al, "C-Reactive Protein Concentration as a Guide to Antibiotic Therapy in Acute Leukemia," *J Clin Pathol*, 1982, 35:866-9.

Shaw AC, "Serum C-Reactive Protein and Neopterin Concentrations in Patients With Viral or Bacterial Infection," *J Clin Pathol*, 1991, 44(7):596-9.

Thimsen DA, Tong GK, and Gruenberg JC, "Prospective Evaluation of C-Reactive Protein in Patients Suspected to Have Acute Appendicitis," *Am J Surg*, 1989, 55(7):466-8.

(Continued)

C-Reactive Protein *(Continued)*

Van Lente F, "The Diagnostic Utility of C-Reactive Protein," *Hum Pathol*, 1982, 13:1061-3.

Crossmatch, Lymphocyte *see* Tissue Typing *on page 757*

CRP *see* C-Reactive Protein *on previous page*

Cryoglobulin, Qualitative, Serum

CPT 82595

Related Information

Cryofibrinogen *on page 416*
Kidney Profile *on page 268*
Rheumatoid Factor *on page 740*

Patient Care **PREPARATION:** Patient should be fasting.

Specimen Serum **CONTAINER:** Red top tube **COLLECTION:** Specimen must be drawn in a prewarmed syringe and kept at 37°C while clotting. **STORAGE INSTRUCTIONS:** Separate serum from cells, recentrifuge serum, pour into clean test tube, and refrigerate. Specimen should be held 7 days at 4°C before cryoglobulins are excluded. **CAUSES FOR REJECTION:** Specimen not allowed to clot at 37°C.

Interpretive **REFERENCE RANGE:** Negative **USE:** Cryoglobulins may be present in macroglobulinemia of Waldenström, myeloma, chronic lymphocytic leukemia, lupus, chronic active hepatitis, and viral infections **METHODOLOGY:** Precipitation of cryoglobulin at 4°C **ADDITIONAL INFORMATION:** These are proteins which precipitate from blood at low temperatures. A precipitate from serum which forms overnight at 4°C and dissolves at 37°C is called a cryoglobulin.

Cryoglobulins may be divided into three classes. **Type I** are monoclonal immunoglobulins and are usually associated with lymphoproliferative disorders. **Type II** are mixtures of a monoclonal IgM and polyclonal IgG, and are associated with macroglobulinemia and chronic active hepatitis. **Type III** are mixtures of polyclonal IgM and polyclonal IgG. These are found in a wide variety of disorders.

A high percentage of patients with cryoglobulinemia have clinical symptoms, and of these the most common are vascular (ie, purpura and digital necrosis). Raynaud's phenomenon is also common.

Patients with SLE who are rheumatoid factor negative but cryoglobulin positive are more likely to develop renal disease than those who are rheumatoid factor positive and cryoglobulin negative.

References

Howard TW, Iannini MJ, Burge JJ, et al, "Rheumatoid Factor, Cryoglobulinemia, Anti-DNA, and Renal Disease in Patients With Systemic Lupus Erythematous," *J Rheumatol*, 1991, 18(6):826-30.
Keren DF and Warren JS, *Diagnostic Immunology*, Baltimore, MD: Williams & Wilkins, 1992, 270-2.
Winfield JB, "Cryoglobulinemia," *Hum Pathol*, 1983, 14:350-4.

Cryptococcosis, IFA *see Cryptococcus* Antibody Titer *on this page*

Cryptococcosis, Indirect Fluorescent Antibody Titer *see Cryptococcus* Antibody Titer *on this page*

Cryptococcus Antibody Titer

CPT 86641

Related Information

Biopsy or Body Fluid Fungus Culture *on page 780*
Cerebrospinal Fluid Fungus Culture *on page 800*
Cryptococcal Antigen Titer, Serum or Cerebrospinal Fluid *on page 805*
Fungus Smear, Stain *on page 813*
India Ink Preparation *on page 822*
Sputum Fungus Culture *on page 853*
Urine Fungus Culture *on page 883*

Synonyms Cryptococcosis, IFA; Cryptococcosis, Indirect Fluorescent Antibody Titer

Test Commonly Includes Detection of antibody titer to *Cryptococcus neoformans* in patient's serum

Specimen Serum **CONTAINER:** Red top tube **SPECIAL INSTRUCTIONS:** Sequential assays may be desirable.

Interpretive **REFERENCE RANGE:** Negative **USE:** Useful in the diagnosis and prognosis of cryptococcal infections **LIMITATIONS:** A negative test result does not rule out infection as an antibody response may be masked by circulating antigen. **METHODOLOGY:** Tube agglutination, indirect fluorescent antibody (IFA) **ADDITIONAL INFORMATION:** Agglutination titers ≥1:2 are suggestive of infection with *Cryptococcus neoformans*. Agglutinins may be detected early in the course of the disease, but if the disease progresses, excess antigen may be produced which renders antibodies undetectable. With effective chemotherapy, the antigen titer declines and antibody may once again be demonstrated. Antibodies may persist for long periods even after cessation of chemotherapy. A positive IFA reaction, as indicated by a 2+ or greater staining intensity at a 1:16 dilution, is presumptive evidence for active cryptococcosis. See Cryptococcal Antigen Titer, Serum listing.

References

Kaufman L and Reiss E, "Serodiagnosis of Fungal Diseases," *Manual of Clinical Laboratory Immunology*, 4th ed, Vol 2, Chapter 78, Rose NR, Conway de Macario E, Fahey JL, et al, eds, Washington, DC: American Society for Microbiology, 1992, 506-28.

CSF *see* VDRL, Cerebrospinal Fluid *on page 761*

CSF Electrophoresis *see* Cerebrospinal Fluid Protein Electrophoresis *on page 661*

CSF Gamma G *see* Cerebrospinal Fluid Immunoglobulin G *on page 656*

CSF IgG *see* Cerebrospinal Fluid Immunoglobulin G *on page 656*

CSF IgG/CSF α_2-Macroglobulin *see* Cerebrospinal Fluid IgG Ratios and IgG Index *on page 653*

CSF IgG/CSF Albumin Ratio *see* Cerebrospinal Fluid IgG Ratios and IgG Index *on page 653*

CSF IgG/CSF Total Protein Ratio *see* Cerebrospinal Fluid IgG Ratios and IgG Index *on page 653*

CSF Immunoglobulin *see* Cerebrospinal Fluid Immunoglobulin G *on page 656*

CSF Myelin Basic Protein *see* Cerebrospinal Fluid Myelin Basic Protein *on page 657*

CSF VDRL *see* VDRL, Cerebrospinal Fluid *on page 761*

Cysticercosis Titer

CPT 86317

Related Information

Ova and Parasites, Stool *on page 836*
Parasite Antibodies *on page 729*

Abstract Eggs of *Taenia solium*, the pork tapeworm acquired from contact with contaminated feces, lead to cysticercosis. Cysticercosis is found in Mexico, portions of South America, and Africa.

Specimen Serum, cerebrospinal fluid **CONTAINER:** Red top tube

Interpretive **REFERENCE RANGE:** Negative **USE:** Establish the diagnosis of cysticercosis, which is most commonly found in the cerebrum. It occurs in almost any tissue. **LIMITATIONS:** Cross reactions in patients with tapeworm or *Echinococcus* **METHODOLOGY:** Indirect fluorescent antibody (IFA), enzyme-linked immunosorbent assay (ELISA), hemagglutination, immunoelectrophoresis (IEP), enzyme-linked immunoelectrotransfer blot (EITB) **ADDITIONAL INFORMATION:** The tapeworms (Cestodes) include *Taenia solium* (the pork tapeworm). In >80% of proven cases of cysticercosis, serum and CSF titers of hemagglutinating antibodies are high. After complete cyst removal, antibodies disappear in a few months. Ninety-four percent of patients with two or more lesions were successfully detected at the CDC by EITB, however, only 28% of patients with a single lesion were identified by this procedure.

References

Ash LR and Orihel TC, *Atlas of Human Parasitology*, 3rd ed, Chicago, IL: ASCP Press, 1990, 224-5.

Jones TC, "Cestodes (Tapeworms)," *Principles and Practice of Infectious Diseases*, 3rd ed, Mandell GL, Douglas RG Jr, and Bennett JE, eds, New York, NY: Churchhill Livingstone, 1990, 2151-7.

(Continued)

Cysticercosis Titer *(Continued)*

Kagan IG and Maddison SE, "Serodiagnosis of Parasitic Diseases," *Manual of Clinical Laboratory Immunology*, 4th ed, Vol 2, Chapter 79, Rose NR, Conway de Macario E, Fahey JL, et al, eds, Washington, DC: American Society for Microbiology, 1992, 529-43.

Wilson M, Bryan RT, Fried JA, et al, "Clinical Evaluation of the Cysticercosis Enzyme-Linked Immunoelectrotransfer Blot in Patients With Neurocysticeriosis," *J Infect Dis*, 1991, 164(5):1007-9.

Cytomegalic Inclusion Virus Titer *see* Cytomegalovirus Antibody *on this page*

Cytomegalovirus Antibody

CPT 86644; 86645 (IgM)

Related Information

Bronchial Washings Cytology *on page 485*
Bronchoalveolar Lavage *on page 793*
Bronchoalveolar Lavage Cytology *on page 487*
Cytomegalic Inclusion Disease Cytology *on page 496*
Cytomegalovirus Culture *on page 1175*
Cytomegalovirus Isolation, Rapid *on page 1176*
Risks of Transfusion *on page 1093*
Sputum Cytology *on page 510*
TORCH *on page 758*

Synonyms CMV-IFA; CMV Titer; Cytomegalic Inclusion Virus Titer

Applies to CMV-IFA, IgG; CMV-IFA, IgM

Test Commonly Includes IgG and IgM testing of acute sera in neonates, patients suspected of post-transfusion CMV infection, immunosuppressed patients, and maternity cases; IgG testing of convalescent sera

Abstract The most common intrauterine infection is congenital cytomegalovirus infection. It is also an important problem in adult immunocompromised subjects and others.

Specimen Serum **CONTAINER:** Red top tube **SAMPLING TIME:** Acute and convalescent sera drawn 10-14 days apart are required. **STORAGE INSTRUCTIONS:** Store serum at 4°C. **SPECIAL INSTRUCTIONS:** Neonatal specimens, and specimens with very high IgG titers should be analyzed for specific IgM antibody after treatment on a chromatographic column which can separate IgG from IgM.

Interpretive **REFERENCE RANGE:** IgM: <1:8 is considered nondiagnostic, IgG: <1:16. A fourfold increase in titer in paired sera drawn 10-14 days apart is usually indicative of acute infection. **USE:** Establish diagnosis of cytomegalovirus infection **LIMITATIONS:** Heterophil antibodies and presence of rheumatoid factor may cause false-positive IgM results. Fetal IgM antibody to maternal IgG may also cause false-positive results. Because of high levels of "background" antibody in adult populations, a single antibody determination is not useful. For rapid confirmation of new CMV infection, rapid shell vial culture is superior to serology. **METHODOLOGY:** Indirect fluorescent antibody (IFA), enzyme immunoassay (EIA) **ADDITIONAL INFORMATION:** Intrauterine transmission of CMV can occur whether or not prior maternal immunity exists. However, the presence of maternal antibody prior to conception does provide a significant degree of protection against neonatal damage of congenital CMV infection. Sequellae of congenital CMV infections are more severe in primary maternal infections occurring during pregnancy.[1]

A single titer is rarely significant if past history is unknown. A fourfold or greater rise in CMV titer between acute and convalescent specimens is evidence of infection. A single IgM specific titer >1:8 is also excellent evidence of acute infection. CMV causes an infectious mononucleosis syndrome clinically indistinguishable from heterophil positive mononucleosis, a very common entity. Significant CMV titers are found almost universally in patients with AIDS. CMV is a significant cause of postcardiotomy, post-transplant and postpump hepatitis syndromes.

Although serology is a useful method to detect CMV infections, the newer shell vial culture can more reliably identify symptomatic CMV infections in immunocompromised patients.

Several new EIA tests agree well with the IFA serology and provide a more objective measure of infection status than the subjective IFA test.

See Related Information at the beginning of this listing for further perspective tests relevant to CMV.

Footnotes

1. Fowler KB, Stagno S, Pass RF, et al, "The Outcome of Congenital Cytomegalovirus Infection in Relation to Maternal Antibody Status," *N Engl J Med*, 1992, 326(10):663-7.

References

Bryan JA, "The Serologic Diagnosis of Viral Infections," *Arch Pathol Lab Med*, 1987, 111:1015-23.
Elder BL, Shelley CD, and Smith TF, "Evaluation of Quaternary Aminoethyl-Sephadex A50 Column Chromatography for Detection of Anticytomegalovirus Immunoglobulin M," *Mayo Clin Proc*, 1987, 62:345-50.
Fenoglio CM, Oster MW, and Lo Gerfo P, "Kaposi's Sarcoma Following Chemotherapy for Testicular Cancer in a Homosexual Man: Demonstration of Cytomegalovirus RNA in Sarcoma Cells," *Hum Pathol*, 1982, 13:955-9.
Hughes JH, "Physical and Chemical Methods for Enhancing Rapid Detection of Viruses and Other Agents," *Clin Microbiol Rev*, 1993, 6(2):150-75.
Marsano L, Perrillo RP, Flye MW, et al, "Comparison of Culture and Serology for the Diagnosis of Cytomegalovirus Infection in Kidney and Liver Transplant Recipients," *J Infect Dis*, 1990, 161(3):454-61.
Paya CV, Smith TF, Ludwig J, et al, "Rapid Shell Vial Culture and Tissue Histology Compared With Serology for the Rapid Diagnosis of Cytomegalovirus Infection in Liver Transplantation," *Mayo Clin Proc*, 1989, 64(6):670-5.
Reed EC and Meyers JD, "Treatment of Cytomegalovirus Infection," *Clin Lab Med*, 1987, 7:831-52.
Van Enk RA, James KK, and Thompson KD, "Evaluation of Three Commercial Enzyme Immunoassays for *Toxoplasma* and Cytomegalovirus Antibodies," *Am J Clin Pathol*, 1991, 95(3):428-34.

Davidsohn Differential *replaced by* Infectious Mononucleosis Screening Test *on page 713*

Delta Agent Serology *see* Hepatitis D Serology *on page 691*

Delta Hepatitis Serology *see* Hepatitis D Serology *on page 691*

Dermatitis Herpetiformis Antibodies *see* Immunofluorescence, Skin Biopsy *on page 708*

Diphtheria Neutralizing Antibody *see* Bacterial Serology *on page 644*

DNA Antibody *see* Anti-DNA *on page 634*

Dysgammaglobulinemia *see* Immunoelectrophoresis, Serum or Urine *on page 706*

Dysgammaglobulinemia Evaluation *see* Immunofixation Electrophoresis *on page 707*

Eastern Equine Encephalitis Virus Serology

CPT *86652*

Related Information

California Encephalitis Virus Titer *on page 651*
St Louis Encephalitis Virus Serology *on page 749*
Western Equine Encephalitis Virus Serology *on page 765*

Synonyms Encephalitis Virus Titer, Eastern Equine

Test Commonly Includes Detection of antibody specific for Eastern equine encephalitis virus in patient's serum

Abstract This is a low incidence disease. It occurs in the summer. There is a 50% to 70% fatality rate.

Specimen Serum **CONTAINER:** Red top tube **SAMPLING TIME:** Acute and convalescent sera drawn 10-14 days apart are required.

Interpretive **REFERENCE RANGE:** Less than a fourfold increase in titer in paired sera; hemagglutinating titer: <1:10 **USE:** Support the diagnosis of Eastern equine encephalitis virus infection **METHODOLOGY:** Complement fixation (CF), hemagglutination inhibition (HAI), enzyme-linked immunosorbent assay (ELISA). Alphaviruses share antigenic relationships. **ADDITIONAL INFORMATION:** Eastern equine encephalitis virus is an alphavirus carried by a mosquito vector. It causes an acute illness which is either fatal or self-limited; chronic illness should suggest a different diagnosis. Syndromes include headache with fever, meningitis, and meningoencephalitis. The other alphavirus agents causing disease in the U.S. are Western equine encephalitis and Venezuelan equine encephalitis. These have been classified as group A arboviruses.

References

Center for Disease Control, "Eastern Equine Encephalitis Virus – Florida," *JAMA*, 1992, 267(10):1324.
Monath TP, "Alphavirus (Eastern, Western, and Venezuelan Equine Encephalitis)," *Principles and Practice of Infectious Diseases*, 3rd ed, Mandell GL, Douglas RG Jr, and Bennett JE, eds, New York, NY: Churchill Livingstone, 1990, 1241-2.
Tsai TF, "Arboviruses," *Manual of Clinical Laboratory Immunology*, 4th ed, Vol 2, Chapter 91, Rose NR, Conway de Macario E, Fahey JL, et al, eds, Washington, DC: American Society for Microbiology, 1992, 606-18.

Eaton Agent Titer *see Mycoplasma* Serology *on page 727*

EBNA *see* Epstein-Barr Virus Serology *on page 676*

EB Nuclear Antigen *see* Epstein-Barr Virus Serology *on page 676*

EB Virus Titer *see* Epstein-Barr Virus Serology *on page 676*

EBV Titer *see* Epstein-Barr Virus Serology *on page 676*

Echinococcosis Serological Test

CPT *86171 (complement fixation); 86403 (agglutination)*

Related Information

Ova and Parasites, Stool *on page 836*
Parasite Antibodies *on page 729*

Synonyms *Echinococcus granulosus* Serological Test; *Echinococcus multilocularis* Serological Test; Hydatid Disease Serological Test

Abstract Echinococcosis is a cestode parasitic disease important in livestock-raising areas. The cause of hydatid disease is a larval form of *Echinococcus granulosus*. The cause of alveolar disease is a larval form of *E. multilocularis*.

Specimen Serum **CONTAINER:** Red top tube

Interpretive **REFERENCE RANGE:** Indirect hemagglutination: 1:2-1:64 **USE:** Support a diagnosis of echinococcosis **LIMITATIONS:** Serum from 50% of patients with cysticercosis cross react in this assay. False-positives in some patients with cirrhosis and lupus; false-negatives with some large cysts or dead cysts. Sensitivity of serological testing is 60% to 90%. **METHODOLOGY:** Complement fixation (CF), bentonite flocculation assay (BFA), indirect hemagglutination (IHA), latex agglutination (LA), enzyme-linked immunosorbent assay (ELISA) **ADDITIONAL INFORMATION:** Peripheral blood eosinophilia occurs but is not always found. After surgical removal of the cyst, there is generally a rapid decline in antibody within a year; failure to observe the decline indicates incomplete cyst removal. Cysts in the liver are more likely to elicit an immune response than cysts in the lungs. The newer ELISA tests are more sensitive than the more traditional hemagglutination and latex assays.

References

Ash LR and Orihel TC, *Atlas of Human Parasitology*, 3rd ed, Chicago, IL: ASCP Press, 1990, 233-5.

Kagan IG and Maddison SE, "Serodiagnosis of Parasitic Diseases," *Manual of Clinical Laboratory Immunology*, 4th ed, Vol 2, Chapter 79, Rose NR, Conway de Macario E, Fahey JL, et al, eds, Washington, DC: American Society for Microbiology, 1992, 529-43.

Moir IL and Ho Yen DO, "The Use of Serology in Patients With Suspected Hydatid Diseases," *Scott Med J*, 1989, 34(3):466-8.

***Echinococcus granulosus* Serological Test** *see* Echinococcosis Serological Test *on this page*

***Echinococcus multilocularis* Serological Test** *see* Echinococcosis Serological Test *on this page*

Electrophoresis, Protein, Urine *see* Protein Electrophoresis, Urine *on page 737*

Electrophoresis, Serum *see* Protein Electrophoresis, Serum *on page 734*

EMA *see* Endomysial Antibodies *on this page*

Encephalitis Virus Titer, California *see* California Encephalitis Virus Titer *on page 651*

Encephalitis Virus Titer, Eastern Equine *see* Eastern Equine Encephalitis Virus Serology *on previous page*

Encephalitis Virus Titer, Western Equine *see* Western Equine Encephalitis Virus Serology *on page 765*

Endomysial Antibodies

CPT *86255 (screen); 86256 (titer)*

Related Information

Immunofluorescence, Skin Biopsy *on page 708*

Synonyms EMA

Test Commonly Includes Detection of antibodies to endomysin using immunofluorescence

Specimen Serum CONTAINER: Red top tube

Interpretive REFERENCE RANGE: No IgA endomysial antibody demonstrated USE: Diagnose dermatitis herpetiformis and gluten-sensitive enteropathy (nontropical sprue, celiac disease); follow response to gluten-free diet LIMITATIONS: Sprue patients with IgA deficiency may show IgG antibodies instead of IgA METHODOLOGY: Indirect fluorescent antibody (IFA) ADDITIONAL INFORMATION: Dermatitis herpetiformis is a bullous skin disorder closely associated with gluten-sensitive enteropathy (celiac sprue, celiac disease). Strict observation of a gluten-free diet often induces remission of both the skin and bowel abnormalities. The presence of circulating IgA antibodies to endomysin (the reticular investment of muscle fibers) has excellent sensitivity (80%) and specificity (96%) for dermatitis herpetiformis and sprue. There is no cross reaction with other bullous skin diseases. Further, these antibodies are not seen in control serum. Antibody titers and clinical findings respond to gluten-free diet. Antibodies reappear if the patient is challenged with a gluten-containing diet.

References

Beutner EH, Kumar V, and Chorzelski TP, "Screening for Celiac Disease," *N Engl J Med*, 1989, 320(16):1087-9.

Kapuscinska A, Zalewski T, and Chorzelski TP, "Disease Specificity and Dynamics of Changes in IgA Class Antiendomysial Antibodies in Celiac Disease," *J Pediatr Gastroenterol Nutr*, 1987, 6:529-34.

Kumar V, Hemedinger E, Chorzelski TP, et al, "Reticulin and Endomysial Antibodies in Bullous Diseases: Comparison of Specificity and Sensitivity," *Arch Dermatol*, 1987, 123:1179-82.

Volta U, Molinaro N, Fusconi M, et al, "IgA Antiendomysial Antibody Test. A Step Forward in Celiac Disease Screening," *Dig Dis Sci*, 1991, 36(6):752-6.

Entamoeba histolytica Serological Test

CPT *86171 (complement fixation); 86256 (immunofluorescence); 86329 (immunodiffusion)*

Related Information

Blood Culture, Aerobic and Anaerobic *on page 784*
Ova and Parasites, Stool *on page 836*
Parasite Antibodies *on page 729*
Stool Culture *on page 858*
Viral Culture, Stool *on page 1205*

Synonyms Amebiasis Serological Test

Test Commonly Includes Detection of antibodies to *Entamoeba histolytica* in serum

Patient Care PREPARATION: Fasting blood sample required

Specimen Serum CONTAINER: Red top tube

Interpretive REFERENCE RANGE: IHA titer: <1:128; CF titer: <1:8; immunodiffusion test: negative USE: Establish the diagnosis of systemic amebiasis. Serologic testing for amebiasis is the best single test to distinguish between the two major types of liver abscesses: amebic and pyogenic. The other major test in this differential diagnosis is blood culture. Since pyogenic liver abscesses usually require surgical drainage and prolonged intravenous antibiotic therapy, this differential diagnosis is a critical one. Overall mortality rates for pyogenic liver abscesses are about 40%, while the mortality rate for properly diagnosed and treated amebic liver abscess should approach 0%.[1] LIMITATIONS: Sensitivity is highest in extraintestinal amebiasis, lower in amebic dysentery, and lowest in asymptomatic carriers. Some false-positives occur in patients with ulcerative colitis. Recently a serine-rich recombinant *Entamoeba histolytica* protein has proven to be a useful antigen to assist in the serodiagnosis of *Entamoeba* which has disseminated.[2] The utility of the serologic marker is diminished in those parts of the world in which amebiasis is highly endemic and antibodies persist; *vide infra.* METHODOLOGY: Complement fixation (CF), indirect hemagglutination (IHA), immunodiffusion (ID), indirect fluorescent antibody (IFA), enzyme-linked immunosorbent assay (ELISA) ADDITIONAL INFORMATION: Indirect hemagglutination is positive in 87% to 100% of patients with amebic liver abscesses and >85% of patients with acute amebic dysentery. Fewer than 6% of uninfected individuals react in the test. Amebic serology when negative is strong evidence against amebic liver abscess. IHA titers ≥1:128 are considered to be clinically significant, and a fourfold rise in titer is firmer diagnostic evidence. It should be noted that although titers will decrease over time, serology may remain positive for as long as 2 years, even after curative therapy.

Footnotes

1. Pitt HA, "Surgical Management of Hepatic Abscesses," *World J Surg*, 1990, 14(4):498-504.
2. Stanley SL Jr, Jackson TF, Reed SL, et al, "Serodiagnosis of Invasive Amebiasis Using a Recombinant *Entamoeba histolytica* Protein," *JAMA*, 1991, 266(14):1984-6.

References

Garcia LS, "Comparison of Indirect Fluorescent Antibody Amebic Serology and Counter Immunoelectrophoresis and Indirect Hemagglutination Amebic Serologies," *J Clin Microbiol*, 1982, 15:603-6.

(Continued)

Entamoeba histolytica Serological Test *(Continued)*

Kagan IG, "Serodiagnosis of Parasitic Diseases," *Manual of Clinical Laboratory Immunology*, 4th ed, Vol 2, Rose NR, Conway de Macario E, Fahey JL, et al, eds, Washington, DC: American Society for Microbiology, 1992, 467-70.

Mathews HM, Walls KW, and Huong AY, "Microvolume Kinetic-Dependent Enzyme-Linked Immunosorbent Assay for Ameba Antibodies," *J Clin Microbiol*, 1984, 19:221-4.

Epstein-Barr Early Antigens *see* Epstein-Barr Virus Serology *on this page*

Epstein-Barr Viral Capsid Antigen *see* Epstein-Barr Virus Serology *on this page*

Epstein-Barr Virus Serology

***CPT** 86663 (early antigen); 86664 (nuclear antigen); 86665 (viral capsid antigen)*

Related Information

Epstein-Barr Virus Culture *on page 1179*

Heterophil Agglutinins *on page 694*

Infectious Mononucleosis Screening Test *on page 713*

Synonyms EB Virus Titer; EBV Titer

Applies to EBNA; EB Nuclear Antigen; Epstein-Barr Early Antigens; Epstein-Barr Viral Capsid Antigen; VCA; VCA Titer; Viral Capsid Antigen

Test Commonly Includes Titers on all patients' serum exhibiting a positive reaction at a 1:10 dilution

Abstract Since Epstein-Barr virus was found in a Ugandan child with Burkitt's lymphoma nearly 30 years ago, a role for the virus has been shown or postulated for diseases additional to infectious mononucleosis. These include hairy leukoplakia (a disorder of the tongue), carcinoma of the nasopharynx, and lymphomas in patients following transplantation and with AIDS. Possible relationships to some T-cell lymphomas and to Hodgkin's disease are discussed in an editorial aptly titled, "Epstein-Barr Virus: Culprit or Consort?".[1]

Specimen Serum **CONTAINER:** Red top tube

Interpretive **REFERENCE RANGE:** See table. **USE:** Diagnose Epstein-Barr virus infection, heterophil-negative mononucleosis, hereditary sex-linked lymphadenopathy **LIMITATIONS:** Despite much publicity, these tests are neither sensitive nor specific for chronic fatigue syndrome **CONTRAINDICATIONS:** **The Epstein-Barr viral test need not be done on patients who have heterophil antibodies with the symptoms, physical findings and lymphocyte morphology consistent with infectious mononucleosis.** **METHODOLOGY:** Indirect fluorescent antibody (IFA), enzyme-linked immunosorbent assay (ELISA) **ADDITIONAL INFORMATION:** Epstein-Barr virus is a herpes group virus which is almost ubiquitous. It is the cause of classic infectious mononucleosis, and is causally implicated in the pathogenesis of Burkitt's lymphoma, some nasopharyngeal carcinomas, lymphoproliferative disorders in immunocompromised patients, and rare hereditary lymphoproliferative disorders. The serologic response to EB virus includes antibody to early antigen, which is usually short lived, IgM and IgG antibodies to viral capsid antigen (VCA), and antibodies to nuclear antigen (EBNA).

Epstein–Barr Virus Serology

	Uninfected	Previous Infection
IgG anti–VCA	<1:10	≥1:10
IgM anti–VCA*	<1:10	≤1:10
Anti–EBNA	<1:5	≥1:5

*IgM anti–VCA indicates a recent primary infection.

Although most cases of infectious mononucleosis can be diagnosed on the basis of clinical findings, blood count and morphology, and a positive test for heterophil antibody, as many as 20% may be heterophil-negative, at least at presentation (heterophil may become positive when repeated in a few days). In some of these cases, a test for Epstein-Barr virus antibodies may be useful.

Of the numerous antibodies that may be assayed, **viral capsid antibody** is the most useful. A high presenting titer is good evidence for EB virus infection. Since titers are generally high by the time a patient is symptomatic, it may not be possible to demonstrate the fourfold rise in titer usually recommended. Even a very high titer may be due to past infection, so IgA and IgM titers should be measured to establish acute infection. Persistent absence of antibody to viral capsid is good evidence against EB virus infection.

Antibody to EB virus nuclear antigen (EBNA) usually develops 4-6 weeks after infection, so its presence early during an acute illness should lead one to consider diagnosis other than EB virus infectious mononucleosis.

Patients with nonkeratinizing squamous carcinoma of the nasopharynx may have elevated levels of IgG antibody to EB early antigen, but the rarity of this condition and the 10% to 20% false-positive rate vitiate its usefulness for screening. Such patients may also have IgA antibodies to VCA.

The most controversial use of EBV serology is in chronic fatigue syndrome, a complaint predominantly but not exclusively of young to middle-aged women, characterized by long persistent debilitating fatigue and a panoply of usually mild somatic complaints. In the initial reports of this illness, chronic infection with EBV was suggested as the cause, and EBV serology suggested as a diagnostic tool. In the past several years, although the legitimacy of a chronic fatigue syndrome seems to have been established, the inappropriateness of EBV serology for diagnosis has been realized. The high levels of EBV antibodies in the general population, their long persistence, and the poor correlation of antibody titers with symptoms combine to make EBV serology useless in diagnosing, following, or ruling out chronic fatigue syndrome.

IgG antibody to early antigen occurs in patients with Hodgkin's disease in higher titer than expected. This observation suggests the possibility that EB virus activation plays a pathogenetic role in Hodgkin's disease. EB viral DNA has been detected in both Hodgkin's lymphoma and non-Hodgkin's lymphomas by *in situ* hybridization and DNA amplification. The EB virus seems to be associated with non-Hodgkin's lymphomas in AIDS patients and transplant patients.[2,3] EBV-associated post-transplantation lymphoproliferative disease is found in 1% to 10% of transplant recipients.[4]

The pathogenesis of hemophagocytic syndrome remains uncertain. Detection of EBV RNA in some (but not all) cases is recently reported.[5]

See Epstein-Barr Virus Culture in the Virology chapter.

Footnotes

1. Pagano JS, "Epstein-Barr Virus: Culprit or Consort?" *N Engl J Med*, 1992, 327(24):1750-2, (editorial).
2. Borisch B, Finke J, Hennig I, et al, "Distribution and Localization of Epstein-Barr Virus Subtypes A and B in AIDS-Related Lymphomas and Lymphatic Tissue of HIV-Positive Patients," *J Pathol*, 1992, 168(2):229-36.
3. Telenti A, Marshall WF, and Smith TF, "Detection of Epstein-Barr Virus by Polymerase Chain Reaction," *J Clin Microbiol*, 1990, 28(10):2187-90.
4. Randhawa PS, Jaffe R, Demetris AJ, et al, "Expression of Epstein-Barr Virus-Encoded Small RNA (by the EBER-1 Gene) in Liver Specimens From Transplant Recipients With Post-Transplantation Lymphoproliferative Disease," *N Engl J Med*, 1992, 327(24):1710-4.
5. Gaffey MJ, Frierson HF Jr, Medeiros LJ, et al, "The Relationship of Esptein-Barr Virus to Infection-Related (Sporadic) and Familial Hemophagocytic Syndrome and Secondary (Lymphoma-Related) Hemophagocytosis: An *In Situ* Hybridization Study," *Hum Pathol*, 1993, 24(6):657-67.

References

Ballow M, Seely J, Purtilo DT, et al, "Familial Chronic Mononucleosis," *Ann Intern Med*, 1982, 97:821-5.

Erlich KS, "Laboratory Diagnosis of Herpesvirus Infections," *Clin Lab Med*, 1987, 7:771-3.

Jones JF, Ray CG, Minnich LL, et al, "Evidence for Active Epstein-Barr Virus Infection in Patients With Persistent, Unexplained Illnesses: Elevated Antiearly Antigen Antibodies," *Ann Intern Med*, 1985, 102:1-7.

Matheson BA, Chisholm SM, Ho-Yen DO, "Assessment of Rapid ELISA Test for Detection of Epstein-Barr Virus Infection," *J Clin Pathol*, 1990, 43(8):691-3.

Matthews DA, Lane TJ, and Manu P, "Antibodies to Epstein-Barr Virus in Patients With Chronic Fatigue," *South Med J*, 1991, 84(7):832-40.

Merlin T, "Chronic Mononucleosis: Pitfalls in the Laboratory Diagnosis," *Hum Pathol*, 1986, 17:2-8.

Mueller N, Evans A, Harris NL, et al, "Hodgkin's Disease and Epstein-Barr Virus. Altered Antibody Pattern Before Diagnosis," *N Engl J Med*, 1989, 320(11):689-95.

Okano M, Thiele GM, Davis JR, et al, "Epstein-Barr Virus and Human Diseases: Recent Advances in Diagnosis," *Clin Microbiol Rev*, 1988, 1:300-12.

Espundia Serological Test *see* Leishmaniasis Serological Test *on page 717*

Esterase Inhibitor *see* C1 Esterase Inhibitor, Serum *on page 648*

Esterase, Subunit of C1 *see* C1 Esterase Inhibitor, Serum *on page 648*

Extractable Nuclear Antigens *see* Antinuclear Antibody *on page 638*

Factor B

CPT 86160 (antigen); 86161 (functional activity)

Related Information

C3 Complement, Serum *on page 649*
C4 Complement, Serum *on page 650*
Complement Components *on page 665*
Complement, Total, Serum *on page 667*
Kidney Biopsy *on page 68*

Synonyms C3 Activator; C3 Proactivator; Properdin

Applies to Alternate Complement Pathway

Abstract Properdin factor B occupies a critical position in the alternative pathway for complement activation. Comparison of its level before and after a clinical episode is useful in implicating activation of the alternative pathway in the clinical process.

Specimen Serum **CONTAINER:** Red top tube **STORAGE INSTRUCTIONS:** Allow sample to clot 15-30 minutes at room temperature, then 30-60 minutes at 4°C. Store serum at -70°C.

Interpretive **REFERENCE RANGE:** 180-400 μg/mL **USE:** Decreased values are seen when the alternate pathway of complement is activated **LIMITATIONS:** Single values may be difficult or impossible to interpret. **METHODOLOGY:** Immunodiffusion (ID), isoelectric focusing/ immunofixation **ADDITIONAL INFORMATION:** Assay of factor B helps distinguish activation of the alternate from the classical complement pathway. Examples of conditions associated with alternate pathway activation are diffuse intravascular coagulation, systemic lupus erythematosus, subacute bacterial endocarditis, bacteremia with shock, paroxysmal nocturnal hemoglobinuria, sickle cell disease, and hypocomplementemic chronic glomerulonephritis. Complement proteins are acute phase reactants and have very short half-lives. Their serum levels are a balance of synthesis and catabolism. Thus, serial measurements may be more informative than single values.

References

Kerr LD, Adelsberg BR, Schulman P, et al, "Factor B Activation Products in Patients With Systemic Lupus Erythematosus. A Marker of Severe Disease Activity," *Arthritis Rheum*, 1989, 32(11):1406-13.

Ruddy S, "Complement," *Manual of Clinical Laboratory Immunology*, 4th ed, Vol 2, Chapter 18, Rose NR, Conway de Macario E, Fahey JL, et al, eds, Washington, DC: American Society for Microbiology, 1992, 114-23.

Shur PH, "Complement Studies of Sera and Other Biologic Fluids," *Hum Pathol*, 1983, 14:338-42.

FANA *see* Antinuclear Antibody *on page 638*

Farmer's Lung Disease *see* Hypersensitivity Pneumonitis Serology *on page 704*

FA Smear for *Legionella pneumophila* *see Legionella pneumophila* Direct FA Smear *on page 715*

Febrile Agglutinins, Serum

CPT 86000 (early antigen)

Related Information

Brucellosis Agglutinins *on page 647*
Rocky Mountain Spotted Fever Serology *on page 741*
Salmonella Titer *on page 744*
Tularemia Agglutinins *on page 760*
Weil-Felix Agglutinins *on page 764*

Synonyms Agglutinins, Febrile

Test Commonly Includes Detection of antibody titer to specific bacterial antigens such as *Salmonella* H antigens – *S. typhi* d, *S. paratyphi* a, b, and c; testing patient's serum with *Salmonella* O antigens – *Salmonella* A, B, C, D and E; *Proteus* antigens – OX-19, OX-K, and OX-2; *Brucella* antigen; and *Francisella tularensis* antigen

Abstract Febrile agglutinins are scientifically obsolescent in most cases and are not cost effective.

Specimen Serum **CONTAINER:** Red top tube **SAMPLING TIME:** Acute and convalescent sera drawn 10-14 days apart are recommended.

Interpretive **REFERENCE RANGE:** Less than a fourfold increase in titer in paired sera. **Titers on a single sample are not diagnostically significant.** **USE:** Screening tests to identify agglutinins in sera of patients suspected of having infectious bacterial diseases characterized by persistent fever **LIMITATIONS:** Many cross reactions; high background levels of antibody make interpretation difficult; requires two patient specimens obtained several weeks apart **METHODOLOGY:** Agglutination **ADDITIONAL INFORMATION:** Febrile antigen agglutination tests have no utility when performed on only one serum specimen. Serum specimens taken over the course of several weeks during the acute and convalescent phases of an infection should be tested, and a titer rise of at least fourfold, of only one antibody, should be interpreted as significant. With the development of better culture methods, and more specific serologic procedures, these rough screening tests are usually not recommended.

Filariasis Serological Test

CPT 86256 (immunofluorescence); 86403 (agglutination)

Related Information

Microfilariae, Peripheral Blood Preparation *on page 571*
Ova and Parasites, Stool *on page 836*
Ova and Parasites, Urine *on page 839*
Parasite Antibodies *on page 729*

Synonyms Microfilariae Serological Test

Applies to *Acanthocheilonema perstans* Serology; *Loa loa* Serology; *Onchocerca volvulus* Serology; *Wuchereria bancrofti* Serology

Abstract Filarial nematodes live in body cavities, subcutaneous tissue, or as adults, in the lymphatics of the host. Microfilariae (embryos) are ingested by bloodsucking arthropods and develop to an infective phase. It is the microfilaria that are accessible for diagnosis.

Specimen Serum **CONTAINER:** Red top tube

Interpretive **REFERENCE RANGE:** Varies with laboratory and methodology **USE:** Used to support a diagnosis of filariasis, microfilariasis **LIMITATIONS:** Because purified species-specific antigens have not been made, testing lacks sensitivity and specificity. Tests measuring IgG_4 subclass antibodies may eliminate some cross reactions. **METHODOLOGY:** Bentonite flocculation assay (BFA), indirect fluorescent antibody (IFA), indirect hemagglutination (IHA), enzyme immunoassay (EIA) **ADDITIONAL INFORMATION:** For screening, an antigen prepared from *Dirofilaria immitis* will detect antibody responses to several clinically significant microfilariae. However, sensitivity and specificity are poor. Testing with antigen prepared from a specific filaria is more sensitive to the homologous antibody, but is less practical for screening. Morphologic examination of a blood film remains the bedrock of diagnosis. Patients with other diseases or other types of parasites (helminths) may have antibodies, as may patients with eosinophilic infiltrates in the lungs, perhaps because of unrecognized dirofilariasis. These cross reactions may be due to antibodies to phosphocholine, a molecule present in many organisms. IgG_4 antibodies are not developed to phosphocholine; antibodies of this class are specific for filaria.

References

Ash LR and Orihel TC, *Atlas of Human Parasitology*, 3rd ed, Chicago, IL: ASCP Press, 1990, 22-5.

Kagan IG and Maddison SE, "Serodiagnosis of Parasitic Diseases," *Manual of Clinical Laboratory Immunology*, 4th ed, Vol 2, Chapter 79, Rose NR, Conway de Macario E, Fahey JL, et al, eds, Washington, DC: American Society for Microbiology, 1992, 529-43.

Lal RB and Ottesen EA, "Enhanced Diagnostic Specificity in Human Filariasis by IgG_4 Antibody Assessment," *J Infect Dis*, 1988, 158:1034-37.

Ro J, Tsakalakis PJ, White VA, et al, "Pulmonary Dirofilariasis: The Great Imitator of Primary or Metastatic Lung Tumor," *Hum Pathol*, 1989, 20(8):69-76.

Weil GJ, Ogunrinade AF, Chandrashekar R, et al, "IgG_4 Subclass Antibody Serology for Onchocerciasis," *J Infect Dis*, 1990, 161(3):549-54.

Flukes *see* Schistosomiasis Serological Test *on page 745*

Fluorescent Treponemal Antibody-Absorption *see* FTA-ABS, Serum *on next page*

Francisella tularensis **Antibodies** *see* Tularemia Agglutinins *on page 760*

Frei Test *replaced by* Lymphogranuloma Venereum Titer *on page 722*

FTA-ABS, Cerebrospinal Fluid

CPT 86781

Related Information

Cerebrospinal Fluid Analysis *on page 527*
Cerebrospinal Fluid Culture *on page 798*
(Continued)

FTA-ABS, Cerebrospinal Fluid *(Continued)*

Cerebrospinal Fluid Protein *on page 659*
Darkfield Examination, Syphilis *on page 808*
FTA-ABS, Serum *on this page*
VDRL, Cerebrospinal Fluid *on page 761*

Synonyms *Treponema pallidum* Antibodies, CSF

Test Commonly Includes CSF specimens are absorbed (FTA-ABS) and tested.

Abstract Syphilis has again become more common than it was between 1955-85. It is epidemiologically linked with HIV infection and the use of illegal drugs, especially crack cocaine.

Specimen Cerebrospinal fluid **CONTAINER:** Clean, sterile CSF tube **CAUSES FOR REJECTION:** Bloody specimen

Interpretive **REFERENCE RANGE:** Nonreactive **USE:** Confirm the presence of *Treponema pallidum* antibodies; establish the diagnosis of neurosyphilis. Although the use of the FTA-ABS in analysis of CSF is not uniformly accepted, a negative CSF FTA-ABS eliminates the diagnostic possibility of neurosyphilis.[1] **LIMITATIONS:** The interpretation of FTA results on CSF is not clearly defined. False-positive results may occur particularly if the specimen is not absorbed prior to testing. VDRL on cerebrospinal fluid is recommended by the Center for Disease Control to help establish the diagnosis of neurosyphilis. However, while a positive CSF VDRL is strong evidence for active neurosyphilis, a negative does not rule it out. A FTA-ABS on CSF can be positive in cases of neurosyphilis when CSF VDRL is negative. Unfortunately, the CSF FTA-ABS test is less specific than CSF VDRL for distinguishing currently active neurosyphilis from past syphilis infection. Therefore, a correlation of the clinical facts with the serologic findings is essential for each case. One useful guide when screening for neurosyphilis is to first detect a serum FTA-ABS and/or a VDRL or RPR. **METHODOLOGY:** Indirect fluorescent antibody (IFA) **ADDITIONAL INFORMATION:** Neurosyphilis encompasses a heterogeneous group of entities spanning all of the stages of lues. It includes syphilitic meningitis, gumma, general paresis, and tabes dorsalis.

Footnotes

1. Hook EW 3d and Marra CM, "Acquired Syphilis in Adults," *N Engl J Med*, 1992, 326(16):1060-9, (review).

References

Davis LE and Schmitt JW, "Clinical Significance of Cerebrospinal Fluid Tests for Neurosyphilis," *Ann Neurol*, 1989, 25(1):50-5.

Young H, Moyes A, McMillan A, et al, "Enzyme Immunoassay for Antitreponemal IgG: Screening or Confirmatory Test?," *J Clin Pathol*, 1992, 45(1):37-41.

FTA-ABS, Serum

CPT 86781

Related Information

Automated Reagin Test *on page 642*
Darkfield Examination, Syphilis *on page 808*
FTA-ABS, Cerebrospinal Fluid *on previous page*
MHA-TP *on page 724*
RPR *on page 742*
VDRL, Serum *on page 762*

Synonyms Fluorescent Treponemal Antibody-Absorption

Applies to Serologic Test for Syphilis

Test Commonly Includes Serum specimen is absorbed and then tested with immunofluorescence for antibody to *Treponema pallidum*

Abstract The FTA-ABS is a specific treponemal test. Although more sensitive than the reaginic tests, it is more expensive and more technically sophisticated. (Quantitative nontreponemal or reaginic tests include the VDRL and RPR.)[1]

Patient Care **PREPARATION:** Patient should be fasting if possible.

Specimen Serum **CONTAINER:** Red top tube

Interpretive **REFERENCE RANGE:** Nonreactive **USE:** Confirm presence of *Treponema pallidum* antibodies; establish the diagnosis of syphilis **LIMITATIONS:** FTA-ABS test for syphilis has been reported to be positive in the treponemal diseases pinta, yaws and bejel, and falsely positive in patients with diseases associated with increased or abnormal globulins, antinuclear antibodies, lupus erythematosus (beaded pattern), pregnancy, and drug addiction (although drug addicts are likely to have true positives as well). Lyme disease, leprosy, malaria, infectious mononucleosis, relapsing fever, and leptospirosis are also listed as potential causes of false-positive FTA-ABS.[1] As many as 2% of the general population may have a false-positive. Borderline results are inconclusive and cannot be interpreted; they may indicate a very low level of treponemal antibody or may be due to nonspecific factors. Further follow-up and serological confirmation with the treponemal immobilization test may be helpful. **METHODOLOGY:** Indirect fluorescent antibody (IFA) of killed *Treponema* after serum absorption **ADDITIONAL INFORMATION:** FTA-ABS is the most sensitive test in all stages of syphilis, and is the best confirmatory test for a serum reactive to a screening test such as ART or VDRL. Occasionally, patients with ocular (uveitis) syphilis or otosyphilis will have a negative VDRL while their FTA-ABS is positive. FTA-ABS cannot be used to follow disease activity or response to treatment, since it will remain high for life. A modification of the test can detect IgM specific antibodies, which may distinguish true congenital syphilis from placental transfer of maternal antibodies. When a positive serum FTA-ABS is required before performing CSF VDRL examination, the specificity of the CSF test is markedly improved. Although not officially recommended for testing cerebrospinal fluid, the FTA test, unabsorbed, can be performed on some spinal fluids with excellent specificity. At present this application of the test should be restricted to reference laboratories. See prior listing.

Footnotes

1. Hook EW 3d and Marra CM, "Acquired Syphilis in Adults," *N Engl J Med*, 1992, 326(16):1060-9, (review).

References

Albright RE Jr, Christenson RH, Emlet JL, et al, "Issues in Cerebrospinal Fluid Management. CSF Venereal Disease Research Laboratory Testing," *Am J Clin Pathol*, 1991, 95(3):397-401.

Birdsall HH, Baughn RE, and Jenkins HA, "The Diagnostic Dilemma of Otosyphilis. A New Western Blot Assay," *Arch Otolaryngol Head Neck Surg*, 1990, 116(5):617-21.

Davis LE and Schmitt JW, "Clinical Significance of Cerebrospinal Fluid Tests for Neurosyphilis," *Ann Neurol*, 1989, 25(1):50-5.

Farnes SW and Setness PA, "Serologic Tests for Syphilis," *Postgrad Med*, 1990, 87(3):37-41, 45-6.

Hart G, "Syphilis Tests in Diagnostic and Therapeutic Decision Making," *Ann Intern Med*, 1986, 104:368-76.

Tamesis RR and Foster CS, "Ocular Syphilis," *Ophthalmology*, 1990, 97(10):1281-7.

Gag Gene of HIV *see* p24 Antigen *on page 727*

Gamma G, CSF *see* Cerebrospinal Fluid Immunoglobulin G *on page 656*

GBM *see* Glomerular Basement Membrane Antibody *on this page*

German Measles Serology *see* Rubella Serology *on page 743*

Globulin, Serum *see* Protein Electrophoresis, Serum *on page 734*

Globulins, Urine *see* Protein Electrophoresis, Urine *on page 737*

Glomerular Basement Membrane Antibody

CPT 88346

Related Information

Antineutrophil Cytoplasmic Antibody *on page 636*
Kidney Biopsy *on page 68*
Kidney Profile *on page 268*

Synonyms Anti-GBM; Antiglomerular Basement Membrane Antibody; GBM; Goodpasture's Antibody

Specimen Serum or tissue (lung or kidney biopsy) **CONTAINER:** Red top tube **STORAGE INSTRUCTIONS:** Specimen requirements vary; check local laboratory **SPECIAL INSTRUCTIONS:** Tissue for immunofluorescence should be transported frozen in liquid nitrogen.

Interpretive **REFERENCE RANGE:** Negative **USE:** Detect presence of circulating glomerular basement membrane antibodies in Goodpasture's syndrome; quantitation may be useful in monitoring treatment. This test is often used in conjunction with the antineutrophil cytoplasmin antibody (ANCA) test for Wegener's granulomatosis and vasculitis. **LIMITATIONS:** 10% to 20% false-negatives **METHODOLOGY:** Direct (DFA) or indirect fluorescent antibody (IFA), enzyme immunoassay (EIA) **ADDITIONAL INFORMATION:** The two principal mechanisms of autoimmune renal disease are immune complex deposition with complement activation and specific antibody mediated damage to renal glomerular basement membrane. Antibody can be demonstrated by immunofluorescence in glomeruli, in renal tubular basement membranes, and in pulmonary capillary basement membranes. The stimulus to the production of these antibodies is unknown, but the M2 subunit of type IV collagen appears to be the major antigen. Note that the presence of immune complexes is **not** needed for the diagnosis of anti-GBM nephritis. Further, the presence of immune complexes does not negate the significance of anti-GBM antibodies.

(Continued)

Glomerular Basement Membrane Antibody *(Continued)*

References

Burkholder PM, "Immunopathology of Renal Disease," *Clin Lab Med*, 1986, 6:55-83.
Butkowski RJ, Langeveld JPM, Wieslander J, et al, "Localization of the Goodpasture Epitope to a Novel Chain of Basement Membrane Collagen," *J Biol Chem*, 1987, 262:7874-7.
Harman EM, "Immunologic Lung Disease," *Med Clin North Am*, 1985, 69:705-14.
Savige JA, Dowling J, and Kincaid-Smith P, "Superimposed Glomerular Immune Complexes in Antiglomerular Basement Membrane Disease," *Am J Kidney Dis*, 1989, 14(2):145-53.

Goodpasture's Antibody *see* Glomerular Basement Membrane Antibody *on previous page*

Granulocyte Antibody *see* Antineutrophil Antibody *on page 636*

HAA *see* Hepatitis B Surface Antigen *on page 688*

HANE Assay *see* C1 Esterase Inhibitor, Serum *on page 648*

HAVAB *see* Hepatitis A Antibody, IgM *on next page*

HB_cAb *see* Hepatitis B Core Antibody *on page 684*

HB_eAb *see* Hepatitis B_e Antibody *on page 685*

HB_eAg *see* Hepatitis B_e Antigen *on page 686*

HB_sAb *see* Hepatitis B Surface Antibody *on page 687*

HB_sAg *see* Hepatitis B Surface Antigen *on page 688*

HB_sAg Ab *see* Hepatitis B Surface Antibody *on page 687*

HCV Serology *see* Hepatitis C Serology *on page 690*

Helicobacter pylori Serology

CPT 86677

Related Information

Helicobacter pylori Urease Test and Culture *on page 820*

Synonyms *Campylobacter pylori* Serology

Test Commonly Includes Detection of IgG and IgA antibodies specific for *Helicobacter pylori*

Abstract Patients with peptic ulcer disease associated with *H. pylori* have elevated levels of serum antibody against this bacterium. *H. pylori* is very strongly associated with duodenal ulcer and chronic active gastritis. It is generally accepted as a cause of chronic active gastritis. The evidence does not unequivocally establish *H. pylori* as the causative agent of duodenal ulcer. Patients should be treated with conventional antiulcer therapy.

Specimen Serum **CONTAINER:** Red top tube

Interpretive **REFERENCE RANGE:** Undetectable or lower than cutoff limits in commercial assays **USE:** Increased antibody levels are associated with *H. pylori* infection, chronic active gastritis, and peptic ulcer. Although earlier ELISA tests for IgG antibodies to *H. pylori* had poor specificity, more recent studies have shown both high sensitivity (96%) and high specificity for *H. pylori* associated with chronic gastritis. Indeed, *H. pylori* serology has become a standard tool for investigating the epidemiology of *H. pylori* infections. **LIMITATIONS:** Ubiquitous antibody response in almost all groups studied, both with and without symptoms or histologic abnormalities on gastric biopsies, makes clinical utility of these antibodies questionable. There is strain-to-strain antigenic variability in *H. pylori* which makes the test potentially insensitive. Clinical significance may be more closely tied to mucosal antibodies than circulating antibody. **METHODOLOGY:** Enzyme-linked immunosorbent assay (ELISA) **ADDITIONAL INFORMATION:** Large numbers of small, spiral-shaped bacteria, *Helicobacter pylori*, can be cultured from, or seen microscopically (especially with Dieterle or Giemsa stain) in gastric biopsies from most patients with chronic active gastritis and/or peptic ulcers. They can also be found in significant numbers of asymptomatic patients who have histologic gastritis, and from some individuals with no abnormality. Similarly, patients with chronic gastritis usually have elevated titers of IgG antibodies to *H. pylori*. The possible role of *H. pylori* infection in development of carcinoma and primary malignant lymphoma of stomach is addressed in the companion listing, *Helicobacter pylori* Urease Test and Culture in the Microbiology chapter.

References

Blaser MJ, "*Campylobacter pylori* in Gastritis and Peptic Ulcer Disease," New York, NY: Igaku-Shoin, 1989.
Crabtree JE, Shallcross TM, Heatley RV, et al, "Evaluation of a Commercial ELISA for Serodiagnosis of *Helicobacter pylori*," *J Clin Pathol*, 1991, 44(4):326-8.
Dooley CP, Cohen H, Fitzgibbons PL, et al, "Prevalence of *Helicobacter pylori* Infection and Histologic Gastritis in Asymptomatic Persons," *N Engl J Med*, 1989, 321(23):1562-6.

Drumm B, Perez-Perez GI, Blaser MJ, et al, "Intrafamilial Clotting of *Helicobacter pylori* Infection," *N Engl J Med*, 1990, 322(6):359-63.
Graham DY, Malaty HM, Evans PG, et al, "Epidemiology of *Helicobacter pylori* in an Asymptomatic Population in the United States. Effect of Age, Race, and Socioeconomic Status," *Gastroenterology*, 1991, 100(6):1495-501.
Hirschl AM, Rathbone BJ, Wyatt JI, et al, "Comparison of ELISA Antigen Preparation Alone or in Combination for Serodiagnosing *Helicobacter pylori* Infections," *J Clin Pathol*, 1990, 43(6):511-3.
Rabeneck L and Ransohoff DF, "Is *Helicobacter pylori* a Cause of Duodenal Ulcer? A Methodologic Critique of Current Evidence," *Am J Med*, 1991, 91(6):566-72.

Hepatitis A Antibody, IgM

CPT 86296 (IgG and IgM); 86299 (IgM)

Related Information

Hepatitis B DNA Detection *on page 913*

Synonyms Antibody to HAV, IgM; Anti-HAV, IgM; HAVAB

Test Commonly Includes Detection of IgM antibody to hepatitis A virus

Abstract Hepatitis A virus (HAV) is a RNA-containing virus. The IgM antibody is found in acute hepatitis A.

Patient Care PREPARATION: Avoid recent administration of radioisotopes (if assay performed by RIA)

Specimen Serum CONTAINER: Red top tube STORAGE INSTRUCTIONS: Remove serum and freeze

Interpretive REFERENCE RANGE: Negative USE: Differential diagnosis of hepatitis. Presence of IgM antibody to hepatitis A virus is good evidence for acute hepatitis A. METHODOLOGY: Radioimmunoassay (RIA), enzyme-linked immunosorbent assay (ELISA) ADDITIONAL INFORMATION: Hepatitis A is transmitted by the fecal-oral route, usually foodborne. Its incubation period is 2-7 weeks. Hepatitis A virus is a picornavirus, and antibody is made to capsid proteins. Fecal excretion of HAV peaks before symptoms develop. If hepatitis A antibody is IgM, the hepatitis A infection is probably acute. IgM antibody develops within a week of symptom onset, peaks in 3 months, and is usually gone after 6 months. Hepatitis A antibody of IgG type is indicative of old infection, is found in almost half of adults, and is not usually clinically relevant. Many cases of hepatitis A are subclinical, particularly in children. Presence of IgG antibody to HAV does not exclude acute hepatitis B or non-A, non-B hepatitis.

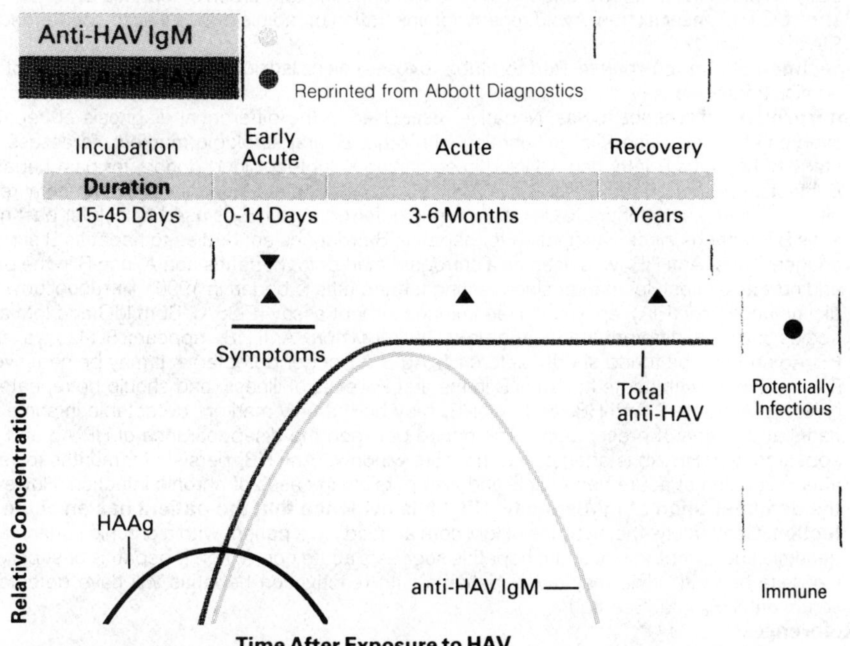

References

Giacoia GP and Kasprisin DO, "Transfusion-Acquired Hepatitis A," *South Med J*, 1989, 82(11):1357-60.
Halliday ML, Kang LY, Zhou TK, et al, "An Epidemic of Hepatitis A Attributable to the Ingestion of Raw Clams in Shanghai, China," *J Infect Dis*, 1991, 164(5):852-9.

(Continued)

Hepatitis A Antibody, IgM *(Continued)*

Lee HS and Vyas GN, "Diagnosis of Viral Hepatitis," *Clin Lab Med*, 1987, 7:741:57.

Mahoney FJ, Farley TA, Kelso KY, et al, "An Outbreak of Hepatitis A Associated With Swimming in A Public Pool," *J Infect Dis*, 1992, 165(4):613-8.

Mbithi JN, Springthorpe VS, Boulet JR, et al, "Survival of Hepatitis A Virus on Human Hands and Its Transfer on Contact With Animate and Inanimate Surfaces," *J Clin Microbiol*, 1992, 30(4):757-63.

Mishu B, Hadler SC, Boaz VA, et al, "Foodborne Hepatitis A: Evidence That Microwaving Reduces Risk?" *J Infect Dis*, 1990, 162(3):655-8.

Summers PL, DuBois DR, Houston Cohen WH, et al, "Solid-Phase Antibody Capture Hemadsorption Assay for Detection of Hepatitis A Virus Immunoglobulin M Antibodies," *J Clin Microbiol*, 1993, 31(5):1299-302.

Hepatitis Associated Antigen *see* Hepatitis B Surface Antigen *on page 688*

Hepatitis B Core Antibody

CPT *86289 (IgG and (IgM); 86290 (IgM)*

Related Information

Hepatitis B DNA Detection *on page 913*
Hepatitis B_e Antibody *on next page*
Hepatitis B_e Antigen *on page 686*
Hepatitis B Surface Antibody *on page 687*
Hepatitis B Surface Antigen *on page 688*
Hepatitis C Serology *on page 690*
Hepatitis D Serology *on page 691*
Polymerase Chain Reaction *on page 927*
Risks of Transfusion *on page 1093*

Synonyms AHBC; Antibody to Hepatitis B Core Antigen; Anti-HB_c; Antihepatitis B Core; Core Antibody; HB_cAb

Applies to Hepatitis B Core Antibody, IgM

Test Commonly Includes Detection of serologic response to hepatitis B infection; specifically, the antibody response to the core protein

Abstract For diagnosis of acute hepatitis, hepatitis B core antibody IgM and HB_sAg are especially helpful. HB_c antibody is found in resolved hepatitis and chronic hepatitis B.

Patient Care PREPARATION: Avoid recent administration of radioisotopes if assay performed by RIA.

Specimen Serum CONTAINER: Red top tube CAUSES FOR REJECTION: Recent radioactive isotope administration if assay is RIA

Interpretive REFERENCE RANGE: Negative USE: Used in the differential diagnosis of hepatitis syndromes. Is also used, in conjunction with other B viral serologic markers, to assess the stage of hepatitis B infection. Utilized in screening volunteer blood donors for past hepatitis B infection. Although the presence of Anti-HB_c usually confers immunity, governmental regulations require such donors to be permanently deferred. Anti-HB_c is used to look for past hepatitis B infections since vaccination for hepatitis B produces antibodies to hepatitis B surface antigen. Thus, Anti-HB_c was used as a surrogate marker for hepatitis non-A, non-B in the past, and now as a "lifestyle" marker since testing for hepatitis C began in 1990. METHODOLOGY: Radioimmunoassay (RIA), enzyme-linked immunosorbent assay (ELISA). Both IgG and IgM antibodies may be differentiated. ADDITIONAL INFORMATION: Anti-HB_c appears 5-14 days after HB_eAg and can be found shortly before HB_sAg is no longer detectable. It may be negative in 9% of patients with acute hepatitis B in the first 2 weeks of illness, and should be repeated if clinically warranted. Anti-HB_c and anti-HB_e may be the only markers detectable in some patients at the time of presentation. The period between the disappearance of HB_sAg and the appearance of HB_sAb is often called the "core window." Anti-HB_c persists for months to years after resolution of acute hepatitis B and also persists in cases of chronic infection. However, **the demonstration of IgM-specific HB_cAb is evidence that the patient has an acute infection**. Conversely, the absence of IgM core antibody in a patient with a chronic surface antigenemia and symptoms of acute hepatitis suggests acute non-A, non-B hepatitis or supervening delta hepatitis. The majority of patients with reactivation hepatitis will have detectable serum anti-HB_c IgM. See figure.

References

AuBuchon JP, Sandler SG, Fang CT, et al, "American Red Cross Experience With Routine Testing for Hepatitis B Core Antibody," *Transfusion*, 1989, 29(3):230-2.

Chambers LA and Popovsky MA, "Decrease in Reported Posttransfusion Hepatitis. Contributions of Donor Screening for Alanine Aminotransferase and Antibodies to Hepatitis B Core Antigen and Changes in the General Population," *Arch Intern Med*, 1991, 151(12):2445-8.

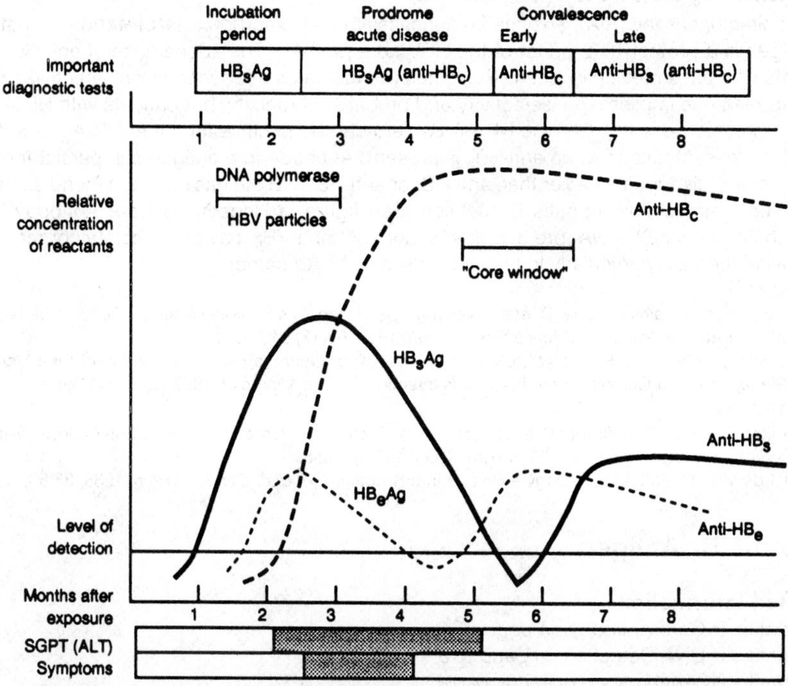

Serologic and clinical patterns observed during acute hepatitis B viral infection. From Hollinger FB and Dreesman GR, *Manual of Clinical Immunology,* 2nd ed, Rose NR and Friedman H, eds, Washington, DC: American Society for Microbiology, 1980, with permission.

Edwards MS, "Hepatitis B Serology – Help in Interpretation," *Pediatr Clin North Am*, 1988, 35:503-15.

Gupta S, Govindarajan S, Fong TL, et al, "Spontaneous Reactivation in Chronic Hepatitis B: Patterns and Natural History," *J Clin Gastroenterol*, 1990, 12(5):562-8.

Lee HS and Vyas GN, "Diagnosis of Viral Hepatitis," *Clin Lab Med*, 1987, 7:741:57.

Mushahwar IK, Dienstag JL, Polesky HF, et al, "Interpretation of Various Serological Profiles of Hepatitis B Virus Infection," *Am J Clin Pathol*, 1981, 76:773-7.

Hepatitis B Core Antibody, IgM *see* Hepatitis B Core Antibody *on previous page*

Hepatitis B$_e$ Antibody

CPT 86295

Related Information

Hepatitis B Core Antibody *on previous page*
Hepatitis B DNA Detection *on page 913*
Hepatitis B$_e$ Antigen *on next page*
Hepatitis B Surface Antibody *on page 687*
Hepatitis B Surface Antigen *on page 688*
Hepatitis C Serology *on page 690*
Hepatitis D Serology *on page 691*
Polymerase Chain Reaction *on page 927*

Synonyms Anti-HB$_e$; HB$_e$Ab

Test Commonly Includes Detection of antibody response to hepatitis e antigen

Patient Care PREPARATION: Avoid recent administration of radioisotopes if assay is RIA.

Specimen Serum CONTAINER: Red top tube CAUSES FOR REJECTION: Radioactive scan within 1 week if assay is RIA

Interpretive REFERENCE RANGE: Negative USE: Used in the differential diagnosis, staging, and prognosis of hepatitis B infection. Anti-HB$_e$ and anti-HB$_c$ together confirm the convalescent stage of hepatitis B after the disappearance of HB surface antigen (HB$_s$Ag). METHODOLOGY: (Continued)

Hepatitis B_e Antibody *(Continued)*

Radioimmunoassay (RIA), enzyme immunoassay (EIA) **ADDITIONAL INFORMATION:** Hepatitis B_e antigen is a proteolytic product of the HBV core protein.[1] The appearance of anti-HB_e in patients who have previously been HB_eAg positive indicates a reduced risk of infectivity. Failure of appearance implies disease activity and probable chronicity, but patients with HB_eAb may have chronic hepatitis. Chronic HB_sAg carriers can be positive for either HB_eAg or anti-HB_e, but are less infectious when anti-HB_e is present. Antibody to e antigen can persist for years, but usually disappears earlier than anti-HB_s or anti-HB_c. HB_eAb has not been found as the sole serologic marker for hepatitis B infection. See figure in Hepatitis B Core Antibody listing. Quantitation of HBV DNA, pre-S antigens, and IgM anti-HB_c may prove helpful for monitoring antiviral therapy, particularly in anti-HB_e-positive HB_sAg carriers.[2]

Footnotes

1. Jean-Jean O, Salhi S, Carlier D, et al, "Biosynthesis of Hepatitis B Virus e Antigen. Directed Mutagenesis of the Putative Aspartyl Protease Site," *J Virol*, 1989, 63(12):5497-500.
2. Zoulim F, Mimms L, Floreani M, et al, "New Assays for Quantitative Determination of Viral Markers in Management of Chronic Hepatitis B Virus Infection," *J Clin Microbiol*, 1992, 30(5):1111-9.

References

Bortolotti F, Calzia R, Cadrobbi P, et al, "Long-Term Evolution of Chronic Hepatitis B in Children With Antibody to Hepatitis B_e Antigen," *J Pediatr*, 1990, 116(4):552-5.

Edwards MS, "Hepatitis B Serology – Help in Interpretation," *Pediatr Clin North Am*, 1988, 35:503-15.

Hepatitis B_e Antigen

CPT 86293

Related Information

Hepatitis B Core Antibody *on page 684*
Hepatitis B DNA Detection *on page 913*
Hepatitis B_e Antibody *on previous page*
Hepatitis B Surface Antibody *on next page*
Hepatitis B Surface Antigen *on page 688*
Hepatitis C Serology *on page 690*
Hepatitis D Serology *on page 691*
Polymerase Chain Reaction *on page 927*

Synonyms HB_eAg

Test Commonly Includes Detection of hepatitis B_e antigen in patient's serum

Abstract Infectivity of a patient with hepatitis can be evaluated with HB_eAg and HB_sAg. Measurement of serum HBV DNA also provides evidence of infectivity.

Patient Care **PREPARATION:** Avoid recent administration of radioisotopes if assay is RIA

Specimen Serum **CONTAINER:** Red top tube **STORAGE INSTRUCTIONS:** Serum must be stored frozen or refrigerated, as HB_eAg is thermolabile **CAUSES FOR REJECTION:** Radioactive scan within 1 week if assay is RIA

Interpretive **REFERENCE RANGE:** Negative **USE:** Differential diagnosis and prognosis of hepatitis B infection. Hepatitis B_e antigen is found during the most infectious period of hepatitis B. It is usually found for only 3-6 weeks. Persistence beyond 10 weeks is evidence of development of the chronic carrier state and likely chronic hepatitis. **METHODOLOGY:** Radioimmunoassay (RIA), enzyme immunoassay (EIA) **ADDITIONAL INFORMATION:** HB_eAg appears in acute B hepatitis with or shortly after HB_sAg, when the patient is most infectious. HB_eAg is a proteolytic product of HB_cAg and is found only in HB_sAg positive sera. During the HB_eAg-positive state, usually 3-6 weeks, hepatitis B patients are at increased risk of transmitting the virus to their contacts, including babies born during this period. Exposure to serum or body fluid positive for HB_eAg and HB_sAg is associated with three to five times greater risk of infectivity than when HB_sAg positivity occurs alone. This is probably related to increased amounts of circulating viral DNA. Persistence of HB_eAg is associated with chronic liver disease. See figures and also Hepatitis B Core Antibody listing.

References

Edwards MS, "Hepatitis B Serology – Help in Interpretation," *Pediatr Clin North Am*, 1988, 35:503-15.

Lee HS and Vyas GN, "Diagnosis of Viral Hepatitis," *Clin Lab Med*, 1987, 7:741-57.

Hepatitis B_s Antibody *see* Hepatitis B Surface Antibody *on next page*

Hepatitis B Serological Profiles

Core Window Identification

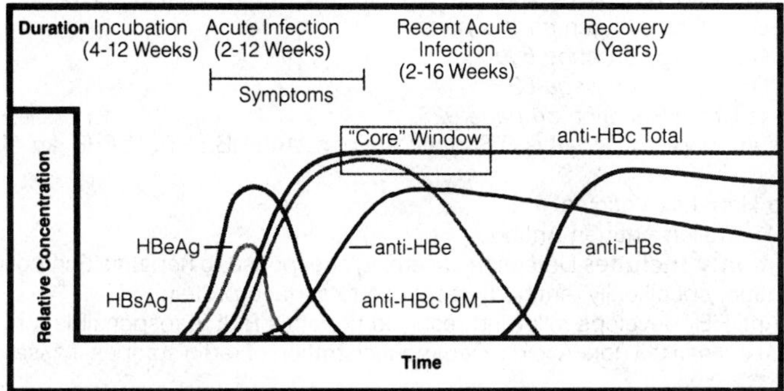

Hepatitis B Chronic Carrier No Seroconversion

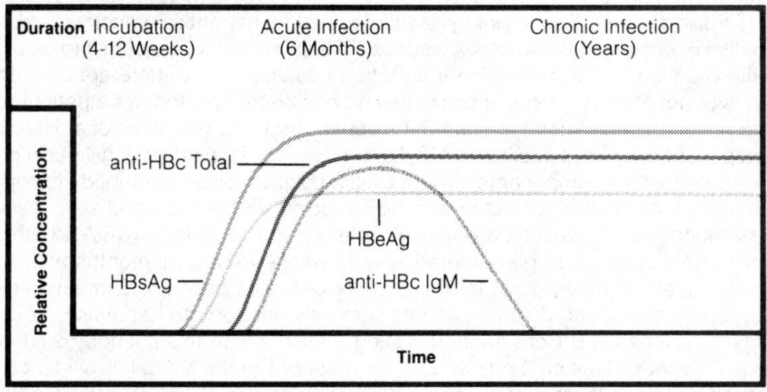

Hepatitis B Chronic Carrier Late Seroconversion

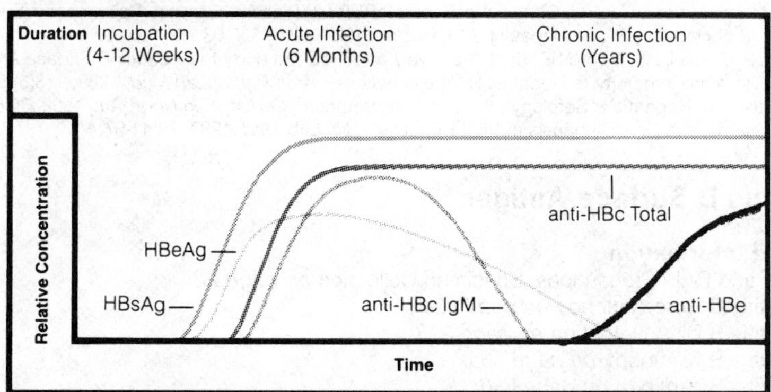

Reprinted from Abbott Diagnostics

Hepatitis B Surface Antibody

CPT 86291

Related Information

Hepatitis B Core Antibody *on page 684*
Hepatitis B DNA Detection *on page 913*
Hepatitis B_e Antibody *on page 685*
Hepatitis B_e Antigen *on page 686*
Hepatitis B Surface Antigen *on this page*
Hepatitis C Serology *on page 690*
Hepatitis D Serology *on page 691*
Polymerase Chain Reaction *on page 927*

Synonyms Antibody to Hepatitis B Surface Antigen; Anti-HB_s; HB_sAb; HB_sAg Ab; Hepatitis B_s Antibody

Applies to Hepatitis Vaccine

Replaces Australian Antigen Antibody

Test Commonly Includes Detection of serologic response to hepatitis B infection or hepatitis B vaccination; specifically, antibody response to surface protein

Abstract Anti-HB_s develops following resolved hepatitis B. It is responsible for immunity.

Patient Care PREPARATION: Avoid recent administration of radioisotopes if assay performed by RIA.

Specimen Serum CONTAINER: Red top tube CAUSES FOR REJECTION: Recently administered radioisotopes if assay performed by RIA

Interpretive REFERENCE RANGE: Varies with clinical circumstance USE: Presence of hepatitis B surface antibody indicates past infection with resolution of previous hepatitis B infection. Evaluate possible immunity in individuals who are at increased risks to further exposure to hepatitis B (ie, hemodialysis unit personnel, phlebotomists, etc). Evaluate need for hepatitis B immune globulin after needlestick injury. Evaluate need for hepatitis B vaccine. Evaluate efficacy of hepatitis B vaccine. LIMITATIONS: Presence of HB_sAb is not an absolute indicator of resolved hepatitis infection, nor of protection from future infection. Since there are different serologic subtypes of hepatitis B virus, it is possible (and has been reported) for a patient to have antibody to one surface antigen type and to be acutely infected with virus of a different subtype. Thus, a patient may have coexisting HB_sAg and HB_sAb. Transfused individuals or hemophiliacs receiving plasma components may give false-positive tests for antibody to hepatitis B surface antigen. Individuals vaccinated with HBV vaccine will have antibodies to the surface protein. METHODOLOGY: Radioimmunoassay (RIA), enzyme immunoassay (EIA) ADDITIONAL INFORMATION: HB_sAb usually can be detected several weeks to several months after HB_sAg is no longer found, and it may persist for many years or for life after acute infection has been resolved. It may disappear in some patients with only antibody to hepatitis B core remaining. See figure in Hepatitis B Core Antibody listing. Patients with this antibody are not overtly infectious. Presence of the antibody without the presence of the antigen is evidence for immunity from reinfection, with virus of the same subtype (*vide supra*). HB_sAb can be induced by vaccination with hepatitis vaccine, now genetically engineered and free of any infective material. This vaccine so far has been safe and effective in protecting recipients from acute hepatitis B.

References

Centers for Disease Control, "Screening Donors of Blood, Plasma, Organs, Tissues, and Semen for Evidence of Hepatitis B and Hepatitis C," *Lab Med*, 1991, 22(8):555-63.

Devine P, Taswell HF, Moore SB, et al, "Passively Acquired Antibody to Hepatitis B Surface Antigen. Pitfall in Evaluating Immunity to Hepatitis B Viral Infections," *Arch Pathol Lab Med*, 1989, 113(5):529-31.

Edwards MS, "Hepatitis B Serology – Help in Interpretation," *Pediatr Clin North Am*, 1988, 35:503-15.

Lee HS and Vyas GN, "Diagnosis of Viral Hepatitis," *Clin Lab Med*, 1987, 7:741-57.

Hepatitis B Surface Antigen

CPT 86287

Related Information

Blood and Fluid Precautions, Specimen Collection *on page 22*
Hepatitis B Core Antibody *on page 684*
Hepatitis B DNA Detection *on page 913*
Hepatitis B_e Antibody *on page 685*
Hepatitis B_e Antigen *on page 686*
Hepatitis B Surface Antibody *on previous page*

Hepatitis C Serology *on next page*
Hepatitis D Serology *on page 691*
Polymerase Chain Reaction *on page 927*
Risks of Transfusion *on page 1093*

Synonyms HAA; HB_sAg; Hepatitis Associated Antigen

Replaces Australian Antigen; Serum Hepatitis Marker

Test Commonly Includes Detection of hepatitis B surface antigen in patient's serum

Abstract For evaluation of acute hepatitis, serologic testing is recommended for HB_sAg, HB_sAb, HB_cAb (IgM), and HAV (IgM). Infectious mononucleosis screening test may be included, especially when the patient is youthful. Cytomegalovirus may cause a hepatitis-like clinical presentation.

Patient Care PREPARATION: Avoid recent administration of radioisotopes if assay is by RIA

Specimen Serum CONTAINER: Red top tube CAUSES FOR REJECTION: Recently administered radioisotopes if assay is by RIA

Interpretive REFERENCE RANGE: Negative USE: Screen blood donors (HB_sAg-positive individuals are rejected); differential diagnosis of hepatitis; evaluate risk in needlestick injuries in healthcare facilities, and guide use of hepatitis B immune globulin Hepatitis B surface antigen is the earliest indicator of acute hepatitis B infection and is found, as well, in chronic carriers. LIMITATIONS: Patients who are negative for HB_sAg may still have acute type B viral hepatitis. There is sometimes a "window" stage when HB_sAg has become negative and the patient has not yet developed the antibody (anti-HB_sAg). On such occasions the anti-HB_cAg (IgM) is usually positive; and the patient should be treated as potentially infectious until anti-HB_sAg is detected, at which time immunity is probable. In cases with strong clinical suspicion of viral hepatitis, serologic testing should not be limited to detecting HB_sAg but should include a battery of tests to evaluate different stages of acute and convalescent hepatitis. These should include a test for hepatitis A antibody (IgM), and HB_sAg, HB_sAb, HB_cAb (IgM), and hepatitis C virus (HCV). METHODOLOGY: Radioimmunoassay (RIA), enzyme immunoassay (EIA) ADDITIONAL INFORMATION: Hepatitis B virus (HBV) is a DNA virus with a protein coat, surface antigen (HB_sAg), and a core consisting of nucleoprotein, (HB_cAg is the core antigen). There are eight different serotypes. Early in infection, HB_sAg, HBV DNA, and DNA polymerase can all be detected in serum.

Transmission is parenteral, sexual or perinatal. The incubation period of hepatitis B is 2-6 months. HB_sAg can be detected 1-7 weeks **before** liver enzyme elevation or the appearance of clinical symptoms. Three weeks after the onset of acute hepatitis about 50% of the patients will still be positive for HB_sAg, while at 17 weeks only 10% are positive. The best available markers for infectivity are HB_sAg and HB_eAg. The presence of HB_sAb and HB_eAb is associated with noninfectivity. The chronic carrier state is indicated by the persistence of HB_sAg and/or HB_eAg over long periods (6 months to years) without seroconversion to the corresponding antibodies. Such a condition has the potential to lead to serious liver damage, but may be an isolated asymptomatic serologic phenomenon. Persistence of HB_sAg, without anti-HB_s, with combinations of positivity of anti-HB_{core}, HB_eAg, or anti-HB_e indicate infectivity and need for investigation for chronic persistent or chronic aggressive hepatitis. See figure in Hepatitis B Core Antibody listing. Chronic carrier states are found in up to 10% of cases. Some remain healthy, but evolution to chronic persistent hepatitis, chronic active hepatitis, cirrhosis, and hepatoma represent major problems of this disease. Prevention of hepatitis B for those at risk is available via vaccination,[1] as well as treatment for some chronic carriers.[2]

Footnotes

1. Mahoney FJ, Burkholder BT, and Matson CC, "Prevention of Hepatitis B Virus Infection," *Am Fam Physician*, 1993, 47(4):865-72.
2. Kaplan MM, "Twelve Questions Physicians Often Ask," *Consultant*, 1993, 33(3):145-52.

References

Edwards MS, "Hepatitis B Serology – Help in Interpretation," *Pediatr Clin North Am*, 1988, 35:503-15.

Jackson JB, "Polymerase Chain Reaction Assay for Detection of Hepatitis B Virus," *Am J Clin Pathol*, 1991, 95(4):442-4.

Lee HS and Vyas GN, "Diagnosis of Viral Hepatitis," *Clin Lab Med*, 1987, 7:741-57.

Repp R, Rhiel S, Heermann KH, et al, "Genotyping by Multiplex Polymerase Chain Reaction for Detection of Endemic Hepatitis B Virus Transmission," *J Clin Microbiol*, 1993, 31(5):1095-102.

Hepatitis C Serology

CPT 86302

Related Information

Hepatitis B Core Antibody *on page 684*
Hepatitis B DNA Detection *on page 913*
Hepatitis B_e Antibody *on page 685*
Hepatitis B_e Antigen *on page 686*
Hepatitis B Surface Antibody *on page 687*
Hepatitis B Surface Antigen *on page 688*
Polymerase Chain Reaction *on page 927*
Risks of Transfusion *on page 1093*

Synonyms HCV Serology

Applies to Anti-HCV (IgM); c100-3; Non-A, non-B Hepatitis; Surrogate Tests

Test Commonly Includes Detection of antibody specific for hepatitis C in patient's serum

Abstract Most cases of post-transfusion non-A, non-B viral hepatitis are caused by HCV. Application of this test has caused a great decrease of post-transfusion hepatitis.

Patient Care PREPARATION: Avoid recent administration of radioisotopes if assay is RIA

Specimen Serum CONTAINER: Red top tube CAUSES FOR REJECTION: Recently administered radioisotopes if assay is RIA

Interpretive REFERENCE RANGE: Negative USE: Differential diagnosis of acute hepatitis; screen blood units for transfusion safety LIMITATIONS: Since as many as 90% of commercial intravenous immunoglobulins test positive for hepatitis C antibody, a false-positive can result briefly after such transfusion. METHODOLOGY: Radioimmunoassay (RIA), enzyme-linked immunosorbent assay (ELISA) ADDITIONAL INFORMATION: Before initiation of hepatitis B surface antigen testing in the 1970's, most significant post-transfusion hepatitis was due to hepatitis B. Following the development of sensitive and specific testing for hepatitis B, greater than 90% of post-transfusion hepatitis became so called "non-A, non-B." Hepatitis C virus is the most common cause of non-A, non-B hepatitis in the United States. Chiron Corporation has isolated a gene product (c100-3) of hepatitis C virus (HCV) and developed an assay for antibodies to it. The assay detects antibody to the flavivirus which is the etiologic agent of hepatitis C. Non-A, non-B, and non-C hepatitis can still occur, probably due to CMV, hepatitis E, and to other viruses that have not been identified.

For blood donors, hepatitis C serology correlates with surrogate tests for non-A, non-B hepatitis (ALT and anti-HB_c). Since hepatitis C serology identifies a broader group of infected individuals than surrogate testing, it reduces risk of HCV during transfusion. Studies in hemophiliacs indicate that antibody to HCV is a reliable marker of HCV. Recently, IgM anti-HCV core has been shown to be a useful acute marker for HCV infection. Transmission is by intravenous drug abuse, dialysis, and other needlesticks. Sexual transmission also occurs. Before screening for hepatitis C antibody was in place, non-A, non-B hepatitis was said to occur in as many as 10% of transfusions. With the introduction of first generation hepatitis C screening tests, the number has fallen to 1 in 3300 units.[1,2,3,4] With a more sensitive second generation hepatitis C test being introduced in 1992, safety has increased even more. Chronic carrier states develop in more than half the patients, and chronic liver disease is a major problem. Substantial risk of chronic active hepatitis and cirrhosis exists in those who develop chronic non-A, non-B hepatitis, of whom, about 80% develop anti-HCV. Of these, a risk of hepatocellular carcinoma exists. A series of patients who developed post-transfusion non-A, non-B hepatitis in the 1970s were followed for up to 15 years after initial diagnosis. It was found that 20% of these patients developed liver failure.[5] Studies are currently being done on the detection of HCV in patient's specimens using reverse transcriptase and PCR.[6]

Footnotes

1. McCullough J, "The Nation's Changing Blood Supply System," *JAMA*, 1993, 269(17):2239.
2. Donahue JG, Muñoz A, Ness PM, et al, "The Declining Risk of Post-Transfusion Hepatitis C Virus Infection," *N Engl J Med*, 1992, 327(6):369-73.
3. Dodd RY, "The Risk of Transfusion-Transmitted Infection," *N Engl J Med*, 1992, 327(6):419-21.
4. Chaudhary RK and Maclean C, "Detection of Antibody to Hepatitis C Virus by Second-Generation Enzyme Immunoassay," *Am J Clin Pathol*, 1993, 99:702-4.
5. Koretz RL, Abbey H, Coleman E, et al, "Non-A, Non-B Post-Transfusion Hepatitis: Looking Back in the Second Decade," *Ann Intern Med* , 1993, 119(2):110-5.
6. François M, Dubois F, Brand D, et al, "Prevalence and Significance of Hepatitis C Virus (HCV) Viremia in HCV Antibody-Positive Subjects from Various Populations," *J Clin Microbiol*, 1993, 31(5):1189-93.

References

Allain JP, Dailey SH, Laurian Y, et al, "Evidence for Persistent Hepatitis C Virus (HCV) Infection in Hemophiliacs," *J Clin Invest*, 1991, 88(5):1672-9.

Alter MJ, Hadler SC, Judson FN, et al, "Risk Factors for Acute Non-A, Non-B Hepatitis in the United States and Association With Hepatitis C Virus Infection," *JAMA*, 1990, 264(17):2231-5.

Alter MJ, Margolis HS, Krawczynski K, et al, "The Natural History of Community-Acquired Hepatitis C in the United States," *N Engl J Med*, 1992, 327(27):1899-905.

Centers for Disease Control, "Screening Donors of Blood, Plasma, Organs, Tissues, and Semen for Evidence of Hepatitis B and Hepatitis C," *Lab Med*, 1991, 22(8):555-63.

Clemens JM, Taskar S, Chau K, et al, "IgM Antibody Response in Acute Hepatitis C Viral Infection," *Blood*, 1992, 79(1):169-72.

Choo Q-L, Kuo G, Weiner AJ, et al, "Isolation of a cDNA Clone Derived From a Blood-Borne Non-A, Non-B Viral Hepatitis Genome," *Science*, 1989, 244(4902):359-62.

Dodd LG, McBride JH, Gitnick GL, et al, "Prevalence of Non-A, Non-B Hepatitis/Hepatitis C Virus Antibody in Human Immunoglobulins," *Am J Clin Pathol*, 1992, 97(1):108-13.

Dodd RY, "Hepatitis C Virus, Antibodies and Infectivity - Paradox, Pragmatism, and Policy," *Am J Clin Pathol*, 1992, 97(1):4-6, (editorial).

Gambino R, "NANB Hepatitis - A New Antibody Test for the Hepatitis C Virus," *Lab Report for Physicians,*™ 1988, 10:89-93.

Hsieh TT, Yao DS, Sheen IS, et al, "Hepatitis C Virus in Peripheral Blood Mononuclear Cells," *Am J Clin Pathol*, 1992, 98(4):392-6.

Kuo G, Choo QL, Alter HJ, et al, "An Assay for Circulating Antibodies to a Major Etiologic Virus of Human Non-A, Non-B Hepatitis," *Science*, 1989, 244(4902):362-4.

Prince AM, Brotman B, Inchauspé G, et al, "Patterns and Prevalence of Hepatitis C Virus Infection in Post-Transfusion Non-A, Non-B Hepatitis," *J Infect Dis*, 1993, 167(6):1296-301.

Richards C, Holland P, Kuramoto K, et al, "Prevalence of Antibody to Hepatitis C Virus in a Blood Donor Population," *Transfusion*, 1991, 31(2):109-13.

Seeff LB, Buskell-Bales Z, Wright EC, et al, "Long-Term Mortality After Transfusion-Associated Non-A, Non-B Hepatitis," *N Engl J Med*, 1992, 327(27):1906-11.

Schiff ER, "Viral Hepatitis Today," *Emerg Med*, 1992, 115-33.

Hepatitis D Serology

CPT 86306 (antigen); 86692 (antibody)

Related Information

Hepatitis B Core Antibody *on page 684*
Hepatitis B DNA Detection *on page 913*
Hepatitis B_e Antibody *on page 685*
Hepatitis B_e Antigen *on page 686*
Hepatitis B Surface Antibody *on page 687*
Hepatitis B Surface Antigen *on page 688*
Polymerase Chain Reaction *on page 927*

Synonyms Delta Agent Serology; Delta Hepatitis Serology

Abstract Hepatitis D virus (HDV) was first recognized in 1977 by Rizzetto and colleagues. HDV always occurs as a simultaneous coinfection with hepatitis B (HBV). Patients coinfected with HDV and HBV have fulminant hepatitis more often than patients infected with HBV alone.[1] Testing for serological markers of HDV should be considered when a patient shows clinical signs of acute or fulminant hepatitis.

Hepatitis D Superinfection

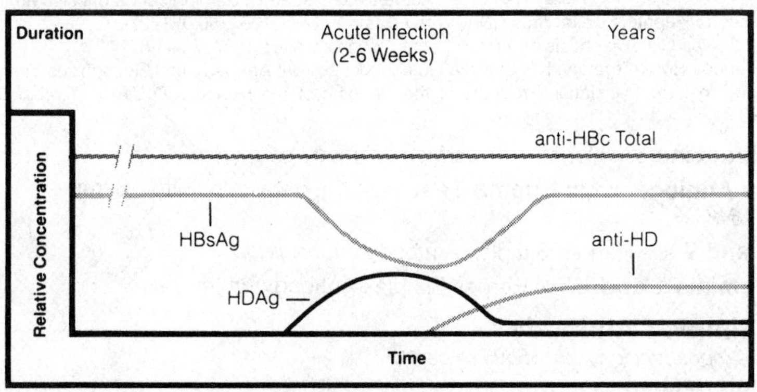

Reprinted from Abbott Diagnostics

(Continued)

Hepatitis D Serology *(Continued)*

Coinfection

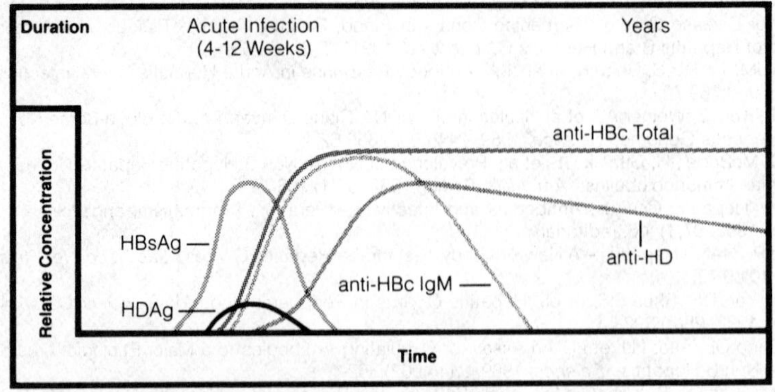

Reprinted from Abbott Diagnostics

Patient Care PREPARATION: Avoid recent administration of radioisotopes

Specimen Serum CONTAINER: Red top tube CAUSES FOR REJECTION: Recently administered radioisotopes

Interpretive REFERENCE RANGE: Negative USE: Differential diagnosis of chronic, recurrent, and acute viral hepatitis METHODOLOGY: Radioimmunoassay (RIA), enzyme-linked immunosorbent assay (ELISA) ADDITIONAL INFORMATION: Hepatitis D virus ("delta" agent) is an incomplete RNA virus, or viroid, that can infect livers already infected by hepatitis B virus. It may occur, therefore, as coinfection with acute HBV hepatitis or super imposed on chronic HBV infection. It cannot occur in an HB_sAg-negative individual. IgG and IgM antibodies to HDV develop 5-7 weeks after infection. IgM antibody is most useful in distinguishing those patients with active liver disease. HDAg can be detected in serum or liver biopsies but is technically demanding and offers little to diagnosis. False-positive EIA results have been reported in patients with lipemia or high titer rheumatoid factor. Studies of liver transplants in patients with end-stage liver disease due to hepatitis B/D have shown, through serial biopsies post-transplant, that HDV viral reinfection occurs within 1 week but without damage. Not until HBV proliferation occurs several weeks to months later does one find histologic and clinical changes.[2,3]

Footnotes

1. Polish LB, Gallagher M, Fields HA, et al, "Delta Hepatitis: Molecular Biology and Clinical and Epidemiological Features," *Clin Microbiol Rev*, 1993, 6(3):211-29.
2. Craig JR, "Hepatitis Delta Virus – No Longer A Defective Virus," *Am J Clin Pathol*, 1992, 98(6):552-3, (editorial).
3. Davies SE, Lau JY, O'Grady JG, et al, "Evidence That Hepatitis D Virus Needs Hepatitis B Virus to Cause Hepatocellular Damage," *Am J Clin Pathol*, 1992, 98(6):554-8.

References

Govindarajan S, Valinluck B, Lake-Bakkar G, "Evaluation of a Commercial Anti-Delta EIA Test for Detection of Antibodies to Hepatitis Delta Virus," *Am J Clin Pathol*, 1991, 95(2):240-1.

Gupta S, Govindarajan S, Cassidy WM, et al, "Acute Delta Hepatitis: Serological Diagnosis With Particular Reference to Hepatitis Delta Virus RNA," *Am J Gastroenterol*, 1991, 86(9):1227-31.

Lee HS and Vyas GN, "Diagnosis of Viral Hepatitis," *Clin Lab Med*, 1987, 7:741-57.

Pohl C, Baroudy BM, Bergmann KF, et al, "A Human Monoclonal Antibody that Recognizes Viral Polypeptides and *In Vitro* Translation Products of the Genome of the Hepatitis D Virus," *J Infect Dis*, 1987, 156:622-9.

Hepatitis Vaccine *see* Hepatitis B Surface Antibody *on page 687*

Hereditary Angioneurotic Edema Test *see* C1 Esterase Inhibitor, Serum *on page 648*

Herpes 1 and 2 *see* Herpes Simplex Antibody *on this page*

Herpes Hominis 1 and 2 *see* Herpes Simplex Antibody *on this page*

Herpes Simplex Antibody

CPT 86694 (nonspecific type); 86695 (type 1)

Related Information

Herpes Cytology *on page 502*

Herpes Simplex Virus Antigen Detection *on page 1181*
Herpes Simplex Virus Culture *on page 1182*
Herpes Simplex Virus Isolation, Rapid *on page 1184*
Herpesvirus Antigen *on this page*
TORCH *on page 758*

Synonyms Herpes 1 and 2; Herpes Hominis 1 and 2; HSV Antibodies

Test Commonly Includes Detection of antibody HSV 1 and 2 in patients' serum

Specimen Serum **CONTAINER:** Red top tube

Interpretive **REFERENCE RANGE:** Interpretation depends on whether episode is initial or reinfection. IgG and IgM specific antibodies may give more useful information about an acute event. **USE:** Determine a patient's exposure to herpes simplex virus 1 or 2 **LIMITATIONS:** Extensive background antibody in the population, and cross reaction of HSV 1 and HSV 2 responses make test useful only in epidemiology **METHODOLOGY:** Indirect fluorescent antibody (IFA), hemagglutination, complement fixation (CF), enzyme immunoassay (EIA) **ADDITIONAL INFORMATION:** A primary HSV 1 or HSV 2 infection will produce a classical rising antibody titer. However, because exposure to herpesvirus is almost universal (50% to 90% of adults have antibodies) the background of antibody makes the serologic response in any particular episode of recurrence difficult to interpret. This is made especially true by the fact the antibody to one virus type may be stimulated by infection with the heterologous virus type. Both false-positives and false-negatives are common with currently licensed enzyme immunoassays. Collecting the requisite paired sera to delineate which titers are rising or stable generally adds nothing to clinical management, and thus herpes serology cannot be recommended in routine clinical cases. However, in research settings or for epidemiologic studies serologic definition of the type of herpes infection have been worthwhile. Herpes serology has not been proved clinically useful in determining whether caesarean delivery should be undertaken in pregnant patients with questionably active herpes. Pap smear or immunochemical demonstration of viral antigen is more useful for this. Nor is herpes serology usually helpful in the differential of a very sick infant with possible congenital herpes. Because of the fulminant course, even early IgM antibody may not be demonstrable in time to contribute to care.

References

Ashley R, Cent A, Maggs U, et al, "Inability of Enzyme Immunoassays to Discriminate Between Infections With Herpes Simplex Virus Types 1 and 2," *Ann Intern Med*, 1991, 115(7):520-6.
Brown ZA, Benedetti J, Ashley R, et al, "Neonatal Herpes Simplex Virus Infection in Relation to Asymptomatic Maternal Infection at the Time of Labor," *N Engl J Med*, 1991, 324(18):1247-52.
Erlich KS, "Laboratory Diagnosis of Herpesvirus Infections," *Clin Lab Med*, 1987, 7:759-76.
Frenkel LM, Garratty EM, Shen JP, et al, "Clinical Reactivation of Herpes Simplex Virus Type 2 Infection in Seropositive Pregnant Women With No History of Genital Herpes," *Ann Intern Med*, 1993, 118(6):414-8.
Johnson RE, Nahmias AJ, Magder LS, et al, "A Seroepidemiological Survey of the Prevalence of Herpes Simplex Virus Type 2 Infection in the United States," *N Engl J Med*, 1989, 321(1):7-12.
Prober CG, Corey L, Brown ZA, et al, "The Management of Pregnancies Complicated by Genital Infections With Herpes Simplex Virus," *Clin Infect Dis*, 1992, 15(6):1031-8.
Whitley R, Arvin A, Prober C, et al, "Predictors of Morbidity and Mortality in Neonates With Herpes Simplex Virus Infections," *N Engl J Med*, 1991, 324(7):450-4.

Herpesvirus Antigen

CPT *87206 (smear, fluorescent); 87207 (smear, special stain)*

Related Information

Herpes Cytology *on page 502*
Herpes Simplex Antibody *on previous page*
Herpes Simplex Virus Antigen Detection *on page 1181*
Herpes Simplex Virus Culture *on page 1182*
Herpes Simplex Virus Isolation, Rapid *on page 1184*

Synonyms HSV Antigen

Test Commonly Includes Testing of appropriate clinical materials for presence of herpesvirus types 1 and 2 antigen

Specimen Appropriate specimens include lesion or vesicle scrapings, conjunctival scrapings, genital lesions, throat swab, bronchial brushings, appropriate autopsy and biopsy specimens **COLLECTION:** Specimen should be received fresh, as quickly as possible, or frozen. Specimen should **not** be in fixative. **TURNAROUND TIME:** 24 hours **SPECIAL INSTRUCTIONS:** Operative biopsy specimens and spinal fluid specimens for fluorescent antibody (FA) testing should be **processed immediately** at any time during the day or night. The laboratory should be **notified in advance** when either or these specimen types will be sent for FA.

(Continued)

Herpesvirus Antigen *(Continued)*

Interpretive **REFERENCE RANGE:** Negative **USE:** Identify herpesvirus types 1 and 2 in clinical specimens **LIMITATIONS:** While the immunofluorescence and immunoperoxidase methods are only about half as sensitive as culture for detecting asymptomatic carriage, recent EIAs have been shown to have a specificity of 96.6% and sensitivity of 93.7% when compared with viral isolation. **METHODOLOGY:** Direct fluorescent antibody (DFA), immunoperoxidase, enzyme immunoassay (EIA) **ADDITIONAL INFORMATION:** When the diagnosis of herpes infection is emergent (herpes encephalitis, or the need to start chemotherapy at once), immunologic techniques are the most rapid and sensitive way to establish the diagnosis if the characteristic cytologic findings of herpes are not present. The procedure may be performed by immunofluorescence on frozen biopsy tissue or smears (see Herpes Simplex Virus, Antigen Detection) by immunoperoxidase technique on fixed and paraffin-embedded material, or with EIA on a variety of specimen types. Some problems in sensitivity have been reported on cervical swabs from pregnant women and necropsy brain material. With appropriate monoclonal antibodies the two HSV serotypes can be differentiated. The use of EIA may be especially important in rapid diagnosis of potentially serious cases.

References

Corey L and Spear PG, "Infections With Herpes Simplex Viruses," *N Engl J Med*, 1986, 314:749-56.
Drew WL, "Diagnostic Virology," *Clin Lab Med*, 1987, 7:721-40.
Erlich KS, "Laboratory Diagnosis of Herpesvirus Infections," *Clin Lab Med*, 1987, 7:759-76.
Sillis M, "Clinical Evaluation of Enzyme Immunoassay in Rapid Diagnosis of Herpes Simplex Infections," *J Clin Pathol*, 1992, 45(2):165-7.

Herpes Zoster Serology *see* Varicella-Zoster Virus Serology *on page 761*

Heterophil Agglutinins

CPT *86308*

Related Information

Epstein-Barr Virus Culture *on page 1179*
Epstein-Barr Virus Serology *on page 676*
Infectious Mononucleosis Screening Test *on page 713*

Test Commonly Includes Differentiation and quantitation of antibodies associated with infectious mononucleosis from the Forssman as well as other heterophil antibodies.

Specimen Serum **CONTAINER:** Red top tube

Interpretive **REFERENCE RANGE:** Negative agglutination **USE:** Detect heterophil antibodies related to infectious mononucleosis. **This test has largely been superseded by rapid screening tests. See Infectious Mononucleosis Screening Test.** **LIMITATIONS:** Rare patients may have positive heterophil agglutinins after a negative screening test. Ten percent of cases of true EBV mononucleosis may have negative heterophil agglutinins. These may be diagnosed with EBV specific tests. **METHODOLOGY:** Differential serum absorption and agglutination of sheep red blood cells **ADDITIONAL INFORMATION:** Heterophil agglutinins clump sheep erythrocytes. They develop in infectious mononucleosis, other conditions, and in some normal individuals. To diagnose infectious mononucleosis, an absorption of serum is done, with guinea pig kidney (which does not bind IgM antibody) and bovine red cells (which do). This differential absorption procedure is the Paul-Bunnell-Davidsohn test. In present usage horse erythrocytes are used in place of sheep cells in many laboratories. In the presumptive test, a positive test in the presence of consistent clinical and/or hematologic findings confirms the diagnosis of infectious mononucleosis. Approximately 10% of mononucleosis syndromes are heterophil-negative. In some of these, antibody to specific Epstein-Barr viral antigen can be demonstrated. See Epstein-Barr Virus Serology. Others may be due to CMV or toxoplasmosis. Although this classic test has excellent specificity, its performance is time consuming. False-positive tests occur and may lead to diagnostic confusion.

References

Fleisher GR, Collins M, and Fager S, "Limitations of Available Tests for Diagnosis of Infectious Mononucleosis," *J Clin Microbiol*, 1983, 17:619-24.
Horwitz CA, Henle W, Henle G, et al, "Persistent Falsely Positive Rapid Tests for Infectious Mononucleosis. Report of Five Cases with 4-6 Year Follow-Up Data," *Am J Clin Pathol*, 1979, 72:807-11.
Ridker PM, Enders GH, and Lifton RP, "False-Positive Mononucleosis Screening Test Results Associated With *Klebsiella* Hepatic Abscess," *Am J Clin Pathol*, 1990, 94(2):222-3.

HHV-6, IgM, IgG *see* Human Herpesvirus 6, IgG and IgM Antibodies, Quantitative *on page 703*

Histocompatibility Testing *see* Tissue Typing *on page 757*

***Histoplasma* Antibodies** *see* Histoplasmosis Serology *on this page*

***Histoplasma capsulatum* Antibody and Antigen** *see* Histoplasmosis Serology *on this page*

Histoplasmosis Immunodiffusion *see* Histoplasmosis Serology *on this page*

Histoplasmosis Serology

CPT 86698

Related Information

Blood Fungus Culture *on page 789*
Fungus Smear, Stain *on page 813*
Sputum Fungus Culture *on page 853*

Synonyms *Histoplasma* Antibodies

Applies to *Histoplasma capsulatum* Antibody and Antigen; Histoplasmosis Immunodiffusion; H Precipitin Bands; Polysaccharide Antigen, *H. capsulatum var capsulatum*

Test Commonly Includes Reaction with yeast and mycelial antigens

Specimen Serum, cerebrospinal fluid (antibody); serum, urine (antigen) **CONTAINER:** Red top tube, sterile CSF tube, plastic urine container **COLLECTION:** Acute and convalescent sera are recommended, especially when acute titers are only presumptive.

Interpretive **REFERENCE RANGE:** Antibody: less than a fourfold change in titer between acute and convalescent samples; titer: <1:4; CSF titer: negative. Antigen: negative. **USE:** Diagnose and evaluate the prognosis of histoplasmosis **LIMITATIONS:** A negative result does not rule out histoplasmosis. Histoplasmin skin testing may interfere with results. Testing with both antigens must be performed. There are cross reactions with other fungi. Anticomplementary sera cannot be tested for complement fixing antibodies. The latex agglutination test gives some false-positives, and must be confirmed with another procedure. **CONTRAINDICATIONS:** Previous skin testing **METHODOLOGY:** Antibody: complement fixation (CF), immunodiffusion (ID), latex agglutination (LA); antigen: radioimmunoassay (RIA), enzyme immunoassay (EIA) **ADDITIONAL INFORMATION:** CF titers of 1:8 or 1:16 are presumptive evidence of histoplasmosis. Titers ≥1:32 are highly suggestive of *H. capsulatum* infection, but cannot be relied on as the sole means of diagnosis. Complement fixation and immunodiffusion each detect about 85% of disease. H and M bands on immunodiffusion indicate active disease. Complement fixation is less sensitive to disseminated or chronic disease. The latex agglutination test detects IgM antibodies and is positive early in disease, but not in late, chronic, or recurrent infection. Tests for fungal antigen are now available and obviate some of the problems of ordinary serology (ie, cross reactions, decreased immune response, need for paired specimens over time). The use of enzyme immunoassay and radioimmunoassay to detect *H. capsulatum* antigen has proven to be a useful approach in the diagnosis of histoplasmosis. Antigenuria or antigenemia is excellent evidence of disseminated disease.

Histoplasmosis immunodiffusion: "H" and "M" precipitin bands are of diagnostic significance and if both are present indicate active infection. "H" identity bands alone are rarely seen; they are always associated with active infection. "M" identity bands alone indicate active infection, recent past infection (within the past year), or recent positive histoplasmin skin test (within past 2 months). The absence of precipitin antibodies does not rule out histoplasmosis.

Unfortunately, because of poorly standardized reagents and inherent biologic cross reactivity, and interference from complement, the general clinical utility of measuring or detecting fungal antibodies is low. For this reason, much effort is now devoted to tests for detecting fungal antigens.

In addition to histoplasmosis in immunologically intact individuals, this fungal infection is a serious opportunistic infection in patients with AIDS (occasionally as its first manifestation). In Kansas City and Indianapolis, histoplasmosis occurs in up to 25% of patients with AIDS.[1]

Footnotes

1. Wheat LJ, Connolly-Stringfield P, Blair R, et al, "Histoplasmosis Relapse in Patients With AIDS: Detection Using *Histoplasma capsulatum* Variety *capsulatum* Antigen Levels," *Ann Intern Med*, 1991, 115(12):936-41.

(Continued)

Histoplasmosis Serology *(Continued)*

References

Kaufman L and Reiss E, "Serodiagnosis of Fungal Diseases," *Manual of Clinical Laboratory Immunology*, 4th ed, Vol 2, Chapter 78, Rose NR, Conway de Macario E, Fahey JL, et al, eds, Washington, DC: American Society for Microbiology, 1992, 506-28.

Wheat LJ, Connolly-Stringfield PA, Baker RL, et al, "Disseminated Histoplasmosis in the Acquired Immune Deficiency Syndrome: Clinical Findings, Diagnosis and Treatment, and Review of the Literature," *Medicine (Baltimore)*, 1990, 69(6):361-74.

Wheat LJ, Kohler RB, and Tewari RP, "Diagnosis of Disseminated Histoplasmosis by Detection of *Histoplasma capsulatum* Antigen in Serum and Urine Specimens," *N Engl J Med*, 1986, 314:83-8.

Zimmerman SE, Stringfield PC, Wheat LJ, et al, "Comparison of Sandwich Solid-Phase Radioimmunoassay and Two Enzyme-Linked Immunosorbent Assays for Detection of *Histoplasma capsulatum* Polysaccharide Antigen," *J Infect Dis*, 1989, 160(4):678-85.

HIV-1/HIV-2 Serology

CPT *86701 (HIV-1); 86702 (HIV-2); 86703 (HIV-1 and HIV-2, single assay)*

Related Information

Beta$_2$-Microglobulin *on page 644*
HTLV-I/II Antibody *on page 702*
Human Immunodeficiency Virus Culture *on page 1185*
Human Immunodeficiency Virus DNA Amplification *on page 915*
Lymphocyte Subset Enumeration *on page 720*
Neisseria gonorrhoeae Culture *on page 831*
Ova and Parasites, Stool *on page 836*
p24 Antigen *on page 727*
Polymerase Chain Reaction *on page 927*
Risks of Transfusion *on page 1093*
Skin Fungus Culture *on page 845*
T- and B-Lymphocyte Subset Assay *on page 750*
Toxoplasmosis Serology *on page 759*
White Blood Count *on page 616*
Zidovudine *on page 1012*

Synonyms Acquired Immune Deficiency Syndrome Serology; AIDS Screen; HIV Antibody; Human Immunodeficiency Virus Serology; RIBA Test for HIV Antibody; Western Blot Test for HIV Antibody

Applies to Recombinant Antigen Immunoblot Assay; RIBA; Western Blot

Test Commonly Includes Detection of antibody to HIV by ELISA and confirmation by Western blot

Patient Care **PREPARATION:** In some states test may not be done or results revealed without express written or informed consent of the patient.

Specimen Serum **CONTAINER:** Red top tube **SPECIAL INSTRUCTIONS:** Blood and body fluid precautions must be observed.

Interpretive **REFERENCE RANGE:** Negative **USE:** Document exposure to HIV-1 and HIV-2; screen blood and blood products for transfusion; screen organ transplant donors **LIMITATIONS:** There is a 2- to 12-week (perhaps much longer) interval after infection before antibody becomes detectable. Positive screening tests must be confirmed by more specific follow up procedures (usually Western blot). If the Western blot for HIV-1 is negative or indeterminate with a positive HIV-1/HIV-2 serology, further testing is required for HIV-2. This may include HIV-2 EIA and HIV-2 Western blot. Antibody is not protective against disease. There are some cross reactions in some test systems due to histocompatibility antigen mismatches (in particular, antibodies to HLA-DR4). Cross reactions have been observed to other viral antigens as well. A recent influenza vaccine can result in reactivity against p24 antigen and give a false-positive enzyme-linked immunosorbent assay.

Because screening tests are neither 100% sensitive nor specific, alone or in combination, a positive result must be interpreted cautiously, considering the prevalence of AIDS in the population being tested. As prevalence decreases compared to high risk groups, false-positives increase, and the predictive value of a positive result decreases.

METHODOLOGY: Enzyme-linked immunosorbent assay (ELISA), Western blot, indirect fluorescent antibody (IFA); radioimmunoprecipitation (RIPA) **ADDITIONAL INFORMATION:** Human immunodeficiency virus (HIV-1, formerly HTLV-III), a lentivirus, is the etiologic agent of AIDS. Acute infection, spread by blood or sexual contact, is usually followed within days by a flu-like illness, or no symptoms. During this time, HIV antigen, usually p24 core protein, may be detectable in serum. This becomes negative in 2 weeks to 1 month. There then follows a period of weeks to months (as long as 35 months) during which an individual is infected with HIV, which may or may not be replicating at a low rate, but screening tests for antibody to HIV are **negative**.[1]

HIV preferentially binds to and infects CD4 (T4, helper) lymphocytes because the viral envelope glycoprotein gp120 binds specifically to the CD4 lymphocyte membrane protein, a key determinant of helper differentiation. HIV also binds to monocytes and macrophages, and infection of bronchial macrophages may explain the frequency of *Pneumocystis* infections in AIDS patients. HIV probably enters the CNS by means of infected monocytes crossing the blood brain barrier.

The HIV RNA genome includes open-reading frames (sor and orf), a transactivator gene (tat), initial and terminal long terminal repeats (LTR), and genes for the viral group specific antigen (gag), the viral envelope (env), and reverse transcriptase (pol). The protein and glycoprotein products of these genes most important in serologic testing are p24, a 24 kD core protein; gp41, a 41 kD envelope glycoprotein; and gp160 and gp120, 160 kD and 120 kD envelope glycoproteins. gp160 is probably the precursor protein of both gp120 and gp41 and is not expressed in intact virus.

Ancillary tests for AIDS include quantitation of CD4 (helper) and CD8 (suppressor) lymphocytes. In AIDS (but **not** diagnostic for it), T4 cells are severely reduced, and the CD4:CD8 ratio is <1. An absolute CD4 count <300/mm^3 is used as an indication for AZT.

Present screening tests for HIV antibodies are ELISA procedures which use recombinant antigen products. Different antibodies are detected. Both the sensitivity and specificity of these tests are extremely high, but positive results on a screen should be repeated; if positive a second time they should be confirmed with a Western blot procedure. Because of the grave implications of a positive result, we recommend that a second sample be assayed to eliminate false-positives due to switched samples or sample contamination.

Some individuals may have reactive screening tests, restricted to one test system, and completely negative Western blots. This may be due to HLA antibodies reacting with residual human cell surface proteins incorporated in the test kit. False-positives have been reported in individuals who have received intravenous gamma globulin. Since these positives are due to antibodies in the transfused gamma globulin, repeat analysis in 3 months (half-life for IgG is about 3 weeks), will show a negative or much weaker EIA result. Sera which test positive by ELISA twice consecutively are subject to confirmatory testing by Western blot technique. Some individuals may have reactive screening tests, restricted to one test system, and completely negative Western blots. This may be due to HLA antibodies reacting with residual human cell surface proteins incorporated in the test kit, cross reactivity of antibodies against other viral antigens, or autoantibodies which react with components of the lysed human substrate cells.

In the Western blot procedure, electrophoretically separated HIV proteins and glycoproteins are overlaid with serum. Antibodies present will bind to the appropriate antigen, which is spatially separated by molecular weight from other viral components. The bound antibody is then visualized by reaction with a labeled (radioisotope or enzyme) antibody to human immunoglobulin or protein A (which binds to the Fc portion of the antibody). Although, early on, several different patterns were used for a positive interpretation, since 1988 two major patterns are used. The Consortium for Retrovirus Serology Standardization recommended that a positive blot have the following bands: p24 or p31 plus gp41 or gp160/120. The standard of the Association of State and Territorial Public Health Laboratory was adopted by the Centers for Disease Control in 1989 and is now the most widely accepted definition of a positive Western blot. This criteria requires the Western blot to contain at least two of the following three bands: p24, gp41, and gp 160/120. The presence of other band patterns is termed indeterminate and should be followed up with subsequent testing. The Western blot is a complex procedure, requiring great technical expertise and informed interpretation. False-positive rates may be in the range of 1% to 2%. False-negative rates are not well established.

The most recent EIA kits allow detection of both HIV-1 and HIV-2 antibodies. Further, recombinant antigens from HIV-1: p24 (gag), p17 (gag), and endonuclease p31 (pol) have been combined with two synthetic peptides from the env genes of HIV-1 and the env gene of HIV-2 to provide a strip-based confirmation assay similar to the Western blot. A similar recombinant antigen immunoblot assay (RIBA) confirmation assay employing HIV-1 p24, p31, p41, and gp120 has been proposed as an alternative confirmation method for HIV-1.

(Continued)

HIV-1/HIV-2 Serology *(Continued)*

Usual serologic response: Within 7-10 days of infection, circulating HIV antigen can be demonstrated. This is short-lived and disappears within 2 weeks. Within 10 days to 2 weeks of infection, IgM antibody to HIV appears; this lasts several weeks. Within 6-16 weeks of infection, IgG antibody becomes detectable by ELISA. These patterns are generalizations and must be interpreted in light of the following information: persistence or reappearance of HIV antigen may signal disease progression; anti-p24 is the first antibody to appear, but may be undetectable in as many as 40% of seropositive patients; anti-gp41 is the most common antibody detected; anti-p24 without anti-gp120 or anti-gp160 is occasionally seen as a false-positive result.

Prolonged latency of HIV has been suggested by several studies. Viral antigens and antibodies can be demonstrated by polymerase chain reaction for as long as 35 months before individuals seroconverted by ELISA testing. Such individuals may have normal numbers of CD4 lymphocytes.

Screening for AIDS infection in low risk populations will be hampered by false-positive results. Although the combined false-positive rate of sequential ELISA and Western blot testing may be very low (0.005% estimated in one article) testing large numbers of individuals in a population with a very low prevalence of disease will generate unmanageable numbers of false-positive results. The predictive value of a positive test will be low, and many individuals will be unnecessarily alarmed. Mass screening is not recommended with tests presently available.

For patients who received blood transfusions or blood products between 1978 and 1985, especially in California, New York City, or Miami, testing with currently available ELISA methodology is satisfactory as an initial procedure to exclude accidental infection via transfusion. Patients who received only Rh immune globulin, or other gamma globulin products, need not be tested unless they fall into some other risk group. "Look back" programs, retrospectively testing blood recipients, and assessing risk of transfusion-associated AIDS, have been undertaken. Now that donor blood is screened for antibodies to HIV-1 (and HTLV-I) the blood supply is acceptably safe; risk is as low as 0.003% per unit. In 1992, testing of blood bank samples by HIV-1 and HIV-2 ELISA became the standard.

Patients in high risk groups (homosexual or bisexual men, I.V. drug abusers and their sexual contacts, male and female prostitutes, hemophiliacs exposed to large amounts of nonheat processed factor VIII) should be tested for diagnosis. This should include an initial ELISA test, and tests for HIV antigen. Repeated testing may be necessary.

TYPICAL SEROLOGICAL PROFILE IN HIV INFECTION

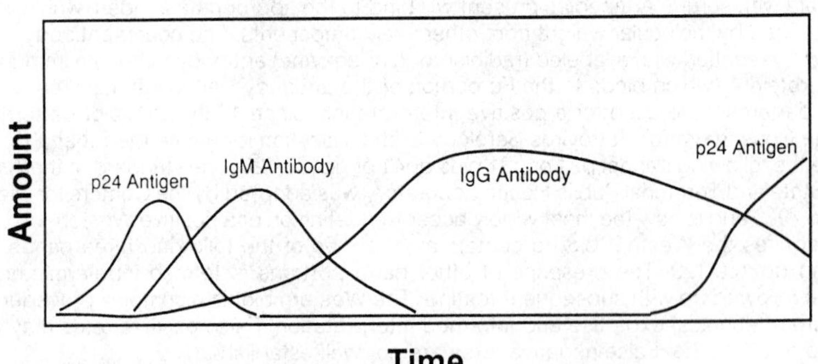

Van de Perre, et al, *Aids Res Hum Retroviruses,* 1992, 8:435.

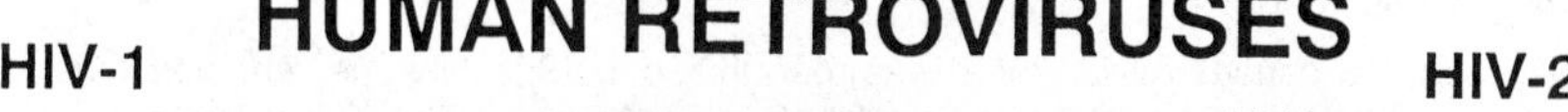

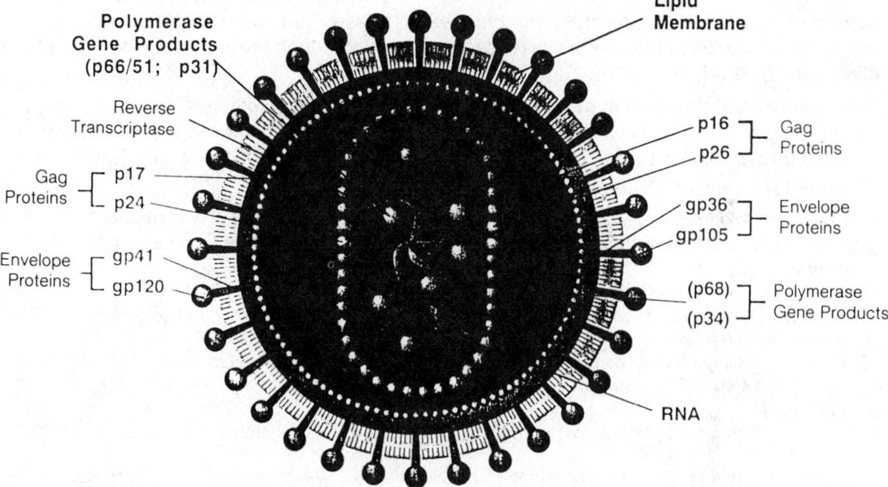

Reprinted from Abbott Diagnostics

HUMAN RETROVIRUSES
HIV-1 Genome

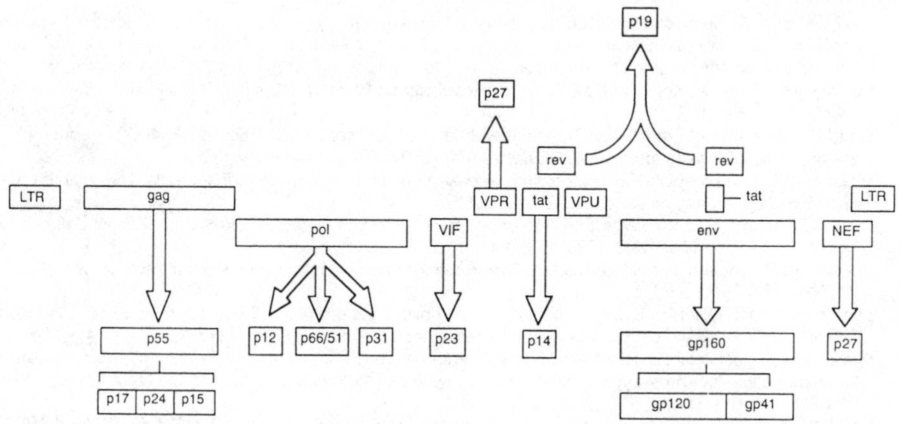

(Continued)

There are no patterns of serologic response to HIV yet known to indicate resolution of disease or loss of infectivity (unlike the situation for hepatitis B virus). A patient in a risk group who has demonstrable antigen or antibody should be assumed to be infected and infectious. See chart on previous page.

Another virus that causes AIDS, HIV-2, was recognized in 1986. HIV-2 is very closely related to HIV-1 with 40% nucleic acid homology. HIV-2 is endemic in West Africa, however, it has spread to other countries. As of September, 1991, 31 cases had been confirmed in the United States.[2] It produces the same clinical disease as HIV-1, although the incubation period before clinical AIDS develops in HIV-2 may be longer than in HIV-1.

Although **central nervous system involvement** is extremely common in AIDS, testing CSF for HIV antigen or antibody lacks both sensitivity and specificity. These tests do not help in differentiating neurologic symptoms secondary to HIV infection from those due to CNS neoplasm or opportunistic infection.

The October 1988 issue of *Scientific American* and July 1993 *Journal of NIH Research* are entirely devoted to a thorough consideration of social, biological and the medical aspects of the AIDS epidemic.

Footnotes

1. Imagawa DT, Lee MH, Wolinsky SM, et al, "Human Immunodeficiency Virus Type 1 Infection in Homosexual Men Who Remain Seronegative for Porlonged Periods," *N Engl J Med*, 1989, 320(22):1458-62.
2. Kloser PC, Mangia AJ, Leonard J, et al, "HIV-2-Associated AIDS in the United States. The First Case," *Arch Intern Med*, 1989, 149(8):1875-7.

References

Blattner WA, "Human T-Lymphotropic Viruses and Diseases of Long Latency," *Ann Intern Med*, 1989, 111(1):4-6.

Burke DS, "Laboratory Diagnosis of Human Immunodeficiency Virus Infection," *Clin Lab Med*, 1989, 9(3):369-92.

Burke DS, Brundage JF, Redfield RR, et al, "Measurement of the False-Positive Rate in a Screening Program for Human Immunodeficiency Virus Infections," *N Engl J Med*, 1988, 319:961-4.

Carlson JR, Yee J, Hinrichs SH, et al, "Comparison of Indirect Immunofluorescence and Western Blot for Detection of Anti-Human Immunodeficiency Virus Antibodies," *J Clin Microbiol*, 1987, 25:494-7.

Centers for Disease Control, "Interpretation and Use of the Western Blot Assay for Serodiagnosis of Human Immunodeficiency Virus Type 1 Infections," *MMWR Morb Mortal Wkly Rep*, 1989, 38(Suppl 7):1-7.

Consortium for Retrovirus Serology Standardization, "Serologic Diagnosis of Human Immunodeficiency Virus Infection by Western Blot Testing," *JAMA*, 1988, 260:674-9.

Cumming PD, Wallace EL, Schorr JB, et al, "Exposure of Patients to Human Immunodeficiency Virus Through the Transfusion of Blood Components That Test Antibody-Negative," *N Engl J Med*, 1989, 321(14):941-6.

Davey RT and Vasudevachari MB, "Serologic Evaluation of Patients With Human Immunodeficiency Virus Infection," *Manual of Clinical Laboratory Immunology*, 4th ed, Vol 2, Rose NR, Conway de Macario E, Fahey JL, et al, eds, Washington DC: American Society for Microbiology, 1992, 364-70.

DeCock KM, Porter A, Konadio J, et al, "Cross-Reactivity on Western Blots in HIV-1 and HIV-2 Infections," *AIDS*, 1991, 5:859-63.

Dodd RY, "The Risk of Transfusion-Transmiteed Infection," *N Engl J Med*, 1992, 327(6):419-21, (editorial).

Haseltine WA, "Silent HIV Infections," *N Engl J Med*, 1989, 320(22):1487-8.

Hollander H, "Cerebrospinal Fluid Normalities and Abnormalities in Individuals Infected With Human Immunodeficiency Virus," *J Infect Dis*, 1988, 158:855-8.

Klatt EC, Shibata D, and Strigle SM, "Postmortem Enzyme Immunoassay for Human Immunodeficiency Virus," *Arch Pathol Lab Med*, 1989, 113(5):485-7.

Krieger JN, "Acquired Immunodeficiency Syndrome Antibody Testing and Precautions," *J Urol*, 1992, 147(3):713-6.

Leitman SF, Klein HG, Melpolder JJ, et al, "Clinical Implications of Positive Tests for Antibodies to Human Immunodeficiency Virus Type 1 in Asymptomatic Blood Donors," *N Engl J Med*, 1989, 321(14):917-24.

MacDonald KL, Jackson JB, Bowman RJ, et al, "Performance Characteristics of Serologic Tests for Human Immunodeficiency Virus Type 1 (HIV-1) Antibody Among Minnesota Blood Donors," *Ann Intern Med*, 1989, 110(8):617-21.

Meyer KB and Pauker SG, "Screening for HIV: Can We Afford the False-Positive Rate?" *N Engl J Med*, 1987, 317:238-41.

O'Gorman MR, Weber D, Landis SE, et al, "Interpretive Criteria of the Western Blot Assay for Serodiagnosis of Human Immunodeficiency Virus Type 1 Infection," *Arch Pathol Lab Med*, 1991, 115(1):26-30.

Quinn TC, "Screening for HIV Infection – Benefits and Costs," *N Engl J Med*, 1992, 327(7):486-8, (editorial).

Rhame FS and Maki DG, "The Case for Wider Use of Testing for HIV Infection," *N Engl J Med*, 1989, 320(19):1248-54.

Sloand EM, Pitt E, Chiarello RJ, et al, "HIV Testing. State of the Art," *JAMA*, 1991, 266(20):2861-6.

Wolinsky SM, Rinaldo CR, Kwok S, et al, "Human Immunodeficiency Virus Type 1 (HIV-1) Infection a Median of 18 Months Before a Diagnostic Western Blot," *Ann Intern Med*, 1989, 111(12):961-72.

HIV Antibody *see* HIV-1/HIV-2 Serology *on page 696*

HIV Core Antigen *see* p24 Antigen *on page 727*

HLA-Antigen B27 *see* HLA-B27 *on this page*

HLA-B27

CPT 86812

Related Information

Tissue Typing *on page 757*

Synonyms B27; HLA-Antigen B27; W27

Test Commonly Includes Human leukocyte antigen testing, to include locus B27

Specimen Leukocytes **CONTAINER:** Green top (heparin) tube **STORAGE INSTRUCTIONS:** Store at room temperature; do not refrigerate **SPECIAL INSTRUCTIONS:** Sample must be tested as soon as possible; testing should be prearranged

Interpretive **REFERENCE RANGE:** Requires clinical correlation **USE:** Evaluate spondyloarthritis and other disorders associated with these loci **LIMITATIONS:** An adequate test requires the presence of viable lymphocytes at the time of testing. Even taking appropriate precautions, an occasional specimen will not be satisfactory for testing. In such cases, fresh blood should be drawn for retesting. **METHODOLOGY:** Incubation of lymphocyte suspensions with antisera to specific B27 locus. If lymphocytes bind the antisera (are B27-positive), they will be killed when complement is added. Live cells can be differentiated from dead ones by supravital dye exclusion. **ADDITIONAL INFORMATION:** HLA-B27 is strongly associated with ankylosing spondylitis (Marie-Strumpell disease). HLA-B27 antigen shares homology with a *Klebsiella* protein, and may imply a bacterial pathogenesis to ankylosing spondylitis. A patient with consistent clinical and radiographic findings who is B27 positive has approximately 100 times greater chance of having or developing ankylosing spondylitis than a negative patient. However, the antigen is not causative, and 10% of normal subjects are B27 positive. **This test should not be considered a screening procedure for ankylosing spondylitis**. The antigen is less strongly associated with Reiter's syndrome and other arthritides than with ankylosing spondylitis. It has been linked with congenital deficiency of C4 and C2, and with adrenal hyperplasia.

References

Braun WE and Zachary AA, "The HLA Histocompatibility System in Autoimmune States," *Clin Lab Med*, 1988, 8:351-72.

Keat A, "Reiter's Syndrome and Reactive Arthritis in Perspective," *N Engl J Med*, 1983, 309:1606-15.

Khan MA and Khan MK, "Diagnostic Value of HLA-B27 Testing in Ankylosing Spondylitis and Reiter's Syndrome," *Ann Intern Med*, 1982, 96:70-5.

Lipsky PE and Taurog JD, "The Second International Simmons Center Conference on HLA-B27-Related Disorders," *Arthritis Rheum*, 1991, 34(11):1476-82.

Yu DT, Choo SY, and Schaack T, "Molecular Mimicry in HLA-B27 Related Arthritis," *Ann Intern Med*, 1989, 111(7):581-91.

HLA Typing *see* Tissue Typing *on page 757*

HLA Typing, Crossmatch *see* Tissue Typing *on page 757*

HLA Typing, Single Human Leukocyte Antigen

CPT 86812

Related Information

Identification DNA Testing *on page 918*
Mixed Lymphocyte Culture *on page 725*
Tissue Typing *on page 757*

Test Commonly Includes Identification of HLA antigens on leukocytes

Specimen Leukocytes **CONTAINER:** Green top (heparin) tube **COLLECTION:** Deliver immediately to the laboratory. **STORAGE INSTRUCTIONS:** Maintain at room temperature. Do not refrigerate. **SPECIAL INSTRUCTIONS:** Should be scheduled in advance, since test requires viable lymphocytes.

Interpretive **REFERENCE RANGE:** Identification of specific leukocyte antigens **USE:** Epidemiologic marker, correlation with disease syndromes, paternity exclusion testing, transplantation candidate matching, among others **LIMITATIONS:** The clinical significance of many of the marker antigens is not well defined **METHODOLOGY:** Use of dye marker to assess leukocyte viability after interaction with numerous monospecific antisera **ADDITIONAL INFORMATION:** The human

(Continued)

HLA Typing, Single Human Leukocyte Antigen *(Continued)*

leukocyte antigen system consists of many alleles in four loci, A-D. Loci A, B, and C control class I genes, with multiple alleles. These are expressed on all nucleated cells and are recognized in concert with foreign antigen by cytotoxic T cells. Locus D controls class II genes, the immune response genes. The D group may be further subdivided into DR, DQ, DP, and DW. These genes exhibit linkage disequilibrium, and occur in certain combinations more often than expected. Many of these antigens have been more or less closely associated statistically with a wide ranging variety of illness, both physical and mental. The most striking association is that of HLA-B27 with ankylosing spondylitis. Another significant association is HLA-B8 and sarcoidosis. Many striking associations with SLE are known, as well as with other autoimmune disorders. However, none of these is an aid to diagnosis. HLA typing is performed to assess potential organ transplants, in conjunction with mixed lymphocyte culture and ABO typing. These cell surface proteins are the targets for rejection of an organ transplant and the more severe graft-vs-host disease. It may also be useful in exclusion of paternity, since the system includes many alleles which can be identified in addition to the many red cell antigenic systems.

References

Bodmer JG, Albert ED, Bodmer WF, et al, "Nomenclature for Factors of the HLA System, 1990," *Immunogenetics*, 1991, 33:301-9.

Braun WE and Zachary AA, "The HLA Histocompatibility System in Autoimmune States," *Clin Lab Med*, 1988, 8:351-72.

Colvin RB, Bhan AK, and McCluskey RT, eds, *Diagnostic Immunopathology*, New York, NY: Raven Press, 1988, 159.

Marsh SG and Bodmer JG, "HLA Class II Nucleotide Sequences, 1991," *Immunogenetics*, 1991, 33(5-6):321-34.

Peter JB and Hawkins BR, "The New HLA," *Arch Pathol Lab Med*, 1992, 116(1):11-5.

Sanfilippo F, "The Influence of HLA and ABO Antigens on Graft Rejection and Survival," *Clin Lab Med*, 1991, 11(3):537-50.

Zemmour J and Parham P, "HLA Class I Nucleotide Sequences, 1991," *Immunogenetics*, 1991, 33(3-5):310-20.

H Precipitin Bands *see* Histoplasmosis Serology *on page 695*

HSV Antibodies *see* Herpes Simplex Antibody *on page 692*

HSV Antigen *see* Herpesvirus Antigen *on page 693*

HTLV-I/II Antibody

CPT *86687 (HTLV-I); 86688 (HTLV-II)*

Related Information

HIV-1/HIV-2 Serology *on page 696*
Polymerase Chain Reaction *on page 927*
Risks of Transfusion *on page 1093*

Synonyms Human T-Cell Leukemia Virus Type I and Type II; Human T-Lymphotropic Virus Type I Antibody

Test Commonly Includes Screening test with confirmation of positives

Abstract Two closely related retroviruses discovered by Dr Robert Gallo in the 1970s. The viruses can cause, after lengthy incubation periods, leukemia and neuromuscular disease.

Specimen Serum **CONTAINER:** Red top tube

Interpretive **REFERENCE RANGE:** Negative **USE:** Screen blood and blood products for transfusion; differential diagnosis of spastic myelopathy for HTLV-I. HTLV-I is also the causative virus for adult T-cell acute lymphoblastic leukemia (ALL). HTLV-II has been associated with chronic neuromuscular diseases. **LIMITATIONS:** The combined assay for Anti HTLV-I/II is used mainly to screen blood donors. The assay cross reacts with only 80% of patients with antibody to HTLV-II.[1] The 20% of blood donors who are not detected by the assay for HTLV-II are not at sufficiently high risk to transmit the disease to warrant a separate assay. **METHODOLOGY:** Screen: enzyme immunoassay (EIA); confirmation: Western blot or radioimmunoprecipitation (RIPA) **ADDITIONAL INFORMATION:** Human T-lymphotropic virus type I (HTLV-I) is a pathogenic retrovirus which is irregularly distributed in the world. Infection is generally uncommon in the U.S. The virus can be asymptomatic for prolonged periods (20 years) but is strongly associated with myelopathies and adult T-cell leukemia. Adult T-cell leukemia is an aggressive malignancy of T-lymphocytes often associated with skin infiltrates and hypercalcemia. The virus is tropic for T4 lymphocytes and is passed by sexual contact, blood products, from mother to fetus, and by breast milk. Pretransfusion testing for antibody to HTLV-I is now mandated by blood banks, in order to avoid transfusion transmitted HTLV-I infection from asymptomatic infected donors. Retrospective studies from the American Red Cross have concluded that about 700 individuals per year received HTLV-I/II blood prior to 1988 when donor testing began. The risk of this is extremely low (0.024% per unit). Early seroconverters have antibodies to the C-terminal region of gp46 (envelope protein) and to gag p19 and p24. The clinical course of HTLV-I infection, and the meaning of a positive serology are not yet well understood. Indeed, a recent study of hemophiliacs who were transfused regularly with plasma or its derivatives found no evidence of HTLV-I/II antibody in 179 patients.

Footnotes

1. CDCP and USPHS Working Group, "Guidelines for Counseling Persons Infected With Human T-Lymphotropic Virus Type I (HTLV-I) and Type II (HTLV-II)," *Ann Intern Med*, 1993, 118(6):448-54.

References

Blattner WA, "Human T-Lymphotropic Viruses and Diseases of Long Latency," *Ann Intern Med*, 1989, 111(1):4-6.

Canavaggio M, Leckie G, Allain JP, et al, "The Prevalence of Antibody to HTLV I/II in United States Plasma Donors and in United States and French Hemophiliacs," *Transfusion*, 1990, 30(9):780-2.

Chen YM, Gomez-Lucia E, Okayama A, et al, "Antibody Profile of Early HTLV-I Infection," *Lancet*, 1990, 336(8725):1214-6.

Cohen ND, Munõz A, Reitz BA, et al, "Transmission of Retroviruses by Transfusion of Screened Blood in Patients Undergoing Cardiac Surgery," *N Engl J Med*, 1989, 320(18):1172-6.

Gessain A and Gout O, "Chronic Myelopathy Associated With Human T-Lymphotropic Virus Type I (HTLV-I)," *Ann Intern Med*, 1992, 117(11):933-46.

Larson CJ and Taswell HF, "Human T-Cell Leukemia Virus Type I (HTLV-I) and Blood Transfusion," *Mayo Clin Proc*, 1988, 63:869-75.

Melief CJM and Goudsmit J, "Transmission of Lymphotropic Retroviruses (HTLV-I and LAV/HTLV-III) by Blood Transfusions and Other Blood Products," *Vox Sang*, 1986, 50:1-11.

Sullivan MT, Williams AE, Fang CT, et al, "Transmission of Human T-Lymphotropic Virus Types I and II by Blood Transfusion," *Arch Intern Med*, 1991, 151(10):2043-8.

Washitani Y, Kuroda N, Shiraki H, et al, "Serological Discrimination Between HTLV-I and HTLV-II Antibodies by ELISA Using Synthetic Peptides as Antigens," *Int J Cancer*, 1991, 49(2):173-7.

Wong-Staal F and Gallo RC, "Human T-Lymphotropic Retroviruses," *Nature*, 1985, 317:395-403.

Human Herpesvirus 6, IgG and IgM Antibodies, Quantitative

CPT 86790

Related Information

Infectious Mononucleosis Screening Test *on page 713*

Synonyms HHV-6, IgM, IgG

Test Commonly Includes Detection and quantitation of antibodies to human herpesvirus 6

Specimen Serum **CONTAINER:** Red top tube or serum separator tube **COLLECTION:** Acute and convalescent specimens are recommended. Specimens should be free from bacterial contamination and hemolysis. **STORAGE INSTRUCTIONS:** Refrigerate serum **CAUSES FOR REJECTION:** Gross lipemia

Interpretive **USE:** IgM HHV-6 may aid in the diagnosis of acute or recent infection with HHV-6. An increase in IgG HHV-6 (fourfold increase in titer) between acute and convalescent samples is evidence of a recent HHV-6 infection. **METHODOLOGY:** Indirect fluorescent antibody (IFA) **ADDITIONAL INFORMATION:** Human herpesvirus 6 (HHV-6) has recently been identified as the agent associated with both pediatric and adult infections. Most children have been infected by 3 years of age. The infection in children is characterized clinically by an acute febrile illness, irritability, inflammation of typanic membranes, and (uncommonly) a rash characteristic of roseola. When acute and convalescent (4-6 weeks later) serum samples are compared, a fourfold rise in HHV-6 IgG titer is typical. In adults, HHV-6 has been associated with chronic fatigue and spontaneously resolving fever resembling a mononucleosis-like illness. During the acute episode an elevated IgM HHV-6 is useful. An increase in IgG HHV-6 between acute and convalescent serum sample is consistent with a recent HHV-6 infection.

References

Buchwald D, Cheney PR, Peterson DL, et al, "A Chronic Illness Characterized by Fatigue, Neurologic and Immunologic Disorders, and Active Human Herpesvirus Type 6 Infection," *Ann Intern Med*, 1992, 116(2):103-13.

Irving WL and Cunningham AL, "Serological Diagnosis of Infection With Human Herpesvirus Type 6," *BMJ*, 1990, 300(6718):156-9.

Pruksananonda P, Hall CB, Insel RA, et al, "Primary Human Herpesvirus 6 Infection in Young Children," *N Engl J Med*, 1992, 326(22):1445-50.

(Continued)

Human Herpesvirus 6, IgG and IgM Antibodies, Quantitative *(Continued)*

Steeper TA, Horwitz CA, Ablashi DV, et al, "The Spectrum of Clinical and Laboratory Findings Resulting From Human Herpesvirus-6 (HHV-6) in Patients With Mononucleosis-Like Illnesses Not Resulting From Epstein-Barr Virus or Cytomegalovirus," *Am J Clin Pathol*, 1990, 93(6):776-83.

Human Immunodeficiency Virus Serology *see* HIV-1/HIV-2 Serology *on page 696*

Human Leukocyte Antigens *see* Tissue Typing *on page 757*

Human T-Cell Leukemia Virus Type I and Type II *see* HTLV-I/II Antibody *on page 702*

Human T-Lymphotropic Virus Type I Antibody *see* HTLV-I/II Antibody *on page 702*

Hydatid Disease Serological Test *see* Echinococcosis Serological Test *on page 674*

Hypersensitivity Pneumonitis Serology

CPT *86329*

Related Information

Sputum Culture *on page 849*

Synonyms Air Conditioner Lung; Allergic Lung Serology; Farmer's Lung Disease; Precipitating Antibodies

Applies to *Aspergillus fumigatus* Precipitating Antibodies; *Aspergillus niger* Precipitating Antibodies; *Micropolyspora faeni* Precipitating Antibodies; *Thermoactinomyces vulgaris* Precipitating Antibodies; *Thermolospora viridis* Precipitating Antibodies

Replaces *Thermoactinomyces* Precipitating Antibodies

Test Commonly Includes *Micropolyspora faeni*; *Aspergillus fumigatus*, *Alternaria* sp, *Aspergillus niger*, *Thermoactinomyces vulgaris*, *Thermolospora viridis* antigen testing by immunodiffusion of combined antigenic extract.

Abstract The diagnostic expression **hypersensitivity pneumonitis** applies to types of interstitial lung disease which are caused by organic dusts derived from living sources: ***vide supra***.

Specimen Serum **CONTAINER:** Red top tube

Interpretive **REFERENCE RANGE:** Negative **USE:** Support the clinical diagnosis of hypersensitivity pneumonitis **LIMITATIONS:** A positive test does not establish the diagnosis of hypersensitivity pneumonitis, nor does the absence of precipitins eliminate the diagnosis. Open lung biopsy may be needed to establish the diagnosis. T cells participate in the alveolitis. **METHODOLOGY:** Immunodiffusion (ID) **ADDITIONAL INFORMATION:** Some individuals in a variety of settings become sensitized to inhaled antigens and develop acute bronchospastic symptoms 4-6 hours following exposure to them. Many of these have been diagnosed with disease names indicating the nature of the exposure (ie, Farmer's lung, silo-filler's disease, maple bark stripper's disease, paprika-slicer's lung, sauna taker's lung). The antigen material is usually an *Aspergillus* sp or one of the thermophilic actinomycetes. Individuals with precipitating antibodies may have no symptoms, and patients with severe symptoms may not show antibody while their disease is inactive. Thus, there must be careful correlation of clinical and laboratory results.

References

Crystal RG, "Interstitial Lung Disease," *Cecil Textbook of Medicine*, Vol 1, 19th ed, Wyngaarden JB, Smith LH Jr, and Bennett JC, eds, Philadelphia, PA: WB Saunders Co, 1992, 396-409.

Hammar SP, "Extrinsic Allergic Alveolitis – Histiocytosis-X," *Pulmonary Pathology*, Dail DH and Hammer SP, eds, New York, NY: Springer-Verlag, 1988, 379-92.

Sharma OP, "Hypersensitivity Pneumonitis," *Dis Mon*, 1991, 37(7):409-71.

I Antigen *see* Cold Agglutinin Titer *on page 664*

i Antigen *see* Cold Agglutinin Titer *on page 664*

IEP, Serum or Urine *see* Immunoelectrophoresis, Serum or Urine *on page 706*

IF Antibody *see* Intrinsic Factor Antibody *on page 714*

IFE *see* Immunofixation Electrophoresis *on page 707*

IgA *see* Immunoglobulin A *on page 709*

IgA Antibodies

CPT 86329

Related Information

Immunoglobulin A *on page 709*
Risks of Transfusion *on page 1093*

Synonyms Anti-immunoglobulin A

Abstract IgA deficient patients may suffer from hypersensitivity reactions to transfused IgA in blood products. Although immunoglobulins including IgA are assayed to evaluate immunity and disease entities such as myeloma, this test measures an antibody to an immunoglobulin antigen.

Specimen Serum **CONTAINER:** Red top tube

Interpretive **REFERENCE RANGE:** Antibody not present **USE:** Evaluate transfusion reaction symptoms as dyspnea, sweating, substernal pain, flushing, laryngeal edema, hypotension, and collapse following infusion of very small quantities of blood.[1] **METHODOLOGY:** Immunodiffusion (ID) **ADDITIONAL INFORMATION:** Approximately 1 in 500-1000 individuals is IgA deficient, either alone or in combination with another immunoglobulin. Such individuals can develop antibodies to IgA, which they recognize as a foreign protein. If such a patient, with antibody to IgA, is transfused with blood, serum, or plasma containing IgA, he/she may experience an anaphylactic reaction. Patients with a history of anaphylactic reaction to blood transfusion should be tested for IgG and IgE antibody to IgA. Frozen washed cells or autologous transfusion should be used for such patients if possible. Unfortunately, laboratory methods to detect IgE and IgG anti-IgA are not standardized. A negative assay does not rule out the possibility of an IgE-mediated anaphylactic event. Some workers have recommended that all IgA-deficient patients receive blood products lacking IgA. At the least, one should have epinephrine and hydrocortisone ready if signs of anaphylaxis appear. Injection of immunoglobulin can cause such reaction because immunoglobulin preparations contain some IgA.[1]

Footnotes

1. Mollison PL, Engelfriet CP, and Contreras M, "Some Unfavorable Effects of Transfusion," *Blood Transfusion in Clinical Medicine*, 9th ed, Oxford, UK: Blackwell Scientific Publications, 1993, 691-3.

References

Keren DF and Warren JS, "Immunodeficiency," *Diagnostic Immunology*, Baltimore, MD: Williams & Wilkins, 1992, 107-8.

IgD *see* Immunoglobulin D *on page 710*

IgE *see* Immunoglobulin E *on page 710*

IgG *see* Immunoglobulin G *on page 710*

IgG_1 *see* Immunoglobulin G Subclasses *on page 711*

IgG_2 *see* Immunoglobulin G Subclasses *on page 711*

IgG_3 *see* Immunoglobulin G Subclasses *on page 711*

IgG_4 *see* Immunoglobulin G Subclasses *on page 711*

IgG Antibodies to Rubella *see* Rubella Serology *on page 743*

IgG, CSF *see* Cerebrospinal Fluid Immunoglobulin G *on page 656*

IgG Ratios and IgG Index, Cerebrospinal Fluid *see* Cerebrospinal Fluid IgG Ratios and IgG Index *on page 653*

IgG Subclasses *see* Immunoglobulin G Subclasses *on page 711*

IgG Synthesis Rate, Cerebrospinal Fluid *see* Cerebrospinal Fluid IgG Synthesis Rate *on page 655*

IgM *see* Immunoglobulin M *on page 712*

IgM Antibodies to Rubella *see* Rubella Serology *on page 743*

Immune Complex Assay

CPT 86332

Related Information

Raji Cell Assay *on page 739*

Applies to Conglutinin Solid-Phase Assay; Immune Complex by C1q Binding; Monoclonal Rheumatoid Factor Inhibition

(Continued)

Immune Complex Assay *(Continued)*

Specimen Serum **CONTAINER:** Red top tube **STORAGE INSTRUCTIONS:** If immune complex by Raji cell is requested, serum must be frozen within 2 hours.

Interpretive **REFERENCE RANGE:** Complexes not detected **USE:** **These are nonspecific assays used in the past for monitoring some autoimmune diseases.** **LIMITATIONS:** Certain cryoglobulins, cold agglutinins, rheumatoid factors, and paraproteins may cause false-positive results. **METHODOLOGY:** C1q and monoclonal rheumatoid factor can bind to immunoglobulins in complexes and then be precipitated and quantitated. Raji cells and conglutinin bind the complement components of the complexes. **ADDITIONAL INFORMATION:** Immune complex assays were once thought to be promising assays to follow patients with autoimmune disease. Due to their lack of specificity and poor correlation with each other, they no longer have diagnostic use. They may be useful in research and epidemiologic settings. **As these tests are expensive, rule nothing in or out, and are poorly standardized, we do not recommend they be used.**

References

Colvin RB, Bhan AK, and McCluskey RT, eds, *Diagnostic Immunopathology*, New York, NY: Raven Press, 1988, 27-9.

Keren DF, "Assays for Circulating Immune Complexes," *Clinical Laboratory Annual*, Batsakis JG and Homburger HA, eds, New York, NY: Appleton-Century-Crofts, 1985, 105.

Keren DF and Warren JS, "Agglutination, Precipitation, and Hemolytic Reactions," *Diagnostic Immunology*, Baltimore, MD: Williams & Wilkins, 1992, 288-90.

Immune Complex Assay by Raji Cell *see* Raji Cell Assay *on page 739*

Immune Complex by C1q Binding *see* Immune Complex Assay *on previous page*

Immune Complex Detection by C1q *see* C1q Immune Complex Detection *on page 649*

Immunodeficiency Profile *see* Lymphocyte Subset Enumeration *on page 720*

Immunoelectrophoresis *see* Protein Electrophoresis, Urine *on page 737*

Immunoelectrophoresis for Myeloma Proteins *see* Immunoelectrophoresis, Serum or Urine *on this page*

Immunoelectrophoresis, Serum *see* Protein Electrophoresis, Serum *on page 734*

Immunoelectrophoresis, Serum or Urine

***CPT** 86320 (serum); 86325 (other fluids)*

Related Information

Immunofixation Electrophoresis *on next page*
Protein Electrophoresis, Serum *on page 734*
Protein Electrophoresis, Urine *on page 737*
Protein, Quantitative, Urine *on page 1145*
Protein, Total, Serum *on page 340*

Synonyms IEP, Serum or Urine; Immunoelectrophoresis for Myeloma Proteins

Applies to Dysgammaglobulinemia; Kappa and Lambda Light Chains Detection; Light Chains; Monoclonal Gammopathy; Paraproteinemia

Replaces Bence Jones Protein Test

Test Commonly Includes Typing of monoclonal proteins for light and heavy chain specificity

Specimen Serum or urine **CONTAINER:** Red top tube or plastic urine container

Interpretive **REFERENCE RANGE:** Interpretation by pathologist **USE:** Diagnose myeloma, macroglobulinemia of Waldenström; evaluate monoclonal gammopathy (M spike) found in serum protein electrophoresis; evaluate amyloidosis; has application to the evaluation of lymphoproliferative diseases (malignant lymphoma and others) and collagen diseases in general; diagnose and characterize immune-deficient and dysgammaglobulinemic states. **LIMITATIONS:** Immunoelectrophoresis is not quantitative. It is being replaced by immunofixation, which is more sensitive and easier to interpret. In most laboratories IgD and IgE specific reagents are not used routinely. Monoclonal gammopathies <300 mg/dL are difficult to detect with IEP. Large molecular weight monoclonal gammopathies (eg, Waldenström's macroglobulinemia) often require treatment with 2-mercaptoethanol prior to IEP or false-negatives will occur. **METHODOLOGY:** Electrophoresis of specimen, followed by immunodiffusion (ID) against monospecific antisera to immunoglobulin and individual heavy and light chains **ADDITIONAL INFORMATION:** Immunoelectrophoresis of serum or urine is most often ordered to evaluate a monoclonal globulin detected in a protein electrophoresis or to delineate a possible lymphoproliferative process, particularly myeloma. This procedure will characterize the specific light and heavy chain components of a monoclonal protein. It may be useful in defining deficiencies of specific immunoglobulins or other serum proteins, however, it is not a quantitative technique and nephelometry of specific immunoglobulins is preferred for detecting immunodeficiencies. Specific identification of abnormal proteins is performed in an increasing number of clinical laboratories by immunofixation (IF). IF combines high resolution electrophoresis with immunoprecipitation. This method is more rapid and sensitive than immunoelectrophoresis.

References

Gochman N and Burke MA, "Electrophoretic Techniques in Today's Clinical Laboratory," *Clin Lab Med*, 1986, 6:403-26.

Keren DF, "Immunofixation Techniques," *High Resolution Electrophoresis and Immunofixation*, Boston, MA: Butterworth's Publishers, 1987, 107-130.

Sun T, *Interpretation of Protein and Isoenzyme Patterns in Body Fluids*, New York, NY: Igaku-Shoin, 1991.

Immunofixation Electrophoresis

CPT 86334

Related Information

Immunoelectrophoresis, Serum or Urine *on previous page*
Immunoglobulin A *on page 709*
Immunoglobulin G *on page 710*
Immunoglobulin M *on page 712*
Protein Electrophoresis, Serum *on page 734*
Protein Electrophoresis, Urine *on page 737*
Protein, Quantitative, Urine *on page 1145*
Protein, Total, Serum *on page 340*
Viscosity, Serum/Plasma *on page 611*

Synonyms IFE

Applies to Bence Jones Protein; Dysgammaglobulinemia Evaluation; Kappa Chains; Lambda Chains; Light Chains; Monoclonal Gammopathy; M Protein; Paraprotein Evaluation

Test Commonly Includes Identification of monoclonal gammopathies, pathologist interpretation

Abstract Immunofixation electrophoresis has become the assay of choice to characterize monoclonal gammopathies.

Specimen Serum, 24-hour urine **CONTAINER:** Red top tube, plastic urine container **COLLECTION:** Urine: See procedure for collection of a 24-hour urine. No preservative required. **STORAGE INSTRUCTIONS:** Separate serum from cells, centrifuge and/or filter urine. **CAUSES FOR REJECTION:** Inadequate specimen identification

Interpretive REFERENCE RANGE: Interpretation by pathologist **USE:** Detect and identify monoclonal immunoglobulin gammopathies **CONTRAINDICATIONS:** Normal serum protein electrophoresis **METHODOLOGY:** High resolution electrophoresis combined with immunoprecipitation **ADDITIONAL INFORMATION:** Immunofixation electrophoresis of serum or urine is most often ordered to evaluate a monoclonal globulin detected in a protein electrophoresis or to delineate a possible lymphoproliferative process, particularly myeloma. It is the assay of choice because it does not suffer from the false-negatives seen in serum IEP. This procedure will characterize the specific light and heavy chain components of a monoclonal protein. Bence Jones proteins are homogeneous urinary light chain protein of kappa or lambda type. IFE is the assay of choice for examining urine for Bence Jones protein. Routine electrophoresis is too insensitive. Although quantification of kappa and lambda chains in urine by nephelometry has been suggested as an alternative, it is too insensitive at the present to be practical. Urinary light chain ladder patterns may be confused with Bence Jones protein.[1]

Footnotes

1. Bailey EM, McDermott TJ, and Bloch KJ, "The Urinary Light-Chain Ladder Pattern: A Product of Improved Methodology That May Complicate the Recognition of Bence Jones Proteinuria," *Arch Pathol Lab Med*, 1993, 117:707-10.

References

Keren DF, "Immunofixation Techniques," *High-Resolution Electrophoresis and Immunofixation: Techniques and Interpretation*, Boston, MA: Butterworth's Publishers, 1987, 107-30.

Keren DF, Warren JS, and Lowe JB, "Strategy to Diagnose Monoclonal Gammopathies in Serum," *Clin Chem*, 1988, 34:2196-202.

(Continued)

Immunofixation Electrophoresis *(Continued)*

Levinson SS, "Studies of Bence Jones Proteins by Immunonephelometry," *Ann Clin Lab Sci*, 1992, 22(2):100-9.

Immunofluorescence, Skin Biopsy

CPT *88346 (each antibody)*

Related Information

Endomysial Antibodies *on page 674*
Oral Cavity Cytology *on page 507*
Pemphigus Antibodies *on page 731*
Skin Biopsies *on page 84*

Synonyms Skin Biopsy Immunofluorescence

Applies to Basement Membrane Antibodies; Dermatitis Herpetiformis Antibodies; Intercellular Antibody Basement Membrane Antibody; LE Antibodies; Lupus Band Test; Skin Biopsy Antibodies; Skin Biopsy For Bullous or Collagen Disease; Skin Biopsy For Pemphigus

Test Commonly Includes Anti-IgG, anti-IgA, anti-IgM, anti-C3, antifibrin immunofluorescence

Abstract Antibodies against specific antigens in skin help distinguish between several autoimmune dermatoses.

Specimen 3 mm^3 skin punch biopsy and serum **CONTAINER:** Covered Petri dish, or screw-cap glass vial; red top tube for blood **COLLECTION:** Take biopsies from the following sites: If pemphigus or bullous pemphigoid is suspected and fresh lesions are present, take a 3 mm biopsy at the edge of the bulla. If only old lesions are available, take biopsy from adjacent area. If dermatitis herpetiformis is suspected or both bullous pemphigoid and dermatitis herpetiformis are suspected, take not only lesion biopsy, but also biopsy of uninvolved area around lesions. Repeated biopsies are sometimes necessary to confirm dermatitis herpetiformis. If systemic lupus erythematosus or discoid LE is suspected, take biopsy of sun-exposed normal skin, preferably of the wrist, for diagnosis of SLE. Biopsies from lesions may be positive in both SLE and discoid LE while normal appearing sun-exposed skin yields positive findings in SLE only. Lesions older than 6 weeks should be biopsied in suspected SLE. In vasculitis lesions for biopsy should be less than 24 hours old. Biopsy must be kept moist on saline soaked gauze or filter paper. Do not put specimen in formalin, Zenker's solution, or other usual fixatives. Deliver to the laboratory on ice immediately upon completion of biopsy. **STORAGE INSTRUCTIONS:** Fixation in N-ethylmaleimide requires subsequent removal of fixative and frozen section. Consult the laboratory prior to obtaining specimen. Background immunofluorescence due to IgG staining is often a problem. It is largely due to deposition of the interstitial IgG and can be considerably reduced by an overnight incubation in phosphate-buffered saline. **CAUSES FOR REJECTION:** Specimen in fixative, drying out of specimen

Interpretive **USE:** Detect immune complexes, complement, and immunoglobulin deposition in SLE, DLE, pemphigus, bullous pemphigoid, and dermatitis herpetiformis; useful in differential diagnosis of bullous skin diseases **LIMITATIONS:** Many skin lesions which may clinically resemble SLE and DLE also have deposits of immunoglobulins at the basement membrane. These include psoriasis, polymorphous light eruption, and drug eruptions. **CONTRAINDICATIONS:** Specimen should not be taken from heavily keratinized body areas if possible. Failure to demonstrate IgG in some biopsies may be due to a secondary change in the tissue due to infection and inflammatory reaction. **METHODOLOGY:** Direct fluorescent antibody (DFA), indirect fluorescent antibody (IFA) **ADDITIONAL INFORMATION:** Distinctive patterns of IgG, IgA, IgM, and complement components in epidermis, basement membrane, and dermal vessels may contribute to the differential diagnosis of bullous skin diseases, and discoid and systemic lupus erythematosus.

- Pemphigus: Fixation of IgG or other immunoglobulin along intercellular bridges of squamous cells; C3 can be fixed.
- Bullous pemphigoid: Fixation of IgG and C3 along epidermal basement membrane.
- Dermatitis herpetiformis: Fixation of IgA immunoglobulin deposits near the epidermal-dermal junction of skin adjacent to bulla.
- Lupus erythematosus: Fixation of IgG or other immunoglobulin deposits and complement along the epidermal-dermal junction. IgG, IgM, and C3 are the most common.

Epidermolysis bullosa acquista may be distinquished from bullous pemphigoid on skin biopsies after separation of the lamina lucida with 1 M sodium chloride. IgG appears on the dermal side of the split specimens in epidermolysis bullosa acquista and mainly or only on the epidermal side in bullous pemphigoid. Serum antibodies to the same skin components can also be demonstrated, using a tissue substrate (usually monkey or guinea pig esophagus), and these may correlate with disease activity. Steroid therapy can convert findings to negative in previously positive patients. In bullous disease antibody levels often reflect disease activity and rising titers may foretell clinical relapse.

References

Alcocer J, Moreno J, Garcia-Torres R, et al, "Immunofluorescent Skin Band Test in the Differential Diagnosis of Systemic Lupus Erythematosus," *J Rheumatol*, 1979, 6:196-203.

Blenkinsopp WK, Clayton RU, and Haffenden GP, "Immunoglobulin and Complement in Normal Skin," *J Clin Pathol*, 1978, 31:1143-6.

Brown C, Lieu TS, and Sontheimer RD, "Correlation Between Dermal Interstitial Immunoglobulin G and Hypergammaglobulinemia," *J Invest Dermatol*, 1991, 97(2):373-7.

Colvin RB, Bhan AK, and McCluskey RT, eds, *Diagnostic Immunopathology*, New York, NY: Raven Press, 1988, 65-82.

Farmer ER and Provost TT, "Immunologic Studies of Skin Biopsy Specimens in Connective Tissue Diseases," *Hum Pathol*, 1983, 14:316-25.

Gammon WR, Kowalewski C, Chorzelski TP, et al, "Direct Immunofluorescence Studies of Sodium Chloride-Separated Skin in the Differential Diagnosis of Bullous Pemphigoid and Epidermolysis Bullosa Acquisita," *J Am Acad Dermatol*, 1990, 22(4):664-70.

Harrist TJ and Mihm MC, "Cutaneous Immunopathology. The Diagnostic Use of Direct and Indirect Immunofluorescence Techniques in Dermatologic Disease," *Hum Pathol*, 1979, 10:625-53.

Izuno GT, "Cutaneous Immunofluorescence," *Clin Lab Med*, 1986, 6:85-102.

Immunoglobulin A

CPT 82784

Related Information

IgA Antibodies *on page 705*
Immunofixation Electrophoresis *on page 707*
Immunoglobulin G Subclasses *on page 711*
Kidney Profile *on page 268*
Protein, Total, Serum *on page 340*
Risks of Transfusion *on page 1093*

Synonyms IgA; Quantitative IgA

Specimen Serum CONTAINER: Red top tube STORAGE INSTRUCTIONS: Samples suspected of having macroglobulins or cryoglobulins should be drawn and held at 37°C. Samples suspected of containing cold agglutinins should not be refrigerated prior to serum separation from clot.

Interpretive REFERENCE RANGE: Adult: 85-385 mg/dL. Pediatric values: cord blood 0 mg/dL; 1-3 months 0-30 mg/dL; 3-6 months 4-55 mg/dL; 6-12 months 10-70 mg/dL; 12-24 months 18-111 mg/dL; 24-36 months 21-98 mg/dL; 3-5 years 30-178 mg/dL; 5-8 years 74-265 mg/dL; 8-12 years 68-333 mg/dL; 12-16 years 68-250 mg/dL. Ranges may vary among laboratories. USE: Evaluate humoral immunity; monitor therapy in IgA myeloma LIMITATIONS: If samples containing macroglobulins, cryoglobulins, or cold agglutinins are handled at incorrect temperatures, false low values may result. METHODOLOGY: Radial immunodiffusion (RID), rate nephelometry ADDITIONAL INFORMATION: Increased monoclonal IgA may be produced in lymphoproliferative disorders, especially multiple myeloma and "Mediterranean" lymphoma involving bowel. An IgA monoclonal peak >2 g/dL is a major criterion for myeloma. It may be elevated in a wide range of conditions affecting mucosal surfaces, where IgA is largely produced. Some clinically significant IgA deficiencies have concomitant deficiencies of IgG_2 and IgG_4. IgA may be decreased in patients with chronic sinopulmonary disease, in ataxia-telangiectasia, or congenitally. Patients with congenital IgA deficiency are prone to autoimmune diseases, and may develop antibody to IgA and anaphylaxis if transfused. IgA levels may rise with exercise and fall during pregnancy.

References

Holbert JM, "Neoplasms of Terminally Differentiated B Lymphocytes," *Clin Lab Med*, 1988, 8:197-210.

Jeske DJ and Capra JD, "Immunoglobulins: Structure and Function," *Fundamental Immunology*, Paul WE, ed, New York, NY: Raven Press, 1984, 131-65.

Kyle RA and Greipp PR, "Immunoglobulins and Laboratory Recognition of Monoclonal Proteins," *Neoplastic Diseases of the Blood*, Wiernik PH, Canellos GP, Kyle RA, et al, eds, New York, NY: Churchill Livingstone, 1985, 431-59.

Wall R and Kuehl M, "Biosynthesis and Regulation of Immunoglobulins," *Annu Rev Immunol*, 1983, 1:393-422.

Immunoglobulin D

CPT 82784

Synonyms IgD; Quantitative IgD

Test Commonly Includes Quantitation of IgD by radial immunodiffusion

Abstract This is a vastly overused test. It provides clinically useful information only in characterizing monoclonal gammopathies.

Specimen Serum **CONTAINER:** Red top tube or two microbilirubin tubes **STORAGE INSTRUCTIONS:** Store serum at 4°C.

Interpretive REFERENCE RANGE: 0-14 mg/dL (SI: 0-140 mg/L) **USE:** Study of patients for IgD myeloma **METHODOLOGY:** Radial immunodiffusion (RID), rate nephelometry **ADDITIONAL INFORMATION:** The significance of IgD in health and disease remains largely obscure. It is not useful as a screening test. When looking for myeloma a serum protein electrophoresis and quantification of IgG, IgA, IgM, kappa and lambda is much more efficient. In cases in which an unexplained restriction is seen which is not explained by the heavy chains obtained, an IgD should be performed. Rare IgD producing myelomas are reported, <1% of reported cases.

References

Bianchi P, MacNamara E, Bergami MR, et al, "Immunochemical Evaluation of Monoclonal Gammopathies: Heavy Chain to Light Chain Ratio Is of Little Practical Value for Detecting IgD Myelomas and Free Light Chains," *Clin Chem*, 1992, 38(2):317-9.

Wall R and Kuehl M, "Biosynthesis and Regulation of Immunoglobulins," *Annu Rev Immunol*, 1983, 1:393-422.

Immunoglobulin E

CPT 82785

Synonyms IgE; Quantitative IgE

Specimen Serum **CONTAINER:** Red top tube

Interpretive REFERENCE RANGE: Newborn: <12 IU/mL; less than 1 year: <50 IU/mL; 2-4 years: <100 IU/mL; 5 years and older: <300 IU/mL. One unit equals 2.4 ng of IgE protein. **USE:** Initial evaluation of atopic disorders **LIMITATIONS:** Normal IgE levels do not exclude allergic phenomena. **CONTRAINDICATIONS:** Recent isotope scan **METHODOLOGY:** Radioimmunosorbent assay **ADDITIONAL INFORMATION:** IgE antibodies do not fix complement, but can bind to basophils and mast cells. When an allergen is then encountered the cells release a variety of bioactive materials, including histamine, prostaglandin D_2, leukotrienes C, D and E, and kallikrein, which can produce symptoms as severe as anaphylaxis. The protective role of such antibodies is not clear. IgE is frequently increased in parasitic infestations and atopic individuals. IgE myeloma is extremely rare and should be sought after abnormal protein electrophoresis (restriction) and/or abnormal kappa/lambda ratio unexplained by IgG, IgA, or IgM.

References

Hamilton RG and Adkinson MF, "Clinical Laboratory Methods for the Assessment and Management of Human Allergic Diseases," *Clin Lab Med*, 1986, 6:117-38.

Jeske DJ and Capra JD, "Immunoglobulins: Structure and Function," *Fundamental Immunology*, Paul WE, ed, New York, NY: Raven Press, 1984, 131-65.

Ownby DR, "Allergy Testing: *In Vitro* Versus *In Vivo*," *Pediatr Clin North Am*, 1988, 35:995-1009.

Van Arsdel PP Jr and Larson EB, "Diagnostic Tests for Patients With Suspected Allergic Disease," *Ann Intern Med*, 1989, 110(4):304-12.

Wall R and Kuehl M, "Biosynthesis and Regulation of Immunoglobulins," *Annu Rev Immunol*, 1983, 1:393-422.

Williams PB, Dolen WK, Koepke JW, "Comparison of Skin Testing and Three *In Vitro* Assays for Specific IgE in the Clinical Evaluation of Immediate Hypersensitivity," *Ann Allergy*, 1992, 68(1):35-45.

Yunginger JW, "Allergens: Recent Advances," *Pediatr Clin North Am*, 1988, 35:981-93.

Immunoglobulin G

CPT 82784

Related Information

Immunofixation Electrophoresis *on page 707*

Immunoglobulin G Subclasses *on next page*

Protein, Total, Serum *on page 340*

Synonyms IgG; Quantitative IgG

Specimen Serum **CONTAINER:** Red top tube **STORAGE INSTRUCTIONS:** Samples suspected of having macroglobulins or cryoglobulins should be drawn and held at 37°C. Samples suspected of containing cold agglutinins should not be refrigerated prior to serum separation from clot. **SPECIAL INSTRUCTIONS:** Requisition must state patient's age.

Interpretive REFERENCE RANGE: Adults: 564-1765 mg/dL. Pediatrics (blood/mg/dL): cord 662-1793; 1-3 months 161-713; 3-6 months 88-563; 6-12 months 296-1004; 12-24 months 135-1106; 24-36 months 517-1346; 3-5 years 570-1592; 5-8 years 757-1686; 8-12 years 851-1805; 12-16 years 767-1752. Subclasses: I 470-1300 mg/dL; II 115-750 mg/dL; III 20-130 mg/dL; IV 2-165 mg/dL. Values may vary in different laboratories. USE: Quantitate IgG in patient's serum to evaluate humoral immunity; monitor therapy in IgG myeloma; evaluate patients, especially children and those with lymphoma, with propensity to infections LIMITATIONS: If samples containing macroglobulins, cryoglobulins, or cold agglutinins are handled at incorrect temperatures, false low values may result. METHODOLOGY: Radial immunodiffusion (RID), rate nephelometry ADDITIONAL INFORMATION: Immunoglobulin G is the major antibody containing protein fraction of blood. There are four subtypes, of which IgG_1 and IgG_2 comprise 85% of the total. IgG_1 and IgG_3 fix complement best; IgG_3 is hyperaggregable and effects serum viscosity disproportionately. With significant decreases in IgG level, on either a congenital or acquired basis, there is an increased susceptibility to infectious processes ordinarily dealt with by humoral antibody (ie, bacterial infection). Thus, patients with repeated infection should have their immunoglobulins, and specifically IgG, measured. Therapy with exogenous gamma globulins may be efficacious in such patients. Conversely, IgG levels will be increased in immunocompetent individuals responding to a wide variety of infections or inflammatory insults (indeed, this represents the basis of the serologic diagnosis of infectious diseases). IgG specific antibody can now be demonstrated for numerous organisms, and when coupled with IgM specific antibody, can give an accurate diagnosis of acute or chronic infection. Today, a major cause for a polyclonal increase in IgG is the acquired immunodeficiency syndrome. Monoclonal IgG can be demonstrated in many cases of multiple myeloma. 3 g/dL of monoclonal IgG is a major diagnostic criterion for myeloma. Oligoclonal IgG can be seen in multiple sclerosis and some instances of chronic hepatitis. Some of these are characterized by features of chronic active hepatitis.

A monoclonal gammopathy may be present when the total IgG value is in the normal range. While many of these patients do not have multiple myeloma, evaluation of these patients for such gammopathy and the presence of Bence Jones protein in urine is important.

The four subclasses of IgG differ in the constant regions of their heavy chains. A patient may have a normal total IgG yet still have a significant decrease in one subclass. IgG_1 deficiencies are associated with EBV infections, IgG_2 with sinorespiratory infections and infections with encapsulated bacteria, IgG_3 with sinusitis and otitis media, and IgG_4 with allergies, ataxia telangiectasia, and sinorespiratory infections.

References

Jacobson DL, McCutchan JA, Spechko PL, et al, "The Evaluation of Lymphadenopathy and Hypergammaglobulinemia are Evidence for Early and Sustained Polyclonal B Lymphocyte Activation During Human Immunodeficiency Virus Infection," *J Infect Dis*, 1991, 163(2):240-6.

Jeske DJ and Capra JD, "Immunoglobulins: Structure and Function," *Fundamental Immunology*, Paul WE, ed, New York, NY: Raven Press, 1984, 131-65.

Ritzmann SE, "Radial Immunodiffusion Revisited, Part 2. Application and Interpretation of RID Assays," *Lab Med*, 1978, 9:27.

Smith AM and Thompson RA, "Paraprotein Estimation: A Comparison of Immunochemical and Densitometric Techniques," *J Clin Pathol*, 1978, 31:1156-60.

Wall R and Kuehl M, "Biosynthesis and Regulation of Immunoglobulins," *Annu Rev Immunol*, 1983, 1:393-422.

Immunoglobulin G, Cerebrospinal Fluid *see* Cerebrospinal Fluid Immunoglobulin G *on page 656*

Immunoglobulin G Subclasses

CPT *82787*

Related Information

Immunoglobulin A *on page 709*
Immunoglobulin G *on previous page*
Protein, Total, Serum *on page 340*

Synonyms IgG_1; IgG_2; IgG_3; IgG_4; IgG Subclasses

Test Commonly Includes Quantitation of IgG subclasses by RID or ELISA

Specimen Serum CONTAINER: Red top tube STORAGE INSTRUCTIONS: Store at 4°C.

Interpretive REFERENCE RANGE: See table. USE: Study of patients with recurrent bacterial infections METHODOLOGY: Radial immunodiffusion (RID), enzyme-linked immunosorbent assay

(Continued)

Immunoglobulin G Subclasses *(Continued)*

(ELISA) **ADDITIONAL INFORMATION:** IgG antibody responses to certain antigens occur to a greater extent in one type of IgG subclass than another. Therefore, some patients with normal total IgG levels may have problems with pyogenic infections because they do not produce IgG_2 or combinations of IgG_2, IgG_3, and/or IgG_4. Some clinically significant IgG subclass deficiencies occur in patients who have IgA deficiency.

IgG Subclass Levels

Age (y)	IgG_1	IgG_2	IgG_3	IgG_4
0–1	190–620	30–140	9–62	6–63
1–2	230–710	30–170	11–98	4–43
2–3	280–830	40–240	6–130	3–120
3–6	350–810	50–310	9–160	5–180
>6	270–1740	30–630	13–320	11–620

References

Keren DF and Warren JS, *Diagnostic Immunology*, Baltimore, MD: Williams & Wilkins, 1992, 109-10.

Shield JP, Strobel S, Levinsky RJ, et al, "Immunodeficiency Presenting as Hypergammaglobulinemia With IgG_2 Subclass Deficiency," *Lancet*, 1992, 340(8817):448-50.

Immunoglobulin M

CPT 82784

Related Information

Immunofixation Electrophoresis *on page 707*

Protein, Total, Serum *on page 340*

Synonyms IgM; Quantitative IgM

Replaces Macroglobulins, Ultracentrifuge Determination

Specimen Serum, cerebrospinal fluid **CONTAINER:** Red top tube, sterile CSF tube **STORAGE INSTRUCTIONS:** Samples suspected of having macroglobulins or cryoglobulins should be drawn and held at 37°C. Samples suspected of containing cold agglutinins should not be refrigerated prior to serum separation from clot. **TURNAROUND TIME:** 3 days

Interpretive **REFERENCE RANGE:** Adult: 53-375 mg/dL. Pediatric (blood/mg/dL): cord 0-19; 1-3 months 7-78; 3-6 months 19-72; 6-12 months 21-104; 12-24 months 19-148; 24-36 months 40-151; 3-5 years 28-142; 5-8 years 30-162; 8-12 years 24-161; 12-16 years 26-221. **USE:** Evaluate humoral immunity; establish the diagnosis and monitor therapy in macroglobulinemia of Waldenström or plasma cell myeloma. IgM levels are used to evaluate likelihood of *in utero* infections or acuteness of infection. **LIMITATIONS:** If samples containing macroglobulins, cryoglobulins, or cold agglutinins are handled at incorrect temperatures, false low values may result. **METHODOLOGY:** Radial immunodiffusion (RID), rate nephelometry **ADDITIONAL INFORMATION:** Immunoglobulin M is a pentamer of 7S gamma globulin, and is an efficient complement binder. It is the antibody type produced initially in the immune response and the first immunoglobulin class to be synthesized by a fetus or newborn. IgM antibodies do not cross the placenta. For these reasons the demonstration of IgM-specific antibody is useful in assessing whether a particular infection is acute (in which case IgM antibodies will be present) or chronic (IgG antibodies will predominate) and whether a newborn has a congenital infection (a newborn with IgM antibody is infected; a newborn with IgG antibody has passively acquired maternal antibody, which simply crossed the placenta). In the hyper-IgM immunodeficiency syndrome, there is an absence of IgG and IgA in serum and a marked increase in IgM. Macroglobulins produced in Waldenström's disease are IgM, and may produce hyperviscosity syndrome. Monoclonal IgM is found in most cases of myeloma and provides a major diagnostic criterion. Increased IgM (with other immunoglobulins) may develop in inflammatory/infectious conditions. IgM is characteristically elevated in primary biliary cirrhosis. The majority of rheumatoid factors are IgM. IgM will be decreased in congenital or acquired hypogammaglobulinemia, and this will be associated with increased, recurrent infection. In patients with bacterial meningitis, CSF IgM is usually elevated along with C-reactive protein.

References

Gougeon ML, Morelet L, Doussau M, et al, "Hyper-IgM Immunodeficiency Syndrome: Influence of Lymphokines on *In Vitro* Maturation of Peripheral B Cells," *J Clin Immunol*, 1992, 12(2):92-100.

Jeske DJ and Capra JD, "Immunoglobulins: Structure and Function," *Fundamental Immunology*, Paul WE, ed, New York, NY: Raven Press, 1984, 131-65.

Jones RG, Aguzzi F, Bienvenu J, et al, "Use of Immunoglobulin Heavy-Chain and Light-Chain Measurements in a Multicenter Trial to Investigate Monoclonal Components: I. Detection," *Clin Chem*, 1991, 37(11):1917-21.

Ribeiro MA, Kimura RT, Irulegui I, et al, "Cerebrospinal Fluid Levels of Lysozyme, IgM, and C-Reactive Protein in the Identification of Bacterial Meningitis," *J Trop Med Hyg*, 1992, 95(2):87-94.

Wall R and Kuehl M, "Biosynthesis and Regulation of Immunoglobulins," *Annu Rev Immunol*, 1983, 1:393-422.

Immunoglobulins *see* Protein Electrophoresis, Serum *on page 734*

Immunophenotyping *see* Lymphocyte Subset Enumeration *on page 720*

IM Serology *see* Infectious Mononucleosis Screening Test *on this page*

Infectious Mononucleosis Screening Test

CPT *86403*

Related Information

Epstein-Barr Virus Culture *on page 1179*
Epstein-Barr Virus Serology *on page 676*
Heterophil Agglutinins *on page 694*
Human Herpesvirus 6, IgG and IgM Antibodies, Quantitative *on page 703*
Lymph Node Biopsy *on page 72*
Peripheral Blood: Differential Leukocyte Count *on page 576*

Synonyms IM Serology; Monospot™ Test; Monosticon® Dri-Dot® Test; Mono Test

Replaces Davidsohn Differential; Paul-Bunnell Test

Test Commonly Includes Screening for the presence of heterophil antibodies

Specimen Serum **CONTAINER:** Red top tube

Interpretive **REFERENCE RANGE:** Negative **USE:** Diagnose infectious mononucleosis **LIMITATIONS:** Correlation with clinical findings is imperative since false-positive and negative results have been reported. About 10% of the adult population with infectious mononucleosis will not develop heterophil antibodies. Failure to develop heterophil antibodies occurs even more frequently in children. In such instances, the presence of Epstein-Barr virus antibodies is relevant. Less than 2% false-positives have been reported with Hodgkin's disease, lymphoma, acute lymphocytic leukemia, infectious hepatitis, pancreatic carcinoma, cytomegalovirus, Burkitt's lymphoma, rheumatoid arthritis, malaria, and rubella. Rare unexplained positive horse cell screening tests have been reported with negative differential absorptions. Overall, the Monospot™ test has 99% specificity and 86% sensitivity. **METHODOLOGY:** Agglutination, immune adherence **ADDITIONAL INFORMATION:** The infectious mononucleosis heterophil antibody appears in the serum of patients by the sixth to tenth day of illness. Highest titers are usually found in the second to third week. Antibody levels may remain detectable for as little as 1 week or persist up to a year; usual persistence is 4-8 weeks. The level of antibody activity is not correlated with the severity of disease or the degree of lymphocytosis. A positive screening or differential test in the appropriate clinical and hematologic setting is sufficient to make the diagnosis of infectious mononucleosis. If there is clinically a mononucleosis syndrome, but the screening test is negative, consider tests for EBV specific antibodies, CMV, HHV-6, and toxoplasmosis antibodies. Consider, as well, repeating this test after a short delay. The peripheral blood smear should be carefully examined.

References

Evans AS and Niederman JC, "EBV-IgA and New Heterophil Antibody Tests in Diagnosis of Infectious Mononucleosis," *Am J Clin Pathol*, 1982, 77:555-60.

Fleisher GR, Collins M, and Fager S, "Limitations of Available Tests for Diagnosis of Infectious Mononucleosis," *J Clin Microbiol*, 1983, 17:619-24.

Horwitz CA, Henle W, Henle G, et al, "Persistent Falsely Positive Rapid Tests for Infectious Mononucleosis. Report of Five Cases with 4-6 Year Follow-Up Data," *Am J Clin Pathol*, 1979, 72:807-11.

Lee CL, Davidsohn I, and Slaby R, "Horse Agglutinins in Infectious Mononucleosis," *Am J Clin Pathol*, 1968, 49:3-11.

Vahlne A, Uertborn M, and Iwarson S, "Mumps Occurring as a Mononucleosis-Like Syndrome With Positive Monospot™ Test," *JAMA*, 1979, 242:711, (letter).

Influenza A and B Antibodies *see* Influenza A and B Titer *on this page*

Influenza A and B Titer

CPT *86710 (each)*

Related Information

Influenza Virus Culture *on page 1186*
Virus, Direct Detection by Fluorescent Antibody *on page 1208*
(Continued)

Influenza A and B Titer *(Continued)*

Synonyms Influenza A and B Antibodies

Test Commonly Includes IgG and IgM antibody titers to influenza A and/or B

Specimen Serum **CONTAINER:** Red top tube **COLLECTION:** Acute and convalescent sera drawn 10-14 days apart are required.

Interpretive **REFERENCE RANGE:** Less than a fourfold increase in titer in paired sera; IgG <1:10, IgM <1:10 **USE:** Establish the diagnosis of influenza virus infection; epidemiologic surveillance and tracking; differentiate type A from B for treatment with amantadine **METHODOLOGY:** Complement fixation (CF), hemagglutination inhibition (HAI), single radial immunodiffusion (RID), enzyme immunoassay (EIA) **ADDITIONAL INFORMATION:** Influenza virus is typed by specifying a neuraminidase and hemagglutinin. Although serologic diagnosis is seldom practical (or necessary) during an influenza epidemic, serologic typing is valuable for epidemiology, and for planning therapy. Since type A influenza can be treated with amantadine, but type B cannot, this distinction may need to be made. Presence of specific IgM antibody indicates acute infection.

References

Bryan JA, "The Serologic Diagnosis of Viral Infections," *Arch Pathol Lab Med*, 1987, 111:1015-23.

Sperber SJ and Hayden FG, "Antiviral Chemotherapy and Prophylaxis of Viral Respiratory Disease," *Clin Lab Med*, 1987, 7:869-96.

Walls H, Harmon MW, Slagle J, et al, "Characterization and Evaluation of Monoclonal Antibodies Developed for Typing Influenza A and Influenza B Viruses," *J Clin Microbiol*, 1986, 23:240-5.

Intercellular Antibody Basement Membrane Antibody *see* Immunofluorescence, Skin Biopsy *on page 708*

Intrinsic Factor Antibody

***CPT** 86340*

Related Information

Folic Acid, Serum *on page 545*
Gastric Analysis *on page 232*
Parietal Cell Antibody *on page 730*
Schilling Test *on page 598*
Vitamin B_{12} *on page 612*
Vitamin B_{12} Unsaturated Binding Capacity *on page 615*

Synonyms IF Antibody

Abstract Patients with pernicious anemia commonly develop antibodies to intrinsic factor.

Specimen Serum **CONTAINER:** Red top tube **CAUSES FOR REJECTION:** Patient having received recent radioactive scan, B_{12} injection within the past 48 hours

Interpretive **REFERENCE RANGE:** None detected **USE:** Differentiate pernicious anemia (PA) from other megaloblastic anemias **METHODOLOGY:** Radioimmunoassay (RIA) **ADDITIONAL INFORMATION:** Antibodies to intrinsic factor are found in very high percentage of children with juvenile pernicious anemia. Approximately 50% to 75% of adult patients have intrinsic factor antibodies. There are two types of antibody. Type I, blocking antibody, the more common, prevents the binding of B_{12} and intrinsic factor, but will not react with complexed intrinsic factor. Type II antibody, or binding antibody, reacts with either free or complexed intrinsic factor. Blocking antibody is extremely specific for PA and is more sensitive than binding antibody. A proportion of patients have IgA intrinsic factor antibody in gastric juice (serum antibody is IgG). Intrinsic factor antibody may be especially useful as an adjunct to serum vitamin B_{12} levels to detect vitamin B_{12} malabsorption in the elderly.

References

Bunting RW, Bitzer AM, Kenney RM, et al, "Prevalence of Intrinsic Factor Antibodies and Vitamin B_{12} Malabsorption in Older Patients Admitted to a Rehabilitation Hospital," *J Am Geriatr Soc*, 1990, 38(7):743-7.

Harty RF and Leibach JR, "Immune Disorders of the Gastrointestinal Tract and Liver," *Med Clin North Am*, 1985, 69:675-704.

Kahn Test *replaced by* RPR *on page 742*

Kahn Test *replaced by* VDRL, Serum *on page 762*

Kala-azar Serological Test *see* Leishmaniasis Serological Test *on page 717*

Kappa and Lambda Light Chains Detection *see* Immunoelectrophoresis, Serum or Urine *on page 706*

Kappa Chains *see* Immunofixation Electrophoresis *on page 707*

Kline Test *replaced by* RPR *on page 742*

Kline Test *replaced by* VDRL, Serum *on page 762*

La Antibodies *see* Sjögren's Antibodies *on page 746*

LaCrosse Virus Titer *see* California Encephalitis Virus Titer *on page 651*

Lambda Chains *see* Immunofixation Electrophoresis *on page 707*

LATS *see* Thyrotropin-Receptor Antibody *on page 756*

LATS Protector *see* Thyrotropin-Receptor Antibody *on page 756*

L. bosemanii *see Legionella pneumophila* Direct FA Smear *on this page*

L. bosemanii *see* Legionnaires' Disease Antibodies *on next page*

L. dumoffii *see Legionella pneumophila* Direct FA Smear *on this page*

L. dumoffii *see* Legionnaires' Disease Antibodies *on next page*

LE Antibodies *see* Immunofluorescence, Skin Biopsy *on page 708*

***Legionella pneumophila* Antibodies** *see* Legionnaires' Disease Antibodies *on next page*

***Legionella pneumophila* Antigen** *see Legionella pneumophila* Direct FA Smear *on this page*

Legionella pneumophila Direct FA Smear

CPT *87206*

Related Information

Legionella Culture *on page 825*
Legionnaires' Disease Antibodies *on next page*
Sputum Culture *on page 849*

Synonyms FA Smear for *Legionella pneumophila*; *Legionella pneumophila* Antigen

Applies to *L. bosemanii*; *L. dumoffii*; *L. gormanii*; *L. jordanis*; *L. longbeachae*; *L. micdadei*

Test Commonly Includes Direct fluorescent antibody (DFA) microscopic examination of specimen smear

Specimen Lung tissue, other body tissue, pleural fluid, other body fluid, transtracheal aspirate, sputum, bronchial washing **CONTAINER:** Sterile container **COLLECTION:** Contamination with normal flora from skin or other body surfaces should be avoided. **CAUSES FOR REJECTION:** Saliva sent rather than sputum specimen

Interpretive **REFERENCE RANGE:** No *Legionella pneumophila* seen in direct FA microscopic examination **USE:** Determine the presence of *Legionella pneumophila* organisms in direct smear of specimen by fluorescent antibody, providing rapid diagnosis **LIMITATIONS:** Staining for several serogroups may be necessary **METHODOLOGY:** Direct fluorescent antibody (DFA) **ADDITIONAL INFORMATION:** Community acquired and nosocomial infections caused by multiple serogroups of *Legionella* are increasingly recognized. Although culture is now possible on buffered charcoal yeast extract agar, the demonstration of organisms in tissue or brushings is the fastest way to make the diagnosis. It also has the advantage of applicability to specimens contaminated with other bacteria. Development of monoclonal antibodies have increased sensitivity and specificity. False-positive reaction has been reported in a case of pleuropulmonary *Tularemia* and in cases of *Campylobacter* infection.[1,2] A combination of both culture and antigen detection is recommended.

Footnotes

1. Andersen LP and Bangsborg J, "Cross Reactions Between *Legionella* and *Campylobacter* Species," *Lancet*, 1992, 340(8813):245.
2. Roy TM, Fleming D, and Anderson WH, "Tularemic Pneumonia Mimicking Legionnaires' Disease With False-Positive Direct Fluorescent Antibody Stains for *Legionella*," *South Med J*, 1989, 82:1429-31.

References

Edelstein PH, Beer KB, Sturge JC, et al, "Clinical Utility of a Monoclonal Direct Fluorescent Reagent Specific for *Legionella pneumophila*: Comparative Study With Other Reagents," *J Clin Microbiol*, 1985, 22:419-21.

Hart CA and Makin T, "*Legionella* in Hospitals: A Review," *J Hosp Infect*, 1991, 18(Suppl A):481-9.

***Legionella pneumophila*, IgM** *see* Legionnaires' Disease Antibodies, IgM *on this page*

***Legionella pneumophila* Titer** *see* Legionnaires' Disease Antibodies *on this page*

Legionnaires' Disease Antibodies

CPT 86713

Related Information

Legionella Culture *on page 825*
Legionella pneumophila Direct FA Smear *on previous page*
Legionnaires' Disease Antibodies, IgM *on this page*
Sputum Culture *on page 849*

Synonyms *Legionella pneumophila* Antibodies; *Legionella pneumophila* Titer; Legionnaires', Indirect Fluorescent Antibody

Applies to *L. bosemanii*; *L. dumoffii*; *L. gormanii*; *L. jordanis*; *L. longbeachae*; *L. micdadei*

Test Commonly Includes Detection of antibody (IgG or IgA) to *Legionella pneumophila*

Specimen Serum **CONTAINER:** Red top tube **COLLECTION:** A convalescent sample is recommended to be drawn 10-14 days after acute sample

Interpretive **REFERENCE RANGE:** Negative. Less than a fourfold change in titer between acute and convalescent samples; <1:256 in a single sample **USE:** Support for the clinical diagnosis of Legionnaires' disease; determine stage of disease **LIMITATIONS:** Testing for multiple serogroups may be necessary. **METHODOLOGY:** Indirect fluorescent antibody (IFA) assay using serogroup 1: Philadelphia, Knoxville, serogroup 2: Togus, serogroup 3: Los Angeles, serogroup 4: Bloomington. When available a polyvalent antigen, which includes serogroup 1-6, is utilized. Latex agglutination (LA). **ADDITIONAL INFORMATION:** A fourfold rise in titer >1:128 from the acute to convalescent phase provides evidence of recent infection. A single titer ≥1:256 is evidence of infection at an undetermined time. However, due to the relatively high prevalence of antibodies to *Legionella pneumophila*, acute and convalescent titers are preferred to a single sample. Demonstration of a high titer in the proper clinical setting may allow timely institution of specific treatment, and may eliminate the need for an invasive procedure to obtain a specimen for culture or direct immunofluorescence. Demonstration of IgM antibody to serogroup I may allow rapid diagnosis. Recent availability of a latex agglutination test with 98.3% specificity and 97.6% sensitivity is well suited as a screening test. Serologic study is also valuable in evaluation of epidemic disease. The presence of IgM in high titer is evidence for acute infection.

References

Holliday MG, "Use of Latex Agglutination Technique for Detecting *Legionella pneumophila* (Serogroup 1) Antibodies," *J Clin Pathol*, 1990, 43(10):860-2.

Nichol KL, Parenti CM, and Johnson JE, "High Prevalence of Positive Antibodies to *Legionella pneumophila* Among Outpatients," *Chest*, 1991, 100(3):663-6.

Wilkinson HW, Reingold AL, Brake BJ, et al, "Reactivity of Serum from Patients With Suspected Legionellosis Against 29 Antigens of Legionellaceae and *Legionella*-Like Organisms by Indirect Immunofluorescence Assay," *J Infect Dis*, 1983, 147:23-31.

Legionnaires' Disease Antibodies, IgM

CPT 86713

Related Information

Legionella Culture *on page 825*
Legionnaires' Disease Antibodies *on this page*
Sputum Culture *on page 849*

Synonyms *Legionella pneumophila*, IgM; Legionnaires' IgM, Indirect Fluorescent Antibody

Test Commonly Includes Legionnaires' IgM by IFA

Specimen Serum **CONTAINER:** Red top tube **COLLECTION:** Acute and convalescent sera drawn 10-14 days apart are recommended.

Interpretive **REFERENCE RANGE:** Titer: <1:256 **USE:** Diagnose acute Legionnaires' disease **METHODOLOGY:** Indirect fluorescent antibody (IFA) **ADDITIONAL INFORMATION:** Since IgM is the initial immunoglobulin produced in the immune response, its presence in high titer is supportive evidence for acute infection. Demonstration of IgM antibody to *Legionella pneumophila* may speed the specific diagnosis of Legionnaires' disease.

References

Zimmerman SE, French MIV, Allen SD, et al, "Immunoglobulin M Antibody Titers in the Diagnosis of Legionnaires' Disease," *J Clin Microbiol*, 1982, 16:1007-11.

Legionnaires' IgM, Indirect Fluorescent Antibody *see* Legionnaires' Disease Antibodies, IgM *on previous page*

Legionnaires', Indirect Fluorescent Antibody *see* Legionnaires' Disease Antibodies *on previous page*

***Leishmania braziliensis* Serological Test** *see* Leishmaniasis Serological Test *on this page*

***Leishmania donovani* Serological Test** *see* Leishmaniasis Serological Test *on this page*

Leishmaniasis Serological Test

CPT *86717*

Related Information

Bone Marrow *on page 524*
Lymph Node Biopsy *on page 72*
Parasite Antibodies *on page 729*
Protein Electrophoresis, Serum *on page 734*
Skin Biopsies *on page 84*

Synonyms Espundia Serological Test; Kala-azar Serological Test; *Leishmania braziliensis* Serological Test; *Leishmania donovani* Serological Test; *Leishmania tropica* Serological Test; Oriental Sore Serological Test

Test Commonly Includes Detection of antibody to the parasite *Leishmania* sp

Abstract Visceral leishmaniasis (kala-azar) is typically caused by *Leishmania donovani*. It parasitizes reticuloendothelial cells, and is found in spleen, bone marrow, liver, and lymph nodes. Cutaneous and mucocutaneous leishmaniasis are the other major types.

Specimen Serum **CONTAINER:** Red top tube

Interpretive **REFERENCE RANGE:** Negative **USE:** Support the clinical diagnosis of visceral leishmaniasis, cutaneous leishmaniasis, and mucocutaneous leishmaniasis **LIMITATIONS:** Cross reactivity with trypanosomiasis; false-positives in malaria **METHODOLOGY:** Indirect hemagglutination (IHA), indirect fluorescent antibody (IFA), complement fixation (CF), enzyme-linked immunosorbent assay (ELISA), immunodot assay **ADDITIONAL INFORMATION:** Serodiagnosis of visceral leishmaniasis is more reliable than serodiagnosis of cutaneous disease, although this has been improved by the use of direct agglutination tests. An ELISA test is positive in 85% of cases. There has been a flurry of reports of visceral leishmaniasis with atypical features in patients with AIDS. Splenomegaly, a major feature in other patients is often absent in AIDS patients. Massive polyclonal IgG gammopathy on serum protein electrophoresis is characteristic of kala-azar. Leukopenia, thrombocytopenia, and anemia are found. Bone marrow aspiration provides diagnostic organisms. *L. tropica*, which usually causes cutaneous disease, produced visceral infection in soldiers returning from Desert Storm.[1]

Footnotes

1. Magill AJ, Grögl M, Gasser RA Jr, et al, "Visceral Infection Caused by *Leishmania tropica* in Veterans of Operation Desert Storm," *N Engl J Med*, 1993, 328(19):1383-7.

References

Borowy NK, Schell D, Schafer C, et al, "Diagnosis of African Trypanosomiasis and Visceral Leishmaniasis Based on the Detection of Anti-Parasite-Enzyme Antibodies," *J Infect Dis*, 1991, 164(2):422-5.

Grimaldi G Jr and Tesh RB, "Leishmaniases of the New World: Current Concepts and Implications for Future Research," *Clin Microbiol Rev*, 1993, 6(3):230-50.

Jones TC, Johnson WD, Banetto AC, et al, "Epidemiology of American Cutaneous Leishmaniasis Due to *Leishmania braziliensis*," *J Infect Dis*, 1987, 156:73-83.

Kagan IG and Maddison SE, "Serodiagnosis of Parasitic Diseases," *Manual of Clinical Laboratory Immunology*, 4th ed, Vol 2, Chapter 79, Rose NR, Conway de Macario E, Fahey JL, et al, eds, Washington, DC: American Society for Microbiology, 1992, 529-43.

Peters BS, Fish D, Golden R, et al, "Visceral Leishmaniasis in HIV Infection and AIDS: Clinical Features and Response to Therapy," *Q J Med*, 1990, 77(283):1101-11.

***Leishmania tropica* Serological Test** *see* Leishmaniasis Serological Test *on this page*

***Leptospira* Agglutination** *see* Bacterial Serology *on page 644*

***Leptospira* Antibodies** *see* *Leptospira* Serodiagnosis *on next page*

Leptospira Serodiagnosis

CPT 86720

Related Information

Darkfield Examination, Leptospirosis *on page 808*
Leptospira Culture, Urine *on page 827*

Synonyms *Leptospira* Antibodies

Test Commonly Includes Testing of patient's serum for antibodies against *Leptospira biflexa* serovar *L. patoc*, and the following serovars of *Leptospira interrogans*: *L. copenhageni*, *L. canicola*, *L. pomona*, *L. autumnalis*, *L. grippotyphosa*, *L. wolffi*, and *L. djatzi*. Supplemental testing may be needed against serovars: *L. poi*, *L. castellonis*, *L. pyrogenes*, *L. borincana*, *L. szwajizak*, *L. bratislava*, *L. tarassovi*, *L. shermani*, *L. panama*, *L. celledoni*, *L. djasiman*, *L. cynopteri*, and *L. louisiana*.

Abstract Leptospirosis is a febrile zoonotic disease occurring in all parts of the world. The disease can be mild to severe with general symptoms of fever, malaise, muscle aches, and headache.

Specimen Serum **CONTAINER:** Red top tube **SAMPLING TIME:** Acute and convalescent sera drawn 10-14 days apart are suggested. **CAUSES FOR REJECTION:** Inadequate labeling, excessive hemolysis, lipemic serum, or gross contamination of the specimen

Interpretive **REFERENCE RANGE:** Negative. A fourfold increase in titer in paired sera is diagnostic of infection. **USE:** Support the diagnosis of leptospirosis **LIMITATIONS:** The antigens used in the test are the ones most commonly causing disease, but there are many other serovars which might not be detected. A battery of antigens should be used. **METHODOLOGY:** Microscopic agglutination test, macroagglutination, complement fixation (CF), hemagglutination, enzyme-linked immunosorbent assay (ELISA) **ADDITIONAL INFORMATION:** Leptospirosis is an acute febrile illness caused primarily by *Leptospira interrogans*, a large spirochete with over 180 serologic variants. Patients with extensive animal contact, either in the wild or with carcasses or excrement, are particularly at risk. Although leptospires can be cultured from blood or urine during the first week of illness, this interval is often missed, and diagnosis must be based on the demonstration of rising antibody titers. Antibody appears at the end of the first week of illness and peaks at 3-4 weeks, after which it slowly disappears. Interestingly there has been an association between patients with leptospirosis and anticardiolipin antibodies which may induce vascular endothelial injury in severe cases.[1]

Footnotes

1. Rugman FP, Pinn G, Palmer MF, et al, "Anticardiolipin Antibodies in Leptospirosis," *J Clin Pathol*, 1991, 44(6):517-9.

References

Larsen SA, Pope V, and Quan TJ, "Immunologic Methods for the Diagnosis of Spirochetal Diseases," *Manual of Clinical Laboratory Immunology*, 4th ed, Vol 2, Chapter 73, Rose NR, Conway de Macario E, Fahey JL, et al, eds, Washington, DC: American Society for Microbiology, 1992, 467-81.

Raoult D, Bres P, and Baranton G, "Serologic Diagnosis of Leptospirosis: Comparison of Line Blot and Immunofluorescence Techniques With the Genus-Specific Microscopic Agglutination Test," *J Infect Dis*, 1989, 160(4):734-5.

Ribeiro MA, Sakata EE, Silva MV, et al, "Antigens Involved in the Human Antibody Response to Natural Infections With *Leptospira interrogans* serovar *copenhageni*," *J Trop Med Hyg*, 1992, 95(4):239-45.

Leptospirosis Antibody Titers *see* Bacterial Serology *on page 644*

L. gormanii *see Legionella pneumophila* Direct FA Smear *on page 715*

L. gormanii *see* Legionnaires' Disease Antibodies *on page 716*

LGV Titer *see* Lymphogranuloma Venereum Titer *on page 722*

Light Chains *see* Immunoelectrophoresis, Serum or Urine *on page 706*

Light Chains *see* Immunofixation Electrophoresis *on page 707*

Light Chains *see* Protein Electrophoresis, Serum *on page 734*

Light Chains, Urine *see* Protein Electrophoresis, Urine *on page 737*

Liver/Kidney Microsomes (LKM) Antibody *see* Smooth Muscle Antibody *on page 747*

L. jordanis *see Legionella pneumophila* Direct FA Smear *on page 715*

L. jordanis *see* Legionnaires' Disease Antibodies *on page 716*

L. longbeachae *see Legionella pneumophila* Direct FA Smear *on page 715*

Lyme Disease Serology

CPT *84181 (western blot); 84182 (immunological probe for ID); 86618 (antibody)*

Related Information

Babesiosis Serological Test *on page 643*

Lyme Disease DNA Detection *on page 920*

Synonyms Lyme Arthritis Serology

Test Commonly Includes Detection of serological response to *Borrelia burgdorferi*

Abstract The diagnosis of Lyme borreliosis is difficult for the clinician and presents problems as well for the clinical laboratory. Clinical and laboratory data require integration.[1] Laboratory capabilities have been frustrating.

Specimen Serum or cerebrospinal fluid **CONTAINER:** Red top tube, sterile CSF tube

Interpretive **REFERENCE RANGE:** Values vary among laboratories **USE:** Diagnose Lyme disease **LIMITATIONS:** Some cases are seronegative; there are cross reactions with antibodies to EB virus, *Rickettsia*, syphilis. There is significant inter- and intralaboratory variation in this assay which highlights the relatively poor assays currently available. Even the Western blot is not considered a definitive assay. Consequently serologic evidence should not be the sole criterion for a diagnosis of Lyme disease. Positive serologic results in apparently healthy subjects are likely to be false-positives. Positive results must be considered critically.[1] **METHODOLOGY:** Screen: enzyme immunoassay (EIA), enzyme-linked immunosorbent assay (ELISA), indirect fluorescent (IFA); confirmation: Western blot **ADDITIONAL INFORMATION:** Lyme disease is a multisystem disorder, with rash and arthritis conspicuous symptoms. It is widespread in the US and is caused by *Borrelia burgdorferi*, a spirochete transmitted by the bite of the tick *Ixodes dammini*, which also transmits *Babesia*. The disease has protean manifestation, can become chronic, and responds to antibiotics; prompt proper diagnosis is therefore important. Assay is available for IgG and IgM antibody in both serum and CSF. In early disease a negative assay does not exclude the diagnosis because sensitivity is 40% to 60% and response may be blunted by antibiotics. All patients with chronic disease will have positive assays. Recent studies using recombinant outer surface protein A and B and flagellin hold out promise for better serologic testing in the near future.[2,3] Patients may harbor *B. burgdorferi* asymptomatically and have positive serology. Such individuals may have symptoms of some other illness incorrectly attributed to Lyme disease and be given inappropriate and ineffective treatment. Antibodies against Lyme disease antigens can interfere with the ANA test.

Cultivation of *B. burgdorferi* from skin lesions suggestive of erythema migrans is recently described as a practical and clinically relevant procedure.[4]

Neurologic manifestations are found in about 15% of subjects. CSF pleocytosis is found in many but not all patients who have cranial nerve or meningeal involvement.[5] *Borrelia*-specific DNA using PCR assay has been compared to conventional serologic testing.[6] See listing in Molecular Pathology chapter, Lyme Disease DNA Detection.

Footnotes

1. Golightly MG, "Laboratory Considerations in the Diagnosis and Management of Lyme Borreliosis," *Am J Clin Pathol*, 1993, 99(2):168-74.
2. Fikrig E, Huguenel ED, Berland R, et al, "Serological Diagnosis of Lyme Disease Using Recombinant Outer Surface Proteins A and B and Flagellin," *J Infect Dis*, 1992, 165(6):1127-32.
3. Robinson JM, Pilot-Matias TJ, Pratt SD, et al, "Analysis of the Humoral Response to the Flagellin Protein of *Borrelia burgdorferi*: Cloning of Regions Capable of Differentiating Lyme Disease From Syphilis," *J Clin Microbiol*, 1993, 31(3):629-35.
4. Mitchell PD, Reed KD, Vandermause MF, et al, "Isolation of *Borrelia burgdorferi* From Skin Biopsy Specimens of Patients With Erythema Migrans," *Am J Clin Pathol*, 1993, 99(1):104-7.
5. Kaslow RA, "Current Perspective on Lyme Borreliosis," *JAMA*, 1992, 267(10):1381-3.

(Continued)

Lyme Disease Serology *(Continued)*

6. Luft BJ, Steinman CR, Neimark HC, et al, "Invasion of the Central Nervous System by *Borrelia burgdorferi* in Acute Disseminated Infection," *JAMA*, 1992, 267(10):1364-7.

References

Bakken LL, Case KL, Callister SM, et al, "Performance of 45 Laboratories Participating in a Proficiency Testing Program for Lyme Disease Serology," *JAMA*, 1992, 268(7):891-5.

Barbour AG, "The Diagnosis of Lyme Disease: Rewards and Perils," *Ann Intern Med*, 1989, 110(7):501-2.

Berardi VP, Weeks, KE, and Steere AC, "Serodiagnosis of Early Lyme Disease: Analysis of IgM and IgG Antibody Responses by Using an Antibody-Capture Enzyme Immunoassay," *J Infect Dis*, 1988, 158:754-60.

Dattwyler RJ, Volkman DJ, Luft BJ, et al, "Seronegative Lyme Disease," *N Engl J Med*, 1988, 319:1441-6.

Duffy J, Mertz LE, Wobig GH, et al, "Diagnosing Lyme Disease: The Contributions of Serologic Testing," *Mayo Clin Proc*, 1988, 63:1116-21.

Lovece S, Stern R, and Kagen LJ, "Effects of Rheumatoid Factor, Antinuclear Antibodies and Plasma Reagin on the Serologic Assay for Lyme Disease," *J Rheumatol*, 1991, 18(12):1813-8.

Magid D, Schwartz B, Craft J, et al, "Prevention of Lyme Disease After Tick Bites: A Cost-Effectiveness Analysis," *N Engl J Med*, 1992, 327(8):534-41.

Magnarelli LA, Anderson JF, and Johnson RC, "Cross Reactivity in Serological Tests for Lyme Disease and Other Spirochetal Infections," *J Infect Dis*, 1987, 156:183-7.

Steere AC, "Lyme Disease," *N Engl J Med*, 1989, 321(9):586-96.

Lymphocyte CD4 Counts *see* Lymphocyte Subset Enumeration *on this page*

Lymphocyte Crossmatch *see* Tissue Typing *on page 757*

Lymphocyte Marker Studies *see* T- and B-Lymphocyte Subset Assay *on page 750*

Lymphocyte Mitogen Response Test *see* Lymphocyte Transformation Test *on page 722*

Lymphocyte Receptor Studies *see* T- and B-Lymphocyte Subset Assay *on page 750*

Lymphocyte Subset Analyses *see* T- and B-Lymphocyte Subset Assay *on page 750*

Lymphocyte Subset Enumeration

CPT 88180

Related Information

Complete Blood Count *on page 533*
HIV-1/HIV-2 Serology *on page 696*
Human Immunodeficiency Virus Culture *on page 1185*
Peripheral Blood: Differential Leukocyte Count *on page 576*
T- and B-Lymphocyte Subset Assay *on page 750*
White Blood Count *on page 616*
Zidovudine *on page 1012*

Synonyms Immunodeficiency Profile; Immunophenotyping; Lymphocyte Typing

Applies to Lymphocyte CD4 Counts

Test Commonly Includes Lymphocyte subpopulation enumeration

Abstract Depletion of $CD4^+$ helper/inducer T lymphocytes is the single most significant surrogate marker to study progression of human immunodeficiency virus disease.[1]

Specimen Whole blood or bone marrow; check with the laboratory performing the assay for volume required. **CONTAINER:** Yellow top (ACD) tube preferred or green top (heparin) tube **STORAGE INSTRUCTIONS:** Blood ideally is delivered to the laboratory immediately, however whole blood may be held for 48 hours at room temperature prior to assay. Do not refrigerate or freeze sample. **SPECIAL INSTRUCTIONS:** Must schedule with laboratory in advance. Laboratory requirements may vary.

Interpretive **REFERENCE RANGE:** Total lymphocytes: 1500-4000/mL; CD20 cells: 64-475/mL; CD3 cells: 876-1900/mL; CD4 cells: 450-1400/mL; CD8 cells: 190-725/mL; CD4/CD8 ratio: 1.0-3.5 **USE:** Follow patients with HIV infection (CD4 cells <200/mL often indicate progression to clinical AIDS); evaluate thymus-dependent or cellular immunocompetence; enumerate T-helper:T-suppressor ratio; study lymphoproliferative disorders for clonality and lineage. CD4 counts are useful in prediction of the clinical course of *Cryptosporidium* infections.[2] **LIMITATIONS:** Values can be abnormal if patient is taking steroids or other immunosuppressives, has a severe intercurrent illness, or has had recent surgery requiring general anesthesia; patterns

Antibodies Commonly Used in Lymphocyte Subset Enumeration

Use	Cluster Designation	Available Antibodies
Pan T	CD2	T11, Leu5
Pan T (T-cell antigen receptor)	CD3	T3, Leu4
T helper/inducer	CD4	T4, Leu3
T suppressor/cytotoxic	CD8	T8, Leu2
T-cell ALL/B-cell CLL	CD5	T1, Leu1
T-cell ALL	CD7	3A1, Leu9
CALLA, ALL	CD10	J5, BA-3
Pan B	CD19	B4, Leu12
B cell specific	CD20	B1, Leu16
Mature B (EBV receptor)	CD21	B2
Myeloid/monocytic	CD13	MY7
Myeloid/monocytic	CD33	MY9
Myeloid adhesion	CD11	Mo1, Mac1
Glycoprotein II b/Ma megakaryocytes	CDw41	J15

of maturation are disordered and inconsistent in lymphomas. **METHODOLOGY:** Flow cytometry (FC); numeration of specific subpopulation with batteries of monoclonal antibodies to lymphocyte, myeloid, and precursor antigens (see table) **ADDITIONAL INFORMATION:** With increased understanding of the functional and immunologic subpopulations of circulating and nodal lymphocytes, and with the commercial availability of monoclonal antibodies to the antigens that define those populations, enumeration of lymphocyte classes has become both possible and clinically important. In the diagnosis and classification of malignant lymphoproliferative disorders, the demonstration of a homogeneous B- or T-lymphocyte population often contributes to prognosis and therapeutic planning. The lineage and stages of development of the proliferating cells can be determined. The demonstration of a reversed T-helper:T-suppressor ratio (<1.0) is important in the diagnosis of acquired immune deficiency syndrome (AIDS) and also helps explain pathogenetically the multiple recurrent opportunistic infections which comprise that illness. The absolute number of T4 cells is crucial in instituting and following treatment with AZT.

Subjects whose CD4 count is <300-400/mm^3, with progressive decline in absolute CD4 count as well as CD4:CD8 ratio less than unity should be intensively worked up for HIV infection and other entities which cause immunodeficiency.

Idiopathic CD4$^+$ T lymphocytopenia is defined by the Centers for Disease Control and Prevention as CD4$^+$ T lymphocytopenia without serologic or virologic evidence of HIV-1 or HIV-2 infection. The diagnosis requires a CD4 count <300/mm^3 on two occasions.[1]

Footnotes

1. Laurence J, "T-Cell Subsets in Health, Infectious Disease, and Idiopathic CD4$^+$ T Lymphocytopenia," *Ann Intern Med*, 1993, 119(1):55-62.
2. Flanigan T, Whalen C, Turner J, et al, "*Cryptosporidium* Infection and CD4 Counts," *Ann Intern Med*, 1992, 116(10):840-2.

References

Calabrese LH, "Autoimmune Manifestations of Human Immunodeficiency Virus (HIV) Infection," *Clin Lab Med*, 1988, 8:269-80.

Colvin RB, Bhan AK, and McCluskey RT, eds, *Diagnostic Immunopathology*, New York, NY: Raven Press, 1988, 275-9.

Davey FR, ed, "Classification, Diagnosis, and Molecular Biology of Lymphoproliferative Disorders," *Clin Lab Med*, 1988, 8:1-252.

Drusano GL, Yuen GJ, Lambert JS, et al, "Relationship Between Dideoxyinosine Exposure, CD4 Counts, and p24 Antigen Levels in Human Immunodeficiency Virus Infection," *Ann Intern Med*, 1992, 116(7):562-6.

Gottlieb MS, Groopman UE, and Weinstein WM, "The Acquired Immunodeficiency Syndrome," *Ann Intern Med*, 1983, 99:208-20.

Keren DF, Hanson CA, and Hurtubise P, "Flow Cytometry in Clinical Diagnosis," Chicago, IL: ASCP Press, 1993, 333-43.

(Continued)

Lymphocyte Subset Enumeration *(Continued)*

Quinnan GV JR, Siegel JP, Epstein JS, et al, "Mechanisms of T Cell Functional Deficiency in the Acquired Immunodeficiency Syndrome," *Ann Intern Med*, 1985, 103:710-4.

Lymphocyte Subset Identification *see* T- and B-Lymphocyte Subset Assay *on page 750*

Lymphocyte Subset Typing *see* T- and B-Lymphocyte Subset Assay *on page 750*

Lymphocyte Surface Immunoglobulin Analysis *see* T- and B-Lymphocyte Subset Assay *on page 750*

Lymphocyte Transformation Test

CPT *86353*

Synonyms Lymphocyte Mitogen Response Test; PHA Stimulation

Test Commonly Includes Phytohemagglutinin, Pokeweed and Concanavalin A mitogen testing by thymidine uptake; comparison to normals

Specimen Whole blood **CONTAINER:** Yellow top (ACD) tube preferred or green top (heparin) tube. Check with the laboratory performing the assay for special instructions. **CAUSES FOR REJECTION:** Old specimen, specimen without viable lymphocytes, specimen refrigerated or frozen **SPECIAL INSTRUCTIONS:** Schedule procedure in advance with laboratory. Specimens to evaluate therapy should include three baseline samples.

Interpretive **REFERENCE RANGE:** Mitogen: phytohemagglutinin (PHA), stimulation index >130; mitogen: pokeweed mitogen (PWM), stimulation index >20; mitogen: concanavalin A (con A), stimulation index >40 **USE:** Study of cellular immune response in congenital immune deficits, histocompatibility testing, immunosuppression **METHODOLOGY:** Lymphocytes transformed by plant mitogens take up tritiated thymidine, flow cytometry measure of S-phase fraction **ADDITIONAL INFORMATION:** With the availability of monoclonal antibodies to a variety of surface antigens, the subjective lymphocyte transformation test has been largely replaced by first performing surface marker analysis. A large proportion of normal lymphocytes undergo blastogenic transformation when exposed to a variety of plant proteins. These are nonspecific, nonimmunologic phenomena. (However, the same changes can be elicited by specific antigens if the lymphocyte has been previously sensitized, and this correlates with delayed hypersensitivity.) Decreased mitogenic response is seen in congenital diseases (DiGeorge syndrome, Wiskott-Aldrich, combined immunodeficiency), and acquired states (sarcoid, lymphoid neoplasms, chemotherapy). Nonspecific events also lower transformation, including burns, surgery and anesthesia, aging, and protein malnutrition.

References

Fletcher MA, Klimas N, Morgan R, et al, "Lymphocyte Proliferation," *Manual of Clinical Laboratory Immunology*, 4th ed, Vol 2, Rose NR, Conway de Macario E, Fahey JL, et al, eds, Washington, DC: American Society for Microbiology, 1992, 213-9.

Lymphocyte Typing *see* Lymphocyte Subset Enumeration *on page 720*

Lymphocyte Typing *see* T- and B-Lymphocyte Subset Assay *on page 750*

Lymphogranuloma Venereum Titer

CPT *86631; 86632 (IgM)*

Related Information

Chlamydia Group Titer *on page 663*
Chlamydia trachomatis Culture *on page 1171*
Chlamydia trachomatis Direct FA Test *on page 1173*
Chlamydia trachomatis DNA Probe *on page 897*

Synonyms LGV Titer

Replaces Frei Test

Abstract LGV is a sexually transmitted disease which causes pronounced regional lymphadenopathy.

Specimen Serum **CONTAINER:** Red top tube **SAMPLING TIME:** Acute and convalescent specimens should be collected 10-14 days apart.

Interpretive **REFERENCE RANGE:** Negative. A fourfold increase in titer in paired sera is usually indicative of acute infection. **USE:** Support the clinical diagnosis of lymphogranuloma venereum **LIMITATIONS:** While a rising titer of antibody supports the diagnosis of LGV, the period of rise is usually missed. Because of the prevalence of antibodies to *Chlamydia*, demonstration of antibody in itself is insufficient to diagnose acute infection. **METHODOLOGY:** Complement fixation (CF), microimmunofluorescence **ADDITIONAL INFORMATION:** LGV is a sexually transmitted disease caused by the L1, L2, and L3 serotypes of *Chlamydia trachomatis*. This disease can produce nongonococcal urethritis in men and women, pelvic inflammatory disease in women, and epididymitis in men. When infants are exposed during delivery, they become vulnerable to pneumonia and conjunctivitis. Serologic study is particularly useful to screen for asymptomatic cases that may act as a reservoir for the disease. The presence of complement fixing antibodies **in the proper clinical setting (lymphadenopathy/rectal strictures)** supports the diagnosis of LGV. However, the increasing prevalence of chlamydial genital infections and the attendant increase in "background" antibody titers are vitiating the role of serology in diagnosis of acute illnesses. Tests for IgM antibody are not as useful as in some other infectious diseases because LGV is chronic, and short-lived IgM may no longer be detectable when the diagnosis is considered. Patients being evaluated for LGV should also have serologic testing for other sexually transmitted diseases. Recently, a commerical PCR kit has become available for the detection of *Chlamydia* in asymptomatic individuals.

References

Buntin DM, Rosen T, Lesher JL Jr, et al, "Sexually Transmitted Diseases: Bacterial Infections," *J Am Acad Dermatol*, 1991, 25(2 Pt 1):287-99.

Martin DH, "Chlamydial Infections," *Med Clin North Am*, 1990, 74(6):1367-87.

Schachter J, "Chlamydiae," *Manual of Clinical Laboratory Immunology*, 4th ed, Vol 2, Chapter 96, Rose NR, Conway de Macario E, Fahey JL, et al, eds, Washington, DC: American Society for Microbiology, 1992, 661-6.

MA Antibody *see* Antinuclear Antibody *on page 638*

Macroglobulins, Ultracentrifuge Determination *replaced by* Immunoglobulin M *on page 712*

Macrophage Migration Inhibition Test *see* Migration Inhibition Test *on next page*

Mazzini *replaced by* RPR *on page 742*

Mazzini *replaced by* VDRL, Serum *on page 762*

MBP Assay *see* Cerebrospinal Fluid Myelin Basic Protein *on page 657*

Measles Antibody

CPT *86765*

Synonyms Rubeola Antibodies

Applies to Rubeola Serology, CSF

Test Commonly Includes Antibodies specific for rubella, IgG and IgM levels, in patient's serum or cerebrospinal fluid

Abstract Measles is a viral disease which involves the respiratory tract and lymphoreticular tissues. It includes a papular eruption, lymphadenopathy, cough, and fever.

Specimen Serum or cerebrospinal fluid **CONTAINER:** Red top tube, sterile CSF tube

Interpretive **REFERENCE RANGE:** Less than fourfold rise in titer, absent or stable IgM titer; hemagglutination inhibition >1:10, neutralization >1:20 indicates immunity **USE:** Differential diagnosis of viral exanthemas, particularly in pregnant women; diagnosis of subacute sclerosing panencephalitis; document adequacy of measles immunization **LIMITATIONS:** Antibody sometimes present in multiple sclerosis **METHODOLOGY:** Hemagglutination inhibition (HAI), viral neutralization (NT), enzyme-linked immunosorbent assay (ELISA) **ADDITIONAL INFORMATION:** Measles (rubeola) is caused by a paramyxovirus, and despite vaccination programs has had several recent local epidemics. Revaccination appears to be of greater value at 11-12 years of age than at 4-6 years of age. Serologic study can be useful in establishing that an individual has effective immunity subsequent to vaccination. In many individuals **detectable** immunity does not persist. In acute illness, hemagglutinating and neutralizing antibody peak 2 weeks after the rash appears. It is necessary to demonstrate rising titers over 2 weeks, or identify IgM antibody. Very high serum titers in the absence of acute illness, or high CSF titer, are seen in subacute sclerosing panencephalitis.

References

Black FL, "Measles and Mumps," *Manual of Clinical Laboratory Immunology*, 4th ed, Vol 2, Chapter 89, Rose NR, Conway de Macario E, Fahey JL, et al, eds, Washington, DC: American Society for Microbiology, 1992, 596-9.

(Continued)

Measles Antibody *(Continued)*

Center for Disease Control and Prevention, "Measles – United States, 1992," *JAMA*, 1993, 269(22):2841-2.
Condorelli F and Ziegler T, "Dot Immunobinding Assay for Simultaneous Detection of Specific Immunoglobulin G Antibodies to Measles Virus, Mumps Virus, and Rubella Virus," *J Clin Microbiol*, 1993, 31(3):717-9.
Markowitz LE, Albrecht P, Orenstein WA, et al, "Persistence of Measles Antibody After Revaccination," *J Infect Dis*, 1992, 166(1):205-8.
Wittler RR, Veit BC, McIntyre S, et al, "Measles Revaccination Response in a School-Age Population," *Pediatrics*, 1991, 88(5):1024-30.

MHA-TP

CPT 86781

Related Information

Automated Reagin Test *on page 642*
FTA-ABS, Serum *on page 680*
RPR *on page 742*
VDRL, Cerebrospinal Fluid *on page 761*
VDRL, Serum *on page 762*

Synonyms Microhemagglutination, *Treponema pallidum*

Applies to Syphilis Serology

Test Commonly Includes Detection of serologic response to *Treponema pallidum*

Abstract A treponemal test for syphilis

Patient Care **PREPARATION:** Patient should be fasting if possible.

Specimen Serum **CONTAINER:** Red top tube **STORAGE INSTRUCTIONS:** Refrigerate serum.

Interpretive **REFERENCE RANGE:** <1:160 **USE:** Confirmatory serologic test for syphilis **LIMITATIONS:** Moderate sensitivity in early (primary) stages of syphilis. False-positives may occur in systemic lupus, infectious mononucleosis, and lepromatous leprosy. **METHODOLOGY:** Hemagglutination **ADDITIONAL INFORMATION:** This is a *Treponema*-specific test and probably should not be used as a screening test. It is as sensitive and specific as FTA-ABS in all stages of syphilis except primary, in which it is less sensitive (but more sensitive than the VDRL). It will be positive with treponemal infections other than syphilis (bejel, pinta, yaws). Like FTA-ABS, MHA-TP once positive remains so, and cannot be used to judge effect of treatment. The test is not applicable to CSF. The reaginic (nontreponemal) tests for syphilis include RPR and VDRL.

References

Hart G, "Syphilis Tests in Diagnostic and Therapeutic Decision Making," *Ann Intern Med*, 1986, 104:368-76.
Huber TW, Storms S, Young P, et al, "Reactivity of Microhemagglutination, Fluorescent Treponemal Antibody Absorption, Venereal Disease Research Laboratory, and Rapid Plasma Reagin Tests in Primary Syphilis," *J Clin Microbiol*, 1983, 17:405-9.
Romanowski B, Sutherland R, Fick GH, et al, "Serologic Response to Treatment of Infectious Syphilis," *Ann Intern Med*, 1991, 114(12):1005-9.

Microfilariae Serological Test *see* Filariasis Serological Test *on page 679*
Microhemagglutination, *Treponema pallidum* *see* MHA-TP *on this page*
***Micropolyspora faeni* Precipitating Antibodies** *see* Hypersensitivity Pneumonitis Serology *on page 704*
Microsomal Antibody *see* Thyroid Antimicrosomal Antibody *on page 755*

Migration Inhibition Test

CPT 86378

Synonyms Macrophage Migration Inhibition Test; Migration Inhibitory Factor

Specimen Whole blood **CONTAINER:** Yellow top (ACD) tube or green top (heparin) tube. Check with the laboratory performing the assay for special instructions. **CAUSES FOR REJECTION:** Old specimen without viable lymphocytes **SPECIAL INSTRUCTIONS:** Blood must be processed on same day as received. Schedule the procedure in advance with the laboratory.

Interpretive **REFERENCE RANGE:** Reported with results; requires interpretation **USE:** Evaluate cellular immune response **LIMITATIONS:** Clinical significance is obscure; test is not widely available; expensive **METHODOLOGY:** Lymphocytes are stimulated by specific antigen to produce macrophage migration inhibitory factor, which is assayed with guinea pig macrophages or human monocytes **ADDITIONAL INFORMATION:** **This is is a highly subjective and poorly stan-**

dardized test which was used to evaluate a variety of infectious diseases and immunodeficiency conditions. With the current availability of newer ELISA tests, DNA probes and surface marker techniques, its use has been diminished greatly. It is based on the observation that immunocompetent lymphocytes will produce several lymphokines when exposed to specific antigens to which they have been sensitized. One of these lymphokines is migration inhibition factor (MIF). This can be assayed by culturing lymphocytes with a specific antigen of interest, and then detecting migration inhibition factor in the culture supernatant by its effect on the migration of macrophages in a capillary tube. Failure of lymphocytes to produce MIF is a manifestation of immunodeficiency, either congenital or acquired (sarcoid, lymphoma, chemotherapy).

References

McCarthy PL Jr and Remold HG, "Production and Assay of Macrophage Migration Inhibitory Factor and Leukocyte Migration Inhibitory Factor," *Manual of Clinical Laboratory Immunology*, 4th ed, Vol 2, Rose NR, Conway de Macario E, Fahey JL, et al, eds, Washington, DC: American Society for Microbiology, 1992, 421-5.

Migration Inhibitory Factor *see* Migration Inhibition Test *on previous page*

Mitochondrial Antibody *see* Antimitochondrial Antibody *on page 635*

Mixed Lymphocyte Culture

CPT 86821

Related Information

HLA Typing, Single Human Leukocyte Antigen *on page 701*
Polymerase Chain Reaction *on page 927*
Tissue Typing *on page 757*

Synonyms Mixed Lymphocyte Reaction; MLC; MLR

Applies to Blood Mononuclear Cells

Test Commonly Includes Blood lymphocytes (and some monocytes) from potential donors and the recipient are cultured together and tested for reactivity against each other.

Specimen Leukocytes **CONTAINER:** Green top (heparin) tube **COLLECTION:** Blood has to be delivered to the laboratory immediately. Check with the laboratory performing the assay for special instructions. **CAUSES FOR REJECTION:** Specimen not collected sterilely in heparin **SPECIAL INSTRUCTIONS:** Blood specimen must be collected fresh on day of test. Test depends on viability of mononuclear lymphocytes.

Interpretive **REFERENCE RANGE:** Response compared with that of simultaneously evaluated normal control; requires interpretation **USE:** Tissue matching for transplantation; evaluate cellular immunocompetence **LIMITATIONS:** Test will be negative if donor or responder cells have a severe cellular immunodeficiency. **METHODOLOGY:** Co-culture of blood mononuclear cells from two different individuals for several days, with addition of ^{3}H thymidine 6 hours prior to harvest as a measure of DNA synthesis. One individual's cells usually pretreated, preferably with irradiation or with mitomycin-C, to prevent them from transforming. **ADDITIONAL INFORMATION:** This is a technique to detect whether a tissue transplant recipient's blood mononuclear cells will react against leukocyte (tissue) antigens from a potential donor. Donor cells pretreated with mitomycin C or radiation (so that they are antigenically effective but cannot undergo blastogenesis) are mixed with untreated recipient cells (which can transform). If the recipient cells "recognize" foreign antigenic determinants they will transform and take up tritiated thymidine. Such data may be predictive of graft survival and be used in selecting possible donors. Genetic analysis of the HLA region is now being investigated for use in typing this region, especially in bone marrow transplants. HLA-DQ is the most used locus for genetic testing.

References

Hansen JA, Mickelson EM, Choo SY, et al, "Clinical Bone Marrow Transplantation: Donor Selection and Recipient Monitoring," *Manual of Clinical Laboratory Immunology*, 4th ed, Vol 2, Chapter 129, Rose NR, Conway de Macario E, Fahey JL, et al, eds, Washington, DC: American Society for Microbiology, 1992, 850-66.

Mixed Lymphocyte Reaction *see* Mixed Lymphocyte Culture *on this page*

MLC *see* Mixed Lymphocyte Culture *on this page*

MLR *see* Mixed Lymphocyte Culture *on this page*

Monoclonal Gammopathies *see* Protein Electrophoresis, Serum *on page 734*

Monoclonal Gammopathy *see* Immunoelectrophoresis, Serum or Urine *on page 706*

Monoclonal Gammopathy *see* Immunofixation Electrophoresis *on page 707*

Monoclonal Gammopathy Work-up *see* Protein Electrophoresis, Urine *on page 737*

Monoclonal Rheumatoid Factor Inhibition *see* Immune Complex Assay *on page 705*

Monospot™ Test *see* Infectious Mononucleosis Screening Test *on page 713*

Monosticon® Dri-Dot® Test *see* Infectious Mononucleosis Screening Test *on page 713*

Mono Test *see* Infectious Mononucleosis Screening Test *on page 713*

***M. pneumoniae* Titer** *see Mycoplasma* Serology *on next page*

M Protein *see* Immunofixation Electrophoresis *on page 707*

Mumps Antibodies *see* Mumps Serology *on this page*

Mumps Serology

CPT 86735

Related Information

Mumps Virus Culture *on page 1187*

Viral Culture, Central Nervous System Symptoms *on page 1199*

Synonyms Mumps Antibodies

Test Commonly Includes Detection of serologic response to mumps infection or vaccination

Specimen Serum **CONTAINER:** Red top tube **SAMPLING TIME:** Acute and convalescent sera drawn 10-14 days apart are required.

Interpretive **REFERENCE RANGE:** A fourfold or greater increase in titer with increasing ratio of V (viral) to S (soluble) titer is indicative of recent mumps infection in complement fixation test; a positive IgM indirect fluorescent test is indicative of infection; an increasing hemagglutination inhibition titer indicates mumps **or another parainfluenza virus** infection; a positive hemolysis-in-gel or neutralization test indicates **immunity** to mumps. **USE:** Support for the diagnosis of mumps virus infection; document previous exposure to mumps virus; document immunity **LIMITATIONS:** Several test systems are not specific for mumps **METHODOLOGY:** Complement fixation (CF), enzyme-linked immunosorbent assay (ELISA), indirect fluorescent antibody (IFA), hemagglutination inhibition (HAI), hemolysis-in-gel, virus neutralization **ADDITIONAL INFORMATION:** Mumps is caused by a paramyxovirus and man is the only known reservoir. In addition to mumps, it is known to cause aseptic meningitis, encephalitis, and inflammation of the testes, pancreas, and ovaries. Serologic study may be undertaken to confirm a diagnosis in acute disease or to demonstrate established immunity. For diagnosis in an acute illness, measuring the ratio of IgG to IgM antibody is simplest and fastest. Immunity depends on neutralizing antibody, which must be demonstrated in tissue culture.

References

Benito RJ, Larrad L, Lasierra MP, et al, "Persistence of Specific IgM Antibodies After Natural Mumps Infection," *J Infect Dis*, 1987, 155:156-7.

Black FL, "Measles and Mumps," *Manual of Clinical Laboratory Immunology*, 4th ed, Vol 2, Chapter 89, Rose NR, Conway de Macario E, Fahey JL, et al, eds, Washington, DC: American Society for Microbiology, 1992, 596-9.

Condorelli F and Ziegler T, "Dot Immunobinding Assay for Simultaneous Detection of Specific Immunoglobulin G Antibodies to Measles Virus, Mumps Virus, and Rubella Virus," *J Clin Microbiol*, 1993, 31(3):717-9.

Costello MJ, Smernoff NT, and Yungbluth M, "Laboratory Diagnosis of Viral Respiratory Tract Infections," *Lab Med*, 1993, 24(3):150.

Harmsen T, Jongerius MC, van der Zwan CW, et al, "Comparison of a Neutralization Enzyme Immunoassay and an Enzyme-Linked Immunosorbent Assay for Evaluation of Immune Status of Children Vaccinated for Mumps," *J Clin Microbiol*, 1992, 30(8):2139-44.

***Mycoplasma* Antibodies** *see Mycoplasma* Serology *on next page*

***Mycoplasma pneumoniae* Titer** *see Mycoplasma* Serology *on next page*

Mycoplasma Serology

CPT *86738*

Related Information

Cold Agglutinin Titer *on page 664*
Mycoplasma pneumoniae Diagnostic Procedures *on page 1188*
Mycoplasma pneumoniae DNA Probe Test *on page 923*

Synonyms Eaton Agent Titer; *M. pneumoniae* Titer; *Mycoplasma* Antibodies; *Mycoplasma pneumoniae* Titer; PPLO Titer

Test Commonly Includes Detection of serologic response to *Mycoplasma pneumoniae* after infection

Specimen Serum **CONTAINER:** Red top tube **SAMPLING TIME:** Acute and convalescent sera drawn 10-14 days apart are required.

Interpretive **REFERENCE RANGE:** Negative. IgG <1:10, IgM <1:10. A fourfold increase in titer in paired sera or a single CF titer >1:256 suggests infection **USE:** Support the diagnosis of *Mycoplasma pneumoniae* infection **LIMITATIONS:** False-positives occur in pancreatitis. **METHODOLOGY:** Complement fixation (CF), indirect fluorescent antibody (IFA), enzyme immunoassay (EIA) **ADDITIONAL INFORMATION:** *Mycoplasma pneumoniae* is the cause of the relatively common "primary atypical pneumonia." *Mycoplasma* is more difficult to culture than ordinary bacteria and thus serologic confirmation of the diagnosis is often desirable. The complement fixation and metabolic inhibition tests detect antibody to a lipid antigen, and are both more specific and more sensitive than the cold agglutinin test. However, both require paired sera, and are thus of limited clinical utility. Demonstration of specific IgG and IgM antibody by immunofluorescence is rapid, sensitive, and specific. IgM antibody indicates acute infection. Recent availability of a DNA probe for *Mycoplasma* has shown a sensitivity of 95% and a specificity of 85% with the stringency of the assay conditions. It may become the method of choice, but currently the test performed with throat swabs seems to have only limited value.

References

Kleemola SR, Karjalainen JE, and Raty RK, "Rapid Diagnosis of *Mycoplasma pneumoniae* Infection: Clinical Evaluation of a Commercial Probe Test," *J Infect Dis*, 1990, 162(1):70-5.

Smith TF, "*Mycoplasma pneumoniae* Infections: Diagnosis Based on Immunofluorescence Titer of IgG and IgM Antibodies," *Mayo Clin Proc*, 1986, 61:830-1.

Myelin Basic Protein, Cerebrospinal Fluid *see* Cerebrospinal Fluid Myelin Basic Protein *on page 657*

Nantucket Fever Serological Test *see* Babesiosis Serological Test *on page 643*

Nasopharyngeal Smear for *Bordetella pertussis* *see Bordetella pertussis* Direct Fluorescent Antibody *on page 646*

n-DNA *see* Anti-DNA *on page 634*

Neutrophil Antibody *see* Antineutrophil Antibody *on page 636*

Non-A, non-B Hepatitis *see* Hepatitis C Serology *on page 690*

Nucleolar Antibody *see* Antinuclear Antibody *on page 638*

Oligoclonal Bands, Cerebrospinal Fluid *see* Cerebrospinal Fluid Oligoclonal Bands *on page 658*

***Onchocerca volvulus* Serology** *see* Filariasis Serological Test *on page 679*

Organ Donor Tissue Typing *see* Tissue Typing *on page 757*

Oriental Sore Serological Test *see* Leishmaniasis Serological Test *on page 717*

p24 Antigen

CPT *86311*

Related Information

HIV-1/HIV-2 Serology *on page 696*
Human Immunodeficiency Virus Culture *on page 1185*
Human Immunodeficiency Virus DNA Amplification *on page 915*
Risks of Transfusion *on page 1093*
T- and B-Lymphocyte Subset Assay *on page 750*

Synonyms HIV Core Antigen

Applies to Gag Gene of HIV

(Continued)

p24 Antigen *(Continued)*

Test Commonly Includes Detection of HIV p24 antigen in serum or cerebrospinal fluid

Specimen Serum or cerebrospinal fluid **CONTAINER:** Red top tube, sterile CSF tube **SPECIAL INSTRUCTIONS:** In some states written or informed patient consent is a prerequisite for the test. Results may need to be kept confidential.

Interpretive **REFERENCE RANGE:** Negative **USE:** Diagnose recent acute infection with HIV; may also be of prognostic significance in AIDS, if antigen becomes positive during infection, after having been negative. (Can also be used to test viral culture supernatants.) **LIMITATIONS:** Test is not as sensitive as culture or polymerase chain reaction for detecting HIV infection. **METHODOLOGY:** Enzyme immunoassay (EIA) **ADDITIONAL INFORMATION:** p24 antigen is a 24 kD protein product of the **gag** gene of HIV. As a viral rather than host product, it appears concomitant with initial infection, and then generally becomes undetectable during periods of viral latency. It reappears with renewed viral replication; the reappearance of p24 antigen in serum generally heralds progression of clinical disease in AIDS. Measuring antigen may also be useful in assessing therapy. It has not been recommended as a further screening test for blood products for transfusion. However, recent studies indicate that an acid dissociation procedure that disrupts the p24 antigen-antibody complexes can increase the sensitivity of the procedure up to fivefold. This may improve its diagnostic utility,[1] especially for neonate testing. It has been suggested that AIDS patients being treated with dideoxyinosine be followed with p24 levels to determine efficacy of treatment.[2]

Footnotes

1. Bollinger RC Jr, Kline RL, Francis HL, et al, "Acid Dissociation Increases the Sensitivity of p24 Antigen Detection for the Evaluation of Antiviral Therapy and Disease Progression in Asymptomatic HIV-Infected Persons," *J Infect Dis*, 1992, 165(5):913-6.
2. Drusano GL, Yuen GJ, Lambert JS, et al, "Relationship Between Dideoxyinosine Exposure, CD4 Counts, and p24 Antigen Levels in Human Immunodeficiency Virus Infection: A Phase I Trial," *Ann Intern Med*, 1992, 116(7):562-6.

References

Goudsmit J, Lange JMA, Paul DA, et al, "Antigenemia and Antibody Titers to Core and Envelope Antigens in AIDS, AIDS-Related Complex, and Subclinical Human Immunodeficiency Virus Infection," *J Infect Dis*, 1987, 155:558-60.

Phair JP and Wolinsky S, "Diagnosis of Infection With the Human Immunodeficiency Virus," *Clin Infect Dis*, 1992, 15(1):13-6.

Wilber JC, "Serologic Testing of Human Immunodeficiency Virus Infection," *Clin Lab Med*, 1987, 7:777-91.

Wittek AE, Phelan MA, Wells MA, et al, "Detection of Human Immunodeficiency Virus Core Protein in Plasma by Enzyme Immunoassay," *Ann Intern Med*, 1987, 107:286-92.

PA *see* Parietal Cell Antibody *on page 730*

Parainfluenza Viral Serology

CPT 86710

Related Information

Parainfluenza Virus Culture *on page 1189*

Viral Culture, Respiratory Symptoms *on page 1204*

Test Commonly Includes Antibody titers to parainfluenza virus types 1, 2, 3, and 4

Specimen Serum **CONTAINER:** Red top tube; capillary puncture: minimum eight full blue tip capillary tubes **SAMPLING TIME:** Acute and convalescent sera drawn 10-14 days apart are recommended. **CAUSES FOR REJECTION:** Inadequate labeling, gross contamination of specimen

Interpretive **REFERENCE RANGE:** A single low titer or less than a fourfold change in titer in paired sera **USE:** Support the diagnosis of parainfluenza virus infection **LIMITATIONS:** Need for convalescent specimen delays diagnosis. Heterotypic rises in parainfluenza titers may occur in infections with other viruses. Infant antibody response may be undetectable. **METHODOLOGY:** Complement fixation (CF), hemagglutination inhibition (HAI), enzyme-linked immunosorbent assay (ELISA) **ADDITIONAL INFORMATION:** Since the demonstration of a fourfold rise in antibody titer requires testing a convalescent specimen, serologic diagnosis is seldom useful in clinical management of an acute illness. This is especially so since the rise may occur even in an infection caused by some other virus. Serologic studies are of value in epidemiology. Rapid diagnosis during acute illness may be accomplished by demonstrating viral antigen in smears or tissue by immunofluorescence. Since parainfluenza virus may respond to ribavirin, prompt accurate diagnosis could become important, particularly in the immunocompromised host.

References

Mufson MA and Belshe RB, "Respiratory Syncytial Virus and the Parainfluenza Viruses," *Manual of Clinical Laboratory Immunology*, 4th ed, Vol 2, Chapter 87, Rose NR, Conway de Macario E, Fahey JL, et al, eds, Washington, DC: American Society for Microbiology, 1992, 582-9.

Sperber SJ and Hayden FG, "Antiviral Chemotherapy and Prophylaxis of Viral Respiratory Disease," *Clin Lab Med*, 1987, 7:869-96.

Paraproteinemia *see* Immunoelectrophoresis, Serum or Urine *on page 706*

Paraprotein Evaluation *see* Immunofixation Electrophoresis *on page 707*

Parasite Antibodies

CPT *86171 (complement fixation); 86280 (hemagglutination inhibition); 86329 (immunodiffusion)*

Related Information

Ascariasis Serological Test *on page 641*
Chagas' Disease Serological Test *on page 662*
Cysticercosis Titer *on page 671*
Echinococcosis Serological Test *on page 674*
Entamoeba histolytica Serological Test *on page 675*
Eosinophil Count *on page 539*
Filariasis Serological Test *on page 679*
Leishmaniasis Serological Test *on page 717*
Malaria Smear *on page 569*
Ova and Parasites, Stool *on page 836*
Ova and Parasites, Urine *on page 839*
Schistosomiasis Serological Test *on page 745*
Toxoplasmosis Serology *on page 759*
Trichinosis Serology *on page 760*

Synonyms Parasite Screen; Parasite Titer

Test Commonly Includes *Echinococcus*, *Entamoeba histolytica*, *Paragonimus*, Toxoplasmosis, Chagas' Disease, Malaria, Filaria, *Schistosoma*, Trichinosis, *Fasciola hepatica*, *Leishmania*, VLM (*Ascaris* and *Toxocara*), *Strongyloides*, cysticercosis, *Taenia solium* and *Taenia saginata*, Trypanosomiasis, *Giardia*, *Onchocerca volvulus*

Specimen Serum **CONTAINER:** Red top tube **SAMPLING TIME:** Acute and convalescent specimens drawn 10-14 days apart are recommended

Interpretive **REFERENCE RANGE:** Negative. A fourfold increase in titer in paired sera is usually indicative of acute infection. **USE:** Support diagnosis of suspected parasitic infestation **METHODOLOGY:** Complement fixation (CF), immunodiffusion (ID), hemagglutination inhibition (HAI), enzyme-linked immunosorbent assay (ELISA) **ADDITIONAL INFORMATION:** "Parasite Screen" is not a specific test as such, but is a service offered by many laboratories, consisting of a battery of procedures to detect antibodies to specific parasites. Which parasites will be screened for by a particular laboratory should be determined depending upon the patient population served and the regional parasites. Antibodies will rarely be present unless tissue invasion has taken place. Because of cross reactions and failures to develop antibody, serologic diagnosis does not replace demonstration of the parasite itself or its eggs as a definitive diagnostic procedure.

Visceral larva migrans is mostly caused by the dog roundworm, *Toxocara canis*, in the U.S. and is found mainly between ages 1 and 4 years. Its characteristics include eosinophilia, hyperglobulinemia, fever, and leukocytosis. An enzyme-linked immunosorbent assay (ELISA) has confirmed the diagnosis in an adult with bronchospasm.[1]

Footnotes

1. Feldman GJ and Parker HW, "Visceral Larva Migrans Associated With the Hypereosinophilic Syndrome and the Onset of Severe Asthma," *Ann Intern Med*, 1992, 116(10):838-40.

References

Kagan IG and Maddison SE, "Serodiagnosis of Parasitic Diseases," *Manual of Clinical Laboratory Immunology*, 4th ed, Vol 2, Chapter 79, Rose NR, Conway de Macario E, Fahey JL, et al, eds, Washington, DC: American Society for Microbiology, 1992, 529-43.

Parasite Screen *see* Parasite Antibodies *on this page*

Parasite Titer *see* Parasite Antibodies *on this page*

Parietal Cell Antibody

CPT 86255 (screen); 86256 (titer)

Related Information

Folic Acid, Serum *on page 545*
Gastric Analysis *on page 232*
Intrinsic Factor Antibody *on page 714*
Phosphorus, Urine *on page 322*
Schilling Test *on page 598*
Vitamin B_{12} *on page 612*
Vitamin B_{12} Unsaturated Binding Capacity *on page 615*

Synonyms Antiparietal Cell Antibody; PA

Specimen Serum CONTAINER: Red top tube

Interpretive REFERENCE RANGE: Negative USE: Useful in the differential diagnosis of pernicious anemia and atrophic gastritis LIMITATIONS: Nonspecific: found in 20% to 30% of patients with a variety of autoimmune disorders and 16% of asymptomatic people older than 60 years of age. In a study of autoantibodies in presumably healthy blood donors, two with antiparietal cell and others with other antibodies were detected. On follow up, no increase in the incidence of autoimmune diseases in such healthy subjects was elicited.[1] METHODOLOGY: Indirect fluorescent antibody (IFA) ADDITIONAL INFORMATION: Antibodies to parietal cells are present in 80% of adults with pernicious anemia and chronic gastritis; they do not correlate with malabsorption of vitamin B_{12}. However, they may participate in the early pathogenesis of parietal cell destruction. They are also present in occasional patients with gastric ulcer or gastric cancer. There is cross positivity of parietal cell and thyroid antibodies in patients with thyroiditis and pernicious anemia. With time, the titer of parietal cell antibodies will decline in some patients with pernicious anemia (possibly related to loss of parietal cells) whereas intrinsic factor antibodies persist.

Footnotes

1. Vrethem M, Skogh T, Berlin G, et al, "Autoantibodies Versus Clinical Symptoms in Blood Donors," *J Rheumatol*, 1992, 19(12):1919-21.

References

Burman P, Kampe O, Kraaz W, et al, "A Study of Autoimmune Gastritis in the Postpartum Period and at a 5-Year Follow-up," *Gastroenterology*, 1992, 103(3):934-42.
Davidson RJ, Atrah HI, and Sewell HF, "Longitudinal Study of Circulating Gastric Antibodies in Pernicious Anemia," *J Clin Pathol*, 1989, 42(10):1092-5.
Harty RF and Leibach JR, "Immune Disorders of the Gastrointestinal Tract and Liver," *Med Clin North Am*, 1985, 69:675-704.

Parvovirus B19 DNA

CPT 83898

Related Information

Parvovirus B19 Serology *on next page*

Test Commonly Includes Detection of parvovirus B19 by DNA hybridization using polymerase chain reaction (PCR)

Specimen Serum CONTAINER: Red top tube

Interpretive USE: Diagnose parvovirus B19 infection. May be positive in immunocompromised patients who do not produce antibodies against parvovirus B19. METHODOLOGY: Polymerase chain reaction (PCR) to detect parvovirus B19 DNA ADDITIONAL INFORMATION: Parvovirus B19 is a DNA virus which can cause a wide spectrum of disease ranging from self-limited erythema infectiosum (Fifth disease) to persistent bone marrow failure and fetal death. In most people, the low titer viremia which begins about 1 week after exposure and persists for 7-10 days is associated with mild symptoms and a subclinical red cell aplasia. Because the virus destroys red blood cell precursors, there is a reduction in erythrocyte production. This transient aplastic crisis may be particularly severe clinically in patients with hemoglobinopathies associated with decreased erythrocyte lifespan (sickle cell disease, spherocytosis, and β-thalassemia). The presence of parvovirus DNA provides definite evidence of recent infection.

References

Koch WC, Massey G, Russell CE, et al, "Manifestations and Treatment of Human Parvovirus B19 Infections in Immunocompromised Patients," *J Pediatr*, 1990, 116(3):355-9.
Kovacs BW, Carlson DE, Shahbahrami B, et al, "Prenatal Diagnosis of Human Parvovirus B19 in Nonimmune Hydrops Fetalis by Polymerase Chain Reaction," *Am J Obstet Gynecol*, 1992, 167(2):461-6.
McOmish F, Yap PL, Jordan A, et al, "Detection of Parvovirus B19 in Donated Blood: A Model System for Screening by Polymerase Chain Reaction," *J Clin Microbiol*, 1993, 31(2):323-8.

Parvovirus B19 Serology

CPT 86747

Related Information

Parvovirus B19 DNA *on previous page*

Synonyms Anti-B19 IgG Antibodies; Anti-B19 IgM Antibodies

Test Commonly Includes Assays for parvovirus B19 IgM and IgG antibodies

Specimen Serum CONTAINER: Red top tube STORAGE INSTRUCTIONS: Separate serum and freeze.

Interpretive USE: Diagnose parvovirus B19 infection METHODOLOGY: Radioimmunoassay (RIA) or immunoblot assay (Western blot) for the detection of IgM and IgG antibodies to parvovirus B19 ADDITIONAL INFORMATION: Parvovirus B19 is a DNA virus and can cause a wide spectrum of disease ranging form outbreaks of self-limiting erythema infectiosum (Fifth disease) to persistent bone marrow failure and fetal death. Intrauterine transfusion has been suggested when there is evidence of B19 parvovirus-associated hydrops and anemia. In most people the low-titer parvovirus B19 viremia, which begins approximately 1 week after exposure and lasts 7-10 days, is associated with mild symptoms and a subclinical red cell aplasia. Because the virus destroys erythroid precursor cells, which leads to a reduction in normal red blood cell production, infection with parvovirus B19 can cause a transient aplastic crisis in patients already at maximum red cell production and in those with increased red cell destruction (sickle cell disease, β-thalassemia, and spherocytosis). In immunocompromised patients, parvovirus B19 infection can cause life-threatening anemia. IgM antibodies are detectable 2 weeks after exposure. IgG antibody production usually occurs 18-24 days after exposure and is probably immune-complex mediated. The presence of IgM antibodies to parvovirus B19 provide definite evidence of recent infection.

References

Patou G and Ayliffe U, "Evaluation of Commercial Enzyme-Linked Immunosorbent Assay for Detection of B19 Parvovirus IgM and IgG," *J Clin Pathol*, 1991, 44(10):831-4.

Rodis JF, Quinn DL, Gary GW Jr, et al, "Management and Outcome of Pregnancies Complicated by Human B19 Parvovirus Infection: A Prospective Study," *Am J Obstet Gynecol*, 1991, 164(4 Pt 1):1363-4.

Paul-Bunnell Test *replaced by* Infectious Mononucleosis Screening Test *on page 713*

Pemphigoid Antibodies *see* Pemphigus Antibodies *on this page*

Pemphigus Antibodies

CPT 86255 (screen); 86256 (titer)

Related Information

Immunofluorescence, Skin Biopsy *on page 708*

Skin Biopsies *on page 84*

Synonyms Pemphigoid Antibodies

Specimen Serum CONTAINER: Red top tube

Interpretive REFERENCE RANGE: Negative USE: Diagnostic test for pemphigus, pemphigoid METHODOLOGY: Indirect fluorescent antibody (IFA) on a substrate of monkey or guinea pig esophagus ADDITIONAL INFORMATION: Pemphigus vulgaris (and its variants) and bullous pemphigoid are blistering diseases of the skin. Although often diagnosed on clinical presentation and routine histologic examination, these diseases may require skin immunofluorescence for differentiation. In pemphigus, antibodies are directed against intercellular material within the epithelium and C3 is found on cell surfaces. Patients with oral lesions may not have circulating antibody. False-positives may be seen in lupus, burns, and drug reactions, but these are usually weak. In pemphigoid, antibody is directed against the basement membrane. Circulating antibody is present in 70% of patients, and 25% will show IgG and C3 basement membrane deposits on skin biopsy. These antibodies correlate with disease activity, and are present in 60% of patients with pemphigoid and 80% of patients with pemphigus.

References

Harrist TJ and Mihm MC, "Cutaneous Immunopathology. The Diagnostic Use of Direct and Indirect Immunofluorescence Techniques in Dermatologic Disease," *Hum Pathol*, 1979, 10:625-53.

Izuno GT, "Cutaneous Immunofluorescence," *Clin Lab Med*, 1986, 6:95-102.

Stanley JR, "Pemphigus. Skin Failure Mediated by Autoantibodies," *JAMA*, 1990, 264(13):1714-7.

Pertussis Serology *see Bordetella pertussis* Serology *on page 647*

Pertussis Titers *see* Bacterial Serology *on page 644*

Phagocytic Cell Immunocompetence Profile

CPT *86160 (C3 and C4); 86384 (NBT)*

Related Information

C3 Complement, Serum *on page 649*
C4 Complement, Serum *on page 650*
Complement Components *on page 665*
Complement, Total, Serum *on page 667*

Test Commonly Includes C3, C4, NBT screen, neutrophil myeloperoxidase, neutrophil chemotaxis, neutrophil phagocytosis, surface adhesion molecule evaluation (Mo-1, LFA-1, p150.95)

Specimen Serum and whole blood **CONTAINER:** C4 and C3: red top tube; NBT: green top (heparin) tube; neutrophil functions: green top (heparin) tube **STORAGE INSTRUCTIONS:** C3 and C4: Store at -20°C; NBT and function studies: cannot be stored. Must be scheduled with and delivered to the laboratory immediately.

Interpretive **REFERENCE RANGE:** C3: 900-2000 μg/mL; C4: 200-800 μg/mL; other tests require interpretation and clinical correlation **USE:** Evaluate complement and phagocytic cell function abnormal in chronic granulomatous disease, C3 and C4 complement component deficiency, hereditary or acquired neutrophil function disorders **LIMITATIONS:** Tests require careful clinical correlation and experienced interpretation. **METHODOLOGY:** C3 and C4: single radial immunodiffusion (RID) or nephelometry; NBT: dye reduction by polymorphonuclear cells after phagocytosis of beads; neutrophil function by skin window and migration assay; myeloperoxidase by cytochemistry; surface marker analysis of surface adhesion molecules **ADDITIONAL INFORMATION:** These tests do not replace but are supplemental to careful clinical assessment and more basic laboratory studies such as complete blood count, protein electrophoresis, and quantitative immunoglobulins. This battery or a variant of it might be applied in the workup of a patient with recurrent infections, particularly with catalase-positive organism (usually *Staphylococcus aureus*) in whom the diagnosis of chronic granulomatous disease is considered. A variety of adhesion deficiencies have been reported. Flow cytometry studies for Mo-1, LFA-1, and p150.95 may be of use as patients with deficiencies of these molecules suffer recurrent infections.

References

Gallin JI, Buescher ES, Seligmann BE, et al, "NIH Conference. Recent Advances in Chronic Granulomatous Disease," *Ann Intern Med*, 1983, 99:657-74.

Keren DF and Warren JS, "Immunodeficiency," *Diagnostic Immunology*, Chapter 7, Baltimore, MD: Williams & Wilkins, 1992.

PHA Stimulation *see* Lymphocyte Transformation Test *on page 722*

Pi Phenotype *see* Alpha$_1$-Antitrypsin Phenotyping *on page 630*

***Pneumocystis carinii* Serology** *see Pneumocystis* Fluorescence *on this page*

Pneumocystis Fluorescence

CPT *86255 (screen); 86256 (titer); 87206 (smear, fluorescent)*

Related Information

Bronchial Washings Cytology *on page 485*
Bronchoalveolar Lavage *on page 793*
Bronchoalveolar Lavage Cytology *on page 487*
Pneumocystis carinii Preparation *on page 508*
Polymerase Chain Reaction *on page 927*
Sputum Culture *on page 849*
Sputum Cytology *on page 510*

Synonyms *Pneumocystis carinii* Serology

Test Commonly Includes Direct and indirect immunofluorescence for detection of antibody to *Pneumocystis carinii* or to detect the organism in clinical specimens

Abstract The most common lung complication in AIDS is pneumonia caused by *Pneumocystis carinii*, but *P. carinii* causes diseases in other patients as well. Many are immunocompromised, but some do not present identifiable risk factors.

Specimen Serum, tissue biopsy, sputum, bronchoalveolar lavage **CONTAINER:** Red top tube, sterile container **SPECIAL INSTRUCTIONS:** Tissue specimens should be received fresh or snap-frozen.

Interpretive **REFERENCE RANGE:** Antibody titer: serum: <1:16; antigen detection: no organisms observed **POSSIBLE PANIC RANGE:** Organisms seen **USE:** Support for the diagnosis of *Pneumocystis carinii* pneumonia; document previous exposure to *Pneumocystis* organism; detect pneumocystosis **LIMITATIONS:** A negative result, either the serum antibody or tissue antigen, does not exclude the diagnosis. **METHODOLOGY:** Indirect (IFA) and direct fluorescent antibody (DFA) **ADDITIONAL INFORMATION:** With the onslaught of the AIDS epidemic *Pneumocystis*, previously an obscure and infrequent pathogen of immunosuppressed cancer and transplant patients, become a common, treatable pathogen. Diagnosis depends primarily on seeing either cysts or trophozoites in tissue or cytology preparations. Silver impregnation stains have been the gold standard (to mix metals if not metaphors) but these are time consuming and may delay treatment. Direct immunofluorescence is more sensitive than silver stain and rapid, although Wright-Giemsa stain to detect foamy exudate is probably even better and faster. One advantage of silver stains, however, is that it will detect fungal infections. Recent studies using PCR detected *P. carinii* in bronchoalveolar lavage and sputum from immunocompromised patients, many of whom did not have evidence of pneumonia. This suggests that this newer, more sensitive PCR technology can detect symptom-free carriers or subclinical infection. PCR will likely soon become the method of choice for detecting this and other infectious agents.[1]

Footnotes

1. Lipschik GY, Gill VJ, Lundgren JD, et al, "Improved Diagnosis of *Pneumocystis carinii* Infection by Polymerase Chain Reaction on Induced Sputum and Blood," *Lancet*, 1992, 340(8813):203-6.

References

Amin MB, Mezger E, and Zarbo RJ, "Detection of *Pneumocystis carinii*. Comparative Study of Monoclonal Antibody and Silver Impregnation," *Am J Clin Pathol*, 1992, 98(1):13-8

Bédos JP, Hignette C, Lucet JC, et al, "Serum Carcinoembryonic Antigen: A Prognostic Marker in HIV-Related *Pneumocystis carinii* Pneumonia," *Scand J Infect Dis*, 1992, 24(3):309-15.

Blumenfeld W and Griffiss JM, "*Pneumocystis carinii* in Sputum," *Arch Pathol Lab Med*, 1988, 112:816-20.

Blumenfeld W, Miller CN, Chew KL, et al, "Correlation of *Pneumocystis carinii* Cyst Density With Mortality in Patients With Acquired Immunodeficiency Syndrome and *Pneumocystis* pneumonia," *Hum Pathol*, 1992, 23(6):612-8.

Coulman CV, Greene I, and Archibald RWR, "Cutaneous Pneumocystosis," *Ann Intern Med*, 1987, 106:396-8.

Homer KS, Wiley EL, Smith AL, et al, "Monoclonal Antibody to *Pneumocystis carinii*: Comparison With Silver Stain in Bronchial Lavage Specimens," *Am J Clin Pathol*, 1992, 97(5):619-24.

Jacobs JL, Libby DM, Winters RA, et al, "A Cluster of *Pneumocystis carinii* Pneumonia in Adults Without Predisposing Illnesses," *N Engl J Med*, 1991, 324(4):246-50.

Kovacs JV, Ng VL, Masur H, et al, "Diagnosis of *Pneumocystis carinii* Pneumonia: Improved Detected in Sputum With Use of Monoclonal Antibodies," *N Engl J Med*, 1988, 318:589-93.

Martin WJ 2d, "Diagnostic Bronchoalveolar Lavage in Immunosuppressed Patients With New Pulmonary Infiltrates," *Mayo Clin Proc*, 1992, 67(3):296-8, (editorial).

Sepkowitz KA, Brown AE, Telzak EE, et al, "*Pneumocystis carinii* Pneumonia Among Patients Without AIDS at a Cancer Hospital," *JAMA*, 1992, 267(6):832-7.

Watts JC and Chandler FW, "*Pneumocystis carinii* Pneumonitis," *Am J Surg Pathol*, 1985, 9:744-51.

Poliomyelitis I, II, III Titer

***CPT** 86658*

Related Information

Enterovirus Culture *on page 1178*

Viral Culture, Stool *on page 1205*

Synonyms Poliovirus Titer

Test Commonly Includes Detection of antibodies to poliovirus in patient's serum

Specimen Serum **CONTAINER:** Red top tube **SAMPLING TIME:** Acute and convalescent sera drawn 10-14 days apart are required

Interpretive **REFERENCE RANGE:** A fourfold increase in titer in paired sera is diagnostic; presence of neutralizing antibody indicates adequate immunization; normal <1:8 **USE:** Support for the diagnosis of poliovirus infection, documentation of previous exposure to poliovirus (complement fixing antibodies); documentation of immunization (neutralizing antibodies) **METHODOLOGY:** Viral neutralization, complement fixation (CF) **ADDITIONAL INFORMATION:** Poliovirus may also be cultured, producing a characteristic cytopathic effect in tissue culture. Culture is more suitable than serology for diagnosis of acute infection.

(Continued)

Poliomyelitis I, II, III Titer *(Continued)*

References

Melnick JL, "Enteroviruses," *Manual of Clinical Laboratory Immunology*, 4th ed, Vol 2, Chapter 93, Rose NR, Conway de Macario E, Fahey JL, et al, eds, Washington, DC: American Society for Microbiology, 1992, 631-3.

Poliovirus Titer *see* Poliomyelitis I, II, III Titer *on previous page*

Polysaccharide Antigen, *H. capsulatum var capsulatum* *see* Histoplasmosis Serology *on page 695*

PPLO Titer *see Mycoplasma* Serology *on page 727*

Precipitating Antibodies *see* Hypersensitivity Pneumonitis Serology *on page 704*

Progressive Systemic Sclerosis Antibody *see* Scleroderma Antibody *on page 745*

Properdin *see* Factor B *on page 678*

Protease Inhibitors *see* Alpha$_1$-Antitrypsin Phenotyping *on page 630*

Proteinase 3 (PR3) *see* Antineutrophil Cytoplasmic Antibody *on page 636*

Protein, Cerebrospinal Fluid *see* Cerebrospinal Fluid Protein *on page 659*

Protein Electrophoresis, Serum

CPT *84165*

Related Information

Albumin, Serum *on page 102*
Alpha$_1$-Antitrypsin Phenotyping *on page 630*
Alpha$_1$-Antitrypsin, Serum *on page 631*
Cerebrospinal Fluid Protein Electrophoresis *on page 661*
Immunoelectrophoresis, Serum or Urine *on page 706*
Immunofixation Electrophoresis *on page 707*
Leishmaniasis Serological Test *on page 717*
Protein Electrophoresis, Urine *on page 737*
Protein, Total, Serum *on page 340*
Viscosity, Serum/Plasma *on page 611*

Synonyms Electrophoresis, Serum; Immunoelectrophoresis, Serum; Serum Protein Electrophoresis; SPE

Applies to Beta-Gamma Bridging; Globulin, Serum; Immunoglobulins; Light Chains; Monoclonal Gammopathies

Test Commonly Includes Serum electrophoresis for quantitation of albumin, alpha$_1$, alpha$_2$, beta, and gamma globulins. A total protein value is needed, since the fractions are otherwise available only as percentages. Used with total protein, the fractions can be expressed as absolute quantities.

Abstract A variable number of the over 100 proteins present in human serum can be separated by an electric field and quantitated.

Specimen Serum **CONTAINER:** Red top tube **STORAGE INSTRUCTIONS:** Refrigerate separated serum.

Interpretive **REFERENCE RANGE:** Values in the table are representative, but variation between methods and laboratories exists. The figures in the table are based on an agarose system. Values in infancy and early childhood are not identical to adult reference ranges. **USE:** The principal use of this test is in the detection of monoclonal gammopathies. These are usually found in association with hematopoietic neoplasms, especially multiple myeloma and macroglobulinemia of Waldenström. They also occur in other benign and malignant conditions. Any such protein detected should be identified by an alternative technique, such as immunofixation or immunoelectrophoresis.

Other applications of serum protein electrophoresis include the following:

- Serum protein evaluation, nutritional status.
- Work-up for **liver disease**, including cirrhosis and chronic active hepatitis. In liver disease albumin is apt to be decreased. Alpha$_2$ may be low. Gamma is often polyclonal (ie, dome-shaped) in many cases of cirrhosis. The normal depression between beta and gamma area may be missing in hepatic cirrhosis; this is called beta-gamma

bridging. No one of these findings is pathognomonic. All rarely are found together, even in patients who have obvious hepatic cirrhosis. Polyclonal gammopathy occurs in a wide range of entities which have in common chronic immunologic stimulation (eg, sarcoidosis, visceral leishmaniasis, and other entities: *vide infra*).

Protein Electrophoresis, Serum

Component	Relative (%) Normal Range	Absolute (g) Normal Range
Total protein		5.90–8.00
Albumin	58.0–74.0	4.00–5.50
$Alpha_1$	2.0–3.5	0.15–0.25
$Alpha_2$	5.4–10.6	0.43–0.75
Beta	7.0–14.0	0.50–1.00
Gamma	8.0–18.0	0.60–1.30
A/G ratio	1.4–2.6	

- The **gamma globulin** may present an isolated increase. The gamma globulin fraction includes IgG, IgA, IgM, IgD, and IgE. Diffuse polyclonal elevation indicates a chronic immunologic process such as that found with liver disease (eg, chronic active hepatitis, cirrhosis), collagen diseases (eg, systemic LE, rheumatoid arthritis), infectious diseases (eg, osteomyelitis, bronchiectasis, visceral leishmaniasis, leprosy), other inflammatory states (eg, sarcoidosis), neoplasms (eg, some instances of Hodgkin's disease), and chronic myelomonocytic leukemia. Several small bands (oligoclonal) are seen in patients with hepatitis, immune complex diseases, acquired immunodeficiency syndrome, and angioimmunoblastic lymphoadenopathy.
- **Monoclonal gammopathy (M protein)** patterns may be benign, especially when small and not increasing, but monoclonal gammopathies relate especially to myeloma, primary amyloidosis, macroglobulinemia of Waldenström, and occasional malignant lymphomas. These are tall, narrow, spire-shaped formations as seen in densitometer tracings. Although small monoclonal gammopathies ("M spots") may be found with benign diseases, they may also be detected with early or evolving plasma cell dyscrasias or malignant lymphoproliferative diseases. Therefore, such small monoclonal gammopathies are regarded as "monoclonal gammopathies of undetermined significance." All patients with monoclonal gammopathies should be followed with periodic serum protein electrophoresis to differentiate stable from increasing M spikes. Increasing M proteins require further evaluation (bone marrow examination, skeletal x-ray studies, urinary protein electrophoresis, immunoelectrophoretic or immunofixation studies and so forth).
- **Low gamma globulin:** Although gamma globulins may decrease slightly with advancing age, any decrease below the normal range if unexplained by obvious causes of protein loss (such as known renal disease), should be further evaluated with urine immunofixation to detect possible monoclonal free light chains (Bence Jones protein) in the urine. Hypogammaglobulinemia is also seen in many patients with B-cell lymphoproliferative disorders such as chronic lymphocytic leukemia. They may be decreased with cytotoxic or immunosuppressive drug therapy (long-term steroid use, antineoplastic chemotherapy), malignant lymphoproliferative diseases, and plasma cell dyscrasias (multiple myeloma), and adult common variable immunodeficiency syndrome. If there is clinical history of susceptibility to infection in the patient or the family, then quantitative immunodiffusion or nephelometric assay for IgG, IgA, and IgM may prove helpful. Attention to lymphocytes in the peripheral blood film, presence or absence of hepatosplenomegaly and in patients older than age 40, presence or absence of light chains in urine immunoelectrophoresis or immunofixation may be relevant (eg, light chain disease).
- **High $alpha_2$**: $Alpha_2$ includes inflammation-reactive fractions, and may be increased with neoplasms (eg, renal cell carcinomas), acute infections, rheumatic fever, arteritis, nephrotic syndromes, and other inflammatory states. $Alpha_2$-macroglobulin is increased in pregnancy and with diabetes mellitus. Healthy children may have higher levels of $alpha_2$-macroglobulin than adults.
- **Low $alpha_2$**: One of the important fractions of $alpha_2$ is haptoglobin. Depression of haptoglobin may indicate hemolysis. $Alpha_2$ globulins may be decreased in hepatocellular damage. Trauma and transfusions may cause a drop in $alpha_2$.
- **$Alpha_1$ globulins** are increased in active inflammatory or neoplastic diseases.
- **Low $alpha_1$ or flat $alpha_1$ curve:** $Alpha_1$-antitrypsin is responsible for 90% of serine antiprotease activity in serum. Its deficiency is due to a genetic abnormality which must be investigated because it leads to emphysema and cirrhosis. If the patient has

(Continued)

Protein Electrophoresis, Serum *(Continued)*

emphysema, a family history of emphysema, or liver disease of uncertain type, $alpha_1$-antitrypsin assay and phenotype may be indicated. See listings $Alpha_1$-Antitrypsin Phenotyping and $Alpha_1$-Antitrypsin, Serum.

- **Albumin** is better measured by electrophoresis than by chemical methods when it is relevant to do so. Electrophoresis permits diagnosis of rare entities such as analbuminemia and bisalbuminemia. Albumin is increased in dehydration and decreased in a wide variety of subacute, subchronic, and chronic diseases including liver, renal, and gastrointestinal diseases, malnutrition, and cachexia.
- **Decreased total protein with essentially normal pattern** might indicate dietary deficiency or hemodilution (eg, I.V. fluid running at time of venipuncture).
- **Significantly elevated total protein with essentially normal pattern** is likely to be secondary to dehydration.
- **Significantly low total protein and albumin, increased $alpha_2$ and low gamma** is prototypical of the nephrotic syndrome.

LIMITATIONS: Serum protein electrophoresis detects some but not all liver disease. Protein electrophoresis and immunoelectrophoresis or immunofixation of urine as well as serum are useful when one is working up a patient for myeloma or macroglobulinemia of Waldenström. Urine studies may be helpful even if serum protein electrophoresis is unremarkable. Light chain disease is found by urine immunoelectrophoresis or immunofixation for light chains (kappa and lambda). **METHODOLOGY:** Cellulose acetate and agarose electrophoresis are widely used methods. Negatively charged particles migrate toward the positive electrode. **ADDITIONAL INFORMATION:** Detection of a significant monoclonal gammopathy should be followed by more specific examinations (serum quantitative immunoglobulins, immunoelectrophoresis, or immunofixation). Further information is provided in this chapter in listings addressing each immunoglobulin.

References

Bernett A, Allerhand J, Efremides AP, et al, "Long-Term Study of Gammopathies. Clinically Benign Cases Showing Transition to Malignant Plasmacytomas After Long Periods of Observation," *Clin Biochem*, 1986, 19:244-9.

Filomena CA, Filomena AP, Hudock J, et al, "Evaluation of Serum Immunoglobulins by Protein Electrophoresis and Rate Nephelometry Before and After Therapeutic Plasma Exchange," *Am J Clin Pathol*, 1992, 98(2):243-8.

Gandara DR and MacKenzie MR, "Differential Diagnosis of Monoclonal Gammopathy," *Med Clin North Am*, 1988, 72:1155-67, (review).

Gerard SK, Chen KH, and Khayam-Bashi H, "Immunofixation Compared With Immunoelectrophoresis for the Routine Characterization of Paraprotein Disorders," *Am J Clin Pathol*, 1987, 88:198-203.

Gertz MA and Kyle RA, "Hepatic Amyloidosis (Primary [AL], Immunoglobulin Light Chain): The Natural History in 80 Patients," *Am J Med*, 1988, 85:73-80.

Heer M, Joller-Jemelka H, Fontana A, et al, "Monoclonal Gammopathy in Chronic Active Hepatitis," *Liver*, 1984, 4:255-63.

Keren DF, "Interpretation of High-Resolution Electrophoresis Patterns in Serum, Urine, and Cerebrospinal Fluid," *High Resolution Electrophoresis and Immunofixation: Techniques and Interpretation*, Boston, MA: Butterworth's Publishers, 1987, 67-106.

Kyle RA, "Benign Monoclonal Gammopathy. A Misnomer?" *JAMA*, 1984, 251:1849-54.

McManamon TG and Lott JA, "Serum Protein Electrophoresis," *Clinical Chemistry – Theory, Analysis, and Correlation*, 2nd ed, Kaplan LA and Pesce AJ, eds, St Louis, MO: Mosby-Year Book Inc, 1989, 1054-7.

Miller RH, Linet MS, Van Natta ML, et al, "Serum Protein Electrophoresis Patterns in Chronic Lymphocytic Leukemia. Clinical and Epidemiologic Correlations," *Arch Intern Med*, 1987, 147:1614-7.

Ng VL, Hwang KM, Reyes GR, et al, "High Titer Anti-HIV Antibody Reactivity Associated With a Paraprotein Spike in a Homosexual Male With AIDS Related Complex," *Blood*, 1988, 71:1397-401.

Tefferi A, Hoagland HC, Therneau TM, et al, "Chronic Myelomonocytic Leukemia: Natural History and Prognostic Determinants," *Mayo Clin Proc*, 1989, 64(10):1246-54.

Tsianos EV, Di Bisceglie AM, Papadopoulos NM, et al, "Oligoclonal Immunoglobulin Bands in Serum in Association With Chronic Viral Hepatitis," *Am J Gastroenterol*, 1990, 85(8):1005-8.

Vladutiu AO, "Prevalence of M-Proteins in Serum of Hospitalized Patients. Physicians' Response to Finding M-Proteins in Serum Protein Electrophoresis," *Ann Clin Lab Sci*, 1987, 17:157-61.

Protein Electrophoresis, Spinal Fluid *see* Cerebrospinal Fluid Protein Electrophoresis *on page 661*

Protein Electrophoresis, Urine

CPT *84175*

Related Information

Immunoelectrophoresis, Serum or Urine *on page 706*
Immunofixation Electrophoresis *on page 707*
Microalbuminuria *on page 1134*
Protein Electrophoresis, Serum *on page 734*
Protein, Quantitative, Urine *on page 1145*
Protein, Semiquantitative, Urine *on page 1147*
Viscosity, Serum/Plasma *on page 611*

Synonyms Electrophoresis, Protein, Urine; Globulins, Urine; Urine Electrophoresis; Urine Protein Electrophoresis

Applies to Immunoelectrophoresis; Light Chains, Urine; Monoclonal Gammopathy Work-up

Replaces Bence Jones Protein

Test Commonly Includes Quantitative total urine protein, urine albumin, urine alpha$_1$, urine alpha$_2$, urine beta, and urine gamma globulin fractions

Abstract Electrophoresis provides separation of proteins, which then can be quantified.

Specimen Urine **CONTAINER:** Plastic urine container **STORAGE INSTRUCTIONS:** Refrigerate. **CAUSES FOR REJECTION:** Total protein too low to measure or to yield usable electrophoretic pattern

Interpretive **REFERENCE RANGE:** No monoclonal gammopathy detected. **USE:** Evaluate patients with known or suspected myeloma, macroglobulinemia of Waldenström, lymphoma, amyloidosis, or with monoclonal protein in serum **LIMITATIONS:** May not detect pathologic light chains due to insufficient sensitivity of this method. Immunoelectrophoretic or immunofixation study performed on concentrated urine, in particular utilizing antisera against kappa and lambda light chain protein is more sensitive. Optimal specimen when looking for a free monoclonal light chain (Bence Jones protein) is either an early morning specimen or a 24-hour collection. Microalbuminuria is defined as albumin excretion in the range of 30-300 mg/24 hours. The sensitivity of dipstick protein estimation is 150-300 mg/L. Following sample concentration, electrophoresis is not sufficiently sensitive to detect clinically relevant but low concentrations of albumin.[1] More sensitive methods are described in the listing Microalbuminuria in the Urinalysis chapter. **METHODOLOGY:** Electrophoresis, cellulose acetate, and agarose substrates are most commonly used. High resolution techniques are available in some laboratory settings. **ADDITIONAL INFORMATION:** A serum protein electrophoresis should be reviewed concurrently if one has not been recently studied. In nonselective glomerular proteinuria, the urine electrophoretic pattern is often a nonspecific one which may be called "mirror image" to that of the serum. Contamination of the urine with blood can give a similar pattern. With selective glomerular permeability, albumin, alpha$_1$ proteins, and transferrin are the predominant proteins identified on the urine protein electrophoresis, with a relative absence of heavier molecular weight proteins (ie, alpha$_2$-macroglobulin and immunoglobulins). With tubular proteinuria, low molecular weight proteins (alpha$_2$- and beta$_2$-microglobulins) are predominant, with trace amounts of albumin. So called "overflow proteinuria" occurs when low molecular weight proteins are filtered through the glomerulus in increased amounts.

Footnotes

1. Shihabi ZK, Konen JC, and O'Connor ML, "Albuminuria vs Urinary Total Protein for Detecting Chronic Renal Disorders," *Clin Chem*, 1991, 37(5):621-4.

References

Brigden ML, Neal ED, McNeely MD, et al, "The Optimum Urine Collections for the Detection and Monitoring of Bence Jones Proteinuria," *Am J Clin Pathol*, 1990, 93(5):689-93.

Deegan MJ, et al, "High Incidence of Monoclonal Proteins in the Serum and Urine of Chronic Lymphocytic Leukemia Patients," *Blood*, 1984, 6:1207-11.

Keren DF, "Interpretation of High-Resolution Electrophoresis Patterns in Serum, Urine, and Cerebrospinal Fluid," *High Resolution Electrophoresis and Immunofixation: Techniques and Interpretation*, Boston, MA: Butterworth's Publishers, 1987, 67-106.

***Proteus* OX-19** *replaced by* Rocky Mountain Spotted Fever Serology *on page 741*

Psittacosis Titer

CPT *86631; 86632 (IgM)*

Related Information

Chlamydia Group Titer *on page 663*

(Continued)

Psittacosis Titer *(Continued)*

Synonyms *Chlamydia psittaci* Antibodies; *Chlamydia psittaci* Titer

Test Commonly Includes Detection of antibody specific for *Chlamydia psittaci*

Abstract Usually presenting as a pneumonia, psittacosis exists in birds including domestic fowl.

Specimen Serum **CONTAINER:** Red top tube **COLLECTION:** Acute and convalescent samples are recommended.

Interpretive **REFERENCE RANGE:** Less than a fourfold increase in titer in paired sera **USE:** Diagnose psittacosis **LIMITATIONS:** Antibody response may be suppressed if patient has been treated with antibiotics. **METHODOLOGY:** Complement fixation (CF), indirect fluorescent antibody (IFA) **ADDITIONAL INFORMATION:** Most patients with psittacosis develop high titers of complement fixing antibody and in some with the proper clinical setting a single very high titer may be strongly supportive of the diagnosis. Specific IgM antibody can sometimes be demonstrated. To detect psittacosis antibody, an antigen specific for *C. psittaci* must be included in the test system. There may be significant antibody titers in veterinarians and patients with Reiter's syndrome.

References

Schachter J, "Chlamydiae," *Manual of Clinical Laboratory Immunology*, 4th ed, Vol 2, Chapter 96, Rose NR, Conway de Macario E, Fahey JL, et al, eds, Washington, DC: American Society for Microbiology, 1992, 661-6.

Q Fever Titer

CPT 86638

Synonyms *Coxiella burnetii* Titer

Test Commonly Includes Detection of antibody specific for *Coxiella burnetii*

Abstract *Coxiella burnetii*, originally called *Rickettsia burneti*, is a member of the family Rickettsiaceae. The primary reservoirs for Q fever are cattle, sheep, and goats. Originally described in Australia, its distribution is worldwide. It is also called Balkan grippe. Its clinical characteristics include fever with interstitial pneumonitis.

Specimen Serum **CONTAINER:** Red top tube **SPECIAL INSTRUCTIONS:** Acute and convalescent samples are recommended.

Interpretive **REFERENCE RANGE:** Titer: <1:2; comparison of acute and convalescent titers is of greatest diagnostic value **USE:** Support the diagnosis of Q fever due to *Coxiella burnetii* **LIMITATIONS:** Reagents prepared from fresh isolates (phase I organisms) react differently from those from multiply-passaged organism (phase II). **METHODOLOGY:** Complement fixation (CF), indirect fluorescent antibody (IFA) **ADDITIONAL INFORMATION:** Q fever shows no reaction in the Weil-Felix test with *Proteus* antigen, so serologic diagnosis must be based on specific rickettsial antigen. Convalescent sera react best with phase II organism (see above), but sera from chronic persistent infection react best with phase I organisms. Cross reactions with *Legionella* have been described.

References

Dwyer DE, Gibbons VL, Brady LM, et al, "Serologic Reaction to *Legionella pneumophila* Group 4 in a Patient With Q Fever," *J Infect Dis*, 1988, 158:499.

Guigno D, Coupland B, Smith EG, et al, "Primary Humoral Antibody Response to *Coxiella burnetii*, the Causative Agent of Q Fever," *J Clin Microbiol*, 1992, 30(8):1958-67.

Hechemy KE, "The Immunoserology of Rickettsiae," *Manual of Clinical Laboratory Immunology*, 4th ed, Vol 2, Chapter 97, Rose NR, Conway de Macario E, Fahey JL, et al, eds, Washington, DC: American Society for Microbiology, 1992, 667-75.

Htwe KK, Yoshida T, Hayashi S, et al, "Prevalence of Antibodies to *Coxiella burnetii* in Japan," *J Clin Microbiol*, 1993, 31(3):722-3.

Reimer LG, "Q Fever," *Clin Microbiol Rev*, 1993, 6(3):193-8.

Quantitative IgA *see* Immunoglobulin A *on page 709*

Quantitative IgD *see* Immunoglobulin D *on page 710*

Quantitative IgE *see* Immunoglobulin E *on page 710*

Quantitative IgG *see* Immunoglobulin G *on page 710*

Quantitative IgM *see* Immunoglobulin M *on page 712*

Rabbit Fever Antibodies *see* Tularemia Agglutinins *on page 760*

Raji Cell Assay

CPT *86332*

Related Information

Immune Complex Assay *on page 705*

Synonyms Immune Complex Assay by Raji Cell

Specimen Serum CONTAINER: Red top tube COLLECTION: Bring directly to the laboratory. STORAGE INSTRUCTIONS: Serum must be frozen within 2 hours.

Interpretive REFERENCE RANGE: Normal: 0-12 μg AHG Eq/mL; borderline: 12-25 μg AHG Eq/mL; abnormal: >25 μg AHG Eq/mL. (AHG Eq – aggregated human gamma globulin equivalents.) USE: Demonstrate circulating immune complexes LIMITATIONS: **All immune complex assays are expensive and nonspecific and such assays do little to elucidate a specific diagnosis.** CONTRAINDICATIONS: Recent radioactive scan METHODOLOGY: Binding of complement components by Raji cells ADDITIONAL INFORMATION: Raji cells are lymphoblastoid cells derived from Burkitt's lymphoma. They have high affinity receptors for C3. Immune complexes can activate complement. The assay is based therefore on the Raji cell's ability to bind complexes through a link of C3. Once this binding has occurred the complexes can be quantitated by tagging with radiolabeled anti-immunoglobulin and comparison with standards of aggregated human globulin. False-positives occur in individuals with antibodies against lymphocytes. Such lymphocytotoxin antibodies are common in autoimmune diseases. This assay is becoming obsolete.

References

Agnello V, "Immune Complex Assays in Rheumatic Diseases," *Hum Pathol*, 1983, 14:343-9.

Endo L, Corman LC, and Panush RS, "Clinical Utility of Assays for Circulating Immune Complexes," *Med Clin North Am*, 1985, 69:623-36.

Keren DF, "Assays for Circulating Immune Complexes," *Clinical Laboratory Annual*, Batsakis JG and Homburger HA, eds, New York, NY: Appleton-Century-Crofts, 1985, 105-23.

Kilpatrick DC and Weston J, "Immune Complex Assays and Their Limitations," *Med Lab Sci*, 1985, 42:178-85.

McDougal JS and McDuffie FC, "Immune Complexes in Man: Detection and Clinical Significance," *Adv Clin Chem*, 1985, 24:1-60.

Theofilopoulos AN and Dixon FJ, "Detection of Immune Complexes: Techniques and Implications," *Hosp Pract*, 1980, 15:107-21.

Rapid Plasma Reagin Test *see* RPR *on page 742*

Receptor Blocking Antibody *see* Acetylcholine Receptor Antibody *on page 628*

Receptor Modulating Antibody *see* Acetylcholine Receptor Antibody *on page 628*

Recombinant Antigen Immunoblot Assay *see* HIV-1/HIV-2 Serology *on page 696*

Respiratory Syncytial Virus Antibodies *see* Respiratory Syncytial Virus Serology *on this page*

Respiratory Syncytial Virus Serology

CPT *86756*

Related Information

Respiratory Syncytial Virus Culture *on page 1190*

Viral Culture, Respiratory Symptoms *on page 1204*

Virus, Direct Detection by Fluorescent Antibody *on page 1208*

Synonyms Respiratory Syncytial Virus Antibodies; RSV Antibodies; RSV Titer

Test Commonly Includes Detection of antibodies specific for RSV

Specimen Serum CONTAINER: Red top tube SPECIAL INSTRUCTIONS: Acute and convalescent specimens are recommended.

Interpretive REFERENCE RANGE: IgG <1:5, IgM <1:5; less than fourfold rise in titer by CF USE: Establish the diagnosis of respiratory syncytial virus infection LIMITATIONS: Children less than 6 months of age may not mount a diagnostic serologic response to infection. METHODOLOGY: Complement fixation (CF), enzyme-linked immunosorbent assay (ELISA) ADDITIONAL INFORMATION: Diagnosis by CF depends on demonstrating a rise in antibody titer over a 2- to 3-week period. As such, the test is seldom useful in planning clinical care in an acute illness. For rapid diagnosis the demonstration of viral antigen in nasopharyngeal washings or of IgM antibody is more useful.

(Continued)

Respiratory Syncytial Virus Serology *(Continued)*

References

Chonmaitree T, Bessette-Henderson BJ, Hepler RE, et al, "Comparison of Three Rapid Diagnostic Techniques for Detection of Respiratory Syncytial Virus from Nasal Wash Specimens," *J Clin Microbiol*, 1987, 25:746-7.

Costello MJ, Smernoff NT, and Yungbluth M, "Laboratory Diagnosis of Viral Respiratory Tract Infections," *Lab Med*, 1993, 24(3):150-1.

Kumar ML, Super DM, Lembo RM, et al, "Diagnostic Efficacy of Two Rapid Tests for Detection of Respiratory Syncytial Virus Antigen," *J Clin Microbiol*, 1987, 25:873-5.

Lauer BA, Masters HA, Wren CG, et al, "Rapid Detection of Respiratory Syncytial Virus in Nasopharyngeal Secretions by Enzyme-Linked Immunosorbent Assay," *J Clin Microbiol*, 1985, 22:782-5.

Meddens MJ, Herbrink P, Lindeman J, et al, "Serodiagnosis of Respiratory Syncytial Virus (RSV) Infection in Children as Measured by Detection of RSV-Specific Immunoglobulins G, M, and A With Enzyme-Linked Immunosorbent Assay," *J Clin Microbiol*, 1990, 28(1):152-5.

Swenson PD and Kaplan MH, "Rapid Detection of Respiratory Syncytial Virus in Nasopharyngeal Aspirates by a Commercial Enzyme Immunoassay," *J Clin Microbiol*, 1986, 23:485-8.

RF *see* Rheumatoid Factor *on this page*

Rheumatoid Factor

CPT 86430

Related Information

Cryoglobulin, Qualitative, Serum *on page 670*
Synovial Fluid Analysis *on page 1158*

Synonyms RF

Applies to Rheumatoid Factor, Synovial Fluid

Replaces Rose-Waaler Test; Singer-Plotz Test

Test Commonly Includes Detection of rheumatoid factor in patient's serum

Specimen Serum **CONTAINER:** Red top tube

Interpretive **REFERENCE RANGE:** Negative **USE:** Help in the differential diagnosis and prognosis of arthritis **LIMITATIONS:** There are numerous interlaboratory and intermethod variations. IgG and IgA rheumatoid factors are not distinguished by most commercial test kits. About 33% of patients with juvenile rheumatoid arthritis are often RF negative. Rheumatoid factor is positive in many diseases besides rheumatoid arthritis (*vide infra*). **METHODOLOGY:** Latex-human IgG agglutination, sheep RBC-rabbit IgG agglutination, rate nephelometry **ADDITIONAL INFORMATION:** Rheumatoid factors are antibodies directed against the Fc fragment of IgG. These are usually IgM antibodies, but may be IgG or IgA. Rheumatoid factor is present in the serum of a majority of patients with rheumatoid arthritis, depending in part on what method is used. Latex beads coated with human IgG will be positive in 70% to 85% (and have significant numbers of false-positives). Sheep RBCs coated with rabbit IgG will be positive in 60% to 70% (and have fewer false-positives). Rheumatoid factor can also be measured quantitatively by laser nephelometry which has good interlaboratory reproducibility.

Many rheumatic conditions and other chronic inflammatory processes also may produce rheumatoid factors. An incomplete list includes bacterial endocarditis, malaria, syphilis, tuberculosis, hepatitis, leprosy, leishmaniasis, sarcoidosis, and infectious mononucleosis. Thus, the presence of rheumatoid factor, especially in low titer, is far from diagnostic for rheumatoid arthritis. Furthermore, people with no clinical illness may have rheumatoid factor.

Statistically, patients with rheumatoid arthritis who have high titer rheumatoid factor are more likely to have severe disease and systemic involvement than other patients. High titers correlate with presence of rheumatoid nodules, and low synovial fluid complement. Rheumatoid factor can be detected in synovial fluid, but contributes little more than a positive serum test. Some rheumatoid factors may behave as cryoglobulins.

The production of RF may be regulated by anti-idiotypic antibodies, IgG antibodies directed against specific sites on Fab fragments.

References

Baumann GP and Hurtubise P, "Anti-Idiotypes and Autoimmune Disease," *Clin Lab Med*, 1988, 8:399-407.

Chandor SB, "Autoimmune Phenomena in Lymphoid Malignancies," *Clin Lab Med*, 1988, 8:373-84.

Colvin RB, Bhan AK, and McCluskey RT, eds, *Diagnostic Immunopathology*, New York, NY: Raven Press, 1988, 89.

Espinoza LR, "Rheumatoid Arthritis: Etiopathogenetic Considerations," *Clin Lab Med*, 1986, 6:27-40.

Shmerling RH and Delbanco TL, "How Useful Is the Rheumatoid Factor? An Analysis of Sensitivity, Specificity, and Predictive Value," *Arch Intern Med*, 1992, 152:2417-20.

Wolfe F, Cathey MA, and Roberts FK, "The Latex Test Revisited Rheumatoid Factor Testing in 8287 Rheumatic Disease Products," *Arthritis Rheum*, 1991, 34(8):951-60.

Rheumatoid Factor, Synovial Fluid *see* Rheumatoid Factor *on previous page*

RIBA *see* HIV-1/HIV-2 Serology *on page 696*

RIBA Test for HIV Antibody *see* HIV-1/HIV-2 Serology *on page 696*

Rickettsial Antibody Titer *see* Bacterial Serology *on page 644*

Rickettsial Disease Agglutinins *see* Weil-Felix Agglutinins *on page 764*

***Rickettsia rickettsii* Serology** *see* Rocky Mountain Spotted Fever Serology *on this page*

RNP Antibody *see* Antinuclear Antibody *on page 638*

Ro Antibodies *see* Sjögren's Antibodies *on page 746*

Rocky Mountain Spotted Fever Serology

CPT *86255 (fluorescent screen); 86256 (titer)*

Related Information

Febrile Agglutinins, Serum *on page 678*

Weil-Felix Agglutinins *on page 764*

Synonyms *Rickettsia rickettsii* Serology

Replaces *Proteus* OX-19

Abstract Transmitted by ticks, this acute, febrile disease is characterized by headache, fever, weakness, and a centipetal macular eruption beginning on hands and feet.

Specimen Serum **CONTAINER:** Red top tube **SPECIAL INSTRUCTIONS:** Acute and convalescent specimens are recommended.

Interpretive **REFERENCE RANGE:** Less than a fourfold increase in titer in paired sera; IgG <1:64, IgM <1:8 **USE:** Establish the diagnosis of Rocky Mountain spotted fever **LIMITATIONS:** Cross reactions in the spotted fever group occurs. False-positive reactions may occur during pregnancy, especially in the last two trimesters. **METHODOLOGY:** Complement fixation (CF), indirect fluorescent antibody (IFA), hemagglutination, enzyme-linked immunosorbent assay (ELISA) **ADDITIONAL INFORMATION:** Rocky Mountain spotted fever occurs primarily in the southeastern and western United States from April through October, but is also endemic on Long Island. It is a disease of variable clinical manifestation (indeed some cases present with few or no "spots"), and since there is good specific therapy, and serious outcome if untreated, all aids to diagnosis are important. Serologic diagnosis may be made promptly enough to direct therapy.

Hemagglutination and immunofluorescent tests are least subject to cross reactions with other *Rickettsia*. The complement fixation test can be used with different concentration of antigen to minimize cross reactions. Tests for IgM specific antibody are helpful in early disease, since they appear in 3-8 days. Patients treated with antibiotics early in illness may not develop serologic responses. A direct fluorescent test is also available to demonstrate the *Rickettsia* in tissue. As many as 71% of patients with Rocky Mountain spotted fever also develop antibodies against cardiolipin and endothelial cells.

References

Durack DT, "*Rus in Urbe* – Spotted Fever Comes to Town," *N Engl J Med*, 1988, 318:1388-90.

Salgo MP, Telzak EE, Currie B, et al, "A Focus of Rocky Mountain Spotted Fever Within New York City," *N Engl J Med*, 1988, 318:1345-8.

Sexton DJ and Corey GR, "Rocky Mountain "Spotless" and "Almost Spotless" Fever: A Wolf in Sheep's Clothing," *Clin Infect Dis*, 1992, 15(3):439-48.

Walker TS and Triplett DA, "Serologic Characterization of Rocky Mountain Spotted Fever. Appearance of Antibodies Reactive With Endothelial Cells and Phospholipids, and Factors That Alter Protein C Activation and Prostacyclin Secretion," *Am J Clin Pathol*, 1991, 95(5):725-32.

Welch KJ, Rumley RL, and Levine JA, "False-Positive Results in Serologic Tests for Rocky Mountain Spotted Fever During Pregnancy," *South Med J*, 1991, 84(3):307-11.

Rose-Waaler Test *replaced by* Rheumatoid Factor *on previous page*

Rotavirus Antibody *see* Rotavirus Serology *on next page*

Rotavirus EIA *see* Rotavirus Serology *on next page*

Rotavirus Serology

CPT 86759

Related Information

Electron Microscopic Examination for Viruses, Stool *on page 1177*
Rotavirus, Direct Detection *on page 1191*

Synonyms Rotavirus Antibody; Rotavirus EIA

Test Commonly Includes Detection of antibody specific for rotaviruses

Specimen Serum **CONTAINER:** Red top tube

Interpretive **REFERENCE RANGE:** Result in terms of positive or negative only; no quantitation is given; IgM antirotavirus is useful to distinguish recent from older infections. **USE:** Aid in the diagnosis of rotavirus infection **METHODOLOGY:** Enzyme-linked immunosorbent assay (ELISA), latex agglutination (LA) **ADDITIONAL INFORMATION:** Rotavirus, of which there are five serogroups, is a common cause of diarrhea, particularly in pediatric population. Although there is no specific treatment for the viral illness, it may be important to establish a viral etiology and exclude some other cause of diarrhea. It may also be important to show that a postviral lactase deficiency is not a reinfection. Stool can be tested directly to demonstrate that virus is present, or blood can be tested to show development of antibody to rotavirus.

References

Bishop RF, Cipriani E, Lund JS, et al, "Estimation of Rotavirus Immunoglobulin G Antibodies in Human Serum Samples By Enzyme-Linked Immunosorbent Assay: Expression of Results as Units Derived From a Standard Curve," *J Clin Microbiol*, 1984, 19:447-52.

Chiba S, Nakata S, Ukae S, et al, "Virological and Serological Aspects of Immune Resistance to Rotavirus Gastroenteritis," *Clin Infect Dis*, 1993, 16(Suppl 2):S117-2.

Nakata S, Estes MK, Graham DY, et al, "Detection of Antibody to Group B Adult Diarrhea Rotaviruses in Humans," *J Clin Microbiol*, 1987, 25:812-8.

Yolken RH, "Enzyme Immunoassay for the Detection of Rotavirus Antigen and Antibody," *Manual of Clinical Laboratory Immunology*, 4th ed, Vol 2, Rose NR, Conway de Macario E, Fahey JL, et al, eds, Washington, DC: American Society for Microbiology, 1992, 651-60.

RPR

CPT 86592

Related Information

Anticardiolipin Antibody *on page 632*
Antinuclear Antibody *on page 638*
Automated Reagin Test *on page 642*
Darkfield Examination, Syphilis *on page 808*
FTA-ABS, Serum *on page 680*
Genital Culture *on page 814*
MHA-TP *on page 724*
Neisseria gonorrhoeae Culture *on page 831*
Risks of Transfusion *on page 1093*
VDRL, Cerebrospinal Fluid *on page 761*
VDRL, Serum *on page 762*

Synonyms Rapid Plasma Reagin Test

Applies to Syphilis Serology

Replaces ART Test; Kahn Test; Kline Test; Mazzini; Wassermann

Test Commonly Includes Reactive specimens may be titered and/or an FTA-ABS test performed

Abstract A screening (reaginic) (nontreponemal) test for syphilis

Specimen Serum **CONTAINER:** Red top tube

Interpretive **REFERENCE RANGE:** Negative **USE:** Screening test for syphilis **LIMITATIONS:** This is a nontreponemal test and is associated with false-positive reactions due to intercurrent infections, pregnancy, drug addiction, autoimmune disease, increased age, autoimmunity, Gaucher's disease, and a number of other entities.[1] **METHODOLOGY:** Agglutination test with reagin antibody **ADDITIONAL INFORMATION:** This is a screening test for syphilis and detects antibodies to reagin. These antibodies usually develop within 4-6 weeks of inoculation, peak during the secondary phase of disease, and then decrease. They also decrease and usually disappear with treatment. The RPR is more sensitive than the VDRL and the ART. Ninety-three percent of patients with primary syphilis will have positive tests. RPR titers are usually higher in HIV-infected patients than in those who do not have HIV infection.

Because of the many causes of false-positive tests, any reactive serum should be tested by a treponemal-specific test, preferably MHA-TP or FTA-ABS. The RPR should not be done on cerebrospinal fluid. False-negative tests may occur at birth in some infants with recently acquired congenital syphilis. Therefore, especially in areas where the disease is prevalent, a serologic test for syphilis should be included in evaluation of febrile infants even if they had a negative screen at birth. False-negatives have also been due to the prozone effect. Therefore, dilution should be performed on serum of pregnant women in areas with high syphilis prevalence when screening tests are negative.

Of 72 mother/newborn pairs, in whom RPR or FTA-ABS was utilized at delivery, positive results were detected in 94% of maternal specimens. The authors concluded that serial serologic testing during pregnancy with maternal and neonatal serologic studies at delivery was desirable for detection of neonates at risk. In instances of negative tests even following dilutions, serology should be repeated within several weeks when suspicion of congenital syphilis exists.[2]

Footnotes

1. Hook EW 3d and Marra CM, "Acquired Syphilis in Adults," *N Engl J Med*, 1992, 326(16):1060-9, (review).
2. Chhabra RS, Brion LP, Castro M, et al, "Comparison of Maternal Sera, Cord Blood, and Neonatal Sera for Detecting Presumptive Congenital Syphilis: Relationship With Maternal Treatment," *Pediatrics*, 1993, 91(1):88-91.

References

Berkowitz K, Baxi L, and Fox HE, "False-Negative Syphilis Serology: The Prozone Phenomenon, Nonimmune Hydrops, and Diagnosis of Syphilis During Pregnancy," *Am J Obstet Gynecol*, 1990, 163(3):975-7.

Dorfman DH and Glaser JH, "Congenital Syphilis Presenting in Infants After the Newborn Period," *N Engl J Med*, 1990, 323(19):1299-302.

Hart G, "Syphilis Tests in Diagnostic and Therapeutic Decision Making," *Ann Intern Med*, 1986, 104:368-76.

Hutchinson CM, Rompalo AM, Reichart CA, et al, "Characteristics of Patients With Syphilis Attending Baltimore STD Clinics. Multiple High-Risk Groups and Interactions With Human Immunodeficiency Virus Infection," *Arch Intern Med*, 1991, 151(3):511-6.

RSV Antibodies *see* Respiratory Syncytial Virus Serology *on page 739*

RSV Titer *see* Respiratory Syncytial Virus Serology *on page 739*

Rubella Antibodies *see* Rubella Serology *on this page*

Rubella Serology

CPT 86762

Related Information

Rubella Virus Culture *on page 1192*

TORCH *on page 758*

Synonyms German Measles Serology; Rubella Antibodies

Applies to IgG Antibodies to Rubella; IgM Antibodies to Rubella

Test Commonly Includes Detection of serologic response to rubella infection or vaccination

Abstract German measles is a viral infection usually characterized by a macular exanthem, an incubation period of 14-21 days and lymphadenopathy, pharyngitis, and conjunctivitis. Severe transplacental infections occur in the first trimester.

Specimen Serum **CONTAINER:** Red top tube

Interpretive **REFERENCE RANGE:** Absence of antibody indicates susceptibility to rubella. Presence of IgM antibody indicates acute infection or vaccination. Presence of IgG antibody requires interpretation. **POSSIBLE PANIC RANGE:** Evidence of susceptibility in a pregnant woman recently exposed to rubella **USE:** Aid in diagnosis of congenital rubella infections; evaluate susceptibility to infections **LIMITATIONS:** Requires clinical correlation and judgment. Low levels of antibody are poorly detected by enzyme immunoassays. **METHODOLOGY:** Indirect fluorescent antibody (IFA), hemagglutination, enzyme-linked immunosorbent assay (ELISA), radioimmunoassay (RIA), hemolysis-in-gel, complement fixation (CF), latex agglutination (LA), enzyme immunoassay (EIA) **ADDITIONAL INFORMATION:** Rubella virus is the cause of German measles, usually a mild exanthem, often subclinical. However, when acquired *in utero*, rubella virus can cause the congenital rubella syndrome, and lead to fetal demise, cataracts, malformation, deafness, and mental retardation. For this reason the federal government and many states support programs to immunize women against rubella before they have children. There has been a resurgence of congenital rubella in the early 1990s and more widespread screening for rubella serology is recommended.

The role of serologic testing for antibodies to rubella is different in different clinical settings. The simplest and most straight forward application is in premarital assessment of immunity.

(Continued)

Rubella Serology *(Continued)*

If a woman has antibodies against rubella, even of low titer, demonstrated by any of multiple methods, she need not worry about infection during subsequent pregnancy. If she is not immune, and is not pregnant, she can receive rubella vaccine.

A second, more complex, role is in the management of a pregnant woman who has been exposed to rubella. Here the questions include susceptibility, present acute infection, and risk to the fetus. Several flowcharts are available to assess these possibilities, utilizing antibody titers, class of antibody, and changes in titer over time. Management of such a case requires individualized expert consultation. Of particular concern is that some enzyme-linked immunoassays are not as sensitive and specific as hemagglutination inhibition.

Still a third role is in the evaluation of an infant born with an illness which may be congenital rubella. Problems here include evaluating whether antibody is present, and whether it represents antibody passively acquired by transplacental passage or is indicative of true neonatal infection. In this setting determining the immunoglobulin class is particularly important; IgM antibody strongly supports congenital infection.

References

Condorelli F and Ziegler T, "Dot Immunobinding Assay for Simultaneous Detection of Specific Immunoglobulin G Antibodies to Measles Virus, Mumps Virus, and Rubella Virus," *J Clin Microbiol*, 1993, 31(3):717-9.

Duverlie G, Roussel C, Driencourt M, et al, "Latex Enzyme Immunoassay for Measuring IgG Antibodies to Rubella Virus," *J Clin Pathol*, 1990, 43(9):766-70.

Fayram SL, Akin S, Aarnaes SL, et al, "Determination of Immune Status in Patients With Low Antibody Titers for Rubella Virus," *J Clin Microbiol*, 1987, 25:178-80.

Lee SH, Ewert DF, Frederick PD, et al, "Resurgence of Congenital Rubella Syndrome in the 1990s. Report on Missed Opportunities and Failed Prevention Policies Among Women of Childbearing Age," *JAMA*, 1992, 267(19):2616-20.

Zhang T, Mauracher CA, Mitchell LA, et al, "Detection of Rubella Virus-Specific Immunoglobulin G (IgG), IgM, and IgA Antibodies by Immunoblot Assays," *J Clin Microbiol*, 1992, 30(4):824-30.

Rubeola Antibodies *see* Measles Antibody *on page 723*

Rubeola Serology, CSF *see* Measles Antibody *on page 723*

Sabin-Feldman Dye Test *replaced by* Toxoplasmosis Serology *on page 759*

***Salmonella* Agglutinins** *see Salmonella* Titer *on this page*

Salmonella Titer

CPT 86768

Related Information

Blood Culture, Aerobic and Anaerobic *on page 784*
Febrile Agglutinins, Serum *on page 678*
Stool Culture *on page 858*

Synonyms *Salmonella* Agglutinins; Typhoid Agglutinins

Applies to Widal Agglutination Test

Test Commonly Includes Agglutination of "O" and/or "H" *Salmonella* antigens for groups A, B, C, or D

Abstract The genus *Salmonella* are gram-negative organisms which fail to ferment lactose. It includes typhoid/paratyphoid bacilli.

Specimen Serum **CONTAINER:** Red top tube **COLLECTION:** Acute and convalescent specimens are recommended

Interpretive **REFERENCE RANGE:** A convalescent titer less than fourfold higher than the acute titer. **Titers on a single specimen are not diagnostically significant.** **USE:** Detect antibodies to specific *Salmonella* antigens **LIMITATIONS:** Numerous false-positives due to cross reacting bacterial antigens and heterospecific anamnestic responses. Clinical correlation is mandatory. **Single determinations are without value. Stool cultures should be obtained.** **METHODOLOGY:** Agglutination, enzyme-linked immunosorbent assay (ELISA) **ADDITIONAL INFORMATION:** The Salmonellacea possess "H" ("Hauch") or flagellar antigens and "O" ("ohne Hauch") or somatic cell wall antigens. The diversity of these is staggering, and screening agglutination tests, even of restricted antigen batteries, are too insensitive and nonspecific to be useful. Misleading titers due to infection with some other organism, false low titers because of partial treatment with antibiotics, and uninterpretable low titers would make the test poor even if it were used correctly, which is almost never the case. Agglutinating titers can only be interpreted if a series of tests are obtained over time, and a single group shows a clear, significant rise. Some of the recently developed EIA techniques may prove more useful than the older agglutination assays. The practice of obtaining a single set of agglutinations with no follow-up is condemned. Stool culture remains the definitive technique for diagnosing bacterial diarrheal disease, supplemented by blood culture. Serologic study may be useful to detect chronic carriers of *S. typhosa*. Such patients have antibody to the Vi antigen of *Citrobacter freundii* and successful treatment lowers the titer.

References

Isomaki O, Vuento R, and Granfors K, "Serological Diagnosis of *Salmonella* Infections by Enzyme Immunoassay," *Lancet*, 1989, 1(8652):1411-4.

Sack RB and Sack DA, "Immunologic Methods for the Diagnosis of Infections by *Enterobacteriaceae* and *Vibrionaceae*," *Manual of Clinical Laboratory Immunology*, 4th ed, Vol 2, Chapter 74, Rose NR, Conway de Macario E, Fahey JL, et al, eds, Washington, DC: American Society for Microbiology, 1992, 482-8.

Schistosomiasis Serological Test

***CPT** 86317 (immunoassay); 88347 (indirect immunofluorescence)*

Related Information

Ova and Parasites, Stool *on page 836*
Ova and Parasites, Urine *on page 839*
Parasite Antibodies *on page 729*

Synonyms Bilharziasis

Applies to Flukes

Test Commonly Includes Detection of serologic response to *Schistosoma* species

Abstract In excess of 200 million people have schistosomiasis (bilharziasis). The three major species of these blood flukes are *Schistosoma haematobium*, *S. mansoni*, and *S. japonicum*.

Specimen Serum CONTAINER: Red top tube

Interpretive REFERENCE RANGE: Negative USE: Support a clinical diagnosis of schistosomiasis LIMITATIONS: Test does not differentiate between recently acquired infection and chronic multiple exposures and so is simply reported as positive or negative. Test does not differentiate between intestinal and vesical schistosomiasis. METHODOLOGY: Indirect fluorescent antibody (IFA) using sections of adult worms; enzyme-linked immunosorbent assay (ELISA) with egg antigen ADDITIONAL INFORMATION: Schistosomiasis worldwide represents one of our greatest public health challenges, and one of the most common diseases (the most common cause of hematuria, for example). Demonstration of eggs in bladder or bowel biopsy is definitive, and the examination of stool and urine for eggs is a mainstay of diagnosis. Serologic diagnosis is now sensitive and specific, but its present role in clinical decision making is not yet established.

References

Ash LR and Orihel TC, *Atlas of Human Parasitology*, 3rd ed, Chicago, IL: ASCP Press, 1990, 206-11.

Kagan IG and Maddison SE, "Serodiagnosis of Parasitic Diseases," *Manual of Clinical Laboratory Immunology*, 4th ed, Vol 2, Chapter 79, Rose NR, Conway de Macario E, Fahey JL, et al, eds, Washington, DC: American Society for Microbiology, 1992, 529-43.

Scl-1 Antibody *replaced by* Scleroderma Antibody *on this page*

Scl-70 *see* Antinuclear Antibody *on page 638*

Scl-70 Antibody *see* Scleroderma Antibody *on this page*

Scleroderma Antibody

***CPT** 86235*

Related Information

Centromere/Kinetochore Antibody *on page 653*
Kidney Biopsy *on page 68*
LE Cell Test *on page 565*

Synonyms Progressive Systemic Sclerosis Antibody; Scl-70 Antibody

Applies to Topoisomerase I

Replaces Scl-1 Antibody

Abstract Systemic sclerosis (scleroderma) is a multisystem disease which includes sclerosis (fibrosis) of skin, gastrointestinal tract, lungs, vessels, heart, and renal parenchyma. Scleroderma may be localized.

Specimen Serum CONTAINER: Red top tube STORAGE INSTRUCTIONS: Refrigerate separated serum.

(Continued)

Scleroderma Antibody *(Continued)*

Interpretive REFERENCE RANGE: Negative USE: Aid the diagnosis of scleroderma (progressive systemic sclerosis) LIMITATIONS: Absence of scleroderma antibody does not exclude diagnosis. METHODOLOGY: Immunodiffusion (ID) ADDITIONAL INFORMATION: The antigen for this autoantibody is topoisomerase I (an enzyme responsible for unwinding supercoiled DNA and creating single-stranded nicks in DNA). In older literature it was referred to as Scl-1. Scl-70 antibody is seen in 20% of patients with scleroderma, and in some patients with CREST syndrome (calcinosis, Raynaud's, esophageal dysfunction, sclerodactyly, telangiectasia). These syndromes are also associated with a high frequency of speckled pattern using immunofluorescent antinuclear antibody tests. Scl-70 may identify a subset of scleroderma patients with severe skin, joint, and lung disease.

References

Colvin RB, Bhan AK, and McCluskey RT, eds, *Diagnostic Immunopathology*, New York, NY: Raven Press, 1988.

Gilliland BC, "Systemic Sclerosis (Scleroderma)," *Harrison's Principles of Internal Medicine*, 12th ed, Vol 1, Wilson JD, Braunwald E, Isselbacher KJ, et al, eds, New York, NY: McGraw-Hill Inc, 1991, 1443-8.

Harmon CE, "Antinuclear Antibodies in Autoimmune Disease," *Med Clin North Am*, 1985, 69:547-63.

Keren DF and Warren JS, *Diagnostic Immunology*, Baltimore, MD: Williams & Wilkins, 1992, 154.

Nakamura RM and Tan EM, "Recent Advances in Laboratory Tests and the Significance of Autoantibodies to Nuclear Antigens in Systemic Rheumatic Diseases," *Clin Lab Med*, 1986, 6:41-53.

Serologic Test for Syphilis *see* Automated Reagin Test *on page 642*

Serologic Test for Syphilis *see* FTA-ABS, Serum *on page 680*

Serum Hepatitis Marker *replaced by* Hepatitis B Surface Antigen *on page 688*

Serum Protein Electrophoresis *see* Protein Electrophoresis, Serum *on page 734*

Serum VDRL *see* VDRL, Serum *on page 762*

Singer-Plotz Test *replaced by* Rheumatoid Factor *on page 740*

Sjögren's Antibodies

CPT 86235

Related Information

Anticardiolipin Antibody *on page 632*

Antinuclear Antibody *on page 638*

LE Cell Test *on page 565*

Synonyms La Antibodies; Ro Antibodies; SS-A Antibodies; SS-B Antibodies

Abstract Sjögren's syndrome is a complex immunologic entity. It includes keratoconjunctivitis, pharyngitis sicca, xerostomia, parotid enlargement, and arthritis. A secondary form is found in patients with other diseases regarded as autoimmune. Lymphoproliferative processes occur. Renal involvement is found in about 40% of those with primary Sjögren's syndrome.[1]

Specimen Serum CONTAINER: Red top tube

Interpretive REFERENCE RANGE: Negative USE: Useful in diagnosis of Sjögren's syndrome (especially with vasculitis) and some forms of lupus; may be present in antiphospholipid antibody syndrome METHODOLOGY: Immunodiffusion (ID) ADDITIONAL INFORMATION: SS-A(Ro) is found in 60% to 70% of patients with Sjögren's syndrome and 30% to 40% of patients with SLE. SS-B(La) is found in 50% to 60% of Sjögren's syndrome and 10% to 15% of SLE. SS-A may be weak or negative by immunofluorescence (it is soluble in the buffers used), but SS-B may be seen as a speckled antinuclear pattern. SS-A and SS-B are particularly useful in "ANA negative" cases of SLE, being present in a majority of such cases. Patients who are ANA positive and who have SS-A but not SS-B are very likely to have nephritis. Antibodies to SS-A are also associated with HLA loci DR3 and DR2 and with hereditary deficiency of C2. Anti-SS-A and anti-SS-B are found in virtually all children with neonatal lupus. Patients with SS-A may also have antibodies to cardiolipin, lupus anticoagulant, and clinical thromboses. This has been termed antiphospholipid antibody syndrome. Biopsy of the lower lip provides minor salivary gland tissue for histopathologic evaluation.

Footnotes

1. Lane HC and Fauci AS, "Sjögren's Syndrome," *Harrison's Principles of Internal Medicine*, 12th ed, Vol 1, Wilson JD, Braunwald E, Isselbacher KJ, et al, eds, New York, NY: McGraw-Hill Inc, 1991, 1449-50.

References

Arnett FC, Hamilton RG, Reveille JD, et al, "Genetic Studies of Ro (SS-A) and La (SS-B) Autoantibodies in Families With Systemic Lupus Erythematosus and Primary Sjögren's Syndrome," *Arthritis Rheum*, 1989, 32(4):413-9.

Colvin RB, Bhan AK, and McCluskey RT, eds, *Diagnostic Immunopathology*, New York, NY: Raven Press, 1988, 100.

Fox RI, Chan EK, and Kang HI, "Laboratory Evaluation of Patients With Sjögren's Syndrome," *Clin Biochem*, 1992, 25(3):213-22.

Nakamura RM and Tan EM, "Recent Advances in Laboratory Tests and the Significance of Autoantibodies to Nuclear Antigens in Systemic Rheumatic Diseases," *Clin Lab Med*, 1986, 6:41-53.

Reichlin M and Wasicek CA, "Clinical and Biologic Significance of Antibodies to Ro/SS-A," *Hum Pathol*, 1983, 14:401-5.

Scully RE, Mark EJ, and McNeely WF, "Case Records of the Massachusetts General Hospital," *N Engl J Med*, 1988, 319:699-712.

Skeletal Muscle Antibody

***CPT** 86255 (screen); 86256 (titer)*

Related Information

Creatine Kinase *on page 196*

Muscle Biopsy *on page 75*

Synonyms Antiskeletal Muscle Antibody

Specimen Serum **CONTAINER:** Red top tube

Interpretive **REFERENCE RANGE:** Negative **USE:** Diagnosis of myopathic disorders **LIMITATIONS:** Clinical applicability not yet established. **METHODOLOGY:** Indirect fluorescent antibody (IFA) **ADDITIONAL INFORMATION:** Immunoglobulins reacting to, or deposited in, muscle can be demonstrated in numerous rheumatic disorders. Sarcolemmal basement membrane, fibers, and vessels may all be involved, individually or in combination. Unfortunately, the variability and inconsistency of patterns reported are such that the test has no clinical application yet.

References

Colvin RB, Bhan AK, and McCluskey RT, eds, *Diagnostic Immunopathology*, New York, NY: Raven Press, 1988, 108-10.

Oxenhandler R and Hart MN, "Skeletal Muscle Immunopathology," *Hum Pathol*, 1983, 14:326-37.

Skin Biopsy Antibodies *see* Immunofluorescence, Skin Biopsy *on page 708*

Skin Biopsy For Bullous or Collagen Disease *see* Immunofluorescence, Skin Biopsy *on page 708*

Skin Biopsy For Pemphigus *see* Immunofluorescence, Skin Biopsy *on page 708*

Skin Biopsy Immunofluorescence *see* Immunofluorescence, Skin Biopsy *on page 708*

SMA *see* Smooth Muscle Antibody *on this page*

Sm Antibody *see* Antinuclear Antibody *on page 638*

Smooth Muscle Antibody

***CPT** 86255 (screen); 86256 (titer)*

Related Information

Antimitochondrial Antibody *on page 635*

LE Cell Test *on page 565*

Synonyms Antismooth Muscle Antibody; SMA

Applies to Liver/Kidney Microsomes (LKM) Antibody; Soluble Liver Antigen (SLA) Antibody

Specimen Serum **CONTAINER:** Red top tube

Interpretive **REFERENCE RANGE:** Negative **USE:** Useful in the differential diagnosis of liver disease. Antismooth muscle antibodies are found mainly in chronic active hepatitis (CAH) (40% to 70% of cases). **LIMITATIONS:** Presence of antinuclear antibody may interfere with the interpretation of smooth muscle antibody. Less than 2% of normal patients have low titer antibody. Antismooth muscle antibody is present, usually at titers <1:80, in 50% of patients with primary biliary cirrhosis, and in occasional cases of cryptogenic cirrhosis, infectious mononucleosis, asthma, and neoplasm. **METHODOLOGY:** Indirect fluorescent antibody (IFA) **ADDITIONAL INFORMATION:** Titers of 1:80-1:320 are characteristic of chronic active hepatitis. When the antibody is present in other conditions it is almost always at titers <1:80. Other laboratory findings sug-

(Continued)

Smooth Muscle Antibody *(Continued)*

gesting chronic active hepatitis include elevated serum transaminases and IgG, and a positive LE preparation with a negative anti-DNA test. Other tests likely to be abnormal in CAH include serum bilirubin, alkaline phosphatase, prothrombin time, and protein electrophoresis. Many patients with chronic active hepatitis (HB_sAg negative) have high titers of antibody to measles, which are not cross reactive with antibody to smooth muscle. SMA are reactive with F-actin. For the best delineation of autoimmune liver disease, SMA should not be done alone, but with assays of antibodies against liver/kidney microsomes (LKM) and soluble liver antigen (SLA). For diagnosis of chronic active hepatitis, liver biopsy is needed to establish diagnosis.

References

Colvin RB, Bhan AK, and McCluskey RT, eds, *Diagnostic Immunopathology*, New York, NY: Raven Press, 1988, 108-10.

Manns MP and Nakamura RM, "Autoimmune Liver Diseases," *Clin Lab Med*, 1988, 8:281-301.

Nakamura RM and Deodhar S, "Laboratory Tests in the Diagnosis of Autoimmune Disorders," Chicago, IL: American Society of Clinical Pathologists, 1976.

Sommer AI and Haukenes G, "Lack of Cross Reactivity Between Antibody Against Smooth Muscle and Antibodies to Measles Virus in Sera From Patients With Chronic Active Hepatitis," *J Clin Pathol*, 1982, 35:1388-91.

Vrethem M, Skogh T, Berlin G, et al, "Autoantibodies Versus Clinical Symptoms in Blood Donors," *J Rheumatol*, 1992, 19(12):1919-21.

Wands JR and Isselbacher KJ, "Chronic Hepatitis," *Harrison's Principles of Internal Medicine*, 12th ed, Vol 1, Wilson JD, Braunwald E, Isselbacher KJ, et al, eds, New York, NY: McGraw-Hill Inc, 1991, 1337-40.

Soluble Liver Antigen (SLA) Antibody *see* Smooth Muscle Antibody *on previous page*

SPE *see* Protein Electrophoresis, Serum *on page 734*

Specific Protein Analysis *see* Alpha$_1$-Antitrypsin, Serum *on page 631*

Spherulin® *see* Coccidioidomycosis Antibodies *on page 664*

Spinal Fluid Electrophoresis *see* Cerebrospinal Fluid Protein Electrophoresis *on page 661*

Spinal Fluid Globulin *see* Cerebrospinal Fluid Immunoglobulin G *on page 656*

Spinal Fluid Immunoglobulin *see* Cerebrospinal Fluid Immunoglobulin G *on page 656*

Spinal Fluid VDRL *see* VDRL, Cerebrospinal Fluid *on page 761*

***Sporothrix* Antibodies** *see* Sporotrichosis Serology *on this page*

Sporothrix schenckii *see* Sporotrichosis Serology *on this page*

Sporotrichosis Serology

CPT 86609

Related Information

Biopsy or Body Fluid Fungus Culture *on page 780*
Fungus Smear, Stain *on page 813*

Synonyms *Sporothrix* Antibodies

Applies to *Sporothrix schenckii*

Test Commonly Includes Detection of serological response to *Sporothrix schenckii*

Abstract Sporotrichosis is a fungal disease classically beginning in the distal extremity, often at a site of inoculation, spreading proximally involving lymphatics. The organisms in tissue and in 37°C culture exist as small structures. They are often difficult or impossible to see in tissue sections. Extracutaneous disease includes monarticular arthritis. Pulmonary sporotrichosis is much less frequently found than osteoarticular infection.

Specimen Serum or cerebrospinal fluid **CONTAINER:** Red top tube; sterile CSF tube

Interpretive **REFERENCE RANGE:** Latex agglutinating titer: <1:4; ELISA: <1:16 in serum, <1:8 in CSF **USE:** Diagnose sporotrichosis, especially extracutaneous disease **LIMITATIONS:** A negative test result does not rule out infection. Serial titers are not prognostically useful. There are occasional low titer false-positives from nonfungal disease. This test is not widely available. **METHODOLOGY:** Tube agglutination, latex agglutination (LA), enzyme-linked immunosorbent assay (ELISA) **ADDITIONAL INFORMATION:** Titer ≥1:4 is presumptive evidence for sporotrichosis. Titers greater than 1:128, rising titers, and persistent elevation are common with pulmonary or systemic disease. Positive reaction in CSF is diagnostic, and is particularly useful in chronic meningitis caused by this organism, which is difficult to culture.

References

Bennett JE, "*Sporothrix schenckii*," *Principles and Practice of Infectious Diseases*, 3rd ed, Mandell GL, Douglas RG Jr, and Bennett JE, eds, New York, NY: Churchill Livingstone, 1990, 1972-5.

Scott EN, Kaufman L, Brown AC, et al, "Serologic Studies in the Diagnosis and Management of Meningitis Due to *Sporothrix schenckii*," *N Engl J Med*, 1987, 317:935-40.

Squamous Cancer *see* TA-4 *on next page*

SS-A Antibodies *see* Sjögren's Antibodies *on page 746*

SS-A/Ro *see* Antinuclear Antibody *on page 638*

SS-B Antibodies *see* Sjögren's Antibodies *on page 746*

SS-B/La *see* Antinuclear Antibody *on page 638*

ss-DNA *see* Anti-DNA *on page 634*

St Louis Encephalitis Virus Serology

CPT 86653

Related Information

California Encephalitis Virus Titer *on page 651*
Eastern Equine Encephalitis Virus Serology *on page 673*
Viral Culture, Central Nervous System Symptoms *on page 1199*
Western Equine Encephalitis Virus Serology *on page 765*

Abstract Most group B arboviruses (family Flaviviridae) are arthropod borne. St Louis encephalitis virus causes fever with headache, aseptic meningitis, and encephalitis. Severity of illness increases with age. Patients over 60 years of age have the highest frequency of encephalitis.

Specimen Serum or cerebrospinal fluid **CONTAINER:** Red top tube, sterile CSF tube **SAMPLING TIME:** Acute and convalescent sera drawn 10-14 days apart are recommended.

Interpretive **REFERENCE RANGE:** Less than a fourfold increase in titer in paired sera; HI titer: <1:10; CF titer: <1:8; plaque reduction: <70%; no IgM antibody in CSF **USE:** Used to support the diagnosis of St Louis encephalitis virus infection **LIMITATIONS:** Cross reactivity between alphavirus group and flavivirus group; false reactions from yellow fever vaccination. (Yellow fever is found in the family Flaviviridae, as is St Louis encephalitis.) **METHODOLOGY:** Complement fixation (CF), hemagglutination inhibition (HAI), plaque reduction neutralization, enzyme-linked immunosorbent assay (ELISA) for IgM **ADDITIONAL INFORMATION:** St Louis encephalitis virus infection can cause fever and headache with meningitis or meningoencephalitis. In the elderly it may be confused with a cerebrovascular accident. Demonstration of IgM antibody in CSF rapidly establishes a diagnosis of arboviral encephalitis. The patient's age, season of the year, place of residence, and exposure are important in the differential diagnosis.

References

Monath TP, "Flavivirus (Yellow Fever, Dengue, and St Louis Encephalitis)," *Principles and Practice of Infectious Diseases*, 3rd ed, Mandell GL, Douglas RG Jr, and Bennett JE, eds, New York, NY: Churchill Livingstone, 1990, 1248-51.

Tsai TF, "Arboviruses," *Manual of Clinical Laboratory Immunology*, 4th ed, Vol 2, Chapter 91, Rose NR, Conway de Macario E, Fahey JL, et al, eds, Washington, DC: American Society for Microbiology, 1992, 606-18.

Streptodornase *see* Antideoxyribonuclease-B Titer, Serum *on page 633*

Streptozyme

CPT 86403

Related Information

Antideoxyribonuclease-B Titer, Serum *on page 633*
Antistreptolysin O Titer, Serum *on page 640*
Kidney Profile *on page 268*
Throat Culture *on page 876*

Test Commonly Includes Screening for anti-NADase, anti-DNase, antistreptokinase (ASK) antistreptolysin O (ASO), antihyaluronidase (AH). Sheep red blood cells are sensitized with the five streptococcal exoenzymes.

Specimen Serum **CONTAINER:** Red top tube

Interpretive **REFERENCE RANGE:** <100 streptozyme units **USE:** Screening for antibodies to

(Continued)

Streptozyme *(Continued)*

streptococcal antigens NADase, DNase, streptokinase, streptolysin O, and hyaluronidase **LIMITATIONS:** A single determination is less useful than a series. May not be as sensitive in children as in adults. **METHODOLOGY:** Hemagglutination **ADDITIONAL INFORMATION:** Streptozyme is a screening test for antibodies to several streptococcal antigens. It has the advantages of detecting several antibodies in a single assay (although which one has been detected cannot be ascertained), of being technically quick and easy, and of being unaffected by several factors producing false-positives in the ASO test. As for other serologic tests, a serially rising titer is more significant than a single determination. A disadvantage of the test is that borderline antibody elevations, which could be clinically significant particularly in children, may not be detected.

References

El-Kholy A, Hafez K, and Krause RM, "Specificity and Sensitivity of the Streptozyme Test for the Detection of Streptococcal Antibodies," *Appl Microbiol*, 1974, 27:748-52.

Washington JA, "Medical Microbiology," *Clinical Diagnosis and Management by Laboratory Methods*, 18th ed, Henry JB, ed, Philadelphia, PA: WB Saunders Co, 1991, 1025-74.

Surrogate Tests *see* Hepatitis C Serology *on page 690*

Synovial Fluid C1q Immune Complexes Detection *see* C1q Immune Complex Detection *on page 649*

Syphilis Screening Test *see* Automated Reagin Test *on page 642*

Syphilis Serology *see* MHA-TP *on page 724*

Syphilis Serology *see* RPR *on page 742*

Syphilis Serology *see* VDRL, Cerebrospinal Fluid *on page 761*

Syphilis Serology *see* VDRL, Serum *on page 762*

TA-4

CPT *86316*

Synonyms Tumor-Antigen 4

Applies to Squamous Cancer

Specimen Serum **CONTAINER:** Red top tube

Interpretive **REFERENCE RANGE:** ≤2.6 ng/mL **USE:** May be useful in diagnosis and management of patients with squamous carcinoma of lung, cervix, or other sites. **LIMITATIONS:** TA-4 is **not** a screening test. **METHODOLOGY:** Radioimmunoassay (RIA), immunoradiometric assay (IRMA) **ADDITIONAL INFORMATION:** TA-4 is a protein (MW 48,000) purified from a cervical squamous carcinoma. Patients with squamous carcinomas, particularly those with advanced disease, have elevated levels of TA-4. Elevation correlates with stage of disease, and rising levels after operation indicate recurrence.

References

Mino N, Atsushi I, and Hamamoto K, "Availability of Tumor-Antigen 4 as a Marker of Squamous Cell Carcinoma of the Lung and Other Organs," *Cancer*, 1988, 62:730-4.

Mino-Miyagawa N, Kimura Y, and Hamamoto K, "Tumor-Antigen 4. Its Immunohistochemical Distribution and Tissue and Serum Concentrations in Squamous Cell Carcinoma of the Lung and Esophagus," *Cancer*, 1990, 66(7):1505-12.

T- and B-Cell Rosettes Studies *see* T- and B-Lymphocyte Subset Assay *on this page*

T- and B-Cell Typing *see* T- and B-Lymphocyte Subset Assay *on this page*

T- and B-Lymphocyte Analysis *see* T- and B-Lymphocyte Subset Assay *on this page*

T- and B-Lymphocyte Assay *see* T- and B-Lymphocyte Subset Assay *on this page*

T- and B-Lymphocyte Subset Assay

CPT *88180*

Related Information

bcl-2 Gene Rearrangement *on page 893*

Gene Rearrangement for Leukemia and Lymphoma *on page 911*
HIV-1/HIV-2 Serology *on page 696*
Human Immunodeficiency Virus DNA Amplification *on page 915*
Immunoperoxidase Procedures *on page 60*
Immunophenotypic Analysis of Tissues by Flow Cytometry *on page 65*
Lymph Node Biopsy *on page 72*
Lymphocyte Subset Enumeration *on page 720*
p24 Antigen *on page 727*
Polymerase Chain Reaction *on page 927*

Synonyms Lymphocyte Marker Studies; Lymphocyte Receptor Studies; Lymphocyte Subset Analyses; Lymphocyte Subset Identification; Lymphocyte Subset Typing; Lymphocyte Surface Immunoglobulin Analysis; Lymphocyte Typing; T- and B-Cell Rosettes Studies; T- and B-Cell Typing; T- and B-Lymphocyte Analysis; T- and B-Lymphocyte Assay

Test Commonly Includes Currently extremely variable. Contact your laboratory to determine what is available on a local and/or referred basis.

Specimen Most procedures call for heparinized whole blood. Methods are available for obtaining suspensions of lymph node, spleen, or bone marrow cells for analysis. Fresh tissue fragments are minced/homogenized to release individual cells into suspension for cell by cell analysis. Fresh tissue may be required to prepare frozen sections for immunofluorescence analysis. Immunoperoxidase methods have been applied with variable results to sections of formalin fixed paraffin imbedded material. Arrangements must be made with your laboratory

Antigenic Profiles of Subtypes of Acute and Chronic Forms of Leukemia

Type of Leukemia	Immunologic Categories With Usual Antigenic Profile	Comments
ALL	Null cell ALL: HLA-DR, TdT, variable CD19	10% of non-T ALL
	Common ALL: HLA-DR, TdT, CD19, CD10, CD20	Most frequent type of ALL (70% of non-T ALL)
	Pre-B ALL: HLA-DR, TdT, CD19, CD10, CD20, cytoplasmic mu	15% to 20% of non-T ALL
	B ALL: HLA-DR, CD19, CD20, SIg	<1% of ALL
	Early thymocyte T ALL: CD7, CD5, T9, CD38, CD2, TdT	15% to 20% of ALL is of T-cell origin
	Common thymocyte T ALL: CD7, CD5, CD38, CD2, CD1, CD3, CD4, CD8, TdT	
	Mature thymocyte T ALL: CD7, CD5, CD38, CD2, CD3, CD4 or CD8	
Chronic lymphoid leukemias	B CLL: weak SIg (often IgM and D), CIg in some cases, HLA-DR, mouse erythrocyte receptor, CD5, CD19, CD20, CD21	CLL phenotype may correlate with prognosis
	T CLL: variable; pan T (E rosette), may have helper or suppressor phenotype	2% CLL of T-cell origin
	B PLL: moderate to strong SIg, HLA-DR, CD19, CD20	80% PLL of B-cell origin
	T PLL: variable; pan T (E rosette), may have helper or suppressor phenotype	20% PLL of T-cell origin
	HCL: SIg, CD11, CD19, CD20, CD25, HLA-DR	Rare cases of T HCL described
ANLL M1, M2	HLA-DR, CD13, CD33 (variable expression of My8, CD11, CD13)	Some association between phenotype and prognosis
M3	CD13, CD33, My8, CD11	
M4	HLA-DR, CD13, CD33, CD14, CD11, My8	
M5	HLA-DR, CD13, CD14, CD11, variable CD33	
M6	Glycophorin A (myeloid precursors react with monoclonals listed for M1, M2)	
M7	Platelet glycoprotein IIb/IIIa, variable Ib	
CML	Blast crisis cells similar in phenotype to corresponding type of acute leukemia	Blast crisis can be of various cell types, although myeloid and lymphoid are most common

(Continued)

Cluster Designations: Third International Workshop, 1987*

Antigen	Distribution†	Molecular Weight•	Representative Monoclonal Antibodies	Comments
CD1a	Thy, LC	49	T6, OKT6, Leu-6	...
CD1b	Thy	45	...	...
CD1c	Thy	43	...	...
CD2	T	50	T11, OKT11, Leu-5b	SRBC receptor
CD3	T	20, 26	OKT3, Leu-4	TCR complex
CD4	T subset	60	(T4), OKT4, Leu-3a	Helper/inducer
CD5	T	67	T1, OKT1, Leu-1	B lineage CLL
CD6	T	120	MBG6, T12	...
CD7	T, NK	40	3A1, Leu-9	FcuR
CD8	T subset	32	T8, OKT8, Leu-2a	Cytotoxic/suppressor
CD9	Pre-B, P, (M)	24	J2	cALL
CD10	Pre-B	100	J5, UL-39	cALL
CD11a	L	180 (95)	...	...
CD11b	M, G, NK, Tc/s	160 (95)	Mo1, OKM1, Leu-15	C3biR
CD11c	M, (G), NK	150 (95)	Leu-M5, Ki-M1	HCL, AML
CDw12	M, G, P	...	M67	...
CD13	G, M	150	My7	...
CD14	M, (G), FDRC	55	My4, Leu-M3	...
CD15	G, M	...	My1, Leu-M1	X hapten
CD16	G, NK	50-60	Leu-11a, Leu-11b, Leu-11c; VEP 13	FcR, low
CD17	G, M, P	...	T5, A7	Lactosyl ceramide
CD18	L	95	60.3, MHM23	LFA β-chain
CD19	B	95	B4, Leu-12	...
CD20	B	35	B1, Leu-16	...
CD21	B, FDRC	140	B2	C3dR
CD22	B	135	Leu-14, TO 15	...
CD23	B	45	PL-13, MHM6	Activation related
CD24	B, G	45, 55, 65	BA-1, HB8	...
CD25	Act-T	55	Tac	IL-2R
CDw26	T	130	4 ELIC7	Activation related
CD27	T, PC, (B)	55	S152, OKT18A	PC cytoplasm
CD28	T subset	44	9.3, KOLT2	...
CDw29	T subset	135	4B4	...
CD30	Act-T, B	130	Ki-1	R-S cells
CD31	M, G, P, (T)	130-140	SG134, TM3	...
CDw32	M, G, P, B	40	2EI, CIKM5	?FcR II
CD33	BMPC	67	My9, L4F3	APL
CD34	Myeloid precursor	115	My10	Leukemia cells
CD35	G, M, FDRC	220	C3bR, CR1	CR1
CD36	M, P	85	5F1, CIMegl	...
CD37	B, (other)	40-45	BL14, HD28	...
CD38	PC, (T), (B)	45	T10, Leu-17	...
CD39	B, M	80	G28-8, G28-10	...
CDw40	B, IRC	50	G28-5	Carcinomas
CDw41	P	130, 155	J15, BC5-C4	gpIIb/IIIa

(continued)

Antigen	Distribution†	Molecular Weight•	Representative Monoclonal Antibodies	Comments
CDw42	P	170	HPL14, AN51	gplb
CD43	L	95	...	Brain
CD44	L	65–85	...	Brain
CD45	L	180–220	4E2, 9.4	T200, LCA
CD45R	B, (T), (M), NK	220, 205	2H4, Leu-18	Restricted T200

*Act-B indicates activated B-cells; Act-T, activated T-cells; AML, acute myelogenous leukemia; APL, acute promyelocytic leukemia; B, B-cells; BMPC, bone marrow precursor cells; cALL, common acute lymphoblastic leukemia; C3biR, receptor for C3bi, C3dR, receptor for C3d; CLL, chronic lymphocytic leukemia; CR1, receptor for C3b; FcR, low, receptor for Fc region of Ig; FcuR, receptor for Fc region of IgM; FDRC, follicular dendritic reticular cells; G, granulocyte; HCL, hairy-cell leukemia; IL-2R, interleukin-2 receptor; IRC, interdigitating reticulum cells; L, leukocytes, not otherwise specified; LC, Langerhans' cells; LCA, leukocyte common antigen; M, monocytes; NK, natural killer cells; P, platelets; PC plasma cells; question mark, questionable; R, red blood cells; R-S, Reed-Sternberg cells; SRBC, sheep red blood cell; T, T-cells; Thy, thymocytes; and TCR, T-cell receptor complex.

†Data in parentheses indicate a lesser degree of certainty or the presence of the antigen on some, but not all, cells of that lineage, ie, weak reactions.

•Two or more values are given because two or more multiple molecular weights have been reported; the values in parentheses for CD11a, b, and c indicate that they share a common 95-kd subunit but are distinguished by their α-subunits that contribute to the variable molecular weights.

preparatory to obtaining material for these specialized studies. **CONTAINER:** Two green top (heparin) tubes **STORAGE INSTRUCTIONS:** Maintain specimen at room temperature. Process within 2-3 hours. There is preliminary evidence that delay and exposure to refrigerator temperatures is related to significant loss of the T4 (inducer/helper) T-lymphocyte subset marker.[1] **SPECIAL INSTRUCTIONS:** Consult laboratory for special arrangements or instructions before collecting specimen.

Interpretive **REFERENCE RANGE:** T cells: 60% to 80%; B cells: 5% to 15%; B-cell surface immunoglobulins FITC polyvalent: 5% to 15% **USE:** Quantitate T and B lymphocytes and lymphocyte subsets; type and classify lymphocytic leukemias and lymphomas; define immunodeficiency states including AIDS **LIMITATIONS:** Method related variables and their effect on normal values are not entirely defined. A lymphocyte subset defined by a monoclonal antibody identified antigen may not be all-inclusive of one functional subset (eg, lymphocytes with T_4 antigens are inducer/helper cells but additional cells of this functional class may exist in the same individual that are T_4 negative). Steroid and immunosuppressive drug therapy may significantly change (usually decreasing) lymphocyte populations. **METHODOLOGY:** Erythrocyte (sheep, mouse, monkey) rosette tests; EA rosette test for detection of Fc receptors; EAC rosette test for detection of complement receptors; immunofluorescence FITC (fluorescein isothiocyanate conjugated) antibody detection of membrane immunoglobulin and other antigens; Immunoperoxidase (variety of methods) detection of membrane immunoglobulin and other antigens; avidin-biotin immunoperoxidase (provides significantly increased sensitivity); Immunobead™ (Quantigen™ - BioRad Laboratories) - T, B, and T-subset immunospecific antibody labeled and color coded microbeads that form rosettes with cells bearing the appropriate membrane antigen;[2] Immunogold monoclonal antibody conjugates for cytohistochemical identification of T/B lymphocyte and subset membrane markers.[3] Result is light microscope analyzed and is automated by use of the Hematrak™ differential counter. Enhanced sensitivity for membrane antigens is achieved using paraffin sections[4,5] and immunogold-silver staining; flow cytometers and fluorescence-activated cell sorter analyzers for which there are currently two major commercial sources. These devices can identify, count, and/or physically separate individual cells that bear a fluorescent labeled immunologically identified antigen. The flow cytometer has become the standard method for immunophenotyping cells with monoclonal antibodies. **ADDITIONAL INFORMATION:** The confluence of prodigious growth in understanding of cell membrane structure, diverse and major role of lymphocyte populations in immunology, and the rapid growth and developments in monoclonal antibody technology has produced a dynamically expanding area of growth for science, medicine, and industry. It is the hope that this new technology will clarify old and often misunderstood disease processes with ultimate important patient benefit. Current application of lymphocyte subset studies include leukemia/lymphoma analysis, diagnosis and classification; a spectrum of autoimmune based diseases; and an equally broad and occasionally overlapping population of immune deficiency states, especially AIDS. The tables evaluate which markers are associated with which disease.[6,7]

Footnotes

1. Weiblen BJ, Debell K, and Valeri CR, "Acquired Immunodeficiency of Blood Stored Overnight," *N Engl J Med*, 1983, 309:793, (letter).

(Continued)

T- and B-Lymphocyte Subset Assay *(Continued)*

2. *Instruction Manual, Quantigen™, T- and B-Cell Enumeration Assay Bulletin* #4238, Bio Rad Laboratories, 1983.
3. De Waele M, De Mey J, Moeremans M, et al, "Cytochemical Profile of Immunoregulatory T-Lymphocyte Subsets Defined by Monoclonal Antibodies," *J Histochem Cytochem*, 1983, 31:471-8.
4. Holgate CS, Jackson P, Lauder I, et al, "Surface Membrane Staining of Immunoglobulins in Paraffin Sections of Non-Hodgkin's Lymphomas Using Immunogold-Silver Staining Technique," *J Clin Pathol*, 1983, 36:742-6.
5. Holgate CS, Jackson P, Cowen PN, et al, "Immunogold-Silver Staining: New Method of Immunostaining With Enhanced Sensitivity," *J Histochem Cytochem*, 1983, 31:938-44.
6. Deegan MJ, "Membrane Antigen Analysis in the Diagnosis of Lymphoid Leukemias and Lymphomas. Differential Diagnosis, Prognosis as Related to Immunophenotype, and Recommendations for Testing," *Arch Pathol Lab Med*, 1989, 113(6):606-18.
7. Foucar K, Chen IM, and Crago S, "Organization and Operation of a Flow Cytometric Immunophenotyping Laboratory," *Semin Diagn Pathol*, 1989, 6(1):13-36.

References

Bowman WP, Melvin S, and Mauer AM, "Cell Markers in Lymphomas and Leukemias," *Adv Intern Med*, 1980, 25:391-425.

Bradley J, "Use of Monoclonal Antibodies in Examining Lymphocyte Populations and Subpopulations in Normal and Leukemic Patients," *Clin Immunol Newslet*, Boston, MA: GK Hall and Co, 1981, 2:43-8.

Gupta S, "Human T-Cell Subpopulations With Receptors for Immunoglobulin Isotypes," Boston, MA: GK Hall and Co, 1981, 2:51-5.

Janossy G, ed, "The Lymphocytes," *Clinics in Haematology*, Philadelphia, PA: WB Saunders Co, 1982, 11:3.

Krause R, Penchansky L, Contis L, et al, "Flow Cytometry in the Diagnosis of Acute Leukemia," *Am J Clin Pathol*, 1988, 89:341-6.

Vogler LB, Grossi CE, and Cooper MD, "Human Lymphocyte Subpopulations," *Prog Hematol*, 1979, 11:1-45.

Whiteside TL, "Cell-Surface Markers in Phenotyping of Human Lymphoproliferative Diseases," *Clin Immunol Newslet*, Boston, MA: GK Hall and Co, 1981, 2:91-4.

Tau Fraction *see* Cerebrospinal Fluid Protein Electrophoresis *on page 661*

Teichoic Acid Antibody

***CPT** 86331 (gel diffusion)*

Related Information

Blood Culture, Aerobic and Anaerobic *on page 784*

Test Commonly Includes Detection of serologic response to teichoic acid from *Staphylococcus aureus*

Specimen Serum **CONTAINER:** Red top tube **COLLECTION:** Acute and convalescent specimens are recommended.

Interpretive **REFERENCE RANGE:** Titer: ≤1:2. Less than a fourfold rise between acute and convalescent serum. (Reference ranges vary among laboratories.) **USE:** Used in assessing therapy in chronic infections caused by *Staphylococcus aureus* **LIMITATIONS:** Clinical significance is not well established; technical variability **METHODOLOGY:** Gel diffusion assay, enzyme-linked immunosorbent assay (ELISA) **ADDITIONAL INFORMATION:** Teichoic acid is a component of the cell wall of gram-positive bacteria. Antibodies to teichoic acid can be demonstrated in some patients with infections due to such organisms, particularly staphylococcal endocarditis and osteomyelitis. Serial determinations of teichoic acid antibodies have been used by some to assess the adequacy of therapy for these conditions, but this or other clinical applications are not yet established.

References

Herzog C, Wood HC, Noel I, et al, "Comparison of a New Enzyme-Linked Immunosorbent Assay Method With Counterimmunoelectrophoresis for Detection of Teichoic Acid Antibodies in Sera From Patients With *Staphylococcus aureus* Infections," *J Clin Microbiol*, 1984, 19:511-15.

Jacob E, Durham LC, Falk MC, et al, "Antibody Response to Teichoic Acid and Peptidoglycan in *Staphylococcus aureus* Osteomyelitis," *J Clin Microbiol*, 1987, 25:122-7.

Tetanus Antibody

***CPT** 86774*

Synonyms Tetanus Immunostatus

Test Commonly Includes Detection of antibodies specific for tetanus toxin

Specimen Serum **CONTAINER:** Red top tube

Interpretive **REFERENCE RANGE:** Hemagglutinating antibody present **USE:** Assess immunocompetence **CONTRAINDICATIONS:** Not valid in an unimmunized individual **METHODOLOGY:** Hemagglutination, enzyme-linked immunosorbent assay (ELISA), *in vivo* mouse neutralization **ADDI-**

TIONAL INFORMATION: Since most individuals have been immunized against tetanus, assessing whether they have antibody to tetanus antigen is a good way of documenting intact humoral immunity. Serologic studies have no place in management of clinical tetanus. The tests are too slow, too insensitive, and do not correlate with the course of disease or response to treatment. Indeed clinical tetanus has been reported in patients with high antitetanus titers.

References

Craig JP, "Immune Response to *Corynebacterium diphtheriae* and *Clostridium tetani*: Diagnostic Methods," *Manual of Clinical Laboratory Immunology*, 4th ed, Vol 2, Chapter 69, Rose NR, Conway de Macario E, Fahey JL, et al, eds, Washington, DC: American Society for Microbiology, 1992, 435-9.

Crone NE and Reder AT, "Severe Tetanus in Immunized Patients With High Anti-Tetanus Titers," *Neurology*, 1992, 42(4):761-4.

Tetanus Immunostatus *see* Tetanus Antibody *on previous page*

***Thermoactinomyces* Precipitating Antibodies** *replaced by* Hypersensitivity Pneumonitis Serology *on page 704*

***Thermoactinomyces vulgaris* Precipitating Antibodies** *see* Hypersensitivity Pneumonitis Serology *on page 704*

***Thermolospora viridis* Precipitating Antibodies** *see* Hypersensitivity Pneumonitis Serology *on page 704*

Thyroglobulin Antibody *see* Thyroid Antithyroglobulin Antibody *on next page*

Thyroid Antimicrosomal Antibody

CPT 86376

Related Information

Free Thyroxine Index *on page 223*
T_3 Uptake *on page 355*
Thyroid Antithyroglobulin Antibody *on next page*
Thyroid Stimulating Hormone *on page 361*
Thyroxine *on page 364*
Thyroxine, Free *on page 368*

Synonyms Antithyroid Microsomal Antibody; Microsomal Antibody; Thyroid Autoantibodies

Test Commonly Includes Titers on all positive specimens

Specimen Serum **CONTAINER:** Red top tube **STORAGE INSTRUCTIONS:** Separated serum stable for 5 days at room temperature

Interpretive **REFERENCE RANGE:** Passive hemagglutination: <1:100; IFA: negative **USE:** Used in differential diagnosis of hypothyroidism and Hashimoto's thyroiditis **LIMITATIONS:** Should be used in conjunction with antithyroglobulin test, since autoimmune thyroiditis may demonstrate a response to antigens other than thyroid microsomes. Other autoimmune disorders such as Sjögren's syndrome, lupus erythematosus, rheumatoid arthritis, pernicious anemia, and others may be positive for antimicrosomal and antithyroglobulin. Patients with myxedema, granulomatous thyroiditis, nontoxic nodular goiter and thyroid carcinoma may occasionally produce thyroid antibodies. Thyroid microsomal antibodies have been reported in drug-induced hypersensitivity reactions to anticonvulsants and sulfonamides resulting in hypothyroidism. **METHODOLOGY:** Passive hemagglutination, indirect fluorescent antibody (IFA), enzyme-linked immunosorbent assay (ELISA) **ADDITIONAL INFORMATION:** Antibodies to thyroid microsomes (thyroid peroxidase) are present in 70% to 90% of patients with chronic thyroiditis. They are also present in smaller percentages of patients with other thyroid diseases. Antibody production may be confined to lymphocytes within the thyroid, and serum may be negative. Small numbers (3%) of people with no evidence of disease may have antibody. This is more frequent in females and increases with age.

References

Baker JR, Saunders NB, Wartofsky L, et al, "Seronegative Hashimoto Thyroiditis With Thyroid Autoantibody Production Localized to the Thyroid," *Ann Intern Med*, 1988, 108:26-30.

Gupta A, Eggo MC, Uetrecht JF, et al, "Drug-Induced Hypothyroidism: The Thyroid as a Target Organ in Hypersensitivity Reactions to Anticonvulsants and Sulfonamides," *Clin Pharmacol Ther*, 1992, 51(1):56-67.

Nakamura RM and Binder WL, "Current Concepts and Diagnostic Evaluation of Autoimmune Disease," *Arch Pathol Lab Med*, 1988, 112:869-77.

Thyroid Antithyroglobulin Antibody

CPT 86800

Related Information

Free Thyroxine Index *on page 223*
T_3 Uptake *on page 355*
Thyroid Antimicrosomal Antibody *on previous page*
Thyroid Stimulating Hormone *on page 361*
Thyroxine *on page 364*
Thyroxine, Free *on page 368*

Synonyms Antithyroglobulin Antibody; Thyroglobulin Antibody

Applies to CA2

Test Commonly Includes Titers on positive specimens

Specimen Serum CONTAINER: Red top tube

Interpretive REFERENCE RANGE: Hemagglutination: <1:400; IFA: negative; values vary with technology used USE: Useful in detection and confirmation of autoimmune thyroiditis, Hashimoto's thyroiditis LIMITATIONS: Must be used in conjunction with antimicrosomal test, since autoimmune thyroiditis may demonstrate a response to antigen other than thyroglobulin. Other autoimmune disorders such as Sjögren's syndrome, SLE, RA, autoimmune hemolytic anemia, may be positive for thyroid antibodies, as may patients with myxedema, granulomatosis, thyroiditis, thyrotoxicosis, nontoxic nodular goiter and thyroid carcinoma. METHODOLOGY: Passive hemagglutination, indirect fluorescent antibody (IFA), enzyme-linked immunosorbent assay (ELISA) ADDITIONAL INFORMATION: Antibodies to thyroglobulin can be detected in 40% to 70% of patients with chronic thyroiditis. Antibodies may also be present in 70% of hypothyroid patients, 40% of patients with Graves' disease, and smaller numbers of patients with other autoimmune conditions, particularly pernicious anemia. Normal individuals, especially elderly females, may have antibody. The immunofluorescent test can detect an additional antibody, to CA2, the "second colloid antigen." A small fraction of patients with thyroiditis will have only antibody to CA2. Rare patients may have antibody production confined to the thyroid gland. A new microparticle nephelometric immunoassay is more sensitive than conventional assays, but the specificity is still not known.

References

Baker JR, Saunders NB, Wartofsky L, et al, "Seronegative Hashimoto Thyroiditis With Thyroid Autoantibody Production Localized to the Thyroid," *Ann Intern Med*, 1988, 108:26-30.

Colvin RB, Bhan AK, and McCluskey RT, eds, *Diagnostic Immunopathology*, New York, NY: Raven Press, 1988, 102-6.

Harchali AA, Montagne P, Cuilliere ML, et al, "Detection of Antithyroglobulin Autoantibodies With Defined Epitopic Specificity by a Microparticle-Enhanced Nephelometric Immunoassay," *Clin Chem*, 1992, 38(9):1859-64.

Nakamura RM and Binder WL, "Current Concepts and Diagnostic Evaluation of Autoimmune Disease," *Arch Pathol Lab Med*, 1988, 112:869-77.

Sakata S, Nakamura S, and Miura K, "Autoantibodies Against Thyroid Hormones or Iodothyronine," *Ann Intern Med*, 1985, 103:579-89.

Takaichi Y, Tamai H, Honda K, et al, "The Significance of Antithyroglobulin and Antithyroidal Microsomal Antibodies in Patients With Hyperthyroidism Due to Graves' Disease Treated With Antithyroid Drugs," *J Clin Endocrinol Metab*, 1989, 68(6):1097-100.

Thyroid Autoantibodies *see* Thyroid Antimicrosomal Antibody *on previous page*

Thyroid Stimulating Autoantibody *see* Thyrotropin-Receptor Antibody *on this page*

Thyroid Stimulating Immunoglobulins *see* Thyrotropin-Receptor Antibody *on this page*

Thyrotropin-Receptor Antibody

CPT 86849

Related Information

Free Thyroxine Index *on page 223*
T_3 Uptake *on page 355*
Thyroid Stimulating Hormone *on page 361*
Thyroxine *on page 364*
Thyroxine, Free *on page 368*

Synonyms Thyroid Stimulating Autoantibody; Thyroid Stimulating Immunoglobulins; TSIG

Applies to LATS; LATS Protector; Long-Acting Thyroid Stimulator

Specimen Serum **CONTAINER:** Red top tube

Interpretive **REFERENCE RANGE:** Negative **USE:** Used to diagnose hyperthyroidism and Graves' disease **LIMITATIONS:** Four percent false-positive rate in normals **METHODOLOGY:** Bioassay, radioreceptor assay **ADDITIONAL INFORMATION:** Thyrotropin-receptor antibody is an autoantibody to the thyroid cell receptor for thyroid stimulating hormone. It can be demonstrated in 90% of patients with Graves' disease, and is the cause of the hyperthyroidism of that condition. The characterization of TRA resolved much confusion about long-acting thyroid stimulator (LATS) and LATS protector, which are both, in fact, thyroid stimulating autoantibodies which simply behaved differently in animal test systems. These antibodies are present in 50% of euthyroid Graves' disease as well as hyperthyroid patients. They play a major role in the pathogenesis of Graves' disease. Detection of these antibodies is useful in prediction of neonatal hyperthyroidism and prediction of relapse of hyperthyroidism.

References

Gupta MK, "Recent Advances in Laboratory Tests for Autoantibodies to Thyrotropin Receptor Protein in Graves' Disease," *Clin Lab Med*, 1988, 303-23.

Gupta MK, "Thyrotropin Receptor Antibodies: Advances and Importance of Detection Techniques in Thyroid Disease," *Clin Biochem*, 1992, 25(3):193-9.

McKenzie JM and Zakarija M, "Clinical Review 3: The Clinical Use of Thyrotropin Receptor Antibody," *J Clin Endocrinol Metab*, 1989, 69(6):1093-6.

Morris JC, Hay ID, Nelson RF, et al, "Clinical Utility of Thyrotropin-Receptor Antibody Assays: Comparison of Radioreceptor and Bioassay Methods," *Mayo Clin Proc*, 1988, 63:707-17.

Nakamura RM and Binder WL, "Current Concepts and Diagnostic Evaluation of Autoimmune Disease," *Arch Pathol Lab Med*, 1988, 112:869-77.

Tissue Typing

***CPT** 86805 (with titration); 86821 (without titration)*

Related Information

HLA-B27 *on page 701*
HLA Typing, Single Human Leukocyte Antigen *on page 701*
Identification DNA Testing *on page 918*
Mixed Lymphocyte Culture *on page 725*
Paternity Studies *on page 1074*

Synonyms Crossmatch, Lymphocyte; Histocompatibility Testing; HLA Typing; HLA Typing, Crossmatch; Human Leukocyte Antigens; Lymphocyte Crossmatch; Organ Donor Tissue Typing; Tissue Typing, Donor; Transplant Tissue Typing; White Cell Crossmatch

Test Commonly Includes Determination of compatibility between recipient and donors for organ or bone marrow transplant

Specimen Heparinized blood from donor, serum from recipient for kidney or bone marrow transplantation **CONTAINER:** Donor: green top (heparin) tube; recipient: red top tube **STORAGE INSTRUCTIONS:** Should be tested immediately. Do **not** refrigerate or freeze.

Interpretive **USE:** Tissue typing aids in determination of compatibility of kidney or bone marrow transplant. HLA-B27 is strongly associated with ankylosing spondylitis (Marie Strümpell disease), especially in the Caucasian population. Other associations include Reiter's syndrome, psoriatic arthritis, and juvenile rheumatoid arthritis. Addison's disease is strongly associated with B8. Juvenile diabetes mellitus, myasthenia gravis and Graves' disease also show association with B8, as does gluten-sensitive enteropathy. A complex relationship exists with multiple sclerosis. **METHODOLOGY:** Lymphocytotoxicity assay, mixed lymphocyte culture (MLC), polymerase chain reaction (PCR) **ADDITIONAL INFORMATION:** HLA antigens are glycoproteins, the product of four closely linked genes on chromosome 6, usually inherited as an intact unit. HLA antigens are the primary determinants of tissue graft acceptance, and thus, the histocompatibility complex. This same HLA region contains genes of importance to complement and immune responses. The HLA loci are HLA-A, B, C, (class I) and DR, DQ, DP, and DW (class II). A, B, and C antigens are expressed on nearly all nucleated human cells, D antigens are restricted to B lymphocytes, monocytes, and possibly endothelial cells. HLA antigens are inherited as two sets of six antigens, one set from each parent and are codominantly expressed. These antigens show linkage disequilibrium, that is certain pairs or triplets occur more frequently than expected by chance.

There is a high occurrence (90%) of HLA-B27 in patients with ankylosing spondylitis, HLA-B8 is found in diseases with immune associations (eg, juvenile diabetes mellitus, Graves' disease and gluten-sensitive enteropathy). Associations with HLA-A and C are rare. Multiple sclerosis is associated with HLA-DRw2 and is an example of linkage disequilibrium being earlier report-

(Continued)

Tissue Typing *(Continued)*

ed to be associated with A3, then B7, and then Dw2, with highest association with DRw2. There is a high incidence of HLA-B27 in patients with reactive arthritis. This has become a quite detailed and complex area of medicine.

Tissue typing is usually undertaken to assess the "match" between donor and recipient of an organ for transplantation. Since these antigens are widely expressed in tissue, mismatches result in graft rejection, or graft-vs-host disease.

References

Braun WE and Zachary AA, "The HLA Histocompatibility System in Autoimmune States," *Clin Lab Med*, 1988, 8:351-72.

Olerup O and Zetterquist H, "HLA-DR Typing by PCR Amplification With Sequence-Specific Primers in 2 Hours: An Alternative to Serological DR Typing in Clinical Practice Including Donor-Recipient Matching in Cadaveric Transplantation," *Tissue Antigens*, 1992, 39(5):225-35.

Perkins HA, "Clinical Applications of HLA Typing," *Clin Lab Med*, 1982, 2:123-35.

Tissue Typing, Donor *see* Tissue Typing *on previous page*

Topoisomerase I *see* Scleroderma Antibody *on page 745*

TORCH

***CPT** 80090*

Related Information

Cytomegalovirus Antibody *on page 672*
Herpes Simplex Antibody *on page 692*
Rubella Serology *on page 743*
Toxoplasmosis Serology *on next page*

Synonyms TORCH Battery; TORCH Screen; TORCH Titer

Test Commonly Includes Toxoplasmosis, rubella, cytomegalovirus, and herpesvirus serology

Specimen Serum **CONTAINER:** Red top tube

Interpretive **REFERENCE RANGE:** Reference ranges provided with report of results **USE:** Screen for serologic response to toxoplasmosis, rubella, cytomegalovirus, and herpesvirus infection, important in newborn infants for evaluation of possible congenital infection **LIMITATIONS:** Even with availability of IgM specific tests, negative results do not exclude diagnosis of congenital viral infection **METHODOLOGY:** Indirect fluorescent antibody (IFA), enzyme-linked immunosorbent assay (ELISA), IgG and IgM specificity **ADDITIONAL INFORMATION:** *Toxoplasma*, rubella, cytomegalovirus, and herpes are all causes of potentially catastrophic congenital infections, which can be quickly fatal or lead to chronic sequelae including hepatitis, encephalitis, and failure to thrive. In the fulminant case serologic diagnosis is of little use since the disease outstrips the immune response and even IgM antibody cannot be demonstrated in time to be clinically useful. However, in the disease which becomes manifest weeks to months after birth, demonstration of IgM antibody or rising titers of IgG antibody can confirm a diagnosis of specific infection. The availability of IgM specific assays also determines whether antibody in cord blood represents passive transfer from the mother (IgG antibody) or signifies congenital infection (IgM antibody). **It should be emphasized that TORCH testing is of very limited usefulness. Results must be interpreted in conjunction with complete clinical information, and such testing in no way substitutes for careful clinical examination and judgment.** TORCH testing should not be applied indiscrimantely to pregnant women or infants with nondescript illnesses.

References

Alford CA Jr, Stagno S, and Reynolds DW, "Diagnosis of Chronic Perinatal Infections," *Am J Dis Child*, 1975, 129:455-63.

Friedman HM, Tustin NB, Hitchings MM, et al, "Comparison of Complement Fixation and Fluorescent Immunoassay (FIAX) for Measuring Antibodies to Cytomegalovirus and Herpes Simplex Virus," *Am J Clin Pathol*, 1981, 76:305-7.

Grossman JH, III, "Viral Infections During Pregnancy," *J Cont Ed Obstet Gynecol*, 1979, 21:11.

Ritzmann SE, "Radial Immunodiffusion Revisited, Part 2. Application and Interpretation of RID Assays," *Lab Med*, 1978, 9:29.

Yolken RH and Leister FJ, "Enzyme Immunoassays for Measurement of Cytomegalovirus Immunoglobulin M Antibody," *J Clin Microbiol*, 1981, 14:427-32.

TORCH Battery *see* TORCH *on previous page*

TORCH Screen *see* TORCH *on previous page*

TORCH Titer *see* TORCH *on previous page*

Total Hemolytic Complement *see* Complement, Total, Serum *on page 667*

***Toxocara canis* Serological Test** *see* Ascariasis Serological Test *on page 641*

***Toxoplasma* Antibodies** *see* Toxoplasmosis Serology *on this page*

Toxoplasmosis Serology

CPT 86777; 86778 (IgM)

Related Information

HIV-1/HIV-2 Serology *on page 696*
Ova and Parasites, Stool *on page 836*
Parasite Antibodies *on page 729*
TORCH *on previous page*

Synonyms *Toxoplasma* Antibodies; Toxoplasmosis Titer

Replaces Sabin-Feldman Dye Test

Test Commonly Includes IgG and IgM antibody specific for *Toxoplasma gondii*

Abstract The most common opportunistic infection of the central nervous system in patients with acquired immunodeficiency syndrome (AIDS) is toxoplasmosis.[1]

Specimen Serum **CONTAINER:** Red top tube **COLLECTION:** Acute and convalescent specimens are recommended.

Interpretive **REFERENCE RANGE:** IFA titer: <1:64; IHA titer: <1:256 **USE:** Support the diagnosis of toxoplasmosis; document past exposure and/or immunity to *Toxoplasma gondii* **LIMITATIONS:** Diagnosis of neonatal infection may be difficult because infection outstrips demonstrable antibody response. Toxoplasmosis occurs in advanced AIDS. The absence in such patients of anti-*Toxoplasma* antibodies on immunofluorescence assay does not exclude the diagnosis.[1] **METHODOLOGY:** Indirect fluorescent antibody (IFA), indirect hemagglutination (IHA), enzyme-linked immunosorbent assay (ELISA) **ADDITIONAL INFORMATION:** *Toxoplasma gondii* is endemic in cats and is excreted by them. Humans are easily exposed to cyst forms, either in caring for pets or in casual environmental contact. The majority of individuals develop antibody without any clinical disease, and a self-limited lymphadenitis is the most common clinical presentation in symptomatic infection. Congenital toxoplasmosis and infection in an immunocompromised host (AIDS) are more serious, and can produce a fatal cerebritis or disseminated illness. **Congenital toxoplasmosis** can now be diagnosed *in utero* by detection of IgM antibody in fetal blood. Diagnosis is supported by high or rising IgG antibody titer, or the demonstration of IgM antibody. The recent availability of IgA anti-*Toxoplasma* may be useful in detection of congenital toxoplasmosis. However, IgM is still the established technique. The median CD4 cell count in subjects with AIDS and toxoplasmosis, at presentation, was 50/mm^3.[1]

Footnotes

1. Porter SB and Sande MA, "Toxoplasmosis of the Central Nervous System in the Acquired Immunodeficiency Syndrome," *N Engl J Med*, 1992, 327(23):1643-8.

References

Bessieres MH, Roques C, Berrebi A, et al, "IgA Antibody Response During Acquired and Congenital Toxoplasmosis," *J Clin Pathol*, 1992, 45(7):605-8.

Cambiaso CL, Galanti LM, Leautaud P, et al, "Latex Agglutination Assay of Human Immunoglobulin M Antitoxoplasma Antibodies Which Uses Enzymatically Treated Antigen-Coated Particles," *J Clin Microbiol*, 1992, 30(4):882-888.

Carlson LG and Plorde JJ, "Evaluation of the FIAX Semiautomatic Fluorescent Immunoassay System for the Detection of IgG Antibodies to *Toxoplasma gondii*," *Diagn Microbiol Infect Dis*, 1983, 1:233-9.

Daffos F, Forestier F, Capella-Pavlovsky M, et al, "Prenatal Management of 746 Pregnancies at Risk for Congenital Toxoplasmosis," *N Engl J Med*, 1988, 318:271-5.

Liu TM, Chin-See MW, Halbert SP, et al, "An Enzyme Immunoassay for Immunoglobulin M Antibodies to *Toxoplasma gondii* Which Is Not Affected by Rheumatoid Factor or Immunoglobulin G Antibodies," *J Clin Microbiol*, 1986, 23:77-82.

Wilson M and McAuley JB, "Laboratory Diagnosis of Toxoplasmosis," *Clin Lab Med*, 1991, 11(3):923-39.

Toxoplasmosis Titer *see* Toxoplasmosis Serology *on this page*

Transplant Tissue Typing *see* Tissue Typing *on page 757*

Transthyretin *see* Cerebrospinal Fluid Protein Electrophoresis *on page 661*

***Treponema pallidum* Antibodies, CSF** *see* FTA-ABS, Cerebrospinal Fluid *on page 679*

***Trichinella* Antibodies** *see* Trichinosis Serology *on this page*

***Trichinella spiralis* Antibodies** *see* Trichinosis Serology *on this page*

Trichinosis Serology

CPT 86784

Related Information

Muscle Biopsy *on page 75*
Ova and Parasites, Stool *on page 836*
Parasite Antibodies *on page 729*

Synonyms *Trichinella* Antibodies

Applies to *Trichinella spiralis* Antibodies

Test Commonly Includes Detection of serologic response to *Trichinella spiralis*

Abstract Ingestion of undercooked pork or other meat containing larvae may lead to myalgias, myocardial infestation, and neurological symptoms.

Specimen Serum CONTAINER: Red top tube

Interpretive REFERENCE RANGE: Negative; <1:16 by ELISA USE: Screen for antibodies to *Trichinella spiralis* to establish the diagnosis of trichinosis LIMITATIONS: Low titers may represent antibody from previous rather than current infection. BFT cannot be used for testing lightly infected pigs. The test may have a high false-negative rate of 15% to 22% during the first period of the infection. METHODOLOGY: Bentonite flocculation test (BFT), indirect fluorescent antibody (IFA), complement fixation (CF), latex agglutination (LA), enzyme-linked immunosorbent assay (ELISA) ADDITIONAL INFORMATION: The bentonite flocculation test is sensitive and specific. Antibody becomes detectable 3 weeks after infection, rises for several weeks, and then declines slowly so that most individuals will test negative in 2-3 years. Immunofluorescence is more sensitive for light infection in pigs. In humans, diagnosis can also be made by finding cysts in a muscle biopsy. As an incidental finding, trichinosis was not infrequently found in pharyngeal striated muscle adhering to tonsillectomy specimens. Peripheral blood eosinophilia is characteristic.

References

Bruschi F, Tassi C, and Pozio E, "Parasite-Specific Antibody Response in *Trichinella* sp Human Infection: A One Year Follow-up," *Am J Trop Med Hyg*, 1990, 43(2):186-93.

Kagan IG and Maddison SE, "Serodiagnosis of Parasitic Diseases," *Manual of Clinical Laboratory Immunology*, 4th ed, Vol 2, Chapter 79, Rose NR, Conway de Macario E, Fahey JL, et al, eds, Washington, DC: American Society for Microbiology, 1992, 529-43.

TSIG *see* Thyrotropin-Receptor Antibody *on page 756*

Tularemia Agglutinins

CPT 86668

Related Information

Bacterial Serology *on page 644*
Febrile Agglutinins, Serum *on page 678*

Synonyms *Francisella tularensis* Antibodies; Rabbit Fever Antibodies

Abstract A single serologic result with a titer of ≥1:160 in a subject having clinical tularemia or a fourfold rise in titer is diagnostic.

Specimen Serum CONTAINER: Red top tube SPECIAL INSTRUCTIONS: Acute and convalescent sera are recommended.

Interpretive REFERENCE RANGE: Agglutination titer: <1:40; ELISA: <1:500 USE: Diagnosis of tularemia LIMITATIONS: Cross reactions with *Brucella*, *Proteus* OX-19. Titers remain elevated for years after exposure; single titers may be misleading. Cell-mediated immunity is also important in host response to *F. tularensis*. METHODOLOGY: Agglutination, hemagglutination, enzyme-linked immunosorbent assay (ELISA) ADDITIONAL INFORMATION: Antibodies to *F. tularensis* develop 2-3 weeks after infection and peak in 4-5 weeks. Although antibodies may cross react with *Brucella* those titers will generally be much lower. Rising titers over 2-week interval are the best indicator of recent infection. Antibody titers may remain elevated for years after infection.

References

Hornick RB, "*Tularemia*," *Cecil Textbook of Medicine*, 19th ed, Wyngaarden JB, Smith LH Jr, and Bennett JC, eds, Philadelphia, PA: WB Saunders Co, 1992, 1712-4.

Stewart SJ, "*Francisella*," *Manual of Clinical Microbiology*, 5th ed, Chapter 43, Balows A, Hausler WJ Jr, Hermann KL, et al, eds, Washington, DC: American Society for Microbiology, 1991, 360-3.

Tumor-Antigen 4 *see* TA-4 *on page 750*
Typhoid Agglutinins *see Salmonella* Titer *on page 744*
Urine Electrophoresis *see* Protein Electrophoresis, Urine *on page 737*
Urine Protein Electrophoresis *see* Protein Electrophoresis, Urine *on page 737*

Varicella-Zoster Virus Serology

***CPT** 86787*

Related Information

Herpes Cytology *on page 502*
Skin Biopsies *on page 84*
Varicella-Zoster Virus Culture *on page 1193*
Varicella-Zoster Virus Culture, Rapid *on page 1194*
Virus, Direct Detection by Fluorescent Antibody *on page 1208*

Synonyms Chickenpox Titer; VZV Serology; Zoster Titer

Applies to Herpes Zoster Serology

Test Commonly Includes Detection of varicella-zoster virus-specific antibody in patient's serum

Specimen Serum **CONTAINER:** Red top tube **SAMPLING TIME:** Acute and convalescent sera drawn 10-14 days apart are recommended.

Interpretive **REFERENCE RANGE:** A single low titer or less than a fourfold increase in titer in paired sera by complement fixation; undetectable antibody by fluorescent antibody to membrane antigen test **USE:** Establish the diagnosis of varicella-zoster infection; determine adult susceptibility to infection **LIMITATIONS:** Complement fixation test is insensitive and has heterologous reactions with herpesvirus **METHODOLOGY:** Fluorescent antibody to membrane antigen (FAMA), hemagglutination, complement fixation (CF), enzyme-linked immunosorbent assay (ELISA) **ADDITIONAL INFORMATION:** Although most cases of varicella or zoster are clinically unambiguous, serology may be occasionally useful in the differential diagnosis of other blistering illnesses or when infection shows an unusual complication, such as hepatitis. It may also be important to establish whether an individual is susceptible when clinical history is unclear, or when varicella immune globulin may be needed, as in the immunocompromised host or cancer patient on toxic chemotherapy. Zoster is more common with aging and may occur in the face of significant antibody titers, demonstrating that cell-mediated immunity is also significant.

References

Brunell PA, Novelli VM, Keller PM, et al, "Antibodies to the Three Major Glycoproteins of Varicella-Zoster Virus: Search for the Relevant Host Immune Response," *J Infect Dis*, 1987, 156:430-5.
Landry ML, Cohen SD, Mayo DR, et al, "Comparison of Fluorescent Antibody to Membrane Antigen Test, Indirect Immunofluorescence Assay, and a Commercial Enzyme-Linked Immunosorbent Assay for Determination of Antibody to Varicella-Zoster Virus," *J Clin Microbiol*, 1987, 25:832-5.
Straus SE, Moderator "Varicella-Zoster Virus Infections: Biology, Natural History, Treatment, and Prevention," *Ann Intern Med*, 1988, 108:221-36.
Weller TH, "Varicella and Herpes Zoster: Changing Concepts of the Natural History, Control, and Importance of a Not-So-Benign Virus," *N Engl J Med*, 1983, 309:1362-8.

VCA *see* Epstein-Barr Virus Serology *on page 676*
VCA Titer *see* Epstein-Barr Virus Serology *on page 676*

VDRL, Cerebrospinal Fluid

***CPT** 86592 (qualitative); 86593 (quantitative titer)*

Related Information

Antinuclear Antibody *on page 638*
Automated Reagin Test *on page 642*
Cerebrospinal Fluid Culture *on page 798*
Cerebrospinal Fluid Protein *on page 659*
Darkfield Examination, Syphilis *on page 808*
FTA-ABS, Cerebrospinal Fluid *on page 679*
(Continued)

VDRL, Cerebrospinal Fluid *(Continued)*

MHA-TP *on page 724*
RPR *on page 742*
VDRL, Serum *on this page*

Synonyms Cerebrospinal Fluid VDRL; CSF; CSF VDRL; Spinal Fluid VDRL; VDRL, CSF

Applies to Syphilis Serology

Test Commonly Includes Titer of reactive specimens

Abstract A reactive CSF VDRL is acceptable to establish the diagnosis of neurosyphilis, but a nonreactive test is inconclusive.

Specimen Cerebrospinal fluid CONTAINER: Clean, sterile CSF container

Interpretive REFERENCE RANGE: Nonreactive USE: Test for syphilis, neurosyphilis; VDRL, CSF is the only laboratory test for neurosyphilis approved by the Center for Disease Control. It is very specific. The sensitivity of the CSF VDRL for the diagnosis of neurosyphilis is approximately 30% to 70%.[1] METHODOLOGY: Flocculation test detects reagin, antibody to nontreponemal antigen ADDITIONAL INFORMATION: Central nervous system syphilis may be asymptomatic. Neurosyphilis includes **meningeal syphilis**, which is usually found within a year of infection. Its characteristics include headache, stiff neck, nausea and vomiting, sometimes with cranial nerve involvement. **Syphilitic meningitis** can be localized (**gumma**). **Meningovascular syphilis** is found 4-7 years after infection. **General paresis** or **tabes dorsalis** occur late, frequently decades after infection. Uveitis, retinitis, luetic optic neuritis may occur with or without syphilitic meningitis. Optic atrophy is usually found with tabes dorsalis.[1]

A positive VDRL in a spinal fluid uncontaminated by serum is essentially diagnostic of neurosyphilis. However, a negative test may occur in 30% of patients with tabes dorsalis. The CSF VDRL may take years to become nonreactive after adequate therapy.

Subjects with HIV, following therapy for syphilis that is usually considered adequate, may develop neurosyphilis. In AIDS patients, serial CSF VDRL determinations may be needed when neurosyphilis is suspected. By requiring either a positive plasma RPR or FTA-ABS, seropositivity of CSF VDRL could increase to 90%.

Footnotes

1. Hook EW 3d and Marra CM, "Acquired Syphilis in Adults," *N Engl J Med*, 1992, 326:1060-9, (review).

References

Albright RE Jr, Christenson RH, Emlet JL, et al, "Issues in Cerebrospinal Fluid Management. CSF Venereal Disease Research Laboratory Testing," *Am J Clin Pathol*, 1991, 95(3):397-401.

Davis LE and Schmitt JW, "Clinical Significance of Cerebrospinal Fluid Tests for Neurosyphilis," *Ann Neurol*, 1989, 25(1):50-5.

Feraru ER, Aronow HA, and Lipton RB, "Neurosyphilis in AIDS Patients: Initial CSF VDRL May Be Negative," *Neurology*, 1990, 40(3 Pt 1):541-3.

Hart G, "Syphilis Tests in Diagnostic and Therapeutic Decision Making," *Ann Intern Med*, 1986, 104:368-76.

VDRL, CSF *see* VDRL, Cerebrospinal Fluid *on previous page*

VDRL, Serum

CPT *86592 (qualitative); 86593 (quantitative)*

Related Information

Anticardiolipin Antibody *on page 632*
Anticoagulant, Circulating *on page 402*
Antinuclear Antibody *on page 638*
Automated Reagin Test *on page 642*
Darkfield Examination, Syphilis *on page 808*
FTA-ABS, Serum *on page 680*
Genital Culture *on page 814*
MHA-TP *on page 724*
Neisseria gonorrhoeae Culture *on page 831*
Risks of Transfusion *on page 1093*
RPR *on page 742*
VDRL, Cerebrospinal Fluid *on previous page*

Synonyms Serum VDRL; Venereal Disease Research Laboratory Test, Serum

Applies to Syphilis Serology

Replaces Kahn Test; Kline Test; Mazzini; Wassermann

Test Commonly Includes Determination of serologic response to *Treponema* infection

Abstract VDRL is a reaginic (nontreponemal) test for syphilis.

Specimen Serum **CONTAINER:** Red top tube

Interpretive **REFERENCE RANGE:** Nonreactive **USE:** Screening test for syphilis. May be used to assess adequacy of treatment. **LIMITATIONS:** Nonspecific positive reactions may be found in malaria, infectious mononucleosis, infectious hepatitis, leprosy, brucellosis, SLE, atypical pneumonia, typhus, and other entities.[1] See table. Reactive tests due to related treponemal

Potential Causes of False-Positive Serologic Tests for Syphilis.*

	Infectious Causes	Noninfectious Causes
Reaginic or nontreponemal tests (RPR, VDRL) Bacterial	Pneumococcal pneumonia Scarlet fever Leprosy Lymphogranuloma venereum Relapsing fever Bacterial endocarditis Malaria Rickettsial disease Psittacosis Leptospirosis Chancroid Tuberculosis Mycoplasmal pneumonia Trypanosomiasis	Pregnancy Chronic liver disease Advanced cancer Intravenous drug use Multiple myeloma Advancing age Connective-tissue disease Multiple blood transfusions
Viral	Vaccinia (vaccination) Chickenpox HIV Measles Infectious mononucleosis Mumps Viral hepatitis	
Treponemal tests (FTA-ABS, MHA-TP)	Lyme disease Leprosy Malaria Infectious mononucleosis Relapsing fever Leptospirosis	Systemic lupus erythematosus

From Hook EW 3d and Marra CM, "Acquired Syphilis in Adults," *N Engl J Med,* 1992, 326:1060-9, with permission.

infections also occur. Other pathogens include *T. pallidum* subspecies *pertenue*, which causes yaws; *T. carateum* which causes pinta and *T. pallidum* subspecies *endemicum*, the cause of nonvenereal or endemic syphilis.

False-positive results may occur in the first few days of postnatal life. False-negative tests due to prozone phenomenon indicates that repeat testing with diluted serum should be performed in individuals who test negative despite high clinical suspicion.

The serum VDRL may be negative in as many as 25% of subjects who have late neurosyphilis. The specific tests (eg, FTA-ABS) remain reactive.[1] Treponemal tests (eg, FTA-ABS) become reactive before nontreponemal (reaginic) tests such as VDRL.[1]

CONTRAINDICATIONS: Positive result in cord blood may be due to passive transfer from mother's blood **METHODOLOGY:** Flocculation procedure detecting the presence of reagin, antibody to nontreponemal cardiolipin antigen **ADDITIONAL INFORMATION:** Despite false-positive results due to now well known causes, VDRL remains an extremely useful screening test for syphilis. VDRL becomes positive starting 2 weeks after the chancre appears, and by 6 weeks, 90% of cases will be positive. By 9-12 weeks, the secondary stage, 100% of patients should be reactive. With therapy the VDRL reverts to negative. Even without treatment the VDRL may become negative years after infection. Thus, in tertiary syphilis, the VDRL may be negative. The VDRL test can be done on CSF and is useful in diagnosis of CNS syphilis (see VDRL, Cerebrospinal Fluid). Positive VDRL tests should have confirmatory testing with a *Treponema*-specific test. The VDRL test is recommended as a screen for uveitis or unexplained ocular inflammation.

Footnotes

1. Hook EW 3d and Marra CM, "Acquired Syphilis in Adults," *N Engl J Med*, 1992, 326:1060-9, (review).

(Continued)

VDRL, Serum *(Continued)*

References

Berkowitz K, Baxi L, and Fox HE, "False-Negative Syphilis Screening: The Prozone Phenomenon, Nonimmune Hydrops, and Diagnosis of Syphilis During Pregnancy," *Am J Obstet Gynecol*, 1990, 163(3):975-7.
Hart G, "Syphilis Tests in Diagnostic and Therapeutic Decision Making," *Ann Intern Med*, 1986, 104:368-76.
Katzmann JA, "Tests for Syphilis," *Mayo Medical Laboratories Communique*, 1984, 4(9).
Tamesis RR and Foster CS, "Ocular Syphilis," *Ophthalmology*, 1990, 97(10):1281-7.

Venereal Disease Research Laboratory Test, Serum *see* VDRL, Serum *on page 762*

Viral Capsid Antigen *see* Epstein-Barr Virus Serology *on page 676*

VLM (Visceral Larva Migrans) Serological Test *see* Ascariasis Serological Test *on page 641*

VZV Serology *see* Varicella-Zoster Virus Serology *on page 761*

W27 *see* HLA-B27 *on page 701*

Wassermann *replaced by* RPR *on page 742*

Wassermann *replaced by* VDRL, Serum *on page 762*

Weil-Felix Agglutinins

CPT *86000*

Related Information

Febrile Agglutinins, Serum *on page 678*
Rocky Mountain Spotted Fever Serology *on page 741*

Synonyms Rickettsial Disease Agglutinins

Test Commonly Includes Titer of serum against *Proteus* OX-19, OX-2, and OX-K antigens

Specimen Serum **CONTAINER:** Red top tube **SAMPLING TIME:** Acute and convalescent specimens drawn 10-14 days apart are recommended.

Interpretive **REFERENCE RANGE:** Titer ≤1:160 **USE:** Support the clinical diagnosis of rickettsial infection **LIMITATIONS:** The absence of agglutinins does not rule out rickettsial disease. False-positives occur in patients with leptospirosis, severe liver disease, *Borrelia* and *Proteus* infections. Some normal sera may possess a titer to *Proteus* antigens. Rickettsial vaccination will result in an antibody titer. Rickettsialpox, Q fever or trench fever do not demonstrate titers when tested. Partial or early treatment with antibiotics may thwart antibody response. **CONTRAINDICATIONS:** Intercurrent infection with *Proteus* **METHODOLOGY:** Agglutination **ADDITIONAL INFORMATION:** This test is based on cross reaction of antibodies to *Rickettsia* with *Proteus* antigens. Rocky Mountain spotted fever, epidemic typhus, and scrub typhus may be distinguished (see table). Antibodies appear 4-5 days after infection and peak a week later. Titers >1:160 are significant, but a fourfold rise in titer is more diagnostic. Specific tests for IgG and IgM rickettsial antibodies may be confirmatory.

Interpretation of Weil–Felix Reaction

Rickettsial Infection	*Proteus* Antigen		
	OX–19	OX–2	OX–K
Rocky Mountain spotted fever	++++ or +	+ or ++++	–
Epidemic typhus	++++	+	–
Murine typhus	++++	+	–
Brill–Zinsser disease*	–	–	–
Scrub typhus	–	–	++++
Rickettsialpox	–	–	–
Q fever	–	–	–

From *Gradwohl's Clinical Laboratory Methods and Diagnosis,* 8th ed, Sonnenwirth AC and Jarett L, eds, Mosby–Year Book Inc, St Louis, MO: 1980, 2311, with permission.

* = A positive OX–19 reaction is occasionally observed.
++++ = Fourfold or greater rise in titer; – = no reaction.

References

Hechemy KE, "The Immunoserology of Rickettsiae," *Manual of Clinical Laboratory Immunology*, 4th ed, Vol 2, Chapter 97, Rose NR, Conway de Macario E, Fahey JL, et al, eds, Washington, DC: American Society for Microbiology, 1992, 667-75.

Western Blot *see* HIV-1/HIV-2 Serology *on page 696*

Western Blot Test for HIV Antibody *see* HIV-1/HIV-2 Serology *on page 696*

Western Equine Encephalitis Virus Serology

CPT 86654

Related Information

California Encephalitis Virus Titer *on page 651*
Eastern Equine Encephalitis Virus Serology *on page 673*
St Louis Encephalitis Virus Serology *on page 749*

Synonyms Encephalitis Virus Titer, Western Equine

Test Commonly Includes Detection of serologic response to Western equine encephalitis virus

Abstract Western equine encephalitis (WEE) is a disease of summer. Its case fatality rate is 3% to 5%. Transmission is via the mosquito vector *Culex tarsalis*. The pathogenesis of WEE resembles that of Eastern equine encephalitis (EEE).

Specimen Serum or cerebrospinal fluid **CONTAINER:** Red top tube, sterile CSF tube **COLLECTION:** Acute and convalescent specimens are recommended.

Interpretive **REFERENCE RANGE:** Less than a fourfold increase in titer in paired sera; HAI titer: <1:10; CF titer: <1:8; no IgM antibody **USE:** Establish the diagnosis of Western equine encephalitis virus infection **LIMITATIONS:** Cross reactions can occur to Eastern equine encephalitis (EEE) virus. **METHODOLOGY:** Complement fixation (CF), hemagglutination inhibition (HAI), neutralization, indirect fluorescent antibody (IFA), enzyme-linked immunosorbent assay (ELISA). Alphaviruses share antigenic relationships. **ADDITIONAL INFORMATION:** Symptoms of this arbovirus infection include fever, aseptic meningitis, and meningoencephalitis. Disease is usually most severe in children. Diagnosis is best established by detecting specific IgM antibody, particularly in CSF.

References

Monath TP, "Alphavirus (Eastern, Western, and Venezuelan Equine Encephalitis)," *Principles and Practice of Infectious Diseases*, 3rd ed, Mandell GL, Douglas RG Jr, and Bennett JE, eds, New York, NY: Churchill Livingstone, 1990, 1241-2.

Tsai TF, "Arboviruses," *Manual of Clinical Laboratory Immunology*, 4th ed, Vol 2, Chapter 91, Rose NR, Conway de Macario E, Fahey JL, et al, eds, Washington, DC: American Society for Microbiology, 1992, 606-18.

White Cell Crossmatch *see* Tissue Typing *on page 757*

Whooping Cough Titers *see* Bacterial Serology *on page 644*

Widal Agglutination Test *see* *Salmonella* Titer *on page 744*

***Wuchereria bancrofti* Serology** *see* Filariasis Serological Test *on page 679*

Yersinia enterocolitica Antibody

CPT 86793

Related Information

Bacterial Serology *on page 644*
Blood Culture, Aerobic and Anaerobic *on page 784*
Risks of Transfusion *on page 1093*
Stool Culture *on page 858*
Viral Culture, Stool *on page 1205*

Abstract Reservoirs of *Y. enterocolitica* include pigs, goats, dogs, and cats. Transmission may include milk, pork, and water. Organisms are ingested, but the infection can be acquired by transfusion. Often the differential diagnosis includes appendicitis.

Specimen Serum **CONTAINER:** Red top tube **COLLECTION:** Acute and convalescent specimens are recommended.

Interpretive **REFERENCE RANGE:** Titer <1:160 **USE:** Useful in diagnosis of *Yersinia enterocolitica* infection, which is characterized by mesenteric lymphadenitis and/or terminal ileitis with abdominal pain, gastroenteritis, and diarrhea. Colitis, arthritis, and other extraintestinal complications may occur. Most infections are self-limited. **METHODOLOGY:** Agglutination with serotypes 03, 08, and 09 **ADDITIONAL INFORMATION:** This test is sensitive and specific, and should be used in conjunction with culture to confirm a diagnosis of yersiniosis. Antibodies may not be detectable for the first week of symptoms, but then rise rapidly to high titers (1:1280 is di-

(Continued)

Yersinia enterocolitica Antibody *(Continued)*

agnostic). After recovery, low titers (1:40 or 1:80) may persist for years. When stool is sent to the laboratory for culture, request for culture of this organism is usually needed so that an enrichment technique can be utilized.

References

Butler T, "*Yersinia* Infections," *Cecil Textbook of Medicine*, 19th ed, Wyngaarden JB, Smith LH Jr, and Bennett JC, eds, Philadelphia, PA: WB Saunders Co, 1992, 1709-12.

Farmer JJ 3d and Kelly MT, "*Enterobacteriaceae*," *Manual of Clinical Microbiology*, 5th ed, Chapter 36, Balows A, Hausler WJ Jr, Herrmann KL, et al, eds, Washington, DC: American Society for Microbiology, 1991, 360-83.

Yersinia pestis Antibody

CPT 86793

Related Information

Blood Culture, Aerobic and Anaerobic *on page 784*
Gram Stain *on page 815*
Viral Culture, Stool *on page 1205*

Abstract The forms of plague include lymphadenitis (bubonic plague), septicemic, pneumonic, cutaneous, and meningeal. This is the disease which caused historical pandemics, including the black death of the fourteenth century. An infection of humans and animals, it is caused by *Yersinia pestis* (*Pasteurella pestis* until 1970). A zoonotic infection, cases continue to appear in a number of areas including portions of the southwestern United States.

Specimen Serum **CONTAINER:** Red top tube **STORAGE INSTRUCTIONS:** Acidified serum may be stored in a refrigerator **SPECIAL INSTRUCTIONS:** In cases of suspected plague, the Center for Disease Control, Atlanta, should be contacted at once. Sera must be inactivated and absorbed with sheep erythrocytes prior to testing.

Interpretive REFERENCE RANGE: Titer <1:16 **USE:** Used to confirm diagnosis of plague **METHODOLOGY:** Passive hemagglutination on acute and convalescent serum **ADDITIONAL INFORMATION:** A hemagglutination titer ≥1:256 is presumptive evidence of an immunologic response to *Yersinia pestis*, the plague bacillus. Diagnosis can also be made by seeing the stained organism in clinical material. Blood, bubo (lymph node) aspiration, and other materials must be cultured.

References

Butler T, "*Yersinia* Infections," *Cecil Textbook of Medicine*, 19th ed, Wyngaarden JB, Smith LH Jr, and Bennett JC, eds, Philadelphia, PA: WB Saunders Co, 1990, 1709-12.

Farmer JJ 3d and Kelly MT, "*Enterobacteriaceae*," *Manual of Clinical Microbiology*, 5th ed, Chapter 36, Balows A, Hausler WJ Jr, Herrmann KL, et al, eds, Washington, DC: American Society for Microbiology, 1991, 360-83.

***Yersinia pestis* Antibody Titer** *see* Bacterial Serology *on page 644*

Zoster Titer *see* Varicella-Zoster Virus Serology *on page 761*

MICROBIOLOGY

Bernard L. Kasten, Jr, MD
Christopher J. Papasian, PhD
Rebecca T. Horvat, PhD
David S. Jacobs, MD

The past decade has witnessed the rapid evolution of medical microbiology as a clinical laboratory discipline. Improved laboratory methods and increased interest in clinical infectious disease have provided stimuli. Efforts at standardization of methods and consensus approaches to common problems have done much to increase the accuracy and relevance of results.

The modern microbiology laboratory is called upon to identify and isolate potential pathogens. In many cases, the laboratory can provide the clinician with therapeutic guidance in the form of antimicrobial susceptibility tests.

The role of the microbiology laboratory begins at a critical point, the acquisition of a representative specimen from the site of infection. Without an appropriately collected and processed specimen, the most sophisticated laboratory procedures are of little value, and the chances of obtaining a meaningful result may be remote. The laboratory is obliged to support the physicians' efforts to establish an accurate and timely diagnosis upon which rational therapy can be based. If the laboratory receives a specimen that is less than optimal because of inappropriate sampling, delays in transit, inadequate volume, or inappropriate transport medium or storage procedures, the physician or medical personnel responsible for the specimen should be contacted regarding the limitations of the specimen and the possibility of obtaining a more adequate specimen. If this is not possible, the limitations of the available specimen are often communicated with the report of the results.

Physicians and other medical personnel should recognize that the efforts to communicate potential limitations of specimens are not efforts to limit the availability of service or avoid work, but are efforts to provide optimal care to patients.

Safety of patients and of medical personnel has become a focus of concern for all involved in healthcare. Obviously, specimens submitted to the laboratory with the outside of the container contaminated are hazardous to laboratory workers and may not be acceptable.

Detailed test listings are provided by body site for aerobic and anaerobic bacterial cultures, fungal cultures, and mycobacterial cultures. Certain fastidious organisms requiring special consideration are listed by name, as are individual diagnostic and susceptibility testing procedures.

Relevant information is available in other chapters, including Immunology and Serology, Molecular Pathology, and Virology.

Abscess, Aerobic and Anaerobic Bacterial Culture

***CPT** 87070 (aerobic); 87075 (anaerobic)*

Related Information

Biopsy or Body Fluid Aerobic Bacterial Culture *on page 778*
Biopsy or Body Fluid Anaerobic Bacterial Culture *on page 778*
Cerebrospinal Fluid Anaerobic Culture *on page 797*
Endometrium Culture *on page 811*
Fine Needle Aspiration, Deep Seated Lesions *on page 498*
Fine Needle Aspiration, Superficial Palpable Masses *on page 499*
Susceptibility Testing, Aerobic and Facultatively Anaerobic Organisms *on page 864*
Susceptibility Testing, Anaerobic Bacteria *on page 866*
Wound Culture *on page 885*

Applies to Aerobic Culture, Abscess; Anaerobic Culture, Abscess

Test Commonly Includes Culture for aerobic and facultative anaerobic organisms. Culture for anaerobic organisms usually must be specifically requested and may require a separate specimen.

Patient Care PREPARATION: The aspiration site is prepared aseptically. The overlying and adjacent areas must be carefully prepared to eliminate isolation of potentially contaminating aerobic and anaerobic bacteria which colonize the skin surfaces.

Specimen Fluid, pus, or other material properly obtained from an abscess for optimal yield. This material should suffice for both aerobic and anaerobic cultures. Specimens for anaerobic culture should be accompanied by a request for aerobic culture from the same site. CONTAINER: The practice of collecting material of this type on swabs should be discouraged. Specimen may be aspirated into a syringe and capped with an airtight stopper; if submitted in this manner, all air should be expelled from the syringe prior to transporting the specimen to the laboratory. Alternatively, clinical material may be transferred from the syringe to commercially available vials that contain anaerobic indicators and maintain anaerobic conditions. Specimens may also be transferred to sterile containers that do not maintain anaerobic conditions, but transport to the laboratory should be expedited to maximize survival of anaerobes. Some laboratories discourage submission of specimens in syringes because of concerns about needlestick injuries. COLLECTION: Significant effort should be made to eliminate the indigenous microbiota from adjacent or overlying normal or necrotic tissue prior to specimen collection. Specimens should be collected from a prepared site using aseptic technique. Some anaerobes will be killed by contact with oxygen for only a few seconds. Ideally, pus obtained by needle aspiration through an intact surface, which has been aseptically prepared, is put directly into anaerobic transport media or transported directly to the laboratory. Sampling of open lesions is enhanced by deep aspiration using a sterile plastic catheter or needle. Curettings of the base of an open lesion may also provide a good yield. If irrigation is necessary, nonbacteriostatic sterile normal saline may be used. Pulmonary samples may be obtained by transtracheal percutaneous needle aspiration by physicians trained in this procedure or by use of a special sheathed catheter. If swabs must be used, two should be collected; one for culture and one for Gram stain. Specimens collected in syringes should be transported to the laboratory within 30 minutes of collection. CAUSES FOR REJECTION: Specimens exposed to air, specimens which have been refrigerated, or have an excessive delay in transit have a less than optimal yield. Rejection of such specimens by a laboratory is impractical if additional clinical material is not readily obtainable, but a comment is usually added to the final report indicating the problem. Specimens from sites which have anaerobic bacteria as normal flora (eg, throat, feces, colostomy stoma, rectal swabs, bronchial washes, cervical-vaginal mucosal swabs, sputums, skin and superficial wounds, voided or catheterized urine) may **not** be acceptable for anaerobic culture because of contamination by the normal flora. TURNAROUND TIME: Preliminary negative reports can be generated for aerobic bacteria within 1 day, and for anaerobic bacteria within 2 days. Final negative results are usually provided after 4-5 days of incubation; if actinomycosis is suspected, however, the specimen may be held for 2 weeks. Positive results may be generated by 18-24 hours (preliminary results for aerobic cultures), but final positive results for anaerobic cultures take at least 4 days, and often take considerably longer if speciation and antimicrobial susceptibilities are required (7-14 days). SPECIAL INSTRUCTIONS: The laboratory should be informed of the specific site of specimen, age of patient, current antibiotic therapy, clinical diagnosis, and time of collection.

Interpretive REFERENCE RANGE: No growth of aerobic or anaerobic bacteria USE: Define the microbial etiology of the abscess and provide a guide for therapy LIMITATIONS: Certain fastidious anaerobes may not be recoverable despite significant efforts to collect and properly submit a specimen. Additionally, any specimen submitted for microbial culture can be contaminated with colonizing organisms that are not contributing to disease. Organisms most likely to contaminate specimens of this type include, but are not limited to, *Corynebacterium* sp and coagulase-negative staphylococci. These organisms are not invariably contaminants, however, and may be pathogenic in certain settings. A Gram stain should always be performed, if sufficient material is obtained, to provide early presumptive information and to help interpret culture results.

Clinical Symptoms Suggestive of Anaerobic Infection

Foul-smelling discharge
Location of infection in proximity to a mucosal surface
Necrotic tissue, gangrene, pseudomembrane formation
Gas in tissues or discharges
Endocarditis with negative routine blood cultures
Infection associated with malignancy or other process producing tissue destruction
Infection related to the use of aminoglycosides (oral, parenteral, or topical)
Septic thrombophlebitis
Bacteremic picture with jaundice
Infection resulting from human or other bites
Black discoloration of blood-containing exudates (may fluoresce red under ultraviolet light in *B. melaninogenicus* infections)
Presence of "sulfur granules" in discharges (actinomycosis)
Classical clinical features of gas gangrene
Clinical setting suggestive for anaerobic infection (septic abortion, infection after gastrointestinal surgery, genitourinary surgery, etc)

From Bartlett JG, "Anaerobic Bacterial Infections of the Lung," *Chest,* 1987, 91:901-9, with permission.

The only sources for specimens with established validity for meaningful anaerobic culture in patients with pleuropulmonary infections are blood, pleural fluid, transtracheal aspirates, transthoracic pulmonary aspirates, specimens obtained at thoracotomy, and fiberoptic bronchoscopic aspirates using the protected brush or sheathed catheter. Pleural fluid is preferred for patients with empyema[1]. Blood cultures yield positive results in <5% of cases of anaerobic pulmonary infection. Specimens received in anaerobic transport containers are not optimal for aerobic fungus cultures.

Frequently, usual laboratory procedure includes screening only for rapidly growing anaerobes (*Bacteroides fragilis*, *Clostridium perfringens*, *Fusobacterium*, and anaerobic gram-positive cocci). Slow-growing *Mycobacterium* sp or *Nocardia* sp which may cause abscesses will **not** be recovered even if present, since extended incubation periods or special media are necessary for their isolation. Cultures for these organisms should be specifically requested.

CONTRAINDICATIONS: Bronchoscopically-obtained specimens are not ideal as the instrument becomes contaminated by organisms normally contaminating the oropharynx during insertion. Culture of specimens from sites harboring endogenous anaerobic organisms or contaminated by endogenous organisms may be misleading with regard to etiology and selection of appropriate therapy. Special sheathed catheters are available to reduce oropharyngeal flora contamination of bronchial aspirate cultures. **METHODOLOGY:** Aerobic and anaerobic culture, usually with broth and solid media. Special handling to maintain anaerobic conditions is required. **ADDITIONAL INFORMATION:** Serious anaerobic infections are often due to mixed flora which are pathologic synergists. Anaerobes frequently recovered from closed postoperative wound infections include *Bacteroides fragilis*, approximately 50%; *Prevotella melaninogenica* (previously *Bacteroides melaninogenicus*), approximately 25%; *Peptostreptococcus prevotii*, approximately 15%; and *Fusobacterium* sp, approximately 25%. Anaerobes are seldom recovered in pure culture (10% to 15% of cultures). Aerobes and facultative bacteria when present are frequently found in lesser numbers than the anaerobes. Anaerobic infection is most commonly associated with operations involving opening or manipulating the bowel or a hollow viscus (eg, appendectomy, cholecystectomy, colectomy, gastrectomy, bile duct exploration, etc). The ratio of anaerobes to facultative species is normally about 10:1 in the mouth, vagina, and sebaceous glands and at least 1000:1 in the colon.

Footnotes

1. Bartlett JG, "Anaerobic Bacterial Infections of the Lung," *Chest*, 1987, 91:901-9.

References

Brook I, "A 12 Year Study of Aerobic and Anaerobic Bacteria in Intra-abdominal and Postsurgical Abdominal Wound Infections," *Surg Gynecol Obstet*, 1989, 169(5):387-92.

Simor AE, Roberts FJ, and Smith JA, "Infections of the Skin and Subcutaneous Tissues," *Cumitech 23*, Smith JA, ed, Washington, DC: American Society for Microbiology, 1988.

(Continued)

Abscess, Aerobic and Anaerobic Bacterial Culture *(Continued)*

Styrt B and Gorbach SL, "Recent Developments in the Understanding of the Pathogenesis and Treatment of Anaerobic Infections," *N Engl J Med*, 1989, 321(5):240-6.

Swenson RM, "Rationale for the Identification and Susceptibility Testing of Anaerobic Bacteria," *Rev Infect Dis*, 1986, 8:809-13.

Acid-Fast Stain

CPT *87206*

Related Information

Acid-Fast Stain, Modified, *Nocardia* Species *on next page*
Biopsy or Body Fluid Mycobacteria Culture *on page 782*
Cerebrospinal Fluid Mycobacteria Culture *on page 801*
Mycobacteria by DNA Probe *on page 921*
Skin Mycobacteria Culture *on page 846*
Skin Test, Tuberculosis *on page 848*
Sputum Mycobacteria Culture *on page 855*
Stool Mycobacteria Culture *on page 863*
Urine Mycobacteria Culture *on page 884*

Synonyms AFB Smear; Atypical *Mycobacterium* Smear; Fluorochrome Stain; Kinyoun Stain; *Mycobacterium* Smear; TB Smear; Ziehl-Neelsen Stain

Applies to Auramine-Rhodamine Stain

Test Commonly Includes Acid-fast stain. For diagnosis, acid-fast stain and culture are usually ordered together.

Abstract Acid-fast bacilli are so called because they are surrounded by a waxy envelope that is resistant to destaining by acid alcohol. Heat (classic Ziehl-Neelsen), prolonged exposure or a detergent (Tergitol™ Kinyoun method) is required to allow carbolfuchsin stain to penetrate the capsule. Once stained, acid-fast bacteria resist decolorization with acid alcohol.[1]

Patient Care PREPARATION: Same as for mycobacteria culture of given site

Specimen The appropriate specimen for an acid-fast smear is the same as for culture. See specific site mycobacteria culture listings for details. CAUSES FOR REJECTION: Insufficient specimen volume, specimen received on a dry swab

Interpretive REFERENCE RANGE: No acid-fast organisms observed. Positive smears are quantitated and reported as 1+ (3-9 bacilli in entire smear), 2+ ($\geq$10 in entire smear), or 3+ (1 or more bacilli per field) acid-fast bacilli seen. USE: Determine the presence of mycobacteria; monitor the course of antimycobacterial therapy; establish the diagnosis of mycobacterial infection in undiagnosed granulomatous disease, fever of unknown origin (FUO), and in patients suspected of having a defect in cellular immunity (eg, AIDS, lymphoma, and so forth) LIMITATIONS: Cultures are significantly more sensitive than smears, therefore, negative acid-fast smears do not adequately exclude a diagnosis of mycobacterial disease. Additionally, acid-fast stains are not specific for *M. tuberculosis*; other species in the genus *Mycobacterium* will stain acid-fast, and other organisms will occasionally stain acid-fast (eg, *Nocardia* sp, *Legionella micdadei*, *Rhodococcus equi*).[2,3] Organisms other than *M. tuberculosis* may be contaminants or may be pathogenic. Some laboratories may guess an organism's identity (eg, *M. tuberculosis* vs atypical *Mycobacterium* sp) by its staining characteristics and morphology, but definitive identification can only be accomplished by culture and subsequent phenotypic or genotypic characterization.[4] The use of the detection of tuberculostearic acid by gas chromatography/mass spectrometry as a rapid and more sensitive method for the diagnosis of mycobacteria is under development and is used by some larger laboratories.[5] METHODOLOGY: Acid-fast stain of concentrated or unconcentrated specimen (Ziehl-Neelsen, Kinyoun, or fluorochrome stain).[1] See diagram. ADDITIONAL INFORMATION: A stat acid-fast smear usually can be performed by many laboratories upon special request. However, concentration procedures are not usually performed on a stat basis and the contribution of stat acid-fast stains to patient care is often equivocal. Very active infection is required to produce a positive without concentration. In extrapulmonary tuberculosis, the acid-fast stain can be useful in yielding a rapid diagnosis. Positive smears were obtained from CSF in 67% of cases of culture-proven tuberculous meningitis, lymph node biopsy in 80% of miliary tuberculosis cases, 75% peritoneal biopsies in peritonitis, and urine in 80% of the cases of renal tuberculosis.[6]

H_2N — C — NH_2 — NH_2

Carbolfuchsin
(triaminotriphenylmethane)

Acid-fast stains performed on gastric aspirate and urine when positive are reliable indicators of true mycobacterial disease. Klotz and Penn have reported the sensitivity, compared to culture, as approximately 30% for gastric aspirates and approximately 50% for urine. False-positives were negligible, <1%.[7]

In a large prospective study, the sensitivity and specificity of acid-fast staining for diagnosing tuberculosis was 53.1% and 99.8%, respectively; the sensitivity and specificity of cultures was 81.5% and 98.4%, respectively.[8]

Footnotes

1. Koneman EW, Allen SD, Janda WM, et al, *Color Atlas and Textbook of Diagnostic Microbiology*, 4th ed, Philadelphia, PA: JB Lippincott Co, 1992, 713-4.
2. Hilton E, Freedman RA, Clintron F, et al, "Acid-Fast Bacilli in Sputum: A Case of *Legionella micdadei* Pneumonia," *J Clin Microbiol*, 1986, 24:1102-3.
3. Harvey RL and Sunstrum JC, "*Rhodococcus equi* Infection in Patients With and Without Human Immunodeficiency Virus Infection," *Rev Infect Dis*, 1991, 13(1):139-45.
4. Dawson DJ, Blacklock ZM, Hayward AJ, et al, "Differential Identification of Mycobacteria in Smears of Sputum," *Tubercle*, 1981, 62:257-62.
5. French GL, Chan CY, Cheung CW, et al, "Diagnosis of Pulmonary Tuberculosis by Detection of Tuberculostearic Acid in Sputum by Using Gas Chromatography – Mass Spectrophotometry," *J Infect Dis*, 1987, 156:356-62.
6. Alvarez S and McCabe WR, "Extrapulmonary Tuberculosis Revisited: A Review of Experience of Boston City and Other Hospitals," *Medicine (Baltimore)*, 1984, 63:25-55.
7. Klotz SA and Penn RL, "Acid-Fast Staining of Urine and Gastric Contents Is an Excellent Indicator of Mycobacterial Disease," *Am Rev Respir Dis*, 1987, 136:1197-8.
8. Levy H, Feldman C, Sacho H, et al, "A Re-evaluation of Sputum Microscopy and Culture in the Diagnosis of Pulmonary Tuberculosis," *Chest*, 1989, 95(6):1193-7.

References

Gordin F and Slutkin G, "The Validity of Acid-Fast Smears in the Diagnosis of Pulmonary Tuberculosis," *Arch Pathol Lab Med*, 1990, 114(10):1025-7.

Wallace RJ Jr, O'Brien R, Glassroth J, et al, "Diagnosis and Treatment of Disease Caused by Nontuberculous Mycobacteria (Official Statement ATS)," *Am Rev Respir Dis*, 1990, 142:940-53.

Acid-Fast Stain, Modified, *Cryptosporidium* *see Cryptosporidium* Diagnostic Procedures, Stool *on page 806*

Acid-Fast Stain, Modified, *Nocardia* Species

CPT 87206

Related Information

Acid-Fast Stain *on previous page*
Actinomyces Culture, All Sites *on next page*
Cryptosporidium Diagnostic Procedures, Stool *on page 806*
Fungus Smear, Stain *on page 813*
Gram Stain *on page 815*
Nocardia Culture, All Sites *on page 835*

Synonyms Hank's Stain; *Nocardia* Species Modified Acid-Fast Stain

Test Commonly Includes Modified acid-fast stain. Culture generally must be ordered specifically as such. The recovery of *Nocardia* sp frequently requires special culture techniques.

Abstract Infections with *Nocardia* sp may resemble many other more common diseases. Because therapy differs, it is important to establish a definitive diagnosis, preferably by culture. The diagnosis of nocardiosis should be considered in unexplained cavitary lung disease, granulomatous lung disease of established cause not responsive to appropriate therapy, brain abscess particularly in the presence of cavitary lung disease, alveolar proteinosis, with mycetoma, and in any patient in whom a disseminated granulomatous disease is considered.

Specimen Appropriate preparation, specimen and container for smear is the same as for culture **CAUSES FOR REJECTION:** Insufficient specimen volume, specimen received on a dry swab

Interpretive **REFERENCE RANGE:** No acid-fast organisms seen **USE:** Determine the presence or absence of *Nocardia* sp which are usually, but not invariably, acid-fast when stained by the modified acid-fast stain. *Actinomyces* and *Streptomyces* sp which may be microscopically similar to *Nocardia* on Gram stain, are negative with the modified acid-fast stain. Establish the etiology of maduromycosis and of fever of unknown origin in patients with suspected defects of cellular immunity (eg, AIDS, Hodgkin's disease, lymphoma, and so forth). **LIMITATIONS:** *Nocardia* sp do not always stain acid-fast by this method, consequently, the presence of branching, gram-positive bacilli on Gram stain may have greater sensitivity. *Nocardia* sp, however,

(Continued)

Acid-Fast Stain, Modified, *Nocardia* Species *(Continued)*

cannot be distinguished from *Actinomyces* sp and other closely related organisms by Gram stain. **METHODOLOGY:** Kinyoun stain followed by light decolorization with 3% acid alcohol (940 mL of 95% ethanol and 60 mL of concentrated HCl)[1] **ADDITIONAL INFORMATION:** Nocardiosis has also been reported with lupus, rheumatoid arthritis, and liver disease. Aggressive diagnostic procedures are often necessary to obtain appropriate specimen for definitive diagnosis. Elements consistent with *Nocardia* sp can be identified presumptively on Gram stain and modified acid-fast stain pending more definitive diagnosis by culture.[2] Examination of sputum with *Nocardia* may show thin, crooked, weakly to strongly gram-positive, modified acid-fast positive, irregularly staining or beaded filaments. Opaque or pigmented sulfur granules may occasionally be present in direct smear of pus. Colonization without apparent infection may occur.

Footnotes

1. Koneman EW, Allen SD, Janda WM, et al, *Color Atlas and Textbook of Diagnostic Microbiology*, 4th ed, Philadelphia, PA: JB Lippincott Co, 1992, 505.
2. Osoagbaka OU and Njoku-Obi AN, "Presumptive Diagnosis of Pulmonary Nocardiosis: Value of Sputum Microscopy," *J Appl Bacteriol*, 1987, 63:27-38.

References

Chazen G, "*Nocardia*," *Infect Control*, 1987, 8:260-3.

Javaly K, Horowitz HW, and Wormser GP, "Nocardiosis in Patients With Human Immunodeficiency Virus Infection. Report of 2 Cases and Review of the Literature," *Medicine (Baltimore)*, 1992, 71(3):128-38.

Laurin JM, Resnik CS, Wheeler D, et al, "Vertebral Osteomyelitis Caused by *Nocardia asteroides*: Report and Review of the Literature," *J Rheumatol*, 1991, 18(3):455-8.

Wilson JP, Turner HR, Kirchner KA, et al, "Nocardial Infections in Renal Transplant Recipients," *Medicine (Baltimore)*, 1989, 68(1):38-57.

Actinomyces Culture, All Sites

CPT 87081

Related Information

Acid-Fast Stain, Modified, *Nocardia* Species *on previous page*
Biopsy or Body Fluid Aerobic Bacterial Culture *on page 778*
Biopsy or Body Fluid Anaerobic Bacterial Culture *on page 778*
Endometrium Culture *on page 811*
Nocardia Culture, All Sites *on page 835*

Synonyms Wound *Actinomyces* Culture

Applies to Intrauterine Device Culture; IUD Culture; Sulfur Granule, Culture

Test Commonly Includes Anaerobic culture for *Actinomyces* sp and direct microscopic examination of Gram stain for sulfur granules and gram-positive branching bacilli

Abstract Actinomycosis is a chronic progressive suppurative disease characterized by the formation of multiple abscesses, draining sinuses, and dense fibrosis. The classic presentations include cervicofacial, thoracic, abdominal, and pelvic infections.

Patient Care **PREPARATION:** Cleanse the skin around the opening of a draining sinus with an alcohol swab, allow to dry, and obtain the specimen from as deep within the sinus as possible.

Specimen Exudate, material from draining sinus **CONTAINER:** Anaerobic specimen transport medium **COLLECTION:** *Actinomyces* sp are fastidious anaerobic organisms. It is, therefore, essential that the specimen be placed into the appropriate anaerobic transport tube and delivered to the laboratory as quickly as possible. If a syringe is used, expel all air before transferring into the tube. Swabs, if used, should be transported in anaerobic transport medium. With a draining sinus, obtain the specimen by passing a swab as far up the sinus as possible. **STORAGE INSTRUCTIONS:** Specimens should be transported immediately to the laboratory and processed as soon as possible. **CAUSES FOR REJECTION:** Specimens exposed to air, specimens which have been refrigerated or have an excessive delay in transit, have a less than optimal yield. Specimens from sites which have anaerobic bacteria as normal flora (eg, throat, feces, colostomy stoma, rectal swabs, bronchial washes, cervical-vaginal mucosal swabs, sputums, skin and superficial wounds, voided or catheterized urine), may **not** be acceptable for anaerobic culture because of contamination by the normal flora. **TURNAROUND TIME:** Preliminary reports are usually available after 7 days. Cultures with no growth may be reported after 14 days. **SPECIAL INSTRUCTIONS:** In tissues, *Actinomyces* sp produce chronic suppuration with formation of multiple draining sinuses. Examination of material from such sinuses often reveals tangled masses of filamentous elements and granules called sulfur granules. The presence of sulfur granules is highly suggestive of *Actinomyces* infection. If actinomycosis is suspected clinically, the laboratory should be informed. The specific site of specimen, current antibiotic therapy, and clinical diagnosis should be provided.

Interpretive **REFERENCE RANGE:** No *Actinomyces* isolated. *A. israelii* is a normal inhabitant of the mouth, oropharynx, and gastrointestinal tract. **USE:** Detect infections due to *Actinomyces* sp; establish the etiology of granulomatous disease, chronic draining sinus, and fever of unknown origin (FUO) particularly in immunocompromised patients **LIMITATIONS:** Inform the laboratory that actinomycosis is clinically suspected, to ensure that cultures will be incubated long enough to permit recovery of *Actinomyces* sp; *Actinomyces* sp are relatively slow growing and will often fail to grow in the period in which most laboratories incubate routine cultures. Additionally, even when incubated appropriately, recovery of *Actinomyces* sp may be hindered by overgrowth with obligate and facultative anaerobic bacteria. **METHODOLOGY:** Anaerobic culture including thioglycolate broth media **ADDITIONAL INFORMATION:** If granules are detected on the gauze pad covering a draining sinus, submit the granules to the laboratory. A Gram stain and culture should be performed on such granules. On smear branching gram-positive rods may be found. They may be similar in appearance to other actinomycetes including species of *Nocardia*, *Streptomyces*, and also *Mycobacterium*.[1] Actinomycetes are not stained by the modified acid-fast stain used for *Nocardia* sp. Several species of *Actinomyces* are responsible for human infection. *Actinomyces israelii* is the most significant. *A. naeslundii*, *A. odontolyticus*, *A. viscosus*, and *Arachnia propionica* also have been reported as human pathogens. Pelvic and perirectal infections have been associated with intrauterine devices (IUDs). A classic presentation of actinomycosis is as a painless lump in the jaw.[2] *Actinomyces* may be found in rare instances of recurrent ventral hernia following appendectomy for appendicitis. The diagnosis of actinomycosis in many settings requires consideration of the possibility followed by persistence on the part of laboratory personnel.

Footnotes

1. Berd D, "Laboratory Identification of Clinically Important Actinomycetes," *Appl Microbiol*, 1973, 25:665-8.
2. Feder HM Jr, "Actinomycosis Manifesting as an Acute Painless Lump of the Jaw," *Pediatrics*, 1990, 85(5):858-64.

References

Bellingan GJ, "Disseminated Actinomycosis," *BMJ*, 1990, 301(6764):1323-4.

Holtz HA, Lavery DP, and Kapila R, "Actinomycetales Infection in the Acquired Immunodeficiency Syndrome," *Ann Intern Med*, 1985, 102:203-5.

Levine LA and Doyle CJ, "Retroperitoneal Actinomycosis: A Case Report and Review of the Literature," *J Urol*, 1988, 140:367-9.

Nahass RG, Scholz P, Mackenzie JW, et al, "Chronic Constrictive Pericarditis, A Case Report and Review of the Literature," *Arch Intern Med*, 1989, 149(5):1202-3.

Persson E, "Genital Actinomycosis and *Actinomyces israelii* in the Female Genital Tract," *Adv Contracept*, 1987, 3:115-23, (review).

Aerobic Culture, Abscess *see* Abscess, Aerobic and Anaerobic Bacterial Culture *on page 768*

Aerobic Culture, Blood *see* Blood Culture, Aerobic and Anaerobic *on page 784*

AFB Culture, Biopsy *see* Biopsy or Body Fluid Mycobacteria Culture *on page 782*

AFB Culture, Sputum *see* Sputum Mycobacteria Culture *on page 855*

AFB Culture, Stool *see* Stool Mycobacteria Culture *on page 863*

AFB Smear *see* Acid-Fast Stain *on page 770*

Airway Lavage *see* Bronchoalveolar Lavage *on page 793*

Amebiasis *see* Ova and Parasites, Stool *on page 836*

Amniotic Fluid Anaerobic Culture *see* Endometrium Culture *on page 811*

Anaerobic Bacterial Susceptibility *see* Susceptibility Testing, Anaerobic Bacteria *on page 866*

Anaerobic Culture, Abscess *see* Abscess, Aerobic and Anaerobic Bacterial Culture *on page 768*

Anaerobic Culture, Biopsy *see* Biopsy or Body Fluid Anaerobic Bacterial Culture *on page 778*

Anaerobic Culture, Blood *see* Blood Culture, Aerobic and Anaerobic *on page 784*

Anaerobic Culture, Body Fluid *see* Biopsy or Body Fluid Anaerobic Bacterial Culture *on page 778*

Anaerobic Culture, Bronchial Aspirate *see* Bronchial Aspirate Anaerobic Culture *on page 792*

Anaerobic Culture, Cerebrospinal Fluid *see* Cerebrospinal Fluid Anaerobic Culture *on page 797*

Anaerobic Culture, Cul-de-sac *see* Endometrium Culture *on page 811*

Anaerobic Culture, Endometrium *see* Endometrium Culture *on page 811*

Anaerobic Culture, Uterus *see* Endometrium Culture *on page 811*

Anergy Testing *see* Skin Test, Tuberculosis *on page 848*

Antibacterial Activity, Serum *see* Serum Bactericidal Test *on page 843*

Antibiotic-Associated Colitis Toxin Test *see Clostridium difficile* Toxin Assay *on page 802*

Antimicrobial Combinations – Test for Synergism and Antagonism *see* Susceptibility Testing, Antimicrobial Combinations *on page 868*

Antimicrobial Drugs *see* Susceptibility Testing, Aerobic and Facultatively Anaerobic Organisms *on page 864*

Antimicrobial Removal Device (ARD) Blood Culture *see* Blood Culture, Aerobic and Anaerobic *on page 784*

ARD, Blood Culture *see* Blood Culture, Aerobic and Anaerobic *on page 784*

Arthropod Identification

CPT 88300 (surgical pathology gross examination)

Related Information

Babesiosis Serological Test *on page 643*

Synonyms Ectoparasite Identification; Insect Identification

Applies to Bed Bugs Identification; Body Lice Identification; *Cimex* Identification; Crab Lice Identification; Deer Tick Identification; Flea Identification; Head Lice Identification; *Ixodes dammini* Identification; Lice Identification; Mite Identification; Nits Identification; *Pediculus humanus* Identification; *Phthirus pubis* Identification; Pubic Lice Identification; Rocky Mountain Spotted Fever, *Dermacentor andersoni*; *Sarcoptes scabiei* Skin Scrapings Identification; Skin Scrapings for *Sarcoptes scabiei* Identification; Tick Identification

Abstract Arthropoda is a phylum which includes Arachnida and Insecta, among other classes. Species include parasites and vectors. Arachnida includes spiders, ticks, mites, and scorpions.

Specimen Gross arthropod, skin scrapings **CONTAINER:** Screw-cap tube or screw-cap jar **COLLECTION:** Arthropods (gross) are to be submitted in alcohol (70%) or formaldehyde in tube or container with secure closure. To establish the diagnosis of scabies, skin scrapings may be collected with a scalpel and a drop of mineral oil. The liquid may be examined directly or alternatively the organism may be teased away from its burrow or papule with a needle or scalpel. **STORAGE INSTRUCTIONS:** Maintain specimen at room temperature. Fill the container with preservative as completely as possible to avoid damage to the specimen by air bubbles in the container. **TURNAROUND TIME:** 1-2 hours; if referral to a state or federal laboratory is required, 2-4 weeks

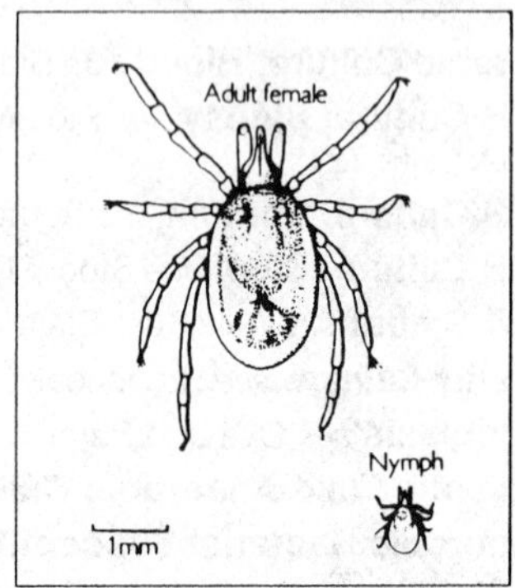

Deer tick (*Ixodes dammini*)

Interpretive **USE:** Identify arthropods affecting man; establish the presence of ectoparasite infestation **METHODOLOGY:** Macroscopic evaluation **ADDITIONAL INFORMATION:** The deer tick (*Ixodes dammini* or *Ixodes ricinus* complex) is recognized as a vector for Lyme disease caused by *Borrelia burgdorferi*, as well as for babesiosis. Thirty percent of ticks collected from patients suffering tick bites in Middletown, Connecticut (1988) were found to be infected with *B. burgdorferi*.[1] The range of *I. dammini* has expanded from the original endemic areas of Long Island, NY and Connecticut.[2]

Footnotes

1. "Is Lyme Disease Prophylaxis Worthwhile," *Emerg Med*, 1989, 49-52, (editorial).

2. White DJ, Chang H-G, Benach JL, et al, "The Geographic Spread and Temporal Increase of the Lyme Disease Epidemic," *JAMA*, 1991, 266(9):1230-6.

References

Agger W, Case KL, Bryant GL, et al, "Lyme Disease: Clinical Features, Classification, and Epidemiology in the Upper Midwest," *Medicine (Baltimore)*, 1991, 70(2):83-90.

Dalton MT and Haldane DJ, "Unusual Dermal Arthropod Infestations," *Can Med Assoc J*, 1990, 143(2):113-4.

Hobbs GD and Harrell RE Jr, "Brown Recluse Spider Bites: A Common Cause of Necrotic Arachnidism," *Am J Emerg Med*, 1989, 7(3):309-12.

Honig PJ, "Bites and Parasites," *Pediatr Clin North Am*, 1983, 30:563-81.

Kaslow RA, "Current Perspective on Lyme Borreliosis," *JAMA*, 1992, 267(10):1381-3.

Moran ME, Ehreth JT, and Drach GW, "Venomous Bites to the External Genitalia: An Unusual Cause of Acute Scrotum," *J Urol*, 1992, 147(4):1085-6.

Pratt HD and Smith JW, "Arthropods of Medical Importance," *Manual of Clinical Microbiology*, 5th ed, Balows A, Hausler WJ Jr, Herrmann KL, et al, eds, Washington, DC: American Society for Microbiology, 1991, 796-810.

Atypical *Mycobacterium* Smear *see* Acid-Fast Stain *on page 770*

Auramine-Rhodamine Stain *see* Acid-Fast Stain *on page 770*

Autoclave Sterility Check *see* Sterility Culture *on page 857*

Bactec® *see* Blood Culture, Aerobic and Anaerobic *on page 784*

Bacterial Antigens by Coagglutination *replaced by* Bacterial Antigens, Rapid Detection Methods *on this page*

Bacterial Antigens by Counterimmunoelectrophoresis *replaced by* Bacterial Antigens, Rapid Detection Methods *on this page*

Bacterial Antigens, CSF *see* Bacterial Antigens, Rapid Detection Methods *on this page*

Bacterial Antigens, Rapid Detection Methods

***CPT** 86403 (each antigen)*

Related Information

Bacteremia Detection, Buffy Coat Micromethod *on page 520*
Cerebrospinal Fluid Analysis *on page 527*
Cerebrospinal Fluid Culture *on page 798*
Cerebrospinal Fluid Fungus Culture *on page 800*
Cerebrospinal Fluid Glucose *on page 176*
Cerebrospinal Fluid Mycobacteria Culture *on page 801*
Cerebrospinal Fluid Protein *on page 659*
Cryptococcal Antigen Titer, Serum or Cerebrospinal Fluid *on page 805*
Group A *Streptococcus* Screen *on page 818*
Group B *Streptococcus* Screen *on page 819*
Viral Culture, Central Nervous System Symptoms *on page 1199*

Synonyms Latex Agglutination for Bacterial Antigens

Applies to Bacterial Antigens, CSF; Bacterial Antigens, Serum; Bacterial Antigens, Urine; Cerebrospinal Fluid Bacterial Antigen Testing

Replaces Bacterial Antigens by Coagglutination; Bacterial Antigens by Counterimmunoelectrophoresis

Test Commonly Includes Qualitative determination of the presence of antigens of *H. influenzae*, *S. pneumoniae*, *N. meningitidis*. Test may also identify subgroups of above organisms and may include testing for group B *Streptococcus* and *E. coli* K1 antigen in neonates. Gram staining and culture should always be done with bacterial antigen testing,[1] and results of Gram staining must be coordinated with antigen testing by knowledgeable laboratory workers.[2]

Abstract Rapid adjunctive tests include latex agglutination, which is more sensitive than coagglutination and counterimmunoelectrophoresis.[3] The newer antigen detection systems useful in meningitis have a level of sensitivity similar to that of the Gram stain;[4] about 80% of cases are diagnosed with either technique.[5] False-negative results occur.[6] Isenberg indicates that **these latex agglutination tests are not intended as a substitute for bacterial culture. Confirmatory diagnosis of bacterial meningitis infection is possible only with appropriate culture procedures.**[7] Similar recommendations are published by others as well.[8,9] Con-

(Continued)

Bacterial Antigens, Rapid Detection Methods *(Continued)*

centration of antigen depends on variables including the number of bacteria, the duration of infection, and the presence or absence of specific antibodies which may prevent antigen detection.[7] A 1992 publication, recognizing their shortcomings, describes the rapid diagnostic tests as not essential but notes that they may be helpful in rapidly establishing an etiologic diagnosis.[10]

Patient Care PREPARATION: Usual aseptic aspiration

Specimen Cerebrospinal fluid, serum, urine CONTAINER: Sterile CSF tube, red top tube, sterile urine container STORAGE INSTRUCTIONS: Keep refrigerated. This differs from the storage requirements for specimens that require culture since the agglutination reaction does not require viable microorganisms. **If culture is requested on the same specimen do not refrigerate.**

Interpretive REFERENCE RANGE: Negative USE: Detect bacterial antigens in CSF for the rapid diagnosis of meningitis. The method may be applied to other body fluids, blood culture supernatants, and urine. LIMITATIONS: May be negative in early meningitis. Such important pathogens as *Staphylococcus aureus* and *Pseudomonas aeruginosa* are not detected by these methods. Most members of the Enterobacteriaceae also fail to react. Antigen detection does not replace Gram stain and culture. Group B *Streptococcus* and the *E. coli* K1 antigen are frequently not tested on infants older than 6 months of age. Nonspecific cross reactions occur. Nonspecific agglutination occurs.[1,3] Antigenic crossover (cross reactions) are seen (eg, *E. coli* K1 and *N. meningitidis* group B). The sensitivity of commercial antigen detection kits remains imperfect;[3,6] the sensitivity differs substantially with various organisms and in various clinical series. The sensitivity of the tests varies from 55% to 100% depending on the reactivity of the antibody and the concentration of antigen in the specimen. False-negative results occur,[1,5,6] especially those taken early in the disease, with low antigen load. Pneumococcal and *Haemophilus* strains not possessing capsular antigens may not be detected by immunological techniques. Pneumococcal antigen is not detected in urine.[7]

Observing that antibiotics are started even when latex tests are negative, Feuerborn et al noted that of five positive latex agglutination tests obtained from CSF, all had positive Gram stains as well. In this series, two cases of bacterial meningitis were described in which the causative organism could not be identified by latex agglutination. They concluded that the CSF white blood cell count and differential were the best predictors of meningitis.[11]

A number of current papers addressing the differential diagnosis of meningitis do not include latex agglutination testing in discussion of laboratory results.[9,12,13,14,15,16] Granoff et al observed that the test had no measurable impact on patient care in patients with bacterial meningitis, since physicians believe that the risks of any error were unacceptable. In this series, the role of rapid antigen testing was confirmation of positive Gram stain results. Culture results rather than antigen testing were used for pivotal decisions. The senior author of the study noted in discussion that one must await the results of culture and concluded that the test may be helpful in selected situations.[17]

Coagglutination and latex agglutination tests may be hampered by nonspecific reactions caused by rheumatoid factor, blood, hemolyzed red cells, and high concentrations of protein. Although boiling specimens can liberate bacterial antigens bound by CSF proteins, meningococcal group B/*E. coli* K1 antigen is heat sensitive and may be more difficult to detect by latex agglutination following exposure to 100°C.[18]

METHODOLOGY: Latex agglutination (LA) ADDITIONAL INFORMATION: Counterimmunoelectrophoresis, coagglutination, or latex agglutination should not replace Gram stain and culture. Bacterial antigens may be detected despite previous antibiotic therapy. Immunologic methods have an advantage over Gram stain in some partially treated cases. The sensitivity ranges for each of the three commercial assays are published for *H. influenzae* type b, *S. pneumoniae*, *Streptococcus* group B, and *N. meningitidis*.[18] They are variable between manufacturers and with differing organisms, but many fall substantially short of 100%.[5,18]

Antigen detection methods should never be substituted for culture and Gram stain. Culture and Gram stain must always have priority when limited quantities of CSF are available,[17] since the sensitivity of antigen detection testing is usually less than that of culture.[19]

The rapid diagnosis of group A and group B *Streptococcus* infection is discussed specifically in Group A *Streptococcus* Screen and Group B *Streptococcus* Screen test listings.

Footnotes

1. Leinonen M, "*Neisseria meningitidis*," *Antigen Detection to Diagnose Bacterial Infections*, Chapter 12, Kohler RB, ed, Boca Raton, FL: CRC Press Inc, 1986, 19-26.
2. Harding SA and Brown DC, "*Streptococcus pneumoniae*," *Antigen Detection to Diagnose Bacterial Infections*, Chapter 13, Kohler RB, ed, Boca Raton, FL: CRC Press Inc, 1986, 27-38.
3. Tilton RC, Dias F, and Ryan RW, "Comparative Evaluation of Three Commercial Products and Counterimmunoelectrophoresis for the Detection of Antigens in Cerebrospinal Fluid," *J Clin Microbiol*, 1984, 231-4.
4. Polito JM II and Stollerman GH, "Aseptic Meningitis: A Case for Clinical Experience," *Hosp Pract Off Ed*, 1992, 27(5A):27-39.
5. Fishman RA, *Cerebrospinal Fluid in Diseases of the Nervous System*, 2nd ed, Philadelphia, PA: WB Saunders Co, 1992, 267.
6. Connolly KJ and Hammer SM, "The Acute Aseptic Meningitis Syndrome," *Infect Dis Clin North Am*, 1990, 4(4):599-622.
7. Isenberg HD, "Bacterial Antigen Detection by Latex Agglutination," *Clinical Microbiology Procedures Handbook*, Washington DC: American Society for Microbiology, 1992, 2:9.2.-9.2.4.
8. Smith AL, "Bacterial Meningitis," *Pediatr Rev*, 1993, 14(1):11-8.
9. Rodewald LE, Woodin KA, Szilágyi PG, et al, "Relevance of Common Tests of Cerebrospinal Fluid in Screening for Bacterial Meningitis," *J Pediatr*, 1991, 119(3):363-9.
10. Feigin RD, McCracken GH Jr, and Klein JO, "Diagnosis and Management of Meningitis," *Pediatr Infect Dis J*, 1992, 11(9):785-814.
11. Feuerborn SA, Capps WI, and Jones JC, "Use of Latex Agglutination Testing in Diagnosing Pediatric Meningitis," *J Fam Pract*, 1992, 34(2):176-9..
12. Hammer SM and Connolly KJ, "Viral Aseptic Meningitis in the United States: Clinical Features, Viral Etiologies, and Differential Diagnosis," *Curr Clin Top Infect Dis*, 1992, 12:1-25.
13. Durand ML, Calderwood SB, Weber DJ, et al, "Acute Bacterial Meningitis in Adults – A Review of 493 Episodes," *N Engl J Med*, 1993, 328(1):21-8.
14. Schaad UB, Suter S, Gianella-Borradori A, et al, "A Comparison of Ceftriazone and Cefuroxime for the Treatment of Bacterial Meningitis in Children," *N Engl J Med*, 1990, 322(3):141-7.
15. Kilpi T, Anttila M, Kallio MJT, et al, "Severity of Childhood Bacterial Meningitis and Duration of Illness Before Diagnosis," *Lancet*, 1991, 338(8764):406-9.
16. Phillips SE and Millan JC, "Reassessment of Microbiology Protocol for Cerebrospinal Fluid Specimens," *Lab Med*, 1991, 22:619-22.
17. Granoff DM, Murphy TV, Ingram DL, et al, "Use of Rapidly Generated Results in Patient Management," *Diagn Microbiol Infect Dis*, 1986, 4:157S-66S.
18. Gray LD and Fedorko DP, "Laboratory Diagnosis of Bacterial Meningitis," *Clin Microbiol Rev*, 1992, 5(2):130-45.
19. Greenlee JE, "Approach to Diagnosis of Meningitis – Cerebrospinal Fluid Evaluation," *Infect Dis Clin North Am*, 1990, 4(4):583-98.

References

Kohler RB, "*Escherichia coli* Somatic Antigens," *Antigen Detection to Diagnose Bacterial Infections*, Chapter 19, Boca Raton, FL: CRC Press Inc, 1986, 97-102.

McIllmurray MB and Moody MD, "Latex Agglutination," *Antigen Detection to Diagnose Bacterial Infections*, Vol II, Applications, Kohler RB, ed, Boca Raton, FL: CRC Press Inc, 1986, 97-102.

Spanos A, Harrell FE Jr, and Durack DT, "Differential Diagnosis of Acute Meningitis. An Analysis of the Predictive Value of Initial Observations," *JAMA*, 1989, 262(19):2700-7.

Bacterial Antigens, Serum *see* Bacterial Antigens, Rapid Detection Methods *on page 775*

Bacterial Antigens, Urine *see* Bacterial Antigens, Rapid Detection Methods *on page 775*

Bacterial Inhibitory Level, Serum *see* Serum Bactericidal Test *on page 843*

Bacterial Smear *see* Gram Stain *on page 815*

BAL *see* Bronchoalveolar Lavage *on page 793*

Bartlett Catheter *see* Bronchial Aspirate Anaerobic Culture *on page 792*

Bed Bugs Identification *see* Arthropod Identification *on page 774*

Beta-Hemolytic Strep Culture, Throat *see* Throat Culture *on page 876*

Beta-Lactamase Production Test *see* Penicillinase Test *on page 840*

Beta-Lactam Ring *see* Penicillinase Test *on page 840*

Beta-Lactam Ring *see* Susceptibility Testing, Aerobic and Facultatively Anaerobic Organisms *on page 864*

Biopsy *Legionella* Culture *see* *Legionella* Culture *on page 825*

Biopsy or Body Fluid Aerobic Bacterial Culture

CPT 87070

Related Information

Abscess, Aerobic and Anaerobic Bacterial Culture *on page 768*
Actinomyces Culture, All Sites *on page 772*
Biopsy or Body Fluid Anaerobic Bacterial Culture *on this page*
Biopsy or Body Fluid Fungus Culture *on page 780*
Biopsy or Body Fluid Mycobacteria Culture *on page 782*
Body Fluid *on page 145*
Body Fluid pH *on page 150*
Body Fluids Analysis, Cell Count *on page 523*
Body Fluids Cytology *on page 482*
Bone Marrow *on page 524*
Cell Wall Defective Bacteria Culture *on page 796*
Fine Needle Aspiration, Deep Seated Lesions *on page 498*
Fine Needle Aspiration, Superficial Palpable Masses *on page 499*
Gram Stain *on page 815*
Histopathology *on page 57*
Synovial Fluid Analysis *on page 1158*
Wound Culture *on page 885*

Synonyms Body Fluid Culture

Applies to Body Fluid Aerobic Culture; Bone Marrow Culture; Synovial Fluid Culture; Tissue Culture

Test Commonly Includes Aerobic culture of biopsy or body fluid specimens

Patient Care PREPARATION: Aseptic preparation of biopsy site

Specimen Surgical tissue, bone marrow, biopsy material from normally sterile site, or aseptically aspirated body fluid CONTAINER: Sterile container with lid, Petri dish, no preservative. Bone marrow aspirates and body fluids may be directly inoculated into blood culture media. COLLECTION: The portion of the biopsy specimen submitted for culture should be separated from the portion submitted for histopathology by the surgeon or pathologist, utilizing sterile technique. STORAGE INSTRUCTIONS: The specimen should be transported immediately to the laboratory. CAUSES FOR REJECTION: Specimens in fixative. Specimens collected on swabs or having excessive travel time to the laboratory may have less than optimal yield. Rejection of such specimens may be impractical if additional clinical material is not readily obtainable, but a comment may be added to the final report indicating the problem. TURNAROUND TIME: Preliminary reports are usually available at 24 hours. Cultures with no growth are usually reported after 2-5 days depending on the laboratory and the specimen type. Final reports on positive specimens usually require a minimum of 48 hours. SPECIAL INSTRUCTIONS: The laboratory should be informed of the specific source of the specimen, current antibiotic therapy, and clinical diagnosis.

Interpretive REFERENCE RANGE: No growth USE: Isolate and identify aerobic organisms causing infections in tissue LIMITATIONS: Any specimen submitted for microbial culture can be contaminated with colonizing organisms that are not contributing to disease. Organisms most likely to contaminate specimens of this type include, but are not limited to, *Corynebacterium* sp and coagulase-negative staphylococci. These organisms are not invariably contaminants, however, and may be pathogenic in certain settings. A Gram stain should always be performed, if sufficient material is obtained, to provide early presumptive information, and to help interpret culture results. If anaerobes are suspected submit a properly collected specimen. METHODOLOGY: Aerobic culture ADDITIONAL INFORMATION: The specimen should be obtained before empiric antimicrobial therapy is started.

References

Simor AE, Roberts FJ, and Smith JA, "Infections of the Skin and Subcutaneous Tissues," *Cumitech 23*, Smith JA, ed, Washington, DC: American Society for Microbiology, 1988, (review).

Biopsy or Body Fluid Anaerobic Bacterial Culture

CPT 87075 (isolation); 87076 (definitive identification)

Related Information

Abscess, Aerobic and Anaerobic Bacterial Culture *on page 768*
Actinomyces Culture, All Sites *on page 772*
Biopsy or Body Fluid Aerobic Bacterial Culture *on this page*
Body Fluid *on page 145*

Synonyms Anaerobic Culture, Biopsy; Anaerobic Culture, Body Fluid

Applies to Body Fluid Anaerobic Culture; Synovial Fluid Anaerobic Culture; Tissue Anaerobic Culture

Test Commonly Includes Isolation and identification of anaerobic organisms. Susceptibility testing may be performed if appropriate.

Patient Care PREPARATION: Aseptic preparation of the biopsy site or site of body fluid aspiration

Specimen Biopsy from normally sterile site or aseptically aspirated body fluid. A specimen for anaerobic culture should always be accompanied by a specimen for aerobic bacterial culture; a single specimen will usually suffice for both aerobic and anaerobic cultures. CONTAINER: Anaerobic transport container, sterile container, no preservative COLLECTION: The specimen must be transported to the laboratory within 30 minutes of collection. Specimens should be collected from a prepared site using sterile technique. Contamination with normal flora from skin, rectum, vagina, or other body surfaces must be avoided. STORAGE INSTRUCTIONS: Do not refrigerate. CAUSES FOR REJECTION: Specimen in fixative. Specimens collected on swabs, exposed to air, or having excessive travel time to the laboratory may have less than optimal yield; rejection of such specimens may be impractical if additional clinical material is not readily obtainable, but a comment may be added to the final report indicating the problem. Specimens from sites which have anaerobic bacteria as normal flora (eg, throat, rectal swabs, bronchial washes, cervical-vaginal mucosal swabs, sputums) are not acceptable for anaerobic culture. TURNAROUND TIME: Cultures showing no bacterial growth can generally be reported after 2 or 3 days. Complete reports of cultures with anaerobic bacteria may take as long as 2 weeks after receipt of culture depending upon the nature of the organisms isolated. SPECIAL INSTRUCTIONS: The laboratory should be informed of the specific source of the specimen, current antibiotic therapy, and clinical diagnosis.

Interpretive REFERENCE RANGE: No growth USE: Anaerobic cultures are indicated particularly when suspected infections are related to gastrointestinal tract, pelvic organs, associated with malignancy, related to use of aminoglycosides; or occur in a setting in which the diagnosis of gas gangrene or actinomycosis is considered. Anaerobic culture is especially indicated when an exudate has a foul odor or if the exudate has a grayish discoloration and is hemorrhagic. Frequently, more than one organism is recovered from an anaerobic infection. LIMITATIONS: Biopsy specimens from chronic infections may be contaminated with anaerobic organisms that may contribute little to the pathologic process. These contaminating organisms may include typical pathogens such as *Bacteroides* and *Peptostreptococcus* sp. In order to enhance the value of cultures of this type, it is necessary to carefully debride the specimen prior to specimen collection and collect viable infected tissue. A Gram stain should always be performed, if sufficient material is obtained, to provide early presumptive information, and to help interpret culture results. Specimens received in anaerobic transport medium are less than optimal for fungal cultures and recovery of certain obligately aerobic bacteria. CONTRAINDICATIONS: Specimens obtained by bronchoscopy are not ideal as the instrument itself becomes contaminated with normal oropharyngeal flora during insertion. METHODOLOGY: Anaerobic culture, usually with broth and solid media ADDITIONAL INFORMATION: See also Abscess Aerobic and Anaerobic Bacterial Culture listing for a table reviewing symptoms suggestive of anaerobic infections. Biopsy culture is particularly useful in establishing the diagnosis of anaerobic osteomyelitis,[1] clostridial myonecrosis, intracranial actinomycosis, and pleuropulmonary infections. Anaerobic infections of soft tissue include anaerobic cellulitis, necrotizing fasciitis, clos-

(Continued)

Biopsy or Body Fluid Anaerobic Bacterial Culture *(Continued)*

tridial myonecrosis (gas gangrene), anaerobic streptococcal myositis or myonecrosis, synergistic nonclostridial anaerobic myonecrosis, and infected vascular gangrene. These infections, particularly clostridial myonecrosis, necrotizing fasciitis, and nonclostridial anaerobic myonecrosis, may be fulminant and are frequently characterized by the presence of gas and foul-smelling necrotic tissue.[2] Empiric therapy based on likely pathogens should be instituted as soon as appropriate cultures are collected. See table.

Principle Types of Anaerobic Infections

Location	Type of Infection
Head and neck	Brain abscess Gingivitis Chronic sinusitis Chronic otitis Odontogenic and oropharyngeal space infections
Respiratory tract	Aspiration pneumonia Necrotizing pneumonia Lung abscess Empyema (adults)
Gastrointestinal tract	Peritonitis Intra–abdominal abscess Liver abscess
Female genital tract	Tubo–ovarian abscess Salpingitis (30% to 50% of cases) Septic abortion and endometritis Bartholin's gland abscess Bacterial vaginosis
Skin and soft tissue	Crepitant cellulitis Necrotizing fascitis Myonecrosis (gas gangrene) Decubitus ulcer Diabetic foot ulcer Bite wounds

From Styrt B and Gorhach SL, "Recent Developments in the Understanding of the Pathogenesis and Treatment of Anaerobic Infections," *N Engl J Med,* 1989, 321:240–6, with permission.

Footnotes

1. Hall BB, Fitzgerald RH Jr, and Rosenblatt JE, "Anaerobic Osteomyelitis," *J Bone Joint Surg*, 1983, 65:30-5.
2. Finegold SM, George LW, and Mulligan ME, "Anaerobic Infections Part II," *Dis Mon*, Vol XXXI, No 11, Chicago, IL: Year Book Medical Publishers Inc, 1985.

References

Gorbach SL, "Treatment of Intra-abdominal Infection," *Am J Med*, 1984, 76:107-10.

Willis AR, "Anaerobic Bacterial Diseases Now and Then. Where Do We Go From Here?" *Rev Infect Dis*, 1984, 1(Suppl):293-9.

Biopsy or Body Fluid Fungus Culture

CPT *87102 (isolation); 87106 (definitive identification)*

Related Information

Aspergillus Serology *on page 641*
Biopsy or Body Fluid Aerobic Bacterial Culture *on page 778*
Blastomycosis Serology *on page 645*
Blood Fungus Culture *on page 789*
Body Fluid *on page 145*
Body Fluid pH *on page 150*
Body Fluids Analysis, Cell Count *on page 523*
Body Fluids Cytology *on page 482*
Bone Marrow *on page 524*
Candida Antigen *on page 652*
Candidiasis Serologic Test *on page 652*
Cerebrospinal Fluid Fungus Culture *on page 800*
Cryptococcus Antibody Titer *on page 670*

Fine Needle Aspiration, Deep Seated Lesions *on page 498*
Fine Needle Aspiration, Superficial Palpable Masses *on page 499*
Fungus Smear, Stain *on page 813*
Histopathology *on page 57*
Skin Fungus Culture *on page 845*
Sporotrichosis Serology *on page 748*
Sputum Fungus Culture *on page 853*
Susceptibility Testing, Fungi *on page 869*
Synovial Fluid Analysis *on page 1158*

Synonyms Body Fluid Fungus Culture; Fungus Culture, Biopsy; Fungus Culture, Body Fluid

Applies to Fungus Culture, Bone Marrow; Synovial Fluid Fungus Culture; Tissue Fungus Culture

Test Commonly Includes Culture and identification of fungal species in body fluid specimens or tissue

Patient Care PREPARATION: Aseptic preparation of biopsy site or site of body fluid aspiration

Specimen Surgical tissue, bone marrow, biopsy material CONTAINER: Sterile container with lid or Petri dish COLLECTION: The portion of the biopsy specimen submitted for culture should be separated from the portion submitted for histopathology by the surgeon or pathologist utilizing sterile technique. The laboratory should be informed of the fungal species suspected. Collect the specimen early in the day if possible so as it may be processed promptly, assuring optimal yield. STORAGE INSTRUCTIONS: Specimens should not be stored or refrigerated. The specimen should be transported to the laboratory as soon as possible after collection. CAUSES FOR REJECTION: Specimen in fixative TURNAROUND TIME: Negatives are usually reported after 4 weeks. SPECIAL INSTRUCTIONS: The laboratory should be informed of the specific source of specimen.

Interpretive REFERENCE RANGE: No growth USE: Establish the diagnosis of localized or disseminated mycosis in patients at risk for fungal infections; isolate and identify fungi to provide guidance for the treatment of fungal infections METHODOLOGY: Culture under aerobic conditions on several media, usually including Sabouraud's and brain heart infusion (BHI), biphasic media with or without lysis concentration technique, frequently incubation at room temperature or at both 30°C and 37°C ADDITIONAL INFORMATION: Optimal isolation of fungi from tissue is accomplished by processing as much tissue as possible. Swabs should be submitted only when adequate tissue is not available. Specimen selection tables are provided in the listings for Sputum Fungus Culture and Skin Fungus Culture. Depending upon the geographic area *Histoplasma capsulatum*, *Blastomyces dermatitidis*, and *Coccidioides immitis*, among the deep pathogenic fungi, are most frequently isolated. *Candida* sp are common opportunistic pathogens in all geographic locations. Immunocompromised patients, transplant patients, and patients with acquired immunodeficiency syndrome (AIDS) are susceptible to opportunistic mycoses.[1] The recovery of a recognized fungal pathogen from a wound culture or draining sinus is significant. Isolates such as *Candida* sp, *Aspergillus* sp, or zygomycetes are often environmental in origin and must be interpreted in the clinical context.

Fungal peritonitis is clinically similar to bacterial peritonitis with pain, fever, and abdominal tenderness. Fungal infections due to *Candida* sp (mostly *Candida albicans* and *Candida parapsilosis*), and rare cases of *Aspergillus fumigatus* and the higher bacterium *Nocardia asteroides*, have been reported in patients undergoing chronic dialysis.[2] In a series of AIDS patients, bone marrow biopsy detected opportunistic fungal or mycobacterial infections in 20%. Eighty percent of the positive biopsies were associated with bone marrow granulomas. Fever, anemia, and neutropenia were often correlated with a positive biopsy.[3] Neutrophil count $<1000/\mu L$ is associated with infection by *Candida*, *Aspergillus*, *Mucor*, *Rhizopus*, *Trichosporon*, and *Fusarium* sp. T-cell defects and/or impaired cell-mediated immunity are associated with infection by *Candida*, *Cryptococcus neoformans*, *Histoplasma capsulatum*, *Coccidioides immitis*, and *Aspergillus* sp. Catheterization (arterial, venous, or urinary) and mechanical disruption of the skin are associated with *Candida* and *Rhodotorula* sp infections. Disruption of the natural barrier of the GI tract and respiratory tree by cytotoxic chemotherapy predispose to *Candida* sp infections.[4]

Footnotes

1. Bodey GP, "Overview of the Problems of Infections in the Immunocompromised Host," *Am J Med*, 1985, 79(Suppl):56-61.
2. Arfania D, Everett DE, Nolph DK, et al, "Uncommon Causes of Peritonitis in Patients Undergoing Peritoneal Dialysis," *Arch Intern Med*, 1981, 141:61-4.
3. Nichols L, Florentine B, Lewis W, et al, "Bone Marrow Examination for the Diagnosis of Mycobacterial and Fungal Infections in the Acquired Immunodeficiency Syndrome," *Arch Pathol Lab Med*, 1991, 115(11):1125-32.

(Continued)

Biopsy or Body Fluid Fungus Culture *(Continued)*

4. Brown AE, "Overview of Fungal Infections in Cancer Patients," *Semin Oncol*, 1990, 17(3 Suppl 6):2-5.

References

Gray LD and Roberts GD, "Laboratory Diagnosis of Systemic Fungal Diseases," *Infect Dis Clin North Am*, 1988, 2:779-803.

Lyons RW, "Fungal Infections of the CNS," *Neurol Clin*, 1986, 4:159-70.

Musial CE, Cockerill FR, and Roberts GD, "Fungal Infections of the Immunocompromised Host: Clinical and Laboratory Aspects," *Clin Microbiol Rev*, Oct 1988, 349-64.

Biopsy or Body Fluid Mycobacteria Culture

***CPT** 87116 (isolation); 87118 (definitive identification)*

Related Information

Acid-Fast Stain *on page 770*
Biopsy or Body Fluid Aerobic Bacterial Culture *on page 778*
Body Fluid *on page 145*
Body Fluid pH *on page 150*
Body Fluids Analysis, Cell Count *on page 523*
Body Fluids Cytology *on page 482*
Bone Marrow *on page 524*
Fine Needle Aspiration, Deep Seated Lesions *on page 498*
Fine Needle Aspiration, Superficial Palpable Masses *on page 499*
Histopathology *on page 57*
Mycobacteria by DNA Probe *on page 921*
Skin Mycobacteria Culture *on page 846*
Sputum Mycobacteria Culture *on page 855*
Susceptibility Testing, Mycobacteria *on page 872*
Synovial Fluid Analysis *on page 1158*

Synonyms AFB Culture, Biopsy; Mycobacteria Culture, Biopsy; TB Culture, Biopsy

Applies to Body Fluid Mycobacteria Culture; Mycobacteria Culture, Tissue; Tissue Mycobacteria Culture

Patient Care PREPARATION: Aseptic preparation of biopsy site

Specimen Surgical tissue, bone marrow, biopsy material CONTAINER: Sterile Petri dish with 0.5 mL sterile saline or sterile water, sterile test tube, sterile container COLLECTION: The portion of the surgical specimen submitted for culture should be separated from the portion submitted for histopathology by the surgeon or pathologist, utilizing sterile technique CAUSES FOR REJECTION: Specimen in fixative TURNAROUND TIME: Negative cultures may be reported after 6-8 weeks. SPECIAL INSTRUCTIONS: The laboratory should be informed of the specific source of specimen, current antibiotic therapy, and clinical diagnosis.

Interpretive REFERENCE RANGE: No growth USE: Isolate and identify mycobacteria; establish the etiology of granulomatous disease, fever of unknown origin (FUO) particularly in immunocompromised patients and others with subtle defects of cellular immunity LIMITATIONS: Transbronchial biopsy cultures may be of assistance in diagnosing tuberculosis in sputum smear negative cases; however, sputum and bronchial washing cultures have a yield.[1,2] In one study, only 2 out of 12 (16%) transbronchial biopsies were positive and in those cases the biopsy was not the only source of culture positive material.[1] *Mycobacterium marinum* may cause a localized cutaneous lesion that may be nodular, verrucous, ulcerative, or sporotrichoid, and which may rarely involve deeper structures. If it is suspected, the laboratory must be notified so that the culture may be incubated at an appropriate temperature (30°C).[3] *Mycobacterium marinum* infection occurs in patients who have been exposed to the organism following cutaneous abrasion or penetrating injury while cleaning aquariums, clearing barnacles, and with other aquatic exposures. METHODOLOGY: Culture on specialized selective media, usually including Löwenstein-Jensen (LJ) and Middlebrook 7H11, incubated at 35°C with 5% to 10% CO_2. Cutaneous and subcutaneous tissues should also be incubated at room temperature to enhance recovery of *M. marinum* and *M. ulcerans*. If *M. haemophilum* is suspected, blood containing medium should be inoculated and incubated at room temperature in 10% CO_2.[4] Mycobacteria are usually definitively identified and may be tested for antimicrobial susceptibility. Radiometric (Bactec®) and DNA probe methods are utilized by some laboratories to provide rapid detection and identification of mycobacteria.

With the emergence of multidrug-resistant *Mycobacterium tuberculosis* strains, most isolates are being submitted for susceptibility testing. A specific request is usually required (see Susceptibility Testing, Mycobacteria). Susceptibility testing of mycobacteria is frequently referred to specialized laboratories.

ADDITIONAL INFORMATION: Occult infections with atypical mycobacteria, particularly *Mycobacterium avium* and *Mycobacterium intracellulare*, occur in patients with acquired immune deficiency syndrome (AIDS).[5] In some institutions, the incidence of isolation of non-*Mycobacterium tuberculosis* species, specifically *M. avium-intracellulare* (*M. avium* complex), may exceed the rate of isolation of *M. tuberculosis*. Mycobacteria have been recovered from culture of Kaposi's sarcoma and bone marrow specimens, in which the characteristic granulomatous reaction has been absent.[6,7] Optimal isolation of mycobacteria from tissue is accomplished by processing as much tissue as possible for culture. Swabs should be submitted only when adequate tissue is not available.

Tuberculous spondylitis represents 50% to 60% of all cases of skeletal tuberculosis. It is seen in children in developing countries and adults older than 50 years of age in the United States and Europe. Frequently, several vertebrae are involved and adjacent psoas muscle abscesses or paravertebral abscesses are not uncommon ("cold abscesses"). Colony counts obtained from bone biopsies are low; however, >90% are culture positive. The diagnosis of vertebral tuberculosis should be considered in all cases of unexplained spondylitis.

Predisposing Clinical Conditions and Site of Involvement of Non-*M. tuberculosis* Mycobacterial Infections

Site	Predisposing Clinical Conditions	Species
Disseminated	Immunodeficiency/malignancy	*M. avium–intracellulare* *M. kansasii*
Gastrointestinal tract/ disseminated	Acquired immunodeficiency syndrome	*M. avium–intracellulare*
Lung	Chronic pulmonary disease	*M. avium–intracellulare* *M. kansasii*
Lymph nodes	Pediatric age group	*M. avium–intracellulare* *M. scrofulaceum*
Peritonitis	Chronic ambulatory peritoneal dialysis	*M. fortuitum* *M. chelonae*
Skeleton	Immunodeficiency/malignancy	*M. avium–intracellulare* *M. kansasii*
Skin and soft tissue	Percutaneous trauma/abrasion	*M. fortuitum* *M. chelonae*
	Immunodeficiency/malignancy	*M. haemophilum*

Cases of sternal wound infection, early prosthetic valve endocarditis, infections complicating mammary augmentation surgery, and other cutaneous/subcutaneous infections have been attributed to rapidly growing mycobacteria.[8,9] *M. fortuitum* is the most commonly implicated *Mycobacterium* in these infections, which are thought to be caused by local environmental strains rather than contaminated commercial surgical materials or devices. Rapidly growing mycobacteria often grow on routine bacterial culture media within the time allotted to incubating routine bacterial cultures. Such organisms may be misidentified as "diphtheroids" and disregarded as contaminants.

Pleural effusions frequently yield positive cultures in cases of pulmonary tuberculosis. The diagnosis of peritoneal tuberculosis is difficult and is usually made at laparotomy or after a considerable delay. Tuberculosis should be considered in any patient with ascitic fluid and chronic abdominal pain.[10] Peritoneal tuberculosis accounted for 11% of a series of cases of extrapulmonary tuberculosis reported by Alvarez and McCabe.[11] Pericardial tuberculosis accounts for <5% of extrapulmonary tuberculosis and frequently requires biopsy for diagnosis. See table.

Footnotes

1. Stenson W, Aranda C, and Bevelagua FA, "Transbronchial Biopsy Culture in Pulmonary Tuberculosis," *Chest*, 1983, 83:883-4.
2. Jett JR, Cortese DA, and Dines DE, "The Value of Bronchoscopy in the Diagnosis of Mycobacterial Disease," *Chest*, 1981, 80:575-8.
3. Brown JW III and Sanders CV, "*Mycobacterium marinum* Infections: A Problem of Recognition, Not Therapy?" *Arch Intern Med*, 1987, 147:817-8, (editorial).
4. Woods GL and Washington JA 2d, "Mycobacteria Other Than *Mycobacterium tuberculosis*: Review of Microbiologic and Clinical Aspects," *Rev Infect Dis*, 1987, 9:275-94.

(Continued)

Biopsy or Body Fluid Mycobacteria Culture *(Continued)*

5. Hawkins CC, Gold JW, Whimbey E, et al, "*Mycobacterium avium* Complex Infections in Patients With the Acquired Immunodeficiency Syndrome," *Ann Intern Med*, 1986, 105:184-8.
6. Cohen RJ, Samoszuk MK, Busch D, et al, "Occult Infections With *M. intracellulare* in Bone Marrow Biopsy Specimens From Patients With AIDS," *N Engl J Med*, 1983, 308:1475-6, (letter).
7. Croxson TS, Ebanks D, and Milduan D, "Atypical Mycobacteria and Kaposi's Sarcoma in the Same Biopsy Specimens," *N Engl J Med*, 1983, 308:1476, (letter).
8. Wallace RJ, Musser JM, Hull SI, et al, "Diversity and Sources of Rapidly Growing Mycobacteria Associated With Infections Following Cardiac Surgery," *J Infect Dis*, 1989, 159(4):708-16.
9. Wallace RJ, Steele LC, Labidi A, et al, "Heterogeneity Among Isolates of Rapidly Growing Mycobacteria Responsible for Infections Following Augmentation Mammoplasty Despite Case Clustering in Texas and Other Southern Coastal States," *J Infect Dis*, 1989, 160(2):281-8.
10. Martin RE and Bradsher RW, "Elusive Diagnosis of Tuberculosis Peritonitis," *South Med J*, 1986, 79:1076-9.
11. Alvarez S and McCabe WR, "Extrapulmonary Tuberculosis Revisited: A Review of Experience at Boston City and Other Hospitals," *Medicine (Baltimore)*, 1984, 63:25-55.

References

Wayne LG and Sramek HA, "Agents of Newly Recognized or Infrequently Encountered Mycobacterial Diseases," *Clin Microbiol Rev*, 1992, 5(1):1-25.

Wolinsky E, "Mycobacterial Diseases Other Than Tuberculosis," *Clin Infect Dis*, 1992, 15(1):1-10.

Biopsy Specimen Culture, Quantitative *see* Burn Culture, Quantitative *on page 794*

Blastocystis hominis *see* Ova and Parasites, Stool *on page 836*

Blood Culture, Aerobic and Anaerobic

CPT *87040*

Related Information

Bacteremia Detection, Buffy Coat Micromethod *on page 520*
Blood Culture, *Brucella on page 788*
Blood Fungus Culture *on page 789*
Buffy Coat Smear Study of Peripheral Blood *on page 526*
Cell Wall Defective Bacteria Culture *on page 796*
Cerebrospinal Fluid Culture *on page 798*
Entamoeba histolytica Serological Test *on page 675*
Leptospira Culture, Urine *on page 827*
Salmonella Titer *on page 744*
Sputum Culture *on page 849*
Stool Culture *on page 858*
Teichoic Acid Antibody *on page 754*
Viral Culture *on page 1195*
Viral Culture, Blood *on page 1197*
Yersinia enterocolitica Antibody *on page 765*
Yersinia pestis Antibody *on page 766*

Synonyms Aerobic Culture, Blood; Anaerobic Culture, Blood; Culture, Blood

Applies to Antimicrobial Removal Device (ARD) Blood Culture; ARD, Blood Culture; Bactec®; Blood Culture, Isolator™; Blood Culture, Lysis Centrifugation; Blood Culture, *Mycobacterium avium-intracellulare*; Blood Culture With Antimicrobial Removal Device (ARD); Blood Mycobacteria Culture; Isolator™ Blood Culture; Mycobacteria Culture, Blood

Test Commonly Includes Isolation of both aerobic and anaerobic microorganisms and susceptibility testing on all significant isolates

Patient Care **PREPARATION:** The major difficulty in interpretation of blood cultures is potential contamination by skin flora. This difficulty can be markedly reduced by careful attention to the details of skin preparation and antisepsis prior to collection of the specimen. After location of the vein by palpation, the venipuncture site should be cleansed with 70% alcohol (isopropyl or ethyl) and then swabbed in a circular motion concentrically from the center outward using tincture of iodine or a povidone iodine solution. The iodine should be allowed to dry before the venipuncture is undertaken. If palpation is required during the venipuncture, the glove covering the palpating finger tip should be disinfected. In iodine sensitive patients, a double alcohol, green soap, or acetone alcohol preparation may be substituted. **AFTERCARE:** Iodine used in the skin preparation should be carefully removed from the skin after venipuncture.

Specimen Venous blood. The yield of positives is not increased by culturing arterial blood even in endocarditis. It is optimal to collect blood specimens from at least two separate venipuncture sites. **CONTAINER:** Bottles of trypticase soy broth or other standard medium, one vented (for aerobes), one unvented (for anaerobes). Recovery may be enhanced by lysis filtration or concentration.[1] **COLLECTION:** Blood cultures should be drawn prior to initiation of antimicrobial therapy. If more than one culture is ordered, the specimens should be drawn from separately prepared sites. A syringe and needle, transfer set, or pre-evacuated set of tubes containing culture media may be used to collect blood. Collection tubes should be held below the level of the venipuncture to avoid reflux. A sample volume of 10-20 mL in adults or 1-5 mL in pediatric patients is usually collected for each set. The likelihood of recovering a pathogen increases as the volume of blood sampled increases. If a syringe and needle or transfer set is used, the top of the blood culture bottles should also be aseptically prepared. See following table.

Blood Culture Collection

Clinical Disease Suspected	Culture Recommendation	Rational
Sepsis, meningitis osteomyelitis, septic arthritis, bacterial pneumonia	Two sets of cultures - one from each of two prepared sites, the second drawn after a brief time interval, then begin therapy.	Assure sufficient sampling in cases of intermittent or low level bacteremia. Minimize the confusion caused by a positive culture resulting from transient bacteremia or skin contamination.
Fever of unknown origin (eg, occult abscess, empyema, typhoid fever, etc)	Two sets of cultures - one from each of two prepared sites, the second drawn after a brief time interval (30 minutes). If cultures are negative after 24–48 hours obtain two more sets, preferably prior to an anticipated temperature rise.	The yield after four sets of cultures is minimal. A maximum of three sets per patient per day for 3 consecutive days is recommended.
Endocarditis:		
Acute	Obtain three blood culture sets within 2 hours, then begin therapy.	95% to 99% of acute endocarditis patients (untreated) will yield a positive in one of the first three cultures.
Subacute	Obtain three blood culture sets on day 1, repeat if negative after 24 hours. If still negative or if the patient had prior antibiotic therapy repeat again.	Adequate sample volume despite low level bacteremia or previous therapy should result in a positive yield.
Immunocompromised host (eg, AIDS):		
Septicemia, fungemia mycobacteremia	Obtain two sets of cultures from each of two prepared sites; consider lysis concentration technique to enhance recovery for fungi and mycobacteria.	Low levels of fungemia and mycobacteremia frequently encountered.
Previous antimicrobial therapy:		
Septicemia, bacteremia; monitor effect of antimicrobial therapy	Obtain two sets of cultures from each of two prepared sites; consider use of antimicrobial removal device (ARD) or increased volume >10 mL/set.	Recovery of organisms is enhanced by dilution, increased sample volume and removal of inhibiting antimicrobials.

Transient bacteremia caused by brushing teeth, bowel movements, etc or by local irritations caused by scratching of the skin may cause positive blood cultures as can contamination by skin flora at the time of collection. Interpretation of results can be enhanced by collecting blood cultures from more than one site and after a time interval (15-30 minutes). Cultures should be taken as early as possible in the course of a febrile episode.

STORAGE INSTRUCTIONS: Specimens collected in tubes with SPS (sodium polyanetholesulfonate) should be processed without delay. The specimen should be transferred to appropriate

(Continued)

Blood Culture, Aerobic and Anaerobic *(Continued)*

culture media to avoid any possible decrease in yield due to storage or prolonged contact with SPS. **CAUSES FOR REJECTION:** Unlabeled bottles are not acceptable. **TURNAROUND TIME:** Common laboratory procedure is to issue a final culture report after 5-10 days. A preliminary culture report based upon Gram stain and primary subculture is usually available at 48 hours. **SPECIAL INSTRUCTIONS:** The requisition should indicate current antibiotic therapy and clinical diagnosis.

Interpretive **REFERENCE RANGE:** Negative **USE:** Isolate and identify potentially pathogenic organisms causing bacteremia, septicemia, enteric fever, meningitis, pneumonia, and other disease states caused by microorganisms **LIMITATIONS:** Three sets of blood cultures in the absence of antimicrobial therapy provide optimal yield for detection of bacteremia; one set is seldom ever sufficient.[2] Prior antibiotic therapy may cause negative blood cultures or delayed growth. Blood cultures from patients suspected of having *Brucella* or *Leptospira* must be requested as special cultures. Consultation with the laboratory for special culture procedures for the recovery of these organisms prior to collection of the specimen is recommended. Yeast often are isolated from routine blood cultures. However, if yeast or other fungi are specifically suspected, a separate fungal blood culture should be drawn along with each of the routine blood culture specimens. See separate listing for proper collection of Blood Fungus Culture. *Mycobacterium avium-intracellulare* (MAI) is frequently recovered from blood of immunocompromised patients, particularly those with acquired immunodeficiency syndrome (AIDS). Special procedures are required for the recovery of these organisms (ie, lysis filtration concentration or use of a special mycobacteria blood culture medium). Radiometric methods facilitate the recovery of mycobacteria from blood.

A substantial fraction of blood culture isolates are not clinically significant. Many of the false-positives involve coagulase-negative staphylococci, however, such organisms can cause serious infections.

Blood culture contamination (ie, false-positives) cause substantial negative financial impact when laboratory costs, hospital stay, and other costs are considered.

CONTRAINDICATIONS: Use of a 2% iodine preparation is contraindicated in patients sensitive to iodine. Green soap may be substituted for the iodine or alcohol acetone alone may be used. **METHODOLOGY:** Early subculture of aerobic bottle; visual, radiometric, or infrared monitoring. Aerobic and anaerobic culture in broth media usually with subculture to blood agar and chocolate agar. The antimicrobial removal device procedure (ARD) includes use of an adsorbent resin in the aerobic bottle. Other vendors also provide resin-containing bottles for use in radiometric or infrared automated detection systems. In the lysis centrifugation procedure, blood is lysed and centrifuged using a Wampole Isolator™ tube or similar method. The sediment is inoculated to media appropriate for growing aerobic and anaerobic bacteria, fungi, and mycobacteria. A new method of continuously monitoring media for increased CO_2 content is available. **ADDITIONAL INFORMATION:** Sequential blood cultures in nonendocarditis patients using a 20 mL sample resulted in an 80% positive yield after the first set, a 90% yield after the second set, and a 99% yield after the third set. Volume of blood cultured seems to be more important than the specific culture technique being employed by the laboratory. The isolation of *Staphylococcus epidermidis* (coagulase-negative *Staphylococcus*) poses a critical and difficult clinical dilemma. Although *S. epidermidis* is the most commonly isolated organism from blood cultures, only a few (6.3%) of the isolates represent "true" clinically significant bacteremia.[3] Conversely, *S. epidermidis* is well recognized as a cause of infections involving prosthetic devices, cardiac valves, CSF shunts, dialysis catheters, and indwelling vascular catheters.[4] Ultimately, the physician is responsible for determination of whether an organism is a contaminant or a pathogen. The decision is based on both laboratory and clinical data. Patient data including patient history, physical examination, body temperatures, clinical course, and laboratory data (ie, culture results, white blood cell count, and differential) are relevant. Clinical experience and judgment may play a significant role in resolution of this clinical dilemma.[5] Various sources of contamination include the patient's own skin flora, transient benign bacteremias, and perhaps, disinfection materials.

The use of a lysis centrifugation system has been reported to increase the recovery rate and decrease the time of fungal recovery compared to traditional or biphasic blood culture systems.[6] Recovery of mycobacteria, atypical mycobacteria, and *Legionella* may also be enhanced by lysis filtration. In patients who have received antimicrobial drugs, four to six blood cultures may be necessary. Any organism isolated from the blood is usually tested for susceptibility.

The use of antimicrobial removal devices (ARD) or resin bottles to attempt to increase the yield of blood cultures drawn from patients on antimicrobial therapy is controversial. Some microorganisms are occasionally not recovered with the use of ARD blood cultures. It is, therefore, advised that at least one culture in a series of three be requested without the use of the ARD bottles. ARD blood cultures are substantially more expensive than routine blood cultures. There is no consensus as to the effectiveness of the ARD cultures in enhancing recovery of organisms. A recent study reports no significant increase in recovery of organisms with the device.[7,8] Selective use of the ARD with consideration of the clinical setting has been recommended.[9]

The diagnosis of bacterial meningitis is accomplished by blood culture as well as culture and examination of the cerebrospinal fluid.[10] Most children with bacterial meningitis are initially bacteremic.[11,12]

Interpretation of Positive Blood Cultures

Virtually **any** organism, including normal flora, **can** cause bacteremia.

A negative culture result does not necessarily rule out bacteremia; false-negative results occur when pathogens fail to grow.

A positive culture result does not necessarily indicate bacteremia; false-positive results occur when contaminants grow.

Gram-negative bacilli, anaerobes, and fungi should be considered pathogens until proven otherwise.

The most difficult interpretation problem is to determine whether an organism that is usually considered normal skin flora is a true pathogen.

From Flournoy DJ and Adkins L, "Understanding the Blood Culture Report," *Am J Infect Control,* 1986, 14:41-6, with permission.

Footnotes

1. Chan R, Munro R, and Tomlison P, "Evaluation of Lysis Filtration as an Adjunct to Conventional Blood Culture," *J Clin Pathol*, 1986, 38:89-92.
2. Aronson MD and Bor DH, "Blood Cultures," *Ann Intern Med*, 1987, 106:246-53.
3. Archer GL, "Coagulase-Negative Staphylococci in Blood Cultures: The Clinician's Dilemma," *Infect Control 6*, 1985, 6:477-8, (editorial).
4. Sheagren JN, "Significance of Blood Culture Isolates of *Staphylococcus epidermidis*," *Arch Intern Med*, 1987, 147:635.
5. Flournoy DJ and Adkins L, "Understanding the Blood Culture Report," *Am J Infect Control*, 1986, 14:41-6.
6. Bille J, Stockman L, Roberts GD, et al, "Evaluation of a Lysis Centrifugation System for Recovery of Yeast and Filamentous Fungi From Blood," *J Clin Microbiol*, 1983, 18:469-74.
7. Lundholm M, "Evaluation of an Antimicrobial Removal Device (ARD) for Detection of Septicemia," *Scand J Infect Dis*, 1986, 18:461-3.
8. Wright AJ, Thompson RL, McLimans CA, et al, "The Antimicrobial Removal Device. A Microbiological and Clinical Evaluation," *Am J Clin Pathol*, 1982, 78:173-7.
9. Munro R, Collignon PJ, Sorrell TC, et al, "Is the Antimicrobial Removal Device a Cost-Effective Addition to Conventional Blood Cultures?" *J Clin Pathol*, 1984, 37:348-51.
10. Francke E, "The Many Causes of Meningitis," *Postgrad Med*, 1987, 82:175-88.
11. Klein JO, Feigin RD, and McCracken GH Jr, "Report of the Task Force on Diagnosis and Management of Meningitis," *Pediatrics*, 1986, 78(5):959-82.
12. Feigin RD, McCracken GH Jr, and Klein JO, "Diagnosis and Management of Meningitis," *Pediatr Infect Dis J*, 1992, 11(9):785-814.

References

MacLowry JD, "Clinical Microbiology of Bacteremia an Overview," *Am J Med*, 1983, 75(1B):2-6.

Mermel LA and Maki DG, "Detection of Bacteremia in Adults: Consequences of Culturing an Inadequate Volume of Blood," *Ann Intern Med*, 1993, 119:270-2.

Murray PR, Traynor P, and Hopson D, "Critical Assessment of Blood Culture Techniques: Analysis of Recovery of Obligate and Facultative Anaerobes, Strict Aerobic Bacteria, and Fungi in Aerobic and Anaerobic Blood Culture Bottles," *J Clin Microbiol*, 1992, 30(6):l462-8.

Salfinger M, Stool EW, Piot D, et al, "Comparison of Three Methods for Recovery of *Mycobacterium avium* Complex From Blood Specimens," *J Clin Microbiol*, 1988, 26:1225-6.

Schifman RB and Pindur A, "The Effect of Skin Disinfection Materials on Reducing Blood Culture Contamination," *Am J Clin Pathol*, 1993, 99(5):536-8.

Wilson ML, Weinstein MP, Reimer LG, et al, "Controlled Comparison of the BacT/Alert™ and Bactec® 660/730 Nonradiometric Blood Culture Systems," *J Clin Microbiol*, 1992, 30(2):323-9.

Blood Culture, *Brucella*

***CPT** 87040; 87163 (addition identification methods)*

Related Information

Blood Culture, Aerobic and Anaerobic *on page 784*
Brucellosis Agglutinins *on page 647*

Synonyms *Brucella* Blood Culture; Undulant Fever, Culture

Applies to Bone Marrow Culture for *Brucella*

Specimen Blood **CONTAINER:** Castañeda bottle, *Brucella* broth and agar, conventional trypticase soy broth (TSB) **COLLECTION:** Should be drawn prior to administration of antibiotics, and before an expected temperature rise. Follow preparation and collection procedures in Blood Culture, Aerobic and Anaerobic listing. **CAUSES FOR REJECTION:** Specimens not received in appropriate bottles will have less than optimal yield. **TURNAROUND TIME:** 6 weeks **SPECIAL INSTRUCTIONS:** The laboratory must be informed of the need for blood culture for *Brucella*. Current antibiotic therapy, clinical diagnosis, and history with other relevant information should be forwarded to the laboratory.

Interpretive **REFERENCE RANGE:** No growth **USE:** Establish the diagnosis of brucellosis **LIMITATIONS:** Blood cultures for *Brucella* are primarily useful in the early acute phase of the disease. Recovery of *Brucella* is limited by the relatively low level of bacteremia and the fastidious nature of the organism. Yield may be increased by culturing larger volumes of blood in a conventional trypticase soy broth or use of a lysis centrifugation concentration technique. **METHODOLOGY:** *Brucella* broth and agar, held at least 21 days with or without lysis concentration. Trypticase soy broth (TSB) cultures yield acceptable results (93% of possible isolates). Blood clot cultures utilizing a variety of methods provide no advantage over more conventional TSB cultures for the isolation of *Brucella melitensis*.[1] The use of a lysis concentration procedure was found to be superior to the use of the Castañeda procedure (biphasic medium) for the recovery of *Brucella* from clinical specimens.[2] *Brucella* may be recovered using the BBL Septi-Chek® system with growth observed on the chocolate section of the paddle. The organism appears as a small, slow-growing white colony. It is a gram-negative coccobacillus. The handling of cultures and specimens as well as the inhalation of dust-containing *Brucella* organisms is dangerous to laboratory workers. A biologic safety cabinet should be used for all suspected isolates.[3] **ADDITIONAL INFORMATION:** Bone marrow culture and serologic testing of acute and convalescent specimens for *Brucella* antibodies may be useful when cultures of peripheral blood are negative. In animals, brucellosis has a bacteremic phase followed by localization in the reproductive tract and reticuloendothelial system. The disease is common worldwide, particularly in the USSR, Mediterranean, Latin America, and Spain. One hundred six cases were reported in the U.S. in 1986.[4] Most brucellosis in the U.S. occurs in abattoir workers, farmers, and rarely veterinarians. Symptoms may be subclinical, subacute, acute, relapsing, and chronic. Undulant fever is most typical of *B. melitensis*. Symptoms may include abdominal pain and may mimic appendicitis or cholecystitis. Unpasteurized milk may be a source of infection. Risk factors raising an index of suspicion include travel, food, and occupation. Six species are recognized: *B. abortus*, *B. melitensis*, *B. suis*, *B. canis*, *B. ovis*, and *B. neotomae*. Serologic confirmation of the diagnosis may be helpful.

Footnotes

1. Escamilla J, Florez-Vgarte H, and Kilpatrick ME, "Evaluation of a Blood Clot Culture for the Isolation of *Salmonella typhi*, *Salmonella paratyphi* A, and *Brucella melitensis*," *J Clin Microbiol*, 1986, 24:388-90.
2. Etemadi H, Raissadt A, Pickett MJ, et al, "Isolation of *Brucella* sp From Clinical Specimens," *J Clin Microbiol*, 1984, 20:586.
3. Olle-Goig JE, Canela-Soler J, "An Outbreak of *Brucella melitensis* Infection by Airborne Transmission Among Laboratory Workers," *Am J Public Health*, 1987, 77:335-8.
4. Center for Disease Control 1987 Annual Summary, *MMWR Morb Mortal Wkly Rep*, 35:51-7.

References

Moyer NP, Holcomb LA, and Hausler WJ, "*Brucella*," *Manual of Clinical Microbiology*, 5th ed, Balows A, Hausler WJ, Herrmann KL, et al, eds, Washington, DC: American Society for Microbiology, 1991, 457-62.

Blood Culture, Isolator™ *see* Blood Culture, Aerobic and Anaerobic *on page 784*

Blood Culture, *Leptospira* *see Leptospira* Culture, Urine *on page 827*

Blood Culture, Lysis Centrifugation *see* Blood Culture, Aerobic and Anaerobic *on page 784*

Blood Culture, *Mycobacterium avium-intracellulare* *see* Blood Culture, Aerobic and Anaerobic *on page 784*

Blood Culture With Antimicrobial Removal Device (ARD) *see* Blood Culture, Aerobic and Anaerobic *on page 784*

Blood Fungus Culture

CPT *87103 (isolation); 87106 (definitive identification)*

Related Information

Amphotericin B *on page 942*
Aspergillus Serology *on page 641*
Biopsy or Body Fluid Fungus Culture *on page 780*
Blood Culture, Aerobic and Anaerobic *on page 784*
Candida Antigen *on page 652*
Candidiasis Serologic Test *on page 652*
Histoplasmosis Serology *on page 695*
Itraconazole *on page 975*
Sputum Culture *on page 849*
Stool Fungus Culture *on page 861*
Susceptibility Testing, Fungi *on page 869*
Urine Fungus Culture *on page 883*

Synonyms Fungus Culture, Blood

Test Commonly Includes Blood culture and inoculation of specific fungal media at time of collection

Patient Care PREPARATION: See preparation for Blood Culture, Aerobic and Anaerobic.

Specimen Blood CONTAINER: Fungal blood culture media (eg, biphasic blood culture media) or lysis centrifugation collecting tubes (Wampole Isolator™) COLLECTION: Remove plastic cap from biphasic bottle, cleanse stoppers with acetone alcohol and 2% iodine, and allow to dry. Collect 8 mL blood in a yellow Vacutainer® tube containing 0.35% sodium polyanethol sulfonate as an anticoagulant. Transfer appropriate volume of blood to biphasic medium to achieve an approximate 1:10 dilution of blood in the broth medium. Alternatively, 10 mL of blood is directly collected in an Isolator™ tube. CAUSES FOR REJECTION: Unlabeled bottles or specimens are not acceptable. TURNAROUND TIME: Preliminary reports are usually available in 1-2 days. Negative cultures are commonly reported at 4-6 weeks. SPECIAL INSTRUCTIONS: The laboratory should be informed of current antibiotic therapy and clinical diagnosis.

Interpretive REFERENCE RANGE: No growth USE: Isolate and identify fungi; establish the diagnosis of fungemia, fungal endocarditis, and disseminated mycosis in patients at risk for fungal infections. Certain yeasts such as *Candida* sp and *Candida glabrata* (*Torulopsis glabrata*) can be isolated from routine bacterial blood cultures; for other agents of systemic mycoses, however, it is essential to perform blood fungal cultures as outlined above. LIMITATIONS: A single (or even multiple) negative fungal blood culture does not exclude disseminated fungal infection. If disseminated or deep fungal infection is strongly suspected despite repeatedly negative blood cultures, biopsy of the appropriate tissue and/or bone marrow aspiration for sections and fungus culture should be considered. METHODOLOGY: Biphasic (broth and agar) blood culture medium, or broth alone with early subculture to solid media, or lysis centrifugation with prompt subculture to solid media are appropriate methodologies. Lysis centrifugation appears to produce higher yields and more rapid detection than other methods.[1,2] ADDITIONAL INFORMATION: Fungemia can be a complication of venous or arterial catheterization, hyperalimentation, the acquired immunodeficiency syndrome (AIDS), and therapy with steroids, antineoplastic drugs, radiation, or broad spectrum antimicrobial agents. Intravenous drug abusers are prone to *Candida* endocarditis. Although many fungal species including *Histoplasma capsulatum*, *Coccidioides immitis*, and *Cryptococcus neoformans* are recoverable from blood cultures, the most common cause of fungemia is *Candida albicans* followed by other *Candida* sp including *Candida glabrata* (*Torulopsis glabrata*). Most *Candida* sp will also grow in routine aerobic bacterial blood cultures. Fungemia represents a failure of the host defense system. Fungemia may be precipitated by contamination of an indwelling catheter or, in the critically ill and immunocompromised patient, contamination of the gastrointestinal and less frequently the urinary tract.[3] In a review of 356 patients with neoplastic disease, *Candida* sp was recovered in 7% of neutropenic patients.

In the potentially immunocompromised host, a temperature of 38.5°C (101°F) for more than 2 hours which is not associated with the administration of a pyrogenic drug (chemotherapy) in-

(Continued)

Blood Fungus Culture *(Continued)*

dicates the presence of infection until proven otherwise. In these patients, characteristic signs and symptoms are frequently absent. A careful physical examination including mouth, anus, and genitalia may reveal the site of infection. Therapy must be instituted as soon as appropriate specimens are collected. Most infections in these patients are caused by gram-negative organisms (eg, *E. coli*, *Pseudomonas* sp, *Klebsiella* sp) and by *S. aureus*; however, fungi and other usually nonpathogenic organisms must be considered significant.[4]

Rarely blastospores (budding yeast structures) and pseudohyphae can be seen by examination of Wright's stained venous peripheral blood smears. This technique may allow early diagnosis and therapy before culture results are available.[5]

Footnotes

1. Bille J, Stockman L, Roberts GD, et al, "Evaluation of a Lysis-Centrifugation System for Recovery of Yeasts and Filamentous Fungi From Blood," *J Clin Microbiol*, 1983, 18:469-71.
2. Paya CV, Roberts GD, and Cockerill FR 3d, "Laboratory Methods for the Diagnosis of Disseminated Histoplasmosis: Clinical Importance of the Lysis-Centrifugation Blood Culture Technique," *Mayo Clin Proc*, 1987, 62:480-5.
3. Dyess DL, Garrison RN, and Fry DE, "*Candida* Sepsis. Implications of Polymicrobial Blood-Borne Infection," *Arch Surg*, 1985, 120:345-8.
4. Whimbey E, Kiehn TE, Brannon P, et al, "Bacteremia and Fungemia in Patients With Neoplastic Disease," *Am J Med*, 1987, 82:723-30.
5. Kates MM, Phair JB, Yungbluth M, et al, "Demonstration of *Candida* in Blood Smears," *Lab Med*, 1988, 19:25.

References

Guerra-Romero L, Telenti A, Thompson RL, et al, "Polymicrobial Fungemia: Microbiology, Clinical Features, and Significance," *Rev Infect Dis*, 1989, 11(2):208-12.

Telenti A, Steckelberg JM, Stockman L, et al, "Quantitative Blood Cultures in Candidemia," *Mayo Clin Proc*, 1991, 66(11):1120-3.

Wey SS, Mori M, Pfaller MA, et al, "Risk Factors for Hospital-Acquired Candidemia: A Matched Case-Controlled Study," *Arch Intern Med*, 1989, 149(10):2349-53.

Blood Mycobacteria Culture *see* Blood Culture, Aerobic and Anaerobic *on page 784*

Body Fluid Aerobic Culture *see* Biopsy or Body Fluid Aerobic Bacterial Culture *on page 778*

Body Fluid Anaerobic Culture *see* Biopsy or Body Fluid Anaerobic Bacterial Culture *on page 778*

Body Fluid Culture *see* Biopsy or Body Fluid Aerobic Bacterial Culture *on page 778*

Body Fluid Fungus Culture *see* Biopsy or Body Fluid Fungus Culture *on page 780*

Body Fluid Mycobacteria Culture *see* Biopsy or Body Fluid Mycobacteria Culture *on page 782*

Body Lice Identification *see* Arthropod Identification *on page 774*

Bone Marrow Culture *see* Biopsy or Body Fluid Aerobic Bacterial Culture *on page 778*

Bone Marrow Culture for *Brucella* *see* Blood Culture, *Brucella on page 788*

Bordetella pertussis Nasopharyngeal Culture

***CPT** 87081 (single organism); 87206 (fluorescent smear)*

Related Information

Bacterial Serology *on page 644*
Bordetella pertussis Direct Fluorescent Antibody *on page 646*
Bordetella pertussis Serology *on page 647*
Nasopharyngeal Culture *on page 830*

Synonyms Nasopharyngeal Culture for *Bordetella pertussis*; Pertussis Culture; Whooping Cough Culture

Replaces Cough Plate Culture for Pertussis; Throat Culture for *Bordetella pertussis*

Test Commonly Includes Specific culture and identification of *Bordetella pertussis* and *Bordetella parapertussis*

Patient Care PREPARATION: Patient should not be on antimicrobial therapy prior to the collection of the specimen.

Specimen Nasopharyngeal swab, cough plate optional CONTAINER: Flexible calcium alginate swab (Calgiswab®) and Bordet Gengou plate. Transport medium composed of half strength Oxoid charcoal agar CM19 supplemented with 40 µg/mL cephalexin and 10% hemolyzed defibrinated horse blood may be used.[1] COLLECTION: Shape the flexible swab into the contour of the nares. Pass the swab gently through the nose. Leave swab in place near septum and floor of nose for 15-30 seconds. Rotate and remove. The recovery of the organism depends on collecting an adequate specimen. Inoculate the plate or transport medium directly at the bedside.

The following procedure optimizes the laboratory diagnosis of pertussis.

- Collect nasopharyngeal specimens in the early stage of illness. Providing specimen collection kits facilitates the appropriate specimen collection and transportation.
- For swab collected specimens, use a transport medium consisting of half strength Oxoid charcoal agar supplemented with 10% hemolyzed, defibrinated horse blood, and 40 µg/mL cephalexin.
- Inoculate a selective primary plating medium composed of Oxoid charcoal agar, 10% defibrinated horse blood, and 40 µg/mL cephalexin. A nonselective medium without cephalexin may be used in addition to the selective medium.
- Perform direct fluorescent antibody (DFA) tests on appropriately collected nasopharyngeal secretions with *B. pertussis*- and *B. parapertussis*-conjugated antisera to facilitate an earlier diagnosis.
- After inoculating primary plating media, retain swabs in the original transport medium at room temperature. If cultures become overgrown with indigenous bacterial flora or fungi, use swabs to inoculate additional media.
- Identify suspicious isolates with appropriate cultural and biochemical tests. The DFA test performed on growth from isolated colonies is an excellent procedure for confirmatory or definitive identification.

STORAGE INSTRUCTIONS: The specimen should not be refrigerated. It should be transported to the laboratory as soon as possible after collection. CAUSES FOR REJECTION: Specimen not received on appropriate isolation medium. Excessive delay in transit to the laboratory results in less than optimal yield. TURNAROUND TIME: Preliminary reports are generally available at 24 hours if pathogens other than *B. pertussis* are isolated. Growth of *Bordetella pertussis* takes at least 72 hours to be detected. Cultures with no growth are usually reported after 1 week. Reports on specimens from which *B. pertussis* has been isolated generally require at least 1 week for completion. SPECIAL INSTRUCTIONS: Consult the laboratory prior to collection of the specimen so that the special isolation medium can be obtained. The laboratory should be made aware of the specific request to screen for *Bordetella pertussis* with information relevant to current antibiotic therapy and current diagnosis.

Interpretive REFERENCE RANGE: No *B. pertussis* or *B. parapertussis* isolated USE: Isolate and identify *B. pertussis*, and *B. parapertussis*; establish the diagnosis of whooping cough LIMITATIONS: Cough plates are less reliable than nasopharyngeal specimens. CONTRAINDICATIONS: Lack of clinical symptoms of pertussis; previous antibiotic therapy; history of vaccination is a relative contraindication METHODOLOGY: Culture on selective medium (selective chocolate agar with 10% defibrinated horse blood and 40 µg/mL cephalexin), presumptive confirmation by direct fluorescent antibody (DFA). Culture after enrichment in transport medium for 48 hours increases yield. ADDITIONAL INFORMATION: Direct fluorescent antibody (DFA) procedures provide more rapid results and have been increasingly used in the diagnosis of *B. pertussis* infection. The DFA procedures are most useful in the first 2-3 weeks of the illness. DFA test detected 42 of 164 (26%) of patients who proved culture positive for *B. pertussis* and 8 of 38 (21%) of patients who proved culture positive for *B. parapertussis*. False-negatives may be caused by inadequate specimens having little cellular material (leukocytes and brush border epithelial cells).[1]

Footnotes

1. Young SA, Anderson GL, and Mitchell PD, "Laboratory Observations During an Outbreak of Pertussis," *Clin Microbiol Newslet*, 1987, 9:22, 176-9.

References

Friedman RL, "Pertussis: The Disease and New Diagnostic Methods," *Clin Microbiol Rev*, 1988, 1:365-76.

Halperin SA, Bortolussi R, and Wort AJ, "Evaluation of Culture, Immunofluorescence, and Serology for the Diagnosis of Pertussis," *J Clin Microbiol*, 1989, 27(4):752-7.

Botulism, Diagnostic Procedure

CPT 87001 (animal inoculation); 87081 (culture, single organism)

Synonyms *Clostridium botulinum* Toxin Identification Procedure; Infant Botulism, Toxin Identification; Sudden Death Syndrome

Abstract A neurotoxin, botulin, may be produced by *C. botulinum* in foods which have been improperly preserved. Characteristics of this type of food poisoning include vomiting and abdominal pain, disturbances of vision, motor function and secretion, mydriasis, ptosis, dry mouth, and cough.

Specimen Vomitus, serum, stool, gastric washings, cerebrospinal fluid or autopsy tissue; food samples **CONTAINER:** Sterile wide-mouth, leakproof, screw-cap jar; red top tube **STORAGE INSTRUCTIONS:** Keep refrigerated at 4°C except for unopened food samples. **TURNAROUND TIME:** 3-7 days **SPECIAL INSTRUCTIONS:** The laboratory must be notified prior to obtaining specimen in order to prepare for transport of the specimen to the State Health Laboratory or Center for Disease Control.

Interpretive **REFERENCE RANGE:** No toxin identified, no *Clostridium botulinum* isolated **USE:** Diagnose infant botulism, sudden death syndrome, floppy baby syndrome, classic botulism in adults **LIMITATIONS:** The toxin from *C. botulinum* binds almost irreversibly to individual nerve terminals; thus, serum and cerebrospinal fluid specimens may yield false-negative results. **CONTRAINDICATIONS:** Due to the difficulty in performance of the diagnostic test and because of the extensive epidemiological studies initiated upon receipt of the specimen, State Department of Health Laboratories require specific clinical symptomatology for infant botulism. Therefore, they should be consulted early to optimize handling of the suspect case. **METHODOLOGY:** Toxin neutralization test in mice, isolation of *Clostridium botulinum* from feces **ADDITIONAL INFORMATION:** The classic presentation of **infant botulism** is hypotonia (floppy baby syndrome), constipation, difficulty in feeding, and a weak cry. Some cases of sudden death syndrome have been traced to ingesting honey containing *C. botulinum.* Both *C. botulinum* and *C. butyricum* have been identified as species capable of toxin production.[1] Autointoxication may occur from toxin production during organism growth in tissue, the intestinal tract in both adults and infants, and in wounds. Botulism has been reported with cocaine-associated sinusitis.[2]

Footnotes

1. Gimenez JA and Sugiyama H, "Comparison of Toxins of *Clostridium butyricum* and *Clostridium botulinum* Type E," *Infect Immun*, 1988, 56:926-9.
2. Kudrow DB, Henry DA, Haake DA, et al, "Botulism Associated With *Clostridium botulinum* Sinusitis After Intranasal Cocaine Abuse," *Ann Intern Med*, 1988, 109(12):984-5.

References

Arnon SS, "Infant Botulism: Anticipating the Second Decade," *J Infect Dis*, 1986, 154:201-6.
Bartlett JC, "Infant Botulism in Adults," *N Engl J Med*, 1986, 315:254-5.
Chia JK, Clark JB, Ryan CA, et al, "Botulism in an Adult Associated With Food-Borne Intestinal Infection With *Clostridium botulinum*," *N Engl J Med*, 1986, 315:239-41.
Hatheway CL, "Toxigenic Clostridia," *Clin Microbiol Rev*, 1990, 3(1):66-98.

Bronchial Aspirate Anaerobic Culture

CPT 87075 (isolation); 87076 (definitive identification)

Related Information

Biopsy or Body Fluid Anaerobic Bacterial Culture *on page 778*
Bronchial Washings Cytology *on page 485*
Bronchoalveolar Lavage Cytology *on page 487*
Gram Stain *on page 815*
Sputum Culture *on page 849*
Sputum Cytology *on page 510*
Susceptibility Testing, Aerobic and Facultatively Anaerobic Organisms *on page 864*

Synonyms Anaerobic Culture, Bronchial Aspirate

Applies to Bartlett Catheter; Endotracheal Anaerobic Culture; Percutaneous Transtracheal Anaerobic Culture; Protected Catheter Brush (PCB); Transtracheal Aspirates

Test Commonly Includes Culture and direct Gram stained smear if specimen is adequate and direct smear is requested

Patient Care **PREPARATION:** Aseptic preparation of the aspiration site

Specimen Transtracheal aspirate or bronchoscopically obtained specimen using a protected catheter brush (PCB), called a Bartlett catheter in most settings. **CONTAINER:** Transtracheal aspirates should be submitted in an anaerobic transport tube or sterile capped syringe. Bartlett catheters should be submitted in 1 mL of sterile nonbacteriostatic saline in a sterile container. **COLLECTION:** Collected at bronchoscopy or transtracheal aspiration by a physician skilled in the procedure. Transport the specimen to the laboratory within 1 hour of collection. Avoid contamination with normal flora from oral cavity. **STORAGE INSTRUCTIONS:** The specimen should not be refrigerated or incubated. **CAUSES FOR REJECTION:** Specimens collected on swabs, exposed to air, and those which have been refrigerated, have a less than optimal yield. **TURNAROUND TIME:** Cultures showing no bacterial growth can generally be reported after 2-4 days. Complete reports of cultures with anaerobic bacteria may take as long as 2 weeks after receipt of culture depending upon the nature of the organisms isolated. **SPECIAL INSTRUCTIONS:** The laboratory should be informed of current antibiotic therapy and clinical diagnosis.

Interpretive **REFERENCE RANGE:** No growth of anaerobic bacteria (transtracheal aspirate). For properly submitted Bartlett catheters (in 1 mL of saline), $<10^3$ CFU/mL is within the expected level of contamination. **USE:** Isolate and identify anaerobic organisms causing pulmonary infections **LIMITATIONS:** Specimens received in anaerobe transport containers are less than optimal for aerobic or fungus cultures. It is often difficult to avoid contamination with normal oral flora during bronchoscopy. **METHODOLOGY:** Anaerobic culture with plated and broth media (transtracheal aspirate); semiquantitative cultures on solid media for protected catheter brushes **ADDITIONAL INFORMATION:** The abundant normal anaerobic flora of the mouth makes anaerobic cultures of any specimen contaminated by oral secretions (eg, bronchial washes, sputums) essentially useless for defining the anaerobic bacterial etiology of lower respiratory infection.[1] Only specimens that bypass the mouth should be cultured anaerobically. Transtracheal aspirates meet this need, but in most hospital settings, they are rarely, if ever, collected. They have been replaced by bronchoscopically obtained specimens using a PCB.[2] Specimens obtained by PCB are subject to low level contamination with normal oral flora, however, this can be accounted for by semiquantitative culture.[3,4]

Pleuropulmonary infections caused by anaerobic organisms are most often secondary to aspiration of oropharyngeal contents. They may be caused by septic emboli. Intra-abdominal infections (ie, subphrenic abscess, diverticulitis, appendicitis, and so forth) may give rise to supradiaphragmatic infection. Community acquired aspiration pneumonia, necrotizing pneumonia with multiple small abscesses, frank lung abscess, and pulmonary empyema yield significant anaerobes in 60% to 95% of cases if appropriate culture technique is employed. The characteristic foul-smelling odor of anaerobic infections may not be present early in the course.

Footnotes

1. Bartlett JG, Alexander J, Mayhew J, et al, "Should Fiberoptic Bronchoscopy Aspirates Be Cultured?" *Am Rev Respir Dis*, 1976, 114:73-8.
2. Allen SD and Sider JA, "An Approach to the Diagnosis of Pleuropulmonary Infection," *Clin Lab Med*, 1982, 2:285-303.
3. Broughton WA, Bass JB, and Kirkpatrick MB, "The Technique of Protected Brush Catheter Bronchoscopy," *J Crit Illness*, 1987, 2:63-70.
4. Pollock HM, Hawkins EL, Bonner JB, et al, "Diagnosis of Bacterial Pulmonary Infections With Quantitative Protected Catheter Cultures Obtained During Bronchoscopy," *J Clin Microbiol*, 1983, 17:255-9.

Bronchial Washings Culture *see* Sputum Culture *on page 849*

Bronchoalveolar Lavage

CPT *89050 (cell count with differential)*

Related Information

Bronchial Washings Cytology *on page 485*
Bronchoalveolar Lavage Cytology *on page 487*
Cytomegalic Inclusion Disease Cytology *on page 496*
Cytomegalovirus Antibody *on page 672*
Pneumocystis carinii Preparation *on page 508*
Pneumocystis Fluorescence *on page 732*
Sputum Culture *on page 849*
Sputum Fungus Culture *on page 853*
Sputum Mycobacteria Culture *on page 855*
Viral Culture, Respiratory Symptoms *on page 1204*

Synonyms BAL

Applies to Airway Lavage

(Continued)

Bronchoalveolar Lavage *(Continued)*

Test Commonly Includes Total cell count, differential, volume

Specimen Bronchoalveolar lavage **CONTAINER:** Sterile suction trap **COLLECTION:** The specimen must be transported to the laboratory within 1 hour of collection.

Interpretive **REFERENCE RANGE:** Normal **total cell count**: 4-23 x 10^6; differential: 95% alveolar macrophages, 3% lymphocytes, 1% polymorphonuclear cells, 0.2% eosinophils; $\leq 10^4$ CFU/mL aerobic bacteria **USE:** Identify the etiology of potentially treatable pulmonary infections **LIMITATIONS:** Contamination with oral pharyngeal secretions causes false-positive bacterial cultures; this can be corrected by performing quantitative cultures. The use of bronchoalveolar lavage for defining the etiology of anaerobic pulmonary infections has not been established. Differentiation of colonization versus infection may be difficult with such agents as *Aspergillus* or *Candida* species. **METHODOLOGY:** Following insertion of the bronchoscope, 20 mL of isotonic saline (containing no bacteriostatic agents) is instilled into the suction part of the bronchoscope. After instillation, 50-100 mm Hg suction is applied and the fluid is collected in an 80 mL suction trap. The procedure is repeated five times (100 mL total infusion) with a typical recovery of 40-70 mL. The specimen may then be submitted for acid fast, Calcofluor white, silver, PAS, and Gram stains, cytology, and viral, aerobic bacterial, fungal, mycobacterial, *Legionella*, and *Nocardia* cultures, as required. **ADDITIONAL INFORMATION:** Bronchoalveolar lavage (BAL) has become an established procedure for defining the etiology of pulmonary infections. It is particularly useful for recovering opportunistic pathogens (eg, *Pneumocystis*, *Histoplasma capsulatum*, *Candida* sp, *Aspergillus* sp, *Mycobacterium* sp) from immunocompromised individuals, and in defining the etiology of nosocomial pneumonia in patients undergoing mechanical ventilation.[1,2,3] The procedure has an acceptable morbidity in immunocompromised and thrombocytopenic patients and is often considered as an initial diagnostic procedure in the immunosuppressed. BAL is performed with a catheter wedged into a segmental bronchus. Bronchial washings or airway washings are collected with a nonwedged, more proximally positioned scope tip. Bronchial washings, therefore, preferentially sample airways. Lavage is preferred for the diagnosis of *Pneumocystis* pneumonia, which is primarily an alveolar process. Limiting lavage to one segment reduces the risk of postprocedural respiratory compromise. Quantitative bacterial cultures of BAL specimens have also proven useful for defining the etiology of acute bacterial pneumonia.[4,5]

Footnotes

1. Martin WJ II, Smith TF, Sanderson DR, et al, "Role of Bronchoalveolar Lavage in the Assessment of Opportunistic Pulmonary Infections: Utility and Complications," *Mayo Clin Proc*, 1987, 62:549-57.
2. Gadek JE, "Diagnosing Pulmonary Disease in the Immunocompromised Patient," *Mayo Clin Proc*, 1987, 62:632-3.
3. Guerra LF and Baughman RP, "Use of Bronchoalveolar Lavage to Diagnose Bacterial Pneumonia in Mechanically Ventilated Patients," *Crit Care Med*, 1990, 18(2):169-73.
4. Baselski VS, El-Torky M, Coalson JJ, et al, "The Standardization of Criteria for Processing and Interpreting Laboratory Specimens in Patients With Suspected Ventilator-Associated Pneumonia," *Chest*, 1992, 102(5 Suppl 1):571S-9S.
5. Thorpe JE, Baughman RP, Frame PT, et al, "Bronchoalveolar Lavage for Diagnosing Acute Bacterial Pneumonia," *J Infect Dis*, 1987, 155:855-61.

References

Raskin JA, Collman R, and Daniels RP, "Acquired Immune Deficiency Syndrome and the Lung," *Chest*, 1988, 94:155-64.

Xaubet A, Torres A, Marco F, et al, "Pulmonary Infiltrates in Immunocompromized Patients. Diagnostic Value of Telescoping Plugged Catheter and Bronchoalveolar Lavage," *Chest*, 1989, 95(1):130-5.

Bronchoscopic *Legionella* Culture *see* *Legionella* Culture *on page 825*

Bronchoscopy Culture *see* Sputum Culture *on page 849*

Bronchoscopy Fungus Culture *see* Sputum Fungus Culture *on page 853*

***Brucella* Blood Culture** *see* Blood Culture, *Brucella on page 788*

Burn Culture, Quantitative

CPT *87070 (aerobic culture); 87999 (unlisted procedure for quantitation)*

Related Information

Gram Stain *on page 815*

Wound Culture *on page 885*

Zeta Sedimentation Ratio *on page 617*

Synonyms Quantitative Burn Culture; Skin Burn Culture, Quantitative

Applies to Biopsy Specimen Culture, Quantitative; Quantitative Culture, Biopsy Specimen

Test Commonly Includes Quantitative bacterial counts (colonies/g of tissue) of skin and tissue specimens from burn patients. Identification of bacterial isolates and susceptibility testing when indicated. May also include direct Gram stain smear and histopathology.

Specimen Viable tissue, **not** eschar **CONTAINER:** Sterile container, no fixative **COLLECTION:** Aseptic technique **STORAGE INSTRUCTIONS:** Transport to the laboratory as soon as possible. **CAUSES FOR REJECTION:** Eschar specimen rather than viable tissue, specimen <0.1 g, specimen in fixative **TURNAROUND TIME:** Quantitative bacterial counts are usually available in 24 hours. Identification of bacterial isolates is usually available in 48 hours. **SPECIAL INSTRUCTIONS:** The laboratory should be informed of the specific site of specimen. The laboratory should be contacted prior to collection of the specimens to ascertain availability and specific procedures required.

Interpretive **REFERENCE RANGE:** No growth to $<10^5$ colonies/g of tissue **USE:** Determine bacterial identity and quantity of organism present (colonies/g) in tissue or skin specimen from burn patient **LIMITATIONS:** Predictive value for sepsis is limited. **METHODOLOGY:** Culture is performed after weighing the specimen and disruption in a glass homogenizer. Trypticase soy broth is the diluent. Colony counts are done at 24 and 48 hours of incubation (35°C with CO_2). Fungus cultures are planted on Sabouraud's agar or supplemented Sabouraud's agar and held at 30°C for 5 weeks. **ADDITIONAL INFORMATION:** Major thermal injuries often precipitate a profound multicentric immunologic depression that may predispose patients to sepsis. Impairment of immune function is almost universal in patients with greater than 40% total body surface area burns and in very young or very old patients with far smaller burns.[1] The principal value of quantitative burn-wound biopsies is the demonstration of the predominant burn-wound flora. Agreement of 96% was found between negative culture ($<10^5$ colonies/g of tissue) and the absence of histopathologic invasive infection. Histopathologic invasion was documented in only 36% of cases with positive cultures.[2] Thus, the use of quantitative burn cultures has little value in identifying patients with invasive infection and in differentiating those who are or are not likely to develop burn-wound sepsis. The organism most frequently recovered from burn wounds is *Pseudomonas aeruginosa*.

Quantitative cultures taken from the center and advancing edge of involved areas from patients with untreated cellulitis had a low yield both in terms of positive (18% of 50) and density of microorganisms recovered except from next to the edges of ulcers. Lymphatic compromise was suspected as a major factor contributing to the intensity of inflammation.[3] See tables.

Histopathologic Findings and Organisms Cultured

Histopathologic Finding	Organism Cultured	No. of Cases
Gram-negative rods	*Pseudomonas aeruginosa*	22
	Klebsiella pneumoniae	4
	Pseudomonas fluorescens	1
	Providencia stuartii	1
	Serratia marcescens	1
	Total	29
Gram-positive cocci	*Staphylococcus aureus*	2
Filamentous fungi	*Aspergillus* species	2
	Fusarium species	2
	Rhizopus species	1
	None*	3
	Total	8

From McManus AT, "Opportunistic Infections in Severely Burned Patients," *Am J Med,* 1984, 75:146-54, with permission.

* Not diagnosed by culture.

Potential Mediators of Immunosuppression Following Thermal Injuries

Arachidonic acid metabolites (prostaglandins, leukotrienes)
Interferon
Bacterial endotoxin
Cutaneous burn toxin
Denatured protein
Corticosteroids
Neutrophil products
Histamine
Anaphylatoxins
Suppressive serum proteins
Immunoglobulins (autoantibody)
Immune complexes
Alpha globulin
Alpha fetoprotein
Iatrogenic
Antibiotics
Topical agents
Pain medication (opiates)
Anesthetics
Blood products

From Ninnerman JL, "Trauma, Sepsis, and the Immune Response,"*J Burn Care Rehabil,* 1987, 8:462-8, with permission.

Footnotes

1. Ninnemann JL, "Trauma, Sepsis, and The Immune Response," *J Burn Care Rehabil*, 1987, 8:462-8, (review).

(Continued)

Burn Culture, Quantitative *(Continued)*

2. McManus AT, Kim SH, McManus WF, et al, "Comparison of Quantitative Microbiology and Histopathology in Divided Burn-Wound Biopsy Specimens," *Arch Surg*, 1987, 122:74-6.
3. Duvanel T, Auckenthaler R, and Rohner P, "Quantitative Cultures of Biopsy Specimens From Cutaneous Cellulitis," *Arch Intern Med*, 1989, 149(2):293-6.

References

McManus AT, "Opportunistic Infections in Severely Burned Patients," *Am J Med*, 1984, 75:146-54.
Ninnemann JL, "Clinical and Immune Status of Burn Patients," *Antibiot Chemother*, 1987, 89:16-25, (review).
Robson MC, "Quantitative Bacteriology and the Burned Patient," *Quantitative Bacteriology: Its Role in the Armamentarium of the Surgeon*, Heggers JP and Robson MC, eds, Boca Raton, FL: CRC Press Inc, 1991, 97-108.

Calcofluor White *see* Fungus Smear, Stain *on page 813*

***Campylobacter pylori* Urease Test and Culture** *see Helicobacter pylori* Urease Test and Culture *on page 820*

***Candida* Culture, Genital** *see* Genital Culture *on page 814*

Catheter Tip Culture *see* Intravascular Device Culture *on page 822*

Cefinase (Nitrocefin) Testing *see* Penicillinase Test *on page 840*

Cell Wall Defective Bacteria Culture

***CPT** 87070*

Related Information

Biopsy or Body Fluid Aerobic Bacterial Culture *on page 778*
Blood Culture, Aerobic and Anaerobic *on page 784*

Synonyms L-Form Culture; L-Phase Organism Culture

Applies to Protoplast Culture; Spheroplast Culture

Test Commonly Includes Aerobic culture, antimicrobial susceptibility when indicated

Specimen Body fluid (eg, blood, spinal fluid, pleural fluid or urine) or tissue from suspected site of infection which is normally sterile **CONTAINER:** Blood: contact laboratory for special hypertonic blood culture bottle; other sources: collect in the same type of container used for usual culture from that site **COLLECTION:** For blood specimens, a conventional blood culture should also be collected following the procedure for Blood Culture, Aerobic and Anaerobic. Extreme care should be taken to avoid contamination with saprophytes. **CAUSES FOR REJECTION:** Blood culture specimens not received in special hypertonic blood culture bottle may have a less than optimal yield. **TURNAROUND TIME:** 4 weeks **SPECIAL INSTRUCTIONS:** Consult laboratory prior to collecting the specimen so that appropriate preparations can be made. The laboratory should be informed of the specific request to screen for cell wall defective bacteria, specific source of specimen, age of patient, current antibiotic therapy, and clinical diagnosis. Cell wall defective organisms will not usually grow on routine culture media. L-form culture must be specified in order that appropriate culture media is inoculated.

Interpretive **REFERENCE RANGE:** No growth **USE:** Detect bacteria which have developed a cell wall defective structure due to drug therapy *in vivo* or exposure to adverse environmental conditions *in vivo* or *in vitro*. This test may be indicated when routine cultures are negative, but infection is still highly suspected clinically. Although the methods used are investigative, such techniques may become more common in clinical practice. **LIMITATIONS:** Slow-growing cell wall defective organisms may be overgrown by saprophytes. Thus, sterile tissue and body fluids are optimal specimens. **METHODOLOGY:** Culture in hypertonic medium **ADDITIONAL INFORMATION:** Cell wall defective organisms (L-forms) have been associated with *Haemophilus influenzae*, *Staphylococcus aureus*, Enterobacteriaceae, and other microorganisms. L-form colonies have been induced by exposing bacteria to agents which inhibit cell wall synthesis, such as penicillin and cephalosporin antibiotics, bacteriostatic chemicals, amino acids, lysozyme, phage, muralytic enzymes, and hyperimmune sera. Gram-positive strains usually require a hyperosmolar environment for induction of L-forms, gram-negatives do not. In laboratory settings, most bacteria can or probably could be converted to L-forms under proper conditions. L-forms resemble *Mycoplasma* after partial or complete loss of the cell wall. Stable L-forms are not able to convert to the original form. Unstable L-forms revert to the original form when the inducing stimulus is removed. Spheroplasts and protoplasts, organisms which have lost their cell walls through digestion, cannot reproduce. Culture in high osmolarity media may allow their propagation as L-forms.

To be identified, L-forms must revert to the parent type, following which they may demonstrate the parent's original antimicrobial susceptibility, antigenicity, and/or propensity to produce toxin. The reversion may be only partial and L-forms recovered in one laboratory may differ widely from those recovered in another. L-forms are usually considered to be pathogenic only in the parent form unless toxin production by the L-form is present. Routine attempts at isolation of L-forms are generally not productive in a clinical setting.

References

Madoff S, "Should the Microbiologist Be Concerned About Bacterial L-Forms in Clinical Specimens," *Clin Microbiol Newslet*, 1988, 10:3-6, (editorial).

Pachas WN, "L-Forms and Bacterial Variants in Infectious Disease Processes," *The Bacterial L-Forms*, Madoff S, ed, New York, NY: Marcel Dekker Inc, 1986, 287-318.

Cephalosporinase Production Testing *see* Penicillinase Test *on page 840*

Cerebrospinal Fluid Anaerobic Culture

CPT *87075 (anaerobic culture); 87076 (definitive identification)*

Related Information

Abscess, Aerobic and Anaerobic Bacterial Culture *on page 768*
Biopsy or Body Fluid Anaerobic Bacterial Culture *on page 778*
Cerebrospinal Fluid Culture *on next page*
Cerebrospinal Fluid Cytology *on page 490*
Viral Culture, Central Nervous System Symptoms *on page 1199*

Synonyms Anaerobic Culture, Cerebrospinal Fluid

Test Commonly Includes Anaerobic culture and identification of isolates from cerebrospinal fluid

Patient Care **PREPARATION:** Aseptic preparation of the aspiration site

Specimen Cerebrospinal fluid or aspirate of fluid from intracranial lesion. Specimen for anaerobic culture should be accompanied by request for routine culture from the same site. **CONTAINER:** Sterile CSF tube **COLLECTION:** Tubes should be numbered 1, 2, 3 with tube #1 representing the first portion of the sample collected. Contamination with normal flora from skin or other body surfaces must be avoided. The third tube collected during lumbar puncture is most suitable for culture, as skin contaminants from the puncture usually are washed out with fluid collected in the first two tubes. **STORAGE INSTRUCTIONS:** Specimen should be transported immediately to the laboratory under anaerobic conditions. If the specimen cannot be processed immediately, it should be kept at room temperature or placed in an incubator. **CAUSES FOR REJECTION:** Refrigeration inhibits viability of certain anaerobic organisms and also the common aerobic pathogens, *Neisseria meningitidis* and *Haemophilus influenzae*. **TURNAROUND TIME:** Cultures showing no bacterial growth can be reported after 3 days. Complete reports of cultures with anaerobic bacteria may take as long as 2 weeks after receipt of culture, depending upon the nature of the organisms isolated. **SPECIAL INSTRUCTIONS:** The laboratory should be informed of the specific source of specimen, age of patient, current antibiotic therapy, and clinical diagnosis. Anaerobic transport medium is recommended.

Interpretive **REFERENCE RANGE:** No growth **USE:** Anaerobic culture is indicated only if brain abscess, subdural empyema, or epidural abscess is suspected or in the presence of a primary anaerobic infection at another site which is suspected of involving the central nervous system. Cerebrospinal fluid is not the specimen of choice in this setting, and collection of cerebrospinal fluid may be contraindicated. Common underlying conditions associated with central nervous system anaerobic infections include otitis media, lung and pleural infections, sinusitis, oral infections (ie, tonsillitis, paratonsillar abscess, dental infections), and congenital heart disease. **METHODOLOGY:** Anaerobic culture usually with solid and broth media **ADDITIONAL INFORMATION:** In general, anaerobes are rare in spinal fluid. Most cases of cerebral abscess are polymicrobial.

References

Bartlett JG, "Anaerobic Bacteria: General Concepts," *Principles and Practice of Infectious Diseases*, Mandell GL, Douglas RG, and Bennett JE, eds, 3rd ed, New York, NY: Churchill Livingstone, 1990, 1828-42.

Gray LD and Fedorko DP, "Laboratory Diagnosis of Bacterial Meningitis," *Clin Microbiol Rev*, 1992, 5(2):130-45.

Mathisen GE, Meyer RD, George WL, et al, "Brain Abscess and Cerebritis," *Rev Infect Dis*, 1984, 6:S101-6.

Cerebrospinal Fluid Bacterial Antigen Testing *see* Bacterial Antigens, Rapid Detection Methods *on page 775*

Cerebrospinal Fluid Cryptococcal Latex Agglutination *see* Cryptococcal Antigen Titer, Serum or Cerebrospinal Fluid *on page 805*

Cerebrospinal Fluid Culture

CPT *87070*

Related Information

Bacterial Antigens, Rapid Detection Methods *on page 775*
Blood Culture, Aerobic and Anaerobic *on page 784*
Cerebrospinal Fluid Anaerobic Culture *on previous page*
Cerebrospinal Fluid Analysis *on page 527*
Cerebrospinal Fluid Cytology *on page 490*
Cerebrospinal Fluid Fungus Culture *on page 800*
Cerebrospinal Fluid Glucose *on page 176*
Cerebrospinal Fluid Lactic Acid *on page 178*
Cerebrospinal Fluid LD *on page 179*
Cerebrospinal Fluid Mycobacteria Culture *on page 801*
Cerebrospinal Fluid Protein *on page 659*
FTA-ABS, Cerebrospinal Fluid *on page 679*
Gram Stain *on page 815*
India Ink Preparation *on page 822*
VDRL, Cerebrospinal Fluid *on page 761*
Viral Culture, Central Nervous System Symptoms *on page 1199*

Synonyms CSF Culture; Culture, Cerebrospinal Fluid

Applies to Ventricular Fluid Culture

Test Commonly Includes Aerobic culture and Gram stain (stat) if requested. Gram stain, cell count, differential, glucose, and protein levels are usually requested. Additional fluid if available may be used for additional cultures and/or rapid diagnostic tests, such as those for bacterial or cryptococcal antigen and/or for acid-fast stain.[1,2] Especially in instances of subacute or chronic onset, tuberculosis and cryptococcosis must be considered and appropriate smears and cultures ordered.

Abstract The major test to be performed on the CNS for meningitis is the bacteriologic culture. The "gold standard" for the diagnosis of bacterial meningitis is the isolation of a bacterium from the cerebrospinal fluid.[3] Diagnosis of meningitis is made by examination and culture of CSF.[4] Nucleated blood cell count, differential, Gram stain, CSF glucose, and CSF protein are needed. Blood cultures are often positive with meningitis.

Patient Care PREPARATION: Aseptic preparation of the aspiration site

Specimen Cerebrospinal fluid CONTAINER: Sterile CSF tube COLLECTION: Contamination with normal flora from skin or other body surfaces must be avoided. Risks to the patient of lumbar puncture are described.[1,2] Since blood cultures are usually positive in subjects with bacterial meningitis,[4] blood cultures should be requested as well. Peripheral blood white cell count and differential are usually abnormal in patients with meningitis and represent an important part of the clinical investigation. STORAGE INSTRUCTIONS: The specimen should be transported immediately to the laboratory. If the specimen cannot be processed immediately, it should be kept at room temperature or placed in an incubator. Refrigeration inhibits viability of certain anaerobic organisms and may prevent the recovery of the common aerobic pathogens, *Neisseria meningitidis* and *Haemophilus influenzae*. TURNAROUND TIME: Preliminary reports are usually available at 24 hours. Cultures with no growth can be reported after 72 hours. Reports of cultures from which pathogens are isolated may require a minimum of 48 hours for completion. SPECIAL INSTRUCTIONS: The laboratory should be informed of the specific source of specimen, age of patient, current antibiotic therapy, clinical diagnosis, and time of collection.

Interpretive REFERENCE RANGE: No growth USE: Isolate and identify pathogenic organisms causing meningitis, shunt infection, brain abscess, subdural empyema, cerebral or spinal epidural abscess, bacterial endocarditis with embolism. The time honored Gram and Ziehl-Neelsen stains with cultures of CSF in suspected bacterial meningitis are fundamental to appropriate diagnosis and treatment.[2] LIMITATIONS: Cultures may be negative in partially treated cases of meningitis. Fastidious microorganisms such as *Neisseria meningitidis* and *Haemophilus influenzae* are sensitive to temperature shifts. Refrigeration can inhibit their isolation from the specimen. Gram stains should be interpreted with care; false-positives occur due to contamination of laboratory staining supplies and tubes. Gram-positive organisms may decolorize (ie, stain gram-negative in partially treated cases). **METHODOLOGY:** Aerobic culture **ADDITIONAL INFORMATION:** *Haemophilus influenzae*, *Neisseria meningitidis*, and *Streptococcus* pneumoniae, commonly isolated organisms, can be serotyped if requested. Infections of cerebrospinal fluid shunts pose a difficult clinical problem. Organisms most commonly cultured from shunts include *S. epidermidis*, other coagulase-negative staphylococci, *S. aureus*, *S. viridans*, enterococci, and *H. influenzae*. Culture of CSF or shunt fluid is diagnostic. Removal of the catheter and later replacement are frequently required to eradicate infection.[5]

Bacterial meningitis remains a diagnostic problem. Symptoms suggestive of the diagnosis are those associated with febrile illness (eg, fever, lethargy, and anorexia); meningeal inflammation giving rise to nausea, vomiting, photophobia, and nuchal rigidity, leading to apathy and desire to be left in bed hyperextended in neck and spine; and encephalopathy with headache, confusion, and seizures. Stupor, coma, and focal neurologic signs indicate a poor prognosis if present before start of therapy.[6] **Mortality of bacterial meningitis** reaches 30%. Prognosis is worse in the very young and very old and is worse in the presence of sickle cell disease, asplenia, and with endocarditis.[4] Complications occur in survivors despite early diagnosis and appropriate use of antimicrobial drugs.[7] Developmental or neurologic sequelae were found in 33%[8,9] to 40% of survivors.[10] In a study of long-term outcome of neonatal meningitis, only 8 of 21 survivors were normal. Among six survivors of gram-negative meningitis, two had major sequelae.[11] A Helsinki study concludes that in some settings of childhood bacterial meningitis, diagnostic delay is almost unavoidable.[12]

Factors of bacterial virulence and impaired host defense are relevant to septicemia. Susceptibility to bacterial meningitis is affected by deficiencies in host defense which may be congenital or acquired. Susceptibility relates to age as well.[13] Tullus and colleagues discuss the role of predisposing host factors in neonatal and infantile *E. coli* bacteremia and meningitis in a recent paper.[14]

Footnotes

1. Greenlee JE, "Approach to Diagnosis of Meningitis - Cerebrospinal Fluid Evaluation," *Infect Dis Clin North Am*, 1990, 4(4):583-98.
2. Fishman RA, *Cerebrospinal Fluid in Diseases of the Nervous System*, 2nd ed, Philadelphia, PA: WB Saunders Co, 1992, 266-7.
3. Smith AL, "Bacterial Meningitis," *Pediatr Rev*, 1993, 14(1):11-8.
4. Francke E, "The Many Causes of Meningitis," *Postgrad Med*, 1987, 82:175-88.
5. McLaurin RL and Frame PT, "Treatment of Infections of Cerebrospinal Fluid Shunts," *Rev Infect Dis*, 1987, 9:595-603.
6. Dagbjartsson A and Ludvigsson P, "Bacterial Meningitis Diagnosis and Initial Antibiotic Therapy," *Pediatr Clin North Am*, 1987, 34:219-30.
7. Feigin RD, McCracken GH Jr, and Klein JO, "Diagnosis and Management of Meningitis," *Pediatr Infect Dis J*, 1992, 11(9):785-814.
8. Gray LD and Fedorko DP, "Laboratory Diagnosis of Bacterial Meningitis," *Clin Microbiol Rev*, 1992, 5(2):130-45.
9. Sáez-Llorens X, Ramilo O, Mustafa MM, et al, "Molecular Pathophysiology of Bacterial Meningitis: Current Concepts and Therapeutic Implications," *J Pediatr*, 1990, 116(5):671-84.
10. McCracken GH Jr, "Current Management of Bacterial Meningitis in Infants and Children," *Pediatr Infect Dis J*, 1992, 11(2):169-74.
11. Franco SM, Cornelius VE, and Andrews BF, "Long-Term Outcome of Neonatal Meningitis," *Am J Dis Child*, 1992, 146(5):567-71.
12. Kilpi T, Anttila M, Kallio MJ, et al, "Severity of Childhood Bacterial Meningitis and Duration of Illness Before Diagnosis," *Lancet*, 1991, 338(8764):406-9.
13. Klein JO, Feigin RD, and McCracken GH Jr, "Report of the Task Force on Diagnosis and Management of Meningitis," *Pediatrics*, 1986, 78(5):959-82.
14. Tullus K, Brauner A, Fryklund B, et al, "Host Factors Versus Virulence-Associated Bacterial Characteristics in Neonatal and Infantile Bacteraemia and Meningitis Caused by *Escherichia coli*," *J Med Microbiol*, 1992, 36(3):203-8.

References

Bell WE, "Bacterial Meningitis in Children - Selected Aspects," *Pediatr Clin North Am*, 1992, 39(4):651-68.

Sáez-Llorens X and McCracken GH Jr, "Bacterial Meningitis in Neonates and Children," *Infect Dis Clin North Am*, 1990, 4(4):623-44.

Scheld WM, Whitley RJ, and Durack DT, *Infections of the Central Nervous System*, New York, NY: Raven Press, 1991.

Tunkel AR and Scheld WM, "Pathogenesis and Pathophysiology of Bacterial Meningitis," *Clin Microbiol Rev*, 1993, 6(2):118-36.

Wenger JD, Hightower AW, Facklam RR, et al, "Bacterial Meningitis in the United States, 1986: Report of a Multistate Surveillance Study," *J Infect Dis*, 1990, 162(6):1316-23.

Cerebrospinal Fluid Fungus Culture

CPT *87102 (isolation); 87106 (definitive identification)*

Related Information

Amphotericin B *on page 942*
Bacterial Antigens, Rapid Detection Methods *on page 775*
Biopsy or Body Fluid Fungus Culture *on page 780*
Cerebrospinal Fluid Analysis *on page 527*
Cerebrospinal Fluid Culture *on page 798*
Cerebrospinal Fluid Glucose *on page 176*
Cerebrospinal Fluid Mycobacteria Culture *on next page*
Cerebrospinal Fluid Protein *on page 659*
Cryptococcal Antigen Titer, Serum or Cerebrospinal Fluid *on page 805*
Cryptococcus Antibody Titer *on page 670*
Flucytosine *on page 967*
India Ink Preparation *on page 822*
Itraconazole *on page 975*
Viral Culture, Central Nervous System Symptoms *on page 1199*

Synonyms Fungus Culture, Cerebrospinal Fluid

Test Commonly Includes Culture for fungi, India ink, smear, and cryptococcal antigen test if requested

Abstract Cryptococcal infection of the central nervous system may produce meningitis, meningoencephalitis, or a mass. Candidiasis, *Coccidioides immitis*, *Blastomyces dermatitidis*, and *Histoplasma capsulatum* are also found. In South America and occasionally in North America, *Paracoccidioides brasiliensis* is encountered. Patients suffering from fungal infections of the central nervous system often have an underlying immunosuppressive disorder.

Patient Care PREPARATION: Aseptic preparation of aspiration site

Specimen Cerebrospinal fluid CONTAINER: Sterile CSF tube COLLECTION: Tubes should be numbered 1, 2, 3 with tube #1 representing the first portion of the sample collected. Contamination with normal flora from skin or other body surfaces must be avoided. The third tube collected during lumbar puncture is most suitable for culture, as skin contaminants from the puncture usually are washed out with fluid collected in the first two tubes. STORAGE INSTRUCTIONS: The specimen should be transported immediately to the laboratory. If it cannot be processed immediately, it should be kept at room temperature or placed in an incubator. TURNAROUND TIME: Negative cultures are usually reported after 4 weeks. SPECIAL INSTRUCTIONS: The laboratory should be informed of the specific source of specimen.

Interpretive REFERENCE RANGE: No growth USE: Isolate and identify fungi, particularly *Cryptococcus neoformans*. Diagnosis is established by detection of cryptococcal antigen and/or fungus culture. LIMITATIONS: Recovery of fungi from cerebrospinal fluid is directly related to the volume of cerebrospinal fluid available. A minimum of 10 mL is recommended. *Cryptococcus* can be mistaken for small lymphocytes in the counting chamber. Yield of a single specimen is <100%; culture of additional specimens increases the chance for recovery. METHODOLOGY: Aerobic culture of centrifuged sediment on noninhibitory media usually including Sabouraud's, brain heart infusion agar (BHI), and blood agar and incubated at 25°C to 30°C and also frequently at 37°C. ADDITIONAL INFORMATION: India ink preparations are useful in identifying the presence of *Cryptococcus neoformans*, the most common fungus isolated from cerebrospinal fluid. Cryptococcal antigen titers of serum and cerebrospinal fluid provide rapid diagnosis and have greater sensitivity than India ink preparation. The diagnosis of central nervous system fungal infections is frequently complicated by the overlapping array of signs and symptoms which may accompany other clinical entities such as tuberculous meningitis, pyogenic abscess, brain tumor, hypersensitivity or allergic reactions, collagen vascular disease, leptomeningeal malignancy, chemical meningitis, meningeal inflammation secondary to contiguous suppuration, Behçet's disease, Mollaret's meningitis, and the uveomeningitic syndromes.[1,2]

Cryptococcosis may be indolent to fulminant, terminating in death within 2 weeks.[3] The India ink preparation is positive in 50% to 90% of cases, and the latex agglutination is positive in >95% of cases.[4]

Immunocompromised hosts may have aspergillosis, mucormycosis, and candidiasis in the central nervous system. Infections with species which cause phaeohyphomycosis are described. Nocardiosis can infect the cerebrospinal fluid. *Cryptococcus neoformans* has been isolated in up to 10% of patients with acquired immunodeficiency syndrome (AIDS), an entity in which multiple opportunistic CNS infections occur, including toxoplasmosis.

Footnotes

1. Rek L Jr, "Disorders That Mimic CNS Infections" *Neurol Clin*, 1986, 4:223-48.
2. Ellner JJ and Wilhelm C, "Chronic Meningitis," *Neurol Clin*, 1986, 4:115-45.
3. Fishman RA, *Cerebrospinal Fluid in Diseases of the Nervous System*, 2nd ed, Philadelphia, PA: WB Saunders Co, 1992, 273-7.
4. Chaisson RE and Volberding PA, "Clinical Manifestations of HIV Infection," *Principles and Practice of Infectious Diseases*, 3rd ed, Mandall GL, Douglas RG Jr, and Bennett JE, eds, New York, NY: Churchill Livingstone, 1990, 1078-9.

References

Greenlee JE, "Approach to Diagnosis of Meningitis - Cerebrospinal Fluid Evaluation," *Infect Dis Clin North Am*, 1990, 4(4):583-98.

Tunkel AR, Wispelwey B, and Scheld WM, "Pathogenesis and Pathophysiology of Meningitis," *Infect Dis Clin North Am*, 1990, 4(4):555-81.

Cerebrospinal Fluid India Ink Preparation *see* India Ink Preparation *on page 822*

Cerebrospinal Fluid Mycobacteria Culture

***CPT** 87116 (isolation only); 87118 (definitive identification)*

Related Information

Acid-Fast Stain *on page 770*
Bacterial Antigens, Rapid Detection Methods *on page 775*
Cerebrospinal Fluid Analysis *on page 527*
Cerebrospinal Fluid Culture *on page 798*
Cerebrospinal Fluid Fungus Culture *on previous page*
Cerebrospinal Fluid Glucose *on page 176*
Cerebrospinal Fluid Protein *on page 659*
Cryptococcal Antigen Titer, Serum or Cerebrospinal Fluid *on page 805*
Mycobacteria by DNA Probe *on page 921*
Viral Culture, Central Nervous System Symptoms *on page 1199*

Synonyms Mycobacteria Culture, Cerebrospinal Fluid

Test Commonly Includes Culture for mycobacteria and acid-fast stain if requested

Abstract A culture for mycobacteria is probably indicated if the Gram stain is negative and the white cell count and protein are elevated. Tuberculous meningitis can occur in both children and adults.

Patient Care PREPARATION: Usual sterile preparation

Specimen Cerebrospinal fluid CONTAINER: Sterile CSF tube COLLECTION: The specimen may be divided for fungus culture and India ink preparation, cryptococcal antigen testing, fungus smear, mycobacteria culture and smear, and routine bacterial culture and Gram stain if the specimen is of adequate volume for all tests requested. Transport specimen to the laboratory as soon as possible. STORAGE INSTRUCTIONS: Do not refrigerate. TURNAROUND TIME: Negative cultures are reported after 6-8 weeks.

Interpretive REFERENCE RANGE: No growth USE: Investigate cases of meningitis with subacute/subchronic or chronic onset, cases in which a history exists of contact with a subject with tuberculosis, or cases in which abnormal CSF findings lack other bacterial or viral pathogens. It is useful in immunosuppressed patients with symptoms of central nervous system infection. LIMITATIONS: Recovery of mycobacteria is directly related to the volume of specimen available for culture; 5-10 mL is recommended for optimal yield. Recovery of organisms can require months.[1] Recovery of *M. tuberculosis* in culture falls short of 100%. METHODOLOGY: Culture on selective media usually including Löwenstein-Jensen (LJ) and Middlebrook 7H11. Broth media may also be used with or without radiometric monitoring. ADDITIONAL INFORMATION: Early in the course, neutrophils may predominate in the CSF. Lymphocytes, mononuclear cells, and granulocytes are found later. Rarely does the cell count exceed 1000 cells/mm^3. The CSF is clear and colorless early; later, a pellicle forms on standing.[1] Low CSF glucose, <40 mg/dL, is frequently observed. Increased protein, almost always, is often >300 mg/dL. Measured CSF parameters may differ markedly from those anticipated for a given clinical entity for patients incapable of mounting a "normal" inflammatory response (eg, neonates, HIV-infected individuals). Other factors raising the index of suspicion include subacute or chronic onset, positive tuberculin skin test (evidence of tuberculosis outside the CNS), previous active tuberculosis, significant recent exposure to tuberculosis, and suspicion of tuberculosis on imaging procedures. Acid-fast organisms can be identified on centrifuged sediments in 60% to 80% of cases.[1]

(Continued)

Cerebrospinal Fluid Mycobacteria Culture *(Continued)*

Untreated tuberculous meningitis is fatal, usually within 3 weeks of presentation. Blacks, Hispanics, and the elderly are most frequently affected. Alcohol abuse, drug abuse, steroid therapy, head trauma, pregnancy, and AIDS all may increase risk. Despite therapy, mortality is high, approximately 30%.[2] Evaluation of contacts is recommended. It is now recognized that atypical mycobacteria species can also cause meningitis in immunosuppressed and elderly patients.[3]

Footnotes

1. Fishman RA, *Cerebrospinal Fluid in Diseases of the Nervous System*, 2nd ed, Philadelphia, PA: WB Saunders Co, 1992, 271-2.
2. Ogawa SK, Smith MA, Brennessel DJ, et al, "Tuberculous Meningitis in an Urban Medical Center," *Medicine (Baltimore)*, 1987, 66:317-26, (review).
3. Wayne LG and Sramek HA, "Agents of Newly Recognized or Infrequently Encountered Mycobacterial Diseases," *Clin Microbiol Rev*, 1992, 5(1):1-25.

References

Alvarez S and McCabe WR, "Extrapulmonary Tuberculosis Revisited: A Review of Experience of Boston City and Other Hospitals," *Medicine (Baltimore)*, 1984, 63:25-55.

Behrman RE, Kliegman RM, Nelson WE, et al, "Acute Aseptic Meningitis," *Nelson Textbook of Pediatrics*, 14th ed, Philadelphia, PA: WB Saunders Co, 1992, 664-6.

Bell WE, "Bacterial Meningitis in Children – Selected Aspects," *Pediatr Clin North Am*, 1992, 39(4):651-68.

Berenguer J, Moreno S, Laguna F, et al, "Tuberculous Meningitis in Patients Infected With the Human Immunodeficiency Virus," *N Engl J Med*, 1992, 326(10):668-72.

Vlcek B, Burchill KU, and Gordon T, "Tuberculosis Meningitis Presenting as an Obstructive Myelopathy," *J Neurosurg*, 1984, 60:196-9, (case report).

Wolinsky E, "Mycobacterial Diseases Other Than Tuberculosis," *Clin Infect Dis*, 1992, 15(1):1-10.

Cervical Culture *see* Genital Culture *on page 814*

***Cimex* Identification** *see* Arthropod Identification *on page 774*

***Clostridium botulinum* Toxin Identification Procedure** *see* Botulism, Diagnostic Procedure *on page 792*

Clostridium difficile Toxin Assay

CPT *87081 (culture); 87230 (toxin)*

Related Information

Methylene Blue Stain, Stool *on page 828*
Ova and Parasites, Stool *on page 836*
Stool Culture *on page 858*
Stool Fungus Culture *on page 861*

Synonyms Antibiotic-Associated Colitis Toxin Test; Pseudomembranous Colitis Toxin Assay; Toxin Assay, *Clostridium difficile*

Applies to Toxin A

Test Commonly Includes Toxin detection and, less commonly, culture

Specimen Stool or proctoscopic specimen **CONTAINER:** Plastic stool container (swabs are inadequate because of small volume) **COLLECTION:** Keep specimen **cold** and transport immediately to prevent deterioration of toxin. Specimens can be frozen if transportation will be delayed. **STORAGE INSTRUCTIONS:** If the specimen cannot be processed immediately, it should be refrigerated or frozen. **TURNAROUND TIME:** 1-2 days **SPECIAL INSTRUCTIONS:** When antibiotic-associated colitis is suspected, a toxin assay rather than a *C. difficile* stool culture should initially be ordered.

Interpretive REFERENCE RANGE: Presence of toxin is suggestive of disease. Isolation of organism (*C. difficile*) may occur in a small percentage of normal adults (5% to 21%) and in normal newborns. Isolation of the organism without demonstration of toxin production is a nonspecific finding since all isolates are not toxigenic. **USE:** Diagnose antibiotic-related colitis caused by *C. difficile* toxin **LIMITATIONS:** No microbiologic test for *C. difficile* disease is definitive. Culture using selective media has high sensitivity, but low specificity. Assays for cytotoxin and immunoassays for enterotoxin have sensitivities and specificities varying between approximately 85% and 98%. Latex agglutination is rapid and simple, but is not specific for any of the toxins produced by *C. difficile*, and actually recognizes an antigen produced by several other microbes; as such, this test is particularly likely to provide unreliable results. **METHODOLOGY:** Latex agglutination (LA) test to detect toxin, neutralization test in tissue culture (toxin), selective anaerobic culture (organism), enzyme immunoassay (EIA) (toxin), fluorogenic immunoassay (toxin) **ADDITIONAL INFORMATION:** Antibiotic-associated pseudomembranous colitis is produced primarily by toxigenic *C. difficile*. Toxigenic strains usually produce two toxins: toxin A, an enterotoxin that is responsible for much of the pathology of pseudomembranous colitis; and toxin B, a cytotoxin which is detected by cell culture and whose role in clinical disease is unclear.[1] Not all *C. difficile* strains are toxigenic, and even toxigenic strains may not produce disease if present in insufficient numbers; consequently, culture for *C. difficile*, using selective anaerobic media, often produces false-positive results. The most accurate clinical laboratory test for diagnosis of pseudomembranous colitis still appears to be cell culture assays for toxin B. These assays take 24-48 hours to complete, are labor intensive, and require cell culture facilities. Recently, commercially available enzyme immunoassays for toxin A have been evaluated.[2] These assays are more rapid and accessible than cytotoxin assays and are highly specific (99%) and fairly sensitive (87%).[2] Latex agglutination has been widely utilized because it is fast and easy to use.[3] Unfortunately, the assay detects an antigen produced by many microorganisms other than *C. difficile* and probably should not be relied upon to diagnose *C. difficile* disease.[1]

Pseudomembranous colitis attributable to *C. difficile* is almost always associated with antimicrobial therapy in the preceding 1-2 months.[4] Many antimicrobial agents predispose to *C. difficile* disease; it is not unique to a particular agent or group of agents. *C. difficile* is an important nosocomial pathogen that may be treated by discontinuing antimicrobial therapy, if possible, or initiating oral metronidazole or vancomycin therapy.[5]

Talbot and Price eloquently describe the histopathology of pseudomembranous colitis and antibiotic-associated colitis. (There is no membrane in the latter, and the three histopathologic patterns of pseudomembranous colitis are not found.) They describe toxigenic *C. difficile* in >90% of cases of pseudomembranous colitis, 30% to 40% of instances of antibiotic-associated colitis, and 6% to 10% of cases of antibiotic-associated diarrhea. (A normal biopsy is found in the last.)[6]

Footnotes

1. Lyerly DM, Krivan HC, and Wilkins TD, "*Clostridium difficile*: Its Disease and Toxins," *Clin Microbiol Rev*, 1988, 1:1-18.
2. De Girolami PC, Hanff PA, Eichelberger K, et al, "Multicenter Evaluation of a New Enzyme Immunoassay for Detection of *Clostridium difficile* Enterotoxin A," *J Clin Microbiol*, 1992, 30(5):1085-8.
3. Kelly MT, Champagne SG, Sherlock CH, et al, "Commercial Latex Agglutination Test for Detection of *Clostridium difficile* Associated Diarrhea," *J Clin Microbiol*, 1987, 25:1244-7.
4. Lyerly DM, "Epidemiology of *Clostridium difficile* Disease," *Clin Microbiol Newslet*, 1993, 15:49-52.
5. Talbot RW, Walker RC, and Beart RW Jr, "Changing Epidemiology, Diagnosis and Treatment of *Clostridium difficile* Toxin-Associated Colitis," *Br J Surg*, 1986, 73:457-60.
6. Talbot IC and Price AB, *Biopsy Pathology in Colorectal Disease*, London, England: Chapman and Hall, 1987, 173-9.

References

Gerding DN, "Disease Associated With *Clostridium difficile* Infection," *Ann Intern Med*, 1989, 110(4):255-7.

Gilligan PH, Janda JM, Karmali MA, et al, "Laboratory Diagnosis of Bacterial Diarrhea," *Cumitech 12A*, Nolte FS, ed, Washington, DC: American Society for Microbiology, 1992, (review).

Hatheway CL, "Toxigenic *Clostridia*," *Clin Microbiol Rev*, 1990, 3(1):66-98.

Marler LM, Siders JA, Wolters LC, et al, "Comparison of Five Cultural Procedures for Isolation of *Clostridium difficile* From Stools," *J Clin Microbiol*, 1992, 30(2):514-6.

McFarland LV, Mulligan ME, Kwok RYY, et al, "Nosocomial Acquisition of *Clostridium difficile* Infection," *N Engl J Med*, 1989, 320(4):204-10.

Wexler H, "Diagnosis of Antibiotic-Associated Disease Caused by *Clostridium difficile*," *Clin Microbiol Newslet*, 1989, 11:25-32.

Clue Cells *see* Genital Culture *on page 814*

CMVS Culture *see* Urine Culture, Clean Catch *on page 881*

Coagglutination Test for Group A Streptococci *replaced by* Group A *Streptococcus* Screen *on page 818*

Conjunctival Culture

CPT *87070*

Related Information

Adenovirus Antibody Titer *on page 629*
Adenovirus Culture *on page 1169*
Adenovirus Culture, Rapid *on page 1170*
(Continued)

Conjunctival Culture *(Continued)*

Chlamydia trachomatis Culture *on page 1171*
Chlamydia trachomatis Direct FA Test *on page 1173*
Chlamydia trachomatis DNA Probe *on page 897*
Conjunctival Fungus Culture *on next page*
Fungus Smear, Stain *on page 813*
Gram Stain *on page 815*
Herpes Simplex Virus Antigen Detection *on page 1181*
Herpes Simplex Virus Culture *on page 1182*
Herpes Simplex Virus Isolation, Rapid *on page 1184*
Ocular Cytology *on page 506*
Viral Culture *on page 1195*
Viral Culture, Eye or Ocular Symptoms *on page 1202*

Applies to Corneal Culture; Eye Culture; Ocular Culture

Test Commonly Includes Culture and smears (Gram and Giemsa) if specifically requested

Patient Care PREPARATION: Cleanse skin around eye with mild antiseptic. Gently remove make-up and ointment with sterile cotton and saline.

Specimen Eye swab CONTAINER: Swab with transport media COLLECTION: The specimen should be transported to the laboratory within 2 hours of collection. Collect the specimen by swabbing; pass moistened swab two times over lower inferior tarsal conjunctival fornix. Avoid eyelid border and lashes. (Culture these separately in a similar fashion if indicated.) Scrapings: Use local anesthetic and platinum spatula. Rub the spatula with scrapings gently over small area on slide. If the specimen is too dry, use a very small amount of nonbacteriostatic sterile water. Scraping should be done by a physician. Swab collection has a better yield for bacteria, while scraping enhances yield of filamentous organisms.[1] The laboratory and the referring physician should consult to avoid misunderstanding regarding the collection, labeling, or handling of specimens (OD=right eye, OS=left eye). Inoculation of prewarmed plates at the time of collection of the specimen (C-streak) is a useful adjunct to optimal culture yield because of the low numbers of organisms usually present. STORAGE INSTRUCTIONS: Handle carefully; transport to the laboratory immediately. TURNAROUND TIME: Preliminary reports are usually available at 24 hours. Cultures with no growth are commonly reported after 48 hours. Reports on specimens from which an organism or organisms have been isolated require a minimum of 48 hours for completion. SPECIAL INSTRUCTIONS: The laboratory should be informed of the specific source of the specimen, current antibiotic therapy, and suspected clinical diagnosis, eg, bacterial, fungal, mycobacterial, inclusion bodies (viral or chlamydial), *Neisseria gonorrhoeae*, allergic (vernal). If orbital cellulitis is present or suspected, this should be communicated to the laboratory as well.

Interpretive REFERENCE RANGE: Normal flora of the eye may include *Corynebacterium* sp (diphtheroids), *Staphylococcus epidermidis*, saprophytic fungi, *Moraxella* (*Branhamella*) *catarrhalis*, *Moraxella* sp, *Streptococcus* sp (nonhemolytic), and gram-negative rods (rare). Abnormal ocular flora include *Haemophilus influenzae*, *Haemophilus aegyptius*, *Streptococcus pneumoniae*, *Staphylococcus aureus*, *Pseudomonas aeruginosa*, *Noguchia granulosus*, *Bacillus subtilis*, *Neisseria gonorrhoeae*, and *Mycobacterium chelonei*. USE: Isolate and identify potentially pathogenic organisms LIMITATIONS: The procedure will not detect *Chlamydia*, viruses, or mycobacteria which may cause conjunctivitis and/or keratitis.[2] Scrapings are a more useful specimen than a swab for Gram stain. METHODOLOGY: Aerobic culture on blood and chocolate agar, incubation at 37°C with CO_2 ADDITIONAL INFORMATION: The major modes of transmission of disease to the conjunctiva include the hands, airborne fomites, and spread for adjacent adnexal infections. Eye infections include eyelid infections, blepharitis, dacryocystitis, orbital cellulitis, conjunctivitis, keratitis, endophthalmitis retinitis, and chorioretinitis. Pinkeye is caused by adenovirus. It presents as bilateral conjunctivitis with a sudden onset. Herpes simplex and zoster present as periorbital or corneal infections. Nontuberculous mycobacterial keratitis may occur following trauma or surgery accompanied by the use of local corticosteroids.[3]

Giemsa and Gram stains must specifically be requested. If gonorrhea is suspected, a Thayer-Martin plate should be inoculated. *Acanthamoeba* may be detected with the Calcofluor white stain (see Fungus Smear, Stain test listing for a description of the stain) and grown on nutrient agar overlaid with a lawn of *E. coli*.

Footnotes

1. Benson WH and Lanier JD, "Comparison of Techniques for Culturing Corneal Ulcers," *Ophthalmology*, 1992, 99(5):800-4.

2. Mato BAA, "*Mycobacterium chelonei* Keratitis," *Am J Ophthalmol*, 1987, 103:595-6.
3. Bullington RH Jr, Lanier JD, and Font RL, "Nontuberculous Mycobacterial Keratitis. Report of Two Cases and Review of the Literature," *Arch Ophthalmol*, 1992, 110(4):519-24.

References

Baker AS, "Ocular Infections: Clinical and Laboratory Considerations," *Clin Microbiol Newslet*, 1989, 11:97-101.

Jones DB, Leisegang TJ, and Robinson NM, *Laboratory Diagnosis of Ocular Infections*, Washington JA, coordinating ed, Cumitech 13, Washington, DC: American Society for Microbiology, 1981, (review).

Conjunctival Fungus Culture

***CPT** 87102 (isolation); 87106 (definitive identification)*

Related Information

Conjunctival Culture *on page 803*
Fungus Smear, Stain *on page 813*

Synonyms Fungus Culture, Conjunctiva

Applies to Corneal Fungus Culture; Eye Fungus Culture

Test Commonly Includes Culture, and if specimen is adequate, KOH preparation and PAS smear

Patient Care **PREPARATION:** Avoid contamination with skin flora.

Specimen Scrapings of corneal ulcer, washings of lacrimal duct, two wet swabs of conjunctiva **CONTAINER:** Sterile tube **COLLECTION:** The physician should collect corneal fragments from the edge and base of the ulcer. Swabs are insufficient. **TURNAROUND TIME:** Negative cultures are generally reported after 4 weeks. **SPECIAL INSTRUCTIONS:** The laboratory should be informed of the specific source of the specimen and the clinical diagnosis.

Interpretive **REFERENCE RANGE:** No growth **USE:** Establish the presence of keratomycosis **LIMITATIONS:** A single negative culture does not rule out the presence of fungal infection. **METHODOLOGY:** Culture on appropriate media usually including Sabouraud's medium, brain heart infusion (BHI), and blood agar incubation at 37°C and 25°C to 30°C **ADDITIONAL INFORMATION:** The more common causes of keratomycosis include *Fusarium solanae*, *Candida albicans*, *Aspergillus fumigatus*, *Curvularia* sp, *Aspergillus flavus*, other species of *Aspergillus*, *Penicillium*, *Paecilomyces*, *Fusarium*, and many other species.[1] A keratomycosis-like clinical presentation may also be encountered caused by *Nocardia asteroides* and *Mycobacterium fortuitum*. Keratomycosis is a rare complication of contact lens use.[2] Direct microscopic observation provides a higher yield than culture for the diagnosis of keratomycosis.[3]

Footnotes

1. Rebell GC and Foster RK, "Fungi of Keratomycosis," *Manual of Clinical Microbiology*, 3rd ed, Lennette EH, Balows AL, Hausler WJ, et al, eds, Washington, DC: American Society for Microbiology, 1980.
2. White GL Jr, Thiese SM, and Lundergan MK, "Contact Lens Care and Complications," *Am Fam Physician*, 1988, 37(4):187-92.
3. Ishibashi Y, Hommura S, and Matsumoto Y, "Direct Examination vs Culture of Biopsy Specimens for the Diagnosis of Keratomycosis," *Am J Ophthalmol*, 1987, 103:636-40.

Corneal Culture *see* Conjunctival Culture *on page 803*

Corneal Fungus Culture *see* Conjunctival Fungus Culture *on this page*

***Corynebacterium diphtheriae* Culture, Throat** *see* Throat Culture for *Corynebacterium diphtheriae on page 878*

Cough Plate Culture for Pertussis *replaced by Bordetella pertussis* Nasopharyngeal Culture *on page 790*

Counterimmunoelectrophoresis for Group B Streptococcal Antigen *replaced by* Group B *Streptococcus* Screen *on page 819*

Crab Lice Identification *see* Arthropod Identification *on page 774*

Cryptococcal Antigen Titer, Serum or Cerebrospinal Fluid

***CPT** 86403*

Related Information

Bacterial Antigens, Rapid Detection Methods *on page 775*
Cerebrospinal Fluid Fungus Culture *on page 800*
Cerebrospinal Fluid Mycobacteria Culture *on page 801*
Cryptococcus Antibody Titer *on page 670*
(Continued)

Cryptococcal Antigen Titer, Serum or Cerebrospinal Fluid *(Continued)*

Fungus Smear, Stain *on page 813*
India Ink Preparation *on page 822*
Sputum Fungus Culture *on page 853*

Synonyms Cerebrospinal Fluid Cryptococcal Latex Agglutination; *Cryptococcus* Antigen, Blood; *Cryptococcus* Latex Antigen Agglutination

Test Commonly Includes Testing patient's serum or CSF for the presence of cryptococcal antigen with rheumatoid factor control

Abstract Cryptococcal antigen testing is the single most useful diagnostic test for cryptococcal meningitis.[1]

Specimen Serum or cerebrospinal fluid **CONTAINER:** Red top tube, sterile CSF tube

Interpretive **REFERENCE RANGE:** Negative **CRITICAL VALUES:** Positive **USE:** Work up subacute or chronic meningitis; investigate CSF-containing cells without Gram stain positivity for bacteria (in such instances, smear of centrifuged CSF for AFB, culture for AFB, and cytology for carcinoma deserve consideration as well); establish the diagnosis of *Cryptococcus neoformans* infection; follow response to therapy **LIMITATIONS:** False-positive results may be seen in patients with rheumatoid arthritis. Less frequently positive in serum than in CSF. Disseminated cryptococcal infections usually produce a positive serum test. False-negatives occur. **METHODOLOGY:** Latex agglutination (LA) with rheumatoid factor control and in some laboratories pronase pretreatment[2,3] **ADDITIONAL INFORMATION:** Presence of cryptococcal capsular polysaccharide is indicative of cryptococcosis. Samples should either be treated to remove rheumatoid factor or tested to distinguish between positivity due to cryptococcal antigen and that due to rheumatoid factor. If this distinction cannot be made, the test cannot be interpreted. Pretreatment of the specimen with pronase reduces false-positives and increases the sensitivity of the method.[2]

The cryptococcal antigen test is positive in about 85% to 90% of patients with cryptococcal meningitis.[1] The India ink test is positive in only about 50% of cases of cryptococcal meningitis. Culture of cerebrospinal fluid for fungus should be performed in patients who are suspected of having cryptococcosis, but very large volumes of CSF are requested for optimal fungus culture.[1]

Footnotes

1. Greenlee JE, "Approach to Diagnosis of Meningitis – Cerebrospinal Fluid Evaluation," *Infect Dis Clin North Am*, 1990, 4(4):583-98.
2. Gray LD and Roberts GD, "Experience With the Use of Pronase to Eliminate Interference Factors in the Latex Agglutination Test for Cryptococcal Antigen," *J Clin Microbiol*, 1988, 26:2450-1.
3. Stockman L and Roberts GD, "Specificity of the Latex Test for Cryptococcal Antigen: A Rapid Simple Method for Eliminating Interference Factors," *J Clin Microbiol*, 1983, 17:945-7.

References

Berlin L and Pincus JH, "Cryptococcal Meningitis: False-Negative Antigen Test Results and Cultures in Nonimmunosuppressed Patients," *Arch Neurol*, 1989, 46(12):1312-6.

Temstet A, Roux P, Poirot JL, et al, "Evaluation of a Monoclonal Antibody-Based Latex Agglutination Test for Diagnosis of Cryptococcosis: Comparison With Two Tests Using Polyclonal Antibodies," *J Clin Microbiol*, 1992, 30(10):2544-50.

***Cryptococcus* Antigen, Blood** *see* Cryptococcal Antigen Titer, Serum or Cerebrospinal Fluid *on previous page*

***Cryptococcus* Latex Antigen Agglutination** *see* Cryptococcal Antigen Titer, Serum or Cerebrospinal Fluid *on previous page*

Cryptosporidium Diagnostic Procedures, Stool

CPT 87015 (concentration); 87206 (fluorescent stain); 87207 (special stain)

Related Information

Acid-Fast Stain, Modified, *Nocardia* Species *on page 771*
Fungus Smear, Stain *on page 813*
Methylene Blue Stain, Stool *on page 828*
Ova and Parasites, Stool *on page 836*
Stool Culture *on page 858*

Synonyms Acid-Fast Stain, Modified, *Cryptosporidium*

Test Commonly Includes Examination of stool for the presence of *Cryptosporidium* by phase contrast microscopy and/or modified acid-fast stain, or fluorescent labeled antibody

Abstract *Cryptosporidium*, a parasite, may cause severe diarrhea, predominantly in immunocompromised individuals.

Specimen Fresh stool; stool preserved with 10% formalin or sodium acetate-acetic acid formalin preservative **CONTAINER:** Plastic stool container **COLLECTION:** Transport fresh specimen to the laboratory promptly following collection. Specimen on outside of container poses excessive risk of contamination to laboratory personnel. **SPECIAL INSTRUCTIONS:** Procedures for the detection of *Cryptosporidium* in humans have recently become available in most clinical laboratories. Consult the laboratory regarding availability of the procedure and specific specimen collection instructions before collecting the specimen.

Interpretive **REFERENCE RANGE:** Negative **USE:** A part of the differential work-up of diarrhea, particularly in immunocompromised hosts and suspected AIDS patients; establish the diagnosis of cryptosporidiosis by demonstration of the oocysts. A recent outbreak in healthy individuals from a contaminated water supply was noted. **LIMITATIONS:** *Cryptosporidium* is not detected by standard methods used to examine stool specimens for other ova and parasites; special stains are required for its detection, and in many laboratories, must be specifically requested. The organisms are most readily demonstrated in diarrheal stools. Forms of *Blastocystis hominis* may cause confusion if Giemsa stain is used. Most recommended procedures cannot be performed on polyvinyl alcohol (PVA) preserved specimens. **METHODOLOGY:** Phase contrast microscopy after floatation concentration technique (Sheather's); modified acid-fast stain on air-dried, methanol-fixed smears (decolorization with 1% H_2SO_4).[1] Auramine and carbol-fuchsin stain is used by some laboratories for screening.[2] A technique utilizing formalin-ethyl acetate and floatation over hypertonic saline is reported to enhance detection of *Cryptosporidium* oocysts.[3] Fluorescent-labeled anti-*Cryptosporidium* antibodies are commercially available.[4] **ADDITIONAL INFORMATION:** *Cryptosporidium* is a coccidian parasite of the intestines and respiratory tract of many animals including mice, sheep, snakes, turkeys, chickens, cows, monkeys, and domestic cats. It is a cause of severe and chronic diarrhea in patients with hypogammaglobulinemia and the acquired immune deficiency syndrome.[5] The organism is widely recognized as a disease of the immunocompromised patient, however, it can also cause disease in immunocompetent subjects. Animal contact, travel to endemic areas, living in a rural environment, and day care attendance by toddlers have been recognized as risk factors for the development of cryptosporidiosis.[6] Perinatal infection has been reported.[7] Children are more prone to develop infection than are adults. In these patients, the disease is a self-limited gastroenteritis, but in immunocompromised patients, a profound enteropathy results. A seasonal variation in incidence exists with the highest frequency reported in summer and autumn. The organism can be demonstrated in biopsies of small bowel and colon, adherent to surface of the epithelial cells (Giemsa stain) and by demonstration in feces by floatation with modified acid-fast stain or smear. Most therapeutic regimens for cryptosporidiosis are not successful unless immunosuppression is reversed.

Footnotes

1. Koneman EW, Allen SD, Janda WM, et al, *Color Atlas and Textbook of Diagnostic Microbiology*, 4th ed, Philadelphia, PA: JB Lippincott Co, 1992.
2. Casemore DP, Armstrong M, Sands RL, et al, "Laboratory Diagnosis of Cryptosporidiosis," *J Clin Pathol*, 1985, 38:1337-41.
3. Weber R, Bryan RT, and Juranek DD, "Improved Stool Concentration Procedure for Detection of *Cryptosporidium* Oocysts in Fecal Specimens," *J Clin Microbiol*, 1992, 30(11):2869-73.
4. Garcia LS, Shum AC, and Bruckner DA, "Evaluation of a New Monoclonal Antibody Combination Reagent for Direct Fluorescence Detection of *Giardia* Cysts and *Cryptosporidium* Oocysts in Human Fecal Specimens," *J Clin Microbiol*, 1992, 30(12):3255-7.
5. Koch KL, et al, "Cryptosporidiosis in a Patient With Hemophilia, Common Variable Hypogammaglobulinemia and the Acquired Immunodeficiency Syndrome," *Ann Intern Med*, 1983, 99:337-40.
6. Kocoshis SA, "Diagnosis and Treatment of Cryptosporidiosis in Children," *Compr Ther*, 1986, 12:56-61.
7. Dale BA, Gordon G, Thomson R, et al, "Perinatal Infection With *Cryptosporidium*," *Lancet*, 1987, 1042-3, (letter).

References

Baron EJ, Schenone C, and Tanenbaum B, "Comparison of Three Methods for Detection of *Cryptosporidium* Oocysts in a Low-Prevalence Population," *J Clin Microbiol*, 1989, 27(1):223-4.

Current WL, "The Biology of *Cryptosporidium*," *ASM News*, 1988, 54:605-11, (review).

Garcia LS, "Incidence of *Cryptosporidium* in All Patients Submitting Stool Specimens for Ova and Parasite Examination: Monoclonal Antibody IFA Method," *Diagn Microbiol Infect Dis*, 1988, 11:25-7.

Petersen C, "Cryptosporidiosis in Patients Infected With the Human Immunodeficiency Virus," *Clin Infect Dis*, 1992, 15(6):903-9.

(Continued)

Cryptosporidium Diagnostic Procedures, Stool *(Continued)*

Soave R and Armstrong D, "*Cryptosporidium* and Cryptosporidiosis," *Rev Infect Dis*, 1986, 8:1012-21, (review).

Crystal Violet *see* Gram Stain *on page 815*

CSF Culture *see* Cerebrospinal Fluid Culture *on page 798*

Cul-de-sac Anaerobic Culture *see* Endometrium Culture *on page 811*

Culture, Blood *see* Blood Culture, Aerobic and Anaerobic *on page 784*

Culture, Cerebrospinal Fluid *see* Cerebrospinal Fluid Culture *on page 798*

Culture, Ear *see* Ear Culture *on page 810*

Culture for *Leptospira*, Urine *see* *Leptospira* Culture, Urine *on page 827*

Darkfield Examination, Leptospirosis

CPT *87164*

Related Information

Leptospira Culture, Urine *on page 827*
Leptospira Serodiagnosis *on page 718*

Synonyms Darkfield Microscopy, *Leptospira*; Leptospirosis, Darkfield Examination

Test Commonly Includes Examination of serum, urine, or CSF for organisms

Abstract The general term leptospirosis is preferred to the synonyms, Weil's disease and canicola fever. It is a widespread zoonosis. Culture and serology are recommended for diagnosis; darkfield examination is not.[1]

Specimen Urine, serum, cerebrospinal fluid **CONTAINER:** Sterile plastic urine container, red top tube, or sterile CSF tube **CAUSES FOR REJECTION:** Specimen dried out

Interpretive **USE:** Determine the presence of *Leptospira* for the diagnosis of Weil's syndrome, hemorrhagic fever with renal syndrome, atypical pneumonia syndrome, aseptic meningitis, and myocarditis including cardiac arrhythmias. Special features are found in pediatric patients.[1] Failure to detect leptospires does not rule out their presence. **LIMITATIONS:** The concentration of leptospires in blood and CSF is low. Therefore, concentration by centrifugation with sodium oxalate or heparin can be useful. The incidence of false-positives is increased because fibrils and cellular extrusions can be mistaken for organisms. **Dr Jay Sanford recommends that direct examination of blood or urine by darkfield methods frequently results in failure or misdiagnosis and should not be used.**[1] **METHODOLOGY:** A very small drop of fluid is distributed in a thin layer between a glass coverslip and slide. Positives should be confirmed by serologic or cultural methods. The typical morphology helicoidal, flexible organisms 6-20 μm long and 0.1 μm in diameter usually with semicircular hooked ends should be observed before a presumptive diagnosis is made. **ADDITIONAL INFORMATION:** *Leptospira* are present in blood early in course of disease (first week only). After 10-14 days, they may be found in the urine. Artifacts are common. Urine must be neutral or alkaline. Culture has much greater value for diagnosis. Saprophytic strains as well as pathogenic ones exist. Darkfield microscopy is best used to demonstrate leptospires in specimens in which a high concentration of organisms is present, ie, tissue from animals (guinea pig or hamster), inoculation including blood, peritoneal fluid, or liver suspensions. Urine or kidney suspensions from swine, dogs, and domestic animals may also yield positive darkfield examination.

Footnotes

1. Sanford JP, "Leptospirosis," *Harrison's Principles of Internal Med*, 12th ed, Chapter 130, Wilson JD, Braunwald E, Isselbacher KJ, et al, eds, New York, NY: McGraw-Hill Inc, 1991, 663-6.

References

Alexander AD, "*Leptospira*," *Manual of Clinical Microbiology*, 5th ed, Balows A, Hausler WJ Jr, Herrmann KL, et al, eds, Washington, DC: American Society for Microbiology, 1991, 554-9.

Faine S, "Leptospirosis," *Laboratory Diagnosis of Infectious Diseases: Principles and Practice*, Vol 1, New York, NY: Springer-Verlag, 1988, 344-52.

Darkfield Examination, Syphilis

CPT *87164*

Related Information

Automated Reagin Test *on page 642*
FTA-ABS, Cerebrospinal Fluid *on page 679*

FTA-ABS, Serum *on page 680*
RPR *on page 742*
VDRL, Cerebrospinal Fluid *on page 761*
VDRL, Serum *on page 762*

Synonyms Darkfield Microscopy, Syphilis; Syphilis, Darkfield Examination; *Treponema pallidum* Darkfield Examination

Test Commonly Includes Cleansing of chancre, procurement of specimen, and darkfield examination

Abstract *Treponema pallidum* is a thin organism that cannot be visualized by conventional light microscopy. Darkfield examination is appropriate for the evaluation of chancre (primary lues) and condylomata lata (secondary syphilis)

Patient Care PREPARATION: The surface of the chancre or condyloma is cleansed by the physician with a swab moistened with saline. This removes exudate and excess bacteria contamination. Serum is then collected from the surface of the chancre using a small pipette. The serum is placed on a slide or coverslip. Alternatively, the specimen can be collected by directly touching the slide to the lesion. The objective is to obtain clear serum exudate from the subsurface of the lesion. It is then examined by darkfield microscopy.

Specimen Moist serum from the base of a cleansed, unhealed chancre or condyloma. The youngest lesion available is best. The chance of identification of treponemes decreases with the age of the lesion as it dries and locally heals. *Treponema pallidum* can be found by lymph node aspiration in the secondary stage of lues. CAUSES FOR REJECTION: Healed chancre, previous treatment, ointment, dried-up specimen

Interpretive REFERENCE RANGE: *Treponema pallidum* has a rapid and purposeful motion as it travels across the microscopic field. The organisms appear as a tight corkscrew, characterized by 6-14 coils. The organisms are 1-1.5 times the diameter of an RBC in length (0.10-0.18 μm by 6-20 μm).[1] USE: Determine the presence of characteristic spirochetes in lesions suspected of being syphilis LIMITATIONS: Darkfield examination is of limited value in oral and rectal lesions because of the normal presence of other, nonpathogenic spirochetes. Dry or bloody specimens render this examination worthless. The specimen should be examined within 15 minutes of collection because the organisms lose motility with decrease in temperature. Serologic diagnosis is described in the Immunology and Serology chapter. CONTRAINDICATIONS: Antibiotic therapy prior to the darkfield examination. The organisms are rapidly cleared following therapy. METHODOLOGY: Darkfield microscopy. Motile organisms are observed to rotate around their long axis and to bend, snap, and flex along their length at 90 degree angles. A smooth translational back and forth directed movement is also apparent. Nonpathogenic mucosal treponemes are often irregularly coiled, longer than *T. pallidum*, and are characterized by a different kind of motility.[1] ADDITIONAL INFORMATION: *Treponema* can be found in skin lesions and lymph nodes in secondary syphilis but are more plentiful in primary chancres. They cannot be grown in culture. The Centers for Disease Control (CDC) and others use fluorescent microscopy with monoclonal or polyclonal anti-*T. pallidum* antibodies for examination of exudates.[1]

Footnotes

1. Hook EW 3d and Marra CM, "Acquired Syphilis in Adults," *N Engl J Med*, 1992, 326(16):1060-9.

References

Fitzgerald TJ, "*Treponema*," *Manual of Clinical Microbiology*, 5th ed, Balows A, Hausler WJ Jr, Herrmann KL, et al, eds, Washington, DC: American Society for Microbiology, 1991, 568-9.

Larsen SA, "Syphilis," *Clin Lab Med*, 1989, 9(3):545-57.

Darkfield Microscopy, *Leptospira* *see* Darkfield Examination, Leptospirosis *on previous page*

Darkfield Microscopy, Syphilis *see* Darkfield Examination, Syphilis *on previous page*

Deer Tick Identification *see* Arthropod Identification *on page 774*

Dermatophyte Fungus Culture *see* Skin Fungus Culture *on page 845*

Diphtheria Culture *see* Throat Culture for *Corynebacterium diphtheriae* *on page 878*

DNA Probe *Legionella* *see Legionella* Culture *on page 825*

Ear Culture

CPT 87070 (aerobic)

Related Information

Gram Stain *on page 815*

Synonyms Culture, Ear

Applies to Middle Ear Culture; Outer Ear Culture; Tympanocentesis Culture

Test Commonly Includes Gram stain and culture for aerobic bacteria

Patient Care PREPARATION: Cleanse the site to reduce the background contamination level

Specimen Aspirate (tympanocentesis) for otitis media; moist swab for otitis externa. In cases of otitis media in which the eardrum has ruptured, a swab may be used to collect the exudate. CONTAINER: Sterile tube or Culturette® COLLECTION: Specimen should be transported to the laboratory as soon as possible. TURNAROUND TIME: Preliminary reports are usually available after 24 hours; negative cultures are usually reported after 48 hours. SPECIAL INSTRUCTIONS: When ear cultures for obligate anaerobic bacteria are needed, consultation with the laboratory may be helpful. If a specific agent such as *Pseudomonas*, *Haemophilus*, or *Candida* is suspected, the laboratory should be informed.

Interpretive REFERENCE RANGE: Normal flora of the skin of the healthy ear includes *Staphylococcus epidermidis*, *Corynebacterium* sp, and *Staphylococcus aureus* USE: Determine the etiologic agent of otitis externa or otitis media LIMITATIONS: Superficial swab specimens are insensitive and nonspecific for definition of the etiology of otitis media; their use for this purpose should be discouraged. Initial therapy of this condition should be empiric. CONTRAINDICATIONS: The presence of topical ointments or drugs in or on the site to be cultured METHODOLOGY: Aerobic and anaerobic bacterial culture of specimens obtained by tympanocentesis; aerobic cultures, only, of swab specimens ADDITIONAL INFORMATION: Correlation of nasopharyngeal cultures with results of tympanocentesis culture is poor and lacks predictive value in identification of the causative agent of otitis media. Bodor[1,2] and associates have described the good correlation between conjunctival cultures and cultures obtained by tympanocentesis and have described the simultaneous occurrence of conjunctivitis and otitis as a clinical syndrome in children. In decreasing order of frequency, the following organisms have been recovered from tympanocentesis: *S. pneumoniae* (50% to 75%), *H. influenzae* (10% to 30%), *Moraxella* (*Branhamella*) *catarrhalis* (5% to 10%), *Streptococcus pyogenes* (5% to 10%), *Staphylococcus aureus* (1% to 5%), *Pseudomonas aeruginosa* (0.1% to 1%). *E. coli*, *Klebsiella pneumoniae*, *Pseudomonas aeruginosa* may be isolated from neonates. In therapeutic failures, *S. aureus*, and *P. aeruginosa* are most frequently recovered.[3] In a series of 908 cases, *H. influenzae* made up 49.7% of them. The incidence of *H. influenzae* peaked at 2 years of age and fell off markedly after 6 years of age.[4] Tympanocentesis is not usually required in primary infections. It is to be considered in treatment failures and neonates. *Candida* superinfection may complicate therapy for recurring ear infections and may be a cause of persistent otorrhea.[5] Otitis externa is frequently caused by *P. aeruginosa* and less frequently by *Candida* sp, *Proteus* sp, *S. aureus*, and *Trichophyton* sp.

Footnotes

1. Bodor FF, Marchant CD, and Shurin PA, "Bacterial Etiology of Conjunctivitis-Otitis Media Syndrome," *Pediatrics*, 1985, 76:26-8.
2. Bodor FF, "Conjunctivitis-Otitis Syndrome," *Pediatrics*, 1982, 69:695-8.
3. Bland RD, "Otitis Media in the First Six Weeks of Life. Diagnosis Bacteriology and Management," *Pediatrics*, 1972, 187-97.
4. Calhoun KH, Norris WB, and Hokanson JA, "Bacteriology of Middle Ear Effusions," *South Med J*, 1988, 81(3):332-6.
5. Cohen SR and Thompson JW, "Otitic Candidiasis in Children: An Evaluation of the Problem and Effectiveness of Ketoconazole in 10 Patients," *Ann Otol Rhinol Laryngol*, 1990, 99(6 Pt 1):427-31.

References

Kligman EW, "Treatment of Otitis Media," *Am Fam Physician*, 1992, 45(1):242-50.

Macknin ML, "Respiratory Infections in Children. What Helps and What Doesn't?" *Postgrad Med*, 1992, 92(2):235-8, 243, 247-50.

Randall DA, Fornadley JA, and Kennedy KS, "Management of Recurrent Otitis Media," *Am Fam Physician*, 1992, 45(5):2117-23.

***E. coli*: 0157:H7 Culture** *see* Stool Culture, Diarrheagenic *E. coli on page 860*

Ectoparasite Identification *see* Arthropod Identification *on page 774*

Endocervical Anaerobic Culture *see* Endometrium Culture *on next page*

Endocervical Culture *see* Genital Culture *on page 814*

Endometrium Culture

CPT *87070 (aerobic); 87075 (anaerobic isolation); 87076 (definitive identification, each anaerobic organism)*

Related Information

Abscess, Aerobic and Anaerobic Bacterial Culture *on page 768*
Actinomyces Culture, All Sites *on page 772*
Biopsy or Body Fluid Anaerobic Bacterial Culture *on page 778*
Chlamydia trachomatis Culture *on page 1171*
Chlamydia trachomatis DNA Probe *on page 897*
Genital Culture for *Ureaplasma urealyticum on page 1180*

Synonyms Amniotic Fluid Anaerobic Culture; Anaerobic Culture, Cul-de-sac; Anaerobic Culture, Endometrium; Anaerobic Culture, Uterus; Cul-de-sac Anaerobic Culture; Endocervical Anaerobic Culture; Genitourinary Anaerobic Culture, Female; Uterus Anaerobic Culture

Applies to Intrauterine Device Culture; IUD Culture

Test Commonly Includes Culture and direct smear if requested

Patient Care PREPARATION: Aseptic preparation of the aspiration site

Specimen Scrapings, aspirates, or swabs taken from endometrium or endocervix without contamination with vaginal or exocervical flora. Protected or sheathed swabs are useful in reducing contamination. Use of an unprotected swab is reported to significantly increase the recovery of both aerobic and anaerobic bacteria commonly regarded as potential pathogens.[1] Specimens for anaerobic culture should be accompanied by a specimen for routine culture from the same site. CONTAINER: Anaerobic transport tube; sterile tube or swab COLLECTION: Disinfect cervix and attempt to aspirate material through the cervical os, expel air bubbles from the syringe, and inject into an anaerobic transport vial. Transport the specimen to the laboratory as soon as possible after collection. STORAGE INSTRUCTIONS: Do not refrigerate or incubate. CAUSES FOR REJECTION: Specimens which have been refrigerated or have an excessive delay in transit have a less than optimal yield TURNAROUND TIME: Negative cultures are reported after 7-10 days. SPECIAL INSTRUCTIONS: The laboratory should be informed of the specific source of the specimen, current antibiotic therapy, and clinical diagnosis

Interpretive REFERENCE RANGE: No growth USE: Isolate and identify aerobic and anaerobic organisms LIMITATIONS: Unprotected swab cultures are invariably contaminated with cervicovaginal flora. Specimens received in anaerobic transport containers are not optimal for routine or fungus culture. ADDITIONAL INFORMATION: Actinomycosis has been reported in association with endometritis and pelvic infection associated with intrauterine devices.[2]

Anaerobic Infections of the Female Genital Tract

Abscesses in glands	Peritonitis
Abscesses in soft tissues	Postoperative infections
Endocervicitis	Pyometra
Endometritis	Salpingitis
IUD (intrauterine device) associated infections	Septic abortion
Pelvic abscess	Tubo-ovarian abscess
Pelvic actinomycosis	Vaginitis, nonspecific

Clinical findings associated with anaerobic infections include proximity of the infection to a mucosal surface, foul-smelling discharge, gas in the tissues, and abscess formation. The most common isolates are of anaerobic gram-positive cocci (*Peptostreptococcus*) and *Bacteroides* sp. Infections are frequently polymicrobic. Aggressive antimicrobial therapy including beta-lactamase resistant antimicrobials[3] and surgical procedures (curettage, incision, and drainage) are frequently required. *Chlamydia* and *Ureaplasma* are often implicated in endometrial and pelvic infections.[4]

In a large series of patients with obstetric and gynecologic infections, the most frequently isolated aerobic and facultative organisms were *Lactobacillus* sp, *E. coli*, *N. gonorrhoeae*, *S. aureus*, and group B *Streptococcus*. The most commonly isolated anaerobic organisms were *Bacteroides* sp; anaerobic gram-positive cocci, and *Fusobacterium* sp were also recovered. Eighteen percent of the isolates were beta-lactamase producing.[4]

Footnotes

1. Martens MG, Faro S, Hammill HA, et al, "Transcervical Uterine Cultures With a New Endometrial Suction Curette: A Comparison of Three Sampling Methods in Postpartum Endometritis," *Obstet Gynecol*, 1989, 74(2):273-6.
2. Gupta PK and Woodruff JD, "*Actinomyces* in Vaginal Smears," *JAMA*, 1982, 247:1175-6.
3. Brook I, Frazier EH, and Thomas RL, "Aerobic and Anaerobic Microbiologic Factors and Recovery of Beta-Lactamase Producing Bacteria From Obstetric and Gynecologic Infection," *Surg Gynecol Obstet*, 1991, 172(2):138-44.

(Continued)

Endometrium Culture *(Continued)*

4. Watts DH, Eschenbach DA, and Kenny GE, "Early Postpartum Endometritis: The Role of Bacteria, Genital *Mycoplasmas*, and *Chlamydia trachomatis*," *Obstet Gynecol*, 1989, 73(1):52-60.

References

Gibbs RS, "Severe Infections in Pregnancy," *Med Clin North Am*, 1989, 73(3):713-21.

Pensson E, "Genital Actinomycosis and *Actinomyces israelii* in the Female Genital Tract," *Adv Contracyst*, 1987, 3:115-23, (review).

Endotracheal Anaerobic Culture *see* Bronchial Aspirate Anaerobic Culture *on page 792*

Enteric Pathogens Culture, Routine *see* Stool Culture *on page 858*

***Enterobius vermicularis* Preparation** *see* Pinworm Preparation *on page 841*

Enterohemorrhagic *E. coli*, Stool Culture *see* Stool Culture, Diarrheagenic *E. coli* *on page 860*

Enteropathogenic *E. coli*, Stool Culture *see* Stool Culture, Diarrheagenic *E. coli* *on page 860*

Enterotoxigenic *E. coli*, Stool Culture *see* Stool Culture, Diarrheagenic *E. coli* *on page 860*

Enzyme Immunoassay for Group A *Streptococcus* Antigen *see* Group A *Streptococcus* Screen *on page 818*

E-Test *see* Susceptibility Testing, Unusual Isolates/Fastidious Organisms *on page 873*

Eye Culture *see* Conjunctival Culture *on page 803*

Eye Fungus Culture *see* Conjunctival Fungus Culture *on page 805*

Fecal Leukocyte Stain *see* Methylene Blue Stain, Stool *on page 828*

Flagellates *see* Ova and Parasites, Stool *on page 836*

Flea Identification *see* Arthropod Identification *on page 774*

Fluorochrome Stain *see* Acid-Fast Stain *on page 770*

Fractional Bactericidal Concentration (FBC) *see* Susceptibility Testing, Antimicrobial Combinations *on page 868*

Fractional Inhibitory Concentration (FIC) *see* Susceptibility Testing, Antimicrobial Combinations *on page 868*

Fungi Susceptibility Testing *see* Susceptibility Testing, Fungi *on page 869*

Fungus Culture, Biopsy *see* Biopsy or Body Fluid Fungus Culture *on page 780*

Fungus Culture, Blood *see* Blood Fungus Culture *on page 789*

Fungus Culture, Body Fluid *see* Biopsy or Body Fluid Fungus Culture *on page 780*

Fungus Culture, Bone Marrow *see* Biopsy or Body Fluid Fungus Culture *on page 780*

Fungus Culture, Cerebrospinal Fluid *see* Cerebrospinal Fluid Fungus Culture *on page 800*

Fungus Culture, Conjunctiva *see* Conjunctival Fungus Culture *on page 805*

Fungus Culture, Gastric Aspirate *see* Sputum Fungus Culture *on page 853*

Fungus Culture, Skin, Hair and Nail *see* Skin Fungus Culture *on page 845*

Fungus Culture, Sputum *see* Sputum Fungus Culture *on page 853*

Fungus Culture, Stool *see* Stool Fungus Culture *on page 861*

Fungus Culture, Urine *see* Urine Fungus Culture *on page 883*

Fungus Smear, Stain

CPT *87205*

Related Information

Acid-Fast Stain, Modified, *Nocardia* Species *on page 771*
Biopsy or Body Fluid Fungus Culture *on page 780*
Blastomycosis Serology *on page 645*
Candida Antigen *on page 652*
Candidiasis Serologic Test *on page 652*
Coccidioidomycosis Antibodies *on page 664*
Conjunctival Culture *on page 803*
Conjunctival Fungus Culture *on page 805*
Cryptococcal Antigen Titer, Serum or Cerebrospinal Fluid *on page 805*
Cryptococcus Antibody Titer *on page 670*
Cryptosporidium Diagnostic Procedures, Stool *on page 806*
Gram Stain *on page 815*
Histoplasmosis Serology *on page 695*
India Ink Preparation *on page 822*
KOH Preparation *on page 825*
Skin Biopsies *on page 84*
Skin Fungus Culture *on page 845*
Sporotrichosis Serology *on page 748*
Sputum Fungus Culture *on page 853*
Susceptibility Testing, Fungi *on page 869*
Urine Fungus Culture *on page 883*

Applies to Calcofluor White; GMS Stain; Gomori Methenamine Silver Stain; Periodic Acid Schiff (PAS)

Test Commonly Includes Smear only; fungus culture and KOH preparation must usually be ordered separately

Patient Care PREPARATION: Avoid contamination with skin flora. Specimen should be obtained by physician only.

Specimen The same specimen as required for fungal culture of the specific site. For conjunctiva or cornea, scrapings of corneal ulcer or wet swabs of conjunctiva. CONTAINER: Glass microscope slide CAUSES FOR REJECTION: Insufficient specimen volume, no cellular material on slide SPECIAL INSTRUCTIONS: The laboratory should be informed of the specific site of specimen and clinical diagnosis. In many laboratories, these procedures are performed by the histology or cytology sections rather than the Microbiology Laboratory.

Interpretive REFERENCE RANGE: No yeast or hyphal elements seen USE: Aid in the diagnosis of fungal disease; used in combination with fungus culture LIMITATIONS: A negative smear does not rule out the presence of fungal infection. METHODOLOGY: Periodic acid Schiff (PAS) stain, Calcofluor white, and Gomori methenamine silver stain (GMS) are used to identify fungal structures. ADDITIONAL INFORMATION: Calcofluor white stain and KOH preparation may be more sensitive than culture in detecting keratomycosis. Calcofluor white dye binds to cellulose and chitin and fluoresces with longwave UV light and shortwave visible light. Fungal elements viewed under UV light demonstrate a brilliant apple green fluorescence that stands out from cells, tissue debris, and background. The preparations can subsequently be overstained with PAS or GMS.[1] *Acanthamoeba* keratitis can be documented by use of Calcofluor white stain.[2]
Caution: Do not fix with ethanol as the *Acanthamoeba* cysts will be desiccated and will not adhere adequately to the direct preparation slides. The PAS stain with a light green counterstain demonstrates the yeast forms, spores and the hyphae of fungi as pinkish red on a green background. The filaments of *Actinomyces* and *Nocardia* are not satisfactorily shown but do stain with Gram stain. *Nocardia* is modified acid-fast positive.

Footnotes

1. Hageage GJ and Harrington BJ, "Use of Calcofluor White in Clinical Mycology," *Lab Med*, 1984, 15:109-11.
2. Marines HM, Osato MS, and Font RL, "The Value of Calcofluor White in the Diagnosis of Mycotic and *Acanthamoeba* Infections of the Eye and Ocular Adnexa," *Ophthalmology*, 1987, 94:23-6.

References

Gray LD and Roberts GD, "Laboratory Diagnosis of Systemic Fungal Diseases," *Infect Dis Clin North Am*, 1988, 2:779-803.

Koneman EW and Roberts GD, *Practical Laboratory Mycology*, 3rd ed, Baltimore, MD: Williams & Wilkins, 1985, 21.

Gastric Biopsy Culture for *Helicobacter pylori* *see Helicobacter pylori* Urease Test and Culture *on page 820*

GC Culture *see Neisseria gonorrhoeae* Culture *on page 831*

GC Smear *see Neisseria gonorrhoeae* Smear *on page 834*

Genital Culture

CPT *87070*

Related Information

Chlamydia trachomatis Culture *on page 1171*
Chlamydia trachomatis Direct FA Test *on page 1173*
Chlamydia trachomatis DNA Probe *on page 897*
Genital Culture for *Ureaplasma urealyticum on page 1180*
Group B *Streptococcus* Screen *on page 819*
Herpes Simplex Virus Antigen Detection *on page 1181*
Herpes Simplex Virus Culture *on page 1182*
Neisseria gonorrhoeae Culture *on page 831*
RPR *on page 742*
Trichomonas Preparation *on page 879*
VDRL, Serum *on page 762*
Viral Culture, Urogenital *on page 1207*

Applies to *Candida* Culture, Genital; Cervical Culture; Clue Cells; Endocervical Culture; Prostatic Fluid Culture; Vaginal Culture

Test Commonly Includes Culture for aerobic organisms, *Candida* sp, and *Neisseria gonorrhoeae*. *Gardnerella* and *Mobiluncus*, Gram stain, and KOH preparation may require separate requests.

Specimen Swab of vagina, cervix, discharge, aspirated endocervical, endometrial, prostatic fluid, or urethral discharge **CONTAINER:** Sterile tube or Culturette® **COLLECTION:** The specimen should be transported to the laboratory within 2 hours of collection. Do not refrigerate. **TURNAROUND TIME:** Preliminary reports are usually available at 24 hours. Cultures from which pathogens are isolated usually require a minimum of 48 hours for completion. **SPECIAL INSTRUCTIONS:** The laboratory should be informed of the specific source of specimen, age of patient, current antibiotic therapy, clinical diagnosis, and time of collection.

Interpretive **REFERENCE RANGE:** Normal flora; properly collected prostatic fluid and endocervical cultures are normally sterile. **CRITICAL VALUES:** Recovery of *Neisseria gonorrhoeae*, herpes simplex virus, and perhaps *Streptococcus agalactiae* (beta-hemolytic group B strep) during pregnancy **USE:** Primarily used to isolate and identify potentially pathogenic bacteria and yeasts. Infectious causes of abnormal vaginal discharge or vulvovaginitis recognizable by these procedures include *Neisseria gonorrhoeae*, *Gardnerella vaginalis*, *Candida* sp, *Staphylococcus* sp, and members of the family *Enterobacteriaceae*. Agents not detected by these procedures include *Treponema pallidum*, *Trichomonas vaginalis*, *Mobiluncus* sp, *Mycoplasma hominis*, *Ureaplasma urealyticum*, *Chlamydia trachomatis*, herpes simplex virus, human papillomavirus, *Enterobius vermicularis* (pinworms), *Giardia lamblia*, and anaerobic bacteria of all types (if anaerobic cultures are not performed); *Haemophilus ducreyi* (chancroid) may be detected, but it is prudent to inform the laboratory if chancroid is suspected. May also be used to document the presence of *Staphylococcus aureus* in cases of suspected toxic shock syndrome and to screen for genital carriage of *Streptococcus agalactiae* during pregnancy. **LIMITATIONS:** As many of the organisms recovered from the female genital tract can be either pathogens or normal flora (eg, *Gardnerella vaginalis*, *Candida* sp, *Staphylococcus* sp, *Enterobacteriaceae*), it is extremely difficult to determine their clinical significance. Most laboratories do not (and should not) culture specimens of this type for anaerobes. **METHODOLOGY:** Aerobic culture with selective (Thayer-Martin) and nonselective media incubated at 35°C to 37°C with CO_2 **ADDITIONAL INFORMATION:** Rapid-growing aerobic organisms which predominate are usually identified. Susceptibility testing can be performed if indicated. Appropriate cultures often include screening for *N. gonorrhoeae*, *Candida albicans*, *Staphylococcus aureus*, group B streptococci, and *Gardnerella vaginalis*. Normal flora of the vagina is dependent upon age, glycogen content, pH, exogenous hormone therapy, etc. Normal vaginal flora includes numerous anaerobes, corynebacteria, enteric gram-negative rods, enterococci, lactobacilli, *Moraxella* sp, staphylococci, streptococci (alpha and nonhemolytic), *Mycobacterium smegmatis*. The laboratory should be consulted to arrange for special toxin identification procedures if toxic shock syndrome is suspected and *Staphylococcus aureus* is recovered.

Vaginitis is one of the most commonly encountered complaints of female patients. A significant portion of these appear to be due to specific etiologic agents such as *Candida* sp or *Trichomonas vaginalis*. Nonspecific vaginitis, also called bacterial vaginosis, is characterized by an excessive malodorous vaginal discharge associated with a decrease in the number of lactobacilli and an increase in the number of *Gardnerella vaginalis* and other bacteria such as *Bacteroides* sp, *Prevotella* sp, and *Peptostreptococcus* sp.[1] Additionally, curved, motile, anaerobic gram-negative bacilli identified as *Mobiluncus* sp have been associated with bacterial vaginosis. Presently, bacterial cultures contribute little to the diagnosis of bacterial vaginosis. Minimum diagnostic requirements for bacterial vaginosis include three of the following signs:

- excessive vaginal discharge
- vaginal pH >4.5
- "clue" cells (vaginal epithelial cells covered by small gram-negative rods)
- a fishy amine-like odor in the KOH test (10% KOH added to vaginal discharge)

Candida sp are frequently present as normal flora in vagina. A saline wet mount may demonstrate yeast cells or pseudohyphae and may provide rapid diagnostic information. The most common clinical presentation is a characteristic clumpy white cottage cheese appearance with vaginal or vulvar itching. Vaginitis and balanitis caused by *Candida albicans* are more common than is generally perceived. Vaginitis frequently complicates pregnancy and diabetes and is seen with broad spectrum antibiotic therapy, as well as, in conditions which lower host resistance. Both *Candida* vaginitis and balanitis may, under some circumstances, be deemed sexually transmitted diseases.[2]

Footnotes

1. Catlin BW, "*Gardnerella vaginalis*: Characteristics, Clinical Considerations, and Controversies," *Clin Microbiol Rev*, 1992, 5(3):213-37.
2. Lossick JG, "Sexually Transmitted Vaginitis," *Urol Clin North Am*, 1984, 11:141-53.

References

Committee on Technical Bulletins of the American College of Obstetricians and Gynecologists, "Vulvovaginitis," *ACOG Technical Bulletin*, No 135, Washington, DC: American College of Obstetricians and Gynecologists, 1989, (review).

Faro S, "Bacterial Vaginitis," *Clin Obstet Gynecol*, 1991, 34(3):582-6.

Frangos DH and Nyberg LM Jr, "Genitourinary Fungal Infections," *South Med J*, 1986, 79:455-9.

Hill LUH and Embil JA, "Vaginitis: Current Microbiological and Clinical Concepts," *Can Med Assoc J*, 1986, 134:321-33.

Sobel JD, "Vaginal Infections in Adult Women," *Med Clin North Am*, 1990, 74(6):1573-602.

Thomason JL, Gelbart SM, and Scaglione NJ, "Bacterial Vaginosis: Current Review With Indications for Asymptomatic Therapy," *Am J Obstet Gynecol*, 1991, 165(4 Pt 2):1210-7.

Genitourinary Anaerobic Culture, Female *see* Endometrium Culture *on page 811*

Giardia *see* Ova and Parasites, Stool *on page 836*

GMS Stain *see* Fungus Smear, Stain *on page 813*

Gomori Methenamine Silver Stain *see* Fungus Smear, Stain *on page 813*

Gonorrhea Culture *see Neisseria gonorrhoeae* Culture *on page 831*

Gonorrhea Smear *see Neisseria gonorrhoeae* Smear *on page 834*

Gram Stain

CPT *87205*

Related Information

Acid-Fast Stain, Modified, *Nocardia* Species *on page 771*
Biopsy or Body Fluid Aerobic Bacterial Culture *on page 778*
Biopsy or Body Fluid Anaerobic Bacterial Culture *on page 778*
Body Fluids Cytology *on page 482*
Bronchial Aspirate Anaerobic Culture *on page 792*
Burn Culture, Quantitative *on page 794*
Cerebrospinal Fluid Analysis *on page 527*
Cerebrospinal Fluid Culture *on page 798*
Cerebrospinal Fluid Glucose *on page 176*
Cerebrospinal Fluid Lactic Acid *on page 178*
Cerebrospinal Fluid Protein *on page 659*
(Continued)

Gram Stain *(Continued)*

Conjunctival Culture *on page 803*
Ear Culture *on page 810*
Fungus Smear, Stain *on page 813*
KOH Preparation *on page 825*
Neisseria gonorrhoeae DNA Probe Test *on page 924*
Neisseria gonorrhoeae Smear *on page 834*
Skin Biopsies *on page 84*
Sputum Culture *on page 849*
Synovial Fluid Analysis *on page 1158*
Throat Culture *on page 876*
Urine Culture, Clean Catch *on page 881*
Yersinia pestis Antibody *on page 766*

Synonyms Bacterial Smear; Smear, Gram Stain

Applies to Crystal Violet; Safranin

Abstract Gram stain is a differential stain used to demonstrate the staining properties of bacteria of all types. Gram-positive bacteria retain crystal violet dye after decolorization and appear deep blue. Gram-negative bacteria are not capable of retaining the crystal violet dye after decolorization and are counterstained red by safranin dye. Gram staining characteristics may be atypical in very young, old, dead, or degenerating cultures.[1] The Gram stain confirms the presence of bacteria and their cell type. In meningitis and other settings, the Gram stain confirms the cell count. With culture, it has priority over latex agglutination procedures.

Patient Care PREPARATION: Same as for routine culture of specific site

Specimen Duplicate of specimen appropriate for routine culture of the specific site CONTAINER: Sterile specimen container, sterile tube, or appropriate tube for swab COLLECTION: Collection procedure same as for routine culture of the specific site. Specimen must be collected to avoid contamination with skin, adjacent structures, and nonsterile surfaces. STORAGE INSTRUCTIONS: Same as for a culture of the specimen CAUSES FOR REJECTION: Insufficient specimen volume TURNAROUND TIME: Usually same day SPECIAL INSTRUCTIONS: The laboratory should be informed of the specific site of specimen, age of patient, current antibiotic therapy, and clinical diagnosis.

Interpretive REFERENCE RANGE: Depends on site of specimen USE: Determine the presence or absence of bacteria, yeast, neutrophils, and epithelial cells; establish the presence of potentially pathogenic organisms. The Gram stain is essential in evaluation of all suspected cases of bacterial meningitis.[2] LIMITATIONS: Organism isolation and identification will usually be performed only if culture is requested. Request for Gram stain will not lead to stain for mycobacteria (TB). For detection of tubercle bacilli, an acid-fast stain must also be requested. Certain organisms do not stain or do not stain well with Gram stain (eg, *Legionella pneumophila*). As many as 20% to 30% of cases of bacterial meningitis have a negative Gram stain. Gram stain is **not** reliable for diagnosis of cervical, rectal, pharyngeal, or asymptomatic urethral gonococcal infection. In acute bacterial meningitis in adults, the most frequent error was misidentification of *Listeria* as *Streptococcus pneumoniae* in smears.[3] METHODOLOGY: Gram stain technique:

- Make a thin smear of the material for study and allow to air dry.
- Fix the material to the slide by passing the slide three or four times through the flame of a Bunsen burner so that the material does not wash off during the staining procedure. Some workers now recommend the use of alcohol for the fixation of material to be Gram stained (flood the smear with methanol or ethanol for a few minutes or warm for 10 minutes at 60°C on a slide warmer).
- Place the smear on a staining rack and overlay the surface with crystal violet solution.
- After 1 minute (less time may be used with some solutions) of exposure to the crystal violet stain, wash thoroughly with distilled water or buffer.
- Overlay the smear with Gram's iodine solution for 1 minute. Wash again with water.
- Hold the smear between the thumb and forefinger and flood the surface with a few drops of the acetone-alcohol decolorizer until no violet color washes off. This usually takes 10 seconds or less.
- Wash with running water and again place the smear on the staining rack. Overlay the surface with safranin counterstain for 1 minute. Wash with running water.
- Place the smear in an upright position in a staining rack, allowing the excess water to drain off and the smear to dry.

- Examine the stained smear under the 100x (oil) immersion objective of the microscope. Gram-positive bacteria stain dark blue; gram-negative bacteria appear pink-red.[1] See diagram.

ADDITIONAL INFORMATION: Gram stains are usually scanned for the presence or absence of white blood cells (indicative of infection) and squamous epithelial cells (indicative of mucosal contamination). A sputum specimen showing >25 squamous epithelial cells per low power field, regardless of the number of white blood cells, indicates that the specimen is grossly contaminated with saliva and bacterial culture should not be performed. Additional sputum specimens should be submitted to the laboratory if evidence of contamination by saliva is revealed. The Gram stain can be a reliable indicator to guide initial antibiotic therapy in community acquired pneumonia. It is imperative that a valid sputum specimen be obtained for Gram stain. In a well designed trial, valid expectorated sputum was obtained in 41% (59 of 144) of patients. The Gram stain is reliable but not infallible. Its principal limitations in the diagnosis of pulmonary infections are in detection of *H. influenzae* and in differentiating polymicrobic pneumonia from background contamination of the specimen by oropharyngeal flora.[4] Although mycobacteria have classically been considered to be gram-positive or faintly gram-positive, they are more correctly characterized as "gram-neutral" on routine stains.[5] A careful search for mycobacteria should be undertaken when purulent sputum without stainable organisms is encountered.

$N(CH_3)_2$ $(CH_3)_2N$ C NH_2

Crystal Violet (hexamethylpararosanilin)

H_3C N N CH_3 NH_2

Safranin (dimethyl phenosafranin)

Gram stains revealing an occasional bacterium per high powered field in an uncentrifuged urine specimen suggest a colony count of 10,000 bacteria/mL. Bacteria in the majority of fields suggests >100,000 bacteria/mL, a level associated with significant bacteriuria.

Gram stain is the most valuable diagnostic test in bacterial meningitis that is immediately available.[6] Organisms are detectable in 60% to 80% of patients who have not been treated and in 40% to 60% of those who have been given antibiotics.[6] Its sensitivity relates to the number of organisms present. The sensitivity of the Gram stain is greater in gram-positive infections and is only positive in half of the instances of gram-negative meningitis. It is positive even less frequently with listeriosis meningitis or with anaerobic infections.[6] Culture and Gram stain should have priority over antigen detection methods if only a small volume of CSF is available.[7]

Footnotes

1. Koneman EW, Allen SD, Janda WM, et al, *Color Atlas and Textbook of Diagnostic Microbiology*, 4th ed, Philadelphia, PA: JB Lippincott Co, 1992, 21, 24.
2. Fishman RA, *Cerebrospinal Fluid in Diseases of the Nervous System*, 2nd ed, Philadelphia, PA: WB Saunders Co, 1992, 346-8.
3. Durand ML, Calderwood SB, Weber DJ, et al, "Acute Bacterial Meningitis in Adults – A Review of 493 Episodes," *N Engl J Med*, 1993, 328(1):21-8.
4. Gleckman R, DeVita J, Hibert D, et al, "Sputum Gram Stain Assessment in Community-Acquired Bacteremic Pneumonia," *J Clin Microbiol*, 1988, 26:846-9.
5. Hinson JM, Bradsher RW, and Bodner SJ, "Gram Stain Neutrality of *Mycobacterium tuberculosis*," *Am Rev Respir Dis*, 1981, 123:365-6.
6. Greenlee JE, "Approach to Diagnosis of Meningitis – Cerebrospinal Fluid Evaluation," *Infect Dis Clin North Am*, 1990, 4(4):583-98.
7. Gray LD and Fedorko DP, "Laboratory Diagnosis of Bacterial Meningitis," *Clin Microbiol Rev*, 1992, 5(2):130-45.

References

Granoff DM, Murphy TV, Ingram DL, et al, "Use of Rapidly Generated Results in Patient Management," *Diagn Microbiol Infect Dis*, 1986, 4:157S-66S.

Provine H and Gardner P, "The Gram Stained Smear and Its Interpretation," *Hosp Pract*, 1974, 9:85-91.

Riccardi NB and Felman YM, "Laboratory Diagnosis in the Problem of Suspected Gonococcal Infection," *JAMA*, 1979, 242:2703-5.

Smith AL, "Bacterial Meningitis," *Pediatr Rev*, 1993, 14(1):11-8.

Gram Stain, Stool *see* Methylene Blue Stain, Stool *on page 828*

Group A Beta-Hemolytic *Streptococcus* Culture, Throat *see* Throat Culture *on page 876*

Group A *Streptococcus* Screen

***CPT** 86588 (direct)*

Related Information

Antistreptolysin O Titer, Serum *on page 640*
Bacterial Antigens, Rapid Detection Methods *on page 775*
Group B *Streptococcus* Screen *on next page*
Throat Culture *on page 876*

Synonyms *Streptococcus* Group A Latex Screen; Throat Swab for Group A Streptococcal Antigen

Applies to Enzyme Immunoassay for Group A *Streptococcus* Antigen

Replaces Coagglutination Test for Group A Streptococci

Test Commonly Includes Latex agglutination test for group A *Streptococcus* (GAS) antigen

Specimen Throat swab; many laboratories request two swabs, one for culture if the rapid screen is negative **CONTAINER:** Rayon or dacron swabs rather than cotton swabs enhance the chance of detection.[1] **COLLECTION:** Rigorous swabbing of the tonsillar pillars and posterior throat increases the probability of detection of streptococcal antigen. **SPECIAL INSTRUCTIONS:** Some laboratories favor submission of dry swabs for antigen testing. Consult the laboratory for their specific recommendations.

Interpretive **USE:** Screen for the presence of group A streptococcal antigen **LIMITATIONS:** Many reviews have indicated a sensitivity of 75% to 80% and a specificity of 95% to 98% for the rapid methods. Sensitivity varies between manufacturers. Some kits are capable of detecting 10^5 colony forming units (CFUs) while others require 10^6-10^7 CFU/mL. Specimens which yield less than 10 colonies on culture usually are negative by rapid method. Adequate specimen collection on younger patients may be difficult, and thus, contribute to the false-negative rate. A positive result can be relied upon as a rational basis to begin therapy. **A negative result is only presumptive, and a culture should be performed to reasonably exclude the diagnosis of group A streptococcal infection.** Careful attention to the details of the method and the use of appropriate controls are required to assume adequate performance. Group A streptococcal antigen disappears rapidly following antibiotic therapy. Thus a history of prior therapy should be sought when assessing pharyngitis.[2] **CONTRAINDICATIONS:** The test may become negative 4 hours after therapy has been started. **METHODOLOGY:** The streptococcal group carbohydrate antigen is extracted from the swab used for collection by use of acid or enzyme reagents. The extraction mixture is added to particles coated with antistreptococcal antibody. If the streptococcal antigen is present, visible agglutination occurs due to antigen cross-links with antibody-coated latex within 10 minutes. Enzyme immunoassay methods (EIA) are also used. **ADDITIONAL INFORMATION:** Rheumatic fever remains a concern in the United States and serious complications including sepsis, soft tissue invasion, and toxic shock-like syndrome have been reported to be increasing in frequency.[3] Therefore, timely diagnosis and early institution of appropriate therapy remains important. Timely therapy may reduce the acute symptoms and overall duration of streptococcal pharyngitis. The sequelae of poststreptococcal glomerulonephritis and rheumatic fever are diminished by early therapy.

Footnotes

1. Berkowitz CD, Anthony BF, Kaplan EL, et al, "Cooperative Study of Latex Agglutination to Identify Group A Streptococcal Antigen on Throat Swabs in Patients With Acute Pharyngitis," *J Pediatr*, 1985, 107:89-92.
2. Beach PS, Balfour LC, and Lucia HL, "Group A Streptococcal Rapid Test. Antigen Detection After 18-24 Hours of Penicillin Therapy," *Clin Pediatr (Phila)*, 1989, 28(1):6-10.
3. Givner LB, Abramson JS, and Wasilauskas B, "Apparent Increase in the Incidence of Invasive Group A Beta-Hemolytic Streptococcal Disease in Children," *J Pediatr*, 1991, 118(3):341-6.

References

Facklam RR, "Specificity Study of Kits for Detection of Group A Streptococci Directly From Throat Swabs," *J Clin Microbiol*, 1987, 25:504-8.

Kaplan EL, "The Rapid Identification of Group A Beta-Hemolytic Streptococci in the Upper Respiratory Tract - Current Status," *Pediatr Clin North Am*, 1988, 35:535-42, (review).

Nadler HL, "Group A Strep Detection," *Diagn Clin Test*, 1989, 27:3:35-41, (review of rapid methods).

"Rapid Diagnostic Tests for Group A Streptococcal Pharyngitis," *Med Lett Drugs Ther*, 1991, 33(843):40-1.

Veasy LG, "Resurgence of Acute Rheumatic Fever in the Intermountain Area of the United States," *N Engl J Med*, 1987, 316:421-7.

Group B *Streptococcus* Screen

***CPT** 86588 (direct)*

Related Information

Bacterial Antigens, Rapid Detection Methods *on page 775*
Genital Culture *on page 814*
Group A *Streptococcus* Screen *on previous page*

Synonyms *Streptococcus agalactiae* Latex Screen; *Streptococcus* Group B Latex Screen

Replaces Counterimmunoelectrophoresis for Group B Streptococcal Antigen

Test Commonly Includes Latex screen for group B beta *Streptococcus* antigen

Specimen Cerebrospinal fluid, blood, urine, endocervical, endometrial material, or amniotic fluid **CONTAINER:** Sterile container, red top tube **STORAGE INSTRUCTIONS:** Set up cultures. If a specimen for antigen detection cannot be tested immediately, it may be stored at 2°C to 8°C for 1 day or frozen at -20°C for longer storage. Storage is inconsistent with the role of the test for rapid diagnosis. **TURNAROUND TIME:** About 1 hour stat

Interpretive USE: Rapid detection of group B *Streptococcus* antigen in body fluids. Early intrapartum detection of group B *Streptococcus* antigen is usually an indication for chemoprophylaxis.[1] Latex testing may be useful in instances in which there has been prior antibiotic therapy. Cultures are needed. **LIMITATIONS:** Latex screens have greater sensitivity than CIE procedures. Sensitivity is relatively low, 15% to 21%, for rapid group B streptococcal antigen tests;[2] 5 x 10^6 colony forming units were required to be present for antigenic detection. Concentrated urine may be used for screening. Testing CSF and serum, as well as, culture for the organism should be considered. Shortcomings of latex detection are addressed in the listing, Bacterial Antigens, Rapid Detection Methods. **METHODOLOGY:** Polystyrene latex particles coated with antibodies specific for the group B *Streptococcus* antigen agglutinate in the presence of the homologous antigen. Controls for nonspecific agglutination of latex particles are generally used. See package insert directions relevant to heat inactivation. Urine may be concentrated to increase sensitivity of the method. Infection can be diagnosed by detection of group B specific carbohydrate antigen of bacterial cell wall, which may be present in body fluids, serum and cerebrospinal fluid and which is excreted in urine. Counterimmunoelectrophoresis (CIE) has been a method for detection of the group B *Streptococcus* antigen. Alternatively, swab specimens collected during antepartum visits may be cultured on appropriate media. **ADDITIONAL INFORMATION:** Group B *Streptococcus* is currently one of the most significant human pathogens in the neonatal period. The most common mode of acquisition by the neonate is exposure to the maternal genital flora *in utero* through ruptured membranes or by contamination during passage through the birth canal. Rapid identification of group B *Streptococcus* carriers is important in management of premature rupture of the membranes because the effectiveness of intrapartum prophylactic ampicillin may be compromised by awaiting the results of conventional cultures.[3] Infection is manifested in two major forms, early onset septicemic infection manifest in the first few days of life and late onset meningitis which occurs during the first few months of life.

Increased isolation of strains of group B *Streptococcus* resistant to erythromycin (9%) or intermediate susceptible clindamycin (9.5%) and cefoxitin (15.3%) have been reported. Nineteen percent exhibited a multiple antibiotic resistance pattern. Penicillinase production and resistance to ampicillin were not encountered in the particular series. Susceptibility testing may be useful in selecting alternate antibiotic regimens.[4]

Footnotes

1. Tuppurainen N and Hallman M, "Prevention of Neonatal Group B Streptococcal Disease: Intrapartum Detection and Chemoprophylaxis of Heavily Colonized Parturients," *Obstet Gynecol*, 1989, 73(4):583-7.
2. Skoll MA, Mercer BM, Baselski V, et al, "Evaluation of Two Rapid Group B Streptococcal Antigen Tests in Labor and Delivery Patients," *Obstet Gynecol*, 1991, 77(2):322-6.
3. Newton ER and Clark M, "Group B *Streptococcus* and Preterm Rupture of Membranes," *Obstet Gynecol*, 1988, 71(2):198-202.
4. Berkowitz K, Regan JA, and Greenberg E, "Antibiotic Resistance Patterns of Group B Streptococci in Pregnant Women," *J Clin Microbiol*, 1990, 28(1):5-7.

References

Brady K, Duff P, Schilhab JC, et al, "Reliability of a Rapid Latex Fixation Test for Detecting Group B Streptococci in the Genital Tract of Parturients at Term," *Obstet Gynecol*, 1989, 73(4):678-81.

Stiller RJ, Blair E, Clark P, et al, "Rapid Detection of Vaginal Colonization With Group B Streptococci by Means of Latex Agglutination," *Am J Obstet Gynecol*, 1989, 160(3):566-8.

Haemophilus influenzae Susceptibility Testing *see* Penicillinase Test *on page 840*

Hanging Drop Mount for *Trichomonas* *see Trichomonas* Preparation *on page 879*

Hank's Stain *see* Acid-Fast Stain, Modified, *Nocardia* Species *on page 771*

Head Lice Identification *see* Arthropod Identification *on page 774*

Helicobacter pylori Urease Test and Culture

CPT *43600 (gastric biopsy); 87081 (culture single organism); 87205 (Gram stain); 88104 (cytopathology smears with interpretation)*

Related Information

Gastric Analysis *on page 232*
Gastrin, Serum *on page 234*
Helicobacter pylori Serology *on page 682*

Synonyms *Campylobacter pylori* Urease Test and Culture; Gastric Biopsy Culture for *Helicobacter pylori*; Urease Test and Culture, *Helicobacter pylori*

Test Commonly Includes Screening for the presence of urease activity indirectly indicating the presence of *Helicobacter pylori*, culture of the organism from gastric biopsy specimens

Abstract *H. pylori* is a gram-negative microaerophilic spiral-shaped bacillus which has been implicated as a frequent cause of gastritis[1] and other inflammatory gastroduodenal lesions. Its urease activity is important in detection and identification of this organism. Culture with biopsy is the gold standard for identification of *H. pylori*[1] (formerly, *Campylobacter pylori*). Culture without biopsy may allow occult neoplasm to go unrecognized.

Specimen Gastric mucosal biopsy **CONTAINER:** Sterile container, **no fixative** for these microbiologic tests **STORAGE INSTRUCTIONS:** If specimen cannot be transported immediately to the laboratory, it should be placed in 0.5 mL transport medium (normal saline). **TURNAROUND TIME:** 24 hours for urease final report; up to 7 days for culture

Interpretive **REFERENCE RANGE:** Negative for urease activity, negative culture, biopsy negative for gastritis and negative for *H. pylori* **USE:** Establish the presence and possible etiologic role of *Helicobacter pylori* in cases of chronic gastric ulcer, chronic active gastritis, and a relationship with duodenal ulcers **LIMITATIONS:** Culture and urease testing alone, without biopsies, may allow occult neoplasms to go undetected. **METHODOLOGY: Urease test**: Gastric biopsies are incubated on slightly buffered medium. A change of phenol red to alkaline (pink color) persisting more than 5 minutes is considered positive and presumptively indicative of the presence of *Helicobacter pylori* even if the organism cannot be grown in culture. Specimens negative at 30 minutes should be re-examined periodically up to 24 hours. The sensitivity of urease testing leaves something to be desired. It was only 62% at 24 hours in a 1991 report. It also is characterized by false-positive results.[2]

Culture: Culture media may include enriched chocolate, Thayer-Martin with antibiotics, brain heart infusion (BHI) with 7% horse blood, and Mueller-Hinton with 5% sheep blood. Nichols et al describe horse blood agar plate (Columbia agar base), then a 5% sheep blood agar plate (trypticase soy base), and finally a plate of Skirrow medium.[2] The organism is microaerophilic and grows best in a reduced O_2 atmosphere or in a Campy-Pak™ system at 35°C. Cultures are usually observed for 7 days before being reported as negative.

Cytology: Touch cytology preparations (ie, imprints from biopsies) may provide a rapid diagnosis and preserve the biopsy specimen for histopathology or culture.

Smear: A direct smear can be Gram stained.[2]

Sensitivity of methods for detection of *H. pylori*:

- 24-hour urease: 62%
- direct Gram stain: 69%
- culture: 90%
- histology: 93%[2]

ADDITIONAL INFORMATION: *Helicobacter pylori* is a major cause of chronic active gastritis. Its importance and etiologic relationship with duodenal ulcer requires further study. It is known that 78% to 100% of subjects who have duodenal ulcer have *H. pylori* infection, but 3% to 70% of patients without duodenal ulcer have *H. pylori* as well.[3,4] The organism may be seen in biopsies stained with Gram stain,[2] hematoxylin-eosin (H & E), Giemsa or Warthin-Starry silver stain. It is most often recognized in biopsies of the antrum but may also be seen in the fundic mucosa, metaplastic gastric mucosa of esophagus (Barrett's esophagus), or duodenum.[1] Biopsy may also establish the diagnosis of carcinoma or lymphoma. *H. pylori* was not found in the gastric mucosa of Meckel's diverticula.[5] Gram stains performed by a reuse imprint technique on biopsies from both the antrum and fundus yielded positives in 100% of 32 culture positive cases.[6]

Most peptic ulcers related to *H. pylori* infection are reported as curable.[4,7]

Breath isotope methods measuring bacterial urease by detection of labeled CO_2 and serologic tests for the detection of antibody are also useful if available. The breath test is preferred as a means of documenting presence of active infection and eradication of infection after therapy in the absence of endoscopy.

The serologic tests are limited because they remain positive for months following therapy. Use of specific IgA enhances the value of serology in monitoring therapy. See *Helicobacter pylori* Serology listing in the Immunology and Serology chapter.

Past *H. pylori* infection increases risk of carcinoma of stomach. Chronic atrophic gastritis and intestinal metaplasia are related to *H. pylori* infection, which induces as well development of lymphoid tissue in the gastric mucosa. The possible role of *H. pylori* in development of primary malignant lymphoma of stomach was recently discussed.[8,9]

Footnotes

1. Peterson WL, "*Helicobacter pylori* and Peptic Ulcer Disease," *N Engl J Med*, 1991, 324(15):1043-8.
2. Nichols L, Sughayer M, DeGirolami PC, et al, "Evaluation of Diagnostic Methods for *Helicobacter pylori* Gastritis," *Am J Clin Pathol*, 1991, 95(6):769-73.
3. Shocket ID, "*Helicobacter pylori* and Duodenal Ulcer: A Review," *Ann Intern Med*, 1992, 116(Suppl 2):61.
4. Graham DY, "Treatment of Peptic Ulcers Caused by *Helicobacter pylori*," *N Engl J Med*, 1993, 328(5):349-50, (editorial).
5. Fich A, Talley NJ, Shorter RG, et al, "Does *Helicobacter pylori* Colonize the Gastric Mucosa of Meckel's Diverticulum?" *Mayo Clin Proc*, 1990, 65(2):187-91.
6. Parsonnet J, Welch K, Compton C, et al, "Simple Microbiologic Detection of *Campylobacter pylori*," *J Clin Microbiol*, 1988, 26:948-9.
7. Graham DY, Lew GM, Klein PD, et al, "Effect of Treatment of *Helicobacter pylori* Infection on the Long-Term Recurrence of Gastric or Duodenal Ulcer," *Ann Intern Med*, 1992, 116(9):705-8.
8. Isaacson PG and Spencer J, "Is Gastric Lymphoma an Infectious Disease?" *Hum Pathol*, 1993, 24(6):569-70, (editorial).
9. Genta RM, Hamner HW, and Graham DY, "Gastric Lymphoid Follicles in *Helicobacter pylori* Infection: Frequency, Distribution, and Response to Triple Therapy," *Hum Pathol*, 1993, 24(6):577-83.

References

Chan WY, Hui PK, Chan JK, et al, "Epithelial Damage by *Helicobacter pylori* in Gastric Ulcers," *Histopathology*, 1991, 19(1):47-53.

Clearfield HR, "*Helicobacter pylori*: Aggressor or Innocent Bystander?" *Med Clin North Am*, 1991, 75(4):815-29.

Debongnie JC, Delmee M, Mainguet P, et al, "Cytology: A Simple, Rapid, Sensitive Method in the Diagnosis of *Helicobacter pylori*," *Am J Gastroenterol*, 1992, 87(1):20-3.

Dooley CP and Cohen H, "The Clinical Significance of *Campylobacter pylori*," *Ann Intern Med*, 1988, 108:70-9.

Drumm B, Perez-Perez GI, Blaser MJ, et al, "Intrafamilial Clustering of *Helicobacter pylori* Infection," *N Engl J Med*, 1990, 322:359-63.

Eastham EJ, Elliott TS, Berkeley D, et al, "*Campylobacter pylori* Infection in Children," *J Infect*, 1988, 16:77-9.

Marshall BJ, "Rapid Urease Test in the Management of *Campylobacter pyloridis*-Associated Gastritis," *Am J Gastroenterol*, 1987, 82:200-10.

Marshall BJ, "Should We Now, Routinely, Be Examining Gastro Biopsies for *Campylobacter pylori*? Gastric Mucosal Biopsy: An Essential Investigation in Patients With Dyspepsia," *Am J Gastroenterol*, 1988, 83:479-81.

Popovic-Uroic T, Patton CM, Wachsmuth IK, et al, "Evaluation of an Oligonucleotide Probe for Identification of *Campylobacter* Species," *Lab Med*, 1991, 22:533-9.

Taylor DN and Blaser MJ, "The Epidemiology of *Helicobacter pylori* Infection," *Epidemiol Rev*, 1991, 13:42-59.

Veenendaal RA, Pena AS, Meijer JL, et al, "Long-Term Serological Surveillance After Treatment of *Helicobacter pylori* Infection," *Gut*, 1991, 32(11):1291-4.

Helminths *see* Ova and Parasites, Stool *on page 836*

Hemovac® Tip Culture *see* Intravascular Device Culture *on next page*

Histoplasmin Skin Test *see* Skin Test, Tuberculosis *on page 848*

Hyperalimentation Line Culture *see* Intravascular Device Culture *on next page*

India Ink Preparation

CPT *87210*

Related Information

Cerebrospinal Fluid Culture *on page 798*
Cerebrospinal Fluid Fungus Culture *on page 800*
Cryptococcal Antigen Titer, Serum or Cerebrospinal Fluid *on page 805*
Cryptococcus Antibody Titer *on page 670*
Fungus Smear, Stain *on page 813*
KOH Preparation *on page 825*

Synonyms Cerebrospinal Fluid India Ink Preparation

Test Commonly Includes Staining of CSF sediment with India ink to detect the polysaccharide capsule surrounding the yeast

Patient Care PREPARATION: Same as for culture of specific site

Specimen Appropriate specimen is the same as for culture of a given site. See Fungus Culture of specific site for details. CONTAINER: Same as for culture of specific site COLLECTION: The specimen may be divided for fungal culture, mycobacteria culture and smear, and conventional bacterial culture and Gram stain, as well as, cerebrospinal fluid analysis (cell count), glucose, protein, and cryptococcal antigen titer. STORAGE INSTRUCTIONS: Do **not** refrigerate. CAUSES FOR REJECTION: Insufficient specimen volume

Interpretive REFERENCE RANGE: No *Cryptococcus* identified USE: Establish the presence of *Cryptococcus* sp or other fungi LIMITATIONS: This technique is only 30% to 50% sensitive in cases of cryptococcal meningitis. Cultures and rapid latex agglutination (LA) methods are more sensitive than direct preparations; therefore, the India ink preparation may be negative when the culture or LA test is positive. Immunologic tests for *Cryptococcus* antigen have a sensitivity of 90% to 100%. Many laboratories have abandoned the use of the India ink preparation in favor of LA. METHODOLOGY: Wet mount with India ink (nigrosin) for contrast. Centrifugation may concentrate organisms and improve sensitivity (10-20 minutes at 1500 g). ADDITIONAL INFORMATION: *Cryptococcus neoformans* is the most common central nervous system fungus in both normal hosts and patients with the acquired immunodeficiency syndrome (AIDS). Skin, lungs, spleen, kidneys, liver, and/or bone may also be infected. Pigeon droppings act as a year-round vector for dispersion of encapsulated yeast cells.

References

Berlin L and Pincus JH, "Cryptococcal Meningitis. False-Negative Antigen Test Results and Cultures in Nonimmunosuppressed Patients," *Arch Neurol*, 1989, 46(12):1312-6.
Ellis DH and Pfeiffer TJ, "Ecology, Life Cycle, and Infectious Propagule of *Cryptococcus neoformans*," *Lancet*, 1990, 336(8720):923-5.

Infant Botulism, Toxin Identification *see* Botulism, Diagnostic Procedure *on page 792*

Insect Identification *see* Arthropod Identification *on page 774*

Intrauterine Device Culture *see Actinomyces* Culture, All Sites *on page 772*

Intrauterine Device Culture *see* Endometrium Culture *on page 811*

Intravascular Device Culture

CPT *87070 (aerobic); 87075 (anaerobic); 87076 (definitive ID); 87102 (fungi isolation); 87106 (fungi definitive identification)*

Synonyms Catheter Tip Culture; Hemovac® Tip Culture; Hyperalimentation Line Culture; Intravenous Catheter Culture; Swan-Ganz Tip Culture

Applies to Quantitative Tip Culture (QTC)

Test Commonly Includes Quantitative or semiquantitative culture of an intravascular catheter or blood specimen collected through the catheter; organism identification, and antimicrobial susceptibilities if appropriate

Abstract Intravascular devices are used to provide continuous vascular access for a variety of therapeutic and diagnostic purposes. Their use in individuals with serious underlying illness and the fact that they penetrate the integument places patients at significant risk for infection.

Specimen I.V. catheter tip, foreign body, blood collected through catheter CONTAINER: Sterile container COLLECTION: Clean the insertion site with an iodophor and alcohol, and aseptically remove the cannula after the alcohol has dried. If purulent material is present at the exit site, it should be submitted for culture and Gram stain. If the catheter is short, the entire cannula should be submitted following removal of the hub with sterile scissors or other sterile device. For longer catheters, two 2-3 cm segments should be submitted, one from the proximal transcutaneous segment and the other from the distal intravascular tip. Alternatively, blood for comparative quantitative cultures may be collected simultaneously from a peripheral vein and from the central venous catheter. A procedure for accomplishing this is as follows:

A blood sample, 0.5-1 mL, is drawn from a peripheral blood vessel and from the central catheter. Aseptic technique at the peripheral site includes three applications of povidone-iodine followed by one application of 70% isopropyl alcohol to the skin. A butterfly needle and a sterile syringe are used for phlebotomy. Aseptic technique at the catheter is as follows.

- The catheter is clamped and the needle adapter removed.
- The end of the catheter is swabbed three times with povidone-iodine and once with 70% isopropyl alcohol.
- A sterile needle adapter is inserted into the end of the catheter.
- The clamp is removed and 2 mL of blood is drawn through a sterile syringe to clear the catheter.
- The blood for culture is then subsequently obtained in a separate sterile syringe.
- The catheter adapter is reattached to the intravenous tubing.

The paired blood specimens are placed in separate lysis centrifugation tubes after the stopper is swabbed three times with povidone-iodine.[1] See also Blood Culture, Aerobic and Anaerobic test listing.

STORAGE INSTRUCTIONS: Specimens should be transported to the laboratory within 1 hour of collection for optimal results. However, if specimens cannot be collected and delivered to the laboratory during regular hours, specimen may be refrigerated overnight. **CAUSES FOR REJECTION:** Foley catheters are unacceptable specimens because they are invariably contaminated with environmental flora.

Interpretive **REFERENCE RANGE:** Roll plate semiquantitative cultures yielding <15 colonies, sonicated specimens yielding $<10^4$ colonies of coagulase-negative staphylococci (cutoffs for other organisms are less clear), and comparative quantitative cultures yielding a ratio of <10:1 (central venous catheter vs peripheral vein cultures) or <100 CFU/mL (central venous catheter only) suggests that the catheter should not be strongly considered as the cause of sepsis.[1,2] **USE:** Culture of intravascular devices should be limited to patients who have laboratory confirmed bacteremia or who appear clinically septic but have no apparent source of infection. In this situation, the intravascular device is investigated as the possible origin of infection by the methods described. Randomly culturing patients who are not bacteremic or who are not clinically septic is unwarranted. **LIMITATIONS:** Results of intravascular device cultures contribute to the work-up of patients with bloodstream infections who lack an obvious source. These results do not stand alone, however, and all methods described give a significant number of false-positive and false-negative results. The sonication and comparative quantitative culture methods are still evolving. **METHODOLOGY:** **Roll plate semiquantitative cultures:** Aseptically roll the catheter tip on a blood and/or chocolate agar plate.

Quantitative sonication method: Place catheter segment in 10 mL of tryptic soy broth, sonicate for 1 minute, then vortex for 15 seconds (original specimen). Add 0.1 mL of this specimen to 9.9 mL of saline (diluted specimen) and inoculate separate blood agar plates with 0.1 mL of the original and diluted specimens. Perform colony counts and multiply by 10^2 (original specimen) or 10^4 (diluted specimen) to determine the number of organisms on the catheter.

Comparative quantitative cultures: Follow procedures for collection listed above and process as you would blood cultures using the lysis centrifugation method. Perform colony counts on both specimens.

ADDITIONAL INFORMATION: Infections complicating therapy with indwelling central venous catheters pose a difficult problem. Catheter-related sepsis is defined when:

- positive blood cultures collected through the central venous catheter show a tenfold or greater colony count compared with peripheral quantitative blood culture or >100 CFU/mL if only central venous catheter blood culture is available
- no obvious clinical or microbiologic source for the infection is apparent

Exit site infections are defined as purulent drainage or erythema at the catheter exit site. Tunnel infection is defined as spreading cellulitis with erythema, tenderness, and swelling of the skin surrounding the subcutaneous tunnel tract of the catheter. Successful therapy of catheter-related infection with antibiotics and local care was reported by Benezra et al. However,

(Continued)

Intravascular Device Culture *(Continued)*

they noted that catheter removal was required to achieve cure particularly in *Pseudomonas* tunnel infections. *Staphylococcus aureus* and polymicrobial infections also were more difficult to eradicate.[1] Intraluminal culture correlate well with catheter tip cultures (87.5% identical) while skin puncture sites were less frequently identical (37.5%).[3] See table.

Summary of Results of Prospective Studies Using Semiquantitative Techniques to Diagnose Vascular-Access Infections

Organism	No. With Same Organism in Semiquantitative Catheter Culture and Blood Culture
Coagulase-negative staphylococci	27
Staphylococcus aureus	26
Yeast	17
Enterobacter	7
Serratia	5
Enterococcus	5
Klebsiella	4
Streptococcus viridans group	3
Pseudomonas species	2
Proteus	2
Others *Pseudomonas aeruginosa* *Yersinia*	1 each

From Hampton A and Sheretz RJ, "Vascular-Access Infections in Hospitalized Patients," *Surg Clin North Am*, 1988, 68:57-72, with permission.

Footnotes

1. Benezra D, Kiehn TE, Gold JWM, et al, "Prospective Study of Infections in Indwelling Central Venous Catheter Using Quantitative Blood Cultures," *Am J Med*, 1988, 85(4):495-8.
2. Sherertz RJ, Raad II, Belani A, et al, "Three-Year Experience With Sonicated Vascular Catheter Cultures in a Clinical Microbiology Laboratory," *J Clin Microbiol*, 1990, 28(1):76-82.
3. Jakobsen CJ, Hansen V, Jensen JJ, et al, "Contamination of Subclavian Vein Catheters: An Intraluminal Culture Method," *J Hosp Infect*, 1989, 13(3):253-60.

References

Andremont A, Paulet R, Nitenberg G, et al, "Value of Semiquantitative Cultures of Blood Drawn Through Catheter Hubs for Estimating the Risk of Catheter Tip Colonization in Cancer Patients," *J Clin Microbiol*, 1988, 26:2297-9.

Damen J, "Positive Tip Cultures and Related Risk Factors Associated With Intravascular Catheterization in Pediatric Cardiac Patients," *Crit Care Med*, 1988, 16:221-7.

Flynn PM, Shenep JL, and Barrett FF, "Differential Quantitation With a Commercial Blood Culture Tube for Diagnosis of Catheter-Related Infection," *J Clin Microbiol*, 1988, 26:1045-6.

Mosca RM, Curtas S, Forbes B, et al, "The Benefits of Isolator Cultures in the Management of Suspected Catheter Sepsis," *Surgery*, 1987, 102:718-22.

Raad II and Bodey GP, "Infectious Complications of Indwelling Vascular Catheters," *Clin Infect Dis*, 1992, 15(2):197-208.

Ramanathan R and Durand M, "Blood Cultures in Neonates With Percutaneous Central Venous Catheters," *Arch Dis Child*, 1987, 62:621-3.

Intravenous Catheter Culture *see* Intravascular Device Culture *on page 822*

Isolator™ Blood Culture *see* Blood Culture, Aerobic and Anaerobic *on page 784*

IUD Culture *see Actinomyces* Culture, All Sites *on page 772*

IUD Culture *see* Endometrium Culture *on page 811*

***Ixodes dammini* Identification** *see* Arthropod Identification *on page 774*

Kinyoun Stain *see* Acid-Fast Stain *on page 770*

Kirby-Bauer Susceptibility Test *see* Susceptibility Testing, Aerobic and Facultatively Anaerobic Organisms *on page 864*

KOH Preparation

CPT *87220*

Related Information

Fungus Smear, Stain *on page 813*
Gram Stain *on page 815*
India Ink Preparation *on page 822*
Skin Biopsies *on page 84*
Skin Fungus Culture *on page 845*
Sputum Fungus Culture *on page 853*

Synonyms Potassium Hydroxide Preparation

Test Commonly Includes Potassium hydroxide, (KOH) hydrolysis of proteinaceous debris, cells, etc. Microscopic examination under 10x and 40x.

Patient Care PREPARATION: Same as for culture of specific site

Specimen Appropriate specimen for KOH preparation is the same as for culture, see specific site fungus culture listing for details CONTAINER: Same as for culture of specific site SPECIAL INSTRUCTIONS: The laboratory should be informed of the specific source of the specimen and the clinical diagnosis.

Interpretive REFERENCE RANGE: No fungus elements identified USE: Determine the presence of fungi in skin, nails, or hair LIMITATIONS: Cultures are usually more sensitive than smears; therefore, the KOH preparation may be negative when culture is positive; *vide infra*. The test may require overnight incubation for complete disintegration of hair, nail, or skin debris. METHODOLOGY: 10% KOH with gentle heat, alternately 20% KOH or 10% KOH and 40% dimethyl sulfoxide (DMSO)[1] ADDITIONAL INFORMATION: Exudates from abscesses, sinus tracts, aspirates, etc, should be examined by KOH preparation and also smeared for Gram stain. Cerebrospinal fluid should be cultured for fungi and tested for *Cryptococcus* antigen. See the specimen selection tables provided in the Skin Fungus Culture and Sputum Fungus Culture test listings. For the diagnosis of keratomycosis, direct examination may have a higher yield than culture because of the presence of dead organisms in the corneal tissue.[2] Recent reports have emphasized the changing pattern of tinea capitis, particularly the fact that infection due to *Trichophyton tonsurans* has become increasingly common. When present it causes a less discrete, more diffuse pattern of alopecia. It is negative by Wood's light examination. The "black dot", a remnant of a broken infected hair shaft, is a good source for diagnostic material which should be sought with a magnifying glass and collected with forceps. Scale and pulled hairs are also useful specimens.[3] Diagnostic specimens should be collected before antifungal therapy is instituted. Topical steroids should not be prescribed until fungal infection is excluded.[4]

Footnotes

1. Stein DH, "Superficial Fungal Infections," *Pediatr Clin North Am*, 1983, 30:545-61.
2. Ishibashi Y, Hommura S, and Matsumoto Y, "Direct Examination vs Culture of Biopsy Specimens for the Diagnosis of Keratomycosis," *Am J Ophthalmol*, 1987, 103:636-40.
3. Krowchuk DP, Lucky AW, Primmer SI, et al, "Current Status of the Identification and Management of Tinea Capitis," *Pediatrics*, 1983, 72:625-31.
4. Pariser DM, "Superficial Fungal Infections. A Practical Guide for Primary Care Physicians," *Postgrad Med*, 1990, 87(5):205-14.

References

Cohn MS, "Superficial Fungal Infections. Topical and Oral Treatment of Common Types," *Postgrad Med*, 1992, 91(2):239-44, 249-52.

Gray LD and Roberts GD, "Laboratory Diagnosis of Systemic Fungal Diseases," *Infect Dis Clin North Am*, 1988, 2:779-803.

Hebert AA and Burton-Esterly N, "Bacterial and Candidal Cutaneous Infections in the Neonate," *Dermatol Clin*, 1986, 4:3-21.

Latex Agglutination for Bacterial Antigens *see* Bacterial Antigens, Rapid Detection Methods *on page 775*

Latex Agglutination *Legionella pneumophila* *see Legionella* Culture *on this page*

Legionella Culture

CPT *87081 (culture single organism); 87163 (additional identification methods)*

Related Information

Legionella pneumophila Direct FA Smear *on page 715*

(Continued)

Legionella Culture *(Continued)*

Legionnaires' Disease Antibodies *on page 716*
Legionnaires' Disease Antibodies, IgM *on page 716*
Sputum Culture *on page 849*

Synonyms Legionnaires' Disease Agent

Applies to Biopsy *Legionella* Culture; Bronchoscopic *Legionella* Culture; DNA Probe *Legionella*; Latex Agglutination *Legionella pneumophila*; Pleural Fluid, *Legionella* Culture; Transtracheal Aspiration *Legionella* Culture

Test Commonly Includes Culture and frequently direct fluorescent antibody (DFA) smear for *Legionella pneumophila*

Infections Caused by *Legionella*

Culture proven

Pneumonia
Empyema
Sinusitis
Prosthetic valve endocarditis
Wound infection
Associated with pneumonia
- Bowel abscesses
- Brain abscesses
- Empyema
- Lung abscesses
- Myocarditis
- Pericarditis
- Peritonitis
- Renal abscesses/pyelonephritis
- Vascular graft infections

Strong seroepidemiological evidence

Pontiac fever

Weak seroepidemiological evidence

Encephalopathy without pneumonia
Myocarditis without pneumonia
Pericarditis without pneumonia

From Edelstein PH, "Laboratory Diagnosis of Infections Caused by*Legionella*," *Eur J Clin Microbiol,* 1987, 6:4-10, with permission.

Clinical Clues to the Diagnosis of Legionnaires' Disease

- Gram's stain of respiratory secretions reveals numerous neutrophils, but few organisms
- Presence of hyponatremia (serum sodium ≤130 mEq/L)
- Failure to respond to β-lactam and aminoglycoside antibiotics
- Occurrence in hospital where potable water system is known to be contaminated with *Legionella*
- History of smoking and alcohol use
- Pleuritic chest pain
- Fever malaise, myalgia, headache

From Harrison TG and Taylor AG, "Timing of Seroconversion in Legionnaires' Disease," *Lancet,* Oct 1988, 795, with permission.

Abstract The family Legionellaceae are ubiquitous, gram-negative, motile, fastidious, aerobic bacilli. During an American Legion Convention in Philadelphia in 1976, an epidemic of pneumonia caused 34 deaths. A single genus, *Legionella*, exists in the the family Legionellaceae.

Specimen Lung tissue, other body tissue, pleural fluid, other body fluid, transtracheal aspiration, bronchoalveolar lavage, bronchial brushing, sputum **CONTAINER:** Sterile container **COLLECTION:** Contamination with normal flora from skin or other body surfaces should be avoided. **TURNAROUND TIME:** Positive results are usually generated between 2-5 days. Primary plates are often held for 7-14 days before a final negative report is issued.

Interpretive **REFERENCE RANGE:** No *Legionella* recovered **USE:** Isolate and identify *Legionella* sp **LIMITATIONS:** Sputum (expectorated), bronchial aspirates, and other specimens having normal flora are subject to bacterial overgrowth and are not as desirable as transtracheal aspirates, pleural fluid, and biopsy material for culture. Sensitivity of cultures is relatively low (50%

to 80%), however, specificity is 100%. A direct fluorescent antibody smear without culture can be done to detect *Legionella*. Cross reactions with *B. fragilis*, *Pseudomonas fluorescens*, and other species occur. Newer approaches utilizing monoclonal antibodies have enhanced the yield of fluorescent procedures. **METHODOLOGY:** Culture on selective and nonselective media (buffered charcoal yeast extract). *Legionella* requires L-cysteine and ferric salt supplementation of growth media **ADDITIONAL INFORMATION:** Acute and convalescent sera for *Legionella* antibodies should also be considered to increase the likelihood for documentation of diagnosis. A fourfold rise to a titer of 1:128 is a diagnostic standard criterion. Seroconversion may be detected in many patients in the first weeks. Seroconversion 0-7 days after onset, 16%; 0-14 days, 52%; 0-21 days, 66%; 0-28 days, 71%. Twenty-five percent of patients did not have diagnostic titers.[1] DNA probes are being developed to improve sensitivity and specificity of detection methods for *Legionella*. Methods to detect *Legionella* antigens in urine include radioimmunoassay, enzyme immunoassay, and latex agglutination. Sensitivity of these methods can be up to 80% under ideal conditions.[1,2] Consult the laboratory regarding availability and selection of the most appropriate method. Nosocomial infections have been recognized with reservoirs in the water distribution systems, cooling systems, and hot water systems of hospitals being reported.[3,4,5] Over 34 species in the Legionellaceae family of bacteria have been discovered since *Legionella pneumophila* was first recognized. Thirteen species have been implicated as causes of human pneumonia.[6] See tables.

Footnotes

1. Harrison TG and Taylor AG, "Timing of Seroconversion in Legionnaires' Disease," *Lancet*, 1988, 2(8614):795.
2. Kohler RB, "Antigen Detection for the Rapid Diagnosis of *Mycoplasma* and *Legionella pneumoniae*," *Diagn Microbiol Infect Dis*, 1986, 4(Suppl):47S-59S.
3. Hoge CW and Brieman RF, "Advances in the Epidemiology and Control of *Legionella* Infections," *Epidemiol Rev*, 1991, 13:329-40.
4. Hart CA and Makin T, "*Legionella* in Hospitals: A Review," *J Hosp Infect*, 1991, 18(Suppl A):481-9.
5. Nguyen ML and Yu VL, "*Legionella* Infection," *Clin Chest Med*, 1991, 12(2):257-68.
6. Fang GD, Yu VL, and Vickers RM, "Disease Due to the Legionellaceae (Other Than *Legionella pneumophila*). Historical, Microbiological, Clinical, and Epidemiological Review," *Medicine (Baltimore)*, 1989, 68(2):116-32.

References

Winn WC Jr, "Legionnaires' Disease: Historical Perspective," *Clin Microbiol Rev*, 1988, 60-81.

Legionnaires' Disease Agent *see Legionella* Culture *on page 825*

***Leptospira* Culture, Blood** *see Leptospira* Culture, Urine *on this page*

Leptospira Culture, Urine

CPT *87081 (culture single organism); 87163 (additional identification methods)*

Related Information

Blood Culture, Aerobic and Anaerobic *on page 784*
Darkfield Examination, Leptospirosis *on page 808*
Leptospira Serodiagnosis *on page 718*

Synonyms Culture for *Leptospira*, Urine

Applies to Blood Culture, *Leptospira*; *Leptospira* Culture, Blood

Abstract Weil's disease (leptospirosis) is best worked up with culture and serology. Special culture media is needed.

Patient Care **PREPARATION:** Thoroughly instruct the patient in the proper collection technique for a midvoid urine specimen; avoid contamination with skin flora. See also Urine Culture, Clean Catch and Blood Culture, Aerobic and Anaerobic test listings for detailed instructions.

Specimen Urine, indicate midvoid, catheter or suprapubic puncture specimen; blood and cerebrospinal fluid may also be cultured **CONTAINER:** Sterile, urine container; for blood, purple top (EDTA) Vacutainer® or green top (heparin) Vacutainer® **COLLECTION:** Specimen should be transported to the laboratory within 1 hour of collection. For midvoid urine culture, patient should be instructed to clean skin thoroughly, do not collect first portion of stream, collect midportion of stream, and do not collect final portion of stream. Catheter or suprapubic puncture specimen may also be used. **STORAGE INSTRUCTIONS:** Specimens should not be refrigerated. They should be left at room temperature. Urine with an acid pH should be alkalinized if it cannot be set up immediately. **CAUSES FOR REJECTION:** Specimens delayed in transit to the laboratory have suboptimal yield. **TURNAROUND TIME:** 4-8 weeks **SPECIAL INSTRUCTIONS:** The labora-

(Continued)

Leptospira Culture, Urine *(Continued)*

tory should be informed of the specific request for *Leptospira* culture, collection time, current antibiotic therapy, and date of onset of illness. Urine must be alkaline; *Leptospira* do not survive in acid urine. Repeated cultures may be required.

Interpretive REFERENCE RANGE: No *Leptospira* isolated USE: Investigate possible leptospirosis (Weil's disease) LIMITATIONS: Specimen will be screened for *Leptospira*; other organisms are not isolated or identified. METHODOLOGY: Urine or blood is inoculated onto specially prepared media containing rabbit serum or albumin and fatty acids. Incubation is for 4-6 weeks in the dark at 28°C to 29°C. Cultures are examined with darkfield or phase microscopy for motile leptospires at weekly intervals; growth occurs 1-3 cm below the surface. ADDITIONAL INFORMATION: Leptospirosis in humans is usually associated with occupational exposure. Veterinarians, dairymen, swineherds, abattoir workers, miners, fish and poultry processors and those who work in a rat-infested environment are at increased risk. During the first week of disease, the most reliable means of detecting leptospires is by direct culture of blood or spinal fluid on appropriate media.[1] Urine does not become positive for *Leptospira* until the second week of disease and then can remain positive for several months. Concentration of *Leptospira* in human urine is low and shedding may be intermittent. Therefore, repeated isolation attempts should be made. Serology (acute and early convalescent) is recommended. Darkfield examination is no longer recommended.

Footnotes

1. Sperber SJ and Schleupner CJ, "Leptospirosis: A Forgotten Cause of Aseptic Meningitis and Multisystem Febrile Illness," *South Med J*, 1989, 82(10):1285-8.

References

Alexander AD, "*Leptospira*," *Manual of Clinical Microbiology*, 5th ed, Balows A, Hausler WJ Jr, Herrmann KL, et al, eds, Washington, DC: American Society for Microbiology, 1991, 554-9.

Faine S, "Leptospirosis," *Laboratory Diagnosis of Infectious Diseases: Principles and Practice*, Vol 1, New York, NY: Springer-Verlag, 1988, 344-52.

Raoult D, Bres P, and Baranton G, "Serologic Diagnosis of Leptospirosis: Comparison of Line Blot and Immunofluorescence Techniques With the Genus-Specific Microscopic Agglutination Test," *J Infect Dis*, 1989, 160:734-5.

Sanford JP, "Leptospirosis," *Harrison's Principles of Internal Med*, 12th ed, Chapter 130, Wilson JD, Braunwald E, Isselbacher KJ, et al, eds, New York, NY: McGraw-Hill Inc, 1991, 663-6.

Leptospirosis, Darkfield Examination *see* Darkfield Examination, Leptospirosis *on page 808*

L-Form Culture *see* Cell Wall Defective Bacteria Culture *on page 796*

Lice Identification *see* Arthropod Identification *on page 774*

L-Phase Organism Culture *see* Cell Wall Defective Bacteria Culture *on page 796*

Maximum Bactericidal Dilution *see* Serum Bactericidal Test *on page 843*

MBC *see* Susceptibility Testing, Minimum Bactericidal Concentration *on page 871*

MBD *see* Serum Bactericidal Test *on page 843*

Methylene Blue Stain, Stool

CPT 87205

Related Information

Clostridium difficile Toxin Assay *on page 802*
Cryptosporidium Diagnostic Procedures, Stool *on page 806*
Stool Culture *on page 858*
Stool Culture, Diarrheagenic *E. coli* *on page 860*
Stool Fungus Culture *on page 861*

Synonyms Fecal Leukocyte Stain; Gram Stain, Stool; Stool for White Cells; White Cells, Stool; Wright's Stain, Stool

Test Commonly Includes Methylene blue, Gram, or Wright's stain of stool smear

Patient Care PREPARATION: Collect specimen prior to barium procedures if possible.

Specimen Fresh random stool, rectal swab CONTAINER: Plastic stool container or Culturette® COLLECTION: Transport specimen to the laboratory as soon as possible after collection. Significant deterioration of the specimen occurs with prolonged storage. STORAGE INSTRUCTIONS: Refrigerate

Interpretive **REFERENCE RANGE:** No predominance of yeast, cocci in clusters, or leukocytes **USE:** Assist in the differential diagnosis of diarrheal disease. Used by some laboratories to screen for invasive enteric pathogens; the test should not be used to exclude specimens from culture. **LIMITATIONS:** Ten percent to 15% of stools which yield an invasive bacterial pathogen have an absence of fecal leukocytes. Fecal leukocytes are present in idiopathic inflammatory bowel disease. **METHODOLOGY:** Smear of stool (preferably mucus) with one drop methylene blue, coverslip, and observe the presence of leukocytes. See diagram. **ADDITIONAL INFORMATION:** Conditions associated with marked fecal leukocytes, blood, and mucus include diffuse antibiotic-associated colitis, ulcerative colitis, shigellosis, salmonellosis, *Helicobacter*, and *Yersinia* infection. *Salmonella typhi* may evoke a monocyte response. Conditions associated with modest numbers of fecal leukocytes include early shigellosis involving small bowel, antibiotic-associated colitis and amebiasis. Conditions associated with an absence of fecal leukocytes include toxigenic bacterial infection, giardiasis, and viral infections. The methylene blue stain for polymorpholeukocytes has a high sensitivity (85%) and specificity (88%) for bacterial diarrhea (*Shigella*, *Salmonella*, *Helicobacter*). Positive predictive value is 59%. Negative predicative value is 97%. Combined with a history of abrupt onset, more than four stools per day, and no vomiting before the onset of diarrhea, the stool methylene blue stain for fecal polymorphonuclear leukocytes is a very effective presumptive diagnostic test for bacterial diarrhea.[1] A positive occult blood test may also be suggestive of acute bacterial diarrhea but lacks specificity. Neither method is sufficiently sensitive or specific to pre-empt the use of culture.[2] Similar findings including a sensitivity of 81% and specificity of 74% were observed when both tests were positive.[3]

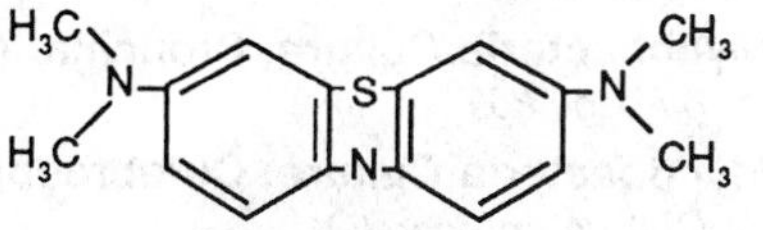

Tetramethyl thionin (methylene blue)

Footnotes

1. DeWitt TG, Humphrey KF, and McCarthy P, "Clinical Predictors of Acute Bacterial Diarrhea in Young Children," *Pediatrics*, 1985, 76:551-6.
2. Paccagnini S, Ceriani R, Galli L, et al, "Occult Blood and Faecal Leukocyte Tests in Acute Infectious Diarrhea of Children," *Lancet*, 1987, 1:442.
3. Seigel D, Cohen PT, Neighbor M, et al, "Predictive Value of Stool Examination in Acute Diarrhea," *Arch Pathol Lab Med*, 1987, 111:715-8.

References

Bishop WP and Ulshen MH, "Bacterial Gastroenteritis," *Pediatr Clin North Am*, 1988, 35:69-87, (review).
Gilligan PH, Janda JM, Karmali MA, et al, "Laboratory Diagnosis of Bacterial Diarrhea," *Cumitech 12A*, Nolte FS, ed, Washington, DC: American Society for Microbiology, 1992, (review).

MIC *see* Susceptibility Testing, Aerobic and Facultatively Anaerobic Organisms *on page 864*

MIC, Anaerobic Bacteria *see* Susceptibility Testing, Anaerobic Bacteria *on page 866*

MIC, Fastidious Organisms, Unusual Isolates *see* Susceptibility Testing, Unusual Isolates/Fastidious Organisms *on page 873*

Middle Ear Culture *see* Ear Culture *on page 810*

Midstream Urine Culture *see* Urine Culture, Clean Catch *on page 881*

Minimal Bactericidal Concentration (MBC) *see* Susceptibility Testing, Antimicrobial Combinations *on page 868*

Minimal Inhibitory Concentration (MIC) *see* Susceptibility Testing, Antimicrobial Combinations *on page 868*

Minimum Bactericidal Concentration *see* Susceptibility Testing, Minimum Bactericidal Concentration *on page 871*

Minimum Inhibitory Concentration Susceptibility Test *see* Susceptibility Testing, Aerobic and Facultatively Anaerobic Organisms *on page 864*

Minimum Inhibitory Concentration, Unusual Isolates *see* Susceptibility Testing, Unusual Isolates/Fastidious Organisms *on page 873*

Minimum Lethal Concentration *see* Susceptibility Testing, Minimum Bactericidal Concentration *on page 871*

Mite Identification *see* Arthropod Identification *on page 774*

MLC *see* Susceptibility Testing, Minimum Bactericidal Concentration *on page 871*

Mycobacteria Culture, Atypical, Skin *see* Skin Mycobacteria Culture *on page 846*

Mycobacteria Culture, Biopsy *see* Biopsy or Body Fluid Mycobacteria Culture *on page 782*

Mycobacteria Culture, Blood *see* Blood Culture, Aerobic and Anaerobic *on page 784*

Mycobacteria Culture, Bronchial Aspirate *see* Sputum Mycobacteria Culture *on page 855*

Mycobacteria Culture, Cerebrospinal Fluid *see* Cerebrospinal Fluid Mycobacteria Culture *on page 801*

Mycobacteria Culture, Gastric Aspirate *see* Sputum Mycobacteria Culture *on page 855*

Mycobacteria Culture, Sputum *see* Sputum Mycobacteria Culture *on page 855*

Mycobacteria Culture, Stool *see* Stool Mycobacteria Culture *on page 863*

Mycobacteria Culture, Tissue *see* Biopsy or Body Fluid Mycobacteria Culture *on page 782*

Mycobacteria Culture, Urine *see* Urine Mycobacteria Culture *on page 884*

Mycobacteria, DNA Probe *see* Sputum Mycobacteria Culture *on page 855*

Mycobacteria Susceptibility Testing *see* Susceptibility Testing, Mycobacteria *on page 872*

***Mycobacterium marinum* Culture, Skin** *see* Skin Mycobacteria Culture *on page 846*

***Mycobacterium* Smear** *see* Acid-Fast Stain *on page 770*

Nasopharyngeal Culture

CPT *87060*

Related Information

Bordetella pertussis Nasopharyngeal Culture *on page 790*

Nasopharyngeal Culture for *Staphylococcus aureus* Carriers *on next page*

Specimen Nasopharyngeal swab **CONTAINER:** Sterile wire swab expressed into transport medium or transported directly to the laboratory **COLLECTION:** Use special nasopharyngeal wire swabs/Calgiswab®. Gently insert swab through nose to posterior nasopharynx; allow to remain for a few seconds and gently remove wire. The specimen should be transported to the laboratory as soon as possible. Swabs must be collected carefully, taking care not to touch the skin. **TURNAROUND TIME:** Reports on specimens from which pathogens are isolated often require 48 hours. **SPECIAL INSTRUCTIONS:** The laboratory should be informed of current antibiotic therapy.

Interpretive **REFERENCE RANGE:** Normal nasopharyngeal flora **USE:** Isolate and identify potentially pathogenic organisms. Nasopharyngeal culture may reflect infection of tonsils, oropharynx, nasopharynx, and sinuses. Useful in identifying carriers of *S. aureus* and *N. meningitidis*. **LIMITATIONS:** Results suggesting primary nasopharyngeal infection must be interpreted with caution, because of the variety of potentially pathogenic normal flora and the potential presence of infection in adjacent sites. **METHODOLOGY:** Aerobic culture **ADDITIONAL INFORMATION:** Presence or absence of normal flora is usually reported. Normal flora of the nose includes *S. epidermidis* (coagulase-negative *Staphylococcus*), *S. aureus*, *S. pneumoniae*, *H. influenzae*, *S. pyogenes*, *M. catarrhalis*, and *Neisseria* sp. Consequently, nasal cultures for bacteria rarely provide useful clinical information.

References

Godley FA, "Chronic Sinusitis: An Update," *Am Fam Physician*, 1992, 45(5):2190-9.

Oppenheimer RW, "Sinusitis. How to Recognize and Treat It," *Postgrad Med*, 1992, 91(5):281-6, 289-92.

Wald ER, "Sinusitis in Children," *N Engl J Med*, 1992, 326(5):319-23.

Nasopharyngeal Culture for *Bordetella pertussis* *see Bordetella pertussis* Nasopharyngeal Culture *on page 790*

Nasopharyngeal Culture for *Corynebacterium diphtheriae* *see* Throat Culture for *Corynebacterium diphtheriae on page 878*

Nasopharyngeal Culture for *Staphylococcus aureus* Carriers

CPT *87081 (screen); 87163 (additional identification methods)*

Related Information

Nasopharyngeal Culture *on previous page*

Synonyms *Staphylococcus aureus* Nasal Culture

Specimen Nasal swab, nasopharyngeal swab **CONTAINER:** Sterile Culturette® **COLLECTION:** For detection of *S. aureus* carriers, the anterior nares should be swabbed. The specimen should be transported to the laboratory within 6 hours of collection. **TURNAROUND TIME:** Reports on specimens from which *Staphylococcus aureus* has been recovered may be generated within 24 hours; if antimicrobial susceptibilities are required (eg, to identify methicillin-resistant *Staphylococcus aureus*), an additional day is usually required. Negative cultures are usually reported after 48 hours. **SPECIAL INSTRUCTIONS:** Objectives of the program should be clearly defined because of the relatively high frequency of carriers in the normal population. The laboratory should be informed of the specimen request to screen for *Staphylococcus aureus*, the collection time, date, specific source of specimen, age of patient, current antibiotic therapy, and clinical diagnosis.

Interpretive REFERENCE RANGE: No *Staphylococcus aureus* isolated **USE:** Determine if a patient is a carrier of *Staphylococcus aureus*. Screen hospital personnel while investigating specific nosocomial outbreaks. **LIMITATIONS:** Culture is usually screened for *Staphylococcus aureus* only, no other potential pathogens are identified. **ADDITIONAL INFORMATION:** The anterior nares are a recognized major reservoir for *S. aureus*. Nasal carriage has been implicated as a source for *S. aureus* in drug addicts with endocarditis, bacteremia in dialysis patients, postoperative wound infections, and recurrent furunculosis. In particular, use of cocaine, topical decongestants, and steroid sprays have a statistically higher rate of carriage than nonusers. Carriage of toxin-capable isolates was reported in 40%.[1] Treatment for the carrier state has included rifampin therapy[2] and replacement of potentially pathogen *S. aureus* with the "low virulence" 502 A strain.[3]

Routine screening for *S. aureus* is not recommended, as up to 30% of normal individuals harbor *S. aureus*. The procedure is very useful in following up on outbreaks once infection control surveillance has identified a potential outbreak. Isolates from an outbreak may be analyzed by phage typing or plasmid typing which is particularly useful in outbreaks of methicillin-resistant *S. aureus* (MRSA).[4]

Footnotes

1. Gittelman PD, Jacobs JB, Lebowitz AS, et al, "*Staphylococcus aureus* Nasal Carriage in Patients With Rhinosinusitis," *Laryngoscope*, 1991, 101(7 Pt 1):733-7.
2. Wheat LJ, Kohler RB, Luft FC, et al, "Long-Term Studies of the Effect of Rifampin on Nasal Carriage of Coagulase-Positive Staphylococci," *Rev Infect Dis*, 1983, 5(Suppl):S459-62.
3. Hedstrom SA, "Treatment and Prevention of Recurrent Staphylococcal Furunculosis: Clinical and Bacteriological Follow-Up," *Scand J Infect Dis*, 1985, 17:55-8.
4. Zuccarelli AJ, Roy I, Harding GP, et al, "Diversity and Stability of Restriction Enzyme Profiles of Plasmid DNA From Methicillin-Resistant *Staphylococcus aureus*," *J Clin Microbiol*, 1990, 28(1):97-102.

References

Mayer LW, "Use of Plasmid Profiles in Epidemiologic Surveillance of Disease Outbreaks and in Tracing Transmission of Antibiotic Resistance," *Clin Microbiol Rev*, 1988, 1:228-43.

Neisseria gonorrhoeae Culture

CPT *87081; 87082 (commercial kit)*

Related Information

Cervical/Vaginal Cytology *on page 491*
Chlamydia trachomatis DNA Probe *on page 897*
Genital Culture *on page 814*
Genital Culture for *Ureaplasma urealyticum on page 1180*
Herpes Simplex Virus Culture *on page 1182*
HIV-1/HIV-2 Serology *on page 696*
Neisseria gonorrhoeae DNA Probe Test *on page 924*
(Continued)

Neisseria gonorrhoeae Culture *(Continued)*

Neisseria gonorrhoeae Smear *on page 834*
Penicillinase Test *on page 840*
RPR *on page 742*
VDRL, Serum *on page 762*

Synonyms GC Culture; Gonorrhea Culture

Patient Care PREPARATION: Preparation same as for clean catch urine. See Urine Culture, Clean Catch for detailed information. *Neisseria gonorrhoeae* is very sensitive to lubricants and disinfectants. If possible avoid collecting urethral specimens until at least 1 hour after urination.

Specimen Body fluid, discharge, pus, swab of genital lesions, urethral discharge (best when available for men); endocervix (best when available for female); throat swab, rectal swab; sediment of first 10 mL of centrifuged urine collected at least 2 hours after last micturition or first few drops of urine voided into a sterile cup for "first voided urine specimen" for asymptomatic males, or first void overnight urine, centrifuged. CONTAINER: Swab with transport medium, sterile container, direct planting on Transgrow, Jembec™, or Thayer-Martin medium COLLECTION:

Urethral discharge: Collect male urethral discharge by endourethral swab after stripping toward the orifice to express exudate.

Rectal swab: Collect anorectal specimens from the crypts just inside the anal ring. Direct visualization with anoscopy is useful. Insert the swab past the anal sphincter. Move the swab circumferentially around the anal crypts. Allow 15-30 seconds for organisms to adsorb onto the swab. Replace the swab and crush the media compartment.

Prostatic fluid yields fewer positives than does culture of urethral discharge.

Urethral or vaginal cultures are indicated from females when endocervical culture is not possible.

Urethra in women: Massage the urethra against the pubic symphysis to express discharge or use endourethral swab.

Vagina: Obtain the specimen from the vaginal vault. Allow 15-30 seconds for organisms to adsorb onto the swab.

Endocervical/cervical: Gently compress cervix between speculum blades to express any endocervical exudate. Swab in a circular pattern.

Bartholin gland: Express exudate from duct. Abscesses should be aspirated with needle and syringe.

Specimens should be transported to the laboratory within 1 hour of collection.

STORAGE INSTRUCTIONS: **Specimen should not be refrigerated or exposed to a cold environment.** If the specimen is directly inoculated on Thayer-Martin medium, it should be transported to the laboratory as soon as possible and placed directly in CO_2 incubator or candle jar. CAUSES FOR REJECTION: Growth of the organism is less likely following refrigeration. TURNAROUND TIME: Cultures with no growth are commonly reported after 48-72 hours. Cultures from which *N. gonorrhoeae* is isolated require a minimum of 48 hours for completion. SPECIAL INSTRUCTIONS: The laboratory should be informed of specific site of specimen, current antibiotic therapy, and clinical diagnosis.

Interpretive REFERENCE RANGE: No *Neisseria gonorrhoeae* isolated CRITICAL VALUES: Positive culture for *Neisseria gonorrhoeae* during pregnancy USE: Isolate and identify *Neisseria gonorrhoeae*; establish the diagnosis of gonorrhea LIMITATIONS: See table. Cultures are usually screened only for *Neisseria gonorrhoeae*. No other organisms are usually identified. Overgrowth by *Proteus* and yeast may make it impossible to rule out presence of *N. gonorrhoeae*. The vancomycin in Thayer-Martin media may inhibit some strains of *N. gonorrhoeae*.

Nongonococcal urethritis may be caused by *Ureaplasma urealyticum*, *Corynebacterium genitalium* type 1, *Trichomonas vaginalis*, *Chlamydia trachomatis*, herpes simplex virus, and rarely, *Candida albicans*.

METHODOLOGY: Culture on selective medium, Thayer-Martin, or NYC. DNA probes, monoclonal antibodies, enzyme immunoassays (EIA), and chromogenic substrate assays are used as alternatives or adjuncts to culture in some laboratories. Advantages of the newer methods over traditional culture and smear techniques are not universally recognized. ADDITIONAL INFORMA-

Selection of Culture Sites for the Isolation of *Neisseria gonorrhoeae*

Culture Site	Diagnostic Sensitivity (%)
Women (nonhysterectomized) Primary site Endocervical canal	86–96
Secondary sites Vagina	55–90
Urethra	60–86
Anal canal	70–85
Oropharynx	50–70
Women (hysterectomized) Primary site Urethra	88.9
Secondary sites Vagina	55.7
Anal canal	40.7
Men (heterosexuals) Primary site Urethra	94–98 (symptomatic) 84 (asymptomatic)
Men (homosexuals) Primary sites Urethra	60–98
Anal canal	40–85
Oropharynx	50–70

From Ehret JM and Knapp JS, "Gonorrhea," *Clin Lab Med,* 1989, 9:445-80, with permission.

TION: In a study of 1001 women consecutively seen at a venereal disease clinic, endocervical culture was positive in 88.4%, urine sediment 72%, and anal canal 22.8%. The prevalence of gonorrhea in the study population was 28.5%[1] A serologic test for syphilis (VDRL, RPR, or ART), HIV, and Cervical/Vaginal Cytology should be considered in patients suspected of having gonorrhea. Throat culture for GC was found to have little contribution to the further recovery of *N. gonorrhoeae* over culture of the urethra, cervix, and anus.[2] Thayer-Martin medium and transport systems are available in most laboratories.

Laboratories may presumptively identify *Neisseria gonorrhoeae* from clinical specimens if the following criteria are met:

- specimen is from a genital source
- patient is presumed to be sexually active
- organism grows on selective medium, is oxidase positive, and is morphologically consistent with *Neisseria gonorrhoeae* (ie, gram-negative diplococci with adjacent sides flattened)

If any of these criteria are not met, the organism must be definitively identified using stricter definitions. **Thus, organisms from the throat or rectum, or isolates from nonsexually active (eg, infants or young children) individuals should never be presumptively identified using the criteria listed above.**[3,4] Similarly, many of the rapid biochemical methods for identifying *Neisseria gonorrhoeae* based on three or four biochemical reactions and a very limited database are only acceptable for genital specimens from sexually active patients.

Footnotes

1. Chapel TA and Smeltzer M, "Culture of Urinary Sediment for the Diagnosis of Gonorrhea in Women," *Br J Vener Dis*, 1975, 51:25-7.
2. Brown RT, Lossick JG, Mosure DJ, et al, "Pharyngeal Gonorrhea Screening in Adolescents: Is It Necessary?" *Pediatrics*, 1989, 84(4):623-5.
3. Knapp J, "Historical Perspectives and Identification of *Neisseria* and Related Species," *Clin Microbiol Rev*, 1988, 1:415-31.
4. Whittington WL, Rice RJ, Biddle JW, et al, "Incorrect Identification of *Neisseria gonorrhoeae* From Infants and Children," *Pediatr Infect Dis J*, 1988, 7:3-10.

References

Judson FN, "Gonorrhea," *Med Clin North Am*, 1990, 74(6):1353-66.

(Continued)

Neisseria gonorrhoeae Culture *(Continued)*

Rajasekariah GR, Edward S, Shapira D, et al, "Direct Detection of *Neisseria gonorrhoeae* With Monoclonal Antibodies Characterized by Serotyping Reagents," *J Clin Microbiol*, 1989, 27(7):1700-3.

Roongpisuthipong A, Lewis JS, Kraus SJ, et al, "Gonococcal Urethritis Diagnosed From Enzyme Immunoassay of Urine Sediment," *Sex Transm Dis*, 1988, 15:192-5.

Schoone GJ, Cornelissen WJ, Veenhuijsen PC, et al, "Comparison of Dot Blot With *In Situ* Hybridization for the Detection of *Neisseria gonorrhoeae* in Urethral Exudate," *J Appl Bacteriol*, 1989, 66(5):401-5.

Thomason JL, Gelbart SM, Sobieski VJ, et al, "Effectiveness of Gonozyme for Detection of Gonorrhea in Low-Risk Pregnant and Gynecologic Populations," *Sex Transm Dis*, 1989, 16(1):28-31.

Young H and Moyes A, "Utility of Monoclonal Antibody Coagglutination to Identify *Neisseria gonorrhoeae*," *Genitourin Med*, 1989, 65(1):8-13.

Neisseria gonorrhoeae Smear

CPT *87205*

Related Information

Chlamydia trachomatis DNA Probe *on page 897*
Gram Stain *on page 815*
Neisseria gonorrhoeae Culture *on page 831*
Neisseria gonorrhoeae DNA Probe Test *on page 924*

Synonyms GC Smear; Gonorrhea Smear

Specimen Urethral swab from males, specimens from any normally sterile site (eg, joint fluid). Gram stains of specimens from the upper respiratory tract or rectum are not reliable for diagnosis of gonorrhea and should not be used for this purpose. Specimens from the female genital tract may or may not be accepted for this procedure, depending on laboratory policy. **CAUSES FOR REJECTION:** Specimen from an inappropriate site, insufficient specimen volume **TURNAROUND TIME:** Approximately 30 minutes after specimen is received in laboratory for stat specimens

Interpretive **REFERENCE RANGE:** Negative **USE:** Detect gram-negative intracellular diplococci resembling *N. gonorrhoeae* **LIMITATIONS:** The diagnosis of gonorrhea cannot be excluded without culture. See table.

Sensitivity and Specificity of Gram Stains for Diagnosis of Gonorrhea

Specimen Source	Sensitivity (%)	Specificity (%)
Women		
Endocervical canal	45–65	90–97
Vagina	Not studied	—
Urethra	16	—
Anal canal	Not recommended	—
Pharynx	Not recommended	—
Men		
Urethra (symptomatic)	95–99	97–98
Urethra (asymptomatic)	50–70	86
Anal canal (with mucopurulent discharge)	40–80	87–100
Pharynx	Not recommended	—

From Ehret JM and Knapp JS, "Gonorrhea," *Clin Lab Med,* 1989, 9:445–80, with permission.

METHODOLOGY: Gram stain with demonstration of intracellular gram-negative diplococci oriented with their broad edges adjacent **ADDITIONAL INFORMATION:** Gram stain smear has a high sensitivity in a symptomatic male with urethral discharge (95% to 99%). Endocervical Gram stain is of little value in the female as the sensitivity is lower (50%), and endemic normal flora have a similar morphologic appearance causing false-positives. Cervical and/or anal and throat cultures are recommended for female patients. Cervical cultures have a sensitivity of 80% to 90%. Although demonstration of gram-negative diplococci in leukocytes in a urethral smear from a symptomatic male is presumptive evidence of gonorrhea and is sufficiently diagnostic to initiate therapy, cultural confirmation should be considered if available. The Gram stain smear will detect 75% of gonococcal conjunctivitis and 10% to 20% of gonococcal skin lesions. It is of no value in pharyngitis.

References

Bowie WR, "Approach to Men With Urethritis and Urologic Complications of Sexually Transmitted Diseases," *Med Clin North Am*, 1990, 74(6):1543-57.

***Neisseria gonorrhoeae* Susceptibility Testing** *see* Penicillinase Test *on page 840*

Nits Identification *see* Arthropod Identification *on page 774*

Nocardia Culture, All Sites

CPT 87081

Related Information

Acid-Fast Stain, Modified, *Nocardia* Species *on page 771*
Actinomyces Culture, All Sites *on page 772*
Sputum Fungus Culture *on page 853*
Sputum Mycobacteria Culture *on page 855*

Applies to Sputum *Nocardia* Culture

Test Commonly Includes Culture for *Nocardia* sp and direct microscopic examination of Gram stain for branching gram-positive bacilli, modified acid-fast stain

Abstract *Nocardia asteroides*, *N. brasiliensis*, and *N. caviae* cause two disease entities, nocardiosis and mycetoma. The latter relates to trauma.

Specimen Pus, tissue, cerebrospinal fluid or other body fluid, aspirate, sputum. The usual portal of entry is the lung. **COLLECTION:** Refer to listing for culture of specific site for complete collection and storage instructions (eg, Biopsy or Body Fluid Culture, Sputum Culture, and Wound Culture). **TURNAROUND TIME:** Negative cultures are reported after 2-4 weeks. **SPECIAL INSTRUCTIONS:** Consultation with laboratory prior to collection of the specimen is recommended when nocardiosis is suspected clinically. Culture should be specifically ordered as Culture for *Nocardia*.

Interpretive **REFERENCE RANGE:** No *Nocardia* sp isolated **CRITICAL VALUES:** *Nocardia* sp recovered from a central nervous system specimen **USE:** Establish the diagnosis of nocardiosis or mycetoma; identify its pathogenic agent **LIMITATIONS:** *Nocardia* sp will not be recovered by routine culture techniques because of its relatively slow growth. Growth of *Nocardia* may be obscured by overgrowth of other organisms in mixed culture (ie, sputum). The diagnosis may not be made unless the laboratory is advised of the clinical suspicion of nocardiosis. *Nocardia* sp are not strongly gram-positive, but their branching pattern when visible is helpful. A modified acid-fast stain (described elsewhere in this chapter) is needed, since *Nocardia* are weakly acid-fast and may not be found with conventional acid-fast staining. Staining may be positive when cultures fail. **METHODOLOGY:** Aerobic culture on blood agar and Löwenstein-Jensen (LJ) media with no antibiotics. Recent data supports the use of *Legionella* culture media (selective and nonselective buffered charcoal yeast agar) for recovery of *Nocardia*.[1,2] *Nocardia* sp can also be cultured on noninhibitory fungal media. Cultures are usually held for 10-30 days. **ADDITIONAL INFORMATION:** *Nocardia* sp are aerobic, gram-positive bacteria which are filamentous, relatively slow growing, and variably acid fast. Human infection is seen most frequently in patients whose immune systems are suppressed by HIV infection, lymphoreticular malignancy, or chemotherapy. Nocardiosis frequently affects debilitated hosts and has been implicated in cases of infections in renal transplant patients, osteomyelitis, in patients on long-term steroid therapy and with peritonsillar abscess, and in cutaneous infections.[3,4,5,6] The clinical picture may be similar to that observed with systemic mycobacterial or fungal infections. Infections may be acute, subacute, or chronic; and they may be disseminated or localized to cutaneous sites or the respiratory tract.[7] Hematogenous dissemination occurs. Metastatic infection in brain, bone, skin, or subcutaneous infection in the presence of pulmonary involvement is suggestive of nocardiosis. *Nocardia asteroides* is the species most commonly recovered from clinical specimens and is usually associated with the respiratory tract; this species is phenotypically heterogeneous, and it has been proposed that the species be considered a complex which is subdivided.[8] *Nocardia brasiliensis* and *Nocardia caviae* also produce human infections; of the two, *Nocardia brasiliensis* is far more common. The species found in mycetoma is usually *N. brasiliensis*.

Nocardia sp are variably acid-fast and may be frequently confused with *Actinomyces* sp or saprophytic fungi in Gram stains of clinical specimens. Prognosis is dependent on early diagnosis, treatment with appropriate antimicrobials, and the course of the underlying disease.

(Continued)

Nocardia Culture, All Sites *(Continued)*

Footnotes

1. Vickers RM, Rihs JD, and Yu VL, "Clinical Demonstration of Isolation of *Nocardia asteroides* on Buffered Charcoal-Yeast Extract Media," *J Clin Microbiol*, 1992, 30(1):227-8.
2. Kerr E, Snell H, Black BL, et al, "Isolation of *Nocardia asteroides* From Respiratory Specimens by Using Selective Buffered Charcoal-Yeast Extract Agar," *J Clin Microbiol*, 1992, 30(5):1320-2.
3. Hellyar AG, "Experience With *Nocardia asteroides* in Renal Transplant Recipients," *J Hosp Infect*, 1988, 12(1):13-8.
4. Schwartz JG and Tio FO, "Nocardial Osteomyelitis: A Case Report and Review of the Literature," *Diagn Microbiol Infect Dis*, 1987, 8:37-46, (review).
5. Adair JC, Amber IJ, and Johnston JM, "Peritonsillar Abscess Caused by *Nocardia asteroides*," *J Clin Microbiol*, 1987, 25:2214-5.
6. Kalb RE, Kaplan MH, and Grossman ME, "Cutaneous Nocardiosis. Case Reports and Review," *J Am Acad Dermatol*, 1985, 13:125-33.
7. McNeil MM, Brown JM, Jarvis WR, et al, "Comparison of Species Distribution and Antimicrobial Susceptibility of Aerobic Actinomycetes From Clinical Specimens," *Rev Infect Dis*, 1990, 12(5):778-83.
8. Wallace RJ Jr, Brown BA, Tsukamura M, et al, "Clinical and Laboratory Features of *Nocardia nova*," *J Clin Microbiol*, 1991, 29(11):2407-11.

References

Bennett JE, "Actinomycosis and Nocardiosis," *Harrison's Principles of Internal Medicine*, 12th ed, Chapter 152, Wilson JD, Braunwald E, Isselbacher KJ, et al, eds, New York, NY: McGraw-Hill Inc, 1991, 752-3.

Chazen G, "*Nocardia*," *Infect Control*, 1987, 8:260-3.

Javaly K, Horowitz HW, and Wormser GP, "Nocardiosis in Patients With Human Immunodeficiency Virus Infection. Report of 2 Cases and Review of the Literature," *Medicine (Baltimore)*, 1992, 71(3):128-38.

Wilson JP, Turner HR, Kirchner KA, et al, "Nocardial Infections in Renal Transplant Recipients," *Medicine (Baltimore)*, 1989, 68(1):38-57.

***Nocardia* Species Modified Acid-Fast Stain** *see* Acid-Fast Stain, Modified, *Nocardia* Species *on page 771*

Ocular Culture *see* Conjunctival Culture *on page 803*

Outer Ear Culture *see* Ear Culture *on page 810*

Ova and Parasites, Stool

CPT *87177*

Related Information

Ascariasis Serological Test *on page 641*
Bile Fluid Examination *on page 1109*
Chagas' Disease Serological Test *on page 662*
Clostridium difficile Toxin Assay *on page 802*
Cryptosporidium Diagnostic Procedures, Stool *on page 806*
Cysticercosis Titer *on page 671*
Echinococcosis Serological Test *on page 674*
Entamoeba histolytica Serological Test *on page 675*
Enterovirus Culture *on page 1178*
Eosinophil Count *on page 539*
Filariasis Serological Test *on page 679*
HIV-1/HIV-2 Serology *on page 696*
Ova and Parasites, Urine *on page 839*
Parasite Antibodies *on page 729*
Pinworm Preparation *on page 841*
Rotavirus, Direct Detection *on page 1191*
Schistosomiasis Serological Test *on page 745*
Stool Culture *on page 858*
Toxoplasmosis Serology *on page 759*
Trichinosis Serology *on page 760*

Synonyms Parasites, Stool; Parasitology Examination, Stool; Stool for Ova and Parasites

Applies to Amebiasis; *Blastocystis hominis*; Flagellates; *Giardia*; Helminths

Test Commonly Includes Gross appearance, direct wet mounts, saline and iodine, concentration procedure, hematoxylin smear or trichrome smear

Abstract Parasitology is an entire discipline, about which major texts are available.

Patient Care PREPARATION: Specimens obtained with a warm saline enema or Fleet Phospho®-Soda are acceptable. Specimens obtained with mineral oil, bismuth, or magnesium compounds are unsatisfactory. Wait 1 week or more after barium procedures or laxative administration before collecting stools for examination. **AFTERCARE:** **Warning**: Any stool collected by or from the patient may harbor pathogens which are **immediately infective.** Use extreme caution when *Entamoeba histolytica*, *Hymenolepis nana*, *Cryptosporidium*, and *Taenia* sp are suspected or reported.

Specimen Fresh or preserved random stool or duodenal aspirate. If pinworm is suspected, a Scotch® Tape preparation should be submitted to the laboratory instead of stool. **CONTAINER:** Plastic stool container. If transport to the laboratory will take more than 1 hour, it is preferable to preserve the stool specimen. Preservative systems are commercially available from several sources; the most useful consist of two separate containers, one of which contains polyvinyl alcohol, the other contains formalin. When collected properly and transferred to these containers, ova and parasites will be adequately preserved; this is particularly important with diarrheal stools that contain protozoan trophozoites, since these forms degenerate rapidly. **COLLECTION:** The specimen should be delivered to the laboratory within 1 hour of collection. Direct wet preparation exams for motile trophozoite observation can be performed on stools which arrive in the laboratory not longer than 1 hour after collection. For most laboratories, it is best to plan for specimen receipt early in the working day, Monday through Friday, when experienced staff are likeliest to be available. The recommended screening procedure is three random stool specimens; one collected every other day. Specimens may be preserved in polyvinyl alcohol (PVA) fixative which is suitable for the preparation of permanent stains and formalin or merthiolate-iodine-formalin (MIF), which is suitable for concentration preparations and direct examination. If specimens are submitted in preservative, they may be transported to the laboratory at a more leisurely pace since organisms will not degenerate. **STORAGE INSTRUCTIONS:** Liquid specimens should be brought directly to the laboratory. Wet mounts should be performed immediately, and the specimen placed in PVA and/or MIF preservatives to maintain ova and trophozoite states when applicable. **CAUSES FOR REJECTION:** Because of risk to laboratory personnel, specimens sent on diaper or tissue paper, specimen contaminating outside of transport container may not be acceptable to the laboratory. Specimen containing interfering substances (eg, castor oil, bismuth, Metamucil®, barium, specimens delayed in transit, and those contaminated with urine) will not have optimal yield. **TURNAROUND TIME:** Variable, depending on method **SPECIAL INSTRUCTIONS:** Geographic history is needed by the Parasitology Laboratory.

Interpretive **REFERENCE RANGE:** No parasites seen **USE:** Establish the diagnosis of parasitic infestation **LIMITATIONS:** **Note**: One negative result does not rule out the possibility of parasitic infestation. Stool examination for *Giardia* may be negative in early stages of infection, in patients who shed organisms cyclically, and in chronic infections.[1] The sensitivity of microscopic methods for the detection of *Giardia* range from 46% to 95%.[2] Tests for *Giardia* antigen may have a much higher yield.[3] **CONTRAINDICATIONS:** Administration of barium, bismuth, Metamucil®, castor oil, mineral oil, tetracycline therapy, administration of antiamebic drugs within 1 week prior to test. Purgation contraindicated for pregnancy, ulcerative colitis, cardiovascular disease, child younger than 5 years of age, appendicitis or possible appendicitis. **METHODOLOGY:** Wet mount and trichrome stain after concentration, immunofluorescence (IF), counterimmunoelectrophoresis (CIE), or enzyme-linked immunosorbent assay (ELISA) for the detection of *Giardia* antigens. The use of pooled preserved specimens to contain costs is warranted.[4] **ADDITIONAL INFORMATION:** Amebas and certain other parasites cannot be seen in stools containing barium. Optimal diagnostic yield is obtained by the examination of fresh, warm stool by an experienced technologist, during usual laboratory hours. Amebic cysts, *Giardia* cysts, and helminth eggs can be recovered from formed stools. Mushy or liquid stools (either normally passed or obtained by purgation) often yield trophozoites. Purgation does not enhance the yield of *Giardia*. Stools which can be processed by the laboratory in less than 1 hour need not be preserved. Mushy, loose, or watery stools which cannot reach the laboratory within 1 hour should be preserved in formalin or merthiolate-iodine-formalin (MIF) and/or polyvinyl alcohol (PVA). Formalin will preserve protozoan cysts and larvae and the eggs of helminths. It is used for concentration procedures. PVA will preserve the trophozoite stage of protozoa. A trichrome-stained smear may be prepared from PVA fixed material. Specimens submitted in PVA cannot be concentrated; therefore, they should always be accompanied by a portion of the specimen in formalin. Formed stools may be preserved in formalin or refrigerated in a secure container until they can be transported to the laboratory. The MIF kit will preserve protozoan cysts, helminth eggs and larvae. It is intended to be sent home with the patient and mailed back to the laboratory.

Parasites identified in the stool of immunocompromised subjects (eg, AIDS patients) include *Cryptosporidium*, Microsporidia, *Entamoeba histolytica*, *Giardia lamblia*, *Isospora belli*, and

(Continued)

AMEBAE							
	Entamoeba histolytica	*Entamoeba hartmanni*	*Entamoeba coli*	*Entamoeba polecki*[1]	*Endolimax nana*	*Iodamoeba bütschlii*	*Dientamoeba fragilis*[2]
Trophozoite							
Cyst							No cyst

[1]Rare, probably of animal origin
[2]Flagellate

Scale: 0 5 10 μm

Amebae found in human stool specimens.

	CILIATE	COCCIDIA			BLASTOCYSTIS
	Balantidium coli	*Isospora belli*	*Sarcocystis* spp.	*Cryptosporidium* spp.	*Blastocystis hominis*
Trophozoite		immature oocyst	mature oocyst	mature oocyst	
Cyst	0 20 40 μm	mature oocyst	single sporocyst		Scale: 0 10 20 μm

Coccidia scale: 0 10 20 30 μm

Ciliate, coccidia, and *B. hominis* found in human stool specimens.

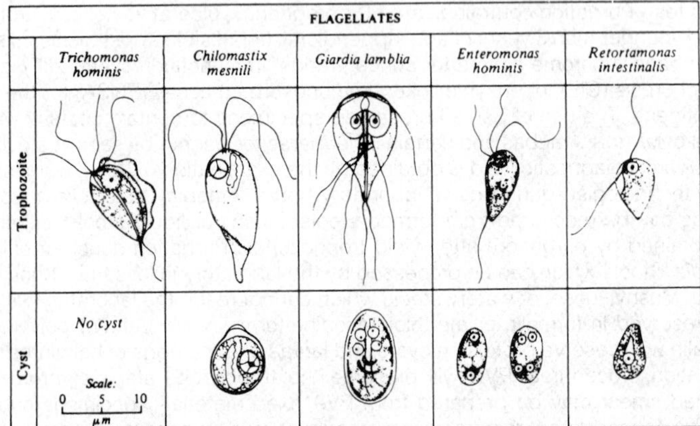

Flagellates found in human stool specimens. From Brooke and Melvin

Strongyloides stercoralis.[5,6] Microsporidia are obligate intracellular spore-forming protozoa. *Enterocytozoon bieneusi*, a Microsporidia sp, is a cause of diarrhea in HIV-positive persons.[7] Its diagnosis is facilitated by duodenal pinch biopsies.[8]

Blastocystis hominis which is commonly observed in stool of healthy and symptomatic patients is not currently deemed to be pathogenic. A review of the literature by Miller and Minshew indicated that there was no convincing proof of a causal relationship between *B. hominis* and symptoms, that there was no correlation between resolution of symptoms with therapy or with the disappearance of the organism from stool, and that treatment directed at the indication of *B. hominis* is not indicated.[9]

Doyle et al have observed a role for *Blastocystis* in acute and chronic gastroenteritis but are unable to conclude whether the role is one of association or causation.[10]

In a large children's hospital study of nosocomial diarrhea, rotavirus, *C. difficile*, and enteric adenovirus were recovered. Stool for ova and parasites and bacterial stool cultures yielded no pathogens.[11]

Footnotes

1. Brooke MM and Melvin DM, *Morphology of Diagnostic Stages of Intestinal Parasites of Humans*, 2nd ed, U.S. Department of Health and Human Services, Publication No 84-8116, Atlanta, GA: Centers for Disease Control, 1984.
2. Janoff EN, Craft CJ, and Pickering LK, "Diagnosis of *Giardia lamblia* Infections by Detection of Parasite-Specific Antigens," *J Clin Microbiol*, 1989, 27(3):431-5.
3. Chappell CL and Matson CC, "*Giardia* Antigen Detection in Patients With Chronic Gastrointestinal Disturbances," *J Fam Pract*, 1992, 35(1):49-53.
4. Peters CS, Hernandez L, Sheffield N, et al, "Cost Containment of Formalin-Preserved Stool Specimens for Ova and Parasites From Outpatients," *J Clin Microbiol*, 1988, 26:1584-5.
5. Garcia LS and Shimizu R, "Diagnostic Parasitology: Parasitic Infections and the Compromised Host," *Lab Med*, 1993, 24:205-15.
6. Curry A, Turner AJ, and Lucas S, "Opportunistic Protozoan Infections in Human Immunodeficiency Virus Disease: Review Highlighting Diagnostic and Therapeutic Aspects," *J Clin Pathol*, 1991, 44(3):182-93.
7. Weber R, Bryan RT, Owen RL, et al, "Improved Light-Microscopical Detection of Microsporidia Spores in Stool and Duodenal Aspirates. The Enteric Opportunistic Infections Working Group," *N Engl J Med*, 1992, 326(3):161-6.
8. Peacock CS, Blanshard C, Tovey DG, et al, "Histological Diagnosis of Intestinal Microsporidiosis in Patients With AIDS," *J Clin Pathol*, 1991, 44(7):558-63.
9. Miller RA and Minshew BH, "*Blastocystis hominis*: An Organism in Search of a Disease," *Rev Infect Dis*, 1988, 10:930-8, (review).
10. Doyle PW, Helgason MM, Mathias RG, et al, "Epidemiology and Pathogenicity of *Blastocystis hominis*," *J Clin Microbiol*, 1990, 28(1):116-21.
11. Brady MT, Pacini DL, Budde CT, et al, "Diagnostic Studies of Nosocomial Diarrhea in Children: Assessing Their Use and Value," *Am J Infect Control*, 1989, 17(2):77-82.

References

Ash LR and Orihel TC, *Atlas of Human Parasitology*, 3rd ed, Chicago, IL: ASCP Press, 1990.

Reed SL, "Amebiasis: An Update," *Clin Infect Dis*, 1992, 14(2):385-93.

Reitano M, Masci JR, and Bottone EJ, "Amebiasis: Clinical and Laboratory Perspective," *Crit Rev Clin Lab Sci*, 1991, 28(5-6):357-85.

René E, Marche C, Regnier B, et al, "Intestinal Infections in Patients With Acquired Immunodeficiency Syndrome: A Prospective Study in 132 Patients," *Dig Dis Sci*, 1989, 34(5):773-80.

Senay H and MacPherson D, "Parasitology: Diagnostic Yield of Stool Examination," *Can Med Assoc J*, 1989, 140(11):1329-31.

Wolfe MS, "Giardiasis," *Clin Microbiol Rev*, 1992, 5(1):93-100.

Ova and Parasites, Urine

CPT *87177*

Related Information

Blood, Urine *on page 1112*
Eosinophil Count *on page 539*
Eosinophils, Urine *on page 1117*
Filariasis Serological Test *on page 679*
Hemoglobin, Qualitative, Urine *on page 1122*
Ova and Parasites, Stool *on page 836*
Parasite Antibodies *on page 729*
Pinworm Preparation *on page 841*
Schistosomiasis Serological Test *on page 745*

(Continued)

Ova and Parasites, Urine *(Continued)*

Urine Cytology *on page 513*

Synonyms Parasites, Urine; Urine for Parasites; Urine for *Schistosoma haematobium*

Applies to Schistosomiasis

Test Commonly Includes Wet preparation and concentration procedure

Specimen Freshly voided urine **CONTAINER:** Sterile, plastic urine container **COLLECTION:** The specimen should be less than 4 hours old and not refrigerated. The recommended screening procedure is to submit three first morning urines on successive days. **STORAGE INSTRUCTIONS:** Do **not** refrigerate. Transport to the laboratory as soon as possible after collection. **CAUSES FOR REJECTION:** Excessive delay in transit to the laboratory may result in less than optimal yield. **TURNAROUND TIME:** 24 hours **SPECIAL INSTRUCTIONS:** The laboratory should be informed of the parasite clinically suspected. Geographic history is needed.

Interpretive **REFERENCE RANGE:** No parasites identified **USE:** Detect parasitic infestation, particularly *Trichomonas* or *Schistosoma haematobium*. Eggs of *Enterobius vermicularis* are sometimes present in urine as the result of fecal contamination, but are best investigated as described under Pinworm Preparation listing. **LIMITATIONS:** A single negative result does not rule out the possibility of parasitic infestation. **ADDITIONAL INFORMATION:** Immunodiagnostic tests including enzyme-linked immunosorbent assay and immunoblot tests have been used to diagnose schistosomiasis in some centers.[1] Patient should have a geographic history consistent with schistosomiasis to warrant undertaking screening the urine.

Footnotes

1. Tsang VC and Wilkins PP, "Immunodiagnosis of Schistosomiasis. Screen With FAST-ELISA and Confirm With Immunoblot," *Clin Lab Med*, 1991, 11(4):1029-39.

References

Ash LR and Orihel TC, *Atlas of Human Parasitology*, 3rd ed, Chicago, IL: ASCP Press, 1990.

Parasites, Stool *see* Ova and Parasites, Stool *on page 836*

Parasites, Urine *see* Ova and Parasites, Urine *on previous page*

Parasitology Examination, Stool *see* Ova and Parasites, Stool *on page 836*

***Pediculus humanus* Identification** *see* Arthropod Identification *on page 774*

Penicillinase *see* Susceptibility Testing, Aerobic and Facultatively Anaerobic Organisms *on page 864*

Penicillinase-Producing Organisms Susceptibility Testing *see* Penicillinase Test *on this page*

Penicillinase Test

***CPT** 87999*

Related Information

Neisseria gonorrhoeae Culture *on page 831*
Susceptibility Testing, Aerobic and Facultatively Anaerobic Organisms *on page 864*
Susceptibility Testing, Anaerobic Bacteria *on page 866*

Synonyms Beta-Lactamase Production Test; Cefinase (Nitrocefin) Testing; Cephalosporinase Production Testing; Penicillinase-Producing Organisms Susceptibility Testing

Applies to Beta-Lactam Ring; *Haemophilus influenzae* Susceptibility Testing; *Neisseria gonorrhoeae* Susceptibility Testing

Test Commonly Includes Rapid testing of isolated bacterial colonies for the production of beta-lactamase

Abstract Certain bacteria produce enzymes that inactivate beta-lactam antibiotics. Some enzymes can hydrolyze penicillin (penicillinases); others hydrolyze cephalosporins (cephalosporinases). In either case the detection of enzyme production by bacterial isolates is essential in determination of appropriate therapy.

Specimen *Haemophilus influenzae*, *Moraxella* (*Branhamella*) *catarrhalis*, *Neisseria gonorrhoeae*, enterococci, *Staphylococcus aureus*, or gram-negative anaerobic rods including *Bacteroides fragilis*

Interpretive **USE:** Rapid detection of beta-lactamase production from isolated colonies of *Haemophilus influenzae*, *Neisseria gonorrhoeae*, *Moraxella catarrhalis*, *S. aureus*, and enterococci sp. This test can be used to predict resistance to penicillins and some cephalosporins. Most isolates of *Staphylococcus aureus* produce beta-lactamases and thus, are often treated as beta-lactamase positive without testing for enzyme production. **METHODOLOGY:** The acidimetric method uses pH color indicators to detect increased acidity that results when the beta-lactam ring of penicillin is cleaved to yield a penicilloic acid. Penicilloic acid can also reduce iodine that can be detected as the decolorization of a starch-iodine mixture. This method is referred to as the iodometric method. The most commonly used method is the use of a chromogenic cephalosporin reagent. The hydrolysis of the beta-lactam ring results in a color change that is quickly detected. The chromogenic assay can detect both penicillinases and cephalosporinases. **ADDITIONAL INFORMATION:** The nitrocefin method is favored for anaerobes because it can detect both the cephalosporinases produced by *Bacteroides fragilis* and *Prevotella melaninogenica* (*Bacteroides melaninogenicus*), as well as, the penicillinases produced by other anaerobes.[1] This is also the method recommended for testing *M. catarrhalis* and *S. aureus* isolates.

Plasmid-mediated production of beta-lactamase occurs in 5% to 15% of clinical isolates of *H. influenzae* type b. However, other mechanisms of resistance have also been reported.[2] Routine testing of *H. influenzae* for beta-lactamase production is performed by most laboratories. Strains of *N. gonorrhoeae* producing beta-lactamase have been linked to contacts of patients acquiring the infection outside the United States and in prostitutes and sexual contacts of drug users.[3] Incidence of penicillinase-producing *N. gonorrhoeae* has increased drastically in Florida, California, and New York. Routine testing of *N. gonorrhoeae* for beta-lactamase production is not routinely necessary in many parts of the United States, but should be considered in treatment failure cases and in areas in which resistance is endemic.

Footnotes

1. Rosenblatt JE, "Susceptibility Testing of Anaerobic Bacteria," *Clin Lab Med*, 1989, 9(2):239-54, (review).
2. Bell SM and Plowman, "Mechanisms of Ampicillin Resistance in *Haemophilus influenzae* From Respiratory Tract," *Lancet*, 1980, 1:279-80.
3. Handsfield HH, Rice RJ, Roberts MC, et al, "Localized Outbreak of Penicillinase-Producing *Neisseria gonorrhoeae* Paradigm for Introduction and Spread of Gonorrhea in a Community," *JAMA*, 1989, 261(16):2357-61.

References

Stratton CW and Cooksey RC, "Susceptibility Tests: Special Tests," *Manual of Clinical Microbiology*, 5th ed, Balows A, Hausler WJ Jr, Herrmann KL, et al, eds, Washington, DC: American Society for Microbiology, 1991, 1153-65.

Percutaneous Transtracheal Anaerobic Culture *see* Bronchial Aspirate Anaerobic Culture *on page 792*

Percutaneous Transtracheal Culture *see* Sputum Culture *on page 849*

Periodic Acid Schiff (PAS) *see* Fungus Smear, Stain *on page 813*

Pertussis Culture *see Bordetella pertussis* Nasopharyngeal Culture *on page 790*

***Phthirus pubis* Identification** *see* Arthropod Identification *on page 774*

Pinworm Preparation

CPT *87208*

Related Information

Ova and Parasites, Stool *on page 836*
Ova and Parasites, Urine *on page 838*

Synonyms *Enterobius vermicularis* Preparation; Scotch® Tape Test

Test Commonly Includes Detection of pinworm eggs from the perianal region

Specimen Scotch® Tape slide preparation of perianal region **CONTAINER:** Scotch® Tape slide must be submitted in a covered container. Commercial kit products are also available for collection of pinworm specimens. **Caution**: Pinworm eggs are very infectious. **COLLECTION:** The specimen is best obtained a few hours after the patient has retired (ie, 10 or 11 PM), or early in the morning before a bowel movement or bath. This collection procedure is essential if valid results are expected. Clear Scotch® Tape should be used. The nontransparent type is unsatisfactory. An 8 cm (3 in) piece of cellophane tape is placed over the end of a glass slide sticky side out. The anal folds are spread apart and the mucocutaneous junction is firmly pressed in all four quadrants. The tape is then pressed over the slide and the specimen is transported to the laboratory in a carefully sealed container. Refer to diagram. It is important to provide clear instructions, because these specimens are often collected at home. **CAUSES FOR REJECTION:**

(Continued)

Pinworm Preparation *(Continued)*

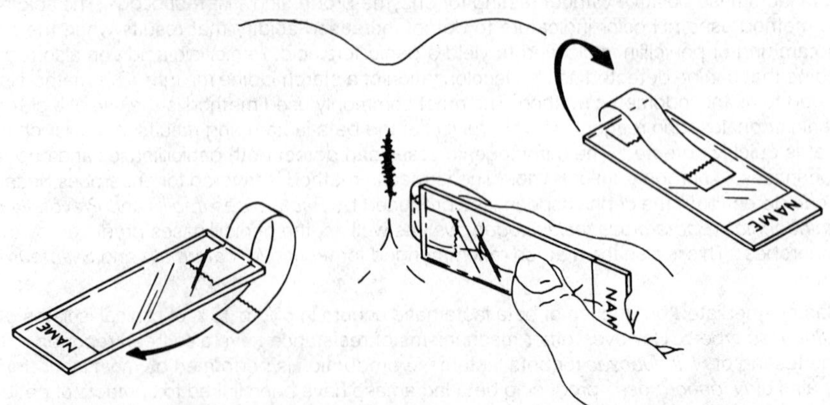

Cellophane tape slide preparation. Attach 3" piece of cellophane tape to undersurface of clear end of microscope slide, which has previously been identified (ground–glass end). Press sticky surface of tape against perianal skin. Then roll back tape onto slide, sticky surface down. Wash hands and nails well. From Bauer JD, *Clinical Laboratory Methods,* 9th ed, Mosby–Year Book Inc, St Louis, MO: 1982, 989, with permission.

Use of nontransparent Scotch® Tape, Scotch® Tape on both sides of the slide, specimen which is not inside a covered container, use of frosted slide, tape sent sticky side up. Specimens which are not properly contained pose excessive risk to laboratory personnel and may not be acceptable to the laboratory.

Interpretive **REFERENCE RANGE:** No pinworm eggs (*Enterobius vermicularis*) identified. Positives reported as few, moderate, or many eggs identified. **USE:** Detect cases of pinworm infestation (enterobiasis), *Enterobius vermicularis* parasitic infestation **LIMITATIONS:** Examination for pinworm only. One negative result does not rule out possibility of parasitic infestation. Examinations on multiple days may be required to diagnose infection. Stool specimens are not usually satisfactory for pinworm studies. **CONTRAINDICATIONS:** Specimen collection at improper time **METHODOLOGY:** Microscopy **ADDITIONAL INFORMATION:** The most satisfactory means of diagnosing pinworm infection is by the recovery of eggs or female worms from the perianal region. Only 5% to 10% of infected persons have demonstrable eggs in their stools. If fecal material is submitted for examination, only the surface should be sampled. Enterobiasis often is present in multiple family members. Therefore, it is recommended that all members of the family be tested. The responsible parent should be instructed how to collect samples, using one kit per individual. Female worms or parts of them may be demonstrated on the tape by microscopic examination. The proportion of positive specimens correlate with severity of disease. Eggs, if present, may be immature, embryonated (with viable or dead larvae), or (if the specimen is several days or more old) empty egg shells will be present. *Enterobius vermicularis* has been reported as a rare cause of appendicitis, salpingitis, epididymitis, and hepatic granuloma. Diagnosis at colonoscopy has been reported.

References

Mondou EN and Gnepp DR, "Hepatic Granuloma Resulting From *Enterobius vermicularis*," *Am J Clin Pathol*, 1989, 91(1):97-100.

Russell LJ, "The Pinworm, *Enterobius vernicularis*," *Prim Care*, 1991, 18(1):13-24.

Schnell VL, Yandell R, Van Zandt S, et al, "*Enterobius vermicularis* Salpingitis: A Distant Episode From Precipitating Appendicitis," *Obstet Gynecol*, 1992, 80(3 Pt 2):553-5.

Sun T, Schwartz NS, Sewell C, et al, "*Enterobius* Egg Granuloma of the Vulva and Peritoneum: Review of the Literature," *Am J Trop Med Hyg*, 1991, 45(2):249-53.

Pleural Fluid, *Legionella* Culture *see* *Legionella* Culture *on page 825*

Potassium Hydroxide Preparation *see* KOH Preparation *on page 825*

PPD Skin Test *see* Skin Test, Tuberculosis *on page 848*

Prostatic Fluid Culture *see* Genital Culture *on page 814*

Protected Catheter Brush (PCB) *see* Bronchial Aspirate Anaerobic Culture *on page 792*

Protoplast Culture *see* Cell Wall Defective Bacteria Culture *on page 796*

Pseudomembranous Colitis Toxin Assay *see Clostridium difficile* Toxin Assay *on page 802*

Pubic Lice Identification *see* Arthropod Identification *on page 774*

Quantitative Burn Culture *see* Burn Culture, Quantitative *on page 794*

Quantitative Culture, Biopsy Specimen *see* Burn Culture, Quantitative *on page 794*

Quantitative Tip Culture (QTC) *see* Intravascular Device Culture *on page 822*

Rectal Swab Culture *see* Stool Culture *on page 858*

Rocky Mountain Spotted Fever, *Dermacentor andersoni* *see* Arthropod Identification *on page 774*

Safranin *see* Gram Stain *on page 815*

***Sarcoptes scabiei* Skin Scrapings Identification** *see* Arthropod Identification *on page 774*

Schistosomiasis *see* Ova and Parasites, Urine *on page 839*

Schlichter Test *see* Serum Bactericidal Test *on this page*

Scotch® Tape Test *see* Pinworm Preparation *on page 841*

Screening Culture for Group A Beta-Hemolytic *Streptococcus* *see* Throat Culture *on page 876*

Sensitivity Testing, Aerobic and Facultatively Anaerobic Organisms *see* Susceptibility Testing, Aerobic and Facultatively Anaerobic Organisms *on page 864*

Serum Antibacterial Titer *see* Serum Bactericidal Test *on this page*

Serum Bactericidal Level *see* Serum Bactericidal Test *on this page*

Serum Bactericidal Test

CPT *87197*

Related Information

Amikacin *on page 938*
Antibiotic Level, Serum *on page 942*
Chloramphenicol *on page 952*
Gentamicin *on page 970*
Susceptibility Testing, Aerobic and Facultatively Anaerobic Organisms *on page 864*
Susceptibility Testing, Antimicrobial Combinations *on page 868*
Tobramycin *on page 1004*
Vancomycin *on page 1009*

Synonyms Antibacterial Activity, Serum; Bacterial Inhibitory Level, Serum; Maximum Bactericidal Dilution; MBD; Schlichter Test; Serum Antibacterial Titer; Serum Bactericidal Level; Serum Inhibitory Titer; Susceptibility Testing, Serum Bactericidal Dilution Method

Applies to Serum Inhibitory Dilution; SID

Patient Care PREPARATION: Sterile aspiration of body fluid

Specimen Peak and trough serum from patient and bacterial isolate causing infection (prepared by laboratory) CONTAINER: Red top tube; sterile tube for body fluid SAMPLING TIME: The peak level for intravenously (I.V.) administered drugs is obtained 30-60 minutes after the drug is given to allow for absorption and distribution. The trough level is obtained within 30 minutes or less of the next dose. For intramuscularly (I.M.) administered drugs and oral (P.O.) drugs, the peak should be drawn later at 2-4 hours. Vancomycin peak is drawn 2 hours postdose. COLLECTION: Specimen should be transported to the laboratory within 1 hour of collection. If this is not possible, the sample should be frozen at -70°C and transported on dry ice. STORAGE INSTRUCTIONS: Separate serum using aseptic technique and freeze at -70°C. Imipenem is inactivated at -20°C. CAUSES FOR REJECTION: Isolate discarded before request for testing, serum specimen allowed to sit at room temperature for more than 2 hours TURNAROUND TIME: 2-3 days SPECIAL INSTRUCTIONS: If a serum bactericidal test is desired, the physician should request that the laboratory save the patient's isolate within 48 hours of submission of the specimen for initial culture. **If the isolate has not been saved, the test cannot be performed.**

(Continued)

Serum Bactericidal Test *(Continued)*

The laboratory should be informed of current antibiotic therapy including date and time of last dosage, route of administration on all antimicrobial agents patient is receiving, and clinical diagnosis. Time of specimen collection should be indicated on requisition.

Interpretive **REFERENCE RANGE:** Peak bactericidal activity should be observed at ≥1:8 dilution, trough at ≥1:2 **USE:** Determine the maximum bactericidal dilution (MBD) or serum bactericidal dilution (SBD) of serum or body fluid after administration of antibiotic(s). This is the last serum/body fluid dilution which is bactericidal for the patient's infecting organism. This titer is useful in monitoring total therapeutic effect. Frequently it is used to evaluate therapy in endocarditis, osteomyelitis, and suppurative arthritis. Serum bactericidal titers of ≥1:8 are often recommended for the optimal treatment of these infections. **LIMITATIONS:** Results will reflect the combined *in vitro* effect of all antimicrobial agents present in the patient's serum or body fluid on his/her infecting organism(s). Results are accurate to ±1 dilution and are not necessarily equivalent to a serum assay. Maximum inhibitory dilution (MID) or serum inhibitory dilution (SID) may also be reported. An apparently adequate ratio may represent a highly susceptible organism responding to a relatively low blood level or a moderately resistant organism responding to an unexpectedly high blood level. A serum inhibitory titer might suggest an adequate therapeutic level but would give no clue to potential toxicity, when an extremely narrow margin exists between a therapeutically adequate dose and a possibly toxic one (eg, aminoglycosides). The serum bactericidal assay has many ill-defined variables (ie, no widely accepted standard procedure, no consensus as to whether dilutions should be performed with serum or broth, the unknown inhibitory effect of serum if used as a diluent, etc). The use of pooled serum diluent may not accurately predict actual bactericidal titers in patients with abnormal protein binding. An ultrafiltrate may prove more useful.[1] **CONTRAINDICATIONS:** The bacterium isolated from patient is not available or fails to grow for the serum bactericidal test. **METHODOLOGY:** Serial dilution of patient's serum with Mueller-Hinton broth, 1:1 final ratio recommended, supplemented if necessary. Each dilution is incubated with a standard inoculum of the patient's isolate. **ADDITIONAL INFORMATION:** It is preferable to run this test with paired specimens, one obtained approximately 15 minutes before an antibiotic dose (predose trough), and one obtained 30-60 minutes after an antibiotic dose (postdose peak).

In patients with chronic osteomyelitis, the observation of peak levels <1:16 and trough levels <1:2 accurately predicted treatment failure. In acute osteomyelitis, peak levels >1:16 and trough >1:2 accurately predicted medical cure. The serum bactericidal test alone is not sufficient to predict outcome in endocarditis. The therapeutic outcome of endocarditis depends on many clinical factors including cardiac status, underlying medical disease, embolic complications, and clinical management of patient. In granulocytopenic patient, titers ≥1:8-1:16 in patients on combination therapy were associated with a more favorable outcome.

The serum bactericidal test has been applied experimentally to detect antimicrobial activity in cerebrospinal fluid, joint fluid, and amniotic fluid.[2,3] It is also useful in determining whether serum antimicrobial activity remains adequate after a shift from parenteral to oral therapy. Serum bactericidal titers are useful in evaluating synergy between antibiotics after administration of the drugs.[4]

Footnotes

1. Leggett JE, Wolz SA, and Craig WA, "Use of Serum Ultrafiltrate in the Serum Dilution Test," *J Infect Dis*, 1989, 160(4):616-23.
2. Viladrich PF, Gudiol F, Liñares J, et al, "Evaluation of Vancomycin for Therapy of Adult Pneumococcal Meningitis," *Antimicrob Agents Chemother*, 1991, 35(12):2467-72.
3. Nix DE, Goodwin SD, Peloquin CA, et al, "Antibiotic Tissue Penetration and Its Relevance: Impact of Tissue Penetration on Infection Response," *Antimicrob Agents Chemother*, 1991, 35(10):1953-9.
4. Van der Auwera P, "*Ex Vivo* Study of Serum Bactericidal Titers and Killing Rates of Daptomycin (LY 146032) Combined or Not Combined With Amikacin Compared With Those of Vancomycin," *Antimicrob Agents Chemother*, 1989, 33(10):1783-90.

References

MacLowry JD, "Perspective: The Serum Dilution Test," *J Infect Dis*, 1989, 160(4):624-6.

Moore RD, Lietman PS, and Smith CR, "Clinical Response to Aminoglycoside Therapy: Importance of the Ratio of Peak Concentration to Minimal Inhibitory Concentration," *J Infect Dis*, 1987, 155:93-9.

Peterson LR and Shanholtzer CJ, "Tests for Bactericidal Effects of Antimicrobial Agents: Technical Performance and Clinical Relevance," *Clin Microbiol Rev*, 1992, 5(4):420-32.

Rosenblatt JE, "Laboratory Tests Used to Guide Antimicrobial Therapy," *Mayo Clin Proc*, 1991, 66(9):942-8.

Stratton CW, "Serum Bactericidal Test," *Clin Microbiol Rev*, Jan 1988, 19-26, (review).

Wolfson JS and Swartz MN, "Serum Bactericidal Activity as a Monitor of Antibiotic Therapy," *N Engl J Med*, 1985, 312:968-75.

Serum Inhibitory Dilution *see* Serum Bactericidal Test *on page 843*

Serum Inhibitory Titer *see* Serum Bactericidal Test *on page 843*

SID *see* Serum Bactericidal Test *on page 843*

Skin Burn Culture, Quantitative *see* Burn Culture, Quantitative *on page 794*

Skin Fungus Culture

CPT 87101 (isolation); 87106 (definitive identification)

Related Information

Amphotericin B *on page 942*
Biopsy or Body Fluid Fungus Culture *on page 780*
Fungus Smear, Stain *on page 813*
HIV-1/HIV-2 Serology *on page 696*
KOH Preparation *on page 825*
Skin Biopsies *on page 84*
Skin Mycobacteria Culture *on next page*
Stool Fungus Culture *on page 861*
Susceptibility Testing, Fungi *on page 869*

Synonyms Dermatophyte Fungus Culture; Fungus Culture, Skin, Hair and Nail

Test Commonly Includes Detection of superficial fungal infections of the skin or hair

Patient Care PREPARATION: Select hairs which are broken off and appear diseased, and pluck them with sterile forceps. If diseased hair stubs are not apparent, scrape the edges of a scalp lesion with a sterile scalpel. Cleanse skin lesions first with 70% alcohol to reduce bacteria and saprophytic fungi. Scrape from the outer edges of skin lesions. In infections of the nails, scrape out the friable material beneath the edge of the nails, or scrape or clip off portions of abnormal appearing nail and submit for examination and culture.

Specimen Skin scrapings, exudates, nail clippings, whole nail, debris under nail, hair CONTAINER: Sterile Petri dish, sterile urine container, envelope COLLECTION: Enclose hair specimens, skin scrapings, or nail clippings or scrapings in clean paper envelopes, sterile urine container, or Petri dish. Label the specimen with the patient's name. Enclose these envelopes in larger heavy paper envelopes. Do not put specimens in cotton-plugged tubes, because the specimen may become trapped among the cotton fibers and lost. Do not put specimen into closed containers, such as rubber-stoppered tubes, because this keeps the specimen moist and allows overgrowth of bacteria and saprophytic fungi. The laboratory should be informed of the fungal species suspected. STORAGE INSTRUCTIONS: Keep specimen at room temperature until delivered to the laboratory TURNAROUND TIME: Cultures positive for *Candida* sp are usually reported within 1 week. Cultures positive for dermatophytes are usually reported within 2-3 weeks. Negative cultures are usually reported after 1 month. Cultures in which suspicion of systemic fungal infection has been indicated are usually reported upon becoming positive or negative after 4 weeks. SPECIAL INSTRUCTIONS: Careful choice of specimens for laboratory study is important. See following table. A Wood's lamp is useful in the collection of specimens in tinea capitis infections, since hairs infected by some members of the genus *Microsporum* exhibit fluorescence under a Wood's lamp. However, in tinea capitis due to *Trichophyton* sp, infected hairs usually do not fluoresce. The laboratory should be informed of the specific site of the specimen.

Interpretive REFERENCE RANGE: No growth USE: Isolate and identify fungi LIMITATIONS: A single negative specimen does not rule out fungal infections. If infection with mycobacteria or aerobic organisms cannot be excluded clinically, a separate culture should be submitted for fungal identification and culture. METHODOLOGY: Aerobic culture on selective media usually including nonselective Sabouraud's agar incubated at 25°C to 30°C; some laboratories also incubate these cultures at 35°C to 37°C. ADDITIONAL INFORMATION: *Candida* sp may colonize skin. Clinical diagnosis of *Candida* infection involves consideration of predisposing factors such as occlusion, maceration altered cutaneous barrier function. Signs of *Candida* infection include bright erythema, fragile papulopustules, and satellite lesions.[1] Patients with defects in T-lymphocyte responses, such as AIDS patients or individuals being treated with antineoplastic drugs, are especially susceptible to many fungal infections including superficial mycoses.[2,3] Most cutaneous fungal infections can be treated with the antifungal azole drugs like ketoconazole, itraconazole, and fluconazole. Severe infections should be treated with intravenous amphotericin B.[4]

(Continued)

Skin Fungus Culture *(Continued)*

Selection of Specimens for the Diagnosis of Superficial Mycosis and Dermatomycosis

Diagnosis	Specimen of Choice
Superficial mycoses	
Piedra	Hair
Tinea nigra	Skin scraping
Tinea versicolor	Skin scraping
Dermatomycoses (cutaneous mycoses)	
Onychomycosis	Nail scraping
Tinea capitis	Hair (black dot)
Tinea corporis	Skin scraping
Tinea pedis	Skin scraping
Tinea cruris	Skin scraping
Candidiasis	
Thrush	Scraping of oral white patches
Diaper dermatitis	Scraping of pustules at margin
Paronychia	Scraping skin around nail
Cutaneous candidiasis	Scraping of pustules at margin
Erosio interdigitalis blastomycetia (coinfection with gram-negative rods)	Scrapings of interdigital space (routine culture also)
Congenital candidiasis	Scraping of scales, pustules and cutaneous debris, cultures of umbilical stump, mouth, urine and stool
Mucocutaneous candidiasis	Scraping of affected area

Footnotes

1. McKay M, "Cutaneous Manifestations of Candidiasis," *Am J Obstet Gynecol*, 1988, 158(4):991-3.
2. Herrod HG, "Chronic Mucocutaneous Candidiasis in Childhood and Complications of Non-*Candida* Infection: A Report of the Pediatric Immunodeficiency Collaborative Group," *J Pediatr*, 1990, 116(3):377-82.
3. Diamond RD, "The Growing Problem of Mycoses in Patients Infected With the Human Immunodeficiency Virus," *Rev Infect Dis*, 1991, 13(3):480-6.
4. Hector RF, "Compounds Active Against Cell Walls of Medically Important Fungi," *Clin Microbiol Rev*, 1993, 6(1):1-21.

References

Cohn MS, "Superficial Fungal Infections. Topical and Oral Treatment of Common Types," *Postgrad Med*, 1992, 91(2):239-44, 249-52.

Ginsburg CM, "*Tinea capitis*," *Pediatr Infect Dis J*, 1991, 10(1):48-9.

Hay RJ, "Fungal Skin Infections," *Arch Dis Child*, 1992, 67(9):1065-7.

Meyer RD, "Cutaneous and Mucosal Manifestations of the Deep Mycotic Infections," *Acta Derm Venereol Suppl (Stockh)*, 1986, 121:57-72.

Rasmussen JE, "Cutaneous Fungus Infections in Children," *Pediatr Rev*, 1992, 13(4):152-6.

Rezabek GH and Friedman AD, "Superficial Fungal Infections of the Skin Diagnosis and Current Treatment Recommendations," *Drugs*, 1992, 43(5):674-82.

Skin Mycobacteria Culture

***CPT** 87116 (isolation); 87118 (definitive identification)*

Related Information

Acid-Fast Stain *on page 770*

Biopsy or Body Fluid Mycobacteria Culture *on page 782*

Mycobacteria by DNA Probe *on page 921*

Skin Biopsies *on page 84*

Skin Fungus Culture *on previous page*

Sputum Mycobacteria Culture *on page 855*

Stool Mycobacteria Culture *on page 863*

Susceptibility Testing, Mycobacteria *on page 872*
Urine Mycobacteria Culture *on page 884*

Synonyms Mycobacteria Culture, Atypical, Skin; TB Culture, Skin

Applies to *Mycobacterium marinum* Culture, Skin

Test Commonly Includes Culture and identification of acid-fast bacteria. This may include a direct acid-fast smear of specimen.

Abstract Due to the increased number of patients with immunosuppressed conditions such as AIDS, transplants, and neoplastic disorders, the number of atypical mycobacteria isolated in clinical laboratories has increased. The recognition of these atypical pathogenic mycobacteria has led to a deeper understanding of the diseases associated with the bacteria and the appropriate use of antibiotic therapy. Most atypical mycobacteria show variable resistance to antituberculous drugs, and it is recommended that isolates be tested for antibiotic sensitivity.

Specimen Scrapings or biopsy of skin or lesions, not in formalin or another fixative. Do not send swabs. **CONTAINER:** Sterile tube containing 0.5 mL sterile saline **STORAGE INSTRUCTIONS:** Transport the specimen directly to the laboratory. **TURNAROUND TIME:** Negative cultures are usually reported after 6-8 weeks.

Interpretive **REFERENCE RANGE:** No growth **USE:** Isolate and identify mycobacteria **LIMITATIONS:** For optimal yield, scrapings, curettings, or biopsy tissue rather than swabs of lesions should be submitted to the laboratory. The yield on cultures is proportional to the volume of specimen submitted. **METHODOLOGY:** Culture on selective media, usually including Löwenstein-Jensen (LJ) and Middlebrook 7H11 media; incubation at 30°C (*M. marinum* will not grow at 37°C on primary isolation.) Identification is based on growth rate, colony morphology (rough vs smooth), development of pigment, color of pigment, and whether or not the pigment is induced by light. Other biochemical and nucleic acid tests can be used to confirm the identification. **ADDITIONAL INFORMATION:** *Mycobacterium marinum* is frequently responsible for granulomatous cutaneous lesions acquired from heated swimming pools and fish tanks. Lesions are similar to those seen with sporotrichosis and follow lymphatics. *Mycobacterium fortuitum* and *Mycobacterium chelonei* complex organisms are saprophytic mycobacteria which can cause cutaneous abscesses and osteomyelitis in trauma victims and debilitated hosts. The organisms are not fastidious and may grow well on usual blood or chocolate agar. The key clinical feature is that symptoms of infection, localized cellulitis, or abscess formation appear 4-6 weeks after traumatic injury. *Mycobacterium ulcerans* causes a chronic granulomatous skin lesion called Buruli ulcer. *M. ulcerans* may also be saprophytic, colonizing cutaneous ulcers associated with circulatory insufficiency and diabetes. *M. ulcerans* is uncommon in North America. It is most frequently isolated in Australia and Africa. Diagnosis of *Mycobacterium marinum* infection is frequently delayed. A careful clinical history addressing occupational or recreational activities usually yields important clues to the diagnosis, eg, swimming pool or seawall abrasions, barnacle scrapes, fish fin punctures, and exposure to tropical fish tanks (salt water).[1] Isolates of *Mycobacterium avium-intracellulare* (MAI) have been reported from skin and Kaposi's sarcoma lesions of patients with the acquired immunodeficiency syndrome (AIDS).[2,3] Cutaneous tuberculosis has been found in patients with neoplastic disease.[4,5]

Subcutaneous nodules which break down and drain are observed in immunocompromised hosts including those on high dose corticosteroid therapy and in association with cases of rheumatoid arthritis and lupus.

The atypical or environmental mycobacteria are frequently resistant to oral antituberculosis therapy. There is wide variation in susceptibility within species. Susceptibility testing should be considered.[6]

Footnotes

1. Brown JW III and Sanders CV, "*Mycobacterium marinum* Infections: A Problem of Recognition, Not Therapy?" *Arch Intern Med*, 1987, 147:817-8, (editorial).
2. Croxson TS, Ebanks D, and Mildvan D, "Atypical Mycobacteria and Kaposi's Sarcoma in the Same Biopsy Specimens," *N Engl J Med*, 1983, 308:1476, (letter).
3. Hawkins CC, Gold JW, Whimbey E, et al, "*Mycobacterium avium* Complex Infections in Patients With the Acquired Immunodeficiency Syndrome," *Ann Intern Med*, 1986, 105:184-8.
4. Asnis DS and Bresciani AR, "Cutaneous Tuberculosis: A Rare Presentation of Malignancy," *Clin Infect Dis*, 1992, 15(1):158-60.
5. Beyt BE, Ortbals DW, Santa Cruz DJ, et al, "Cutaneous Mycobacteriosis: Analysis of 34 Cases With a New Classification of the Disease," *Med*, 1980, 60:95-109.
6. Wallace RJ Jr, Swenson JM, Silcox VA, et al, "Treatment of Nonpulmonary Infections Due to *Mycobacterium fortuitum* and *Mycobacterium chelonei* Based on *In Vitro* Susceptibility," *J Infect Dis*, 1985, 152:500-14.

(Continued)

Skin Mycobacteria Culture *(Continued)*

References

Hamrick HJ, Maddux DW, and Lowry EK, "*Mycobacterium chelonei* Facial Abscess: Case Presentation and Review of Cutaneous Infection Due to Runyon Group IV Organisms," *Pediatr Infect Dis J*, 1984, 3:335-40.

Wallace RJ Jr, "Recent Clinical Advances in Knowledge of the Nonleprous Environmental Mycobacteria Responsible for Cutaneous Disease," *Arch Dermatol*, 1987, 123:337-9.

Wayne LG and Sramek HA, "Agents of Newly Recognized or Infrequently Encountered Mycobacterial Diseases," *Clin Microbiol Rev*, 1992, 5(1):1-25.

Wolinsky E, "Mycobacterial Diseases Other Than Tuberculosis," *Clin Infect Dis*, 1992, 15(1):1-10.

Skin Scrapings for *Sarcoptes scabiei* Identification *see* Arthropod Identification *on page 774*

Skin Test, Tuberculosis

***CPT** 86580 (intradermal); 86585 (tine)*

Related Information

Acid-Fast Stain *on page 770*
Sputum Mycobacteria Culture *on page 855*
Stool Mycobacteria Culture *on page 863*
Urine Mycobacteria Culture *on page 884*

Synonyms PPD Skin Test; Tuberculin Skin Test

Applies to Anergy Testing; Histoplasmin Skin Test

Test Commonly Includes Intradermal injection of tuberculin PPD (purified protein derivative)

Patient Care PREPARATION: Following preparation of the skin by alcohol swab, the test is performed by intradermal injection of 0.1 mL of diluent containing the desired amount of PPD.

Specimen TURNAROUND TIME: 48-72 hours

Interpretive REFERENCE RANGE: No reaction. PPD_{int} (5TU) giving 5-10 mm of induration should be repeated. Reactions ≥10 mm are considered positive. In patients with HIV infection and suspected tuberculosis, a >5 mm reaction to PPD should be considered indicative of tuberculosis infection. The reaction is read after 48-72 hours by outlining the area of induration and measuring the maximum diameter of induration. Erythema frequently occurs with induration, however, interpretation of positivity should be based on objective measurement of induration. Arthus reactions which are inflammatory and edematous are soft to the touch. They usually subside by 48 hours and are not interpreted as positives. Wheal and flare reactions also occur; they subside rapidly and are not interpreted as positive. USE: Test for delayed hypersensitivity reaction to tuberculin LIMITATIONS: A negative skin test does not rule out disease. Immunocompromised patients and patients with advanced tuberculosis may be anergic. BCG vaccinated patients will have a positive tuberculin test. Anergic patients may give a false-negative skin test reaction in the presence of active tuberculosis. Thus, a negative skin test should not be the sole criterion for exclusion of the diagnosis of tuberculosis. A negative reaction to first strength PPD followed by a positive reaction to second strength may indicate infection with atypical mycobacteria. CONTRAINDICATIONS: Patients suspected of having tuberculosis should have a 5 tuberculin unit PPD applied. Known positives should not be retested without consultation. ADDITIONAL INFORMATION: Tuberculin skin testing with 5 tuberculin units should be performed in all HIV-infected patients with suspected tuberculosis. Many patients with advanced HIV infection may be anergic, 33% to 50% of patients with AIDS and tuberculosis have a <10 mm reaction to PPD. Fifty percent to 80% of HIV-seropositive patients with tuberculosis but without AIDS react to PPD.[1,2] A >2 mm reaction for definition of positive in HIV-seropositive patients has been proposed in order to reduce misclassification.[3] The relative equivalents of the various skin tests are shown in the table.

Skin Test for Tuberculosis

Tuberculin Units (TU)	Strength	PPD Type
1.0	First	1st
5.0	Intermediate	Int/5
250.0	Second	2nd/250

The use of skin testing with multiple antigens is often used to evaluate delayed and cutaneous hypersensitivity (DCH). A common battery includes the following antigens: tetanus, diphtheria, *Streptococcus*, old tuberculin, *Candida*, *Trichophyton*, and *Proteus*. Premeasured standardized doses and an applicator for the battery of antigens are available commercially (Merieux Institute Inc, Miami, FL). Less than 1% of healthy adults are anergic when tested with the battery. Seven percent of elderly nursing home patients were reported to be anergic.[4] The incidence of positive delayed cutaneous hypersensitivity reactions to individual antigens decreases with age.

The use of the **histoplasmin skin test** has declined because application of the skin test antigen interferes with interpretation of serologic tests. Culture if possible and serology are recommended to establish the diagnosis of histoplasmosis. The usefulness of histoplasmin in an anergy battery is limited because of the restricted geographic area for previous exposure to histoplasmosis (ie, central United States, Mississippi river basin).

Footnotes

1. Chaisson RE and Slutkin G, "Tuberculosis and Human Immunodeficiency Virus Infection," *J Infect Dis*, 1989, 159(1):96-108.
2. Johnson MP, Coberly JS, Clermont HC, et al, "Tuberculin Skin Test Reactivity Among Adults Infected With Human Immunodeficiency Virus," *J Infect Dis*, 1992, 166(1):194-8.
3. Graham NM, Nelson KE, Solomon L, et al, "Prevalence of Tuberculin Positivity and Skin Test Anergy in HIV-1 Seropositive and Seronegative Intravenous Drug Users," *JAMA*, 1992, 267(3):369-73.
4. Delafuente JC, Meuleman JR, and Nelson RC, "Anergy Testing in Nursing Home Residents," *J Am Geriatr Soc*, 1988, 36(8):733-5.

References

Bianco NE, "The Immunopathology of Systemic Anergy in Infectious Diseases: A Reappraisal and New Perspectives," *Clin Immunol Immunopathol*, 1992, 62(3):253-7.

Center for Disease Control, "Diagnosis and Management of Mycobacterial Infections in Persons With Human T-Lymphotropic Virus Type III/Lymphadenopathy Associated Infection," *MMWR Morb Mortal Wkly Rep*, 1986, 35:488-52.

Chaparas SD, Vandiviere HM, Melvin I, et al, "Tuberculin Test: Variability With the Mantoux Procedure," *Am Rev Respir Dis*, 1985, 132:175-7.

Delafuente JC, "Immunosenescence: Clinical and Pharmacologic Considerations," *Med Clin North Am*, 1985, 69:475-86.

Smear, Gram Stain *see* Gram Stain *on page 815*

Spheroplast Culture *see* Cell Wall Defective Bacteria Culture *on page 796*

Sputum Culture

CPT *87070 (aerobic); 87205 (Gram stain)*

Related Information

Blood Culture, Aerobic and Anaerobic *on page 784*
Blood Fungus Culture *on page 789*
Bordetella pertussis Serology *on page 647*
Bronchial Aspirate Anaerobic Culture *on page 792*
Bronchial Washings Cytology *on page 485*
Bronchoalveolar Lavage *on page 793*
Bronchoalveolar Lavage Cytology *on page 487*
Gram Stain *on page 815*
Hypersensitivity Pneumonitis Serology *on page 704*
Legionella Culture *on page 825*
Legionella pneumophila Direct FA Smear *on page 715*
Legionnaires' Disease Antibodies *on page 716*
Legionnaires' Disease Antibodies, IgM *on page 716*
Mycoplasma pneumoniae Diagnostic Procedures *on page 1188*
Pneumocystis Fluorescence *on page 732*
Sputum Cytology *on page 510*
Sputum Fungus Culture *on page 853*
Sputum Mycobacteria Culture *on page 855*
Viral Culture, Respiratory Symptoms *on page 1204*

Applies to Bronchial Washings Culture; Bronchoscopy Culture; Percutaneous Transtracheal Culture; Tracheal Aspirate Culture

Test Commonly Includes Culture of aerobic organisms and usually Gram stain

Patient Care PREPARATION: The patient should be instructed to remove dentures, rinse mouth, and gargle with water. The patient should then be instructed to cough deeply and expectorate sputum into proper container.

Specimen Sputum, first morning specimen preferred; tracheal aspiration, bronchoscopy specimen, or transtracheal aspirate CONTAINER: Sterile sputum container, sputum trap, sterile tra-

(Continued)

Sputum Culture *(Continued)*

cheal aspirate or bronchoscopy aspirate tube **COLLECTION:** Specimen collected, at time of bronchoscopy, by aspiration or by transtracheal aspiration by a physician skilled in the procedure. The specimen should be transported to the laboratory within 1 hour of collection for processing. **STORAGE INSTRUCTIONS:** Refrigerate if the specimen cannot be promptly processed. **CAUSES FOR REJECTION:** Specimens contaminated on the outside of the container pose excessive risk to laboratory personnel. **TURNAROUND TIME:** Preliminary reports are usually available at 24 hours. Cultures with no growth or normal flora are usually reported after 48 hours. Reports on specimens from which pathogens are isolated may require at least 48 hours for completion. **SPECIAL INSTRUCTIONS:** The laboratory should be informed of the specific site of specimen, the age of patient, current antibiotic therapy, clinical diagnosis, and time of collection.

Interpretive **REFERENCE RANGE:** Normal upper respiratory flora. Tracheal aspirate and bronchoscopy specimens can be contaminated with normal oral flora. Transtracheal aspiration should have no growth. **USE:** Isolate and identify potentially pathogenic organisms present in the lower respiratory tract; identify isolates responsible for pneumonia, bronchitis, bronchiectasis. Presence or absence of normal upper respiratory flora is often reported. **LIMITATIONS:** An adequate sputum specimen should contain many neutrophils and few to no squamous epithelial cells. The latter are indicative of contamination with saliva. Results obtained by culture without evaluation for contamination may be noncontributory or misleading.[1] A Gram stain from a carefully collected specimen, with neutrophils and lancet-shaped diplococci staining gram-positive, which are intracellular or encapsulated, can provide strong support to the clinical diagnosis of pneumococcal pneumonia.[2]

In bronchoscopy and aspirated specimens reduction of contamination may be accomplished by a head-down position to reduce gravitational flow of saliva, when combined with quantitative culture techniques. Oral contamination may successfully be reduced by using a telescoping double catheter with a plug to protect the brush or a sheathed brush. The use of the telescoping plugged catheter (TPC) and bronchoalveolar lavage (BAL) increases the overall diagnostic yield, however, a high frequency of false-positives, circa 25%, is a drawback. Quantitation aids interpretation. Bronchial washings are unfortunately commonly diluted with topical anesthetics, which are bacteriostatic, and with irrigating solutions. If anaerobic bacteria are suspected in a transtracheal aspiration, a properly collected specimen for anaerobic culture should be submitted.

Culture of expectorated sputum in subjects with bacteremia and pneumococcal pneumonia does not always identify the pathogen.

Sputum is contaminated by oropharyngeal flora. Such flora contaminates bronchoscopy instruments during their introduction. Transtracheal aspiration involves serious risks.

See Bronchial Aspirate Anaerobic Culture for detailed instructions pertaining to transtracheal aspirate anaerobic culture.

METHODOLOGY: Aerobic culture following appropriate specimen selection. The most important step in the evaluation is to be certain that the secretions that are examined are the product of the inflammatory process in the bronchi and not oropharyngeal material. This can be accomplished by a simple microscopic evaluation of the sputum specimen. A promising (thick) portion should be separated from the sputum sample and placed on a microscopic slide. This selection is easier if the sputum is poured into one-half of a Petri dish and viewed against a dark background so that a likely plug can be identified. The specimen placed on the slide is scanned under low magnification. The most productive material is that which represents bronchial secretions. Frequently, they are present as a plug or cast of the infected bronchus. The identified portions are selected and inoculated on selective and nonselective media. **ADDITIONAL INFORMATION:** See table.

Potential pathogens recovered by usual sputum culture methods include *Staphylococcus aureus*, *Haemophilus influenzae*, *Streptococcus pneumoniae*, *Neisseria meningitidis*, *Haemophilus parainfluenzae*, *Pseudomonas aeruginosa*, *Escherichia coli*, *Proteus* sp, *Moraxella* (*Branhamella*) *catarrhalis*, and rarely many other organisms. *Haemophilus* sp and *Neisseria* sp may not be routinely isolated and identified. Thus, if their presence is clinically suspected, they should be specifically requested.

Agents such as *Bordetella pertussis*, *Chlamydia pneumoniae* TWAR strain, *Corynebacterium diphtheriae*, *Legionella pneumophila*, *Mycoplasma pneumoniae*, and *Mycobacterium tuberculosis* require special laboratory measures for isolation. Clinical suspicion of involvement by these agents should be communicated to the laboratory. See also listings for the specific agents.

Bacterial Species Recovered From Sputa in 103 Acute Bronchitic Exacerbations

	Number	Percent of All Types Cultured	Percent of Sputa Cultured
H. influenzae	41	24.0	39.8
H. parainfluenzae	29	17.0	28.2
S. pneumoniae	34	19.9	33.0
M. catarrhalis	19	11.1	18.4
N. meningitidis	5	2.9	4.9
K. pneumoniae	8	4.7	7.8
P. aeruginosa	4	2.3	3.9
Other possible pathogens	14	8.2	13.6
Unlikely pathogens	17	9.9	16.5

From Chodosh S, "Acute Bacterial Exacerbations in Bronchitis and Asthma, *Am J Med,* 1987, 82(Suppl 4A):154-63, with permission.

The critical criteria for the diagnosis of acute bacterial infection of the bronchi are obtained from examination and culture of the sputum. The presence of bacteria in numbers greater than when the patient's condition is stable and a significant increase (ie, doubling) in the numbers of neutrophils present are essential laboratory criteria for the diagnosis of an acute bronchitic exacerbation. Gram stain results more closely reflect the clinical outcome and along with the criterion of the number of neutrophils in the sputum should be laboratory basis for determination of success.[3] Other commonly recognized agents causing pneumonia are reviewed in the following tables.

Community-Acquired Bacterial Pneumonias: Frequency of Various Pathogens	**%**
Streptococcus pneumoniae	40–60
Haemophilus influenzae	2.5–20
Gram-negative bacilli	6-37
Staphylococcus aureus	2–10
Anaerobic infections	5–10
Legionella	0–22.5
Mycoplasma pneumoniae	5–15
Nosocomial Pneumonias: Frequency of Various Pathogens	**%**
Klebsiella	13
Pseudomonas aeruginosa	10–12
Staphylococcus aureus	3–10.6
Escherichia coli	4–7.2
Enterobacter	6.2
Group D *Streptococcus*	1.3
Proteus and *Providencia*	6
Serratia	3.5
Pneumococcus	10–20
Aspiration pneumonia anaerobic pneumonia*	5–25
*Legionella**	0–15

From Verghese A and Berk SL, "Bacterial Pneumonia in the Elderly Medicine," 1983, 62:271–85, with permission.

* The specific incidence of pneumonias caused by *Mycoplasma, Legionella,* and anaerobes is difficult to document because of the technical problems in isolating the organisms.

(Continued)

Sputum Culture *(Continued)*

Spectrum of Frequent Etiologic Agents in Pneumonia

Aerobic Bacteria	Anaerobes	Fungi
Gram-positive aerobes *Streptococcus pneumoniae* *Staphylococcus aureus* *Streptococcus pyogenes* Gram-negative aerobes *Haemophilus influenzae* *Legionella pneumophila* *Escherichia coli* *Klebsiella pneumoniae* *Pseudomonas aeruginosa*	*Bacteroides melaninogenicus* *Fusobacterium* *Peptostreptococcus* *Bacteroides fragilis* *Actinomyces israelii*	*Aspergillus* *Coccidioides immitis* *Histoplasma capsulatum* *Blastomyces dermatitidis* *Cryptococcus neoformans* Zygomycetes
Viruses	**Parasites**	**Other**
Respiratory syncytial virus Parainfluenza virus Influenza virus Adenovirus Enterovirus Rhinovirus Measles virus Varicella-zoster virus Rickettsia *Coxiella burnetii* Cytomegalovirus	*Pneumocystis carinii* *Ascaris lumbricoides* *Toxocara canis* and *catis* *Filaria* *Strongyloides stercoralis* Hookworms *Paragonimus* *Echinococcus* Schistosomes	*Mycoplasma pneumoniae* *Chlamydia trachomatis* *Chlamydia psittaci* *Mycobacterium tuberculosis* *Chlamydia* TWAR strains *Nocardia*

From Cohen GJ, "Management of Infections of the Lower Respiratory Tract in Children," *Pediatr Infect Dis,* 1987, 6:317-23, with permission.

Footnotes

1. Barrett-Connor E, "The Nonvalue of Sputum Culture in the Diagnosis of Pneumococcal Pneumonia," *Am Rev Respir Dis*, 1971, 103:845-8.
2. Boerner DF and Zwadyk P, "The Value of the Sputum Gram's Stain in Community Acquired Pneumonia," *JAMA*, 1982, 247:642-5.
3. Chodosh S, "Acute Bacterial Exacerbations in Bronchitis and Asthma," *Am J Med*, 1987, 82:154-63.

References

Plorde JJ, "The Diagnosis of Infectious Diseases," *Harrison's Principles of Internal Medicine*, 12th ed, Chapter 80, New York, NY: McGraw-Hill Inc, 1991, 454-9.

Stratton CW, "Bacterial Pneumonias - An Overview With Emphasis on Pathogenesis, Diagnosis, and Treatment," *Heart Lung*, 1986, 15:226-44.

Wijnands GJ, "Diagnosis and Interventions in Lower Respiratory Tract Infections," *Am J Med*, 1992, 92(4SA):91S-7S.

Sputum Fungus Culture

CPT *87102 (isolation); 87106 (definitive identification)*

Related Information

Amphotericin B *on page 942*
Aspergillus Serology *on page 641*
Biopsy or Body Fluid Fungus Culture *on page 780*
Blastomycosis Serology *on page 645*
Bronchial Washings Cytology *on page 485*
Bronchoalveolar Lavage *on page 793*
Bronchoalveolar Lavage Cytology *on page 487*
Candidiasis Serologic Test *on page 652*
Coccidioidomycosis Antibodies *on page 664*
Cryptococcal Antigen Titer, Serum or Cerebrospinal Fluid *on page 805*
Cryptococcus Antibody Titer *on page 670*
Fungus Smear, Stain *on page 813*
Histoplasmosis Serology *on page 695*
KOH Preparation *on page 825*
Nocardia Culture, All Sites *on page 835*

Sputum Culture *on page 849*
Sputum Cytology *on page 510*
Sputum Mycobacteria Culture *on page 855*
Stool Fungus Culture *on page 861*
Susceptibility Testing, Fungi *on page 869*
Throat Culture *on page 876*
Urine Fungus Culture *on page 883*
Viral Culture, Respiratory Symptoms *on page 1204*

Synonyms Fungus Culture, Sputum

Applies to Bronchoscopy Fungus Culture; Fungus Culture, Gastric Aspirate

Patient Care PREPARATION: The patient should be instructed to remove dentures, rinse mouth with water, and cough deeply expectorating sputum into the sputum collection cup.

Specimen First morning sputum, gastric aspirate, induced sputum, aspirated sputum, bronchial aspirate, tracheal aspirate, transtracheal aspirate. See table. CONTAINER: Sterile sputum cup, sputum trap, sterile tracheal aspirate or bronchoscopy tube COLLECTION: Collect the specimen early in the day so that it may be processed by the laboratory for optimal recovery. A recommended screening procedure is three first morning specimens submitted on successive days. The specimen can be divided for fungus culture and KOH preparation, mycobacteria culture and smear, and routine bacterial culture and Gram stain if the specimen is of adequate volume. STORAGE INSTRUCTIONS: Refrigerate the specimen if storage is in excess of 1 hour CAUSES FOR REJECTION: Specimens contaminated on the outside of the container pose excessive risk to laboratory personnel and may not be acceptable to the laboratory. TURNAROUND TIME: Negative cultures are reported after 4 weeks SPECIAL INSTRUCTIONS: The laboratory should be informed of the specific source of specimen and the suspected clinical diagnosis.

Selection of Specimens for the Diagnosis of Systemic and Subcutaneous Mycosis

Diagnosis	Specimen of Choice in Order of Usefulness	Diagnosis	Specimen of Choice in Order of Usefulness
Systemic Mycoses		**Systemic Mycoses *(continued)***	
Aspergillosis	Sputum Bronchial aspirate Biopsy (lung)	Mycomycosis/ phycomycosis	Sputum Bronchial aspirate Biopsy (lung)
Blastomycosis	Skin scrapings Abscess drainage (pus) Urine Sputum Bronchial aspirate	Paracoccidioidomycosis (South American blastomycosis)	Skin scrapings Mucosal scrapings Biopsy (lymph nodes) Sputum Bronchial aspirate
Candidiasis	Sputum Bronchial aspirate Blood Cerebrospinal fluid Urine Stool	**Subcutaneous Mycoses**	
		Chromoblastomycosis	Skin scrapings Biopsy (skin) Drainage (pus)
Coccidioidomycosis	Sputum Bronchial aspirate Cerebrospinal fluid Urine Skin scrapings Abscess drainage (pus)	Maduromycosis (mycetoma)	Drainage (pus) Abscess drainage Biopsy (lesion)
		Sporotrichosis	Drainage (pus) Abscess drainage Biopsy (skin, lymph node)
Cryptococcosis	Cerebrospinal fluid Sputum Abscess drainage (pus) Skin scraping Urine		

See Skin Fungus Culture test listing for Superficial and Cutaneous Mycoses Specimen Selection.

Interpretive REFERENCE RANGE: No growth; normal flora such as yeast from the oropharynx may be present. USE: Establish the presence and identity of potentially pathogenic fungi (eg, *Aspergillus* sp) LIMITATIONS: The yield may be reduced by bacterial overgrowth during storage or on standing; therefore, fresh sputum is preferred. A single negative culture does not

(Continued)

Sputum Fungus Culture *(Continued)*

rule out the presence of fungal infection. If two specimens are received simultaneously, many laboratories will pool them and process them as one specimen unless specific instructions are provided. **METHODOLOGY:** Culture on selective media usually including supplemented Sabouraud's agar and brain heart infusion (BHI) with antibiotics to reduce bacterial overgrowth **ADDITIONAL INFORMATION:** Deeply coughed sputum, transtracheal aspirate, bronchial washing or brushing, or deep tracheal aspirate are preferred specimens. Oncology patients, transplant patients, and patients with the acquired immunodeficiency syndrome (AIDS) are particularly prone to infection with fungi.[1]

Primary fungal pulmonary infections include *Histoplasma capsulatum*, *Coccidioides immitis*, *Cryptococcus neoformans*, and *Blastomyces dermatitidis*. The incidence is largely related to geographic exposure and cases can occur in seemingly normal hosts. Numbers of reports of opportunistic fungal pulmonary infections due to a variety of etiologic agents which are ubiquitous in the environment are being published. Definitive diagnosis depends upon the presence of clinical signs of pulmonary infection, a chest x-ray revealing abnormality such as granuloma; laboratory isolation of a potentially significant organism from a suitable specimen; histologic documentation of tissue invasion by the isolated organism. A list of etiologic agents of pulmonary fungal disease has been compiled.[2] See table.

Common Pulmonary Fungal Infections

Endemic Fungi	Opportunistic Fungi
Histoplasma capsulatum	*Candida albicans*
Blastomyces dermatitidis	*Candida tropicalis*
Coccidioides immitis	*Aspergillus niger*
Paracoccidioides brasiliensis	*Aspergillus fumigatus*
	Mucor
	Rhizopus
	Absidia
	Cryptococcus neoformans

From Haque AK, "Pathology of Common Pulmonary Fungal Infections," *J Thorac Imaging,* 1992, 7:1–11, with permission.

In practice a diagnosis sufficient for therapy can frequently be established by observation of hyphae, pseudohyphae, or yeast cells in tissue sections; recovery of the organism from a normally sterile site; repeated isolation of the same suspect organism from the same or different sites; seroconversion (ie, the development of an immune response to the suspected organism).[3] *Candida* and *Aspergillus* sp are the most frequently isolated fungal organisms. However, they are frequently present as the result of contamination from the patient's normal flora or airborne sources. Their presence may represent colonization rather than invasion. Recovery of *Candida* from blood (see Blood Fungus Culture) is a major adjunct to definitive diagnosis. Even without invasion *Aspergillus* may cause IgE mediated asthma, allergic alveolitis cell mediated hypersensitivity, mucoid impaction, and bronchocentric granulomatosis.[4] Fungal tracheobronchitis has recently been recognized as a pseudomembranous form involving the circumference of the bronchial wall or as multiple or discrete plaques. The plaques or pseudomembranes are composed of necrotic tissue exudate and fungal hyphae.[5]

Footnotes

1. Diamond RD, "The Growing Problem of Mycoses in Patients Infected With the Human Immunodeficiency Virus," *Rev Infect Dis*, 1991, 13:480-6.
2. Haque AK, "Pathology of Common Pulmonary Fungal Infections," *J Thorac Imaging*, 1992, 7(4):1-11.
3. Boyars MC, Zwischenberger JB, and Cox CS Jr, "Clinical Manifestations of Pulmonary Fungal Infections," *J Thorac Imaging*, 1992, 7(4):12-22.
4. Fraser RS, "Pulmonary Aspergillosis: Pathologic and Pathogenetic Features," *Pathol Annu*, 1993, 28(Pt 1):231-77.
5. Clarke A, Skelton J, and Fraser RS, "Fungal Tracheobronchitis. Report of 9 Cases and Review of the Literature," *Medicine (Baltimore)*, 1991, 70(1):1-14.

References

Batra P, "Pulmonary Coccidioidomycosis," *J Thorac Imaging*, 1992, 7(4):29-38.

Gray LD and Roberts GD, "Laboratory Diagnosis of Systemic Fungal Diseases," *Med Clin North Am*, 1988, 2:779-803.

Saral R, "*Candida* and *Aspergillus* Infections in Immunocompromised Patients: An Overview," *Rev Infect Dis*, 1991, 13(3):487-92.

Schuyler MR, "Allergic Bronchopulmonary Aspergillosis," *Clin Chest Med*, 1983, 4:15-22.

Tang CM and Cohen J, "Diagnosing Fungal Infections in Immunocompromised Hosts," *J Clin Pathol*, 1992, 45(1):1-5.

Wheat LJ, "Histoplasmosis," *Med Clin North Am*, 1988, 2:841-59.

Sputum Mycobacteria Culture

CPT *87116 (isolation); 87117 (concentration plus isolation); 87118 (definitive identification)*

Related Information

Acid-Fast Stain *on page 770*
Biopsy or Body Fluid Mycobacteria Culture *on page 782*
Bronchial Washings Cytology *on page 485*
Bronchoalveolar Lavage *on page 793*
Bronchoalveolar Lavage Cytology *on page 487*
Mycobacteria by DNA Probe *on page 921*
Nocardia Culture, All Sites *on page 835*
Skin Mycobacteria Culture *on page 846*
Skin Test, Tuberculosis *on page 848*
Sputum Culture *on page 849*
Sputum Cytology *on page 510*
Sputum Fungus Culture *on page 853*
Stool Mycobacteria Culture *on page 863*
Susceptibility Testing, Mycobacteria *on page 872*
Urine Mycobacteria Culture *on page 884*
Viral Culture, Respiratory Symptoms *on page 1204*

Synonyms AFB Culture, Sputum; Mycobacteria Culture, Sputum; TB Culture, Sputum

Applies to Mycobacteria Culture, Bronchial Aspirate; Mycobacteria Culture, Gastric Aspirate; Mycobacteria, DNA Probe

Test Commonly Includes Mycobacteria (AFB) stain, culture, and identification

Patient Care PREPARATION: The patient should be instructed to remove dentures, rinse mouth with water, and then cough deeply expectorating sputum into the sputum collection cup.

Specimen First morning sputum or induced sputum, fasting gastric aspirate, bronchial aspirate, tracheal aspirate, transtracheal aspirate CONTAINER: Sputum cup, sputum trap, sterile tracheal aspirate or bronchoscopy tube SAMPLING TIME: In children, the gastric aspirate should be done early in the morning as the child awakens before the stomach empties. COLLECTION: A recommended screening procedure is three first morning specimens submitted on successive days. The patient should be instructed to brush his/her teeth and/or rinse their mouth well with water before attempting to collect the specimen, to reduce the possibility of contamination of the specimen with food particles, oropharyngeal secretions, etc. After the specimen has been collected, it should be examined to make sure it contains a sufficient quantity (at least 5 mL) of thick mucus (**not saliva**). If a two-part collection system has been used, only the screw-cap tube should be submitted to the laboratory. (The outer container is considered contaminated and its transport through the hospital constitutes a health hazard!) The specimen should be properly labeled and accompanied by properly completed requisition. The specimen can be divided in the laboratory for fungal, mycobacterial, and routine cultures. STORAGE INSTRUCTIONS: The specimen should be refrigerated if it cannot be promptly processed. If a gastric aspirate cannot be processed immediately, its pH should be neutralized for storage. CAUSES FOR REJECTION: Specimens contaminated on the outside of the container pose excessive risk to laboratory personnel and may not be acceptable to the laboratory. Specimens left at room temperature for more than 1 hour may have an overgrowth of contaminating bacteria. TURNAROUND TIME: Negative cultures are reported after 6-8 weeks. SPECIAL INSTRUCTIONS: Early morning specimen is preferred. Since at least 5 mL of sputum (**not saliva**) is required, the specimen may be collected over a 1- to 2-hour period in order to obtain sufficient quantity. However, specimens that are 24 hours old are unacceptable because of bacterial overgrowth.

Interpretive REFERENCE RANGE: No growth USE: Diagnose pulmonary tuberculosis or other *Mycobacterium* sp from expectorated sputum, induced sputum, nasotracheal aspiration, or, if necessary, gastric aspiration or bronchoscopy LIMITATIONS: Bronchial washings are frequently diluted with topical anesthetics and irrigating fluids, but bronchoscopy still provides a high yield of positive specimens. Postbronchoscopy expectorated specimens may provide a better yield of organisms than those obtained during the procedure. Gastric aspirates yield organisms in <50% of cases of *M. tuberculosis* infection in children. Acid-fast stain of gastric aspirate has a sensitivity of 30% and provides a useful clinical diagnosis if positive.[1] Separate Cytology specimens must be submitted. Transbronchial biopsy cultures were positive in only

(Continued)

Sputum Mycobacteria Culture *(Continued)*

16% of cases reviewed by Stensen et al.[2] The yield of prebronchoscopy sputum was 75%, bronchial washings 66%, and postbronchoscopy sputum 58%. Bronchoscopy can, however, be an important adjunct to serial sputum collection in the definitive diagnosis of pulmonary infection due to mycobacteria. **METHODOLOGY:** Concentration and decontamination by exposure to acid or alkaline agents, mycolytic agents, and centrifugation. Culture on selective media usually including Löwenstein-Jensen (LJ) and Middlebrook 7H11 with and without antibiotics. DNA probe technology using chemiluminescent-labeled DNA probes complementary to the ribosomal RNA of the *M. tuberculosis* complex which includes *M. tuberculosis*, *M. bovis*, BCG, *M. africanum*, and *M. microti* are available for culture confirmation. Probes are also available for *M. avium-intracellulare* complex, *M. gordonae*, and *M. kansasii*. The probes can provide more rapid confirmation of the species of mycobacteria isolated. Mycobacteria in clinical specimens can be detected by the radiometric Bactec® system which detects production of $^{14}CO_2$ from ^{14}C-labeled palmitic acid supplemented Middlebrook 7H12 medium.[3] Detection times are more rapid than with conventional culture methods. Gas-liquid chromatography (GLC) can also be used to rapidly speciate mycobacterial colonies. The detection and identification of mycobacterial organisms directly in clinical specimens is improving with the development of a test that amplifies specific mycobacterial DNA.[4] **ADDITIONAL INFORMATION:** Tuberculosis decreased in incidence in the United States in the 1970s and 1980s, but the incidence of tuberculosis in the United States has increased since 1986. High incidence populations exist in depressed inner city areas, some rural areas, amongst new immigrants, in prison inmates, and in HIV-positive patients. The emergence of *M. tuberculosis* and *M. avium-intracellulare* infections complicating the acquired immunodeficiency syndrome has been striking. When tuberculosis occurs as a first or case-defining opportunistic infection, 75% to 100% of patients of HIV-positive patients have pulmonary disease. After the diagnosis of AIDS has been made, 25% to 70% of HIV-associated tuberculosis patients have an extrapulmonary site of infection.[5]

In an ambulatory inner city population, two specimens processed for acid-fast stain and culture identified all cases of active tuberculosis within the time required for culture. The most infective cases were identified immediately by the acid-fast stain. Tuberculin tests and chest x-rays were also performed but did not significantly increase the number of cases identified in this population.[6] See also Acid-Fast Stain, Biopsy or Body Fluid Mycobacteria Culture, and Skin Test Tuberculosis listings for additional discussion of mycobacterial disease in patients with the acquired immunodeficiency syndrome (AIDS).

M. kansasii is uncommon as an environmental contaminant. Implication of *M. avium-intracellulare* as a pathogen usually requires at least one of the following criteria:

- clinical evidence of a disease process that can be explained by atypical mycobacterial infection
- repeated isolation of the same mycobacterial species from sputum over a period of weeks to months
- exclusion of other possible etiologies
- biopsy demonstrating acid-fast bacilli or diagnostic histopathologic changes[7]

Endobronchial tuberculosis has been increasingly recognized because of its incidence in association with the acquired immunodeficiency syndrome and because it may mimic carcinoma.[8,9]

Nosocomial transmission of multidrug-resistant *Mycobacterium tuberculosis* has been noted to occur from patient to patient and from patient to healthcare worker. Acid-fast bacilli isolation precautions and adherence to appropriate infection control procedures is recommended.[10,11]

While *M. tuberculosis* is contagious and is usually transmitted from person to person, most of the other disease-causing mycobacteria are not characterized by person-to-person spread, are found in the environment, and are considered opportunistic pathogens. They may be called potentially pathogenic environmental (PPE) mycobacteria. They include *M. avium*, *M. intracellulare*, *M. asiaticum*, *M. flavescens*, *M. fortuitum* complex, *M. gordonae*, *M. haemophilum*, *M. kansasii*, *M. malmoense*, *M. marinum*, *M. scrofulaceum*, *M. simiae*, *M. smegmatis*, and *M. xenopi*. They are correlated with HIV.[7]

Footnotes

1. Klotz SA and Penn RL, "Acid-Fast Staining of Urine and Gastric Contents Is An Excellent Indicator of Mycobacterial Disease," *Am Rev Respir Dis*, 1987, 136:1197-8.

2. Stenson W, Aranda C, and Bevelaqua FA, "Transbronchial Biopsy Culture in Pulmonary Tuberculosis," *Chest*, 1983, 83:883-4.
3. Stager CE, Libonati JP, Siddigi SH, et al, "Role of Solid Media When Using in Conjunction With the Bactec® System for Mycobacterial Isolation and Identification," *J Clin Microbiol*, 1991, 29(1):154-7.
4. Kolk AH, Schuitema AR, Kuijper S, et al, "Detection of *Mycobacterium tuberculosis* in Clinical Samples by Using Polymerase Chain Reaction and a Nonradioactive Detection System," *J Clin Microbiol*, 1992, 30(10):2567-75.
5. Chaisson RE and Slutkin G, "Tuberculosis and Human Immunodeficiency Virus Infection," *J Infect Dis*, 1989, 159(1):96-100.
6. Tenover FC, Crawford JT, Huebner RE, et al, "The Resurgence of Tuberculosis: Is Your Laboratory Ready?" *J Clin Microbiol*, 1993, 31(4):767-70.
7. Wayne LG and Sramek HA, "Agents of Newly Recognized or Infrequently Encountered Mycobacterial Diseases," *Clin Microbiol Rev*, 1992, 5(1):1-25.
8. Smith LS, Schillaci RF, and Sarlin RF, "Endobronchial Tuberculosis Serial Fiberoptic Bronchoscopy and Natural History," *Chest*, 1987, 91:644-7.
9. Maguire GP, Delorenzo LJ, and Brown RB, "Case Report: Endobronchial Tuberculosis Simulating Bronchogenic Carcinoma in a Patient With the Acquired Immunodeficiency Syndrome," *Am J Med Sci*, 1987, 294:42-4.
10. Pearson ML, Jereb JA, Frieden TR, et al, "Nosocomial Transmission of Multidrug-Resistant *Mycobacterium tuberculosis*. A Risk to Patients and Healthcare Workers," *Ann Intern Med*, 1992, 117(3):191-6.
11. Iseman MD, "A Leap of Faith. What Can We Do to Curtail Intrainstitutional Transmission of Tuberculosis?" *Ann Intern Med*, 1992, 117(3):251-3.

References

Barnes PF and Barrows SA, "Tuberculosis in the 1990s," *Ann Intern Med*, 1993, 119:400-10.

Beck-Sague C, Dooley SW, Hutton MD, et al, "Hopsital Outbreak of Multidrug-Resistant *Mycobacterium tuberculosis* Infections. Factors in Transmission to Staff and HIV-Infected Patients," *JAMA*, 1992, 268(10):1280-6.

Mehta JB and Morris F, "Impact of HIV Infection on Mycobacterial Disease," *Am Fam Physician*, 1992, 45(5):2203-11.

Musial CE and Roberts GD, "Rapid Detection and Identification Procedures for Acid-Fast Organisms," *Clin Microbiol Newslet*, 1987, 9:89-96.

Pitchenik AE, "Tuberculosis Control and AIDS Epidemic in Developing Countries," *Ann Intern Med*, 1990, 113(2):89-90.

Wolinsky E, "Mycobacterial Diseases Other Than Tuberculosis," *Clin Infect Dis*, 1992, 15(1):1-10.

Sputum *Nocardia* Culture *see* *Nocardia* Culture, All Sites *on page 835*

***Staphylococcus aureus* Nasal Culture** *see* Nasopharyngeal Culture for *Staphylococcus aureus* Carriers *on page 831*

Sterility Culture

CPT *87070*

Synonyms Autoclave Sterility Check; Sterilizer Function Check

Specimen Three strips (one control and two test strips) **CONTAINER:** Sterility test envelope **COLLECTION:** The two test strips should be placed separately in the center of the two largest packs, in the largest loads or in areas of the load that is least likely to come up to sterilizing temperature. Do not place the strips on open shelves, on the peripheral, or the exterior surface of a pack. **CAUSES FOR REJECTION:** Strips not received in the proper envelope, appropriate number of strips not received, improperly labeled envelope **SPECIAL INSTRUCTIONS:** One strip (control strip) must not be autoclaved or steam sterilized. The two other strips (test strips) must be sterilized.

Interpretive **REFERENCE RANGE:** No growth in test strips; growth in control strip **USE:** Confirm that adequate sterilization conditions have been attained **LIMITATIONS:** Manufacturers instructions should be followed carefully. It may be necessary to add water (500 mL) to sealed plastic biohazard bags. See bag manufacturer's instructions. **METHODOLOGY:** Indicator strips impregnated with spores of *Bacillus stearothermophilus* are used with steam autoclaves, and *Bacillus subtilis* variety *niger* are used for ethylene oxide sterilizers. **ADDITIONAL INFORMATION:** Biological indicators must be used at least once weekly with the steam autoclaves and with every load with the ethylene oxide sterilizer.

Sterilizer Function Check *see* Sterility Culture *on this page*

Stool Culture

CPT 87045

Related Information

Blood Culture, Aerobic and Anaerobic *on page 784*
Clostridium difficile Toxin Assay *on page 802*
Cryptosporidium Diagnostic Procedures, Stool *on page 806*
Electron Microscopic Examination for Viruses, Stool *on page 1177*
Entamoeba histolytica Serological Test *on page 675*
Enterovirus Culture *on page 1178*
Methylene Blue Stain, Stool *on page 828*
Ova and Parasites, Stool *on page 836*
Rotavirus, Direct Detection *on page 1191*
Salmonella Titer *on page 744*
Stool Culture, Diarrheagenic *E. coli on page 860*
Stool Fungus Culture *on page 861*
Stool Mycobacteria Culture *on page 863*
Viral Culture, Stool *on page 1205*
Yersinia enterocolitica Antibody *on page 765*

Synonyms Enteric Pathogens Culture, Routine; Stool for Culture

Applies to Rectal Swab Culture

Test Commonly Includes Screening culture for *Campylobacter*, *Salmonella*, *Shigella*, and, if requested, *Staphylococcus*, *Yersinia*, and *Vibrio*.

Specimen Fresh random stool, rectal swab **CONTAINER:** Plastic stool container, Culturette® **COLLECTION:** If stool is collected in a clean bedpan, it must not be contaminated with urine, residual soap, or disinfectants. Swabs of lesions of the rectal wall during proctoscopy or sigmoidoscopy are preferred.

Rectal swab: Insert the swab past the anal sphincter, move the swab circumferentially around the rectum. Allow 15-30 seconds for organisms to adsorb onto the swab. Withdraw swab, place in Culturette® tube, and crush media compartment.

STORAGE INSTRUCTIONS: Refrigerate if the specimen cannot be processed promptly. **CAUSES FOR REJECTION:** Because of risk to laboratory personnel, specimens sent on diaper or tissue paper, or specimen contaminating outside of transport container may not be acceptable to the laboratory. Specimen containing interfering substances (eg, castor oil, bismuth, Metamucil®, barium), specimens delayed in transit and those contaminated with urine may not have optimal yield. **TURNAROUND TIME:** Minimum 48 hours if negative; 72 hours if identification of *Yersinia* is required **SPECIAL INSTRUCTIONS:** The laboratory should be informed of the specific pathogen suspected if not *Salmonella*, *Shigella*, or *Campylobacter*.

Interpretive **REFERENCE RANGE:** Negative for *Campylobacter*, *Salmonella*, *Shigella*, *Yersinia*, *Vibrio*, and large numbers of *Staphylococcus*. In endemic areas the isolation of a pathogen may not indicate the cause or only cause of diarrhea. **USE:** Screen for pathogenic bacterial organisms in the stool; diagnose typhoid fever, enteric fever, bacillary dysentery, *Salmonella* infection.

Indications for stool culture include:[1]

- bloody diarrhea
- fever
- tenesmus
- severe or persistent symptoms
- recent travel to a third world country
- known exposure to a bacterial agent
- presence of fecal leukocytes

LIMITATIONS: *Yersinia* sp and *Vibrio parahaemolyticus* may not be isolated **unless specifically requested**. These organisms are fastidious and have very specific requirements for growth. Routine stool cultures are among the least cost effective procedures performed. The cost per positive result is $900 to $1200 (*Salmonella*, *Shigella*, *C. jejuni*, or *Yersinia*).[2] Thus, some laboratories may use careful history and application of the methylene blue stain in patient selection for stool culture. **CONTRAINDICATIONS:** A rectal swab culture is not as effective as a stool culture for detection of the carrier state. **METHODOLOGY:** Aerobic culture on selective media **ADDITIONAL INFORMATION:** In enteric fever caused by *Salmonella typhi*, *S. choleraesuis*, or *S. enteritidis*, blood culture may be positive before stool cultures, and blood cultures are indicated early; urine cultures may also be helpful.

Diarrhea is common in patients with the acquired immunodeficiency syndrome (AIDS). It is frequently caused by the classic bacterial pathogens, as well as, unusual opportunistic bacterial pathogens and parasitic infestation. (*Giardia*, *Cryptosporidium*, and *Entamoeba histolytica* frequently reported.) *Cryptosporidium* and *Pneumocystis* can occur with AIDS.[3] Rectal swabs

Diarrhea Syndromes Classified by Predominant Features

Syndrome (anatomic site)	Features	Characteristic Etiologies
Gastroenteritis (stomach)	Vomiting	Rotavirus Norwalk virus Staphylococcal food poisoning *Bacillus cereus* food poisoning
Enteritis (small bowel)	Watery diarrhea Large–volume stools, few in number	Enterotoxigenic *Escherichia coli* *Vibrio cholerae* Any enteric microbe
Dysentery, colitis (colon)	Small–volume stools containing blood and/or mucus and many leukocytes	*Shigella* *Campylobacter* *Salmonella* Invasive *E. coli* *Plesiomonas shigelloides* *Aeromonas hydrophila* *Vibrio parahaemolyticus* *Clostridium difficile* *Entamoeba histolytica* Inflammatory bowel disease

are useful for the diagnosis of *Neisseria gonorrhoeae* and *Chlamydia* infections. AIDS patients are also subject to cytomegalovirus, *Salmonella*, *Campylobacter*, *Shigella*, *C. difficile*, herpes, and *Treponema pallidum* gastrointestinal tract involvement.

In acute or subacute diarrhea, three common syndromes are recognized: gastroenteritis, enteritis, and colitis (dysenteric syndrome). With colitis, patients have fecal urgency and tenesmus. Stools are frequently small in volume and contain blood, mucus, and leukocytes. External hemorrhoids are common and painful. Diarrhea of small bowel origin is indicated by the passage of few large volume stools. This is due to accumulation of fluid in the large bowel before passage. Leukocytes indicate colonic inflammation rather than a specific pathogen. Bacterial diarrhea may be present in the absence of fecal leukocytes, and fecal leukocytes may be present in the absence of bacterial or parasitic agents (ie, idiopathic inflammatory bowel disease).[4] See table. Although most bacterial diarrhea is transient (1-30 days), cases of persistent symptoms (10 months) have been reported. The etiologic agent in the reported case was *Shigella flexneri* diagnosed by culture of rectal swab.[5] Infants younger than 1 year of age with a history of blood in the stool, more than 10 stools in 24 hours, and temperature greater than 39°C have a high probability of having bacterial diarrhea.[6,7] Diarrhea is also a common side effect of long-term antibiotic treatment. Although often associated with *Clostridium difficile*, other bacteria and yeasts have been implicated.[8]

Footnotes

1. Bishop WP and Ulshen MH, "Bacterial Gastroenteritis," *Pediatr Clin North Am*, 1988, 35(1):69-87, (review).
2. Guerrant RL, Wanke CA, Barrett LJ, et al, "A Cost-Effective and Effective Approach to the Diagnosis and Management of Acute Infectious Diarrhea," *Bull N Y Acad Med*, 1987, 63:484-99, (review).
3. Greenson JK, Belitsos PC, Yardley JH, et al, "AIDS Enteropathy: Occult Enteric Infections and Duodenal Mucosal Alterations in Chronic Diarrhea," *Ann Intern Med*, 1991, 114(5):366-72.
4. DuPont HL, "Subacute Diarrhea to Treat or to Wait?" *Hosp Pract [Off]*, 1989, 24(3A)111-8.
5. Clements D, Ellis CJ, and Allan RN, "Persistent Shigellosis - Case Report," *Gut*, 1988, 29(9):1277-8.
6. Finkelstein JA, Schwartz JS, Torrey S, et al, "Common Clinical Features as Predictors of Bacterial Diarrhea in Infants," *Am J Emerg Med*, 1989, 7(5):469-73.
7. Cohen MB, "Etiology and Mechanisms of Acute Infectious Diarrhea in Infants in the United States," *J Pediatr*, 1991, 118(4 Pt 2):S34-9.
8. Bartlett JG, "Antibiotic-Associated Diarrhea," *Clin Infect Dis*, 1992, 15(4):573-81.

References

DeWitt TG, "Acute Diarrhea in Children," *Pediatr Rev*, 1989, 11(1):6-13.

Farmer RG, "Infectious Causes of Diarrhea in the Differential Diagnosis of Inflammatory Bowel Disease," *Med Clin North Am*, 1990, 74(1):29-38.

(Continued)

Stool Culture *(Continued)*

Guerrant RL, "Nausea, Vomiting, and Noninflammatory Diarrhea," *Principles and Practice of Infectious Diseases*, 3rd ed, Chapter 82, Mandell GL, Douglas RG Jr, and Bennett JE, eds, New York, NY: Churchill Livingstone, 1990, 851-63.

Guerrant RL, Hughes JM, Lima NL, et al, "Diarrhea in Developed and Developing Countries: Magnitude, Special Settings, and Etiologies," *Rev Infect Dis*, 1990, 12(Suppl 1):541-50.

Pickering LK, "Therapy for Acute Infectious Diarrhea in Children," *J Pediatr*, 1991, 118(4 Pt 2):S118-28.

Stool Culture, Diarrheagenic *E. coli*

***CPT** 87081*

Related Information

Methylene Blue Stain, Stool *on page 828*

Stool Culture *on page 858*

Applies to *E. coli*: 0157:H7 Culture; Enterohemorrhagic *E. coli*, Stool Culture; Enteropathogenic *E. coli*, Stool Culture; Enterotoxigenic *E. coli*, Stool Culture; Verocytotoxin Producing *E. coli*, Stool Culture

Test Commonly Includes Culture and/or identification of *E. coli* associated with diarrhea

Specimen Rectal swab, fresh stool **CONTAINER:** Plastic stool container, Culturette® **COLLECTION:** If stool is collected in sterile bedpan, it must not be contaminated with urine or residual soap or disinfectants. Swabs of lesions of the rectal wall during proctoscopy or sigmoidoscopy are preferred.

Rectal swab: Insert the swab past the anal sphincter, move the swab circumferentially around the anus. Allow 15-30 seconds for organisms to adsorb onto the swab. Withdraw swab, place in Culturette® tube, and crush media compartment.

STORAGE INSTRUCTIONS: Do not refrigerate **CAUSES FOR REJECTION:** Because of risk to laboratory personnel, specimen sent on diaper or tissue paper or specimen contaminating outside of transport container may not be acceptable to the laboratory. Specimen containing interfering substances (eg, castor oil, bismuth, Metamucil®, barium), specimens delayed in transit, and those contaminated with urine may not have optimal yield. **TURNAROUND TIME:** Preliminary report available at 24 hours; minimum 72 hours for final reports **SPECIAL INSTRUCTIONS:** Stool culture is usually performed on all requests for enteropathogenic *E. coli*

Interpretive **REFERENCE RANGE:** Normal colonic flora **USE:** Establish diarrheagenic *E. coli* as the cause of clinical illness **LIMITATIONS:** Many laboratories are not equipped to perform elaborate diagnostic procedures needed to definitively characterize and type diarrheagenic *E. coli*. Clinical diagnosis, use of methylene blue stain, and exclusion of other more readily characterized pathogens form the practical basis of presumptive diagnosis of diarrheagenic *E. coli* illness.[1] **METHODOLOGY:** Cultures may be screened for sorbitol negative (colorless) colonies on sorbitol-MacConkey agar; enterohemorrhagic *E. coli* (EHEC) is confirmed by serotyping.[2] Culture filtrate can be incubated with Vero cells. Changes observed in the presence of toxin include rounding up at 36 hours and destruction of the monolayer with detachment at 72 hours. Verocytotoxin is most frequently associated with the 0157:H7 serotype. Counterimmunoelectrophoresis (CIE) was reported to be 86% sensitive and 94% specific for the detection of verotoxin in stool filtrates.[3] DNA probes have recently been developed for the detection of verotoxin.[4] **ADDITIONAL INFORMATION:** See table. Factors common to diarrheagenic *E. coli* include the presence of critical virulence factors encoded in plasmids, characteristic interaction with intestinal mucosa, production of enterotoxin or cytotoxin, and the observation that within each category the strains fall into certain O:H serotypes.

Hemorrhagic colitis can be differentiated from other causes of diarrhea by its progression from watery to bloody diarrhea over a few days time. Fecal leukocytes are markedly increased. See also Methylene Blue Stain, Stool test listing. Fever is usually absent. The disease is mediated by the production of a shiga-like toxin which interferes with colonic brush border cells, protein synthesis, and ultimately causes cell death. Enterohemorrhagic *E. coli* (EHEC) differ from other strains of bacteria in the large amount of toxin they produce. Virtually all 0157:H7 organisms produce this toxin.

Enterotoxigenic *E. coli* (ETEC) infection is acquired by ingestion of contaminated food or water. The organisms colonize the proximal small intestine and there they elaborate enterotoxins. Clinical features of ETEC infection include watery diarrhea, nausea, abdominal cramps, and low-grade fever.[1] Enterotoxigenic *E. coli* is the most common agent of travelers diarrhea. Symptoms start early in the visit, typically on day 3. The illness may typically last 3-4

Four Major Categories of Diarrheagenic *E. coli*

Category	Abbreviation	Clinic Manifestation
Enterotoxigenic	ETEC	Travelers diarrhea and infant diarrhea in less developed countries
Enteropathogenic	EPEC	Infant diarrhea
Enterohemorrhagic	EHEC	Hemorrhagic colitis Hemolytic uremic syndrome Thrombotic thrombocytopenia purpura
Enteroinvasive	EIEC	Dysentery

days. The illness is mild with 4% of travelers consulting a local physician and less than 1% being hospitalized. Occurrence rates vary from 5.8% of Europeans visiting the U.S. to 34% when visiting the tropics.[5]

Enteropathogenic *E. coli* (EPEC) produce a cytotoxin similar or identical to that produced by *Shigella dysenteriae* type 1. The clinical symptoms of EPEC illness include fever, malaise, vomiting, and diarrhea with large amounts of mucus but not grossly bloody. EPEC diarrhea in infants may persist for more than 14 days and is frequently severe. The incidence of diarrhea due to EPEC has declined in developed countries over the past 10 years.[6]

Enteroinvasive *E. coli* (EIEC) invade and proliferate within epithelial cells and cause eventual cell death, like *Shigella*. Clinical illness is characterized by fever, severe abdominal cramps, malaise, toxemia, and watery diarrhea. The illness progresses to gross dysentery with scant stools consisting of blood and mucus. The methylene blue stain of stool reveals sheets of leukocytes.[1]

Recently DNA probes have been developed to provide a rapid and accurate diagnosis of diarrheagenic *E. coli*.[7] Although these are currently experimental, they may soon be incorporated into routine screening for diarrhea.

Footnotes

1. Levine MM, "*Escherichia coli* That Cause Diarrhea: Enterotoxigenic, Enteropathogenic, Enteroinvasive, Enterohemorrhagic, and Enteroadherent," *J Infect Dis*, 1987, 155:377-89.
2. Sack RB, "Enterohemorrhagic *Escherichia coli*," *N Engl J Med*, 1987, 317:1535-7, (editorial).
3. Maniar AC, Williams T, Anand CM, et al, "Detection of Verotoxin in Stool Specimens," *J Clin Microbiol*, 1990, 28(1):134-5.
4. Smith HR, Willshaw GA, Thomas A, et al, "Applications of DNA Probes for Vero Cytotoxin-Producing *Escherichia coli*," *J Hosp Infect*, 1991, 18(Suppl A):438-42.
5. Bishop WP and Ulshen MH, "Bacterial Gastroenteritis," *Pediatr Clin North Am*, 1988, 35(1):69-87, (review).
6. Morris KJ and Rao GG, "Conventional Screening for Enteropathogenic *Escherichia coli* in the UK. Is It Appropriate or Necessary?" *J Hosp Infect*, 1992, 21(3):163-7.
7. Gicquelais KG, Baldini MM, Martinez J, et al, "Practical and Economical Method for Using Biotinylated DNA Probes With Bacterial Colony Blots to Identify Diarrhea-Causing *Escherichia coli*," *J Clin Microbiol*, 1990, 28(11):2485-90.

References

Donnenberg MS and Kaper JB, "Enteropathogenic *Escherichia coli*," *Infect Immun*, 1992, 60(10):3953-61.

Doyle MP, "Pathogenic *Escherichia coli*, *Yersinia enterocolitica*, and *Vibrio parahaemolyticus*," *Lancet*, 1990, 336(8723):1111-5.

Griffin PM, Ostroff SM, and Tauxe RV, "Illness Associated With *Escherichia coli* 0157:H7 Infections – A Broad Clinical Spectrum," *Ann Intern Med*, 1988, 109:705-12.

Okhuysen PC and Ericsson CD, "Traveler's Diarrhea Prevention and Treatment," *Med Clin North Am*, 1992, 76(6):1357-73.

Stool for Culture *see* Stool Culture *on page 858*

Stool for Ova and Parasites *see* Ova and Parasites, Stool *on page 836*

Stool for White Cells *see* Methylene Blue Stain, Stool *on page 828*

Stool Fungus Culture

***CPT** 87102 (isolation); 87106 (definitive identification)*

Related Information

Amphotericin B *on page 942*

(Continued)

Stool Fungus Culture *(Continued)*

Blood Fungus Culture *on page 789*
Candida Antigen *on page 652*
Candidiasis Serologic Test *on page 652*
Clostridium difficile Toxin Assay *on page 802*
Methylene Blue Stain, Stool *on page 828*
Skin Fungus Culture *on page 845*
Sputum Fungus Culture *on page 853*
Stool Culture *on page 858*

Synonyms Fungus Culture, Stool

Specimen Freshly passed stool, rectal swab **CONTAINER:** Plastic stool container or Culturette® **COLLECTION:** The specimen can be divided for fungus culture and KOH preparation if the specimen is of adequate volume. Specify fungal species suspected. **STORAGE INSTRUCTIONS:** Refrigerate if the specimen cannot be promptly processed. **CAUSES FOR REJECTION:** Because of risk to laboratory personnel, specimen sent on diaper or tissue paper or specimen contaminating outside of transport container may not be acceptable to the laboratory. Specimen containing interfering substances (eg, castor oil, bismuth, Metamucil®, barium), specimens delayed in transit, and those contaminated with urine may not have optimal yield. **TURNAROUND TIME:** Negative cultures are usually reported after 1 week. If suspicion of systemic fungus infection has been indicated, the culture is usually observed for 4 weeks.

Interpretive **REFERENCE RANGE:** No growth **USE:** Establish the presence of fungi, particularly *Candida* sp in debilitated hosts, patients receiving antimicrobial chemotherapeutic agents, and hyperalimentation **LIMITATIONS:** Use of this test is generally limited to screening for *Candida.* Stool cultures have a low yield and are not recommended for the isolation of systemic fungi, however, *Histoplasma capsulatum* is frequently recovered from the stool of AIDS patients with disseminated infection. See Sputum Fungus Culture and Skin Fungus Culture listings for fungus culture specimen selection and Blood Fungus Culture listing for additional discussion of appropriate specimens. **METHODOLOGY:** Culture on selective media usually including Sabouraud's agar with antibiotics **ADDITIONAL INFORMATION:** *Candida* can be isolated in up to 30% of oropharyngeal cultures and 65% of stool cultures; thus, it is a common saprophyte.[1] Neonates and adults may develop watery diarrhea due to intestinal overgrowth by yeast which readily responds to specific therapy. *Candida* may become disseminated in patients with leukopenia, immunosuppressive therapy, AIDS, corticosteroid therapy, phagocytic defects, hyperalimentation, use of broad spectrum antibiotics, and oral contraceptives. Travelers in endemic areas with poor sanitation have also experienced intestinal overgrowth with *Candida*, although the specific mechanism causing diarrhea is unknown. Serology, particularly immunodiffusion for *Candida* antigens, may help document the presence of invasive candidiasis.[2]

Candida-associated diarrhea is predominantly of the secretory type, characterized by frequent watery stools, usually without blood, mucus, tenesmus, or abdominal pain.[3] Overgrowth of *Candida* sp should be considered when evaluating *Clostridium difficile* negative cases of antibiotic-associated colitis.[4]

Footnotes

1. Cohen R, Roth FJ, Delgado E, et al, "Fungal Flora of Normal Human Small and Large Intestine," *N Engl J Med*, 1969, 280; 638-41.
2. Chretien JH and Garagusi VF, "Current Management of Fungal Enteritis," *Med Clin North Am*, 1982, 66:675-87.
3. Gupta TP and Ehrinpreis MN, "*Candida*-Associated Diarrhea in Hospitalized Patients," *Gastroenterology*, 1990, 98(3):780-5.
4. Sanderson PJ and Bukhari SS, "*Candida* spp and *Clostridium difficile* Toxin-Negative Antibiotic-Associated Diarrhoea," *J Hosp Infect*, 1991, 19(2):142-3.

References

Anaissie EJ, Bodey GP, and Kantarjian H, "A New Spectrum of Fungal Infections in Patients With Cancer," *Rev Infect Dis*, 1989, 11(3):369-78.

Danna PL, Urban C, Bellin E, et al, "Role of *Candida* in Pathogenesis of Antibiotic-Associated Diarrhoea in Elderly Inpatients," *Lancet*, 1991, 337(8740):511-4.

Ullrich R, Heise W, Bergs C, et al, "Gastrointestinal Symptoms in Patients Infected With Human Immunodeficiency Virus: Relevance of Infective Agents Isolated From Gastrointestinal Tract," *Gut*, 1992, 33(8):1080-4.

Stool Mycobacteria Culture

CPT *87116 (isolation); 87118 (definitive identification)*

Related Information

Acid-Fast Stain *on page 770*
Mycobacteria by DNA Probe *on page 921*
Skin Mycobacteria Culture *on page 846*
Skin Test, Tuberculosis *on page 848*
Sputum Mycobacteria Culture *on page 855*
Stool Culture *on page 858*
Susceptibility Testing, Mycobacteria *on page 872*
Urine Mycobacteria Culture *on page 884*

Synonyms AFB Culture, Stool; Mycobacteria Culture, Stool; TB Culture, Stool

Specimen Stool **CONTAINER:** Plastic stool container **STORAGE INSTRUCTIONS:** If the specimen cannot be processed immediately by the laboratory, it should be refrigerated. **CAUSES FOR REJECTION:** Because of risk to laboratory personnel, specimen sent on diaper or tissue paper or specimen contaminating outside of transport container may not be acceptable to the laboratory. **TURNAROUND TIME:** Negative cultures are usually reported after 8 weeks.

Interpretive REFERENCE RANGE: No growth **USE:** Isolate and identify mycobacteria **LIMITATIONS:** Isolation of mycobacteria from feces does not necessarily imply intestinal tuberculosis. Mycobacteria in feces are most likely from sputum swallowed by patient with pulmonary disease. The recovery of *M. gordonae*, "the tap water bacillus," from stool occurs occasionally. The recovery of mycobacteria from stool is technically limited by the rapid overgrowth of normal intestinal bacterial flora. **Stool is rarely the specimen of choice** for the primary diagnosis of mycobacterial infection. **METHODOLOGY:** Culture on selective media usually including Löwenstein-Jensen (LJ) and Middlebrook 7H11 media with antibiotics after decontamination of the specimen by a procedure similar to that used for sputum cultures. Many laboratories screen by smear before culturing. In such circumstances, if the smear is negative, culture is not performed. **ADDITIONAL INFORMATION:** The increasing recognition of mycobacterial infections in patients with the acquired immunodeficiency syndrome (AIDS) has resulted in increased awareness of the potential to recover clinically significant mycobacteria from stool. Seven of 132 AIDS patients studied for intestinal infection were found to harbor *M. avium-intracellulare.*[1] Isolation of mycobacteria from stool indicates disseminated disease, and cultures from blood, bone marrow, and lymph nodes are usually also positive for the same mycobacterial isolate.[2]

Footnotes

1. René E, Marche C, Regnier B, et al, "Intestinal Infections in Patients With Acquired Immunodeficiency Syndrome: A Prospective Study in 132 Patients," *Dig Dis Sci*, 1989, 34(5):773-80.
2. Wolinsky E, "Mycobacterial Diseases Other Than Tuberculosis," *Clin Infect Dis*, 1992, 15(1):1-10.

References

Claydon EJ, Coker RJ, and Harris JR, "*Mycobacterium malmoense* Infection in HIV Positive Patients," *J Infect*, 1991, 23(2):191-4.

Gradon JD, Timpone JG, and Schnittman SM, "Emergence of Unusual Opportunistic Pathogens in AIDS: A Review," *Clin Infect Dis*, 1992, 15(1):134-57.

Yajko DM, Nassos PS, Sanders CA, et al, "Comparison of Four Decontamination Methods for Recovery of *Mycobacterium avium* Complex From Stools," *J Clin Microbiol*, 1993, 31(2):302-6.

Strep Throat Screening Culture *see* Throat Culture *on page 876*

***Streptococcus agalactiae* Latex Screen** *see* Group B *Streptococcus* Screen *on page 819*

***Streptococcus* Group A Latex Screen** *see* Group A *Streptococcus* Screen *on page 818*

***Streptococcus* Group B Latex Screen** *see* Group B *Streptococcus* Screen *on page 819*

Streptococcus pyogenes *see* Throat Culture *on page 876*

Sudden Death Syndrome *see* Botulism, Diagnostic Procedure *on page 792*

Sulfur Granule, Culture *see Actinomyces* Culture, All Sites *on page 772*

Susceptibility Testing, Aerobic and Facultatively Anaerobic Organisms

CPT *87181 (agar diffusion, each antibiotic); 87184 (disk method, each antibiotic); 87186 (MIC microtiter); 87188 (macrotube dilution, each antibiotic)*

Related Information

Abscess, Aerobic and Anaerobic Bacterial Culture *on page 768*
Amikacin *on page 938*
Antibiotic Level, Serum *on page 942*
Bronchial Aspirate Anaerobic Culture *on page 792*
Chloramphenicol *on page 952*
Gentamicin *on page 970*
Penicillinase Test *on page 840*
Serum Bactericidal Test *on page 843*
Susceptibility Testing, Antimicrobial Combinations *on page 868*
Susceptibility Testing, Fungi *on page 869*
Susceptibility Testing, Minimum Bactericidal Concentration *on page 871*
Susceptibility Testing, Mycobacteria *on page 872*
Susceptibility Testing, Unusual Isolates/Fastidious Organisms *on page 873*
Tobramycin *on page 1004*
Vancomycin *on page 1009*

Synonyms Kirby-Bauer Susceptibility Test; MIC; Minimum Inhibitory Concentration Susceptibility Test; Sensitivity Testing, Aerobic and Facultatively Anaerobic Organisms

Applies to Antimicrobial Drugs; Beta-Lactam Ring; Penicillinase

Test Commonly Includes Qualitative or quantitative determination of antimicrobial susceptibility of an isolated organism

Abstract The purpose of antimicrobial susceptibility testing is to determine the antibacterial activity of antimicrobial agents against specific pathogens. These susceptibility assays have been standardized for use in clinical laboratories by the National Committee for Clinical Laboratory Standards (NCCLS).[1,2] Standards include the use of quality control microorganisms to ensure that results are reliable and the use of standard agar and broth media to diminish variability between laboratories.

Specimen Viable pure culture of a rapidly growing aerobic or facultatively anaerobic organism **TURNAROUND TIME:** Usually 1 day after isolation from a clinical specimen

Interpretive **REFERENCE RANGE:** Minimal inhibitory concentration (MIC) reported. Results may be qualitatively reported as susceptible (S), intermediate (I), or resistant (R). **USE:** Determine antimicrobial susceptibility of organisms involved in infectious processes when the susceptibility of the organism cannot be predicted from its identity. The pattern of antibiotic susceptibility is sometimes used to monitor nosocomial infections such as methicillin-resistant *Staphylococcus aureus* and to evaluate or follow the development of resistance to new antimicrobial drugs.[3,4] **METHODOLOGY:** Disk diffusion (qualitative) broth dilution, microbroth dilution, or agar dilution (quantitative), or antimicrobial concentrations are selected to correspond to therapeutically relevant levels. Several automated instruments have been developed to perform routine susceptibility testing of microorganisms.[5] **ADDITIONAL INFORMATION:** Effective antimicrobial therapy is usually selected with intent to achieve a peak level two to four times the MIC at the site of infection. An antimicrobial level 10 times the MIC is usually sought in urinary tract infections. The "breakpoints" indicate MICs above which organisms are moderately or very resistant and would not be expected to respond to readily achievable levels of antimicrobial therapy.

Susceptible: This category implies that an infection due to the strain may be appropriately treated with the dosage of antimicrobial agent recommended for that type of infection and infecting species, unless otherwise contraindicated.

Intermediate: This category provides a "buffer zone," which should prevent small, uncontrolled, technical factors from causing major discrepancies in interpretations, (eg, species that should have few or no endpoints in this range, or drugs with *in vitro* results affected by media variation or drugs with narrow pharmacotoxicity margins).

Resistant: Strains falling in this category are not inhibited by the usually achievable systemic concentrations of the agent with normal dosage schedules and/or fall in the range where specific microbial resistance mechanisms are likely (eg, beta-lactamases), and clinical efficacy has not been reliable in treatment studies. See table.

Major Mechanisms of Bacterial Antimicrobial Resistance

Enzymatic inactivation or modification of drug

- β-lactamase hydrolysis of β-lactam ring with subsequent inactivation of β-lactam antibiotics
- Modification of aminoglycosides by acetylating, adenylating, or phosphorylating enzymes
- Modification of chloramphenicol by chloramphenicol acetyltransferase

Decreased drug uptake or accumulation

- Intrinsic or acquired lack of outer membrane permeability
- Faulty or lacking antibiotic uptake and transport system
- Antibiotic efflux system (eg, tetracycline resistance)

Altered or lacking antimicrobial target

- Altered penicillin-binding proteins (β-lactam resistance)
- Altered ribosomal target (eg, aminoglycoside, macrolide, and lincomycin resistance)
- Altered enzymatic target (eg, sulfonamide, trimethoprim, rifampin, and quinolone resistance)

Circumvention of drug action consequences

- Hyperproduction of drug targets or competitive substrates (eg, sulfonamide and trimethoprim resistance)

Uncoupling of antibiotic attack and cell death

- Bacterial tolerance and survival in presence of usually bactericidal drugs (eg, β-lactams and vancomycin)

A MIC to penicillin >0.1 μg/mL for *S. aureus* indicates resistance due to penicillinase production.

Footnotes

1. National Committee for Clinical Laboratory Standards, "Performance Standards for Antimicrobial Disk Susceptibility Tests," Approved Standard M2-A4, 4th ed, Villanova, PA: National Committee for Clinical Laboratory Standards, 1990.
2. National Committee for Clinical Laboratory Standards, "Methods for Dilution Susceptibility Tests for Bacteria That Grow Aerobically." Approved Standard M7-A2, 2nd ed, Villanova, PA: National Committee for Clinical Laboratory Standards, 1990.
3. Grayson ML and Eliopoulos GM, "Antimicrobial Resistance in the Intensive Care Unit," *Semin Respir Infect*, 1990, 5(3):204-14.
4. Parry MF, "Epidemiology and Mechanisms of Antimicrobial Resistance," *Am J Infect Control*, 1989, 17(5):286-94.
5. Stager CE and Davis JR, "Automated Systems for Identification of Microorganisms," *Clin Microbiol Rev*, 1992, 5(3):302-27.

References

Gill VJ, Witebsky FG, and MacLowry JD, "Multicategory Interpretive Reporting of Susceptibility Testing With Selected Antimicrobial Concentrations. Ten Years of Laboratory and Clinical Experience," *Clin Lab Med*, 1989, 9(2):221-38.

Hindler JA and Thrupp LD, "Interpretive Guidelines for Antimicrobial Susceptibility Test Results: What Do They Mean?" *Clin Microbiol Newslet*, 1989, 17:129-36.

National Committee for Clinical Laboratory Standards, "Performance Standards for Antimicrobial Susceptibility Testing," Fourth Information Supplement NCCLS Document M100-S4, Villanova, PA: National Committee for Clinical Laboratory Standards, 1992.

Rosenblatt JE, "Laboratory Tests Used to Guide Antimicrobial Therapy," *Mayo Clin Proc*, 1991, 66(9):942-8.

Sherris JC, "Antimicrobic Susceptibility Testing. A Personal Perspective," *Clin Lab Med*, 1989, 9(2):191-202.

Silver LL and Bostian KA, "Discovery and Development of New Antibiotics: The Problem of Antibiotic Resistance," *Antimicrob Agents Chemother*, 1993, 37(3):377-83.

Wilkowske CJ, "General Principles of Antimicrobial Therapy," *Mayo Clin Proc*, 1991, 66(9):931-41.

Susceptibility Testing, Anaerobic Bacteria

CPT *87181 (agar dilution, each antibiotic); 87188 (tube dilution, each antibiotic)*

Related Information

Abscess, Aerobic and Anaerobic Bacterial Culture *on page 768*
Penicillinase Test *on page 840*
Susceptibility Testing, Antimicrobial Combinations *on page 868*
Susceptibility Testing, Unusual Isolates/Fastidious Organisms *on page 873*

Synonyms Anaerobic Bacterial Susceptibility; MIC, Anaerobic Bacteria

Specimen A pure culture of the isolated organism to be tested, prepared by the laboratory **TURNAROUND TIME:** 2-5 days from time organism is isolated and identified **SPECIAL INSTRUCTIONS:** The laboratory should be consulted regarding appropriateness and scope of anaerobic susceptibility testing in a particular clinical setting.

Interpretive **REFERENCE RANGE:** See table. **USE:** Susceptibility test results are usually reported on anaerobic bacterial isolates only on special request to the laboratory. Susceptibility testing of anaerobes is usually done on individual patient isolates when the infection does not respond to empiric therapy. In this event, the selection of an appropriate therapeutic agent is critical. Selection of antibacterial agents to treat these infections can be difficult and often affect the outcome of disease. Certain infections which may require determination of anaerobic susceptibility include brain abscess, endocarditis, osteomyelitis, joint infection, infection of prosthetic devices, or vascular grafts.[1] **LIMITATIONS:** Breakpoints are not well defined or universally accepted for categorization of susceptible and resistant. Methods are still being developed to standardize testing, reporting, and interpretation of anaerobic susceptibility tests for the broth disk elution and microdilution methods. Anaerobic infections are frequently polymicrobial, involving aerobic and anaerobic flora. Thus, the predictive value of an anaerobic susceptibility test for a successful clinical outcome may be limited by the complexity of the clinical infection. **CONTRAINDICATIONS:** Anaerobic bacterial isolate from patient is not available or fails to give adequate growth for susceptibility testing. **METHODOLOGY:** Broth microdilution, macrobroth dilution, and agar dilution technique; beta-lactamase testing **ADDITIONAL INFORMATION:** At present, routine susceptibility testing of anaerobic isolates is not recommended.[2] Infections involving anaerobes frequently contain mixed flora, and appropriate drainage rather than antimicrobial therapy seems to be the most crucial factor in the successful treatment of these infections.

Indications for anaerobic susceptibility testing include:

- determination of susceptibility of anaerobes to new antimicrobial agents
- monitoring susceptibility patterns by geographic area
- monitoring susceptibility patterns in local hospitals
- assisting in the management of selected individual patients; ***vide supra, vide infra***

Some anaerobes have predictable *in vitro* susceptibility patterns but grow so slowly that by the time isolation and susceptibility testing are completed (6-14 days), such results are of little clinical value. Thus, susceptibility testing is generally performed only on anaerobic isolates from blood, pleural fluid, peritoneal fluid, and CSF. In cases of chronic anaerobic infections (septic arthritis, osteomyelitis, etc), susceptibility testing may be done by special request. The physician should contact the laboratory regarding the specific antibiotic(s) to be tested and the testing method available.

Organisms that are recognized as virulent such as *Bacteroides fragilis* group, pigmented *Prevotella* sp, *Porphyromonas* sp (formerly *Bacteroides gracilis*), certain *Fusobacterium*, *Clostridium perfringens*, and *Clostridium ramosus*, may also be considered for testing.[3]

The E test is a new method under investigation for testing antimicrobial susceptibility of anaerobic organisms. It has recently been approved by the FDA, and initial studies show that it correlates well with the reference methods.[4] The advantages of the E test would be to provide a quick, reliable susceptibility test that is not labor intensive.

Footnotes

1. Finegold SM and The National Committee for Clinical Laboratory Standards Working Group on Anaerobic Susceptibility Testing, "Minireview," *J Clin Microbiol*, 1988, 1253-6.
2. National Committee for Clinical Laboratory Standards, "Methods for Antimicrobial Susceptibility Testing of Anaerobic Bacteria," Approved Standard, M11-A2, Villanova, PA: National Committee for Clinical Laboratory Standards, 1990.
3. Styrt B and Gorbach SL, "Recent Developments in the Understanding of the Pathogenesis and Treatment of Anaerobic Infections," *N Engl J Med*, 1989, 321(5):298-302, (review).
4. Citron DM, Ostovari MI, Karlsson A, et al, "Evaluation of the E Test for Susceptibility Testing of Anaerobic Bacteria," *J Clin Microbiol*, 1991, 29(10):2197-203.

Typical Sensitivities of Important Anaerobic Pathogens to Major Classes of Antibiotics

Antibiotic	*B. fragilis* Group	*B. melanino-genicus* Group	*Fusobacterium*	*Clostridium*	*Propioni-bacterium*	*Actinomyces*	*Peptostrepto-coccus*
Penicillin G	- to +	- to +++	++	+ to ++	+++	+++	+++
Antipseudomonal penicillins	++ to +++	+ to +++	+++	+++	+++	+++	+++
Cefoxitin	++	+++	++ to +++	- to ++	+++	+++	+++
Imipenem-cilastatin	+++	+++	++	+++	+++	+++	+++
Combinations of beta-lactam and beta-lactamase inhibitor	+++	+++	+++	+++	+++	+++	+++
Clindamycin	++ to +++	+++	+++	++	+++	+++	+++
Chloramphenicol	+++	+++	+++	+++	+++	+++	+++
Metronidazole	+++	+++	+++	+++	—	—	++ to +++

From Styrt B and Gorbach SL, "Recent Developments in the Understanding of the Pathogenesis and Treatment of Anaerobic Infections," *N Engl J Med,* 1989, Part I, 321:240–6 and Part II, 321:298–302, (review), with permission.

- denotes that <50% of the strains were susceptible.
+ denotes that 50% to 70% of the strains were susceptible.
++ denote that 70% to 90% of the strains were susceptible.
+++ denote that >90% of the strains were susceptible.

(Continued)

Susceptibility Testing, Anaerobic Bacteria *(Continued)*

References

Amsterdam D, "Dilemmas of Antimicrobial Susceptibility Testing of Anaerobic Bacteria," *Antimicrob Newslet*, 1990, 7:5-7.

Rosenblatt JE, "Susceptibility Testing of Anaerobic Bacteria," *Clin Lab Med*, 1989, 9(2):239-54, (review).

Zebransky RJ, "Revisiting Anaerobe Susceptibility Testing," *Clin Microbiol Newslet*, 1989, 11:185-92.

Susceptibility Testing, Antimicrobial Combinations

CPT *87184 (disk method, each antibiotic); 87186 (MIC, any number of antibiotics)*

Related Information

Serum Bactericidal Test *on page 843*
Susceptibility Testing, Aerobic and Facultatively Anaerobic Organisms *on page 864*
Susceptibility Testing, Anaerobic Bacteria *on page 866*
Susceptibility Testing, Unusual Isolates/Fastidious Organisms *on page 873*

Synonyms Antimicrobial Combinations - Test for Synergism and Antagonism; Synergistic Studies, Antimicrobial

Applies to Fractional Bactericidal Concentration (FBC); Fractional Inhibitory Concentration (FIC); Minimal Bactericidal Concentration (MBC); Minimal Inhibitory Concentration (MIC)

Test Commonly Includes MICs of both antibiotics against patient's organism, determination of synergistic or antagonistic antimicrobial effect of drug combination

Specimen A pure culture of the isolated organism to be tested, prepared by the laboratory **CAUSES FOR REJECTION:** Organism discarded prior to request for test by physician, organism fails to grow on subculture or is too fastidious to grow under usual conditions of testing **TURNAROUND TIME:** 2-4 days (depends on antimicrobials assayed and procedure used) **SPECIAL INSTRUCTIONS:** Notify the laboratory to retain organism needed for test.

Interpretive **REFERENCE RANGE:** Additive effect, synergism or antagonism **USE:** Determine whether the addition of a second antibiotic (B) will increase or decrease the known sensitivity of an organism to antibiotic (A). Some antibiotics have well established synergistic activity such as a cell wall active agent (ie, penicillin and vancomycin) and an aminoglycoside.[1,2] This is recommended for serious infections due to enterococci. Other antibacterial agents are tested for their ability to inhibit each other. This is usually done for experimental purposes during development of new antibiotics. **LIMITATIONS:** This test procedure is usually available only from specialized laboratories. Predicated upon availability of antibiotic standard for testing. Test cannot be run if organism fails to grow. The clinical relevance of synergy studies and standardized methods is still being defined. **METHODOLOGY:** Checkerboard titration, time-kill technique, double diffusion testing **ADDITIONAL INFORMATION:** Laboratory should be notified 24 hours in advance of time when test is to be performed. Patient's organism must be saved at request of physician. Physician must specify antimicrobials to be tested in combination culture, site of isolated organism, and culture date. The MICs of antibiotics to be tested must be known or performed.

Combinations of antimicrobials are often used with intent of achieving a synergistic effect (ie, a demonstrated inhibitory or bactericidal activity that is greater than the sum of the activities of the agents alone). The use of combination therapy is also often undertaken to reduce potential toxicity. A lower dose of each agent may be used (eg, aminoglycosides and a cephalosporin or penicillin). Also the use of combinations prevents or minimizes the emergence of resistant strains (eg, usual antituberculosis therapy).

Several methods, checkerboard titration, time-kill technique, and diffusion tests, are used in research settings. In usual clinical practice, testing of the enterococci and viridans streptococci isolated from patients with serious infections for high level aminoglycoside resistance is adequate to predict the potential presence or absence of synergism when these agents are combined with cell wall active agents (eg, cephalosporins, penicillins). Fixed-dose combinations, trimethoprim-sulfamethoxazole and beta-lactam/beta-lactamase inhibitor combinations (eg, amoxicillin-clavulanate or ticarcillin-clavulanate) can be tested because of the standard availability of combination disks and commercially prepared microtiter susceptibility panels which include the combinations. A clear consensus regarding the usefulness of synergy studies has not yet emerged, primarily because of organism strain differences in response and lack of consensus on choice of laboratory methods. The greatest potential for clinical usefulness exists in patients with sustained profound neutropenia and in patients with endocarditis. The serum bactericidal test (Schlichter test) has efficacy in determining the potential clinical effects of antimicrobial combinations, particularly in endocarditis and osteomyelitis.

Definition of Technical Terms

* **Minimal Inhibitory Concentration (MIC)**: The lowest concentration of drug that **inhibits** growth of >99% of the bacterial population.

* **Minimal Bactericidal Concentration (MBC)**: The lowest concentration of drug that **kills** >99.9% of the bacterial population in a broth culture. The MIC/MBC ratio is the standard for expressing the bactericidal potency of the drug.

* **Fractional Inhibitory Concentration (FIC)**: An interaction coefficient indicating whether the combined inhibitory (bacteriostatic) effect of drugs is synergistic (FIC ≤0.5), additive (FIC = 1), or antagonistic (FIC ≥4) ("a" and "b" are drugs):

$$\text{FIC} = \frac{\text{MIC}_a \text{ in combination}}{\text{MIC}_a \text{ alone}} + \frac{\text{MIC}_b \text{ in combination}}{\text{MIC}_b \text{ alone}}$$

* **Fractional Bactericidal Concentration (FBC)**: An interaction coefficient indicating whether the combined bactericidal effect of drugs is synergistic, additive, or antagonistic:[3]

$$\text{FBC} = \frac{\text{MBC}_a \text{ in combination}}{\text{MBC}_a \text{ alone}} + \frac{\text{MBC}_b \text{ in combination}}{\text{MBC}_b \text{ alone}}$$

Footnotes

1. Sahm DF and Torres C, "High-Content Aminoglycoside Disks for Determining Aminoglycoside-Penicillin Synergy Against *Enterococcus faecalis*," *J Clin Microbiol*, 1988, 26:257-60.
2. Winstanley TG and Hastings JG, "Penicillin-Aminoglycoside Synergy and Postantibiotic Effect for Enterococci," *J Antimicrob Chemother*, 1989, 23(2):189-99.
3. Heifets L, "Qualitative and Quantitative Drug Susceptibility Test in Mycobacteriology," *Am Rev Respir Dis*, 1988, 137(5):1217-22.

References

Amsterdam D, "Evaluating the *In Vitro* Efficacy of Antimicrobic Combination," *Antimicrob Newslet*, 1989, 6:41-3.

Edberg SC, "Antibiotic Interaction Tests Should They Be Performed," *Clin Microbiol Newslet*, 1988, 10:77-8.

Eliopoulos GM and Eliopoulos CT, "Antibiotic Combinations Should They Be Tested," *Clin Microbiol Rev*, 1988, 1:139-56, (review).

Rand KH, Houck HJ, Brown P, et al, "Reproducibility of the Microdilution Checkerboard Method for Antibiotic Synergy," *Antimicrob Agents Chemother*, 1993, 37(3):613-5.

Susceptibility Testing, Fungi

CPT *87192 (each drug)*

Related Information

Amphotericin B *on page 942*
Biopsy or Body Fluid Fungus Culture *on page 780*
Blood Fungus Culture *on page 789*
Fungus Smear, Stain *on page 813*
Itraconazole *on page 975*
Ketoconazole *on page 975*
Skin Fungus Culture *on page 845*
Sputum Fungus Culture *on page 853*
Susceptibility Testing, Aerobic and Facultatively Anaerobic Organisms *on page 864*
Susceptibility Testing, Unusual Isolates/Fastidious Organisms *on page 873*

Synonyms Fungi Susceptibility Testing

Test Commonly Includes Broth dilution, agar dilution and disk diffusion testing of antifungal agents. Results may be quantitative or qualitative.

Specimen A pure culture of the isolated organism to be tested, prepared by the laboratory **CAUSES FOR REJECTION:** Organism disposed of prior to request for testing. **SPECIAL INSTRUCTIONS:** Consult the laboratory to determine availability and choice of methods.

Interpretive **REFERENCE RANGE:** See table. **USE:** Determine susceptibility of isolated fungi to available therapeutic agents, predict probable clinical response, explain observed or suspected therapeutic failures, determine if primary or secondary resistance is present **LIMITATIONS:** This test procedure is usually available only from specialized laboratories. Proposed methods for fungal susceptibility testing have recently been standardized.[1] Stability and solubility of some of the agents cause technical difficulty. **METHODOLOGY:** Standardized methods

(Continued)

In vitro Antifungal Activities of Four Antifungal Agents Against Pathogenic Fungi*

Organism	Amphotericin B		Flucytosine (5–FC)		Miconazole		Ketoconazole
	MIC (μg/mL)	MFC (μg/mL)	MIC (μg/mL)	MFC (μg/mL)	MIC (μg/mL)	MFC (μg/mL)	MIC (μg/mL)
Pathogenic yeasts							
Cryptococcus neoformans	0.05–0.78†	0.1–12.5	0.10–100#	0.39–>100	0.05–3.13	0.05–25	0.1–32
Candida albicans	0.2–0.78•	0.39–0.78	0.05–12.5#	0.10–>100	0.1–2.0•	0.1–10	<0.1–128
Candida sp not *C. albicans*	0.2–1.56•	0.39–6.25	0.10–50#	0.20–>100	<0.1–2.0	0.1–>10	<0.1–64
Torulopsis glabrata	0.1–0.4	0.2–0.78	0.05–1.56	0.4–>100	0.5–10	2–10	1–64
Trichosporon sp	0.78–3.13	1.56–3.13	25–100	>100	0.2–25	0.2–>100	
Geotrichum sp	0.4–1.56	0.78–3.13	1.56–12.5	25–>100	0.1–2	0.5–>10	
Filamentous fungi							
Pseudallescheria (Petrillidium) boydii	1.56–>100#	>100	Resistant		0.5§	0.05	0.1–4#
Aspergillus sp including *A. fumigatus*	0.05–8	6.25–>100	0.2–1.56#	>100	0.4–>100	0.8–>100	0.1–100
Blastomyces dermatitidis	0.05–0.2	0.1–0.4	Resistant		≤0.25	ND	0.1–2
Xylohypha bautiano	3.13–>100	3.13–>100	3.13–12.5#	12.5–>100	0.5–>64	ND	0.1–64
Coccidioides immitis	0.1–0.78	0.70–1.56	Resistant		0.25–1.0	ND	0.1–0.8
Histoplasma capsulatum	0.05–1.0	0.05–0.2	Resistant		≤0.25	ND	0.1–0.5
Phialophora sp and other dematiaceous fungi	0.05–>128	6.25–>128	Variable susceptibility	Resistant	0.05–32	ND	0.1–64
Sporothrix schenckii	1.56–12.5	3.13–>100	Resistant		1–2	ND	0.1–16
Zygomycetes	0.78–1.56	1.56–>100	Variable susceptibility	Resistant			
Control organisms							
S. cerevisiae ATCC 36375, etc	0.1	0.2	0.05	0.10	0.20	0.39	0.20
C. pseudotropicalis ATCC 28838			0.05	0.10	0.10	0.20	0.05

From Shadomy S and Pfaller MA, "Laboratory Studies With Antifungal Agents: Susceptibility Tests and Quantitation in Body Fluids," *Manual of Clinical Microbiology,* 5th ed, Washington, DC, American Society for Microbiology, 1991, 1173–83, with permission.

*Based upon both data obtained at the Medical College of Virginia, Virginia Commonwealth University, Richmond, and a review of the literature. *In vitro* data for nystatin is not included because of the narrow clinical spectrum of this agent; however, most isolates of *Candida* species and *Torulopsis* species should be clinically susceptible (MIC of ≤10 μg/mL) to nystatin. MFC, minimal fungicidal concentration; ND, not determined.

†Expected ranges of MICs and MFCs.

#Resistance not uncommon.

•Resistance reported but rare.

§Only limited data available.

‡*In vitro* susceptibility of *Aspergillus* sp to ketoconazole is highly species dependent.

are proposed for the susceptibility testing of yeasts. The availability of a choice of therapeutic agents will continue to cause laboratories to attempt to provide susceptibility data with a useful predictive value for clinicians.[2] **ADDITIONAL INFORMATION:** Interpretation of *in vitro* susceptibility data for antifungal drugs has been hindered by the absence of standardized test criteria. Thus, it has been extremely difficult to identify a clear relation between *in vitro* minimal inhibitory concentrations and clinical outcome. However, some recent reports suggest that clinically significant resistance exists in some important fungal strains.[3,4] The situation appears more readily resolvable for yeast-like than for filamentous fungi since the former are more easily quantified by standardized microbiologic techniques.[5,6]

Footnotes

1. National Committee for Clinical Laboratory Standards, "Reference Method for Broth Dilution Antifungal Susceptibility Testing for Yeasts," Proposed Standard Document M-27-P, Villanova, PA: National Committee for Clinical Laboratory Standards, 1992.
2. Shadomy S and Pfaller MA, "Laboratory Studies With Antifungal Agents Susceptibility Tests and Bioassays," *Manual of Clinical Microbiology*, 5th ed, Balows A, Hausler WJ Jr, Herrmann KL, et al, eds, Washington, DC: American Society for Microbiology, 1991, 1173-83.
3. McIlroy MA, "Failure of Fluconazole to Suppress Fungemia in a Patient With Fever, Neutropenia, and Typhlitis," *J Infect Dis*, 1991, 163(2):420-1.
4. Willocks L, Leen CL, Brettle RP, et al, "Fluconazole Resistance in AIDS Patient," *J Antimicrob Chemother*, 1991, 28(6):937-9.
5. Drutz DJ, "*In Vitro* Antifungal Susceptibility Testing and Measurement of Levels of Antifungal Agents in Body Fluids," *Rev Infect Dis*, 1987, 9:392-7.
6. Hector RF and Schaller K, "Positive Interaction of Nikkomycins and Azoles Against *Candida albicans In Vitro* and *In Vivo*," *Antimicrob Agents Chemother*, 1992, 36(6):1284-9.

References

Bennett JE, "Antifungal Agents," *Principles and Practice of Infectious Diseases*, New York, NY: John Wiley and Sons, 1985, 263-70.

Fromtling RA, "Overview of Medically Important Antifungal Azole Derivatives," 1988, 1:187-217.

Fromtling RA, Galgiani JN, Pfaller MA, et al, "Multicenter Evaluation of a Broth Macrodilution Antifungal Susceptibility Test for Yeasts," *Antimicrob Agents Chemother*, 1993, 37(1):39-45.

Hector RF, "Compounds Active Against Cell Walls of Medically Important Fungi," *Clin Microbiol Rev*, 1993, 6:1-21.

Saag MS and Dismukes WE, "Azole Antifungal Agents: Emphasis on New Triazoles," *Antimicrob Agents Chemother*, 1988, 32:1-8.

Susceptibility Testing, Minimum Bactericidal Concentration

***CPT** 87187 (MBC); 87188 (macrotube dilution)*

Related Information

Susceptibility Testing, Aerobic and Facultatively Anaerobic Organisms *on page 864*

Synonyms MBC; Minimum Bactericidal Concentration; Minimum Lethal Concentration; MLC

Applies to Tolerance Testing, Antimicrobial

Abstract The minimum bactericidal concentration (MBC) is the concentration of an antibiotic that kills 99%, 99.9%, or 100% of a standardized bacterial inoculum.

Specimen A pure culture of the isolated organism to be tested, prepared by the laboratory **CAUSES FOR REJECTION:** Organism discarded prior to request by physician to save the organism for MBC, organism fails to grow on subculture from original plates **TURNAROUND TIME:** 48 hours after isolation of bacterium to be tested **SPECIAL INSTRUCTIONS:** In order to perform an MBC test, an isolate of the organism of interest must be saved at the request of the physician often within 48 hours of submission of specimen for initial culture. If the isolate has not been saved, the test cannot be performed. The laboratory should be informed by the physician of the specific source of the culture, culture date, as well as, the specific bacterial isolate to be tested and the antimicrobial agent to be tested.

Interpretive **REFERENCE RANGE:** End points may be reported as MBC 99% of colonies killed, MBC 99.9% of colonies killed, and MBC 100% of colonies killed; the latter being of interest in debilitated hosts with leukopenia. **USE:** Determine minimum bactericidal concentration, MBC, of an antimicrobial agent. Frequently utilized in endocarditis and osteomyelitis in immunocompromised hosts. **LIMITATIONS:** Results are accurate to plus or minus one dilution. However, technical factors including inoculum, medium, incubation, growth phase, tube type, mixing, etc, are a significant influence on results. **CONTRAINDICATIONS:** Bacterium isolated from patient is not available or fails to grow for susceptibility testing. **METHODOLOGY:** Macrodilution or microdilution technique with subculture. Twofold dilutions of antibiotics are added to broth media that is then inoculated with a standard number of bacteria. After incubation, bacterial growth is monitored. The MIC of the isolate is determined by visually inspecting broth media, while

(Continued)

Susceptibility Testing, Minimum Bactericidal Concentration *(Continued)*

the MBC is determined by plating a portion of each well/tube onto solid media and performing colony counts to determine the percent survival. **ADDITIONAL INFORMATION:** Tolerance, defined as inhibition of growth without killing, is manifested in the laboratory as an MBC (minimum bactericidal concentration) 32 or more times the MIC (minimum inhibitory concentration). Tolerance is most frequently observed with vancomycin and beta-lactam antibiotics against gram-positive organisms.[1] Although tolerance is frequently observed in the laboratory, it is not often associated with clinical treatment failure. The selection of an endpoint of 99.9% killing is used to avoid the problem of the "persistent phenomenon" where a few highly resistant organisms persist regardless of the concentration of the antimicrobial agent.

Footnotes

1. Bradley HE, Wetmur JG, and Hodes DS, "Tolerance in *Staphylococcus aureus*: Evidence for a Bacteriophage Role," *J Infect Dis*, 1980, 2:233-7.

References

James PA, "Comparison of Four Methods for the Determination of MIC and MBC of Penicillin for Viridans Streptococci and the Implications for Penicillin Tolerance," *J Antimicrob Chemother*, 1990, 25(2):209-16.

Peterson LR and Shanholtzer CJ, "Tests for Bactericidal Effects of Antimicrobial Agents: Technical Performance and Clinical Relevance," *Clin Microbiol Rev*, 1992, 5(4):420-32.

Sherris JC, "Problems in the *In Vitro* Determination of Antibiotic Tolerance in Clinical Isolates," *Antimicrob Agents Chemother*, 1986, 30:633-7.

Susceptibility Testing, Mycobacteria

***CPT** 87190 (each drug)*

Related Information

Biopsy or Body Fluid Mycobacteria Culture *on page 782*
Skin Mycobacteria Culture *on page 846*
Sputum Mycobacteria Culture *on page 855*
Stool Mycobacteria Culture *on page 863*
Susceptibility Testing, Aerobic and Facultatively Anaerobic Organisms *on page 864*
Susceptibility Testing, Unusual Isolates/Fastidious Organisms *on next page*
Urine Mycobacteria Culture *on page 884*

Synonyms Mycobacteria Susceptibility Testing

Test Commonly Includes Panel of antimycobacterial agents tested against clinical isolates at appropriate concentrations

Antimicrobials Commonly Used for Mycobacterial Susceptibility Testing

Antituberculosis Drugs	
Primary	**Secondary**
Ethambutol	Capreomycin
Isoniazid	Ciprofloxacin
Pyrazinamide	Cycloserine
Rifampin	Ethionamide
Streptomycin	Kanamycin
Other Mycobacterial Isolates*	
Primary	**Secondary**
Amikacin	Azithromycin
Ciprofloxacin	Clarithromycin
Ethambutol	Clofazimine
Isoniazid	Doxycycline
Rifampin	
Streptomycin	
Sulfonamides	
Tobramycin	

From Wolinsky E, Mycobacterial Diseases Other Then Tuberculosis," *Clin Infect Dis,* 1992, 15:1–12, with permission.
*Drug regimens will depend on the mycobacterial species identified.

Specimen A pure culture of the isolated organism to be tested, prepared by the laboratory **CAUSES FOR REJECTION:** Specimen not available for testing. **TURNAROUND TIME:** 4-6 weeks after organism is isolated

Interpretive **USE:** Determine the susceptibility of the isolated organism to a panel of antimycobacterial agents **LIMITATIONS:** Susceptibilities cannot be reported if the organism fails to grow on test media. **METHODOLOGY:** Disk diffusion, agar containing antibiotic, or broth containing antibiotic. Quantitative methods may be required to accurately assess the clinical value of susceptibility data provided when atypical species, particularly *M. avium*, is tested. See table. **ADDITIONAL INFORMATION:** Susceptibilities are performed on the first organism isolated from a patient and at 3- to 6-month intervals if that organism continues to be isolated while the patient is on therapy. Susceptibility tests should be performed in patients with recurrent tuberculosis as resistant strains are common in recurrent infection. In the United States, the rate of newly diagnosed tuberculosis cases has increased 18.4% since 1985.[1] More alarming is the increased number of nosocomial outbreaks of multidrug-resistant tuberculosis (MDR-TB). Since 1990, over 200 patients have been reported to CDC. These outbreaks have occurred in healthcare workers, prison inmates, and prison employees.[2,3] Failure to take all drugs in a multidrug regimen can lead to a shift toward resistant organisms and treatment failure. Atypical or environmental mycobacteria, particularly strains of the *M. avium* complex, have variable susceptibility within species. Frequently, they are resistant to oral therapy.[4]

Footnotes

1. Centers for Disease Control, "Tuberculosis Morbidity – United States, 1991," *MMWR Morb Mortal Wkly Rep*, 1992, 41:240.
2. Beck-Sague C, Dooley Sw, Hutton MD, et al, "Hospital Outbreak of Multidrug-Resistant *Mycobacterium tuberculosis* Infections. Factors in Transmission to Staff and HIV-Infected Patients," *JAMA*, 1992, 268(10):1280-6.
3. Dooley SW, Villarino ME, Lawrence M, et al, "Nosocomial Transmission of Tuberculosis in a Hospital Unit for HIV-Infected Patients," *JAMA*, 1992, 267(19):2632-4.
4. Wolinsky E, "Mycobacterial Diseases Other Than Tuberculosis," *Clin Infect Dis*, 1992, 15(1):1-10.

References

Heifets L, "Qualitative and Quantitative Drug Susceptibility Tests in Mycobacteriology," *Am Rev Respir Dis*, 1988, 137:1217-22.

Mor N and Heifets L, "MICs and MBCs of Clarithromycin Against *Mycobacterium avium* Within Human Macrophages," *Antimicrob Agents Chemother*, 1993, 37(1):111-4.

Rastogi N and Goh KS, "Effect of pH on Radiometric MICs of Clarithrombycin Against 18 Species of Mycobacteria," *Antimicrob Agents Chemother*, 1992, 36(12):2841-2.

Van Scoy RE and Wilkowske CJ, "Antituberculous Agents," *Mayo Clin Proc*, 1992, 67(2):179-87.

Susceptibility Testing, Serum Bactericidal Dilution Method *see* Serum Bactericidal Test *on page 843*

Susceptibility Testing, Unusual Isolates/Fastidious Organisms

***CPT** 87181 (agar dilution, each antibiotic); 87184 (disk method, each antibiotic); 87186 (microtiter); 87188 (tube dilution, each antibiotic)*

Related Information

Susceptibility Testing, Aerobic and Facultatively Anaerobic Organisms *on page 864*
Susceptibility Testing, Anaerobic Bacteria *on page 866*
Susceptibility Testing, Antimicrobial Combinations *on page 868*
Susceptibility Testing, Fungi *on page 869*
Susceptibility Testing, Mycobacteria *on previous page*

Synonyms MIC, Fastidious Organisms, Unusual Isolates; Minimum Inhibitory Concentration, Unusual Isolates

Applies to E-Test

Specimen A pure culture of the isolated organism to be tested, prepared by the laboratory **CAUSES FOR REJECTION:** Organism disposed of prior to request by physician to save the organism for susceptibility testing. Certain isolates are too fastidious (eg, some anaerobes, some streptococci) to perform susceptibility testing. **TURNAROUND TIME:** 24-48 hours after isolation of bacterium **SPECIAL INSTRUCTIONS:** An isolate of the organism of interest must be saved at the request of the physician. The request usually must be received by the laboratory within 48 hours of submission of specimen for initial culture in order to perform an MIC test. If the isolate has not been saved, the test cannot be performed. Broth dilution minimum inhibitory concen-

(Continued)

Susceptibility Testing, Unusual Isolates/Fastidious Organisms *(Continued)*

tration (MIC) susceptibility can be requested for drugs not in the routine panels. The laboratory should be informed by the physician of the specific source of the culture, culture date, the specific bacterial isolate to be tested, and the antimicrobial agent to be tested.

Interpretive **REFERENCE RANGE:** Minimal inhibitory concentration reported. Results may be qualitatively reported as susceptible (S), intermediate (I), and resistant (R). **USE:** Determine minimum inhibitory concentration (MIC) susceptibility of a given organism to an antimicrobial therapeutic agent **LIMITATIONS:** Determination of MIC on fastidious organisms may be attempted. If the organism of interest fails to grow, it will usually be reported out as unable to grow for MIC. A disk diffusion susceptibility test (Kirby-Bauer susceptibility) is usually reported (susceptible, intermediate, resistant) if interpretive criteria exist. **CONTRAINDICATIONS:** The test cannot be performed if the organism isolated from the patient is not available or fails to grow for susceptibility test. The test cannot be interpreted if criteria for interpretation do not exist. **METHODOLOGY:** Microtiter or macrotiter broth dilution technique, disk diffusion. Special methods are required for individual species. These generally include addition of supplement and/or alteration of incubation atmosphere. **ADDITIONAL INFORMATION:** The terms "fastidious or unusual isolates" refer to organisms which do not grow well on Mueller-Hinton medium or are unusual in that there is insufficient data to document that reliable susceptibility testing can be performed by routine methods. Organisms such as *Haemophilus influenzae* and *Neisseria gonorrhoeae* have developed resistance to beta-lactam antibiotics by plasmid or chromosomal genes mediating the production of beta-lactamase.[1,2] See table. Other organisms, such as

Susceptibility of *H. influenzae* to Commonly Used Antimicrobials

Uniformly active	Third-generation cephalosporins Fluoroquinolones
<1% resistance	Amoxicillin/clavulanate Ampicillin/sulbactam Cefonicid Cefuroxime Rifampin Trimethoprim/sulfamethoxazole
1% to 5% resistance	Aztreonam Cefaclor Imipenem Tetracycline
>50% resistance	Erythromycin Erythromycin/sulfisoxazole

From Doern GV, "Antimicrobial Resistance Among Clinical Isolates of *Haemophilus influenzae* and *Branhamella catarrhalis*," *Clin Microbiol Newslet*, 1989, 10:185, with permission.

Streptococcus pneumoniae, have developed chromosomal gene mediated alteration of the penicillin-binding proteins. Because of the emergence of resistance, empiric therapy with penicillin or ampicillin can no longer be relied upon, and susceptibility testing for those "fastidious" organisms may be necessary. Susceptibility testing for group A streptococci is still not necessary because the organism remains highly susceptible to penicillin, which is the drug of choice. Rare resistant strains have been reported.

The following organisms generally require special susceptibility testing procedures: anaerobes, *Moraxella*, (*Branhamella*) *catarrhalis*, *Helicobacter* sp, *Corynebacterium* sp, *Francisella tularensis*, *Haemophilus influenzae*, *Legionella* sp, *Listeria monocytogenes*, *Neisseria meningitidis*, *Neisseria gonorrhoeae*, *Nocardia* sp, nonfermentative bacteria, *Streptococcus pneumoniae*, *Streptococcus* sp, *Streptococcus* sp peridoxal dependent, *Enterococcus* sp.

The susceptibility testing of *Staphylococcus aureus* also is a concern because of the special conditions (35°C incubation for 24 hours) required to demonstrate methicillin resistance (usually tested with oxacillin). Resistance may be intrinsic or may be beta-lactamase mediated.

Methods for the susceptibility testing of the above organisms are reasonably well defined and are designed to vary as little as possible from the well established methods used for rapidly growing "nonfastidious" aerobic organisms.[3]

Breakpoint broth microdilution methods in which two concentrations of antimicrobials are tested, one below the breakpoint and one above, are frequently used. These methods allow the testing of more individual drugs than is possible with a complete minimum inhibitory concentration (MIC) series in which six to eight concentrations of each drug are tested. A full MIC or minimum bactericidal concentration (MBC) may also assist in selection of appropriate antimicrobial agents. Antimicrobial agents not routinely available for testing on routine MIC panels are often available as breakpoint determinations.

The E test is a new *in vitro* susceptibility testing method now being used for quantitative determination of susceptibility to antimicrobial agents.[4,5] This test uses a defined continuous antimicrobial gradient on a thin plastic strip. When the E-strip is placed on a confluent lawn of bacteria on agar media, the antimicrobial agent diffuses producing an organism inhibition ellipse. The intercept of the ellipse with the graded test strip indicates MICs. This testing procedure provides a reliable method for assessing antimicrobial sensitivity of fastidious isolates.

Footnotes

1. Barry AL, Fuchs PC, and Pfaller MA, "Susceptibilities of β-Lactamase-Producing and -Nonproducing Ampicillin-Resistant Strains of *Haemophilus influenzae* to Ceftibuten, Cefaclor, Cefuroxine, Cefixime, Cefotaxime, and Amoxicillin-Clavulanic Acid," *Antimicrob Agents Chemother*, 1993, 37(1):14-8.
2. Fuchs PC, Barry AL, Baker CN, et al, "Proposed Interpretive Criteria and Quality Control Parameters for Testing Susceptibility of *Neisseria gonorrhoeae* to β-Lactam-Clavulanate Combinations," *J Clin Microbiol*, 1992, 30(8):2191-4.
3. National Committee for Clinical Laboratory Standards, "Performance Standards for Antimicrobial Testing," Fourth Information Supplement NCCLS Document M100-S4 (M7-A2 Aerobic Dilution), Table 7, Villanova, PA: National Committee for Clinical Laboratory Standards, 1992.
4. Sanchez ML, Barrett MS, and Jones RN, "The E-Test Applied to Susceptibility Tests for Gonococci, Multiply Resistant Enterococci and *Enterobacterioceae* Producing Potent Beta-Lactamases," *Diagn Microbiol Infect Dis*, 1992, 15(5):459-64.
5. Sanchez ML, Barrett MS, and Jones RN, "Use of the E-Test to Predict High-Level Resistance to Aminoglycosides Among Enterococci," *J Clin Microbiol*, 1992, 30(11):3030-2.

References

Doern GV, "*In Vitro* Susceptibility Testing of *Haemophilus influenzae*: Review of New National Committee for Clinical Laboratory Standards Recommendations," *J Clin Microbiol*, 1992, 30(12):3035-8.

Doern GV and Jones RN, "Antimicrobial Susceptibility Testing of *Haemophilus influenzae*, *Branhamella catarrhalis*, and *Neisseria gonorrhoeae*," *Antimicrob Agents Chemother*, 1988, 12:1747-53.

Jorgensen JH, Doern GV, Maher LA, et al, "Antimicrobial Resistance Among Respiratory Isolates of *Haemophilus influenzae*, *Moraxella catarrhalis*, and *Streptococcus pneumoniae* in the United States," *Antimicrob Agents Chemother*, 1990, 34(11):2075-80.

Powell MD, McVey MH, Kassim MH, et al, "Antimicrobial Susceptibility of *Streptococcus pneumoniae*, *Haemophilus influenzae*, and *Moraxella* (*Branhamella catarrhalis*) Isolated in the UK From Sputa," *J Antimicrob Chemother*, 1991, 28(2):249-59.

Thornsberry C, Swenson JM, Baker CN, et al, "Susceptibility Testing of Fastidious and Unusual Pathogens," *Antimicrobic Newslet*, 1987, 4:47-56, (review).

Swan-Ganz Tip Culture *see* Intravascular Device Culture *on page 822*

Synergistic Studies, Antimicrobial *see* Susceptibility Testing, Antimicrobial Combinations *on page 868*

Synovial Fluid Anaerobic Culture *see* Biopsy or Body Fluid Anaerobic Bacterial Culture *on page 778*

Synovial Fluid Culture *see* Biopsy or Body Fluid Aerobic Bacterial Culture *on page 778*

Synovial Fluid Fungus Culture *see* Biopsy or Body Fluid Fungus Culture *on page 780*

Syphilis, Darkfield Examination *see* Darkfield Examination, Syphilis *on page 808*

TB Culture, Biopsy *see* Biopsy or Body Fluid Mycobacteria Culture *on page 782*

TB Culture, Skin *see* Skin Mycobacteria Culture *on page 846*

TB Culture, Sputum *see* Sputum Mycobacteria Culture *on page 855*

TB Culture, Stool *see* Stool Mycobacteria Culture *on page 863*

TB Culture, Urine *see* Urine Mycobacteria Culture *on page 884*

TB Smear *see* Acid-Fast Stain *on page 770*

Throat Culture

CPT 87060

Related Information

Antideoxyribonuclease-B Titer, Serum *on page 633*
Antihyaluronidase Titer *on page 635*
Antistreptolysin O Titer, Serum *on page 640*
Bacterial Serology *on page 644*
Gram Stain *on page 815*
Group A *Streptococcus* Screen *on page 818*
Sputum Fungus Culture *on page 853*
Streptozyme *on page 749*
Throat Culture for *Corynebacterium diphtheriae on page 878*

Synonyms Beta-Hemolytic Strep Culture, Throat; Group A Beta-Hemolytic *Streptococcus* Culture, Throat; Screening Culture for Group A Beta-Hemolytic *Streptococcus*; Strep Throat Screening Culture; *Streptococcus pyogenes*

Applies to Throat Culture, *Candida albicans*; Throat Culture for Group A Beta-Hemolytic *Streptococcus*

Test Commonly Includes Screening for group A beta-hemolytic streptococci, *Candida* sp, presence or absence of normal flora

Patient Care PREPARATION: Do not swab throat in cases of acute epiglottitis unless provisions to establish an alternate airway are readily available.

Specimen Throat swab CONTAINER: Sterile Culturette®; cotton, dacron, or alginate swabs are acceptable. COLLECTION: The specimen should be transported to the laboratory promptly. Both tonsillar pillars and the oropharynx should be swabbed. The tongue should be depressed while the tonsillar pillars and the oropharynx are swabbed. Exudates should be swabbed, and the tongue and uvula should be avoided. STORAGE INSTRUCTIONS: Refrigerate TURNAROUND TIME: Preliminary reports are available at 24 hours. Cultures with no beta-hemolytic streptococci are usually reported after 24 hours. Reports on specimens from which beta-hemolytic streptococci group A have been isolated require a minimum of 24-48 hours for completion. Cultures with no growth are usually reported after 48 hours. SPECIAL INSTRUCTIONS: The laboratory should be informed of the specific site of the specimen, the age of patient, current antibiotic therapy, and clinical diagnosis.

Interpretive REFERENCE RANGE: See table.

Throat Culture

Organisms Implicated in Infections of the Oropharynx	Organisms Commonly Present in the Normal Oropharynx	
*Bordetella pertussis**†	*Actinomyces israelii* (tonsils)	*Hemophilus parainfluenzae*
Candida albicans	*Bacteroides* sp (tonsils)	*Klebsiella* sp
Corynebacterium diphtheriae†	*Candida albicans*	*Neisseria meningitidis*
Leptotrichia buccalis†	*Candida* sp	Nonhemolytic streptococci
Neisseria gonorrhoeae†	*Corynebacterium* sp (diphtheroids)	*Proteus* sp
Respiratory viruses:†	*E. coli*	*Staphylococcus aureus*
Adenovirus	Enterococci	*Staphylococcus epidermidis*
Enterovirus	*Fusobacterium* sp (tonsils)	*Streptococcus pneumoniae*
Epstein-Barr virus	*Hemophilus influenzae*	*Streptococcus pyogenes*
Parainfluenza virus		*Veillonella* sp
Reovirus		
Rhinovirus		
Streptococcus pyogenes		

* Rare because of vaccination.
† Not recovered by routine culture.

USE: Isolate and identify potentially pathogenic organisms from throat; evaluate pharyngitis LIMITATIONS: Beta-hemolytic streptococci are the only bacteria that should be routinely reported on throat culture. Interpretation requires a significant level of experience and technical proficiency in order to avoid false-positives and false-negatives.[1] Many other etiologic agents not isolated by routine bacterial culture can be responsible for pharyngitis (see table).[2] **This procedure does not usually include screening for *Neisseria gonorrhoeae* or *Corynebacterium diphtheriae*.** See listing, Throat Culture for *Corynebacterium diphtheriae*. Cultures for *Candida albicans* are usually held for about 1 week; thus, fungi other than *Candida albicans* will not be recovered. *Candida* sp frequently do not adhere well to swabs, therefore, scraping may have a higher yield.[3] Anaerobic organisms which are frequently implicated in chronic infection of the tonsils and adenoids are not recovered by aerobic culture methods. **METHODOLOGY:** Aerobic culture including blood agar medium **ADDITIONAL INFORMATION:** A saline wet preparation, Gram stain, or KOH preparation demonstrating yeast cells or pseudohyphae may also be useful in rapidly establishing the diagnosis of oral or mucocutaneous candidiasis. Thrush, oral candidiasis, and *Candida* esophagitis frequently complicate antineoplastic therapy, hyperalimentation, transplantation immunosuppression, pregnancy, and the acquired immunodeficiency syndrome (AIDS). Routine throat cultures will detect group A *Streptococcus*, however, a specific culture can be requested for detection of beta-hemolytic *Streptococcus* only.

Streptococcus pyogenes (group A beta-hemolytic strep) is generally susceptible to penicillin and its derivatives, therefore, susceptibility need not be routinely determined. The principal reason for considering an alternative drug for individual patients is allergy to penicillin. Erythromycin, a cephalosporin, or clindamycin might be substituted in these cases. Patients allergic to penicillins may also be allergic to cephalosporins.

Use of latex agglutination screening tests and enzyme-linked immunoassay tests provide rapid confirmation of the presence of group A streptococci.[4] The sensitivity of the rapid methods is as high as 96% in overt clinical pharyngitis and/or scarlet fever. Confirmation of negatives by culture is recommended.[4] Lieu et al recommend both antigen testing and culture as the most clinically effective strategy giving consideration to the complications of therapy for those who do not have streptococcal infection and the relative lack of sensitivity of antigen tests as compared to culture.[5]

In the late 1980s, a resurgence of serious *Streptococcus pyogenes* infection was observed. Complications including rheumatic fever, sepsis, severe soft tissue invasion, and toxic shock-like syndrome (TSLS) are reported to be most common with the M1 serotype and that a unique invasive clone has become the predominant cause of severe streptococcal infections.[6]

Footnotes

1. Bibler MR and Ronan GW, "Cryptogenic Group A Streptococcal Bacteremia: Experience at an Urban General Hospital and Review of the Literature," *Rev Infect Dis*, 1986, 8:941-51.
2. Lang SD and Singh K, "The Sore Throat, When to Investigate and When to Prescribe," *Drugs*, 1990, 40(6):854-62.
3. Gray LD and Roberts GD, "Laboratory Diagnosis of Systemic Fungal Diseases," *Infect Dis Clin North Am*, 1988, 2:779-803.
4. Tenjarla G, Kumar A, and Dyke JW, "TestPack Strep A Kit for the Rapid Detection of Group A Streptococci on 11,088 Throat Swabs in a Clinical Pathology Laboratory," *Am J Clin Pathol*, 1991, 96(6):759-61.
5. Lieu TA, Fleisher GR, and Schwartz JS, "Cost-Effectiveness of Rapid Latex Agglutination Testing and Throat Culture for Streptococcal Pharyngitis," *Pediatrics*, 1990, 85(3):246-56.
6. Cleary PP, Kaplan EL, Handley JP, et al, "Clonal Basis for Resurgence of Serious *Streptococcus pyogenes* Disease in the 1980s," *Lancet*, 1992, 339(8792):518-21.

References

Brodsky L, "Modern Assessment of Tonsils and Adenoids," *Pediatr Clin North Am*, 1989, 36(6):1551-69.

Brook I, "The Clinical Microbiology of Waldeyer's Ring," *Otolaryngol Clin North Am*, 1987, 20:259-73.

Epstein JB, Truelove EL, and Izutzu KT, "Oral Candidiasis: Pathogenic and Host Defense," *Rev Infect Dis*, 1984, 6:96-106.

Gregory DW, "*Candida* Infections," *South Med J*, 1982, 75:339-45.

Givner LB, Abramson JS, and Wasilauskas B, "Apparent Increase in the Incidence of Invasive Group A Beta-Hemolytic Streptococcal Disease in Children," *J Pediatr*, 1991, 118(3):341-6.

Kaplan EL, "The Rapid Identification of Group A Beta-Hemolytic Streptococci in the Upper Respiratory Tract," *Pediatr Clin North Am*, 1988, 35:535-42.

Meyer RD, "Cutaneous and Mucosal Manifestations of the Deep Mycotic Infections," *Acta Derm Venereol (Stockh)*, 1986, 121(Suppl):57-72.

Wheeler MC, Roe MH, Kaplan EL, et al, "Outbreak of Group A *Streptococcus* Septicemia in Children: Clinical, Epidemiologic, and Microbiological Correlates," *JAMA*, 1991, 266(4):533-7.

Wright JM, Taylor PP, Allen EP, et al, "A Review of the Oral Manifestations of Infections in Pediatric Patients," *Pediatr Infect Dis*, 1984, 3:80-8.

Throat Culture, *Candida albicans* *see* Throat Culture *on previous page*

Throat Culture for *Bordetella pertussis* *replaced by* *Bordetella pertussis* Nasopharyngeal Culture *on page 790*

Throat Culture for *Corynebacterium diphtheriae*

CPT 87060 (culture); 87163 (additional identification methods)

Related Information

Bacterial Serology *on page 644*

Throat Culture *on page 876*

Synonyms *Corynebacterium diphtheriae* Culture, Throat; Diphtheria Culture

Applies to Nasopharyngeal Culture for *Corynebacterium diphtheriae*

Abstract Diphtheria causes pseudomembranes. It may be found in the anterior nasal mucosa, but classically it is a disease of the oropharynx. It may spread to or begin in the larynx and can involve the tracheobronchial tree. The major effects of the exotoxin are on the heart and nervous system.

Patient Care **AFTERCARE:** Observe for laryngospasm following collection of specimen.

Specimen Throat swab, nasopharyngeal swab **CONTAINER:** Sterile Mini-Tip Culturette® or flexible calcium alginate swab, Calgiswab®, is recommended for obtaining nasopharyngeal culture. **COLLECTION:** The tongue should be depressed while both the tonsillar crypts and nasopharynx and throat lesions are swabbed. If a pseudomembrane is present, the swab should be taken from the membrane and beneath its edge if possible. Separate swabs for throat and nasopharynx are desirable. Avoid swabbing the tongue and uvula. Specimen must be transported to the laboratory immediately following collection. **STORAGE INSTRUCTIONS:** Refrigerate the specimen if it cannot be promptly processed. **TURNAROUND TIME:** Preliminary reports are usually available at 24 hours. Cultures with no growth are usually reported after 72 hours. Final reports on specimens from which *C. diphtheriae* has been isolated usually take at least 4 days. **SPECIAL INSTRUCTIONS:** **The laboratory should be notified before collection of specimens so that special isolation media can be made available.** The laboratory should be informed of the specific site of specimen, age of patient, current antibiotic therapy, and clinical diagnosis.

Interpretive **REFERENCE RANGE:** No *C. diphtheriae* isolated **USE:** Isolate *C. diphtheriae* from patients suspected of having diphtheria. The organisms remain superficial in the respiratory tract and skin, but the potent exotoxin is responsible for the virulence of the disease. **LIMITATIONS:** Cultures should be taken from nasopharynx, as well as, the throat; culture of both sites increases the chance of recovery of the organism. Stain results are presumptive and are commonly reported out as "gram-positive pleomorphic bacilli suggestive of *C. diphtheriae*". Definitive diagnosis depends on isolation of the organism because of the similar appearance of other organisms commonly found in the oropharynx. **CONTRAINDICATIONS:** Lack of clinical symptoms or signs of diphtheria, valid history of immunization **METHODOLOGY:** Culture on selective medium (Löeffler's), cystine tellurite agar, and blood agar smear stained with Löeffler's methylene blue stain and/or Gram stain. *C. diphtheriae* may appear as V, Y, or L figures. Metachromatic granules which stain deep blue may also be seen. **ADDITIONAL INFORMATION:** Routine throat culture should be ordered in addition. *C. diphtheriae* may occasionally cause skin infections, wound infections, pulmonary infections, and endocarditis and may be recovered from the oropharynx of healthy carriers. *C. diphtheriae* is spread through respiratory secretions by convalescent and healthy carriers. The clinical presentation includes a grayish pseudomembrane, overlying superficial ulcers in the oropharynx. The organism is noninvasive, however, the exotoxin elaborated in the throat affects primarily the heart and nervous system. Mortality is 10% to 30%. Only strains of *C. diphtheriae* infected by B-phage are capable of producing toxin. Nontoxigenic strains are commonly recovered and are capable of producing pharyngitis. Confirmation of exotoxin production requires animal testing and is rarely done for clinical testing. *C. ulcerans* may also produce a diphtheria-like disease.

References

Farizo KM, Strebel PM, Chen RT, et al, "Fatal Respiratory Disease Due to *Corynebacterium diphtheriae*: Case Report and Review of Guidelines for Management, Investigation, and Control," *Clin Infect Dis*, 1993, 16(1):59-68.

Larsson P, Brinkhoff B, and Larsson L, "*Corynebacterium diphtheriae* in the Environment of Carriers and Patients," *J Hosp Infect*, 1987, 10:282-6.

MacGregor RR, "*Corynebacterium diphtheriae*," *Principles and Practice of Infectious Diseases*, 3rd ed, Chapter 183, Mandell GL, Douglas RG Jr, and Bennett JE, eds, New York, NY: Churchill Livingstone, 1990, 1574-81.

Rappuoli R, Perugini M, and Falsen E, "Molecular Epidemiology of the 1984-1986 Outbreak of Diphtheria in Sweden," *N Engl J Med*, 1988, 318:12-4.

Walters RF, "Diphtheria Presenting in the Accident and Emergency Department," *Arch Emerg Med*, 1987, 4:47-51.

Throat Culture for Group A Beta-Hemolytic *Streptococcus* *see* Throat Culture *on page 876*

Throat Swab for Group A Streptococcal Antigen *see* Group A *Streptococcus* Screen *on page 818*

Tick Identification *see* Arthropod Identification *on page 774*

Tissue Anaerobic Culture *see* Biopsy or Body Fluid Anaerobic Bacterial Culture *on page 778*

Tissue Culture *see* Biopsy or Body Fluid Aerobic Bacterial Culture *on page 778*

Tissue Fungus Culture *see* Biopsy or Body Fluid Fungus Culture *on page 780*

Tissue Mycobacteria Culture *see* Biopsy or Body Fluid Mycobacteria Culture *on page 782*

Tolerance Testing, Antimicrobial *see* Susceptibility Testing, Minimum Bactericidal Concentration *on page 871*

Toxin A *see Clostridium difficile* Toxin Assay *on page 802*

Toxin Assay, *Clostridium difficile* *see Clostridium difficile* Toxin Assay *on page 802*

Tracheal Aspirate Culture *see* Sputum Culture *on page 849*

Transtracheal Aspirates *see* Bronchial Aspirate Anaerobic Culture *on page 792*

Transtracheal Aspiration *Legionella* Culture *see Legionella* Culture *on page 825*

***Treponema pallidum* Darkfield Examination** *see* Darkfield Examination, Syphilis *on page 808*

***Trichomonas* Culture** *see Trichomonas* Preparation *on this page*

***Trichomonas* Pap Smear** *see Trichomonas* Preparation *on this page*

Trichomonas Preparation

CPT 87210 (wet mount); 87211 (wet and dry mount)

Related Information

Cervical/Vaginal Cytology *on page 491*
Genital Culture *on page 814*

Synonyms Hanging Drop Mount for *Trichomonas*; *Trichomonas vaginalis* Wet Preparation

Applies to *Trichomonas* Culture; *Trichomonas* Pap Smear; Urethral *Trichomonas* Smear; Urine *Trichomonas* Wet Mount

Test Commonly Includes Wet mount and microscopic examination. Pap smear and/or culture may also be performed.

Specimen Vaginal, cervical, or urethral swabs, prostatic fluid, urine sediment **CONTAINER:** Sterile tube containing 1 mL of sterile nonbacteriostatic saline **COLLECTION:** The specimen should be collected using a speculum without lubricant. The mucosa of the posterior vagina may be swabbed, or the secretions may be collected with a pipette. The swab should be expressed into saline for transport. The specimen should be examined as soon as possible. **STORAGE INSTRUCTIONS:** Do not refrigerate. Transport immediately to the laboratory so that viable motile organisms may be obtained. **CAUSES FOR REJECTION:** Specimen dried out **TURNAROUND TIME:** Same day; 48 hours if culture in Kupferberg's medium **SPECIAL INSTRUCTIONS:** Provide the specific source of the specimen to the laboratory.

Interpretive **REFERENCE RANGE:** Negative: no trichomonads identified; positive: demonstration of actively motile flagellates, positive culture **USE:** Establish the presence of *Trichomonas vaginalis* **LIMITATIONS:** The specimen is examined for *Trichomonas vaginalis* only. A separate swab (Culturette®) must be collected for culture of bacteria or fungus cultures, if required. One negative result does not rule out the possibility of *Trichomonas vaginalis* infection. The wet mount is negative in 30% to 50%[1] of women with trichomoniasis. Culture is not available in many laboratories. **CONTRAINDICATIONS:** Douching within 3 days prior to specimen collection **METHODOLOGY:** Wet mount microscopic examination, Pap smear, culture in Kupferberg's liquid medium or Hirsch charcoal agar, direct immunofluorescent technique with monoclonal antibody **ADDITIONAL INFORMATION:** The absence of the classical yellow, frothy discharge does not exclude trichomoniasis. Culture may yield positive results when wet preparations are negative. Cultures are expensive and have limited availability.[2] The high rate of false-negatives,

(Continued)

Trichomonas Preparation *(Continued)*

48.4%, and false-positives observed with stained preparations (Pap smears) requires that confirmation by wet mount or culture be considered when the reported results are inconsistent with the clinical findings.[3] Culture provides similar sensitivity to wet mount methods,[4] although other studies have reported wet mount/cytology sensitivity of about 60%.[5] Immunofluorescence tests are being adopted which have increased sensitivity. The false-positives observed when immunofluorescent methods are compared to culture may represent failure of culture in patients with few organisms.

In a series of 600 "high risk" women, 88 *Trichomonas* infected patients were observed. Co-infection was noted as follows: *Ureaplasma urealyticum* 96%, *Gardnerella vaginalis* 91%, *Mycoplasma hominis* 89%, bacterial vaginosis 57%, *Neisseria gonorrhoeae* 29%, and *Chlamydia trachomatis* 15%. *Candida albicans* and other *Candida* sp are frequently implicated in vulvovaginitis.[1] A vaginal pH >5 is suggestive of *Trichomonas*.

In males, a milky white fluid discharge and urethral irritation present for more than 4 weeks is frequently associated with urethritis caused by *T. vaginalis*.

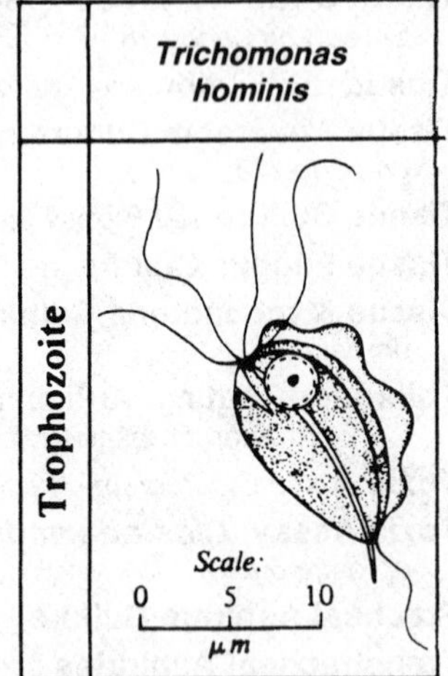

From Brooks MM and Melvin DM, *Morphology of Diagnostic Stages of Intestinal Parasites of Humans*, 2nd ed, Atlanta, GA: U.S. Department of Health and Human Services, Publication No. 84-8116, Centers for Disease Control, 1984, with permission.

Footnotes

1. Bennett JR, "The Emergency Department Diagnosis of *Trichomonas vaginalis*," *Ann Emerg Med*, 1989, 18(5):564-6.
2. Spence MR, Hollander DH, Smith J, et al, "The Clinical and Laboratory Diagnosis of *Trichomonas vaginalis* Infections," *Sex Transm Dis*, 1980, 7:168-71.
3. Borchardt KA, Hernandez V, Miller S, et al, "A Clinical Evaluation of Trichomoniasis in San Jose, Costa Rica Using the In Pouch TV Test," *Genitourin Med*, 1992, 68(5):328-30.
4. Bickley LS, Krisher KK, Ponsalang A Jr, et al, "Comparison of Direct Fluorescent Antibody, Acridine Orange, Wet Mount, and Culture for Detection of *Trichomonas vaginalis* in Women Attending a Public Sexually Transmitted Diseases Clinic," *Sex Transm Dis*, 1989, 16(3):127-31.
5. Krieger JN, Tam MR, Stevens CE, et al, "Diagnosis of Trichomoniasis. Comparison of Conventional Wet-Mount Examination With Cytologic Studies, Cultures, and Monoclonal Antibody Staining of Direct Specimens," *JAMA*, 1988, 259:1223-7.

References

Clay JC, Veeravahu M, and Smyth RW, "Practical Problems of Diagnosing Trichomoniasis in Women," *Genitourin Med*, 1988, 64:115-7.

Latif AS, Mason PR, and Marowa E, "Urethral Trichomoniasis in Men," *Sex Transm Dis*, 1987, 14:9-11.

Lossick JG, "The Diagnosis of Vaginal Trichomoniasis," *JAMA*, 1988, 259:1230, (editorial).

Moldwin RM, "Sexually Transmitted Protozoal Infections. *Trichomonas vaginalis*, *Entamoeba histolytica*, and *Giardia lamblia*," *Urol Clin North Am*, 1992, 19(1):93-101.

Sobel JD, "Vaginal Infections in Adult Women," *Med Clin North Am*, 1990, 74(6):1573-602.

Thomason JL and Gelbart SM, "*Trichomonas vaginalis*," *Obstet Gynecol*, 1989, 74(3 Pt 2):536-41.

Wolner-Hanssen P, Krieger JN, Stevens CE, et al, "Clinical Manifestations of Vaginal Trichomoniasis," *JAMA*, 1989, 261:571-6.

***Trichomonas vaginalis* Wet Preparation** *see* *Trichomonas* Preparation *on previous page*

Tuberculin Skin Test *see* Skin Test, Tuberculosis *on page 848*

Tympanocentesis Culture *see* Ear Culture *on page 810*

Undulant Fever, Culture *see* Blood Culture, *Brucella* *on page 788*

Urease Test and Culture, *Helicobacter pylori* *see* *Helicobacter pylori* Urease Test and Culture *on page 820*

Urethral *Trichomonas* Smear *see* *Trichomonas* Preparation *on previous page*

Urine Anaerobic Culture, Suprapubic Puncture *see* Urine Culture, Suprapubic Puncture *on page 882*

Urine Culture, Clean Catch

CPT *87086 (quantitative culture); 87088 (identification)*

Related Information

Chlamydia trachomatis Culture *on page 1171*
Gram Stain *on page 815*
Kidney Stone Analysis *on page 1129*
Leukocyte Esterase, Urine *on page 1131*
Nitrite, Urine *on page 1137*
Urine Culture, Suprapubic Puncture *on next page*
Urine Fungus Culture *on page 883*
Urine Mycobacteria Culture *on page 884*
Viral Culture, Urine *on page 1207*

Synonyms CMVS Culture; Midstream Urine Culture

Applies to Urine Culture, Foley Catheter

Patient Care PREPARATION: Instruct patient for proper collection of "clean catch" specimen. Wash hands thoroughly. Wash penis or vulva using downward strokes four times with four soapy sponges, then once with sponge wet with warm water. Urethral meatus and perineum must be washed. Each sponge must be discarded after one use. Urinate about 30 mL (1 ounce) of urine directly into toilet or bedpan **- stop -** position container and take middle portion of urine sample. Screw cap securely on container without touching the inside rim. Apply the completed patient label to the specimen cup. Most patients, with instruction, do better with privacy than with an attendant.

Specimen Random urine CONTAINER: Plastic urine container or sterile tube COLLECTION: Early morning specimens yield highest bacterial counts from overnight incubation in the bladder. Forced fluids dilute the urine and may cause reduced colony counts. Hair from perineum will contaminate the specimen. The stream from a male may be contaminated by bacteria from beneath the prepuce. Bacteria from vaginal secretions, vulva, or distal urethra may also contaminate the specimen as may organisms from hands or clothing. Receptacle must be sterile. Provide time and date of urine collection. STORAGE INSTRUCTIONS: Refrigerate the specimen if it cannot be promptly processed. A transport stabilizer may be used to preserve the specimen if refrigeration is not available.[1] CAUSES FOR REJECTION: Unrefrigerated specimen more than 2 hours old may be subject to overgrowth of bacteria and may yield false-positive results. TURNAROUND TIME: Preliminary reports are usually available at 24 hours. Cultures with no growth are usually reported after 24 hours. Reports on specimens from which an organism or organisms have been isolated require a minimum of 48 hours for completion.

Interpretive REFERENCE RANGE: No growth. Significant bacteriuria is usually considered to be 10^5 CFU/mL (colony forming units). A break point of 10^2 maximizes diagnostic sensitivity.[2] USE: Isolate and identify potentially pathogenic organisms causing urinary tract infection LIMITATIONS: Bacteria present in numbers <1000 organisms/mL may not be detected by routine methods. Contamination during collection (particularly in women) may cause colony counts of 10^3 or 10^4; thus, a breakpoint of 10^2 CFU/mL causes inclusion of a large number of normal women without significant bacteriuria.[3] METHODOLOGY: Quantitative aerobic culture; usually plated at a 0.001 dilution, allowing detection of organisms in enumeration of 10^3 CFU/mL or greater ADDITIONAL INFORMATION: A single culture is about 80% accurate in the female; two containing the same organism with count of 10^5 or more represents 95% chance of true bacteriuria; three such specimens mean virtual certainty of true bacteriuria. Recent studies have shown that a Gram stain from 0.2 mL of urine cytocentrifuged onto a slide is a very sensitive method of screening for bacteriuria.[4] Rapid detection of bacteriuria is helpful in the early treatment of patients. Several other methods have also been described for the rapid detection of bacteriuria, growth-photometric, bioluminescence, measurement of bacterial adenosine triphosphate, and acridine orange stain.

Urinary tract infection is significantly higher in women who use diaphragm-spermicide contraception, perhaps secondary to increased vaginal pH and a higher frequency of vaginal colonization with *E. coli*.[5] A single, clean-voided specimen from an adult male may be considered diagnostic with proper preparation and care in specimen collection. If the patient is receiving antimicrobial therapy at the time the specimen is collected, any level of bacteriuria may be significant. When more than two organisms are recovered, the likelihood of contamination is high; thus, the significance of definitive identification of the organisms and susceptibility testing in this situation is severely limited. A repeat culture with proper specimen collection including patient preparation is often indicated. Periodic screening of diabetics and pregnant women for asymptomatic bacteriuria has been recommended.[6] Institutionalized patients, es-

(Continued)

Urine Culture, Clean Catch *(Continued)*

pecially elderly individuals, are prone to urinary tract infections which can be severe.[7] Cultures of specimens from Foley catheters yielding multiple organisms with high colony counts may represent colonization of the catheter and not true significant bacteriuria. Most laboratories limit the number of organisms which will be identified when recovered from urine to two. Similarly, most do not routinely perform susceptibility tests on isolates from presumably contaminated specimens.

Failure to recover aerobic organisms from patients with pyuria or positive Gram stains of urinary sediment may indicate the presence of mycobacteria or anaerobes.

Footnotes

1. Williams JD, "Criteria for Diagnosis of Urinary Tract Infection and Evaluation of Therapy," *Infection*, 1992, 4(20 Suppl 4):S257-60.
2. Johnson JR and Stamm WE, "Urinary Tract Infections in Women: Diagnosis and Treatment," *Ann Intern Med*, 1989, 111(11):906-17.
3. Hooton TM and Stamm WE, "Management of Acute Uncomplicated Urinary Tract Infection in Adults," *Med Clin North Am*, 1991, 75(2):339-57.
4. Olson ML, Shanholtzer CJ, Willard KE, et al, "The Slide Centrifuge Gram Stain as a Urine Screening Method," *Am J Clin Pathol*, 1991, 96(4):454-8.
5. Stamm WE, Hooton TM, Johnson JR, et al, "Urinary Tract Infections: From Pathogenesis to Treatment," *J Infect Dis*, 1989, 159(3):400-6, (review).
6. Andriole VT, "Urinary Tract Infections in the 90s: Pathogenesis and Management," *Infection*, 1992, 4(20 Suppl 4):S251-6.
7. Nicolle LE, "Urinary Tract Infection in the Elderly: How to Treat and When?" *Infection*, 1992, 4(20 Suppl 4):S261-5.

References

Clarridge JE, Pezzlo MT, and Vosti KL, "Laboratory Diagnosis of Urinary Tract Infections," *Cumitech 2*, Weissfeld AS, ed, Washington, DC: American Society for Microbiology, March 1987.

Ronald AR, Nicolle LE, and Harding GKM, "Standards of Therapy for Urinary Tract Infections in Adults," *Infection*, 1992, 20(Suppl 3):S164-70.

Stamm WE, "Criteria for the Diagnosis of Urinary Tract Infection and for the Assessment of Therapeutic Effectiveness," *Infection*, 1992, 20(Suppl 3):S151-9.

Urine Culture, Foley Catheter *see* Urine Culture, Clean Catch *on previous page*

Urine Culture, Straight Catheter *see* Urine Culture, Suprapubic Puncture *on this page*

Urine Culture, Suprapubic Puncture

***CPT** 87086 (quantitative culture); 87088 (identification)*

Related Information

Urine Culture, Clean Catch *on previous page*
Urine Fungus Culture *on next page*
Urine Mycobacteria Culture *on page 884*

Applies to Urine Anaerobic Culture, Suprapubic Puncture; Urine Culture, Straight Catheter

Abstract Suprapubic aspiration of the urinary bladder is only indicated infrequently.

Patient Care PREPARATION: Aseptic preparation of the aspiration site. Collect the specimen to avoid contamination with normal skin flora. Fluids should be forced prior to collection of the specimen to distend the bladder. Successful suprapubic collection requires a distended bladder; 6-10 hours may be required for the bladder to fill.

Specimen Label the specimen as urine obtained by suprapubic puncture CONTAINER: Sterile, plastic urine container COLLECTION: After aseptic preparation of the skin, the specimen is aspirated in a sterile syringe by a physician skilled in the technique. STORAGE INSTRUCTIONS: **To optimize the recovery of fastidious organisms, the specimen should be transported to the laboratory as soon as possible after collection.** Refrigerate the specimen if it cannot be promptly processed. CAUSES FOR REJECTION: Unrefrigerated specimen more than 2 hours old may be subject to overgrowth of microorganisms. TURNAROUND TIME: Preliminary reports are usually available at 24 hours. Cultures with no growth are usually reported after 24 hours. Reports on specimens from which an organism or organisms have been isolated require 48 hours for completion. SPECIAL INSTRUCTIONS: The laboratory should be informed of the specific site of specimen (ie, that the specimen is a "suprapubic puncture"), age of patient, current antibiotic therapy, clinical diagnosis, and time of collection.

Interpretive REFERENCE RANGE: No growth. Any organisms recovered are considered significant if the specimen has been properly obtained. USE: Isolate and identify pathogenic organisms causing urinary tract infection; useful infrequently to obtain sterile urine specimens on newborns. Suprapubic aspiration may allow isolation of organisms which are too fastidious to be recovered by culture of voided urine. **LIMITATIONS:** Bacteria present in numbers <1000 organisms/mL may not be detected by routine methods. Mycobacteria will not be identified unless a mycobacteria culture is requested. **METHODOLOGY:** Quantitative aerobic culture. All rapid-growing, nonfastidious aerobic bacteria will usually be isolated and identified. Antimicrobial susceptibility testing is usually performed if indicated, regardless of colony count when obtained by suprapubic puncture. This is the only acceptable urine specimen for isolation of anaerobic organisms. Anaerobic organisms may be recovered if anaerobic culture is requested. Special culture procedures must be undertaken to recover *Ureaplasma urealyticum*, *Gardnerella vaginalis*, and *Mycoplasma hominis*, which are the most frequently encountered fastidious species.[1] The cultures are usually plated at a 0.01 dilution, allowing detection of organisms in a concentration of 10^2 CFU/mL or greater. **ADDITIONAL INFORMATION:** Fairley and Birch, studying male and female patients with acute urinary tract symptoms, found 31% (561/1817) females and 12% (36/300) males culture positive.[2] Seventy percent of the isolates were "fastidious" bacteria which are not usually recovered by conventional techniques. The organisms recovered were frequently (67%) present in $<10^5$ CFU/mL. Thirty-four percent of females but none of the males had polymicrobic isolates which usually included a fastidious organism. Many cases of negative culture in females with acute urinary symptoms may represent cases of low count 10^2 to 10^4 CFU/mL cystitis. Suprapubic puncture can be used to document ascending infection (ie, cystitis) due to *Neisseria gonorrhoeae*.[3] Specimens for *N. gonorrhoeae* culture should not be refrigerated and should be transported to the laboratory quickly.

Footnotes

1. Gilbert GL, Garland SM, and Fairley KF, "Bacteriuria Due to *Ureaplasma* and Other Fastidious Organisms During Pregnancy," *Pediatr Infect Dis*, 1986, 5:S239.
2. Fairley KF and Birch DF, "Detection of Bladder Bacteriuria in Patients With Acute Urinary Symptoms," *J Infect Dis*, 1989, 159:226-31.
3. Péc J Jr, Moravćik P, Kliment J, et al, "Isolation of *Neisseria gonorrhoeae* for Urine Obtained by Suprapubic Puncture of Bladders of Men With Gonococcal Urethritis," *Genitourin Med*, 1988, 64:156-8.

References

Komaroff AL, "Urinalysis and Urine Culture in Women With Dysuria," *Ann Intern Med*, 1986, 104:212-8.
Stamm WE, Hooton TM, Johnson JR, et al, "Urinary Tract Infections: From Pathogenesis to Treatment," *J Infect Dis*, 1988, 159:400-6, (review).

Urine for Parasites *see* Ova and Parasites, Urine *on page 839*

Urine for *Schistosoma haematobium* *see* Ova and Parasites, Urine *on page 839*

Urine Fungus Culture

***CPT** 87102 (isolation); 87106 (definitive identification)*

Related Information

Blastomycosis Serology *on page 645*
Blood Fungus Culture *on page 789*
Candidiasis Serologic Test *on page 652*
Cryptococcus Antibody Titer *on page 670*
Fungus Smear, Stain *on page 813*
Sputum Fungus Culture *on page 853*
Urine Culture, Clean Catch *on page 881*
Urine Culture, Suprapubic Puncture *on previous page*
Urine Cytology *on page 513*
Urine Mycobacteria Culture *on next page*

Synonyms Fungus Culture, Urine

Abstract Use of antibacterial, antineoplastic, and immunosuppressive drugs, corticosteroids, urinary indwelling catheters, urinary tract obstruction, or the presence of diseases such as diabetes mellitus predispose to funguria. *C. albicans* is reported to cause up to 59% of positive urinary fungal cultures. *Torulopsis glabrata* and other *Candida* species account for many of the remainder.[1]

Patient Care **PREPARATION:** Usual preparation for clean catch midvoid urine specimen collection. See Urine Culture, Clean Catch listing.

Specimen Urine **CONTAINER:** Sterile, plastic urine container **COLLECTION:** The specimen should be transported to the laboratory within 2 hours of collection if not refrigerated. The patient

(Continued)

Urine Fungus Culture *(Continued)*

must be instructed to thoroughly cleanse skin and collect midstream specimen. **CAUSES FOR REJECTION:** Unrefrigerated specimen more than 2 hours old may be subject to overgrowth of microorganisms and may not yield valid results **SPECIAL INSTRUCTIONS:** Inform the laboratory of the specific source of the specimen, and if possible, the fungal species suspected.

Interpretive **REFERENCE RANGE:** No growth **USE:** Detect and identify yeasts and fungi in urine specimens **LIMITATIONS:** A single negative culture does not rule out the presence of fungal infection. **METHODOLOGY:** Specimen is cultured on selective media such as supplemented Sabouraud's agar and/or brain heart infusion (BHI) with antibiotics. **ADDITIONAL INFORMATION:** Asymptomatic funguria often ultimately clears spontaneously. However, candiduria with >15,000 colony forming units/mL of urine and with such evidence of dissemination as elevated serum precipitin antibody titers, is associated with increased mortality.[1] Patients with candiduria may or may not have candidemia; positive urine culture for fungi often may be followed by positive blood culture for fungi. Ascending infections occur in patients with diabetes, prolonged antimicrobial therapy, or following instrumentation. Urinary obstruction due to "fungus balls" may occur in diabetes and following renal transplantation. Candiduria associated with hematogenous infections is observed in patients with granulocytopenia, corticosteroid therapy, and with immunosuppression. The source is frequently the gastrointestinal tract or indwelling catheters particular with hyperalimentation.[2] A blood fungus culture is useful to define invasive disease. However, proof of invasive *Candida* infection requires direct cystoscopic or operative visualization, fungus balls, pyelonephritis, or histological evidence of mucosa invasion. Urine is a useful specimen for culture in cryptococcosis, blastomycosis, and candidiasis. See table for fungus culture specimen selection in Sputum Fungus Culture listing. The incidence of genitourinary fungal infections is increasing. They are usually associated with broad spectrum antibiotic therapy, corticosteroid therapy, underlying general debility, and AIDS. In addition to *Candida*, opportunistic pathogens in the genitourinary tract include *Aspergillus* and *Cryptococcus*. Endemic pathogens such as *Histoplasma*, *Blastomyces*, and *Coccidioides* are also encountered.[3]

Footnotes

1. Wong-Beringer A, Jacobs RA, and Guglielmo BJ, "Treatment of Funguria," *JAMA*, 1992, 267(20):2780-5.
2. Kunin CM, and Lipsky BA, "Treatment of Candiduria," *JAMA*, 1989, 262:691-2, (question and answer).
3. Frangos DN and Nyberg LM Jr, "Genitourinary Fungal Infections," *South Med J*, 1986, 79:455-9.

References

Roy JB, Geyer JR, and Mohr JA, "Urinary Tract Candidiasis: An Update," *Urology*, 1984, 23:533-7.
"Urinary Tract Candidosis," *Lancet*, 1988, 2:1000-2, (review).

Urine Mycobacteria Culture

***CPT** 87116 (isolation); 87117 (concentration plus isolation); 87118 (definitive identification)*

Related Information

Acid-Fast Stain *on page 770*
Mycobacteria by DNA Probe *on page 921*
Skin Mycobacteria Culture *on page 846*
Skin Test, Tuberculosis *on page 848*
Sputum Mycobacteria Culture *on page 855*
Stool Mycobacteria Culture *on page 863*
Susceptibility Testing, Mycobacteria *on page 872*
Urine Culture, Clean Catch *on page 881*
Urine Culture, Suprapubic Puncture *on page 882*
Urine Fungus Culture *on previous page*

Synonyms Mycobacteria Culture, Urine; TB Culture, Urine

Test Commonly Includes Concentration of specimen, culture, and identification of mycobacterial species

Abstract Active extragenitourinary tuberculosis is found in fewer than 10% of subjects who have genitourinary tuberculosis.

Patient Care **PREPARATION:** Usual preparation for clean catch midvoid urine specimen collection. See Urine Culture, Clean Catch for detailed information.

Specimen First morning voided urine **CONTAINER:** Sterile, plastic urine container **COLLECTION:** Three first morning voided urine specimens should be submitted. The specimen may be divided for fungus culture and KOH preparation, mycobacteria culture and AFB stain, and routine bacterial culture and Gram stain if the specimen is of adequate volume for all tests requested. **STORAGE INSTRUCTIONS:** Refrigerate the specimen if it cannot be promptly processed. **CAUSES**

FOR REJECTION: Unrefrigerated specimen more than 2 hours old may be subject to overgrowth and may not yield valid results. Twenty-four hour specimens are not usually acceptable because of bacterial contamination. **TURNAROUND TIME:** Negatives are reported after 6-8 weeks. **SPECIAL INSTRUCTIONS:** Inform the laboratory of the specific source of the specimen.

Interpretive **REFERENCE RANGE:** No growth **USE:** Isolate and identify mycobacteria from the urinary tract. Most patients with genitourinary tuberculosis have symptoms of urinary tract disease, but some are asymptomatic. **LIMITATIONS:** Positive acid-fast stained smears are not diagnostic, because of the presence of *Mycobacterium smegmatis* in genital secretions of normal patients. **CONTRAINDICATIONS:** A 24-hour urine collection is less valuable because of increased chance of bacterial contamination. **ADDITIONAL INFORMATION:** If mycobacteria are cultured, isolates can be definitively identified, and susceptibility testing performed on request. Although it has been thought that tuberculosis of the urinary tract should be suspected when hematuria and pyuria (sterile pyuria) occur without recovery by routine culture of usual urinary tract pathogens, concomitant infections with ordinary pathogens are not rare. Mycobacteria cultures of the urine are approximately 90% sensitive. The kidney is the most frequent site of infection; prostate, salpinx, and endometrial involvement also occurs. Continuing tuberculous bacilluria may cause cystitis with frequency. Genitourinary infections with atypical mycobacteria, particularly *M. kansasii* and *M. avium-intracellulare*, occur.[1] Mycobacterial genitourinary tract infections represented about 20% of extrapulmonary tuberculosis cases.[2] This proportion will probably increase as more infections with *M. tuberculosis* and *M. avium-intracellulare* are identified in patients with the acquired immunodeficiency syndrome (AIDS). Urine cultures were reported positive in 77% of HIV-positive patients with extrapulmonary tuberculosis.[3] The direct detection of mycobacterial DNA in urine is being investigated. Specific DNA sequences can be amplified from patient specimens.[4]

Footnotes

1. Wayne LG and Sramek HA, "Agents of Newly Recognized or Infrequently Encountered Mycobacterial Diseases," *Clin Microbiol Rev*, 1992, 5(1):1-25.
2. Alvarez S and McCabe WR, "Extrapulmonary Tuberculosis Revisited: A Review of Experience at Boston City and Other Hospitals," *Medicine (Baltimore)*, 1984, 63:25-55.
3. Shafer RW, Kim DS, Weiss JP, et al, "Extrapulmonary Tuberculosis in Patients With Human Immunodeficiency Virus Infection," *Medicine (Baltimore)*, 1991, 70(6):384-97.
4. Kolk AH, Schuitema AR, Kuijper S, et al, "Detection of *Mycobacterium tuberculosis* in Clinical Samples by Using Polymerase Chain Reaction and a Nonradioactive Detection System," *J Clin Microbiol*, 1992, 30(10):2567-75.

References

Des Prez RM and Heim CR, "Mycobacterium Tuberculosis," *Principles and Practice of Infectious Diseases*, 3rd ed, Chapter 229, Mandell GL, Douglas RG Jr, and Bennett JE, eds, New York, NY: Churchill Livingstone, 1990, 1877-906.

Urine *Trichomonas* Wet Mount *see Trichomonas* Preparation *on page 879*

Uterus Anaerobic Culture *see* Endometrium Culture *on page 811*

Vaginal Culture *see* Genital Culture *on page 814*

Ventricular Fluid Culture *see* Cerebrospinal Fluid Culture *on page 798*

Verocytotoxin Producing *E. coli*, Stool Culture *see* Stool Culture, Diarrheagenic *E. coli on page 860*

White Cells, Stool *see* Methylene Blue Stain, Stool *on page 828*

Whooping Cough Culture *see Bordetella pertussis* Nasopharyngeal Culture *on page 790*

Wound *Actinomyces* Culture *see Actinomyces* Culture, All Sites *on page 772*

Wound Culture

CPT 87070

Related Information

Abscess, Aerobic and Anaerobic Bacterial Culture *on page 768*
Biopsy or Body Fluid Aerobic Bacterial Culture *on page 778*
Biopsy or Body Fluid Anaerobic Bacterial Culture *on page 778*
Burn Culture, Quantitative *on page 794*

Test Commonly Includes Culture for aerobic organisms and usually Gram stain

Patient Care **PREPARATION:** Sterile preparation of the aspiration site

(Continued)

Wound Culture *(Continued)*

Specimen Pus or other material properly obtained from a wound site or abscess **CONTAINER:** Sterile tube or Culturette® swab **COLLECTION:** The specimen should be transported to the laboratory as soon as possible after collection. Contamination with normal flora from skin, rectum, vaginal tract, or other body surfaces should be avoided. If anaerobes are suspected, a properly collected specimen for anaerobic culture should also be submitted. **STORAGE INSTRUCTIONS:** Refrigerate the specimen if it cannot be promptly processed. **CAUSES FOR REJECTION:** Specimens delayed in transit to the laboratory may have less than optimal yields. **TURNAROUND TIME:** Preliminary reports are usually available at 24 hours. Cultures with no growth are usually reported after 72 hours. Reports on specimens from which pathogens are isolated require a minimum of 48 hours for completion. **SPECIAL INSTRUCTIONS:** The laboratory should be informed of the specific site of specimen, the age of patient, current antibiotic therapy, clinical diagnosis, and time of collection. The submission of biopsy specimens or specimens from normally sterile sites should be clearly indicated to the laboratory. Procedures for laboratory work-up of wound cultures which may contain contamination from the skin surface are different than those from sites which are expected to be sterile. Drainage cultured by aspiration away from a sinus tract may provide more useful information.

Interpretive **REFERENCE RANGE:** No growth. A simultaneous Gram stain should always be performed to facilitate interpretation. Gram-negative organisms frequently colonize wounds, and mixed culture results are common. **USE:** Isolate and identify potentially pathogenic organisms from wounds or biopsy/aspiration material **LIMITATIONS:** Only rapid-growing, nonfastidious aerobic organisms can be recovered and identified by routine methods. Often only organisms which predominate will be completely identified. Unless specifically requested by the physician or mandated by the specimen source (ie, genital specimen), fastidious organisms such as *N. gonorrhoeae* may not be isolated. Anaerobic, fungal, and mycobacterial pathogens should be considered, and appropriate cultures requested if indicated. **CONTRAINDICATIONS:** Culture of contaminated open wounds which have not been cleansed or debrided **METHODOLOGY:** Culture of material on routine media and identification of organisms isolated **ADDITIONAL INFORMATION:** See table. Susceptibility testing is usually performed, if indicated. The majority

Classification of Soft–Tissue Infections

Tissue Level	Common Surgical Pathogens				
	S. pyogenes	*S. aureus*	*C. perfringens*	Mixed Bacteria	
				Staph & Strep	Enteric
Epidermis	Ecthyma contagiosum	Scalded–skin syndrome		Possibly impetigo	
Dermis and subdermis	Erysipelas/cellulitis	Folliculitis/abscess	Abscess/cellulitis	Meleny's ulcer (synergistic gangrene)	Tropical ulcer
Fascial planes	Strep gangrene	Carbuncle	Fasciitis	Necrotizing fasciitis	
Muscle tissue	Strep myositis	Muscular abscess/ pyomyositis	Myonecrosis	Nonclostridial myonecrosis	

From Ahrenholz DH, "Necrotizing Soft Tissue Infections," *Surg Clin North Am,* 1988, 68:198–214, with permission.

of bacteria infecting surgical wounds are common airborne microorganisms.[1] Effective treatment of wound infection usually includes drainage, removal of foreign bodies, infected prosthetic devices, and retained foreign objects such as suture material. Suction irrigation may be helpful in resolving wound infections. Species commonly recovered from wounds include *Escherichia coli*, *Proteus* sp, *Klebsiella* sp, *Pseudomonas* sp, *Enterobacter* sp, enterococci, other streptococci, *Bacteroides* sp, *Prevotella* sp, *Clostridium* sp, *Staphylococcus aureus*, and *Staphylococcus epidermidis* (coagulase-negative *Staphylococcus*).

Footnotes

1. Whyte W, Hambraeus A, Laurell G, et al, "The Relative Importance of the Routes and Sources of Wound Contamination During General Surgery. II. Airborne," *J Hosp Infect*, 1992, 22(1):41-54.

References

Cheadle WG, "Current Perspectives on Antibiotic Use in the Treatment of Surgical Infections," *Am J Surg*, 1992, 164(4A Suppl):44S-47S.

Goldstein EJ, "Management of Human and Animal Bite Wounds," *J Am Acad Dermatol*, 1989, 21(6):1275-9.

Pollack AV and Evans M, "Microbiologic Prediction of Abdominal Surgical Wound Infection," *Arch Surg*, 1987, 122:33-6.

Wright's Stain, Stool *see* Methylene Blue Stain, Stool *on page 828*

Ziehl-Neelsen Stain *see* Acid-Fast Stain *on page 770*

MOLECULAR PATHOLOGY

Rebecca T. Horvat, PhD

Over the past few decades remarkable progress has been made in the field of molecular biology. This new technology is rapidly being translated into new diagnostic tests. Molecular biology has revealed much about the nature of the mechanisms involved in cancer and genetic diseases. Nucleic acid analysis has also aided in the identification of infectious microorganisms, especially those microorganisms that require tedious isolation or cannot be cultured. The progress in this area of diagnostic testing continues to grow with the advent of nucleic acid amplification technology. The most frequently used amplification procedure is the polymerase chain reaction (PCR), which is able to amplify a specific DNA target sequence in a short period of time. Subsequently, several other amplification methods have been developed. These new amplification methods will allow greater usage of molecular detection in the clinical laboratory.

The cytogenetic analysis of cancer cells has lead to the identification of translocations, amplifications, deletions, and insertions associated with certain cancers. This has lead to the identification of oncogenes, antioncogenes, and genetic aberrations that are central to the process of malignant transformation. Genetic analysis is now used to study the DNA abnormalities associated with human tumors. Used diagnostically, these DNA studies can detect amplified oncogenes, translocations, mutations, deletions, and clonal rearrangements that can aid in the diagnosis and prognosis of several types of tumors. Likewise, cytogenetic analysis has identified certain mutations associated with inherited diseases such as fragile X syndrome and muscular dystrophy. These observations eventually led to the identification of the genes involved in these genetic abnormalities. These genetic diseases can now be detected by using DNA analysis. Several other genetic diseases can currently be detected by molecular analysis while many others are under investigation. Molecular biology will become a major facet in the future detection of inherited defects and analysis of tumors.

Another major area of diagnostic testing that has benefited from molecular technology is the identification of infectious microorganisms. Most infectious agents, both bacterial and viral, are present in specimens in very limited quantities unless they are first cultured. Some infectious microorganisms cannot be cultured or require long tedious incubations before they can be identified. The use of nucleic acid-based detection tests provide a distinct advantage in the diagnosis of infectious agents in that it provides a quick, accurate result. Future use of molecular techniques in infectious disease will aid in detection of antibiotic resistance, epidemiology, rapid assessment of bacteremia and meningitis, detection of bacteriuria, and rapid detection of more viral infections. Eventually, nucleic acid-based tests will become automated and will displace or supplement many current methods of detecting infectious agents.

Adult Polycystic Kidney Disease DNA Detection

CPT *83890 (molecular isolation or extraction); 83894 (separation); 83896 (nucleic acid probe, each)*

Synonyms Adult Polycystic Kidney Disease Inheritance Determination With DNA Restriction Fragment Length Polymorphism Probes; Genetic Detection of Presymptomatic Adult Polycystic Kidney Disease; Molecular Diagnosis of Polycystic Kidney Disease; Polycystic Kidney Disease, Prenatal Diagnosis

Test Commonly Includes This test can detect DNA linkage association with the major genetic mutation (autosomal dominant polycystic kidney disease locus 1, ADPKD1) on chromosome 16. This gene is tightly associated with adult polycystic kidney disease, presently designated autosomal dominant PKD.

Abstract Autosomal dominant polycystic kidney disease (adult PKD) is a disorder characterized by the development of myriads of renal cysts. Although the biochemical nature of this disease is not known, DNA technology has been applied to families affected with this progressive disease. A linkage has been established in a large number of families with a gene on chromosome 16. The abnormal gene on the short arm of chromosome 16 is found in >95% of individuals with adult (autosomal dominant) polycystic disease. Individuals in families affected with this entity can now have genetic studies performed to determine their risk for developing the disease. Patients at high risk can then be followed closely. Such testing must be done only with genetic counseling.

Specimen Blood, amniotic fluid, chorionic villus, or tissue **CONTAINER:** Blood should be collected in yellow top (ACD) Vacutainer® tube; amniotic fluid and chorionic villus should be collected in a sterile manner and transferred to a sterile tube for transport or to a T25 culture flask; amniotic cells can be sent after culturing or can be sent directly to the laboratory. **SAMPLING TIME:** Amniotic fluid should be collected between the 17th and 18th week of pregnancy. Chorionic villus specimens should be collected between the 8th and 12th week of gestation. **STORAGE INSTRUCTIONS:** All specimens should be sent to the laboratory **immediately** after collection, preferably by overnight delivery. All specimens should be kept at room temperature or refrigerated, never frozen. **CAUSES FOR REJECTION:** Any amniotic fluid specimen that is bloody may be contaminated with maternal blood and is unsuitable for this test, any specimen that has been frozen before processing cannot be tested, specimens unlabeled or mislabeled **TURNAROUND TIME:** Results are usually available after 3 weeks.

Interpretive **REFERENCE RANGE:** The laboratory generally provides an interpretive report that includes a risk analysis. **USE:** This test is indicated for a family with history of autosomal dominant polycystic disease. For this purpose it is necessary to have a family pedigree that includes all medical histories. Test is also indicated for prenatal diagnosis in couples known to be carriers of the much less common recessive form of polycystic kidney disease, which has been called infantile PKD and is strongly associated with hepatic fibrosis and pulmonary maldevelopment. This test requires genetic testing of several family members (often as many as seven or eight) to determine the characteristic of the mutation. **LIMITATIONS:** DNA linkage analysis for polycystic kidney disease can detect the inheritance pattern associated with one of the major genes responsible for the disease. However, a negative result does not rule out the possibility that an individual may carry another mutation causing polycystic kidney disease or even be affected with polycystic kidney disease. However, the test can greatly lower that probability. Such testing is available only in a few reference laboratories. **METHODOLOGY:** DNA is isolated from the specimen. Several regions on chromosome 16 close to and flanking the ADPKD1 gene are examined using Southern blotting techniques. Restriction enzyme sites on the DNA close to the disease gene are examined. Genetic linkage analysis uses specific DNA probes to follow the inheritance of a gene associated with disease. This requires testing several members of a family, including both affected and unaffected individuals, preferably from several generations. The DNA probes used to follow the gene must be located very close to the disease gene and must show differences in the size of DNA that results from restriction enzyme digestion (polymorphic) between individuals from the same family (see figure). This allows for distinction between all the possible different chromosomes 16s that an individual could inherit; it can be determined from this information which chromosome is associated with disease. If these polymorphic sites are located very close to the disease gene then they are called "informative". The accuracy of genetic linkage analysis is greater if DNA probes on both sides of the disease gene are informative. The genetic linkage analysis for polycystic kidney disease uses flanking markers very closely associated with ADPKD1, the gene associated with the disease.[1] Thus, in families in which this mutation is found, linkage analysis can very accurately predict inheritance of the disease gene (ADPKD1). **ADDITIONAL INFORMATION:** Auto-

(Continued)

Adult Polycystic Kidney Disease DNA Detection *(Continued)*

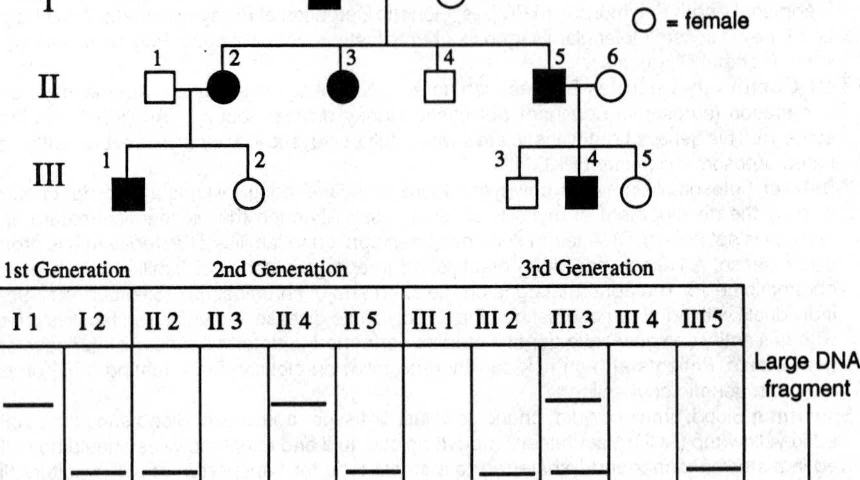

DNA is digested with restriction enzymes to make smaller pieces of DNA. This DNA is then electrophoresed in an agarose gel to separate DNA of different sizes (large to small). After transfer to a membrane, the DNA is hybridized with a radioactive DNA probe and hybridized DNA bands are visible with autoradiography. Inheritance patterns are noted that associate with disease (—✳—). Open symbols are normal individuals and shaded symbols are affected individuals.

somal dominant polycystic kidney disease is a common fatal inherited disorder which affects approximately 1 in 1000 people. Thus, each child born of an affected parent has a 50% chance of inheritance of the disease gene. Polycystic kidney disease is characterized by progressive increase and enlargement of numerous fluid-filled renal cysts. The growth of such cysts causes progressive impairment which usually leads to irreversible renal failure in middle age. In 40% to 70% of patients, cysts are also present in the liver. They are encountered sporadically in the pancreas, spleen, subarachnoid space, and pineal gland, and other abnormalities are described as well. The mechanism of cyst formation and the biochemical defect of the disease are currently not known. Genetic linkage studies with a large number of families (more than 50) have localized a disease-associated gene to the short arm of chromosome 16. The gene was designated autosomal dominant polycystic kidney disease locus 1 (ADPKD1).[2] Because the ADPKD1 gene has not been cloned, the nature of the exact genetic mutation is not known. Therefore, genetic analysis depends on indirect inference from linkage analysis. Individuals within a family with a history of autosomal dominant PKD must be analyzed in the context of the entire family to determine linkage. The family should be referred to a genetic counselor for advice in this regard. Several affected families have been described that show no linkage to this gene and no diagnosis would be possible using this test.[3,4]. Therefore, patients should be made aware that this test is not indicated for all affected families. A review of autosomal dominant polycystic kidney disease has recently been published.[5]

Footnotes

1. Reeders ST, Keith T, Green P, et al, "Regional Localisation of the Autosomal Dominant Polycystic Kidney Disease Locus," *Genomics*, 1988, 3:150-5.
2. Reeders ST, Breuning MH, Davies KE, et al, "A Highly Polymorphic DNA Marker Linked to Adult Polycystic Disease on Chromosome 16," *Nature*, 1985, 317:542-4.
3. Kimberling WJ, Fain PR, Kenyon JB, et al, "Linkage Heterogeneity of Autosomal Dominant Polycystic Kidney Disease," *N Engl J Med*, 1988, 319(14):913-8.
4. Romeo G, Costa G, Catizone L, et al, "A Second Genetic Locus for Autosomal Dominant Polycystic Kidney Disease," *Lancet*, 1988, 2(8601):8-11.
5. Gabow PA, "Autosomal Dominant Polycystic Kidney Disease," *N Engl J Med*, 1993, 329:332-42.

References

Bear JC, Parfrey PS, Morgan JM, et al, "Autosomal Dominant Polycystic Kidney Disease: New Information for Genetic Counseling," *Am J Med Genet*, 1992, 43(3):548-53.

Grantham JJ, "Polycystic Kidney Disease," *The Principles and Practice of Nephrology*, Jacobson HR, Striker GE, and Klahr S, eds, Philadelphia, PA: BC Decker Inc, 1991, 370-3.

Kimberling WJ, Pieke-Dahl SA, and Kumar S, "The Genetics of Cystic Diseases of the Kidney," *Semin Nephrol*, 1991, 11(6):596-606.

Reeders ST, Germino GG, and Gillespie GA, "Mapping the Locus of Autosomal Dominant Polycystic Kidney Disease: Diagnostic Application," *Clin Chem*, 1989, 35(7 Suppl):B13-6.

Ye M and Grantham JJ, "The Secretion of Fluid by Renal Cysts From Patients With Autosomal Dominant Polycystic Kidney Disease," *N Engl J Med*, 1993, 329:310-3.

Adult Polycystic Kidney Disease Inheritance Determination With DNA Restriction Fragment Length Polymorphism Probes *see* Adult Polycystic Kidney Disease DNA Detection *on page 889*

Amniotic Fluid, Chromosome and Genetic Abnormality Analysis

***CPT** 88235 (culture); 88267 (chromosome analysis); 88283 (specialized banding technique)*

Related Information

Alpha$_1$-Fetoprotein, Amniotic Fluid *on page 114*
Amniotic Fluid Analysis for Erythroblastosis Fetalis *on page 122*
Amniotic Fluid Creatinine *on page 123*
Amniotic Fluid Cytology *on page 482*
Amniotic Fluid Lecithin/Sphingomyelin Ratio and Phosphatidylglycerol *on page 124*
Amniotic Fluid Pulmonary Surfactant *on page 126*
Chromosome Analysis, Blood or Bone Marrow *on page 898*
Chromosome *In Situ* Hybridization *on page 901*
Cystic Fibrosis DNA Detection *on page 903*
Duchenne/Becker Muscular Dystrophy DNA Detection *on page 908*
Fragile X DNA Detection *on page 910*
Polymerase Chain Reaction *on page 927*
Tests for Uncommon Inherited Diseases of Metabolism and Cell Structure *on page 605*

Synonyms Chromosome Karyotype, Amniotic Fluid; Chromosome Studies, Amniotic Fluid

Test Commonly Includes Examination of chromosome karyotype in amniotic cells to determine abnormalities

Patient Care PREPARATION: The patient should be placed on her abdomen for approximately 20 minutes prior to the amniocentesis. The pregnancy should be at least 16 weeks gestation. Ultrasound studies (to verify fetal life, detect multiple gestation, confirm age, localize placenta, and detect fetal/uterine/adnexal pathology) have usually been carried out.

Specimen Amniotic fluid CONTAINER: Sterile container COLLECTION: Using strict aseptic technique, collect specimen in a 20 mL sterile syringe. Pass stylet several times through the needle before drawing fluid to avoid maternal cell contamination. Collect first few mL separately, draw sample into two additional syringes, and transfer quickly to sterile tubes.[1] Cap the hub to maintain sterility. Pertinent medical findings should accompany request, including age, reason for study, relevant history, medication history, transfusion history, note of any virus infection or previous radiation therapy, number of pregnancies and miscarriages, gestational age by sonography if available, and suspected diagnosis. In case of twins or triplets, amniotic fluid must be collected separately from each amniotic sac. STORAGE INSTRUCTIONS: Maintain speci-

(Continued)

Amniotic Fluid, Chromosome and Genetic Abnormality Analysis *(Continued)*

men at room temperature. **CAUSES FOR REJECTION:** Specimen frozen or clotted (due to excessive contamination with blood) **TURNAROUND TIME:** Patient and family should be advised that 3-4 weeks may be needed to process material and before results will be available.

Interpretive **REFERENCE RANGE:** Twenty-two sets of normal autosomal chromosomes and normal number and appearance of sex chromosomes (XX for female, XY for male). Interpretive information is usually included. **USE:** Prenatal detection of chromosome abnormalities, especially Down syndrome, in groups of pregnant women at risk. Such groups include women age 35 years or older, previous child having chromosome abnormality or multiple congenital abnormalities, three or more previous spontaneous abortions, chromosome abnormality in parental history of current gestation, known familial Down syndrome or other chromosome abnormality, or known carrier of an X-linked disorder. Paternal age past 55 might also be considered an indication. While amniotic fluid sample for chromosome analysis is being obtained, samples for inherited metabolic disorders (enzyme deficiency analyses on cultured cells) or neural tube defects (alpha-fetoprotein analysis) can be obtained. **LIMITATIONS:** Failure of cells to grow in culture and/or contamination (eg, by *Mycoplasma*) precludes analysis. Overall culture success rate has been reported as 97% with a fetal loss (within 4 weeks of the amniocentesis) of 1.2%. **CONTRAINDICATIONS:** Environment lacking capability in ultrasonography, genetic counseling, amniocentesis, amniotic fluid culturing, and chromosome analysis techniques **METHODOLOGY:** Cell culturing of fetal cells, subsequent harvesting and chromosome analysis with Giemsa staining or Quinacrine and/or Giemsa banding techniques **ADDITIONAL INFORMATION:** A 1.4% incidence of abortions and stillbirths has been found following amniocentesis. Mean risk of 1.4% was within the range of spontaneous abortion expected for the stage of pregnancy. More recent studies have shown that chorionic villus sampling (CVS) is also a safe and acceptable procedure for early prenatal diagnosis of cytogenetic abnormalities.[2,3] The risk of miscarriage with CVS is 1% to 1.5% but the risk of maternal infection appears to be higher with CVS than with amniocentesis.[4] Cytogenetic analyses using such samples allow rapid turnaround time (24-72 hours) and a level of sensitivity approaching 100%.[5] Current developments for harvesting fetal cells from the maternal circulation with enrichment by flow cytometry followed by application of sensitive analytic methods (eg, polymerase chain reaction and fluorescent *in situ* hybridization) will increase the accuracy and use of prenatal testing.[6]

Chromosomal aberration was found in 4.6% of fetuses in women older than 38-40 years of age. Trisomy 21 was the most common abnormality (62%). Klinefelter's syndrome (11%) and Edward's syndrome, trisomy 18, (11%) were next most frequent in the cases of advanced maternal age. Some 2% to 5% of live newborns have a birth defect or genetic disorder.[4]

Prenatal diagnosis is possible for more than 1000 inherited diseases, including inborn errors of metabolism. See table for some of the most common disorders. Most are inherited in an autosomal recessive manner. Many disorders can be detected with metabolic/biochemical tests. Antenatal diagnosis using gene probes has become available for cystic fibrosis, muscular dystrophy, sickle cell anemia, hemophilia, fragile X syndrome, and many other genetic abnormalities.[7] This can be done by either using cultured amniotic fluid cells or direct chorionic villous sampling. The techniques require isolation of DNA with subsequent digestion of DNA using certain restriction endonucleases. The DNA is electrophoresed, transferred to nitrocellulose, and hybridized with specific DNA probes which bind to or very near (restriction fragment length polymorphisms) the genes of interest. The patterns obtained after development of the blot can determine, with a high degree of certainty, the presence or absence of disease in the fetus.[8]

Footnotes

1. Milbeck R, "Cytogenetic Examination: Specimen Acquisition and Handling," *Lab Med*, 1982, 13:416-9.
2. Ledbetter DH, Zachary JM, Simpson JL, et al, "Cytogenetic Results From the U.S. Collaborative Study on CVS," *Prenat Diagn*, 1992, 12(5):317-45.
3. Desnick RJ, Schuette JL, Golbus MS, et al, "First-Trimester Biochemical and Molecular Diagnoses Using Chorionic Villi: High Accuracy in the U.S. Collaborative Study," *Prenat Diagn*, 1992, 12(5):357-72.
4. DiLiberti JH, Greenstein MA, and Rosengren SS, "Prenatal Diagnosis," *Pediatr Rev*, 1992, 13(9):334-43.
5. Simpson JL, "Chronic Villus Sampling," *Semin Perinatol*, 1990, 14(6):446-55.
6. Chueh J and Golbus MS, "Prenatal Diagnosis Using Fetal Cells in the Maternal Circulation," *Semin Perinatol*, 1990, 14(6):471-82.
7. Beaudet AL, Scriver CR, Sty WS, et al, "Genetics and Biochemistry of Variant Human Phenotypes," *The Metabolic Basis of Inherited Disease*, 6th ed, Chapter 1, New York, NY: McGraw-Hill Inc, 1989, 3-163.
8. Kiechle FL and Quattrociocchi-Longe TM, "The Role of the Molecular Probe Laboratory in the 21st Century," *Lab Med*, 1992, 23:758-63.

Methods for Prenatal Diagnosis of Genetic Disorders

Biochemical Analysis

Adenosine deaminase deficiency	Lesch-Nyhan disease
Argininosuccinic aciduria	Mannosidosis
Batten disease	Maple syrup urine disease
Citrullinemia	Menkes' disease
Cystinosis	Methylmalonic aciduria
Fabry's disease	Mucopolysaccharidosis (I, II, III, VI, VII)
Farber's disease	Niemann-Pick
Fucosidosis	Orotic aciduria
Galactosemia	Pyruvate decarboxylate deficiency
Gaucher's disease	Refsum's disease
Generalized gangliosidosis	Sandhoff's disease
Glycogen storage disease (II, III, IV)	Steroid sulfatase deficiency
Homocystinuria	Tay-Sachs disease
I-cell disease	Wolman's disease
Krabbe's disease	

Cytogenic Analysis

Cri Du Chat syndrome (deletion 5)	**Chromosome Instability**
Down syndrome (trisomy 21)	Ataxia telangiectasia
Edwards' syndrome (trisomy 18)	Bloom's syndrome
Klinefelter's syndrome (XXY)	Fanconi's anemia
Miller-Dieker syndrome (trisomy 13) (deletion 17)	Fragile X syndrome
Prader-Willi syndrome (deletion 15)	
Retinoblastoma (deletion 13)	
Wiedemann-Beckwith syndrome (deletion 11)	
Wilms' tumor (deletion 11)	
XXX syndrome (XXX)	

Genetic Analysis

Adult polycystic kidney disease	Lesch-Nyhan syndrome
Alpha$_1$-antitrypsin deficiency	Multiple endocrine neoplasia (types 1 and 2a)
Alpha-thalassemia	Myotonic muscular dystrophy
Beta-thalassemia	Neurofibromatosis I
Carbamyl phosphate synthetase I deficiency	Norrie's disease
Congenital adrenal hyperplasia	Ornithine transcarbamylase deficiency
Cystic fibrosis	Osteogenesis imperfecta
Duchenne/Becker muscular dystrophy	Phenylketonuria
Ehlers-Danlos syndrome	Retinoblastoma
Familial amyloidosis	Sickle cell disease
Fragile X-associated mental retardation	Tay-Sachs disease
Friedrich ataxia	Wiskott-Aldrich syndrome
Hemophilias A and B	X-linked lymphoproliferative disease
Huntington disease	

References

Antonarakis SE, "Diagnosis of Genetic Disorders at the DNA Level," *N Engl J Med*, 1988, 320:153-63.

Schauer GM, Kalousek DK, and Magee JF, "Genetic Causes of Stillbirth," *Semin Perinatol*, 1992, 16(6):341-51.

Shapiro LJ, Gross I, and Hill HR, "Advances in Human Genetics: Current Applications and Prospects for the Future," *Semin Perinatol*, 1991, 15(Suppl 1):1-56.

Barr Bodies *see* Buccal Smear for Sex Chromatin Evaluation *on page 896*

Base Pairs *see* Chromosome Analysis, Blood or Bone Marrow *on page 898*

B-Cell Lymphomas *see* bcl-2 Gene Rearrangement *on this page*

bcl-2 Gene Analysis *see* bcl-2 Gene Rearrangement *on this page*

bcl-2 Gene Rearrangement

***CPT** 83890 (molecular isolation or extraction); 83892 (enzymatic digestion); 83894 (separation); 83896 (nucleic acid probe, each)*

Related Information

Gene Rearrangement for Leukemia and Lymphoma *on page 911*
Lymph Node Biopsy *on page 72*
Polymerase Chain Reaction *on page 927*

(Continued)

bcl-2 Gene Rearrangement *(Continued)*

T- and B-Lymphocyte Subset Assay *on page 750*

Synonyms bcl-2 Gene Analysis; Southern Blot of bcl-2 Gene Rearrangement

Applies to B-Cell Lymphomas

Test Commonly Includes Identification of unique DNA bands associated with the bcl-2 oncogene rearrangement in B-cell lymphomas

Abstract The bcl-2 oncogene codes for a unique protein that is located in the mitochondria of the cell. The bcl-2 protein regulates cell death and when it is overexpressed the cell is resistant to the "natural" death cycle, called apoptosis. The rearrangement of the bcl-2 gene with the B-cell receptor genes are found in a number of different B-cell lymphomas. This translocation can be identified cytogenetically as t14;18 in follicular lymphomas or large diffuse lymphomas.[1]

Specimen 0.1 g or more of frozen tissue, specifically from the involved area of the lymph node or tumor **CONTAINER:** Tissue must be shipped on dry ice or in 95% ethanol. **COLLECTION:** Tissue must be carefully cut from the surgically removed tumor and contain at least 10% of tumor cells from the involved area. **STORAGE INSTRUCTIONS:** Tissue can be stored in a -70°C freezer until shipped. **CAUSES FOR REJECTION:** Tissue samples that have thawed during transit cannot be used for DNA analysis. DNA cannot be isolated from tissue that has been fixed in formalin or paraffin. **TURNAROUND TIME:** Results are usually available 10 days to 2 weeks after the sample is received in the laboratory.

Interpretive **REFERENCE RANGE:** No rearrangement of bcl-2 is the normal result. **USE:** Detect bcl-2 rearrangement in B-cell lymphomas. The bcl-2 rearrangement is found in follicular lymphomas, large diffuse B-cell lymphomas, and undifferentiated lymphomas. Usually this rearrangement also involves a reciprocal translocation with the J_H region on chromosome 14, thus forming t14;18. **LIMITATIONS:** Rearrangement will not be found if the tissue is not from the involved tumor. Tissue samples that are too small will not yield enough DNA to do an accurate Southern blot analysis. **METHODOLOGY:** DNA is extracted from the clinical sample and digested with restriction enzymes. The digested fragments of DNA are electrophoresed in an agarose gel and then transferred to a nylon membrane. The DNA on the nylon membrane is hybridized with a radioactive DNA probe specific for the bcl-2 gene. Hybridization of the bcl-2 probe is detected using autoradiography. Clinical samples are always compared to a normal control sample that does not have a bcl-2 rearrangement. Hybridization to a DNA fragment different from the control sample indicates a rearranged bcl-2 gene. **ADDITIONAL INFORMATION:** The protein coded for by the oncogene, bcl-2, acts by suppressing the cell death program or apoptosis.[2] Apoptosis occurs in all cells but is especially important in immune and hematopoietic cells, which have a high cell turnover rate. When the bcl-2 gene is overexpressed, it will act to prevent apoptosis and possibly may render cells resistant to cell death by irradiation and certain chemotherapeutic agents.[3,4] A translocation between immunoglobulin genes (heavy chain or light chain genes) and bcl-2 results in the overexpression of bcl-2 protein and thus the expansion of B cells due to halting cell death. This type of translocation is found in 80% to 90% of follicular lymphomas, 30% of large diffuse lymphomas, and 50% of undifferentiated lymphomas.[1]

Footnotes

1. Weiss LM, Warnke RA, Sklar J, et al, "Molecular Analysis of the t(14;18) Translocation in Malignant Lymphomas," *N Engl J Med*, 1987, 317:1185.
2. Cohen JJ, "Programmed Cell Death in the Immune System," *Adv Immunol*, 1991, 50:55-85.
3. Strasser A, Harris AW, and Cory S, "bcl-2 Transgene Inhibits T-Cell Death and Perturbs Thymic Self-Censorship," *Cell*, 1992, 67(5):889-99.
4. Sentman CL, Shutter JR, Hockenbery D, et al, "bcl-2 Inhibits Multiple Forms of Apoptosis but Not Negative Selection in Thymocytes," *Cell*, 1992, 67(5):879-88.

References

Chaganti RSK, Doucette LA, Offit K, et al, "Specific Translocations in non-Hodgkin's Lymphoma: Incidence, Molecular Detection, and Histological and Clinical Correlations," *Cancer Cells*, Vol 7, Furth ME and Greaves MF, eds, 1989, 33-6.

Yanis JJ, "bcl-2 Oncogene Rearrangement in Follicular and Diffuse Large-Cell and Mixed-Cell Lymphoma," *Cancer Cells*, Vol 7, Furth ME and Greaves MF, eds, 1989, 37-40.

Borrelia burgdorferi DNA Assay

see Lyme Disease DNA Detection *on page 920*

***Borrelia burgdorferi* DNA Probe Test** *see* Lyme Disease DNA Detection *on page 920*

Breakpoint Cluster Rearrangement *see* Breakpoint Cluster Region Rearrangement in CML *on this page*

Breakpoint Cluster Region Rearrangement in CML

CPT *83890 (molecular isolation or extraction); 83892 (enzymatic digestion); 83894 (separation); 83896 (nucleic acid probe, each)*

Related Information

Bone Marrow *on page 524*
Chromosome Analysis, Blood or Bone Marrow *on page 898*
Leukocyte Alkaline Phosphatase *on page 566*
Leukocyte Cytochemistry *on page 567*
Polymerase Chain Reaction *on page 927*

Synonyms Breakpoint Cluster Rearrangement; Chronic Myelogenous Leukemia; Gene Rearrangement, BCR

Applies to Philadelphia Chromosome

Test Commonly Includes DNA detection of chromosomal translocation associated with chronic myelogenous leukemia (CML)

Abstract Chronic myelogenous leukemia (CML) is a myeloproliferative disorder characterized by the transformation of pluripotent hematopoietic stem cells. Ninety percent to 95% of the CML cases have a translocation between chromosome 9 and chromosome 22. This chromosomal translocation results in an abnormal gene rearrangement that can be detected using nucleic acid technology. This rearrangement has been extensively studied and analysis of DNA is now widely used in the diagnosis and monitoring of patients with CML.

Specimen Blood or bone marrow **CONTAINER:** Blood should be collected in a lavender top (EDTA) Vacutainer® tube; bone marrow should be collected in a syringe with heparin or transferred to a green top (heparin) tube or lavender top (EDTA) tube. **TURNAROUND TIME:** 1-2 weeks

Interpretive **REFERENCE RANGE:** No rearrangement observed **USE:** Characterize and monitor chronic myelogenous leukemia (CML) **METHODOLOGY:** Leukocyte DNA is extracted, cut with restriction enzymes, electrophoresed in agarose, and then transferred to membranes using the Southern blot method. The membrane is hybridized with a gene probe that will bind only to the target bcr gene on the membrane. The banding pattern is developed by autoradiography or color detection methods depending on the system used. In normal patients, there is one band in each lane digest. In patients with CML, there are two bands in the lanes because the movement of genes from one chromosome to another produces new restriction endonuclease sites.[1] **ADDITIONAL INFORMATION:** Chronic myelogenous leukemia (CML) is characterized by a reciprocal translocation between chromosomes 9 and 22 producing the Philadelphia chromosome. The translocation involves a gene rearrangement of the breakpoint cluster region (bcr) gene located on chromosome 22 with the c-abl oncogene on chromosome 9.[2] The hybrid bcr/c-abl gene is transcribed into an abnormal messenger RNA which is translated into an abnormal tyrosine kinase of 210,000 molecular weight instead of the normal 160,000 molecular weight protein. More than 90% of patients with CML have the Philadelphia chromosome by cytogenetic analysis as well as the rearrangement of the bcr/c-abl. Most patients with clinically documented CML that lack the Philadelphia chromosome still have the bcr/c-abl rearrangement. A small number of patients do not have the Philadelphia chromosome as the bcr/c-abl rearrangement. During reassessment many of these patients have a myelodysplastic syndrome, usually chronic myelomonocytic leukemia. A very small number of patients with clinical CML remain both Philadelphia chromosome negative and bcr/c-abl negative. This test is used for the confirmation of CML along with bone marrow examination, cytogenetics, and leukocyte alkaline phosphatase score.

Cytogenetically the Philadelphia chromosome has been found in 20% to 25% of patients with acute lymphoblastic leukemia (ALL) and 2% of patients with acute myelogenous leukemia (AML).[3] The Philadelphia chromosome from ALL cases appears similar to CML Philadelphia chromosomes in cytogenetic analysis. However, the two chromosomes result from distinct molecular rearrangements that can be analyzed and detected with DNA analysis. Some ALL Philadelphia chromosomes have been found to be identical to the CML Philadelphia chromosome even at the molecular level. These ALL cases are generally regarded as the blast crisis of CML.[4]

(Continued)

Breakpoint Cluster Region Rearrangement in CML *(Continued)*

The bcr/c-abl rearrangement assay is clinically useful for:

- confirmation of Philadelphia chromosome-positive CML
- diagnosis of Philadelphia-negative CML
- diagnosis and monitoring of CML blast crisis during and after chemotherapy as bone marrow transplantation
- detection of remission or early detection of relapse

Some specialty laboratories now provide a DNA amplification assay (PCR) for detection of this translocation. This is helpful in the detection of minimal residual disease.[5]

Footnotes

1. Tilzer LL and Concepcion EG, "Detection of the Gene Rearrangement in Chronic Myelogenous Leukemia With Biotinylated Gene Probes," *Am J Clin Pathol*, 1989, 91(4):464-7.
2. Groffen J, Stephenson JR, Heisterkamp N, et al, "Philadelphia Chromosome Breakpoints Are Clustered Within a Limited Region, bcr, on Chromosome 22," *Cell*, 1984, 36:93-9.
3. Kurzrock R, Gutterman J, and Talpaz M, "The Molecular Genetics of Philadelphia Chromosome-Positive Leukemias," *N Engl J Med*, 1988, 319(15):990-8.
4. Saikevych I, Timson L, Denny C, et al, "Philadelphia Chromosome Positive (Ph^+) Leukemias With p210 BCR-abl and p185 BCR-abl May Be Distinct Disorders," *Blood*, 1989, 74:79a.
5. Lee MS, Chang KS, Freireich EJ, et al, "Detection of Minimal Residual bcr/abl Transcripts by a Modified Polymerase Chain Reaction," *Blood*, 1988, 72(3):893-7.

References

Crisan D and Carr ER, "BCR/abl Gene Rearrangement in Chronic Myelogenous Leukemia and Acute Leukemias," *Lab Med*, 1992, 23:730-6.

Groffen J, Hermans A, Grosveld G, et al, "Molecular Analysis of Chromosome Breakpoints," *Prog Nucleic Acid Res Mol Biol*, 1989, 36:281-300.

Watson JD, Hopkin NA, Roberts JW, et al, *Molecular Biology of the Gene*, 4th ed, Menlo Park, CA: Benjamin/Cummings, 1987, 1058-94.

Buccal Smear for Sex Chromatin Evaluation

***CPT** 88130*

Related Information

Chromosome Analysis, Blood or Bone Marrow *on page 898*

Chromosome *In Situ* Hybridization *on page 901*

Oral Cavity Cytology *on page 507*

Synonyms Barr Bodies; Sex Chromatin

Test Commonly Includes Cell count of Barr bodies under oil immersion; fluorescent Y chromosome examination

Patient Care PREPARATION: Rinse mouth prior to obtaining specimens for adults. In infants, collection should be performed between feedings. AFTERCARE: Usually not needed but saline rinses may be used. Any bleeding should be reported to a nurse.

Specimen Scrape of buccal mucosa (right and left sides submitted separately) COLLECTION: Scrape buccal mucosa with tongue depressor and **discard**. Then firmly scrape again with **clean** tongue depressor and spread evenly on frosted side of glass slides; fix immediately in 95% ethanol. Label frosted slide with patient's name. Label bottle with patient's name, hospital number, and room number. CAUSES FOR REJECTION: Improper fixation, air drying, no clinical history, too few cells, unlabeled slides SPECIAL INSTRUCTIONS: Include age, phenotype, sex, and pertinent clinical information including tentative diagnosis on the requisition.

Interpretive REFERENCE RANGE: For practical purposes, the presence of ≥4% cells in which clear sex chromatin bodies are found is diagnostic of XX chromosomal constitution.[1] USE: Confirm the presence or absence of sex chromatin and the presence or absence of fluorescent portion of the "Y" chromosome LIMITATIONS: Chromatin testing of newborn infants should be deferred for 1 week. The incidence of chromatin-positive cells may fall in both the mother and in a normal female infant; thus, the buccal smear of an infant female may be erroneously interpreted as chromatin negative in the first few days of life. The incidence of chromatin-positive nuclei rises slowly to reach normal ranges within 3-4 days. **This is a screening test only.** It is subject to marked technical variability in interpretation. It is also unable to detect chimeric states reliably. For complete sex chromatin evaluation, a formal karyotype should be obtained. CONTRAINDICATIONS: Mouth lesions, bleeding abnormalities ADDITIONAL INFORMATION: In a phenotypic mature female, vaginal wall scrapings are suitable and possibly more accurate than buccal scrapings.

Footnotes

1. Koss LG, ed, *Diagnostic Cytology and Its Histopathologic Bases*, 4th ed, Philadelphia, PA: JB Lippincott Co, 1992, 867.

***Chlamydia trachomatis* DNA Detection Test** *see Chlamydia trachomatis* DNA Probe *on this page*

Chlamydia trachomatis DNA Probe

CPT *87179*

Related Information

Chlamydia Group Titer *on page 663*
Chlamydia trachomatis Culture *on page 1171*
Chlamydia trachomatis Direct FA Test *on page 1173*
Conjunctival Culture *on page 803*
Endometrium Culture *on page 811*
Genital Culture *on page 814*
Lymphogranuloma Venereum Titer *on page 722*
Neisseria gonorrhoeae Culture *on page 831*
Neisseria gonorrhoeae DNA Probe Test *on page 924*
Neisseria gonorrhoeae Smear *on page 834*
Polymerase Chain Reaction *on page 927*
Viral Culture, Eye or Ocular Symptoms *on page 1202*
Viral Culture, Urogenital *on page 1207*

Synonyms *Chlamydia trachomatis* DNA Detection Test; DNA Hybridization Test for *Chlamydia trachomatis*; DNA Test for *Chlamydia trachomatis*; PACE2®

Test Commonly Includes Direct detection of *Chlamydia trachomatis* nucleic acid in swab specimens

Abstract Sexually transmitted diseases are a major infectious disease problem in the United States and Europe. Many of the sexually transmitted diseases like, *Chlamydia trachomatis*, remain undetected in asymptomatic carriers. Likewise, other sexually transmitted infectious agents such as *Neisseria gonorrhoeae* are often isolated from the same individuals infected with *C. trachomatis*.[1,2] Many of the nucleic acid tests available for the detection of *C. trachomatis* will also detect *N. gonorrhoeae* from the same specimen.[2] Thus, the screening for these sexually transmitted infectious agents becomes more cost-effective if a single specimen can be collected and tested for two agents. These DNA probe tests have become fairly simple and inexpensive to offer and will soon become incorporated in routine hospital clinical laboratories.

Patient Care **PREPARATION:** When taking urethral specimens the patient should not have urinated for 1 hour prior to collection.

Specimen Swab specimen collected from the genitourinary site of a male or female patient **CONTAINER:** Special DNA transport medium is provided by the laboratory and should not be substituted. A kit containing a swab and special transport media is made by Gen-Probe Inc, and is recommended for this test. **COLLECTION:** Currently the DNA test for *Chlamydia trachomatis* is only FDA approved for genitourinary and eye specimens, but not for rectal or nasopharyngeal specimens.

For a male, the urethra is swabbed by rotating the swab 2-3 cm into the urethra. This should provide enough epithelial cells from the infected site to detect *C. trachomatis*. The swab is then placed in the transport tube for shipping to the laboratory.

For females, the commercial kit provides two swabs. The cervix or endocervix should be swabbed with one swab first to clean the area and the second swab is used to collect the specimen. The swab is inserted 2-3 cm into the endocervix and then rotated to collect the epithelial cells from the infected site. The swab is then put immediately into the transport tube and shipped to the laboratory.

STORAGE INSTRUCTIONS: The specimens should be maintained at room temperature or refrigerated. Specimens are stable up to 1 week after collection. **CAUSES FOR REJECTION:** Contamination with urine **TURNAROUND TIME:** Results are available usually within 24 hours of receipt of the specimen.

Interpretive **REFERENCE RANGE:** The normal test should be negative for *Chlamydia trachomatis* DNA. A sexually active, asymptomatic individual may harbor *C. trachomatis* in rates ranging from 0% to 7%. **USE:** This test provides for the rapid detection of *C. trachomatis* in clinical specimens. **LIMITATIONS:** DNA detection test cannot be done in child abuse cases. Cell culture is the only approved test in these circumstances. However, this test can be used to confirm culture-positive tests. **METHODOLOGY:** This test detects *C. trachomatis*-specific nucleic acid di-

(Continued)

Chlamydia trachomatis DNA Probe *(Continued)*

rectly from swab specimens. This requires denaturation of the DNA/RNA in the specimens by heating, hybridization with a specific DNA probe, and detection of bound probe after several washing steps. Detection can be done by using a radioactive DNA probe, however a positive sample is now commonly detected with chemiluminescence. In July 1993, a *Chlamydia* assay by polymerase chain reaction (PCR) was approved for use by the Food and Drug Administration. This is the first clinical assay by PCR approved in the U.S. **ADDITIONAL INFORMATION:** Approximately 4,000,000 cases of *C. trachomatis* occur annually in the United States[3], and it is considered a serious sexually transmitted disease problem. The detection of *C. trachomatis* DNA provides a diagnostic test that has several advantages over the traditional culture method. The turnaround time is shorter, it is less labor intensive, and it provides an objective result that makes interpretation easier.[4] The DNA detection test for *C. trachomatis* has been proven to have an equivalent sensitivity as the antibody-based tests (EIA and fluorescent antibody detection) and to have a greater specificity than these tests.[5,6] However, at the present time this test cannot be used exclusively in cases of child abuse. These cases must be detected with a cell culture test.

Footnotes

1. Thomson SE and Washington AE, "Epidemiology of Sexually Transmitted *Chlamydia trachomatis* Infections," *Epidemiol Rev*, 1983, 5:96-123.
2. Limberger RL, Biega R, Evancoe A, et al, "Evaluation of Culture and the Gen-Probe PACE2® Assay for Detection of *Neisseria gonorrhoeae* and *Chlamydia trachomatis* in Endocervical Specimens Transported to a State Health Laboratory," *J Clin Microbiol*, 1992, 30(5):1162-6.
3. Centers for Disease Control, "*Chlamydia trachomatis* Infections. Policy Guidelines for Prevention and Control," *MMWR Morb Mortal Wkly Rep*, 1985, 35:535-74.
4. Dean D, Palmer L, Pant CR, et al, "Use of a *Chlamydia trachomatis* DNA Probe for Detection of Ocular Chlamydiae," *J Clin Microbiol*, 1989, 27(5):1062-7.
5. Iwen PC, Blair TMH, and Woods GL, "Comparison of the Gen-Probe PACE2® System, Direct Fluorescent Antibody, and Cell Culture for Detecting *Chlamydia trachomatis* in Cervical Specimens," *Am J Clin Pathol*, 1991, 95(4):578-82.
6. LeBar W, Herschman B, Jemal C, et al, "Comparison of DNA Probe, Monoclonal Antibody Enzyme Immunoassay and Cell Culture for the Detection of *Chlamydia trachomatis*," *J Clin Microbiol*, 1989, 27(5):826-8.

References

Barnes RC, "Laboratory Diagnosis of Human Chlamydial Infections," *Clin Microbiol Rev*, 1989, 2(2):119-36.
Dembry LM and Zervos MJ, "Molecular Biologic Techniques: Applications to the Clinical Microbiology Laboratory," *Lab Med*, 1992, 23:743-51.
Ehret JM and Judson FN, "Genital *Chlamydia* Infections," *Clin Lab Med*, 1989, 9(3):481-500.
Peterson EM, Oda R, Alexander R, et al, "Molecular Techniques for the Detection of *Chlamydia trachomatis*," *J Clin Microbiol*, 1989, 27(10):2359-63.

Chromosome Analysis, Blood or Bone Marrow

***CPT** 88230 (culture, lymphocytes); 88237 (culture, bone marrow); 88262 (chromosome analysis)*

Related Information

Amniotic Fluid, Chromosome and Genetic Abnormality Analysis *on page 891*
Bone Marrow *on page 524*
Breakpoint Cluster Region Rearrangement in CML *on page 895*
Buccal Smear for Sex Chromatin Evaluation *on page 896*
Chromosome *In Situ* Hybridization *on page 901*
Lymph Node Biopsy *on page 72*
Oral Cavity Cytology *on page 507*
White Blood Count *on page 616*

Synonyms Chromosome Karyotype, Blood; Chromosome Studies; Cytogenetics; Karyotype

Applies to Base Pairs; Inherited Disorders; Mosaicism; Philadelphia Chromosome; Translocation

Test Commonly Includes Buccal smear Barr body (X chromatin body) analysis. The number of metaphase spreads prepared, karyotypes included in the study, and banding techniques applied, if any, will vary with the specimen studied (blood, marrow, tissue culture) and between institutions.

Abstract The first description and enumeration of human chromosomes was in 1956 and shortly afterward the first constitutional chromosome change (trisomy 21) was described. Banding patterns were then found to be associated with certain chromosomes after trypsin treatment and staining, which allowed for numbering the chromosomes. From this starting point research has progressed rapidly to identify cytogenetic abnormalities in neoplastic cells. Many

Some Common Leukemia Related Chromosome Abnormalities

Disease	Chromosome Abnormality	% of Cases With Abnormality
Chronic myelogenous leukemia (CML)	Ph[1] chromosome t (9q+, 22q-)	>90%
Blast crisis CML	Abnormalities additional to Ph[1], commonly duplication of Ph[1] trisomy 8	75%–80%
Acute myelogenous leukemia	Translocation part of 8–21 (long arms) t (8q-, 21q+). Prognosis correlates directly with number of cells having abnormal chromosomes.	About 50%
Acute promyelocytic leukemia	Translocation 17–15 (portion of long arms). Presence of this abnormality correlates with worse prognosis.	40%–50%
Postchemotherapy leukemia	Deletion of 5 and/or 7 and hypodiploidy	Nearly 100%
Preleukemia	Changes similar to those in acute myelogenous leukemia	
Lymphoproliferative disorders	Translocation part of long arms 8 to long arms of 14 (14q+ anomaly)	
Chronic lymphocytic leukemia	Trisomy 12 and 14q+	

of the genetic changes in malignant cells were found to be characteristic changes associated with certain malignancies. See table.

A classic example is the translocation between chromosome 9 and chromosome 22 in chronic myelogenous leukemia. This chromosomal translocation resulted in the chromosome known as the Philadelphia chromosome. Since the discovery of human chromosomes and banding patterns, molecular techniques have identified oncogenes and antioncogenes at chromosomal regions often involved in translocation. However, the translocations identified in malignant cells (especially leukemias and lymphomas) continue to be analyzed cytogenetically to establish diagnoses, assess prognosis, and monitor disease during chemotherapy.

Patient Care **PREPARATION:** A 3-hour fast before the test is preferable. Abstinence from fatty foods for 12 hours before this test is advised.

Specimen Whole blood, bone marrow **CONTAINER:** Green top (sodium heparin) tube for blood, heparinized (20-25 units/mL of marrow) syringe for bone marrow. If specimen is put into a heparinized vacuum tube, vacuum should be released after specimen is in tube. EDTA, citrate, or lithium heparin anticoagulants should not be used. **COLLECTION:** Sterile technique with 12 mL syringe, 21-gauge needle **STORAGE INSTRUCTIONS:** Specimen should be delivered to the laboratory **immediately**. Maintain bone marrow at room temperature. **CAUSES FOR REJECTION:** Clotted or hemolyzed specimen, specimen more than 24 hours old, use of improper anticoagulant **SPECIAL INSTRUCTIONS:** Call laboratory so that test can be arranged and scheduled. Include with request, clinical and family history, indication for study, medication history, transfusion history, radiation exposure, viral history, and important CBC parameters, including presence of any circulating blasts.

Interpretive **REFERENCE RANGE:** Interpretation is usually provided with report. **USE:** Evaluate congenital anomaly (birth defect), mental retardation, growth retardation, infertility, cryptorchidism, hypogonadism, amenorrhea (primary), abnormal/ambiguous genitalia, myeloproliferative diseases, chronic myelogenous leukemia; predict and confirm leukemic remission/relapse; study preleukemic state, neoplasia, recurrent miscarriage, prenatal diagnosis in cases of advanced maternal age, Turner's syndrome, Klinefelter's syndrome, Down syndrome (trisomy 21), and other suspected chromosomal disorders **LIMITATIONS:** Cells may fail to grow in culture. Banding studies require a high level of technical expertise, specialized equipment, and may not be reproducible and/or successful. Banding studies generally require a research environment. Availability of different types of banding techniques vary between institutions.

(Continued)

Chromosome Analysis, Blood or Bone Marrow *(Continued)*

Chromosome analysis is expensive. **METHODOLOGY:** Lymphocyte culture, phytohemagglutinin or other mitogen stimulation, colchicine arrest of cells in metaphase, methanol/acetic acid fixation, spread preparation using hypotonic solution, banding of chromosomes (see Additional Information), photography, chromosome analysis with determination of modal number and preparation and analysis of karyotype. "Direct harvest" technique is used with bone marrow specimens. Analysis of cells undergoing spontaneous mitoses is desired so a mitogen (eg, phytohemagglutinin) is not used to stimulate lymphocytes (as in the procedure using peripheral blood). **ADDITIONAL INFORMATION:** Cytogenetics has become a broad and complex field with a large body of knowledge embodying descriptive detail of each of the 22 different chromosomes (autosomes), X and Y chromosomes, deletions, reduplications, translocations, mosaicism, etc. The haploid genome is formed of about 3 billion base pairs of DNA in which some 50,000-100,000 genes are distributed. Some of the early discoveries (late 1950s) remain as the most common and useful clinical applications. These include such sex chromosome anomalies as Turner's and Klinefelter's syndromes and the nearly constant association of the Philadelphia chromosome with **chronic myelogenous leukemia** (see Breakpoint Cluster Region Rearrangement in CML entry). Nearly 0.65% of live born infants have a chromosomal abnormality.[1] Some 3000 of the over 50,000 human genes have undergone mutation. Instances of multiple congenital defects with delayed growth and neuromotor development in infancy may have an autosomal abnormality. Individuals with disturbance of gonadal development or function or impaired reproductive ability may have a sex chromosome defect. Gene maps of the autosomal, X, and Y chromosomes and a comprehensive table of disease states and their chromosomal genesis is given by Beaudet et al.[2]

Turner syndrome (female with poorly developed secondary sexual characteristics, primary amenorrhea or sterility) may be associated with the classical XO finding or with XO/XX or XO/XXX mosaic forms or such symptoms may relate to trisomy X.

Klinefelter's syndrome (male hypogonadism with small testicles and sterility) occurs in about 1 of 700 live male births. In some 80% of cases there is an XXY constitution. About 15% are mosaics and the remaining 5% are XXYY, XXXY, or XXXXY Klinefelter variants. These latter are the "X chromatin-positive testicular dysgenesis" cases and are usually sterile. There is a 1 in 50 chance of having a chromosomally defective child in mothers between the ages 35 and 39, 1 in 30 for mothers 40-44 years of age. There is an increased frequency of autosomal trisomy (especially trisomy 21, Down syndrome) and sex chromosome aneuploidy (XXX, XXY, XYY). Children with (or parents of children with) Down syndrome or other chromosome defects should have cytogenetic studies.

Chromosome studies in the hematologic diseases can be performed on peripheral blood lymphocytes (stimulated with a mitogen), on bone marrow aspirate cells undergoing spontaneous mitosis (unstimulated), or on unstimulated peripheral blood if many leukemic cells are present. Chromosome analysis has practical value in the diagnosis and treatment of chronic myelogenous leukemia. Some 90% of patients with CML who have t9:22 translocation respond more favorably to treatment and have longer mean survival than patients without this defect. Later in the course of CML, a change in karyotype of a Ph^1 may indicate onset of acute or blast phase. Ph^1 chromosome has been found in a few patients with acute lymphocytic leukemia and acute nonlymphocytic leukemia. Variable chromosome defects occur with acute myelogenous leukemia (AML), but 40% of such patients have normal karyotype. Patients with AML and a normal karyotype have approximately an 87% rate of remission and a mean survival of 8 months. Patients with an abnormal karyotype have 20% remission rate and 2-month mean survival time.[3] Such statistics, however, are likely to vary with the therapeutic regimen in use and to change with the addition of new chemotherapeutic agents and combinations of agents.

Individual identification of chromosomes by banding techniques has added an additional dimension to chromosome analysis in hematology. These techniques, applied to malignant diseases, have revealed a broader ferment of chromosomal abnormality than was previously suspect. Application of banding allowed identification of a consistent chromosome abnormality in chronic myelogenous leukemia (Ph^1, a translocation from the long arm of chromosome 22 to the long arm of chromosome 9.) Currently, a variety of banding techniques are applied.

Detection of **sister chromatid exchange** (SCE) is another technique of cytogenetic analysis. SCE involves a four-stranded exchange in DNA during the cell cycle. The number of SCEs per cell reflects DNA damage and provides a test for chromosomal effects of mutagenic/

Chromosome Analysis, Blood

Q	Quinacrine banding QFQ technique (Q bands by fluorescence using quinacrine)	Bands are visible only by fluorescence microscopy. Y chromosome fluoresces brightly and is readily identified.
G	Giemsa banding	Produces permanently stained slides once G banded, application of other banding techniques is difficult. Same bands produced as with Q banding.
R	Reverse banding (RHG, RFA)	Produces reverse of Q and G bands. May use Giemsa or acridine orange (fluorescent) to stain the bands.
C	Constitutive heterochromatin banding (CBG technique)	Stains all centromeres, some heterochromatic areas and distal long arms of Y chromosome. Alternative to Q banding for Y identification.
Others:	T (terminal banding), G-11 banding, silver banding (NSG), DAPI technique	

carcinogenic agents. The method involves growing cells in a medium with 5-bromo-2'-deoxyuridine (BrdU). DNA strands that have incorporated BrdU will fluoresce brighter than other strands of DNA. Thus, exchange of DNA between sister chromosomes can be detected by the difference in the intensity of fluorescence. Spontaneous chromatid exchange between sister chromosomes occurs as a normal event in the cell cycle; however, certain disease states have an increased incidence of SCE (ie, Bloom's syndrome, leukemia, Fanconi's anemia). This technique is also used to test various substances for mutagenic effects.[3,4]

Footnotes

1. Hsu LYF, "Prenatal Diagnosis of Chromosome Abnormalities," *Genetic Disorders and the Fetus*, Chapter 5, New York, NY: Plenum Publishing Co, 1986, 115-83.
2. Beaudet AL, Scriver CR, Sty WS, et al, "Genetics and Biochemistry of Variant Human Phenotypes," *The Metabolic Basis of Inherited Disease,* 6th ed, Chapter 1, New York, NY: McGraw-Hill Inc, 1989, 3-163.
3. Wulf HC, Niebuhr E, and Lundgren K, "Extremely High Sister Chromatid Exchange Baseline Levels in Normal, Healthy Individuals," *Hereditary*, 1987, 106:115-8.
4. Cengiz K, Block AW, Hossfeld DK, et al, "Sister Chromatid Exchange and Chromosome Abnormalities in Uremic Patients," *Cancer Genet Cytogenet*, 1988, 36:55-67.

References

Davey FR and Nelson DA, "Leukocytic Disorders," *Clinical Diagnosis and Management by Laboratory Methods*, 18th ed, Chapter 27, Henry JB, ed, Philadelphia, PA: WB Saunders Co, 1991.

McKusik VA, *Mendelian Inheritance in Man*, 8th ed, Baltimore, MD: John Hopkins Press, 1988.

Rowley JD, Golomb HM, and Vardiman JW, "Nonrandom Chromosome Abnormalities in Acute Leukemia and Dysmyelopoietic Syndromes in Patients With Previously Treated Malignant Disease," *Blood*, 1981, 58:759-67.

Sandberg AA, "Methods in Cytogenetics," *The Chromosomes in Human Cancer and Leukemia*, 2nd ed, Chapter 5, New York, NY: Elsevier Science Publishing Co Inc, 1990, 100-19.

Chromosome *In Situ* Hybridization

***CPT** 88365*

Related Information

Alpha$_1$-Fetoprotein, Amniotic Fluid *on page 114*
Amniotic Fluid, Chromosome and Genetic Abnormality Analysis *on page 891*
Bone Marrow *on page 524*
Buccal Smear for Sex Chromatin Evaluation *on page 896*
Chromosome Analysis, Blood or Bone Marrow *on page 898*

Synonyms Fluorescent *in situ* Hybridization; *In situ* Chromosome Hybridization; Molecular Cytogenetics

Applies to Detection of Aneuploidy in Tumor Metaphases; Detection of Extra Chromosomes or Loss of Chromosomes in Leukemias; Detection of Trisomies of Chromosomes 8, 13, 18, and 21; Detection of X and Y Chromosome

Abstract Chromosome *in situ* hybridization is the use of labeled nucleic acid probes (DNA or RNA) to detect DNA targets in metaphase chromosome spreads or interphase nuclei. Labeled chromosome probes are available commercially and can be used to detect either numerical chromosomal abnormalities or translocations. Chromosome probes will bind to specific cen-

(Continued)

Chromosome *In Situ* Hybridization *(Continued)*

tromeric regions of the chromosomes or to specific genes on the chromosome. The sensitivity of this technique is such that detection requires many copies of the target (oncogene amplification or centromere region) or an enlarged chromosome probe that carries more detection reagents on the DNA probe (yeast artificial chromosome probes).[1] The technique of chromosome *in situ* hybridization will eventually revolutionize chromosome analysis by reducing the amount of time required to detect chromosomal abnormalities.

Specimen The specimen required will depend on the reason the test is requested. Leukemia samples would require peripheral blood or bone marrow. This test can also be performed on amniotic fluid cells and chorionic villi. **CONTAINER:** Blood should be collected in a green top (sodium heparin) tube, 5 mL minimum; bone marrow should be collected in a heparinized syringe (20-25 units heparin), 1-2 mL minimum; amniotic fluid should be collected in a sterile syringe used to draw the fluid from the patient, 10-20 mL minimum. See Amniotic Fluid, Chromosome and Genetic Abnormality Analysis listing for more collection information. **STORAGE INSTRUCTIONS:** All specimens must be sent to the laboratory **immediately** after collection. Maintain at room temperature. **CAUSES FOR REJECTION:** Specimen more than 24 hours old, or specimen clotted or hemolyzed due to the use of improper anticoagulant will yield suboptimal result. Specimens that are unlabeled or mislabeled are not acceptable. **TURNAROUND TIME:** Usually 48-72 hours are required.

Interpretive **REFERENCE RANGE:** Normal chromosome number. Interpretation is usually provided with the report. **USE:** *In situ* hybridization of chromosomes is useful in prenatal diagnosis of chromosomal abnormalities such as those with trisomies, Turner's syndrome, or Klinefelter's syndrome. These studies are useful in pregnant women who are at risk for having an offspring with chromosomal abnormalities. It is currently recommended that all *in situ* hybridization studies be done in conjunction with standard cytogenetic studies. **LIMITATIONS:** Specimen must be received in the laboratory as soon as possible after collection to assure viability of the cells. Some techniques of chromosome *in situ* hybridization does not require a metaphase spread and therefore does not require culture. Freezing or heating the sample can cause cell lysis. **METHODOLOGY:** Cells from the specimen are first immobilized on a microscope slide and fixed with a methanol:acetic acid fixative. The DNA in the cells is then denatured to make it available for hybridization with the specific probe. A denatured, labeled probe (biotin or fluorescent) is added to the cells and allowed to hybridize. The complementary sequences in the target DNA (cells from the specimen) will bind the probe. After washing the cells to remove the excess probe, the specifically bound DNA probe is then detected using a series of fluorescein-labeled reagents and a fluorescent microscope. **ADDITIONAL INFORMATION:** Chromosome *in situ* hybridization is a recently introduced specialized procedure, but is rapidly becoming an important offering of cytogenetic laboratories. Since chromosome *in situ* hybridization does not always require a cell to be in metaphase, results are more rapidly available than with standard cytogenetic tests, which usually require cell culture and extensive examination of banding patterns. Therefore, use of this technique provides more rapid results in a variety of situations such as prenatal diagnosis of trisomies[2,3], determination of fetal sex[4], or studies for aneuploidy in tumors or leukemias.[5] Recently chromosome painting DNA probes have been utilized to examine an entire chromosome. Such new probe techniques should find increasing application in the detection of translocations, trisomies, and the identification of marker chromosomes.[6,7,8]

Footnotes

1. Kearney L, Bower M, Gibbons B, et al, "Chromosome 11q23 Translocations in Both Infant and Adult Acute Leukemias Are Detect by *In Situ* Hybridization With a Yeast Artificial Chromosome," *Blood*, 1992, 80(7):1659-65.
2. Cremer T, Landegent J, Bruckner A, et al, "Detection of Chromosome Aberrations in the Human Interphase Nucleus by Visualization of Specific Target DNAs With Radioactive and Nonradioactive *In Situ* Hybridization: Diagnosis of Trisomy 18 With Probe L1.84," *Hum Genet*, 1986, 74:346-52.
3. Julien C, Bazin A, Guyot B, et al, "Rapid Prenatal Diagnosis of Down Syndrome With *In Situ* Hybridization of Fluorescent DNA Probes," *Lancet*, 1986, ii:863-4.
4. Burns J, Chan VTW, Jonasson JA, et al, "Sensitive System for Visualizing Biotinylated DNA Probes Hybridized *In Situ*: Rapid Sex Determination of Intact Cells," *J Clin Pathol*, 1985, 38:1085-92.
5. Eastmond DA and Pinkel D, "Aneuploidy Detection by Analysis of Interphase Nuclei Using Fluorescence *In Situ* Hybridization With Chromosome-Specific Probes," *Prog Clin Biol Res*, 1989, 318:277-84.
6. Cremer T, Lichter P, Borden J, et al, "Detection of Chromosome Aberrations in Metaphase and Interphase Tumor Cells by *In Situ* Hybridization Using Chromosome-Specific Library Probes," *Hum Genet*, 1988, 80:235-46.
7. Kraker WJ, Borell TJ, Schad CR, et al, "Fluorescent *In Situ* Hybridization: Use of Whole Chromosome Paint Probes to Identify Unbalanced Chromosome Translocations," *Mayo Clin Proc*, 1992, 67(7):658-62.

8. Jenkins RB, Le Beau MM, Kraker WJ, et al, "Fluorescence *In Situ* Hybridization: A Sensitive Method for Trisomy 8 Detection in Bone Marrow Specimens," *Blood*, 1992, 79(12):3307-15.

References

Pinkel D, Straume T, and Gray JW, "Cytogenetic Analysis Using Quantitative, High-Sensitivity Fluorescence Hybridization," *Proc Natl Acad Sci U S A*, 1986, 83:2934-8.

Trask BJ, "Fluorescence *In Situ* Hybridization: Applications in Cytogenetics and Gene Mapping," *Trends Genet*, 1991, 7(5):149-54.

Chromosome Karyotype, Amniotic Fluid *see* Amniotic Fluid, Chromosome and Genetic Abnormality Analysis *on page 891*

Chromosome Karyotype, Blood *see* Chromosome Analysis, Blood or Bone Marrow *on page 898*

Chromosome Studies *see* Chromosome Analysis, Blood or Bone Marrow *on page 898*

Chromosome Studies, Amniotic Fluid *see* Amniotic Fluid, Chromosome and Genetic Abnormality Analysis *on page 891*

Chronic Myelogenous Leukemia *see* Breakpoint Cluster Region Rearrangement in CML *on page 895*

Constant Region of T-Cell Receptor *see* Gene Rearrangement for Leukemia and Lymphoma *on page 911*

Cystic Fibrosis Carrier Detection *see* Cystic Fibrosis DNA Detection *on this page*

Cystic Fibrosis DNA Detection

CPT *83890 (molecular isolation or extraction); 83892 (enzymatic digestion); 83894 (separation); 83898 (nucleic acid probe with amplification)*

Related Information

Alpha$_1$-Fetoprotein, Amniotic Fluid *on page 114*
Amniotic Fluid, Chromosome and Genetic Abnormality Analysis *on page 891*
Amniotic Fluid Pulmonary Surfactant *on page 126*
Chloride, Sweat *on page 183*
Polymerase Chain Reaction *on page 927*
Tryptic Activity, Stool *on page 1161*

Synonyms Cystic Fibrosis Carrier Detection; Cystic Fibrosis, Prenatal Diagnosis; Genetic Detection of Cystic Fibrosis; Molecular Diagnosis of Cystic Fibrosis; Mutation Test for Cystic Fibrosis

Test Commonly Includes Detection of the major genetic mutations responsible for causing cystic fibrosis

Abstract Recent developments have identified the gene defects responsible for cystic fibrosis (CF).[1,2,3] The defective gene was discovered in 1989. Until the cystic fibrosis gene was identified there was no information on the biochemical basis of CF. Since the discovery of the gene numerous studies have clarified the function of both the normal CF gene product and the defective gene product responsible for disease. Genetic studies can be done on both carriers and patients to identify the defect and risk of disease. A list of common mutations can be found in the table. Some mutations are associated with milder forms of cystic fibrosis. This information will be useful in the management of disease and as a diagnostic tool.

Specimen 10-20 mL amniotic fluid, 10-15 mL whole blood, 30-50 mg wet chorionic villus **CONTAINER:** Blood should be collected in a yellow top (ACD) Vacutainer® tube; blood collected in a lavender top (EDTA) Vacutainer® tube is also acceptable. Amniotic fluid and chorionic villus should be collected in a sterile manner and transferred to a sterile tube for transport or to a T25 culture flask. **SAMPLING TIME:** Amniotic fluid should be collected between the 17th and 18th week of pregnancy. Chorionic villus specimens should be collected between the 8th and 12th week of gestation. **COLLECTION:** All specimens should be sent to the laboratory **immediately** after collection preferably by overnight delivery. **STORAGE INSTRUCTIONS:** All specimens should be maintained at room temperature or refrigerated, never frozen. **CAUSES FOR REJECTION:** Any amniotic fluid specimen that is bloody may be contaminated with maternal blood and is unsuitable for this test. Specimens that are unlabeled or mislabeled are not acceptable. **TURNAROUND TIME:** Times vary from 10-21 days before results are available.

(Continued)

Cystic Fibrosis DNA Detection *(Continued)*

Mutations Identified With the Cystic Fibrosis Disease Gene

Name	Mutation	Location	Footnote	Frequency
delF508	3 bp deletion	Exon 10	5	70%–73%
D110H	G →C (460)	Exon 4	10	NA
R117H	G →A (482)	Exon 4	10	0.4%
621+1	G →T (621)	Exon 4	15	0.6%
R347P	C →G (1173)	Exon 7	10	1.1%
A455E	C →A (1496)	Exon 9	7	NA*
Q493X	C →T (1609)	Exon 10	7	NA
dell507	3 bp deletion	Exon 10	7	0.4%
1717-1	G →A (1717-1)	Intron 10	7	0.6%
G542X	G →T (1756)	Exon 11	7	2.2%
S549N	G →A (1778)	Exon 11	6	0.1%
S549I	G →T (1778)	Exon 11	7	NA
S549R	T →G (1779)	Exon 11	7	NA
G551D	G →A (1784)	Exon 11	6	2.4%
R553X	C →T (1789)	Exon 11	6	1.1%
A559T	G →A (1807)	Exon 11	6	NA
R560T	G →C (1811)	Exon 11	7	1.0%
Y563N	T →A (1819)	Exon 12	7	NA
P574H	C →A (1853)	Exon 12	7	NA
2566insAT	AT insertion (2566)	Exon 13	11	NA
W846X	G →A (2670)	Exon 14a	12	NA
Y913C	A →G (2870)	Exon 15	12	NA
3659delC	C deletion (3659)	Exon 19	7	NA
S1255X	C →A (3896)	Exon 20	13	NA
W1282X	G →A (3978)	Exon 20	12	1.6%
N1303K	C →G (4041)	Exon 21	14	1.7%

*NA means that this information is not available on the mutation.

Interpretive REFERENCE RANGE: The laboratory usually provides an interpretive report which includes a risk analysis. USE: This test is indicated for a family with history of cystic fibrosis. For this purpose it is helpful to have a complete family pedigree that includes all medical histories. This test is also indicated for prenatal diagnosis in couples known to be carriers. It is helpful in diagnosing neonates in whom cystic fibrosis is suspected, but who have had equivocal sweat tests. The American Society of Human Genetics has recently published guidelines for the use of genetic testing of cystic fibrosis carriers.

Recommendations: Although the sensitivity of carrier testing for CF has improved and pilot studies are under way, CF testing is not recommended, at this time, for individuals or couples who do not have a family history of CF. Individuals with a positive family history of CF or who have a blood relative identified as a CF carrier should be offered CF testing with appropriate education and counseling. Optimally, carrier testing should be offered prior to conception, to provide a couple the broadest range of reproductive options.

When indicated, CF counseling and testing should adhere to the following guidelines.

- Screening should be voluntary, and confidentiality must be ensured.
- Screening requires informed consent. Pretest education should explain the benefits and hazards (eg, stigmatization and possible loss of insurability).
- Providers of screening services have the obligation to ensure that adequate post-test counseling is provided.
- Quality control of all aspects of laboratory testing, including systemic proficiency testing, is required.

- As with all indicated healthcare services, there should be equal access to testing.

Efforts should be expanded to educate healthcare providers and the public, regarding the complexities of CF screening in particular and issues involved in genetic healthcare services in general.[4]

LIMITATIONS: The estimated carrier rate for cystic fibrosis in the United States is 1 in 25. The current technology will detect 10-20 of the most common cystic fibrosis mutations, however, other mutations are also responsible for this disease. An extensive list can be found in footnote 15. Individuals found to be negative for the known mutations reduce their chance of being cystic fibrosis carriers to 1 in 250. Thus, a negative result does not rule out the possibility that an individual is a cystic fibrosis carrier but can lower that probability. **METHODOLOGY:** DNA is isolated from the specimen and several regions on chromosome 7 are amplified using the polymerase chain reaction. Several of the most common cystic fibrosis mutations are detected within the amplified regions of DNA. The presence of these mutations results in a smaller amplified DNA product or a DNA product which reflects a change in restriction enzyme sites. These changes can be detected visually after digestion with appropriate restriction enzymes and gel electrophoresis. Some laboratories will assay for cystic fibrosis mutations by directly examining the specimen DNA using Southern blot techniques. These assays require a longer turnaround time and are rapidly being replaced by the amplification technique. **ADDITIONAL INFORMATION:** Cystic fibrosis is inherited as an autosomal recessive disorder and affects approximately 1 in 2500 Caucasians.[5] The disease locus was initially mapped to chromosome 7q31.[6] The gene responsible for the disease has recently been identified and was found to have over 250 kilobases and codes for a protein that contains 1480 amino acids. This protein was found to be a transmembrane protein that regulated the conduction of ions across epithelial cell membranes.[1,2] The most common mutation causing the disease has been identified in the tenth exon of this gene as a deletion of three nucleotides. The loss of these nucleotides removes a phenylalanine codon at position 508 (delF508) in the first ATP binding domain.[3] This mutation accounts for approximately 70% of all cystic fibrosis chromosomes, while the remaining 30% of cystic fibrosis chromosomes are made up of numerous heterogeneous mutations.[7,8] Over 150 of these less common mutations have now been identified. Several of these mutations occur with reasonable frequency, while the others are rare (see table). A special NIH Workshop on Population Screening for the Cystic Fibrosis Gene in March 1990 recommended that the delF508 test "be offered to all individuals and couples with a family history of cystic fibrosis".[9] Currently these tests have a total detection rate >84% in Caucasian North American populations with European ancestry.[10]

Footnotes

1. Rommens JM, Iannuzzi MC, Kerem B-S, et al, "Identification of the Cystic Fibrosis Gene: Chromosome Walking and Jumping," *Science*, 1989, 245(4922):1059-65.
2. Riordan JR, Rommens JM, Kerem B-S, et al, "Identification of the Cystic Fibrosis Gene: Cloning and Characterization of Complementary DNA," *Science*, 1989, 245(4922):1066-73.
3. Kerem B-S, Rommens JM, Buchanan JA, et al, "Identification of the Cystic Fibrosis Gene: Genetic Analysis," *Science*, 1989, 245(4922):1073-80.
4. ASHG Ad Hoc Committee on Cystic Fibrosis Carrier Screening, "Statement of the American Society of Human Genetics on Cystic Fibrosis Carrier Screening," *Am J Hum Genet*, 1992, 51(6):1443-4.
5. Boat TF, Welsh MJ, and Beaudet AL, "Cystic Fibrosis", *The Metabolic Basis of Inherited Disease*, 6th ed, Scriver CR, Beaudet AL, Sly WS, et al, eds, New York, NY: McGraw-Hill Inc, 1989, 2649-80.
6. Tsui L-C, Buchwald M, Barker D, et al, "Cystic Fibrosis Locus Defined by a Genetically Linked Polymorphic DNA Marker," *Science*, 1985, 230:1054-7.
7. Cutting GR, Kasch LM, Rosenstein BJ, et al, "A Cluster of Cystic Fibrosis Mutations in the First Nucleotide-Binding Fold of the Cystic Fibrosis Conductance Regulator Protein," *Nature*, 1990, 346(6282):366-9.
8. Kerem B-S, Zielenski J, Markiewicz D, et al, "Identification of Mutations in Regions Corresponding to the Two Putative Nucleotide (ATP)-Binding Folds of the Cystic Fibrosis Gene," *Proc Natl Acad Sci U S A*, 1990, 87(21):8447-51.
9. Workshop on Population Screening for the Cystic Fibrosis Gene, "Statement From the National Institutes of Health Workshop on Population Screening for the Cystic Fibrosis Gene," *N Engl J Med*, 1990, 323(1):70-1.
10. Romeo G and Devoto M, "Population Analysis of the Major Mutation in Cystic Fibrosis," *Hum Genet*, 1990, 85:391-445.
11. Dean M, White MB, Amos J, et al, "Multiple Mutations in Highly Conserved Residues Are Found in Mildly Affected Cystic Fibrosis," *Cell*, 1990, 61(5):863-70.
12. White MB, Amos J, Hsu JMC, et al, "A Frame-Shift Mutation in the Cystic Fibrosis Gene," *Nature*, 1990, 344(6267):665-7.
13. Vidaud M, Fanen P, Martin J, et al, "Three Point Mutations in the CFTR Gene in French Cystic Fibrosis Patients: Identification by Denaturing Gradient Gel Electrophoresis," *Hum Genet*, 1990, 85(4):446-9.
14. Cutting GR, Kasch LM, Rosenstein BJ, et al, "Two Patients With Cystic Fibrosis, Nonsense Mutations in Each Cystic Fibrosis Gene and Mild Pulmonary Disease," *N Engl J Med*, 1990, 323(24):1685-9.

(Continued)

Cystic Fibrosis DNA Detection *(Continued)*

15. Tsui L-C and Buchwald M, "Biochemical and Molecular Genetics of Cystic Fibrosis," *Adv Hum Genet*, 1991, 20:153-266, 311-2.

References

Beaudet AL, "Carrier Screening for Cystic Fibrosis," *Am J Hum Genet*, 1990, 47(14):603-5.
Davies K, "Cystic Fibrosis. Complementary Endeavours," *Nature*, 1990, 348(6297):110-1.
Smith DR, Fulton TR, Swain P, et al, "Cystic Fibrosis: Diagnostic Testing and the Search for the Gene," *Clin Chem*, 1989, 35(7 Suppl):B17-20.
Weinberger SE, "Recent Advances in Pulmonary Medicine," *N Engl J Med*, 1993, 328(19):1389-97.

Cystic Fibrosis, Prenatal Diagnosis *see* Cystic Fibrosis DNA Detection *on page 903*

Cytogenetics *see* Chromosome Analysis, Blood or Bone Marrow *on page 898*

Detection of Aneuploidy in Tumor Metaphases *see* Chromosome *In Situ* Hybridization *on page 901*

Detection of Extra Chromosomes or Loss of Chromosomes in Leukemias *see* Chromosome *In Situ* Hybridization *on page 901*

Detection of Trisomies of Chromosomes 8, 13, 18, and 21 *see* Chromosome *In Situ* Hybridization *on page 901*

Detection of X and Y Chromosome *see* Chromosome *In Situ* Hybridization *on page 901*

DNA Amplification *see* Polymerase Chain Reaction *on page 927*

DNA Amplification Assay *see* Mycobacteria by DNA Probe *on page 921*

DNA Amplification of N-myc *see* N-myc Amplification *on page 925*

DNA Analysis for Parentage Evaluation *see* Identification DNA Testing *on page 918*

DNA Banking

CPT *83890*

Synonyms DNA Storage

Test Commonly Includes Isolation and storage of DNA specimens for future diagnostic testing

Abstract Understanding of the molecular basis of disease is proceeding at a rapid rate and will continue to progress into the next century. The sequencing of human genes has largely been due to the federally-supported Human Genome Project. One of the greatest advances expected from this project is the increase in diagnostic tests for inherited diseases and genetic abnormalities associated with cancers. This information will also elucidate the influence of the environment on genetic material. Thus, the storage of DNA from individuals or tumors will be invaluable both to scientists and to individuals interested in their family history of disease.

Specimen Whole blood, tissue, or cultured cells **CONTAINER:** Blood should be collected in yellow top (ACD) tubes; tissue should be frozen at -70°C; amniotic cells, fibroblasts, or lymphocytes should be grown in appropriate media in T25 tissue culture flasks. **COLLECTION:** A 0.1-1 g of tissue should be obtained. The specimen should then be put into a sealable plastic freezer bag and frozen at -70°C. The specimen should be kept frozen until shipped to the laboratory. Cell cultures should be grown to confluency and tightly sealed before shipping. **STORAGE INSTRUCTIONS:** Store tissue at -70°C or on dry ice. Peripheral blood should be stored and shipped at 4°C. Do **not** freeze blood. **CAUSES FOR REJECTION:** If the tissue specimen thaws out during transport to the laboratory or before shipping, DNA may not be obtained from the specimen; if less than 0.1 g of tissue is sent to the laboratory, it may not yield enough DNA for analysis; blood samples that have been frozen and thawed will yield low quality DNA. **TURNAROUND TIME:** Samples can be stored for an unlimited amount of time.

Interpretive **USE:** The storage of DNA isolated from individuals provides purified genetic material that can be used either for identification or for future diagnostic testing. **LIMITATIONS:** Failure to obtain DNA from the blood, tissue, or cultured cells due to inappropriate shipping or processing (as mentioned above) **METHODOLOGY:** DNA is released and isolated from the white blood cells, tissue, or cultured cells by lysing the cells and extracting the cell lysate with phenol and chloroform. Purified, intact DNA is precipitated with salt in the presence of alcohol.

The DNA is then stored indefinitely at -70°C usually at two separate facilities. **ADDITIONAL INFORMATION:** There has been remarkable progress recently in the field of diagnostic molecular biology. Rapid advances are expected to continue. The new tests currently being developed will analyze DNA for the diagnosis of genetic diseases and may facilitate the genetic testing of future generations.[1] This would enable individuals to have access to their genetic heritage which could be crucial to future family testing. Some of the other tests being developed will be able to diagnose certain cancers;[2] thus, it can sometimes be prudent to bank DNA from certain unusual cancers. Tissue from such cancers can be used to isolate DNA that can be stored for years at -70°C. This would allow investigation of the genetics of these cancers in the future. Stored DNA is always the property of the person from whom it was isolated. When family testing for either a genetic disease or cancer diagnosis is desired, signed permission is usually required before the sample is released. If the person owning the DNA is deceased then its disposition is under the control of a legal guardian or heir. All information received from DNA tests performed on any DNA sample is completely confidential and will be released only to the individual requesting the test (through an appropriate medical professional).

Footnotes

1. Katayama S, "Molecular Biological Approaches to Genetic Disorders in Prenatal Diagnosis," *Early Hum Dev*, 1992, 29(1-3):149-53.
2. Bishop JM, "The Molecular Genetics of Cancer," *Science*, 1987, 235:305-11.

References

Antonarakis SE, "Recombinant DNA Technology in the Diagnosis of Human Genetic Disorders," *Clin Chem*, 1989, 35(7 Suppl):B4-6.

Caskey CT, "Disease Diagnosis by Recombinant DNA Methods," *Science*, 1987, 236:1223-4.

Landegren V, Kaiser R, Caskey CT, et al, "DNA Diagnostic: Molecular Techniques and Automation," *Science*, 1988, 242:229-37.

DNA Fingerprinting *see* Identification DNA Testing *on page 918*

DNA Hybridization Test for *Borrelia burgdorferi* *see* Lyme Disease DNA Detection *on page 920*

DNA Hybridization Test for *Chlamydia trachomatis* *see Chlamydia trachomatis* DNA Probe *on page 897*

DNA Hybridization Test for HBV *see* Hepatitis B DNA Detection *on page 913*

DNA Hybridization Test for HPV *see* Human Papillomavirus DNA Probe Test *on page 916*

DNA Hybridization Test for Mycobacteria *see* Mycobacteria by DNA Probe *on page 921*

DNA Hybridization Test for *Mycoplasma pneumoniae* *see Mycoplasma pneumoniae* DNA Probe Test *on page 923*

DNA Hybridization Test for *Neisseria gonorrhoeae* *see Neisseria gonorrhoeae* DNA Probe Test *on page 924*

DNA Probe Test for HBV *see* Hepatitis B DNA Detection *on page 913*

DNA Probe Test for HPV *see* Human Papillomavirus DNA Probe Test *on page 916*

DNA Probe Test for Lyme Disease *see* Lyme Disease DNA Detection *on page 920*

DNA Storage *see* DNA Banking *on previous page*

DNA Test for *Chlamydia trachomatis* *see Chlamydia trachomatis* DNA Probe *on page 897*

DNA Test for Mycobacteria *see* Mycobacteria by DNA Probe *on page 921*

DNA Test for *Mycoplasma pneumoniae* *see Mycoplasma pneumoniae* DNA Probe Test *on page 923*

DNA Test for *Neisseria gonorrhoeae* *see Neisseria gonorrhoeae* DNA Probe Test *on page 924*

Duchenne/Becker Muscular Dystrophy Carrier Detection *see* Duchenne/Becker Muscular Dystrophy DNA Detection *on next page*

Duchenne/Becker Muscular Dystrophy DNA Detection

CPT *83890 (molecular isolation or extraction); 83892 (enzymatic digestion); 83894 (separation); 83896 (nucleic acid probe, each)*

Related Information

Alpha$_1$-Fetoprotein, Amniotic Fluid *on page 114*
Amniotic Fluid, Chromosome and Genetic Abnormality Analysis *on page 891*
Muscle Biopsy *on page 75*
Polymerase Chain Reaction *on page 927*

Synonyms Duchenne/Becker Muscular Dystrophy Carrier Detection; Duchenne/Becker Muscular Dystrophy, Prenatal Diagnosis; Genetic Detection of Duchenne/Becker Muscular Dystrophy; Molecular Diagnosis of Duchenne/Becker Muscular Dystrophy; Mutation Test for Duchenne/Becker Muscular Dystrophy

Applies to Dystrophin Protein

Test Commonly Includes This test can detect many of the major genetic deletions and insertions responsible for causing Duchenne or Becker muscular dystrophy.

Abstract Recent molecular biology advances have identified the muscular dystrophy gene on the short arm of the X chromosome. This information showed for the first time that Duchenne muscular dystrophy (DMD) and Becker muscular dystrophy (BMD) are actually allelic disorders. Allelic disorders are diseases caused by different mutation on the same gene. These molecular advances have increased the understanding of the biochemical defect in DMD and BMD and will enable the clinician to make a diagnosis based on molecular analysis. Currently, DNA studies for muscular dystrophy are offered by several DNA diagnostic laboratories, either private companies or associated with academic medical centers.

Specimen Whole blood, amniotic fluid, chorionic villus **CONTAINER:** Blood should be collected in yellow top (ACD) Vacutainer® tubes, blood collected in lavender top (EDTA) Vacutainer® tubes is also acceptable; amniotic fluid and chorionic villus should be collected in a sterile manner and transferred to a sterile tube for transport or to a T25 culture flask. **SAMPLING TIME:** Amniotic fluid should be collected between the 17th and 18th week of pregnancy. Chorionic villus specimens should be collected between the 8th and 12th week of gestation. **STORAGE INSTRUCTIONS:** All specimens should be sent to the laboratory **immediately** after collection, preferably by overnight delivery. All specimens should be kept at room temperature or refrigerated, never frozen. **CAUSES FOR REJECTION:** Any amniotic fluid specimen that is bloody may be contaminated with maternal blood and is unsuitable for this tests. Any specimen that has been frozen cannot be tested. Specimens that are unlabeled or mislabeled are not acceptable. **TURNAROUND TIME:** 10-21 days

Interpretive **REFERENCE RANGE:** The laboratory usually provides an interpretive report which includes a risk analysis. **USE:** This test is indicated for families with history of Duchenne or Becker muscular dystrophy. For this purpose it is helpful to have a complete family pedigree that includes all medical histories. This test is also indicated for prenatal diagnosis in females known to be carriers. It is also helpful in diagnosing neonates suspected of having Duchenne or Becker muscular dystrophy. **LIMITATIONS:** DNA analysis for Duchenne or Becker muscular dystrophy can only detect 65% of the deletions or insertions responsible for the disease. Thus, a negative result does not rule out the possibility that an individual is a muscular dystrophy carrier or affected, but it can lower that probability. **METHODOLOGY:** DNA is isolated from the specimen and several regions within the dystrophin gene are detected using Southern blotting techniques. Restriction enzyme digestion of the DNA in each exon can be examined for deletion or duplication. Because of the large size of the gene, as many as seven different Southern blots are required. Multiplex polymerase chain reaction (PCR) can be used to detect many of the most common deletions found at the 5' end of the gene. Several of the DNA regions can be amplified in the same PCR and a change (either loss or varied mobility) in the DNA fragments indicates a deletion or insertion. These changes can be detected visually after gel electrophoresis and staining with ethidium bromide. PCR cannot be used to detect the carrier status of females in affected families. To detect carrier status in females, a Southern blot is required with careful analysis to distinguish the copy number of particular regions of the DNA. In affected families in which there is no detectable deletion, linkage analysis can be done using Southern blotting to detect linkage to several known mutations.[1,2] **ADDITIONAL INFORMATION:** **Duchenne's muscular dystrophy**, the most common of the childhood dystrophies, is a severe crippling muscle disorder. **Becker muscular dystrophy** is a milder form with a similar clinical course followed at a much slower rate.[3] These are inherited as X-linked recessive disorders with an incidence of approximately 1 in 3500 male births. The gene responsible for these disorders has recently been cloned and the protein product has been identified as the dystrophin protein, a muscle cytoskeletal protein. This protein was found to be 400 kilodalton (kD) and the gene identified was very large, with a 14 kilobase (kb) transcript encoding more than 70 exons spread over 2500 kb of genomic DNA.[4,5] The polymerase chain reaction (PCR) and Southern blotting can both be used to detect alterations of the dystrophin gene. Approximately 65% of muscular dystrophy patients have detectable deletions or duplications that can be detected using Southern blots. In these families, females can be tested to detect carrier status and prenatal diagnosis can be done on either chorionic villus sampling or amniotic cells.[1,2] Many of the deletions in the dystrophin gene are found within two "hot-spot" regions at the 5' end of the gene.[6] Taking advantage of the clustering of deletions, the multiplex PCR analysis amplifies such particular DNA regions and compares them with normal DNA. Genetic deletions are detected as specimens missing one or more DNA bands when compared with DNA bands amplified from normal DNA.[7] The advantage of the PCR test over Southern blotting is the decreased turnaround time (1-2 days versus 1-2 weeks) and the increased sensitivity (as little as 0.5 mL of blood) which may be useful in prenatal diagnosis. However, this test cannot be used for carrier detection because the female carrier usually has a normal X chromosome that masks the deletion when the DNA is amplified. In cases with a positive family history but with no detectable mutation, a more intensive search using restriction fragment length polymorphism (RFLP)-linkage analysis can be done to determine the existence of known point mutations or alterations not detected by the other assay. This requires the participation of several family members (at least seven or eight) both affected and unaffected to correlate the inheritance pattern of the RFLPs with inheritance of disease. In many laboratories DNA analysis on a patient or prenatal diagnosis is performed first with PCR, and then, if negative, by Southern blot and then, if family history indicates, by the RFLP-linkage analysis.

Footnotes

1. Davies KE, Pearson PL, Harper PS, et al, "Linkage Analysis of Two Cloned DNA Sequences Flanking the Duchenne Muscular Dystrophy Locus on the Short Arm of the Human X Chromosome," *Nucleic Acids Res*, 1983, 11:2303-12.
2. Kingston HM, Sarfarazi M, Thomas NST, et al, "Localization of the Becker Muscular Dystrophy Gene on the Short Arm of the X Chromosome by Linkage to Cloned DNA Sequences," *Hum Genet*, 1984, 67:6-17.
3. Koenig M, Beggs AH, Moyer M, et al, "The Molecular Basis for Duchenne Versus Becker Muscular Dystrophy: Correlation of Severity With Type of Deletion," *Am J Hum Genet*, 1989, 45(4):498-506.
4. Monaco AP, Neve R, Colletti-Feener C, et al, "Isolation of Candidate cDNAs for Portions of the Duchenne Muscular Dystrophy Gene," *Nature*, 1986, 323:646-50.
5. Burghes AHM, Logan C, Hu X, et al, "A cDNA Clone From the Duchenne/Becker Muscular Dystrophy Gene," *Nature* (London), 1987, 328:434-7.
6. Forrest SM, Cross GS, Speer A, et al, "Preferential Deletion of Exons in Duchenne and Becker Muscular Dystrophies," *Nature* (London), 1987, 329:638-40.
7. Chamberlain JS, Gibbs RA, Ranier JE, et al, "Deletion Screening of the Duchenne Muscular Dystrophy Locus Via Multiplex DNA Amplification," *Nucleic Acids Res*, 1988, 16:11141-56.

References

Beggs AH and Kunkel LM, "Improved Diagnosis of Duchenne/Becker Muscular Dystrophy," *J Clin Invest*, 1990, 85(3):613-9.

Clemens PR, Fenwick RG, Chamberlain JS, et al, "Carrier Detection and Prenatal Diagnosis in Duchenne and Becker Muscular Dystrophy Families, Using Dinucleotide Repeat Polymorphisms," *Am J Hum Genet*, 1991, 49(5):951-60.

Darras BT, "Molecular Genetics of Duchenne and Becker Muscular Dystrophy," *J Pediatr*, 1990, 117(1 Pt 1):1-15.

Kunkel LM, Beggs AH, and Hoffman EP, "Molecular Genetics of Duchenne and Becker Muscular Dystrophy: Emphasis on Improved Diagnosis," *Clin Chem*, 1989, 35(7 Suppl):B21-4.

Duchenne/Becker Muscular Dystrophy, Prenatal Diagnosis *see* Duchenne/Becker Muscular Dystrophy DNA Detection *on previous page*

Dystrophin Protein *see* Duchenne/Becker Muscular Dystrophy DNA Detection *on previous page*

Fluorescent *in situ* Hybridization *see* Chromosome *In Situ* Hybridization *on page 901*

Fragile X, Carrier Detection *see* Fragile X DNA Detection *on next page*

Fragile X DNA Detection

CPT *83890 (molecular isolation or extraction); 83892 (enzymatic digestion); 83894 (separation); 83896 (nucleic acid probe, each)*

Related Information

Amniotic Fluid, Chromosome and Genetic Abnormality Analysis *on page 891*

Synonyms Fragile X, Carrier Detection; Fragile X, Prenatal Diagnosis; Genetic Detection of Fragile X Syndrome; Molecular Diagnosis of Fragile X; Mutation Test for Fragile X

Test Commonly Includes This test can detect the major genetic insertions responsible for causing fragile X mental retardation.

Abstract Fragile sites are chromosome loci where breaks occur frequently. One of these fragile sites on the X chromosome is linked to a heritable mental retardation syndrome associated with specific physical characteristics. This fragile site was first identified by cytogenetic analysis and has recently been characterized at the DNA level. An unstable region of DNA has been identified on the X chromosome that defines the cytogenetic fragile site. Insertions of DNA repeat sequences within this region of the chromosome make the chromosomal structure unstable and interrupts the expression of a gene, FMR-1. Genetic studies can now be done to determine the presence of this fragile site in both patients affected with fragile X mental retardation and in female carriers of the unstable X chromosome.

Specimen Whole blood, amniotic fluid, chorionic villus **CONTAINER:** Blood should be collected in yellow top (ACD) Vacutainer® tubes, blood collected in lavender top (EDTA) Vacutainer® tubes is also acceptable; amniotic fluid and chorionic villus should be collected in a sterile manner and transferred to a sterile tube for transport or to a T25 culture flask. Some laboratories prefer that amniotic cells are cultured prior to shipping, therefore it is advisable to contact the laboratory before collecting the sample. **SAMPLING TIME:** Amniotic fluid should be collected between the 17th and 18th week of pregnancy. Chorionic villus specimens should be collected between the 8th and 12th week of gestation. **STORAGE INSTRUCTIONS:** All specimens should be sent to the laboratory **immediately** after collection, preferably by overnight delivery. If amniotic cells need to be cultured the specimen should be transferred quickly to T25 flasks with culture media. All other specimens should be kept at room temperature or refrigerated, never frozen. **CAUSES FOR REJECTION:** Any amniotic fluid specimen that is bloody may be contaminated with maternal blood and is unsuitable for this tests. Any specimen that has been frozen cannot be tested. Specimens that are unlabeled or mislabeled are not acceptable. **TURNAROUND TIME:** 10-21 days

Interpretive **REFERENCE RANGE:** The laboratory usually provides an interpretive report which includes a risk analysis. **USE:** This test is indicated for a family with a history of fragile X syndrome. For this purpose it is helpful to have a complete family pedigree that includes all medical histories. This test is also indicated for prenatal diagnosis in females known to be carriers of the fragile X premutation. It is also helpful in diagnosis of neonates suspected of the fragile X syndrome. Genetic testing of several family members to determine the characteristic of the mutation is sometimes required. **LIMITATIONS:** DNA analysis for fragile X syndrome can detect >98% of the insertions and premutations responsible for the disease. A negative result does not completely rule out the possibility that an individual is a fragile X carrier or an affected individual, but the test can greatly lower that probability. **METHODOLOGY:** DNA is extracted from the specimen and then digested with restriction enzymes, electrophoresed, and blotted onto a solid support using Southern blotting technique. This DNA is then probed with a radiolabeled DNA probe to the fragile X region of the X chromosome (Xq27.3). This region contains an unstable repeated sequence that can amplify in length with successive generations. Such insertions can be identified with this technique and will distinguish individuals at risk for being carriers of the premutation.[1] Recently an individual was identified with a deletion within the same region who showed a clinical phenotype of fragile X syndrome.[2] The same technique was able to identify this deletion as well. **ADDITIONAL INFORMATION:** Fragile X syndrome is the most common form of inherited mental retardation in humans. It is characterized by mental retardation, macro-orchidism, and characteristic facial dysmorphy. The disease segregates as an X-linked dominant disorder with variable penetrance. Individuals of either sex can exhibit characteristics of the disease.[3] Cytogenetically this syndrome is associated with a fragile site at Xq27.3, which appears as a chromosomal gap on metaphase chromosomal preparations from patients.[4] Recently, a gene, FMR-1, with an unstable region has been identified at the fragile X locus. This unstable region contains a trinucleotide repeat $p(CCG)_n$ which shows variable copy number. In families affected with fragile X, this sequence shows amplification and the length of this region correlates with clinical fragile X expression. There is a direct relationship between increased $p(CCG)_n$ copy number and manifestation of fragile X syndrome phenotype.[5] Thus, current experimental evidence indicates that this unstable region represents the molecular basis of the fragile X syndrome. To date, all families showing the cytogenetic fragile X site in chromosomal preparations also show the premutation and amplifications of this site in DNA analysis. Studies are currently underway to identify other mutations in the FMR-1 gene that associate with the fragile X syndrome.

Footnotes

1. Yu S, Pritchard M, Kremer E, et al, "Fragile X Genotype Characterized by an Unstable Region of DNA," *Science*, 1991, 252(5010):1179-81.
2. Wohrle D, Kotzot D, Hirst MC, et al, "A Microdeletion of Less Than 250 kb, Including the Proximal Part of the FMR-1 Gene and the Fragile X Site, in a Male With the Clinical Phenotype of Fragile X Syndrome," *Am J Hum Genet*, 1992, 51(2):299-306.
3. Sutherland GR, "The Enigma of the Fragile X Chromosome," *Trends Genet*, 1985, 1:108-12.
4. Sutherland GR and Baker E, *Am J Med Genet*, 1986, 23:409-19.
5. Poustka A, Dietrich A, Langenstein G, et al, "Physical Map of Human Xq27-qter: Localizing the Region of the Fragile X Mutation," *Proc Natl Acad Sci U S A*, 1991, 88(19):8302-6.

References

Bell MV, Hirst MC, Nakahori Y, et al, "Physical Mapping Across the Fragile X: Hypermethylation and Clinical Expression of the Fragile X Syndrome," *Cell*, 1991, 64(4):861-6.

Hirst MC, Nakahori Y, Knight SJ, et al, "Genotype Prediction in the Fragile X Syndrome," *J Med Genet*, 1991, 28(12):824-9.

Richards RI, Shen Y, Holman K, et al, "Fragile X Syndrome: Diagnosis Using Highly Polymorphic Microsatellite Markers," *Am J Hum Genet*, 1991, 48(6):1051-7.

Fragile X, Prenatal Diagnosis *see* Fragile X DNA Detection *on previous page*

Gene Rearrangement, BCR *see* Breakpoint Cluster Region Rearrangement in CML *on page 895*

Gene Rearrangement for Leukemia and Lymphoma

CPT *83890 (molecular isolation or extraction); 83892 (enzymatic digestion); 83894 (separation); 83896 (nucleic acid probe, each)*

Related Information

bcl-2 Gene Rearrangement *on page 893*
Body Fluids Cytology *on page 482*
Bone Marrow *on page 524*
Histopathology *on page 57*
Immunoperoxidase Procedures *on page 60*
Immunophenotypic Analysis of Tissues by Flow Cytometry *on page 65*
Lymph Node Biopsy *on page 72*
Skin Biopsies *on page 84*
T- and B-Lymphocyte Subset Assay *on page 750*

Synonyms Leukemia Gene Rearrangement; Lymphocyte T-Cell Receptor Gene Rearrangement; Lymphoma Gene Rearrangement

Applies to Constant Region of T-Cell Receptor; Joining Region of B-Cell Receptor; Kappa Light Chains; Lambda Light Chains

Test Commonly Includes Detection of unique DNA rearrangements associated with T- and B-cell leukemias and lymphomas

Abstract New molecular biology techniques allow for detection of receptor genes rearrange from germline DNA to that in maturing T or B cells. As lymphoid cells mature they go through rearrangements of variable, joining, and constant DNA coding regions of immunoglobulin or T-cell receptors. Such recombinations allow for almost unlimited diversity of immune responses allowing response to literally millions of antigens. Lymphoma and lymphocytic leukemia are neoplastic disorders, diagnosis of which requires the demonstration of clonal expansion of lymphoid cells. In the typical case, demonstration of clonality may be satisfied immunophenotypically by demonstration of surface T- and B-cell markers. When immunophenotypic methods fail to demonstrate clonality, the detection of T-cell and B-cell receptor gene rearrangements may be an invaluable adjunct study.

Specimen Use **peripheral whole blood** for leukemia or lymphoma cells in the blood. Buffy coat is isolated by centrifugation. If large contamination with normal cells exists, Ficoll-Hypaque is used to separate the leukemia or lymphoma cells from normal granulocytes. **Lymph node biopsy** of suspected lymphoma is obtained during surgery for histological diagnosis, immunophenotyping, and gene rearrangement assay. Other tissue such as skin biop-

(Continued)

Gene Rearrangement for Leukemia and Lymphoma *(Continued)*

sies, gastrointestinal tissue, and bone marrow may also be studied for gene rearrangement. **CONTAINER:** Lavender top (EDTA) tube or green top (heparin) tube **STORAGE INSTRUCTIONS:** Isolated white cells, lymph nodes, or tissue can be frozen at -70°C until DNA is extracted. **CAUSES FOR REJECTION:** Insufficient DNA isolated. Muscle tissue yields little DNA for analysis. **TURNAROUND TIME:** 10 days to 3 weeks

Interpretive **REFERENCE RANGE:** No unique rearrangement of T- and B-cell receptors is found in normal white blood cells. An interpretive report is usually included with results. **USE:** Gene rearrangement may be used to supplement and complement conventional histopathology and immunophenotyping in the diagnosis of lymphoid leukemia and lymphoma. Gene rearrangement studies have revealed that most lymphoid leukemias are pre-B cells and not non-B, non-T. Such leukemic cells have rearrangements of genes coding for B-cell receptors, but are too immature to express cytoplasmic or surface immunoglobulins. Occasionally, lymphoid leukemia and lymphoma are of T-cell phenotype, which may be confirmed using probes designed to detect rearrangements of genes coding for T-cell receptors. Rarely, lymphoid neoplasms may have rearrangements of both T- and B-cell genes.[1,2]

Lymphoproliferative Disease and Gene Rearrangements*

Lymphoproliferative Disease	Rearrangement, % of Cases				
	Immunoglobulin			T-Cell Receptor	
	IgH	κ	λ	β	γ
B-cell					
Precursor B ALL	100	40	20	10–30	40
B CLL; B follicular lymphoma	100	100	30	<20	<10
Diffuse lymphoma — large cell, Burkitt's, and undifferentiated	100	100	30	0	0
Hairy cell leukemia	100	100	75	...	...
T-cell					
Precursor T ALL	10–20	0	0	90	95
Diffuse lymphoma	0	0	0	100	...
MF/Sèzary syndrome	2	0	0	100	...
T CLL	0	0	0	100	...
Tλ LPD	0	0	0	60	...
ATL	0	0	0	100	...
Lymphomatoid papulosis	0	0	0	66	...
Other					
Hodgkin's disease	30–60	30–60	...	50	...
AILD	40	40	...	100	...
AML	5	...	...	10	30

From Crossman J, Uppenkamp M, Sundeen J, et al, "Molecular Genetics and the Diagnosis of Lymphoma," *Arch Pathol Lab Med,* 1988, 112:120, with permission.

*ALL = acute lymphocytic leukemia
CLL = chronic lymphocytic leukemia
MF = mycosis fungoides LPD, lymphoproliferative disorder
ATL = adult T cell leukemia/lymphoma
AILD = angioimmunoblastic lymphadenopathy with dysproteinemia
AML = acute myelogenous leukemia

LIMITATIONS: Some tissue yield little DNA or DNA that is degraded. Lymph nodes with <1% tumor cells cannot provide evidence of gene rearrangements. **METHODOLOGY:** Genomic DNA is extracted from the nuclei of leukemic or lymphomatous nuclei with removal of protein and lipids using detergent (sodium dodecyl sulfate), and proteolytic enzymes followed by extraction in phenol:chloroform. DNA is precipitated with alcohol and resuspended in low salt buffer. It is then digested with restriction endonucleases that recognize specific nucleotide sequences and cut DNA at such specific points (as though the enzymes were specialized scissors). Digested DNA is electrophoresed in agarose gel to separate DNA fragments by size and is then transferred to nitrocellulose or nylon filters by Southern blotting. DNA is permanently immobilized to the filter and is exposed to labeled gene probes. Such probes anneal to immobilized DNA according to the exact base pairing of target and probe. The match must essentially be highly specific to bind under the conditions of hybridization. Specificity of most probes **is nearly perfect**. Detection of rearrangements thus may help to demonstrate clonality (neoplastic nature) of an atypical lymphoid lesion. Filters containing hybridized DNA-probe complexes are examined for bands after autoradiography or color detection to ascertain if germline or unique gene rearrangements are present. Guidelines for interpretation and use of gene rearrangements in the diagnosis of lymphomas and leukemias have recently been published.[3] **ADDITIONAL INFORMATION:** This procedure is useful in determining whether T- or B-cell gene rearrangements exist in lymphoid neoplasms. A list of various tumors and gene rearrangements can be seen in the table. Most commonly used probes are for the joining region of B-cell receptors (J_H) and the constant region of the T-cell receptor (C_BT). B-cell maturation may be further categorized by determining if kappa and/or lambda light chain genes have undergone rearrangement, using probes directed against their constant or joining DNA regions. Gene rearrangements may be detected in minute quantities of tissue, sometimes as little as 200 mg. The assay is so sensitive that gene rearrangements may be detected in larger specimens even if the percentage of cancer cells is 1%. Gene rearrangement studies are invaluable adjunctive tests that may provide evidence of clonality in an atypical lymphoid infiltrate when other methods fail. They may become a standardized diagnostic modality, should results of these studies with greater experience be found useful for therapeutic or prognostic purposes.

Footnotes

1. Farkas DH, "The Southern Blot: Application to the B- and T-Cell Gene Rearrangement Test," *Lab Med*, 1992, 23:723-9.
2. Cossman J, Uppenkamp M, Sundeen J, et al, "Molecular Genetics and the Diagnosis of Lymphoma" *Arch Pathol Lab Med*, 1988, 112(2):117-27.
3. Cossman J, Zehnbauer B, Garrett CT, et al, "Gene Rearrangements in the Diagnosis of Lymphoma/ Leukemia: Guidelines for Use Based on a Multi-institutional Study," *Am J Clin Pathol*, 1991, 95(3):347-54.

References

Harrington DS, "Molecular Gene Rearrangement Analysis in Hematopathology," *Am J Clin Pathol*, 1990, 93(4 Suppl 1):S38-43.

Korsmeyer SJ, Arnold A, Bakhshi A, et al, "Immunoglobulin Gene Rearrangement and Cell Surface Antigen Expression in Acute Lymphocytic Leukemias of T-Cell and B-Cell Precursor Origins," *J Clin Invest*, 1983, 71:301-13.

Genetic Detection of Cystic Fibrosis *see* Cystic Fibrosis DNA Detection *on page 903*

Genetic Detection of Duchenne/Becker Muscular Dystrophy *see* Duchenne/ Becker Muscular Dystrophy DNA Detection *on page 908*

Genetic Detection of Fragile X Syndrome *see* Fragile X DNA Detection *on page 910*

Genetic Detection of Presymptomatic Adult Polycystic Kidney Disease *see* Adult Polycystic Kidney Disease DNA Detection *on page 889*

Genetic Identification by DNA Fingerprinting *see* Identification DNA Testing *on page 918*

Gen-Probe® Rapid Diagnostic System for *Mycoplasma pneumoniae* *see* *Mycoplasma pneumoniae* DNA Probe Test *on page 923*

HBV DNA *see* Hepatitis B DNA Detection *on this page*

HBV DNA Probe Test *see* Hepatitis B DNA Detection *on this page*

Hepatitis B DNA Detection

***CPT** 83890 (molecular isolation or extraction); 83892 (enzymatic digestion); 83894 (separation); 83896 (nucleic acid probe, each)*

Related Information

Hepatitis A Antibody, IgM *on page 683*
Hepatitis B Core Antibody *on page 684*
Hepatitis B_e Antibody *on page 685*
Hepatitis B_e Antigen *on page 686*
Hepatitis B Surface Antibody *on page 687*
Hepatitis B Surface Antigen *on page 688*
(Continued)

Hepatitis B DNA Detection *(Continued)*

Hepatitis C Serology *on page 690*
Hepatitis D Serology *on page 691*
Viral Culture, Tissue *on page 1206*

Synonyms DNA Hybridization Test for HBV; DNA Probe Test for HBV; HBV DNA; HBV DNA Probe Test; Hepatitis B Viral DNA Assay

Test Commonly Includes Use of an HBV specific DNA probe for the detection of HBV viral DNA in serum samples or tissue. Sometimes the HBV DNA is amplified by polymerase chain reaction (PCR).

Abstract Chronic viral hepatitis is due to infection with the human hepadnavirus, hepatitis B (HBV). Infection may result in a long-term carrier state of either mild to severe chronic liver disease. Two weeks after infection with hepatitis B a large excess of viral protein can be detected in serum (surface antigen of HBV) and is followed by an antibody response to the viral proteins (anti-HB_s). The antihepatitis B response will persist in most patients for life. However, about 10% of HBV infections result in a chronic carrier state marked by a lack of seroconversion. Diagnosis in these cases should be supplemented by additional analysis. Hepatitis B viral DNA can be detected in the serum or liver tissue from these individuals. Recent studies on symptomatic individuals with chronic liver disease of unknown etiology show that >90% are positive when tested for HBV DNA;[1] indicating that current serological testing does not detect all infections due to HBV. With the rapid growth of technology in this area, it is expected that DNA testing for HBV will soon be done in routine clinical laboratories.

Specimen Serum or plasma, liver tissue **CONTAINER:** Red top tube or lavender top (EDTA) tube, sterile container **STORAGE INSTRUCTIONS:** Serum or plasma should be transferred to a plastic tube and kept frozen at -20°C. Tissue should be frozen at -70°C. **CAUSES FOR REJECTION:** Samples containing sodium azide cannot be used in this test. **TURNAROUND TIME:** 4-7 days; turnaround time may vary with individual laboratories.

Interpretive **REFERENCE RANGE:** No HBV viral DNA detected **USE:** This test aids clinicians in the diagnosis of HBV versus the other non-B hepatitis entities and helps establish the stage of disease.[2] **METHODOLOGY:** A slot-blot DNA hybridization based assay is used. DNA extracted from serum or plasma is denatured in an alkaline solution and is then filtered through a nylon membrane. The DNA binds to the nylon membrane and specific HBV DNA is detected by using a radiolabeled DNA probe. Hybridization with the HBV DNA probe is detected using autoradiography. **ADDITIONAL INFORMATION:** The DNA probe assay provides a direct measure of HBV in serum or plasma and correlates with infectivity titers. The information provided from this test should be used in conjunction with serologic tests and HBV antigen detection. DNA detection should not replace serologic testing. Amplification of HBV DNA has been reported and may soon replace the currently used DNA blot assay.[3,4]

Footnotes

1. Overby LR and Houghton M, "Hepatitis Viruses," *Laboratory Diagnosis of Viral Infections*, 2nd ed, Chapter 19, Lennette EH, ed, New York, NY: Murcel Dekken Inc, 1992, 403-41.
2. Brechot C, Degos F, Lugassy C, et al, "Hepatitis B Virus DNA in Patients With Chronic Liver Disease and Negative Tests for Hepatitis B Surface Antigen," *N Engl J Med*, 1985, 312:270-6.
3. Larzul D, Guigue F, Sninsky JJ, et al, "Detection of Hepatitis B Virus Sequences in Serum by Using *In Vitro* Enzymatic Amplification," *J Virol Methods*, 1988, 20:227-37.
4. Kaneko S, Feinstone SM, and Miller RH, "Rapid and Sensitive Method for the Detection of Serum Hepatitis B Virus DNA Using the Polymerase Chain Reaction Technique," *J Clin Microbiol*, 1989, 27(9):1930-3.

References

Weller IVD, Fowler MJF, Monjardino J, et al, "The Detection of HBV DNA in Serum by Molecular Hybridisation: A More Sensitive Method for the Detection of Complete HBV Particles," *J Med Virol*, 1982, 9:273-80.

Hepatitis B Viral DNA Assay *see* Hepatitis B DNA Detection *on previous page*

HIV DNA Amplification Assay *see* Human Immunodeficiency Virus DNA Amplification *on next page*

HIV DNA PCR Test *see* Human Immunodeficiency Virus DNA Amplification *on next page*

HPV DNA Probe Test *see* Human Papillomavirus DNA Probe Test *on page 916*

HPV Screen *see* Human Papillomavirus DNA Probe Test *on page 916*

HPV Type *see* Human Papillomavirus DNA Probe Test *on page 916*

Human Immunodeficiency Virus DNA Amplification

***CPT** 83890 (molecular isolation or extraction); 83898 (nucleic acid probe with amplification)*

Related Information

HIV-1/HIV-2 Serology *on page 696*
Human Immunodeficiency Virus Culture *on page 1185*
p24 Antigen *on page 727*
Polymerase Chain Reaction *on page 927*
T- and B-Lymphocyte Subset Assay *on page 750*
Viral Culture, Tissue *on page 1206*

Synonyms HIV DNA Amplification Assay; HIV DNA PCR Test; Human Immunodeficiency Virus (HIV) Proviral DNA by Polymerase Chain Reaction Amplification; PCR for HIV DNA

Test Commonly Includes HIV DNA is detected by amplifying specific proviral DNA sequences from peripheral blood lymphocytes and subsequent hybridization with a specific HIV DNA probe.

Abstract Human immunodeficiency virus (HIV) is the causative agent of acquired immune deficiency syndrome (AIDS). Currently, testing for HIV is based on evidence of circulating antibody to the viral proteins. Commercially available tests are remarkably accurate with a low false-positive rate (1:135,000).[1] However, accuracy of the test is compromised during the time interval between infection and the development of antibody to HIV. The exact time to seroconversion is controversial but certain cases of accidental exposure have shown seroconversion to occur within 2-3 months.[2] Babies born to HIV-infected mothers will be seropositive for HIV due to transplacental antibodies. Studies have shown that only 30% to 50% of babies born to HIV infected mothers are actually infected with the virus.[1] Thus, the serologic test is unreliable for assessing HIV infection in these populations.

This virus contains an RNA genome that will incorporate into host DNA as proviral DNA. The target cells of this virus are the CD4 (T4) T-lymphocytes (helper T cells) and monocytes/macrophage populations; however, during infection, few such peripheral blood cells contain HIV.[3] To detect the incorporated viral genome, the DNA must be amplified. This procedure specifically increases the amount of DNA within the HIV genome, and the amplified DNA product is detected by specific binding to an HIV probe. The DNA detection assay has been useful for the diagnosis of HIV in infants and for monitoring individuals with a known exposure to HIV.

Specimen Peripheral blood lymphocytes from 10-20 mL whole blood **CONTAINER:** Two yellow top (ACD), lavender top (EDTA), or green top (sodium heparin) tubes should be collected. Type of tube is dependent on the laboratory performing the test. **STORAGE INSTRUCTIONS:** Tubes of blood can be sent directly to the laboratory at ambient temperature and should arrive within 48 hours of collection. **CAUSES FOR REJECTION:** Specimens with inadequate volume or more than 48 hours old may be rejected. **TURNAROUND TIME:** 2 weeks is usually required. Turnaround time may vary with individual laboratories.

Interpretive **REFERENCE RANGE:** No HIV viral DNA detected in peripheral blood lymphocytes. **USE:** HIV detection in patients with unusual or indeterminant HIV serology.[4] It may also be useful in patients with immunodeficiency syndromes characterized by a negative HIV serology and Western blot tests. **METHODOLOGY:** DNA amplification is used, polymerase chain reaction (PCR).[5] DNA is extracted from peripheral blood lymphocytes. The proviral HIV DNA is exponentially amplified by using specific primers that bind to regions of the HIV genome. Using a series of denaturation, annealing, and polymerization steps the original proviral DNA can be amplified 10^5 to 10^6 fold (see figure in the Polymerase Chain Reaction listing in this chapter). The amplified HIV DNA is confirmed by hybridization with an HIV specific DNA probe. Hybridization with the HIV DNA probe can be detected using autoradiography or enzymatic detection procedures. **ADDITIONAL INFORMATION:** Currently, the diagnosis of HIV infection is dependent on the detection of specific antibodies.[4] The antibody screening test commonly used is the enzyme linked immunosorbent assay (ELISA) with a confirmatory Western blot or immunoblot. These serologic assays will identify individuals with prior exposure to HIV or passively obtained antibody such as babies born to HIV-positive mothers. In addition, serologic tests may not identify patients with recent active infection. Due to this problem, other tests have also been used to document the presence of HIV, such as viral antigen assays, viral culture, and the detection of viral DNA.[3,5,6] Viral culture of HIV is a prolonged procedure taking 3-4 weeks; it suffers from a lack of sensitivity in that HIV cannot be consistently isolated from seropositive patients.[7] Studies using *in situ* hybridization have shown that few peripheral blood mononuclear cells may actually harbor HIV proviral DNA (1 in 10,000).[3] This makes it difficult to directly assay for HIV proviral DNA. Thus, DNA amplification assays have been developed to detect HIV DNA. The assay most commonly used is the polymerase chain reaction (PCR), which can

(Continued)

Human Immunodeficiency Virus DNA Amplification *(Continued)*

amplify a single copy of DNA by 10^5 to 10^6 fold.[8] The PCR test for HIV DNA is useful in resolution of unsatisfactory HIV antibody test results and in determination of the status of children born to mothers with positive HIV serology[9,10] without the need for viral culture.

Footnotes

1. Wilber JC, "Human Immunodeficiency Viruses: HIV-1 and HIV-2," *Laboratory Diagnosis of Viral Infections*, 2nd ed, Chapter 22, Lennette EH, ed, New York, NY: Marcel Dekker Inc, 1992, 477-94.
2. Bowen PA, Lobel SA, Caruana RJ, et al, "Transmission of Human Immunodeficiency Virus (HIV) by Transplantation: Clinical Aspects and Time Course Analysis of Viral Antigenemia and Antibody Production," *Ann Intern Med*, 1988, 108(1):46-8.
3. Harper ME, Marselle LM, Gallo RC, et al, "Detection of Lymphocytes Expressing Human T-Lymphotropic Virus Type III in Lymph Nodes and Peripheral Blood From Infected Individuals by *In Situ* Hybridization," *Proc Natl Acad Sci U S A*, 1986, 83:772.
4. Burke DS, Brundage JF, Redfield RR, et al, "Measurement of False-Positive Rate in a Screening Program for Human Immunodeficiency Virus Infections," *N Engl J Med*, 1988, 319(15):961-4.
5. Jackson JB, Sannerud KJ, Hopsicker JS, et al, "Hemophiliacs With the HIV Antibody Are Actively Infected," *JAMA*, 1988, 260(15):2236-9.
6. Goudsmit J, Wolfe F, Paul DA, et al, "Expression of Human Immunodeficiency Virus Antigen (HIVOAg) in Serum and Cerebrospinal Fluid During Acute and Chronic Infection," *Lancet*, 1986, 2:177-80.
7. Feorino PM, Kulyanaraman VS, Haverkos HW, et al, "Lymphadenopathy Associated Virus Infection of a Blood Donor-Recipient Pair With Acquired Immunodeficiency Syndrome," *Science*, 1984, 225:69.
8. Saiki RK, Gelfand DH, Stoffel S, et al, "Primer-Directed Enzymatic Amplification of DNA With a Thermostable DNA Polymerase," *Science*, 1988, 239(4839):487-91.
9. Rogers MF, Ou C-Y, Rayfield M, et al, "Use of the Polymerase Chain Reaction for Early Detection of the Proviral Sequences of Human Immunodeficiency Virus in Infants Born to Seropositive Mothers," *N Engl J Med*, 1989, 320(25):1649-54.
10. Imagawa DT, Lee MH, Wolinsky SM, et al, "Human Immunodeficiency Virus Type 1 Infection in Homosexual Men Who Remain Seronegative for Prolonged Periods," *N Engl J Med*, 1989, 320(22):1458-62.

References

Loche M and Mach B, "Identification of HIV-Infected Seronegative Individuals by a Direct Diagnostic Test Based on Hybridisation to Amplified DNA," *Lancet*, 1988, 2:418-21.

Phair JP and Wolinsky S, "Diagnosis of Infection With the Human Immunodeficiency Virus," *Clin Infect Dis*, 1992, 15(1):13-6.

Sheppard HW, Dondero D, Arnon J, et al, "An Evaluation of the Polymerase Chain Reaction in HIV-1 Seronegative Men," *J Acquir Immune Defic Syndr*, 1991, 4(8):819-23.

Human Immunodeficiency Virus (HIV) Proviral DNA by Polymerase Chain Reaction Amplification *see* Human Immunodeficiency Virus DNA Amplification *on previous page*

Human Papillomavirus DNA Probe Test

CPT *83890 (molecular isolation or extraction); 83892 (enzymatic digestion); 83894 (separation); 83896 (nucleic acid probe, each)*

Related Information

Cervical/Vaginal Cytology *on page 491*
Histopathology *on page 57*
Viral Culture, Tissue *on page 1206*
Viral Culture, Urogenital *on page 1207*

Synonyms DNA Hybridization Test for HPV; DNA Probe Test for HPV; HPV DNA Probe Test; HPV Screen; HPV Type; ViraPap®; ViraType®

Test Commonly Includes Screening specimens for the presence of HPV and optional determination of the specific type(s) of HPV present in positive specimens

Abstract Papillomaviruses are nonencapsulated icosahedral viruses which belong to the papovavirus family. The life cycle of HPV is linked to squamous cell differentiation. HPV infection of the uterine cervix is venereally transmitted. It causes koilocytosis, condyloma acuminatum, and cervical intraepithelial neoplasia. Squamous epithelial lesion, SIL, is defined *vida infra*. Many other such viral infections probably have little oncogenic potential.

Patient Care PREPARATION: At least 2 days must elapse between the time acetic acid or iodine preparations are used and the time swab specimens are taken. Biopsies can be taken immediately after the use of acetic acid or iodine.

Specimen Cervical swab, cervical biopsy, vulvar biopsy CONTAINER: **Specific** tubed transport medium provided by the laboratory. Do **not** substitute. SAMPLING TIME: At the time of clinical suspicion of HPV infection COLLECTION: Use **specific** swab provided by the laboratory to collect endocervical and ectocervical cells similar to the manner in which Pap smear cells are taken. Obtain biopsy in usual manner. Biopsies **must** be ≤3 mm. Cervical cells also can be taken by **scraping** the cervix with an appropriate spatula. Place swabs, scrapings, and biopsies into specific transport medium. **Important:** Collection of a sufficiently large number of epithelial cells is mandatory. However, scraping/removal of cells to the point of bleeding should not be done, because visible blood in specimen might reduce the chance of detecting HPV. **STORAGE INSTRUCTIONS:** Freeze biopsies in transport medium immediately. Swab or scrape specimens can be stored at room temperature for several days, but for simplicity, can be frozen immediately. **CAUSES FOR REJECTION:** Some laboratories reject visibly bloody specimens. **TURNAROUND TIME:** Usually 4 days to 2 weeks, but depends on laboratory protocol and lability of radioactive reagents

Interpretive **REFERENCE RANGE:** HPV has been found in genital lesions of both normal and symptomatic persons.[1,2] **USE:** Aid clinicians in making decisions regarding treatment, follow-up visits and tests, management, and prognosis of patients with HPV infections **LIMITATIONS:**

- Detects only 7 of the approximately 57 genotypes of HPV, of which 20 have been isolated from the female genital tract
- Can be negative with accompanying cytological changes
- Can be positive without accompanying cytological changes; by Southern blot hybridization, HPV DNA is found in approximately 15% of morphologically normal cervices
- Viral integration is not always found in invasive carcinoma of the uterine cervix
- Can give false-negative results if specimens are visibly bloody or if an insufficient sample of HPV-infected cells is obtained
- Latent viral infection does not cause morphologic abnormalities
- A wide variety of HPV types is found in CIN 1
- Can give borderline results
- Expensive

Recognizing that HPV plays an important role in the development of SIL, Kurman observes that identification of HPV DNA in the uterine cervix by Southern blot hybridization, *in situ* hybridization, or PCR for clinical diagnosis and management of the preinvasive squamous proliferative lesions represent technologic advances for which the value has not been determined. He indicates (1993) that **the routine use of this test at present is not recommended**.

METHODOLOGY: Disruption and digestion of specimen, attachment of specimen DNA to filters, and probing denatured (HPV) DNA with commercially available RNA probes which are specific for HPV types 6, 11, 16, 18, 31, 33, and 35. **ADDITIONAL INFORMATION:** The presence of HPV types 6/11, 16/18, and 31/33/35 has been associated with "low" (condyloma), "high," and "moderate" risk of development of cervical cancer, respectively.[3,4] HPV 16 is found in 20% of CIN 1, 40% of CIN 2, and 66% of CIN 3 and is found in about 50% of the invasive squamous cell carcinomas of the cervix. HPV 18 is found in about 20% of invasive cervical squamous cell carcinomas. HPV detection in intraepithelial proliferative lesions of the cervix segregate into two morphologic groups. The **Bethesda System** provides **low grade and high grade squamous intraepithelial lesion** (SIL) classifications, in which low grade corresponds to CIN 1. High grade lesions are CIN 2, and 3, moderate and severe dysplasia and carcinoma *in situ*. The utility of HPV typing continues to be studied.

The screening test is FDA-approved, and the typing test currently is pending FDA approval.

Footnotes

1. Meanwell CA, Cox MF, Blackledge G, et al, "HPV 16 DNA in Normal and Malignant Cervical Epithelium: Implications for the Aetiology and Behavior of Cervical Neoplasia," *Lancet*, 1987, 1:703-7.
2. deVilliers EM, Wagner D, Schneider A, et al, "Human Papillomavirus Infections in Women With and Without Abnormal Cervical Cytology," *Lancet*, 1987, 2:703-6.
3. zurHausen H and Schneider A, "The Role of Papillomaviruses in Human Anogenital Cancer," Salzmann NP and Howley PM, eds, *The Papovaviridae*, Vol 2, "The Papillomaviruses," New York, NY: Plenum, 1987, 245-63.
4. Shah KV and Buscema J, "Genital Warts, Papillomaviruses, and Genital Malignancies," *Annu Rev Med*, 1988, 39:371-9.

References

Bauer HM, Ting Y, Greer CE, et al, "Genital Human Papillomavirus Infection in Female University Students as Determined by A PCR-Based Method," *JAMA*, 1991, 265(4):472-7.

Chang F, "Role of Papillomaviruses," *J Clin Pathol*, 1990, 43(4):269-76.

Crum CP and Roche JK, "Molecular Pathology of the Lower Female Genital Tract – The Papillomavirus Model," *Am J Surg Pathol*, 1990, 14(Suppl 1):26-33.

Howley PM and Schlegel R, "The Human Papillomaviruses. An Overview," *Am J Med*, 1988, 85:155-8.

(Continued)

Human Papillomavirus DNA Probe Test *(Continued)*

Kurman RJ, "Current Concepts in the Relationship of HPV Infection to the Pathogenesis and Classification of Precancerous Squamous Lesions of the Cervix," *Current Issues in Surgical Pathology*, XII, University of Texas Southwestern Medical Center at Dallas, May, 1993, (discussion).

Lungu O, Sun XW, Felix J, et al, "Relationship of Human Papillomavirus Type to Grade of Cervical Intraepithelial Neoplasia," *JAMA*, 1992, 267(18):2493-6.

Milde-Langosch K, Schreiber C, Becker G, et al, "Human Papillomavirus Detection in Cervical Adenocarcinoma by Polymerase Chain Reaction," *Hum Pathol*, 1993, 24(6):590-4.

Reid R, ed, "Human Papillomavirus," *Obstet Gynecol Clin North Am*, 1987, 14:329-614.

Roman A and Fife KH, "Human Papillomaviruses: Are We Ready to Type?" *Clin Microbiol Rev*, 1989, 2(2):166-90.

Identification DNA Testing

CPT *83890 (molecular isolation or extraction); 83892 (enzymatic digestion); 83894 (separation); 83896 (nucleic acid probe, each)*

Related Information

HLA Typing, Single Human Leukocyte Antigen *on page 701*
Paternity Studies *on page 1074*
Tissue Typing *on page 757*

Synonyms DNA Analysis for Parentage Evaluation; DNA Fingerprinting; Genetic Identification by DNA Fingerprinting; Parentage Studies; Paternity Testing; RFLP Analysis for Parentage Evaluation

Test Commonly Includes Identification of individuals by using DNA polymorphic regions

Abstract The progress in the field of DNA technology and the ongoing Human Genome Project has resulted in a tremendous store of information about the genetic material that makes each individual unique. The human genome is made up of about 120 million base pairs organized into 46 different chromosomes. Half of an individual's genetic material is "donated" by their mother while the other half is "donated" by their father. The DNA from both maternal and paternal sources may be normal, but will have slight variations in character. These variations can be detected and used to map heredity much like the variations in blood group antigens and the human leukocyte antigen (HLA) system. By using between 20-30 different polymorphic sites on different chromosomes, identity or parentage can be established with up to 99.99% exclusion probability.[1,2]

Patient Care PREPARATION: Patient should receive no transfusions 90 days prior to testing.

Specimen Peripheral whole blood, tissue, semen, or cultured cells CONTAINER: Blood should be collected in a yellow top (ACD) tube or lavender top (EDTA) tube; tissue should be frozen at -70°C; amniotic cells, fibroblasts, or lymphocytes should be grown in appropriate media in T25 tissue culture flasks. COLLECTION: A 0.1-1 g of tissue should be obtained. The specimen should then be put into a sealable plastic freezer bag and frozen at -70°C. The specimen should be kept frozen until shipped to the laboratory. Cell cultures should be grown to confluency and tightly sealed before shipping. STORAGE INSTRUCTIONS: Store tissue at -70°C or on dry ice. Peripheral blood should be stored and shipped at 4°C. Do **not** freeze blood. CAUSES FOR REJECTION: If the tissue specimen thaws out during transport to the laboratory or before shipping, DNA may not be obtained from the specimen; if less than 0.1 g of tissue is sent to the laboratory, it may not yield enough DNA for analysis; blood samples that have been frozen and thawed will yield low quality DNA; specimens inadequately identified will be rejected. TURNAROUND TIME: 2-4 weeks. Samples of DNA can be stored for an unlimited amount of time.

Interpretive REFERENCE RANGE: The laboratory bears an obligation to communicate results in confidence. The test provides a 99.99% exclusion probability. USE: The analysis of highly polymorphic regions of human DNA can clarify the relationships between individuals and verify the identify of unknown individuals (such as suspects in criminal investigations or unidentified victims of murder). LIMITATIONS: Failure to obtain DNA from the blood, tissue, or cultured cells due to inappropriate shipping or processing (as mentioned above) METHODOLOGY: DNA is released and isolated from the white blood cells, tissue, or cultured cells by lysing the cells and extracting the cell lysate with phenol and chloroform. Purified, intact DNA is precipitated with salt in the presence of alcohol. The DNA is then digested with various restriction enzymes and electrophoresed through an agarose gel. DNA is then transferred to a solid support such as a nylon membrane and hybridized with a radioactive DNA probe. After washing the unhybridized DNA probe off the membrane, the target DNA is exposed to x-ray film to detect the polymorphic regions of DNA. All autosomal genes are inherited as a pair. One gene copy is of maternal origin and one copy is of paternal origin. Certain regions of the human genome show a high degree of polymorphism in that >85% of the population show heterogeneity.[3] These regions are highly informative in determining DNA identification. When human DNA in these regions is digested with different restriction enzymes, the size and pattern of the DNA fragments will vary with each individual. This pattern is an inherited trait and if the appropriate family members are tested, the inheritance pattern can be established. This is important in determining the paternity of a child or if a set of twins is heterozygous or monozygous. This can also help establish the identity of an unknown criminal or victim. **ADDITIONAL INFORMATION:** The genetic material of humans is highly polymorphic and an individual's genotype will represent a unique pattern that determines that persons identity and heredity. The only exception to this rule is identical twins, since they are derived from a single fertilized egg and hence have the same DNA profile.[4] As a general rule, DNA is constant in all tissues of the body (even prenatal samples such as amniotic cells and chorionic villi specimens). DNA isolated from any specimen from an individual will be identical, which can prove to be very valuable in forensic evidence.[5]

DNA typing provides a valuable tool for establishing family relationships and associations between forensic specimens (dried blood, semen, hair, skin scrapings, etc) and criminal suspects. Southern blots using a panel of DNA probes specific for several polymorphic DNA regions can produce a composite profile which is unique to an individual and can be traced through families to establish relationships.[1,6] DNA identification can be used for many applications such as paternity identification, identification of military casualties, clarifying parentage of infants possibly switched at birth or abducted, immigration disputes dealing with relationships, determination of sexual abuse and rape, as well as other criminal investigations.[2,7] Healthcare professionals are often involved in collecting specimens. Great care should be taken in the collection and storage of these specimens to prevent contamination and to preserve the evidence which may be crucial to any legal case.[7]

Footnotes

1. Honma M and Ishiyama I, "Application of DNA Fingerprinting to Parentage and Extended Family Relationship Testing," *Hum Hered*, 1990, 40(6):356-62.
2. Jeffreys AJ, Turner M, and Debenham P, "The Efficiency of Multilocus DNA Fingerprint Probes for Individualization and Establishment of Family Relationships, Determined From Extensive Casework," *Am J Hum Genet*, 1991, 48(5):824-40.
3. Nakamura Y, Leppert M, O'Connell P, et al, "Variable Number of Tandem Repeat (VNTR) Markers For Human Gene Mapping," *Science*, 1987, 253:1616-22.
4. Jones L, Thein SL, Jefferys AJ, et al, "Identical Twin Marrow Transplantation for 5 Patients With Chronic Myeloid Leukemia: Role of DNA Fingerprinting to Confirm Monozygosity in 3 Cases," *Eur J Haematol*, 1987, 37:144-7.
5. Gill P, Jefferys AJ, and Werret DJ, "An Evaluation of DNA Fingerprinting for Forensic Purposes," *Electrophoresis*, 1987, 8:38-44.
6. Balazs I, Baird M, Clyne M, et al, "Human Population Genetics Studies of Five Hypervariable DNA Loci," *Am J Hum Genet*, 1989, 44(2):182-90.
7. Lander ES, "Research on DNA Typing Catching Up With Courtroom Application [Invited Editorial]", *Am J Hum Genet*, 1991, 48(5):819-23.

References

McCabe ER, "Application of DNA Fingerprinting in Pediatric Practice," *J Pediatr*, 1992, 120(4 Pt 1):499-509.
Walker RH, "Molecular Biology in Paternity Testing," *Lab Med*, 1992, 23:752-7.
Wolff RK, Nakanura Y, and White R, "Molecular Characterization of a Spontaneously Generated New Allele at VNTR Locus: No Exchange of Flanking DNA Sequences," *Genomics*, 1988, 3:347-51.
Wong Z, Wilson V, Jeffreys AJ, et al, "Cloning a Selected Fragment From a Human DNA Fingerprint: Isolation of an Extremely Polymorphic Minisatellite," *Nucleic Acids Res*, 1986, 14:4605-16.

Inherited Disorders *see* Chromosome Analysis, Blood or Bone Marrow *on page 898*

***In situ* Chromosome Hybridization** *see* Chromosome *In Situ* Hybridization *on page 901*

Joining Region of B-Cell Receptor *see* Gene Rearrangement for Leukemia and Lymphoma *on page 911*

Kappa Light Chains *see* Gene Rearrangement for Leukemia and Lymphoma *on page 911*

Karyotype *see* Chromosome Analysis, Blood or Bone Marrow *on page 898*

Lambda Light Chains *see* Gene Rearrangement for Leukemia and Lymphoma *on page 911*

Leukemia Gene Rearrangement *see* Gene Rearrangement for Leukemia and Lymphoma *on page 911*

Lyme Disease DNA Detection

CPT *87179*

Related Information

Lyme Disease Serology *on page 719*
Polymerase Chain Reaction *on page 927*

Synonyms *Borrelia burgdorferi* DNA Assay; *Borrelia burgdorferi* DNA Probe Test; DNA Hybridization Test for *Borrelia burgdorferi*; DNA Probe Test for Lyme Disease

Test Commonly Includes DNA from the spirochete *Borrelia burgdorferi* is amplified from a patient specimen and specific DNA hybridization is used to detect the amplified product.

Abstract Lyme disease was first recognized in the U.S. in Wisconsin in 1969. Since that time sporadic epidemics of Lyme disease have been reported primarily in the northeastern and upper midwestern United States, California, Georgia, and Texas. Isolated reports have occurred in 46 states. The disease is caused by the spirochete *Borrelia burgdorferi*. Epidemics tend to occur in the spring and fall when the tick vector, *Ixodes ricinus*, is proliferating. The tick transmits the spirochete to humans through bites. The diagnosis of Lyme disease is difficult due to the insensitivity and unreliability of serological tests. Thus, recent developments have made available a DNA based test that can detect *Borrelia burgdorferi* in body fluids such as serum, spinal fluid, synovial fluid, and urine. This test can often establish the diagnosis of Lyme disease when serologic tests are equivocal.

Specimen Serum or plasma, cerebrospinal fluid, synovial fluid, urine **CONTAINER:** Red top tube or lavender top (EDTA) tube for blood samples. Spinal fluid and synovial fluid should be collected in a sterile container. Plastic container is used for urine. **SAMPLING TIME:** Urine should be collected before antibiotic therapy is initiated. **STORAGE INSTRUCTIONS:** All specimens should be sent to the laboratory immediately or kept at 4°C until shipped to the laboratory. Once in the laboratory, serum or plasma should be transferred to a sealed plastic tube. **CAUSES FOR REJECTION:** Samples containing sodium azide cannot be used in this test; samples left at extreme temperature will yield suboptimal results. **TURNAROUND TIME:** 2-3 weeks

Interpretive **REFERENCE RANGE:** Lack of *Borrelia burgdorferi* DNA detection **USE:** Detect the presence of DNA from the spirochete *Borrelia burgdorferi* in patients with signs and symptoms of Lyme disease **METHODOLOGY:** Patient specimens are treated to isolate DNA and rid the sample of substances that inhibit amplification of DNA. The DNA is then amplified using specific primers for *Borrelia burgdorferi* sequences. The amplified DNA is then confirmed to be *B. burgdorferi* by hybridization with a DNA probe. **ADDITIONAL INFORMATION:** Transmission of *Borrelia burgdorferi*, a pathogenic spirochete, to humans occurs primarily by way of infected *Ixodid* ticks, including *I. dammini*, *I. pacificus*, and others, the *Ixodes ricinus* complex. The signs and symptoms of Lyme disease vary, but the most common clinical manifestation following the bite of an infected tick is a distinctive skin lesion, erythema chronicum migrans. This initial stage of Lyme disease is benign and is usually successfully treated with oral antibiotics. Symptoms sometimes persist or reappear after antibiotic treatment and the later stage disease may include chronic progressive encephalomyelitis, chronic severe arthritis, as well as various cardiac manifestations.[1,2,3] Direct microscopic detection of *Borrelia burgdorferi* is difficult, therefore the most widely used indicator of infection is *Borrelia burgdorferi*-specific antibodies. However, serologic studies have limited sensitivity and antibody can be detected in only 40% to 60% of infected patients.[4] Serological testing also appears to suffer from lack of sensitivity, specificity, and reproducibility when examined in a trial proficiency testing program.[5] Thus, a more direct and sensitive method to diagnosis Lyme disease has been needed. Infected patients appear to have spirochetes in their tissues, serum, or spinal fluids. The amplification of *Borrelia burgdorferi* DNA provides the ability to detect the organism in a specific and sensitive assay from patient specimens. A test for direct detection of *Borrelia burgdorferi* DNA would enable the clinician to detect the dissemination of the spirochete early in the course of infection.[2,3,6] Thus, appropriate antibiotic therapy can be initiated. It also allows for monitoring of patients during and after chemotherapy. This is a valuable diagnostic tool since recognition of Lyme disease is often complicated by the variety of clinical signs, and alternative diagnostic tests lack the sensitivity of the DNA detection assay.

Footnotes

1. Steere AC, Schoen RT, and Taylor E, "The Clinical Evolution of Lyme Arthritis," *Ann Intern Med*, 1987, 107:725-31.
2. Reik L, Steere AC, Bartenhagen NH, et al, "Neurologic Abnormalities of Lyme Disease," *Medicine (Baltimore)*, 1979, 58:281-94.

3. Steere AC, Batsford WP, Weinberg M, et al, "Lyme Carditis: Cardiac Abnormalities of Lyme Disease," *Ann Intern Med*, 1980, 93:8-16.
4. Grodzicki RL and Steere AC, "Comparison of Immunoblotting and Indirect Enzyme-Linked Immunosorbent Assay Using Different Antigen Preparations for Diagnosing Early Lyme Diseases," *J Infect Dis*, 1988, 157(4):790-7.
5. Bakker LL, Case KL, Callister SM, et al, "Performance of 45 Laboratories Participating in a Proficiency Testing Program for Lyme Disease Serology," *JAMA*, 1992, 268(7):891-5.
6. Luft BJ, Steinman CR, Neimark HC, et al, "Invasion of the Central Nervous System by *Borrelia burgdorferi* in Acute Disseminated Infection," *JAMA*, 1992, 267(10):1364-7.

References

Guy EC and Stanek G, "Detection of *Borrelia burgdorferi* in Patients With Lyme Disease by the Polymerase Chain Reaction," *J Clin Pathol*, 1991, 44(7):610-1.

Kaslow RA, "Current Perspective on Lyme Borreliosis," *JAMA*, 1992, 267(10):1381-3.

Malloy DC, Nauman RK, and Paxton H, "Detection of *Borrelia burgdorferi* Using the Polymerase Chain Reaction," *J Clin Microbiol*, 1990, 28(6):1089-93.

Rosa PA and Schwan TG, "A Specific and Sensitive Assay for the Lyme Disease Spirochete *Borrelia burgdorferi* Using the Polymerase Chain Reaction," *J Infect Dis*, 1989, 160(6):1018-29.

Steere AC, "*Borrelia burgdorferi* (Lyme Disease, Lyme Borreliosis)," *Principles and Practice of Infectious Diseases*, 3rd ed, Chapter 217, Mandell GL, Douglas RG Jr, and Bennett JE, eds, New York, NY: Churchill Livingstone, 1990, 1819-27.

Lymphocyte T-Cell Receptor Gene Rearrangement *see* Gene Rearrangement for Leukemia and Lymphoma *on page 911*

Lymphoma Gene Rearrangement *see* Gene Rearrangement for Leukemia and Lymphoma *on page 911*

Molecular Cytogenetics *see* Chromosome *In Situ* Hybridization *on page 901*

Molecular Diagnosis of Cystic Fibrosis *see* Cystic Fibrosis DNA Detection *on page 903*

Molecular Diagnosis of Duchenne/Becker Muscular Dystrophy *see* Duchenne/Becker Muscular Dystrophy DNA Detection *on page 908*

Molecular Diagnosis of Fragile X *see* Fragile X DNA Detection *on page 910*

Molecular Diagnosis of Polycystic Kidney Disease *see* Adult Polycystic Kidney Disease DNA Detection *on page 889*

Mosaicism *see* Chromosome Analysis, Blood or Bone Marrow *on page 898*

Mutation Test for Cystic Fibrosis *see* Cystic Fibrosis DNA Detection *on page 903*

Mutation Test for Duchenne/Becker Muscular Dystrophy *see* Duchenne/Becker Muscular Dystrophy DNA Detection *on page 908*

Mutation Test for Fragile X *see* Fragile X DNA Detection *on page 910*

Mycobacteria by DNA Probe

CPT *87179*

Related Information

Acid-Fast Stain *on page 770*
Biopsy or Body Fluid Mycobacteria Culture *on page 782*
Cerebrospinal Fluid Mycobacteria Culture *on page 801*
Skin Mycobacteria Culture *on page 846*
Sputum Mycobacteria Culture *on page 855*
Stool Mycobacteria Culture *on page 863*
Urine Mycobacteria Culture *on page 884*

Synonyms DNA Hybridization Test for Mycobacteria; DNA Test for Mycobacteria; Mycobacteria DNA Detection Test; Mycobacterial Accuprobe®

Applies to DNA Amplification Assay

Test Commonly Includes Direct detection of mycobacterial DNA in patient specimens or after primary culture

Abstract The number of infections due to *Mycobacterium tuberculosis* has risen dramatically in the last few years. This increased frequency of infection is due to patients with acquired immune deficiency syndrome, patients with malignant disorders and immunosuppression, I.V.
(Continued)

Mycobacteria by DNA Probe *(Continued)*

drug users, prison inmates, refugees and immigrants, nursing home residents, and the homeless population.[1,2] The lack of a rapid and unequivocal means of detecting *M. tuberculosis* from patients is a major obstacle in establishing effective infection control. Culture and identification of this organism can take up to 8 weeks and direct staining procedures are insensitive. Thus, the ability to detect specific mycobacterial DNA directly from the patient specimen has a great advantage in diagnosis and treatment of this disease. Nucleic acid tests are also available to determine the species of *Mycobacterium* after isolation by culture. Many of the culture confirmation DNA tests for *Mycobacterium* are available in larger clinical laboratories.

Specimen Whole blood, sputum, pleural fluid, cerebrospinal fluid, bronchial aspirates, urine, and tissue biopsy **CONTAINER:** Blood requires a yellow top (ACD) Vacutainer® tube. Sputum, pleural fluid, and cerebrospinal fluid should be collected and transported in a tightly sealed plastic container such as a sputum cup or a sterile bronchoscopy tube. This container should be transferred into a secondary sealed container for transport. **COLLECTION:** Samples should be collected as for mycobacteria culture. Sputum should be collected as early in the morning as possible, preferably before the morning meal. Urine should be collected in midvoid as for culture. **STORAGE INSTRUCTIONS:** The specimens should be kept refrigerated if not immediately processed. Do not freeze. **CAUSES FOR REJECTION:** Containers contaminated on the outside may be rejected. They pose a risk to laboratory personnel. Samples that are left at room temperature for more than 12 hours may be rejected due to overgrowth of other bacteria. Samples that are frozen will be rejected because of dilution of DNA. **TURNAROUND TIME:** Approximately 4-7 days

Interpretive **REFERENCE RANGE:** No mycobacteria DNA detected **USE:** This test provides for the rapid detection of *Mycobacterium* species in clinical specimens. **METHODOLOGY:** Cells from the patient specimen are lysed and the DNA is denatured by heating. A specific *Mycobacterium* DNA probe is then hybridized to the denatured specimen DNA. After hybridization the excess probe is removed and the bound probe is detected by chemiluminescence, color detection, or autoradiography. (Radioisotopes are less commonly used and are being replaced with chemiluminescence.) **ADDITIONAL INFORMATION:** Mycobacteria are aerobic rod-shaped bacteria noted for their very slow growth. The laboratory diagnosis of mycobacterial disease is currently based on a positive acid-fast stain and on laboratory culture of the mycobacterial organism. The most common isolates in the United States are *Mycobacterium tuberculosis* and species within the *Mycobacterium avium* complex.[3] Because of the long culture periods required and the difficulty of isolation, the detection and identification of mycobacteria to the species level has been difficult. Often clinical and therapeutic decisions are made before a laboratory diagnosis is available. To improve upon the detection of mycobacteria, DNA detection assays have been developed that have increased sensitivity and specificity when compared with culture assays and have a decreased turnaround time.[4,5] Recently, several studies have shown that amplification of mycobacterial DNA in patient specimens is feasible and can provide a rapid and sensitive diagnosis.[6,7] Because of its increased sensitivity, DNA amplification assay for mycobacteria may soon replace DNA detection assay.

Footnotes

1. Center for Disease Control, "A Strategic Plan for the Elimination of Tuberculosis in the United States," *MMWR Morb Mortal Wkly Rep*, 1989, 38(16):269-72.
2. Rieder HL, Cauthen GM, Kelly GD, et al, "Tuberculosis in the United States," *JAMA*, 1989, 262(3):385-9.
3. Good RC, "Opportunistic Pathogens in the Genus *Mycobacterium*," *Annu Rev Microbiol*, 1985, 39:347-69.
4. Eisenach KD, Crawford JT, and Bates JH, "Repetitive DNA Sequences as Probes for *Mycobacterium tuberculosis*," *J Clin Microbiol*, 1988, 26:2240-5.
5. Pao CC, Lin SS, Wu SY, et al, "The Detection of Mycobacterial DNA Sequences in Uncultured Clinical Specimens With Cloned *Mycobacterium tuberculosis* DNA as Probes," *Tubercle*, 1988, 69:27-36.
6. DeWit D, Steyn L, Shoemaker S, et al, "Direct Detection of *Mycobacterium tuberculosis* in Clinical Specimens by DNA Amplification," *J Clin Microbiol*, 1990, 28(11):2437-41.
7. Hance AJ, Grandchamp B, Levy-Frebault V, et al, "Detection and Identification of Mycobacteria by Amplification of Mycobacterial DNA," *Mol Microbiol*, 1989, 3(7):843-9.

References

Brisson-Noel A, Aznar C, Chureau C, et al, "Diagnosis of Tuberculosis by DNA Amplification in Clinical Practice Evaluation," *Lancet*, 1991, 338(8763):364-6.

Patel RJ, Piessens WF, David JR, et al, "A Cloned DNA Fragment for Identification of *Mycobacterium tuberculosis*," *Rev Infect Dis*, 1989, 11(Suppl 2):411-9.

Roberts MC, McMillan C, and Coyle MB, "Whole Chromosomal DNA Probes for Rapid Identification of *Mycobacterium tuberculosis* and *Mycobacterium avium* Complex," *J Clin Microbiol*, 1987, 25:1239-43.

Mycobacteria DNA Detection Test *see* Mycobacteria by DNA Probe *on page 921*

Mycobacterial Accuprobe® *see* Mycobacteria by DNA Probe *on page 921*

***Mycoplasma pneumoniae* DNA Detection Test** *see Mycoplasma pneumoniae* DNA Probe Test *on this page*

Mycoplasma pneumoniae DNA Probe Test

CPT 87179

Related Information

Mycoplasma pneumoniae Diagnostic Procedures *on page 1188*
Mycoplasma Serology *on page 727*

Synonyms DNA Hybridization Test for *Mycoplasma pneumoniae*; DNA Test for *Mycoplasma pneumoniae*; Gen-Probe® Rapid Diagnostic System for *Mycoplasma pneumoniae*; *Mycoplasma pneumoniae* DNA Detection Test

Test Commonly Includes Direct detection of *Mycoplasma pneumoniae* nucleic acids in clinical specimens

Abstract Respiratory infections due to *Mycoplasma pneumoniae* are difficult to assess because current laboratory techniques lack sensitivity or require long periods of time (3 weeks) for results. Serological procedures are the most widely used but require paired acute and convalescent sera to confirm diagnosis.[1] Cold agglutinins are also used to diagnose *M. pneumoniae*; however, only 50% of infected patients become positive.[2] Culture of this microorganism is rarely done due to the difficulty of recovery and the long incubation time required for growth. A rapid and sensitive laboratory diagnosis of *M. pneumoniae* infection is important since effective antibiotic therapy is available. The nucleic acid based test is a sensitive and practical method for rapid diagnosis of respiratory infections of *M. pneumoniae*.

Specimen Sputum, throat swab, bronchial wash, lung biopsy **CONTAINER:** Special DNA transport medium is usually provided by the laboratory. If this is not available, a sterile container is acceptable. Sterile viral swabs can be used to collect throat specimens. **COLLECTION:** Sputum specimens should be collected early in the day so they can be sent directly to the laboratory. **STORAGE INSTRUCTIONS:** The specimens should be maintained at room temperature or refrigerated. Do not freeze. **CAUSES FOR REJECTION:** Specimens that are frozen during storage or shipping are inadequate for assay. **TURNAROUND TIME:** 1-2 days

Interpretive **REFERENCE RANGE:** Negative for *Mycoplasma pneumoniae* **USE:** Rapid detection of *Mycoplasma pneumoniae* in clinical specimens from respiratory sites **LIMITATIONS:** This assay cannot determine whether the microorganism is viable or not. Antibiotic susceptibility cannot be established. **METHODOLOGY:** This test detects *Mycoplasma pneumoniae* rRNA directly from respiratory specimens. It requires lysis of the cells in the specimen and release of the *Mycoplasma pneumoniae*-specific rRNA. The lysed specimens are then hybridized with a specific DNA probe. Detection of the bound probe is assessed after several washing steps. Detection can be done by use of a radioactive DNA probe, but positive samples are now commonly detected with chemiluminescence. **ADDITIONAL INFORMATION:** There is a wide range of clinical manifestations of *Mycoplasma pneumoniae* respiratory infections. These range from mild infection to severe pneumonia.[3,4] This microorganism causes approximately 20% of pneumonias in the general population. Laboratory diagnosis of *Mycoplasma pneumoniae* is usually based on serology of paired sera and/or isolation of the organism by culture. Culture isolation of the fastidious *Mycoplasma pneumoniae* is tedious, labor intensive, and usually requires several weeks.[3] The serological assays are the most commonly used tests. However, they lack sensitivity and specificity and require acute- and convalescent-phase sera, which also may require 2-3 weeks.[1] The DNA detection assay for *Mycoplasma pneumoniae* has been found to have a specificity and sensitivity that matches culture and serology assays.[2,5] The advantage of this test is is the rapid turnaround time, which facilitates the treatment of the patient with appropriate antibiotics.

Footnotes

1. Hirschberg L, Krook A, Petterson CA, et al, "Enzyme-Linked Immunosorbent Assay for Detection of *Mycoplasma pneumoniae* Specific Immunoglobulin M," *Eur J Clin Microbiol Infect Dis*, 1988, 7:420-3.
2. Kleemola SR, Karjalainen JE, and Raty RK, "Rapid Diagnosis of *Mycoplasma pneumoniae* Infection: Clinical Evaluation of a Commercial Probe Test," *J Infect Dis*, 1990, 162(1):70-5.
3. Broughton RA, "Infections Due to *Mycoplasma pneumoniae* in Childhood," *Pediatr Infect Dis J*, 1986, 5:71-85.
4. Murray HW and Tuazon C, "Atypical Pneumonias," *Med Clin North Am*, 1980, 64:507-27.

(Continued)

Mycoplasma pneumoniae DNA Probe Test *(Continued)*

5. Dular R, Kajioka R, and Kasatiya S, "Comparison of Gen-Probe Commercial Kit and Culture Technique for the Diagnosis of *Mycoplasma pneumoniae* Infection," *J Clin Microbiol*, 1988, 26:1068-9.

References

Harris R, Marmion BP, Varkanis G, et al, "Laboratory Diagnosis of *Mycoplasma pneumoniae* Infection," *Epidemiol Infect*, 1988, 101:685-94.

Hata D, Kuze F, Mochizuki Y, et al, "Evaluation of DNA Probe Test for Rapid Diagnosis of *Mycoplasma pneumoniae* Infections," *J Pediatr*, 1990, 116(2):273-6.

Hyman HC, Yogev D, and Razin S, "DNA Probes for Detection and Identification of *Mycoplasma pneumoniae* and *Mycoplasma genitalium*", *J Clin Microbiol*, 1987, 25:726-8.

Neisseria gonorrhoeae DNA Detection Test *see Neisseria gonorrhoeae* DNA Probe Test *on this page*

Neisseria gonorrhoeae DNA Probe Test

***CPT** 87179*

Related Information

Chlamydia trachomatis DNA Probe *on page 897*
Gram Stain *on page 815*
Neisseria gonorrhoeae Culture *on page 831*
Neisseria gonorrhoeae Smear *on page 834*

Synonyms DNA Hybridization Test for *Neisseria gonorrhoeae*; DNA Test for *Neisseria gonorrhoeae*; *Neisseria gonorrhoeae* DNA Detection Test; PACE2®

Test Commonly Includes Direct detection of *Neisseria gonorrhoeae* nucleic acid in clinical specimens from the urogenital site. This test cannot be used in legal cases or child protection cases.

Abstract The new genetic probe test for the detection of *Neisseria gonorrhoeae* significantly reduces the turnaround time required for test results. This is a distinct advantage in the treatment of sexually transmitted diseases. The expedient treatment of individuals positive for any sexually transmitted disease is an important factor in controlling these epidemic diseases. Thus, the use of a quick, reliable, and available laboratory diagnosis is essential. An additional advantage is that many of these tests will detect both *N. gonorrhoeae* and *C. trachomatis* in the same specimen.

Patient Care **PREPARATION:** When taking urethral specimens, the patient should not have urinated for 1 hour prior to collection.

Specimen Swab specimen collected from the genitourinary site of a male or female patient **CONTAINER:** Special DNA transport medium is provided by the laboratory and should not be substituted. A kit containing a swab and special transport media is made by Gen-Probe Inc, and is recommended for this test. **COLLECTION:** Currently the nucleic acid test for *Neisseria gonorrhoeae* is only FDA approved for genitourinary specimens.

For a male, the urethra is swabbed by rotating the swab 2-3 cm into the urethra. This should provide enough specimen from the infected site to detect *N. gonorrhoeae* nucleic acid. The swab is then placed in the transport tube for shipment to the laboratory.

For females, the commercial kit provides two swabs. The cervix or endocervix should be swabbed first with one swab to clean the area and then the second swab is used to collect the specimen. The swab is then put immediately into the transport tube and shipped to the laboratory. This is the same collection kit used for the *C. trachomatis* nucleic acid detection assay. In most cases a single swab specimen from each patient is sufficient to test for both *N. gonorrhoeae* and *C. trachomatis* nucleic acid.

STORAGE INSTRUCTIONS: The specimens should be maintained at room temperature or refrigerated. Specimens are stable up to 1 week at room temperature. **CAUSES FOR REJECTION:** Contamination of specimen with urine **TURNAROUND TIME:** 24 hours

Interpretive **REFERENCE RANGE:** Negative for *Neisseria gonorrhoeae* nucleic acid. A sexually active, asymptomatic female may harbor *N. gonorrhoeae* without overt clinical symptoms. **USE:** This test provides for the rapid detection of *N. gonorrhoeae* in clinical urogenital specimens. **LIMITATIONS:** Genetic probe detection tests cannot be done in child abuse cases. In these cases many laboratories perform more than one confirmatory test after culture of the isolate. In addition to fluorescent antibody testing, coagglutination and enzyme-based tests, the nucleic acid detection assay can be used to confirm culture-positive organisms. Since no microorganism is isolated, antibiotic sensitivity assays cannot be done. **METHODOLOGY:** This test detects *N. gonorrhoeae* nucleic acid directly from swab specimens. This requires denaturation of the ribosomal RNA in the specimens by heating, hybridization with a specific DNA probe, and detection of bound probe after several washing steps. Positive specimens are detected with chemiluminescence. **ADDITIONAL INFORMATION:** Gonorrhea is the most commonly reported sexually transmitted disease in the United States.[1] The disease is manifest as acute urethritis in males and as cervicitis in females. *N. gonorrhoeae* can be isolated from asymptomatic females. Detection and treatment of these individuals is critical because if it is left untreated, gonorrhea can result in serious complications including pelvic inflammatory disease, sterility, and ectopic pregnancy.[2,3]

It is very important to control the spread of this disease between sexual partners; thus, the use of a quick, reliable test system is essential. The DNA based detection system for the presence of *N. gonorrhoeae* provides this type of test. The DNA detection assay has a sensitivity and a specificity equal to traditional methods of organism isolation and identification.[4,5] The current definitive method of detection for *N. gonorrhoeae* is the culture of the microorganism. However, this organism is especially fastidious. It can be difficult to grow in culture, especially when an established laboratory is not available. Many times such specimens are shipped to an off-site microbiology laboratory, often resulting in negative cultures due to loss of viability (especially in extreme weather conditions) and overgrowth of contaminating microorganisms. The DNA detection assay is an alternative method of detection for specimens that must be shipped to laboratories in other locations.

The major disadvantage at the present time is that this test cannot be done exclusively if a child abuse case is involved. These cases must be detected with the microbiologic recovery of *N. gonorrhoeae* organism from the clinical specimen. Antibiotic sensitivity testing cannot be done on these specimens. Guidelines for antibiotic susceptibility testing of *N. gonorrhoeae* have recently been published;[6] however, this microorganism is not routinely tested for antibiotic sensitivities.

Footnotes

1. Dillion JR, Bygdeman SM, and Sandstrom EG, "Serological Ecology of *Neisseria gonorrhoeae* (PPNG and non-PPNG) Strains: Canadian Perspective," *Genitourin Med*, 1987, 63:160-8.
2. Knapp JS, Holmes KK, Bonin P, et al, "Epidemiology of Gonorrhea: Distribution and Temporal Changes in Auxotype/Serovar Classes of *Neisseria gonorrhoeae*," *J Clin Microbiol*, 1990, 28:2340-50.
3. Lind I, "Epidemiology of Antibiotic Resistant *Neisseria gonorrhoeae* in Industrialized and Developing Countries," *Scand J Infect Dis*, 1990, 69(Suppl):77-82.
4. Granato PA and Franz MR, "Evaluation of a Prototype DNA Probe Test for the Nonculture Diagnosis of Gonorrhea," *J Clin Microbiol*, 1989, 27(4):632-5.
5. Lewis JS, Kranig-Brown D, and Trainor DA, "DNA Probe Confirmatory Test for *Neisseria gonorrhoeae*," *J Clin Microbiol*, 1990, 28(10):2349-50.
6. Putnam SD, Lavin BS, Stone JR, et al, "Evaluation of the Standardized Disk Diffusion and Agar Dilution Antibiotic Susceptibility Test Methods by Using Strains of *Neisseria gonorrhoeae* From the United States and Southeast Asia," *J Clin Microbiol*, 1992, 30(4):974-80.

References

Limberger RJ, Biega R, Evancoe A, et al, "Evaluation of Culture and the Gen-Probe PACE2® Assay for Detection of *Neisseria gonorrhoeae* and *Chlamydia trachomatis* in Endocervical Specimens Transported to a State Health Laboratory," *J Clin Microbiol*, 1992, 30(5):1162-6.

Panke ES, Yang LI, Leist PA, et al, "Comparison of Gen-Probe DNA Probe Test and Culture for the Detection of *Neisseria gonorrhoeae* in Endocervical Specimen," *J Clin Microbiol*, 1991, 29:883-8.

N-myc Amplification

CPT *83890 (molecular isolation or extraction); 83896 (nucleic acid probe, each)*

Related Information

Histopathology *on page 57*

Synonyms DNA Amplification of N-myc; N-myc Gene Amplification

Test Commonly Includes Detection of increased N-myc oncogene copy number

Abstract The role of oncogenes in the progression of tumor development has been clarified by recent advances in molecular biology. Neuroblastoma was the first human tumor in which an increased number of copies of a specific oncogene (N-myc) correlated with progression of disease. Patients with amplification of the N-myc oncogene have a worse prognosis than patients whose tumors have a single copy of N-myc gene. The neuroectodermal tumors, neuroepitheliomas, do not have amplification of the N-myc oncogene. This is useful in distinguishing between neuroblastomas and neuroepitheliomas. Thus, detection of N-myc amplification in immature neuroectodermal tumors is helpful in establishing both diagnosis and prognosis.

(Continued)

N-myc Amplification *(Continued)*

Specimen Tissue from neuroblastoma **CONTAINER:** The specimen should be immediately frozen and then shipped to the laboratory on dry ice. **COLLECTION:** A 0.1-1 g of neuroblastoma tissue should be cut from the biopsy. The specimen is then put into a sealable plastic freezer bag and frozen at -70°C. The specimen should be kept frozen until shipped to the laboratory. **STORAGE INSTRUCTIONS:** Store tissue at -70°C or on dry ice. **CAUSES FOR REJECTION:** If the specimen thaws out during transport to the laboratory or before shipping then the specimen must be rejected. If less than 0.1 g of tissue is sent to the laboratory for evaluation it may not yield enough DNA for analysis. **TURNAROUND TIME:** Results require about 3 weeks. **SPECIAL INSTRUCTIONS:** Tumor specimen should be frozen immediately at -70°C or in liquid nitrogen.

Interpretive **REFERENCE RANGE:** An interpretive report usually is included with the results of analysis. **USE:** In neuroblastomas, N-myc amplification is associated with poor prognosis and rapid tumor progression. The poor clinical outcome in these patients seems to be independent of tumor stage. N-myc copy numbers greater than five indicate a poor prognosis. **LIMITATIONS:** Failure to obtain DNA from the tissue sample due to inappropriate shipping or processing (such as freeze/thaw series) **METHODOLOGY:** DNA is released and isolated from the tumor tissue by lysing the cells and extracting cell lysate with phenol and chloroform. Several dilutions of the DNA is then suctioned onto a solid support and hybridized with a specific radioactive N-myc probe. After hybridization, the copy number of N-myc is calculated by extrapolation to a standard curve. The standard curve is generated by using various dilutions of a known N-myc DNA sample, such as a plasmid containing the N-myc gene. After hybridization of the standard dilutions, the hybridized dots of DNA are counted in a beta scintillation counter and plotted as cpm vs copy number. **ADDITIONAL INFORMATION:** A number of studies have shown that an increased copy number of N-myc in neuroblastoma is predictive of a poor prognosis.[1,2,3] Thus, the determination of N-myc copy number provides information that has prognostic significance. This information may direct a more appropriate choice of treatment since N-myc amplification is associated with poor prognosis regardless of clinical stage.[2]

Footnotes

1. Brodeur GM, Seeger RC, Schwab M, et al, "Amplification of N-myc in Untreated Human Neuroblastomas Correlates With Advanced Disease Stage," *Science*, 1984, 224:1121-4.
2. Nakagawara A, Ikeda K, Tsuda T, et al, "Amplification of N-myc Oncogene in Stage II and IVS Neuroblastomas May Be a Prognostic Indicator," *J Pediatr Surg*, 1987, 22:415-8.
3. Seeger RC, Brodeur GM, Sathers H, et al, "Association of Multiple Copies of the N-myc Oncogene With Rapid Progression of Neuroblastomas," *N Engl J Med*, 1985, 313:1111-6.

References

Brodeur GM, "Clinical Significance of Genetic Rearrangements in Human Neuroblastoma," *Clin Chem*, 1989, 35(7 Suppl):B38-42.

Brodeur GM and Fong CT, "Molecular Biology and Genetics of Human Neuroblastoma," *Cancer Genet Cytogenet*, 1989, 41(2):153-74.

N-myc Gene Amplification *see* N-myc Amplification *on previous page*

PACE2® *see Chlamydia trachomatis* DNA Probe *on page 897*

PACE2® *see Neisseria gonorrhoeae* DNA Probe Test *on page 924*

Parentage Studies *see* Identification DNA Testing *on page 918*

Paternity Testing *see* Identification DNA Testing *on page 918*

PCR *see* Polymerase Chain Reaction *on next page*

PCR for HIV DNA *see* Human Immunodeficiency Virus DNA Amplification *on page 915*

Philadelphia Chromosome *see* Breakpoint Cluster Region Rearrangement in CML *on page 895*

Philadelphia Chromosome *see* Chromosome Analysis, Blood or Bone Marrow *on page 898*

Polycystic Kidney Disease, Prenatal Diagnosis *see* Adult Polycystic Kidney Disease DNA Detection *on page 889*

Polymerase Chain Reaction

CPT *83898 (nuclear molecular diagnostics); 87179 (microbial identification by PCR)*

Related Information

Amniotic Fluid, Chromosome and Genetic Abnormality Analysis *on page 891*
bcl-2 Gene Rearrangement *on page 893*
Body Fluids Cytology *on page 482*
Breakpoint Cluster Region Rearrangement in CML *on page 895*
Cerebrospinal Fluid Cytology *on page 490*
Chlamydia trachomatis DNA Probe *on page 897*
Cystic Fibrosis DNA Detection *on page 903*
Duchenne/Becker Muscular Dystrophy DNA Detection *on page 908*
Hepatitis B Core Antibody *on page 684*
Hepatitis B_e Antibody *on page 685*
Hepatitis B_e Antigen *on page 686*
Hepatitis B Surface Antibody *on page 687*
Hepatitis B Surface Antigen *on page 688*
Hepatitis C Serology *on page 690*
Hepatitis D Serology *on page 691*
HIV-1/HIV-2 Serology *on page 696*
HTLV-I/II Antibody *on page 702*
Human Immunodeficiency Virus Culture *on page 1185*
Human Immunodeficiency Virus DNA Amplification *on page 915*
Lyme Disease DNA Detection *on page 920*
Mixed Lymphocyte Culture *on page 725*
Pneumocystis Fluorescence *on page 732*
T- and B-Lymphocyte Subset Assay *on page 750*

Synonyms DNA Amplification; PCR

Test Commonly Includes Amplification of target DNA sequences as much as a millionfold

Abstract The polymerase chain reaction is a new technique developed in molecular biology with unlimited potential use in the medical laboratory. The technique was developed at the Cetus Corporation in Emeryville, California, and was first described for use in the prenatal diagnosis of sickle cell anemia. The technique may become as important as gene cloning itself. The PCR technique permits a millionfold amplification of small pieces of DNA in several hours. The amplification is performed by multiple cycles of DNA polymerizing enzyme in the presence of known sequences, of primer DNA sequences, flanking the region of DNA to be amplified. (See figure.) Thus, the nucleotide sequence of the gene to be amplified must be known so oligonucleotide primers can be constructed on oligonucleotide synthesizers. The method has potential use not only in prenatal diagnosis, but also for cancer and infectious disease detection and diagnosis.

Specimen The specimen for the PCR assay will depend on the type of analysis. For example, prenatal diagnosis will require amniotic fluid or chorionic villous biopsy (see Amniotic Fluid, Chromosome and Genetic Abnormality Analysis), whole blood will be required for human immunodeficiency virus (HIV) detection, other specimens such as cerebrospinal fluid, sputum, serum, biopsies, or discharge from wounds for other infectious agents, or solid tissue by biopsy for cancer diagnosis. **COLLECTION:** Varies with type of specimen

Interpretive **USE:** The use of the technique is limited only by one's imagination. The uses in the laboratory include prenatal diagnosis of sickle cell anemia, hemophilia, cystic fibrosis, and muscular dystrophy, as well as oncogene activation in the case of lymphoma and chronic myelogenous leukemia. Numerous infectious agents such as *Mycobacterium* species, the agent of Lyme disease, and viruses, have been detected using this amplification technique. **LIMITATIONS:** The tests must be carefully monitored with appropriate controls (especially negative controls) due to the great sensitivity of the amplification technique. **METHODOLOGY:** The PCR technique requires knowledge of the base sequence of the gene of interest to be amplified. From the sequence data, oligonucleotide primers 25 nucleotides in length can be constructed using oligonucleotide synthesizers. These primers flank a 100-2000 base sequence of the gene of interest. The primers are constructed so that the primers bind (anneal) to opposite strands of the target double helix. A special DNA polymerase, purified from *Thermus aquaticus* (*Taq*), is used because it can withstand the many denaturing, reannealing, and polymerizing cycles without the need for replenishment. The reaction requires the target DNA, the primers, *Taq* polymerase, and the four deoxynucleotide triphosphates. The mixture is heated several minutes to 95°C to separate the target DNA double strands. The primers are

(Continued)

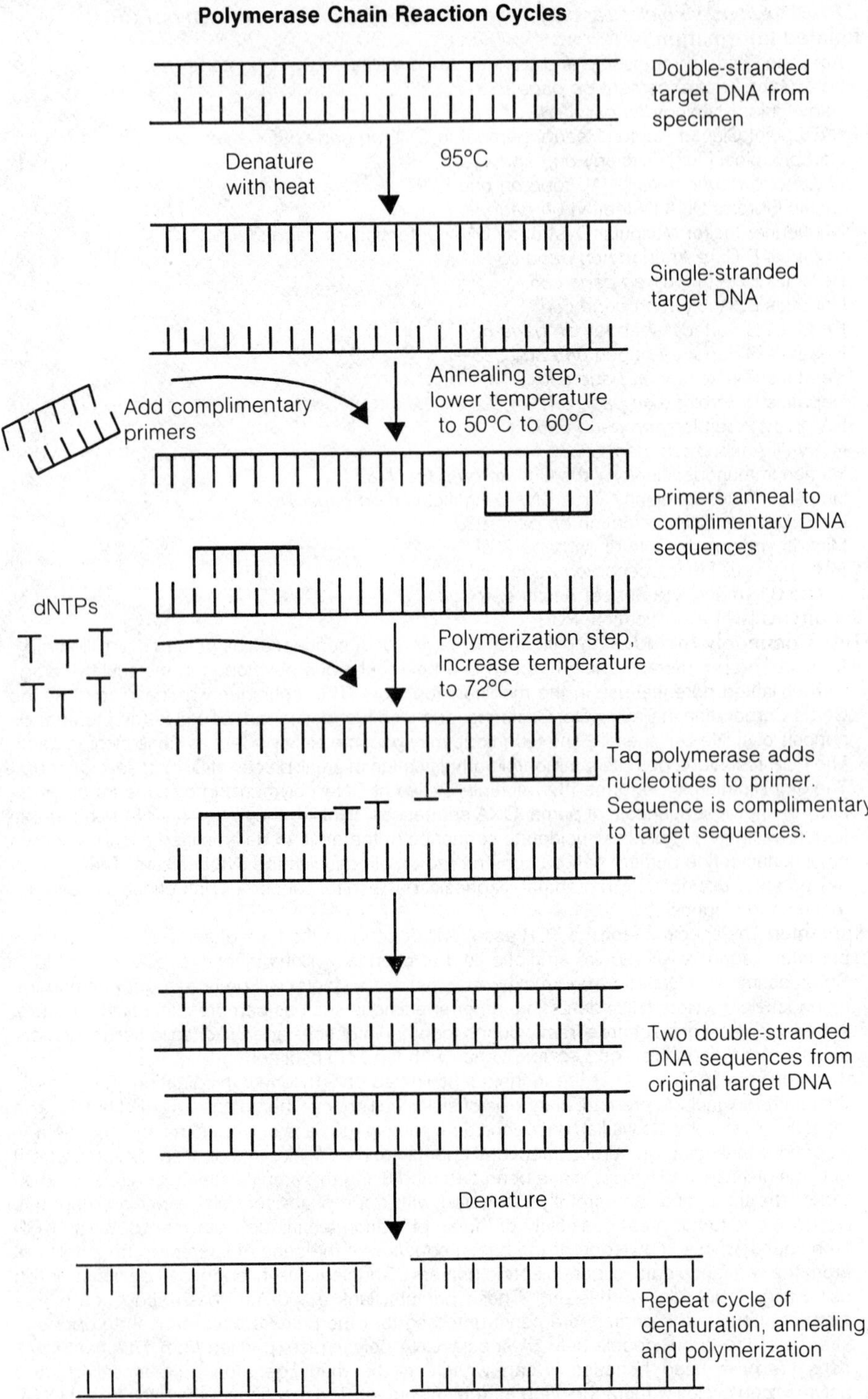
Polymerase Chain Reaction Cycles
Double-stranded target DNA from specimen
Denature with heat
95°C
Single-stranded target DNA
Add complimentary primers
Annealing step, lower temperature to 50°C to 60°C
Primers anneal to complimentary DNA sequences
dNTPs
Polymerization step, Increase temperature to 72°C
Taq polymerase adds nucleotides to primer. Sequence is complimentary to target sequences.
Two double-stranded DNA sequences from original target DNA
Denature
Repeat cycle of denaturation, annealing, and polymerization

then allowed to bind to the target DNA at 50°C to 60°C and the polymerase reaction allowed to proceed for several minutes at 72°C. This cycle of denaturation, annealing, polymerization is repeated over and over as many as 25-35 times amplifying the sequence between the primers hundreds of thousands to millions of times (see figure). The amplified DNA can then be detected by agarose electrophoresis followed by ethidium bromide staining. The amplified bands can be seen with a UV light with and photographed for analysis. **ADDITIONAL INFORMATION:** The technique described is being expanded and refined. The procedure is automated with programmable heating blocks to cycle the reaction automatically. The technique has unprecedented sensitivity, being able to use nanogram quantities of target DNA and could theoretically be used to amplify the DNA from a single cell. Other amplification reactions are also being developed for use in the diagnostic laboratory.

References

Embury SH, Scharf SJ, Saiki RK, et al, "Rapid Prenatal Diagnosis of Sickle Cell Anemia by a New Method of DNA Analysis," *N Engl J Med*, 1987, 316:656-61.

Erlich HA, ed, *PCR Technology: Principles and Applications for DNA Amplification*, New York, NY: Stockton Press, 1989.

Kogan SC, Doherty M, and Gitschier J, "An Improved Method for Prenatal Diagnosis of Genetic Diseases by Analysis of Amplified DNA Sequences: Application to Hemophilia A," *N Engl J Med*, 1987, 317:985-90.

Ou C, Kwok S, and Mitchell SW, "DNA Amplification for Direct Detection of HIV-1 in DNA of Peripheral Blood Mononuclear Cells," *Science*, 1988, 239:295-7.

Saiki RK, Chang, CA, Levenson CH, et al, "Diagnosis of Sickle Cell Anemia and β-Thalassemia With Enzymatically Amplified DNA and Nonradioactive Allele-Specific Oligonucleotide Probes," *N Engl J Med*, 1988, 319: 537-41.

Saiki RK, Gelfand DH, Stoffel S, et al, "Primer-Directed Enzymatic Amplification of DNA With Thermostable DNA Polymerase," *Science*, 1988, 239:487-90.

Saiki RK, Scharf S, and Faloona F, "Enzymatic Amplification of β-Globin Genomic Sequences and Restriction Site Analysis for Diagnosis of Sickle Cell Anemia," *Science*, 1985, 230:1350-4.

Shibata D and Klatt EC, "Analysis of Human Immunodeficiency Virus and Cytomegalovirus Infection by Polymerase Chain Reaction in the Acquired Immunodeficiency Syndrome," *Arch Pathol Lab Med*, 1989, 113(11):1239-44.

RFLP Analysis for Parentage Evaluation *see* Identification DNA Testing *on page 918*

Sex Chromatin *see* Buccal Smear for Sex Chromatin Evaluation *on page 896*

Southern Blot of bcl-2 Gene Rearrangement *see* bcl-2 Gene Rearrangement *on page 893*

Translocation *see* Chromosome Analysis, Blood or Bone Marrow *on page 898*

ViraPap® *see* Human Papillomavirus DNA Probe Test *on page 916*

ViraType® *see* Human Papillomavirus DNA Probe Test *on page 916*

THERAPEUTIC DRUG MONITORING TOXICOLOGY DRUGS OF ABUSE

Harold J. Grady, PhD

Contributing to this chapter are the following authors:

Daniel H. Jacobs, MD — Anticonvulsants

Christopher J. Papasian, PhD — Antibiotics

Therapeutic Drug Monitoring

It has been established that drug dosage regulated through the measurement of serum/plasma drug levels (therapeutic drug monitoring — TDM) is more likely to produce the desired therapeutic effect without toxicity than when empiric dosing alone is used. This finding is consistent with three common assumptions concerning the pharmacological effects of drugs.

- The therapeutic effects are initiated through interaction of the drug with receptors on the cells of the target tissue.
- The therapeutic effects are proportional to the drug concentration at the receptor site.
- Drug concentration at the receptor site is proportional to the serum/plasma drug concentration.

Although many drugs are safely and effectively administered without TDM, it has been found useful to monitor serum/plasma levels when one or more of the following conditions apply.[1]

- The drug has a narrow therapeutic range.
- The drug exhibits large intraindividual variations in utilization and metabolism.
- The drug does not produce the desired therapeutic effect when empiric dosing is used.
- The drug produces toxicity when empiric dosing is used.
- Secondary disease alters drug utilization.
- Noncompliance is suspected.
- Drug interactions are suspected.
- Medicolegal verification of treatment is desired.

Reliable laboratory methods (many of them automated) are available for TDM. It is common practice to use them for many of the drugs in the following classes:

- antibiotics
- antiasthmatics
- anticonvulsants
- antipsychotics and antidepressants
- antiarrhythmics

---

[1] Pippenger CE, "The Rationale of Therapeutic Drug Monitoring," *Interpretations in Therapeutic Drug Monitoring*, Baer DM and Dito WR, eds, Chicago, IL: ASCP Press, 1981, 1-18.

For the most part, laboratory methods for serum/plasma drug levels produce precise and accurate results within a reasonable turnaround time. However, a number of other variables need to be considered to adequately interpret the result. Of prime importance is drawing the first sample only after **steady-state** has been reached. This means that monitoring should not begin until **five to six elimination half-lives** have elapsed after starting a dosage regimen or changing a dosage level. Obviously, this limitation does not apply if loading doses are administered. Of equal importance is the relation of the **sampling time** to the time of the last dose. Many drugs are monitored using only trough values (immediately before the next dose) and when one level only is measured it is the trough value. Other drugs (particularly the aminoglycoside antibiotics) must be monitored at both the trough and the peak (various times shortly after the dose). The following factors may influence the serum/plasma level achieved from a given dosage regimen:

- patient's age
- genetic variability
- nature of the disease
- drug regimen
- compliance
- absorption
- distribution
- metabolism
- excretion
- time of last dose
- drug tolerance
- toxicity

When clinical response is not consistent with the dosage given, one or more of the above should be considered as a possible explanation of the discrepancy.

In the text of drug listings in this chapter, therapeutic ranges are given when TDM is applicable. Separate ranges apply to **peak and trough values** and are so labeled. The optimum sampling time, time to steady-state, and special information concerning toxicity, drug-drug interactions, and other helpful clinical data is presented.

Certain classes of drugs may require specialized knowledge concerning drug interactions and levels of efficacy of the individual members of that group as illustrated by the following discussion of the **antiepileptics**. Antiepileptic drugs (AED) are titrated clinically to prevent seizures and avoid adverse effects. The ranges used in therapeutic monitoring of anticonvulsants are presented as "reference" ranges rather than "normal" ranges. Some patients require levels outside the reference range. Moreover, dosing requirements may, in some cases, be based on the patient's weight rather than the AED level. With drugs of this class, changes in serum/plasma levels must be considered in terms of clinical relevance, since they are not always related to changes in efficacy or toxicity. For example, **phenytoin** and **carbamazepine** may mutually lower the level of the other drug without causing increased seizures.[2] It is also true that certain undesirable interactions and side effects can occur at normal drug levels. Antiepileptics at normal levels can decrease the efficacy of oral contraceptives[2] or cause teratogenesis.[3] For a more complete treatment of the pharmacological and biological effects of antiepileptics other than those relating to serum/plasma levels, readers are referred elsewhere.[4] Desktop automated instrumentation (eg, Seralyzer, Vision, and Ektachem) is now available for the measurement of **phenobarbital**, **phenytoin**, and

[2] Hansten PD and Horn JR, "The Top 40 Drug Interactions," *Drug Interactions Newsletter*, 1991, 11:483-90.

[3] Engel J, *Seizures and Epilepsy*, Contemporary Neurology Series, Philadelphia, PA: FA Davis, 1989.

[4] Levy RH, Dreifuss FE, Mattson, et al, *Antiepileptic Drugs*, 3rd ed, New York, NY: Raven Press, 1989.

carbamazepine. They have been studied and have been found to be reliable.[5,6] The listings that follow will generally be concerned with the larger laboratory automated systems that are well established with respect to acceptable accuracy and precision. Several new anticonvulsants are in clinical trials. Two of them, **felbamate** and **GABA-pentin**, seem to be close to approval and are listed.

Information relevant to **antibiotics**, **cardiac drugs**, and **anticonvulsants** is tabulated in the Appendix of this chapter.

Toxicology

Modern toxicology has three divisions: environmental, clinical, and forensic. All are concerned with poisons and their effect on living organisms but differ with respect to the types of samples involved and the use to which the results will be put. Most hospital laboratory toxicology is concerned with clinical toxicology, namely, the identification of substances involved in acute or chronic poisoning of man. When little or no clue is available concerning the toxin from the history and physical, the laboratory is frequently asked to perform a comprehensive drug screen. The term "comprehensive" is a relative one since no hospital laboratory can truly screen for all possible toxic substances. Two available systems, a thin-layer chromatographic method from Toxi-Lab, Inc, called Toxi-Lab® and an automated high performance liquid chromatographic instrument from Biorad Inc, called Remedi®, can each screen for several hundred drugs. However, they must be supplemented with individual methods to detect the drugs not measured such as salicylates, and for one of the systems, acetaminophen and marijuana. Most of the time qualitative identification of the toxin in a timely manner (1-2 hours) is the most useful, although in a few cases a quantitative response is of value. Quantitative measurement is usually carried out on serum/plasma and is most often used for the following drugs:

- acetaminophen
- salicylate
- carboxyhemoglobin
- digoxin (usually from TDM)
- ethanol
- heavy metals
- iron
- theophylline (usually from TDM)
- phenytoin (usually from TDM)

Of the other anticonvulsants, carbamazepine, primidone, phenobarbital, and valproic acid are most commonly monitored, although others may also be measured.

The laboratory can be most helpful when it has all the information available concerning possible substances involved. The dialogue between the laboratory and the treating physician should be reciprocal and ongoing as the situation develops. Forms designed by the laboratory for requesting toxicological analyses should require as much of this detail as possible to be submitted along with the sample. Toxicology and TDM overlap when drug levels significantly above the therapeutic range are involved. It should be noted that at such levels the usual values for elimination rates (half-lives) may not apply because enzyme systems can become saturated and then the typical first-order kinetics are not valid.

---

[5] Abramowicz M, "Desktop Systems for Office Chemistries," *The Medical Letter*, 1990, 32:96-7.
[6] Leppik IE, *Therapeutic Drug Monitoring*, New York, NY: Raven Press, 1989, 11:73.

Drugs of Abuse

The drugs or drug classes most commonly listed as drugs of abuse are the following:

- amphetamine/methamphetamine
- barbiturates
- benzodiazepines
- cannabinoids (marijuana or THC)
- cocaine
- opiates (heroin, morphine, codeine)
- phencyclidine (PCP)
- methadone
- methaqualone
- propoxyphene

These drugs are measured under one of two circumstances: one, in the overdose situation in which the analysis is treated as any toxicological sample, and two, in testing for the presence of the drug in clinically well persons. Most of the following discussion applies to the latter situation. Analysis for these drugs in clinically-well subjects frequently involves two sequential tests, the first a screening test and the second a confirmatory test performed only on positive screens. The screening test must have good sensitivity but may lack some specificity while the confirmatory test must be both sensitive and specific and involve a different chemical principle than the screen. When used strictly for clinical purposes, the screening test result may be used without confirmation if an occasional false-positive will do no serious harm. However, when medicolegal or forensic application is a possibility, confirmation is essential. It is also extremely important for forensic applications that the sample be accompanied by a chain-of-custody document which will assure the integrity of the sample through the process of collection, delivery, receipt, and analysis. Samples without such a document have no forensic value regardless of the quality of the analysis.

The sample for analysis of drugs of abuse is urine because of the ease of collection and because concentrations of drugs and metabolites are usually higher than in serum/plasma or saliva. Laboratory reports for detection of drugs of abuse in well persons are not quantitative and are usually expressed as "positive" or "negative." For each drug a predetermined threshold or cutoff value has been agreed upon by scientific and regulatory groups and results equal to the cutoff or above are considered positive and all other values negative. Thus, a report of "negative" does not necessarily mean absence of the drug but rather a result less than the cutoff. Cutoff values for a given drug are often different for the screening test than for the confirmatory test. For a few drugs (eg, marijuana) several different cutoff values are in current use. When such specimens are sent to reference laboratories, one must verify that the cutoff they use will satisfy needs. A sample having either a negative screening test or negative confirmatory test is reported as negative. When screening in the overdose situation, quantitative estimates are sometimes given when values are well above the cutoff. In a number of cases metabolites, rather than the parent drug, are the substances actually measured in the screening and confirmatory tests.

The **National Institute on Drug Abuse (NIDA)** (an agency of the Department of Health and Human Services) has set up strict guidelines for sample handling, measurement, and reporting of drugs of abuse in urine. This agency certifies laboratories following a rigorous proficiency testing and inspection procedure. Only NIDA certified laboratories may perform drugs-of-abuse testing for federal agencies or for firms contracting with federal agencies. Only five drugs are on the NIDA panel: amphetamine/methamphetamine, cannabinoids, cocaine, opiates, and PCP. Other drugs are measured by NIDA laboratories but are not part of the certification. The College of American Pathologists (CAP) also certifies laboratories for toxicology and drugs-of-abuse testing using similar proficiency samples and inspection procedures. NIDA and CAP guidelines for all aspects of drugs-of-abuse testing are goals to which all good drug laboratories aspire.

A majority of the laboratories screening for drugs of abuse employ enzyme immunoassay (EIA) which has adequate sensitivity and reasonable specificity in most cases. The amphetamine/ methamphetamine class produces the most problems with false-positives. Thin-layer chromatography (TLC) is occasionally used to screen but is probably inferior because of borderline sensitivity for some drugs. Confirmatory testing may be done by gas chromatography/mass spectrometry (GC/MS) and is clearly the method of choice. Thin-layer chromatography or gas-liquid chromatography may be used for confirmation following EIA screening. For drugs of abuse in the pages that follow, in addition to the usual information, the cutoff values for screening and confirmation will be listed.

Urine collection procedures for drugs-of-abuse testing should incorporate certain checks and precautions to preserve sample integrity. The collection room should not have warm water available, and the stool water should be colored with a dye. The temperature within 4 minutes of collection should be between 90°F and 99°F. Later measurement of pH should be between 5 and 9 and the specific gravity (refractometer) >1.002. Any unusual colors, odors, or physical appearance should be noted.

Serum collection tubes for drugs: Silicones and plasticizers used on stoppers of standard red top tubes interfere with some drug assay procedures. Silicones and plasticizers also interfere with GC assays. Some drugs adsorb to the silicone in the red tops and to tops with plasticizers. Gel separator tubes should not be utilized. Use of navy top Vacutainer® tubes avoids this problem since they are free of these interferents. When a drug screen on serum is contemplated, use of a navy top tube rather than a red top tube is suggested.

Please see the Appendix of this chapter for chain-of-custody protocol and related information.

See also the separate chapter, **Trace Elements**, by Dr Glen R Willie.

References

Amdur MO, Doull J, and Klaasen CD, *Cararett and Doull's Toxicology*, 4th ed, New York, NY: Pergammon Press, 1991.

Baer DM and Dito WR, *Interpretations in Therapeutic Drug Monitoring*, Chicago, IL: ASCP Press, 1981.

Baselt RC and Cravey RH, *Disposition of Toxic Drugs and Chemicals in Man*, 3rd ed, Littleton, MA: Year Book Medical Publishers, 1989.

Bryson PD, *Comprehensive Review in Toxicology*, Rockville, MD: Aspen Publishers, Inc., 1989.

Journal of Analytical Toxicology, Niles, IL: Preston Publications, Inc, 1977.

Journal of Clinical Toxicology, New York, NY: Marcel Dekker Journals, 1968.

Kaplan LA and Pesce AJ, eds, *Methods in Clinical Chemistry*, St Louis, MO: Mosby-Year Book Inc, 1987.

Therapeutic Drug Monitoring, New York, NY: Raven Press, 1979.

Tietz N, ed, *Textbook of Clinical Chemistry*, Philadelphia, PA: WB Saunders Co, 1986.

Toxicology and Applied Pharmacology, New York NY: Academic Press, 1959.

Toxicology Methods, New York, NY: Raven Press, 1991.

Abuse Screen *see* Drugs of Abuse Testing, Urine *on page 962*

Accenon *see* Ethotoin *on page 965*

Acetaminophen, Serum

***CPT** 82003*

Related Information

Lactic Acid, Blood *on page 273*

Liver Profile *on page 282*

Synonyms Anacin-3®; Datril®; Liquiprin®; Panadol®; Panex®; Paracetamol; Phenaphen®; Tempra®; Tylenol®

Abstract Acetaminophen is an analgesic-antipyretic widely used as a replacement for aspirin. It is frequently seen in the deliberate overdose situation.

Specimen Serum **CONTAINER:** Red top tube

Interpretive **REFERENCE RANGE:** Acetaminophen, serum: 20-110 ng/mL (SI: 43-240 nmol) **CRITICAL VALUES:** Toxic: >150 μg/mL (SI: >990 μmol/L) (within 4 hours); >50 μg/mL (SI: >330 μmol/L) (within 12 hours) **USE:** Therapeutic monitoring, evaluate acetaminophen toxicity **METHODOLOGY:** UV spectrophotometry, immunoassay, gas-liquid chromatography (GLC), or high performance liquid chromatography (HPLC) **ADDITIONAL INFORMATION:** Acetaminophen is an analgesic and antipyretic with little anti-inflammatory properties. It is used for headache, fever, relief of pain in patients who cannot tolerate aspirin or those with bleeding disorders or peptic ulcers. Acetaminophen is the analgesic/antipyretic of choice in children 13 years of age or younger due to the association of aspirin with the possible development of Reye's syndrome.

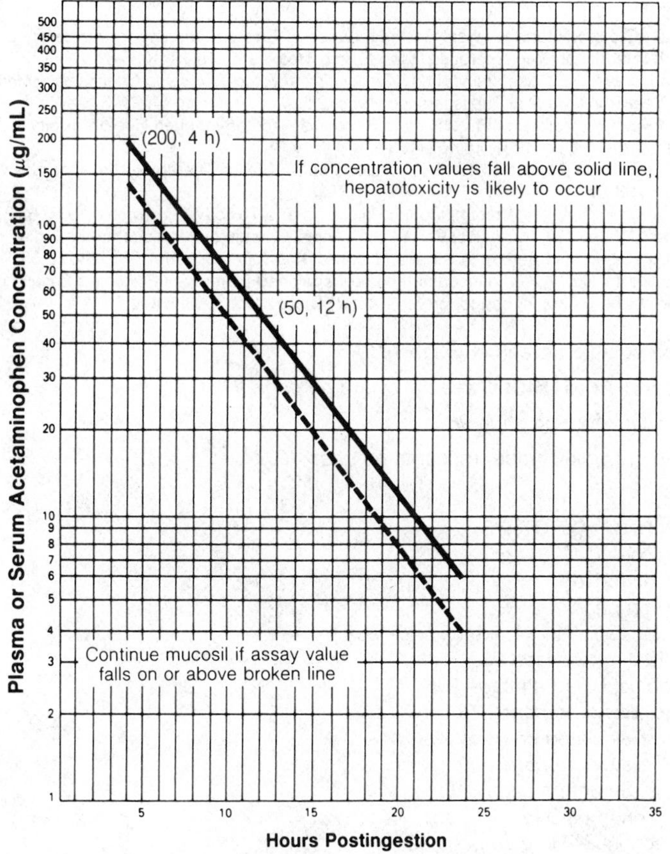

From Rumack BH and Matthews H, "Acetaminophen Poisoning and Toxicity," *Pediatrics*, 1975, 55:871-6, with permission.

(Continued)

Acetaminophen, Serum *(Continued)*

Acetaminophen is rapidly absorbed from the GI tract. Peak plasma concentrations are reached in 30-60 minutes. Steady-state concentrations are reached in 10-20 hours. However, prolonged (more than 10 days in adults; more than 5 days in children) treatment is to be avoided. Acetaminophen is metabolized to several conjugated forms, glucuronide (45% to 55%), sulfate (20% to 30%), and cysteine and mercaptopurine (20%). Acetanilid and phenacetin owe much of their analgesic effect to their metabolite, acetaminophen.

The best indicator of acetaminophen toxicity is to measure the drug half-life by analyzing a blood level taken 6 hours postingestion, then a second level 3-4 hours later. Expected half-life is 1-3 hours. Half-lives exceeding 4 hours are consistent with hepatic necrosis. The Rumack nomogram is useful for estimation of toxicity from serum level at 6 hours or later after ingestion.[1] See nomogram in this listing.

Hepatic toxicity may appear 3-5 days after ingestion of a toxic dose. Toxic levels require monitoring liver function with AST (SGOT), ALT (SGPT), and bilirubin with study also of glucose, creatinine, prothrombin time, and electrolytes. Serum levels drawn before 4 hours may not represent peak levels. The hepatotoxicity of acetaminophen is related to the formation of one or more highly reactive metabolites in the liver. Impaired hepatic metabolism may be found in the elderly. Orally administered N-acetylcysteine (Mucomyst®) has been shown to provide rather dramatic protection against acetaminophen hepatotoxicity. Early treatment is especially recommended in pregnant subjects.[2]

Footnotes

1. Bryson PD, *Comprehensive Review in Toxicology*, 2nd ed, Rockville, MD: Aspen Publishers Inc, 1989, 422.
2. Riggs BS, Bronstein AC, Kulig K, et al, "Acute Acetaminophen Overdose During Pregnancy," *Obstet Gynecol*, 1989, 74(2):247-53.

References

Ashbourne JF, Olson KR, and Khayam-Bashi H, "Value of Rapid Screening for Acetaminophen in All Patients With Intentional Drug Overdose," *Ann Emerg Med*, 1989, 18(10):1035-8.

Baselt RC and Cravey RH, "Acetaminophen," *Disposition of Toxic Drugs and Chemicals in Man*, 3rd ed, Chicago, IL: Year Book Medical Publishers Inc, 1989, 2-5.

Kumar S and Rex DK, "Failure of Physicians to Recognize Acetaminophen Hepatotoxicity in Chronic Alcoholics," *Arch Intern Med*, 1991, 151(6):1189-91.

Montamat SC, Cusack BJ, and Vestal RE, "Management of Drug Therapy in the Elderly," *N Engl J Med*, 1989, 321(5):303-9.

Rumack BH and Matthew H, "Acetaminophen Poisoning and Toxicity," *Pediatrics*, 1975, 55:871-6.

Stewart MJ and Watson ID, "Analytical Reviews in Clinical Chemistry: Methods for the Estimation of Salicylate and Paracetamol in Serum, Plasma, and Urine," *Ann Clin Biochem*, 1987, 24:552-65.

Veltri JC and Rollins DE, "A Comparison of the Frequency and Severity of Poisoning Cases From Ingestion of Acetaminophen, Aspirin, and Ibuprofen," *Am J Emerg Med*, 1988, 6:104-7.

Acetone *see* Volatile Screen *on page 1010*

Acetylsalicylic Acid, Blood *see* Salicylate *on page 999*

Adapin® *see* Doxepin *on page 962*

Adapin® *see* Tricyclic Antidepressants *on page 1007*

Alcohol, Blood or Urine

CPT *82055 (chemical)*

Related Information

Anion Gap *on page 132*
Drugs of Abuse Testing, Urine *on page 962*
Glucose, Fasting *on page 238*
Ketone Bodies, Blood *on page 265*
Lactic Acid, Blood *on page 273*
Osmolality, Calculated *on page 299*
Osmolality, Serum *on page 300*
Phosphorus, Serum *on page 319*
Uric Acid, Serum *on page 378*
Urine Collection, 24-Hour *on page 32*
Venous Blood Collection *on page 32*
Volatile Screen *on page 1010*

Synonyms Ethanol, Blood; Ethyl Alcohol, Blood; EtOH

Abstract Alcohol is the single most abused drug in the United States. Whole blood values are required for legal use.

Patient Care PREPARATION: Do not use alcohol wipe to clean venipuncture site. Hexachlorophene-based, iodine-based, or mercury-based antiseptics not containing alcohol may be used.

Specimen Serum or plasma, urine CONTAINER: Red top tube, gray top (sodium fluoride) tube recommended for medicolegal specimens and prolonged storage; plastic urine container COLLECTION: **Do not prepare venipuncture site with an alcohol swab**. When police agencies bring an individual in for blood alcohol levels, medical and laboratory people should at all times be aware of their state statutes.[1] STORAGE INSTRUCTIONS: Refrigerate in a tightly stoppered tube. SPECIAL INSTRUCTIONS: Concentrations of ethanol are 10% to 15% higher in serum and plasma versus whole blood. For forensic purposes, only whole blood values are used.

Interpretive REFERENCE RANGE: Blood: negative. In most laboratories, values <10 mg/dL (SI: <2 mmol/L) are considered negative. Signs of intoxication can be observed at levels of 50-100 mg/dL (SI: 10.9-21.7 mmol/L). Urine: negative. Less than 10 mg/dL is considered negative. Presence of any level of urine alcohol cannot be used to determine impairment. CRITICAL VALUES: Fatal concentration is usually considered to be >400 mg/dL (SI: >86.8 mmol/L). Whole blood levels of 300 mg/dL (SI: 65.1 mmol/L) are associated with coma. In most states, levels ≥100 mg/dL are considered evidence of impairment for driving. POSSIBLE PANIC RANGE: ≥300 mg/dL (SI: ≥65.1 mmol/L) USE: Quantitation of alcohol level for medical or legal purposes; screen unconscious patients; used to diagnose alcohol intoxication and determine appropriate therapy; screen for alcoholism and monitor ethanol treatment for methanol intoxication. Must be tested as possible cause of coma of unknown etiology since alcohol intoxication may mimic diabetic coma, cerebral trauma, and drug overdose. LIMITATIONS: Certain other alcohols (in high concentration) can interfere with enzymatic methods. The rate of dehydrogenation of isopropanol (2-propanol) is 6% and that of n-propanol (1-propanol) is 36% of that of ethanol. Methanol does not interfere. Gas chromatography is the most specific methodology because it can separate, identify, and quantitate each type of alcohol present. Freezing point osmometry and enzymatic analysis can together determine the presence of volatile intoxicants and can determine causes of metabolic intoxication. METHODOLOGY: Enzymatic analysis (alcohol dehydrogenase), freezing point osmometry, gas chromatography (GC) ADDITIONAL INFORMATION: Ethanol is absorbed rapidly from the GI tract. Peak blood levels usually occur within 40-70 minutes on an empty stomach. Food in the stomach can decrease the absorption of alcohol. Ethanol is metabolized by the liver to acetaldehyde. Once peak blood ethanol levels are reached, disappearance is linear; a 70 kg man metabolizes 7-10 g of alcohol/hour (15±5 mg/dL/hour). The urine/blood ratio is considered to be about 1:35 but is quite variable. The average saliva/blood ratio is 1:20. Symptoms of intoxication in the presence of low alcohol levels could indicate a serious acute medical problem requiring immediate attention. The half-lives and effectiveness of certain drugs (eg, barbiturates, etc) are increased in the presence of ethanol. Urine alcohol can be measured by immunoassay and gas chromatography and is tested for in abused drug screening programs. Only in Europe are urine ethanol levels accepted as legal evidence. Alcohol ingestions are discussed in the Osmolality, Serum, Anion Gap, and Ketone Bodies listings in the Chemistry chapter. Breath alcohol analyzers are used by law enforcement personnel and the results are accepted as legal evidence of intoxication. They must not be used less than 15 minutes after the last alcohol ingestion.[2]

Footnotes

1. Gerson B, "Alcohol," *Clin Lab Med*, 1990, 10(2):355-74.
2. Simpson G, "Accuracy and Precision of Breath Alcohol Measurements," *Clin Chem*, 1987, 33:261-8.

References

Blume SB, "Women and Alcohol," *JAMA*, 1986, 256:1467-70, (review).

Gadsden RH and Terry CS, "Alcohols in Biological Fluids by Gas Chromatography," *Selected Methods of Emergency Toxicology*, Frings CS and Faulkner WR, eds, Washington, DC: American Association of Clinical Chemistry Press, 1986, 40-3.

Lovejoy FH, "Ethanol Intoxication," *Clin Toxicol Rev*, 1981, 4:1-2.

Mendenhall CL and Weesner RE, "Alcoholism," *Clinical Chemistry*, Kaplan LA and Pesce AJ, eds, St Louis, MO: Mosby-Year Book Inc, 1984, 594-610.

Wilkinson PK, "Pharmacokinetics of Ethanol," *Alcohol Clin Exp Res*, 1980, 4:6-21.

Alurate® *see* Barbiturates, Quantitative, Blood *on page 946*

Amikacin

CPT 80150

Related Information

Antibiotic Level, Serum *on page 942*
Creatinine, Serum *on page 202*
Magnesium, Serum *on page 287*
Serum Bactericidal Test *on page 843*
Susceptibility Testing, Aerobic and Facultatively Anaerobic Organisms *on page 864*

Synonyms Amikin®

Applies to Kanamycin (Kantrex®)

Abstract Aminoglycoside antibiotics, including amikacin, are used primarily to treat infections caused by aerobic gram-negative bacilli. Amikacin has a narrow therapeutic window. Its use in life-threatening infections makes it mandatory that effective serum concentrations be achieved without overdosing.

Specimen Serum **CONTAINER:** Red top tube **COLLECTION:** Not more than 30 minutes before the next dose for trough level; for peak level draw 15-30 minutes after completion of infusion or 45-75 minutes following intramuscular injection. Specify dosage, time of dosage, and all other co-administered antimicrobials. For send outs, ship specimen frozen in plastic vial on dry ice. **STORAGE INSTRUCTIONS:** Separate serum within 1 hour of collection, refrigerate or freeze until assayed.

Interpretive **REFERENCE RANGE:** Therapeutic: peak: 15-25 μg/mL (SI: 26-43 μmol/L) (depends in part on the minimal inhibitory concentration of the drug against the organism being treated); trough: <10 μg/mL (SI: <17 μmol/L). **CRITICAL VALUES:** Toxic: peak: >35 μg/mL (SI: >60 μmol/L); trough: >10 μg/mL (SI: >17 μmol/L). See Table B in the Appendix of this chapter. **USE:** Peak levels are necessary to assure adequate therapeutic levels for organism being treated. Trough levels are necessary to reduce the likelihood of nephrotoxicity. **LIMITATIONS:** High peak levels may not have strong correlation with toxicity. **METHODOLOGY:** High performance liquid chromatography (HPLC), fluorescence polarization immunoassay (FPIA), enzyme immunoassay (EIA) **ADDITIONAL INFORMATION:** Amikacin is cleared by the kidney and accumulates in renal tubular cells. **Nephrotoxicity** is most closely related to the length of time that trough levels >10 μg/mL (SI: >17 μmol/L). Creatinine levels should be monitored every 2-3 days as an indicator of impending renal toxicity. The initial toxic result is nonoliguric renal failure that is usually reversible if the drug is discontinued. Continued administration of amikacin may produce oliguric renal failure. Nephrotoxicity may occur in as many as 10% to 25% of patients receiving aminoglycosides; most of this toxicity can be avoided by monitoring levels and adjusting dosing schedules accordingly. Aminoglycosides may also cause irreversible **ototoxicity** that manifests itself clinically as hearing loss. Aminoglycoside ototoxicity is relatively uncommon and clinical trials in which levels were carefully monitored and dosing adjusted failed to show a correlation between auditory toxicity and plasma aminoglycoside levels. In situations where dosing is not adjusted, however, sustained high levels may be associated with ototoxicity. This association is far from clear cut, and new once-daily dosing regimens (and associated high peak serum concentrations) that fail to enhance toxicity further complicates this issue.

References

Beaubien AR, Desjardins S, Ormsby E, et al, "Incidence of Amikacin Ototoxicity: A Sigmoid Function of Total Drug Exposure Independent of Plasma Levels," *Am J Otolaryngol*, 1989, 10(4):234-43.

Contreras AM, Gamba G, Cortes J, et al, "Serial Trough and Peak Amikacin Levels in Plasma as Predictors of Nephrotoxicity," *Antimicrob Agents Chemother*, 1989, 33(6):973-6.

Edson RS and Terrell CL, "The Aminoglycosides," *Mayo Clin Proc*, 1991, 66(11):1158-64.

Gilbert DN, "Once-Daily Aminoglycoside Therapy," *Antimicrob Agents Chemother*, 1991, 35(3):399-405.

Mullins RE, Lampasona V, and Conn RB, "Monitoring Aminoglycoside Therapy," *Clin Lab Med*, 1987, 7:513-29.

Pancoast SJ, "Aminoglycoside Antibiotics in Clinical Use," *Med Clin North Am*, 1987, 72:581-612.

Porter WH, "Therapeutic Drug Monitoring," *Clinical Chemistry*, Taylor EH, ed, New York, NY: John Wiley and Sons, 1989, 217-48.

Amikin® *see* Amikacin *on this page*

Aminophylline *see* Theophylline *on page 1002*

Amiodarone

CPT 80299

Related Information

Liver Profile *on page 282*
Thyroid Stimulating Hormone *on page 361*
Thyroxine *on page 364*

Synonyms Cordarone®

Test Commonly Includes Desethylamiodarone

Abstract Amiodarone is an antiarrhythmic which should be monitored.

Specimen Serum **CONTAINER:** Red top tube **SAMPLING TIME:** At least 12 hours after last dose

Interpretive **REFERENCE RANGE:** 0.5-2.5 mg/L (SI: 1-4 μmol/L) (parent); desethyl metabolite is active and is present in equal concentration to parent drug. **POSSIBLE PANIC RANGE:** Adverse effects at >2.5 mg/L (SI: >4 μmol/L) (parent) and >5 mg/L (SI: >7 μmol/L) (both) **USE:** Therapeutic monitoring and toxicity assessment of an antiarrhythmic drug **CONTRAINDICATIONS:** Amiodarone affects the metabolism of other cardioactive drugs; serum concentrations and pharmacological effects of the following drugs can be increased when taken in combination with amiodarone: digitalis, warfarin-type anticoagulants, quinidine, procainamide, and phenytoin; see PDR. **METHODOLOGY:** High performance liquid chromatography (HPLC) **ADDITIONAL INFORMATION:** Amiodarone is a class III antiarrhythmic agent approved for the treatment of life-threatening ventricular tachyarrhythmias. Because of potential toxicity, the serum level of this drug should be monitored.[1] Its major elimination is by hepatic excretion. Negligible renal excretion occurs. Use of the drug is restricted because of its many side effects, including pulmonary fibrosis, neuromuscular weakness, exacerbation of congestive heart failure, tremor, thyroid dysfunction, and interaction with other drugs. It contains 37% iodine by weight. About 10% of patients on the drug develop hypothyroidism and 5% develop hyperthyroidism. Potassium or magnesium deficiency should be corrected. AST and ALT should be monitored on a regular basis. Elevation of AST and ALT are frequently seen in patients treated with amiodarone. Increased serum concentrations of such enzymes may be three times normal. If serum AST or ALT concentrations go beyond normal or doubles in a patient with an elevated baseline, then reduction of dosage or withdrawal should be considered.[2] When liver biopsy has been performed, the histopathological appearance of the liver has been that of alcoholic hepatitis or cirrhosis.[2]

Footnotes

1. Vrobel TR, Miller PE, Mostow ND, et al, "A General Overview of Amiodarone Toxicity: Its Prevention, Detection, and Management," *Prog Cardiovasc Dis*, 1989, 31(6):393-426.
2. *Physicians Desk Reference* (PDR), 47th ed, Mont Vale, NJ: Medical Economics Data, 1993, 2257-60.

References

Evans SJ, Myers M, Zaher C, et al, "High Dose Oral Amiodarone Loading: Electrophysiologic Effects and Clinical Tolerance," *J Am Coll Cardiol*, 1992, 19(1):169-73.
Falek R, Flores BT, Shaw L, et al, "Relationship of Steady-State Serum Concentrations of Amiodarone and Desethylamiodarone to Therapeutic Efficacy and Adverse Effects," *Am J Med*, 1987, 82:1102-8.
Mason JW, "Amiodarone," *N Engl J Med*, 1987, 316:455-66.

Amitriptyline, Blood

CPT 80152

Related Information

Nortriptyline *on page 989*
Tricyclic Antidepressants *on page 1007*

Synonyms Elavil®; Endep®; Etrafon®; Limbitrol®; Triavil®

Applies to Pamelor®

Test Commonly Includes Nortriptyline levels

Abstract Amitriptyline is a tricyclic antidepressant. Nortriptyline is a major active metabolite.

Specimen Serum or plasma **CONTAINER:** Red top tube, green top (heparin) tube **SAMPLING TIME:** Trough levels at steady-state

Interpretive **REFERENCE RANGE:** Amitriptyline and nortriptyline 100-250 ng/mL (SI: 360-900 nmol/L); nortriptyline 50-150 ng/mL (SI: 190-570 nmol/L). Metabolism may be impaired in the elderly.[1] **CRITICAL VALUES:** >300 ng/mL (SI: >1080 nmol/L) **USE:** Therapeutic monitoring and toxicity assessment **METHODOLOGY:** Immunoassay, high performance liquid chromatography (HPLC), gas chromatography (GC) **ADDITIONAL INFORMATION:** Amitriptyline is a tricyclic antidepressant that blocks the reuptake of serotonin at nerve endings and possesses high anticholinergic activity and cardiovascular toxicity. The drug is extensively metabolized to many polar compounds, the chief of which is nortriptyline. It is also an antidepressant. Both drugs are prescribed for depression and a range of other disorders.

(Continued)

Amitriptyline, Blood *(Continued)*

Amitriptyline has a peak serum concentration 2-6 hours postoral dose, and steady-state is achieved after 3-8 days of chronic oral dosing. The half-life is 17-40 hours and the usual therapeutic range (predose sample at steady-state) includes nortriptyline and is 100-250 ng/mL. Nortriptyline is administered orally, has a half-life of 15-90 hours, and peak serum values 2-6 hours postoral dose. Steady-state is achieved after 4-20 days of chronic dosing. Therapeutic levels of nortriptyline alone are 50-150 ng/mL.

All the tricyclic antidepressants have significant **drug interactions**: hydrocortisone methylphenidate and phenothiazines increase tricyclic levels; barbiturates, chloral hydrate, phenytoin, and glutethimide lower serum tricyclic levels; tricyclics impair the antihypertensive effectiveness of clonidine and guanethidine; tricyclics and alcohol produce additive sedative effects; tricyclics and antiparkinsonism agents have potent anticholinergic side effects; and tricyclics and MAO inhibitors should not be coadministered because of the potential for antihypertensive and CNS crises.

Tricyclics should be avoided in pregnant and lactating women because these drugs have not been established as safe. Geriatric patients are especially prone to postural hypotension, urinary retention, and sedation.[1]

Footnotes

1. Montamat SC, Cusack BJ, and Vestal RE, "Management of Drug Therapy in the Elderly," *N Engl J Med*, 1989, 321(5):303-9.

References

Katz IR, Curlik S, and Lesher EL, "Use of Antidepressants in the Frail Elderly. When, Why and How," *Clin Geriatr Med*, 1988, 4:203-22.

Katz MM, Koslow SH, Maas JW, et al, "Identifying the Specific Clinical Actions of Amitriptyline: Interrelationships of Behavior, Affect, and Plasma Levels in Depression," *Psychol Med*, 1991, 21(3):599-611.

Knudsen K, Ricksten SE, and Heath A, "Clonidine Interaction in Amitriptyline Poisoning," *J Toxicol Clin Toxicol*, 1988, 26:223-32.

Lukey BJ, Jones DR, Wright JH, et al, "Relationships Among Nortriptyline, 10-OH (E) Nortriptyline and 10-OH (Z) Nortriptyline Steady-State Plasma Levels and Nortriptyline Dosage," *Ther Drug Monit*, 1989, 11(3):221-7.

Preskom SH, Dorey RC, and Jerkovich GS, "Therapeutic Drug Monitoring of Tricyclic Antidepressants," *Clin Chem*, 1988, 34:822-8.

Svennson C, Nyberg G, and Martensson E, "High Performance Liquid Chromatography Quantitation of Amitriptyline and Nortriptyline in Dialysate From Plasma or Serum Using On-line Solid Phase Extraction," *J Chromatogr*, 1988, 432:363-9.

Wong SHY, "Measurement of Antidepressants by Liquid Chromatography: A Review of Current Methodology," *Clin Chem*, 1988, 34:848-55.

Amobarb *see* Barbiturates, Qualitative, Urine *on page 945*

Amobarbital *see* Barbiturates, Quantitative, Blood *on page 946*

Amoxapine, Blood

CPT *80299*

Synonyms Asendin®

Test Commonly Includes 8-OH-amoxapine

Abstract Amoxapine is a tricyclic antidepressant.

Specimen Serum or plasma **CONTAINER:** Red top tube or green top (heparin) tube **SAMPLING TIME:** Trough level at steady-state. Time to steady-state is 35-50 hours.

Interpretive **REFERENCE RANGE:** Amoxapine 20-100 ng/mL (SI: 64-319 nmol/L); 8-OH-amoxapine 150-400 ng/mL (SI: 478-1275 nmol/L); both 200-500 ng/mL (SI: 637-1594 nmol/L) **CRITICAL VALUES:** >500 ng/mL (SI: >1594 nmol/L) (both) **USE:** Therapeutic monitoring and toxicity assessment **METHODOLOGY:** High performance liquid chromatography (HPLC), gas chromatography (GC) **ADDITIONAL INFORMATION:** Amoxapine is a tricyclic antidepressant that is chemically distinct from amitriptyline and imipramine. The drug is a demethylated derivative of loxapine, a neuroleptic used to treat schizophrenia. Half-life is 8 hours. Time to peak in blood after dose is 1-2 hours. Amoxapine is metabolized by the liver to 7-hydroxy and 8-hydroxy metabolites. The 8-hydroxy derivative is an active antidepressant with a half-life of 30 hours. The 7-hydroxy derivative has neuroleptic potency. Both acute and chronic toxicities of amoxapine are different from other tricyclics; its cardiotoxicity is very low.

References

Anton RF Jr and Burch EA Jr, "Amoxapine Versus Amitriptyline Combined With Perphenazine in the Treatment of Psychotic Depression," *Am J Psychiatry*, 1990, 147(9):1203-8.

Coccaro EF and Siever LJ, "Second Generation Antidepressants: A Comparative Review," *J Clin Pharmacol*, 1985, 25:241-60.

Osiewicz RJ and Middleburg R, "Detection of a Novel Compound After Overdoses of Aspirin and Amoxapine," *J Anal Toxicol*, 1989, 13(2):97-9.

Amphetamines, Qualitative, Urine

***CPT** 80101 (screen); 80102 (confirmation); 82145 (quantitative)*

Related Information

Drugs of Abuse Testing, Urine *on page 962*

Methamphetamines, Qualitative, Urine *on page 984*

Synonyms Bennies; Crystal; Dexies; Ice; Speed; Uppers

Test Commonly Includes Amphetamine, methamphetamine

Abstract Amphetamine and methamphetamine are major drugs of abuse. They have limited medical use and are DEA schedule II drugs.

Specimen Random urine **CONTAINER:** Plastic urine container **COLLECTION:** If forensic, observe precautions (see Introduction). **STORAGE INSTRUCTIONS:** Refrigerate **CAUSES FOR REJECTION:** If forensic, failure to meet temperature requirements and/or tests for unusual urine dilution (specific gravity or creatinine) or alteration **TURNAROUND TIME:** Usually 1-2 hours for screen if done in-house. Confirmation, 1 day. **SPECIAL INSTRUCTIONS:** If forensic, use Chain-of-Custody form. See the Appendix of this chapter.

Interpretive **REFERENCE RANGE:** Negative (less than cutoff) **CRITICAL VALUES:** Cutoff: screen: 1000 ng/mL; confirmation: 500 ng/mL **USE:** Drug abuse evaluation, toxicity assessment **LIMITATIONS:** Some over-the-counter cold and antiallergy medications may cross react in certain immunoassay screens; confirmation by a different, more sensitive method (eg, GC/MS) is necessary. **METHODOLOGY:** Screen: fluorescence polarization immunoassay (FPIA),[1] radioimmunoassay (RIA), enzyme immunoassay (EIA), gas chromatography (GC), thin-layer chromatography (TLC), high performance liquid chromatography (HPLC); confirmation: gas chromatography/mass spectrometry (GC/MS) **ADDITIONAL INFORMATION:** For the amphetamine class, the material detected is the parent drug. Amphetamines are stimulants that tend to increase alertness and physical activity. Methamphetamine is more frequently the abused drug because its more pronounced central effects are preferred. Some drivers use amphetamines to counteract the drowsiness or "down" feeling caused by sleeping pills or alcohol. In pure form, they are yellowish crystals that are manufactured into tablets or capsules. Abusers also sniff the crystals, make a solution and inject it, or smoke the form known as "ice." Can be detected in urine 3 hours after use. Half-life is 10-20 hours. Usually detectable 24-48 hours after use.

Amphetamines increase the heart and breathing rate and blood pressure, dilate pupils, and decrease appetite. The user can experience a dry mouth, sweating, headache, blurred vision, dizziness, sleeplessness, and anxiety. Extremely high doses can cause people to flush or become pale; they can cause a rapid or irregular heartbeat, tremors, loss of coordination, and even physical collapse. People who use a large dose over a long period of time may develop an amphetamine psychosis: seeing, hearing, and feeling things that do not exist, having irrational thoughts or beliefs and feeling that people are out to get them. People in this extremely suspicious state frequently exhibit bizarre and sometimes violent behavior. Tolerance to the drug is developed after repeated use. Life-threatening overdoses are rare.

Footnotes

1. Turner GJ, Colbert DL, and Chowdry BZ, "A Broad Spectrum Immunoassay Using Fluorescence Polarization for the Detection of Amphetamines in Urine," *Ann Clin Biochem*, 1991, 28(Pt 6):588-94.

References

Bost RD, "3,4 Methylenedioxymethamphetamine (MDMA) and Other Amphetamine Derivatives," *J Forensic Sci*, 1988, 33:576-87.

Ellenhorn MJ and Barceloux DG, "Amphetamines," *Medical Toxicology*, New York, NY: Elsevier, 1988, 625-42.

Gan BK, Baugh D, Liu RH, et al, "Simultaneous Analysis of Amphetamine, Methamphetamine, and 3,4-Methylenedioxymethamphetamine (MDMA) in Urine Samples by Solid-Phase Extraction, Derivatization, and Gas Chromatography/Mass Spectrometry," *J Forensic Sci*, 1991, 36(5):1331-41.

Gillogley KM, Evans AT, Hansen RL, et al, "The Perinatal Impact of Cocaine, Amphetamine, and Opiate Use Detected by Universal Intrapartum Screening," *Am J Obstet Gynecol*, 1990, 163(5 Pt 1):1535-42.

Grinstead GF, "Ranitidine and High Concentrations of Phenylpropanolamine Cross React in the EMIT Monoclonal Amphetamine/Methamphetamine Assay," *Clin Chem*, 1989, 35(9):1998-9.

Hurst PM, "Amphetamines and Driving," *Alcohol, Drugs, and Driving*, 1987, 3:9-11.

Martz W and Schutz HW, "Synthetic Sweetener Cyclamate as a Potential Source of False-Positive Amphetamine Results in the TDx System," *Clin Chem*, 1991, 37(11):2016-7.

Amphetamines, Urine *see* Methamphetamines, Qualitative, Urine *on page 984*

Amphotericin B

CPT 80299

Related Information

Blood Fungus Culture *on page 789*
Cerebrospinal Fluid Fungus Culture *on page 800*
Creatinine, Serum *on page 202*
Itraconazole *on page 975*
Ketoconazole *on page 975*
Skin Fungus Culture *on page 845*
Sputum Fungus Culture *on page 853*
Stool Fungus Culture *on page 861*
Susceptibility Testing, Fungi *on page 869*

Synonyms Fungizone®

Abstract Amphotericin B is a clinically useful but highly toxic antifungal agent. Newer, less toxic agents are available. However, for many serious fungal infections, amphotericin B is the drug of choice despite its toxicity.

Specimen Serum **CONTAINER:** Red top tube

Interpretive **REFERENCE RANGE:** Therapeutic: 1.0-2.0 μg/mL (SI: 1.0-2.2 μmol/L) **USE:** Monitor serum levels for potential toxicity and correlation with *in vitro* susceptibility data **LIMITATIONS:** Assays for amphotericin B are performed only in a few reference laboratories. In routine clinical use, it is probably more prudent to follow serum creatinine, potassium, bicarbonate, and magnesium concentrations and CBC than to perform amphotericin B assays. **METHODOLOGY:** High performance liquid chromatography (HPLC), bioassay **ADDITIONAL INFORMATION:** Amphotericin B therapy frequently induces fever, chills, nausea, and reversible bone marrow suppression. Additionally, approximately 80% of patients develop increased creatinine concentrations, and occasional patients show an acute deterioration in **renal function**; when creatinine levels exceed 3.0 μg/mL it is advisable to withhold amphotericin B for several days and resume therapy at a lower dose. Because the pharmacokinetics and biodistribution of the drug are not clearly defined, it may be useful to correlate serum levels with desired concentrations determined by *in vitro* susceptibility testing. Susceptibility testing, however, is not widely available, not well standardized, and may not accurately predict clinical response. Amphotericin B can increase digitalis toxicity and decrease the anti-*Candida* effect of miconazole. Its toxicities are additive with those of the aminoglycosides.

References

Bodey GP, "Topical and Systemic Antifungal Agents," *Med Clin North Am*, 1988, 72:637-59.
Branch RA, "Prevention of Amphotericin B Induced Renal Impairment," *Arch Intern Med*, 1988, 148:2389-94.
Chabot GG, Pazdur R, Valeriote FA, et al, "Pharmacokinetics and Toxicity of Continuous Infusion Amphotericin B in Cancer Patients," *J Pharm Sci*, 1989, 78(4):307-10.
Christiansen KJ, Bernard EM, Gold JW, et al, "Distribution and Activity of Amphotericin B in Humans," *J Infect Dis*, 1985, 152:1037-43.
Dugoni BM, Gugliemo BJ, and Hollander H, "Amphotericin B Concentration in Cerebrospinal Fluid of Patients With AIDS and Cryptococcal Meningitis," *Clin Pharm*, 1989, 8(3):220-1.
Edmonds LC, Davidson L, and Bertino JS Jr, "Solubility and Stability of Amphotericin B in Human Serum," *Ther Drug Monit*, 1989, 11(3):323-6.
Starke JR, Mason EO, Kramer WG, et al, "Pharmacokinetics of Amphotericin B in Infants and Children," *J Infect Dis*, 1987, 155:766-74.
Terrell CL and Hughes CE, "Antifungal Agents Used for Deep-Seated Mycotic Infections," *Mayo Clin Proc*, 1992, 67(1):69-91.

Amytal® *see* Barbiturates, Quantitative, Blood *on page 946*
Anacin-3® *see* Acetaminophen, Serum *on page 935*
Ancobon® *see* Flucytosine *on page 967*
Angel Dust *see* Phencyclidine, Qualitative, Urine *on page 992*

Antibiotic Level, Serum

CPT 80299 (each drug)

Related Information

Amikacin *on page 938*

Chloramphenicol *on page 952*
Gentamicin *on page 970*
Serum Bactericidal Test *on page 843*
Susceptibility Testing, Aerobic and Facultatively Anaerobic Organisms *on page 864*
Tobramycin *on page 1004*
Vancomycin *on page 1009*

Synonyms Antimicrobial Assay

Abstract Assays for antimicrobial agents in serum are performed for two primary reasons: 1) to ensure therapeutic levels, and 2) to monitor for potentially toxic levels. In most situations, it is not necessary to monitor antimicrobial levels because serum levels are relatively predictable based on dosing; *in vitro* susceptibility testing uses those predictable levels to determine clinical efficacy. Similarly, toxicity is not always related to serum levels. It may be more appropriate to monitor for toxicity by following determinants of hematologic, renal, or hepatic function. In certain situations (eg, aminoglycoside antibiotics which have a narrow therapeutic range and a high potential for toxicity) it is essential to follow serum levels.

Specimen Serum **CONTAINER:** Red top tube **SAMPLING TIME:** Peak: 30 minutes after 30 minute I.V. infusion, 1 hour after I.M. dose; trough: immediately prior to next dose **COLLECTION:** Keep frozen if not assayed immediately. **CAUSES FOR REJECTION:** Incomplete clinical information (eg, specific antimicrobial, dosage and schedule, other concurrent antimicrobials)

Interpretive REFERENCE RANGE: Therapeutic range depends on agent being tested for and minimal inhibitory concentration of drug against organism. Selected ranges in µg/mL are presented as a guide only. See table in this listing and Table B in the Appendix of this chapter. **POSSIBLE PANIC RANGE:** See entries on aminoglycoside drugs (eg, amikacin, gentamicin, and tobramycin). **USE:** Evaluate adequacy of serum antibiotic level; detect toxic levels **LIMITATIONS:** May not be technically possible in a patient taking more than one antibiotic **METHODOLOGY:** Bioassay: cephalosporins, clindamycin, erythromycin, metronidazole, penicillins, polymyxin, tetracycline, trimethoprim; high performance liquid chromatography (HPLC): chloramphenicol, flucytosine, mezlocillin; fluorescence polarization immunoassay (FPIA): amikacin, gentamicin, tobramycin, kanamycin, streptomycin, vancomycin, neomycin, netilmicin **ADDITIONAL INFORMATION:** With the increasing availability of *in vitro* sensitivity testing expressed as the minimal inhibitory or bactericidal concentration of an antibiotic, measurement of serum levels of these drugs has taken on practical clinical importance. This is especially true for agents with narrow therapeutic ranges and significant toxicity. It should be remembered, however, that in most patients, cure of infection depends on numerous host factors as well as on antibiotics. Therefore, antibiotic levels should not be relied on as the sole guide to therapy.

Antibiotic Level, Serum

Drug	Peak		Trough	
	µg/mL	SI: µmol/L	µg/mL	SI: µmol/L
Amikacin	15-25	26-43	<10	<17
Chloramphenicol	25	77		
Flucytosine	100	775		
Gentamicin	4-10	8-21	<2	<4
Netilmicin	4-8	8.0-17.0	1-2	0.7-1.4
Streptomycin	5-20	9-34	<5	<9
Tobramycin	4-10	8-21	<2	<4
Trimethoprim	≥5	17		
Sulfamethoxazole	≥100	395		
Vancomycin	20-40	13.6-27.2	5-10	3.4-6.8

Selected ranges in µg/mL are presented as a guide only.

References

Denowitz GR and Mandell GL, "Beta-Lactam Antibiotics," *N Engl J Med*, 1988, 318:419-26, 490-500.
Dinsmoor MJ and Gibbs RS, "The Role of the Newer Antimicrobial Agents in Obstetrics and Gynecology," *Clin Obstet Gynecol*, 1988, 31:423-34.
Jawetz E, *Basic and Clinical Pharmacology*, Katzung BG, ed, Norwalk, CT: Appleton and Lange, 1987, 509-53.
Smith AL and Opheim E, "Comparison of Methods for Clinical Quantitation of Antibiotics," *Curr Clin Top Infect Dis*, Remington JS and Swartz MN, eds, New York, NY: McGraw-Hill Inc, 1983, 4:333-57.
Wise R, "Antimicrobial Agents: A Widening Choice," *Lancet*, Nov 1987, 1251-4.

Anticoagulants, Oral *see* Warfarin *on page 1011*
Antidepressants *see* Tricyclic Antidepressants *on page 1007*

Antifreeze *see* Ethylene Glycol *on page 965*

Antimicrobial Assay *see* Antibiotic Level, Serum *on page 942*

Aprobarbital *see* Barbiturates, Quantitative, Blood *on page 946*

Arsenic, Blood

CPT 82175

Related Information

Arsenic, Hair, Nails *on this page*
Heavy Metal Screen, Blood *on page 972*
Heavy Metal Screen, Urine *on page 973*

Synonyms Heavy Metal Screen, Arsenic

Applies to Hair Analysis

Abstract Arsenic is a toxic heavy metal. The largest source of human exposure is arsenic in food resulting from broad use of arsenical pesticides.

Specimen Blood, oxalated **CONTAINER:** Trace metal-free container **COLLECTION:** See Blood Collection Methods for Trace Elements in the introduction of the Trace Elements chapter. **CAUSES FOR REJECTION:** Containers not metal-free

Interpretive **REFERENCE RANGE:** <5 μg/dL (SI: <93.5 nmol/g) **CRITICAL VALUES:** 10-50 μg/dL (SI: 133.5-667.5 nmol/g) in chronic poisoning; >60 μg/dL (SI: >801 nmol/g) in acute poisoning **USE:** Blood arsenic is for diagnosis of acute poisoning only **LIMITATIONS:** Short half-life in blood **METHODOLOGY:** Electrothermal atomic absorption spectrometry (AA) **ADDITIONAL INFORMATION:** Heparinized whole blood and serum have been used for arsenic determination. Blood levels of arsenic have a short half-life and are useful only within a few days of exposure. Urine arsenic concentration is a better measure of arsenic poisoning. In addition to pesticides, rodenticides, weed killers, paint, and wood preservatives contain arsenic. See following listing.

References

Bryson PD, "Arsenic," *Comprehensive Review in Toxicology*, 2nd ed, Rockville, MD: Aspen Publishers, 1989, 501-8.

Campbell JP and Alvarez JA, "Acute Arsenic Intoxication," *Am Fam Physician*, 1989, 40(6):93-7.

Goyer RA, "Toxic Effects of Metals," *Casarett and Doull's Toxicology*, 4th ed, Klassen CD, Amdur MO, and Doull J, eds, New York, NY: Macmillan Publishing, 1991, 623-80.

Arsenic, Gastric Content *see* Arsenic, Urine *on next page*

Arsenic, Hair *see* Arsenic, Hair, Nails *on this page*

Arsenic, Hair, Nails

CPT 82175

Related Information

Arsenic, Blood *on this page*
Arsenic, Urine *on next page*
Heavy Metal Screen, Blood *on page 972*
Heavy Metal Screen, Urine *on page 973*

Synonyms Arsenic, Hair; Arsenic, Nails; As, Quantitative

Applies to Hair Analysis

Abstract This is a toxic heavy metal that is incorporated into hair and nails. Its presence there in abnormal concentrations is a sign of chronic poisoning.

Specimen Clean hair or nails **CONTAINER:** Clean envelope or heavy metal-free screw top plastic container **COLLECTION:** Extreme care is necessary to avoid surface contamination; pubic hair is preferable as are toenails. **SPECIAL INSTRUCTIONS:** Hair should be clean, free of oil and tonic; clip close. Nails should be thoroughly washed, dried, and clipped close to cuticle.

Interpretive **REFERENCE RANGE:** Hair: up to 65 μg/100 g (SI: 8.7 nmol/g); nail: 90-180 μg/100 g (SI: 12-24 nmol/g) **CRITICAL VALUES:** Values >100 μg/100 g (SI: >13.4 nmol/g) of hair are considered toxic **USE:** Diagnose chronic arsenic intoxication **LIMITATIONS:** Urine arsenic concentration is a better indication of recent exposure. **METHODOLOGY:** Electrothermal atomic absorption spectrometry (AA), neutron activation analysis **ADDITIONAL INFORMATION:** Arsenic accumulates in bones, hair, and nails and is used to detect chronic exposure, since arsenic is laid down in keratin soon after ingestion. Arsenic binds to protein sulfhydryl groups. Variations in arsenic hair levels may be due to geographic location and exposure to industrial waste and drinking water.

References

Bryson PD, *Comprehensive Review in Toxicology*, 2nd ed, Rockville, MD: Aspen Publishers Inc, 1989, 501-8.

Robertson WO, "Arsenic and Other Heavy Metals," *Clinical Management of Poisoning and Drug Overdose*, Haddad LM and Winchester JF, eds, Philadelphia, PA: WB Saunders Co, 1983, 656-64.

Arsenic, Nails *see* Arsenic, Hair, Nails *on previous page*

Arsenic, Urine

CPT *82175*

Related Information

Arsenic, Hair, Nails *on previous page*
Heavy Metal Screen, Blood *on page 972*
Heavy Metal Screen, Urine *on page 973*

Synonyms As, Quantitative, Urine

Applies to Arsenic, Gastric Content; Hair Analysis

Abstract This toxic heavy metal appears in urine, and its excretion rate is used to determine toxicity.

Specimen 24-hour urine **CONTAINER:** Acid-washed plastic container, no preservative **COLLECTION:** Collect a 24-hour urine specimen, on ice, with care to avoid specimen contact with metal. Container must be securely closed and properly labeled. **STORAGE INSTRUCTIONS:** Refrigerate **CAUSES FOR REJECTION:** Specimen not collected on ice, specimen in contact with metal during collection

Interpretive **REFERENCE RANGE:** Ranges for urine arsenic levels can be variable among different laboratories. A general guideline[1] is given: normal: 0-50 μg/L (SI: 0-0.65 μmol/L); chronic industrial exposure: >100 μg/L (SI: >1.3 μmol/L). The 24-hour urinary excretion rate should be <50 μg/24 hours. **CRITICAL VALUES:** Toxic: >850 μg/L (SI: >11.3 μmol/L). **USE:** Evaluate recent exposure to arsenic, arsenic toxicity **METHODOLOGY:** Atomic absorption spectrometry (AA) **ADDITIONAL INFORMATION:** 25 mL acidified gastric washing is acceptable for arsenic analysis; gastric content normally contains no arsenic. Random urine samples are acceptable.

Footnotes

1. Bryson PD, "Arsenic," *Comprehensive Review in Toxicology*, 2nd ed, Rockville, MD: Aspen Publishers, 1989, 501-8.

References

Amdur MO, Doull J, and Klaasen CD, eds, *Casarett and Doull's Toxicology*, 4th ed, New York, NY: Pergamon Press, 1991, 623-80.

Nixon DE, Mussmann GV, Eckdahl SJ, et al, "Total Arsenic in Urine: Palladium-Persulfate vs Nickel as a Matrix Modifier for Graphite Furnace Atomic Absorption Spectrophotometry," *Clin Chem*, 1991, 37(9):1575-9.

ASA, Blood *see* Salicylate *on page 999*
Asendin® *see* Amoxapine, Blood *on page 940*
Aspirin, Blood *see* Salicylate *on page 999*
As, Quantitative *see* Arsenic, Hair, Nails *on previous page*
As, Quantitative, Urine *see* Arsenic, Urine *on this page*
Athrombin-K® *see* Warfarin *on page 1011*
Aurothioglucose *see* Gold *on page 971*
Aventyl® *see* Nortriptyline *on page 989*
Aventyl® *see* Tricyclic Antidepressants *on page 1007*
Azidothymidine *see* Zidovudine *on page 1012*
AZT *see* Zidovudine *on page 1012*
Barbiturate Screen, Urine *see* Barbiturates, Quantitative, Blood *on next page*

Barbiturates, Qualitative, Urine

CPT *80101*

Synonyms Amobarb; Butalbital; Mephobarb; Pentobarb; Phenobarb; Secobarb

Test Commonly Includes Identification and confirmation of barbiturates in urine

Abstract This test is usually used to detect barbiturate as a drug of abuse.

(Continued)

Barbiturates, Qualitative, Urine *(Continued)*

Specimen Random urine **CONTAINER:** Plastic urine container **COLLECTION:** If forensic, observe precautions (see Introduction). **STORAGE INSTRUCTIONS:** Refrigerate specimen. **CAUSES FOR REJECTION:** If forensic, failure to meet temperature requirements or test for unusual urine dilution **SPECIAL INSTRUCTIONS:** Chain-of-custody documentation required for samples submitted for pre-employment, random employee testing, and forensic purposes. See the Appendix of this chapter.

Interpretive **REFERENCE RANGE:** Less than cutoff **CRITICAL VALUES:** Cutoff: screen: 300 ng/mL, confirmation: 300 ng/mL **USE:** Urine drugs of abuse testing, pre-employment screens, random drug testing **LIMITATIONS:** Short- and intermediate-acting barbiturates can be detected in urine 24-72 hours following ingestion, longer-acting drugs up to 7 days. **METHODOLOGY:** Enzyme immunoassay (EIA), gas chromatography/mass spectrometry (GC/MS) **ADDITIONAL INFORMATION:** Barbiturates are nonselective CNS depressants that may be used as sedative-hypnotics or anticonvulsants. They are capable of producing all levels of CNS mood effects from sedation to hypnosis to deep coma and anesthesia. Sensory cortex functions, cerebellar functions, and motor activity are decreased. Secobarbital and pentobarbital are short-term hypnotics and lose effectiveness after about 2 weeks of continued usage. Withdrawal symptoms from any barbiturate may be severe and may include convulsions and delirium. The presence of barbiturates in urine is presumptively positive at a level >300 ng/mL using secobarbital as a standard and can indicate prescribed or abused intake of this class of drugs. The presence of these drugs should be confirmed.

References

Pesce AJ, "Barbiturates," *Clinical Chemistry - Theory, Analysis, and Correlation*, 2nd ed, Kaplan LA and Pesce AJ, eds, St Louis, MO: Mosby-Year Book Inc, 1989, 1081-7.

Maurer HH, "Identification and Differentiation of Barbiturates and Their Metabolites in Urine," *J Chromatogr*, 1990, 530:307-26.

Barbiturates, Quantitative, Blood

CPT 80102

Related Information

Phenobarbital, Blood *on page 992*

Applies to Alurate®; Amobarbital; Amytal®; Aprobarbital; Barbiturate Screen, Urine; Blue Angels; Butabarbital; Butalbital; Butisol Sodium®; Fiorinal®; Gemonil®; Lotusate®; Luminal®; Mebaral®; Mephobarbital; Metharbital; Nembutal®; Pentobarbital; Phenobarbital; Red Devils; Secobarbital; Seconal™; Talbutal; Yellow Jackets

Test Commonly Includes Quantitation of barbiturates present in blood

Abstract Measurement of barbiturates as a class is usually used for drug-of-abuse testing or as evidence for toxicity.

Specimen Plasma or serum **CONTAINER:** Lavender top (EDTA) tube; green top (heparin) tube; red top tube, avoid serum separator tube for pentobarbital

Interpretive **REFERENCE RANGE:** Negative. Therapeutic: short-acting (secobarbital): 1-5 μg/mL (SI: 4.2-21.0 μmol/L); intermediate-acting (amobarbital): 5-15 μg/mL (SI: 22-66 μmol/L); long-acting (phenobarbital): 15-40 μg/mL (SI: 65-172 μmol/L); for seizure control, phenobarbital therapeutic levels: 10-30 μg/mL (SI: 43-129 μmol/L) **CRITICAL VALUES:** Toxic: short-acting: >10 μg/mL (SI: >43 μmol/L); intermediate-acting: >20 μg/mL (SI: >86 μmol/L); long-acting: >40 μg/mL (SI: >172 μmol/L) **USE:** Evaluate barbiturate toxicity, drug abuse, therapeutic levels; if barbiturates are suspected in a drug overdose, determination of long-, medium-, or short-acting may influence treatment.[1] **LIMITATIONS:** Only barbiturates will be identified and quantitated; individual agents cannot be identified by screening tests, particularly if there has been a mixed ingestion **METHODOLOGY:** Gas chromatography (GC), high performance liquid chromatography (HPLC), immunoassay **ADDITIONAL INFORMATION:** To monitor therapeutic phenobarbital level see listing for Phenobarbital, Blood. Barbiturates are sedative hypnotics and frequent drugs of abuse, alone and in combination with alcohol and/or amphetamines. If overdosage occurs, coma and death may result. The implication of any concentration is more serious for short-acting barbiturates than for phenobarbital. The toxic or lethal blood level varies with many factors and cannot be stated with certainty. Lethal blood levels determined at autopsy may be as low as 60 μg/mL (SI: 258 μmol/L) for long-acting (barbital and phenobarbital) and 10 μg/mL (SI: 43 μmol/L) for intermediate- and short-acting barbiturates (amobarbital, butabarbital, butalbital, pentobarbital, secobarbital). In presence of alcohol or other depressant drugs, the lethal concentrations may be lower. Addicts, however, may tolerate with no ill effect levels which would be acutely toxic to a nonaddicted individual. The long-acting drugs are metabolized slowly and depend primarily on the kidney for elimination, the short- and intermediate-acting drugs are metabolized primarily by the liver and are much less dependent on the kidney for excretion. Except for barbital, all barbiturates are primarily transformed by the liver. Only barbital is dependent mainly on renal excretion for termination of its pharmacological action. Individual barbiturates can be identified and separated from each other by HPLC.

Barbiturates can be assayed in **urine** or **gastric contents**. The presence of barbiturates in urine is presumptively positive at a level ≥300 ng/mL using secobarbital as a standard and can indicate prescribed or abused intake of this class of drugs. The presence of these drugs should be confirmed. The most commonly abused barbiturates are secobarbital (red devils), pentobarbital (yellow jackets), and amobarbital (blue angels). Short and intermediate acting barbiturates can be detected in urine 24-72 hours following ingestion, longer-acting drugs up to 7 days.

Footnotes

1. Blanke RB, "Analysis of Toxic Substance," *Clinical Chemistry*, Tietz NW, ed, New York, NY: WB Saunders Co, 1986, 1670-744.

References

Chen XH, "Solid-Phase Extraction for Screening of Acidic, Neutral, and Basic Drugs in Plasma Using a Single-Column Procedure on Bond Elut Certify," *J Chromatogr*, 1990, 529:161-6.

Pesce AJ, "Barbiturates," *Clinical Chemistry – Theory, Analysis, and Correlation*, 2nd ed, Kaplan LA and Pesce AJ, eds, St Louis, MO: Mosby-Year Book Inc, 1989, 1081-7.

Bennies *see* Amphetamines, Qualitative, Urine *on page 941*

Benzodiazepines, Qualitative, Urine

***CPT** 80101 (screen); 80102 (confirmation)*

Related Information

Chlordiazepoxide, Blood *on page 953*
Clonazepam *on page 954*
Diazepam, Blood *on page 958*
Oxazepam, Serum *on page 990*

Synonyms Tranquilizers (Valium®, Librium®, etc)

Abstract This group of drugs is used as antianxiety agents (tranquilizers). They are used by more Americans than any other single prescription drug.

Specimen Random urine **CONTAINER:** Clean plastic urine container **STORAGE INSTRUCTIONS:** Refrigerate or freeze if not analyzing immediately

Interpretive **REFERENCE RANGE:** None present unless prescribed. When used as drug-of-abuse screen, negative (less than cutoff). **CRITICAL VALUES:** Cutoff: screen: 300 ng/mL (as oxazepam); confirmation: 200 ng/mL **USE:** Drug abuse evaluation, toxicity assessment **METHODOLOGY:** Immunoassay, thin-layer chromatography (TLC), high performance liquid chromatography (HPLC), gas chromatography (GC), gas chromatography/mass spectrometry (GC/MS) **ADDITIONAL INFORMATION:** The benzodiazepines are a class of chemically-related central nervous depressants used as sedative-hypnotics to treat sleep disorders, anxiety, alcohol withdrawal, and seizure disorders. The drug class in low doses can cause sedation, drowsiness, blurred vision, fatigue, mental depression, and loss of coordination. In higher doses or used chronically, they can cause confusion, slurred speech, hypotension, and diminished reflexes. Chronic use may produce a physical dependence and a withdrawal syndrome which can last for weeks. Urine should be screened for benzodiazepines in suspected overdose cases, or as part of an abused drug program. These drugs have a relatively low potential for abuse.[1] They are, however, frequently found with other drugs in emergency room drug screens. Immunoassay screens detect a broad range of drugs and their metabolites in this class using either oxazepam or nordiazepam as positive controls. Using the latter, the test is more specific and more sensitive for detecting flurazepam. Positive screen results (usually >300 ng/mL of urine metabolites) should be confirmed by an alternate technique.

Footnotes

1. Cole JO and Chiarello RJ, "The Benzodiazepines as Drugs of Abuse," *J Psychiatr Res*, 1990, 24(Suppl 2):135-44.

References

Baker MA and Oleen MA, "The Use of Benzodiazepines Hypnotics in the Elderly," *Pharmacotherapy*, 1988, 8:241-7.

Beck O, Lafolie P, Hjemdahl P, et al, "Detection of Benzodiazepine Intake in Therapeutic Doses by Immunoanalysis of Urine: Two Techniques Evaluated and Modified for Improved Performance," *Clin Chem*, 1992, 38(2):271-5.

(Continued)

Benzodiazepines, Qualitative, Urine *(Continued)*

DuPont RL, "Abuse of Benzodiazepines: The Problem and the Solutions," *Am J Drug Alcohol Abuse*, 1988, 14(Suppl 1):1-69.

Jones CE, Wians FH Jr, Martinez LA, et al, "Benzodiazepines Identified by Capillary Gas Chromatography-Mass Spectrometry With Specific Ion Screening Used to Detect Benzophenone Derivatives," *Clin Chem*, 1989, 35(7):1394-8.

Montamat SC, Cusack BJ, and Vestal RE, "Management of Drug Therapy in the Elderly," *N Engl J Med*, 1989, 321(5):303-9.

Smith DE and Landry MJ, "Benzodiazepine Dependency Discontinuation: Focus on the Chemical Dependency Detoxification Setting and Benzodiazepine-Polydrug Abuse," *J Psychiatr Res*, 1990, 24(Suppl 2):145-56.

Blue Angels *see* Barbiturates, Quantitative, Blood *on page 946*

Bromide, Serum

CPT 80299

Related Information

Chloride, Serum *on page 182*

Abstract Inorganic bromide salts were formerly used as antiepileptics. They are no longer available as nonprescription items in the United States.

Specimen Serum **CONTAINER:** Red top tube

Interpretive **REFERENCE RANGE:** Normal: <20 mg/dL (SI: <2.5 mmol/L); therapeutic: 20-120 mg/dL (SI: 2.5-15.0 mmol/L) **CRITICAL VALUES:** Toxic: >120 mg/dL (SI: >15.0 mmol/L) **USE:** Evaluate bromide toxicity. This test is seldom ordered. **LIMITATIONS:** Patients on iodide therapy will have falsely elevated serum bromide levels. A high level of bromide in the serum will falsely elevate the chloride level. **METHODOLOGY:** Reaction of bromide in a protein-free filtrate with gold chloride **ADDITIONAL INFORMATION:** In order to convert mg/dL to mEq/L (the same units in which serum or plasma chlorides are reported), multiply the bromide values in mg/dL by 0.125. Both chloride and bromide react identically to titrimetric chloride methods (chloridometer). Many ion selective chloride electrodes give a response to bromide which is double that for chloride. A reported "chloride" value will equal the true sum of chloride and bromide. Bromism may be suspected in the presence of a history of ingestion of proprietary bromide preparations, fever, skin rash, and neurologic symptoms. Over-the-counter former bromide-containing preparations such as Bromo-Seltzer® and Nervine® have not contained bromide in the U.S. since 1971.

References

Goldfrank LR, Kirstein RH, and Howland MA, "Bromides," *Toxicological Emergencies*, Goldfrank LR, et al, eds, Norwalk, CT: Appleton-Century-Crofts, 1986, 398-403.

Svirbely J, "Bromide," *Methods in Clinical Chemistry*, Pesce AJ and Kaplan LA, eds, St Louis, MO: Mosby-Year Book Inc, 1987, 342-5.

Butabarbital *see* Barbiturates, Quantitative, Blood *on page 946*

Butalbital *see* Barbiturates, Qualitative, Urine *on page 945*

Butalbital *see* Barbiturates, Quantitative, Blood *on page 946*

Butisol Sodium® *see* Barbiturates, Quantitative, Blood *on page 946*

Cadmium, Urine and Blood

CPT 82300

Related Information

Heavy Metal Screen, Blood *on page 972*
Heavy Metal Screen, Urine *on page 973*

Synonyms Cd, Blood; Cd, Urine

Abstract This toxic heavy metal is used in industry in alloys and metal platings

Specimen 24-hour urine is recommended for chronic exposure, whole blood for diagnosis of acute intoxication **CONTAINER:** Plastic (preferably polycarbonate) urine container, acid-washed, no preservative; metal-free tube for blood **COLLECTION:** Blood must be collected into metal-free tubes with a plastic syringe. See Blood Collection Methods for Trace Elements in the introduction of the Trace Elements chapter. A 24-hour urine specimen must be collected in a metal-free container and be properly labeled, capped, and sealed. **STORAGE INSTRUCTIONS:**

Refrigerate urine. **CAUSES FOR REJECTION:** Specimen allowed to contact metal **SPECIAL INSTRUCTIONS:** Requisition must state date and time urine collection started and date and time collection finished.

Interpretive **REFERENCE RANGE:** Nonsmokers: urine: <1 μg/L (SI: <8.9 nmol/L), <1 μg/g creatinine; whole blood: <1 μg/L **POSSIBLE PANIC RANGE:** Levels >10 μg/L (SI: >88.97 μmol/L) in whole blood and 10-20 μg/L (SI: 89-178 μmol/L) in urine probably reflect excessive exposure. **USE:** Evaluate cadmium toxicity in industrial exposure to cadmium fumes or cadmium ingestion **METHODOLOGY:** Flameless atomic absorption spectrophotometry (AA) **ADDITIONAL INFORMATION:** Inhalation of cadmium fumes produces an acute pneumonitis. Long-term exposure may lead to emphysema (with decreased α_1-antitrypsin). Increased cadmium is reported to be associated with hypertension and (perhaps) prostatic cancer. Cadmium ingestion may result from contact of acid foods with metal containers. There is exposure of the general populace to cadmium from food, water, and air contamination. Because of slow excretion and constant exposure cadmium values increase with age. Body cadmium elimination half-life may be as long as 30 years.

References

Baselt RC, *Disposition of Toxic Drugs and Chemicals in Man*, 2nd ed, Davis, CA: Biomedical Publications, 1982, 105-8.

Tonks DB, "Cadmium," *Methods in Clinical Chemistry*, Pesce AJ and Kaplan LA, eds, St Louis, MO: Mosby-Year Book Inc, 1987, 346-61.

Caffeine, Blood

CPT *82486 (chromatography, qualitative); 82491 (chromatography, quantitative)*

Related Information

Theophylline *on page 1002*

Abstract The principle intake is from drinking coffee and tea. Some soft drinks may also contain moderate amounts of caffeine. It is a metabolite of theophylline in infants.

Specimen Serum **CONTAINER:** Red top tube **COLLECTION:** Indicate exact time blood drawn and relationship to last theophylline or caffeine dose on requisition.

Interpretive **REFERENCE RANGE:** None present. Caffeine is one of the most widely used mind-altering substances and is found in numerous beverages (cocoa, coffee, cola, tea) and prescription and nonprescription medications. The therapeutic range in the treatment of neonatal apnea is 8-14 μg/mL (SI: 41-72 μmol/L). **POSSIBLE PANIC RANGE:** Toxic concentration: >30 μg/mL (SI: >155 μmol/L) **USE:** Monitor total xanthine concentration in newborns receiving theophylline **LIMITATIONS:** Not often ordered **METHODOLOGY:** High performance liquid chromatography (HPLC) **ADDITIONAL INFORMATION:** Theophylline is used to treat neonatal apnea. Unlike its metabolism in adults, theophylline in neonates is extensively metabolized to caffeine. Plasma elimination half-life in adults is 3-6 hours. In neonates caffeine has a half-life of 30 hours. Caffeine overdoses are rare. The clinical presentation is similar to that of theophylline.

References

Bryson PD, "Stimulants," *Comprehensive Review in Toxicology*, 2nd ed, Rockville, MD: Aspen Publishers, 1989, 374-9.

Lewin NA, Goldfrank LR, Melinetz M, et al, "Caffeine," *Toxicological Emergencies*, Goldfrank LR, et al, eds, Norwalk, CT: Appleton-Century-Crofts, 1986, 537-44.

Moyer TP, Pippinger CE, Blanke RV, et al, "Therapeutic Drug Monitoring," *Clinical Chemistry*, Tietz NW, ed, New York, NY: WB Saunders Co, 1986, 1647-9.

Calan® *see* Verapamil *on page 1010*

Cannabinoids, Qualitative, Urine

CPT *80101 (screen); 80102 (confirmation)*

Related Information

Chain-of-Custody Protocol *on page 952*
Drugs of Abuse Testing, Urine *on page 962*

Synonyms Cannabis; Carboxy THC; Hashish; Hemp; Marijuana; 11-Nor-9-Carboxy-Delta-9-Tetrahydrocannabinol; Pot; THC (Delta-9-Tetrahydrocannabinol)

Abstract The main active ingredient of marijuana (cannabinoids) is tetrahydrocannabinol (THC). It is metabolized to THC-carboxylic acid which is detected in the urine. The name comes from the source of marijuana, the plant *Cannabis sativa*. It is a DEA schedule I drug and a widely used drug of abuse.

(Continued)

Cannabinoids, Qualitative, Urine *(Continued)*

Specimen Random urine **CONTAINER:** Plastic urine container **COLLECTION:** For employee screening or forensic purpose, use precautions during collection (see Introduction). **CAUSES FOR REJECTION:** Evidence of urine dilution or alteration **TURNAROUND TIME:** 1-2 hours, if in-house **SPECIAL INSTRUCTIONS:** If forensic, use chain-of-custody protocol and form. See test entry Chain-of-Custody Protocol and the Appendix of this chapter.

Interpretive **REFERENCE RANGE:** Negative (less than cutoff) **CRITICAL VALUES:** Cutoff: screen (NIDA): 100 ng/mL. Some laboratories use 50 ng/mL and a few use 20 ng/mL; confirmation: 15 ng/mL. **USE:** Drug abuse evaluation, toxicity assessment **LIMITATIONS:** Cannabinoids are rapidly metabolized from blood. Urine is the best specimen for screening although blood (serum or plasma) and saliva have been used. Cannabinoids can adhere to plastic. **METHODOLOGY:** Enzyme immunoassay (EIA), fluorescence polarization immunoassay (FPIA), thin-layer chromatography (TLC), gas chromatography/mass spectrometry (GC/MS) **ADDITIONAL INFORMATION:** A positive screen for cannabinoids indicates the presence of cannabinoid metabolites, 11-nor-9-carboxy-delta-9-THC is the major one (carboxy THC), in urine but is not related to source, time of exposure, amount, or impairment. Unless the screen is confirmed by GC/MS, a positive result is presumptive and an unconfirmed screen should not be used to test employees. Urine may contain carboxy THC for a week or 10 days after light or moderate use and as long as a month to 6 weeks after heavy use. Elimination half-life of carboxy THC is 35-40 hours. Rapid storage of THC metabolites in body fat occurs after use. These substances are then released from storage sites slowly over time.

A marijuana cigarette is made form the dried particles of the plant, *Cannabis sativa*. The immediate effects of smoking marijuana include a faster heartbeat and pulse rate, bloodshot eyes, and a dry mouth and throat. The drug can impair or reduce short-term memory, alter sense of time, and reduce the ability to do things which require concentration, swift reactions and coordination, such as driving and operating machinery.

Driving experiments show that marijuana affects a wide range of skills needed for safe driving. Thinking and reflexes are slowed, making it hard for drivers to respond to sudden unexpected events. Furthermore, a driver's ability to "track" through curves, brake quickly, and maintain speed and proper distance between vehicles is affected. Research shows that these skills are impaired for at least 4-6 hours after smoking a single marijuana cigarette. If a driver drinks alcohol along with using marijuana, the risks of a vehicular collision greatly increase.

References

Chiang CN and Barnett G, "Marijuana Pharmacokinetics and Pharmacodynamics," *Cocaine, Marijuana, Designer Drugs: Chemistry, Pharmacology and Behavior*, Redda KK, Walker CA, and Barnell G, eds, Boca Raton, FL: CRC Press, 1989, 113-26.

ElSohly MA and ElSohly HN, "Marijuana: Analysis and Detection of Use Through Urinalysis," *Cocaine, Marijuana, Designer Drugs: Chemistry, Pharmacology and Behavior*, Redda KK, Walker CA, and Barnett G, eds, Boca Raton, FL: CRC Press, 1989, 145-62.

Hawks RL and Chiang CN, "Examples of Specific Drug Assays: Marijuana/Cannabinoids," *Urine Testing for Drugs of Abuse*, NIDA Research Monograph 73, Rockville, MD, 1986, 85-92.

Schucket MA, "Cannabinols," *Drug and Alcohol Abuse*, New York, NY: Plenum, 1989, 143-57.

Wells DJ and Barnhill MT Jr, "Comparative Results With Five Cannabinoid Immunoassay Systems at the Screening Threshold of 100 Micrograms/L," *Clin Chem*, 1989, 35(11):2241-3.

Zuckerman B, Frank DA, Hingson R, et al, "Effects of Maternal Marijuana and Cocaine Use on Fetal Growth," *N Engl J Med*, 1989, 320(12):762-8.

Cannabis *see* Cannabinoids, Qualitative, Urine *on previous page*

Carbamazepine

CPT *80156*

Related Information

Carbamazepine-10,11-Epoxide *on next page*
Theophylline *on page 1002*
Valproic Acid *on page 1008*
Verapamil *on page 1010*
Warfarin *on page 1011*

Synonyms Tegretol®

Applies to P-450 System Inhibitor

Abstract Carbamazepine is a first-line antiepileptic drug for generalized and partial seizures. It is used for control of pain in trigeminal neuralgia and in treatment of bipolar affective disorder.

Patient Care PREPARATION: Levels should be drawn before next oral dose with patient at steady-state.

Specimen Serum CONTAINER: Red top tube SAMPLING TIME: A consistent sampling time, ideally a trough level, should be used to monitor patients on chronic therapy.

Interpretive REFERENCE RANGE: 8-12 μg/mL (SI: 25-51 μmol/L). Low level: The most common cause of a low level is noncompliance. The addition of anticonvulsants which induce the P-450 system, such as phenytoin, primidone, and phenobarbital, may decrease carbamazepine levels without causing seizures. (The P-450 system is a liver enzymatic system which degrades drugs.) The withdrawal of phenytoin from the regimen of a patient on carbamazepine may lower the level and cause seizures. Because of autoinduction of metabolism, patients in the first 2 months of therapy may have diminishing levels and be at risk for seizures. Occasionally, patients may have toxicity when levels are within the reference range. High level: Drugs which inhibit the P-450 system, including isoniazid, fluoxetine, propoxyphene, verapamil, and stiripentol can cause a precipitous rise in carbamazepine levels and clinical toxicity, usually within 48 hours. Danazol may cause a delayed toxicity. The addition of cimetidine, erythromycin, lithium, triacetyloleandomycin, and valproic acid also can cause toxicity. POSSIBLE PANIC RANGE: Central nervous system toxicity occurs progressively with levels near or above high end of reference range. USE: Monitor for compliance, efficacy, or possible toxicity LIMITATIONS: See Carbamazepine-10,11-Epoxide listing. CONTRAINDICATIONS: Half-life of warfarin is shortened; monoamine oxidase inhibitors not recommended. METHODOLOGY: Enzyme immunoassay (EIA), gas-liquid chromatography (GLC), high performance liquid chromatography (HPLC) ADDITIONAL INFORMATION: Leukopenia may be dose related and necessitates stopping the drug if the absolute neutrophil count falls <1000/mm³.[1] Hyponatremia may occur, especially in older patients. Patients in the first month of pregnancy are at increased risk of neural tube defects. Carbamazepine may interfere with the actions of theophylline, oral contraceptives, oral anticoagulants, or doxycycline. See Table A in the Appendix of this chapter.

Footnotes

1. Engel J, *Seizures and Epilepsy*, Contemporary Neurology Series, Philadelphia, PA: FA Davis Co, 1989.

References

Bertilsson L and Tomson T, "Clinical Pharmacokinetics and Pharmacological Effects of Carbamazepine and Carbamazepine-10-11-Epoxide," *Clin Pharmacokinet*, 1986, 11:177-98.

Grimsley SR, Jann MW, Carter JG, et al, "Increased Carbamazepine Concentrations After Fluoxetine Coadministration," *Clin Pharmacol Ther*, 1991, 50(1):10-5.

Levy RH, Dreifuss FE, Mattson RH, et al, *Antiepileptic Drugs*, 3rd ed, New York, NY: Raven Press, 1989.

Perry PJ, Alexander B, and Liskow BI, *Psychotropic Drug Handbook*, Cincinnati, OH: Harvey Whitney Books, 1988.

Carbamazepine-10,11-Epoxide

CPT 80156

Related Information

Carbamazepine *on previous page*

Synonyms Carbamazepine Metabolite

Test Commonly Includes Carbamazepine and carbamazepine-10,11-epoxide

Abstract Occasional cases of carbamazepine toxicity occur with normal levels of carbamazepine due to accumulation of the active metabolite, 10,11-epoxide.[1,2]

Specimen Serum CONTAINER: Red top tube

Interpretive REFERENCE RANGE: 0.8-3.2 mg/L. High level: In patients on chronic carbamazepine therapy, the addition of valpromide or progabide produces clinical toxicity with high levels of metabolite and normal levels of parent compound.[3] LIMITATIONS: Valproic acid, a compound chemically related to valpromide, may increase the epoxide/carbamazepine ratio by eliminating excretion of the epoxide. Since most cases of fatal valproate hepatotoxicity occur in young children on multiple anticonvulsants, the combination of valproate and carbamazepine is not recommended. Phenytoin may also increase the ratio of epoxide/parent compound.[4] METHODOLOGY: High performance liquid chromatography (HPLC), fluorescence polarization immunoassay (FPIA) ADDITIONAL INFORMATION: Carbamazepine-10,11-epoxide has been shown to be pharmacologically active in animals.[5]

Footnotes

1. Pisani F, Fazio A, Oteri G, et al, "Sodium Valproate and Valpromide: Differential Interaction With Carbamazepine in Epileptic Patients," *Epilepsia*, 1986, 27:548-52.
2. Kutt H, Solomon GE, Dhar AK, et al, "Effects of Progabide on Carbamazepine Epoxide and Carbamazepine Concentrations in Plasma," *Epilepsia*, 1984, 25:674.
3. Meijer JWA, Binnie CD, Debets RMC, et al, "Possible Hazard of Valpromide-Carbamazepine Combination Therapy in Epilepsy," *Lancet*, 1984, 802.

(Continued)

Carbamazepine-10,11-Epoxide *(Continued)*

4. Theodore WH, Narang PK, Holmes MD, et al, "Carbamazepine and its Epoxide: Relation of Plasma Levels to Toxicity and Seizure Control," *Ann Neurol*, 1989, 25:194-6.
5. Albright PS and Bruni J, "Effects of Carbamazepine and its Epoxide Metabolite on Amygdala-Kindled Seizures in Rats," *Neurology*, 1984, 34:1383-6.

Carbamazepine Metabolite *see* Carbamazepine-10,11-Epoxide *on previous page*

Carboxy THC *see* Cannabinoids, Qualitative, Urine *on page 949*

Cardioquin® *see* Quinidine, Serum *on page 999*

Cd, Blood *see* Cadmium, Urine and Blood *on page 948*

Cd, Urine *see* Cadmium, Urine and Blood *on page 948*

Cerebrospinal Fluid Methotrexate *see* Methotrexate *on page 985*

Chain-of-Custody Protocol

Related Information

Blood Collection Tube Information *on page 26*
Drugs of Abuse Testing, Urine *on page 962*
Specimen Identification Requirements *on page 30*
Venous Blood Collection *on page 32*

Synonyms Specimen Chain-of-Custody Protocol

Applies to Medical Legal Specimens

Abstract A procedure to ensure sample integrity from collection through transport, receipt, sampling, and analysis. It is associated with a Chain-of-Custody form. See the Appendix of this chapter.

Specimen COLLECTION: See Introduction for collection precautions. **CAUSES FOR REJECTION:** Sample cup or bag containing sample cup not sealed

Interpretive REFERENCE RANGE: Normal: all seals intact and Chain-of-Custody form completed. USE: Chain-of-custody is a legal term that describes a method to maintain sample integrity in the collection, handling, and storage of urine samples. ADDITIONAL INFORMATION: The chain-of-custody protocol is a clerical and custodial service offered by the laboratory to document specimen transfer and provide for extended specimen storage. A written record of specimen transfer from patient, to analyst, to storage and disposal is maintained on all specimens covered by chain-of-custody. All drug screens, blood alcohols, or any other tests that have medicolegal significance should be accompanied by Chain-of-Custody and a written release form.

References

Smith ML, Bronner WE, Shimomura ET, et al, "Quality Assurance in Drug Testing Laboratories," *Clin Lab Med*, 1990, 10(3):503-16.

Chloramphenicol

CPT 82415

Related Information

Antibiotic Level, Serum *on page 942*
Serum Bactericidal Test *on page 843*
Susceptibility Testing, Aerobic and Facultatively Anaerobic Organisms *on page 864*

Synonyms Chloromycetin®; Mychel-S®

Abstract The use of the antimicrobial agent, chloramphenicol, has been greatly reduced in recent years because of the introduction of a wide variety of less toxic alternative agents. It is still appropriately used to treat certain rickettsial infections or penicillin-allergic patients with bacterial meningitis. Life-threatening bone marrow toxicity is not closely associated with high serum levels.

Specimen Serum CONTAINER: Red top tube SAMPLING TIME: Collect for trough level immediately before next dose; for peak level about 2 hours after oral dose, 30 minutes after I.V. dose (time to peak can be variable) STORAGE INSTRUCTIONS: Freeze processed specimen

Interpretive REFERENCE RANGE: Therapeutic: 10-25 μg/mL (SI: 31-77 μmol/L), trough <5 μg/mL (SI: <15 μmol/L) CRITICAL VALUES: Toxic: >25 μg/mL (SI: >77 μmol/L) USE: Monitor drug therapy; monitoring for potential toxicity. See Table B in the Appendix of this chapter. LIMITATIONS: Reversible dose related bone marrow depression may occur when serum/plasma concentration >25 μg/mL (SI: >77 μmol/L). Idiosyncratic bone marrow aplasia is a rare event that usually occurs weeks to months after completion of therapy, but approximately 25% occur during the course of therapy. Hematologic studies should be performed before and during therapy. **METHODOLOGY:** High performance liquid chromatography (HPLC), gas-liquid chromatography (GLC), immunoassay **ADDITIONAL INFORMATION:** Chloramphenicol is an extremely effective antibacterial agent which unfortunately has both idiosyncratic and dose-related toxicities. Half-life is 1.6-3.3 hours longer in infants and patients with hepatic and renal disease. The dose related toxicity is, in adults, bone marrow suppression. "Gray syndrome," a type of circulatory collapse, occurs primarily in infants whose livers are unable to metabolize chloramphenicol effectively. Idiosyncratic aplastic anemia occurs in between 1 in 20,000 and 1 in 40,000 exposures. There are a number of chloramphenicol drug interactions since chloramphenicol can inhibit hepatic microsomal metabolism, increasing the serum concentration of phenytoin, tolbutamide, and dicumarol. Phenobarbital may be elevated in the presence of chloramphenicol.

References

Baselt RC, *Analytical Procedures for Therapeutic Drug Monitoring and Emergency Toxicology*, Davis, CA: Biomedical Publications, 1980, 71-5.

deLouvois J, Mulhall A, and Hurley R, "Comparison of Methods Available for Assay of Chloramphenicol in Clinical Specimens," *J Clin Pathol*, 1980, 33:575-80.

Miceli J, "Chloramphenicol and Vancomycin," *Clin Lab Med*, 1987, 7:531-40.

Mulhall A, deLouvois J, and Hurley R, "Chloramphenicol Toxicity in Neonates; Its Incidence and Prevention," *Br Med J [Clin Res]*, 1983, 287:1424-7.

Peuell DA and Nahatz MC, "Chloramphenicol: New Perspectives on an Old Drug," *Drug Intell Clin Pharm*, 1982, 16:295-300.

Smilack JD, Wilson WR, and Cockerill FR 3d, "Tetracyclines, Chloramphenicol, Erythromycin, Clindamycin, and Metronidazole," *Mayo Clin Proc*, 1991, 66(12):1270-80.

Chlordiazepoxide, Blood

CPT *80154*

Related Information

Benzodiazepines, Qualitative, Urine *on page 947*

Synonyms Librax®; Librium®

Abstract This is a benzodiazepine drug used as a sedative-hypnotic (tranquilizer). It is widely prescribed.

Specimen Serum **CONTAINER:** Red top tube **SAMPLING TIME:** Collect for trough level prior to next dose; collect for peak level 4 hours after oral dosing. **STORAGE INSTRUCTIONS:** Process immediately; avoid exposure to light; freeze if not analyzed immediately.

Interpretive **REFERENCE RANGE:** Therapeutic: 0.1-3.0 μg/mL (SI: 0-10 μmol/L) **CRITICAL VALUES:** Toxic (stupor): >20 μg/mL (SI: >77 μmol/L) **USE:** Monitor therapeutic drug level, determine toxic level **METHODOLOGY:** High performance liquid chromatography (HPLC), thin-layer chromatography (TLC), gas chromatography (GC), fluorometry **ADDITIONAL INFORMATION:** This drug is an antianxiety agent commonly used in suicide attempts. Chlordiazepoxide is slowly absorbed and may take several hours to reach a peak plasma level. Distribution after intramuscular administration is poor. Drug half-life in blood ranges from 16-27 hours. The drug is highly (90%) protein bound. Overdosage with the benzodiazepines is frequent, but serious sequelae are rare. However, there is an additive effect when used with other CNS depressants (eg, ethanol). If a patient is comatose after a drug ingestion, chlordiazepoxide **alone** is not a sufficient explanation. Metabolism results in the production of four active metabolites.

References

Baselt RC, *Disposition of Toxic Drugs and Chemicals in Man*, 3rd ed, Davis, CA: Biomedical Publications, 1989, 155.

Minder EI, "Toxicity in a Case of Acute and Massive Overdose of Chlordiazepoxide and its Correlation to Blood Concentration," *J Toxicol Clin Toxicol*, 1989, 27(1-2):117-27.

Chloromycetin® *see* Chloramphenicol *on previous page*

Chlorpromazine *see* Methamphetamines, Qualitative, Urine *on page 984*

Chlorpromazine *see* Phenothiazines, Serum *on page 993*

Chlorpromazine, Urine

CPT *84022*

Synonyms Thorazine®

Applies to Phenothiazines

Abstract This is an aliphatic phenothiazine used as an antipsychotic and sedative.

(Continued)

Chlorpromazine, Urine *(Continued)*

Specimen Urine **CONTAINER:** Plastic urine container **COLLECTION:** Freshly voided random urine **STORAGE INSTRUCTIONS:** Refrigerate

Interpretive **REFERENCE RANGE:** Negative unless on therapeutic regimen **USE:** Screen for chlorpromazine in urine; evaluate possibility of chlorpromazine poisoning or drug toxicity **LIMITATIONS:** Test is not specific for chlorpromazine and will detect other phenothiazines if present. **METHODOLOGY:** Gas-liquid chromatography (GLC); thin-layer chromatography (TLC) **ADDITIONAL INFORMATION:** Due to the complex metabolism of this drug, the pharmacokinetics are variable and follow a multiphasic pattern. Attempts to correlate drug levels with clinical responses have not been successful. Antipsychotic drugs are nonaddicting. Deaths from accidental poisonings are rare. Chlorpromazine may have endocrinopathic, hematologic, and hepatic consequences. Endocrinopathic consequences may include blocked ovulation with increased urinary estrogens and decreased urinary gonadotropins and progestins. Other endocrinopathic consequences may be associated with decreased serum growth hormone, increased metabolism by hepatic microsomes (decreased thyroxine, T_4), increased metabolism and decreased organ uptake of norepinephrine (increased VMA), altered steroid metabolism (increased 17-ketosteroids), or an inhibition of the hypothalamus and decreased ACTH secretion (decreased 17-ketosteroids and 17-OH corticosteroids). Hematologic consequences may be associated with hemolytic anemia (decreased serum haptoglobin and decreased blood hematocrit, hemoglobin, and red cell count) as well as occasional neutropenia, agranulocytosis, leukopenia, and granulocytopenia. A recent study shows that some patients on this drug have an increase in antiphospholipid antibodies. However, no predisposition to thromboembolism was noted.[1] Also, increase in antinuclear antibodies has been noted.[2] Hepatic sensitivity may occur in 2% of patients and may be associated with increased alkaline phosphatase, AST, bilirubin, and in increased eosinophils, often a precursor of jaundice. False-positive pregnancy tests may occur in patients on chlorpromazine.

Footnotes

1. Lillicrap DP, Pinto M, Benford K, et al, "Heterogeneity of Laboratory Test Results for Antiphospholipid Antibodies in Patients Treated With Chlorpromazine and Other Phenothiazines," *Am J Clin Pathol*, 1990, 93(6):771-5.
2. Zucker S, Zarrabi HM, Schubach WH, et al, "Chlorpromazine-Induced Immunopathy: Progressive Increase in Serum IgM," *Medicine (Baltimore)*, 1990, 69(2):92-100.

References

Baselt RC and Cravey RH, *Disposition of Toxic Drugs and Chemicals in Man*, Chicago, IL: Year Book Medical Publishers Inc, 1989, 177-82.

Chrysotherapy *see* Gold *on page 971*

Clonazepam

CPT 80154

Related Information

Benzodiazepines, Qualitative, Urine *on page 947*

Synonyms Klonopin™; Rivatril®

Abstract The drug is in the class of benzodiazepines which are used as tranquilizers.

Specimen Serum **CONTAINER:** Red top tube **STORAGE INSTRUCTIONS:** Separate serum and freeze. Protect from sunlight.

Interpretive **REFERENCE RANGE:** Therapeutic: 10-50 ng/mL (SI: 32-158 nmol/L) **CRITICAL VALUES:** Serum values >100 ng/mL **POSSIBLE PANIC RANGE:** Toxic: >100 ng/mL (SI: >317 nmol/L) **USE:** Monitor drug level and toxicity **METHODOLOGY:** Gas-liquid chromatography (GLC) **ADDITIONAL INFORMATION:** Serum peak levels occur approximately 2 hours after oral administration. The apparent half-life after a single oral dose is 20-40 hours. Active metabolites have longer half-lives than the parent drug. Half-lives are increased in the elderly. Therapeutic effect is not well correlated with serum levels. Effect of CNS depressants may be augmented by concomitant use of this agent. This drug is used as an anticonvulsant. It is useful in reducing tardive dyskinesia.[1] See Table A in the Appendix of this chapter.

Footnotes

1. Thaker GK, Nguyen JA, Strauss ME, et al, "Clonazepam Treatment of Tardive Dyskinesia: A Practical GABAmimetic Strategy," *Am J Psychiatry*, 1990, 147(4):445-51.

References

Baselt RC and Cravey RH, *Disposition of Toxic Drugs and Chemicals in Man*, Chicago, IL: Year Book Medical Publishers Inc, 1989, 199-201.

CN⁻ *see* Cyanide, Blood *on next page*

Cocaine (Cocaine Metabolite), Qualitative, Urine

***CPT** 80101 (screen); 80102 (confirmation)*

Related Information

Chain-of-Custody Protocol *on page 952*
Drugs of Abuse Testing, Urine *on page 962*
Myoglobin, Qualitative, Urine *on page 1135*

Synonyms Coke; Crack; Snow

Test Commonly Includes Cocaine is detected in urine as its metabolite, benzoylecgonine.

Abstract A prominent metabolite of cocaine is benzoylecgonine, which is the substance measured in urine to detect the presence of cocaine. Cocaine is a heavily abused drug which has legitimate medical uses in some ENT procedures.

Specimen Urine **CONTAINER:** Plastic urine container **COLLECTION:** If forensic, observe precautions concerning surreptitious dilution or alteration. **STORAGE INSTRUCTIONS:** Refrigerate **CAUSES FOR REJECTION:** If forensic, failure to meet temperature requirements immediately after collection and/or tests for unusual dilution (specific gravity, urine creatinine) or alteration. **SPECIAL INSTRUCTIONS:** If forensic, use chain-of-custody protocol and form. See test entry Chain-of-Custody Protocol and the Appendix of this chapter.

Interpretive **REFERENCE RANGE:** Negative (less than cutoff) **CRITICAL VALUES:** Cutoff: screen: 300 ng/mL; confirmation: 150 ng/mL **USE:** Evaluate cocaine use **METHODOLOGY:** Screen: immunoassay, fluorescence polarization immunoassay (FPIA), thin-layer chromatography (TLC); confirmation: gas chromatography/mass spectrometry (GC/MS) **ADDITIONAL INFORMATION:** Cocaine is a highly abused drug which is most frequently detected in the urine as the metabolite, benzoylecgonine and usually as part of a multiclass drug panel. In pre-employment drug screening, the presence of cocaine (benzoylecgonine) should be confirmed by GC/MS.

Cocaine is a central nervous system stimulant. It usually appears as a fine crystal-like powder which is the hydrochloride or sulfate salt and as such is "snorted" (inhaled through the nose). When mixed with sodium bicarbonate and converted to free base, it appears as hard pieces called "crack" which can be smoked. This is currently a very prevalent form of the drug.

The effects of the drug begin within minutes and peak within 15-20 minutes. These effects include dilated pupils, increase in blood pressure, heart rate, breathing rate, and body temperature. The dangers of cocaine use vary, depending on how the drug is taken, the dose, and the individual. Some regular users report feelings of restlessness, irritability, anxiety, and sleeplessness. In some people even low doses of cocaine may create psychological problems. People who use high doses of cocaine over a long period of time may become paranoid or experience what is called a cocaine psychosis. This may include hallucinations of touch, sight, taste, and smell. Cocaine itself has a half-life of 1-2 hours while benzoylecgonine has a half-life of 7-9 hours. Benzoylecgonine is detectable in urine within 2-3 hours and for a period of 2-3 days after a single use.

References

Cone EJ, "Validity Testing of Commercial Urine Cocaine Metabolite Assays: III. Evaluation of an Enzyme-Linked Immunosorbent Assay (ELISA) for Detection of Cocaine and Cocaine Metabolite," *J Forensic Sci*, 1989, 34(4):991-5.

Cone EJ, Menchen SL, Paul BD, et al, "Validity Testing of Commercial Urine Cocaine Metabolite Assays: I. Assay Detection Times, Individual Excretion Patterns, and Kinetics After Cocaine Administration to Humans," *J Forensic Sci*, 1989, 34(1):15-31.

Cone EJ and Mitchell J, "Validity Testing of Commercial Urine Cocaine Metabolite Assays: II. Sensitivity, Specificity, Accuracy, and Confirmation by Gas Chromatography/Mass Spectrometry," *J Forensic Sci*, 1989, 34(1):32-45.

Gawin FH and Ellinwood EH Jr, "Cocaine and Other Stimulants," *N Engl J Med*, 1988, 318:1173-82.

Karch SB, "The History of Cocaine Toxicity," *Hum Pathol*, 1989, 20(11):1037-9.

Zuckerman B, Frank DA, Hingson R, et al, "Effects of Maternal Marijuana and Cocaine Use on Fetal Growth," *N Engl J Med*, 1989, 320(12):762-8.

Codeine, Urine

***CPT** 80101 (screen); 80102 (confirmation); 82101 (quantitative)*

Related Information

Chain-of-Custody Protocol *on page 952*
Opiates, Qualitative, Urine *on page 989*
(Continued)

Codeine, Urine *(Continued)*

Applies to Opiates, Urine

Test Commonly Includes Part of opiate screen

Abstract Codeine occurs naturally in opium but is produced commercially by 3-O-methylation of morphine. It is used as a narcotic analgesic. It is present in numerous proprietary preparations combined with non-narcotic analgesics and antihistamines. It is a drug of abuse.

Specimen Urine **CONTAINER:** Plastic urine container **SAMPLING TIME:** Random **STORAGE INSTRUCTIONS:** Refrigerate specimen **SPECIAL INSTRUCTIONS:** If forensic, use precautions in collection and Chain-of-Custody form. See test entry Chain-of-Custody Protocol and the Appendix of this chapter.

Interpretive **REFERENCE RANGE:** Negative (below cutoff) **CRITICAL VALUES:** Cutoff: screen: 300 ng/mL (for drug-of-abuse screen), confirmation: 300 ng/mL **USE:** Evaluate codeine toxicity; detect drug-of-abuse **METHODOLOGY:** Enzyme immunoassay (EIA); thin-layer chromatography (TLC) **ADDITIONAL INFORMATION:** Codeine, made by the methylation of morphine, is similar to morphine in uses, actions, contraindications, and adverse reactions. About $1/6$ to $1/10$ as potent as morphine, it is used to manage mild to moderate pain. In low doses, it is an antitussive. After oral dose, the onset of action is 15-30 minutes, and peak levels are reached in 1-1.5 hours. The half-life is 2.5-4 hours. Codeine is excreted mainly in the urine as norcodeine and free and conjugated morphine. Adverse effects of codeine include miosis, increased intracranial pressure, antidiuretic hormone release, and physical and psychological dependence.

References

Barson W, "Narcotic Agents," *Ann Emerg Med*, 1986, 15:1019-20.

Blanke RV and Decker WJ, "Analysis of Toxic Substances," *Textbook of Clinical Chemistry*, Tietz NW, ed, Philadelphia, PA: WB Saunders Co, 1986, 1735-9.

Coke *see* Cocaine (Cocaine Metabolite), Qualitative, Urine *on previous page*

Comatose Profile *see* Toxicology Drug Screen, Blood *on page 1005*

Compazine® *see* Phenothiazines, Serum *on page 993*

Cordarone® *see* Amiodarone *on page 939*

Coumadin® *see* Warfarin *on page 1011*

Crack *see* Cocaine (Cocaine Metabolite), Qualitative, Urine *on previous page*

Crystal *see* Amphetamines, Qualitative, Urine *on page 941*

Crystal *see* Methamphetamines, Qualitative, Urine *on page 984*

Crystodigin® *see* Digitoxin *on page 959*

Cyanide, Blood

CPT 82600

Related Information

Hemoglobin *on page 554*

Synonyms CN⁻; Hydrocyanic Acid; Potassium or Sodium Cyanide

Abstract This highly toxic substance is one of the oldest poisons known. It binds to cytochrome oxidase and prevents cellular respiration.

Specimen Whole blood or serum **CONTAINER:** Lavender top (EDTA) tube or red top tube **STORAGE INSTRUCTIONS:** Fill tube to capacity and keep tightly closed; analyze as soon as possible. Refrigerate whole blood, gastric contents or tissue.

Interpretive **REFERENCE RANGE:** Whole blood: nonsmoker: 20 ng/mL, smoker: 40 ng/mL; plasma: nonsmoker: 4 ng/mL, smoker: 6 ng/mL **CRITICAL VALUES:** In whole blood, values >1.0 μg/mL are potentially fatal although subjects with higher values have survived. **POSSIBLE PANIC RANGE:** Toxic: >1 μg/mL (SI: >77 μmol/L); >2 μg/mL (SI: >115 μmol/L) is lethal **USE:** Establish the diagnosis of cyanide poisoning **METHODOLOGY:** Conway diffusion, color reaction, ion specific potentiometry **ADDITIONAL INFORMATION:** Cyanide is present in insecticides, rodenticides, vermicides, metal polishes, and electroplating baths. Symptoms of toxicity include headache, agitation, vomiting, and confusion. A scent of bitter almonds is suggestive, but not all individuals can detect it. Treatment with nitrites is effective. Nitrites produce methemoglobin which binds cyanide ions and thus removes them from cytochrome oxidase. Half-life of cyanide in whole blood is 45-65 hours. Cyanide is metabolized by rhodanase to thiocyanate. Thiosulfate is given along with nitrites to promote the conversion of cyanide to thiocyanate which is much less toxic and is excreted. Cyanide itself blocks cellular metabolism by inhibiting cytochrome oxidase.

References

Lundquist P and Sorbo B, "Rapid Determination of Toxic Cyanide Concentrations in Blood," *Clin Chem*, 1989, 35(4):617-9.

Moore SJ, Ho IK, and Hume AS, "Severe Hypoxia Produced by Concomitant Intoxication With Sublethal Doses of Carbon Monoxide and Cyanide," *Toxicol Appl Pharmacol*, 1991, 109(3):412-20.

Cyclosporine

CPT 80158

Related Information

Magnesium, Serum *on page 287*

Synonyms Sandimmune®

Applies to Cyclosporine A

Abstract This drug is widely used as an immunosuppressant, especially after organ transplants.

Specimen Whole blood, plasma, or serum **CONTAINER:** Lavender top (EDTA) tube (whole blood), green top (heparin) tube (plasma), red top tube (serum) **SAMPLING TIME:** Trough levels should be obtained 12-18 hours after oral dose (chronic usage), 12 hours after intravenous dose, or immediately prior to next dose.

Interpretive REFERENCE RANGE: RIA: immediately following transplant: 150-250 ng/mL (SI: 125-210 nmol/L) (plasma levels), 450-750 ng/mL (SI: 374-624 nmol/L) (whole blood levels). Maintenance levels months after transplant: 50-150 ng/mL (SI: 40-125 nmol/L) (plasma levels), 150-450 ng/mL (SI: 125-375 nmol/L) (whole blood levels). Reference ranges are method dependent and specimen dependent. **USE:** Monitor blood level in management of immunosuppression of organ transplant recipients. **LIMITATIONS:** Results are method dependent – some measure multiple metabolites as well as parent drug. It is not yet clearly established whether whole blood or plasma/serum levels are clinically most appropriate. Single assays are not as informative as a series over time. **METHODOLOGY:** Radioimmunoassay (RIA), high performance liquid chromatography (HPLC), fluorescence polarization immunoassay (FPIA) **ADDITIONAL INFORMATION:** Cyclosporine is an immunosuppressive agent derived from *Tolypocladium inflatum gams*, a fungus originally isolated from a Norwegian soil sample. The agent is used extensively to control rejection of organ transplants, especially of liver, heart, or kidney. The exact mechanism of action of the drug is not known, but it appears to interfere with T-helper cell function and secretion of lymphokines. It is not myelosuppressive.

Monitoring of blood levels is imperative because the pharmacokinetics of cyclosporine are not only complex, but vary over time in the same patient; thus, blood levels cannot be well predicted from dosing schedules. Furthermore, this drug has a narrow therapeutic window and significant toxicity at levels above that range.

Renal toxicity with eventual renal failure is the most severe complication. Other assays to assess renal function (ie, BUN, creatinine clearance) should be ordered along with cyclosporine level, since toxicity may begin even with "acceptable" blood levels. Other toxicities include hypertension, convulsions, tremors, pulmonary edema, and an increased risk of lymphoma.

Drugs which enhance the potential toxicity of cyclosporine, and which are also likely to be administered to a transplant recipient, include aminoglycoside antibiotics, cephalosporins, trimethoprim-sulfa, amphotericin B, acyclovir, ketoconazole, and furosemide. Agents which raise cyclosporine levels by decreasing biotransformation include methylprednisolone, amphotericin B, cimetidine, and erythromycin. Drugs which increase hepatic metabolism and thus lower cyclosporine levels include phenobarbital, phenytoin, rifampin, and trimetheprim-sulfa.

Because results will vary depending on whether the assay is done on whole blood or serum/plasma and on the method and cyclosporine antibody employed (monospecific or polyspecific), it is best for a given patient's specimens to be analyzed at a single laboratory to eliminate as many assay-dependent variables as possible. If switching of laboratories is unavoidable, it is advisable to have a few specimens run in parallel in the second laboratory prior to changing.

The clinical use of cyclosporine is difficult and requires experience and judgment. A drug blood level is only one of many pieces in the puzzle of transplant medicine.

References

Cannafax DM and Ascher NL, "Cyclosporine Immunosuppression," *Clin Pharm*, 1983, 2:515-24.

Frey FJ, Horber FF, and Frey BM, "Trough Levels and Concentration Time Curves of Cyclosporine in Patients Undergoing Renal Transplantation," *Clin Pharmacol Ther*, 1988, 43:55-62.

Gerson B, "Cyclosporine Controversies," *Clin Lab Med*, 1987, 7:669-86.

(Continued)

Cyclosporine *(Continued)*

Giesbrecht, EE, Soldin SJ, and Wong PY, "A Rapid, Reliable High Performance Liquid Chromatographic Micromethod for the Measurement of Cyclosporine in Whole Blood," *Ther Drug Monit*, 1989, 11(3):332-36.

Hayashi Y, Shibata N, Minouchi T, et al, "Evaluation of Fluorescence Polarization Immunoassay for Determination of Cyclosporine in Plasma," *Ther Drug Monit*, 1989, 11(2):205-9.

Hooks MA, Millikan WJ, Henderson JM, et al, "Comparison of Whole-Blood Cyclosporine Levels Measured by Radioimmunoassay and Fluorescence Polarization in Patients Post Orthotropic Liver Transplant," *Ther Drug Monit*, 1989, 11(3):304-9.

Kahan BD, "Cyclosporine," *N Engl J Med*, 1989, 321(25):1725-38.

Kahan BD, "Individualization of Cyclosporine Therapy Using Pharmacokinetics and Pharmacodynamic Parameters," *Transplantation*, 1985, 40:457-76.

Lindholm A and Henricsson S, "Simultaneous Monitoring of Cyclosporine in Blood and Plasma With Four Analytical Methods: A Clinical Evaluation," *Transplant Proc*, 1989, 21(1 Pt 2):1472-4.

Martinez L, Foradori A, Vaccarezza A, et al, "Monitoring of Cyclosporine Blood Levels With Polyclonal and Monoclonal Assays During Episodes of Renal Graft Dysfunction," *Transplant Proc*, 1989, 21(1 Pt 2):1490-1.

McBride JH, Rodgerson DO, Allin RE, et al, "Comparison of Four Immunoassays for the Measurement of Cyclosporine and Metabolites in Plasma," *Clin Chem*, 1988, 34:1259.

Moyer TP, Johnson P, Faynor SM, et al, "Cyclosporine: A Review of Drug Monitoring Problems and Presentation of a Simple, Accurate Liquid Chromatographic Procedure That Solves These Problems," *Clin Biochem*, 1986, 19:83-9.

Ptachinski R, Venkataramanan R, and Burkart GJ, "Clinical Pharmacokinetics of Cyclosporine," *Clin Pharmacokinet*, 1986, 11:107-32.

Sanghvi A, Diven W, Seltman H, et al, "Abbott's Fluorescence Polarization Immunoassay for Cyclosporine and Metabolites Compared With the Sandoz "Sandimmune®" RIA," *Clin Chem*, 1988, 34:1904-6.

Terreros DA and Coombs J, "Cyclosporine Nephropathy: Inhibition of Osmoregulatory Renal Cell Transport," *Ann Clin Lab Sci*, 1989, 19(5):337-44, (abstract).

Cyclosporine A *see* Cyclosporine *on previous page*

Dalmane® *see* Flurazepam *on page 969*

Darvocet-N® *see* Propoxyphene, Blood or Urine *on page 997*

Darvon® *see* Propoxyphene, Blood or Urine *on page 997*

Datril® *see* Acetaminophen, Serum *on page 935*

DAU *see* Drugs of Abuse Testing, Urine *on page 962*

DAU-10 *see* Drugs of Abuse Testing, Urine *on page 962*

Delta Aminolevulinic Acid Dehydratase *see* Lead, Blood *on page 976*

Demerol® *see* Meperidine, Urine *on page 981*

Depakene® *see* Valproic Acid *on page 1008*

Depakote® (Enteric-Coated Divalproex-Sodium) *see* Valproic Acid *on page 1008*

Depamide® *see* Valproic Acid *on page 1008*

Desipramine *see* Imipramine *on page 974*

Desipramine *see* Tricyclic Antidepressants *on page 1007*

Desoxyn® *see* Methamphetamines, Qualitative, Urine *on page 984*

Desyrel® *see* Trazodone *on page 1006*

Dexies *see* Amphetamines, Qualitative, Urine *on page 941*

Diazepam, Blood

CPT 80154

Related Information

Benzodiazepines, Qualitative, Urine *on page 947*

Synonyms Valium®

Abstract This is a benzodiazepine used as a sedative-hypnotic (tranquilizer).

Specimen Serum **CONTAINER:** Red top tube **SAMPLING TIME:** For peak level, 1 hour after oral dose or 15 minutes after I.V. **STORAGE INSTRUCTIONS:** Do not freeze

Interpretive **REFERENCE RANGE:** Diazepam: therapeutic: 0.2-1.5 μg/mL (SI: 0.7-5.3 μmol/L); N-desmethyldiazepam (nordiazepam): therapeutic: 0.1-0.5 μg/mL (SI: 0.35-1.8 μmol/L) **CRITICAL**

VALUES: Toxic: sum of diazepam plus N-desmethyldiazepam >3.0 μg/mL **POSSIBLE PANIC RANGE:** Total of diazepam and nordiazepam >5 μg/mL (SI: >18 μmol/L) is toxic. **USE:** Therapeutic monitoring and toxicity assessment **METHODOLOGY:** Enzyme immunoassay (EIA), high performance liquid chromatography (HPLC), UV spectrophotometry, gas-liquid chromatography (GLC) **ADDITIONAL INFORMATION:** Diazepam is a muscle relaxant and antianxiety drug. Peak blood levels are achieved within an hour after oral dose. Half-life in adults is 21-37 hours. The major metabolite (N-desmethyldiazepam) has a half-life in adults of 50-99 hours. It is the major metabolite also of Tranxene® and prazepam. Diazepam may exhibit synergism with barbiturates, tricyclic antidepressants, and amine oxidase inhibitors. Toxicity may be additive with other central nervous system depressants, and ethanol enhances the absorption of diazepam itself. Many cases of overdose are seen but few fatalities result from use of this drug alone. A frequent finding is a combination of this drug and ethanol.

References

Greenblatt DJ, Ehrenberg BL, Gunderman J, et al, "Pharmacokinetic and Electroencephalographic Study of Intravenous Diazepam, Midazolam, and Placebo," *Clin Pharmacol Ther*, 1989, 45(4):356-65.

Digitalis *see* Digitoxin *on this page*

Digitoxin

CPT 80299

Synonyms Crystodigin®; Digitalis; Lanotoxin®; Purodigin®

Abstract One of a group of plant glycosides used in the treatment of congestive heart failure, digitoxin is infrequently used compared to digoxin. It must not be confused with digoxin when serum levels are ordered.

Specimen Serum **CONTAINER:** Red top tube **SAMPLING TIME:** 6-12 hours after dose **STORAGE INSTRUCTIONS:** Separate serum and store in refrigerator.

Interpretive **REFERENCE RANGE:** Therapeutic: 20-35 ng/mL (SI: 26-46 nmol/L). **CRITICAL VALUES:** Levels >35 ng/mL (SI: >46 nmol/L) are associated with clinical toxicity in 80% of patients. **USE:** Therapeutic monitoring and toxicity assessment. See Table C in the Appendix of this chapter. **LIMITATIONS:** **Do not order digitoxin level on a patient receiving digoxin**. Digitoxin is not commonly used. **CONTRAINDICATIONS:** Patient on **digoxin**; recent radioactive tracer **METHODOLOGY:** Radioimmunoassay (RIA), gas-liquid chromatography (GLC), high performance liquid chromatography (HPLC) **ADDITIONAL INFORMATION:** Optimal sampling time after dosage is 6 hours. Optimal resampling time after change in dosage is 48-96 hours. Elimination half-life is 5-7 days. Be sure the patient is not on digoxin instead of digitoxin. There is cross reactivity between the two drugs and the levels reported will not be valid, and in fact could be misleading and catastrophic. Digitalis leaf has both digoxin and digitoxin as active components. Digitoxin is the best test for evaluation of toxicity in a patient taking digitalis leaf, but neither test is truly satisfactory. There is considerable overlap in the upper therapeutic ranges with levels which may be toxic. **Digitoxin levels must be correlated with clinical and other chemical data.** Numerous factors modify the effect of cardiac glycosides, including serum potassium, calcium, magnesium, and cardiac blood flow. Hypokalemia, hypomagnesemia, and hypercalcemia all potentiate toxicity from cardiac glycosides. Agents with significant interactions with digitoxin include cholestyramine, heparin, phenobarbital, phenytoin, rifampin, and possibly quinidine.

References

Bayer MJ, "Recognition and Management of Digitalis Intoxication: Implications for Emergency Medicine," *Am J Emerg Med*, 1991, 9(2 Suppl 1):29-34.

Kulick DL and Rahimtoola SH, "Current Role of Digitalis Therapy in Patients With Congestive Heart Failure," *JAMA*, 1991, 265(22):2995-7.

Digoxin

CPT 80162

Related Information

Creatinine, Serum *on page 202*
Flecainide *on page 967*
Magnesium, Serum *on page 287*
Quinidine, Serum *on page 999*
Verapamil *on page 1010*
(Continued)

Digoxin *(Continued)*

Synonyms Lanoxin®

Abstract Digoxin is a widely used cardiac glycoside and should be monitored. Samples for serum assay usually are not drawn less than 6 hours after last dose.

Patient Care PREPARATION: Avoid radioactivity prior to collection of specimen if analysis is by radioimmunoassay.

Specimen Serum CONTAINER: Red top tube SAMPLING TIME: Blood specimen must be drawn at least 6 hours after the administration of the last dose; additionally, just before next dose if steady-state estimate is needed. The steady-state is usually attained in 5 days. STORAGE INSTRUCTIONS: Separate serum and refrigerate. CAUSES FOR REJECTION: Patient on a cardiac glycoside other than digoxin, recently administered radioisotopes SPECIAL INSTRUCTIONS: **Be sure patient is not on DIGITOXIN**.

Interpretive REFERENCE RANGE: Adults: <0.5 ng/mL (SI: <0.6 nmol/L) probably indicates underdigitalization unless there are special circumstances. Therapeutic: 1.0-2.0 ng/mL (SI: 1.3-2.6 nmol/L) CRITICAL VALUES: Toxic: >2.0 ng/mL (SI: >2.6 nmol/L). POSSIBLE PANIC RANGE: >3.0 ng/mL (SI: >3.8 nmol/L). See Table C in the Appendix of this chapter. USE: Diagnose and prevent digoxin toxicity; prevent underdosage; monitor therapeutic drug level; prevention and therapy of cardiac arrhythmias, patients with implanted pacemaker, especially patients on digoxin who are elderly, and/or who have renal failure, and/or who have been given quinidine. See Quinidine, Serum listing. LIMITATIONS: **Digitoxin** should not be confused with **digoxin**. Since there is cross reactivity between the two drugs, results will not be valid if digoxin is measured when the patient is taking digitoxin. All other digitalis derivatives will also cross react with this test and give invalid results. Toxic levels of digitoxin when assayed as digoxin give low results. The elimination half-life in normal subjects is 37 hours. Patients with renal failure may have an endogenous digoxin-like material in their serum which makes digoxin measurements unreliable. METHODOLOGY: Radioimmunoassay (RIA), enzyme immunoassay (EIA), fluorescence polarization immunoassay (FPIA) ADDITIONAL INFORMATION: Be sure the patient is not on digitoxin instead of digoxin. Digitoxin is also an active component of digitalis leaf. Ninety percent of nontoxic patients have levels ≤2.0 ng/mL (SI: ≤2.6 nmol/L), 87% of toxic patients have levels >2.0 ng/mL. Levels >3.0 ng/mL in adults are strongly suggestive of overdosage. However, **digitalis levels must always be interpreted in light of clinical and chemical data**. Older, smaller patients require less digoxin. Proportionally lower loading doses are advocated in the elderly.[1] The primary cause of digoxin toxicity in the aged is decreased renal function. Maintenance doses should be adjusted to the glomerular filtration rate.[1] Renal failure, hypercalcemia, alkalosis, myxedema, hypomagnesemia, recent MI and other acute heart disease, hypokalemia, and hypoxia may increase sensitivity to the toxic effects of digoxin.

Quinidine may cause elevation of digoxin level by decreasing its excretion.[2,3] It is recommended that serum digoxin concentration be measured before initiation of quinidine therapy and again in 4-6 days.

When confronted with unexpectedly low digoxin levels, consider thyroid disease, malabsorption, cholestyramine, colestipol, kaolin, pectin, neomycin, sulfasalazine, anticholinergic drug effects, and reduced intestinal blood flow from mesenteric arteriosclerosis. Consider as well congestive failure when low digoxin levels are encountered. Falsely normal or low levels with toxic reactions may occur in patients recently given radioactive isotopes, when the method used is radioimmunoassay. At one time this was the predominant method, but it has largely been replaced by EIA and FPIA methods.

Patients with **digitalis resistance** may require larger doses and higher than usual serum levels (eg, patients with hyperthyroidism).

The probability that a patient will take a drug exactly as the physician has prescribed it (compliance) has been shown to be hardly better than half. Probability of compliance is further decreased in elderly patients treated with a large number of medications. Measure trough serum concentrations because of variability of peak interval.

FAB fragments of digoxin-specific sheep antibodies are available for the treatment of digoxin toxicities but should be limited to potentially life-threatening overdoses.

Compounds with "digoxin-like" immunoreactivity are present in a variety of clinical states associated with salt and fluid retention (eg, renal failure, pregnancy third trimester, congestive heart failure) and are also present during the first 2 weeks of neonatal life. These compounds (DLF – digoxin-like factors, etc) cross react with digoxin-specific immunoassays and give falsely elevated plasma digoxin concentrations. Laboratories must evaluate new antibody preparations for cross reactivity with such factors.

Footnotes

1. Montamat SC, Cusack BJ, and Vestal RE, "Management of Drug Therapy in the Elderly," *N Engl J Med*, 1989, 321(5):303-9.
2. Leakey EB, "Digoxin-Quinidine Interaction: Current Status," *Ann Intern Med*, 1980, 93:775-6, (editorial).
3. Mungall DR, Robichaux RP, Perry W, et al, "Effects of Quinidine on Serum Digoxin Concentration: A Prospective Study," *Ann Intern Med*, 1980, 93:689-93.

References

Antman EM, Wenger TL, Butler VP Jr, et al, "Treatment of 150 Cases of Life-Threatening Digitalis Intoxication With Digoxin-Specific Fab Antibody Fragments. Final Report of a Multicenter Study," *Circulation*, 1990, 81(6):1744-52.

Cohen AF, Kroon R, Schoemaker R, et al, "Influence of Gastric Acidity on the Bioavailability of Digoxin," *Ann Intern Med*, 1991, 115(7):540-5.

Graves BW, "Endogenous Digitalis-Like Factors," *Crit Rev Clin Lab Sci*, 1986, 23:177.

Haddy FJ, "Endogenous Digitalis-Like Factor or Factors," *N Engl J Med*, 1987, 316:621-3.

Howanitz PJ and Steindel SJ, "Digoxin Therapeutic Drug Monitoring Practices – A College of American Pathologists Q-Probes Study of 666 Institutions and 18,679 Toxic Levels," *Arch Pathol Lab Med*, 1993, 117:684-90.

Smith TW, "Digoxin in Heart Failure," *N Engl J Med*, 1993, 329(1):51-3.

Stone JA and Soldin SJ, "An Update on Digoxin," *Clin Chem*, 1989, 35(7):1326-31.

Tsang P and Gerson B, "Digoxin Monitoring in the Geriatric Patient," *Drug Monitoring and Toxicology*, 1991, 12.

Tsang P and Gerson B, "Understanding Digoxin Use in the Elderly Patient," *Clin Lab Med*, 1990, 10(3):479-92.

Vine DL, "What Is the Practical Value of Digitalis in CHF?" *Kans Med*, 1992, 93(7):231-2.

Withering W, "An Account of the Foxglove," Birmingham, Printed by M Swinney for GGJ and J Robinson, London, England: Paternoster-Row, 1785.

Woolf AD, Wenger T, Smith TW, et al, "The Use of Digoxin-Specific Fab Fragments for Severe Digitalis Intoxication in Children," *N Engl J Med*, 1992, 326(26):1739-44.

Dilantin® *see* Phenytoin *on page 994*

Diphenylhydantoin *see* Phenytoin *on page 994*

Disopyramide

***CPT** 80299*

Synonyms Norpace®

Abstract Disopyramide is an antiarrhythmic agent which is frequently monitored.

Specimen Serum or plasma **CONTAINER:** Red top tube, green top (heparin) tube, or lavender top (EDTA) tube **SAMPLING TIME:** Collect specimen 2-3 hours after an oral dose of disopyramide for peak. Draw trough just before next dose. Trough level is the best guide for dosing. **SPECIAL INSTRUCTIONS:** Specify other cardiac medications on requisition.

Interpretive **REFERENCE RANGE:** Therapeutic: 2-5 μg/mL (SI: 5.9-14.7 μmol/L) **CRITICAL VALUES:** Fatalities are seen with concentrations >20 μg/mL. **POSSIBLE PANIC RANGE:** Toxic: >7 μg/mL (SI: >20.6 μmol/L) **USE:** Therapeutic monitoring. See Table C in the Appendix of this chapter. **LIMITATIONS:** Arrhythmias may occur at low levels **METHODOLOGY:** Enzyme immunoassay (EIA), high performance liquid chromatography (HPLC) **ADDITIONAL INFORMATION:** Disopyramide shares electrophysiologic properties with quinidine and procainamide. Up to 80% of oral dose is absorbed. Half-life is 4-10 hours. Eighty percent of the drug is excreted in the urine. Dosage must be modified (dosage intervals prolonged) in patients with renal failure. Serious toxic effects are depression of myocardial contractility and disturbances in myocardial conduction. Other effects include dry mouth, constipation, urinary hesitancy, and blurred vision. Metabolite N-desisopropyl disopyramide is also pharmacologically active. Concomitant treatment with phenytoin may lead to decreased serum levels of disopyramide. There may be cumulative effects with other class I antiarrhythmic drugs (lidocaine, procainamide).

References

Duff HJ, Mitchell LB, Nath CF, et al, "Concentration-Response Relationships of Disopyramide in Patients With Ventricular Tachycardia," *Clin Pharmacol Ther*, 1989, 45(5):542-7.

Ragosta M, Weihl AC, and Rosenfeld LE, "Potentially Fatal Interaction Between Erythromycin and Disopyramide," *Am J Med*, 1989, 86(4):465-6.

d-Methamphetamine *see* Methamphetamines, Qualitative, Urine *on page 984*

Doe *see* Methamphetamines, Qualitative, Urine *on page 984*

Dolophine® *see* Methadone, Urine *on page 983*

Doriden® *see* Glutethimide *on page 970*

Doxepin

CPT 80166

Synonyms Adapin®; Sinequan®

Test Commonly Includes Desmethyldoxepin

Abstract This is a tricyclic antidepressant. It is not a drug of abuse.

Specimen Serum or plasma **CONTAINER:** Red top tube or green top (heparin) tube **SAMPLING TIME:** Trough levels at steady-state

Interpretive **REFERENCE RANGE:** Doxepin and desmethyldoxepin 110-250 ng/mL (SI: 4-9 nmol/L) **CRITICAL VALUES:** >300 ng/mL (SI: >11 nmol/L). Fatal cases associated with values >10,000 ng/mL. **USE:** Therapeutic monitoring and toxicity assessment **METHODOLOGY:** High performance liquid chromatography (HPLC), gas chromatography (GC) **ADDITIONAL INFORMATION:** Doxepin, a tricyclic antidepressant, is a tertiary amine structural analog of amitriptyline with similar but less potent neurotransmitter effects and considerably less cardiotoxicity. Doxepin is metabolized to the active metabolite desmethyldoxepin (nordoxepin); its half-life is 45 hours. Doxepin serum levels peak at 2-6 hours after an oral dose and the half-life is 8-25 hours (average is 15 hours). The parent drug has a low bioavailability and steady-state is reached in 2-8 days. Geriatric patients respond well to doxepin.

References

Ereshefsky L, Tran-Johnson T, Davis CM, et al, "Pharmacokinetic Factors Affecting Antidepressant Drug Clearance and Clinical Effect: Evaluation of Doxepin and Imipramine – New Data and Review," *Clin Chem*, 1988, 34:863-80.

Milstein S, Buetikofer J, Dunnigan A, et al, "Usefulness of Disopyramide for Prevention of Upright Tilt-Induced Hypotension-Bradycardia," *Am J Cardiol*, 1990, 65(20):1339-44.

Drug Screen, Comprehensive Panel or Analysis *see* Toxicology Drug Screen, Blood *on page 1005*

Drug Screen, Comprehensive Panel or Analysis, Urine *see* Toxicology Drug Screen, Urine *on page 1006*

Drugs of Abuse Testing, Urine

CPT 80100 (screen); 80102 (confirmation, each procedure)

Related Information

Alcohol, Blood or Urine *on page 936*
Amphetamines, Qualitative, Urine *on page 941*
Cannabinoids, Qualitative, Urine *on page 949*
Chain-of-Custody Protocol *on page 952*
Cocaine (Cocaine Metabolite), Qualitative, Urine *on page 955*
Methadone, Urine *on page 983*
Methamphetamines, Qualitative, Urine *on page 984*
Methaqualone *on page 985*
Morphine, Urine *on page 987*
Opiates, Qualitative, Urine *on page 989*
Phencyclidine, Qualitative, Urine *on page 992*
Propoxyphene, Blood or Urine *on page 997*
Urine Collection, 24-Hour *on page 32*

Synonyms Abuse Screen; DAU; DAU-10; Pre-employment Drug Screen

Test Commonly Includes Screens for common classes of abused drugs – amphetamines, barbiturates, benzodiazepines, cannabinoids, cocaine, methadone, methaqualone, opiates, phencyclidine, propoxyphene. In some laboratories, urine ethanol is included.

Abstract The usual drug-of-abuse screening panel consists of the 10 drugs listed above under "test includes".

Specimen Urine **CONTAINER:** Plastic urine container **COLLECTION:** If forensic, observe precautions. **STORAGE INSTRUCTIONS:** Refrigerate **CAUSES FOR REJECTION:** If forensic, failure to meet temperature requirements and tests for unusual urine dilution or alteration **TURNAROUND TIME:** Screen: 1-2 hours if done in-house; confirmation: 1-2 days **SPECIAL INSTRUCTIONS:** Specify the drug or drugs suspected in an emergency situation. If forensic, use chain-of-custody protocol and form. See test entry Chain-of-Custody Protocol and the Appendix of this chapter.

Interpretive REFERENCE RANGE: Negative (less than cutoff) CRITICAL VALUES: See individual drug entries for cutoff values. USE: Screen for drug overdose and toxicity; screen for the presence of drugs of abuse LIMITATIONS: This test provides only **qualitative** detection of drugs. Quantitation of drug levels is not included and is not recommended because urine levels are time and clearance dependent and are not directly related to toxic symptoms seen clinically. In a nonclinical setting (eg, pre-employment drug screening, etc), the sample should be collected under chain-of-custody, and all positive screens must be confirmed by a different, more sensitive method, preferably GC/MS. The transportation industry [Department of Transportation (DOT)] tests certain employees by screening for five classes of drugs only (amphetamines, cannabinoids, cocaine, opiates, phencyclidine) and confirms all positive results with GC/MS. National Institute on Drug Abuse (NIDA) certification required to perform tests for DOT. (See Federal Register 54(230), December 1, 1989.) Any agent identified in a screening test **should be confirmed** by a test specific for that drug (usually GC/MS). METHODOLOGY: Screen: immunoassay, gas chromatography (GC), thin-layer chromatography (TLC), high performance liquid chromatography (HPLC); confirmation: gas chromatography/mass spectrometry (GC/MS) ADDITIONAL INFORMATION: For specific drug classes see the listing by specific drug name.

References

Caplan YH, "Drug Testing in Urine," *J Forensic Sci*, 1989, 34:1417-21.

Council on Scientific Affairs, "Alcohol and the Driver," *JAMA*, 1986, 255:522-7.

De Cresce R, Mazura A, Lifshitz M, et al, *Drug Testing in the Workplace*, Chicago, IL: ASCP Press, 1989.

Hawks RL and Chiang CN, "Urine Testing for Drugs of Abuse," NIDA Research Monograph 73, 1986.

McBay AJ and Mason AP, "Forensic Science Identification of Drugs of Abuse," *J Forensic Sci*, 1989, 34:1471-6.

Schwartz RH, "Urine Testing in the Detection of Drugs of Abuse," *Arch Intern Med*, 1988, 148:2407-12.

Simpson D, Jarvie DR, and Heyworth R, "An Evaluation of Six Methods for the Detection of Drugs of Abuse in Urine," *Ann Clin Biochem*, 1989, 26(Pt 2):172-81.

Wells VE, Halperin W, Thun M, "The Estimated Predictive Value of Screening for Illicit Drugs in the Workplace," *Am J Public Health*, 1988, 78:817-9.

Elavil® *see* Amitriptyline, Blood *on page 939*

Elephant Tranquilizers *see* Phencyclidine, Qualitative, Urine *on page 992*

Elixophyllin® *see* Theophylline *on page 1002*

Encainide

***CPT** 80299*

Synonyms Enkaid®

Test Commonly Includes 3-methoxy-O-desmethylencainide (MODE), O-desmethylencainide (ODE)

Abstract Encainide is an antiarrhythmic used to suppress premature ventricular contractions and ventricular tachycardia. It undergoes extensive metabolism to two very active metabolites, which must also be measured.

Specimen Serum CONTAINER: Red top tube STORAGE INSTRUCTIONS: Centrifuge, separate, and freeze if not analyzing immediately.

Interpretive REFERENCE RANGE: At steady-state encainide: 50-85 μg/L (SI: 130-220 nmol/L); ODE: 180-220 μg/L (SI: 460-565 nmol/L); MODE: 140-185 μg/L (SI: 360-475 nmol/L) (normal phenotype) POSSIBLE PANIC RANGE: Not well established; side effects at ODE levels of 300-500 μg/L (SI: 770-1285 nmol/L) USE: Therapeutic monitoring and toxicity assessment CONTRAINDICATIONS: Cimetidine significantly increases serum concentration of parent and metabolites METHODOLOGY: High performance liquid chromatography (HPLC) ADDITIONAL INFORMATION: Encainide is a class 1C antiarrhythmic drug approved for the suppression of premature ventricular contractions and life-threatening ventricular tachycardia. It undergoes extensive first-pass metabolism. The metabolites O-desmethyl (ODE) and 3-methoxy-O-desmethylencainide (MODE) have greater activity than the parent drug. In normal metabolizers, therapeutic effect correlates with combined concentration of two metabolites and the parent drug; in poor metabolizers there are small amounts of metabolites and effect correlates with parent drug concentration. Drug can worsen arrhythmias or induce new tachycardias. Minor side effects (dizziness and blurred vision) can be minimized by administering drug with food. Coadministration with other cardioactive drugs is well tolerated. Can cause adverse effects in patients with severe chronic heart failure.[1]

(Continued)

Encainide *(Continued)*

Footnotes

1. Gottlieb SS, Kukin ML, Yushak M, et al, "Adverse Hemodynamic and Clinical Effects of Encainide in Severe Chronic Heart Failure," *Ann Intern Med*, 1989, 110(7):505-9.

References

Bartek MD, "Analysis of Encainide and Metabolites in Plasma and Urine by High Performance Liquid Chromatography," *Ther Drug Monit*, 1988, 10:446-51.

Fish FA, Gillette PC, and Benson DW Jr, "Proarrhythmia, Cardiac Arrest and Death in Young Patients Receiving Encainide and Flecainide. The Pediatric Electrophysiology Group," *J Am Coll Cardiol*, 1991, 18(2):356-65.

Roden DM and Woosley RL, "Clinical Pharmacokinetics of Encainide," *Clin Pharmacokinet*, 1988, 14:141-7.

Turgeon J and Roden DM, "Pharmacokinetic Profile of Encainide," *Clin Pharmacol Ther*, 1989, 45(6):692-4.

Woosley RL, "Encainide," *N Engl J Med*, 1988, 318:1107-15.

Endep® *see* Amitriptyline, Blood *on page 939*

Enkaid® *see* Encainide *on previous page*

Enphenemalum *see* Methylphenobarbital *on page 986*

Epilim® *see* Valproic Acid *on page 1008*

Equagesic® *see* Meprobamate *on page 982*

Equanil® *see* Meprobamate *on page 982*

Ergenyl® *see* Valproic Acid *on page 1008*

Eskalith® *see* Lithium *on page 979*

1,2-Ethanediol *see* Ethylene Glycol *on next page*

Ethanol *see* Volatile Screen *on page 1010*

Ethanol, Blood *see* Alcohol, Blood or Urine *on page 936*

Ethchlorvynol

CPT 82690

Synonyms Placidyl®

Abstract This is a sedative hypnotic which is considered dangerous if not carefully monitored.

Specimen Serum or plasma **CONTAINER:** Red top tube or green top (heparin) tube **SAMPLING TIME:** The peak blood level is attained in 1.5 hours

Interpretive **REFERENCE RANGE:** 2-8 μg/mL (SI: 14-55 μmol/L) **POSSIBLE PANIC RANGE:** Toxic: levels >20 μg/mL (SI: >138 μmol/L) are associated with severe sedation, coma, respiratory depression, hypotension, bradycardia, and hypothermia **USE:** Monitor therapeutic drug level **METHODOLOGY:** High performance liquid chromatography (HPLC), gas chromatography (GC), spectrophotometry **ADDITIONAL INFORMATION:** Ethchlorvynol is a nonbarbiturate sedative-hypnotic drug. The peak blood level is attained in 1.5 hours. The half-life is 10-20 hours and increases to 100 hours when high levels of drug are present. Most of the drug is metabolized in the liver. Exaggerated hypnotic effects occur if taken with ethanol. Can be detected in urine but only small amounts of the parent drug are present. Should be used cautiously in combination with oral anticoagulants. Effect is potentiated by alcohol.

References

Baselt RC, *Disposition of Toxic Drugs and Chemicals in Man*, 3rd ed, Davis, CA: Biomedical Publications, 1989, 326.

Gomolin I, "Ethchlorvynol," *Clin Toxicol Rev*, 1980, 2:1-2.

Winek CL, Wahba WW, and Winek CL Jr, "Body Distribution of Ethchlorvynol," *J Forensic Sci*, 1989, 34(3):687-90.

Yell RP, "Ethchlorvynol Overdose," *Am J Emerg Med*, 1990, 8(3):246-50.

Ethosuximide

CPT 80168

Synonyms Suxinutin®; Zarontin®; Zartalin®

Abstract Ethosuximide is a drug of choice for absence seizures not accompanied by other seizure types.

Specimen Serum or plasma **CONTAINER:** Red top tube or green top (heparin) tube **SAMPLING TIME:** Peak or trough levels may be used to monitor therapy because blood levels are fairly constant.

Interpretive REFERENCE RANGE: 40-100 μg/mL (SI: 284-710 μmol/L) POSSIBLE PANIC RANGE: >100 μg/mL (SI: >710 μmol/L); toxicity may manifest with lethargy or psychotic behavior; significant drug interactions are uncommon. See Table A in the Appendix of this chapter. USE: Monitor for compliance, efficacy, or possible toxicity LIMITATIONS: Ethosuximide has relatively few serious adverse effects with chronic administration. Dose-related adverse effects, including photophobia and lethargy, sometimes may be avoided by slowly titrating the drug to effective levels. Blood dyscrasias may occur and respond to decreasing dose or stopping the drug. If patients have other seizure types in addition to absence seizures, ethosuximide may exacerbate the other seizure types. Therefore, valproic acid is the drug of choice in that situation.[1] Other succinimides, notably methsuximide and phensuximide, have been used adjunctively for absence seizures but are less effective and more toxic.[2] METHODOLOGY: Enzyme immunoassay (EIA), gas-liquid chromatography (GLC), high performance liquid chromatography (HPLC)

Footnotes

1. Engel J, *Seizures and Epilepsy*, Contemporary Neurology Series, Philadelphia, PA: FA Davis Co, 1989.
2. Chang T, "Ethosuximide: Chemistry and Methods of Determination," *Antiepileptic Drugs*, 3rd ed, Levy RH, Dreifuss FE, Mattson RH, et al, eds, New York, NY: Raven Press, 1989.

References

Baselt RC and Cravey RH, "Ethosuximide," *Disposition of Toxic Drugs and Chemicals in Man*, 3rd ed, Chicago, IL: Year Book Medical Publishers Inc, 1989, 332-4.

Ethotoin

CPT 80299

Synonyms Accenon; Peganone®

Test Commonly Includes Ethotoin. Antiepileptic activity is due to parent compound.

Abstract Ethotoin is occasionally used as an adjunctive anticonvulsant. Patients suffer dose-related gingival hyperplasia and hirsutism less often than with phenytoin.

Specimen Serum CONTAINER: Red top tube

Interpretive REFERENCE RANGE: 14-34 μg/mL LIMITATIONS: Most common side effect is a bitter taste. ADDITIONAL INFORMATION: Like phenytoin, ethotoin has zero-order kinetics and small dosage changes may produce large changes in clinical response. Teratogenicity may occur, particularly since ethotoin is usually combined with other anticonvulsants. The half-life of ethotoin is approximately 5 hours, necessitating four times daily dosing.

References

Carter CA, Helms RA, and Boehm R, "Ethotoin in Seizures of Childhood and Adolescence," *Neurology*, 1984, 34:791-5.

Kupferberg HJ, "Other Hydantoins: Mephenytoin and Ethotoin," *Antiepileptic Drugs*, 3rd ed, Levy RH, Dreifuss FE, Mattson RH, et al, eds, New York, NY: Raven Press, 1989, 257-65.

Ethyl Alcohol, Blood *see* Alcohol, Blood or Urine *on page 936*

Ethyl and Methyl Thiocyanate (Thanite® and Lethane®) *see* Thiocyanate, Blood or Urine *on page 1003*

Ethylene Glycol

CPT 82693

Related Information

Anion Gap *on page 132*
Osmolality, Calculated *on page 299*
Osmolality, Serum *on page 300*
Oxalate, Urine *on page 303*
Urinalysis *on page 1162*

Synonyms 1,2-Ethanediol

Applies to Antifreeze

Test Commonly Includes Propylene glycol

Abstract A commercial chemical used as a radiator antifreeze and for commercial chemical synthesis.

Specimen Serum or plasma CONTAINER: Red top tube or green top (heparin) tube

Interpretive REFERENCE RANGE: Negative POSSIBLE PANIC RANGE: Values between 0.3-4.0 g/L have been observed in fatal cases; levels at 0.5 g/L indicate hemodialysis. USE: Detect and quantitate ingestion of ethylene glycol METHODOLOGY: Gas-liquid chromatography (GLC), pho-

(Continued)

Ethylene Glycol *(Continued)*

tometry, fluorometry, enzymatic assay (automated)[1] **ADDITIONAL INFORMATION:** Ethylene glycol is a colorless, odorless, sweet tasting compound used commercially in antifreeze. It has been utilized in suicide attempts, as a substitute for ethanol, and in accidental poisonings in both children and domestic pets. 100 mL is lethal; rapid treatment can prevent damage. Half-life is 3-5 hours. Toxicity is manifested by CNS depression (1-12 hours after ingestion), cardiopulmonary symptoms (12-24 hours after ingestion), and renal damage (24-72 hours after ingestion). Oxalate is a minor metabolite of ethylene glycol and crystals are commonly seen in urine. In addition to blood levels of ethylene glycol, hypocalcemia, anion gap metabolic acidosis, and osmolal gap elevation are observed. See the following listings in the Chemistry chapter: Anion Gap; Osmolality, Calculated; and Osmolality, Serum. **Precaution:** Toxicity may be manifested without osmolal gap changes and osmolal and anion gap increases can be present with very low levels of glycol.

Footnotes

1. Standefer J and Blackwell N, "Enzymatic Method for Measuring Ethylene Glycol With a Centrifugal Analyzer," *Clin Chem*, 1991, 37(10 Pt 1):1734-6.

References

Burkhart KK and Kulig KW, "The Other Alcohols. Methanol, Ethylene Glycol, and Isopropanol," *Emerg Med Clin North Am*, 1990, 8(4):913-28.

Cheng JT, Beysolow TD, Kaul B, et al, "Clearance of Ethylene Glycol by Kidneys and Hemodialysis," *Clin Toxicol*, 1987, 25:95-108.

Jarvie DR and Simpson D, "Simple Screening Tests for the Emergency Identification of Methanol and Ethylene Glycol in Poisoned Patients," *Clin Chem*, 1990, 36(11):1957-61.

Ochs ML, Glick MR, Ryder KW, et al, "Improved Method for Emergency Screening for Ethylene Glycol in Serum," *Clin Chem*, 1988, 34:1507-8.

Porter GA, "The Treatment of Ethylene Glycol Poisoning Simplified," *N Engl J Med*, 1988, 319:109-10.

EtOH *see* Alcohol, Blood or Urine *on page 936*

Etrafon® *see* Amitriptyline, Blood *on page 939*

Etrafon® *see* Phenothiazines, Serum *on page 993*

Etrafon® *see* Tricyclic Antidepressants *on page 1007*

5-FC *see* Flucytosine *on next page*

Felbamate

CPT *80299*

Synonyms Felbamyl; Felbatol™

Abstract Felbamate is a new anticonvulsant which is undergoing clinical trials for the treatment of partial and generalized seizures. It may be especially useful for patients with the Lennox-Gastaut syndrome, with multiple seizure types.

Specimen Serum **CONTAINER:** Red top tube **SAMPLING TIME:** Consistent sampling point

Interpretive **REFERENCE RANGE:** Levels of 20-80 μg/mL have been obtained without serious toxicity. **CRITICAL VALUES:** No critical value is established. Serum levels have varied considerably in published trials. **USE:** Evaluate efficacy, compliance, and possibly toxicity **METHODOLOGY:** High performance liquid chromatography (HPLC) **ADDITIONAL INFORMATION:** The most common adverse effects, anorexia and headache, may respond to lowering the dose or stopping the drug. Toxicity is more common in patients on more than one anticonvulsant. Significant interactions: If felbamate is added to the regimen of patients taking either phenytoin or valproic acid, the dose of the other drug should be lowered to prevent toxicity. The blood level of carbamazepine may be lowered, but the level of its metabolite, 10,11-epoxide is raised.

References

"Efficacy of Felbamate in Childhood Epileptic Encephalopathy (Lennox-Gastaut Syndrome)," *N Engl J Med*, 1993, 328(1):29-33.

Leppik IE, Dreifuss FE, Pledger GW, et al, "Felbamate for Partial Seizures: Results of a Controlled Clinical Trial," *Neurology*, 1991, 41(11):1785-9.

Theodore WH, Raubertas RF, Porter RJ, et al, "Felbamate: A Clinical Trial for Complex Partial Seizures," *Epilepsia*, 1991, 32(3):392-7.

Felbamyl *see* Felbamate *on this page*

Felbatol™ *see* Felbamate *on this page*

Fiorinal® *see* Barbiturates, Quantitative, Blood *on page 946*

Flecainide

CPT 80299

Related Information

Digoxin *on page 959*

Synonyms Tambocor®

Abstract An antiarrhythmic drug not significantly metabolized. When coadministered can affect activity of other antiarrhythmic drugs.

Specimen Serum or plasma **CONTAINER:** Red top tube (preferred) or green top (heparin) tube; do not use serum separator tube **SAMPLING TIME:** Draw sample 3 hours after last dose. **STORAGE INSTRUCTIONS:** Separate serum or plasma within 2 hours of specimen draw. **SPECIAL INSTRUCTIONS:** Draw immediately prior to next dose for trough levels.

Interpretive REFERENCE RANGE: Therapeutic: 0.2-0.8 μg/mL (SI: 0.4-2.0 μmol/L) **POSSIBLE PANIC RANGE:** >1.0 μg/mL (SI: >2.0 μmol/L) **USE:** Therapeutic monitoring and toxicity assessment (toxic effects – hypotension, asystole – proportional to dose and concentration) **METHODOLOGY:** High performance liquid chromatography (HPLC), fluorescence polarization immunoassay (FPIA) **ADDITIONAL INFORMATION:** Flecainide is a class 1C antiarrhythmic drug approved for the suppression of ventricular arrhythmias. The drug is well absorbed orally. Plasma half-life averages 20 hours (range 12-27 hours) in adults although in children it has been reported to be 8 hours.[1] Steady-state concentrations are achieved in 3-5 days. Since 10% to 50% of the drug is eliminated in the urine as unchanged drug, impaired renal function will significantly prolong the plasma half-life. Clearance of flecainide can be accelerated by phenobarbital and rifampin. There are no significant metabolites of flecainide. Coadministration with digoxin increases serum digoxin by 20%; coadministration with propranolol increases both by 20% in serum and creates an additive pharmacological effect.

Footnotes

1. Till JA, Shinebourne EA, Rowland E, et al, "Pediatric Use of Flecainide in Supraventricular Tachycardia: Clinical Efficacy and Pharmacokinetics," *Br Heart J*, 1989, 62(2):133-9.

References

Perry JC, McQuinn RL, Smith RT Jr, et al, "Flecainide Acetate for Resistant Arrhythmias in the Young: Efficacy and Pharmacokinetics," *J Am Coll Cardiol*, 1989, 14(1):185-93.

Rosen DM and Woosely RL, "Drug Therapy. Flecainide," *N Engl J Med*, 1986, 315:36-41.

Flucytosine

CPT 80299

Related Information

Cerebrospinal Fluid Fungus Culture *on page 800*

Synonyms Ancobon®; 5-FC; 5-Fluorocytosine

Abstract Flucytosine is an antifungal agent often used in conjunction with amphotericin B for treatment of fungal (primarily cryptococcal) meningitis. Bone marrow toxicity is occasionally seen in patients being treated with flucytosine.

Specimen Serum **CONTAINER:** Red top tube **SAMPLING TIME:** 2 hours after dose

Interpretive REFERENCE RANGE: Therapeutic: 50-100 μg/mL (SI: 390-775 μmol/L) **POSSIBLE PANIC RANGE:** 100-125 μg/mL (SI: 775-970 μmol/L) **USE:** Monitor for bone marrow toxicity; evaluate weekly if patient has normal renal function, more often if renal function is abnormal. **LIMITATIONS:** Serum levels do not correlate well with clinical toxicity **METHODOLOGY:** High performance liquid chromatography (HPLC), gas chromatography/mass spectrometry (GC/MS) **ADDITIONAL INFORMATION:** Clinical use of flucytosine is associated with significant frequency of life-threatening bone marrow suppression which occurs most often when blood levels are >100 μg/mL (SI: >775 μmol/L) for 2 or more weeks. The bone marrow suppression is usually reversible and is most likely to occur in patients with underlying hematologic disorders or in patients undergoing myelosuppressive therapy.

References

Bodey GP, "Topical and Systemic Antifungal Agents," *Med Clin North Am*, 1988, 72:637-59.

Gerson B, "Flucytosine," *Clin Lab Med*, 1987, 7:541-4.

Terrell CL and Hughes CE, "Antifungal Agents Used for Deep-Seated Mycotic Infections," *Mayo Clin Proc*, 1992, 67(1):69-91.

Fluoride, Serum

CPT 82735

Synonyms Sodium Fluoride

Abstract Fluoride is added at low levels to toothpaste and is added to drinking water in many areas at a level of 1 ppm. It is present in high concentrations in insecticides and rodenticides.

Specimen Serum **CONTAINER:** Red top tube

Interpretive **REFERENCE RANGE:** Diet dependent, approximately 1.9-7.6 μg/dL (SI: 1-4 μmol/L) **POSSIBLE PANIC RANGE:** Toxic concentration: >28.5 μg/dL (SI: >15 μmol/L) **USE:** Evaluate fluoride toxicity; work up ant poison, roach poison intoxication **METHODOLOGY:** Fluoride-specific electrode **ADDITIONAL INFORMATION:** Fluoride poisoning can occur from ingestion of ant or roach poisons; death is usually from cardiovascular collapse. Fatal dose is 5-10 g orally. Half-life is 2-9 hours.

References

Frink EJ Jr, Ghantous H, Malan TP, et al, "Plasma Inorganic Fluoride With Sevoflurane Anesthesia: Correlation With Indices of Hepatic and Renal Function," *Anesth Analg*, 1992, 74(2):231-5.

Gruber HE and Baylink DJ, "The Effects of Fluoride on Bone," *Clin Orthop*, 1991, 267:264-77.

Whitford GM, "The Physiological and Toxicological Characteristics of Fluoride," *J Dent Res*, 1990, 69:539-49.

5-Fluorocytosine *see* Flucytosine *on previous page*

Fluoxetine

CPT 80299

Synonyms Prozac®

Test Commonly Includes Fluoxetine and norfluoxetine

Abstract This is a new nontricyclic antidepressant with a long half-life and an active metabolite.

Specimen Serum or plasma **CONTAINER:** Red top tube or green top (heparin) tube; do not use serum separator tube **SAMPLING TIME:** Trough just prior to next dose

Interpretive **REFERENCE RANGE:** Fluoxetine 100-800 ng/mL (SI: 289-2314 nmol/L); norfluoxetine 100-600 ng/mL (SI: 289-1735 nmol/L) **CRITICAL VALUES:** >2000 ng/mL (SI: >5784 nmol/L) (fluoxetine and norfluoxetine) **USE:** Therapeutic monitoring and toxicity assessment **METHODOLOGY:** High performance liquid chromatography (HPLC), gas chromatography (GC) **ADDITIONAL INFORMATION:** Fluoxetine is a new antidepressant that is a potent, selective inhibitor of serotonin reuptake. It is metabolized via demethylation to the active norfluoxetine. The parent drug has a long half-life of 24-96 hours which facilitates maintenance of steady-state concentrations (2-6 weeks to steady-state). The therapeutic efficiency as an antidepressant is comparable to the tricyclics but not for the relief of sleep disorders. The overall toxicity of the drug is considerably less than that of the tricyclics.

References

Benfield P, Heel RC, and Lewis SP, "Fluoxetine: A Review of its Pharmacodynamic and Pharmacokinetic Properties and Therapeutic Efficacy in Depressive Illness," *Drugs*, 1986, 32:481-508.

Bergstrom RF, Lemberger L, Fared NA, et al, "Clinical Pharmacology and Pharmacokinetics of Fluoxetine: A Review," *Br J Psychiatry*, 1988, 153(Suppl 3):47-50.

Borys DJ, Setzer SC, Ling LJ, et al, "The Effects of Fluoxetine in the Overdose Patient," *J Toxicol Clin Toxicol*, 1990, 28(3):331-40.

Pary R, Tobias CR, and Lippmann S, "Fluoxetine: Prescribing Guidelines for the Newest Antidepressant," *South Med J*, 1989, 82(8):1005-9.

Tacke U, "Fluoxetine: An Alternative to the Tricyclics in the Treatment of Major Depression?" *Am J Med Sci*, 1989, 298(2):126-9.

Fluphenazine

CPT 80299

Related Information

Phenothiazines, Serum *on page 993*

Synonyms Permitil®; Prolixin®

Abstract Fluphenazine is a phenothiazine antipsychotic active at low dosage.

Specimen Serum **CONTAINER:** Red top tube

Interpretive **REFERENCE RANGE:** 5-20 ng/mL (SI: 10-40 nmol/L) **CRITICAL VALUES:** >50 ng/mL (SI: >98 nmol/L) **USE:** Therapeutic monitoring and toxicity assessment **METHODOLOGY:** High performance liquid chromatography (HPLC), gas chromatography (GC), radioimmunoassay (RIA) **ADDITIONAL INFORMATION:** Fluphenazine is a phenothiazine derivative (piperazine) used in the treatment of psychotic disorders. Its dose in milligrams equivalent to 100 mg of chlorpromazine is 0.6-1.2 mg. As a high potency antipsychotic it may have a high potential for causing extrapyramidal side effects. This would be in addition to the usual adverse effects of antipsychotic drugs (neurologic, anticholinergic, hypotension). Elderly patients should be observed for these occurrences. The half-life of fluphenazine is formulation-dependent. (The decanoate is 5-12 days; the hydrochloride 12-60 hours.) Fluphenazine is also used to alleviate pain and in childhood development disorders.

References

Chouinard G, Annable L, and Campbell W, "A Randomized Clinical Trial of Haloperidol Decanoate and Fluphenazine Decanoate in the Outpatient Treatment of Schizophrenia," *J Clin Psychopharmacol*, 1989, 9(4):247-53.

Cooper JK, Hawes EM, Hubbard JW, et al, "An Ultrasensitive Method for the Measurement of Fluphenazine in Plasma by High Performance Liquid Chromatography With Coulometric Detection," *Ther Drug Monit*, 1989, 11(3):354-60.

Levinson DF, Simpson GM, Singh H, et al, "Fluphenazine Dose, Clinical Response, and Extrapyramidal Symptoms During Acute Treatment," *Arch Gen Psychiatry*, 1990, 47(8):761-8.

Marder SR, Midha KK, Van Putten T, et al, "Plasma Levels of Fluphenazine in Patients Receiving Fluphenazine Decanoate. Relationship to Clinical Response," *Br J Psychiatry*, 1991, 158:658-65.

Mendel CM, Klein RF, Chappell DA, et al, "A Trial of Amitriptyline and Fluphenazine in the Treatment of Painful Diabetic Neuropathy," *JAMA*, 1986, 255:637-9.

Midha KK, McKay G, Edom R, et al, "Kinetics of Oral Fluphenazine Disposition in Human Plasma," *Comm Psychopharm*, 1980, 4:107-14.

Flurazepam

CPT *82742*

Synonyms Dalmane®

Abstract This drug is a sedative-hypnotic of the benzodiazepine class with a rather wide therapeutic window.

Specimen Serum **CONTAINER:** Red top tube

Interpretive **REFERENCE RANGE:** Therapeutic: 0-4 ng/mL (SI: 0-9 nmol/L); metabolite N-desalkylflurazepam: 20-110 ng/mL (SI: 43-240 nmol/L) **POSSIBLE PANIC RANGE:** Toxic: 2000 ng/mL (SI: 4300 nmol/L) **USE:** Monitor therapeutic drug level (rarely), toxicity assessment **METHODOLOGY:** Thin-layer chromatography (TLC), high performance liquid chromatography (HPLC) **ADDITIONAL INFORMATION:** Half-life of parent drug is 2-3 hours. Half-life of active metabolite, N-desalkylflurazepam, is 50-100 hours. Most common side effect is daytime drowsiness. The major urinary metabolite is N-1-hydroxyethyl flurazepam.

References

Greenblatt DJ, Harmatz JS, Engelhardt N, et al, "Pharmacokinetic Determinants of Dynamic Differences Among Three Benzodiazepine Hypnotics. Flurazepam, Temazepam, and Triazolam," *Arch Gen Psychiatry*, 1989, 46(4):326-32.

Kales A, "Benzodiazepine Hypnotics and Insomnia," *Hosp Pract Off Ed*, 1990, 25(Suppl 3):7-23.

Free Phenytoin *see* Phenytoin, Free *on page 995*

Fungizone® *see* Amphotericin B *on page 942*

GABA Pentin

CPT *80299*

Synonyms Neurontin

Abstract GABA pentin is a GABAergic, novel anticonvulsant with a broad spectrum of activity and minor side effects. It is undergoing clinical trials for the treatment of partial seizures.

Interpretive **ADDITIONAL INFORMATION:** Therapeutic monitoring is not required with GABA pentin. GABA pentin has no reported interactions with other anticonvulsants. Toxicity (not dose related) includes somnolence, dizziness, ataxia, headache, diplopia, tremor, and weight gain. GABA pentin is cleared by the kidney and may accumulate in clinical situations associated with decreased creatinine clearance.

References

Sivenius J, Kalviainen R, Ylinen A, et al, "Double Blind Study of Gabapentin in the Treatment of Partial Seizures," *Epilepsia*, 1991, 32(4):539-42.

Garamycin® *see* Gentamicin *on next page*

Gardenal® *see* Phenobarbital, Blood *on page 992*

Gemonil® *see* Barbiturates, Quantitative, Blood *on page 946*

Gentamicin

***CPT** 80170*

Related Information

Antibiotic Level, Serum *on page 942*
Beta$_2$-Microglobulin *on page 644*
Creatinine, Serum *on page 202*
Magnesium, Serum *on page 287*
Serum Bactericidal Test *on page 843*
Susceptibility Testing, Aerobic and Facultatively Anaerobic Organisms *on page 864*

Synonyms Garamycin®

Abstract Aminoglycoside antibiotics, including gentamicin, are used primarily to treat infections caused by aerobic gram-negative bacilli. Additionally, when used in combination with penicillins, they may have synergistic bactericidal activity against gram-positive cocci such as *Staphylococcus aureus* and *Enterococcus faecalis*. Gentamicin has a narrow therapeutic window and is potentially ototoxic and nephrotoxic. Its use in life-threatening infections makes it mandatory that effective levels be achieved without overdosage.

Specimen Serum **CONTAINER:** Red top tube **SAMPLING TIME:** Peak: 30-60 minutes after end of 30-minute I.V. infusion or 60 minutes post I.M. dose; trough: immediately prior to next dose. Specimens should be drawn at steady-state, usually after fifth dose, if drug given every 8 hours, or after third dose, if drug given every 12 hours. **STORAGE INSTRUCTIONS:** Separate within 1 hour of collection and refrigerate or freeze until assayed. Must be frozen if a β-lactam antibiotic is also present because of potential inactivation of aminoglycosides.

Interpretive **REFERENCE RANGE:** Therapeutic: peak: 4-10 μg/mL (SI: 8-21 μmol/L) (depends in part on the minimal inhibitory concentration of the drug against the organism being treated); trough: <2 μg/mL (SI: <4 μmol/L) **POSSIBLE PANIC RANGE:** Toxic: peak: >12 μg/mL (SI: >25 μmol/L); trough: >2 μg/mL (SI: >4 μmol/L). See Table B in the Appendix of this chapter. **USE:** Peak levels are necessary to assure adequate therapeutic levels for organism being treated. Trough levels are necessary to evaluate the likelihood of nephrotoxicity. **LIMITATIONS:** High peak levels may not have strong correlation with toxicity. **METHODOLOGY:** Enzyme immunoassay (EIA), fluorescence polarization immunoassay (FPIA), high performance liquid chromatography (HPLC) **ADDITIONAL INFORMATION:** Gentamicin is cleared by the kidney and accumulates in renal tubular cells. Nephrotoxicity is most closely related to the length of time that trough levels are >2 μg/mL (SI: >4 μmol/L). Creatinine levels should be monitored every 2-3 days as an indicator of impending renal toxicity. The initial toxic result is nonoliguric renal failure that is usually reversible if the drug is discontinued. Continued administration of gentamicin may produce oliguric renal failure. Nephrotoxicity may occur in as many as 10% to 25% of patients receiving aminoglycosides; most of this toxicity can be avoided by monitoring levels and adjusting dosing schedules accordingly. Aminoglycosides may also cause irreversible ototoxicity that manifests itself clinically as hearing loss. Aminoglycoside ototoxicity is relatively uncommon and clinical trials where levels were carefully monitored and dosing adjusted failed to show a correlation between auditory toxicity and plasma aminoglycoside levels. In situations where dosing is not monitored and adjusted, however, sustained high levels may be associated with ototoxicity. This association is far from clear cut, and new once-daily dosing regimens (and associated high peak serum concentrations) that fail to enhance toxicity further complicate this issue.

References

Crisan D, Cadoff EM, and Howrie DL, "Use of Pharmacokinetics in Optimizing Aminoglycoside Therapy," *ASCP Check Sample®*, Chicago, IL: American Society of Clinical Pathologists, 1989, 10.

Desai TK and Tsang T-K, "Aminoglycoside Nephrotoxicity in Obstructive Jaundice," *Am J Med*, 1988, 85:47-50.

Dipersio JR, "Gentamicin and Other Aminoglycosides," *Clinical Chemistry – Theory, Analysis, and Correlation*, 2nd ed, Kaplan LA and Pesce AJ, eds, St Louis, MO: Mosby-Year Book Inc, 1989, 1102-8.

Edson RS and Terrell CL, "The Aminoglycosides," *Mayo Clin Proc*, 1991, 66(11):1158-64.

Gilbert DN, "Once-Daily Aminoglycoside Therapy," *Antimicrob Agents Chemother*, 1991, 35(3):399-405.

Pancoast SJ, "Aminoglycoside Antibiotics in Clinical Use," *Med Clin North Am*, 1987, 72:581-612.

Glutethimide

***CPT** 82980*

Synonyms Doriden®; Loads

Abstract This drug is a sedative hypnotic which has been in use for some time. The pharmacological effect is similar to that of barbiturates.

Specimen Serum CONTAINER: Red top tube

Interpretive REFERENCE RANGE: Therapeutic: 5 μg/mL (variable) (SI: 23 μmol/L) POSSIBLE PANIC RANGE: Toxic: >10 μg/mL (SI: >46 μmol/L). Fatalities have occurred with serum levels between 10-100 μg/mL (average, 50 μg/mL). USE: Monitor therapeutic drug level, determine toxic level LIMITATIONS: Serum levels obtained during dialysis may not reflect tissue levels METHODOLOGY: Gas-liquid chromatography (GLC), high performance liquid chromatography (HPLC), thin-layer chromatography (TLC). A spot test is described.[1] ADDITIONAL INFORMATION: Glutethimide is a nonbarbiturate sedative-hypnotic. The drug is erratically absorbed from the gastrointestinal tract and undergoes extensive metabolism to pharmacologically active and inactive metabolites. An important active metabolite in 4-hydroxy-2-ethyl-2-phenylglutarimide. This metabolite has twice the potency of glutethimide and a longer half-life. Peak blood levels are at 2-3 hours postingestion. The half-life is biphasic, ranging from 5-22 hours. The average plasma half-life is 10 hours. Serious toxic effects are respiratory depression and circulatory collapse. Glutethimide and codeine ("packs" or "loads") in combination are frequently used by drug abusers.

Footnotes

1. Blanke RV and Decker WJ, "Analysis of Toxic Substances," *Fundamentals of Clinical Chemistry*, 3rd ed, Tietz NW, ed, Philadelphia, PA: WB Saunders Co, 1987, 869-905.

References

Bailey DN and Shaw RF, "Blood Concentrations and Clinical Findings in Nonfatal and Fatal Intoxications Involving Glutethimide and Codeine," *Clin Toxicol*, 1985, 23:557-70.

Gold

CPT 80172

Synonyms Aurothioglucose; Chrysotherapy; Gold Sodium Thiomalate; Myochrysine®; Solganal®

Abstract Gold is used as a treatment for rheumatoid arthritis, but its value is being questioned.

Specimen Serum, urine CONTAINER: Red top tube for blood, acid-washed polyethylene container for urine

Interpretive REFERENCE RANGE: Normal: 0-0.1 μg/mL (SI: 0-0.5 μmol/L); therapeutic: 1-3 μg/mL (SI: 5.1-15.2 μmol/L); urine <0.1 μg/24 hours LIMITATIONS: Blood levels do not correlate with therapeutic or toxic effects. No relationship between serum gold levels and efficacy is established. Serum gold concentrations have not been helpful in monitoring adverse reactions.[1] A relationship is not recognized between urinary gold and response to therapy. Hair and nail gold concentrations have not been helpful.[1] METHODOLOGY: Atomic absorption spectrometry (AA) ADDITIONAL INFORMATION: Complex gold compounds are used in the treatment of severe, progressive rheumatoid arthritis which is not controlled by other medical therapy. It is also used selectively for juvenile rheumatoid arthritis and for psoriatic arthritis affecting peripheral joints.[1] The mechanism of action is not clear, but may be due to reticuloendothelial system blockade, and/or effects on lymphocyte proliferation and antibody production. Elimination is mainly renal and the half-life is 5.5 days. Gold toxicity may be manifested by dermatitis, pruritus, stomatitis, metallic taste, eosinophilia, leukopenia, anemia, thrombocytopenia, hematuria, proteinuria, nephrosis, and bone marrow suppression, among other possible effects. Discussing the pharmacokinetics and clinical-pharmacologic correlates, Gottlieb provides recommendations for monitoring chrysotherapy.[1]

Footnotes

1. Gottlieb NL, "Gold Compounds," *Textbook of Rheumatology*, 2nd ed, Vol 1, Kelley WN, Harris ED, Ruddy S, et al, eds, Philadelphia, PA: WB Saunders Co, 1985, 789-809.

References

Bendix G and Bjelle A, "Outcome of Parenteral Gold Therapy in RA Patients: A Comparison Between Two Periods Using Life-Table Analysis," *Br J Rheumatol*, 1991, 30(6):407-12.

Epstein WV, Henke CJ, Yelin EH, et al, "Effect of Parenterally Administered Gold Therapy on the Course of Adult Rheumatoid Arthritis," *Ann Intern Med*, 1991, 114(6):437-44.

Gold Sodium Thiomalate *see* Gold *on this page*

GX *see* Lidocaine *on page 978*

Hair Analysis *see* Arsenic, Blood *on page 944*

Hair Analysis *see* Arsenic, Hair, Nails *on page 944*

Hair Analysis *see* Arsenic, Urine *on page 945*

Hair Analysis *see* Heavy Metal Screen, Urine *on next page*

Hair Analysis *see* Mercury, Blood *on page 982*

Haldol® *see* Haloperidol *on this page*

Haloperidol

CPT 80299

Synonyms Haldol®

Abstract This drug is an antipsychotic agent which is extensively metabolized and should be monitored.

Specimen Serum or plasma **CONTAINER:** Red top tube or green top (heparin) tube

Interpretive **REFERENCE RANGE:** 5-15 ng/mL (SI: 10-40 nmol/L) (psychotic disorders – less for Tourette's and mania) **CRITICAL VALUES:** >50 ng/mL (SI: >130 nmol/L) (variable) **USE:** Therapeutic monitoring and toxicity assessment **METHODOLOGY:** High performance liquid chromatography (HPLC), gas chromatography (GC) **ADDITIONAL INFORMATION:** Half-life is 15-40 hours. Haloperidol is an antipsychotic tranquilizer used to control acute and chronic psychotic disorders, for the control of Tourette's syndrome, and for the treatment of severe behavior problems in hyperactive children. Haloperidol is metabolized by dealkalization, oxidation, and conjugation; the hydroxy derivative is active but concentrations are very low. Haloperidol should be monitored to assess and optimize dosing regimens and maintenance therapy since the relationship between dosage and serum levels at steady-state can be highly variable. The drug should also be monitored to assess adverse reactions and changes associated with coadministered drugs. Haloperidol may increase serum tricyclic concentrations, increase the toxicity of lithium, inhibit hypertensive action, and antagonize the stimulant effect of amphetamines.

References

Cannon DJ, McMillan DE, Newton JEO, et al, "Serum Haloperidol and Neuroleptic Receptor Levels in Chronic Psychosis," *Ann Clin Lab Sci*, 1988, 18:378-83.

Derlet RW, Albertson TE, and Rice P, "The Effect of Haloperidol in Cocaine and Amphetamine Intoxication," *J Emerg Med*, 1989, 7(6):633-7.

Goff DC, Midha KK, Brotman AW, et al, "Elevation of Plasma Concentrations of Haloperidol After the Addition of Fluoxetine," *Am J Psychiatry*, 1991, 148(6):790-2.

Hemstrom CA, Evans RL, and Lobeck FG, "Haloperidol Decanoate: A Depot Antipsychotic," *Drug Intell Clin Pharm*, 1988, 22:290-95.

Rifkin A, Doddi S, Karajgi B, et al, "Dosage of Haloperidol for Schizophrenia," *Arch Gen Psychiatry*, 1991, 48(2):166-70.

Volavka J and Cooper TB, "Review of Haloperidol Blood Levels and Clinical Response," *J Clin Psychopharmacol*, 1987, 7:25-30.

Hashish *see* Cannabinoids, Qualitative, Urine *on page 949*

Heavy Metal Screen, Arsenic *see* Arsenic, Blood *on page 944*

Heavy Metal Screen, Blood

CPT 83015 (screen); 83018 (quantitative, each)

Related Information

Aluminum, Serum *on page 1019*
Arsenic, Blood *on page 944*
Arsenic, Hair, Nails *on page 944*
Arsenic, Urine *on page 945*
Cadmium, Urine and Blood *on page 948*
Chromium, Serum *on page 1021*
Chromium, Urine *on page 1023*
Copper, Serum *on page 1024*
Copper, Urine *on page 1027*
Heavy Metal Screen, Urine *on next page*
Lead, Blood *on page 976*
Lead, Urine *on page 977*
Manganese, Blood *on page 1029*
Manganese, Urine *on page 1031*
Mercury, Blood *on page 982*
Mercury, Urine *on page 983*
Selenium, Serum *on page 1033*

Synonyms Metals, Blood; Poisonous Metals, Blood; Toxic Metals, Blood

Test Commonly Includes Antimony, arsenic, bismuth, boron, cadmium, cobalt, copper, lead, mercury, selenium, tellurium, thallium, zinc

Abstract Used principally to detect arsenic, cadmium, mercury, and lead poisoning.

Specimen Whole blood (EDTA) plus serum **CONTAINER:** Special metal-free tube and red top tube **STORAGE INSTRUCTIONS:** Refrigerate: do not spin down. **SPECIAL INSTRUCTIONS:** Check with laboratory performing the assay to determine what elements will be detected and for any special instructions.

Interpretive **REFERENCE RANGE:** Varies with metal detected. See individual listings. **USE:** Screen for heavy metal poisoning **METHODOLOGY:** Atomic absorption spectrometry (AA) **ADDITIONAL INFORMATION:** See individual test listings in this chapter and the Trace Elements chapter for further information.

References

Gerson B, "Lead," *Clin Lab Med*, 1990, 10(3):441-73.
Malachowski ME, "An Update on Arsenic," *Clin Lab Med*, 1990, 10(3):459-72.

Heavy Metal Screen, Urine

***CPT** 83015 (screen); 83018 (quantitative, each)*

Related Information

Synonyms Metal Screen; Metals, Toxic; Poisonous Metals, Urine; Toxic Metals, Urine

Applies to Hair Analysis

Test Commonly Includes Arsenic, mercury, lead (could also include nickel and cadmium)

Abstract Used to detect arsenic, mercury, lead, and cadmium poisoning

Specimen 24-hour urine **CONTAINER:** Plastic, acid-washed urine container (preferably polyethylene), no preservative, 20-25 mL 6N HCl (low metal content) **COLLECTION:** 24-hour collection **STORAGE INSTRUCTIONS:** Refrigerate **SPECIAL INSTRUCTIONS:** Include volume of urine

Interpretive **REFERENCE RANGE:** Arsenic: <50 μg/L; lead: <80 μg/L; mercury: <20 μg/L; nickel: <25 μg/L; cadmium: <10 μg/L **USE:** Screen for heavy metal poisoning and toxic exposure; urine lead analysis is useful for organic lead exposure and to monitor chelation. Blood is preferred for inorganic lead exposure monitoring. **LIMITATIONS:** **Hair analysis** should be used for arsenic and mercury poisoning or exposure especially if one is interested in determining chronic exposure. Hair should be clean, free of oil, and clipped (0.5 g for As; 2 g for Hg) as close as possible. Recent ingestion of seafood can cause misleading increases of urine arsenic. **METHODOLOGY:** Atomic absorption spectrometry (AA) **ADDITIONAL INFORMATION:** Please see the test listings Heavy Metal, Screen, Blood for further information. See also the Trace Elements chapter.

(Continued)

Heavy Metal Screen, Urine *(Continued)*

References

Gerson B, "Lead," *Clin Lab Med*, 1990, 10(3):441-73.

Malochowski ME, "An Update on Arsenic," *Clin Lab Med*, 1990, 10(3):459-72.

Hemp *see* Cannabinoids, Qualitative, Urine *on page 949*

Heroin *see* Opiates, Qualitative, Urine *on page 989*

Heroin Metabolite, Urine *see* Morphine, Urine *on page 987*

Hg, Blood *see* Mercury, Blood *on page 982*

Hg, Urine *see* Mercury, Urine *on page 983*

Hog *see* Phencyclidine, Qualitative, Urine *on page 992*

Hydrocyanic Acid *see* Cyanide, Blood *on page 956*

Ice *see* Amphetamines, Qualitative, Urine *on page 941*

Imipramine

CPT 80174

Related Information

Tricyclic Antidepressants *on page 1007*

Synonyms Presamine®; Tofranil®

Applies to Desipramine; Norpramin®; Pertofrane®

Test Commonly Includes Desipramine levels

Abstract This drug is a tricyclic antidepressant. It has an active metabolite which should also be monitored.

Specimen Serum or plasma **CONTAINER:** Red top tube or green top (heparin) tube **SAMPLING TIME:** Trough levels at steady-state

Interpretive **REFERENCE RANGE:** Imipramine and desipramine 150-250 ng/mL (SI: 530-890 nmol/L); desipramine 150-300 ng/mL (SI: 560-1125 nmol/L). Metabolism may be impaired in geriatric patients.[1] **CRITICAL VALUES:** >300 ng/mL (SI: >1070 nmol/L) **POSSIBLE PANIC RANGE:** 1000 ng/mL (SI: 3570 nmol/L) **USE:** Therapeutic monitoring and toxicity assessment **METHODOLOGY:** Immunoassay, high performance liquid chromatography (HPLC), gas chromatography (GC) **ADDITIONAL INFORMATION:** Imipramine is a tertiary tricyclic antidepressant prescribed for the treatment of various depressive disorders. Imipramine is metabolized to desipramine which is pharmacologically active and marketed separately. Both drugs have anticholinergic and antihistamine effects and are cardiotoxic. Imipramine reaches a peak serum concentration in 1-2 hours (desipramine 2-6 hours), has a half-life of 9-24 hours (desipramine 12-54 hours) and reaches steady-state levels in 2-5 days (desipramine 3-11 days). Drug interactions and effects in geriatric patients[1] are the same as listed under amitriptyline.

Footnotes

1. Montamat SC, Cusack BJ, and Vestal RE, "Management of Drug Therapy in the Elderly," *N Engl J Med*, 1989, 321(5):303-9.

References

Amsterdam JD, Brunswick DJ, Potter L, et al, "Desipramine and 2-Hydroxydesipramine Plasma Levels in Endogenous Depressed Patients," *Arch Gen Psychiatry*, 1985, 42:361-4.

Ereshefsky L, Tran-Johnson T, Davis CM, et al, "Pharmacokinetic Factors Affecting Antidepressant Drug Clearance and Clinical Effect: Evaluation of Doxepin and Imipramine – New Data and Review," *Clin Chem*, 1988, 34:863-80.

Gawin FH, Kleber HD, Byck R, et al, "Desipramine Facilitation of Initial Cocaine Abstinence," *Arch Gen Psychiatry*, 1989, 46(2):117-21.

Siegel DM, "Bulimia, Tricyclic Antidepressants and Mania," *Clin Pediatr (Phila)*, 1989, 28(3):123-6.

Inderal® *see* Propranolol, Blood *on page 998*

Isopropanol *see* Volatile Screen *on page 1010*

Isoptin® *see* Verapamil *on page 1010*

Itraconazole

CPT 80299

Related Information

Amphotericin B *on page 942*
Blood Fungus Culture *on page 789*
Cerebrospinal Fluid Fungus Culture *on page 800*
Susceptibility Testing, Fungi *on page 869*

Synonyms Sporanox

Abstract Itraconazole is a new orally administered antifungal agent with a broad spectrum of activity. As of this writing it has not been released in the United States, though it is available in several other countries. Similarly, its role in clinical medicine is still evolving. It appears likely that this agent will become widely accepted due to its low toxicity compared with other antifungal agents and its broad spectrum of activity. The role for monitoring of serum levels has not been established.

Specimen Serum **CONTAINER:** Red top tube **SAMPLING TIME:** 4 hours after oral dose and approximately 1-2 weeks after therapy has begun so that a steady-state is achieved

Interpretive **REFERENCE RANGE:** Therapeutic: varies with methodology; see Additional Information. **USE:** May be useful to ensure therapeutic levels if poor absorption is suspected, or in cases of therapeutic failure or relapse **LIMITATIONS:** *In vitro* susceptibility testing of fungi against itraconazole is method dependent and may not accurately predict clinical success. Consequently, monitoring levels and adjusting dosage to attain therapeutic concentrations as determined by minimum inhibitory concentrations may not be helpful. Assays for itraconazole are performed only in a few reference laboratories. **METHODOLOGY:** Bioassay, high performance liquid chromatography (HPLC) **ADDITIONAL INFORMATION:** Serum levels as determined by bioassay are approximately 10 times the levels determined by HPLC, presumably because bioassay also detects an active metabolite. Consequently therapeutic levels vary with method. Concentrations >5 μg/mL (bioassay) were predictive of therapeutic success in invasive aspergillosis, whereas serum concentrations <1 μg/mL (bioassay) predicted therapeutic failure in cases of cryptococcal meningitis. Concentrations <0.25 μg/mL (HPLC) predicted failure to prevent aspergillosis in granulocytopenic patients. Absorption is often depressed in bone marrow transplant and in AIDS patients.

References

Bodey GP, "Topical and Systemic Antifungal Agents," *Med Clin North Am*, 1988, 72:637-59.
British Society for Antimicrobial Chemotherapy Working Party, "Laboratory Monitoring of Antifungal Chemotherapy," *Lancet*, 1991, 337(8769):1577-80.
Terrell CL and Hughes CE, "Antifungal Agents Used for Deep-Seated Mycotic Infections," *Mayo Clin Proc*, 1992, 67(1):69-91.

Kanamycin (Kantrex®) *see* Amikacin *on page 938*

Ketoconazole

CPT 80299

Related Information

Amphotericin B *on page 942*
Susceptibility Testing, Fungi *on page 869*

Synonyms Nizoral

Abstract Ketoconazole is an orally administered antifungal agent that is appropriately used for a variety of nonlife-threatening fungal infections. Determining serum levels rarely contributes significantly to patient care. Performed in only a few reference laboratories.

Specimen Serum **CONTAINER:** Red top tube **SAMPLING TIME:** 2 hours after administration

Interpretive **REFERENCE RANGE:** Therapeutic: 5-20 μg/mL (SI: 9-30 μmol/L), dependent on dose **USE:** Monitoring is usually not necessary. May be useful to ensure therapeutic levels if poor absorption is suspected, or in cases of therapeutic failure or relapse. **LIMITATIONS:** *In vitro* susceptibility testing of fungi against ketoconazole is method dependent and may not accurately predict clinical success. Consequently, monitoring levels and adjusting dosage to attain therapeutic concentrations as determined by minimum inhibitory concentrations may not be helpful. Assays for ketoconazole are performed only in a few reference laboratories. **METHODOLOGY:** Bioassay, high performance liquid chromatography (HPLC) **ADDITIONAL INFORMATION:** Approximately 5% to 10% of patients receiving ketoconazole develop abnormally elevated serum transaminases, a transient and reversible state. Rarely, patients develop symptomatic hepatitis which is idiosyncratic and not dependent upon serum concentrations. Absorption is often depressed in bone marrow transplant and AIDS patients.

(Continued)

Ketoconazole *(Continued)*

References

Bodey GP, "Topical and Systemic Antifungal Agents," *Med Clin North Am*, 1988, 72:637-59.

British Society for Antimicrobial Chemotherapy Working Party, "Laboratory Monitoring of Antifungal Chemotherapy," *Lancet*, 1991, 337(8769):1577-80.

Terrell CL and Hughes CE, "Antifungal Agents Used for Deep-Seated Mycotic Infections," *Mayo Clin Proc*, 1992, 67(1):69-91.

Killer Weed *see* Phencyclidine, Qualitative, Urine *on page 992*

Klonopin™ *see* Clonazepam *on page 954*

Lanotoxin® *see* Digitoxin *on page 959*

Lanoxin® *see* Digoxin *on page 959*

Lead, Blood

CPT 83655

Related Information

Delta Aminolevulinic Acid, Urine *on page 207*
Heavy Metal Screen, Blood *on page 972*
Heavy Metal Screen, Urine *on page 973*
Porphobilinogen, Qualitative, Urine *on page 325*
Protoporphyrin, Free Erythrocyte *on page 341*
Protoporphyrin, Zinc, Blood *on page 342*
Uric Acid, Serum *on page 378*

Synonyms Pb, Blood

Applies to Delta Aminolevulinic Acid Dehydratase

Abstract Blood lead concentrations are used to detect recent lead exposure. Does not necessarily measure lead body burden from chronic exposure in the past.

Specimen Whole blood **CONTAINER:** Special lead-free tube with heparin **COLLECTION:** See Blood Collection Methods for Trace Elements in the Trace Elements chapter. **STORAGE INSTRUCTIONS:** Do not separate red cells. **SPECIAL INSTRUCTIONS:** Avoid contact with leaded glass during collection

Interpretive **REFERENCE RANGE:** <20 μg/dL (whole blood) (SI: <0.97 μmol/L). See accompanying CDC chart for evaluating blood lead concentrations in children.

CDC Classification of Blood Lead in Children

Class	Blood Lead Level* (μg/dL)	Comment
I	<10	Not lead–poisoned
IIA	10–14	Rescreen frequently and consider prevention activities
IIB	15–19	Institute nutritional and educational interventions
III	20–44	Evaluate environment and consider chelation therapy
IV	45–69	Institute environmental intervention and chelation therapy
V	>69	A medical emergency

*Due to possible contamination during collection, elevated levels should be confirmed with a second specimen before action is instituted.

POSSIBLE PANIC RANGE: >80 μg/dL (SI: >3.86 μmol/L) in acute lead poisoning; toxicity at lower levels in chronic poisoning **USE:** Evaluate lead toxicity, poisoning **LIMITATIONS:** Lead poisoning is not ruled out by normal blood levels; clinical findings and heme synthetic enzymes must also be evaluated. **METHODOLOGY:** Electrothermal atomic absorption spectrometry (AA), photometry, anodic stripping voltammeter **ADDITIONAL INFORMATION:** Great care is required to avoid contamination in the collection of specimens for lead analysis. Lead can be measured in tissue and urine. Another test that may be used to evaluate lead intoxication is **free erythrocyte protoporphyrin (FEP)**. FEP concentrations >35 μg/dL are consistent with undue absorption of lead. However, FEP is also elevated in iron deficiency, sickle cell anemia, and chronic infection. **Erythrocyte zinc protoporphyrin** is a more specific indicator of lead toxicity and, therefore, superior to FEP. Normal values for erythrocyte zinc protoporphyrin are <100 ng/dL. Inhibition of erythrocyte **delta aminolevulinic acid dehydratase** is a very sensitive measure of lead toxicity. However, a blood lead assay is the definitive test for recent acute exposure if sample collection is meticulous. Blood lead concentrations are evidence of **recent** exposure but do not indicate the body burden from past exposure. Saturnine gout is mentioned in the Uric Acid, Serum listing.

References

Bernard BP and Becker CF, "Environmental Lead Exposure and the Kidney," *Clin Toxicol*, 1988, 26:1-34.

Braithwaite RA and Brown SS, "Clinical and Subclinical Lead Poisoning: A Laboratory Perspective," *Hum Toxicol*, 1988, 7:503-13.

Goyer RA, "Mechanisms of Lead and Cadmium Nephrotoxicity," *Toxicol Lett* 1989, 46(1-3):153-62.

Markowitz ME and Rosen JF, "Need for the Lead Mobilization Test in Children With Lead Poisoning," *J Pediatr*, 1991, 119(2):305-10.

Mushak P, Davis JM, Crocetti AF, et al, "Prenatal and Postnatal Effects of Low-Level Lead Exposure: Integrated Summary of a Report to the U.S. Congress on Childhood Lead Poisoning," *Environ Res*, 1989, 50(1):11-36.

Rempel D, "The Lead-Exposed Worker," *JAMA*, 1989, 262(4):532-4.

Staessen JA, Lauwerys RR, Buchet J-P, et al, "Impairment of Renal Function With Increasing Blood Lead Concentrations in the General Population," *N Engl J Med*, 1992, 327(3):151-6.

Lead Excretion Ratio *see* Lead, Urine *on this page*

Lead, Urine

CPT 83655

Related Information

Delta Aminolevulinic Acid, Urine *on page 207*
Heavy Metal Screen, Blood *on page 972*
Heavy Metal Screen, Urine *on page 973*
Protoporphyrin, Free Erythrocyte *on page 341*
Uric Acid, Urine *on page 380*

Synonyms Pb, Urine

Applies to Lead Excretion Ratio

Abstract This test is used to assess lead body burden (lead mobilization test), not to diagnose lead poisoning.

Patient Care PREPARATION: Patient should be instructed to use a specially cleaned plastic urinal or bedpan

Specimen Random or 24-hour urine CONTAINER: Plastic (preferably polyethylene) acid-washed urine container STORAGE INSTRUCTIONS: Record total volume. Acidify to pH 2 with concentrated HCl or add 20 mL 6N HCl to the 24-hour volume. CAUSES FOR REJECTION: Specimen allowed to contact glass or metal, specimen not collected in acid-washed containers SPECIAL INSTRUCTIONS: Indicate if a chelating agent has been administered

Interpretive REFERENCE RANGE: ≤ 80 μg/24 hours (SI: ≤ 0.39 μmol/day) POSSIBLE PANIC RANGE: >125 μg/24 hours (SI: >0.60 μmol/day) is considered excessive and associated with toxicity; values of 80-125 μg/24 hours (SI: 0.39-0.60 μmol/day) are inconclusive USE: Evaluate lead toxicity and chelation therapy METHODOLOGY: Electrothermal atomic absorption (AA) ADDITIONAL INFORMATION: Lead is poorly excreted and is found in lower concentrations in urine versus blood. Urine is not the specimen for screening potential toxicity. Urine lead mobilization tests (postchelation therapy) are good indicators of lead body burden. Children with blood lead levels between 25-40 μg/dL should be evaluated by a lead mobilization test to determine need for chelation therapy. Those with levels >40 μg/dL should receive chelation therapy.[1] A lead mobilization test is carried out by giving Ca EDTA and measuring the lead excreted in the next 24-hour urine. The lead excretion ratio (LER) is calculated by dividing the amount of lead excreted (in μg/24 hours) by the amount of Ca EDTA given (in mg). A ratio >0.60 is considered positive for the LER. Unstimulated urinary excretion at rates >0.19 μg lead/mg creatinine may also be used to indicate need for chelation therapy.[2]

Footnotes

1. Markowitz ME and Rosen JF, "Need for the Lead Mobilization Test in Children With Lead Poisoning," *J Pediatr*, 1991, 119(2):305-10.
2. Berger OG, Gregg DJ, and Succop PA, "Using Unstimulated Lead Excretion to Assess the Need for Chelation in the Treatment of Lead Poisoning," *J Pediatr*, 1990, 116(1):46-51.

(Continued)

Lead, Urine *(Continued)*

References

Bryson PD, *Comprehensive Review in Toxicology*, 2nd ed, Rockville, MD: Aspen Publishers Inc, 1989, 487-500.

Cory-Slechta DA, "Lead Exposure During Advanced Age: Alterations in Kinetics and Biochemical Effects," *Toxicol Appl Pharmacol*, 1990, 104(1):67-78.

D'Haese PC, Lamberts LV, Liang L, et al, "Elimination of Matrix and Spectral Interferences in the Measurement of Lead and Cadmium in Urine and Blood by Electrothermal Atomic Absorption Spectrometry With Deuterium Background Correction," *Clin Chem*, 1991, 37(9):1583-8.

Librax® *see* Chlordiazepoxide, Blood *on page 953*

Librium® *see* Chlordiazepoxide, Blood *on page 953*

Lidocaine

CPT *80176*

Related Information

Monoethylglycinexylidide *on page 987*

Tocainide *on page 1004*

Synonyms Lignocaine; Xylocaine®

Applies to GX; MEGX

Abstract Lidocaine is a local anesthetic which more recently has been used as an antiarrhythmic. The most active metabolite is MEGX.

Specimen Serum or plasma **CONTAINER:** Red top tube, green top (heparin) tube, or lavender top (EDTA) tube **SAMPLING TIME:** Draw specimens 12 hours after initiating therapy for arrhythmia prophylaxis, then every 24 hours thereafter. Obtain specimens every 12 hours when cardiac or hepatic insufficiency exists. **COLLECTION:** Avoid collection tubes with stoppers containing the plasticizer, TBEP.

Interpretive **REFERENCE RANGE:** Therapeutic: 1.5-5.0 μg/mL (SI: 6.4-21.4 μmol/L), up to 6.0 μg/mL (SI: 25.6 μmol/L) if necessary.[1] **POSSIBLE PANIC RANGE:** At levels >6.0 μg/mL (SI: >25.6 μmol/L), there may be seizure activity. See Table C in the Appendix of this chapter. **USE:** Monitor therapeutic drug level. Lidocaine is used especially in acute arrhythmias. **LIMITATIONS:** Cross reactions with other drugs occur. Certain blood collection tubes have been shown to lead to falsely low results. See Collection above. **METHODOLOGY:** Enzyme immunoassay (EIA), gas-liquid chromatography (GLC), high performance liquid chromatography (HPLC) **ADDITIONAL INFORMATION:** This drug is used in therapy of ventricular but not supraventricular arrhythmias. Following initial parenteral administration of a bolus, lidocaine is rapidly cleared with a short half-life of approximately 10 minutes (first-pass effect). After approximately 30 minutes, there is a slower elimination phase about 90 minutes long. With continuous intravenous administration, a half-life of about 1.5-2 hours may be achieved, hence, prolonged administration by the I.V. route is often necessary to achieve the desired therapeutic result. Time to reach steady-state by I.V. is 6-12 hours. In most cases, a relatively constant plasma level may be maintained by slow intravenous infusion administered over a period of 6-10 hours. Blood levels are also elevated by impaired cardiac or hepatic function. The drug is metabolized by the liver to two active metabolites, monoethylglycinexylidide (MEGX) and glycinexylidide (GX). Both accumulate and MEGX most likely contributes to toxicity. Toxic symptoms may include confusion, respiratory depression, seizures, dizziness, drowsiness, paresthesias, hypotension, bradycardia, and double vision. Convulsions, cardiac and respiratory arrest may occur. Barbiturates and phenytoin seem to enhance drug metabolism and lower serum levels, whereas propranolol, cimetidine, and norepinephrine increase levels. Lidocaine is approximately 70% bound to plasma proteins, especially $alpha_1$ acid glycoprotein (the concentration of which is variable) and to albumin.

Footnotes

1. Blanke RV and Decker WJ, "Analysis of Toxic Substances," *Fundamentals of Clinical Chemistry*, 3rd ed, Tietz NW, ed, Philadelphia, PA: WB Saunders Co, 1987, 869-905.

References

Gumucio CA, Bennie JB, Fernando B, et al, "Plasma Lidocaine Levels During Augmentation Mammoplasty and Suction-Assisted Lipectomy," *Plast Reconstr Surg*, 1989, 84(4):624-7.

Montamat SC, Cusack BJ, and Vestal RE, "Management of Drug Therapy in the Elderly," *N Engl J Med*, 1989, 321(5):303-9.

Palmisano JM, Meliones JN, Crowley DC, et al, "Lidocaine Toxicity After Subcutaneous Infiltration in Children Undergoing Cardiac Catheterization," *Am J Cardiol*, 1991, 67(7):647-8.

Lidocaine Metabolite *see* Monoethylglycinexylidide *on page 987*

Lignocaine *see* Lidocaine *on previous page*

Limbitrol® *see* Amitriptyline, Blood *on page 939*

Liquiprin® *see* Acetaminophen, Serum *on page 935*

Lithium

CPT 80178

Related Information

Thyroid Stimulating Hormone *on page 361*
Thyroxine *on page 364*
Verapamil *on page 1010*

Synonyms Eskalith®; Lithonate®

Abstract Lithium is used in the treatment of depression and particularly for manic-depressive psychosis. It should be monitored.

Patient Care **AFTERCARE:** Follow urine osmolality, ECGs, thyroid profile, BUN, creatinine, and sodium. Avoid sodium depletion.

Specimen Serum **CONTAINER:** Red top tube **COLLECTION:** Collect at a standard time from last dose, 6-12 hours recommended. **STORAGE INSTRUCTIONS:** Refrigerate a minimum of 2 mL serum. Serum specimens are stable for 24 hours at room temperature. Separate serum immediately. **CAUSES FOR REJECTION:** Specimen collected in tube containing lithium heparin, hemolysis **TURNAROUND TIME:** 1-2 hours if in-house

Interpretive **REFERENCE RANGE:** Therapeutic: 0.6-1.2 mEq/L (SI: 0.6-1.2 mmol/L), for acute mania; 0.8-1.0 mEq/L (SI: 0.8-1.0 mmol/L) for protection against future episodes in most patients with bipolar disorder. A higher rate of relapse is described in subjects who are maintained at levels <0.4 mEq/L (SI: 0.4 mmol/L).[1] **POSSIBLE PANIC RANGE:** Toxic: >1.5 mEq/L (SI: >1.5 mmol/L). Toxicity can become serious when levels rise to levels ≥2.0 mEq/L (SI: ≥2.0 mmol/L). Levels >4.0 mEq/L (SI: >4.0 mmol/L) are associated with coma, death. A narrow therapeutic index exists for lithium.[2] **USE:** Monitor therapeutic drug level, evaluate coma **LIMITATIONS:** Lithium toxicity can occur with normal serum lithium levels. Thiazides can cause significant rise in serum lithium. **METHODOLOGY:** Flame photometry, atomic absorption spectrophotometry (AA), ion-selective electrode (ISE) **ADDITIONAL INFORMATION:** Lithium as lithium carbonate is used as a psychoactive agent in the treatment of manic depressive disorders. Lithium therapy demands daily monitoring of serum lithium levels until the proper dose schedule is determined. Serum half-life ranges from 20-60 hours. Insomnia in a low-range group is described. Tremor, gastrointestinal symptoms, urinary frequency, and weight gain were less frequent at lower levels.[1] Intoxication never occurs suddenly. Several days to a week before full-blown symptoms develop, a patient will experience lethargy, drowsiness, tremor, muscle twitching, dysarthria, anorexia and vomiting or diarrhea. A fully developed case of intoxication shows coma to semicoma, rigidity, hyperactive reflexes and seizures at times. There is a high incidence of pulmonary complications. It is advisable to perform periodic plasma sodium determinations. Low plasma sodium levels are associated with lithium retention; high levels with lithium elimination. Varying degrees of nephrogenic diabetes insipidus have been reported to occur in 33% of lithium treated patients. Lithium significantly inhibits antidiuretic-hormone-induced water transport in kidney. Lithium interferes with solute and water absorption from the gastrointestinal system producing nausea, vomiting, diarrhea, and abdominal pain. These symptoms may occur at any time, at any serum level. They most commonly occur during early treatment stages and usually clear spontaneously or by adjustment of dosage. Chronic lithium administration has a goitrogenic effect on 4% of lithium-treated patients, with or without hypothyroidism. In general, lithium administration results in slightly decreased serum T_4 levels and transiently elevated levels of TSH in nearly 33% of these patients. Lithium affects the cardiac conduction system by incomplete substitution for other cations, especially sodium and potassium. These electrolyte changes account for the usually unimportant and reversible T-wave depressions observed in 10% to 20% of patients on lithium therapy.

Footnotes

1. Gelenberg AJ, Kane JM, Keller MB, et al, "Comparison of Standard and Low Serum Levels of Lithium for Maintenance Treatment of Bipolar Disorder," *N Engl J Med*, 1989, 321(22):1489-93.
2. Ritschel WA, "Therapeutic Drug Monitoring," *Clinical Chemistry Theory, Analysis, and Correlation*, Kaplan LA and Pesce AJ, eds, St Louis, MO: Mosby-Year Book Inc, 1989, 795-807.

References

Chamberlain S, Hahn PM, Casson P, et al, "Effect of Menstrual Cycle Phase and Oral Contraceptive Use on Serum Lithium Levels After a Loading Dose of Lithium in Normal Women," *Am J Psychiatry*, 1990, 147(7):907-9.

(Continued)

Lithium *(Continued)*

Krishel S and Jackimczyk K, "Cyclic Antidepressants, Lithium, and Neuroleptic Agents. Pharmacology and Toxicology," *Emerg Med Clin North Am*, 1991, 9(1):53-86.

Manji HK, Hsiao JK, Risby ED, et al, "The Mechanisms of Action of Lithium. I. Effects on Serotoninergic and Noradrenergic Systems in Normal Subjects," *Arch Gen Psychiatry*, 1991, 48(6):505-12.

Murray RL, "Lithium," *Clinical Chemistry – Theory Analysis, and Correlation*, 2nd ed, Kaplan LA and Pesce AJ, eds, St Louis, MO: Mosby-Year Book Inc, 1989, 1108-10.

Schweyen DH, Sporka MC, and Burnakis TG, "Evaluation of Serum Lithium Concentration Determinations," *Am J Hosp Pharm*, 1991, 48(7):1536-7.

Lithonate® *see* Lithium *on previous page*

l-Methamphetamine *see* Methamphetamines, Qualitative, Urine *on page 984*

Loads *see* Glutethimide *on page 970*

Lotusate® *see* Barbiturates, Quantitative, Blood *on page 946*

Lude® *see* Methaqualone *on page 985*

Ludiomil® *see* Maprotiline *on this page*

Luminal® *see* Barbiturates, Quantitative, Blood *on page 946*

Luminal® *see* Phenobarbital, Blood *on page 992*

Majsolin® *see* Primidone *on page 996*

Maprotiline

***CPT** 80299*

Synonyms Ludiomil®

Abstract Maprotiline is a tetracyclic antidepressant with a long half-life.

Specimen Serum **CONTAINER:** Red top tube **STORAGE INSTRUCTIONS:** Separate serum from clot and refrigerate.

Interpretive **REFERENCE RANGE:** 200-600 ng/mL (SI: 721-2163 nmol/L) **CRITICAL VALUES:** >1000 ng/mL (SI: >3605 nmol/L) **USE:** Evaluate toxicity and therapeutic drug monitoring **METHODOLOGY:** High performance liquid chromatography (HPLC), gas chromatography (GC) **ADDITIONAL INFORMATION:** Maprotiline is a tetracyclic antidepressant prescribed for depression, chronic schizophrenia, idiopathic pain, and potentially for drug abuse withdrawal. Maprotiline is often used in patients who do not respond to tricyclics. The drug is taken orally at an average adult dose of 75-300 mg/day (50-75 mg/day in elderly patients). Peak serum values are reached in 12 hours and steady-state is achieved in 20-24 days; half-life is 27-58 hours. Maprotiline is a very potent inhibitor of the reuptake of norepinephrine to the presynaptic nerve terminal. The drug possesses moderate anticholinergic activity and cardiovascular toxicity. It also may lower seizure control. It should not be given in combination with MAO inhibitor.[1] Overdoses (coma, convulsions, dysrhythmias, hypotension) are exacerbated by its long half-life.

Footnotes

1. Craig CR and Stitzel RE, *Modern Pharmacology*, 3rd ed, Boston, MA: Little, Brown and Co, 1990, 479-81.

References

Drebit R, Baker GB, and Dewhurst WG, "Determination of Maprotiline and Desmethylmaprotiline in Plasma and Urine by Gas Chromatography With Nitrogen-Phosphorus Detection," *J Chromatogr*, 1988, 432:334-9.

Tollefson GD, Montaque-Clouse J, Lesan T, et al, "Pharmacokinetic Properties of Maprotiline in Geriatric Depression," *J Clin Psychopharmacol*, 1989, 9(4):313-5.

Yamagami S and Soejima K, "Effect of Maprotiline Combined With Conventional Neuroleptics Against Negative Symptoms of Chronic Schizophrenia," *Drugs Exp Clin Res*, 1989, 15(4):171-6.

Marijuana *see* Cannabinoids, Qualitative, Urine *on page 949*

MDMA *see* Methamphetamines, Qualitative, Urine *on page 984*

Mebaral® *see* Barbiturates, Quantitative, Blood *on page 946*

Mebaral® *see* Methylphenobarbital *on page 986*

Medical Legal Specimens *see* Chain-of-Custody Protocol *on page 952*

MEGX *see* Lidocaine *on page 978*

MEGX *see* Monoethylglycinexylidide *on page 987*

Mellaril® *see* Phenothiazines, Serum *on page 993*

Meperidine, Urine

CPT 83925

Related Information

Chain-of-Custody Protocol *on page 952*

Synonyms Demerol®

Test Commonly Includes This test is included in the comprehensive Urine Drug Screen.

Abstract Meperidine is a synthetic narcotic analgesic with about one-tenth the potency of morphine. It is a drug of abuse.

Specimen Urine **CONTAINER:** Plastic urine container **STORAGE INSTRUCTIONS:** Refrigerate **SPECIAL INSTRUCTIONS:** If forensic, use chain-of-custody protocol and form. See test entry Chain-of-Custody Protocol in this chapter and the Appendix of this chapter. When evaluating drug of abuse, order Toxicology Drug Screen, Blood.

Interpretive **REFERENCE RANGE:** Negative. Patients with therapeutic blood levels can have up to 10 μg/mL in urine. **USE:** Evaluate toxicity; detect an abused drug **LIMITATIONS:** Therapeutic levels not detected by enzyme-multiplied immunoassay technique (EMIT), thin-layer chromatography, and enzyme immunoassay. Use HPLC methods to detect therapeutic concentrations. **METHODOLOGY:** Thin-layer chromatography (TLC) and enzyme immunoassay (EIA); gas chromatography (GC), high performance liquid chromatography (HPLC) **ADDITIONAL INFORMATION:** Meperidine is a synthetic morphine-like compound used in the management of moderate to severe pain and as an adjunct to anesthesia and preoperative sedation. Analgesic effects after oral ingestion or I.M. injection peak in 1 hour. The half-life is 2.4-4 hours. Adverse effects include tachycardia, CNS and respiratory depression, nausea and vomiting, hypotension, bradycardia, miosis, increased intracranial pressure, and physical and psychological dependence. When evaluating therapeutic levels, order Meperidine, Blood. Usual therapeutic range in serum, 50-250 ng/mL (SI: 200-1010 nmol/L).

References

Belgrade MJ, Ling LJ, Schleevogt MB, et al, "Comparison of Single-Dose Meperidine, Butorphanol, and Dihydroergotamine in the Treatment of Vascular Headache," *Neurology*, 1989, 39(4):590-2.

Johnson MD, Hurley RJ, Gilbertson LI, et al, "Continuous Microcatheter Spinal Anesthesia With Subarachnoid Meperidine for Labor and Delivery," *Anesth Analg*, 1990, 70(6):658-61.

Mephenytoin

CPT 80299

Related Information

Phenytoin *on page 994*

Synonyms Mesantoin®; Sedantoinal®

Applies to Nirvanol®

Abstract Mephenytoin has a pharmacologic effect similar to that of phenytoin. Mephenytoin has serious toxicity but less dose-related effects compared to phenytoin.

Specimen Serum **CONTAINER:** Red top tube **SAMPLING TIME:** Consistent sampling time

Interpretive **REFERENCE RANGE:** 10-40 μg/mL for drug and Nirvanol® metabolite, which is usually present at a higher level than the parent compound **POSSIBLE PANIC RANGE:** Toxic level about 50 μg/mL (SI: 230 μmol/L). See Table A in the Appendix of this chapter. **USE:** Monitor for compliance, efficacy, and possible toxicity **LIMITATIONS:** Unlike phenytoin, cognitive side effects, cerebellar symptoms, gingival hypertrophy, and hirsutism do not occur as commonly with increasing dosage. The main active metabolite, 5-ethyl-5-phenylhydantoin, is a biologically active anticonvulsant with a half-life of 100 hours. **METHODOLOGY:** Gas chromatography (GC) **ADDITIONAL INFORMATION:** Mephenytoin, like phenytoin, has zero-order kinetics so that small changes in dosage may produce large changes in clinical response. Acute overdosage results in sedation and eventually coma. Most adverse effects are not dose-related, but are due to the accumulation of arene-oxide intermediates. They include rash, hepatotoxicity, blood dyscrasias, systemic lupus erythematosus, periarteritis nodosa, and fever. Mephenytoin may be suited for patients who respond to phenytoin but who cannot tolerate dose-related side effects. The drug is considered more highly toxic than other hydantoins. The half-life of the parent compound is 7 hours, but that of the metabolites is close to 100 hours.

References

Engel J, *Seizures and Epilepsy*, Contemporary Neurology Series, Philadelphia, PA: FA Davis Co, 1989.

Kupferberg HJ, "Other Hydantoins: Mephenytoin and Ethotoin," *Antiepileptic Drugs*, 3rd ed, Levy RH, Dreifuss FE, Mattson RH, et al, eds, New York, NY: Raven Press, 1989, 257-65.

Mephobarb *see* Barbiturates, Qualitative, Urine *on page 945*

Mephobarbital *see* Barbiturates, Quantitative, Blood *on page 946*

Mephobarbital *see* Methylphenobarbital *on page 986*

Mephobarbitone *see* Methylphenobarbital *on page 986*

Meprobamate

CPT 83805

Synonyms Equagesic®; Equanil®; Meprospan®; Miltown®

Abstract Meprobamate is a sedative-anxiolytic producing effects similar to the benzodiazepines and barbiturates.

Specimen Serum **CONTAINER:** Red top tube

Interpretive **REFERENCE RANGE:** Sedative dose: 8-24 μg/mL (SI: 37-110 μmol/L) **POSSIBLE PANIC RANGE:** Toxic: >50 μg/mL (SI: >229 μmol/L); lethal: 200 μg/mL (SI: 916 μmol/L) **USE:** Therapeutic monitoring and toxicity assessment **METHODOLOGY:** Gas-liquid chromatography (GLC) **ADDITIONAL INFORMATION:** Meprobamate is a propanediol carbamate sedative and tranquilizer, having pharmacological effects similar to barbiturates. It is well absorbed from the gastrointestinal tract and reaches its peak concentration in 2-3 hours. Its half-life is 6-15 hours. Respiratory depression, coma, and cardiovascular collapse characterize overdosage. It may also be detected in urine or gastric juice.

References

Bertino J and Reed M, "Barbiturate and Nonbarbiturate Sedative Hypnotic Intoxication in Children," *Pediatr Clin North Am*, 1986, 33:703-22.

Dennison J, Edwards JN, and Volans GN, "Meprobamate Overdosage," *Hum Toxicol*, 1985, 4:215-7.

Meprospan® *see* Meprobamate *on this page*

Mercury, Blood

CPT 83825

Related Information

Heavy Metal Screen, Blood *on page 972*

Heavy Metal Screen, Urine *on page 973*

Synonyms Hg, Blood

Applies to Hair Analysis

Abstract This metal is toxic in any of its three forms: elemental, inorganic, and organic. The mode of entry into the body varies among the three forms.

Specimen Whole blood **CONTAINER:** Special metal-free EDTA tube **COLLECTION:** See Blood Collection Methods for Trace Elements in the introduction of the Trace Elements chapter. **SPECIAL INSTRUCTIONS:** Whole blood is analyzed.

Interpretive **REFERENCE RANGE:** 0.020-0.080 μg/mL (SI: 0.10-0.80 μmol/L) **POSSIBLE PANIC RANGE:** >0.10 μg/mL **USE:** Evaluate for mercury toxicity, neurological findings related to organic mercurials, inhalation of mercury vapors **LIMITATIONS:** Methyl mercury must be measured in whole blood or erythrocytes. **METHODOLOGY:** Electrothermal atomic absorption (AA), gold electrode deposition, gas chromatography (GC) **ADDITIONAL INFORMATION:** Organic methyl mercury is a new important environmental mercurial contaminant. It was discovered that inorganic mercurial industrial wastes dumped into Minimata Bay (Japan) could be organified by plankton and incorporated into fish, and thus, the human food chain. Ingestion of mercury-laden fish leads to severe neurologic deficits. Inhalation of mercury vapors can lead to pneumonitis. Inorganic mercurials deposit in kidneys, liver, heart, striated muscle, marrow, brain, and lungs. Gastrointestinal symptoms, stomatitis, colitis, anemia, and peripheral neuritis can relate to mercury poisoning. Ingestion of inorganic mercurials results in a serious medical emergency. Mercury exposure from a brand of interior latex paint was recently described.[1] Half-life of inorganic mercury is 24 days and of methyl mercury (organic mercury) is 54 days. Hair analysis can be used for poisoning or exposure. It should be clean and clipped as close to the scalp as possible.

Footnotes

1. Agocs MM, Etzel RA, Parrish RG, et al, "Mercury Exposure From Interior Latex Paint," *N Engl J Med*, 1990, 323(16):1096-101.

References

Bryson PD, *Comprehensive Review in Toxicology*, 2nd ed, Rockville, MD: Aspen Publishers Inc, 1989, 477-86.

Snapp KR, Boyer DB, Peterson LC, et al, "The Contribution of Dental Amalgam to Mercury in Blood," *J Dent Res*, 1989, 68(5):780-5.

Mercury, Urine

***CPT** 83825*

Related Information

Heavy Metal Screen, Blood *on page 972*
Heavy Metal Screen, Urine *on page 973*

Synonyms Hg, Urine

Abstract This metal is toxic in elemental, inorganic, and organic forms. Urine mercury is used for evaluation of inorganic and possibly elemental forms.

Specimen 24-hour urine **CONTAINER:** Plastic (preferably polyethylene) acid-washed container, no preservative **STORAGE INSTRUCTIONS:** Store in special metal-free container

Interpretive **REFERENCE RANGE:** 10-50 μg/24 hours (SI: 0.05-0.25 μmol/day) **POSSIBLE PANIC RANGE:** >100 μg/24 hours (SI: >0.50 μmol/day) **USE: Inorganic** mercury toxicity is best evaluated by urine mercury levels. **LIMITATIONS: Organic** mercury is found mostly in red cells; see Mercury, Blood listing. Urine mercury would not be useful for organic mercury poisoning. **METHODOLOGY:** Electrothermal atomic absorption (AA), gold electrode deposition, gas chromatography (GC) **ADDITIONAL INFORMATION:** Industrial and agricultural exposure includes inhalation of vapor and ingestion.

References

Bryson PD, *Comprehensive Review in Toxicology*, 2nd ed, Rockville, MD: Aspen Publishers Inc, 1989, 477-86.

Gothe CJ, Langworth S, Carleson R, et al, "Biological Monitoring of Exposure to Metallic Mercury," *Clin Toxicol*, 1985, 23:381-9.

Piikivi L and Ruokonen A, "Renal Function and Long-Term Low Mercury Vapor Exposure," *Arch Environ Health*, 1989, 44(3):146-9.

Mesantoin® *see* Mephenytoin *on page 981*

Mesoridazine *see* Phenothiazines, Serum *on page 993*

Metabolites of Primidone *see* Primidone *on page 996*

Metals, Blood *see* Heavy Metal Screen, Blood *on page 972*

Metal Screen *see* Heavy Metal Screen, Urine *on page 973*

Metals, Toxic *see* Heavy Metal Screen, Urine *on page 973*

Methadone, Urine

***CPT** 83840*

Related Information

Chain-of-Custody Protocol *on page 952*
Drugs of Abuse Testing, Urine *on page 962*

Synonyms Dolophine®

Abstract This drug is a synthetic opiate agonist used during World War II as a morphine substitute. It is used for detoxification of opiate addicts. It is a drug of abuse.

Specimen Urine **CONTAINER:** Plastic urine container **STORAGE INSTRUCTIONS:** Refrigerate **SPECIAL INSTRUCTIONS:** If forensic, use chain-of-custody protocol and form. See test entry Chain-of-Custody Protocol and the Appendix of this chapter.

Interpretive **REFERENCE RANGE:** Negative (less than cutoff); when used therapeutically for pain, plasma levels are in the range of 0.05-0.10 μg/mL. **CRITICAL VALUES:** Cutoff for screening: 300 ng/mL; confirmation: 200 ng/mL **USE:** Evaluate toxicity and detection as drug of abuse **METHODOLOGY:** Thin-layer chromatography (TLC) and enzyme immunoassay (EIA) for screening; gas chromatography/mass spectrometry (GC/MS) for confirmation **ADDITIONAL INFORMATION:** Methadone is a synthetic diphenylheptane derivative. It produces less sedation and euphoria than morphine and its effects are cumulative. Methadone is highly addictive, but the withdrawal symptoms are less intense. This drug is used in the management of severe pain and in narcotic detoxification maintenance programs. Onset of action is 30-60 minutes after oral dose and 10-20 minutes following parenteral administration. The half-life is 15-25 hours. Adverse effects include marked sedation after repeated administration, CNS and respiratory depression, nausea and vomiting, bradycardia, hypotension, increased intracranial pressure, miosis, antidi-

(Continued)

Methadone, Urine *(Continued)*

uretic hormone release, and physical and psychological dependence. Methadone is a drug of abuse and is included in most drug-of-abuse screening panels. Patients on methadone maintenance protocols will test above cutoff in urine drug screens.

References

Baselt RC and Cravey RH, *Disposition of Toxic Drugs and Chemicals in Man*, 3rd ed, Chicago, IL: Year Book Medical Publishers Inc, 1989, 512-5.

Bryson PD, *Comprehensive Review in Toxicology*, 2nd ed, Rockville, MD: Aspen Publishers Inc, 1989, 329.

Calsyn DA, Saxon AJ, and Barndt DC, "Urine Screening Practices in Methadone Maintenance Clinics. A Survey of How the Results Are Used," *J Nerv Ment Dis*, 1991, 179(4):222-7.

Wolff K, Hay AW, and Raistrick D, "Plasma Methadone Measurements and Their Role in Methadone Detoxification Programs," *Clin Chem*, 1992, 38(3):420-5.

Wolff K, Sanderson M, Hay AW, et al, "Methadone Concentrations in Plasma and Their Relationship to Drug Dosage," *Clin Chem*, 1991, 37(2):205-9.

Methamphetamines, Qualitative, Urine

CPT *80101 (screen); 80102 (confirmation)*

Related Information

Amphetamines, Qualitative, Urine *on page 941*
Chain-of-Custody Protocol *on page 952*
Drugs of Abuse Testing, Urine *on page 962*

Synonyms Crystal; Desoxyn®; Doe; Methedrine®; Speed

Applies to Amphetamines, Urine; Chlorpromazine; d-Methamphetamine; l-Methamphetamine; MDMA; Methylenedioxymethamphetamine; Phentermine; Phenylpropanolamine; Pseudoephedrine; Ranitidine

Test Commonly Includes Amphetamine

Abstract The d-isomer of this drug is used therapeutically as an anorectic agent and for treatment of hyperactive children. It is also a drug of abuse.

Specimen Random urine **CONTAINER:** Plastic urine container **COLLECTION:** If forensic, observe precautions. **STORAGE INSTRUCTIONS:** Refrigerate **CAUSES FOR REJECTION:** If forensic, failure to meet temperature check and reasonable urine creatinine concentration **TURNAROUND TIME:** Usually 1-2 hours if done in-house **SPECIAL INSTRUCTIONS:** If forensic, use chain-of-custody protocol and form. See test entry Chain-of-Custody Protocol and the Appendix of this chapter.

Interpretive **REFERENCE RANGE:** Negative (less than cutoff) **CRITICAL VALUES:** Cutoff: screen: 1000 ng/mL; confirmation: 500 ng/mL **USE:** Evaluate for drug abuse, assess toxicity **LIMITATIONS:** Screening test may give false-positives with common cold and antiallergy medications. Qualitative results only (positive or negative). **METHODOLOGY:** Screening: enzyme immunoassay (EIA), fluorescence polarization immunoassay (FPIA), thin-layer chromatography (TLC); confirmation: gas chromatography/mass spectrometry (GC/MS), gas-liquid chromatography (GLC), high performance liquid chromatography (HPLC) **ADDITIONAL INFORMATION:** The most abused drug in this class is d-methamphetamine. The optical isomer, l-methamphetamine, has less pronounced central effects and is used as a nasal decongestant in Vicks Inhaler® (legal, over-the-counter). Amphetamine isomers are present in Dexedrine® and Benzedrine®. These drugs are self-administered orally, I.V., or by smoking. Half-life is 10-20 hours and it can be detected in urine within 3 hours of use. The parent drugs are the substances detected by the screening tests. Over-the-counter medication for colds and allergies (Contac®, Dimetapp®, Sine-Off®, Sudafed®) contain phenylpropanolamine or pseudoephedrine which give a positive EIA screening test when the polyclonal antibody is used. This antibody also detects methylenedioxymethamphetamine (MDMA), a controlled substance classed as an hallucinogen and "designer" drug.[1] With the monoclonal EIA test, the above medications are not detected, but phentermine (Adipex®, Fastin®), ranitidine (Zantac®), and chlorpromazine (Thorazine®) give a positive test. Confirmation by GC/MS rules out these false-positives. In order to rule out the false-positive given by l-methamphetamine (legal nasal decongestant), a chiral column or procedure, which separates the "l" and "d" isomers, must be used in the GC/MS confirmation. See Amphetamine listing in this chapter for discussion of physiological effects.

Methamphetamine is a sympathomimetic amine chemically related to ephedrine and amphetamine. It is used in the management of obesity, to treat certain depressive reactions, and as adjunctive therapy for narcolepsy, epilepsy, attention deficit disorders, and postencephalitic parkinsonism. Methamphetamine is readily absorbed by the GI tract and the effects last from 6-12 hours. Adverse effects include tremor, insomnia, nervousness, anxiety, euphoria or dysphoria, hyper- or hypotension, arrhythmias, circulatory collapse, and nausea and vomiting.

Footnotes

1. Bost RD, "3,4-Methylenedioxymethamphetamine (MDMA) and Other Amphetamine Derivatives," *J Forensic Sci*, 1988, 33(2):576-87.

References

Baselt RC and Cravey RH, *Disposition of Toxic Drugs and Chemicals in Man*, 3rd ed, Chicago, IL: Year Book Medical Publishers Inc, 1989, 516-9.

Bryson PD, *Comprehensive Review in Toxicology*, 2nd ed, Rockville, MD: Aspen Publishers Inc, 1989, 369-79.

DePace A, Verebey K, and elSohly M, "Capillary Gas-Liquid Chromatography Separation of Phenethylamines in Amphetamine-Positive Urine Samples," *J Forensic Sci*, 1990, 35(6):1431-5.

Derlet RW and Heischober B, "Methamphetamine. Stimulant of the 1990s?" *West J Med*, 1990, 153(6):625-8.

Ellenhorn MJ and Barceloux DG, "Amphetamines," *Medical Toxicology*, New York, NY: Elsevier, 1988, 625-42.

Gan BK, Baugh D, Liu RH, et al, "Simultaneous Analysis of Amphetamine, Methamphetamine, and 3,4-Methylenedioxymethamphetamine (MDMA) in Urine Samples by Solid-Phase Extraction, Derivatization, and Gas Chromatography/Mass Spectrometry," *J Forensic Sci*, 1991, 36(5):1331-41.

Grinstead GF, "Ranitidine and High Concentrations of Phenylpropanolamine Cross React in the EMIT Monoclonal Amphetamine/Methamphetamine Assay," *Clin Chem*, 1989, 35(9):1998-9.

Methanol *see* Volatile Screen *on page 1010*

Methaqualone

***CPT** 80101 (screen); 80102 (confirmation)*

Related Information

Chain-of-Custody Protocol *on page 952*
Drugs of Abuse Testing, Urine *on page 962*

Synonyms Lude®

Abstract This drug is a sedative-hypnotic but is currently a DEA schedule II drug. It is a drug of abuse.

Specimen Serum, urine **CONTAINER:** Red top tube, plastic urine container **SPECIAL INSTRUCTIONS:** If forensic, use chain-of-custody protocol and form. See test entry Chain-of-Custody Protocol and the Appendix of this chapter.

Interpretive **REFERENCE RANGE:** Urine: negative (less than cutoff); serum: 1-5 μg/mL (SI: 4-20 nmol/L) **CRITICAL VALUES:** Cutoff for urine: screen: 300 ng/mL; confirmation: 200 ng/mL **POSSIBLE PANIC RANGE:** Serum values >8 μg/mL (SI: >32 nmol/L) associated with unconsciousness; toxic: >10 μg/mL (SI: >40 nmol/L) **USE:** Evaluate for toxicity, evaluate for drug abuse **METHODOLOGY:** Immunoassay, gas-liquid chromatography (GLC), UV spectrophotometry, fluorometry **ADDITIONAL INFORMATION:** Methaqualone is a nonbarbiturate sedative-hypnotic. It is rapidly absorbed from the GI tract. Hyperexcitability, coma, and cardiovascular and respiratory depression characterize overdosage. It is a common drug of abuse, and "street" preparations may be adulterated with other pharmacoactive substances. Half-life is 20-60 hours. It is extensively metabolized and screening methods must detect metabolites. Enzyme-multiplied immunoassay technique (EMIT) detects four of the most common metabolites.

References

Baselt RC and Cravey RH, *Disposition of Toxic Drugs and Chemicals in Man*, 3rd ed, Chicago, IL: Year Book Medical Publishers Inc, 1989, 524-7.

Beebe DK and Walley E, "Substance Abuse: The Designer Drugs," *Am Fam Physician*, 1991, 43(5):1689-98.

Buckner JC and Mandell W, "Risk Factors for Depressive Symptomatology in a Drug Using Population," *Am J Public Health*, 1990, 80(5):580-5.

Metharbital *see* Barbiturates, Quantitative, Blood *on page 946*

Methedrine® *see* Methamphetamines, Qualitative, Urine *on previous page*

Methotrexate

***CPT** 80299*

Synonyms Mexate®; MTX, Blood

Applies to Cerebrospinal Fluid Methotrexate; Methotrexate, CSF

Abstract This is a widely used anticancer drug acting as an antimetabolite in DNA synthesis. It must be monitored.

Specimen Serum or plasma **CONTAINER:** Red top tube, green top (heparin) tube, or lavender top (EDTA) tube **SAMPLING TIME:** Will vary according to dosing protocol **STORAGE INSTRUCTIONS:** Separate and freeze **SPECIAL INSTRUCTIONS:** Advise laboratory if patient is also on trimethoprim.

(Continued)

Methotrexate *(Continued)*

Interpretive REFERENCE RANGE: Therapeutic range is dependent upon therapeutic approach. "High dose" regimens produce drug levels between 10^{-6} M and 10^{-7} M 24-72 hours after drug infusion. POSSIBLE PANIC RANGE: >2.27 μg/mL (SI: >5 μmol/L) 24 hours after high dose therapy USE: Monitor therapeutic drug level of methotrexate, evaluate potential toxicity METHODOLOGY: Enzyme immunoassay (EIA), radioimmunoassay (RIA), high performance liquid chromatography (HPLC) ADDITIONAL INFORMATION: Methotrexate is an antimetabolite that combines with dihydrofolate reductase and therefore interferes with the synthesis of tetrahydrofolic acid necessary for DNA synthesis. From 40% to 50% of a small dose and up to 90% of a larger dose is excreted unchanged in the urine in 48 hours, a major portion of it during the first 8 hours. Toxicity consists of bone marrow depression with megaloblastosis. Concomitant salicylate administration increases incidence of toxicity, due to diminished renal tubular excretion. The effect of methotrexate on normal cells may be reversed by administration of 5-formyltetrahydrofolate, also called citrovorum factor or leucovorin. This "rescue" makes possible administration of much higher doses of methotrexate than the body would otherwise survive. The initial half-life is 2-4 hours but the total body clearance (terminal) half-life is 8-15 hours.

References

Brooks PJ, Spruill WJ, Parish RC, et al, "Pharmacokinetics of Methotrexate Administered by Intramuscular and Subcutaneous Injections in Patients With Rheumatoid Arthritis," *Arthritis Rheum*, 1990, 33(1):91-4.

Fossa SD, Heilo A, and Bormer O, "Unexpectedly High Serum Methotrexate Levels in Cystectomized Bladder Cancer Patients With an Ileal Conduit Treated With Intermediate Doses of the Drug," *J Urol*, 1990, 143(3):498-501.

Moore MJ and Erlichman C, "Therapeutic Drug Monitoring in Oncology," *Clin Pharmacokinet*, 1987, 13:205-27.

Olsen EA, "The Pharmacology of Methotrexate," *J Am Acad Dermatol*, 1991, 25(2 Pt 1):306-18.

Wallace CA, Bleyer WA, Sherry DD, et al, "Toxicity and Serum Levels of Methotrexate in Children With Juvenile Rheumatoid Arthritis," *Arthritis Rheum*, 1989, 32(6):677-81.

Wernick R and Smith DL, "Central Nervous System Toxicity Associated With Weekly Low-Dose Methotrexate Treatment," *Arthritis Rheum*, 1989, 32(6):770-5.

Methotrexate, CSF *see* Methotrexate *on previous page*

Methylenedioxymethamphetamine *see* Methamphetamines, Qualitative, Urine *on page 984*

Methylphenobarbital

CPT *80299*

Related Information

Phenobarbital, Blood *on page 992*

Synonyms Enphenemalum; Mebaral®; Mephobarbital; Mephobarbitone

Abstract Mephobarbital is metabolized to phenobarbital, which accounts for most pharmacologic effects, but has slightly different pharmacokinetics than phenobarbital.

Specimen Serum SAMPLING TIME: Consistent sampling time

Interpretive REFERENCE RANGE: In humans, most drug is converted to phenobarbital, and many methods of determination have difficulty distinguishing between the drug and metabolite. Determination of total phenobarbital then gives an approximation of antiepileptic drug (AED) level of the parent compound. Very little data exists on reference values for methylphenobarbital. CRITICAL VALUES: See Phenobarbital, Blood. METHODOLOGY: Gas-liquid chromatography (GLC), gas chromatography/mass spectrometry (GC/MS) ADDITIONAL INFORMATION: Methylphenobarbital has a more linear response between dosage and blood phenobarbital level than does phenobarbital. The limitations and adverse effects of the two drugs are likely to be very similar.

Methyl Salicylate *see* Salicylate *on page 999*

Mexate® *see* Methotrexate *on previous page*

Mexiletine

CPT *80299*

Synonyms Mexitil®

Abstract Mexiletine is an antiarrhythmic used to treat ventricular arrhythmia.

Specimen Serum CONTAINER: Red top tube SAMPLING TIME: Draw 2-4 hours after last dose for peak level. Draw immediately prior to next dose for trough levels.

Interpretive REFERENCE RANGE: Therapeutic 0.75-2.00 μg/mL (SI: 4-9 μmol/L) POSSIBLE PANIC RANGE: >2.00 μg/mL (SI: >9 μmol/L) USE: Therapeutic monitoring and toxicity assessment METHODOLOGY: Fluorometry, high performance liquid chromatography (HPLC), gas chromatography (GC) ADDITIONAL INFORMATION: Mexiletine is a class I antiarrhythmic approved for treatment of ventricular arrhythmias. It has no active metabolites. Toxic effects include dizziness, vomiting, confusion, tremor, bradycardia, and hypotension. Metabolism of mexiletine is accelerated by rifampin, phenobarbital, and phenytoin and retarded by cimetidine and ketoconazole. Half-life is 8-17 hours and is urine pH dependent. Acidic urine accelerates elimination.

References

Gottlieb SS and Weinberg M, "Comparative Hemodynamic Effects of Mexiletine and Quinidine in Patients With Severe Left Ventricular Dysfunction," *Am Heart J*, 1991, 122(5):1368-74.

Grech-Belanger O, Barbeau G, Kishka P, et al, "Pharmacokinetics of Mexiletine in the Elderly," *J Clin Pharmacol*, 1989, 29(4):311-5.

Manolis AS, Deering TF, Cameron J, et al, "Mexiletine: Pharmacology and Therapeutic Use," *Clin Cardiol*, 1990, 13(5):349-59.

Skluth H, Grauer K, and Gums J, "Ventricular Arrhythmias. An Assessment of Newer Therapeutic Agents," *Postgrad Med*, 1989, 85(6):137-8, 141-8, 153.

Mexitil® *see* Mexiletine *on previous page*

Miltown® *see* Meprobamate *on page 982*

Monoethylglycinexylidide

CPT *80299*

Related Information

Lidocaine *on page 978*

Synonyms MEGX

Applies to Lidocaine Metabolite

Test Commonly Includes This is the major active metabolite of lidocaine and is monitored along with lidocaine as an antiarrhythmic agent.

Abstract Monitored along with lidocaine as an antiarrhythmic agent. May also be used to assess donor organ liver function.

Specimen Serum CONTAINER: Red top tube SAMPLING TIME: 15 minutes after subtherapeutic, intravenous dose of 1 mg/kg lidocaine

Interpretive REFERENCE RANGE: >50 μg/L (SI: >170 nmol/L) USE: Used as a liver function test in assessing donor organ function and as a potential function test in the post transplant period METHODOLOGY: High performance liquid chromatography (HPLC), gas chromatography (GC), fluorescence polarization immunoassay (FPIA) ADDITIONAL INFORMATION: MEGX is the major metabolite of lidocaine and is used to assess donor and recipient liver function in transplantation of this organ in adults and children. Plasma half-life is 2 hours.

References

Estes NA 3d, Manolis AS, Greenblatt DJ, et al, "Therapeutic Serum Lidocaine and Metabolite Concentrations in Patients Undergoing Electrophysiologic Study After Discontinuation of Intravenous Lidocaine Infusion," *Am Heart J*, 1989, 117(5):1060-4.

Oellerich M, Rande E, Burdelski M, et al, "Monoethylglycinexylidide Formation Kinetics: A Novel Approach to Assessment of Liver Function," *J Clin Chem Clin Biochem*, 1987, 25:845-53.

Schroeder TJ, "A Novel Approach to the Diagnosis of Acute Rejection in Pediatric Liver Allograft Recipients," *J Hepatol*, 1989, 10:616-24.

Schroeder TJ, Tasset JJ, and Pesce AJ, "Lidocaine Metabolism," *Clin Chem News*, 1989, 15:5.

Morphine, Urine

CPT *83925*

Related Information

Chain-of-Custody Protocol *on page 952*

Drugs of Abuse Testing, Urine *on page 962*

Opiates, Qualitative, Urine *on page 989*

Oral Cavity Cytology *on page 507*

Synonyms Heroin Metabolite, Urine

Test Commonly Includes Codeine, Demerol®, heroin, hydromorphone (Dilaudid®), morphine, and morphine glucuronide

Abstract This drug is widely used therapeutically as an analgesic. Morphine itself is not an extensively used drug of abuse but two derivatives, heroin and codeine, are.

(Continued)

Morphine, Urine *(Continued)*

Specimen Urine **CONTAINER:** Plastic urine container **STORAGE INSTRUCTIONS:** Refrigerate sample **SPECIAL INSTRUCTIONS:** If forensic, use chain-of-custody protocol and form. See test entry Chain-of-Custody Protocol and the Appendix of this chapter.

Interpretive **REFERENCE RANGE:** Negative (less than cutoff) **CRITICAL VALUES:** Cutoff: screen (total opiates): 300 ng/mL; confirmatory: 300 ng/mL **USE:** Evaluate toxicity or detect drug of abuse. Heroin is metabolized to morphine, therefore morphine detection may suggest heroin use. To **prove** heroin use, 6-O-acetyl morphine must be identified in the urine. **METHODOLOGY:** Gas-liquid chromatography (GLC) **ADDITIONAL INFORMATION:** Morphine, the major phenanthrene alkaloid of powdered opium, is used for relief of moderate to severe acute and chronic pain after non-narcotic analgesics have failed. It is also used as preanesthetic medication, to relieve the pain of myocardial infarction and to relieve the dyspnea of acute left ventricular failure and pulmonary edema. Peak analgesia is achieved 50-90 minutes after subcutaneous administration and 20 minutes after I.V. injection. The half-life is 2.5-3 hours. Ninety percent of morphine is found in the urine after 24 hours, either free, or the majority in the glucuronide conjugated form. Adverse effects include CNS depression, nausea and vomiting, hypotension, bradycardia, histamine release, increased intracranial pressure, miosis, antidiuretic hormone release, and physical and psychological dependence. Naloxone is a specific antidote.

References

Baselt RC and Cravey RH, *Disposition of Toxic Drugs and Chemicals in Man*, 3rd ed, Chicago, IL: Year Book Medical Publishers Inc, 1989, 575-9.

McQuay HJ, Carroll D, Faura CC, et al, "Oral Morphine in Cancer Pain: Influences on Morphine and Metabolite Concentration," *Clin Pharmacol Ther*, 1990, 48(3):236-44.

Osborne R, Joel S, Trew D, et al, "Morphine and Metabolite Behavior After Different Routes of Morphine Administration: Demonstration of the Importance of the Active Metabolite Morphine-6-Glucuronide," *Clin Pharmacol Ther*, 1990, 47(1):12-9.

Portenoy RK, Khan E, Layman M, et al, "Chronic Morphine Therapy for Cancer Pain: Plasma and Cerebrospinal Fluid Morphine and Morphine-6-Glucuronide Concentrations," *Neurology*, 1991, 41(9):1457-61.

Portenoy RK, Thaler HT, Inturrisi CE, et al, "The Metabolite Morphine-6-Glucuronide Contributes to the Analgesia Produced by Morphine Infusion in Patients With Pain and Normal Renal Function," *Clin Pharmacol Ther*, 1992, 51(4):422-31.

Sear JW, Hand CW, Moore RA, et al, "Studies on Morphine Disposition: Influence of Renal Failure on the Kinetics of Morphine and its Metabolites," *Br J Anaesth*, 1989, 62(1):28-32.

"Toxicity and Pharmacokinetics of Morphine and Morphine-6-Glucuronide," *Br J Anaesth*, 1991, 67(3):362-3.

Zakowski MI, Ramanathan S, Sharnick S, et al, "Uptake and Distribution of Bupivacaine and Morphine After Intrathecal Administration in Parturients: Effects of Epinephrine," *Anesth Analg*, 1992, 74(5):664-9.

MTX, Blood *see* Methotrexate *on page 985*

Mychel-S® *see* Chloramphenicol *on page 952*

Mylepsin® *see* Primidone *on page 996*

Myochrysine® *see* Gold *on page 971*

Mysoline® *see* Primidone *on page 996*

N-Acetyl Procainamide *see* Procainamide *on page 996*

NAPA *see* Procainamide *on page 996*

Narcotics *see* Opiates, Qualitative, Urine *on next page*

Narcotics Drug Screen, Urine *see* Toxicology Drug Screen, Urine *on page 1006*

Nebcin® *see* Tobramycin *on page 1004*

Nembutal® *see* Barbiturates, Quantitative, Blood *on page 946*

Neurontin *see* GABA Pentin *on page 969*

Nipride® *see* Thiocyanate, Blood or Urine *on page 1003*

Nirvanol® *see* Mephenytoin *on page 981*

Nitroprusside *see* Thiocyanate, Blood or Urine *on page 1003*

Nizoral *see* Ketoconazole *on page 975*

11-Nor-9-Carboxy-Delta-9-Tetrahydrocannabinol *see* Cannabinoids, Qualitative, Urine *on page 949*

Norpace® *see* Disopyramide *on page 961*

Norpramin® *see* Imipramine *on page 974*

Norpramin® *see* Tricyclic Antidepressants *on page 1007*

Norpropoxyphene *see* Propoxyphene, Blood or Urine *on page 997*

Nortriptyline

CPT *80182*

Related Information

Amitriptyline, Blood *on page 939*
Tricyclic Antidepressants *on page 1007*

Synonyms Aventyl®; Pamelor®

Abstract This is a tricyclic antidepressant.

Specimen Serum **CONTAINER:** Red top tube **COLLECTION:** Collect specimen immediately prior to next dose unless specified otherwise. **STORAGE INSTRUCTIONS:** Separate serum and refrigerate.

Interpretive **REFERENCE RANGE:** Therapeutic: 50-150 ng/mL **CRITICAL VALUES:** Toxic: >1000 ng/mL **USE:** Monitor therapeutic drug level; evaluate toxicity **LIMITATIONS:** Results not valid if patient receiving imipramine or desipramine **METHODOLOGY:** High performance liquid chromatography (HPLC) **ADDITIONAL INFORMATION:** Nortriptyline, a tricyclic antidepressant, is a derivative and metabolite of amitriptyline and is used to treat endogenous depression. The half-life of nortriptyline is 20-80 hours. Nortriptyline may be associated with cholestasis and cholestatic jaundice. Hematological consequences include agranulocytosis, purpura, and thrombocytopenia. Other side effects include a host of GI, endocrinologic, allergic, anticholinergic, cardiovascular, and neurologic disorders.

References

Baselt RC and Cravey RH, *Disposition of Toxic Drugs and Chemicals in Man*, 3rd ed, Chicago, IL: Year Book Medical Publishers Inc, 1989, 613-5.

Brasfield KH, "Practical Psychopharmacologic Considerations in Depression," *Nurs Clin North Am*, 1991, 26(3):651-63.

Shapiro PA, "Nortriptyline Treatment of Depressed Cardiac Transplant Recipients," *Am J Psychiatry*, 1991, 148(3):371-3.

Norverapamil *see* Verapamil *on page 1010*

Oil of Wintergreen *see* Salicylate *on page 999*

Opiates, Qualitative, Urine

CPT *80101 (screen); 80102 (confirmation)*

Related Information

Chain-of-Custody Protocol *on page 952*
Codeine, Urine *on page 955*
Drugs of Abuse Testing, Urine *on page 962*
Morphine, Urine *on page 987*

Applies to Heroin; Narcotics; Poppy Seeds

Test Commonly Includes Morphine, codeine, hydrocodone (Hycodan®), hydromorphone (Dilaudid®)

Abstract The qualitative detection of urine opiates is used almost exclusively to show presence of drugs of abuse in this class. Morphine and codeine are used therapeutically for pain.

Specimen Random urine **CONTAINER:** Plastic urine container **COLLECTION:** If forensic, observe precautions (see Introduction). **STORAGE INSTRUCTIONS:** Refrigerate **SPECIAL INSTRUCTIONS:** If forensic, use chain-of-custody protocol and form. See test entry Chain-of-Custody Protocol and the Appendix of this chapter.

Interpretive **REFERENCE RANGE:** Negative (less than cutoff) **CRITICAL VALUES:** Cutoff: screen: 300 ng/mL; confirmation: 300 ng/mL of specific opiates **USE:** Evaluate drug abuse; assess toxicity **LIMITATIONS:** In most immunoassays a number of narcotic drugs can cross react to give a positive screen. Every effort should be made to confirm, by an analytically different and more sensitive method, all presumptive, positive opiate screens. See Test Commonly Includes above. **METHODOLOGY:** Screening: immunoassay, thin-layer chromatography (TLC), high performance liquid chromatography (HPLC), gas chromatography (GC); confirmation: gas chromatography/mass spectrometry (GC/MS) **ADDITIONAL INFORMATION:** A qualitative urine screen for opiates is performed in suspected overdose cases or as part of a drugs-of-abuse program. The test is most sensitive for morphine and codeine, but other drugs will

(Continued)

Opiates, Qualitative, Urine *(Continued)*

cross react in an immunoassay and give positive results (eg, hydrocodone, hydromorphone). All presumptive positive assays should be confirmed, preferably by GC/MS. Morphine is a prescribed drug for pain relief, a metabolite of heroin, a metabolite of codeine, and a constituent of poppy seeds. Its presence in urine, even after confirmation, must be interpreted very carefully. Ingestion of poppy seeds (bagels, Danish) can cause positive opiate screens at a 300 ng/mL cutoff.[1] The intake of heroin by the user can only be proved by the detection of 6-O-acetyl morphine by the urine confirmatory test.

Opiates in general are a group of drugs (commonly referred to as narcotics) which are used medically to relieve pain, but which also have a high potential for abuse. Some opiates come from a resin taken from the seed pod of the Asian poppy. This group of drugs includes opium, morphine, and codeine. Other opiates are synthesized or manufactured (eg, heroin). Opium appears as dark brown chunks or as a powder, and is usually smoked or eaten. Heroin can be a white or brownish powder which is usually dissolved in water and injected.

Opiates tend to relax the user. When the opiates are injected, the user feels an immediate "rush." Other initial and unpleasant effects include restlessness, nausea, and vomiting. The user may go "on the nod," going back and forth from feeling alert to drowsy. With very large doses, the user cannot be awakened, pupils become smaller, and the skin becomes cold, moist, and bluish in color. Furthermore, breathing slows down and death may occur. Clearance may be slower in geriatric patients.

Footnotes

1. Selavka CM, "Poppy Seed Ingestion as a Contributing Factor to Opiate-Positive Urinalysis Results: The Pacific Perspective," *J Forensic Sci*, 1991, 36(3):685-96.

References

Barsan W, "Narcotic Agents," *Ann Emerg Med*, 1986, 15:1019-20.

Gillogley KM, Evans AT, Hansen RL, et al, "The Perinatal Impact of Cocaine, Amphetamine, and Opiate Use Detected by Universal Intrapartum Screening," *Am J Obstet Gynecol*, 1990, 163(5 Pt 1):1535-42.

Kulburg A, "Substance Abuse: Clinical Identification and Management," *Pediatr Clin North Am*, 1986, 33:325-61.

Montamat SC, Cusack BJ, and Vestal RE, "Management of Drug Therapy in the Elderly," *N Engl J Med*, 1989, 321(5):303-9.

Pettitt BC, Dyszel SM, and Hood LVS, "Opiates in Poppy Seed," *Clin Chem*, 1987, 33:1251-2.

Opiates, Urine *see* Codeine, Urine *on page 955*

Oxazepam, Serum

***CPT** 80154*

Related Information

Benzodiazepines, Qualitative, Urine *on page 947*

Synonyms Serax®

Abstract Oxazepam is a benzodiazepine used as an antianxiety agent. It is an active metabolite of several other benzodiazepines that are used therapeutically.

Specimen Serum **CONTAINER:** Red top tube **SAMPLING TIME:** Collect specimen immediately prior to next dose unless specified otherwise. **STORAGE INSTRUCTIONS:** Separate serum and refrigerate.

Interpretive **REFERENCE RANGE:** 0.5-2.5 μg/mL **USE:** Monitor therapeutic drug level; evaluate toxicity **METHODOLOGY:** Gas-liquid chromatography (GLC) **ADDITIONAL INFORMATION:** Oxazepam, a benzodiazepine derivative, is related to chlordiazepoxide and shares many of its qualities. It does, however, have a shorter duration of action and causes fewer adverse effects. It is rapidly eliminated by urinary excretion as a glucuronide conjugate. Oxazepam is used to manage tension and anxiety and to aid in the control of acute withdrawal symptoms in chronic alcoholism. Peak plasma levels are achieved in 2-4 hours and the half-life is 4-12 hours. Adverse effects are mild and infrequent. They include drowsiness, vertigo, ataxia, headache, tremor, slurred speech, nausea, hypotension, and leukopenia. Simultaneous alcohol ingestion potentiates some of the effects of benzodiazepines.

References

Baselt RC and Cravey RH, *Disposition of Toxic Drugs and Chemicals in Man*, Chicago, IL: Year Book Medical Publishers Inc, 1989, 622-3.

Craig CR and Stitzel RE, *Modern Pharmacology*, 3rd ed, Boston, MA: Little, Brown and Co, 1990, 440-6.

Oxazolidinediones

CPT 80299

Synonyms Paradione®; Tridione®; Trimedone

Test Commonly Includes Trimethadione and paramethadione

Abstract Trimethadione and paramethadione can be considered for absence seizures in patients unable to take other medications. However, oxazolidinediones are less effective and have clear teratogenic effects.

Specimen Serum **CONTAINER:** Red top tube

Interpretive **REFERENCE RANGE:** Therapeutic monitoring of trimethadione is achieved by measurement of its active metabolite, dimethadione. Reference range: 50-1200 μg/mL. Reference ranges for paramethadione and its metabolites have not been determined. There are no relevant drug interactions reported. Low levels of dimethadione may occur in the first 2 weeks of administration as the metabolite reaches plateau levels. **POSSIBLE PANIC RANGE:** Dose dependent, reversible adverse effects include hemeralopia (night blindness), photophobia, sedation, fatigue, dizziness, and ataxia **USE:** Monitor for compliance, efficacy, and possible toxicity **METHODOLOGY:** High performance liquid chromatography (HPLC), gas-liquid chromatography (GLC), infrared spectrophotometry **ADDITIONAL INFORMATION:** Dimethadione has a half-life of 6-13 days. Close monitoring during administration is indicated.

P-450 System Inhibitor *see* Carbamazepine *on page 950*

Pamelor® *see* Amitriptyline, Blood *on page 939*

Pamelor® *see* Nortriptyline *on page 989*

Pamelor® *see* Tricyclic Antidepressants *on page 1007*

Panadol® *see* Acetaminophen, Serum *on page 935*

Panex® *see* Acetaminophen, Serum *on page 935*

Panwarfin® *see* Warfarin *on page 1011*

Paracetamol *see* Acetaminophen, Serum *on page 935*

Paradione® *see* Oxazolidinediones *on this page*

Pb, Blood *see* Lead, Blood *on page 976*

Pb, Urine *see* Lead, Urine *on page 977*

PCP *see* Phencyclidine, Qualitative, Urine *on next page*

Peace Pills *see* Phencyclidine, Qualitative, Urine *on next page*

Peganone® *see* Ethotoin *on page 965*

PEMA *see* Primidone *on page 996*

Pentobarb *see* Barbiturates, Qualitative, Urine *on page 945*

Pentobarbital *see* Barbiturates, Quantitative, Blood *on page 946*

Permitil® *see* Fluphenazine *on page 968*

Pertofrane® *see* Imipramine *on page 974*

Pertofrane® *see* Tricyclic Antidepressants *on page 1007*

Phenacemide

CPT 80299

Synonyms Phenurone®

Abstract Phenacemide is used as an antiepileptic drug of last resort for patients with uncontrollable seizures.

Specimen Serum **CONTAINER:** Red top tube

Interpretive **REFERENCE RANGE:** 16-75 μg/mL[1] **POSSIBLE PANIC RANGE:** Signs of hepatic, renal, or psychiatric problems regardless of level **METHODOLOGY:** High performance liquid chromatography (HPLC) **ADDITIONAL INFORMATION:** The half-life is 40 hours with chronic administration. Fatal bone marrow depression, hepatotoxicity, and renal toxicity are reported. Depression and psychotic reactions, including a risk of suicide, are reported with phenacemide. Close medical supervision with administration is required.

Footnotes

1. Coker SB, Holmes EW, and Egel RT, "Phenacemide Therapy of Complex Partial Epilepsy in Children: Determination of Plasma Drug Concentrations," *Neurology*, 1987, 37:1861-6.

(Continued)

Phenacemide *(Continued)*

References

Engel J, *Seizures and Epilepsy*, Contemporary Neurology Series, Philadelphia, PA: FA Davis Co, 1989.

Phenaphen® *see* Acetaminophen, Serum *on page 935*

Phencyclidine, Qualitative, Urine

CPT *80101 (screen); 80102 (confirmation, each procedure); 83992 (quantitative)*

Related Information

Chain-of-Custody Protocol *on page 952*
Drugs of Abuse Testing, Urine *on page 962*

Synonyms Angel Dust; Elephant Tranquilizers; Hog; Killer Weed; PCP; Peace Pills; Rocket Fuel

Abstract This is a widely used drug of abuse which was formerly sold as a veterinary tranquilizer. All legal manufacture and sale has been stopped. It is classified by DEA as a Schedule II controlled substance.

Specimen Random urine **CONTAINER:** Plastic urine container **COLLECTION:** If forensic, observe precautions (see Introduction). **SPECIAL INSTRUCTIONS:** If forensic, use chain-of-custody protocol and form. See test entry Chain-of-Custody Protocol and the Appendix of this chapter.

Interpretive **REFERENCE RANGE:** Negative (less than cutoff) **CRITICAL VALUES:** Cutoff: screen: 25 ng/mL; confirmation: 25 ng/mL **USE:** Evaluate presence of phencyclidine, drug abuse, PCP toxicity; determine phencyclidine involvement in unexplained psychoses **METHODOLOGY:** Immunoassay, thin-layer chromatography (TLC), gas chromatography (GC), gas chromatography/mass spectrometry (GC/MS). Immunoassays are very specific and detect PCP at 25 ng/mL (SI: 100 nmol/L) **ADDITIONAL INFORMATION:** Phencyclidine is most often called "angel dust." It was first developed as an anesthetic in the 1950s. It was taken off the market for human use because it sometimes caused hallucinations. PCP is available in a number of forms. It can be a pure white crystal-like powder, a tablet or capsule, and it can be swallowed, smoked (alone or with marijuana), sniffed, or injected. Although PCP is illegal, it is easily manufactured.

Effects depend on how much of the drug is taken, the way it is used, and the individual. Small amounts act as a stimulant, speeding up body functions. For many users, PCP changes how they see their own bodies and things around them. Speech, muscle coordination, and vision are affected; sense of touch and pain are dulled; and body movements are slowed. Time seems to "space out." Effects include increased heart rate and blood pressure, flushing, sweating, dizziness, and numbness. When large doses are taken, effects include drowsiness, convulsions, and coma. Taking large amounts of PCP can also cause death from repeated convulsions, heart and lung failure, or ruptured blood vessels in the brain. PCP can be detected for 7 days after administration; 2-4 weeks in chronic users. Half-life is 7-46 hours.

References

Ellenhorn MJ and Barceloux DG, "Phencyclidine," *Medical Toxicology*, New York, NY: Elsevier, 1988, 763-78.

Milhorn HT Jr, "Diagnosis and Management of Phencyclidine Intoxication," *Am Fam Physician*, 1991, 43(4):1293-302.

Wessinger WD and Owens SM, "Phencyclidine Dependence: The Relationship of Dose and Serum Concentrations to Operant Behavioral Effects," *J Pharmacol Exp Ther*, 1991, 258(1):207-15.

Phenemal *see* Phenobarbital, Blood *on this page*

Phenemalum *see* Phenobarbital, Blood *on this page*

Phenobarb *see* Barbiturates, Qualitative, Urine *on page 945*

Phenobarb *see* Phenobarbital, Blood *on this page*

Phenobarbital *see* Barbiturates, Quantitative, Blood *on page 946*

Phenobarbital *see* Valproic Acid *on page 1008*

Phenobarbital, Blood

CPT *80184*

Related Information

Barbiturates, Quantitative, Blood *on page 946*
Methylphenobarbital *on page 986*

Primidone *on page 996*
Valproic Acid *on page 1008*

Synonyms Gardenal®; Luminal®; Phenemal; Phenemalum; Phenobarb; Phenobarbitone; Stental Extentabs®

Abstract Phenobarbital is indicated for generalized tonic-clonic and partial seizures.

Specimen Serum or plasma **CONTAINER:** Red top tube, green top (heparin) tube, or lavender top (EDTA) tube **SAMPLING TIME:** Consistent sampling time is desirable but less important than for other anticonvulsants due to its long half-life.

Interpretive **REFERENCE RANGE:** Infants and children: 15-30 μg/mL (SI: 65-129 μmol/L); adults: 20-40 μg/mL (SI: 86-172 μmol/L). See Table A in the Appendix of this chapter. Low level: Most common cause is noncompliance. Other causes include drug interactions, including antipsychotic medication, chloramphenicol, acetazolamide, and phenytoin. Some patients are fast metabolizers, such as infants and children. High level: addition of valproic acid to regimen inhibits phenobarbital metabolism (parahydroxylation) and should be accompanied by a cut in phenobarbital dosage. Newborns, unlike older infants, have very long half-lives which may be associated with high levels. **CRITICAL VALUES:** Toxic: >40 μg/mL (SI: >172 μmol/L) but if given intravenously, life-threatening side effects can occur with much lower levels, and patients should be monitored. Toxic effects are mostly neurologic. Adults present with lethargy and coma; children may present with irritability or hyperactivity. **USE:** Monitor patients for compliance, efficacy, and possible toxicity. Mephobarbital and primidone are metabolized to phenobarbital and, therefore, patients taking these drugs will have detectable levels of phenobarbital on therapeutic monitoring. **METHODOLOGY:** Enzyme immunoassay (EIA), gas-liquid chromatography (GLC), high performance liquid chromatography (HPLC) **ADDITIONAL INFORMATION:** Phenobarbital has a half-life of 84-108 hours. Phenobarbital can affect the metabolism of phenytoin, ethosuximide, and increase the clearance and elimination of chloramphenicol, theophylline, oral anticoagulants (warfarin), cyclosporine, and oral contraceptives; where appropriate, the use of these drugs in patients on phenobarbital should be monitored clinically and through the laboratory.

References

Bertino J and Reed M, "Barbiturate and Nonbarbiturate Sedative-Hypnotic Intoxication in Children," *Pediatr Clin North Am*, 1986, 33:703-22.

Kutt H, "Phenobarbital: Interactions With Other Drugs," *Antiepileptic Drugs*, 3rd ed, Levy RH, Dreifuss FE, Mattson RH, et al, eds, New York, NY: Raven Press, 1989, 313-27.

Phenobarbitone *see* Phenobarbital, Blood *on previous page*

Phenothiazines *see* Chlorpromazine, Urine *on page 953*

Phenothiazines, Serum

CPT *80101 (screen); 80102 (confirmation, each procedure); 84022 (quantitative)*

Related Information

Fluphenazine *on page 968*

Applies to Chlorpromazine; Compazine®; Etrafon®; Mellaril®; Mesoridazine; Prochlorperazine; Prolixin®; Serentil®; Stelazine®; Thioridazine; Thorazine®; Trifluoperazine

Abstract The drugs in this class are used as antipsychotic agents and tranquilizers.

Specimen Serum **CONTAINER:** Red top tube **SAMPLING TIME:** Obtain serum at least 3 hours after last dose.

Interpretive **REFERENCE RANGE:** Chlorpromazine; therapeutic: 30-50 ng/mL (SI: 100-160 nmol/L) **POSSIBLE PANIC RANGE:** Toxic: chlorpromazine >750 ng/mL (SI: >2350 nmol/L); thioridazine >500 ng/mL (SI: >1350 nmol/L); trifluoperazine >50 ng/mL (SI: >104 nmol/L) **USE:** Evaluate phenothiazine toxicity **LIMITATIONS:** Less than optimal assay accuracy and number of drug metabolites make clinical application infrequent. These drugs are not usually monitored because the correlation between serum level and antipsychotic effect is not good. **METHODOLOGY:** Thin-layer chromatography (TLC), gas-liquid chromatography (GLC), radioimmunoassay (RIA), high performance liquid chromatography (HPLC), spectrophotometry **ADDITIONAL INFORMATION:** Phenothiazines are tranquilizers frequently used in the treatment of psychoses. They may act by antagonizing postsynaptic dopamine receptors. There are three different classes of phenothiazines: aliphatic (chlorpromazine), piperidine (thioridazine), and piperazine (fluphenazine). All are effective in therapy in appropriate doses, but differ in frequency, type, and severity of side effects. Side effects include drowsiness, ataxia, respiratory depression, hypotension, tachycardia, cardiac arrest, bone marrow depression. There is also a "dysphoric" re-

(Continued)

Phenothiazines, Serum *(Continued)*

sponse by some patients. Half-life is usually in the range of 18-30 hours. The efficacy in therapy of psychosis of measuring phenothiazine blood levels is not firmly established. The piperazine prochlorperazine (Compazine®) is widely used as an antiemetic. Phenothiazines can also be measured in urine and gastric contents.

References

Knight M and Roberts R, "Phenothiazine and Butyrophenone Intoxication in Children," *Pediatr Clin North Am*, 1986, 33:299-305.

Krishel S and Jackimczyk K, "Cyclic Antidepressants, Lithium, and Neuroleptic Agents. Pharmacology and Toxicology," *Emerg Med Clin North Am*, 1991, 9(1):53-86.

Ryan PM, "Epidemiology, Etiology, Diagnosis, and Treatment of Schizophrenia," *Am J Hosp Pharm*, 1991, 48(6):1271-80.

Phentermine *see* Methamphetamines, Qualitative, Urine *on page 984*

Phenurone® *see* Phenacemide *on page 991*

Phenylethylmalonamide *see* Primidone *on page 996*

Phenylpropanolamine *see* Methamphetamines, Qualitative, Urine *on page 984*

Phenytoin

CPT 80185

Related Information

Mephenytoin *on page 981*
Phenytoin, Free *on next page*
Quinidine, Serum *on page 999*
Valproic Acid *on page 1008*

Synonyms Dilantin®; Diphenylhydantoin

Abstract Phenytoin is effective for generalized tonic-clonic and partial seizures.

Specimen Serum or plasma **CONTAINER:** Red top tube or lavender top (EDTA) tube **SAMPLING TIME:** In monitoring patients maintained on chronic therapy, a trough level or consistent sampling time should be used.

Interpretive **REFERENCE RANGE:** 10-20 μg/mL (SI: 40-79 μmol/L). Patients treated for status epilepticus should have levels at or slightly above the upper limit of range. Low level: The most common cause of a low level is noncompliance. Absorption problems are most important in young infants (younger than 3 months) or occasionally in patients given phenobarbital, charcoal, or antacids at the same time as the phenytoin. Pediatric and some adult patients (fast metabolizers), who have breakthrough seizures at the end of the day, require more than once daily dosing. Some formulations other than Kapseals® may require more than once daily dosing, and changing formulations can cause changes in levels. Pregnancy or intercurrent illness such as mononucleosis can cause subtherapeutic levels with seizures. The addition of carbamazepine to a patient taking phenytoin can lower or raise phenytoin level but usually does not cause seizures. Disulfiram administration can increase phenytoin metabolism, lower levels, and may cause seizures. Patients can have lower than expected values if intravenous formulations are given with fluids containing glucose, which precipitates in solution with phenytoin. High levels: In patients chronically controlled on phenytoin who become clinically toxic without a change in dose, toxicity can be brought on by a change in formulation, drug interaction, or intercurrent infection. Drugs which can precipitate phenytoin toxicity include chloramphenicol, tricyclic antidepressants, fluconazole, and levodopa. Small dose changes or changes in formulation (including change from one brand to another or to a generic) can cause large changes in antiepileptic drug (AED) levels and toxicity, because phenytoin manifests zero-order kinetics. **POSSIBLE PANIC RANGE:** Toxicity may manifest progressively outside reference range (or occasionally within it) with ataxia, dizziness, nystagmus, and diplopia. Patients can have life-threatening complications with intravenous administration with normal levels; such patients should be placed on a cardiac monitor during intravenous administration of drug. **USE:** Monitor for compliance, efficacy, and possible toxicity **LIMITATIONS:** See Phenytoin, Free **METHODOLOGY:** Routine: Enzyme multiplied immunoassay technique (EMIT), enzyme-linked immunosorbent assay (ELISA), and fluorescence polarization immunoassay (FPIA). For physician's office testing, apoenzyme reactive immunoassay (ARIS; Ames Seralyzer®) is rapid, accurate, and may become increasingly important. **ADDITIONAL INFORMATION:** Ninety percent of phenytoin is bound to serum proteins. Only the unbound fraction is biologically active. Primary site of action is thought to be the motor cortex, where the promotion of a sodium "efflux" from neurons probably stabilizes the threshold of the neuron against hyperexcitibility. Most of a dose of phenytoin is excreted into the bile as inactive metabolites which are then reabsorbed from the intestines and excreted into the urine. Despite normal levels, phenytoin may interfere with the actions of other drugs, including cyclosporine, oral anticoagulants, oral contraceptives, and theophylline; appropriate laboratory monitoring of some of these agents is advised. The half-life of phenytoin in adults is 20-40 hours; in children, it is around 10 hours. Teratogenic effects of phenytoin have been proposed but not confirmed; the risks in women of childbearing age should be balanced against the risks of increased seizures.[1]

Footnotes

1. Dalessio D, "Current Concepts: Seizure Disorders and Pregnancy," *N Engl J Med*, 1985, 312:559-63.

References

Engel J, *Seizures and Epilepsy*, Contemporary Neurology Series, Philadelphia, PA: FA Davis Co, 1989.

Phenytoin, Free

CPT *80186*

Related Information

Phenytoin *on previous page*

Synonyms Free Phenytoin

Abstract Measurement of free phenytoin may be clinically important in situations associated with altered binding of phenytoin.

Specimen Serum or plasma **CONTAINER:** Red top tube or lavender top (EDTA) tube

Interpretive **REFERENCE RANGE:** 1-2 μg/mL (SI: 4-8 μmol/L) **POSSIBLE PANIC RANGE:** Toxicity may be progressive >2 μg/mL. **ADDITIONAL INFORMATION:** Phenytoin is 90% bound to serum proteins, but only the free fraction circulates through plasma membranes and is biologically active. Because of rapid equilibration between free and bound portions of drugs, free levels are potentially important only in antiepileptic drugs (AEDs) that are highly bound (ie, phenytoin but not carbamazepine). Measurement of the free fraction is not cost-effective on a routine outpatient basis, but may be clinically relevant in exceptional circumstances associated with alterations in the binding of phenytoin.[1] Binding kinetics may be altered in uremia, hepatic disease, late pregnancy or postpartum, cases of head injury associated with a hypermetabolic state, and certain instances of polypharmacy, described below.[2,3,4] Determination of free levels may also be helpful in overdosages, since only the free portion can be cleared by dialysis.

Most phenytoin is excreted into bile as inactive metabolites which are then reabsorbed by the intestines and excreted into the urine. In renal disease, total phenytoin levels may generate falsely high values, leading to inadequate dosage. Dialysis may increase the amount of free phenytoin available.[5] In hepatic disease, phenytoin competes with endogenous bilirubin for binding sites,[6] and thus the need for a free level may be greatest if the total bilirubin level is high and albumin low. Available liver function tests are not predictive of free phenytoin levels in patients with liver disease.[4]

Drugs which compete for binding sites on albumin and which may displace phenytoin include valproic acid, acetazolamide, high doses of salicylic acid, phenylbutazone, ceftriaxone, nafcillin, and sulfamethoxazole.[7] In a clinical setting in which one of these drugs is used with phenytoin and toxicity is suspected despite normal phenytoin levels, a free level may be useful.

The free phenytoin level can be approximated by the total phenytoin level in cerebrospinal fluid or saliva or other body fluids that are albumin-poor.

Footnotes

1. Theodore W, Yu L, Price B, et al, "The Clinical Value of Free Phenytoin Levels," *Ann Neurol*, 1985, 18:90-3.
2. Levy RH, Dreifuss FE, Mattson RH, et al, *Antiepileptic Drugs*, 3rd ed, New York, NY: Raven Press, 1989.
3. Griebel ML, Kearns GL, Fiser DH, et al, "Phenytoin Protein Binding in Pediatric Patients With Acute Traumatic Injury," *Crit Care Med*, 1990, 18(4):385-91.
4. Dasgupta A, Dennen DA, Dean R, et al, "Prediction of Free Phenytoin Levels Based on Total Phenytoin/Albumin Ratios," *Am J Clin Pathol*, 1991, 95(2):253-6.
5. Dasgupta A and Abu-Alfa A, "Increased Free Phenytoin Concentrations in Predialysis Serum Compared to Postdialysis Serum in Patients With Uremia Treated With Hemodialysis: Role of Uremic Compounds," *Am J Clin Pathol*, 1992, 98(1):19-25.
6. Hooper W, Sutherland J, Bochner F, et al, "Plasma Protein Binding of Diphenylhydantoin. Effects of Sex Hormones, Renal and Hepatic Disease," *Clin Pharmacol Ther*, 1973, 15:276-82.
7. Dasgupta A, Dennen DA, Dean R, et al, "Displacement of Phenytoin From Serum Protein Carriers by Antibiotics: Studies With Ceftriaxone, Nafcillin, and Sulfamethoxazole," *Clin Chem*, 1991, 37(1):98-100.

Placidyl® *see* Ethchlorvynol *on page 964*

Poisonous Metals, Blood *see* Heavy Metal Screen, Blood *on page 972*

Poisonous Metals, Urine *see* Heavy Metal Screen, Urine *on page 973*

Poppy Seeds *see* Opiates, Qualitative, Urine *on page 989*

Pot *see* Cannabinoids, Qualitative, Urine *on page 949*

Potassium or Sodium Cyanide *see* Cyanide, Blood *on page 956*

Potassium Thiocyanate (KCN) *see* Thiocyanate, Blood or Urine *on page 1003*

Pre-employment Drug Screen *see* Drugs of Abuse Testing, Urine *on page 962*

Presamine® *see* Imipramine *on page 974*

Presamine® *see* Tricyclic Antidepressants *on page 1007*

Primidone

CPT 80188

Related Information

Phenobarbital, Blood *on page 992*

Valproic Acid *on page 1008*

Synonyms Majsolin®; Mylepsin®; Mysoline®; Prysolin®

Applies to Metabolites of Primidone; PEMA; Phenylethylmalonamide

Test Commonly Includes Phenobarbital, PEMA

Abstract Primidone is indicated for generalized tonic-clonic and partial seizures.

Specimen Serum or plasma **CONTAINER:** Red top tube, green top (heparin) tube, or lavender top (EDTA) tube **SAMPLING TIME:** Trough or consistent sampling time. Levels of phenobarbital and PEMA can be measured simultaneously.

Interpretive **REFERENCE RANGE:** Children younger than 5 years of age: 7-10 μg/mL (SI: 32-46 μmol/L); adults: 5-12 μg/mL. Phenobarbital concentration can also be used to guide dosing. **CRITICAL VALUES:** At levels >12 μg/mL (SI: >55 μmol/L) primidone produces CNS depression, vertigo, visual disturbances, areflexia, somnolence, and lethargy. Clinical toxicity correlates with primidone rather than metabolite concentrations. In overdosage, a biphasic peak may be seen with highest toxicity a few hours after ingestion and again 48 hours afterwards. Crystalluria is a feature of overdosage. **POSSIBLE PANIC RANGE:** >12 μg/mL (SI: >55 μmol/L). See Table A in the Appendix of this chapter. **USE:** Monitor efficacy, compliance, and possible toxicity **METHODOLOGY:** Enzyme immunoassay (EIA), gas-liquid chromatography (GLC), high performance liquid chromatography (HPLC) **ADDITIONAL INFORMATION:** Plasma half-life of primidone usually ranges from 6-8 hours with rapid elimination (24-40 hours). Since phenobarbital requires a longer interval (48 hours) to achieve therapeutic blood levels, checking both levels can be used to determine chronic compliance. The phenobarbital/primidone ratio normally is 2.5, can be higher (4.3 mean) in patients on other anticonvulsants (phenytoin, carbamazepine) and lower than normal among patients discontinued from those medicines or who are chronically noncompliant. Primidone decreases the effects of oral anticoagulants.

References

Kutt H, "Phenobarbital: Interactions With Other Drugs," *Antiepileptic Drugs*, 3rd ed, Levy RH, Dreifuss FE, Mattson RH, et al, eds, New York, NY: Raven Press, 1989, 313-27.

Schafer H, "Primidone: Chemistry and Methods of Determination," *Antiepileptic Drugs*, 3rd ed, Levy RH, Dreifuss FE, Mattson RH, et al, eds, New York, NY: Raven Press, 1989, 379-90.

Procainamide

CPT 80190

Related Information

Quinidine, Serum *on page 999*

Synonyms Pronestyl®

Applies to N-Acetyl Procainamide; NAPA

Test Commonly Includes Procainamide and its metabolite, N-acetyl procainamide (NAPA)

Abstract This drug is an antiarrhythmic with an active metabolite, N-acetyl procainamide. Both should be measured when TDM is used.

Specimen Serum **CONTAINER:** Red top tube **SAMPLING TIME:** Oral treatment: peak: 75 minutes after dose; trough: immediately before next dose. I.V. treatment: immediately after loading dose; 2, 6, 12, and 24 hours after starting I.V. maintenance. **SPECIAL INSTRUCTIONS:** One sample is an inadequate basis for evaluating dosing. Three steady-state levels should be obtained during one dosing interval. For therapeutic drug monitoring, consistently use the same time interval between sampling and dose administration when comparing results from serial samples.

Interpretive REFERENCE RANGE: Therapeutic: procainamide: 4.0-10.0 μg/mL (SI: 17-42 μmol/L); sum of procainamide and N-acetyl procainamide: <30 μg/mL (SI: <127 μmol/L). Optimal ranges must be ascertained for individual patients with ECG monitoring. POSSIBLE PANIC RANGE: Toxic: procainamide: >20 μg/mL[1] (SI: >84.7 μmol/L); sum of procainamide and N-acetyl procainamide: >30 μg/mL (SI: >127 μmol/L). See Table C in the Appendix of this chapter. USE: Monitor therapeutic drug level LIMITATIONS: Severely hemolyzed, lipemic, or icteric specimens interfere with methods other than HPLC and GC.[1] **Evaluation of toxicity must be made with consideration of patient's clinical status**. METHODOLOGY: Enzyme immunoassay (EIA), fluorescence polarization immunoassay (FPIA), enzyme-multiplied immunoassay (EMIT); high performance liquid chromatography (HPLC), gas chromatography (GC) ADDITIONAL INFORMATION: The cardiac actions of this drug are similar to those of quinidine. It is used in a variety of arrhythmias. Procainamide usually is rapidly absorbed from the gastrointestinal tract. Peak blood levels are reached within 1 hour. Optimal plasma sampling time after oral dosage is 1-2 hours. Optimal sampling time after I.V. administration of dose is 30 minutes. The drug is converted by the liver to its active metabolite, N-acetyl procainamide (NAPA). The half-life of procainamide is 2-6 hours and for NAPA is 8 hours. Rate of metabolism is genetically determined (slow and fast acetylator types) contributing to significant interindividual variability. Impairment of renal function has pronounced effect on drug disposition, especially for NAPA. Patients with severe renal dysfunction generally have prolonged and highly variable half-life characteristics. Elimination half-life may be prolonged in geriatric subjects.[2]

Footnotes

1. Sherwin JE, "Procainamide and N-Acetylprocainamide," *Clinical Chemistry Theory, Analysis, and Correlation*, 2nd ed, Kaplan LA and Pesce AJ, eds, St Louis, MO: Mosby-Year Book Inc, 1989, 1110-3.
2. Montamat SC, Cusack BJ, and Vestal RE "Management of Drug Therapy in the Elderly," *N Engl J Med*, 1989, 321(5):303-9.

References

Funck-Brentano C, Light RT, Lineberry MD, et al, "Pharmacokinetic and Pharmacodynamic Interaction of N-Acetyl Procainamide and Procainamide in Humans," *J Cardiovasc Pharmacol*, 1989, 14(3):364-73.

Gottlieb SS, Kukin ML, Medina N, et al, "Comparative Hemodynamic Effects of Procainamide, Tocainide, and Encainide in Severe Chronic Heart Failure," *Circulation*, 1990, 81(3):860-4.

Interian A Jr, Zaman L, Velez-Robinson E, et al, "Paired Comparisons of Efficacy of Intravenous and Oral Procainamide in Patients With Inducible Sustained Ventricular Tachyarrhythmias," *J Am Coll Cardiol*, 1991, 17(7):1581-6.

Yamaji A, Kataoka K, Oishi M, et al, "Simultaneous Determination of Procainamide and N-Acetylprocainamide in Serum by Gas Chromatography," *J Chromatogr*, 1987, 415:143-7.

Prochlorperazine *see* Phenothiazines, Serum *on page 993*

Prolixin® *see* Fluphenazine *on page 968*

Prolixin® *see* Phenothiazines, Serum *on page 993*

Pronestyl® *see* Procainamide *on previous page*

Propoxyphene, Blood or Urine

CPT *80101 (screen); 80102 (confirmation, each procedure)*

Related Information

Chain-of-Custody Protocol *on page 952*

Drugs of Abuse Testing, Urine *on page 962*

Synonyms Darvocet-N®; Darvon®

Applies to Norpropoxyphene

Test Commonly Includes Quantitation of propoxyphene and metabolite norpropoxyphene

Abstract Propoxyphene is a narcotic analgesic and is also a drug of abuse.

Specimen Serum (TDM), urine (DAU) CONTAINER: Red top tube, plastic urine container SPECIAL INSTRUCTIONS: If forensic, use chain-of-custody protocol and form. See test entry Chain-of-Custody Protocol and the Appendix of this chapter.

Interpretive REFERENCE RANGE: Therapeutic: serum: 0.1-0.4 μg/mL (SI: 0.3-1.2 μmol/L) (therapeutic ranges published vary between laboratories and may not correlate with clinical effect); urine (for DAU): negative (less than cutoff) CRITICAL VALUES: Cutoff for urine: screen: 300 ng/

(Continued)

Propoxyphene, Blood or Urine *(Continued)*

mL; confirmation: 200 ng/mL **POSSIBLE PANIC RANGE:** Toxic: serum: >0.5 μg/mL (SI: >1.5 μmol/L); minimal fatal: 1.0 μg/mL (SI: 2.9 μmol/L) **USE:** Therapeutic monitoring, toxicity assessment, and drug-of-abuse testing **METHODOLOGY:** Immunoassay, gas chromatography (GC), high performance liquid chromatography (HPLC) **ADDITIONAL INFORMATION:** Propoxyphene is an analgesic structurally similar to methadone. Its metabolite, norpropoxyphene is also pharmacologically active. Toxic effects include nausea, vomiting, and progressive central nervous system depression. Toxicity is additive with ethanol. Toxicity can be neutralized by narcotic antagonists. Peak serum level occurs 2 hours postoral dose, half-life is 8-24 hours. Propoxyphene can also be measured in urine as part of a drug of abuse screen.

References

Gilman AG, Goodman LS, Rall TW, et al, *The Pharmacological Basis of Therapeutics*, 7th ed, New York, NY: Macmillan Publishing, 1985, 519-20.

Hartmann B, Miyada DS, Pirkle H, et al, "Serum Propoxyphene Concentrations in a Cohort of Opiate Addicts on Long-Term Propoxyphene Maintenance Therapy," *J Anal Toxicol*, 1988, 12:25-9.

Kurlan R, Majumdar L, Deeley C, et al, "A Controlled Trial of Propoxyphene and Naltrexone in Patients With Tourette's Syndrome," *Ann Neurol*, 1991, 30(1):19-23.

Oles KS, Mirza W, and Penry JK, "Catastrophic Neurologic Signs Due to Drug Interaction: Tegretol® and Darvon®," *Surg Neurol*, 1989, 32(2):144-51.

Propranolol, Blood

CPT 84600

Synonyms Inderal®

Abstract A relatively short-acting beta blocker. Propranolol is used as an antiarrhythmic and antihypertensive.

Specimen Serum **CONTAINER:** Red top tube **SAMPLING TIME:** Trough: immediately prior to next dose **SPECIAL INSTRUCTIONS:** The stoppers of some blood collection tubes contain TBEP plasticizers that affect drug distribution in sample. Check with local laboratory.

Interpretive **REFERENCE RANGE:** Therapeutic: 50-100 ng/mL (SI: 190-390 nmol/L) at end of dose interval **POSSIBLE PANIC RANGE:** >1000 ng/mL (SI: >3860 nmol/L). See Table C in the Appendix of this chapter. **USE:** Monitor therapeutic drug level in patients with cardiac arrhythmias, angina pectoris, and hypertension; evaluate for potential toxicity **METHODOLOGY:** Fluorometry, fluorescence polarization immunoassay (FPIA), enzyme immunoassay (EIA), gas-liquid chromatography (GLC), high performance liquid chromatography (HPLC) **ADDITIONAL INFORMATION:** Propranolol is well absorbed after oral administration. Its plasma half-life is 2-4 hours. For therapeutic drug monitoring, consistently use the same time interval between sampling and dose administration when comparing results from serial samples. A number of metabolites have been identified with at least one, 4-hydroxyl propranolol, having pharmacologic activity. Adverse effects of this drug include precipitation of heart failure, bronchospasm, bradycardia, and hypoglycemia. Hyperthyroidism exerts an age-dependent inducing effect on the metabolism of propranolol.[1]

Footnotes

1. Montamat SC, Cusack BJ, and Vestal RE, "Management of Drug Therapy in the Elderly," *N Engl J Med*, 1989, 321(5):303-9.

References

Hall ST, Harding SM, Hassani H, et al, "The Pharmacokinetic and Pharmacodynamic Interaction Between Lacidipine and Propranolol in Health Volunteers," *J Cardiovasc Pharmacol*, 1991, 18(Suppl 11):S13-7.

Nace GS and Wood AJJ, "Pharmacokinetics of Long-Acting Propranolol," *Clin Pharmacokinet*, 1987, 13:51-64.

Walle T, Walle UK, Cowart TD, et al, "Pathway-Selective Sex Differences in the Metabolic Clearance of Propranolol in Human Subjects," *Clin Pharmacol Ther*, 1989, 46(3):257-63.

Protriptyline *see* Tricyclic Antidepressants *on page 1007*

Prozac® *see* Fluoxetine *on page 968*

Prysolin® *see* Primidone *on page 996*

Pseudoephedrine *see* Methamphetamines, Qualitative, Urine *on page 984*

Purodigin® *see* Digitoxin *on page 959*

Quinidex® *see* Quinidine, Serum *on next page*

Quinidine, Serum

CPT *80194*

Related Information

Digoxin *on page 959*
Phenytoin *on page 994*
Procainamide *on page 996*

Synonyms Cardioquin®; Quinidex®; Quinora®

Abstract Quinidine is an antiarrhythmic that is frequently monitored.

Specimen Serum **CONTAINER:** Red top tube. The stoppers on some tubes contain plasticizers which affect measured drug levels. **SAMPLING TIME:** Collect just before next dose. **SPECIAL INSTRUCTIONS:** Serum concentration **must be correlated** with patient's clinical status.

Interpretive **REFERENCE RANGE:** Therapeutic: 2-5 μg/mL (SI: 6.2-15.4 μmol/L). Patient dependent therapeutic response occurs at levels of 3-6 μg/mL (SI: 9.2-18.5 μmol/L). Optimal therapeutic level is method dependent.[1] **POSSIBLE PANIC RANGE:** Toxic: >8 μg/mL (SI: >24.7 μmol/L).[1] See Table C in the Appendix of this chapter. **USE:** Therapeutic monitoring for quinidine is to provide documentation for adequate dosage[1] as well as toxicity assessment. **LIMITATIONS:** An assay method should be used which also detects active metabolites, in particular dihydroquinidine. Cross reactions occur with EMIT and fluorescence polarization methods.[1] **METHODOLOGY:** Enzyme-multiplied immunoassay technique (EMIT), fluorometry, high performance liquid chromatography (HPLC), gas chromatography (GC) **ADDITIONAL INFORMATION:** Optimal resampling time after change in dosage is 1-2 days. Biologic half-life is about 6-8 hours. **Doses >250 mg/day of quinidine result in increased serum digoxin concentrations about 2.5 times the digoxin concentration before quinidine was added.** The new steady-state of digoxin concentration occurs in 7-14 days, with signs of toxicity beginning to appear in 3-7 days after initiation of quinidine therapy. Therefore, **serum digoxin concentrations should be measured before initiation of quinidine therapy and again in 4-6 days.** Measure trough because of variability of peak interval. **Renal failure** prolongs apparent half-life, perhaps through accumulation of fluorescent metabolites. Severe heart failure also prolongs half-life, as does liver disease. Concomitant administration of **phenytoin** increases hepatic metabolism, and therefore decreases half-life and serum quinidine concentrations. Clearance may be diminished in the elderly.[2]

Footnotes

1. Moyer TP, Pippenger CE Jr, Blanke RV, et al, "Therapeutic Drug Monitoring," *Fundamentals of Clinical Chemistry*, 3rd ed, Tietz NW, ed, Philadelphia, PA: WB Saunders Co, 1987, 842-68.
2. Montamat SC, Cusack BJ, and Vestal RE, "Management of Drug Therapy in the Elderly," *N Engl J Med*, 1989, 321(5):303-9.

References

Giardina EG and Wechsler ME, "Low Dose Quinidine-Mexiletine Combination Therapy Versus Quinidine Monotherapy for Treatment of Ventricular Arrhythmias," *J Am Coll Cardiol*, 1990, 15(5):1138-45.

Kavanagh KM, Wyse DG, Mitchell LB, et al, "Contribution of Quinidine Metabolites to Electrophysiologic Responses in Human Subjects," *Clin Pharmacol Ther*, 1989, 46(3):352-8.

Kessler KM, Wozniak PM, McAuliffe D, et al, "The Clinical Implication of Changing Unbound Quinidine Levels," *Am Heart J*, 1989, 118(1):63-9.

Quinora® *see* Quinidine, Serum *on this page*

Ranitidine *see* Methamphetamines, Qualitative, Urine *on page 984*

Red Devils *see* Barbiturates, Quantitative, Blood *on page 946*

Retrovir® *see* Zidovudine *on page 1012*

Rivatril® *see* Clonazepam *on page 954*

Rocket Fuel *see* Phencyclidine, Qualitative, Urine *on page 992*

Salicylate

CPT *80196*

Related Information

Anion Gap *on page 132*
Lactic Acid, Blood *on page 273*

Synonyms Acetylsalicylic Acid, Blood; ASA, Blood; Aspirin, Blood; Salicylic Acid, Blood

Applies to Methyl Salicylate; Oil of Wintergreen

Abstract This is the active product produced from aspirin (acetylsalicylic acid) in the body. It is an analgesic, antipyretic, and anti-inflammatory drug.

(Continued)

Salicylate *(Continued)*

Specimen Serum or plasma **CONTAINER:** Red top tube or lavender top (EDTA) tube

Interpretive **REFERENCE RANGE:** Therapeutic: <10 mg/dL (SI: <0.72 mmol/L) for analgesic; 15-20 mg/dL (SI: 1.09-1.45 mmol/L) for anti-inflammatory **POSSIBLE PANIC RANGE:** Mild toxicity: 30 mg/dL (SI: 2.17 mmol/L) (tinnitus, dizziness); severe toxicity: >80 mg/dL (SI: >3.62 mmol/L) (CNS effects) **USE:** Monitor therapeutic drug level, evaluate aspirin toxicity **LIMITATIONS:** Bilirubin (at concentrations of 5-20 mg/dL) has been shown to depress salicylate results by 1-5 mg/dL. Sodium azide will increase results significantly; anticoagulants interfere. **METHODOLOGY:** Photometry, fluorometry, high performance liquid chromatography (HPLC), gas-liquid chromatography (GLC) **ADDITIONAL INFORMATION:** Optimal sampling time after dosage is 2-6 hours. Serum half-life is 2-3 hours on low dose therapy, 15-30 hours on high dose treatment. Optimal resampling time after change in dosage is 6 hours. In patients on chronic therapy, small dose changes may produce disproportionate changes in serum level. Use of antacids, which increase renal excretion, can lower serum levels. Steady-state concentrations for an individual patient are not adequately predicted from nomograms or standard dose schedules. In salicylate poisoning the following symptoms may occur: initial alkalosis followed by acidosis in the blood, ketosis, and possible elevated plasma glucose. Glucose should be measured when levels >25 mg/dL (SI: >1.81 mmol/L) are detected. Salicylate can be done on urine or gastric juice. The Done nomogram is used to estimate blood level and prognosis following a single dose ingestion. See nomogram. The level measured 4 hours or more following ingestion is plotted. Specimens drawn earlier may not reflect the peak. The nomogram is not useful when accumulation over several ingestions exists. Urine pH and volume hourly is advocated with plasma pH, potassium and other electrolytes, prothrombin time, AST, ALT, serum bilirubin and arterial blood gases for care of serious pediatric salicylate poisoning. Salicylate hepatitis, usually at blood levels of 20-25 mg/dL (1.45-1.81 mmol/L), occurs. Salicylates are believed to play a role in the hepatonecrosis of Reye's syndrome in children. They are no longer recommended for use in children.

Serum Salicylate Level and Severity of Intoxication

Single Dose Acute Ingestion Nomogram

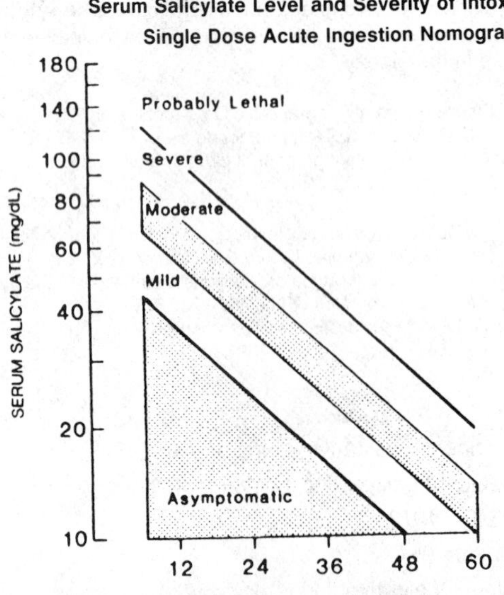

Nonogram relating serum salicylate concentration and expected severity of intoxication at varying intervals following the ingestion of a single dose of salicylate.
From Done AK, "Aspirin Overdosage: Incidence, Diagnosis, and Management," *Pediatrics*, 1978, 62:890–7, with permission.

References

Bailey RB and Jones SR, "Chronic Salicylate Intoxication. A Common Cause of Morbidity in the Elderly," *J Am Geriatr Soc*, 1989, 37(6):556-61.

Chapman BJ and Proudfoot AT, "Adult Salicylate Poisoning: Deaths and Outcome in Patients With High Plasma Salicylate Concentrations," *Q J Med*, 1989, 72(268):699-707.

Done AK, "Aspirin Overdosage: Incidence, Diagnosis, and Management," *Pediatrics*, 1978, 62:890-7.

Mayer AL, Sitar DS, and Tenenbein M, "Multiple-Dose Charcoal and Whole-Bowel Irrigation Do Not Increase Clearance of Absorbed Salicylate," *Arch Intern Med*, 1992, 152(2):393-6.

Pierce RP, Gazewood J, and Blake RL Jr, "Salicylate Poisoning From Enteric-Coated Aspirin. Delayed Absorption May Complicate Management," *Postgrad Med*, 1991, 89(5):61-2, 64.

Sallis RE, "Management of Salicylate Toxicity," *Am Fam Physician*, 1989, 39(3):265-70.

Sullivan J and Lander D, "Planning an Effective Therapeutic Strategy in Salicylate Poisoning," *Emerg Med*, 1986, 7:89-96.

Salicylic Acid, Blood *see* Salicylate *on page 999*

Sandimmune® *see* Cyclosporine *on page 957*

Secobarb *see* Barbiturates, Qualitative, Urine *on page 945*

Secobarbital *see* Barbiturates, Quantitative, Blood *on page 946*

Seconal™ *see* Barbiturates, Quantitative, Blood *on page 946*

Sedantoinal® *see* Mephenytoin *on page 981*

Serax® *see* Oxazepam, Serum *on page 990*

Serentil® *see* Phenothiazines, Serum *on page 993*

Sinequan® *see* Doxepin *on page 962*

Sinequan® *see* Tricyclic Antidepressants *on page 1007*

Slo-Phyllin® *see* Theophylline *on next page*

Snow *see* Cocaine (Cocaine Metabolite), Qualitative, Urine *on page 955*

Sodium Fluoride *see* Fluoride, Serum *on page 968*

Solganal® *see* Gold *on page 971*

Specimen Chain-of-Custody Protocol *see* Chain-of-Custody Protocol *on page 952*

Speed *see* Amphetamines, Qualitative, Urine *on page 941*

Speed *see* Methamphetamines, Qualitative, Urine *on page 984*

Sporanox *see* Itraconazole *on page 975*

Stelazine® *see* Phenothiazines, Serum *on page 993*

Stental Extentabs® *see* Phenobarbital, Blood *on page 992*

Sustaire® *see* Theophylline *on next page*

Suxinutin® *see* Ethosuximide *on page 964*

TAD *see* Tricyclic Antidepressants *on page 1007*

Talbutal *see* Barbiturates, Quantitative, Blood *on page 946*

Tambocor® *see* Flecainide *on page 967*

TCA *see* Tricyclic Antidepressants *on page 1007*

Tegretol® *see* Carbamazepine *on page 950*

Tempra® *see* Acetaminophen, Serum *on page 935*

Tetracyclic Antidepressants *see* Tricyclic Antidepressants *on page 1007*

Thallium, Urine or Blood

CPT 82190

Related Information

Heavy Metal Screen, Blood *on page 972*

Heavy Metal Screen, Urine *on page 973*

Abstract Thallium salts are components of insecticides and rodenticides.

Patient Care PREPARATION: The patient should be instructed to use a plastic bedpan or urinal if necessary

Specimen 24-hour urine, serum CONTAINER: Plastic urine container, red top tube CAUSES FOR REJECTION: Specimen allowed to contact metal

Interpretive REFERENCE RANGE: Urine: <10 μg/24 hours; serum: <10 ng/mL (SI: <49 nmol/L) USE: Diagnose thallium toxicity in patients exposed to insecticides and rat poisons METHODOL-

(Continued)

Thallium, Urine or Blood *(Continued)*

OGY: Atomic absorption spectrometry (AA) **ADDITIONAL INFORMATION:** Thallium salts have been used in the past as a depilatory. Alopecia may occur several weeks after poisoning. Thallium is an ingredient in rodenticides and insecticides. Poisoning causes GI symptoms, rash, polyneuritis, encephalitis, delirium, convulsions, shock, and coma. Lethal dose is 1 g. Half-life is 2 days.

References

Baselt RC and Cravey RH, *Disposition of Toxic Drugs and Chemicals in Man*, 3rd ed, Chicago, IL: Year Book Medical Publishers Inc, 1989, 786-8.

THC (Delta-9-Tetrahydrocannabinol) *see* Cannabinoids, Qualitative, Urine *on page 949*

Theo-Dur® *see* Theophylline *on this page*

Theolair™ *see* Theophylline *on this page*

Theophylline

CPT 80198

Related Information

Caffeine, Blood *on page 949*
Carbamazepine *on page 950*

Synonyms Aminophylline; Elixophyllin®; Slo-Phyllin®; Sustaire®; Theo-Dur®; Theolair™; Theo-span®

Abstract Theophylline is an antiasthmatic which is frequently monitored.

Specimen Serum **CONTAINER:** Red top tube **SAMPLING TIME:** Measure **trough** (just before the next dose) and **peak**. Ideally, to measure peak serum theophylline **no** missed doses for previous 48 hours; blood drawn at 2 hours after most recent dose for rapid dissolution preparations; 4-6 hours after sustained release preparations. **STORAGE INSTRUCTIONS:** Refrigerate (do not freeze) a minimum of 0.5 mL serum. **CAUSES FOR REJECTION:** Stored specimen not refrigerated

Interpretive **REFERENCE RANGE:** Therapeutic: 10-20 μg/mL (SI: 56-111 μmol/L) **POSSIBLE PANIC RANGE:** >20 μg/mL (SI: >111 μmol/L); >10 μg/mL (SI: >56 μmol/L) in neonates. High probability of seizures when levels are >40 μg/mL. **USE:** Monitor therapeutic drug level; detect noncompliance and subtherapeutic levels; attempt to predict theophylline toxicity if possible **METHODOLOGY:** Enzyme immunoassay (EIA), high performance liquid chromatography (HPLC), gas chromatography (GC) **ADDITIONAL INFORMATION:** Theophylline is prescribed for bronchial asthma, for chronic obstructive pulmonary disease, and for newborn apnea. The drug is extensively metabolized with peak serum levels reached 4 hours after oral dose. Troleandomycin and erythromycin may slow theophylline elimination. Heart failure, liver disease, prolonged fever, certain infections, and obesity may have similar effects. Prolonged half-life occurs in premature infants. **Dosage should be reduced in these situations.**

By contrast, half-life is shortened in smokers, variable with phenobarbital administration; higher doses tolerated also in acidemia. Smokers on the average are reported to need 1.5 to 2 times as much of the drugs as nonsmokers to achieve the same effects. Optimal resampling time after change in dosage is 48 hours for adults, 1-2 days for children. The half-life of theophylline is from 3-10 hours for adults and 1.4-7.9 hours for children, but varies between individuals.

Studying serum concentrations and toxic effects, Bertino et al found toxicity with peak theophylline concentrations as low as 19.4 mg/L (SI: 108 μmol/L). Recognizing theophylline toxicity over a wide range of theophylline levels, these authors questioned the association between the severity of toxic effects and serum concentrations.[1] Aitken and Martin also found lack of correlation between serum theophylline level and toxic effects.[2]

Blood levels should be interpreted in light of the patient's clinical status and use of other medications.

Toxic effects include nausea, vomiting, diarrhea, headache, atrial and ventricular arrhythmias, tremors, and convulsions.

Footnotes

1. Bertino JS Jr and Walker JW, "Reassessment of Theophylline Toxicity: Serum Concentrations, Clinical Course, and Treatment," *Arch Intern Med*, 1987, 147:757-60.

2. Aitken ML and Martin TR, "Life-Threatening Theophylline Toxicity Is Not Predictable by Serum Levels," *Chest*, 1987, 91:10-4.

References

Anderson W, Youl B, and Mackay IR, "Acute Theophylline Intoxication," *Ann Emerg Med*, 1991, 20(10):1143-5.

Bryson PD, "Theophylline," *Comprehensive Review in Toxicology*, 2nd ed, Rockville, MD: Aspen Publications, 1989, 105-16.

Butts JD, Secrest B, and Berger R, "Nonlinear Theophylline Pharmacokinetics. A Preventable Cause of Iatrogenic Theophylline Toxic Reactions," *Arch Intern Med*, 1991, 151(10):2073-7.

Emerman CL, Devlin C, and Connors AF, "Risk of Toxicity in Patients With Elevated Theophylline Levels," *Ann Emerg Med*, 1990, 19(6):643-8.

Greenberger PA, Cranberg JA, Ganz MA, et al, "A Prospective Evaluation of Elevated Serum Theophylline Concentrations to Determine if High Concentrations are Predictable," *Am J Med*, 1991, 91(1):67-73.

Meatheral R and Ford A, "Isoeratic Liquid Chromatographic Determination of Theophylline, Acetaminophen, Caffeine, Chloramphenicol, Anticonvulsants and Barbiturates in Serum," *Ther Drug Monit*, 1988, 10:101-15.

Paloucek FP and Rodrold KA, "Evaluation of Theophylline Overdoses and Toxicities," *Ann Emerg Med*, 1988, 17:135-44.

Poe RH and Utell MJ, "Theophylline in Asthma and COPD: Changing Perspectives and Controversies," *Geriatrics*, 1991, 46(4):55-6, 61-5.

Rowe DJF, Walson ID, and Williams J, "The Clinical Use and Measurement of Theophylline," *Ann Clin Biochem*, 1988, 25:4-6.

Ruff F, Santais MC, Callens E, et al, "Effect of Temafloxacin on the Pharmacokinetics of Theophylline," *Am J Med*, 1991, 91(6A):76S-80S.

Sessler CN, "Theophylline Toxicity: Clinical Features of 116 Consecutive Cases," *Am J Med*, 1990, 88(6):567-76.

Tsiu SJ, Self TH, and Burns R, "Theophylline Toxicity: Update," *Ann Allergy*, 1990, 64(2 Pt 2):241-57.

Theospan® *see* Theophylline *on previous page*

Thiocyanate, Blood or Urine

CPT *84430*

Synonyms Ethyl and Methyl Thiocyanate (Thanite® and Lethane®); Potassium Thiocyanate (KCN)

Applies to Nipride®; Nitroprusside

Abstract Thiocyanate is a metabolite of the antihypertensive drug, nitroprusside. It is also a product of cyanide metabolism.

Specimen Serum or plasma, urine **CONTAINER:** Red top tube, lavender top (EDTA) tube, plastic urine container

Interpretive **REFERENCE RANGE:** Serum, therapeutic: 1-4 μg/mL (SI: 0.02-0.07 mmol/L), smokers: 3-12 μg/mL (SI: 0.05-0.21 mmol/L); urine: 1-4 mg/24 hours, smokers: 7-17 mg/24 hours **POSSIBLE PANIC RANGE:** Serum: >35 μg/mL (SI: >0.60 mmol/L); 200 μg/mL (SI: 3.44 mmol/L) is lethal **USE:** Evaluate thiocyanate toxicity, nitroprusside poisoning, smoking. Toxic manifestations are psychotic behavior, agitation, and convulsions. **LIMITATIONS:** **Because of rapid metabolism of the drug, results are usually meaningless in the clinical setting by the time they are reported.** **METHODOLOGY:** Photometry/chromatography **ADDITIONAL INFORMATION:** Thiocyanate is a major metabolite of cyanide produced in the liver by the enzyme rhodanase. Thiocyanate is present in healthy subjects. It is a component of cigarette smoke, and it can arise from the drug nitroprusside.

References

Balistreri WF, A-Kader HH, Setchell KD, et al, "New Methods for Assessing Liver Function in Infants and Children," *Ann Clin Lab Sci*, 1992, 22(3):162-74.

Hall A and Rumack B, "Clinical Toxicology of Cyanide," *Ann Emerg Med*, 1986, 15:1067-74.

Thioridazine *see* Phenothiazines, Serum *on page 993*

Thorazine® *see* Chlorpromazine, Urine *on page 953*

Thorazine® *see* Phenothiazines, Serum *on page 993*

Tobramycin

CPT *80200*

Related Information

Antibiotic Level, Serum *on page 942*
Creatinine, Serum *on page 202*
Magnesium, Serum *on page 287*
Serum Bactericidal Test *on page 843*
Susceptibility Testing, Aerobic and Facultatively Anaerobic Organisms *on page 864*

Synonyms Nebcin®

Abstract Aminoglycoside antibiotics, including tobramycin, are used primarily to treat infections caused by aerobic gram-negative bacilli. Tobramycin has a narrow therapeutic window, and its use in life-threatening infections makes it mandatory that effective levels be achieved without overdosing. It is potentially ototoxic and nephrotoxic.

Specimen Serum **CONTAINER:** Red top tube **SAMPLING TIME:** Peak: 30 minutes after I.V. infusion; trough: immediately before next dose. Levels should be drawn at steady-state, usually 24-36 hours after starting treatment, depending on dosing schedule. See Table B in the Appendix of this chapter. **STORAGE INSTRUCTIONS:** Separate serum and refrigerate; must be frozen if a β-lactam is also present

Interpretive **REFERENCE RANGE:** Therapeutic: peak: 4-10 μg/mL (SI: 8-21 μmol/L) (depends in part on the minimal inhibitory concentration of the drug against the organism being treated); trough: <2 μg/mL (SI: <4 μmol/L) **POSSIBLE PANIC RANGE:** Toxic: peak: >12 μg/mL (SI: >25 μmol/L); trough: >2 μg/mL (SI: >4 μmol/L) **USE:** Peak levels are necessary to assure adequate therapeutic levels for organism being treated. Trough levels are necessary to reduce the likelihood of nephrotoxicity. **LIMITATIONS:** High peak levels may not have strong correlation with toxicity. **METHODOLOGY:** Immunoassay, fluorescence polarization immunoassay (FPIA) **ADDITIONAL INFORMATION:** Tobramycin is cleared by the kidney and accumulates in renal tubular cells. Nephrotoxicity is most closely related to the length of time that trough levels exceed 2 μg/mL (SI: >4 μmol/L). Creatinine levels should be monitored every 2-3 days as this serves as a useful indicator of impending renal toxicity. The initial toxic result is nonoliguric renal failure that is usually reversible if the drug is discontinued. Continued administration of tobramycin may produce oliguric renal failure. Nephrotoxicity may occur in as many as 10% to 25% of patients receiving aminoglycosides; most of this toxicity can be eliminated by monitoring levels and adjusting dosing schedules accordingly.

Aminoglycosides may also cause irreversible ototoxicity that manifests itself clinically as hearing loss. Aminoglycoside ototoxicity is relatively uncommon and clinical trials where levels were carefully monitored and dosing adjusted failed to show a correlation between auditory toxicity and plasma aminoglycoside levels. In situations in which dosing is not adjusted, sustained high levels may be associated with ototoxicity. The association is far from clear cut, and new once-daily dosing regimens (and associated high peak serum concentrations) that fail to enhance toxicity further complicate this issue.

References

Edson RS and Terrell CL, "The Aminoglycosides," *Mayo Clin Proc*, 1991, 66(11):1158-64.

Gilbert DN, "Once-Daily Aminoglycoside Therapy," *Antimicrob Agents Chemother*, 1991, 35(3):399-405.

Lane JR, Murray WE, Willenborg NL, et al, "Controlled Release Infusion Kinetics of Tobramycin," *Ther Drug Monit*, 1989, 11(3):264-8.

Slaughter RL, "Probability Assessment Approach to Therapeutic Drug Monitoring: Tobramycin," *DICP*, 1989, 23(3):240-4.

Townsend PL, Fink MP, Stein KL, et al, "Aminoglycoside Pharmacokinetics: Dosage Requirements and Nephrotoxicity in Trauma Patients," *Crit Care Med*, 1989, 17(2):154-7.

Tocainide

CPT *80299*

Related Information

Lidocaine *on page 978*

Synonyms Tonocard®

Abstract Tocainide is an antiarrhythmic closely related to lidocaine.

Specimen Serum or plasma **CONTAINER:** Red top tube or green top (heparin) tube; avoid serum separator tube **SAMPLING TIME:** Peak: 1-1.5 hours after administration; trough: just before next dose

Interpretive **REFERENCE RANGE:** Therapeutic: 4-10 μg/mL (SI: 18-43 μmol/L) **POSSIBLE PANIC RANGE:** >12 μg/mL (SI: >52 μmol/L) **USE:** Therapeutic monitoring and toxicity assessment

METHODOLOGY: High performance liquid chromatography (HPLC), gas chromatography (GC) ADDITIONAL INFORMATION: Tocainide is an analog of lidocaine used in the treatment of ventricular antiarrhythmias (class 1B). Adverse effects of tocainide are mainly neurological (faintness, tremor) and following overdose coma, seizures, edema and respiratory arrest can occur. Tocainide has a plasma half-life of 12-18 hours and metabolites are inactive.

References

Gottlieb SS, Kukin ML, Medina N, et al, "Comparative Hemodynamic Effects of Procainamide, Tocainide, and Encainide in Severe Chronic Heart Failure," *Circulation*, 1990, 81(3):860-4.

Manolis AS, Smith E, Payne D, et al, "Randomized Double-Blind Study of Intravenous Tocainide Versus Lidocaine for Suppression of Ventricular Arrhythmias After Cardiac Surgery," *Clin Cardiol*, 1990, 13(3):177-81.

Roden DM and Woosley RL, "Drug Therapy: Tocainide," *N Engl J Med*, 1986, 315:41-4.

Sperry K, Wohlenberg N, and Standefer JC, "Fatal Intoxication by Tocainide," *J Forensic Sci*, 1987, 32:1440-6.

Tofranil® *see* Imipramine *on page 974*

Tofranil® *see* Tricyclic Antidepressants *on page 1007*

Tonocard® *see* Tocainide *on previous page*

Toxic Metals, Blood *see* Heavy Metal Screen, Blood *on page 972*

Toxic Metals, Urine *see* Heavy Metal Screen, Urine *on page 973*

Toxicology Drug Screen, Blood

CPT 80100 (screen); 80102 (confirmation, each procedure)

Related Information

Ketone Bodies, Blood *on page 265*

Toxicology Drug Screen, Urine *on next page*

Synonyms Drug Screen, Comprehensive Panel or Analysis

Applies to Comatose Profile

Test Commonly Includes Amobarbital, butabarbital, butalbital, chlordiazepoxide, diazepam, ethchlorvynol, glutethimide, meprobamate, methaqualone, pentobarbital, phenobarbital, secobarbital, ethanol, methanol, acetone, isopropanol, acetaminophen, phenytoin, salicylates, tricyclics, other drugs could also be analyzed.

Abstract This toxicology screen is carried out by performing individual quantitative tests for each drug. Many times urine qualitative screening is faster and more useful in toxicologic emergencies but both may be needed. Recent introduction of systems such as the Remedi® make an automated approach to this screen possible.

Specimen Serum or plasma CONTAINER: Red top tube or lavender top (EDTA) tube CAUSES FOR REJECTION: Specimen collected in heparinized tube SPECIAL INSTRUCTIONS: Do **not** collect blood in heparinized tubes.

Interpretive REFERENCE RANGE: See individual drug listing for therapeutic and toxic ranges. USE: Monitor toxic/overdose situations; most desirable to analyze in conjunction with urine toxicology testing; used to quantitate drug identified qualitatively in urine LIMITATIONS: Evidence for presence of a drug/drug metabolite (screening, qualitative) in the case of most groups of therapeutic agents and drugs of abuse will be found in urine rather than serum. See Toxicology, Drug Screen, Urine. **All agents identified in a screening test should be confirmed with a specific test.** METHODOLOGY: Immunoassay, thin-layer chromatography (TLC), gas chromatography (GC), high performance liquid chromatography (HPLC), colorimetry, spectrophotometry ADDITIONAL INFORMATION: If only documentation of exposure to toxic drugs or drugs of abuse is desired, a urine drug screen is the most economical approach. See listing for Toxicology Drug Screen, Urine. When Toxicology Drug Screen, Blood is ordered, the individual drugs are quantitated in serum. When Toxicology Drug Screen, Urine is ordered, qualitative identification is carried out.

References

Bryson PD, *Comprehensive Review in Toxicology*, 2nd ed, Rockville, MD: Aspen Publishers Inc, 1989, 43-52.

Helper B, Sutheimer C, and Sunshine I, "Role of the Toxicology Laboratory in Suspected Ingestions," *Pediatr Clin North Am*, 1986, 33:245-60.

Puopolo PR, Volpicelli SA, Johnson DM, et al, "Emergency Toxicology Testing (Detection, Confirmation, and Quantification) of Basic Drugs in Serum by Liquid Chromatography With Photodiode Array Detection," *Clin Chem*, 1991, 37(12):2124-30.

(Continued)

Toxicology Drug Screen, Blood *(Continued)*

Schwartz JG, Zollars R, Okorodudu AO, et al, "Accuracy of Common Drug Screen Tests," *Am J Emerg Med*, 1991, 9(2):166-70.

Toxicology Drug Screen, Urine

CPT 80100 (screen); 80102 (confirmation, each procedure)

Related Information

Toxicology Drug Screen, Blood *on previous page*

Synonyms Drug Screen, Comprehensive Panel or Analysis, Urine

Applies to Narcotics Drug Screen, Urine

Test Commonly Includes A variety of qualitative screens are in use. Sensitivity and specificity vary and are method dependent. Screens should detect drugs (qualitatively) in the following classes: amphetamines, analgesics, anticonvulsants, antidepressants, antihistamines, cardiacs, narcotics, sedative/hypnotics, tranquilizers, volatiles, and drugs of abuse.

Abstract This is a qualitative screen which in the case of thin-layer chromatography or automated high performance liquid chromatography can detect any of several hundred drugs.

Specimen Random urine. The use of meconium samples from newborns has been shown to be useful.[1] **CONTAINER:** Plastic urine container **STORAGE INSTRUCTIONS:** Keep refrigerated **SPECIAL INSTRUCTIONS:** Specify the drug or drugs suspected.

Interpretive **REFERENCE RANGE:** None detected or negative (less than cutoff for drugs of abuse) **USE:** Screen for drug abuse, drug toxicity alone or in conjunction with serum/plasma testing **LIMITATIONS:** Test provides **only** qualitative detection of drugs, unless laboratory automatically confirms and quantitates drugs detected as a part of the "screening" procedure. Quantitation of urine drug levels is usually not included and is not recommended because urine levels are time and clearance dependent and are not directly related to toxic symptoms seen clinically. Some drugs and/or metabolites are not detected or optimally detected in urine, again relating to method. Serum may be preferable because of clinical and at times technical/kinetic factors (eg, barbiturates, phenytoin). Sensitivity is of the order of 0.5-1.0 μg/mL for TLC of urine. Some substances should be quantitated in blood or serum (eg, iron overdose, methanol, acetaminophen, salicylate, carbon monoxide, ethanol, digoxin, lithium, theophylline, and methemoglobin). **METHODOLOGY:** A variety of methods or combination of methods are in fairly common use and include thin-layer chromatography (TLC), colorimetry/spectrophotometry, enzyme immunoassay technique (EIA), enzyme-multiplied immunoassay technique (EMIT), gas chromatography (GC), gas chromatography/mass spectrometry (GC/MS), high performance liquid chromatography (HPLC). **ADDITIONAL INFORMATION:** For specific drug blood levels see the listing by specific generic drug name for drug desired. Some toxins (eg, metals, volatiles, gaseous compounds) may require specific methodology (eg, atomic absorption spectrophotometry, gas chromatography). Also see Toxicology, Drug Screen, Blood test listing.

Footnotes

1. Maynard EC, Amoruso LP, and Oh W, "Meconium for Drug Testing," *Am J Dis Child*, 1991, 145(6):650-2.

References

Bryson PD, *Comprehensive Review in Toxicology*, 2nd ed, Rockville, MD: Aspen Publishers Inc, 1989, 43-52.

Osterloh JD, "Utility and Reliability of Emergency Toxicologic Testing," *Emerg Med Clin North Am*, 1990, 8(3):693-723.

Osterloh JD and Lee BL, "Urine Drug Screening in Mothers and Newborns," *Am J Dis Child*, 1989, 143(7):791-3.

Toxicology, Volatiles *see* Volatile Screen *on page 1010*

Tranquilizers (Valium®, Librium®, etc) *see* Benzodiazepines, Qualitative, Urine *on page 947*

Trazodone

CPT 80299

Synonyms Desyrel®

Abstract This drug is an antidepressant chemically unrelated to the tricyclic or tetracyclic antidepressants.

Specimen Serum or plasma **CONTAINER:** Red top tube or green top (heparin) tube **SAMPLING TIME:** Trough: just before next dose

Interpretive **REFERENCE RANGE:** Therapeutic: 0.5-2.0 μg/mL (SI: 1-4.8 μmol/L) **CRITICAL VALUES:** >2.5 μg/mL (SI: >6 μmol/L) **POSSIBLE PANIC RANGE:** 4 μg/mL (SI: 10 μmol/L) **USE:** Therapeutic monitoring and toxicity assessment **METHODOLOGY:** High performance liquid chromatography (HPLC), gas chromatography (GC) **ADDITIONAL INFORMATION:** Trazodone is a structurally unique antidepressant that is pharmacologically different from other drugs of this class. The toxicities observed in tricyclic overdose (neuro and cardiotoxicity and respiratory depression) are not seen with trazodone. Chronic toxicity is very low with trazodone although it does have unique side effects including akathisia, allergic reactions, chest pain, delayed urine flow, early and delayed menses, hypersalivation and hypomania, among others. The half-life of trazodone is 4-7 hours, peak plasma concentrations with average daily dosing is reached in 2-4 hours.

References

Aranow AB, Hudson JI, Pope HG Jr, et al, "Elevated Antidepressant Plasma Levels After Addition of Fluoxetine," *Am J Psychiatry*, 1989, 146(7):911-3.

Carson CC and Mino RD, "Priapism Associated With Trazodone Therapy," *J Urol*, 1988, 139:369-70.

Fabre LF, "United States Experience and Perspectives With Trazodone," *Clin Neuropharmacol*, 1989, 12(Suppl 1):511-7.

Spar JE, "Plasma Trazodone Concentrations in Elderly, Depressed Inpatients: Cardiac Effects and Short-Term Efficacy," *J Clin Psychopharmacol*, 1987, 7:406-9.

Triavil® *see* Amitriptyline, Blood *on page 939*

Tricyclic Antidepressants

***CPT** 80101 (screen); 80102 (confirmation, each procedure)*

Related Information

Amitriptyline, Blood *on page 939*
Imipramine *on page 974*
Nortriptyline *on page 989*

Synonyms Antidepressants; TAD; TCA; Tetracyclic Antidepressants

Applies to Adapin®; Aventyl®; Desipramine; Etrafon®; Norpramin®; Pamelor®; Pertofrane®; Presamine®; Protriptyline; Sinequan®; Tofranil®; Vivactil®

Abstract Drugs in this class are widely used as antidepressants. They are frequently involved in suicidal ingestion and responsible for a large percentage of drug-related deaths.

Specimen Serum or plasma **CONTAINER:** Red top tube, green top (heparin) tube; avoid serum separator tubes and the plasticizer, TBEP **SAMPLING TIME:** Steady-state specimen after 1 week of dose schedule; draw specimen 12 hours after the last dose. **STORAGE INSTRUCTIONS:** Remove serum within 2 hours of drawing; refrigerate or freeze if not analyzed immediately. **SPECIAL INSTRUCTIONS:** Order individual drug level or tricyclic overdose screen

Interpretive **REFERENCE RANGE:** Therapeutic: amitriptyline: 100-250 ng/mL (SI: 360-900 nmol/L); amoxapine: 50-400 ng/mL; desipramine: 150-300 ng/mL (SI: 563-1126 nmol/L); doxepin: 100-200 ng/mL (SI: 360-720 nmol/L); imipramine: 75-250 ng/mL (SI: 279-890 nmol/L); maprotiline: 150-400 ng/mL (SI: 541-1442 nmol/L); nortriptyline: 50-150 ng/mL (SI: 190-570 nmol/L); protriptyline: 50-150 ng/mL (SI: 190-570 nmol/L); trazodone: 300-1600 ng/mL **POSSIBLE PANIC RANGE:** >500 ng/mL; toxicity observed at ≥300 ng/mL **USE:** Therapeutic monitoring and toxicity assessment **LIMITATIONS:** Immunoassays for tricyclic antidepressants (toxic overdose) do not distinguish between parent compounds and active metabolites. Immunoassays are available for amitriptyline, nortriptyline, desipramine, and imipramine. Drug-drug interactions occur; hydrocortisone, neuroleptics, methylphenidate, cimetidine, and oral contraceptives produce higher levels by inhibiting metabolism of tricyclics by the liver. Barbiturates, chloral hydrate, and glutethimide lower plasma tricyclic levels by stimulating liver microsomal activity. Cigarette smoking also lowers steady-state plasma levels, apparently by a similar hepatic enzyme induction mechanism. **CONTRAINDICATIONS:** Patient taking more than one tricyclic antidepressant, patient taking phenothiazines or monoamine oxidase inhibitors **METHODOLOGY:** Immunoassay, gas chromatography (GC), gas chromatography/mass spectrometry (GC/MS), high performance liquid chromatography (HPLC) **ADDITIONAL INFORMATION:** Tricyclic antidepressants (TADs) are metabolized to secondary active compounds. These agents are useful in treating clinical depression, and enuresis (imipramine). However, they show a narrow therapeutic window, and great individual variations in blood levels associated with dosage. Blacks usually have 50% greater blood level than whites for same dose schedule. Symptoms of overdose may mimic those of condition for which agent was prescribed. The most important of the more serious or toxic effects of TADs is cardiotoxicity. Arrhythmias and conduction defects with precipitation of congestive heart failure and possibly myocardial infarction are common at combined levels >1000 ng/mL. Widening of the QRS interval to >100 msec is highly suggestive of a TAD overdose.

(Continued)

Tricyclic Antidepressants *(Continued)*

Tricyclic antidepressant drugs represent a frequent and serious problem in both unintentional and intentional overdosage. Reports of poor correlations between plasma levels and toxic clinical manifestations indicate that QRS duration >100 msec may provide the most reliable indicator of toxicity. It has been reported that levels of parent to metabolite (P/M) ratios >2 are associated with acute overdosage. In contrast, P/M ratios <2 are more consistent with high steady-state plasma levels following "therapeutic" dosages although ECG or other clinical evidence of toxicity may be present. Variations in blood levels between doses are comparatively small. Peak levels occur 4-8 hours after oral ingestion. A level dose of medication should be prescribed for at least 2 weeks to obtain steady plasma levels. Monitoring of tricyclic antidepressant plasma levels is useful in a number of situations. Older patients may develop higher steady-state plasma levels than younger individuals. In geriatric patients conventional doses may lead to toxic levels. Toxic plasma levels of tricyclic drugs may be dangerous in cardiac disease patients. Recommended lower and higher plasma levels for the different tricyclic drugs are evolving and are discussed in the literature. A recent study of tricyclic levels in children and adolescents has emphasized the lack of correlation between oral dose and plasma concentration and has found that the incidence of side effects and therapeutic effect in treatment of enuresis relates to concentration of circulating drug.

References

Beaumont G, "The Toxicity of Antidepressants," *Br J Psychiatry*, 1989, 154:454-8.

Bergstrom RF, Peyton AL, and Lemberger L, "Quantification and Mechanism of the Fluoxetine and Tricyclic Antidepressant Interaction," *Clin Pharmacol Ther*, 1992, 51(3):239-48.

Brasfield KH, "Practical Psychopharmacologic Considerations in Depression," *Nurs Clin North Am*, 1991, 26(3):651-63.

Frommer DA, Kulig KW, Marx JA, et al, "Tricyclic Antidepressant Overdose: A Review," *JAMA*, 1987, 257:521-6.

Hantsen PH, *Drug Interactions*, 5th ed, Philadelphia, PA: Lea & Febiger, 1985, 366-7.

Krishel S and Jackimczyk K, "Cyclic Antidepressants, Lithium, and Neuroleptic Agents. Pharmacology and Toxicology," *Emerg Med Clin North Am*, 1991, 9(1):53-86.

Lavoie FW, Gansert GG, and Weiss RE, "Value of Initial ECG Findings and Plasma Drug Levels in Cyclic Antidepressant Overdose," *Ann Emerg Med*, 1990, 19(6):696-700.

Tridione® *see* Oxazolidinediones *on page 991*

Trifluoperazine *see* Phenothiazines, Serum *on page 993*

Trimedone *see* Oxazolidinediones *on page 991*

Tylenol® *see* Acetaminophen, Serum *on page 935*

Uppers *see* Amphetamines, Qualitative, Urine *on page 941*

Valium® *see* Diazepam, Blood *on page 958*

Valproic Acid

CPT *80164*

Related Information

Ammonia, Blood *on page 120*
Carbamazepine *on page 950*
Phenobarbital, Blood *on page 992*
Phenytoin *on page 994*
Primidone *on page 996*

Synonyms Depakene®; Depakote® (Enteric-Coated Divalproex-Sodium); Depamide®; Epilim®; Ergenyl®

Applies to Phenobarbital

Abstract Valproic acid is a first-line anticonvulsant for absence seizures. It is useful for many other seizure types, including primary generalized tonic-clonic, myoclonic, atonic, and mixed seizures.[1,2] It is the drug of choice for mixed absence and generalized seizures and for the epileptic syndromes of juvenile myoclonic epilepsy and generalized tonic-clonic seizures on awakening.

Specimen Serum or plasma **CONTAINER:** Red top tube or green top (heparin) tube **SAMPLING TIME:** Trough values drawn just before next dose or consistent sampling time in chronic monitoring

Interpretive **REFERENCE RANGE:** 50-100 μg/mL (SI: 350-690 μmol/L). Low levels: The most important cause is noncompliance. Phenytoin, phenobarbital, primidone, and carbamazepine decrease the half-life of valproic acid. High levels: Carbamazepine and phenytoin can increase the level of valproic acid. **CRITICAL VALUES:** Toxic concentration >200 μg/mL (SI: >1390 μmol/L). Seizure control may improve at levels >100 μg/mL (SI: >690 μmol/L), but toxicity may occur at levels of 100-150 μg/mL (SI: 690-1040 μmol/L). See Table A in the Appendix of this chapter. **USE:** Monitor for compliance, efficacy, and possible toxicity **LIMITATIONS:** Since valproic acid is highly bound, drugs that compete for protein binding sites can increase the amount of free valproic acid (biologically active fraction). These include dicumarol, high dose salicylates, and phenylbutazone. If toxicity is suspected, a free valproic acid level should be obtained. **METHODOLOGY:** Enzyme immunoassay (EIA), gas-liquid chromatography (GLC), high performance liquid chromatography (HPLC) **ADDITIONAL INFORMATION:** Hepatic failure has occurred during the first 6 months of therapy. Hepatotoxicity may be preceded by nonspecific symptoms such as malaise, weakness, lethargy, anorexia, and vomiting. Hepatotoxicity may be fatal, but is idiosyncratic and not preventable by routinely monitoring liver enzymes. Hepatotoxicity occurs in very young children, most often those on multiple anticonvulsants.[3] Valproate-induced cytopenias may be dose-related and warrant monitoring of complete blood counts during therapy.[4] Encephalopathy with hyperammonemia without liver function test abnormalities may occur.[5] Pregnant women in first month are at risk for neural tube defects.

Footnotes

1. Penry JK and Dean JC, "Valproate Monotherapy in Partial Seizures," *Am J Med*, 1988, 84(1A):14-6.
2. Dean JC and Penry JK, "Valproate Monotherapy in 30 Patients With Partial Seizures," *Epilepsia*, 1988, 29(2):140-4.
3. Dreifuss FE, Santilli N, Langer DH, et al, "Valproic Acid Hepatic Fatalities: A Retrospective Review," *Neurology*, 1987, 37:379-85.
4. Watts RG, Emanuel PD, Zuckerman KS, et al, "Valproic Acid-Induced Cytopenias: Evidence for a Dose-Related Suppression of Hematopoesis," *J Pediatr*, 1990, 117(3):495-9.
5. Zaret BS, Beckner RR, Marini AM, et al, "Sodium Valproate-Induced Hyperammonemia Without Clinical Hepatic Dysfunction," *Neurology*, 1982, 32(2):206-8.

References

Engel J, *Seizures and Epilepsy*, Contemporary Neurology Series, Philadelphia, PA: FA Davis Co, 1989.
Levy RH, Dreifuss FE, Mattson RH, et al, *Antiepileptic Drugs*, 3rd ed, New York, NY: Raven Press, 1989.

Vancocin® *see* Vancomycin *on this page*

Vancomycin

***CPT** 80202*

Related Information

Antibiotic Level, Serum *on page 942*
Serum Bactericidal Test *on page 843*
Susceptibility Testing, Aerobic and Facultatively Anaerobic Organisms *on page 864*

Synonyms Vancocin®

Abstract Vancomycin is an antimicrobial agent with potent activity against most gram-positive bacteria. Its use has occasionally been associated with nephrotoxicity and/or ototoxicity, though the frequency of these toxicities has decreased as vancomycin preparations have become more purified.

Specimen Serum, body fluid **CONTAINER:** Red top tube, sterile fluid container **SAMPLING TIME:** Peak: 30 minutes following dose; trough: immediately prior to next dose **STORAGE INSTRUCTIONS:** Separate serum using aseptic technique and place in freezer **CAUSES FOR REJECTION:** Specimen more than 4 hours old

Interpretive **REFERENCE RANGE:** Therapeutic concentration: peak: 20-40 μg/mL (SI: 14-27 μmol/L) (depends in part on minimum inhibitory concentration of organism being treated); trough: 5-10 μg/mL (SI: 3.4-6.8 μmol/L) **POSSIBLE PANIC RANGE:** Toxic: >80 μg/mL (SI: >54 μmol/L). See Table B in the Appendix of this chapter. **USE:** Monitor therapeutic levels and potential toxicities, particularly in patients with impaired renal function and in patients also being treated with aminoglycoside antibiotics **METHODOLOGY:** High performance liquid chromatography (HPLC), gas-liquid chromatography (GLC), immunoassay **ADDITIONAL INFORMATION:** Vancomycin is currently being used in its intravenous form to treat a variety of gram-positive bacterial infections, particularly those due to methicillin-resistant staphylococci. Additionally, vancomycin is often used in its oral form to treat pseudomembranous colitis due to *Clostridium difficile*. When administered orally, serum vancomycin levels are undetectable due to poor absorption from the gastrointestinal tract. When administered intravenously, vancomycin may be ototoxic and nephrotoxic, though nephrotoxicity is rare with newer preparations. Ototoxici-

(Continued)

Vancomycin *(Continued)*

ty is seen primarily in patients with extremely high serum concentrations (80-100 μg/mL; SI: 54-68 μmol/L) and rarely occurs when serum concentrations are maintained at ≤30 μg/mL (SI: ≤20 μmol/L). Both oto- and nephrotoxicity is enhanced by concurrent administration of aminoglycosides.

References

Fogarty KA and McClain WJ, "Vancomycin: Current Perspectives and Guidelines for Use in the NICU," *Neonatal Netw*, 1989, 7(5):31-5.

Ingerman MJ and Santoro J, "Vancomycin. A New Old Agent," *Infect Dis Clin North Am*, 1989, 3(3):641-51.

Levine JF, "Vancomycin: A Review," *Med Clin North Am*, 1987, 71:1135-45.

Miceli J, "Chloramphenicol and Vancomycin," *Clin Lab Med*, 1987, 7:531-40.

Wilhelm MP, "Vancomycin," *Mayo Clin Proc*, 1991, 66(11):1165-70.

Verapamil

CPT *80299*

Related Information

Carbamazepine *on page 950*

Digoxin *on page 959*

Lithium *on page 979*

Synonyms Calan®; Isoptin®

Applies to Norverapamil

Test Commonly Includes Verapamil and norverapamil (metabolite levels)

Abstract Verapamil is an antihypertensive, antiarrhythmic drug with an active metabolite.

Specimen Serum or plasma **CONTAINER:** Red top tube (preferred) or green top (heparin) tube. Do not use serum separator tubes. **SAMPLING TIME:** Peak: 1-2 hours after last dose **STORAGE INSTRUCTIONS:** Centrifuge, separate, and freeze serum (plasma) in a plastic container. **SPECIAL INSTRUCTIONS:** Include the following information with the request: time specimen drawn, date of last dose, time of last dose, amount of dose, and route administered.

Interpretive **REFERENCE RANGE:** Therapeutic: 50-200 ng/mL (SI: 100-410 nmol/L) for parent; under normal conditions norverapamil concentration is the same as parent drug. **POSSIBLE PANIC RANGE:** >400 ng/mL (SI: >815 nmol/L); toxicity proportional to verapamil concentration **USE:** Therapeutic monitoring and toxicity assessment **METHODOLOGY:** Fluorometry, high performance liquid chromatography (HPLC), gas chromatography (GC) **ADDITIONAL INFORMATION:** Verapamil is an antiarrhythmic, antihypertensive drug whose main metabolite is norverapamil, which has about 20% of the activity of the parent drug. Verapamil is a calcium channel blocker with a half-life of 6-9 hours. Coadministration of verapamil and beta-blockers should be approached with caution. Verapamil increases serum digoxin concentrations 50% to 70%. Toxicity may result when verapamil is used with carbamazepine or lithium.

References

Hla KK, Latham AN, and Henry JA, "Influence of Time of Administration on Verapamil Pharmacokinetics," *Clin Pharmacol Ther*, 1992, 51(4):366-70.

Hosie J, Hosie G, and Meredith PA, "The Effects of Age on the Pharmacodynamics and Pharmacokinetics of Two Formulations of Verapamil," *J Cardiovasc Pharmacol*, 1989, 13(Suppl 4):S60-2.

Pritza DR, Bierman MH, and Hammeke MD, "Acute Toxic Effects of Sustained-Release Verapamil in Chronic Renal Failure," *Arch Intern Med*, 1991, 151(10):2081-4.

Schwartz JB, "Aging Alters Verapamil Elimination and Dynamics: Single Dose and Steady-State Responses," *J Pharmacol Exp Ther*, 1990, 255(1):364-73.

Vivactil® *see* Tricyclic Antidepressants *on page 1007*

Volatile Screen

CPT *80101 (screen, single drug class); 80102 (confirmation, each procedure); 84600 (quantitative)*

Related Information

Alcohol, Blood or Urine *on page 936*

Anion Gap *on page 132*

Ketone Bodies, Blood *on page 265*

Ketones, Urine *on page 1128*

Osmolality, Serum *on page 300*

Synonyms Toxicology, Volatiles

Applies to Acetone; Ethanol; Isopropanol; Methanol

Test Commonly Includes Determination of volatiles by GLC including acetone, ethanol, isopropanol, and methanol

Abstract This screening profile measures ethanol and other possible volatiles.

Specimen Serum or plasma, urine, gastric fluid **CONTAINER:** Red top tube, gray top (sodium fluoride) tube; tightly stoppered container for urine and gastric fluid **COLLECTION:** All containers should be tightly stoppered and transported on ice. The gray (oxalate/fluoride) tube top is recommended for medicolegal collections and if storage is prolonged. Sodium fluoride (50 mg) can be added as a preservative to urine and gastric samples. Other anticoagulants (eg, heparin EDTA) are acceptable. **CAUSES FOR REJECTION:** Specimen leakage

Interpretive **REFERENCE RANGE:** None detected **POSSIBLE PANIC RANGE:** Blood: acetone, methanol, isopropanol >500 μg/mL (SI: acetone: >8610 μmol/L, methanol: >15.6 mmol/L, isopropanol: >8.32 mmol/L), ethanol: >2000 μg/mL (SI: >43.4 mmol/L); urine: acetone, methanol, isopropanol >500 μg/mL (SI: acetone: >8610 μmol/L, methanol: >15.6 mmol/L, isopropanol: 8.32 mmol/L), ethanol: >1600 μg/mL (SI: >34.7 mmol/L) **USE:** Evaluate methanol and isopropanol toxicity, and alcohol drug abuse **METHODOLOGY:** Gas-liquid chromatography (GLC) **ADDITIONAL INFORMATION:** Both methanol and isopropanol are more intoxicating than ethanol. Methanol is converted to formaldehyde and formic acid which causes retinal damage leading to blindness and metabolic acidosis. Isopropanol is converted to acetone.

References

Burkhart KK and Kulig KW, "The Other Alcohols. Methanol, Ethylene Glycol, and Isopropanol," *Emerg Med Clin North Am*, 1990, 8(4):913-28.

Jarvie DR and Simpson D, "Simple Screening Tests for the Emergency Identification of Methanol and Ethylene Glycol in Poisoned Patients," *Clin Chem*, 1990, 36(11):1957-61.

Lacouture PG, Heldreth DD, Shannon M, et al, "The Generation of Acetonemia/Acetonuria Following Ingestion of a Subtoxic Dose of Isopropyl Alcohol," *Am J Emerg Med*, 1989, 7(1):38-40.

Litovitz T, "The Alcohols: Ethanol, Methanol, Isopropanol, Ethylene Glycol," *Pediatr Clin North Am*, 1986, 33:311-23.

Warfarin

CPT *80299*

Related Information

Carbamazepine *on page 950*

Prothrombin Time *on page 468*

Synonyms Athrombin-K®; Coumadin®; Panwarfin®

Applies to Anticoagulants, Oral

Abstract Warfarin is an oral anticoagulant. Serum warfarin concentrations are seldom used to manage therapy; rather, typically, prothrombin time is used.

Specimen Serum or plasma **CONTAINER:** Red top tube, lavender top (EDTA) tube

Interpretive **REFERENCE RANGE:** Therapeutic: 2-5 μg/mL (SI: 6.5-16.2 μmol/L) **POSSIBLE PANIC RANGE:** Toxic: >10 μg/mL (SI: >32.4 μmol/L) **USE:** Therapeutic monitoring and toxicity assessment **LIMITATIONS:** This test **does not** measure bishydroxycoumarin and should not be used to monitor this drug. **METHODOLOGY:** High performance liquid chromatography (HPLC), gas-liquid chromatography (GLC), UV spectrophotometry **ADDITIONAL INFORMATION:** Warfarin is used for chronic oral anticoagulation in a variety of clinical settings. Management of warfarin therapy is usually done by following the **prothrombin time**, rather than by measuring serum drug concentrations. Warfarin is subject to a bewildering number and variety of drug interactions, producing increased or decreased clinical effect of itself or other drugs. See Prothrombin Time entry in Coagulation chapter for additional discussion and table. Many of these effects are due to changes in protein binding or hepatic metabolism. Reductions in dosage may be indicated for aging subjects treated for venous thromboembolic or coronary arterial disease, but not in those with peripheral vascular disease, deep vein thrombosis, or valvular heart disease.[1,2]

Footnotes

1. Montamat SC, Cusack BJ, and Vestal RE, "Management of Drug Therapy in the Elderly," *N Engl J Med*, 1989, 321(5):303-9.
2. James AH, Britt RP, Raskino CL, et al, "Factors Affecting the Maintenance Dose of Warfarin," *J Clin Pathol*, 1992, 45(8):704-6.

References

Bick RL, "Antithrombolytic Therapy," *Disorders of Thrombosis and Hemostasis: Clinical Laboratory Practice*, Chapter 14, Chicago, IL: ASCP Press, 1992, 291-312.

Mortensen M, "Management of Acute Childhood Poisonings Caused By Selected Insecticides and Herbicides," *Pediatr Clin North Am*, 1986, 33:421-45.

(Continued)

Warfarin *(Continued)*

Redwood M, Taylor C, Bain BJ, et al, "The Association of Age With Dosage Requirement for Warfarin," *Age Ageing*, 1991, 20(3):217-20.

Schreiber TL, Miller DH, Silvasi D, et al, "Superiority of Warfarin Over Aspirin Long-Term After Thrombolytic Therapy for Acute Myocardial Infarction," *Am Heart J*, 1990, 119(6):1238-44.

Xylocaine® *see* Lidocaine *on page 978*

Yellow Jackets *see* Barbiturates, Quantitative, Blood *on page 946*

Zarontin® *see* Ethosuximide *on page 964*

Zartalin® *see* Ethosuximide *on page 964*

Zidovudine

***CPT** 80299*

Related Information

Beta$_2$-Microglobulin *on page 644*
HIV-1/HIV-2 Serology *on page 696*
Human Immunodeficiency Virus Culture *on page 1185*
Lymphocyte Subset Enumeration *on page 720*

Synonyms Azidothymidine; AZT; Retrovir®

Abstract Azidothymidine (AZT) is the first FDA approved drug for the treatment of human immunodeficiency virus (HIV) infection, the cause of AIDS. The drug is a competitive inhibitor of HIV reverse transcriptase; it is incorporated into the viral DNA in place of thymidine and interrupts viral replication because the DNA can no longer elongate.

Specimen Serum or plasma **CONTAINER:** Red top tube preferred, green top (heparin) tube acceptable **SAMPLING TIME:** Trough level, just before next dose **COLLECTION:** Volume needed is method dependent (0.1-1 mL) **CAUSES FOR REJECTION:** Incorrect specimen sampling time

Interpretive **REFERENCE RANGE:** Not established **USE:** Not established for routine clinical use. Monitoring should probably be limited to studies on pharmacokinetics and efficacy of antiretroviral therapy. **METHODOLOGY:** High performance liquid chromatography (HPLC), radioimmunoassay (RIA), fluorescence polarization immunoassay (FPIA) **ADDITIONAL INFORMATION:** Zidovudine is usually administered at a total daily dose of 500 mg (100 mg orally, every 4 hours while the patient is awake); optimal dosing, however, has not been established. Peak serum concentrations are attained within 30-40 minutes after ingestion. The drug has a half-life of approximately 1 hour; the main metabolite is a glucuronide derivative with no antiviral activity that is excreted by the kidneys. The major toxicity associated with zidovudine use is hematologic suppression which may manifest as anemia, leukopenia, and/or granulocytopenia. Monitoring hematologic parameters is the most reasonable approach toward evaluating toxicity; serum levels currently contribute little to evaluating toxic effects of zidovudine. Coadministration of probenecid results in increased serum levels due to competition for glucuronidation pathways. Hepatic and renal failure increases serum levels.

References

Amin NM, "Zidovudine for Treating AIDS. What Physicians Need to Know," *Postgrad Med*, 1989, 86(1):195-6, 201-8.

Collins JM and Unadket JD, "Clinical Pharmacokinetics of Zidovudine. An Overview of Current Data," *Clin Pharmacokinet*, 1989, 17(1):1-9.

Langtry HD and Campoli-Richards DM, "Zidovudine. A Review of its Pharmacodynamic and Pharmacokinetic Properties, and Therapeutic Efficacy," *Drugs*, 1989, 37(4):408-50.

THERAPEUTIC DRUG MONITORING/ TOXICOLOGY/DRUGS OF ABUSE APPENDIX

The following form is a combination requisition and external chain-of-custody form. The strip at the bottom peels off and is used to seal the urine specimen cup. The number on the strip appears on all 5 copies of the form and serves to positively associate the form with the sample. An internal chain-of-custody form (used in the laboratory and not illustrated here) appears on the back of copy 1.

I.

ACCOUNT NAME AND ADDRESS

ROCKHILL MEDICAL LABORATORY

TOXICOLOGY

LIS NO.

ACC NO.

II

COLLECTOR IDENTIFICATION	LOCATION	MEDICAL REVIEW OFFICER
	MEDICATIONS WITHIN LAST 30 DAYS	

III

REASON FOR TESTING:

1 ☐ PRE-EMPLOYMENT
2 ☐ PERIODIC
3 ☐ REASONABLE CAUSE
4 ☐ BLOOD (PROBABLE SUSPICION)
5 ☐ POST-ACCIDENT
6 ☐ RANDOM
7 ☐ OTHER (SPECIFY) ________

PROFILES

- ☐ DRUGS OF ABUSE SCREEN (THIN LAYER CONFIRMATION)
- ☐ DRUGS OF ABUSE SCREEN-5 (GC/MS* CONFIRMATION)
- ☐ DRUGS OF ABUSE SCREEN-10 (GC/MS* CONFIRMATION)
- ☐ BLOOD ALCOHOL
- ☐ URINE ALCOHOL

★ GAS CHROMATOGRAPHY/MASS SPECTROMETRY

IV

TEMPERATURE

SPECIMEN TEMPERATURE Has been read within 4 minutes ☐ Yes ☐ No

TEMPERATURE IS WITHIN RANGE OF 32.5°-37.7°C/90.5°-99.8°F ☐ Yes ☐ No—*If NOT, record actual temp:* ________ °

V

TO BE COMPLETED BY COLLECTOR

NAME ____________________ LOCATION ____________________

I CERTIFY THAT THE SPECIMEN IDENTIFIED ON THIS FORM IS THE SPECIMEN PRESENTED TO ME BY THE APPLICANT/EMPLOYEE SIGNING THIS FORM, AND THAT THE SPECIMEN BEARS AN IDENTIFICATION NUMBER IDENTICAL TO THE NUMBER BELOW, AND THAT IT HAS BEEN COLLECTED, LABELED, AND SEALED WITH THE SECURITY LABEL PROVIDED ON THIS FORM IN THE DONOR'S PRESENCE, AS REQUIRED BY THE INSTRUCTIONS.

SIGNATURE ________ DATE/TIME ________ PHONE ________

VI

TO BE COMPLETED BY DONOR

I HEREBY CONSENT TO HAVE A SPECIMEN OF MY URINE AND/OR BLOOD TAKEN, AND I UNDERSTAND THAT IT WILL BE USED FOR DRUG ANALYSIS BY ROCKHILL MEDICAL LABORATORY. THE RESULTS OF THE TESTS ON MY SPECIMEN WILL THEN BE MADE AVAILABLE TO THE ABOVE NAMED COMPANY/EMPLOYER FOR EMPLOYMENT EVALUATION ONLY. I HEREBY RELEASE ALL PHYSICIANS, MEDICAL FACILITIES, TESTING FACILITIES, THE ABOVE NAMED EMPLOYER/COMPANY, CLINICS, AND THEIR EMPLOYEES, AGENTS AND REPRESENTATIVES FROM ANY AND ALL LIABILITY ARISING FROM THE RELEASE OF THE INFORMATION DISCOVERED FROM MY TEST. IN ADDITION, I HEREBY ACKNOWLEDGE THAT THE SPECIMEN LABELED WITH THE IDENTIFICATION NUMBER BELOW IS MY OWN, AND THE SPECIMEN WAS LABELED AND SEALED IN MY PRESENCE.

SIGNATURE OF APPLICANT ____________________ TIME/DATE: ________

VII

CHAIN OF CUSTODY

COLLECTOR REASON FOR CUSTODY CHANGE	RELEASED BY: SIGNATURE/PRINT NAME	RECEIVED BY: SIGNATURE/PRINT NAME	DATE/TIME
PROVIDE SPECIMEN FOR TESTING	DONOR XXXX		
SHIP TO LABORATORY			

VIII

LAB USE ONLY

SEAL INTACT YES NO	VOLUME	SPECIMEN IS: ☐ ACCEPTED ☐ NOT SUITABLE FOR ANALYSIS
COMMENTS:		

IX

X ____________________ COLLECTOR'S SIGNATURE

________ DONOR'S INITIAL ________ DATE

PLACE OVER CAP

TOXICOLOGY COPY-1

____________________ NAME OR I.D. NUMBER OF DONOR

002576

Reprinted with permission from Baptist Medical Center, Kansas City, MO.

Table A. Class of Drug — Anticonvulsants

Name of Drug	Therapeutic Range	Toxic Level	Half-Life	Time to Sample	Protein Binding %	Active Metabolites	Route of Excretion	Major Drug Interactions
Carbamazepine	8–12 μg/mL	>12 μg/mL	30 h	7–12 d	60–73	10,11–N–epoxide	Hepatic	
Clonazepam	10–50 ng/mL	>100 μg/mL	20–40 h	5–6 d	40–70	7–Amino		
Ethosuximide	40–100 μg/mL	>100 μg/mL	40–60 h	10–13 d	0		Hepatic	
Mephenytoin	15–40 μg/mL	>50 μg/mL	8 h		20–50	5–Ethyl, 5–phenyl-hydantoin		
Phenobarbital	15–35 μg/mL	>40 μg/mL	48–96 h	20 d	50		Hepatic	Hydantoin Valproic acid
Primidone	5–12 μg/mL	>12 μg/mL	10–12 h	5 d	0–30	Phenobarbital		
Valproic acid	50–100 μg/mL	>100 μg/mL	6–18 h	4 d	90		Renal	Phenobarbital Phenytoin

Table B. Class of Drug — Antibiotics

Name of Drug	Therapeutic Range	Toxic Level (peak)	Half-Life	Time to Sample (after starting)	Protein Binding %	Route of Excretion
Amikacin	P: 15–25 μg/mL; T: <10 μg/mL	T: >10 μg/mL	2–3 h	15 h	4	Renal
Chloramphenicol	P: 25 μg/mL; T: <5 μg/mL	P: >25 μg/mL	1.5–5 h	10–15 h*	50–60	Renal†
Gentamicin	P: 4–10 μg/mL; T: <2 μg/mL	T: >2 μg/mL	2–3 h	15 h	10	Renal
Tobramycin	P: 4–10 μg/mL; T: <2 μg/mL	T: >2 μg/mL	2–3 h	15 h	10	Renal
Vancomycin	P: 20–40 μg/mL; T: 5–10 μg/mL	P: >80 μg/mL	4 h	24 h	55	Renal

P = peak, T = trough.
*Varies substantially with age.
†Hepatic inactivation very important.

Table C. Class of Drug — Cardiac Drugs

Name of Drug	Therapeutic Range	Toxic Level	Half-Life	Time to Sample	Protein Binding %	Active Metabolites	Route of Excretion	Major Drug Interactions
Digitoxin	20–35 ng/mL	>35 ng/mL	>30 h		88	Digoxin	Hepatic	
Digoxin	1–2 ng/mL	>2 ng/mL	>30 h	5 d	20–30		Renal	Quinidine
Disopyramide	2–5 μg/mL	>7 μg/mL	5–6 h	30 h	30–70	N-desisopropyl	Renal	
Lidocaine	2–5 μg/mL	>6 μg/mL	2 h	5–10 h	40–60	MEGX	Hepatic	Phenobarbital
Procainamide	4–10 μg/mL	>20 μg/mL	2 h	20 h	10–20	N-acetylprocainamide	Renal	
Propranolol	50–100 ng/mL	>1000 ng/mL	2–6 h	30 h	90	4-Hydroxy-	Hepatic	
Quinidine	2–5 μg/mL	>8 μg/mL	4–7 h	24 h	90	3-Hydroxy-	Hepatic	Digitalis

TRACE ELEMENTS

Glen R. Willie, MD

Knowledge of trace elements in human toxicity, nutrition, and trace element-related disease states has lagged behind similar knowledge in veterinary medicine, but there have recently been substantial advances.

All trace elements are toxic if given in excessive amounts, and some metals such as thallium, lead, mercury, and arsenic are classically known as "heavy metals" and are covered in the chapter, "Therapeutic Drug Monitoring/Toxicology/Drugs of Abuse." Other elements have major additional aspects of clinical interest and are included in this chapter, drawn together by the common thread of either heir being essential to human health or by the need to monitor them on a regular basis in certain clinical situations (aluminum: patients with chronic renal failure with potential aluminum exposure).

Many essential trace elements have specific binding proteins, and all bind nonspecifically to various serum proteins. Knowledge of these binding characteristics is often essential to properly interpret trace element analyses.

Acknowledgment is given for helpful advice from Phillip H. Stoltenberg, MD,[1] for review of the entries for serum copper and urine copper; and to H. Ray Adams, PhD[2] and Edward D. Harris, PhD,[3] for review of the entire chapter.

Blood Collection Methods for Trace Elements

Since at least 1971, reports have appeared detailing trace metal contamination or alteration of blood and serum samples by blood collection needles, syringes, and vacuum tubes. Problems have included the leaching of chromium or manganese from metal needles; the contamination of the sample by the glass or the rubber parts of syringes or by the rubber stopper; or the adsorption with time of selenium or lead onto ordinary glass blood tubes, leading to falsely low levels for these elements.

Because of these problems, the gold-standard method that evolved was to:

- draw the sample through a plastic catheter preplaced in the vein
- use a syringe (acid-leached, all plastic) that allowed centrifugation in the syringe, or transfer of the blood to a plastic centrifuge tube, and
- transfer or store serum sample or blood in a special acid-leached plastic vial

Although these methods provide reliable results, they are sufficiently cumbersome for clinical practice that alternative methods have been sought.

---

[1] Phillip H. Stoltenberg, MD, Associate Professor of Medicine, Chief of Endoscopy, Division of Gastroenterology, Texas A&M University Health Science Center College of Medicine, Scott & White Clinic, and Memorial Hospital, Temple, Texas.

[2] H. Ray Adams, PhD, Chief of General Chemistry and Toxicology, Department of Pathology, Texas A&M University Health Science Center College of Medicine, Scott & White Clinic, and Memorial Hospital, Temple, Texas.

[3] Edward D. Harris, PhD, Professor of Biochemistry and Biophysics, Texas A&M University, Bryan-College Station, Texas.

For several years, Becton Dickinson has marketed a "trace metal" royal blue top tube which has been found satisfactory for most analyses, **but not for chromium, manganese, aluminum, and selenium**. Recently, Sherwood Medical Company has marketed a trace metal evacuated blood collection tube that, for clinical purposes, has been found satisfactory for aluminum, arsenic, cadmium, copper, chromium, iron, lead, magnesium, manganese, mercury, selenium, and zinc. Although slight alterations in lead, aluminum, and manganese were noted over a 24-hour period of time of contact, these tubes appear satisfactory for usual clinical practice where brief contact time is anticipated, and are recommended for these analyses.

Specifically, if using a vacuum device for drawing blood, we recommend the BD #5175 20-gauge stainless steel needle and a Sherwood Monoject™ trace element blood collection tube, #8881-307006, as a clot tube for serum or #8881-307022 EDTA tube for whole blood. If several tubes of blood are to be drawn together, draw all trace metal tubes first so as not to contaminate the needle by puncture of the ordinary Vacutainer® stoppers. (Vacutainer® rubber stoppers are heavily contaminated by several trace metals.)

If a "butterfly" type needle is needed for a difficult venipuncture, Terumo or Abbot butterfly needles have been found not to contribute trace metals to the sample.

Not reliable are ordinary "red top" clot tubes or the use of needles with metal hubs or syringes with rubber plungers. Directions for obtaining blood samples are briefly summarized for each specific test.

References

Moody JR and Lindstrom RM, "Selection and Cleaning of Plastic Containers for Storage of Trace Element Samples," *Anal Chem*, 1977, 49:2264-7.

Moyer TP, Mussmann GV, and Nixon DE, "Blood-Collection Device for Trace and Ultra-Trace Metal Specimens Evaluated," *Clin Chem*, 1991, 37:709-14.

Pragay DA, Howard SF, and Chilcote ME, "Inorganic Ion Contamination in Vacutainer® Tubes and Micropipets Used for Blood Collection," *Clin Chem*, 1971, 17:350-1.

Aluminum, Bone

CPT 82108

Related Information

Aluminum, Serum *on next page*
Calcium, Serum *on page 160*
Desferrioxamine Infusion Test *on page 1028*
Histopathology *on page 57*

Applies to Histomorphometry

Test Commonly Includes Aluminum measured on anterior iliac crest bone biopsy specimen

Patient Care PREPARATION: Tetracycline and Declomycin® fluoresce differently under ultraviolet light and can be separately distinguished under the microscope so as to indicate the amount of bone formed between the two tetracycline labels. Tetracycline and Declomycin® should be taken between meals, and all antacids (such as Maalox®, Gelusil®, Amphojel®, Basaljel®, Tums®, Os-Cal®, Citracal®, PhosLo®, Phos-Ex®) should be avoided on the days when these labels are taken. Days 1, 2 (2 days): tetracycline 500 mg twice daily, midmorning and midafternoon, days 3-12: no tetracycline; days 13, 14, 15, 16 (4 days): Declomycin® 300 mg twice daily, midmorning and midafternoon; days 17, 18 (2 days): no tetracycline; day 19, 20, or 21: do bone biopsy. The exact time should be recorded and submitted with the specimen to facilitate interpretation.

Specimen The patient's skeleton is prelabeled with tetracycline (see below). The day of the biopsy is critical to standardize the time between tetracycline labels (which appear fluorescent in the bone) and the day of biopsy. The biopsy specimen is a 0.8 cm diameter core of bone taken under local or general anesthesia from the anterior iliac crest in a standardized fashion with a hollow bone biopsy instrument so as to obtain both layers of cancellous bone as well as the internal trabecular bone. CONTAINER: Acid-washed plastic vial containing 95% ethanol. (**The surgeon should be requested not to fix the specimen in formalin**.) SPECIAL INSTRUCTIONS: Bone aluminum is usually measured in concert with bone histomorphometry and is performed by prearrangement with a reference laboratory specializing in bone histomorphometry. These instructions assume bone histomorphometry will also be performed in parallel with bone aluminum determination.

Interpretive REFERENCE RANGE: Bone aluminum: <15 μg/g dry weight[1] (see figure) .

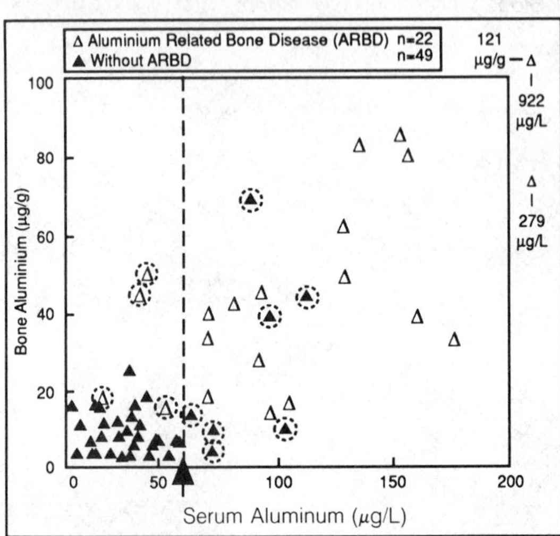

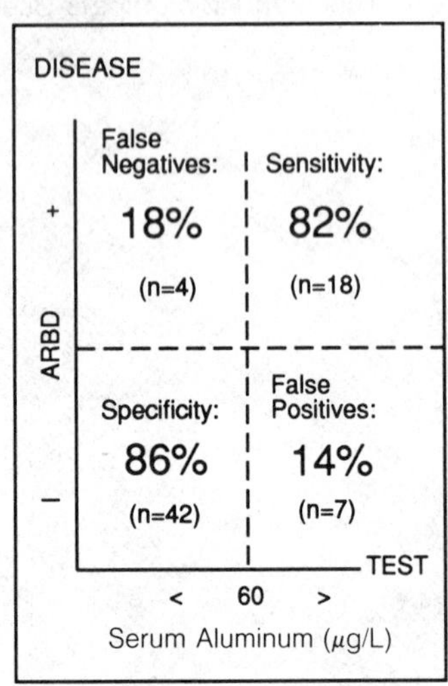

Relationship between serum aluminum, bone aluminum, and ARBD. The sensitivity and specificity of a serum aluminum value of 60 μg/L (↑) in the detection of ARBD is illustrated. ▲ without ARBD; Δ with ARBD as diagnosed by histochemistry, histology, and bulk analysis; (▲) false-positives; (Δ) false-negatives.

Bone aluminum relates to total body burden of aluminum, whereas **serum aluminum** may be only recently elevated in heavy exposure and may not correlate with aluminum related bone disease (ARBD).

Histomorphometry:[2]

- Trabecular bone: 3% unmineralized, 97% mineralized
- Osteoid covers 25% bone surface, lined with osteoblasts
- Osteoclasts 4% of trabecular surface

Variations from normal histomorphometry are interpreted by the pathologist as compatible with pure osteitis fibrosa, pure osteomalacia, aplastic bone disease, or mixed bone disease. The measured distance between the two tetracycline labels allows calculation of bone formation rate, which is reduced in aluminum related bone disease. Many feel that an aluminum stain, however, is most specific for aluminum related bone disease if the aluminum is detected on the mineralization front, blocking calcium deposition and resulting in osteomalacia.[3] The rate of bone formation has been found to be inversely related to the amount of aluminum present.[4]

USE: Diagnose or confirm aluminum related bone disease in patients with renal failure (with or without dialysis) or receiving parenteral nutrition. Aluminum bone disease is much less of a clinical problem recently as nutritional products for intravenous use are more pure. Intravenous albumin products may still be a significant source of aluminum. Patients with aluminum related bone disease may have coexisting other types of bone disease from hyperparathyroidism or osteomalacia related to lack of vitamin D. **LIMITATIONS:** Histomorphometry does not always correlate with total bone aluminum content. Secondary hyperparathyroidism relatively protects from clinical aluminum bone disease, despite the presence of substantial aluminum stored in bone. Stainable aluminum at the osteoid mineralization front is taken by some authors as most sensitive for aluminum bone disease, but this is present in many aluminum exposed patients who are without symptoms. Bone aluminum correlates best with aluminum bone disease, but not as well with aluminum related microcytic anemia or encephalopathy, other forms of aluminum toxicity. **CONTRAINDICATIONS:** Bone biopsy should be done with caution in the presence of a coagulopathy; history of allergy to tetracyclines precludes tetracycline labeling. **METHODOLOGY:** Atomic absorption (AA), graphite furnace flameless atomic absorption **ADDITIONAL INFORMATION:** Aluminum interferes with normal bone formation by several mechanisms including direct reduction of osteoblast function and population; reduction of parathyroid hormone (PTH) release, thereby down-regulating bone turnover; and in the presence of citrate, direct inhibition of calcium phosphate crystal growth. Bone serves as a major store of aluminum, and aluminum from bone can be released back to the blood and other tissues during stress, illness, hyperthyroidism, or failed renal transplant, precipitating aluminum encephalopathy.

Footnotes

1. D'Haese PC, Clement JP, Elseviers MM, et al, "Value of Serum Aluminum Monitoring in Dialysis Patients: A Multicentre Study," *Nephrol Dial Transplant*, 1990, 5(11):45-53.
2. Visser WJ and Van de Vyver FL, "Aluminum-Induced Osteomalacia in Severe Chronic Renal Failure (SCRF)," *Clin Nephrol*, 1985, 24(1 Suppl):S30-6.
3. McCarthy JT, Kurtz SB, and McCall JT, "Elevated Bone Aluminum Content in Dialysis Patients Without Osteomalacia," *Mayo Clin Proc*, 1985, 60:315-20.
4. Ott SM, Maloney NA, Coburn JW, et al, "The Prevalence of Bone Aluminum Deposition in Renal Osteodystrophy and Its Relation to the Response to Calcitriol Therapy," *N Engl J Med*, 1982, 307:709-13.

References

Wills MR and Savory J, "Aluminum and Chronic Renal Failure: Sources, Absorption, Transport, and Toxicity," *Crit Rev Clin Lab Sci*, 1989, 27(1):59-107.

Aluminum, Serum

***CPT** 82108*

Related Information

Aluminum, Bone *on previous page*
Calcium, Serum *on page 160*
Desferrioxamine Infusion Test *on page 1028*
Heavy Metal Screen, Blood *on page 972*
Heavy Metal Screen, Urine *on page 973*
Red Blood Cell Indices *on page 592*

Specimen Serum, dialysis fluid, urine, cerebrospinal fluid **CONTAINER:** Special metal-free Sherwood Monoject™ trace element blood collection tube #8881-307006 for serum separation; acid-washed plastic vials for other samples. See introduction to this chapter. **COLLECTION:** Use B-D #5175 20-gauge stainless steel needle, or Terumo or Abbot butterfly needle. Draw any trace metal tube prior to any other type of blood sample to prevent contamination of needle

(Continued)

Aluminum, Serum *(Continued)*

by regular rubber stoppers. **CAUSES FOR REJECTION:** Contamination by aluminum contact, dust, or ordinary collection tubes or stoppers. Urine must not be contaminated by stool. **TURNAROUND TIME:** Samples are usually sent to a reference laboratory. **SPECIAL INSTRUCTIONS:** The patient should take no aluminum containing antacids or medicines (such as Basaljel®, Gelusil®, Maalox®, Amphojel®, Sucralfate) for 24 hours prior to blood test.

Interpretive **REFERENCE RANGE:** Serum (normal patient): 0-6 ng/mL (SI: 0-0.22 μmol/L) (may vary with laboratory); serum (dialysis patients): up to 40 ng/mL (SI: <1.48 μmol/L) without apparent acute effects, >100 ng/mL (SI: >3.7 μmol/L) possible CNS toxicity, >200 ng/mL (SI: >7.4 μmol/L) probable multisystem toxicity; urine: 0-32 ng/day (SI: 0-1.2 μmol/day); dialysate: <0.01 mg/L (AAMI standards)[1] **USE:** Monitor patients for prior and ongoing exposure to aluminum. Patients at risk include:

- infants on parenteral fluids, particularly parenteral nutrition
- burn patients through administration of intravenous albumin, particularly with coexisting renal failure
- adult and pediatric patients with chronic renal failure, who accumulate aluminum readily from medications and dialysate
- adult parenteral nutrition patients (less so, recently)
- patients with industrial exposure

Monitor dialysate and water to prepare dialysate to prevent aluminum toxicity in dialysis patients. Research use: investigation of amyotrophic lateral sclerosis (in Guam) and Alzheimer's disease.

LIMITATIONS: Serum levels rise and fall after each dose of aluminum-containing phosphate binder or sucralfate. If renal function is normal, renal clearance of aluminum is prompt with urine levels rising quickly after a course of aluminum-containing antacid is begun and elevated levels persisting for over a week. Urine levels rise after a dose of desferrioxamine given for any reason. The degree of rise in serum aluminum after desferrioxamine is regarded as reflecting total body aluminum burden (see Desferrioxamine Infusion test). **METHODOLOGY:** Atomic absorption (AA), inductively coupled plasma atomic emission spectrometry **ADDITIONAL INFORMATION:** Aluminum toxicity has been recognized in many settings where exposure is heavy or prolonged, where renal function is limited, or where a previously accumulated bone burden is released in stress or illness. Toxicity may include:

- encephalopathy (stuttering, gait disturbance, myoclonic jerks, seizures, coma, abnormal EEG)
- osteomalacia or aplastic bone disease (associated with painful spontaneous fractures, hypercalcemia, tumorous calcinosis)
- proximal myopathy
- increased risk of infection
- increased left ventricular mass and decreased myocardial function
- microcytic anemia
- with very high levels, sudden death

Aluminum is ubiquitous in our environment; it is the third most prevalent element in the earth's crust. The gastrointestinal tract is relatively impervious to aluminum, absorption normally being only about 2%. Aluminum is absorbed by a mechanism related to that for calcium. Gastric acidity and oral citrate favors absorption, and H_2-blockers reduce absorption. As is true for several trace elements, transferrin is the primary protein binder and carrier for aluminum in the plasma, where 80% is protein bound and 20% is free or complexed to small molecules such as citrate. Cells appear to take up aluminum from transferrin rather than from citrate. Purified preparations of ferritin from brain and liver have been found to contain aluminum. It is not known if ferritin has a specific binding site for aluminum. Factors regulating the migration of aluminum across the blood-brain barrier are not well understood. Serum aluminum correlates with encephalopathy; red cell aluminum correlates with microcytic anemia;[2] and bone aluminum correlates with aluminum bone disease. Basal PTH when elevated appears to protect bone and thereby favor CNS toxicity. Other factors favoring one form of toxicity over another are not well understood. Aluminum toxicity has been reported to impair the formation and release of parathyroid hormone. The parathyroid glands concentrate aluminum above levels in surrounding tissues. Treatment of aluminum toxicity in renal failure patients often reactivates hyperparathyroidism, which to a certain extent is helpful for bone remodeling and healing.

Footnotes

1. Recommended Maximum Promulgated by the Association for Advancement of Medical Instrumentation, 1990, 33330 Washington Blvd, Suite 400, Arlington, VA 22201.

2. Abreo K, Brown ST, Sella M, et al, "Application of An Erythrocyte Aluminum Assay in the Diagnosis of Aluminum-Associated Microcytic Anemia in Patients Undergoing Dialysis and Response to Deferoxamine Therapy," *J Lab Clin Med*, 1989, 113(1):50-7.

References

Alfrey AC, LeGendre GR, and Kaehny WD, "The Dialysis Encephalopathy Syndrome: Possible Aluminum Intoxication," *N Engl J Med*, 1976, 294:184-8.

Chappuis P, Poupon J, and Rousselet F, "A Sequential and Simple Determination of Zinc, Copper, and Aluminum in Blood Samples by Inductively Coupled Plasma Atomic Emission Spectrometry," *Clin Chim Acta*, 1992, 206(3):155-65.

Ellenberg R, King AL, Sica DA, et al, "Cerebrospinal Fluid Aluminum Levels Following Deferoxamine," *Am J Kidney Dis*, 1990, 16(2):157-9.

Gruskin AB, "Aluminum: A Pediatric Overview," *Adv Pediatr*, 1988, 35:281-330.

Klein GL, "Aluminum in Parenteral Products: Medical Perspective on Large and Small Volume Parenterals," *J Parenter Sci Technol*, 1989, 43(3):120-4.

Monteagudo FS, Cassidy MJ, and Folb PI, "Recent Developments in Aluminum Toxicology," *Med Toxical Adverse Drug Exp*, 1989, 4(1):1-16.

Tzamaloukas AH, "Diagnosis and Management of Bone Disorders in Chronic Renal Failure and Dialyzed Patients," *Med Clin North Am*, 1990, 74(4):961-74.

Wills MR and Savory J, "Aluminum and Chronic Renal Failure: Sources, Absorption, Transport, and Toxicity," *Crit Rev Clin Lab Sci*, 1989, 27(1):59-107.

Chromium, Serum

CPT *82495*

Related Information

Heavy Metal Screen, Blood *on page 972*

Heavy Metal Screen, Urine *on page 973*

Synonyms Cr, Serum

Abstract Determination of the amount of chromium in the serum or urine of normal persons is extremely difficult, due to the very low levels present. Levels observed are in the 0.1 ng/mL range, equivalent to one part in 10 billion. Extreme caution must be taken to avoid contamination by dust (from skin, leather, cloth) and contact with steel (which contains chromium). Chromium is felt to be an essential element in the human, with chromium III purported to be an integral part of "glucose tolerance factor," a partially characterized complex that has been suggested to contain two molecules of nicotinic acid and a small oligopeptide complexed to chromium III. This organic moiety is thought necessary for insulin action on the cell surface. Deficiency of chromium can cause an acquired insulin resistance or diabetes mellitus with associated hyperlipidemia in otherwise well-nourished patients. The classic cases, however, were reported prior to the availability of accurate serum levels of chromium, and reported levels then in "deficiency" were tenfold or more higher than we now know to be "normal". Chromium deficiency with associated glucose intolerance and fasting hypoglycemia has been most often observed during refeeding of malnourished individuals after famine starvation in relief programs. In infants, one or more oral doses of chromium, 250 μg, have been curative. Chromium deficiency with associated glucose intolerance has also been observed in long-term parenteral nutrition when inadequate chromium was included.[1] Neuropathy, encephalopathy, and abnormalities of amino acid profile (serum low in branched-chain amino acids and high in aromatic amino acids) have been noted in conjunction with this condition.[2]

With regard to toxicity, pure metallic chromium is nontoxic. Chromium III is poorly absorbed, and much less toxic than chromium VI. Industrial monitoring for toxicity in the past has relied on air samples largely for total and hexavalent chromium, the major species of concern. Workers are potentially exposed in tanneries, mines, and industries for metal plating, welding, photography, paint, dye, and explosives. Skin exposure may lead to dermatitis, and respiratory exposure to bronchitis, asthma, and lung cancer. Hair contains 1000-fold more chromium than serum or urine, and hair chromium content does correlate with industrial exposure, but more data are needed before hair chromium monitoring can replace industrial air monitoring and samples of blood and urine in cases of suspected toxicity[3] or deficiency. Acute systemic chromate toxicity may cause acute tubular necrosis, acute hepatitis, convulsions, and coma. Acute respiratory or gastrointestinal symptoms relate to the locus of absorption. Intermediate levels of long-term exposure may cause tubular proteinuria in industrial workers.[4]

Chromium supplementation has been shown by some workers to improve glucose tolerance and improve insulin efficiency in glucose intolerant (but not in normal or overtly diabetic) patients on diets equivalent to the lower quartile of ordinary chromium intake in the United States.[5] The implication is that many individuals in the U.S. population have a marginal chro-

(Continued)

Chromium, Serum *(Continued)*

mium intake. We may, therefore, anticipate increased self-medication and supplementation in the future, and greater medical interest in this trace metal. The literature regarding chromium was for many years confused due to difficulties with analysis and contamination. Much old work needs to be repeated, and this field is still very much in flux.

Patient Care **PREPARATION:** The patient should be fasting for basal level.

Specimen Serum **CONTAINER:** Special metal-free, Sherwood Monoject™ trace element blood collection tube #8881-307006. See the introduction to this chapter. **SAMPLING TIME:** In the nocturnal total parenteral nutrition patient, the sample will be drawn "fasting" in the afternoon, before the nocturnal solution is started for the evening. **COLLECTION:** Follow specific instructions of laboratory to which sample will be submitted. Contact with steel, dust, ordinary glassware, or plastic is to be avoided. Draw blood through indwelling plastic intracath needle. Some siliconized stainless steel needles have also been found to be acceptable as is the B-D #5175 20-gauge stainless steel needle, or the Terumro or Abott butterfly needles. Draw trace metal sample prior to any other blood samples. Remove serum with an all-plastic pipette (no internal metal parts) and store serum in plastic vial. Leeching plastic containers in 10% nitric acid for 48 hours removes trace metal contamination if special purpose vials are not available. The containers are then rinsed three times with twice distilled water and air dried in a dust-free environment prior to use. **STORAGE INSTRUCTIONS:** Some reference laboratories request specimens to be frozen and sent on dry ice. **CAUSES FOR REJECTION:** Improper collection or storage with contact by steel, dust, or ordinary Vacutainer® tubes **TURNAROUND TIME:** Samples are usually sent to a reference laboratory.

Interpretive **REFERENCE RANGE:** 0.05-0.15 ng/mL (SI: 1-3 nmol/L).[6] Some laboratories report much higher "normals" because the methods they use or the collection technique is not adequate to prevent substantial contamination. If a laboratory reports "<1 ng/mL" or some similar figure without a lower level for normal, the value can be relied upon to discover toxic states, perhaps, but not deficiency states. Serum levels of 10 ng/mL correspond to short-term atmospheric exposure limit of 0.1 mg/m^3 of chromium trioxide.[7] Serum levels even higher would be expected in acute systemic toxicity. Almost a twofold diurnal variation is noted in serum chromium levels, with the level highest in the morning and falling after each meal as insulin levels rise. Serum chromium levels are about 60% of normal in diabetic patients, which overlaps the normal range. **USE:** Evaluate suspected chromium toxicity or exposure; follow patients receiving chromium in their parenteral nutrition; evaluate acquired glucose intolerance in refeeding programs, or in parenteral or enteral nutrition; evaluate insulin resistance in the nonseptic patient during parenteral nutrition **LIMITATIONS:** Extreme attention to detail is needed to achieve reliable results; for many laboratories even now a high serum level more often reflects sample contamination rather than excess chromium exposure. **METHODOLOGY:** Any reported levels in biological materials prior to about 1979 are suspect, as the available methods did not have the sensitivity to separate normal values from the "blank." Reported levels were tenfold or more too high. Accurate and independently verified values have been reported with:

- stable isotope dilution, isotope ratio mass spectroscopy
- graphite furnace atomic absorption spectroscopy

All pipettes must have plastic tips and no exposed internal metal parts. Work is done in the laboratory under a laminar flow class 100 work station, free from exposed stainless steel to avoid airborne contamination. This is essential to reduce contamination sufficiently to detect "normal levels" in human serum or urine. Even with these precautions, different laboratories report different normal values.

ADDITIONAL INFORMATION: Iron competitively inhibits the binding of chromium III to transferrin. Iron overloaded patients with hemochromatosis poorly retain a radioactive tracer dose of chromium III. It has been suggested that chromium deficiency at a cellular level may play a role in the development of diabetes in hemochromatosis.[8]

Footnotes

1. Jeejecbhoy KN, Chu RC, Marliss EB, et al, "Chromium Deficiency, Glucose Intolerance, and Neuropathy Reversed by Chromium Supplementation, in a Patient Receiving Long-Term Total Parenteral Nutrition," *Am J Clin Nutr*, 1977, 30:531-8.
2. Freund H, Atamian S, and Fischer JE, "Chromium Deficiency During Total Parenteral Nutrition," *JAMA*, 1979, 241:496-8.
3. Randall JA and Gibson RS, "Hair Chromium as an Index of Chromium Exposure of Tannery Workers," *Br J Ind Med*, 1989, 46(3):171-5.
4. Wedeen RP and Qian L, "Chromium-Induced Kidney Disease," *Environ Health Perspect*, 1991, 92:71-4.
5. Anderson RA, Polansky MM, Bryden NA, et al, "Supplemental-Chromium Effects on Glucose, Insulin, Glucagon, and Urinary Chromium Losses in Subjects Consuming Controlled Low-Chromium Diets," *Am J Clin Nutr*, 1991, 54(5):909-16.

6. Chappuis P, Poupon J, Deschamps JF, et al, "Physiological Chromium Determination in Serum by Zeeman Graphite Furnace Atomic Absorption Spectrometry. A Serious Challenge," *Biol Trace Elem Res*, 1992, 32:85-91.
7. Baruthio F, "Toxic Effects of Chromium and Its Compounds," *Biol Trace Elem Res*, 1992, 32:145-53.
8. Sargent T, Lim TH, and Jenson RL, "Reduced Chromium Retention in Patients With Hemochromatosis, A Possible Basis of Hemochromatotic Diabetes," *Metabolism*, 1979, 28:70-9.

References

Brown RO, Forloines-Lynn S, Cross RE, et al, "Chromium Deficiency After Long-Term Total Parenteral Nutrition," *Dig Dis Sci*, 1986, 31:661-4.

Hopkins LL Jr, Ransome-Kuti O, and Majaj AS, "Improvement of Impaired Carbohydrate Metabolism by Chromium (III) in Malnourished Infants," *Am J Clin Nutr*, 1968, 21:203-11.

Morris BW, Blumsohn A, Mac Neil S, et al, "The Trace Element Chromium – A Role in Glucose Homeostasis," *Am J Clin Nutr*, 1992, 55(5):989-91.

Schermaier AJ, O'Connor LH, and Pearson KH, "Semiautomated Determination of Chromium in Whole Blood and Serum by Zeeman Electrothermal Atomic Absorption Spectrophotometry," *Clin Chim Acta*, 1985, 152:123-34.

Veillon C, "Chromium," *Methods Enzymol*, 1988, 158:334-43.

Chromium, Urine

CPT 82495

Related Information

Heavy Metal Screen, Blood *on page 972*
Heavy Metal Screen, Urine *on page 973*
Urine Collection, 24-Hour *on page 32*

Synonyms Cr, Urine

Abstract Urine chromium levels are extremely low, and until recently, not reliable. Urine chromium assay is used to look for chromium toxicity in cases of potential exposure. As testing becomes more reliable, new applications of the test will arise to determine chromium III nutritional adequacy or deficiency states. There are also potential uses in the follow-up of patients with mild glucose intolerance. See listing, Chromium, Serum for signs and symptoms of toxicity and deficiency states, and for additional references.

Specimen 24-hour urine **CONTAINER:** Plastic metal-free container. To prepare, leech 48 hours in 10% nitric acid and wash with distilled water that has had no contact with metal. Dry in quiet air in a metal-free environment. **COLLECTION:** Care must be taken to avoid contact with metal. Use plastic urinal, prepared as above. Stool contamination must be avoided. **CAUSES FOR REJECTION:** Improper collection, contact with metal, ordinary containers, or stool contamination

Interpretive **REFERENCE RANGE:** <1 μg/24 hours[1]. Levels vary with the laboratory and have declined with improved methods of avoiding contamination. Levels two- to threefold above this may reflect supplementation or excess losses. Levels elevated tenfold and higher have been seen in exposed asymptomatic tannery workers. Spot levels of chromium in urine of 30 ng/g creatinine correspond to the short-term atmospheric exposure limit of 0.1 mg/m^3 of chromium trioxide in industrial exposure situations.[2] **USE:** Evaluate industrial exposure, suspected toxicity; or in conjunction with serum levels, to attempt to detect suspected chromium deficiency, especially in a recent onset of glucose intolerance **LIMITATIONS:** Levels are so low in normal people (on the order of one part in 10 billion in urine) that many laboratories are not able to detect the lower limit of normal, and thus report "less than" some set level as being normal. Thus, for many laboratories, the test can only be used to detect toxicity. Contamination of the specimen may result in a tenfold or more increase in urine concentration being reported, making potential contamination the major limiting factor in the test. **METHODOLOGY:** Atomic absorption (AA) or neutron activation **ADDITIONAL INFORMATION:** The main excretory pathway for chromium III is renal. Estimated safe and adequate, oral intake recommended by the U.S. National Academy of Sciences range from 50-200 μg/day,[3] but in the U.S. 90% of people eat less, the mean intake being 25-33 μg/day. Such intake recommendations likely derive from the 1980s when average estimated intake was determined to be 50-100 μg/day. With increasingly accurate assays, new recommended ranges may be set lower. Absorption of chromium III is on the order of 0.5%, by radioisotope studies. One hospital pharmacy supplies 12 μg of chromium from MTE5® trace mineral parenteral nutrition supplement per day. We are unaware of a large survey.

As improved methods have progressively reduced the lower level of detection, urine chromium levels have been found to be related to glucose metabolism. Recent studies[4] have demonstrated the metabolic relationships between serum insulin, serum glucose, and serum chromium III in the fasting and postprandial states and the relationship of the postprandial state to

(Continued)

Chromium, Urine *(Continued)*

urine chromium concentration. Briefly, diabetic patients lose threefold more chromium in the urine than nondiabetics, and despite increased intestinal absorption, diabetic patients on ordinary diets develop and maintain lower serum levels. Chromium loss is not specifically related to micro- or macroalbuminuria and precedes the onset of diabetic nephropathy. Urine chromium rises threefold 40 minutes after a carbohydrate meal and more so with carbohydrates that stimulate higher insulin levels. Serum levels fall after a meal, more so than can be explained by urine loss. Thus, glucose stimulates insulin to take chromium to a cellular location, which favors increased renal excretion.

Footnotes

1. Jacob RA, "Trace Elements," *Textbook of Clinical Chemistry*, Tietz NA, ed, Philadelphia, PA: WB Saunders Co, 1986, 965-96.
2. Baruthio F, "Toxic Effects of Chromium and Its Compounds," *Biol Trace Elem Res*, 1992, 32:145-53.
3. National Research Council, *Recommended Dietary Allowances*, 10th ed, National Academy of Sciences.
4. Morris BW, Blumsohn A, Mac Neil S, et al, "The Trace Element Chromium – A Role in Glucose Homeostasis," *Am J Clin Nutr*, 1992, 55(5):989-91.

Copper, Serum

CPT *82525*

Related Information

Ceruloplasmin *on page 180*
Copper, Urine *on page 1027*
Heavy Metal Screen, Blood *on page 972*
Heavy Metal Screen, Urine *on page 973*

Synonyms Cu, Serum

Applies to Metallothiomein; Transcuprein

Abstract Copper is an essential trace element in human nutrition and a component of many metalloenzymes including:

- cytochrome C oxidase
- superoxide dismutase
- tyrosinase
- dopamine-β-hydroxylase
- lysyl oxidase
- clotting factor V
- an unknown enzyme that crosslinks keratin in hair
- ceruloplasmin, a ferroxidase in serum which also seems to serve as a major transport protein for copper

Inorganic copper is very reactive and therefore a cellular toxin. Its metabolism is complicated. Copper is absorbed in the stomach and duodenum by a process regulated by the metallothionein concentration in intestinal mucosal cells. The more metallothionein present, the more copper is trapped in the mucosal cell and is sloughed into the gastrointestinal lumen to be lost in the stool unabsorbed. Thus, copper absorption is partially self-limiting.

Tissue levels of metallothionein are induced by either copper or zinc. Zinc is more poorly bound by metallothionein than copper, but zinc is the better inducing agent; so, small excesses of zinc in the food stream markedly inhibit copper absorption by stimulating high levels of metallothionein. Cadmium and iron can also inhibit copper absorption, possibly through a similar mechanism. Molybdenum decreases absorption by forming insoluble copper-molybdenum-sulfur compounds. In ruminants, this interaction is an important cause of copper deficiency, which is economically important. This interaction has been used to advantage in detoxification of certain patients with Wilson's disease.

After absorption, copper appears to be initially transported, partly by loose binding to albumin and probably as copper-histidine, and carried to the liver and other organs, where the copper is taken up by membrane-bound ligands and transferred into cells. Linder has isolated a 270,000 dalton protein ("transcuprein") which may also serve to transport copper from the intestine to the liver. In the liver, copper is used to synthesize ceruloplasmin, which, in a few hours, appears in the blood stream containing six atoms of copper per molecule. The transport to various organs depends on the amount of copper in the blood that is incorporated into ceruloplasmin as opposed to that loosely bound to histidine or albumin. About 65% of the copper in peripheral blood is in the form of ceruloplasmin – earlier estimates had been much higher.

Copper is stored in the liver and secreted in the bile. Biliary excretion increases when copper stores are plentiful. Copper has an enterohepatic circulation, but that amount of copper secreted in the bile formed in ceruloplasmin fragments resists digestion and is carried out in the stool, little reabsorbed by the more distal small bowel. Renal tubular reabsorption of filtered copper is efficient, so normally only a small fraction of copper is lost in the urine. Abnormal urine losses occur in burns, I.V. administration of amino acids, Menkes' syndrome, Wilson's disease, and with chelating drugs.

This complicated metabolic pathway explains many features of known human diseases involving copper. Oral zinc administration inhibits absorption of copper and may cause copper deficiency states. Oral zinc can be used to treat copper excess states including Wilson's disease[1] or can inadvertently cause copper deficiency[2] by stimulating excess metallothionein synthesis. Even after oral zinc therapy is discontinued, high total body zinc stores continue to block oral copper absorption through the metallothionein mechanism. Failure of ceruloplasmin synthesis (Wilson's disease) leads to higher free and loosely albumin-bound copper which abnormally deposits copper in and damages brain tissue. The reduced ceruloplasmin synthesis simultaneously decreases biliary excretion of copper[3] and thereby leads to excess hepatic copper which is stored in and damages the liver. In a later acute hepatitis syndrome, the liver can release so much copper to the blood (unbound to ceruloplasmin) that acute red blood cell hemolysis and acute renal failure may result.

Copper deficiency causes markedly reduced ceruloplasmin synthesis rates and blood levels, and a microcytic or normocytic anemia due to blocks in iron metabolism. This anemia fails to respond to oral or I.V. iron, but brisk reticulocytosis follows copper administration. Copper deficiency can cause a scurvy-like bone disease (probably due to lysyl oxidase deficiency), depigmentation (probably due to tyrosinase deficiency), growth failure, and neutropenia.

Menkes' disease is a severe X-linked copper deficiency syndrome of infants which involves copper malabsorption, increased renal copper loss due to failure of renal tubular reabsorption, and abnormal distribution of copper in tissues. Effects are noted in bone, pigmentation, CNS development, growth, and arterial connective tissue, all apparently due to copper deficiency on a cellular level. Oral or I.V. inorganic copper is ineffective in treatment, and the condition is usually fatal, but a recent report[4] of I.V. copper-histidine (plus intermittent penicillamine to prevent copper overload) is encouraging.

Acute copper toxicity causes gastrointestinal irritation or bleeding (locally) and systemically leads to intravascular hemolysis, hepatic and renal tubular necrosis. Chronic copper toxicity, particularly in children, causes Indian childhood cirrhosis (ICC), a potentially fatal liver disease not at all confined to India where it was first described. ICC is predominantly a condition of young boys ages 3-7 years exposed to copper through excess copper in the food or water supply. The copper load has been usually related to the corrosive effects of water in copper pipes (usually from a home well) or, in India, to milk or food boiled in brass vessels.

Ceruloplasmin synthesis is stimulated by copper intake, and ordinarily ceruloplasmin carries about 65% of serum copper. Serum copper and serum ceruloplasmin usually parallel each other in the healthy patient and, therefore, do not provide independent information. Red blood cell copper has a similar value to serum, so hemolysis does not interfere with serum copper determination.

There are at least two situations in which ceruloplasmin may not reflect so closely the total serum copper. In acute copper toxicity, there may not yet have been time for ceruloplasmin synthesis, so free (or loosely bound) copper is elevated, total serum copper may be elevated, and ceruloplasmin may still be normal. In Wilson's disease, with chronic low levels of ceruloplasmin, more copper in serum may be loosely bound and (total) serum copper may even be normal (10% incidence) rather than low. In this situation, it is especially important to measure both total serum copper and ceruloplasmin as an aid to diagnosis. High urine copper is also a feature of Wilson's disease. Because no combination of noninvasive tests has proven 100% sensitive and specific for Wilson's disease, molecular genetics has recently been proposed to aid in diagnosis within families.

Liver tissue copper level remains the gold standard for diagnosis of Wilson's disease, although even this, though sensitive, is not 100% specific. It remains diagnostic in sibships because Wilson's disease is an inherited disorder, and other etiologies of excess liver copper are rarely in the differential diagnosis within a family where one patient has firmly diagnosed Wilson's disease.

Specimen Serum, cerebrospinal fluid, tissue **CONTAINER:** Royal blue top tube which contains no anticoagulant. Alternate is the Sherwood trace metal tube #8881-307006. See introduction (Continued)

Copper, Serum *(Continued)*

to this chapter. **COLLECTION:** Use a stainless steel needle (B-D #5175). Draw tube prior to any other blood samples. After centrifugation, pour serum into a metal-free vial for transport to reference laboratory. CSF can be transferred directly to a royal blue top tube. For liver tissue, follow directions of reference laboratory. **TURNAROUND TIME:** Samples are usually sent to a reference laboratory.

Interpretive **REFERENCE RANGE:** Serum: Approximately 0.7-1.5 μg/mL (SI: 11-24 μmol/L). Mean levels are slightly higher in women and children. There is diurnal variation with peak levels in the morning. Cerebrospinal fluid: 6-35 ng/mL.[5] Levels in CSF are elevated up to threefold in the neurotoxicity of Wilson's disease. Liver tissue: 9-45 ng/g dry weight. Ceruloplasmin levels rise dramatically in the last 2 weeks of pregnancy, and therefore copper levels rise then also. **USE:** It is used, along with serum ceruloplasmin and urine copper to screen for Wilson's disease and more often, in monitoring the nutritional adequacy of parenteral or enteral nutrition, especially when copper deficiency may be suspected because of ongoing gastrointestinal losses of the element (see table). The test is done in suspected copper toxicity in premature infants when they are acutely ill and may not be able to assimilate the copper in their prescribed nutrition; in acute copper intoxications; or in "Indian childhood cirrhosis," an illness not limited to Indian children.[6] Serum copper is low in Menkes' syndrome. Copper in the CSF is reported to mirror the neurotoxicity of copper in Wilson's disease.[5] Liver copper is used to confirm Wilson's disease and Menkes' syndrome and may be measured in liver disease of uncertain etiology. It can confirm ICC in the right setting. Liver copper rises with time in biliary cirrhosis, but does not confirm the diagnosis.

Copper, Serum

	Deficiency, Nutritional	Menkes' Syndrome	Acute Copper Toxicity	ICC and Chronic Copper Toxicity	Wilson's Disease	Smoking, Inflammatory Conditions, Pregnancy, Estrogens
Serum copper	↓	↓	↑, ↑↑	↑	N or ↓	↑, ↑↑
Serum ceruloplasmin	↓	↓	N (early)	↑	Usually ↓; may be N in children	↑, ↑↑
Urine copper	↓	↑	↑	↑	↑, ↑↑	N
CSF copper					N or ↑	N
Liver copper	↓	↓	N (early)	↑, ↑↑	↑↑	N

N = normal, ↑ = increase, ↑↑ = large increase, ↓ = decrease.

LIMITATIONS: Serum ceruloplasmin is an acute-phase reactant type protein, and since it binds a large portion of serum copper, both serum copper and ceruloplasmin increase under the influence of inflammatory conditions and estrogen. Serum copper is therefore elevated in pregnancy, in patients on estrogens and estrogen-containing contraceptive drugs, in rheumatoid arthritis, and a number of other pathologic entities. It may be low with low serum proteins as in nephrosis, malabsorption, and malnutrition without necessarily reflecting inadequate liver copper stores. It is reduced under the influence of ACTH or glucocorticoids, or valproate[7] therapy. Although serum copper levels are usually ordered to work up possible cases of Wilson's disease, Menkes' syndrome, and ICC, serum copper alone is of only limited value. Elevations in liver tissue copper are found in Wilson's disease but may occur also in other types of liver disease, especially primary biliary cirrhosis.[4] **METHODOLOGY:** Atomic absorption (AA), inductively coupled plasma atomic emission spectrometry. **ADDITIONAL INFORMATION:** The demand for sensitive noninvasive tests for Wilson's disease, especially for children in families where the disease is known to occur, has stimulated search for newer indices of copper metabolism. Urine copper after penicillamine load has recently been proposed.[8]

Footnotes

1. Brewer GJ, Hill GM, Dick RD, et al, "Treatment of Wilson's Disease With Zinc: III. Prevention of Reaccumulation of Hepatic Copper," *J Lab Clin Med*, 1987, 109:526-31.
2. Hoffman HN II, Phyliky RL, and Fleming CR, "Zinc-Induced Copper Deficiency," *Gastroenterology*, 1988, 94(2):508-12.
3. Lee HH, Hill GM, Sikha VKN, et al, "Pancreaticobiliary Secretion of Zinc and Copper in Normal Persons and Patients With Wilson's Disease," *J Lab Clin Med*, 1990, 116(3):283-8.

4. Nadal D and Baerlocher K, "Menkes' Disease: Long-Term Treatment With Copper and D-Penicillamine," *Eur J Pediatr*, 1988, 147:621-5.
5. Weisner B, Hartard C, and Dieu C, "CSF Copper Concentration: A New Parameter for Diagnosis and Monitoring Therapy of Wilson's Disease With Cerebral Manifestation," *J Neurol Sci*, 1987, 79:229-37.
6. Weiss M, Müller-Höcker J, Wiebecke B, et al, "First Description of "Indian Childhood Cirrhosis" in A Non-Indian Infant in Europe," *Acta Paediatr Scand*, 1989, 78(1):152-6.
7. Kaji M, Ito M, Okuno T, et al, "Serum Copper and Zinc Levels in Epileptic Children With Valproate Treatment," *Epilepsia*, 1992, 33(3):555-7.
8. Martins da Costa C, Baldwin D, Portmann B, et al, "Value of Urinary Copper Excretion After Penicillamine Challenge in the Diagnosis of Wilson's Disease," *Hepatology*, 1992, 15(4):609-15.

References

"A Unified Hypothesis of Copper Transport and Uptake," *Nutr Rev*, 1988, 46:332-3.
Clayton BE, "Clinical Chemistry of Trace Elements," *Adv Clin Chem*, 1980, 21:147-76.
Danks DM, "Copper Deficiency in Humans," *Annu Rev Nutr*, 1988, 8:235-57.
Danks DM, "Disorders of Copper Transport," *The Metabolic Basis of Inherited Disease*, 6th ed, Scriver CR, Beaudet AL, Sly WS, et al, eds, New York, NY: McGraw-Hill Inc, 1989, 1411-31.
Davidoff GN, Votaw ML, Coon WW, et al, "Elevations in Serum Copper, Erythrocytic Copper, and Ceruloplasmin Concentrations in Smokers," *Am J Clin Pathol*, 1978, 70:790-2.
Pereira GR and Zucker AH, "Nutritional Deficiencies in the Neonate," *Clin Perinatol*, 1986, 13:175-89.
Prasad AS, "Trace Elements: Biochemical and Clinical Effects of Zinc and Copper," *Am J Hematol*, 1979, 6:77-87.
Scheinberg IH, "Wilson's Disease and the Physiological Chemistry of Copper," *Inorg Chem in Biol and Med*, 1980, 21:373-80.
Wachnik A, "The Physiological Role of Copper and the Problems of Copper Nutritional Deficiency," *Die Nahrung*, 1988, 32:755-65.
Youssef AAR, Wood B, and Baron DN, "Serum Copper: A Marker of Disease Activity in Rheumatoid Arthritis," *J Clin Pathol*, 1983, 36:14-7.
Yuzbasiyan-Gurkan V, Johnson V, and Brewer GJ, "Diagnosis and Characterization of Presymptomatic Patients With Wilson's Disease and the Use of Molecular Genetics to Aid in the Diagnosis," *J Lab Clin Med*, 1991, 118(5):458-65.

Copper, Urine

CPT 82525

Related Information

Ceruloplasmin *on page 180*
Copper, Serum *on page 1024*
Heavy Metal Screen, Blood *on page 972*
Heavy Metal Screen, Urine *on page 973*
Urine Collection, 24-Hour *on page 32*

Synonyms Cu, Urine

Abstract Copper is an essential trace element in human nutrition and a component of many metalloenzymes. Urine copper may be used as an aid to detect Wilson's disease, Menkes' syndrome, and chronic or acute copper toxicity.

Patient Care **PREPARATION:** If a bedpan or urinal is necessary for collection, it should be made of plastic. Stool contamination must be avoided.

Specimen 24-hour urine **CONTAINER:** Plastic urine container, no preservative **COLLECTION:** Collect in acid-washed plastic container, preferably polyethylene. Acidify to pH 2 with hydrochloric or nitric acid. **CAUSES FOR REJECTION:** Specimen allowed to contact metal or stool **TURNAROUND TIME:** Samples are usually sent to a reference laboratory.

Interpretive **REFERENCE RANGE:** 15-60 μg/24 hours (SI: 0.22-0.9 μmol/day). See following figure. **USE:** Increased urinary copper is found in Wilson's disease, Menkes' syndrome, and in chronic and acute copper toxicity states including "Indian childhood cirrhosis" (ICC). The test is used to follow the effectiveness of chelation therapy for Wilson's disease, or to check copper balance in patients with Wilson's disease on oral zinc therapy. Copper excretion by the kidneys is abnormally increased with high dose intravenous histidine or mixed amino acids, as in total parenteral nutrition. Captopril and other medications may chelate copper and increase urinary excretion (usually only a tiny fraction of total daily balance). For comparison of urine copper in Wilson's disease sibships, see figure. Over time, biliary cirrhosis leads to copper accumulation, and since biliary excretion is partly blocked, urinary excretion rises and is usually elevated, leading to diagnostic confusion with Wilson's disease. Serum ceruloplasmin and liver biopsy can distinguish these. **LIMITATIONS:** Increased urinary copper excretion may occur in ICC or with chronic active hepatitis; Wilson's disease and chronic active hepatitis may also resemble one another; thus, parameters in addition to urinary copper excretion, such as ceruloplasmin and serum copper, are needed. **METHODOLOGY:** Atomic absorption, inductively coupled plasma atomic emission spectrometry

(Continued)

Copper, Urine *(Continued)*

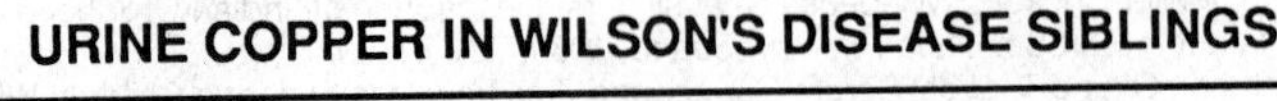

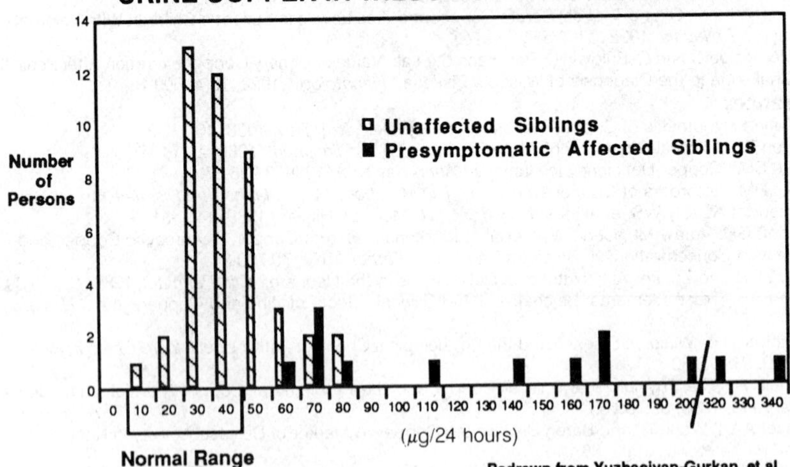

References

Yuzbasiyan-Gurkan V, Johnson V, and Brewer GJ, "Diagnosis and Characterization of Presymptomatic Patients With Wilson's Disease and the Use of Molecular Genetics to Aid in the Diagnosis," *J Lab Clin Med*, 1991, 118(5):458-65.

Cr, Serum *see* Chromium, Serum *on page 1021*

Cr, Urine *see* Chromium, Urine *on page 1023*

Cu, Serum *see* Copper, Serum *on page 1024*

Cu, Urine *see* Copper, Urine *on previous page*

Desferrioxamine Infusion Test

CPT 82108 (plus charge for desferrioxamine administration)

Related Information

Aluminum, Bone *on page 1018*
Aluminum, Serum *on page 1019*

Test Commonly Includes Determination of serum aluminum prior to and 48 hours postinfusion of desferrioxamine

Abstract A controversial test of disputed benefit sometimes used to screen patients with known aluminum exposure who lack diagnostically elevated serum aluminum concentrations

Specimen Serum **CONTAINER:** Special metal-free Sherwood Monoject™ trace element blood collection tube #8881-307006. See introduction to this chapter. **COLLECTION:** Use B-D #5175 20-gauge stainless steel needle, or Terumo or Abbot butterfly needle. Draw any trace metal tubes prior to collecting other blood samples. Serum is separated, and stored or submitted to reference laboratory in special acid-washed plastic vial. **SPECIAL INSTRUCTIONS:** Most patients for whom this test is indicated are on dialysis, and the test is done in conjunction with their dialysis procedure (hemodialysis or peritoneal dialysis). The patient is instructed to stop any aluminum-containing antacids 3 days prior to the test. The first blood sample is obtained, then 0.5 g desferrioxamine is administered in 100 mL 0.9% sodium chloride intravenously during the last 2 hours of dialysis through the venous blood line. Forty-eight hours later, prior to the next hemodialysis, a second blood sample is drawn. The timing is the same for peritoneal dialysis patients, for whom peritoneal dialysis is halted during the 48-hour period.

Interpretive **REFERENCE RANGE:** The test is considered positive if the second sample more than triples the first, or exceeds it by 150 ng/mL (SI: 5.6 μmol/L)[1,2] **CRITICAL VALUES:** Serum levels >200 ng/mL (SI: >7.4 μmol/L) can be associated with development of aluminum neurotoxicity. **USE:** Screen patients with known aluminum exposure and abnormal (but not diagnostically elevated) serum aluminum levels for high body burden of aluminum, which is known to be correlated with aluminum bone disease. Patients with serum aluminum levels ≤75 ng/mL are less likely to benefit from the test[3], and patients with persistent serum aluminum levels >150 ng/mL should probably go directly to bone biopsy for confirmation of bone aluminum burden. **LIMITATIONS:** Use of this test is controversial. Originally proposed as a 2 g desferrioxamine infusion test,[4] complications have been reported, including permanent visual disturbances after a single 2 g dose.[5,6] Due to multiple reported complications (ocular, auditory, anaphylaxis, hematopoietic, infectious) of high dose desferrioxamine therapy for iron overload in thalassemia and for aluminum overload and toxicity in chronic renal failure, therapeutic doses have generally been reduced. The 0.5 g dose infusion test[2] has so far not been reported to cause complications. Some authors endorse the use of an infusion test,[7] others do not. By restricting its use to patients with moderate but not extreme body burdens of aluminum, the test will help select patients needing further study by bone biopsy, a more invasive procedure. **CONTRAINDICATIONS:** When there is a heavy bone burden of aluminum, often reflected by high basal levels of aluminum, the serum aluminum may acutely rise to toxic levels after desferrioxamine dose is given as "challenge" test or as treatment, and encephalopathy may worsen. In cases of actual or anticipated intolerance to desferrioxamine, hemoperfusion over specially treated charcoal (an aluminum removal device) would be an alternative treatment modality. **METHODOLOGY:** Atomic absorption (AA), inductively coupled plasma atomic emission spectrometry

Footnotes

1. Yaqoob M, Ahmad R, Roberts N, et al, "Low-Dose Desferrioxamine Test for the Diagnosis of Aluminum-Related Bone Disease in Patients on Regular Haemodialysis," *Nephrol Dial Transplant*, 1991, 6(1):484-6.
2. De Broe ME, D'Haese PC, Elseviers MM, et al, "Aluminum and End Stage Renal Failure," *Nephrology*, 1988, 2:1086-116.
3. de Vernejoul MC, Marchais S, London G, et al, "Deferoxamine Test and Bone Disease in Dialysis Patients With Mild Aluminum Accumulation," *Am J Kidney Dis*, 1989, 14(2):124-30.
4. Milliner DS, Nebeker HG, Ott SM, et al, "Use of the Deferoxamine Infusion Test in the Diagnosis of Aluminum-Related Osteodystrophy," *Ann Intern Med*, 1984, 101:775-80.
5. Bene C, Manzler A, Bene D, et al, "Irreversible Ocular Toxicity From Single "Challenge" Dose of Deferoxamine," *Clin Nephrol*, 1989, 31(1):45-8.
6. Ravelli M, Scaroni P, Mombelloni S, et al, "Acute Visual Disorders in Patients on Regular Dialysis Given Desferrioxamine as a Test," *Nephol Dial Transplant*, 1990, 5(11):945-9.
7. McCarthy JT, Milliner DS, and Johnson WJ, "Clinical Experience With Desferrioxamine in Dialysis Patients With Aluminum Toxicity," *Q J Med*, 1990, 74(275):257-76.

References

Monteagudo FS, Cassidy MJ, and Folb PI, "Recent Developments in Aluminum Toxicology," *Med Toxicol Adverse Drug Exp*, 1989, 4(1):1-16.

Wills MR and Savory J, "Aluminum and Chronic Renal Failure: Sources, Absorption, Transport, and Toxicity," *Crit Rev Clin Lab Sci*, 1989, 27(1):59-107.

Histomorphometry *see* Aluminum, Bone *on page 1018*

Hypoxanthine, Urine *see* Molybdenum, Blood *on page 1032*

Manganese, Blood

***CPT** 83785*

Related Information

Heavy Metal Screen, Blood *on page 972*

Heavy Metal Screen, Urine *on page 973*

Synonyms Mn, Serum

Abstract Manganese is essential to life in many species and is part of many human enzyme systems. For this reason, it is considered essential for human nutrition, even though no well-documented example of a manganese deficiency state has been found in humans.[1] Manganese is routinely included in parenteral and enteral nutrition formulae, in a "multiple trace metals" additive for the former. As in several trace metals that are concentrated in the cellular elements of blood, whole blood manganese or red blood cell manganese may better reflect total body manganese stores than do serum levels in healthy individuals. Because, up to 30% of the blood manganese content is contained in the tiny "buffy coat" consisting of white blood cells and platelets,[2] and because leukocytosis occurs in many clinical situations, serum levels may be more practical than whole blood manganese in clinical situations (in which leukocytosis may or may not be present) as opposed to research use.

(Continued)

Manganese, Blood *(Continued)*

Manganese is implicated as a cofactor in many important cellular enzyme systems, especially mitochondrial superoxide dismutase. *In vitro*, magnesium or even cobalt, iron, calcium, or zinc may substitute for manganese in some of these enzyme systems. From animal studies, manganese deficiency is involved in osteoporosis and skeletal deformities. In humans, low levels are associated with epilepsy[3] (regardless of type of anticonvulsant) and reported with the skeletal deformities of Perthes' disease.[4] Some have argued that the late hip dislocations in infants may be related to the low manganese content in cow's milk. A single case of suspected inadvertent experimental deficiency was reported to cause hair changes and coagulopathy.

Manganese toxicity causes nausea, vomiting, headache, and psychiatric disturbances with central nervous system damage manifested by disorientation, memory loss, anxiety, and compulsive laughing or crying. In the more chronic form, manganese toxicity resembles Parkinson's disease with akinesia, rigidity, tremors, and mask-like faces. Normalization of serum levels later may not completely reverse the neurological damage. Recent reports, however, of slow chelation therapy in patients with chronic manganese toxicity, have documented neurological improvement (not cure) in patients in whom therapy was delayed by over 20 years from the time of exposure.[5]

Several medications are thought to chelate manganese, including valproate and hydralazine. Dialysis lowers manganese levels, and patients on hemodialysis usually have lower basal serum levels. Ninety-nine percent of manganese excretion occurs in the feces, from the bile. When intake is limited, excretion in the urine and feces may fall more than tenfold. Manganese levels rise to two to four times normal (without signs of toxicity) in children given standard amounts in their parenteral nutrition when jaundice occurs. High, potentially toxic levels have been seen after liver transplantation. Recommendations have been made[6] that supplemental manganese be withheld from parenteral nutrition solutions if serum levels cannot be followed in the presence of cholestatic jaundice (some manganese is still present in the ingredients of parenteral nutrition on a contaminant basis). Manganese is present in very small quantities in biological samples. Published normal levels have fallen by more than tenfold with better methods of avoiding contamination and improvements in analytic methods.

Specimen Serum, whole blood **CONTAINER:** Special metal-free Sherwood Monoject™ trace element blood collection tube #8881-307006. For whole blood, use #8881-307022 EDTA tube. See introduction to this chapter. **COLLECTION:** Use B-D #5175 20-gauge stainless steel needle; or Terumo or Abbot butterfly needle; draw directly into the trace metal vacuum tube. Draw this and any other trace metal blood sample first before using needle to perforate ordinary rubber stopper of ordinary blood tube. For isolation of serum, allow clotting and centrifuge. Carefully pour serum into special plastic metal-free vial or transfer with acid-washed all-plastic pipet, being careful not to disturb the clot, or any buffy coat. Store sample frozen if it is to be transported to reference laboratory. One author has suggested the use of an aluminum needle, not widely available. **TURNAROUND TIME:** Samples are usually sent to a reference laboratory.

Interpretive **REFERENCE RANGE:** Serum: 0.43-0.76 ng/mL (SI: 7.8-13.8 nmol/L)[7]; whole blood: 10-11 ng/mL (SI: 190-200 nmol/L).[2] In a recent report, exposed manganese workers who developed signs of manganese toxicity had whole blood manganese levels of 20-400 ng/mL when measured during on-going exposure.[8] One worker who left the company had a whole blood level of 10 ng/mL 6 months after exposure. **USE:** Follow manganese therapy in parenteral nutrition, especially in liver disease, or when there are excessive gastrointestinal losses; evaluate suspected manganese toxicity or exposure, especially neurological syndromes and movement disorders **LIMITATIONS:** In evaluating toxicity, the serum level may have returned to normal while the neurological damage persists. In evaluating possible deficiency states, the human deficiency syndrome is poorly defined, making interpretation difficult. Levels are reportedly reduced mildly in epilepsy, and raised in hepatitis or jaundice. Manganese levels are 60% lower than normal in hemodialysis patients. **METHODOLOGY:** Neutron activation is the most sensitive but does not lend itself to clinical testing. Atomic absorption spectrophotometry (AA) with Zeeman background correction is currently the preferred method. **ADDITIONAL INFORMATION:** Toxic exposure may occur from dry cells, fungicide (maneb), and in the steel industry or chemical industry. Manganese is present in the coloring agents for glass and soap, in paints, varnish and enamel, and in linoleum. It is used in the manufacture of chlorine gas and now in lead-free gasoline. Industrial manganese poisoning has been recognized since 1837. Some water supplies are sufficiently contaminated by manganese that endemic psychiatric and neurological disease is present. Manganese levels in tears are 50-fold higher than in serum.

Footnotes

1. "Manganese Deficiency in Humans: Fact or Fiction?" *Nutr Rev*, 1988, 46(10):348-52.
2. Milne DB, Sims RL, and Ralston NVC, "Manganese Content of the Cellular Components of Blood," *Clin Chem*, 1990, 36(3):450-2.
3. Carl GF, Keen CL, Gallagher BB, et al, "Association of Low Blood Manganese Concentrations With Epilepsy," *Neurology*, 1986, 36:1584-7.
4. Hall AJ, Margetts BM, Barker DJ, et al, "Low Blood Manganese Levels in Liverpool Children With Perthes' Disease," *Paediatr Perinat Epidemiol*, 1989, 3(2):131-6.
5. Ky SQ, Deng HS, Xie PY, et al, "A Report of Two Cases of Chronic Serious Manganese Poisoning Treated With Sodium Para-aminosalicylic Acid," *Br J Ind Med*, 1992, 49(1):66-9.
6. Hambidge KM, Sokol RJ, Fidanza SJ, et al, "Plasma Manganese Concentrations in Infants and Children Receiving Parenteral Nutrition," *J Parenter Enteral Nutr*, 1989, 13(2):168-71.
7. Neve J and Leclercq N, "Factors Affecting Determinations of Manganese in Serum by Atomic Absorption Spectrometry," *Clin Chem*, 1991, 37(5):723-8.
8. Wang JD, Huang CC, Hwang YH, et al, "Manganese Induced Parkinsonism: An Outbreak Due to an Unrepaired Ventilation Control System in a Ferromanganese Smelter," *Br J Ind Med*, 1989, 46(12):856-9.

References

Barlow PJ and Sylvester PE, "Hip Dislocation and Manganese Deficiency," *Lancet*, 1983, 2:685.

Falbe WJ, Brown RO, Luther RW, et al, "Individualized Manganese Supplementation in Patients Receiving Total Parenteral Nutrition," *Clin Pharm*, 1987, 6:226-9.

Ferraz HB, Bertolucci PHF, Pereira JS, et al, "Chronic Exposure to the Fungicide Maneb May Produce Symptoms and Signs of CNS Manganese Intoxication," *Neurology*, 1988, 38:550-3.

Kondakis XG, Makris N, Leotsinidis M, et al, "Possible Health Effects of High Manganese Concentration in Drinking Water," *Arch Environ Health*, 1989, 44(3):175-8.

Kurkus J, Alcock NW, and Shils ME, "Manganese Content of Large-Volume Parenteral Solutions and of Nutrient Additives," *J Parenter Enteral Nutr*, 1984, 8:254-7.

Manganese, Urine

CPT 83785

Related Information

Heavy Metal Screen, Blood *on page 972*
Heavy Metal Screen, Urine *on page 973*
Urine Collection, 24-Hour *on page 32*

Synonyms Mn, Urine

Abstract Urine manganese is used in conjunction with serum manganese to evaluate possible toxicity or deficiency of manganese,[1] an essential mineral which, in high concentration, can cause neurological damage similar to Parkinson's disease. See Manganese, Serum for signs and symptoms of deficiency and toxicity, and for additional references.

Specimen 24-hour or random ("spot") urine. Consider simultaneous determination of urine creatinine, especially on "spot" samples. **CONTAINER:** Acid-washed plastic urine container, avoid contamination by stool, dust, and metal. **CAUSES FOR REJECTION:** Contamination by metal, stool, or dust **TURNAROUND TIME:** Samples are usually sent to a reference laboratory.

Interpretive **REFERENCE RANGE:** <2.0 μg/L (SI: <36 nmol/L) (97.5% confidence).[2] Varies with laboratory. Level may fall to 0.2 μg/L (tenfold) in experimental deficiency.[1] Some of the best data on industrial exposure have been normalized to the creatinine content of urine or to μg/hour excretion due to the impracticality of 24-hour urine samples in the industrial setting.[3] Ten free-living, nonexposed young men in Wisconsin had urinary excretion varying from approximately 0.17-0.66 μg/g creatinine.[2] Levels higher than this but <9.0 μg/g creatinine may reflect increased exposure, not necessarily at a toxic level.[4] Another group of factory workers exposed to manganese, some of whom were symptomatic with parkinsonian signs, had urine levels of manganese varying from 11.2-216.0 μg/L.[5] Bile and feces are the main routes of excretion, accounting for 99% of excretion when intake is low, and excretion rather than absorption appears to be regulated. Urine losses appear to be overflow losses, representing a higher fraction of total loss when intake is high. **USE:** Confirm manganese exposure, toxicity, or poisoning by documenting excessive urine excretion of the metal. Also used to individualize manganese dosing in long-term parenteral nutrition, especially in liver disease, when biliary excretion is low, or when there is excessive gastrointestinal losses, such as in short bowel syndrome. Has been used to follow the success of chelation therapy with para-aminosalicylate sodium in manganism. **LIMITATIONS:** Levels in urine are so low that considerable error may be introduced by contamination. Manganese toxicity may leave residual neurologic damage after serum and urine levels have returned to normal, masking the original cause. **METHODOLOGY:** Atomic absorption (AA) **ADDITIONAL INFORMATION:** As much as twofold diurnal variation is present in urine manganese, especially in workers exposed to manganese during their time at work.

(Continued)

Manganese, Urine *(Continued)*

Footnotes

1. "Manganese Deficiency in Humans: Fact or Fiction?" *Nutr Rev*, 1988, 46(10):348-52.
2. Greger JL, Davis CD, Suttie JW, et al, "Intake, Serum Concentrations, and Urinary Excretion of Manganese by Adult Males," *Am J Clin Nutr*, 1990, 51(3):457-61.
3. Roels HA, Ghyselen P, Buchet JP, et al, "Assessment of the Permissible Exposure Level to Manganese in Workers Exposed to Manganese Dioxide Dust," *Br J Ind Med*, 1992, 49(1):25-34.
4. Siqueira ME, Hirata MH, and Adballa DS, "Studies on Some Biochemical Parameters in Human Manganese Exposure," *Med Lav*, 1991, 82(6):504-9.
5. Hua MS and Huang CC, "Chronic Occupational Exposure to Manganese and Neurobehavioral Function," *J Clin Exp Neuropsychol*, 1991, 13(4):495-507.

References

Jacob RA, "Trace Elements," *Textbook of Clinical Chemistry*, Tietz NA, ed, Philadelphia, PA: WB Saunders Co, 1986, 965-96.

Metallothiomein *see* Copper, Serum *on page 1024*

Metallothionein *see* Zinc, Serum *on page 1036*

Methionine, Serum *see* Molybdenum, Blood *on this page*

Mn, Serum *see* Manganese, Blood *on page 1029*

Mn, Urine *see* Manganese, Urine *on previous page*

Mo, Blood *see* Molybdenum, Blood *on this page*

Molybdenum, Blood

CPT *82190*

Synonyms Mo, Blood

Applies to Hypoxanthine, Urine; Methionine, Serum; Molybdopterin; S-Sulfocysteine, Urine; Sulfite, Urine; Xanthine, Urine

Abstract Molybdenum is vital to human health through its essential inclusion in at least three human enzymes: xanthine oxidase, aldehyde oxidase, and sulfite oxidase. The active site of each of these binds molybdenum in the form of a cofactor "molybdopterin," a pterin ring similar to folic acid which tightly complexes molybdenum.[1]

Molybdenum interferes with copper metabolism, especially in the presence of dietary sulfides, by the formation of insoluble copper thiomolybdenates in the gut lumen; absorbed thiomolybdenates may also interfere with copper metabolism. Copper deficiency on this basis is common in ruminant animals but so far has not been reported in man. High levels of tungsten in the diet compete with molybdenum in experimental animals so that total body molybdenum deficiency can be created by loading with tungsten. So far this has not been reported to occur in humans, but there is no reason not to anticipate molybdenum deficiency should chronic tungsten exposure occur. The clinical syndromes so far reported for humans involving molybdenum include:

1. **Molybdenum cofactor deficiency**: This is a recessively inherited error of metabolism involving failure to synthesize molybdopterin. It is diagnosed by noting combined xanthine oxidase deficiency (low serum uric acid <1 mg/dL, increased urine hypoxanthine and xanthine) and sulfite oxidase deficiency (marked by increased urinary sulfite, decreased to absent urine inorganic sulfate, increased urinary S-sulfocysteine). These patients have severe neurologic abnormalities from infancy on the basis of the sulfite oxidase deficiency including seizures, anterior lens dislocations, opisthotonos, decreased brain weight, decreased brain myelin, and usually death prior to age 1 year.[2] Molybdenum is virtually absent from the liver of such patients, suggesting that molybdopterin is an important storage form of molybdenum in soft tissues. Molybdenum may not be retained at all in soft tissue without molybdenum cofactor. Serum molybdenum in this disease is reported to be normal.
2. **Parenteral nutrition-associated molybdenum deficiency**: One case of molybdenum deficiency has been reported in this setting in a 24-year-old man with Crohn's disease.[3] Biochemical abnormalities were only corrected by the addition of molybdenum to the total parenteral nutrition (TPN). The biochemical abnormalities were essentially similar to those listed above for molybdenum cofactor deficiency: increased urinary sulfate, thiosulfate, xanthine, and hypoxanthine; decreased urinary sulfate and uric acid. In addition, unlike reported cases of molybdenum cofactors deficiency,

this patient showed increased serum levels of methionine. The patient suffered night blindness, tachycardia, tachypnea, central scotomata, and irritability leading to coma over 24-48 hours while on TPN. These symptoms disappeared when amino acid administration was stopped, but the symptoms recurred with either amino acid infusion or bisulfite infusion until molybdenum was added to the TPN. Unfortunately, serum or whole blood molybdenum was not reported for this case, so we do not know at what reduced level of serum or whole blood molybdenum a patient might become symptomatic. The patient refused liver biopsy to assess hepatic stores of molybdenum.

3. **Molybdenum toxicity**: This has only rarely been reported. Two situations are known to expose human populations chronically to excess molybdenum: industrial exposure and through the food chain in areas of the world with high local soil molybdenum. Two villages in Armenia have a high frequency of patients with hepatosplenomegaly, "kidney disease," and an inflammatory arthritis of the knees and small joints of hands and feet, associated with joint erythema, edema, and deformity. Serum levels of uric acid are modestly elevated and whole blood molybdenum is markedly elevated: 310 ± 20 ng/mL vs 60 ± 10 ng/mL control. Dietary intake for these patients is estimated to be 10-15 mg/day vs 0.15-0.5 mg/day recommended. Asymptomatic subjects in the same villages also with high molybdenum intakes have lower but still markedly elevated blood molybdenum levels of 170 ± 10 ng/mL.[1]

Specimen Whole blood **CONTAINER:** In lieu of authoritative recommendations regarding potential molybdenum contamination from blood-drawing vacuum containers and stoppers, the same methods for containers and blood collection for other trace metals should be employed, that is, use the Sherwood Monoject™ trace metal blood collection tube with EDTA #8881-307022 and draw through a B-D #5175 20-gauge stainless steel needle. If other samples are to be collected at the same blood draw, draw the trace metal tube first so as not to contaminate the needle by puncture through ordinary rubber stoppers. See introduction to this chapter.

Interpretive **REFERENCE RANGE:** Whole blood molybdenum: <60 ng/mL; lower limit not established. Blood level parallels molybdenum intake. Apparently normal individuals vary from each other by over a 100-fold from 0.5-60 ng/mL, depending on molybdenum intake. 170 ng/mL appears to border on the toxic level based on the report above. Seventy-five percent of people in the United States have levels ≤5 ng/mL, but some geographical areas show 70% of the population >5 ng/mL. **LIMITATIONS:** Data are new and sketchy for this trace metal, and clinical syndromes poorly defined. Serum or plasma molybdenum norms are still being developed. Levels in apparently healthy people vary enormously based on intake, and blood levels are only significant when extremely high or extremely low levels (yet undefined) are encountered. **METHODOLOGY:** Neutron activation, graphite furnace atomic absorption spectrophotometry (AA) after extraction into 8-hydroxyquinoline[4]

Footnotes

1. Rajagopalan KV, "Molybdenum: An Essential Trace Element in Human Nutrition," *Annu Rev Nutr*, 1988, 8:401-27.
2. Johnson JL, Waud WR, Rajagopalan KV, et al, "Inborn Errors of Molybdenum Metabolism: Combined Deficiencies of Sulfite Oxidase and Xanthine Dehydrogenase in a Patient Lacking the Molybdenum Cofactor," *Proc Natl Acad Sci U S A*, 1980, 77:3715-9.
3. Abumrad NN, Schneider AJ, Steel D, et al, "Amino Acid Intolerance During Prolonged Total Parenteral Nutrition Reversed by Molybdate Therapy," *Am J Clin Nutr*, 1981, 34:2551-9.
4. Morrice PC, Humphries WR, and Bremner I, "Determination of Molybdenum in Plasma Using Graphite Furnace Atomic Absorption Spectrometry," *Analyst*, 1989, 114(12):1667-9.

References

Bougle D, Foucault D, Voirin J, et al, "Molybdenum in the Premature Infant," *Biol Neonate*, 1991, 59(4):201-3.
Bougle D, Voirin J, Bureau F, et al, "Molybdenum: Normal Plasma Values at Delivery in Mothers and Newborns," *Acta Paediatr Scand*, 1989, 78(2):319-20.

Molybdopterin *see* Molybdenum, Blood *on previous page*
Penicillamine *see* Zinc, Serum *on page 1036*

Selenium, Serum

CPT *84255*

Related Information

Heavy Metal Screen, Blood *on page 972*
Heavy Metal Screen, Urine *on page 973*
(Continued)

Selenium, Serum *(Continued)*

Synonyms Se, Serum

Abstract The essential nature of selenium in human nutrition is beyond dispute. The element is part of the enzyme that converts T_4 to the active thyroid hormone T_3. It is also part of selenium-dependant glutathione peroxidase, an important antioxidant in blood and tissue. Multiple cases of selenium deficiency have been reported, mostly among patients given parenteral nutrition with no added selenium. Deficiency also occurs endemically in places where soil selenium is low, and low levels are thus present throughout the food chain. Endemic cretinism,[1,2] Balkan nephropathy,[3] Keschan disease[4] (endemic dilated cardiomyopathy), and Kashin-Bek disease[5] (endemic deforming osteoarthritis) are probably all caused by endemic selenium deficiency conditioning the host to poorly tolerate an additional environmental stress (cretinism: iodine deficiency; the others: unknown local toxins). Simple deficiency is marked by whitening of the nailbeds, erythrocyte macrocytosis, cardiomyopathy, painful weak muscles, skin and hair depigmentation, and elevations of transaminase and creatinine kinase.[5,6,7] The cardiomyopathy may be mild and asymptomatic or fulminant and fatal. Selenium toxicity can occur endemically, again due to high soil levels, or through accidental or industrial exposure. Symptoms include garlic breath, odor, thick brittle fingernails, dry brittle hair, red swollen skin of the hands and feet, and nervous system abnormalities of numbness, convulsions, or paralysis.

Specimen Serum **CONTAINER:** Sherwood Monoject™ trace element blood collection tube #8881-307006 or #8881-307022 with EDTA for whole blood. See introduction to this chapter. **COLLECTION:** Draw blood through B-D #5175 stainless steel needle into special trace metal vacuum tube. Centrifuge and pour serum into special plastic metal-free vial for transport. **TURNAROUND TIME:** Samples are usually sent to a reference laboratory.

Interpretive **REFERENCE RANGE:** Serum: 95-165 ng/mL. Approximately 40% higher for whole blood. Serum reflects recent intake; red cells reflect more remote intake. Whole blood therefore reflects an average of recent and remote intake of selenium. (Selenium-dependent glutathione peroxidase activity reflects selenium available for enzyme synthesis – see below.) Levels are depressed in HIV infection,[8] critical illness,[9] kwashiorkor, inflammatory bowel disease,[10] renal failure, hemodialysis status, low protein diet, phenylketonuria, maple syrup urine disease, (possibly all in part related to poor protein intake), low birth weight,[11] and premature infants with inadequate selenium intake. Levels are increased mostly with the use of glucocorticoids.[12] Levels >500 ng/mL are associated with toxicity. **USE:** Monitor selenium nutritional status in long-term parenteral nutrition. Studies have indicated no factor or factors that can accurately predict serum selenium levels to preclude need for measurement. May be used diagnostically in cardiomyopathy of unknown cause, especially where nutritional factors are suspected. **LIMITATIONS:** Some controversy exists regarding the "best" marker for selenium status. Since selenium as selenomethionine is incorporated nonspecifically into protein, serum and whole blood selenium concentration increases with increasing selenium intake to different degrees depending on inorganic or organic sources of selenium. Glutathione peroxidase activity is more sensitive to deficiency but the test is not well standardized and therefore not reproducible from laboratory to laboratory. Hair selenium may be contaminated by selenium-containing shampoo. Serum selenium level correlates best with intake and therefore with both deficiency and toxicity states, but a wide range of serum levels is compatible with apparent good health. **METHODOLOGY:** Atomic absorption, fluorometric methods[13] **ADDITIONAL INFORMATION:** Selenium is excreted in feces from the bile, in sweat and skin losses, and the remaining 50% to 70% in the urine. Significant breath losses occur only in toxic states. Dosages in renal failure need not be modified. The deficiency syndrome may be rapidly induced under surgery or other stress after a long asymptomatic phase.

Footnotes

1. Arthur JR, "The Role of Selenium in Thyroid Hormone Metabolism," *Can J Physiol Pharmacol*, 1991, 69(11):1648-52.
2. Contempré B, Vanderpas J, and Dumont JE, "Cretinism, Thyroid Hormones and Selenium," *Mol Cell Endocrinol*, 1991, 81(1-3):C193-5.
3. Maksimović ZJ, "Selenium Deficiency and Balkan Endemic Nephropathy," *Kidney Int Suppl*, 1991, 34:S12-4.
4. Lockitch G, Taylor GP, Wong LTK, et al, "Cardiomyopathy Associated With Nonendemic Selenium Deficiency in a Caucasian Adolescent," *Am J Clin Nutr*, 1990, 52(3):572-7.
5. Levander OA, "A Global View of Human Selenium Nutrition," *Annu Rev Nutr*, 1987, 7:227-50.
6. Kien CL and Ganther HE, "Manifestations of Chronic Selenium Deficiency in a Child Receiving Total Parenteral Nutrition," *Am J Clin Nutr*, 1983, 37:319-28.
7. Brown MR, Cohen HJ, Lyons JM, et al, "Proximal Muscle Weakness and Selenium Deficiency Associated With Long-Term Parenteral Nutrition," *Am J Clin Nutr*, 1986, 43:549-54.

8. Cirelli A, Ciardi M, De Simone C, et al, "Serum Selenium Concentration and Disease Progress in Patients With HIV Infection," *Clin Biochem*, 1991, 24(2):211-4.
9. Hawker FH, Stewart PM, and Snitch PJ, "Effects of Acute Illness on Selenium Homeostasis," *Crit Care Med*, 1990, 18(4):442-6.
10. Fernández-Bañares F, Mingorance MD, Esteve M, et al, "Serum Zinc, Copper, and Selenium Levels in Inflammatory Bowel Disease: Effect of Total Enteral Nutrition on Trace Element Status," *Am J Gastroenterol*, 1990, 85(12):1584-9.
11. Lockitch G, Jacobson B, Quigley G, et al, "Selenium Deficiency in Low Birth Weight Neonates: An Unrecognized Problem," *J Pediatr*, 1989, 114(5):865-70.
12. Marano G, Fischioni P, Graziano C, et al, "Increased Serum Selenium Levels in Patients Under Corticosteroid Treatment," *Pharmacol Toxicol*, 1990, 67(2):120-2.
13. Sheehan TMT and Gao M, "Simplified Fluorometric Assay of Total Selenium in Plasma and Urine," *Clin Chem*, 1990, 36(12):2124-6.

References

Edmonds DK and Letchworth AT, "Selenium Deficiency in Kwashiorkor," *Lancet*, 1982, 1:1312-3.

Fleming CR, Lie JT, McCall JT, et al, "Selenium Deficiency and Fatal Cardiomyopathy in A Patient on Home Parenteral Nutrition," *Gastroenterology*, 1982, 83:689-93.

Kòller LD and Exon JH, "The Two Faces of Selenium – Deficiency and Toxicity – Are Similar in Animals and Man," *Can J Vet Res*, 1986, 50:297-306.

Pentel P, Fletcher D, and Jentzen J, "Fatal Acute Selenium Toxicity," *J Forensic Sci*, 1985, 30:556-62.

Vinton NE, Dahlstrom KA, Strobel CT, et al, "Macrocytosis and Pseudoalbinism: Manifestations of Selenium Deficiency," *J Pediatr*, 1987, 111:711-7.

Selenium, Urine

***CPT** 84255*

Related Information

Heavy Metal Screen, Blood *on page 972*
Heavy Metal Screen, Urine *on page 973*
Urine Collection, 24-Hour *on page 32*

Synonyms Se, Urine

Abstract Urine selenium is used in conjunction with serum selenium to assess selenium nutrition or potential toxic exposure. Like any other 24-hour urine collection of an essential element, this reflects recent intake, assuming the patient is in selenium balance. In the case of selenium, skin and stool losses are significant and amount to 30% to 50% of total losses; nevertheless, urine losses often represent overflow losses and can help indicate whether recent intake has been adequate or possibly toxic. When selenium intake is low to normal, less than approximately 140 μg/day, 24-hour urine may not reflect the 24-hour intake of the previous day. This is especially true when the body stores are low and selenium is retained to fill body stores.[1] At higher levels of intake, the 24-hour urine is well correlated with intake and can be used as evidence of excess intake, adequate intake, or prior toxic exposure. Twenty-four hour urine selenium reflects recent intake. When selenium supplementation normalizes serum selenium and whole blood selenium, and then selenium supplementation is stopped, urine selenium falls back toward baseline much faster than blood or serum levels.[2] Urine selenium has recently been found to be correlated with 24-hour urine urea in critically ill patients. This probably reflects catabolism of protein and release of body stores of selenium, though details of the selenium intake of the patients (proportional to protein intake in tube-fed patients) were not provided.[3]

Specimen 24-hour urine **CONTAINER:** Acid-washed plastic urine container **COLLECTION:** Avoid contamination by hair since some patients use selenium-containing shampoos. **TURNAROUND TIME:** A specified aliquot of the urine is usually sent to a reference laboratory.

Interpretive **REFERENCE RANGE:** Levels <15 μg/L or >150 μg/L probably represent unusually low or high intake without necessarily representing illness. Values vary widely and in apparently healthy U.S. citizens they have been reported to vary from 7 μg/L (24-hour sample) to 231 μg/L. Intake is partly determined by local soil content of selenium and use of local vegetables as food. Healthy persons in New Guinea have been reported with levels as low as 0.9 μg/L but similar patients have rapidly developed symptomatic selenium deficiency when placed on total parenteral nutrition lacking selenium. Urine levels of 7 μg/L have been reported from China in areas where selenium deficiency is symptomatic. Levels >880 μg/L have been seen in chronic selenosis and >600 μg/L during the first 24 hours after acute selenium intoxication. Levels >500 μg/L probably represent toxicity. See the comprehensive review by Robberecht and Deelstra.[1] Some authors or laboratories report as μg/day. **USE:** Monitor nutritional therapy, especially parenteral nutrition; monitor potential toxic exposure **LIMITATIONS:** Selenomethionine is incorporated into body protein nonspecifically as methionine, so it is not as

(Continued)

Selenium, Urine *(Continued)*

quickly excreted in the urine as inorganic selenium (selenite). Thus, the form of selenium ingested will affect short-term balance estimates. Spot urine selenium is of little value, as urine selenium goes up after each meal related to selenium intake and probably other factors, and dilution in spot urine samples varies. **METHODOLOGY:** Fluorometry, atomic absorption (AA) **ADDITIONAL INFORMATION:** In addition to serum and urine levels of selenium, red cell glutathione peroxidase can be monitored as an example of the activity of a seleno-enzyme. Levels will be depressed in deficiency but will not monitor toxicity.

Footnotes

1. Robberecht HJ and Deelstra HA, "Selenium in Human Urine: Concentration Levels and Medical Implications," *Clin Chim Acta*, 1984, 136:107-20.
2. Välimäki M, Alfthan G, Vuoristo M, et al, "Effects of Selenium Supplementation on Blood and Urine Selenium Levels and Liver Function in Patients With Primary Biliary Cirrhosis," *Clin Chim Acta*, 1991, 196(1):7-15.
3. Hawker FH, Stewart PM, and Snitch PJ, "Effects of Acute Illness on Selenium Homeostasis," *Crit Care Med*, 1990, 18(4):442-6.

References

Edmonds DK and Letchworth AT, "Selenium Deficiency in Kwashiorkor," *Lancet*, 1982, 1:1312-3.
Levander OA, "A Global View of Human Selenium Nutrition," *Annu Rev Nutr*, 1987, 7:227-50.
Pentel P, Fletcher D, and Jentzen J, "Fatal Acute Selenium Toxicity," *J Forensic Sci*, 1985, 30:556-62.
Thomson CD, "Clinical Consequences and Assessment of Low Selenium Status," *N Z Med J*, 1991, 104(919):376-7.

Se, Serum *see* Selenium, Serum *on page 1033*
Se, Urine *see* Selenium, Urine *on previous page*
S-Sulfocysteine, Urine *see* Molybdenum, Blood *on page 1032*
Sulfite, Urine *see* Molybdenum, Blood *on page 1032*
Thymulin Assay *see* Zinc, Serum *on this page*
Transcuprein *see* Copper, Serum *on page 1024*
Xanthine, Urine *see* Molybdenum, Blood *on page 1032*

Zinc, Serum

CPT 84630

Related Information

Albumin, Serum *on page 102*
Heavy Metal Screen, Blood *on page 972*
Heavy Metal Screen, Urine *on page 973*

Synonyms Zn, Serum

Applies to Metallothionein; Penicillamine; Thymulin Assay

Abstract Zinc nutrition has been widely studied over the past 30 years and many potential markers have been examined in the search for an index of zinc status. The simplest of these is serum zinc, which is reduced in moderate to severe zinc deficiency, but is not sensitive to mild zinc deficiency states. The problem is that it is also reduced in many other clinical states. Other more sensitive tests each have their own problems in clinical use.[1,2,3] Serum zinc remains useful if knowledge of zinc metabolism is applied in the interpretation of the test.

Nutritional deficiency, both primary and conditioned, is fairly common worldwide, as well as in the United States, and has been described in a large variety of clinical situations: in premature infants born with low hepatic stores; in breast fed premature and full-term infants[4] whose mother's milk is lower than normal in zinc; in growing children, especially boys, whose height velocity has increased while under zinc therapy; in prepubertal boys who display delayed sexual maturity, especially in association with diets low in animal protein and high in phytates from grains[5] (which reduce gastrointestinal zinc absorption); in malabsorption and diarrheal states;[6] in diabetes, nephrotic syndrome, cirrhosis (in each of these hyperzincuria occurs), in AIDS and ARC;[7] in burn patients,[8] and those receiving high doses of oral histidine or I.V. amino acids[9] especially cysteine or histidine associated with hyperzincuria; and in geophagia[5] (where zinc absorption is reduced). The most severe cases of zinc deficiency occurred in the early days of total parenteral nutrition,[10] when zinc was not specifically included in the formulation.

Zinc is absorbed in the small bowel facilitated by small organic molecules, probably citrate and/or picolinic acid. Picolinic acid is a molecule synthesized by the pancreas from tryptophan and also present in human milk more so than cow's milk.

Babies with the disease of zinc malabsorption known as acrodermatitis enteropathica usually first develop their characteristic facial and diaper rash when weaned.[11] Untreated, symptoms progress and include growth retardation, diarrhea, impaired T-cell immunity, poor wound healing, infections, delayed testicular development in adolescence, and early death. Parenteral or enteral zinc corrects the condition. The classic disease is associated with low serum and urine zinc, but some cases have a normal serum zinc.[12] These cases nevertheless respond to zinc supplementation.

Zinc absorption in the human appears regulated, through the metallothionein mechanism which is shared with copper. (See Copper, Serum.) Zinc excretion in normal subjects is also regulated. When oral intake of zinc falls, stool excretion, sweat excretion, and eventually urinary excretion of zinc all are down regulated.[3] Normally, urine losses are a small proportion of total losses; but under certain situations, high urinary losses are not regulated and can serve to promote the deficiency state. High urine losses have been reported in diabetes mellitus, cirrhosis, nephrosis, total parenteral nutrition, penicillamine therapy, and in burn patients. When there are no excessive losses, normal healthy adults come into zinc balance with 3-20 mg oral zinc and positive zinc balance with 3 mg I.V. zinc per day.[3]

Assessment of Zinc Status*

Reduced pool size	Low plasma zinc + Low plasma metallothionein
Tissue redistribution	Low plasma zinc + High plasma metallothionein

*Differentiation of declines in plasma zinc due to decreases in pool size from tissue redistribution.
From King JC, "Assessment of Zinc Status," *J Nutr,* 1990, 120:(Suppl 11):1474-9, with permission.

Recently, it has been proposed to use serum zinc together with serum metallothionein to distinguish reductions in serum zinc due to redistribution (sepsis, stress) from that due to nutritional inadequacy.[3] See table. Alternatively, the thymulin assay (a zinc dependent thymic hormone) has been proposed to serve as a marker for zinc status.[13] Further work is needed. It is unlikely that any single marker by itself will be appropriate in most situations. In the meanwhile, serum zinc, when low in an apparently healthy (nonstressed, nonseptic) patient who has normal serum albumin, can be taken as evidence for low zinc stores, especially if urine zinc is also low, or there is known excessive unregulated zinc loss (diarrhea, nephrotic syndrome, etc.). One should not take a normal serum zinc as evidence for adequate zinc stores, however. Zinc deficiency in adolescents and adults is marked by slow growth or weight loss, altered taste, delayed puberty, dwarfism, impaired dark adaptation, central scotomata, alopecia, emotional instability, tremors, cerebellar ataxia, and a bullous-pustular rash over acral areas. Candidiasis reflects impaired T-cell function. Thymulin apo-hormone is present but inactive due to lack of zinc. Lymphopenia may occur and death usually follows overwhelming infection.

Specimen Serum **CONTAINER:** Avoid hemolysis or stasis. Use B-D #5175 stainless steel needle. Avoid contact with rubber. Separate serum and store in metal-free plastic vial. See introduction to this chapter. **CAUSES FOR REJECTION:** Improper collection

Interpretive **REFERENCE RANGE:** 66-110 μg/dL (SI: 10.0-16.8 μmol/L) **USE:** Evaluate suspected nutritional inadequacy, especially in enteral or parental nutrition, critically ill or burn patients; cases of diabetes or delayed would healing; growth retardation; follow therapy, for example when higher intravenous zinc doses are used to balance excessive ongoing GI losses in long-term total parenteral nutrition; follow oral zinc therapy in Wilson's disease; confirm acrodermatitis enteropathica and follow therapy; evaluate possible zinc toxicity or metal fume fever in possible exposure situations (poisoning, industrial exposure) **LIMITATIONS:** Levels may be low in fever, sepsis, estrogen therapy, stress, or myocardial infarction – reflecting mobilization from serum to the liver by interleukin. Levels are usually low in uremia with normal tissue levels. Levels may be high in familial hyperzincemia without toxicity or high zinc stores. **ADDITIONAL INFORMATION:** Chronic oral zinc supplementation interferes with copper absorption and may precipitate copper deficiency. Albumin is the primary zinc binding protein: zinc levels should be interpreted with awareness of serum albumin level.

Footnotes

1. Peretz A, Nève J, Jeghers O, et al, "Interest of Zinc Determination in Leukocyte Fractions for the Assessment of Marginal Zinc Status," *Clin Chim Acta*, 1991, 203(1):35-46.

(Continued)

Zinc, Serum *(Continued)*

2. "Assessment of Zinc Nutriture," *J Lab Clin Med*, 1991, 118:299-300, (editorial).
3. King JC, "Assessment of Zinc Status," *J Nutr*, 1990, 120(Suppl 11):1474-9.
4. Khoshoo V, Kjarsgaard J, Krafchick B, et al, "Zinc Deficiency in A Full-Term Breast-Fed Infant: Unusual Presentation," *Pediatrics*, 1992, 89(6 Pt 1):1094-5.
5. Prasad AS, Miale A Jr, Farid Z, et al, "Clinical and Experimental: Zinc Metabolism in Patients With the Syndrome of Iron Deficiency Anemia, Hepatosplenomegaly, Dwarfism, and Hypogonadism," *J Lab Clin Med*, 1963, 61:537-49.
6. MacMahon RA, Parker ML, and McKinnon MC, "Zinc Treatment in Malabsorption," *Med J Aust*, 1968, 210-2.
7. Odeh M, "The Role of Zinc in Acquired Immunodeficiency Syndrome," *J Intern Med*, 1992, 231(5):463-9.
8. Boosalis MG, Solem LD, Cerra FB, et al, "Increased Urinary Zinc Excretion After Thermal Injury," *J Lab Clin Med*, 1991, 118(6):538-45.
9. Zlotkin SH, "Nutrient Interactions With Total Parenteral Nutrition: Effect of Histidine and Cysteine Intake on Urinary Zinc Excretion," *J Pediatr*, 1989, 114(5):859-64.
10. Kay RG, Tasman-Jones C, and Pybus J, "A Syndrome of Acute Zinc Deficiency During Total Parenteral Alimentation in Man," *Ann Surg*, 1976, 183:331-40.
11. Moynahan EJ, "Acrodermatitis Enteropathica: A Lethal Inherited Human Zinc-Deficiency Disorder," *Lancet*, 1974, 2:399-400.
12. Smith JC Jr, Zeller JA, Brown ED, et al, "Elevated Plasma Zinc: A Heritable Anomaly," *Science*, 1976, 193:496-8.
13. Prasad AS, Meftah S, Abdallah J, et al, "Serum Thymulin in Human Zinc Deficiency," *J Clin Invest*, 1988, 82(4):1202-10.

References

Alfrey AC, "Essential Trace Elements," *The Kidney: Physiology and Pathophysiology*, 2nd ed, Seldin DW and Giebisch G, eds, New York, NY: Raven Press, 1992, 2993-3003.

Mack D, Koletzko B, Cunnane S, et al, "Acrodermatitis Enteropathica With Normal Serum Zinc Levels: Diagnostic Value of Small Bowel Biopsy and Essential Fatty Acid Determination," *Gut*, 1989, 30(10):1426-9.

Ruz M, Cavan KR, Bettger WJ, et al, "Development of a Dietary Model for the Study of Mild Zinc Deficiency in Humans and Evaluation of Some Biochemical and Functional Indices of Zinc Status," *Am J Clin Nutr*, 1991, 53(5):1295-303.

Zinc, Urine

***CPT** 84630*

Related Information

Heavy Metal Screen, Blood *on page 972*
Heavy Metal Screen, Urine *on page 973*
Urine Collection, 24-Hour *on page 32*

Synonyms Zn, Urine

Specimen 24-hour urine **CONTAINER:** Plastic urine container, no preservative **STORAGE INSTRUCTIONS:** Keep on ice or refrigerated. Laboratory will measure and record volume and remove aliquot for analysis. **CAUSES FOR REJECTION:** Specimen allowed to contact rubber. **TURNAROUND TIME:** Samples are usually sent to a reference laboratory. **SPECIAL INSTRUCTIONS:** Avoid contact with rubber during collection such as through rubber catheter. If a urinary catheter is absolutely essential, as in burn patients, consider the use of a silicone catheter, which has been shown to release less zinc than other types. Most catheters contribute zinc to the collection, some to a substantial degree. For critical or research cases, it is advisable to document acceptability of the catheter prior to use.[1]

Interpretive **REFERENCE RANGE:** 0.14-0.8 mg/24 hours **USE:** Evaluate zinc toxicity; evaluate low serum zinc levels; evaluate compliance in oral zinc therapy of Wilson's disease.[2] Low urine zinc levels in the presence of depressed serum zinc tend to confirm zinc deficiency. **LIMITATIONS:** Zinc deficiency is usually accompanied by decreased urine zinc excretion. Zinc deficiency, however, may be in part due to excess urine losses, especially in cirrhosis, hemolytic anemias, sickle cell disease, alcoholism, diabetes, or chronic renal diseases. **METHODOLOGY:** Atomic absorption spectrometry (AA)

Footnotes

1. de Haan KEC and Woroniecka UD, "Bladder Catheters and Zinc Contamination of Urine," *Clin Chem*, 1989, 35(5):888.
2. Milanino R, Marrella M, Moretti U, et al, "Oral Zinc Sulphate as Primary Therapeutic Intervention in A Child With Wilson Disease," *Eur J Pediatr*, 1989, 148(7):654-5.

Zn, Serum *see* Zinc, Serum *on page 1036*

Zn, Urine *see* Zinc, Urine *on this page*

TRANSFUSION SERVICE (BLOOD BANK)

Douglas W. Huestis, M.D.

Contributing to this chapter:

Lowell Tilzer, MD, PhD

Albumin
Factor VIII Concentrate
Factor IX Concentrate
Plasma Protein Fraction

Dread of AIDS and worry about other transfusion-related infectious diseases have led to public reluctance to permit the use of donor blood and its components. Physicians and surgeons, re-examining their usage of blood, have gradually come to realize that blood transfusions and the maintenance of arbitrary hemoglobin levels are not as important as they were once thought to be. These trends have also led to some diminution in the use of blood and components, and to increasing demands for the use of autologous blood, and other alternatives to conventional allogeneic transfusion.

As a result, physicians now must explain to their patients why transfusions of blood and components may be necessary, the risks involved (in appropriate perspective), and ways of reducing the risks. Obviously, such information should be available to the patient well ahead of the anticipated event so that there will be time to arrange alternatives to address the patient's concerns. Many blood services now have informative brochures about blood transfusion, its risks, and the alternatives. These materials can be placed in clinics and physicians' offices to provide a basis for informed consent for blood transfusion.

Important: The availability of such brochures does not absolve the physician from responsibility to obtain and document informed consent.

Preparation for Transfusion

1. **Sample Collection.** Ask the patient his or her name and check this against the information on the identification band. If the Transfusion Service uses a special transfusion wristband, label it with the patient's full name, hospital number, and date, and apply it appropriately. At the patient's bedside, label the sample tube with at least the patient's full name, hospital number, and date. Other information may be locally required. The same identification must be on the requisition form, plus the initials of the phlebotomist who certifies that the patient's identity has been properly verified.

   Information on the patient's identification plate must agree fully with that on the wristband or the sample should not be drawn. Adjust procedures for emergencies or disasters with great care to avoid the increased likelihood of mixups that is inherent in such situations.

   - The patient's identification band (or bands, if the Transfusion Service uses an additional one) must be attached to an accessible part of the patient's body, not taped to the bed or chart. If the bands have been removed for any reason, the identification procedure must be repeated and another sample obtained.

   - Any identification discrepancies or problems must be corrected promptly.

Clerical error is the most common cause of blood incompatibility and resultant hemolytic transfusion reactions. Full and correct labeling **at the bedside** is essential for all samples of blood drawn for the Transfusion Service. Wax pencil marking is not acceptable. The Blood Bank must not be permitted to accept unlabeled tubes or those with unattached or loose identification, no matter who presents them. Specimen identification requirements are outlined in a listing bearing that name in the specimen collection chapter.

2. **Issuing Blood.** Unless there is some good reason to do otherwise, the oldest unit crossmatched for a patient is dispensed first. But if a patient has autologous and/or directed as well as allogeneic (homologous) units, issue them in this order: first autologous, then directed, and last allogeneic.

   Remove the selected unit from the refrigerator. Carefully inspect for clots, hemolysis, or discoloration. Quarantine any unit of abnormal appearance.

   Two responsible persons (eg, nurse and technologist) should jointly compare the identifying information on the transfusion request form and on the blood bag. This information includes at least the following:

   - patient's name, hospital number, other identifying data
   - patient's ABO and Rh type
   - donor blood ABO and Rh type
   - donor number, expiration date, component being issued
   - crossmatch result (if applicable)
   - result of antibody screen

   Resolve any discrepancies before releasing blood.

   The nurse and technologist, after verifying all information, should certify in writing that they have done so, and enter the date and time of issue.

   With some exceptions (emergencies, major surgery), issue only one unit of blood at a time for a patient receiving elective transfusions. Otherwise, the second unit may remain at room temperature for an extended period.

   Personnel should never be allowed to pick up two units for two or more different patients at the same time.

Administration of Blood and Blood Components

1. Except in urgent situations, avoid starting transfusions at night for three reasons. First, hospital staffing is thinner at night, making it harder to keep a close watch on patients being transfused. Second, patients need sleep. Third, any untoward reaction will awaken the patient and create turmoil on the ward.

2. If possible, before picking up the blood from the Blood Bank, start an I.V. with a Y-type blood-recipient set having a standard clot filter, using isotonic saline and a needle of 19-gauge or bigger. Smaller needles and special sets may be necessary in pediatrics. Run the saline at a slow drip. With an already existing I.V., check the needle gauge and the I.V. site. Change the I.V. tubing if necessary. If solutions other than isotonic saline have been running, flush with saline.

   Do not use any other solution which may be incompatible with stored blood. Ringer's, for example, causes formation of small clots that may block the needle, while hypotonic solutions, particularly those containing dextrose, may cause decreased post-transfusion survival of transfused red cells. For the same reasons of pharmacologic compatibility, add no medications to stored blood. The same applies to the tubing containing blood, unless it is flushed with saline before and after the medication.

Check other I.V. medications that may have to be given and try to reschedule them before or after the blood transfusion. If necessary, other I.V.s can be given into another extremity.

3. Correctly identify the intended recipient.
    - Compare all information on the transfusion form with that on the patient's identification band or bands, and on the donor blood unit. Make sure that everything conforms.
    - The wristband or bands must be attached to the patient's body, not elsewhere. Otherwise, the transfusion should not be given until a new sample has been obtained and crossmatching repeated.
4. Inspect the blood unit looking for hemolysis or other abnormal appearance. In the case of anything out of the ordinary, consult the Blood Bank before starting the transfusion.
5. Record the vital signs, including temperature.
6. Do not attempt to vent plastic blood containers.
7. Once the blood is obtained from the Blood Bank or Transfusion Service, it should be mixed thoroughly by repeatedly inverting the bag, and started at once. Return the blood to the Blood Bank without delay if anything interferes with starting the transfusion.
8. **Do not store blood**, even temporarily, in conventional refrigerators on nursing stations, O.R., ER, or anywhere other than in blood storage units that are specially and continuously monitored. To do so is contrary to all accreditation standards, including federal regulations.
9. Hang the blood.
    - Mix gently.
    - Carefully insert the plastic cannula of the infusion set to avoid puncturing the wall of the bag.
    - In the case of red blood cells, lower the unit and allow 50-100 mL of saline to run into the bag. This allows easier and faster infusion.
10. Special blood filters may be indicated for some patients. See Filters for Blood listing.
11. Note the time the blood is started.
12. Remain with and observe the patient for at least the first 5 minutes. Take vital signs again at 15 minutes and at the end of the transfusion. Check the patient frequently.
13. Try not to exceed 2 hours for one unit of RBCs. If there is danger of pulmonary edema or congestive heart failure, or if there is a possible immunologic problem or a history of reactions, the time may be extended to 4 hours. If circumstances require even slower transfusion, it may be better to divide the unit in half and give it as two transfusions.
14. After the transfusion, return the empty blood bags to the Blood Bank. The residual small amounts of blood can be very useful in the event of a reaction.

Release of Blood Set Up for Transfusion Then Not Used

1. Blood issued for transfusion and then not used can be used for another patient as long as:
   - the unit has not been entered or punctured
   - the unit has not been warmed
   - the unit has been returned to the Blood Bank within 30 minutes of the time it was issued (its temperature must not exceed 10°C)
   - the unit has not been stored in an unmonitored refrigerator

2. When blood has been set up for a patient but not used, most hospitals limit the time it can be held for that patient. Otherwise, there is a likelihood the blood would be held indefinitely and would outdate because someone forgot to notify the Blood Bank that the patient no longer needed a transfusion. The time limit may vary according to the needs of the institution, but is usually 24-48 hours, or 24 hours after an indicated surgical procedure.

   The foregoing policy should be automatic, but not absolute. Clinicians must have the option of requesting that units be held longer for specific clinical indications, provided that those indications do not violate immunologic principles and thus lead to increased risk of transfusion reactions.

   Another exception, at the Blood Bank's option, may be when antigen-negative units have been obtained (often with great difficulty) for a patient with a particular blood group antibody. The likelihood of a continuing need will dictate that such units be reserved for the patient.

3. Patients receiving a series of transfusions are at particular risk of forming blood group antibodies that could cause future transfusion reactions. Because such antibodies can form quickly and unpredictably, standards require that a crossmatch sample be valid only for 3 days, after which a new one must be obtained. This is particularly important in patients who have either been pregnant or had transfusions within the past 3 months. The rule may be waived for those who have not had either such event, but the Blood Bank seldom has such knowledge.

   Both the foregoing rules (ie, the 1-day hold of blood and the 3-day hold of crossmatch samples) are best written into the Blood Bank's standard policies so as to form part of the operating routine. Requests for exceptions should be the onus of the clinical physician, referred to the Blood Bank physician if necessary.

Transfusions in Trauma and Other Emergencies

Transfusions may be needed at once in an emergency where delay may result in loss of life. In such a case, somewhat different procedures are essential and some steps, such as the crossmatch, may have to be dispensed with in the interest of time. All abbreviated procedures increase the risk to the patient, but to varying degrees.

In this discussion, understand that "blood" usually means red blood cells (previously also known as "packed cells"). Whole blood may be the preferred transfusion medium in acute blood loss or in hypovolemic shock, but it is seldom available nowadays. Experience in the past 20 or so years has shown that emergencies and massive surgical procedures can be as effectively treated with red blood cells and appropriate plasma expanders as has been the case historically with whole blood.

The following procedures are suggested for different periods of time available.

1. **No sample, blood needed now.** Give type O Rh-negative red cells (packed cells) without delay. Request blood sample. If O Rh-negative blood is in short supply, inform the physician and issue O Rh-positive red cells (packed cells). Better a live, immunized patient than a dead one without antibodies. As soon as the patient's own blood type is known, issue type-specific units.

2. **Blood sample provided, blood needed in 5-10 minutes.** Give blood of the patient's own type without crossmatch. If any blood is needed before the typing is finished, give out two units of O Rh-negative red cells (packed cells) immediately, with type-specific to follow.

   In both the foregoing situations, it is important for all persons involved to understand that **blood issued in this manner may turn out to be incompatible with the recipient.**

3. **Blood sample provided, blood needed in 15-30 minutes.** It may be possible to complete crossmatches within this time, depending on the technique used. It will probably not be possible to complete the antibody screening test on the patient's serum.

4. **Afterwards.** When the emergency is over, finish the antibody screening test and all the crossmatches so that the patient's record will be complete. The Blood Bank physician may add a note to the patient's chart as to the departures from normal transfusion routine and on whose authority they were carried out. Many hospitals require an emergency release form to document the original request. Because of the increased risks, this is a good idea.

5. **Additional thoughts.** Blood Bank and Emergency Room should work out their policies and procedures together, so that surprises do not turn up during emergencies. This should include the importance of sample pickup, identification, and the principles of blood selection. In times of blood shortage, notify the ER so they will be prepared.

   A foolproof blood sample identification system is vital in all emergencies, since some of the usual precautions will not be used. The system must also be applicable to the multiple trauma situation (imagine dealing with 4 or 5 people from an accident, all with the same surname) and to the mass casualty disaster.

   Remember that blood samples do not clot immediately, and there may be difficulty with fibrin shreds in incompletely clotted samples.

   Do not use up the community's supply of O Rh-negative blood on a massive trauma case. It is reasonable to switch to Rh-positive early, particularly in the case of a male or older female patient, in whom the effects of immunization are more manageable. Remember that even Rh-negative patients often do not become immunized in that setting. This, too, can be part of an understanding between the Blood Bank and the Emergency Room. The Blood Bank physician should always make sure that such decisions are appropriately documented with the names of the deciding parties.

   See Uncrossmatched Blood, Emergency listing.

Guidelines for Outpatient Transfusion

With some minor exceptions, mostly concerning the timing of the blood sample and crossmatch, outpatient transfusions are handled the same as for inpatients. The precautions are the same, and if the hospital clinic staff are not accustomed to dealing with transfusions, they must be trained to do so.

1. **Informed consent.** The patient must give informed consent for any transfusion. This is the responsibility of the patient's physician. One consent may be understood to cover a series of transfusions, although it may be well to consult legal counsel on that point.

2. **Pretransfusion testing.** Because all these transfusions are elective, the patient should come in the day before (or within 3 days of) the transfusion. The same strictures apply to sample collection, identification, and banding as for inpatients. Be sure the bands used are waterproof, otherwise washing or bathing may obliterate the identification.

3. **Quantity to be transfused.** Since most of these patients have chronic conditions, and many are elderly, it may not be possible to give their units fast. Also, they must take up a bed in the clinic until the transfusions and an observation period are over. For these reasons, it is seldom practical to give more than two units in 1 day.

4. **Observation.** Observe the patient continuously for the first 15 minutes, frequently thereafter. After the transfusion is over, the patient should remain in the clinic under observation for at least 30 minutes. It is better that a relative or friend be available to accompany the patient home.

   Report any untoward reaction at once to the clinic physician or the patient's physician. In such a case, stop the transfusion and allow a saline drip to continue. Notify the Blood Bank.

5. **Instructions.** It is potentially useful to have a set of printed instructions to give the patient, or an informative brochure.

6. **Follow-up.** The patient's physician should inform the Blood Bank of any delayed untoward reactions to the transfusion, or of any evidence of transfusion-associated infectious disease. It may be helpful to see that the physician gets a copy of the Red Cross-AABB *Circular of Information for the Use of Human Blood and Blood Components*, the latest version, which should be obtainable from the community blood center or hospital transfusion service.

Summary Chart of Blood Components

Component	Major Indications	Action	Not Indicated for —	Special Precautions	Hazards	Rate of Infusion
Whole blood	Symptomatic anemia with large volume deficit	Restoration of oxygen-carrying capacity, restoration of blood volume	Condition responsive to specific component	Must be ABO-identical Labile coagulation factors deteriorate within 24 hours after collection	Infectious diseases; septic/toxic, allergic, febrile reactions; circulatory overload	For massive loss, fast as patient can tolerate
Red blood cells	Symptomatic anemia	Restoration of oxygen-carrying capacity	Pharmacologically treatable anemia Coagulation deficiency	Must be ABO-compatible	Infectious diseases; septic/toxic, allergic, febrile reactions	As patient can tolerate but less than 4 hours
Red blood cells, leukocytes removed	Symptomatic anemia, febrile reactions from leukocyte antibodies	Restoration of oxygen-carrying capacity	Pharmacologically treatable anemia Coagulation deficiency	Must be ABO-compatible	Infectious diseases; septic/toxic, allergic reaction (unless plasma also removed, eg, by washing)	As patient can tolerate but less than 4 hours
Red blood cells, adenine-saline added	Symptomatic anemia with volume deficit	Restoration of oxygen-carrying capacity	Pharmacologically treatable anemia Coagulation deficiency	Must be ABO-compatible	Infectious diseases; septic/toxic, allergic, febrile reactions; circulatory overload	As patient can tolerate but less than 4 hours
Fresh frozen plasma	Deficit of labile and stable plasma coagulation factors and TTP	Source of labile and nonlabile plasma factors	Condition responsive to volume replacement	Should be ABO-compatible	Infectious diseases; allergic reactions; circulatory overload	Less than 4 hours
Liquid plasma and plasma	Deficit of stable coagulation factors	Source of nonlabile factors	Deficit of labile coagulation factors or volume replacement	Should be ABO-compatible	Infectious diseases, allergic reactions	Less than 4 hours
Cryoprecipitated AHF	Hemophilia A, von Willebrand's disease, hypofibrinogenemia, factor XIII deficiency	Provides factor VIII, fibrinogen, vWF, factor XIII	Conditions not deficient in contained factors	Frequent repeat doses may be necessary	Infectious diseases, allergic reactions	Less than 4 hours
Platelets	Bleeding from thrombocytopenia or platelet function abnormality	Improves hemostasis	Plasma coagulation deficits and some conditions with rapid platelet destruction (eg, ITP)	Should not use microaggregate filters	Infectious diseases; septic/toxic, allergic, febrile reactions	Less than 4 hours
Granulocytes	Neutropenia with infection	Provides granulocytes	Infection responsive to antibiotics	Preferably ABO-compatible, do not use microaggregate filters	Infectious diseases; allergic, febrile reactions	One apheresis unit over 2- to 4-hour period — closely observe for reactions

Modified from *Circular of Information for the Use of Human Blood and Blood Components*, American Red Cross, Council of Community Blood Centers, and American Association of Blood Banks, 1992, with permission.

ABO Group and Rh Type

CPT *86900 (ABO); 86901 (Rh(D))*

Related Information

Rh Genotype *on page 1090*
Rh_o(D) Typing *on page 1093*

Synonyms Blood Grouping and Rh Typing; Type and Rh

Patient Care PREPARATION: Patient should be wearing a wristband.

Specimen Blood CONTAINER: Red top tube COLLECTION: At the patient's bedside, ask the patient to give his or her name. Compare with the hospital wristband. Label the Transfusion Service wristband (if there is one) with the patient's full name, hospital number, date, and initials of the collector. Label sample tube with the same information, including identification number from the wristband. Label requisition form with identification number. The collector signs the requisition, verifying the patient's identity with hospital wristband and Transfusion Service wristband. Some hospitals require additional information. It is always best to stamp the requisition with the patient's identification plate to avoid transcription errors. CAUSES FOR REJECTION: Gross hemolysis, sample placed in a serum separator tube, specimen tube not properly labeled

Interpretive USE: Determine blood type before transfusion; performed on expectant mothers and on newborn blood samples to detect possible ABO or Rh hemolytic disease of the newborn[1]; as part of Type and Screen and Type and Crossmatch; protect mother or surgical patient in case of obstetric or other hemorrhage LIMITATIONS: Abnormal plasma proteins, cold autoagglutinins, positive direct antiglobulin test, and in some cases, bacteremia may interfere. ADDITIONAL INFORMATION: Only Rh_o(D) is usually tested in the Rh system. The other Rh antigens are identified generally only on indication, such as the presence of an antibody against another Rh antigen. If spherocytes are present in the newborn's peripheral smear, and the mother is type O and the baby is type A or B, the diagnosis of ABO hemolytic disease of the newborn should be considered. The direct antiglobulin test may be positive or negative in ABO hemolytic disease of the newborn. ABO and Rh typing can each be ordered alone.

Footnotes

1. Chan-Shu S and Blair O, "ABO Hemolytic Disease of the Newborn," *Am J Clin Pathol*, 1979, 71:677-9.

References

Cooper ES, Ryden SE, Hill JR, et al, "The 1987 Comprehensive Blood Bank Survey of the College of American Pathologists," *Arch Pathol Lab Med*, 1989, 113(9):969-74.

Walker RH, ed, *Technical Manual*, 10th ed, Arlington, VA: American Association of Blood Banks, 1990, 173-88.

Absorption-Elution Techniques *see* Antibody Identification, Red Cell *on next page*

Acid Eluate *see* Antibody Identification, Red Cell *on next page*

AHF, Lyophilized *see* Factor VIII Concentrate *on page 1064*

Albumin for Infusion

CPT *36430*

Related Information

Plasma Protein Fraction (Human) *on page 1079*

Synonyms Normal Serum Albumin (Human)

Abstract Commercially prepared human albumin is 96% pure. Heat inactivation for 10 hours at 60°C destroys viruses. Albumin is available as either 5% or 25% (weight/volume). For volume expansion alone, hydroxyethyl starch can often be substituted.

Patient Care AFTERCARE: Follow blood pressure after rapid administration.

Interpretive USE: Volume expander used mostly for replacement of colloid in emergencies such as burns, pancreatitis, shock due to trauma, hemorrhage, or surgery; adult respiratory distress syndrome; with removal of ascitic fluid and for hypotension related to hemodialysis.[1] Used as standard replacement in therapeutic plasma exchange (q.v.). The 25% albumin is used in patients who are not dehydrated, but it may be used with large volumes of normal saline or lactated Ringer's solution. LIMITATIONS: Does not contain components of the clotting mechanism of blood or plasma; brief retention; less effective for nutritional objectives than amino acid solutions. **Side effects and hazards**: Fast administration can cause fluid overload, especially with the hyperosmotic 25 g/dL albumin.[2] Additional saline must be given to patients who are dehydrated.[2] Bacterial contamination has occurred on rare occasions.[3] CON-

TRAINDICATIONS: Severely anemic patients presumably need transfused erythrocytes; patients with cardiac failure **ADDITIONAL INFORMATION:** Supplied as 25% and as 5% solutions. Sodium content is 100-160 mmol/L; thus, the expression "salt poor" is inappropriate; it has been applied to the 25 g/dL dose. A colloid solution that lacks hepatitis risk. Antibodies are not present. Albumin costs the pharmacy about $140/L. Some of the albumin can be replaced with saline, for instance, in plasma exchange.

Footnotes

1. Alexander MR, Alexander B, Mustion AL, et al, "Therapeutic Use of Albumin: 2," *JAMA*, 1982, 247:831-3.
2. Huestis DW, Bove JR, and Case J, *Practical Blood Transfusion*, 4th ed, Boston, MA: Little, Brown and Co, 1988, 315.
3. Swisher SN and Petz LD, "Clinical Use of Blood Substitutes," *Clinical Practice of Blood Transfusion*, 2nd ed, New York, NY: Churchill Livingstone, 1989, 746-56.

References

Walker RH, ed, *Technical Manual*, 10th ed, Arlington, VA: American Association of Blood Banks, 1990, 359-60.

Allogeneic Blood Transfusion *replaced by* Autologous Transfusion, Intraoperative Blood Salvage *on page 1052*

Alloimmunization, Leukocyte *see* Filters for Blood *on page 1066*

Antibody Identification, Elution Technique *see* Antibody Identification, Red Cell *on this page*

Antibody Identification Panel *see* Antibody Identification, Red Cell *on this page*

Antibody Identification, Red Cell

***CPT** 86870 (each panel)*

Related Information

Antiglobulin Test, Indirect *on page 1051*
Cold Agglutinin Screen *on page 1056*
Cold Autoabsorption *on page 1057*
Hemolytic Disease of the Newborn, Antibody Identification *on page 1070*
Type and Crossmatch *on page 1100*

Synonyms Absorption-Elution Techniques; Antibody Identification, Elution Technique; Antibody Identification Panel; Panel; Red Cell Antibody Identification

Applies to Acid Eluate; Elution; Ether Eluate; Heat Eluate; Red Cell Antigen Typing

Test Commonly Includes Cold autoabsorption may be necessary to remove cold autoagglutinins in order to determine whether or not an unexpected antibody is present. Antibodies identified during prenatal testing and known to cause hemolytic disease of the newborn may be titrated.

Specimen Blood **CONTAINER:** One red top tube and one lavender top (EDTA) tube **CAUSES FOR REJECTION:** Gross hemolysis, sample placed in a serum separator tube, specimen tube not properly labeled **TURNAROUND TIME:** 1 hour, or substantially more **SPECIAL INSTRUCTIONS:** Provide Blood Bank with diagnosis, history of pregnancies and/or transfusions, and list of medications taken by patient.

Interpretive USE: Panel testing is done on serum of patients who have a positive antibody screening test to identify unexpected antibody(ies). It is also done on eluates from red cells that have a positive direct antiglobulin test. Antibody identification is necessary before transfusion, if antibody screen is positive. Test is useful to work up obstetric patient's positive antibody screen for antenatal diagnosis of possible hemolytic disease of the newborn and to work up hemolytic anemia when direct or indirect antiglobulin test is positive. **LIMITATIONS:** Antibody may be too weak to be detected or identified. Antibodies to low incidence antigens may not be detected. **CONTRAINDICATIONS:** When a positive antibody screen is due to cold autoagglutination, autoabsorption of the serum in the cold (4°C) can eliminate the autoagglutinins. The absorbed serum can then be tested against a cell panel in the usual way to detect alloantibodies of clinical importance, such as Rh antibody. In the case of warm autoagglutination, autoabsorption should be done only if the patient has not been transfused for 3-4 months, to avoid the likelihood of removing significant alloantibodies. See also Cold Agglutinin Screen and Cold Autoabsorption test listings. **METHODOLOGY:** Panel of separate, selected red cell samples, each of known antigenic composition, exposed to patient's serum or to eluate. Serum may be absorbed with certain test red cells, followed by a repeat panel with the absorbed serum or with antibody eluted from the absorbing cells. Auto controls are extremely

(Continued)

Antibody Identification, Red Cell *(Continued)*

important to rule out autoagglutination. **ADDITIONAL INFORMATION:** Such immunization to red cell antigens may present crossmatch problems. When a panel seems to identify an antibody in a patient's serum, make sure that the patient's red cells lack the corresponding antigen. If the antibody is clinically significant (see table), donor units must also lack this corresponding antigen. Elution and testing the eluate against a panel may identify the antibody causing a positive direct antiglobulin test. Compatible donor blood must then be sought.

Clinically Significant Blood Group Antibodies	
General	Antibodies that react by immediate spin Antibodies that react at 37°C and by antiglobulin, that show hemolysis *in vitro,* and that have been reported to cause hemolytic reactions
Examples	Anti-A and anti-B; antibodies of the Rh, Kell, Duffy, Kidd systems; also anti-S, -s, -U, and some others reacting as above
Clinically Unimportant Blood Group Antibodies	
General	Antibodies reacting only at room temperature or below, which do not show hemolysis
Examples*	Antibodies of the Lewis, P, MN systems; high-titer low-avidity antibodies; cold agglutinins

*Rare exceptions exist, usually when activity extends to 37°C.

Antibody Screen *see* Antiglobulin Test, Indirect *on page 1051*

Antibody Titer

CPT 86886

Related Information

Prenatal Screen, Immunohematology *on page 1085*

Synonyms Atypical Antibody Titer; Irregular Antibody Titer; Rh Titer; Titer, Irregular Antibodies in Transfusion Service; Titer of Anti-Rh_0(D); Titer of Unexpected Antibody

Applies to Hemolytic Disease of the Newborn, Antibody Titer

Test Commonly Includes Antibody detection and identification must be done first; if an antibody is present, then it may be titrated in antenatal work-up.

Specimen Serum **CONTAINER:** Red top tube **STORAGE INSTRUCTIONS:** Freeze remaining serum in case subsequent parallel titers are required. **CAUSES FOR REJECTION:** Gross hemolysis, sample placed in a serum separator tube, specimen tube not properly labeled

Interpretive **POSSIBLE PANIC RANGE:** An increase of at least two tube dilutions during pregnancy indicates consideration for amniocentesis. **USE:** Detection of titer of a red cell antibody in antenatal maternal serum when antibody screen is positive. Commonly involves Rh antibody titers in Rh_0(D)-negative mothers. Follow the course of Rh or other antibody formation in cases of potential maternal-fetal blood incompatibility to predict hemolytic disease of the newborn. Among other criteria, used to evaluate need for amniocentesis. **LIMITATIONS:** Although correlations do exist between titer and severity of erythroblastosis, titers do not reflect the condition of an unborn child. False-negatives and false-positives occur. First-time appearance of antibody or rise of at least two tubes in titer usually means the fetus has the corresponding antigen. Failure of titer to rise is not meaningful. There is an inherent error of plus or minus one tube dilution in test performance within a given laboratory and more between different laboratories. Some laboratories use enhancement techniques such as low ionic strength saline (LISS) or enzymes. **Consistency is extremely important and the same laboratory should be used throughout.** Even in the same laboratory, the red cells used as target antigen cannot be kept absolutely constant. **Many laboratories freeze a sample of serum to compare to a subsequent sample;** this is an extremely helpful practice. **CONTRAINDICATIONS:** No antibody detected; biologic father lacking corresponding antigen; antibody identified is not implicated in hemolytic disease of newborn (eg, Lewis) **METHODOLOGY:** Serial dilution with saline, enzyme, or low ionic strength saline followed by antiglobulin. Expressed as reciprocal of highest dilution still giving agglutination visible without a microscope. **ADDITIONAL INFORMATION:** Although an indirect antiglobulin titer of 16-32 or higher has been considered significant for

$Rh_0(D)$, such figures are not necessarily applicable to other alloantibodies. A rising titer of an antibody capable of causing hemolytic disease of the newborn is more significant than a single assay. Specific phenotype determinations on the father's red cells may be helpful.

References

Walker RH, ed, *Technical Manual*, 10th ed, Arlington, VA: American Association of Blood Banks, 1990, 312-3, 467-9.

Antiglobulin Test, Direct

***CPT** 86880*

See Also Anemia Flowchart in the Hematology Appendix

Related Information

Cold Agglutinin Screen *on page 1056*
Cold Autoabsorption *on page 1057*
Cord Blood Screen *on page 1057*
Transfusion Reaction Work-up *on page 1098*
Type and Crossmatch *on page 1100*
Type and Screen *on page 1102*

Synonyms Anti-human Globulin Test, Direct; Anti-human Serum Test, Direct; Broad Spectrum Direct Antiglobulin; Coombs' Test, Direct; DAT; Direct Antiglobulin Test; Direct Coombs'; Polyspecific Direct Antiglobulin

Test Commonly Includes Direct antiglobulin testing with polyspecific anti-human globulin serum. It may include use of monospecific reagents (anti-IgG, anticomplement) when indicated. Eluates from coated red cells may be prepared for antibody identification (eg, specimens from cord bloods, recently transfused patients, hemolytic anemia work-up).

Specimen Blood **CONTAINER:** One lavender top (EDTA) tube and one red top tube **CAUSES FOR REJECTION:** Gross hemolysis, sample placed in a serum separator tube, specimen tube not properly labeled **SPECIAL INSTRUCTIONS:** Indicate diagnosis, transfusion history, and pertinent medications on the requisition form.

Interpretive **REFERENCE RANGE:** Negative **USE:** Polyspecific antiglobulin serum detects immunoproteins, IgG or complement on red cells (ie, detection of sensitization of erythrocytes *in vivo*). Coated red cells are said to be "sensitized." Used to detect autoimmune hemolytic anemias caused by antibody and/or complement components being bound to patient's red cells (including drug-induced), transfusion reaction, and erythroblastosis fetalis (hemolytic disease of the newborn). In warm autoimmune hemolytic anemias, the antibody is usually IgG. In cold hemolytic anemias, the cell coating is usually with complement components. **LIMITATIONS:** False-positives may occur with cold agglutinins. See also Cold Agglutinin Screen and Cold Autoabsorption test listings. Use of red top tubes or serum separator tubes may cause false-positive reactions particularly if tubes have been refrigerated. Newborn's cells may have negative direct antiglobulin test in ABO hemolytic disease. Wharton's jelly from cord samples can cause problems. Technical factors can cause false-positive and false-negative reactions; lists of technical causes of misleading results are published[1,2] and include saline stored improperly, cold autoagglutinins, and contaminated glassware. **METHODOLOGY:** Antiglobulin serum. In the **direct antiglobulin test**, one examines for antibody attached to the patient's red cells *in vivo*. In the **indirect antiglobulin test**, the antigen-antibody reaction occurs *in vitro* and one tests patient's serum for antibody with reagent red cells (the antigen). **ADDITIONAL INFORMATION:** Drugs, including the penicillins and cephalosporins, α-methyldopa, levodopa, quinidine, insulin, mefenamic acid, sulfonamides, tetracycline, and others may cause positive direct antiglobulin tests.[2] Many positive direct antiglobulin tests are due to methyldopa. Methyldopa antibodies are predominantly IgG; about 1% of patients on methyldopa develop hemolytic anemia, but as many as 15% develop a positive DAT. Although drugs and alloantibodies may cause a positive direct antiglobulin test, the majority have no such association. It is unusual to find a significant antibody in the eluate from a positive direct antiglobulin test. Broad spectrum or polyspecific antisera contain both anti-IgG and anti-C3d. Anti-IgG may be used to determine if the cells are coated with IgG. If indicated, an indirect test and antibody identification are included in the work-up of a positive direct antiglobulin test. In cases of autoimmune hemolytic anemia, an eluate from the patient's red cells can indicate antibody specificity. Elution is also indicated when the DAT on the patient's red cells is positive within 14 days of transfusion and in newborns.

Footnotes

1. Canadian Red Cross Society, *Serological and Immunological Methods of the Canadian Red Cross Blood Transfusion Service*, 8th ed, Toronto: The Canadian Red Cross Society, 1980.

(Continued)

Antiglobulin Test, Direct *(Continued)*

2. Walker RH, ed, *Technical Manual*, 10th ed, Arlington, VA: American Association of Blood Banks, 1990, 147-57.

References

Freedman J, "False-Positive Antiglobulin Tests in Healthy Subjects and in Hospital Patients," *J Clin Pathol*, 1979, 32:1014-8.

Garratty G, "The Clinical Significance (and Insignificance) of Red-Cell-Bound IgG and Complement," *Current Applications and Interpretations of the Direct Antiglobulin Test*, Arlington, VA: American Association of Blood Banks, 1988.

Huh YO, Liu FJ, Rogge K, et al, "Positive Direct Antiglobulin Test and High Serum Immunoglobulin G Values," *Am J Clin Pathol*, 1988, 89:197-200.

Judd WJ, Barnes BA, Steiner EA, et al, "The Evaluation of a Positive (Autocontrol) in Pretransfusion Testing Revisited," *Transfusion*, 1986, 26:220-4.

Snyder EL and Falast GA, "Significance of the Direct Antiglobulin Test," *Lab Med*, 1985, 16:89-96.

Antiglobulin Test, Direct, Complement

***CPT** 86880*

Synonyms Complement Direct Coombs' Test; Coombs', Direct, Complement; Coombs', Non-gamma; DAT, Complement; Direct Antiglobulin Test, Complement

Test Commonly Includes Antiglobulin test using anticomplement

Specimen Blood **CONTAINER:** One lavender top (EDTA) tube and one red top tube **STORAGE INSTRUCTIONS:** Do not refrigerate specimen. **CAUSES FOR REJECTION:** Gross hemolysis, sample placed in a serum separator tube, specimen tube not properly labeled **SPECIAL INSTRUCTIONS:** Indicate diagnosis and **all** medications received by patient before and after admission to the hospital.

Interpretive **REFERENCE RANGE:** Negative **USE:** Determine if a positive direct antiglobulin is due to complement coating the patient's red blood cells; this should be evaluated in instances of any autoimmune hemolytic anemia.[1] About 10% to 13% of instances of warm autoimmune hemolytic anemias react only to complement DAT.[1] The complement DAT is used in work-up of the cold agglutinin syndrome and in paroxysmal cold hemoglobinuria.[1] Work-up of drug-induced antibodies, cold autoimmune hemolytic anemia, cold agglutinin disease, paroxysmal cold hemoglobinuria, collagen disease may include complement-active antiglobulin testing. **LIMITATIONS:** Serum separator tubes and red top tubes may cause false-positives due to *in vitro* sensitization with complement. Harmless cold autoagglutinins coating previously refrigerated patient red cells may give weak positive results with such antiglobulin serum. Only a small number of clinically significant antibodies are found by anticomplement. Many transfusion services keep broad spectrum and IgG antiglobulins but not anticomplement. **METHODOLOGY:** Antiglobulin serum, C3 **ADDITIONAL INFORMATION:** Usually done only upon special request or particular indication. A positive polyspecific antiglobulin with a negative IgG implies that the positive direct test is due to complement. IgG DAT alone, without complement DAT, is found in 20% to 40% of instances of warm-reactive autoimmune hemolytic anemia and about 50% or more of such patients have both IgG and complement coating their erythrocytes.[1]

Drug therapy: Some drugs causing antiglobulin positivity (eg, quinidine and phenacetin) are commonly characterized by positivity of complement DAT.[1] Positivity of complement-active direct antiglobulin in a patient on methyldopa is evidence that methyldopa is probably not the only problem.

Footnotes

1. Petz LD and Swisher SN, "Blood Transfusion in Acquired Hemolytic Anemias," *Clinical Practice of Blood Transfusion*, 2nd ed, New York, NY: Churchill Livingstone, 1989, 549-82.

References

Garratty G, "The Clinical Significance (and Insignificance) of Red-Cell-Bound IgG and Complement," *Current Applications and Interpretations of the Direct Antiglobulin Test*, Arlington, VA: American Association of Blood Banks, 1988.

Snyder EL and Falast GA, "Significance of the Direct Antiglobulin Test," *Lab Med*, 1985, 16:89-96.

Antiglobulin Test, Direct, IgG

***CPT** 86880*

Synonyms Coombs', Direct, IgG; DAT, IgG; Gamma Anti-human Globulin Test; Gamma Direct Coombs'

Test Commonly Includes Direct antiglobulin test using anti-IgG

Specimen Blood **CONTAINER:** One lavender top (EDTA) tube and one red top tube **CAUSES FOR REJECTION:** Gross hemolysis, sample placed in a serum separator tube, specimen tube not properly labeled **SPECIAL INSTRUCTIONS:** On the request form give diagnosis, transfusion history, and **all** medications received by patient before and after admission to the hospital.

Interpretive **REFERENCE RANGE:** Negative **USE:** Determine if the patient's positive direct antiglobulin is due to an IgG antibody, as commonly occurs with warm autoimmune hemolytic anemias, transfusion reactions, erythroblastosis fetalis (hemolytic disease of the newborn), chronic lymphocytic leukemia, some drugs (eg, penicillins, cephalosporin drugs, methyldopa). **LIMITATIONS:** Positive DAT requires at least 100-300 IgG molecules per red cell. Some instances of autoimmune hemolytic anemia have a negative direct antiglobulin test. **METHODOLOGY:** Antiglobulin serum, IgG **ADDITIONAL INFORMATION:** Done when a positive direct antiglobulin is encountered with a polyspecific anti-human globulin reagent.

Antiglobulin Test, Indirect

CPT 86886

Related Information

Antibody Identification, Red Cell *on page 1047*
Bilirubin, Neonatal *on page 138*
Hemolytic Disease of the Newborn, Antibody Identification *on page 1070*
Prenatal Screen, Immunohematology *on page 1085*
Type and Crossmatch *on page 1100*
Type and Screen *on page 1102*

Synonyms Antibody Screen; Atypical Antibodies; Coombs', Indirect; IAT; Indirect Antiglobulin Test; Indirect Anti-human Globulin Test; Indirect Coombs'

Specimen Blood **CONTAINER:** Red top tube **COLLECTION:** If for crossmatch, see Type and Crossmatch. **CAUSES FOR REJECTION:** Gross hemolysis, sample placed in a serum separator tube, specimen tube not properly labeled

Interpretive **REFERENCE RANGE:** Negative **USE:** Detect sensitization of erythrocytes *in vitro* (ie, screen for unknown antibodies in serum by use of known red cells). Such detection of antibody in patient's serum by normal reagent red blood cells is in very wide use, especially to screen for unexpected antibodies in pretransfusion testing and the first trimester of pregnancy, in Rh_o(D)-positive as well as in Rh_o(D)-negative expectant mothers. Evaluate potential cause of hemolysis. The indirect antiglobulin test is used in panels, in titers, and in full crossmatches. In addition to its use in investigation of unknown antibodies in serum, the indirect antiglobulin test is also the means of antibody identification with elution techniques when antibody is eluted from coated red cells. When the indirect antiglobulin test is used in the crossmatch, neither antigens nor antibodies are known. **LIMITATIONS:** Abnormal proteins and cold autoagglutinins may interfere and cause delays in interpretation. Test will not detect all antibodies (eg, antibodies in low titer, antibodies to low-incidence antigens). In some instances of autoimmune hemolytic anemia, the antibody may be completely adsorbed onto the erythrocytes and not detectable by the indirect antiglobulin test. **METHODOLOGY:** Antiglobulin serum **ADDITIONAL INFORMATION:** The antibody screen is the "screen" portion of the "type and screen." It is done routinely with compatibility testing (crossmatch) and on mother's serum during prenatal care and at the time of delivery. A positive indirect antiglobulin test must be followed up with antibody identification. The **indirect antiglobulin** is done on patient serum with red cells of known antigenic type. The **direct antiglobulin** is done on patient red cells. A common **drug cause** of positive indirect antiglobulin tests is methyldopa, which causes as much as 25% of positive DAT reactions in hospital patients. It causes positive indirect reactions in 15% of such patients.[1] Levodopa and mefenamic acid are among other drugs known to cause positive indirect reactions. For management of such problems, see Footnote 1.

Footnotes

1. Snyder EL and Spivack M, "Clinical and Serological Management of Patients With Methyldopa-Induced Positive Antiglobulin Tests," *Transfusion*, 1979, 19:313-6.

References

Walker RH, ed, *Technical Manual*, 10th ed, Arlington, VA: American Association of Blood Banks, 1990, 147-57.

Antihemophilic Factor, Cryoprecipitated *see* Cryoprecipitate *on page 1058*
Antihemophilic Factor (Human) *see* Factor VIII Concentrate *on page 1064*
Anti-human Globulin Test, Direct *see* Antiglobulin Test, Direct *on page 1049*

Anti-human Serum Test, Direct *see* Antiglobulin Test, Direct *on page 1049*

Antiplatelet Antibody *see* Platelet Antibody, Immunohematologic *on page 1080*

Anti-Rh Globulin *see* Rh_o(D) Immune Globulin (Human) *on page 1091*

Atypical Antibodies *see* Antiglobulin Test, Indirect *on previous page*

Atypical Antibody Titer *see* Antibody Titer *on page 1048*

Autologous Stem Cells *see* Peripheral Blood Stem Cells, Autologous *on page 1074*

Autologous Transfusion, Intraoperative Blood Salvage

CPT 86891

Related Information

Autologous Transfusion, Preoperative Deposit *on this page*

Synonyms Blood Salvage, Intraoperative Autologous Transfusion

Replaces Allogeneic Blood Transfusion

Specimen SPECIAL INSTRUCTIONS: With automated systems, it is usually necessary to reserve or schedule use of the equipment beforehand. In some regions, this service is offered by the community blood center.

Interpretive METHODOLOGY: Although preoperative autologous blood collection is the best-known way of avoiding a transfusion of homologous blood, a patient's own blood may be saved and returned during the operation or immediately afterwards.

Three procedures are available:

- Intraoperative hemodilution: Blood is withdrawn from the patient after the induction of anesthesia but before the surgical incision is made. Crystalloid may be given to the patient to support the blood volume.
- Intraoperative cell salvage: This procedure is only cost-effective if two or more units of shed blood can be salvaged during surgery. Some red cell savers process the blood in a semicontinuous manner. They wash the blood in normal saline. Most of the plasma and platelets and other debris are removed. A reinfusion bag contains the saline-suspended red cells, which can be transfused back to the patient using a standard filter. The cycle of removal, washing, and resuspension takes about 10 minutes. A specially trained operator is required.

Other systems usually involve collection of shed blood into a container from which it is given back to the patient through a filter. Without a wash step, such systems risk transfusing thromboplastic debris with the collected blood.

- Postoperative cell salvage: The blood from mediastinal drainage and from other sterile operative sites is saved, defibrinogenated, and returned to the patient. The blood collected in this way may be washed and spun down so as to get rid of any microaggregates. The procedure appears to be safe, but the quantities salvaged are often too small to be cost-effective. Infection has not been a problem.

References

Council on Scientific Affairs, "Autologous Blood Transfusions – Council Report," *JAMA*, 1986, 256:2378-80.

Dzik WH and Sherburne B, "Intraoperative Blood Salvage: Medical Controversies," *Transfus Med Rev*, 1990, 4:208-35.

Johnson RG, Rosenkrantz KR, Daggett WM, et al, "The Efficacy of Postoperative Autotransfusion in Patients Undergoing Cardiac Operations," *Ann Thorac Surg*, 1983, 36:173-9.

Autologous Transfusion, Preoperative Deposit

CPT 86890 (collection processing and storage); 86985 (splitting of blood or blood products, each unit)

Related Information

Autologous Transfusion, Intraoperative Blood Salvage *on this page*

Donation, Blood *on page 1061*

Donation, Blood, Directed *on page 1062*

Synonyms Autotransfusion; Transfusion, Autologous; Transfusion, Autologous, Predeposit

Test Commonly Includes Removal of blood or components from a donor for subsequent autologous transfusion. ABO and Rh typing of blood.[1] It is best to use distinctively colored blood bag labels and wristbands. Autologous transfusion serves to alleviate concern about the safety and availability of blood for transfusion. Blood from a given patient is returned to that person for elective surgery. There is no risk of transmission of hepatitis, AIDS, or other donor infectious disease, nor of reaction to serum protein or red cell antigens. Alloimmunization cannot occur. But risks do exist, namely those of identification mixup, bacterial contamination, volume overload, plus the possibility of donation reactions and excessive anemia. The patient's bone marrow is usually stimulated to produce red cells faster (increased erythropoietin production).

Categories of autologous programs are recognized:

- preoperative phlebotomy (the principal type discussed in this summary)
- immediate preoperative phlebotomy with hemodilution
- intraoperative cell salvage
- postoperative salvage
- combinations of techniques; especially the first and third types are used together successfully.

Patient Care PREPARATION: Donor should be in generally good health. AFTERCARE: Replacement of iron is essential. Fluid intake on the days of donation should be increased. Immediately after donating blood, the patient is kept lying down for a few minutes. When moved to a chair **with assistance**, the donor/patient should remain seated for 15-30 minutes. The bandage can be removed 2-4 hours after applied.

Specimen CONTAINER: Blood bag, which must be labeled "for autologous use only". A donor classification label or tag is required, "Autologous Donation".[1] COLLECTION: The blood unit is collected as for regular blood donation (see Donation, Blood), although the patient/donor qualifications will obviously have to allow for some exceptions. In elderly patients or children, who might otherwise suffer hypovolemia on blood withdrawal, an effective preventive measure is to infuse about 500 mL of isotonic saline (less for children) immediately before phlebotomy (isovolemic blood donation). STORAGE INSTRUCTIONS: Blood unit is kept in a monitored Blood Bank refrigerator for up to 42 days, when collected in the AS-1 system. For longer storage, blood may be frozen within 5 days of collection if such facilities are available. CAUSES FOR REJECTION: Criteria for disqualification of the proposed autologous donor are variable among hospitals and blood banks. Those for whom elective orthopedic procedures are planned, with intact cardiorespiratory and other systems, are ideal candidates for autologous donation. Some persons who have been disqualified as candidates for homologous donation, for instance those with a history of cancer, may still be candidates for autologous donation.

Widely accepted **criteria for disqualification** of a proposed autologous donor include:

- anemia (hematocrit <33%)
- possibility of bacteremia. Patients should be off antibiotics for 48-72 hours. Dental work in the prior 72 hours is a contraindication for fear of low-grade bacteremia and contamination of the unit.
- unstable angina
- aortic or subaortic stenosis
- cardiac failure
- recent infarct of myocardium
- significant ventricular arrhythmia
- atrioventricular block
- uncontrolled epilepsy

Other possible criteria for rejection of a proposed autologous donor include:

- pregnancy – autologous or any other transfusion is seldom indicated in uncomplicated pregnancy. Thus, lacking some specific problem, autologous blood donation is usually unnecessary. Nevertheless, it is a reasonably safe procedure, even in pregnancy. Some legal questions exist.
- uncontrolled hypertension

SPECIAL INSTRUCTIONS: Usually by appointment with Blood Bank. There is often a charge for the donation. Physician should write out a prescription giving the date of the intended surgery, how many units are to be drawn, and indicating that the patient has been given a prescription for oral iron. An order for Type and Screen is essential to cover unanticipated blood needs that might exceed the amount of autologous blood.

Interpretive USE: Usually for elective surgery. Eliminates risks of alloimmunization, of transmission of infectious diseases, and of a number of other hazards. Autologous blood may be the only suitable source of blood/components for patients who react adversely to homologous

(Continued)

Autologous Transfusion, Preoperative Deposit *(Continued)*

blood, patients of extremely rare blood types, patients who have antibodies to high incidence antigens, or who have multiple antibodies. **LIMITATIONS:** Phlebotomy hemoglobin concentration should be ≥11.0 g/dL or the hematocrit ≥33%.

Technical problems may prevent return of the donated autologous blood (eg, accidental puncture of the bag, clot formation, or discoloration leading to concern about bacterial growth). Surgery may require use of additional, homologous units. Hypovolemic and vasovagal reactions may occur. Preoperative donations diminish presurgical hemoglobin. Identification procedures are important throughout.

There is usually a charge for each unit of blood collected, even though it may not be transfused.

Blood, which is not used by the autologous donor, usually cannot be used for anyone else for the following reasons.

a. The donor, by the nature of his/her illness, may not qualify as a regular donor, and the donor history for an autologous donor may not meet the requirements for conventional (allogeneic) donation.
b. Some of the units collected may not meet the requirements for donor blood (eg, hematocrit).
c. A hospital collecting autologous blood for its own patients need not do the infectious disease screening tests. In that case, the blood may be used **only** by the patient/donor, may not be released for other patients, and may not be shipped to other facilities.

METHODOLOGY: Similar to conventional blood donation **ADDITIONAL INFORMATION:** Some general considerations of an autologous blood program follow.

- "Your own blood is the best blood."
- Donors/patients generally should meet the general requirements of a regular blood donor, except that the hematocrit may be as low as 33%; the patient's age may be younger than 17 at the discretion of the Blood Bank physician.
- The patient should be taking iron for at least 1 week before the first donation. This is especially important if a series of 3 or 4 units are to be drawn.
- Units of blood are normally drawn at weekly intervals. The last unit must be drawn not less than 72 hours before the intended operation.
- Autologous donation is a stimulus to increased erythropoietin production.
- The use of recombinant human erythropoietin may make autologous donation easier for patients with a marginal hemoglobin level.
- Predonated autologous blood for elective surgery has the potential to provide as much as 10% of all red cell transfusions.[2,3]
- Elderly persons are not necessarily excluded.[4,5]
- Autologous donations in preteen and adolescent patient/donors are described as safe and effective.[6] If donor weighs less than 100 pounds, the amount of anticoagulant should be adjusted.
- An old technique called "leapfrog" can be useful if surgery is delayed after some autologous units have already been collected. To prevent the first unit or units from outdating, give the oldest unit back to the patient then collect two fresh ones at the same session. This can be repeated but has obvious limitations.

Except under special circumstances, donations should be no more frequent than every 3 days and not within 72 hours of major surgery.[1] However, in usual practice, weekly intervals may be more desirable.

Should autologous blood be transfused on the same strict clinical indications as donor blood? This is a pertinent topic for a hospital blood utilization committee.[7] Most authorities say it should. On the other hand, some surgeons and patients feel that, because autologous blood is the patient's own, it may be transfused postoperatively even if the usual criteria do not hold. Whereas it is axiomatic that a treatment not indicated is contraindicated, whether desired by the patient or not, the risks of autologous blood are clearly less than homologous. So it seems reasonable that the criteria could be eased for autologous. It is important that there be some **clinical** reason for any transfusion and that reason must be documented in the patient's record.

In addition to elective autologous transfusion previously outlined, intraoperative blood salvage procedures are now commonly used.

Footnotes

1. Widmann FK, ed, *Standards for Blood Banks and Transfusion Services*, 15th ed, Bethesda, MD: Committee on Standards, American Association of Blood Banks, 1993, 35-8.
2. Toy PT, Strauss RG, Stehling LC, et al, "Predeposited Autologous Blood for Elective Surgery," *N Engl J Med*, 1987, 316:517-20.
3. Owings DV, Kruskall MS, Thurer RL, et al, "Autologous Blood Donations Prior to Elective Cardiac Surgery. Safety and Effect on Subsequent Blood Use," *JAMA*, 1989, 262(14):1963-8.
4. Haugen RK and Hill GE, "A Large-Scale Autologous Blood Program in a Community Hospital," *JAMA*, 1987, 257:1211-4.
5. Pindyck J, Avorn J, Kuriyan M, et al, "Blood Donation by the Elderly," *JAMA*, 1987, 257:1186-8.
6. Silvergleid AJ, "Safety and Effectiveness of Predeposit Autologous Transfusions in Preteen and Adolescent Children," *JAMA*, 1987, 257:3403-4.
7. Simon TL and Stehling L, "Indications for Autologous Transfusions," *JAMA*, 1992, 267(19):2669.

References

Axelrod FB, Pepkowitz SH, and Goldfinger D, "Establishment of a Schedule of Optimal Preoperative Collection of Autologous Blood," *Transfusion*, 1989, 29(8):677-80.

Dzik WH and Sherburne B, "Intraoperative Blood Salvage: Medical Controversies," *Transfus Med Rev*, 1990, 4(3):208-35.

Goodnough LT, Rudnick S, Price TH, et al, "Increased Preoperative Collection of Autologous Blood With Recombinant Human Erythropoietin Therapy," *N Engl J Med*, 1989, 321(17):1163-8.

Huestis DW, Bove JR, and Case J, *Practical Blood Transfusion*, 4th ed, Boston, MA: Little, Brown and Co, 1988.

Kruskall MS, "Autologous Transfusions – Past, Present, and Future," *Mayo Clin Proc*, 1992, 67(4):392-3, (editorial).

Moore SB, Swenke PK, Foss ML, et al, "Simplified Enrollment for Autologous Transfusion: Automatic Referral of Presurgical Patients for Assessment for Autologous Blood Collections," *Mayo Clin Proc*, 1992, 67(4):323-7.

National Blood Resource Education Program Expert Panel, "The Use of Autologous Blood," *JAMA*, 1990, 263(3):414-7.

Popovsky MA, "Autologous Blood Transfusion in the 1990s. Where Is It Heading?" *Am J Clin Pathol*, 1992, 97(3):297-300.

Surgenor DM, "The Patient's Blood Is the Safest Blood," *N Engl J Med*, 1987, 316:542-4.

Autotransfusion *see* Autologous Transfusion, Preoperative Deposit *on page 1052*

Blood Donation *see* Donation, Blood *on page 1061*

Blood Donation, Designated *see* Donation, Blood, Directed *on page 1062*

Blood Fractions, Irradiated *see* Irradiated Blood Components *on page 1071*

Blood Grouping and Rh Typing *see* ABO Group and Rh Type *on page 1046*

Blood Salvage, Intraoperative Autologous Transfusion *see* Autologous Transfusion, Intraoperative Blood Salvage *on page 1052*

Bone Marrow, Autologous

CPT 86915

Related Information

Peripheral Blood Stem Cells, Autologous *on page 1074*

Synonyms Bone Marrow Transplant, Autologous; Marrow Transplant, Autologous; Pluripotential Stem Cells, Bone Marrow

Test Commonly Includes Aspiration of bone marrow from leukemia or cancer patient in remission, frozen storage, and autologous transfusion after tumoricidal therapy that has bone-marrow-ablative side effect

Abstract Patient is in remission from cancer or leukemia, without evidence of residual disease in bone marrow. Marrow aspiration is an operating room procedure. A single session usually produces enough marrow for restoration of normal marrow function. The standard is a minimum of 2 x 10^8 nucleated cells per kg patient's body weight (in at least 75% of collections); total volume aspirated is less than 1500 mL.

Patient Care **PREPARATION:** Because of blood loss in marrow collection, it is customary to collect two units of autologous red cells in preparation.

Specimen **STORAGE INSTRUCTIONS:** Marrow is concentrated, resuspended in dimethyl sulfoxide, and frozen at a controlled rate in liquid nitrogen. Label as comparable autologous blood component. Unless red cells are removed by various techniques, marrow contains a substantial amount of blood. No formal expiration date has been set. **CAUSES FOR REJECTION:** Malignant in-

(Continued)

Bone Marrow, Autologous *(Continued)*

volvement of bone marrow; fibrosis of marrow at usual sites of collection, such as might be caused by prior radiation therapy of the pelvis **SPECIAL INSTRUCTIONS:** Available on scheduled basis only after consultation with Blood Bank physician.

Interpretive **USE:** Collection and storage of autologous bone marrow make it possible to treat malignant disease with heavy doses of chemotherapy and/or irradiation that would otherwise destroy the patient's marrow function. After such treatment, marrow is repopulated from the stored autologous supply. **LIMITATIONS:** Repopulation of marrow depends on the number of pluripotent stem cells in the stored collection. This can be evaluated only by stem cell culture, which is thus the primary quality control method. Inadequacy of stem cells will mean failure of repopulation. **METHODOLOGY:** The patient/donor is under general or spinal anesthesia. Multiple aspirations of bone marrow from the posterior superior iliac crests are made by means of special needles and syringes until, under cell-count control, enough nucleated cells have been collected. The total volume is usually less than 1500 mL and contains substantial amounts of blood. Blood loss usually requires transfusion of the units of autologous blood that were collected before the procedure. After marrow collection, the harvest is filtered to remove clots and bony spicules. **ADDITIONAL INFORMATION:** Label the aspirated bone marrow with the same care needed in the preparation of other autologous blood components.

References

Areman EM and Sacher RA, "Bone Marrow Processing for Transplantation," *Transfus Med Rev*, 1991, 5(3):214-27.

Bone Marrow Transplant, Autologous *see* Bone Marrow, Autologous *on previous page*

Broad Spectrum Direct Antiglobulin *see* Antiglobulin Test, Direct *on page 1049*

Cold Agglutinin Screen

CPT 86940 (auto, screen, each); 86941 (incubated)

Related Information

Antibody Identification, Red Cell *on page 1047*
Antiglobulin Test, Direct *on page 1049*

Specimen Blood **CONTAINER:** Red top tube **CAUSES FOR REJECTION:** Gross hemolysis, sample placed in a serum separator tube, specimen tube not properly labeled

Interpretive **REFERENCE RANGE:** Negative; titer <32 **USE:** Usually done when the antibody screen or panel indicates that a cold autoagglutinin may be present, interfering with examination for irregular antibodies **METHODOLOGY:** 4°C and room temperature testing **ADDITIONAL INFORMATION:** A cold agglutinin titer is another serologic test not directly related to transfusion but used as an aid in diagnosis of primary atypical pneumonia and certain hemolytic anemias. When present, cold autoagglutinins may have to be removed to detect a clinically significant unexpected antibody, masked by the cold agglutinins. See following listing. Cold hemagglutinins are found in everybody's serum. They react most strongly at 4°C. They are not normally seen in the room temperature crossmatch. When cold agglutinins are present at 20°C or higher they are said to be of "wide thermal amplitude." Such cold agglutinins may cause pain in the extremities, thrombosis, agglutination, and hemolysis. Cold autoagglutinins are usually of I specificity. Their presence may follow an infection, such as *Mycoplasma pneumoniae*. Cold hemagglutination (autoagglutination) can also occur during cardiac surgery when the temperature of the perfusate may be between 15°C and 32°C.[1,2]

Footnotes

1. Leach AB, Van Hasselt GL, and Edwards JC, "Cold Agglutinins and Deep Hypothermia," *Anaesthesia*, 1983, 38:140-3.
2. Diaz JH, Cooper ES, and Ochsner JL, "Cold Hemagglutination Pathophysiology. Evaluation and Management of Patients Undergoing Cardiac Surgery With Induced Hypothermia," *Arch Intern Med*, 1984, 144:1639-41.

References

Heddle NM, "Acute Paroxysmal Cold Hemoglobinuria," *Transfus Med Rev*, 1989, 3(3):219-29.
Roelcke D, "Cold Agglutination," *Transfus Med Rev*, 1989, 3(2):140-66.

Cold Autoabsorption

CPT *86975*

Related Information

Antibody Identification, Red Cell *on page 1047*
Antiglobulin Test, Direct *on page 1049*

Test Commonly Includes Detection of cold autoagglutinin, removal of antibody by absorption at 4°C with autologous RBCs

Specimen Blood **CONTAINER:** One red top tube and one lavender top (EDTA) tube **CAUSES FOR REJECTION:** Gross hemolysis, sample placed in a serum separator tube, specimen tube not properly labeled **TURNAROUND TIME:** Up to 48 hours

Interpretive **REFERENCE RANGE:** Negative antibody screen after absorption **USE:** Removes cold autoagglutinins in order to determine whether or not an unexpected antibody, such as Rh_o(D), is present in the serum of patients needing transfusion, particularly when the cold autoagglutinin is active at 37°C, and to permit identification of such antibody. **LIMITATIONS:** Potent autoagglutinins may not readily absorb out of patient's serum. **ADDITIONAL INFORMATION:** Often done when there is a positive antibody screen due to cold autoagglutinins, to rule out clinically significant unexpected antibodies, such as Rh antibodies. Such antibodies can be masked by cold autoagglutinins. Cold autoabsorption is a common cause of delay in the availability of compatible blood. In the case of high-titered cold autoagglutinins, prolonged or repeated absorption may be needed. Repeated absorptions are best. Absorb the serum with the patient's washed RBCs for 30 minutes, remove the supernatant, wash the red cells in warm saline, then repeat using the same red cells, until the absorbed serum no longer agglutinates the cells at 4°C. **Warm** autoabsorption is addressed briefly under Antibody Identification, Red Cell. An important alternative is to do crossmatching at 37°C.[1]

Footnotes

1. Petz LD and Swisher SN, "Blood Transfusion in Acquired Hemolytic Anemias," *Clinical Practice of Blood Transfusion*, 2nd ed, New York, NY: Churchill Livingstone, 1989, 549-82.

References

Mollison PL, Engelfriet CP, and Contreras M, *Blood Transfusion in Clinical Medicine*, 9th ed, Oxford, UK: Blackwell Scientific Publications, 1992, 284-92.

Compatibility Testing *see* Type and Crossmatch *on page 1100*

Complement Direct Coombs' Test *see* Antiglobulin Test, Direct, Complement *on page 1050*

Complications of Transfusion *see* Whole Blood *on page 1106*

Coombs', Direct, Complement *see* Antiglobulin Test, Direct, Complement *on page 1050*

Coombs', Direct, IgG *see* Antiglobulin Test, Direct, IgG *on page 1050*

Coombs', Indirect *see* Antiglobulin Test, Indirect *on page 1051*

Coombs', Nongamma *see* Antiglobulin Test, Direct, Complement *on page 1050*

Coombs' Test, Direct *see* Antiglobulin Test, Direct *on page 1049*

Cord Blood Screen

CPT *86880 (antiglobulin, direct); 86900 (ABO); 86901 (Rh(D))*

Related Information

Amniotic Fluid Analysis for Erythroblastosis Fetalis *on page 122*
Antiglobulin Test, Direct *on page 1049*
Bilirubin, Neonatal *on page 138*
Hemolytic Disease of the Newborn, Antibody Identification *on page 1070*
Newborn Crossmatch and Transfusion *on page 1072*
Prenatal Screen, Immunohematology *on page 1085*
Rh Genotype *on page 1090*
Rh_o(D) Immune Globulin (Human) *on page 1091*
Rh_o(D) Typing *on page 1093*

Synonyms Type and Coombs', Cord Blood

Applies to Hemolytic Disease of the Newborn, Cord Blood Screen

Test Commonly Includes ABO group, Rh type, direct antiglobulin test on cord blood sample

Specimen Cord blood **CONTAINER:** One lavender top (EDTA) tube and one red top tube **COL-**

(Continued)

Cord Blood Screen *(Continued)*

LECTION: Do not overfill lavender top tube with cord blood. Mix well. Patient's identity must be verified and recorded on label and request form. **CAUSES FOR REJECTION:** Gross hemolysis, sample placed in a serum separator tube, specimen tube not properly labeled

Interpretive USE: Determine ABO group and Rh type of the newborn. The direct antiglobulin test detects maternal antibody bound to fetal cells in cases of hemolytic disease of the newborn. A negative direct antiglobulin test on Rh_o(D)-positive baby's cells when the mother has not received antenatal Rh_o(D) immune globulin and is Rh_o(D)-negative, is an indication that the mother is a candidate for Rh_o(D) immune globulin (human). **LIMITATIONS:** Wharton's jelly may interfere with testing; cells heavily coated with maternal IgG antibodies may give misleading results with many antisera. Accurate results may be impossible if the cord blood specimen is contaminated with maternal red cells. Positive direct antiglobulin results due to anti-D are not a contraindication to postdelivery Rh_o(D) immune globulin, when the mother has been given an antenatal dose of this material. **ADDITIONAL INFORMATION:** Further investigation may be indicated based on results of this screen. Rh_o(D) immunization is not the only cause of fetal hemolytic disease. In addition to anti-A and anti-B, any blood group antibody of IgG class (especially of subclass 1 and 3) can cross the placenta and cause hemolytic disease. But, other than the ABO situation, these are uncommon.[1]

Footnotes

1. Whittle MJ, "Rhesus Haemolytic Disease," *Arch Dis Child*, 1992, 67(1 Spec No):65-8.

Crossmatch *see* Type and Crossmatch *on page 1100*

Cryoprecipitate

***CPT** 36430 (transfusion); 86965 (pooling)*

Related Information

Anticoagulant, Circulating *on page 402*
Bleeding Time, Mielke *on page 411*
Factor VIII *on page 424*
Factor VIII Concentrate *on page 1064*
Fibrin Breakdown Products *on page 433*
Fibrinogen *on page 435*
Fibrin Split Products, Protamine Sulfate *on page 439*
Partial Thromboplastin Time *on page 450*
Plasma, Fresh Frozen *on page 1078*
Prothrombin Time *on page 468*
Thrombin Time *on page 474*
von Willebrand Factor Antigen *on page 476*
von Willebrand Factor Assay *on page 478*
von Willebrand Factor Multimer Assay *on page 478*

Synonyms Antihemophilic Factor, Cryoprecipitated; Cryoprecipitated Antihemophilic Factor

Applies to Fibrinogen Therapy; Hemophilia A Therapy; von Willebrand's Disease Therapy

Test Commonly Includes Cryoprecipitate is a labile component containing factor VIII, von Willebrand's factor, fibrinogen, and factor XIII

Abstract Cryoprecipitate is the only available source of fibrinogen for patients with clinical deficiencies of that fraction, eg, disseminated intravascular coagulation (DIC). In the right clinical conditions, it can also be useful in hemophilia A, in von Willebrand's disease, and for making fibrin glue.

Patient Care PREPARATION: Prothrombin time, PTT, and fibrinogen assay to document indication (eg, hemophilia). Patient should have transfusion wristband for checking against component container label before administration.

Dosage and administration: Rapid administration of about 10 mL of diluted cryoprecipitate per minute is used as a loading dose for hemophilia, followed by a smaller dose at 12-hour intervals,[1] depending on clinical circumstances. In pooling, single containers are washed with 0.9% saline, so that the volume of six units of cryoprecipitate is 100-150 mL. In the presence of circulating anticoagulants, larger doses or other special measures may be indicated.[1]

A 70 kg patient should have an increase of about 2.5% AHF for each bag of cryoprecipitate given.[2] For minor bleeding, dosage raising the patient's level to 30% to 50% may be used. For major surgical procedures, a preoperative dose sufficient to raise the level to 80% to 100%, followed by postoperative maintenance calculated to keep the level constantly >50% for 10-14 days.

Factor VIII activity should be greater than 80 units/bag.[3]

In treatment of von Willebrand's disease, smaller amounts given less often will usually suffice.[1] When using cryoprecipitates, the factor VIII levels achieved from a calculated dose will vary.

Cryoprecipitate must be given through a filter.

To treat hypofibrinogenemia, one bag can be expected to raise plasma fibrinogen level about 7-10 mg/dL. A bag of cryoprecipitate provides at least 250 mg of fibrinogen.[3]

Cryoprecipitate may also be used as a topical "fibrin glue," which can stop local bleeding especially in cardiothoracic surgery.[4] Topical thrombin and calcium chloride convert the fibrinogen in the cryoprecipitate to fibrin. The volume of the individual units of cryoprecipitate used for the fibrin glue should not exceed 15 mL.

AFTERCARE: Factor VIII assay[1] and activated partial thromboplastin time can serve as controls in therapy of hemophilia A and von Willebrand's disease, and fibrinogen levels[1] and thrombin time when hypofibrinogenemia is being treated. Bleeding time measurements can also be useful in some cases of von Willebrand's disease.

Specimen Blood **STORAGE INSTRUCTIONS:** (For blood component) Cryoprecipitate may be stored for up to 1 year, preferably at -30°C or below, but not above -18°C. It must be stored frozen without thawing. Before infusion, thaw (but do not warm) for up to 15 minutes in a water bath at 37°C in a plastic overwrap, so that the precipitate is dissolved. Multiple units are pooled before administration. Once thawed, store at room temperature. Transfuse cryoprecipitate ideally within 2 hours or less. It should be used within 6 hours after thawing if the container has not been entered.[1] Pooled cryoprecipitates should be used within 4 hours. Once thawed it cannot be reissued by the Blood Bank. **CAUSES FOR REJECTION:** (Of patient sample): Gross hemolysis, sample placed in a serum separator tube, specimen tube not properly labeled

Interpretive **USE:** Treatment of deficiency of coagulation factor VIII (hemophilia A), von Willebrand's disease, and hypofibrinogenemic states. Replacement of fibrinogen should be considered when levels decrease to <100 mg/dL and patient is bleeding. The physician making such decisions should be aware of the coefficient of variation for fibrinogen levels in the laboratory being used. Prolongation of the thrombin time may support indications for infusion of fibrinogen as cryoprecipitate. Cryoprecipitate rather than antihemophilic factor concentrate should serve for treatment of von Willebrand's disease. Classical hemophilia usually requires factor VIII concentrate, but cryoprecipitate may be suitable when the need for treatment is only occasional. Cryoprecipitate is useful as a temporary treatment of bleeding tendency in uremia.[4] It also provides factor XIII. Cryoprecipitate may also help remove renal stones ("gravel"). Use 25 mL of cryoprecipitate, 4 mL of topical bovine thrombin, 1 mL of 10% $CaCl_2$. Administer using a #8 Foley catheter with a 22-gauge needle.[5] **LIMITATIONS:** There is considerable variation from bag to bag in factor VIII levels, but a "pool" of six units will help to iron out the variation. Cryoprecipitate is a poor source of factors II, V, IX, X, and XI.[3] **CONTRAINDICATIONS:** Do not use unless laboratory or clinical studies indicate a specific coagulation defect for which cryoprecipitate is appropriate. **ADDITIONAL INFORMATION:** A crossmatch is not necessary. Many units are sometimes needed. One concentrate per 5 kg body weight may serve as a rough guide to initial dosage. Fresh frozen plasma contains coagulation factors, but none of them are concentrated. The larger fluid volumes can create circulatory overload. **Hazards**: The risk of hepatitis and other viral infections is less than that of AHF concentrate because each bag comes from a single donor. Febrile and allergic reactions may occur.[1] Large volumes of ABO incompatible cryoprecipitate may result in a positive direct antiglobulin test with mild hemolysis.[1] Presence of acquired inhibitors to factor VIII makes treatment with cryoprecipitate difficult or impossible. Factor VIII concentrates will be needed for such patients.

Footnotes

1. *Circular of Information for the Use of Human Blood and Blood Components*, American Red Cross, Council of Community Blood Centers, American Association of Blood Banks, 1992, 21-3.
2. Huestis DW, Bove JR, and Case J, *Practical Blood Transfusion*, 4th ed, Boston, MA: Little, Brown and Co, 1988, 320-1.
3. Ness PM and Perkins HA, "Cryoprecipitate as a Reliable Source of Fibrinogen Replacement," *JAMA*, 1979, 241:1690-1.
4. Lupinetti FM, Stoney WS, Alford WC, et al, "Cryoprecipitate – Topical Thrombin Glue," *J Thorac Cardiovasc Surg*, 1985, 90:502-5.
5. Janson PA, Jubelirer SJ, Weinstein MJ, et al, "Treatment of the Bleeding Tendency in Uremia With Cryoprecipitate," *N Engl J Med*, 1980, 303:1318-22.

References

Code of Federal Regulations, Food and Drugs, Title 21, Parts 640.50-640.56, 1991.

Goodnight SH, "Cryoprecipitate and Fibrinogen," *JAMA*, 1979, 241:1716-7, (editorial).

(Continued)

Cryoprecipitate *(Continued)*

Widmann FK, ed, *Standards for Blood Banks and Transfusion Services*, 15th ed, Bethesda, MD: American Association of Blood Banks, 1993, 10-1.

Cryoprecipitated Antihemophilic Factor *see* Cryoprecipitate *on page 1058*

Cytapheresis, Therapeutic

CPT 36520

Related Information

Plasma Exchange *on page 1076*
Platelets, Apheresis, Donation *on page 1083*
Sickle Cell Tests *on page 600*

Synonyms Cytoreduction; Therapeutic Cytapheresis

Applies to Erythrocytapheresis; Granulocytapheresis; Leukapheresis, Therapeutic; Red Cell Exchange; Stem Cell Collection; Therapeutic Leukapheresis

Test Commonly Includes Selective removal of platelets or granulocytes with subsequent return of plasma and red cells to the patient, removal of red cells in the treatment of hemoglobinopathies

Patient Care PREPARATION: Excellent vascular access is essential. AFTERCARE: Monitor patient's vital signs, watch for hypovolemia resulting from removal of large volumes of buffy coat. It is common to process as much as 10 L of patient's blood. Some albumin replacement is sometimes necessary.

Specimen COLLECTION: Carried out by Blood Bank personnel in apheresis area or patient's room CAUSES FOR REJECTION: Moribund patient, or one who cannot withstand establishment of an extracorporeal circuit; lack of specific indication for procedure. Decision to do this form of blood manipulation is shared between clinical and Blood Bank physicians. SPECIAL INSTRUCTIONS: Usually on scheduled basis, but can be emergent. Consult with Blood Bank physician.

Interpretive USE: Reduce platelets in thrombocythemic patient or leukocytes in hyperleukocytic leukemia; remove abnormal RBC and replace with normal RBCs in sickle cell disease with crisis. See table. LIMITATIONS: The extent of each procedure will be determined by the Blood Bank physician in consultation with the attending physician. When clinical circumstances so indicate, 10 L or more of patient's blood may be processed. Depends on blood cell separator used. ADDITIONAL INFORMATION: Therapeutic cytapheresis or cytoreduction, the removal of excessive blood cells, is carried out to correct extraordinarily increased leukocytes in various leukemias or platelets in severe thrombocytosis. This procedure is a stopgap method for immediate reduction of these two elements when there is risk of hemorrhage, thrombosis, or pulmonary or cerebral leukostasis. The body's tumor burden can thus be reduced while chemotherapy is initiated. Guidelines are given in the table. Red cell exchange is used to remove defective red cells and replace these with healthy red cells. This procedure is used predominantly to treat sickle cell anemia during pregnancy or before surgery. Peripheral blood stem cell (PBSC) collection is being used to supplement or replace bone marrow transplants in patients with leukemia, lymphoma, and certain solid tumors.

Indications for Therapeutic Cytapheresis

Leukapheresis Clinical indication	Evidence of vascular insufficiency (leukostasis), especially pulmonary or cerebral
WBC count (x 10^3/mm^3)	<100: seldom necessary 100–200: occasionally* >200: often urgent* (except in chronic lymphocytic leukemia)
Platelet Apheresis Clinical indication	Thrombosis or hemorrhage
Platelet count (/mm^3)	>1,500,000 spleen present, not in reactive thrombocytosis
Red Cell Exchange	Sickle cell crisis, pregnancy

*Particularly when there is a high proportion of blasts.
From Huestis DW, Bove JR, and Case J, *Practical Blood Transfusion*, 4th ed, Boston, MA: Little, Brown and Co, 1988, 383, with permission.

References

Hester J, "Therapeutic Cytapheresis," *Therapeutic Hemapheresis*, Vol II, MacPherson J and Kasprisin DO, eds, Boca Raton, FL: CRC Press, 1985, 143-53.

Cytoreduction *see* Cytapheresis, Therapeutic *on previous page*

DAT *see* Antiglobulin Test, Direct *on page 1049*

DAT, Complement *see* Antiglobulin Test, Direct, Complement *on page 1050*

DAT, IgG *see* Antiglobulin Test, Direct, IgG *on page 1050*

D Factor *see* Rh_o(D) Typing *on page 1093*

Direct Antiglobulin Test *see* Antiglobulin Test, Direct *on page 1049*

Direct Antiglobulin Test, Complement *see* Antiglobulin Test, Direct, Complement *on page 1050*

Direct Coombs' *see* Antiglobulin Test, Direct *on page 1049*

Directed Blood Donation *see* Donation, Blood, Directed *on next page*

Donation, Blood

CPT 86890 (collection processing and storage)

Related Information

Alanine Aminotransferase *on page 100*
Autologous Transfusion, Preoperative Deposit *on page 1052*
Phlebotomy, Therapeutic *on page 1075*
Whole Blood *on page 1106*

Synonyms Blood Donation; Phlebotomy, Blood Donor

Test Commonly Includes Donor phlebotomy, ABO grouping, Rh typing, antibody screen, HB_sAg, hepatitis core antibody, hepatitis C antibody, HIV-1 antibody, HTLV-I antibody, and ALT (SGPT)

Patient Care PREPARATION: Donors should be at least 18 years of age. Depending on state law, donors between 17 and 18 may donate with parental consent. The upper age limit usually is decided by the Blood Bank physician. Donor should weigh at least 110 pounds, should have a light meal before donation, no alcoholic beverages for 12 hours, **be in generally good health**, and afebrile. AFTERCARE: Activities are restricted for certain hazardous occupations for 24 hours. Donor reactions occur, rarely severe.[1,2]

Specimen Blood CONTAINER: Blood bag of appropriate configuration COLLECTION: Drawn by Blood Bank personnel CAUSES FOR REJECTION: History of hepatitis, history of HB_sAg positivity, drug addiction involving injection, homosexuality, diabetes requiring insulin, coronary heart disease permanently disqualify. Temporary disqualifications include hypotension, hypertension, anemia, positive syphilis serology (STS), travel to malaria endemic areas, exposure to hepatitis, pregnancy, recent childbirth, recent surgery, recent transfusion, tattoo within 6 months, inmate of penal or mental institution, and certain other medical conditions. Donors who have taken penicillin should be excluded from donation for 7 days. Use of vitamins, thyroid preparations, or oral contraceptives does **not** disqualify donors. Blood Banks now must present would-be donors with educational materials explaining the risk of AIDS in blood transfusion and encouraging self-deferment by those at risk of AIDS. They should also ask donors directly (face to face) about sexual behavior that might place donors at risk of AIDS (ie, male homosexual activity, I.V. drug use, prostitution, or exchange of sex for drugs or money). The aim is to discourage donors at risk from donating blood as a means of getting an AIDS test.

Interpretive USE: Obtain blood and its components for transfusion to patients. LIMITATIONS: Once per 8 weeks. Donations not to exceed six in any 12-month period. Truthful information must be provided by the prospective donor. METHODOLOGY: Donor blood must be tested for ABO and Rh type, screen for unexpected antibodies, HB_sAg, HB core antibody, hepatitis C antibody, ALT, STS (a serological test for syphilis), anti-HIV-1 and -2, and anti-HTLV-I and -II ADDITIONAL INFORMATION: Increasing use of blood and components requires more donations to assure adequate supplies for transfusion. Questions often arise as to acceptance or disqualification of would-be blood donors taking various medications.[1,3]

Footnotes

1. Huestis DW, Bove JR, and Case J, *Practical Blood Transfusion*, 4th ed, Boston, MA: Little, Brown and Co, 1988, 1-54.
2. Kasprisin DO, Glynn SH, Taylor F, et al, "Moderate and Severe Reactions in Blood Donors," *Transfusion*, 1992, 32(1):23-6.

(Continued)

Donation, Blood *(Continued)*

3. Ferner RE, Chaplin S, Dunstan JA, et al, "Drugs in Donated Blood," *Lancet*, 1989, 2(8654):93-4.

References

Sayers MH, "Duties to Donors," *Transfusion*, 1992, 32(5):465-6.
Walker RH, ed, *Technical Manual*, 10th ed, Arlington, VA: American Association of Blood Banks, 1990, 1-18.

Donation, Blood, Directed

CPT 36430 (transfusion); 86999

Related Information

Autologous Transfusion, Preoperative Deposit *on page 1052*
Irradiated Blood Components *on page 1071*

Synonyms Blood Donation, Designated; Directed Blood Donation; Recipient-Selected Transfusions

Test Commonly Includes Donor phlebotomy, ABO grouping, Rh typing, antibody screen, HB_sAg, HB core antibody, ALT (SGPT) (alanine aminotransferase), hepatitis C antibody, HIV-1 antibody, and HTLV-I antibody

Abstract Designation of a friend or relative to provide blood donation. Siblings, parents, and children are most likely to provide compatible blood.

Patient Care PREPARATION: Donors must meet all the requirements of a regular blood donor. AFTERCARE: Activities are restricted for certain hazardous occupations for 24 hours. Donor reactions occur occasionally.

Specimen Blood CONTAINER: Blood bag COLLECTION: Commonly drawn at a regional blood center. CAUSES FOR REJECTION: History of hepatitis, history of HB_sAg positivity, drug addiction involving injection, homosexuality, diabetes requiring insulin, coronary heart disease permanently disqualify. Temporary disqualifications include hypotension, hypertension, anemia, positive syphilis serology (STS), travel to malaria endemic areas, exposure to hepatitis, pregnancy, recent childbirth, recent surgery, recent transfusion, tattoo within 6 months, inmate of penal or mental institution, and certain other medical conditions. Donors who have taken penicillin should be excluded from donation for 7 days. Use of vitamins, thyroid preparations, or oral contraceptives does **not** disqualify donors. Blood Banks now must present would-be donors with educational materials explaining the risk of AIDS in blood transfusion and encouraging self-deferment by those at risk of AIDS. They should also ask donors directly (face to face) about sexual behavior that might place donors at risk of AIDS (ie, male homosexual activity, I.V. drug use, prostitution, or exchange of sex for drugs or money). The aim is to discourage donors at risk from donating blood as a means of getting an AIDS test.

Interpretive USE: Obtain blood or components for later use by a designated patient LIMITATIONS: Donors recruited by the family and friends of the patient may not be eligible to give blood. They must not have donated blood within the past 8 weeks, they must be in good health, and they must pass all the tests.

The following other limitations should also be considered.

- Directed donations cannot supply blood in an emergency.
- Blood from directed donations generally cannot be available in less than 72 hours.
- No evidence exists that potential blood recipients can select their blood donors any better than the community blood bank can. On the other hand, directed donors have not been shown to be any more dangerous than regular donors.
- Administrative costs increase when directed donors are requested. Telephone calls and unproductive visits to the blood center take up secretarial and technologists' time.
- Directed donors lose the anonymous position of the conventional (homologous) donor and may become subject to legal complications.
- More units may be needed than the directed donor(s) can provide.
- Rh negative recipients may have difficulty in obtaining all blood needs from directed donors unless such donors know their blood type.[1]
- Husband-to-wife transfusions incur increased likelihood of both hemolytic disease of the newborn and transfusion reactions. The reason is that blood group immunization may take place or may already have taken place.
- Graft-versus-host disease (GVHD) occurs rarely in immunocompetent recipients of directed donations from first degree family members. In this setting, such donated blood should be irradiated with at least 1500 rad (1500 cGy). Increased potassium occurs in irradiated blood.

- Although, as pointed out above, there is little logic in directed donations for general purposes (eg, surgery); the Blood Bank physician should not take too rigid an attitude to this. First, directed donors have been and continue to be used to provide platelets for cancer and leukemia patients, for somewhat different reasons. Second, many patients have a highly emotional fixation about it and are not moved by logic. Finally, although the procedure is an administrative nuisance, it does make the patient feel better about transfusions.

METHODOLOGY: Contact the blood center and the hospital Blood Bank to make the arrangements. Send a prescription giving the name of the patient, the number of units of blood requested, the date of surgery, and the name of the hospital.

Footnotes

1. Kanter M, Selvin S, and Myhre BA, "The Probability of Finding Suitable Directed Donors," *Arch Pathol Lab Med*, 1989, 113(2):174-6.

References

Aubuchon JP, "Autologous Transfusion and Directed Donations: Current Controversies and Future Directions," *Transfus Med Rev*, 1989, 3(4):290-306.

Hillyer CD, Tiegerman KO, and Berkman EM, "Evaluation of the Red Cell Storage Lesion After Irradiation in Filtered Packed Red Cell Units," *Transfusion*, 1991, 31(6):497-9.

Starkey JM, MacPherson JL, Bolgiano DC, et al, "Markers for Transfusion-Transmitted Disease in Different Groups of Blood Donors," *JAMA*, 1989, 262(24):3452-4.

Thaler M, Shamiss A, Orgad S, et al, "The Role of Blood From HLA-Homozygous Donors in Fatal Transfusion-Associated Graft-Versus-Host Disease After Open Heart Surgery," *N Engl J Med*, 1989, 321(1):25-8.

Donor Blood *see* Red Blood Cells *on page 1087*

Donor Plasmapheresis *see* Plasmapheresis, Donor *on page 1079*

Donor Units *see* Type and Crossmatch *on page 1100*

D^u

CPT *86901*

Related Information

Hemolytic Disease of the Newborn, Antibody Identification *on page 1070*
Kleihauer-Betke *on page 563*
Prenatal Screen, Immunohematology *on page 1085*
Rh Genotype *on page 1090*
Rh_o(D) Immune Globulin (Human) *on page 1091*
Rh_o(D) Typing *on page 1093*
Rosette Test for Fetomaternal Hemorrhage *on page 1097*

Synonyms Rh_o Variant; Weak D (D^u)

Applies to Prenatal Testing; Rh; Rosette Test (Erythrocyte)

Test Commonly Includes Rh_o(D); rosette test (in some laboratories)

Specimen Blood **CONTAINER:** One red top tube and one lavender top (EDTA) tube **CAUSES FOR REJECTION:** Gross hemolysis, sample placed in a serum separator tube, specimen tube not properly labeled

Interpretive **USE:** Determine candidacy for Rh immune globulin and detect massive fetal-maternal bleeds in Rh-negative mothers; distinguish Rh-negative from Rh-positive donor blood **LIMITATIONS:** Does not detect all massive fetal-maternal bleeds (the Kleihauer-Betke and the rosetting tests are superior for this purpose). Contaminating antibodies in anti-Rh_o reagent may cause weak false-positive reactions. D^u typing is not dependable in newborn babies who have concomitant positive DAT due to ABO incompatibility. D^u cells from newborns are not easily detectable by the rosette test. A Kleihauer-Betke test should be performed on the maternal specimen when the infant types D^u positive. **METHODOLOGY:** Read microscopically **ADDITIONAL INFORMATION:** Some people are weakly Rh_o(D)-positive and are called type "D^u".[1] Do test before and after delivery on Rh-negative mothers. If a woman is D^u-negative antepartum but appears D^u-positive immediately postpartum, sufficient fetal Rh-positive RBCs have escaped into her circulation to cause the mother to appear transiently D^u-positive. This is an indication to do a Kleihauer-Betke immediately. Although all antepartum Rh-negative patients should be tested for D^u, the D^u run postpartum misses a significant number of fetal-maternal bleeds for which one dose of Rh_o(D) immune globulin (human) is insufficient. Thus, Rh immunization may still occur, uncommonly, in postpartum women who have had Rh immune globulin

(Continued)

D^u *(Continued)*

in an inadequate dose. In the erythrocyte rosetting test, the endpoint of rosetted red cells detects fetomaternal hemorrhages of 10-15 mL of fetal blood cells.[2,3] See Rosette Test for Fetomaternal Hemorrhage.

Footnotes

1. Szymanski IO and Araszkiewicz P, "Quantitative Studies on the D Antigen of Red Cells With the D^u Phenotype," *Transfusion*, 1989, 29(2):103-5.
2. Stedman CM, Baudin JC, White CA, et al, "Use of the Erythrocyte Rosette Test to Screen for Excessive Fetomaternal Hemorrhage in Rh-Negative Women," *Am J Obstet Gynecol*, 1986, 154:1363-9.
3. Taswell HF and Reisner RK, "Prevention of Rh_0 Hemolytic Disease of the Newborn: The Rosette Method – a Rapid, Sensitive Test," *Mayo Clin Proc*, 1983, 58:342-3.

Elution *see* Antibody Identification, Red Cell *on page 1047*

Emergency Blood *see* Uncrossmatched Blood, Emergency *on page 1104*

Emergency Issue of Uncrossmatched Blood *see* Uncrossmatched Blood, Emergency *on page 1104*

Emergency Transfusion *see* Uncrossmatched Blood, Emergency *on page 1104*

Erythrocytapheresis *see* Cytapheresis, Therapeutic *on page 1060*

Ether Eluate *see* Antibody Identification, Red Cell *on page 1047*

Exchange Transfusion *see* Hemolytic Disease of the Newborn, Antibody Identification *on page 1070*

Exchange Transfusion *see* Newborn Crossmatch and Transfusion *on page 1072*

Exclusion of Parentage *see* Paternity Studies *on page 1074*

Exsanguinating Emergency *see* Uncrossmatched Blood, Emergency *on page 1104*

Factor VIII Concentrate

***CPT** 36430*

Related Information

Anticoagulant, Circulating *on page 402*
Cryoprecipitate *on page 1058*
Factor VIII *on page 424*
Partial Thromboplastin Time *on page 450*
Plasma, Fresh Frozen *on page 1078*

Synonyms AHF, Lyophilized; Antihemophilic Factor (Human)

Patient Care **PREPARATION:** Factor VIII levels, prothrombin time, and PTT should be determined prior to calculation of dosage if time permits; factor VIII levels are often run prior to dose.

Interpretive **REFERENCE RANGE:** Half-life of factor VIII is 8-12 hours[1] in the absence of inhibitors. **USE:** Treatment of acute bleeding and sometimes, prophylaxis, in patients with deficiency of clotting factor VIII (hemophilia A) and with acquired factor VIII inhibitors. **LIMITATIONS:** Cryoprecipitate is a better source of von Willebrand's factor and fibrinogen, with a relatively low risk of virus transmission. Heat-treated, solvent-detergent-treated, monoclonal-antibody-purified, and recombinant factor VIII concentrates are purer and cause less immune stimulation than the older concentrates.[1] These newer preparations, though much more expensive, are a great deal safer from the point of view of virus contamination.[1,2] The presence of inhibitors to factor VIII make treatment more difficult; refer to physicians experienced in the treatment of such cases. **CONTRAINDICATIONS:** Normal coagulation studies. Cryoprecipitate is preferable for treatment of von Willebrand's disease. **ADDITIONAL INFORMATION:** The activated partial thromboplastin time is useful for both hemophilia and von Willebrand's disease and may be more readily available than are factor assays. All these tests can guide therapy, as can the clinical response of the patient.

Calculation of dosage: Each bottle is labeled with the number of AHF units it contains. One AHF unit is defined as the activity in 1 mL of normal pooled human plasma less than 1 hour old (100% AHF level). One factor VIII unit per kilogram may raise the level by 2%.[1] The dose required may vary from 10-50 units/kg.[1] In general, deeper hemorrhage and hemarthrosis need higher levels of activity. Still greater levels are necessary for retropharyngeal and retroperitoneal bleeds, even 100% activity for head injuries.[1]

Hazards: Since lyophilized AHF concentrate is a derivative of pooled plasma, the risk of transmitting hepatitis, HIV, and other viral infections is present.[3] Treatment of the product by heat for a prolonged period of time has greatly reduced the risk of transmitting viruses.[1] AHF contains anti-A and anti-B; when large or frequent doses are needed, monitor patients of group A, B, or AB for signs of intravascular hemolysis. Infrequent allergic reactions may occur. See table.

Therapeutic Factor VIII and Factor IX Concentrates

	Demonstrated Viral Disease Transmission?	
	Non-A, Non-B Hepatitis	**Human Immunodeficiency Virus**
Factor VIII		
Cryoprecipitate	Yes	Yes
"Dry" heat	Yes	Yes
"Wet" heat (pasteurized)	No	No
Monoclonal antibody-purified		
"Dry" heat	No	No
Solvent/detergent-treated	No	No
"Wet" heat in organic solvent	Yes	No
Detergent/solvent-treated	No	No
Factor IX		
"Dry" heat	Yes	?
"Wet" heat in organic solvent	?	No

From Menitove JE, "Preparation and Clinical Use of Plasma and Plasma Fractions", *Hematology,* 4th ed, Williams WJ, Beutler E, Erslev AJ, et al, eds, New York, NY: McGraw-Hill, 1990, 1659-73, with permission.

Footnotes

1. Menitove JE, "Preparation and Clinical Use of Plasma and Plasma Fractions," *Hematology*, 4th ed, Williams WJ, Beutler E, Erslev AJ, et al, eds, New York, NY: McGraw-Hill Inc, 1990, 1659-73.
2. Aronson DL, "The Development of the Technology and Capacity for the Production of Factor VIII for the Treatment of Hemophilia A," *Transfusion*, 1990, 30(8):748-58.
3. Thomas DP, "Reducing the Risk of Virus Transmission by Blood Products," *Br J Haematol*, 1988, 70(4):393-5.

References

Goedert JJ, Kessler CM, Aledort LM, et al, "A Prospective Study of Human Immunodeficiency Virus Type 1 Infection and the Development of AIDS in Subjects With Hemophilia," *N Engl J Med*, 1989, 321(17):1141-8.

Pierce GF, Lusher JM, Brownstein AP, et al, "The Use of Purified Clotting Factor Concentrates in Hemophilia: Influence of Viral Safety, Cost, and Supply on Therapy," *JAMA*, 1989, 261(23):3434-7.

Roberts HR, "The Treatment of Hemophilia: Past Tragedy and Future Promise," *N Engl J Med*, 1989, 321(17):1188-90.

Schimpf K, Brackmann HH, Kreuz W, et al, "Absence of Anti-Human Immunodeficiency Virus Types 1 and 2 Seroconversion After the Treatment of Hemophilia A or von Willebrand's Disease With Pasteurized Factor VIII Concentrate," *N Engl J Med*, 1989, 321(17):1148-52.

Factor IX Complex (Human)

***CPT** 36430*

Related Information

Anticoagulant, Circulating *on page 402*
Factor VIII *on page 424*
Factor IX *on page 426*
Partial Thromboplastin Time *on page 450*
Plasma, Fresh Frozen *on page 1078*

Synonyms Prothrombin Complex Concentrates

Test Commonly Includes Factor IX concentrate is a preparation containing high levels of the vitamin K-dependent factors, factor II (prothrombin), VII, IX (PTC, Christmas factor), and X (Stuart-Prower factor).

Abstract A plasma fraction for treatment of hemophilia B (factor IX deficiency) and hemophilia A with inhibitor

(Continued)

Factor IX Complex (Human) *(Continued)*

Patient Care PREPARATION: Identification of the deficiency as one of factor II or IX is essential before administration of factor IX complex. Follow manufacturers' instructions on package insert.

Interpretive USE: **High risk fraction** for patients with severe Christmas disease, hemophilia B (inherited factor IX deficiency) during episodes of traumatic or spontaneous bleeding, or in conjunction with surgery; it may also control deficiency of factor II, VII, X, or factor VIII with inhibitor. **Fresh frozen or aged plasma should be used instead**, if possible, unless patient cannot tolerate the larger fluid volumes necessary.[1,2] LIMITATIONS: **Hazards:** Heat- and solvent-detergent-treatment have reduced the once high risk of hepatitis. Disseminated intravascular coagulation and thrombosis are among the risks. Inhibitors may occur. CONTRAINDICATIONS: Do not use in liver disease. Do not use in vitamin K deficiency, for which vitamin K preparations are appropriate, or in patients with overdose of coumarin. See Plasma, Fresh Frozen listing.

Footnotes

1. Menitove JE, "Preparation and Clinical Use of Plasma and Plasma Fractions," *Hematology*, 4th ed, Williams WJ, Beutler E, Erslev AJ, et al, eds, New York, NY: McGraw-Hill Inc, 1990, 1659-73.
2. Walker RH, ed, *Technical Manual*, 10th ed, Arlington, VA: American Association of Blood Banks, 1990, 357.

References

Goedert JJ, Kessler CM, Aledort LM, et al, "A Prospective Study of Human Immunodeficiency Virus Type 1 Infection and the Development of AIDS in Subjects With Hemophilia," *N Engl J Med*, 1989, 321(17):1141-8.

Huestis DW, Bove JR, and Case J, *Practical Blood Transfusion*, 4th ed, Boston, MA: Little, Brown and Co, 1988, 320-6.

Febrile Transfusion Reaction *see* Filters for Blood *on this page*

Febrile Transfusion Reaction *see* Red Blood Cells, Washed *on page 1089*

Fetalscreen™ *see* Rosette Test for Fetomaternal Hemorrhage *on page 1097*

FFP *see* Plasma, Fresh Frozen *on page 1078*

Fibrinogen Therapy *see* Cryoprecipitate *on page 1058*

Filters for Blood

CPT 86999

Related Information

Platelet Concentrate, Donation and Transfusion *on page 1081*

Red Blood Cells, Washed *on page 1089*

Synonyms Filters, Microaggregate; Leukocyte Removal

Applies to Alloimmunization, Leukocyte; Febrile Transfusion Reaction; Transfusion Reaction, Febrile

Specimen SPECIAL INSTRUCTIONS: Regular and special blood filters are available, as a rule, at hospital transfusion services or from pharmacy and supplies services.

Interpretive USE: Clots may form in any unit of blood and are readily removed by the clot filters in all regular blood infusion sets. Microaggregate filters remove debris composed of platelets with admixed granulocytes and fibrin in massive transfusions of older stored units of blood. This common usage remains controversial. Leukocyte filters help reduce, but do not eliminate febrile nonhemolytic reactions. Two consecutive febrile reactions may be an indication for leukocyte-poor blood. Leukocyte filters also reduce the likelihood of HLA alloimmunization, CMV transmission, and graft-versus-host disease. LIMITATIONS: Do **not** use microaggregate filters for platelet or granulocyte transfusions. Filters other than regular clot filters diminish flow when rapid infusion of red cells is necessary. Newer filters remove white cells even though microaggregates have not yet formed. Leukocyte filtration after various periods of storage of RBCs or platelets may not be as effective as at the time of collection. ADDITIONAL INFORMATION: There are several types of blood filters:

Clot filter (170 micron pore size): All blood and components must be given through this filter, intended to remove clots and fibrin shreds.

Microaggregate filters (20-40 microns pore size).[1] These filters have been recommended to remove the microaggregates of leukocytes and platelets that form in stored blood, particularly for massively transfused patients. The aim is to prevent microembolization and respiratory distress syndrome. This use remains controversial.[1,2] A volume of literature has developed with regard to best use of microaggregate filters. They did not provide demonstrable benefits in a series of patients with pulmonary dysfunction.[3]

Leukocyte-depletion filters (3-100 micron pore size).[4,5,6] These remove up to 99.9% of WBCs from platelets or RBCs, the intention being to prevent febrile reactions and alloimmunization to leukocyte antigens or to prevent transmission of viruses carried by donor leukocytes (eg, cytomegalovirus). For such purposes, it appears that filtration must be so efficient that platelet or RBC concentrates contain no more than 5 x 10^6 WBCs per transfusion. Since electronic particle counters are grossly inaccurate in those count ranges, quality control requires special techniques. Furthermore, the efficacy of filtration is in part inversely proportional to the initial WBC count of the concentrate.[6] There is little question that leukocyte removal is advantageous for many patients, but the cost and other practical matters are still evolving. An obvious question, for example, is whether cellular components should be filtered at the time of collection, or whether filtration should be done at the bedside for those patients needing leukocyte-depleted components. For optimal effect, most leukocyte-depleting filters must be carefully used according to the manufacturer's instructions.

Footnotes

1. International Forum, "When Is Microfiltration of Whole Blood and Red Cell Concentrates Essential? When Is It Superfluous?" *Vox Sang*, 1986, 50:54-64.
2. Snyder EL, Hezzey A, Barash PG, et al, "Microaggregate Blood Filtration in Patients With Compromised Pulmonary Function," *Transfusion*, 1982, 22:21.
3. Steneker I, van Luyn MJ, van Wachem PB, et al, "Electronmicroscopic Examination of White Cell Reduction by Four White Cell-Reduction Filters," *Transfusion*, 1992, 32(5):450-7.
4. Dzik WH, "White Cell-Reduced Blood Components: Should We Go With The Flow?" *Transfusion*, 1991, 31(9):789-91.
5. Wenz B, "Clinical and Laboratory Precautions That Reduce the Adverse Reactions, Alloimmunization, Infectivity, and Possibly Immunomodulation Associated With Homologous Transfusions," *Transfus Med Rev*, 1990, 4(4 Suppl 1):3-7.
6. Freedman J, Blanchette V, Hornstein S, et al, "White Cell Depletion of Red Cell and Pooled Random-Donor Platelet Concentrates by Filtration and Residual Lymphocyte Subset Analysis," *Transfusion*, 1991, 31(5):433-40.

References

Andreu G, Dewailly J, Leberre C, et al, "Prevention of HLA Immunization With Leukocyte-Poor Packed Red Cells and Platelet Concentrates Obtained by Filtration," *Blood*, 1988, 72:964-9.

Hill RC, Middaugh RE, Menk EJ, et al, "Clinical Evaluation of Commonly Used Blood Administration Sets," *J Emerg Med*, 1989, 7(2):103-7.

Snyder EL and Bookbinder M, "Role of Microaggregate Blood Filtration in Clinical Medicine," *Transfusion*, 1983, 23:460-70.

Filters, Microaggregate *see* Filters for Blood *on previous page*

Fresh Blood *see* Whole Blood *on page 1106*

Fresh Frozen Plasma *see* Plasma, Fresh Frozen *on page 1078*

Frozen Blood *see* Frozen Red Blood Cells *on this page*

Frozen Red Blood Cells

***CPT** 86930 (preparation for freezing); 86931 (with thawing); 86932 (with freezing and thawing)*

Synonyms Frozen Blood; Frozen, Washed Red Cells; Red Blood Cells, Deglycerolized; Red Blood Cells, Frozen

Test Commonly Includes ABO, Rh, antibody screen, and crossmatch. Glycerol serves as a cryoprotective agent when added to reasonably fresh red blood cells, which can then be frozen at -80°C or lower. After thawing and deglycerolization by washing, some 80% to 90% of the original red cells remain, as a more or less pure suspension in isotonic saline.[1] The hematocrit is usually about 60%. Platelets, leukocytes (except for a few lymphocytes), and plasma constituents are almost completely removed during processing. Frozen storage time can be up to 10 years, although some data support even longer periods.[2,3] Post-thaw storage time is 24 hours at 1°C to 6°C. Volume and hematocrit vary between institutions.[1]

Patient Care PREPARATION: As for transfusion of whole blood or red blood cells

Specimen Blood CONTAINER: As in Donation, Blood, for obtaining unit; one red top tube and one lavender top (EDTA) tube for patient testing COLLECTION: A unit of red blood cells is prepared in the usual way from whole blood. The method of transfer to a special freezing container and the addition and concentration of glycerol vary according to the method used. Freezing

(Continued)

Frozen Red Blood Cells *(Continued)*

may be in mechanical freezers or in liquid nitrogen. **STORAGE INSTRUCTIONS:** Deglycerolized red blood cells must be transfused within 24 hours after thawing or be discarded. **CAUSES FOR REJECTION:** If a crack is found in the frozen plastic of the container or if there is evidence of leakage, the unit should be discarded.[1] **TURNAROUND TIME:** Long processing time is a severe disadvantage in emergency settings. **SPECIAL INSTRUCTIONS:** After issue from the transfusion service, blood must be transfused within 2 hours; blood cannot be returned to the Blood Bank.

Interpretive USE: Restores red cell volume. Prevents leukocyte-mediated febrile transfusion reaction. About 99% of PMNs are removed in washing, but some lymphocytes remain viable. There is less immunization to histocompatibility antigens. Frozen red cells are essentially free of plasma proteins; about 0.025% of the original plasma is present. Such properties have more to do with the washing, than with the freezing process itself. Frozen red cells are useful particularly for patients with very rare red cell types and antibodies to high frequency antigens or combinations of antigens.[1]

Autologous cells depot.

Rare donor red cell depot.

LIMITATIONS: About 10% to 15% of the original red cells are lost in processing; expensive – about two to three times the cost of a unit of conventional red blood cells; short dating after thawing – 24-hour shelf-life;[1] not always available even in larger cities; slow and complex **CONTRAINDICATIONS:** Sickling hemoglobinopathies and G-6-PD deficiency in donors are contraindications to freezing, since red cell recovery in these conditions has been poor.[1] Regarding recipients, frozen red cells should generally not be used when anemia and/or hypoxia can be corrected with specific products (eg, iron, B_{12}, folic acid). Not suitable for correction of coagulation deficiencies. **METHODOLOGY:** A number of methods for freezing and thawing red cells are in use. **ADDITIONAL INFORMATION:** Red blood cells must be ABO and Rh compatible. A crossmatch is necessary. Hepatitis and some other infectious diseases remain a hazard. Infuse within 2 hours; more rapidly in urgent situations.

Footnotes

1. Chaplin H Jr, "Clinical Uses of Frozen-Stored Red Blood Cells," *Clinical Practice of Blood Transfusion*, Petz LD and Swisher SN, eds, New York, NY: Churchill-Livingstone, 1989, 315-25.
2. Umlas J, Jacobson M, and Kevy SV, "Suitable Survival and Half-Life of Red Cells After Frozen Storage in Excess of 10 Years," *Transfusion*, 1991, 31(7):648-9.
3. Valeri CR, Pivacek LE, Gray AD, et al, "The Safety and Therapeutic Effectiveness of Human Red Cells Stored at -80°C for as Long as 21 Years," *Transfusion*, 1989, 29(5):429-37.

References

Circular of Information for the Use of Human Blood and Blood Components, American Red Cross, Council of Community Blood Centers, American Association of Blood Banks, 1992.

Walker RH, ed, *Technical Manual*, 10th ed, Arlington, VA: American Association of Blood Banks, 1990, 92-9.

Frozen, Washed Red Cells *see* Frozen Red Blood Cells *on previous page*

Gamma Anti-human Globulin Test *see* Antiglobulin Test, Direct, IgG *on page 1050*

Gamma Direct Coombs' *see* Antiglobulin Test, Direct, IgG *on page 1050*

Genetic Studies *see* Paternity Studies *on page 1074*

Genotype, Immigration *see* Paternity Studies *on page 1074*

Genotype, Rh *see* Rh Genotype *on page 1090*

Granulocytapheresis *see* Cytapheresis, Therapeutic *on page 1060*

Granulocytes, Apheresis, Donation

CPT 36520 (leukapheresis)

Synonyms Leukapheresis, Automated; Leukocytes, Apheresis

Test Commonly Includes As for regular blood donation

Patient Care PREPARATION: The more granulocytes, the more effective the transfusions. To achieve maximal yields, it is best to stimulate the donor with corticosteroids (eg, three doses of prednisone, 20 mg each, given respectively at about 18, 12, and 2 hours before donation). Steroid given at the beginning of leukapheresis is useless. The best qualification of a donor for leukapheresis is a history of uneventful regular blood donation.

Specimen Donor granulocytes including therapeutic doses of platelets **COLLECTION:** Collection of granulocytes is by means of a blood cell separator. Most makes are satisfactory. Methods of collecting granulocytes from fresh whole blood units have been published, but the numbers obtainable this way appear to be too small even for infants. Anticoagulation is by a citrated macromolecular agent, usually hydroxyethyl starch (HES, Hetastarch, Hespan®). "Pentastarch," which has a shorter half-life, is now also available. Without such an agent, separation of granulocytes from RBCs is poor and yields are unacceptably low. The final concentrate must contain at least 10^{10} granulocytes. To attain this minimum, collections will need to **average** about twice that, as considerable variation occurs. Each concentrate also contains at least 15 mL RBCs and 3-8 x 10^{11} platelets. **CAUSES FOR REJECTION:** As for regular blood donation. A history of successful regular blood donation is the best qualifying criterion. **SPECIAL INSTRUCTIONS:** Donors selected for this procedure are often family members (best motivation). ABO and Rh compatibility are desirable but not essential, as RBCs can readily be removed. HLA compatibility is desirable in the case of alloimmunized recipients but is seldom practical. Screening and testing are as for regular blood donations.

Interpretive **USE:** Granulocytes for transfusion of septic patients with severe neutropenia (ie, granulocyte count $<500/mm^3$) **LIMITATIONS:** Donation not exceeding twice a week with a 48-hour interval between procedures unless otherwise determined by Blood Bank physician. **CONTRAINDICATIONS:** Donors with intolerance of HES; donors with conditions that might be exacerbated by prednisone (eg, diabetes, history of tuberculosis, peptic ulcer, hypertension) **METHODOLOGY:** Continuous or intermittent flow centrifugation. Exact method depends on separator used. **ADDITIONAL INFORMATION:** Crossmatch may be desirable if recipient has a positive antibody screen, since most concentrates include considerable RBCs.

References

Hinkley MH and Huestis DW, "Premedication for Optimal Granulocyte Collection," *Plasma Ther Transfus Technol*, 1981, 2:149-52.

Huestis DW, "Technical Aspects of Cell Collection - Donor Considerations," *Clin Chem*, 1983, 2:529-47.

Mishler JM IV, *Pharmacology of Hydroxyethyl Starch. Use in Therapy and Blood Banking*, Oxford, UK: Oxford University Press, 1982.

Granulocytes, Transfusion

CPT 86950

Synonyms Leukocyte Concentrate; Leukocytes, Transfusion; White Cells, Transfusion

Test Commonly Includes Preparations of granulocytes generally contain platelets and red blood cells, as well as granulocytes. ABO and Rh type, antibody screen, antibody identification if indicated, and crossmatch.

Patient Care **PREPARATION:** Unit should preferably be ABO and Rh compatible. Red cell compatibility test is needed, since most units contain sufficient red cells to cause red cell transfusion reaction. However, in case of incompatibility, it is relatively easy to remove almost all the red cells. HLA compatibility is seldom practical. Family members may be the most suitable. **Dosage and administration:** Granulocytes are usually given for at least 4 days and Mollison's 1993 text recommends functioning granulocytes twice daily for 4-7 days.[1] Use clot filter but not microaggregate filter. During infusion, patient should be carefully monitored. Administer as soon as possible after collection.

Specimen Blood from recipient and donor **CONTAINER:** Red top tube from recipient **COLLECTION:** (Of sample from intended recipient): As for other red-cell-containing blood components. **STORAGE INSTRUCTIONS:** Storage should be at 20°C to 24°C, without agitation, for a maximum of 24 hours. **CAUSES FOR REJECTION:** (Of patient sample): Gross hemolysis, sample placed in a serum separator tube, specimen tube not properly labeled **SPECIAL INSTRUCTIONS:** Expiration date is 24 hours.

Interpretive **USE:** Temporary therapy for severely neutropenic patients, especially newborns, with infection nonresponsive to antibiotic therapy. Criteria for granulocyte transfusion: Absolute granulocyte count $\leq 500/mm^3$ in at least two counts; sepsis or severe local infection; infection caused by gram-negative organism or suspicion of gram-negative infection, in patient with profound granulocytopenia not responding to at least 3 days of conventional therapy. Use in gram-positive and fungal infections has not been well studied. Granulocyte transfusion is never used as the sole form of therapy. Prophylactic use is not recommended. **LIMITATIONS:** Expensive. HLA selection may be indicated for alloimmunized recipients. High incidence of febrile and other reactions, which are not necessarily cause for stopping the transfusion. Granulocyte transfusions are seldom now used in adults.[2] However, in septic newborns with poor marrow granulocyte production, granulocytes (even a single large infusion) may be lifesaving. **CONTRAINDICATIONS:** Not indicated for infections that can be managed successfully with antibiotics. Stop infusion of granulocytes in the presence of pulmonary distress and give hydrocorti-

(Continued)

Granulocytes, Transfusion *(Continued)*

sone.[1] Given with amphotericin B, there may be a risk of severe pulmonary reaction.[1] **METHODOLOGY:** Cytapheresis, using hydroxyethyl starch with steroid premedication of donor **ADDITIONAL INFORMATION:** Transfusions are administered at a slower rate than whole blood or red blood cells to prevent reactions. **Hazards**: Chills, fever, allergic reactions, including urticaria; immunization to HLA antigens. Graft-versus-host reactions may occur in immunodeficient or immunosuppressed patients.[1] Units may be irradiated to prevent graft-versus-host disease.[3] **Hazards of transfusion**. Risks of viral hepatitis and other microbiologic hazards exist. Since red cells are present in granulocyte units, evolution of red cell antibodies and hemolysis can occur.

Footnotes

1. Mollison PL, Engelfriet CP, and Contreras M, "The Transfusion of Platelets, Leukocytes, Hematopoietic Cells, and Plasma Components," *Blood Transfusion in Clinical Medicine*, 9th ed, Oxford, UK: Blackwell Scientific Publications, 1993, 651-2.
2. Lazarus HM, "Granulocyte Transfusions: Have We Learned Anything?" *J Lab Clin Med*, 1990, 115(3):271-2.
3. Walker RH, ed, *Technical Manual*, 10th ed, Arlington, VA: American Association of Blood Banks, 1990, 24, 243-4, 390.

References

Dahlke MB, Keashen M, Alavi JB, et al, "Granulocyte Transfusions and Outcome of Alloimmunized Patients With Gram-Negative Sepsis," *Transfusion*, 1982, 22:374-8.

Huestis DW, Bove JR, and Case J, *Practical Blood Transfusion*, 4th ed, Boston, MA: Little, Brown and Co, 1988, 337-41.

Schiffer CA, "Granulocyte Transfusions: An Overlooked Therapeutic Modality," *Transfus Med Rev*, 1990, 4(1):2-7.

Hazards of Transfusion *see* Risks of Transfusion *on page 1093*

Heat Eluate *see* Antibody Identification, Red Cell *on page 1047*

Hemolytic Disease of the Newborn, Antibody Identification

***CPT** 86870 (panel); 86886 (screen)*

Related Information

Antibody Identification, Red Cell *on page 1047*
Antiglobulin Test, Indirect *on page 1051*
Bilirubin, Neonatal *on page 138*
Cord Blood Screen *on page 1057*
D^u *on page 1063*
Fetal Hemoglobin *on page 542*
Newborn Crossmatch and Transfusion *on page 1072*
Rh Genotype *on page 1090*

Synonyms Newborn/Maternal Antibody Work-up

Applies to Exchange Transfusion

Test Commonly Includes Infant ABO, Rh, and antiglobulin test, direct; mother's ABO, Rh, and antiglobulin test, indirect; antibody identification, red cell, if indicated

Specimen Blood from mother and newborn **CONTAINER:** Red top tube and lavender top (EDTA) tube **CAUSES FOR REJECTION:** Gross hemolysis, sample placed in a serum separator tube, specimen tube not properly labeled

Interpretive **USE:** Diagnose erythroblastosis fetalis (hemolytic disease of the newborn) and provide the safest possible donor blood for potential exchange transfusion. Panel for identification of irregular antibodies is run on mother's serum when her indirect antiglobulin test (antibody screen) is positive. **LIMITATIONS:** If mother is Rh negative, the specimen must be drawn before Rh immune globulin is given if it is indicated. **ADDITIONAL INFORMATION:** Newborn's antibody is from mother. Hemolytic disease caused by fetomaternal ABO incompatibility is common, often subclinical, usually mild and rarely requires exchange transfusion; the direct antiglobulin test may be positive or negative, spherocytes are often found in the peripheral blood film, and in uncomplicated ABO incompatibility, the maternal serum lacks irregular antibodies.

Unlike Rh incompatibility, where much of the antibody is bound to the red cells, in ABO incompatibility there is often a marked quantitative discrepancy between the maternal and cord anti-A or anti-B antibody. The difference may be explained by the absorption of anti-A or anti-B on to A and B sites other than those on the red cells.[1] The usual situation is an O mother with an A baby. Serologically, diagnosis is not difficult (see table). Whether or not the serologic findings are clinically significant is determined by clinical means. Blood group antibodies other than ABO and Rh can also cause fetal hemolytic disease and may be even more dangerous because of being unsuspected.[2] The severity of hemolytic disease probably depends more on the biochemical characteristics of the antibody than on its serologic specificity.

Rh hemolytic disease of the newborn is largely preventable[1] but still occurs occasionally. The cause of death *in utero* is anemia. It is now possible to transfuse the baby directly into the umbilical vein under ultrasound monitoring.[3] However, it takes skill and experience to transfuse a baby *in utero*.[4] The more usual treatment for intrauterine disease when the baby cannot survive to maturity is intrauterine transfusion into the fetal abdominal cavity.

Blood Grouping Results in a Typical Case of ABO Erythroblastosis

	Known Serums, Anti-			Known Red Cells			Direct Antiglobulin Test
	A	B	A, B	A	B	O	
Mother	0	0	0	+*	+	0	0
Baby	+	0	+	+	Weak	0	+
Eluate from baby's cells				+	0 or +	0	

*Hemolysis

Note that the mother has hemolytic anti–A and that anti–A was eluted from the baby's red cells. Incompatible maternal anti–A, as well as some anti–B, are present in the baby's serum, an important diagnostic point.

From Huestis DW, Bove JR, and Case J, *Practical Blood Transfusion,* 4th ed, Boston MA: Little, Brown and Co, 1988, 364, with permission.

Footnotes

1. Chavez GF, Mulinare J, and Edmonds LD, "Epidemiology of Rh Hemolytic Disease of the Newborn in the United States," *JAMA*, 1991, 265(24):3270-4.
2. Bowman JM, Pollock JM, Manning FA, et al, "Maternal Kell Blood Group Alloimmunization," *Obstet Gynecol*, 1992, 79(2):239-44.
3. Grannum PA, Copel JA, Plaxe SC, et al, "*In Utero* Exchange Transfusion by Direct Intravascular Injection in Severe Erythroblastosis Fetalis," *N Engl J Med*, 1986, 314:1432-4.
4. Queenan JT, "Erythroblastosis Fetalis: Closing the Circle," *N Engl J Med*, 1986, 314:1448-9.

Hemolytic Disease of the Newborn, Antibody Titer *see* Antibody Titer *on page 1048*

Hemolytic Disease of the Newborn, Cord Blood Screen *see* Cord Blood Screen *on page 1057*

Hemolytic Disease of the Newborn, Crossmatch *see* Newborn Crossmatch and Transfusion *on next page*

Hemolytic Reaction to Transfusion *see* Transfusion Reaction Work-up *on page 1098*

Hemophilia A Therapy *see* Cryoprecipitate *on page 1058*

IAT *see* Antiglobulin Test, Indirect *on page 1051*

Indirect Antiglobulin Test *see* Antiglobulin Test, Indirect *on page 1051*

Indirect Anti-human Globulin Test *see* Antiglobulin Test, Indirect *on page 1051*

Indirect Coombs' *see* Antiglobulin Test, Indirect *on page 1051*

Irradiated Blood Components

CPT 36430 (transfusion); 86945 (irradiation of blood product, each unit)

Related Information

Donation, Blood, Directed *on page 1062*
Platelet Concentrate, Donation and Transfusion *on page 1081*

Applies to Blood Fractions, Irradiated; Whole Blood, Irradiated

Test Commonly Includes Irradiation of blood components with a gamma radiation source, usually cesium-137 or cobalt-60

Patient Care PREPARATION: Patient must be banded with name and Blood Bank number. Usual pretransfusion testing.

(Continued)

Irradiated Blood Components *(Continued)*

Interpretive USE: Avoid graft-versus-host disease in immunodeficient recipients METHODOLOGY: Irradiation of blood leads to nonviability of donor lymphocytes. Although 1500 rad has been the dose generally used, at least 2500 may be best. ADDITIONAL INFORMATION: Graft-versus-host disease (GVHD) occurs when viable lymphocytes are transfused into severely immunosuppressed patients. The patient is unable to destroy these incoming lymphocytes, and they attack the host cells, recognizing them as foreign. GVHD also occurs after allogeneic bone marrow transplantation. GVHD may occur in immunocompetent patients if they receive blood from a close relative who is homozygous for an HLA haplotype for which the patient is heterozygous. Preventive irradiation is a wise resort in the case of directed donations from close relatives, even if the HLA types are unknown. Irradiation of blood products prevents GVHD by rendering lymphocytes no longer viable. It has little effect on RBCs and none on platelets. Currently there is no means to prevent GVHD following bone marrow transplantation.

References

Linden JV and Pisciotto PT, "Transfusion-Associated Graft-Versus-Host Disease and Blood Irradiation," *Transfus Med Rev*, 1992, 6(2):116-23.

Thorp JA, Plapp FV, Cohen GR, et al, "Hyperkalemia After Irradiation of Packed Red Blood Cells: Possible Effects With Intravascular Fetal Transfusion," *Am J Obstet Gynecol*, 1990, 163(2):607-9.

Irregular Antibody Titer *see* Antibody Titer *on page 1048*

Leukapheresis, Automated *see* Granulocytes, Apheresis, Donation *on page 1068*

Leukapheresis, Therapeutic *see* Cytapheresis, Therapeutic *on page 1060*

Leukocyte Concentrate *see* Granulocytes, Transfusion *on page 1069*

Leukocyte-Poor Washed Red Cells *see* Red Blood Cells, Washed *on page 1089*

Leukocyte Removal *see* Filters for Blood *on page 1066*

Leukocytes, Apheresis *see* Granulocytes, Apheresis, Donation *on page 1068*

Leukocytes, Transfusion *see* Granulocytes, Transfusion *on page 1069*

Major Screen *see* Type and Crossmatch *on page 1100*

Marrow Transplant, Autologous *see* Bone Marrow, Autologous *on page 1055*

Massive Acute Blood Loss *see* Uncrossmatched Blood, Emergency *on page 1104*

Massive Transfusions *see* Whole Blood *on page 1106*

Neonatal Transfusion *see* Newborn Crossmatch and Transfusion *on this page*

Newborn Crossmatch and Transfusion

CPT *36450 (exchange transfusion, blood, newborn); 86921 (incubation technique); 86922 (antiglobulin technique)*

Related Information

Cord Blood Screen *on page 1057*
Hemolytic Disease of the Newborn, Antibody Identification *on page 1070*
Rh Genotype *on page 1090*
Rh_o(D) Immune Globulin (Human) *on page 1091*
Rh_o(D) Typing *on page 1093*
Rosette Test for Fetomaternal Hemorrhage *on page 1097*

Synonyms Exchange Transfusion; Neonatal Transfusion; Newborn Transfusion; Transfusion, Neonatal; Type and Crossmatch for Exchange Transfusion of Newborn

Applies to Hemolytic Disease of the Newborn, Crossmatch

Test Commonly Includes Reasonably fresh donor blood, preferably in storage less than 5 days, compatible with mother's serum. ABO and Rh type of mother and infant, antibody screen on mother's blood, antibody identification if indicated, crossmatch of mother's serum and donor cells. If mother's blood is not available, crossmatch may use newborn's serum and/or eluate from cord red cells.

Patient Care PREPARATION: Blood should be passed through a warming device to raise the temperature of the blood to about 37°C during administration. Do not infuse unfiltered blood.

Donor blood must lack the antigen corresponding to the mother's antibody (eg, in $Rh_o(D)$ erythroblastosis, donor blood must be $Rh_o(D)$-negative). It may be desirable to transfuse blood known to lack hemoglobin S. When mother and baby are the same ABO type, use group-specific donor blood.[1] Type O Rh-negative donor packed cells are usually used, not whole blood. **AFTERCARE:** Citrate toxicity, hypocalcemia, and other metabolic effects may occur. Postexchange serum calcium levels are useful. When exchange transfusion is completed, determinations of hematocrit, electrolytes, calcium, direct antiglobulin test, and bilirubin are often useful.[1]

Specimen Blood from mother and infant **CONTAINER:** 10 mL red top tube from mother; 15-20 blue tip capillaries from baby **COLLECTION:** (Of sample from mother): As for regular type and crossmatch. Similarly, verify identity of baby and prepare appropriate labels. **CAUSES FOR REJECTION:** (Of patient sample): Gross hemolysis, sample placed in a serum separator tube, specimen tube not properly labeled **SPECIAL INSTRUCTIONS:** Mother's blood is best, if available, for crossmatch. Advance notice permits collection of appropriate donor blood into a bag with multiple satellites (quad packs). The advantage of such satellite bags is that multiple small transfusions can be given to the infant from the same donor, without exposure of the baby to multiple risks of viral hepatitis. Another way of accomplishing the same end is by subdividing donor blood units by means of a sterile-connecting device. This permits multiple transfusions from a regular blood unit without affecting the dating and at lower cost than quad-pack sets. CMV negative blood should be provided for babies who weigh less than 1200 g if the mother is also CMV negative or if her status is unknown. There are unresolved questions about transfusions to newborns of blood stored in extended-storage media. It is unlikely that any risk attaches to small-volume supplementary transfusions of such blood. But the situation may be different in premature babies with liver or kidney damage or in massive transfusions, such as exchange transfusion. Even lacking clinical data on harmful effects, the use of unmodified extended-storage blood in such patients might be unwise. Removal of the supernatant and substitution of saline or albumin might be a more prudent course.

Interpretive **REFERENCE RANGE:** Compatible **USE:** Hemolytic disease of the newborn is due to transplacental passage of maternal antibodies – ABO, Rh (D, C, c), Kell, Duffy, Kidd, or other blood group system antibodies.

Immediate exchange laboratory criteria of Sacher and Lenes for term infants include cord blood direct antiglobulin positive, cord hemoglobin <14 g/dL, cord bilirubin >4 mg/dL, bilirubin increasing rapidly, reticulocytosis >8%, normoblastosis >10/100 WBCs.[1] Other published criteria include cord hemoglobin <12 g/dL, cord bilirubin >5 mg/dL, capillary hemoglobin <12 g/dL and dropping. Consult pediatric literature for more detailed criteria and procedure.[2]

Exchange transfusion is indicated in full-term infants with an indirect bilirubin level of ≥20 mg/dL. At this level, brain damage may occur. However, in premature babies or in babies with other complications, brain damage may occur at lower levels of bilirubin.[1] An exchange transfusion may then be done at levels <20 mg/dL. Other causes of severe bilirubinemia may also occur with hepatic failure, disseminated intravascular coagulopathy,[1] and in the respiratory distress syndrome. In the latter disorder, the aim is to shift the oxygen dissociation curve to the right by replacing hemoglobin F with hemoglobin A.

LIMITATIONS: Clots in the cord blood tube may occur; when present, they will generate misleading cord hemoglobin and hematocrit. Relatively mild jaundice beginning 1-2 days after delivery with a weakly positive direct antiglobulin test in a baby of type A or B and a mother of type O usually indicates ABO hemolytic disease. Anti-A or anti-B incompatible with the baby's own RBCs is usually detected. A more definitive test is to elute antibody from the baby's RBCs and test it against A_1, B, and O red cells. Exchange transfusion is seldom necessary in ABO hemolytic disease. Complications of exchange transfusion have been compiled.[1] **CONTRAINDICATIONS:** Units for exchange transfusion should lack hemoglobin S.[3]

Footnotes

1. Sacher RA and Lenes BA, "Exchange Transfusion," *Clinics Laboratory Medicine: 1. Symposium on Perinatal Diagnosis*, Wenk RE, ed, Philadelphia, PA: WB Saunders Co, 1981, 265-83.
2. Klemperer M, "Perinatal and Neonatal Transfusion," *Clinical Practice of Transfusion Medicine*, Petz LD and Swisher SN, eds, New York, NY: Churchill Livingstone, 1989, 615-34.
3. Widmann, FK, ed, *Standards for Blood Banks and Transfusion Services*, 15th ed, Bethesda, MD: American Association of Blood Banks, 1993, 26-7.

References

Luban NLC, Strauss RG, and Hume HA, "Commentary on the Safety of Red Cells Preserved in Extended Storage Media for Neonatal Transfusions," *Transfusion*, 1991, 31(3):229-35.

Sayers MH, Anderson KC, Goodnough LT, et al, "Reducing the Risk for Transfusion-Transmitted Cytomegalovirus Infection," *Ann Intern Med*, 1992, 116(1):55-62.

Newborn/Maternal Antibody Work-up *see* Hemolytic Disease of the Newborn, Antibody Identification *on page 1070*

Newborn Transfusion *see* Newborn Crossmatch and Transfusion *on page 1072*

Normal Serum Albumin (Human) *see* Albumin for Infusion *on page 1046*

O Negative Blood *see* Uncrossmatched Blood, Emergency *on page 1104*

Packed Red Cells, Transfusion *see* Red Blood Cells *on page 1087*

Panel *see* Antibody Identification, Red Cell *on page 1047*

Parentage Studies *see* Paternity Studies *on this page*

Paternity Studies

CPT *86910*

Related Information

Identification DNA Testing *on page 918*
Tissue Typing *on page 757*

Synonyms Exclusion of Parentage; Genetic Studies; Genotype, Immigration; Parentage Studies; Paternity Testing

Specimen Blood; legal chain-of-custody problems exist **CONTAINER:** Red top tube for red cell antigens; containers for other systems as laboratory requests **COLLECTION:** Witnesses are required during collection of blood samples from mother, baby, and presumptive father. Identification procedures of persons are often required before samples are drawn. These should include a photograph of mother, father, and child. All samples must be appropriately labeled. **CAUSES FOR REJECTION:** All parties usually must be at the laboratory at the same time, and appointments are required. When a single individual appears for venipuncture for paternity studies, many transfusion centers and blood centers will decline to draw a specimen for logical legal reasons of need for mutual identification. **SPECIAL INSTRUCTIONS:** Exclusion of parentage is a highly specialized area of forensic medicine. It is not a field for amateurs, nor is it part of the procedures involved in the diagnosis or treatment of disease. For these reasons, those without special forensic training are wise to refer paternity studies to experts.

Interpretive **USE:** Determine chance of paternity or nonpaternity in cases of disputed paternity; establish blood relationship of potential immigrant, possible exchange of infants in nursery, and kidnapped child; it can also be used to estimate the chance of monozygosity and dizygosity of twins **LIMITATIONS:** Paternity studies have only ruled out parentage. Although they have not previously proved parentage, the likelihood of paternity can be admitted as evidence in some courts. **METHODOLOGY:** Red cell antigens including ABO, MN, Rh, Duffy, Kell, and Kidd systems, serum protein markers, RBC enzymes, and HLA typing **ADDITIONAL INFORMATION:** In the future, restriction endonuclease fragment-length polymorphisms and computers are predicted to provide near certainty in paternal identity.[1,2] See Identification DNA Testing in the Molecular Pathology chapter.

Footnotes

1. Markowicz KR, Tonelli LA, Anderson MB, et al, "Use of Deoxyribonucleic Acid (DNA) Fingerprints for Identity Determination: Comparison With Traditional Paternity Testing Methods," Part II, *J Forensic Sci*, 1990, 35(6):1270-6.
2. Tonelli LA, Markowicz KR, Anderson MB, et al, "Use of Deoxyribonucleic Acid (DNA) Fingerprints for Identity Determination: Comparison With Traditional Paternity Testing Methods," Part I, *J Forensic Sci*, 1990, 35(6):1265-9.

References

Brooks MA, "Paternity Testing," *Modern Blood Banking and Transfusion Practices*, 2nd ed, Harmening D, ed, Philadelphia, PA: FA Davis Co, 1989, 379-89.

Bryant NJ, "Paternity Testing: Current Status and Review," *Transfus Med Rev*, 1988, 2:29-39.

Council on Scientific Affairs, "Guidelines for Reporting Estimates of Probability of Paternity," *JAMA*, 1985, 253:3298.

Paternity Testing *see* Paternity Studies *on this page*

Peripheral Blood Stem Cells, Autologous

CPT *86890*

Related Information

Bone Marrow, Autologous *on page 1055*

Synonyms Autologous Stem Cells; Peripheral Stem Cells; Progenitor Cells

Test Commonly Includes Multiple collections of peripheral stem cells by hemapheresis, frozen storage, and autologous transfusion of stem cells after bone marrow ablative therapy for cancer or leukemia

Abstract Patient first undergoes course of chemotherapy and may also receive hematopoietic growth factor (eg, GM-CSF, G-CSF) stimulation. Using a stem-cell protocol with any suitable blood cell separator, collect 6-8 x 10^8 mononuclears per kg of patient's body weight, by a series of 3- to 4-hour leukapheresis. Three to 12 procedures may be necessary. Procedures are usually done daily.

Specimen COLLECTION: As prescribed by the manufacturer of the blood cell separator used. STORAGE INSTRUCTIONS: Store each collection in liquid nitrogen after concentration and resuspension in dimethyl sulfoxide. Label as for other blood components. CAUSES FOR REJECTION: Cancer or leukemia cells in peripheral blood SPECIAL INSTRUCTIONS: Available on a scheduled basis only after consultation with Blood Bank physician.

Interpretive USE: Patients with malignant disease not responding to conventional therapy. Concept is to collect enough peripheral stem cells to repopulate patient's bone marrow after heavy chemotherapy and/or irradiation sufficient to obliterate marrow function and, it is hoped, also to destroy remaining malignant cells. METHODOLOGY: Depends on blood cell separator used ADDITIONAL INFORMATION: This is a relatively new therapy, involving very close coordination between Hematology/Oncology and laboratory physicians. So far, the results have been encouraging. The reconstitution of bone marrow function in this setting depends on many variables involving the patient and the treatment regimen. We count the mononuclear cells as a means of obtaining an endpoint for the collection of stem cells, but the ultimate quality assurance method would be to count stem cells themselves. Unfortunately, short of actual stem cell culture and quantitation of colony-forming units, there is no quick and reliable way to do this.

References

Inwards D and Kessinger A, "Peripheral Blood Stem Cell Transplantation: Historical Perspective, Current Status, and Prospects for the Future," *Transfus Med Rev*, 1992, 6(3):183-90.

Peripheral Stem Cells *see* Peripheral Blood Stem Cells, Autologous *on previous page*

Phlebotomy, Blood Donor *see* Donation, Blood *on page 1061*

Phlebotomy, Therapeutic

CPT 99195

Related Information

Blood Gases, Arterial *on page 140*
Blood Volume *on page 522*
Donation, Blood *on page 1061*
Erythropoietin, Serum *on page 214*

Synonyms Therapeutic Phlebotomy

Test Commonly Includes Removal of whole blood from patient to reduce red blood cell mass or blood volume

Patient Care PREPARATION: Before the elective removal of blood, the physician should ascertain that an absolute polycythemia actually exists (ie, that a significant absolute increase of red cell mass exists, rather than a decrease of plasma volume). The attending physician must make written request and must specify amount of blood to be drawn. Prephlebotomy and postphlebotomy vital signs should be recorded. AFTERCARE: Advice should be provided to outpatients who have phlebotomy to guard against fainting while driving, working, etc. They should also be told whom to call if they have a reaction at home. Multiple procedures may be needed over a long period.

Specimen CAUSES FOR REJECTION: Anemia, patient with blood pressure <90 mm Hg. Certain conditions may require the presence of the attending physician during phlebotomy (eg, hypertension, cardiac symptoms). The Blood Bank physician may decline to do the procedure if the risk is considered too high. SPECIAL INSTRUCTIONS: Physician should evaluate the patient's hemoglobin, hematocrit, red cell count, platelet count, and blood volume. In primary polycythemia, erythropoietin levels in blood and urine are decreased. Erythropoietin is increased in secondary polycythemia. Arterial blood gases may be helpful, with significantly decreased pO_2 and oxygen saturation pointing to secondary polycythemia.[1,2]

Interpretive USE: Polycythemia vera or secondary polycythemia, with the patient's hematocrit >53%; occasionally in acute cardiac failure for emergency reduction of circulatory volume; id-

(Continued)

Phlebotomy, Therapeutic *(Continued)*

iopathic hemochromatosis, for which ferritin levels and/or serum iron are used as monitors **LIMITATIONS:** No more than 450 mL of whole blood is usually drawn from a patient at one time. The goal is to reduce the hematocrit to <50% for secondary polycythemia. The procedure may be repeated subsequently. **CONTRAINDICATIONS:** Lack of documented increase of red cell mass. Hemoglobinopathies exist in which polycythemia occurs, the abnormal hemoglobin having increased oxygen affinity. Methemoglobinemias may relate to secondary polycythemias. Uncommonly, certain tumors induce erythrocytosis. Renal tumors are the most widely known cause of tumor erythrocytosis. These considerations are the responsibility of the clinical physician. **ADDITIONAL INFORMATION:** Platelet counts as well as hematocrit should be followed; platelet counts over 1 million may require special treatment.[1] Blood viscosity increases significantly when hemoglobin increases from 14 g/dL to 16 g/dL. Phlebotomies for hemochromatosis should lead to decreased serum ferritin, then decreased serum iron.

Footnotes

1. Landaw SA, "Polycythemia Vera and Other Polycythemic States," *Clin Lab Med*, 1990, 10(4):857-71.
2. Chetty KG, Light RW, Stansbury DW, et al, "Exercise Performance of Polycythemic Chronic Obstructive Pulmonary Disease Patients. Effect of Phlebotomies," *Chest*, 1990, 98(5):1073-7.

References

Dostik H and Prasad B, "Coulter S Hematocrit and Microhematocrit in Polycythemic Patients," *Am J Hematol*, 1978, 5:51.

England JM, Walford DM, Waters DA, et al, "Reassessment of the Reliability of the Hematocrit," *Br J Haematol*, 1972, 23:247-56.

Plasma Exchange

***CPT** 36520*

Related Information

Cytapheresis, Therapeutic *on page 1060*

Plasmapheresis, Donor *on page 1079*

Synonyms Plasmapheresis; Plasmapheresis, Therapeutic

Test Commonly Includes Use of blood cell separator to remove pathogenic component from plasma (eg, autoantibody, paraprotein), with simultaneous replacement by protein-containing medium (eg, 5% albumin) and electrolyte solutions

Patient Care **PREPARATION:** Excellent vascular access is essential, as most continuous-flow blood cell separators require two venipunctures and a series of procedures is usual. **AFTERCARE:** Monitor fluid and electrolyte balance. If infection seems to be a risk, it may be necessary to provide immunoglobulins when the replacement fluid has been albumin. Likewise, observe patient carefully for hemorrhage from loss of clotting factors. Both of these potential complications are rare.

Specimen **SPECIAL INSTRUCTIONS:** Generally on scheduled basis, depending on availability of blood cell separator and by consultation with Blood Bank physician. Occasionally emergent; team must be prepared to offer 24-hour, 7-day coverage. Plasma exchange removes the good with the bad in the patient's plasma. This means that blood levels of the patient's medications will be reduced significantly. Adjust medication schedule therefore to allow for effect of plasma exchange. Whenever possible, measure efficacy of exchanges by monitoring levels of some marker that indicates progress or regression of the disease treated (eg, specific antibody, immunoglobulin, abnormal protein). The usual amount of plasma exchanged in a procedure is 40 mL per kg patient's body weight. This figure can be applied to children as well.

Interpretive **USE:** Treatment of blood diseases, primarily autoimmune. The **clinical indications** for plasma exchange are now fairly well established, but it continues to be applied to some conditions for which its scientific basis is not firm. These two groups are given in the table.

CONTRAINDICATIONS: Moribund patient or one who cannot withstand the establishment of an extracorporeal circuit; inadequate vascular access; lack of specific indication for the procedure. The decision to do this form of blood manipulation is shared between clinical and Blood Bank physicians. **METHODOLOGY:** Depends on the blood cell separator used. Most available machines can be used successfully, but **continuous-flow** systems are generally quicker, more efficient, and entail a smaller extracorporeal volume of blood. When plasma is removed in quantity approximating one blood volume (40 mL/kg body weight), it must be replaced with a protein-containing medium. This is usually 5% albumin. For first exchanges, albumin need not be used exclusively, but can make up about half the replacement, with the other half isotonic saline. For further exchanges, particularly when doing a large series at short intervals, in-

Efficacy of Plasma Exchange

Generally Seems To Be Effective*	Efficacy Debatable or Controlled Studies Lacking
Hyperviscosity syndrome	Systemic lupus erythematosus
Myasthenia gravis	Fulminant crescentic nephritis
Goodpasture's syndrome	Rheumatoid arthritis
Thrombotic thrombocytopenic purpura	Multiple sclerosis
Cryoglobulinemia	Rh hemolytic disease of the newborn
Hemophilia with inhibitor	ABO-incompatible bone marrow transplantation
Guillain-Barré syndrome	Renal transplant rejection
Post-transfusion purpura	Hypercholesterolemia (familial)
Refsum's disease	Cold antibody hemolytic anemia

*Effective = producing significant clinical improvement that is better than transitory.
From Huestis DW, Bove JR, and Case J, *Practical Blood Transfusion,* 4th ed, Boston, MA: Little, Brown and Co, 1988, 377-80, with permission.

crease the proportion of albumin to saline, depending on the patient's serum protein values. Electrolyte supplementation is sometimes necessary, as judged by the clinical physician. It might seem logical to use normal plasma for replacement, but plasma causes too many reactions in the volumes used; allergic and citrate reactions are common, and more severe reactions have been reported. Use fresh frozen plasma as a replacement, however, in thrombotic thrombocytopenic purpura, hemolytic uremic syndrome, and other forms of microangiopathic hemolytic anemia where plasma seems to supply normal factors needed in those conditions.
ADDITIONAL INFORMATION: Although, when properly carried out for appropriate indications, plasma exchange is a relatively benign procedure; risks of morbidity and even rarely mortality exist.[1,2] The Blood Bank physician needs to be aware of the risks, as clinical physicians often are not (see table).

Complications of Plasma Exchange

	Vascular Complications	
Hemorrhage, hematoma Sclerosis of veins Thrombosis, embolism	Shunts, fistulas: surgical procedure needed Thrombosis infection, circulatory interference	Catheters: perforation infection
	Procedural Reactions	
Vasovagal reaction Chilling Hemolysis, mechanical Allergy, anaphylaxis Acute pulmonary edema Hypoproteinemia	Citrate effects: tremors, paresthesias Tetany Cardiac arrhythmia, arrest	Volume changes: hypovolemia hypervolemia, overload
	Delayed Complications	
Clotting factor depletion Thrombocytopenia Hemorrhage Hypoproteinemia DIC, thrombosis	Infections: bacterial (sepsis) viral hepatitis	

From Huestis DW, "Risks and Safety in Hemapheresis Procedures," *Arch Pathol Lab Med,* American Medical Association, 1989, 113:273-8, with permission.

Footnotes

1. Huestis DW, "Risks and Safety Practices in Hemapheresis Procedures," *Arch Pathol Lab Med*, 1989, 113(3):273-8.
2. Pohl MA, Lan SP, and Berl T, "Plasmapheresis Does Not Increase the Risk for Infection in Immunosuppressed Patients With Severe Lupus Nephritis. The Lupus Nephritis Collaborative Study Group," *Ann Intern Med*, 1991, 114(11):924-9.

References

Huestis DW, Bove JR, and Case J, *Practical Blood Transfusion*, 4th ed, Boston, MA: Little, Brown and Co, 1988, 367-89.

Plasma, Fresh Frozen

CPT *36430 (transfusion); 86927 (thawing, each unit)*

Related Information

Cryoprecipitate *on page 1058*
Factor V *on page 421*
Factor VII *on page 422*
Factor VIII *on page 424*
Factor VIII Concentrate *on page 1064*
Factor IX *on page 426*
Factor IX Complex (Human) *on page 1065*
Factor X *on page 427*
Factor XI *on page 429*
Factor XII *on page 429*
Factor XIII *on page 430*
Fibrinogen *on page 435*
Partial Thromboplastin Time *on page 450*
Prothrombin Time *on page 468*

Synonyms FFP; Fresh Frozen Plasma; SDFP

Test Commonly Includes ABO type.[1] Plasma from a unit of whole blood separated from the red blood cells within 6 hours of collection and frozen rapidly. The unit has a volume of approximately 150-275 mL. It contains all coagulation factors except platelets, but it is not a concentrate. A severe deficiency of coagulation factors cannot be corrected by giving FFP. Fluid overload may result.

Patient Care PREPARATION: Use coagulation studies as a guide to transfusion of FFP. **Dosage and administration:** FFP should be ABO compatible;[1] it contains anti-A or anti-B. Rh need not be considered. Crossmatch is not necessary. Administer through a filter. The usual unit contains about 200 units of factor VIII,[1] and 250-400 mg of fibrinogen. It contains factor IX as well as other stable and labile coagulation factors. A unit of fresh frozen plasma will raise patient's plasma level of fibrinogen only about 10-13 mg/dL; cryoprecipitate is a better source of fibrinogen. Give FFP at about 10 mL/minute, to a total dose of about 10 mL/kg.[1]

Specimen Blood CONTAINER: Red top tube STORAGE INSTRUCTIONS: Frozen at -18°C or lower, FFP has a shelf-life of 1 year. Examine the frozen plastic bag for cracks, especially the seams. Thaw at 37°C with agitation in a waterbath, using a plastic overwrap.[2] Thawing requires 15-30 minutes depending on the number of units being thawed. Once thawed, store in Blood Bank refrigerator and transfuse within 24 hours.[2] Plasma ideally should be transfused within 2 hours after thawing when the patient requires labile coagulation factors. Once thawed and not transfused, FFP usually cannot be reissued by the Blood Bank. After 24 hours, a thawed unit of FFP is equivalent to a unit of single donor plasma. SPECIAL INSTRUCTIONS: Usually available on request. Requires 15-30 minutes to thaw and issue.

Interpretive USE: Treatment of bleeding caused by labile and stable coagulation factor deficiency,[1] in some instances while awaiting specific concentrates or fractions. FFP is a source of factor V, factor VII, factor X, factor XI, factor XIII, and fibrinogen. Do not use FFP prophylactically to prevent dilutional coagulopathy in large transfusions. Do not use it as a plasma expander (unless it is autologous); albumin is better and safer. Up to a point, FFP may be used to replace factor IX; factor IX concentrates carry a high risk of hepatitis.[2] Used with vitamin K, for bleeding related to vitamin K deficiency; in severe Coumadin® overdosage, uncommonly; for bleeding patients with severe liver disease.[1] Also used as replacement medium in plasma exchange for thrombotic thrombocytopenic purpura or hemolytic-uremic syndrome. LIMITATIONS: Circulatory overload is a hazard of use of FFP in a number of situations. There is little doubt that **fresh frozen plasma is grossly overused.**[3] CONTRAINDICATIONS: FFP is seldom indicated if prothrombin time and partial thromboplastin time are less than 1.5 times normal and in the absence of abnormal bleeding. Coagulopathies are usually better corrected with specific therapy, such as cryoprecipitate or AHF for hemophilia and cryoprecipitate for von Willebrand's disease. ADDITIONAL INFORMATION: **Hazards**: Risk of disease transmission (that of any single unit exposure), plasma volume overload, anaphylaxis in IgA deficient recipient is a remote hazard. FFP contains anti-A or anti-B. Although FFP is basically cell-free, it is not without antigens. Recipients can have mild or severe allergic reactions and sometimes fever. Immunization can take place to soluble constituents as well as to Rh and other red cell antigens,[4] the latter presumably from cell fragments in the plasma. See also Cryoprecipitate listing.

Footnotes

1. *Circular of Information for the Use of Human Blood and Blood Components*, American Red Cross, Council of Community Blood Centers, American Association of Blood Banks, 1992.

2. Walker RH, ed, *Technical Manual*, 10th ed, Arlington, VA: American Association of Blood Banks, 1990, 46-7, 55, 389, 482, 639.
3. National Institutes of Health Consensus Conference, "Fresh Frozen Plasma Indications and Risks," *JAMA*, 1985, 253:551-3.
4. Ching EP, Poon M-C, Neurath D, et al, "Red Blood Cell Alloimmunization Complicating Plasma Transfusion," *Am J Clin Pathol*, 1991, 96(2):201-2.

References

Barnette RE, Fish DJ, and Eisenstaedt RS, "Modification of Fresh-Frozen Plasma Transfusion Practices Through Educational Intervention," *Transfusion*, 1990, 30(3):253-7.

Coffin C, Matz K, and Rich E, "Algorithms for Evaluating the Appropriateness of Blood Transfusion," *Transfusion*, 1989, 29(4):298-303.

"Use of Blood Components," *FDA Drug Bulletin*, 1989, 19:15.

Plasmapheresis *see* Plasma Exchange *on page 1076*

Plasmapheresis, Donor

CPT *36520*

Related Information

Plasma Exchange *on page 1076*

Synonyms Donor Plasmapheresis

Test Commonly Includes Plasmapheresis is a procedure by which whole blood from a donor is subjected to centrifugation, with separation and retention of plasma and return of RBCs to the donor. The procedure may be done manually or using a blood cell separator.

Specimen **COLLECTION:** Blood to be drawn by Blood Bank personnel. **CAUSES FOR REJECTION:** History of hepatitis, history of HB_sAg positivity, drug addiction involving injection, homosexuality, diabetes requiring insulin, coronary heart disease permanently disqualify. Temporary disqualifications include hypotension, hypertension, anemia, positive syphilis serology (STS), travel to malaria endemic areas, exposure to hepatitis, pregnancy, recent childbirth, recent surgery, recent transfusion, tattoo within 6 months, inmate of penal or mental institution, and certain other medical conditions. Donors who have taken penicillin should be excluded from donation for 7 days. Use of vitamins, thyroid preparations, or oral contraceptives does **not** disqualify donors. Blood Banks now must present would-be donors with educational materials explaining the risk of AIDS in blood transfusion and encouraging self-deferment by those at risk of AIDS. They should also ask donors directly (face to face) about sexual behavior that might place donors at risk of AIDS (ie, male homosexual activity, I.V. drug use, prostitution, or exchange of sex for drugs or money). The aim is to discourage donors at risk from donating blood as a means of getting an AIDS test.

Interpretive **USE:** Obtain plasma for transfusion or laboratory use **LIMITATIONS:** Must meet donor criteria specified by AABB and FDA. **METHODOLOGY:** May be separated manually from whole blood collections with return of RBCs to donors or may be prepared by use of mechanical blood cell separators. **ADDITIONAL INFORMATION:** Plasma is used as fresh frozen plasma or the starting material for various blood components. It can be obtained either by direct plasmapheresis or harvested from a single donation of whole blood. The products derived from plasmapheresis include fresh frozen plasma (plasma frozen within 6 hours after phlebotomy to maintain labile coagulation factors V and VIII), cryoprecipitate, and manufactured derivatives, such as plasma protein fraction, albumin, immune globulins (used prophylactically or therapeutically to treat a wide variety of conditions), and clotting factor concentrates.

References

Code of Federal Regulations, 21 CFR 640.60-640.76, 1992.

Plasmapheresis, Therapeutic *see* Plasma Exchange *on page 1076*

Plasma Protein Fraction (Human)

CPT *36430*

Related Information

Albumin for Infusion *on page 1046*
Fibrinogen *on page 435*
Prothrombin Time *on page 468*

Synonyms PPF

Applies to Plasma Substitutes

(Continued)

Plasma Protein Fraction (Human) *(Continued)*

Test Commonly Includes A colloid preparation derived from human blood, containing at least 83% albumin

Abstract A purified plasma albumin fraction interchangeable with albumin

Patient Care PREPARATION: Monitor vital signs throughout infusion.

Specimen Blood TURNAROUND TIME: Plasma protein fraction is usually available immediately.

Interpretive USE: A colloid plasma expander used in **immediate** treatment of hypovolemic shock; a therapy for cases of severe hypoproteinemia. Used for volume expansion while type and crossmatch for transfusion are in progress, in massive acute blood loss, as an interim emergency measure. LIMITATIONS: Coagulation factors, including fibrinogen, are absent. **Hazards**: Avoid rapid infusion (more than 10 mL/minute). Hypotensive episodes rarely follow rapid infusions of PPF. PPF can cause anaphylaxis in IgA deficient recipients who have anti-IgA. CONTRAINDICATIONS: Control of hemorrhage due to coagulation defects, for which fresh frozen plasma and/or other fractions are necessary. Severe anemia, congestive heart failure, or increased blood volume. Plasma protein fraction is not suitable for nutritional support. ADDITIONAL INFORMATION: This colloid contains about 5 g/dL of protein, 130-160 mmol/L sodium, <2 mmol/L potassium.

References

Huestis DW, Bove JR, and Case J, *Practical Blood Transfusion*, 4th ed, Boston, MA: Little, Brown and Co, 1988, 215, 313, 372.

Walker RH, ed, *Technical Manual*, 10th ed, Arlington, VA: American Association of Blood Banks, 1990, 359-60.

Plasma Substitutes *see* Plasma Protein Fraction (Human) *on previous page*

Platelet Antibody, Immunohematologic

CPT 86022

Related Information

Platelet Antibody *on page 462*
Platelet Count *on page 586*

Synonyms Antiplatelet Antibody; Platelet-Bound IgG, Direct; Platelet-Bound IgG, Indirect

Abstract Increase platelet-associated IgG and/or IgM (surface-bound) generally indicates antibody adsorbed to the platelet membrane and is the platelet equivalent of a direct antiglobulin test on RBCs. The corresponding indirect test, using a patient's serum and a substrate of known reagent platelets, is the equivalent of an indirect antiglobulin test on RBCs. Interpretation of results is similar to that of the RBC tests.

Specimen Blood COLLECTION: Depends on method used STORAGE INSTRUCTIONS: Depends on method used SPECIAL INSTRUCTIONS: Must consult with laboratory in advance.

Interpretive REFERENCE RANGE: Consult with laboratory. USE: Test for presumably specific auto- or alloantibodies directed against platelet antigens in cases of thrombocytopenia or apparent clinical refractoriness to platelet transfusions. Can also theoretically be used to select compatible platelets for refractory patients ("platelet crossmatch") LIMITATIONS: Unfortunately, these procedures are not well standardized, and the results do not always conform to the clinical situation or correlate with the presence or absence of cytotoxic antibodies. Furthermore, in thrombocytopenic patients, it may be necessary to collect large amounts of blood to have enough platelets to test. This may make the test impractical. CONTRAINDICATIONS: The quantity of blood required for platelet isolation may make the test impractical in children or anemic adults. METHODOLOGY: Flow cytometry (FC) is the method of choice for the direct test, and may also be suitable for the indirect test. A problem is to find suitable substrate platelets (analogous to reagent red blood cells in the indirect antiglobulin test). A single sample, even pooled from several donors, is seldom satisfactory. A platelet panel would be ideal but putting one together presents formidable obstacles. Another method for indirect testing is solid-phase, binding platelets to wells in a microplate, exposing them to patient serum, then adding an indicator of IgG-coated RBCs. A commercial testing kit for this is available, although it has a very short shelf-life and is costly. But it does seem to be a good system, has its own small panel of typed platelets, and gives clear positive and negative results. ADDITIONAL INFORMATION: Platelet antigen and antibody testing is still in a developmental stage. Those not prepared to put up with the problems of poorly standardized procedures would be wise to consult with reference or research laboratories working in this field. For additional discussion and from the perspective of immune thrombocytopenia see the listing, Platelet Antibody in the Coagulation chapter.

References

Finley PR, Williams RJ, and Fletcher C, "Flow Cytometry Analysis of Platelet Antibodies," *J Clin Lab Anal*, 1988, 2:249-55.

George JN, "Platelet Immunoglobulin G: Its Significance for the Evaluation of Thrombocytopenia and for Understanding the Origin of α-Granule Proteins," *Blood*, 1990, 76(5):859-70.

Rachel JM, Sinor LT, Tawfik OW, et al, "A Solid-Phase Red Cell Adherence Test for Platelet Crossmatching," *Med Lab Sci*, 1985, 42:194.

von dem Borne AE and Décary F, "Nomenclature of Platelet-Specific Antigens," *Hum Immunol*, 1990, 29(1):1-2.

Platelet-Bound IgG, Direct *see* Platelet Antibody, Immunohematologic *on previous page*

Platelet-Bound IgG, Indirect *see* Platelet Antibody, Immunohematologic *on previous page*

Platelet Concentrate, Donation and Transfusion

CPT *36430 (transfusion); 36520 (donation); 86965 (pooling of platelets)*

Related Information

Bleeding Time, Mielke *on page 411*
Factor V *on page 421*
Filters for Blood *on page 1066*
Irradiated Blood Components *on page 1071*
Platelet Count *on page 586*
Platelets, Apheresis, Donation *on page 1083*

Synonyms Platelet Rich Plasma; Platelets; Platelet Transfusion; Pooled Platelets; Random Platelets

Test Commonly Includes ABO and Rh type

Abstract Platelet concentrate consists of platelets, suspended in about 50 mL of plasma, separated from whole blood collected from a single donor. It contains at least 5.5×10^{10} platelets; the average content should be about 7×10^{10}. Storage life is 5 days. It contains stable coagulation factors and labile factors V and VIII. The presence of these factors may be significant, since a common dose is about 1 concentrate per 10 kg body weight.

Patient Care PREPARATION: Patient should have a wristband for checking against component container label before transfusion. A recent platelet count should be completed. It is not unusual for a platelet concentrate to have a pink tinge, indicating the presence of some RBCs. Despite this, a red cell crossmatch is not useful. If the patient is likely to receive many platelet transfusions, it is wise to have the patient HLA-typed early, in case platelet refractoriness occurs. **Dosage and administration:** In a bleeding adult with a platelet count $<20,000/mm^3$, 1 concentrate per 10 kg body weight is a good dose. Use special platelet filters for a leukocyte-poor product. Use a 19-gauge needle or larger for administration. Platelets should be given rapidly, with an average of 10 minutes per platelet concentrate. Isotonic saline may be used to flush the container and filter. Do not warm platelets. Do not add any medications to platelet packs. AFTERCARE: Close clinical/nursing observation for bleeding, petechiae. **To evaluate efficacy of platelet transfusions, get a platelet count within 1 hour after the transfusions are completed.**[1] This is useful in evaluating the response to platelet transfusions and in calculating the corrected count increment (CCI). The latter expresses the platelet increment per 10^{11} platelets transfused per meter of body surface area (BSA). Conventional platelet concentrates contain about 7×10^{10} platelets each. Where post = post-transfusion platelet count $\times 10^3/mm^3$; pre = pretransfusion platelet count; and PTx = number of platelets transfused ($\times 10^{11}$).

Causes of Refractoriness to Platelet Transfusions

Nonimmune	Immune
Infection, sepsis, fever Hemorrhage, purpura, DIC Splenomegaly Antibiotic therapy Amphotericin B Bone marrow transplant	Alloimmunity; prior transfusions, pregnancy, HLA, platelet-specific ABO (uncommon)

$$CCI \times 10^3 = (post-pre) \times BSA/PTx$$

(Continued)

Platelet Concentrate, Donation and Transfusion *(Continued)*

A value above 7.5 is usually considered satisfactory. Thus, a patient with a BSA of 1.5 m^2 receives 6 platelet concentrates with a total of 4.2×10^{11} platelets. The pre- and postcounts are 10×10^3 and 40×10^3 respectively.

$$CCI = (40 - 10) \times 1.5/4.2 = 10.7 \times 10^3$$

That would be considered a good response. This formula is not needed if the raw increment is zero or close to it, or if the response is obviously satisfactory. But it is helpful when the patient is small (eg, a child), or when the post counts appear to show small or moderate increments. Poor response to platelet transfusions (refractoriness) are common.[2] Most of them are due to nonimmune causes (see table). When refractoriness seems to be due to alloimmunization, then it will be necessary to change from regular platelet concentrates to single-donor platelets (platelets, apheresis) and perhaps to select donors according to HLA type. Alloimmunization to platelets seems to be largely caused by contaminating leukocytes in the concentrates and may be prevented by the removal of leukocytes by special filtration[3] (see Filters for Blood), or experimentally by ultraviolet-B irradiation of platelet concentrates.[4]

Specimen Blood **CONTAINER:** Red top tube **STORAGE INSTRUCTIONS:** Store at room temperature with continuous agitation for 5 days. Pooled platelets must be transfused within 4 hours after pooling. Once pooled, they may not be reissued for another patient. **SPECIAL INSTRUCTIONS:** May not be kept "on hold." When ordered, each platelet concentrate usually must be transfused or discarded. Do not refrigerate platelet concentrate.

Interpretive USE: Treatment of bleeding, petechiae, and ecchymoses when platelet count is $<20,000/mm^3$ when platelets are functionally abnormal; prophylaxis against bleeding due to thrombocytopenia when platelet count is $<20,000/mm^3$, especially when platelet count is dropping; in splenectomy for ITP when abnormal bleeding occurs; in acute blood loss with platelet count $<50,000/mm^3$. **LIMITATIONS: Hazards**: Allergic, febrile, and overload transfusion reactions. Platelet concentrates always contain both red and white blood cells, so immunization to any of these antigens may occur. If feasible, Rh-negative girls and women younger than age 50 should receive Rh-negative platelets to avoid Rh immunization. Otherwise, consider giving them Rh immune globulin. The dosage can be calculated by the fact that regular platelet concentrates seldom contain more than 0.1 mL RBC each and single-donor platelets rarely more than 2 mL each. Although the ABO antigens are poorly developed on platelets, ABO-incompatible platelets sometimes have decreased post-transfusion survival.[5] Immunosuppressed patients, and rarely immunocompetent patients, receiving platelets from closely related donors can suffer graft-versus-host disease; this is easily prevented by irradiation of platelet concentrates (see Irradiated Blood Components). As with whole blood and other cellular blood components, viral and other diseases may be transmitted. Bacterial contamination and growth during storage are a real risk, as platelets are stored at room temperature. **CONTRAINDICATIONS:** Not usually useful in idiopathic or immune thrombocytopenia, thrombotic thrombocytopenic purpura or certain stages of disseminated intravascular coagulation. Not to be used if bleeding is not caused by thrombocytopenia or abnormal platelet function. Microaggregate filters may remove platelets. However, leukocytes can be effectively removed from preparations for platelet transfusion using special leukocyte filters.[3] **ADDITIONAL INFORMATION:** A platelet count of not less than $100,000/mm^3$ is desirable for major surgery. One unit of platelet concentrate usually increases the platelet count of an adult with a blood volume of 5000 mL by about $5000/mm^3$.[6] Neonatal **alloimmune thrombocytopenia** may be treated with maternal platelet transfusions.

Alloimmune neonatal thrombocytopenia is usually caused by Pl^{A1} antigen inherited from the father by the baby, who then immunizes the mother so that she makes antibody to the baby's platelet (ie, anti-Pl^{A1}). The mother's platelet count is normal, but the baby's platelet count is low. It may not, however, be sufficiently low to cause symptoms, and so the diagnosis may be missed. The first born child may be affected.[7,8] The most serious complication is intracranial hemorrhage, which may occur during pregnancy, but the risk is probably greatest during delivery. If the diagnosis is made after delivery and the baby is unharmed, remember that later babies are also at risk. The presumptive diagnosis is made with a normal platelet count in the mother and a low platelet count in the baby.

For confirmatory diagnosis, send mother's serum and father's platelets (and the baby's if they can be obtained) to a reference laboratory for antibody test and selection of platelets for transfusion.

Treatment: The most convenient and readily available source of compatible platelets is the mother. A large number of platelets, relative to the baby's size, can be obtained by maternal platelet apheresis. Such platelets should last about 7 or 8 days in the baby. Platelet count should be checked daily. A further collection of platelets from the mother can be done if necessary.

Neonatal **autoimmune thrombocytopenia**, in which maternal thrombocytopenia occurs, is treated by steroids or exchange transfusion.[2]

One thing to remember is that with each 10 units of platelets the patient will also receive 500 mL of fresh plasma (in which the platelets are suspended). This volume may need to be reduced for children.

Footnotes

1. *Circular of Information for the Use of Human Blood and Blood Components*, American Red Cross, Council of Community Blood Centers, American Association of Blood Banks, 1992.
2. Bishop JF, Matthews JP, McGrath K, et al, "The Definition of Refractoriness to Platelet Transfusions," *Transfus Med Rev*, 1992, 2:35-41.
3. van Marwijk-Kooy M, van Prooijen HC, Borghuis L, et al, "Filtration. A Method to Prepare White Cell-Poor Platelet Concentrates With Optimal Preservation of Platelet Viability," *Transfusion*, 1990, 30(1):34-8.
4. Sherman L, Menitove J, Kagen LR, et al, "Ultraviolet-B Irradiation of Platelets: A Preliminary Trial of Efficacy," *Transfusion*, 1992, 32(5):402-7.
5. Lee EJ and Schiffer CA, "ABO Compatibility Can Influence the Results of Platelet Transfusion. Results of a Randomized Trial," *Transfusion*, 1989, 29(5):384-9.
6. Myhre BA and Harris GE, "Blood Components for Hemotherapy," *Clin Lab Med*, 1982, 2:3-20.
7. "Management of Alloimmune Neonatal Thrombocytopenia," *Lancet*, 1989, 1(8630):137-8, (editorial).
8. Mueller-Eckhardt C, Grubert A, Weisheit M, et al, "348 Cases of Suspected Neonatal Alloimmune Thrombocytopenia," *Lancet*, 1989, 1(8634):363-7.

References

Federal Code of Regulations, Title 21, Sections 640.26 K and 640.57 L, 1978.

Gernsheimer T, Stratton J, Ballem PJ, et al, "Mechanisms of Response to Treatment in Autoimmune Thrombocytopenic Purpura," *N Engl J Med*, 1989, 320(15):974-80.

Kickler TS, Ness PM, and Braine HG, "Platelet Crossmatching: A Direct Approach to the Selection of Platelet Transfusions for the Alloimmunized Thrombocytopenic Patient," *Am J Clin Pathol*, 1988, 90:69-72.

National Institutes of Health Consensus Conference, "Platelet Transfusion Therapy," *JAMA*, 1987, 257:1777-80.

Rachel JM, Summers TC, Sinor LT, et al, "Use of a Solid Phase Red Blood Cell Adherence Method for Pretransfusion Platelet Compatibility Testing," *Am J Clin Pathol*, 1988, 90:63-8.

Welch HG, Larson EB, and Slichter SJ, "Providing Platelets for Refractory Patients. Prudent Strategies," *Transfusion*, 1989, 29(3):193-5.

Plateletpheresis *see* Platelets, Apheresis, Donation *on this page*

Platelet Rich Plasma *see* Platelet Concentrate, Donation and Transfusion *on page 1081*

Platelets *see* Platelet Concentrate, Donation and Transfusion *on page 1081*

Platelets, Apheresis, Donation

***CPT** 36520*

Related Information

Cytapheresis, Therapeutic *on page 1060*
Platelet Antibody *on page 462*
Platelet Concentrate, Donation and Transfusion *on page 1081*
Platelet Count *on page 586*

Synonyms Plateletpheresis; Platelets, Pheresis; Single-Donor Platelets

Test Commonly Includes Collection of platelets by cytapheresis, using a blood cell separator. Donor screening, blood typing, and testing for infectious diseases as routinely done in regular blood donation.

Specimen STORAGE INSTRUCTIONS: Storage of platelets is in their native plasma, at 20°C to 24°C, with continuous gentle agitation. Do not refrigerate. **CAUSES FOR REJECTION:** (Of donor): As for regular blood donation. A history of successful regular blood donation is the best qualifying criterion. Platelet concentrates that show any visible aggregation are not suitable for transfusion. **SPECIAL INSTRUCTIONS:** Single-donor platelets are available from most blood centers and larger hospital blood banks on a more or less regular basis. In many institutions they are reserved for patients who regularly receive platelet transfusions, or who may be refractory to regular platelet transfusions. Donors must not (within previous 3 days) have taken any medications that might adversely affect their platelets (eg, aspirin).

(Continued)

Platelets, Apheresis, Donation *(Continued)*

Interpretive USE: Platelet apheresis can be used for any patient needing platelet transfusions. Single-donor platelets have the advantage of providing an entire platelet transfusion for an adult from one donor, hence with a single antigenic combination and a single donor exposure. Furthermore, the donor can be selected (eg, from a patient's relatives or by HLA type). LIMITATIONS: FDA guidelines recommend a maximum of 24 donations per year. This is undoubtedly too much for most donors. It is better to limit donations to the same frequency as regular blood donations (ie, every 2 months). In the case of specially selected donors for a particular patient (eg, relatives), donations can be as often as twice a week for limited periods, but this must be authorized on an individual basis by the Blood Bank physician, with careful monitoring of platelet counts and other variables. Reactions to platelet apheresis donation are given in the table.

Reactions Encountered in Hemapheresis Donations

Reaction	Prevention
Procedural reactions	
Vasovagal	Psychology; friendly, professional atmosphere
Hypovolemia	Avoid excessive extracorporeal volume
Hypervolemia	Control inflow to equal outflow
Citrate	Slow blood flow; decrease citrate proportion; use oral calcium or milk
Hemolysis	Avoid kinks in plastic tubing
Chills	Keep donors warm, use blood warmer
Allergy, anaphylaxis	Not avoidable, be prepared for immediate treatment
Reactions specific to leukapheresis*	
Hypervolemia, edema, skin manifestations, HES† accumulation	Avoid too frequent use of HES (eg, several times/week)
Steroid effect	Avoid excessive dosage and frequency
Perineal pain	Avoid filtration leukapheresis
Priapism	Avoid filtration leukapheresis
Complement activation	Avoid filtration leukapheresis
General reaction	
Donor burnout	Do not overuse donors; keep their interest in program; maintain a warm, friendly atmosphere

*Because of the additional risks to the donor in leukapheresis and the dubious value of transfused leukocytes in many situations, granulocyte transfusions should be given only on impeccable clinical indications.

† HES indicates hydroxyethyl starch.

From Huestis DW, "Risks and Safety Practices in Hemapheresis Procedures," *Arch Pathol Lab Med,* American Medical Association, 1989, 113:273-8, with permission.

METHODOLOGY: Apheresis by continuous- or intermittent-flow centrifugation. Exact procedure depends on the separator used. Platelet apheresis differs from leukapheresis in that a macromolecular agent is not used and there is no need to stimulate the donor with steroids. ADDITIONAL INFORMATION: Single-donor platelets are desirable because of the limitation in donor exposures. But regular platelets are entirely adequate for patients receiving platelets only once or twice (eg, surgical patients). Cancer or leukemia patients, who will receive many transfusions over a long time, may become refractory (ie, fail to show the expected response to regular platelets). Refractoriness has many causes, most of them nonimmune (see Causes for Refractoriness to Platelet Transfusions in Platelet Concentrate, Donation and Transfusion test listing). Patients with **nonimmune platelet refractoriness** are not likely to have a platelet count increase in response to any platelet transfusions. However, **immune refractoriness** sometimes responds to selection of platelet donors from among a patient's blood relatives, or by HLA type, or lacking an antigen corresponding to the patient's antibody. See the following table.

The technology of platelet apheresis is changing rapidly, with increasing emphasis on the reduction or virtual elimination of contaminating leukocytes.[1,2] The aim is to prevent immune refractoriness in patients who must receive repeated platelet transfusions.[2] In the face of existing immune refractoriness, ABO[3] and HLA selection are options. Platelet crossmatching is still a developing field.[4]

Selection of Platelets for Immune-Refractory Patients

1. Change from random (regular) platelets to single-donor.
2. Recruit blood relatives of patient as donors, if available.
3. HLA type patient, if possible.
4. Test patient for cytotoxic antibodies.
5. Test patient for platelet-specific antibodies.
6. Select platelet donors lacking antigens corresponding to any antibodies detected in steps 4 and 5, if feasible.
7. Check whether ABO compatibility affects outcome. Sometimes it does, especially type A platelets to an O patient.
8. Select donors by HLA type. The HLA does not have to be identical; a reasonable match by cross-reacting groups is usually as effective.
9. Recognize that this is a thorny problem. Any or all of the above may work, not necessarily in the order given; or none of them may be effective.

Footnotes

1. van Marwijk Kooy M, van Prooijen HC, et al, "Use of Leukocyte-Depleted Platelet Concentrations for the Prevention of Refractoriness and Primary HLA Alloimmunization: A Prospective, Randomized Trial," *Blood*, 1991, 77(1):201-5.
2. Schiffer CA, "Prevention of Alloimmunization Against Platelets," *Blood*, 1991, 77(1):1-4, (editorial).
3. "ABO Incompatibility and Platelet Transfusion," *Lancet*, 1990, 335(8682):142-3, (editorial).
4. Kieckbusch ME, Moore SB, Koenig VA, et al, "Platelet Crossmatch Evaluation in Refractory Hematologic Patients," *Mayo Clin Proc*, 1987, 62:595-600.

References

Consensus Conference, "Platelet Transfusion Therapy," *JAMA*, 1987, 257:1777-85.
McCullough J, Steeper TA, Connelly DP, et al, "Platelet Utilization in a University Hospital," *JAMA*, 1988, 259:2414-8.
Slichter SJ, "Controversies in Platelet Transfusion Therapy," *Annu Rev Med*, 1980, 31:509-40.

Platelets, Pheresis *see* Platelets, Apheresis, Donation *on page 1083*

Platelet Transfusion *see* Platelet Concentrate, Donation and Transfusion *on page 1081*

Pluripotential Stem Cells, Bone Marrow *see* Bone Marrow, Autologous *on page 1055*

Polyspecific Direct Antiglobulin *see* Antiglobulin Test, Direct *on page 1049*

Pooled Platelets *see* Platelet Concentrate, Donation and Transfusion *on page 1081*

PPF *see* Plasma Protein Fraction (Human) *on page 1079*

Prenatal Screen, Immunohematology

CPT *86880 (antiglobulin test, direct); 86886 (antiglobulin test, indirect); 86900 (ABO); 86901 (D^u); 86901 (Rh(D))*

Related Information

Amniotic Fluid Analysis for Erythroblastosis Fetalis *on page 122*
Antibody Titer *on page 1048*
Antiglobulin Test, Indirect *on page 1051*
Cord Blood Screen *on page 1057*
D^u *on page 1063*
Type and Screen *on page 1102*

Synonyms Prenatal Testing

Test Commonly Includes Initial screen: ABO, Rh, D^u if D negative; antibody screen (indirect antiglobulin test), antibody identification (panel) when screen is positive. Prenatal screen is essentially the same as Type and Screen, except that, when indicated, includes phenotype of father and antibody titers.

Patient Care PREPARATION: Do prenatal screen in the first trimester, at the initial visit, when baselines can be established, in all pregnant women. Repeat antibody screen ideally at about 28 weeks and again as indicated by circumstances[1] in Rh_o(D)-negative women. Multiparity (Continued)

Prenatal Screen, Immunohematology *(Continued)*

and/or history of prior transfusion are factors that indicate a need to follow antibody screens more closely. In patients with antibody, coordinate titers with possible amniocentesis. It is not usually necessary to do titrations and repeat testing in the case of antibodies that are predominantly IgM or otherwise not clinically significant (eg, Lewis, P, or cold autoagglutinins). American College of Obstetrics and Gynecology recommends ABO and Rh type and antibody screen as early as practical and repeat screens at 28, 32, and 36 weeks if subject is D-negative and not immunized to $Rh_o(D)$.[2]

Specimen Blood **CONTAINER:** Red top tube **CAUSES FOR REJECTION:** Improperly labeled tube, gross hemolysis **SPECIAL INSTRUCTIONS:** Considerable variation exists as to schedule of antibody screens. All patients, regardless of Rh status, must have a prenatal screen at the first visit, in the first trimester. History of prior transfusions or presence of antibody may require more frequent studies.

Interpretive **REFERENCE RANGE:** Indirect antiglobulin test (antibody screen): negative **USE:** Prenatal screen for possible maternal-fetal blood incompatibility, to identify women at risk of having a baby affected by hemolytic disease of the newborn and to try to predict risk to the fetus. Rh and D^u to work up for possible administration of Rh immune globulin. Do a D^u on all apparently Rh-negative women. Should a prenatal patient be shown to be D^u-negative, but then immediately after delivery appear D^u-positive, an extremely important observation has been made. There may be a massive fetal-maternal bleed from an Rh-positive baby, and a Kleihauer-Betke stain is strongly indicated. **LIMITATIONS:** Will not detect all maternal-fetal incompatibilities or all antibodies present in a patient's serum **METHODOLOGY:** Antibody screening including antiglobulin testing. Titrate IgG-type antibodies known to be associated with hemolytic disease of the newborn. **ADDITIONAL INFORMATION:** Antibody screen is part of the type and screen and, in most laboratories, is done as part of type and crossmatch. Antibody screen is commonly done for obstetric patients, including those with incomplete abortion or with ectopic pregnancy, including those possibly requiring transfusion. Rh-negative women with miscarriage or ectopic pregnancy are candidates for Rh immune globulin.

Footnotes

1. Huestis DW, Bove JR, and Case J, *Practical Blood Transfusion*, 4th ed, Boston, MA: Little, Brown and Co, 1988.
2. "The Selective Use of $Rh_o(D)$ Immune Globulin (RhIG)," *ACOG Technical Bulletin Update*, November, 1983.

Prenatal Testing *see* D^u *on page 1063*

Prenatal Testing *see* Prenatal Screen, Immunohematology *on previous page*

Prenatal Testing *see* Rh Genotype *on page 1090*

Progenitor Cells *see* Peripheral Blood Stem Cells, Autologous *on page 1074*

Prognosis for Rh Hemolytic Disease of Newborn *see* Rh Genotype *on page 1090*

Prothrombin Complex Concentrates *see* Factor IX Complex (Human) *on page 1065*

Quality Assurance, Transfusion

Synonyms Quality Control

Applies to Transfusion Review Committee

Test Commonly Includes Peer professional review of clinical transfusion practices

Abstract Physicians practicing in hospitals and using blood services are likely to find their transfusion practices monitored by the institutional Transfusion Review Committee. In fact, this is a requirement of the Joint Commission on Accreditation of Healthcare Organizations. The commission requires detailed records of review of transfusion practices, including indications, single-unit transfusions, transfusion reactions, clinical effectiveness, and other aspects. The JCAHO's Accreditation Manual for Hospitals[1] covers blood usage and criteria for transfusion in its sections on medical staff, pathology and clinical laboratory services, surgical and anesthesia services, emergency services, special care units, and quality assessment and improvement. Transfusion Services are also inspected by the Commission on Laboratory Accreditation of the College of American Pathologists and American Association of Blood Banks voluntary peer review programs, the FDA, and by some state agencies.

Interpretive **USE:** Close peer review of all transfusions of blood and components is a fact of modern hospital practice. Maintenance of perfusion, need for replacement in acute hemorrhage, as well as arterial oxygenation, cardiac output, and blood volume are relevant. Many current publications address indications for transfusion. Hemoglobin level <8 g/dL and hematocrit <24% with clinical signs and symptoms of anemia usually justifies red blood cell transfusion. Use of whole blood, platelets, cryoprecipitate, and fresh frozen plasma is monitored by the transfusion committee.[2] However, the important thing is the patient's clinical status; emphasis upon hemoglobin and other laboratory test results, with insufficient bedside assessment, leads to transfusion overuse.[3] **ADDITIONAL INFORMATION:** Current concern over the adverse effects of transfusion and the cost of medical care, as well as the current litigious climate in blood transfusion, all justify an important role for quality assurance procedures. A casual attitude to the use of blood is no longer acceptable. The physician must not only follow established guidelines in blood transfusion but must also include in the patient's clinical records the rationale for using blood or its components in the existing circumstances.

Footnotes

1. Joint Commission on Accreditation of Healthcare Organizations, "1993 Joint Commission Accreditation Manual for Hospitals," *Standards*, Volume 1, Oakbrook Terrace, IL: JCAHO, 1993.
2. Silberstein LE, Kruskall MS, Stehling LC, et al, "Strategies for the Review of Transfusion Practices," *JAMA*, 1989, 262(14):1993-7.
3. Carmel R and Shulman IA, "Blood Transfusion in Medically Treatable Chronic Anemia. Pernicious Anemia as a Model for Transfusion Overuse," *Arch Pathol Lab Med*, 1989, 113(9):995-7.

References

Blanchette VS, Hume HA, Levy GJ, et al, "Guidelines for Auditing Pediatric Blood Transfusion Practices," *Am J Dis Child*, 1991, 145(7):787-96.

Carson JL, Spence RK, Poses RM, et al, "Severity of Anemia and Operative Mortality and Morbidity," *Lancet*, 1988, 727-9.

Goldman RL, "The Reliability of Peer Assessments of Quality of Care," *JAMA*, 1992, 267(7):958-60.

Goodnough LT, Johnston MF, Ramsey G, et al, "Guidelines for Transfusion Support in Patients Undergoing Coronary Artery Bypass Grafting," *Ann Thorac Surg*, 1990, 50(4):675-83.

Grindon AJ, Tomasulo PA, Bergin JJ, et al, "The Hospital Transfusion Committee. Guidelines for Improving Practice," *JAMA*, 1985, 253:540-3.

Mozes B, Epstein M, Ben-Bassat I, et al, "Evaluation of the Appropriateness of Blood and Blood Product Transfusion Using Preset Criteria," *Transfusion*, 1989, 29(6):473-6.

National Institutes of Health Consensus Conference, "Fresh Frozen Plasma Indications and Risks," *JAMA*, 1985, 253:551-3.

National Institutes of Health Consensus Conference, "Perioperative Red Blood Cell Transfusion," *JAMA*, 1988, 260:2700-3.

National Institutes of Health Consensus Conference, "Platelet Transfusion Therapy," *JAMA*, 1987, 257:1777-80.

Salem-Schatz SR, Avorn J, and Soumerai SB, "Influence of Clinical Knowledge, Organizational Context, and Practice Style on Transfusion Decision Making," *JAMA*, 1990, 264(4):471-5.

van Schoonhoven P, Berkman EM, and Lehmann R, *Medical Staff Monitoring Functions-Blood Usage Review*, Fromberg R, ed, Chicago, IL: JCAHO, 1987.

Welch HG, Meehan KR, and Goodnough LT, "Prudent Strategies for Elective Red Blood Cell Transfusion," *Ann Intern Med*, 1992, 116(5):393-402.

Quality Control *see* Quality Assurance, Transfusion *on previous page*

Random Platelets *see* Platelet Concentrate, Donation and Transfusion *on page 1081*

Reaction Work-up *see* Transfusion Reaction Work-up *on page 1098*

Recipient-Selected Transfusions *see* Donation, Blood, Directed *on page 1062*

Red Blood Cells

CPT *36430 (transfusion); 86880 (antiglobulin test, direct); 86886 (antiglobulin test, indirect); 86900 (ABO); 86901 (D^u); 86901 (Rh(D)); 86922 (compatibility test, each unit, antiglobulin)*

Related Information

Hematocrit *on page 552*
Hemoglobin *on page 554*
Risks of Transfusion *on page 1093*
Type and Crossmatch *on page 1100*
Type and Screen *on page 1102*
Whole Blood *on page 1106*

Synonyms Packed Red Cells, Transfusion; Red Cells, Packed; Transfusion, Type and Crossmatch

(Continued)

Red Blood Cells *(Continued)*

Applies to Donor Blood

Test Commonly Includes A unit of red blood cells has a volume of about 230-300 mL. ABO and Rh type, antibody screen, crossmatch, antibody identification when screen is positive (ie, preparation as for other transfusions). Red cells have a hematocrit of approximately 70% and contain the same mass of red cells as does a unit of whole blood, approximately 200 mL. The expiration date with CPDA-1 anticoagulant is 35 days after the date of collection, when stored continuously between 1°C to 6°C until transfused. With additional adenine supplementation after removal of plasma, AS-1 red blood cells have a hematocrit of 55% to 60% and a storage period of 42 days at 1°C to 6°C. If the hermetic seal is broken during preparation, the red blood cells must be infused within 24 hours.

Patient Care PREPARATION: The patient should have an identification wristband. ER may use special or temporary identification. **Dosage and administration:** Red cells must be administered through a standard 170 micron filter. Most transfusions can be given in less than 2 hours per unit, but preferably not more than 4 hours. Speed up the infusion by adding 50-100 mL of sterile isotonic sodium chloride solution, USP, just before administration.[1] **Do not add or transfuse with lactated Ringer's solution, 5% aqueous dextrose, 5% dextrose in 0.225% saline, or other calcium-containing, hypotonic, or glucose-containing fluids through the same tubing, as clumping, hemolysis, or clotting may occur.**[1] AFTERCARE: One unit should raise the hematocrit of an adult about 4 percentage points. Monitor hemoglobin and hematocrit.

Specimen Blood CONTAINER: Red top tube COLLECTION: (Of sample from intended recipient): At the patient's bedside, ask the patient to give his or her name. Compare with hospital wristband. Label the Transfusion Service wristband (if there is one) with the patient's full name, hospital number, date, and initials of collector. Label sample tube with the same information, including identification number from the wristband. Label requisition form with identification number. The collector signs the requisition, verifying the patient's identity with hospital wristband and Transfusion Service wristband. Some hospitals require additional information. It is always best to stamp the requisition with the patient's identification plate to avoid transcription errors. STORAGE INSTRUCTIONS: Store in Transfusion Service monitored refrigerator only until issue. When it is not possible to transfuse immediately after issue, blood must be returned to Transfusion Service within approximately 20 minutes. CAUSES FOR REJECTION: (Of patient sample): Gross hemolysis, sample placed in a serum separator tube, specimen tube not properly labeled TURNAROUND TIME: Red blood cells can be ready for transfusion within 30-45 minutes from the time the Blood Bank gets the type and crossmatch sample, if blood of the appropriate type is on hand. Presence of unexpected antibodies may require hours to a day or two for identification. SPECIAL INSTRUCTIONS: Crossmatched blood is usually held only for 24 hours after which it is released for other patients. There will be some exceptions. The Transfusion Service should be notified as soon as it is known definitely that the patient will not need transfusion, so blood can be used for some other patient.

Interpretive USE: Replace red cell volume;[2] provide oxygen transport; transfusion of patients with heart, liver, or renal disease in whom restriction of plasma volume or of sodium may be desirable, eg, to decrease the likelihood of volume overload (as compared with effect of whole blood); transfusion of patients with chronic anemias; replace blood lost in surgical operations. Type O RBCs may be given in emergencies to recipients of unknown ABO type (RBCs have less anti-A and anti-B than whole blood). When red cells are used for exchange transfusion, they should be 5 days or less in storage, if possible. Indications for transfusion include maintenance of perfusion, arterial oxygenation, cardiac output, and blood volume. Hemoglobin <8 g/dL with signs and symptoms of anemia usually justifies transfusion, but in some patients with chronic anemia, hemoglobin of 7 g/dL or even less may provide adequate oxygen carrying capacity.[3] LIMITATIONS: Red cells prepared in an "open" system expire in 24 hours. Most RBCs, however, are prepared in closed systems with full dating. RBCs often have a slow flow rate, which can be speeded up by adding 50-100 mL of isotonic saline to the bag. CONTRAINDICATIONS: In the past, surgeons and many other physicians have been casual in the use of RBCs. With the AIDS epidemic and increasing knowledge of the risks of transfusion, as well as Transfusion Committee surveillance, a casual attitude to transfusion is no longer acceptable. Blood transfusion is usually contraindicated when anemia and/or hypoxia can be corrected with specific and safer therapy such as iron, B_{12}, or folic acid. For correction of coagulation deficiencies, specific fractions are appropriate. No medications may be added to blood for transfusion. ADDITIONAL INFORMATION: Red blood cells must be ABO and Rh compatible. A crossmatch is necessary unless life-threatening urgency exists. See Risks of Transfusion test listing. Advantage of RBCs is greater safety in treatment of patients likely to suffer complications of volume excess.

Footnotes

1. *Circular of Information for the Use of Human Blood and Blood Components*, American Red Cross, Council of Community Blood Centers, American Association of Blood Banks, 1992.
2. National Institute of Health Consensus Conference, "Perioperative Red Blood Cell Transfusion," *JAMA*, 1988, 260(18):2700-3.
3. "Use of Blood Components," *FDA Drug Bulletin*, 1989, 19:14-5.

References

Carson JL, Spence RK, Poses RM, et al, "Severity of Anemia and Operative Mortality and Morbidity," *Lancet*, 1988, 727-9.

Walker RH, ed, *Technical Manual*, 10th ed, Arlington, VA: American Association of Blood Banks, 1990, 43-5, 344-5.

Red Blood Cells Crossmatch *see* Type and Crossmatch *on page 1100*

Red Blood Cells, Deglycerolized *see* Frozen Red Blood Cells *on page 1067*

Red Blood Cells, Frozen *see* Frozen Red Blood Cells *on page 1067*

Red Blood Cells, Washed

***CPT** 36430 (transfusion); 86985 (splitting of blood products)*

Related Information

Filters for Blood *on page 1066*

Synonyms Leukocyte-Poor Washed Red Cells; Red Cells, Washed; Washed Blood; Washed Cells

Applies to Febrile Transfusion Reaction; Transfusion Reaction, Allergic; Transfusion Reaction, Febrile

Test Commonly Includes ABO and Rh type, antibody screen, crossmatch, and antibody identification when screen is positive are needed, as for other transfusions. Hematocrit is 65% to 85%.[1] Expiration date is 24 hours from washing.

Patient Care **PREPARATION:** Patient should have wristband. **AFTERCARE:** Same as for other RBC transfusions.

Specimen Blood **CONTAINER:** One red top tube and one lavender top (EDTA) tube **COLLECTION:** Of sample from intended recipient: Same as for other RBC transfusions. **CAUSES FOR REJECTION:** (Of patient sample): Gross hemolysis, sample placed in a serum separator tube, specimen tube not properly labeled **SPECIAL INSTRUCTIONS:** Must be used within 24 hours after preparation.

Interpretive **USE:** Reduction of likelihood of febrile transfusion reaction in patients with history of febrile transfusion reactions. Useful also for patients who have severe allergic reaction to conventional transfusion. Prevention of transfusion reaction to plasma proteins, especially IgA, in patients with IgA immunoglobulin deficiency. Washed red cells are usually used for patients with paroxysmal nocturnal hemoglobinuria although some believe this to be a myth.[2] Mollison quotes the latter observation but recommends the use of washed RBCs as the prudent therapy.[3] **LIMITATIONS:** High outdating rate (24 hours). Cannot be ordered "on hold." Time consuming and expensive. There is up to 20% loss of red cells. **METHODOLOGY:** Various methods are available. The best is probably a system using a continuous-flow centrifuge and 2-3 L of isotonic saline per unit. **ADDITIONAL INFORMATION:** This component is comparable to deglycerolized red blood cells, from which 99% of WBCs are removed. The washing process removes most of the plasma proteins, fibrinogen, fibrin, potassium, citrate, ammonia, microaggregates, platelets and leukocytes, including lymphocytes.[3] The effectiveness of washing depends on the method and on the volume of isotonic saline used. Red cells have been shown to have normal survival after washing. See also Filters for Blood test listing. Use of washed RBCs is giving way to leukocyte filters for removal of WBCs, but washed cells are still appropriate for patients who have repeated allergic reactions or who have anti-IgA.

Footnotes

1. *Circular of Information for the Use of Human Blood and Blood Components*, American Red Cross, Council of Community Blood Centers, American Association of Blood Banks, 1992.
2. Sherman L and Taswell H, *Transfusion*, 1977, 17:683, (abstract).
3. Mollison PL, Engelfriet CP, and Contreras M, *Blood Transfusion in Clinical Medicine*, 8th ed, Oxford, UK: Blackwell Scientific Publications, 1987, 599-600.

(Continued)

Red Blood Cells, Washed *(Continued)*

References

Rosse WF, "Transfusion in Paroxysmal Nocturnal Hemoglobinuria - To Wash or Not to Wash?" *Transfusion*, 1989, 29(8):663-4.

Red Cell Antibody Identification *see* Antibody Identification, Red Cell *on page 1047*

Red Cell Antigen Typing *see* Antibody Identification, Red Cell *on page 1047*

Red Cell Exchange *see* Cytapheresis, Therapeutic *on page 1060*

Red Cells, Packed *see* Red Blood Cells *on page 1087*

Red Cells, Washed *see* Red Blood Cells, Washed *on previous page*

Rh *see* D^u *on page 1063*

Rh Factor *see* Rh_o(D) Typing *on page 1093*

Rh Genotype

CPT *86906*

Related Information

ABO Group and Rh Type *on page 1046*
Cord Blood Screen *on page 1057*
D^u *on page 1063*
Hemolytic Disease of the Newborn, Antibody Identification *on page 1070*
Newborn Crossmatch and Transfusion *on page 1072*
Rh_o(D) Immune Globulin (Human) *on next page*
Rh_o(D) Typing *on page 1093*

Synonyms Genotype, Rh; Zygosity, Rh

Applies to Prenatal Testing; Prognosis for Rh Hemolytic Disease of Newborn

Test Commonly Includes Rh typing of male partners of pregnant, Rh-immunized women. Testing of RBCs with anti-Rh_o(D), -rh'(C), -hr'(c), -rh''(E), and sometimes anti-hr''(e).

Specimen **CAUSES FOR REJECTION:** Hemolyzed blood sample **SPECIAL INSTRUCTIONS:** Some antiserums may be hard to get. Antiserums may contain extraneous antibodies brought out by different techniques, so use them strictly according to the manufacturer's instructions.

Interpretive **REFERENCE RANGE:** Frequencies of various Rh phenotypes and genotypes vary significantly in different ethnic groups.[1] Most of the published data are for whites of European descent (see table), so make allowance for other ethnic groups.

Frequencies of the More Common Rh-Positive Genotypes

Phenotype		Genotype		Genotype Frequency in the Total Population (%)	Likelihood of Zygosity (%)*	
CDE	Rh	CDE	Rh		Homozygous	Heterozygous
DCce	Rh_1rh	*DCe/dce*	R^1r	32.0		
		DCe/Dce	R^1R^0	2.0	6	94
DCe	Rh_1Rh_1	*DCe/DCe*	R^1R^1	17.0		
		DCe/dCe	R^1r'	0.8	96	4
DcEe	Rh_2rh	*DcE/dce*	R^2r	11.0		
		DcE/Dce	R^2R^0	0.7	6	94
DcE	Rh_2Rh_2	*DcE/DcE*	R^2R^2	2.0		
		DcE/dcE	R^2r''	0.3	86	14
DCcEe	Rh_z	*DCe/DcE*	R^1R^2	12.0		
		DCe/dcE	R^1r''	1.0	89	11
		dCe/DcE	$r'R^2$	0.3		
		DCE/dce	R^zr	0.2		
Dce	Rh_0	*Dce/dce*	R^0r	2.0		
		Dce/Dce	R^0R^0	0.07	3	97

*The figures given are for the random white population. Among blacks, the *Dce* (R^0) gene is much more common, which will greatly increase the probability of homozygosity, most particularly when the phenotype is DCce (Rh_1rh), DcEe (Rh_2rh), or Dce (Rh_0).

From Huestis DW, Bove JR, and Case J, *Practical Blood Transfusion,* 4th ed, Boston, MA: Little, Brown and CO, 1988, 97, with permission.

LIMITATIONS: Genotype frequencies are given for random populations. Remember that the husbands of Rh-immunized women are a loaded population, with a higher incidence of homozygosity.[2] On the other hand, if any of the children of an Rh-positive/Rh-negative couple is Rh-negative, or if either of the husband's parents is Rh-negative, the husband must be heterozygous. **METHODOLOGY:** Determine the husband's Rh phenotype with the serums mentioned above. Once the phenotype is known, determine the most likely corresponding genotype (and thus the likelihood of homozygosity versus heterozygosity) by consulting a table of known genotype frequencies (such as the table given here). **ADDITIONAL INFORMATION:** When a woman of childbearing age has Rh antibody, it is important for prognostic purposes to know whether the husband is homozygous or heterozygous for the gene determining D. An infant whose father is homozygous will be Rh-positive, but half the babies of a heterozygous man will be Rh-negative. The D genotype must be estimated indirectly, there being no detectable allele of D. One can usually determine the zygosity for Rh factors other than D directly by testing with appropriate serums. For example, in the case of hemolytic disease due to anti-c, if the husband's red cells are positive for both C and c, then he is heterozygous for c. If his cells are negative for C, then he is probably homozygous. There are occasional exceptions. In reporting, it is always wise to express the conclusion as "probable genotype". Mathematical odds can be given to support the conclusion.

Footnotes

1. Mourant AE, Kopec A, and Domaniewska-Sobczak K, "The Distribution of the Human Blood Groups and Other Biochemical Polymorphisms," 2nd ed, Oxford, UK: Oxford University Press, 1976.
2. Kanter MH, "Derivation of New Mathematic Formulas for Determining Whether a D-Positive Father Is Heterozygous or Homozygous for the D Antigen," *Am J Obstet Gynecol*, 1992, 166(1 Pt 1):61-3.

RhIG *see* Rh_o(D) Immune Globulin (Human) *on this page*

Rh Immune Globulin *see* Rh_o(D) Immune Globulin (Human) *on this page*

Rh_o(D) Immune Globulin (Human)

CPT *90742*

Related Information

Cord Blood Screen *on page 1057*
D^u *on page 1063*
Kleihauer-Betke *on page 563*
Newborn Crossmatch and Transfusion *on page 1072*
Rh Genotype *on previous page*
Rosette Test for Fetomaternal Hemorrhage *on page 1097*

Synonyms Anti-Rh Globulin; Rh Immune Globulin; RhIG

Test Commonly Includes Work-up for RhIG: Rh_o(D) type of mother and baby, rosette test, D^u, and antibody screen on mother, direct antiglobulin test on baby. Rh_o(D) immune globulin is an immunoglobulin product, an IgG containing anti-Rh_o(D). A dose of RhIG contains 300 μg anti-D in the U.S. Each U.S. vial of injection is sufficient to prevent immunization by 30 mL of whole blood or 15 mL of red cells.

Patient Care **PREPARATION:** The Kleihauer-Betke test on maternal blood is advisable after delivery to estimate the volume of fetal-maternal hemorrhage. The D^u on maternal blood after delivery, read microscopically, will detect some massive fetal-maternal hemorrhages. It will not detect them all. See Rosette Test for Fetomaternal Hemorrhage test listing.

Specimen Blood from both mother and infant **CONTAINER:** Red top tube or capillary tube; lavender top (EDTA) tube **COLLECTION:** Collected postpartum. Blood required from both mother and newborn. Label each specimen. **CAUSES FOR REJECTION:** (Of patient sample): Gross hemolysis, sample placed in a serum separator tube, specimen tube not properly labeled. RhIG is not indicated for newborn Rh_o(D)-negative, mother Rh_o(D)-positive or D^u-positive, anti-D present in mother's serum when mother has not had prenatal Rh_o(D) immune globulin. The question of using RhIG for women of type D^u remains debatable. Certainly, the likelihood of a D^u mother making anti-Rh is low, and one might expect that passive anti-Rh would be as likely to attach to the mother's RBCs as to any invading fetal cells. But there is evidence that some administered RhIG does remain unbound,[1] so the question remains open. Data as to effectiveness of RhIG in this setting are lacking.

Interpretive **USE:** Given to Rh_o(D), D^u-negative women postpartum, or after termination of pregnancy, abortion, or ectopic pregnancy to prevent development of anti-Rh_o(D) antibody. Such antibody may cause erythroblastosis fetalis (hemolytic disease of the newborn) or years

(Continued)

Rh_o(D) Immune Globulin (Human) *(Continued)*

later lead to transfusion reaction if Rh-positive RBCs are transfused. Occasionally, RhIG is given to Rh_o(D)-negative person who received Rh_o(D)-positive red blood cells accidentally or an Rh_o(D)-positive component (eg, platelets). RhIG has been given to Rh_o(D)-negative women after amniocentesis. This material is given antepartum at 28-32 weeks, in addition to its well accepted application within 3 days of delivery. When it is given antepartum, then following delivery anti-D will be found in the maternal serum. The direct antiglobulin test may be positive on the cord cells; in this setting such findings are not contraindications for a postpartum dose. Give a postpartum dose to the appropriate mother whether or not Rh immune globulin was given antepartum. **LIMITATIONS:** In instances of large fetomaternal hemorrhage, one dose is not sufficient. The D^u test read microscopically will detect some very large bleeds but miss others that require more than one dose. The rosette test is more sensitive. See preparation discussion in the Kleihauer-Betke test. The Kleihauer-Betke test is not needed in amniocentesis, ectopic pregnancy, first or second trimester abortion, or miscarriage. A smaller Rh immune globulin dose may be used after abortion or miscarriage up to 12 weeks gestation, but not beyond; after 12 weeks of gestation a conventional dose is indicated. **Failures** occur. The most common cause of immunization to Rh_o(D) is failure to give RhIG when it is indicated. RhIG is sometimes forgotten in ectopic gestation and in abortion in Rh_o(D)-negative women. However, 1% to 2% of term mothers develop anti-D in spite of postpartum RhIG properly administered. Postpartum failure may be secondary to fetomaternal hemorrhage in the third trimester (for which antenatal doses are recommended)[2] and because of large fetomaternal hemorrhages at delivery (for which the Kleihauer-Betke acid elution test is recommended). If a postpartum blood sample is tested for D^u and thought to be positive, RhIG may be withheld; if the apparent D^u positivity is secondary to a large fetomaternal bleed from an Rh-positive baby to an Rh-negative mother, the mother may falsely appear as a D^u-positive but really needs more than one dose of RhIG. Over 300,000 Rh-negative women deliver Rh-positive babies annually in the United States, of whom relatively few have fetomaternal hemorrhages larger than 15 mL of red cells. Some of these may become immunized.[3] **CONTRAINDICATIONS:** Do not give Rh_o(D) immune globulin to an Rh_o(D)-positive or D^u-positive person, or a person already immunized to the Rh_o(D) blood factor whose serum contains anti-D. (However, if Rh_o(D) immune globulin was given as an antenatal dose to mother, then anti-D detectable in her serum is not a contraindication to postnatal administration of RhIG.) Rh_o(D) immune globulin should not be given to an infant, to the mother of an Rh-negative baby, or when the biological father of the fetus is known with certainty to be Rh negative. **METHODOLOGY:** Read package insert. **ADDITIONAL INFORMATION:** RhIG should be given to Rh_o(D)-negative mother within 72 hours of delivery, miscarriage, or removal of ectopic pregnancy.

The **Kleihauer-Betke** test is a stain that can be done on maternal blood after delivery to estimate the volume of fetal-maternal hemorrhage. The dose of Rh_o immune globulin necessary to protect the mother from stimulation to antibody formation can be estimated as follows.[4]

- Percent of fetal red cells x 50 = mL fetal blood in maternal circulation.
- Give one dose of RhIG for every 25 mL of fetal maternal hemorrhage.
- This is slightly higher than the usually recommended dose of 300 μg of RhIG per 30 mL of fetal blood. There is a tendency to underestimate because of the poor precision of the Kleihauer-Betke test.

Rh-negative mothers with negative screens are always given Rh_o(D) immune globulin when cord blood is not available to be tested (ectopic pregnancies, abortions, etc) unless the father can be shown to be Rh negative. If the patient refuses, she should sign an appropriate statement to that effect. Although **antenatal doses** may have been given at 28-32 weeks, give a postpartum dose anyway. Transmission of viral infections does not occur with this preparation.

Footnotes

1. Lubenko A, Contreras M, and Habash J, "Should Anti-Rh Immunoglobulin Be Given to D Variant Women?" *Br J Haematol*, 1989, 72(3):429-33.
2. Bowman JM, "Antenatal Suppression of Rh Alloimmunization," *Clin Obstet Gynecol*, 1991, 34(2):296-303.
3. Sebring ES and Polesky HF, "Fetomaternal Hemorrhage: Incidence, Risk Factors, Time of Occurrence, and Clinical Effects," *Transfusion*, 1990, 30(4):344-57.
4. Walker RH, ed, *Technical Manual*, 10th ed, Arlington, VA: American Association of Blood Banks, 1990, 381-7.

References

Mittendorf R and Williams MA, "Rh_o(D) Immunoglobulin (RhoGAM™): How It Came Into Being," *Obstet Gynecol*, 1991, 77(2):301-3.

Zimmerman DR, *Rh. The Intimate History of a Disease and Its Conquest*, New York, NY: Macmillan Publishing Co Inc, 1973.

Rh_o(D) Typing

CPT *86901*

Related Information

ABO Group and Rh Type *on page 1046*
Cord Blood Screen *on page 1057*
D^u *on page 1063*
Newborn Crossmatch and Transfusion *on page 1072*
Rh Genotype *on page 1090*
Type and Crossmatch *on page 1100*

Synonyms D Factor; Rh Factor

Test Commonly Includes D typing is included in type and crossmatch. Rh-Hr control may be needed with D typing; see manufacturer's instructions.

Specimen Blood **CONTAINER:** Red top tube **CAUSES FOR REJECTION:** Serum separator tube, gross hemolysis, unlabeled tube

Interpretive **USE:** Rh_o(D) typing is a part of Type and Screen, Type and Crossmatch, and Prenatal Screen, and is done on newborns of Rh-negative mothers as a part of Rh immune globulin work-up **LIMITATIONS:** When a newborn's direct antiglobulin test (DAT) is strongly positive, maternal antibody may be occupying all D sites on the baby's erythrocytes; this can lead to false-negative Rh typing. Rh typing may be invalid in the presence of strongly reactive DAT. **ADDITIONAL INFORMATION:** Rh_o(D) is the most important antigen in the Rh system. Its corresponding antibody has been the most common cause of clinically significant erythroblastosis fetalis. Saline D typing is available. It is used in special situations (eg, when the Rh-Hr control is positive, or in the presence of strongly positive DAT).

References

Agre P and Cartron JP, "Molecular Biology of the Rh Antigens," *Blood*, 1991, 78(3):551-63.
Mollison PL, Engelfriet CP, and Contreras M, "The Rh Blood Group System," *Blood Transfusion in Clinical Medicine*, 9th ed, Chapter 5, Oxford, UK: Blackwell Scientific Publications, 1993.

Rh_o Variant *see* D^u *on page 1063*
Rh Titer *see* Antibody Titer *on page 1048*

Risks of Transfusion

Related Information

Alanine Aminotransferase *on page 100*
Automated Reagin Test *on page 642*
Babesiosis Serological Test *on page 643*
Chagas' Disease Serological Test *on page 662*
Cytomegalovirus Antibody *on page 672*
Hepatitis B Core Antibody *on page 684*
Hepatitis B Surface Antigen *on page 688*
Hepatitis C Serology *on page 690*
HIV-1/HIV-2 Serology *on page 696*
HTLV-I/II Antibody *on page 702*
IgA Antibodies *on page 705*
Immunoglobulin A *on page 709*
p24 Antigen *on page 727*
Red Blood Cells *on page 1087*
RPR *on page 742*
Transfusion Reaction Work-up *on page 1098*
Type and Crossmatch *on page 1100*
VDRL, Serum *on page 762*
Whole Blood *on page 1106*
Yersinia enterocolitica Antibody *on page 765*

Synonyms Hazards of Transfusion; Transfusion Complications; Transfusion Risks

Specimen **SPECIAL INSTRUCTIONS:** All adverse effects of transfusion must be reported at once to the Blood Bank for follow-up and investigation. The physician in charge of transfusion must in

(Continued)

Risks of Transfusion *(Continued)*

turn investigate **all** reported reactions, with interpretation and recommendations recorded in the patient's chart. The FDA requires a report of all fatal transfusion reactions. Any suspected cases of transfusion-associated infectious disease must be reported to the Blood Bank so that implicated donors can be traced and investigated. These are obligations written into federal regulations, AABB standards, and those of other accrediting agencies.

Some Risks of Allogeneic Transfusion

Reactions	Disease Transmission	Other
Hemolytic, immediate, delayed	Hepatitis B, C, etc	Alloimmunization RBC, WBC, etc
Febrile	Cytomegalovirus	Marrow suppression
Allergic, anaphylactic	Syphilis	Immunosuppression
Sepsis	Malaria	Storage changes
Overload	Babesiosis	Graft–vs–host disease
Hypothermia, cold	Brucellosis	Dilutional coagulopathy
Air embolism	Chagas disease	Nonimmune hemolysis
Post–transfusion purpura	AIDS	Iron overload

Interpretive ADDITIONAL INFORMATION:

INCOMPATIBLE BLOOD:

Hemolytic transfusion reactions usually result from clerical and other identification errors involving ABO incompatibility.[1,2] This is why unlabeled or improperly labeled sample tubes are unacceptable to the Transfusion Service. Chills, fever, dyspnea, chest or back pain, headache, abnormal bleeding, or shock can all characterize acute hemolytic reactions. Hemoglobinemia heralds **intravascular** hemolysis, followed by hemoglobinuria, then jaundice. This is usually mediated by anti-A or anti-B or both. **Extravascular** hemolysis takes place mostly in the spleen as a result of the action of IgG antibodies, such as those of the Rh system. With these, hemoglobinemia and hemoglobinuria seldom occur. See listing, Transfusion Reaction Work-up. Renal shutdown, shock, or hemorrhage may be fatal. When this type of reaction occurs, stop the transfusion at once. Treat shock. Give appropriate fluids and diuretics to maintain urinary output. Treat for incipient renal failure, if indicated.

Delayed hemolytic reactions can occur in some patients with other serologically undetectable antibodies (other than anti-A or anti-B).[3] These are noticed when more blood is ordered a few days after an earlier transfusion of apparently compatible blood. There has usually been a poor clinical response to the prior transfusion. The Blood Bank finds a positive direct antiglobulin test and antibody that is now incompatible with the recently transfused RBCs. The antibody may be either in the patient's serum or in an eluate from the red cells. The diagnosis is easily missed. Delayed hemolytic reactions are not uncommon; they are usually mild, rarely severe.

Remember that **nonimmune hemolysis** can also occur and may be mistaken for an incompatible blood reaction. Some causes include inappropriate I.V. solutions run in the same tubing with blood (eg, hypotonic or dextrose-containing solutions – even water has been used this way); overheating; accidental freezing (eg, packing RBCs in a box with dry ice); irrigation of bleeding surgical surfaces with water (eg, in bladder surgery); accidental infusion of water instead of saline; bacterial contamination of blood; and, rarely, G-6-PD deficiency (either in donor or patient).

Other immune reactions include **febrile nonhemolytic** reactions,[4] usually in patients with antibodies to donor leukocytes, occurring in as many as 1% of transfusions. They are treated symptomatically with antipyretics, and may be prevented by passing RBCs or platelets through leukocyte-removing filters, or by using washed RBCs. **Allergic transfusion reactions** are about equally frequent and usually appear in the form of hives (urticaria). Treatment and prevention is with antihistaminics (given to the patient, not put into the blood container).[1] fortunately rare.

TRANSFUSION-ASSOCIATED INFECTIOUS DISEASES:

Viral hepatitis, the incidence of which is changing rapidly.[5,6] Type A is very rare, B now uncommon, and C decreasing significantly.

Cytomegalovirus infection, significant in premature newborns and immunosuppressed adults, including transplant recipients.[7,8] For the latter and for babies weighing less than 1200 g and having CMV-seronegative mothers, use blood from CMV-seronegative donors. Removal of WBCs may reduce and perhaps prevent CMV infections.

Bacterial contamination of blood or components, usually with gram-negatives.[9] This can cause septic shock and death and must be vigorously treated if observed. Currently, there is concern over contamination with *Yersinia enterocolitica*, particularly in platelets.[10] The following infections are occasionally seen, but should be considered rare: syphilis, malaria (rare in the U.S.), babesiosis (endemic in some areas of the east coast), brucellosis, Chagas' disease (trypanosomiasis, rare in the US, common in parts of South America), and, of course, AIDS.

In the case of **AIDS**, we are dealing with a transfusion-transmitted infection that is statistically rare,[5,11] but regarded by the public as a terrifying risk of transfusion. Fear of AIDS gives it a prominence in the public eye that is out of all proportion to the real risk, but this is the perception transfusionists must face. Most recipients of HIV-infected blood or components will become seropositive and will in time progress to clinical AIDS. Since the onset of testing for anti-HIV-1 in 1985, very few cases of transfusion-associated AIDS have occurred.[12] These depend, for the most part, on donations by persons recently infected with HIV who have not yet formed detectable antibody.

Bone marrow suppression of RBC production will occur after the transfusion of RBCs, another reason to avoid giving transfusions to patients whose anemia might respond to conventional medication.

Immunosuppression of varying degree follows allogeneic transfusion.[13] Just as transfusion improves the survival of kidney allografts, so also does it depress the body's natural immunity and resistance. Patients who get transfusions at surgery to remove malignancies are more likely to have the tumor recur than those who were not transfused.[14] Presumably for the same reason, transfused patients are more likely to have postoperative infections.[15] This phenomenon does not seem to occur with autologous transfusion.

Transfusion-related acute lung injury ("TRALI"). Clinically similar to adult respiratory distress syndrome, seems to be related to leukocyte antibodies in donor plasma, reacting with recipient's antigens, perhaps with release of complement.[16] Unlike ARDS, the condition usually improves quickly with pulmonary support.

Simple **volume overload** of the recipient's circulation may cause pulmonary edema without leukocyte antibodies.

Air embolism can result from any admission of air into intravenous tubing and can have serious consequences.

Anaphylactic reaction: See IgA Antibodies and Immunoglobulin A listings in Immunology and Serology chapters.

Graft-versus-host disease (GVHD) can result from transfusion of blood components containing living donor lymphocytes. Normally, these would be rapidly eliminated by the host's immune response. But in immunocompromised patients (transplant recipients, patients receiving immunosuppressive chemotherapy and, rarely, premature newborns), the donor lymphocytes are able to attack the host tissues, sometimes with fatal results.[17] GVHD occasionally occurs in immunocompetent recipients, which is harder to understand. This seems to be rare in the U.S., but not uncommon in Japan, where the population is more homogeneous and where homozygous HLA phenotypes are more common. It requires a donor, usually a close relative, who is homozygous for an HLA haplotype for which the recipient is heterozygous. Thus, the recipient does not recognize the donor lymphocytes as foreign, while the donor cells are able to survive and attack the recipient. In general, GVHD is preventable by irradiation of the blood or component to be transfused to a patient at risk[18] (see Irradiated Blood Components). AABB advises irradiation of directed donations from first-degree relatives of any patient to prevent this rare complication.

Complications of massive transfusion: **Hemorrhagic diathesis** due to dilution and washout (dilutional coagulopathy) of coagulation factors and platelets.[19] DIC can also occur in the settings in which massive transfusions are given. Rapid laboratory evaluation of hemostasis

(Continued)

Risks of Transfusion *(Continued)*

Approximate Frequency of Some Transfusion Complications Compared to a Large Study of Hospitalized Patients*

Complication	Approximate Frequency per Unit Transfused
Hepatitis C	1:3300
Hepatitis B	1:200,000
HIV-1 (AIDS)	1:225,000
HTLV-I	1:50,000
Transfusion-associated infections (overall)	3 per 10,000 patients
Febrile or allergic reaction	1:100
Hemolytic transfusion reaction	1:6000
Fatal hemolytic reaction	1:100,000
Accidental and preventable deaths in hospital	6 per 1000 patients

*From Dodd RY, "The Risk of Transfusion-Transmitted Infections", *N Eng J Med*, 1992, 327:419-21, with permission.

can be vital. Treatment of abnormal bleeding in this situation is primarily with platelet concentrates, sometimes also with FFP, and less often cryoprecipitate. If fluid balance is not carefully observed, fluid overload or adult respiratory distress syndrome may occur. 2,3-DPG depletion of stored RBCs is a theoretic problem, rarely of any clinical significance. Hypothermia caused by cold blood banked can be prevented with blood warmers (see Warming, Blood). With massive transfusions, particularly in trauma, there is often tumult and confusion, which makes an ideal setup for clerical errors and increased likelihood of incompatible blood transfusion. Avoiding errors in such settings is vital and requires great care and alertness on the part of all.

Footnotes

1. Huestis DW, Bove JR, and Case J, *Practical Blood Transfusion*, 4th ed, Boston, MA: Little, Brown and Co, 1988, 249-68.
2. Mollison PL, Engelfriet CP, and Contreras M, *Blood Transfusion in Clinical Medicine*, 9th ed, chapters 10, 11, 15, 16, Oxford, UK: Blackwell Scientific Publications, 1993, 499-542, 677-785.
3. Ness PM, Shirey RS, Thoman SK, et al, "The Differentiation of Delayed Serologic and Delayed Hemolytic Transfusion Reactions: Incidence, Long-Term Serologic Findings, and Clinical Significance," *Transfusion*, 1990, 30(8):688-93.
4. Brubaker DB, "Clinical Significance of White Cell Antibodies in Febrile Nonhemolytic Transfusion Reactions," *Transfusion*, 1990, 30(8):733-7.
5. Dodd RY, "The Risk of Transfusion-Transmitted Infection," *N Engl J Med*, 1992, 327(6):419-21.
6. Donahue JG, Muñoz A, Ness PM, et al, "The Declining Risk of Post-transfusion Hepatitis C Virus Infection," *N Engl J Med*, 1992, 327(6):369-73.
7. Eisenfeld L, Silver H, McLaughlin J, et al, "Prevention of Transfusion-Associated Cytomegalovirus Infection in Neonatal Patients by the Removal of White Cells From Blood," *Transfusion*, 1992, 32(3):205-9.
8. Sayers MH, Anderson KC, Goodnough LT, et al, "Reducing the Risk for Transfusion-Transmitted Cytomegalovirus Infection," *Ann Intern Med*, 1992, 116(1):55-62.
9. Goldman M and Blajchman MA, "Blood Product-Associated Bacterial Sepsis," *Transfus Med Rev*, 1991, 5(1):73-83.
10. Morrow JF, Braine HG, Kickler TS, et al, "Septic Reactions to Platelet Transfusions. A Persistent Problem," *JAMA*, 1991, 266(4):555-8.
11. Carson JL, Russell LB, Taragin MI, et al, "The Risks of Blood Transfusion: The Relative Influence of Acquired Immunodeficiency Syndrome and Non-A, Non-B Hepatitis," *Am J Med*, 1992, 92(1):45-52.
12. Conley LJ and Holmberg SD, "Transmission of AIDS From Blood Screened Negative for Antibody to the Human Immunodeficiency Virus," *N Engl J Med*, 1992, 326(22):1499-1500, (letter).
13. Brunson ME and Alexander JW, "Mechanisms of Transfusion-Induced Immunosuppression," *Transfusion*, 1990, 30(7):651-8.
14. Wobbes T, Joosen KH, Kuypers HH, et al, "The Effect of Packed Cells and Whole Blood Transfusions on Survival After Curative Resection for Colorectal Carcinoma," *Dis Colon Rectum*, 1989, 32(9):743-8.
15. Triulzi DJ, Vanek K, Ryan DH, et al, "A Clinical and Immunologic Study of Blood Transfusion and Postoperative Bacterial Infection in Spinal Surgery," *Transfusion*, 1992, 32(6):517-24.
16. Popovsky MA, Chaplin HC Jr, and Moore SB, "Transfusion-Related Acute Lung Injury: A Neglected, Serious Complication of Hemotherapy," *Transfusion*, 1992, 32(6):589-91.

17. Holland PV, "Prevention of Transfusion-Associated Graft-vs-Host Disease," *Arch Pathol Lab Med*, 1989, 113(3):285-91.
18. Anderson KC, Goodnough LT, Sayers M, et al, "Variation in Blood Component Irradiation Practice: Implications for Prevention of Transfusion-Associated Graft-Versus-Host Disease," *Blood*, 1991, 77(10):2096-102.
19. Sohmer PR, "Transfusion Therapy in Surgery," *Clinical Practice of Transfusion Medicine*, Petz LD and Swisher SN, eds, New York, NY: Churchill-Livingstone, 1989, 363-400.

References

Leslie SD and Toy PT, "Laboratory Hemostatic Abnormalities in Massively Transfused Patients Given Red Blood Cells and Crystalloid," *Am J Clin Pathol*, 1991, 96(6):770-3.

Rosette Test (Erythrocyte) *see* D^u *on page 1063*

Rosette Test for Fetomaternal Hemorrhage

CPT 86999

Related Information

D^u *on page 1063*
Kleihauer-Betke *on page 563*
Newborn Crossmatch and Transfusion *on page 1072*
Rh_0(D) Immune Globulin (Human) *on page 1091*

Synonyms Fetalscreen™

Test Commonly Includes A postdelivery Rh-negative maternal specimen is screened for the presence of Rh_0(D)-positive fetal cells.

Specimen Blood **CONTAINER:** One red top tube and one lavender top (EDTA) tube **CAUSES FOR REJECTION:** Specimen grossly hemolyzed **SPECIAL INSTRUCTIONS:** Specimen used for testing must be a postdelivery specimen.

Interpretive **USE:** Determine if fetal maternal hemorrhage of more than 15 mL red cells has occurred **LIMITATIONS:** This is a screening test for the detection of fetal D-positive cells in D-negative maternal blood. An acid-elution test should follow a positive screen to quantify the number of fetal cells present. May be unreliable if the newborn is a D^u variant. **METHODOLOGY:** Anti-D is added to the Rh-negative maternal blood and incubated. D-positive cells are then added to the maternal cell-anti-D mixture. Antibody coating is not strong enough to cause direct agglutination, but rosette formation occurs in positive specimens after addition of the D-positive cells.

References

Mollison PL, Engelfriet CP, and Contreras M, *Blood Transfusion in Clinical Medicine*, 9th ed, Oxford, UK: Blackwell Scientific Publications, 1993, 546-53.

SDFP *see* Plasma, Fresh Frozen *on page 1078*

Single-Donor Platelets *see* Platelets, Apheresis, Donation *on page 1083*

Stem Cell Collection *see* Cytapheresis, Therapeutic *on page 1060*

Therapeutic Cytapheresis *see* Cytapheresis, Therapeutic *on page 1060*

Therapeutic Leukapheresis *see* Cytapheresis, Therapeutic *on page 1060*

Therapeutic Phlebotomy *see* Phlebotomy, Therapeutic *on page 1075*

Titer, Irregular Antibodies in Transfusion Service *see* Antibody Titer *on page 1048*

Titer of Anti-Rh_0(D) *see* Antibody Titer *on page 1048*

Titer of Unexpected Antibody *see* Antibody Titer *on page 1048*

Transfusion *see* Type and Crossmatch *on page 1100*

Transfusion, Autologous *see* Autologous Transfusion, Preoperative Deposit *on page 1052*

Transfusion, Autologous, Predeposit *see* Autologous Transfusion, Preoperative Deposit *on page 1052*

Transfusion Complications *see* Risks of Transfusion *on page 1093*

Transfusion, Neonatal *see* Newborn Crossmatch and Transfusion *on page 1072*

Transfusion Reaction, Allergic *see* Red Blood Cells, Washed *on page 1089*

Transfusion Reaction, Febrile *see* Filters for Blood *on page 1066*

Transfusion Reaction, Febrile *see* Red Blood Cells, Washed *on page 1089*

Transfusion Reaction Work-up

***CPT** 86880 (antiglobulin test, direct); 86900 (ABO); 86901 (Rh(D))*

Related Information

Antiglobulin Test, Direct *on page 1049*

Risks of Transfusion *on page 1093*

Synonyms Hemolytic Reaction to Transfusion; Reaction Work-up; Transfusion Review

Test Commonly Includes If there is any evidence of significant reaction other than mild urticaria, **stop the transfusion** but keep normal saline dripping in slowly to keep the I.V. open. Report reaction to Blood Bank. Examine label on blood container(s) and all clerical work and records for possible error, and review possible mirror image or other-side-of-the-coin error (is there a roommate also getting blood? If one unit is infused into a wrong patient, what has be-

Schedule of Investigation of Reported Transfusion Reactions

A. All reported reactions

1. Specimens needed
   - a. Pretransfusion blood of recipient
   - b. Post-transfusion blood of recipient
2. Investigation (letters refer to specimens listed above)
   - Check donor and patient identification and crossmatch report
   - Repeat ABO and Rh typing (b, and donor bag, if indicated)
   - Direct antiglobulin test (b, if indicated)
   - Examine for visible hemolysis (b); if necessary, compare (b) with (a)

If these procedures reveal no evidence of incompatibility or hemolysis, and there is no additional information to arouse suspicion, no further investigation is needed. Otherwise, proceed as follows:

B. If there is evidence of hemolysis or incompatible transfusion

1. Specimens needed
   - a. Pretransfusion blood of recipient
   - b. Post-transfusion blood of recipient
   - c. Pilot samples of donor blood
   - d. Blood from container implicated in reaction (if available)
   - e. Post-transfusion urine
2. Immunologic investigation
   - Repeat ABO, Rh, and direct antiglobulin test (a, c, d)
   - Repeat crossmatch (a, b, c; d, if indicated) (major; minor only if indicated)
   - Repeat antibody screen (a, b, c) (special, sensitive techniques if necessary)
   - Identification of any unexpected antibody or incompatibility
3. Other procedures as indicated
   - Serum haptoglobin (a, b)
   - Bacteriologic smear and culture (d)
   - Serum urea and bilirubin (a, b)
   - Urine hemoglobin (e)
   - Urine hemosiderin (e)
4. Investigation of nonimmune causes of hemolysis

From Huestis DW, Bove JR, and Case J, *Practical Blood Transfusion*, 4th ed, Boston, MA: Little, Brown and Co, 1988, 268, with permission.

come of the other unit crossmatched?) Examination of prereaction and postreaction serum or plasma for hemolysis or jaundice. This should be begun by examination of the postreaction blood sample sent very promptly to the Blood Bank.

Direct antiglobulin test on postreaction specimen.

Repeat ABO and Rh typing on patient and donor blood; compare with previous reports.

If the above are negative, additional tests are not essential for moderate febrile reaction. If actual hemolysis is suspected, the following may be done.

Hemoglobin and hematocrit: Look for expected increase from amount of blood infused or lack of increase... was there an appropriate rise? (But in the bleeding patient, for instance, the hemoglobin may not rise anyway.)

Urinalysis for free hemoglobin: A red supernatant in the centrifuged urine specimen, positive for hemoglobin. Watch for brown as well as red urine. Urine dipsticks also provide reactions for bilirubin and urobilinogen. Follow urine output and record it.

Blood container, attached transfusion set, and intravenous solutions must be sent to Transfusion Service.

Serum bilirubin

Culture of remaining donor blood, especially if the patient has fever and shock.

BUN and creatinine

Repeat crossmatch and antibody screen on donor and recipient.

Antibody identification if indicated.

Test for haptoglobin in recipient (but haptoglobin may decrease even following uneventful transfusions).

In case of possible DIC (disseminated intravascular coagulation), baseline studies include platelet count, prothrombin time, PTT, fibrin split products, fibrinogen, and thrombin time. Oozing from venipuncture site or sites or from a surgical wound is an indication for as many of these tests as can be done stat; preferably, all of them. Such microvascular bleeding has often been the only clue to a hemolytic reaction occurring during surgery.

Patient Care AFTERCARE: As investigation is in progress in the laboratory, those caring for the patient must monitor for evidence of shock, renal shutdown, and/or evidence of DIC (ie, look for oozing, petechiae, or ecchymoses). Vigorous treatment may be needed for any or all of these manifestations, possibly including additional transfusions.

Specimen Blood, urine CONTAINER: Red top tube, lavender top (EDTA) tube, and plastic urine container CAUSES FOR REJECTION: (Of patient sample): Specimen tube not properly labeled TURNAROUND TIME: Examination of pretransfusion and current serum or plasma for hemolysis can be done very rapidly. A repeat ABO and Rh, direct antiglobulin test, and clerical check can be done in minutes. SPECIAL INSTRUCTIONS: If patient develops chills, fever exceeding 1.5°C, hypotension, dyspnea, nausea, etc, stop the transfusion, notify physician and Transfusion Service immediately. **If in doubt about any possible reaction, stop transfusion immediately. Notify physician and Transfusion Service immediately**. Return blood bag to Transfusion Service. If a hemolytic transfusion reaction is suspected, send all I.V. solutions and concurrent medications to Transfusion Service. Report patient's diagnosis, medications, pretransfusion and post-transfusion vital signs to the patient's physician and to the Transfusion Service. Keep I.V. needle open with slowly infusing normal saline, pending physician's instructions. **Blood container**, attached transfusion set, and intravenous solutions must be sent to the Transfusion Service.

Interpretive USE: Investigate cause of possible transfusion reactions. Symptoms and signs of transfusion reaction may include chills, temperature elevation, dyspnea, nausea, pain in lower back, shock, urticaria, and/or hematuria. LIMITATIONS: The transfusion reaction work-up will mainly detect those reactions caused by red cell incompatibility and with culture, those caused by bacterial contamination of the infused unit. The conventional investigation may not detect reactions to white cells, platelets, or to plasma proteins such as IgA reactions. CONTRAINDICATIONS: The two most common complications of transfusion are urticaria and fever. **Urticaria** (hives, rash, itching) occurs in about 1% of transfusions and does not call for a full reaction work-up. An antihistamine by mouth or by vein usually relieves such symptoms. The patient's physician may decide to continue the transfusion after symptomatic medication, bearing in mind the risk of giving more allergen to a demonstrably allergic patient. **Fevers and chills** (a sharp rise of at least 1°C, not sustained, without other causes of fever) indicates a **fe-**

(Continued)

Transfusion Reaction Work-up *(Continued)*

brile nonhemolytic transfusion reaction. Most such reactions are caused by a recipient's antibody to donor leukocytes and respond to symptomatic antipyretic medication. Since true hemolytic reactions may start with fever, the investigation must rule out hemolysis. The time needed to do this usually precludes restarting transfusion of the unit implicated. If a patient has repeated febrile reactions, provide washed red cells or filter the blood through special leukocyte filters. Culture of the unit is not indicated. If a patient has sustained high fever, bloody emesis, diarrhea, or signs of **sepsis, toxemia, or "red shock,"** suspect bacteremia or endotoxic shock from contaminated blood. Immediate, intensive treatment is essential for this very dangerous reaction. A Gram stained smear and culture from the suspected unit and blood culture from the patient will be diagnostic. **ADDITIONAL INFORMATION: Most fatal transfusion reactions involve clerical (labeling) error and incompatibility in the ABO system, with intravascular hemolysis**.

Hemolytic transfusion reactions are characterized by fever, flushing, a feeling of apprehension, chest or back pain, chills, nausea, vomiting, and in severe cases, shock, oliguria, hemoglobinuria, bleeding, and renal failure. If a hemolytic transfusion reaction is suspected, the transfusion must be discontinued immediately, the Transfusion Service or Blood Bank notified at once, and appropriate clinical measures taken to support circulation, renal failure, and coagulation.

Bacterial pyrogens, circulatory overload, air embolism, faulty blood warming apparatus, inappropriate storage of blood or components before infusion, and medications added to the blood unit or infusion tubing are other causes of transfusion reactions. These are not always detected by the transfusion reaction work-up. Most are prevented by careful transfusion technique.

Delayed transfusion reactions are often missed. They may be detected by unexplained anemia, by a positive direct antiglobulin test, or by the detection of an unexplained antibody, which was absent when the type and screen were done.

Report any case of unexplained **liver dysfunction** occurring 2 weeks to 6 months after transfusion to the Transfusion Service because they may be secondary to post-transfusion hepatitis (hepatitis C, cytomegalovirus, or now rarely, hepatitis B).

See Risks of Transfusion test listing.

By federal regulations, all suspected transfusion reactions must be reported to the Transfusion Service and all must be investigated and reported to the patient's physician. Any fatal reaction must be reported to the FDA.

References

Huestis DW, Bove JR, and Case J, *Practical Blood Transfusion*, 4th ed, Boston, MA: Little, Brown and Co, 1988, 249-85.

Mollison PL, Engelfriet CP, and Contreras M, *Blood Transfusion in Clinical Medicine*, 9th ed, Chapters 10 and 11, Oxford, UK: Blackwell Scientific Publications, 1993.

Walker RH, ed, *Technical Manual*, 10th ed, Arlington, VA: American Association of Blood Banks, 1990, 411-32.

Widmann FK, ed, *Standards for Blood Banks and Transfusion Services*, 15th ed, Bethesda, MD: American Association of Blood Banks, 1993, 33-4.

Transfusion Review *see* Transfusion Reaction Work-up *on page 1098*

Transfusion Review Committee *see* Quality Assurance, Transfusion *on page 1086*

Transfusion Risks *see* Risks of Transfusion *on page 1093*

Transfusion, Type and Crossmatch *see* Red Blood Cells *on page 1087*

Type and Coombs', Cord Blood *see* Cord Blood Screen *on page 1057*

Type and Crossmatch

CPT *36430 (transfusion); 86880 (antiglobulin test, direct); 86886 (antiglobulin test, indirect); 86900 (ABO); 86901 (D^u); 86901 (Rh(D)); 86922 (compatibility test, each unit, antiglobulin)*

Related Information

Antibody Identification, Red Cell *on page 1047*

Antiglobulin Test, Direct *on page 1049*
Antiglobulin Test, Indirect *on page 1051*
Red Blood Cells *on page 1087*
Rh_o(D) Typing *on page 1093*
Risks of Transfusion *on page 1093*
Type and Screen *on next page*

Synonyms Compatibility Testing; Crossmatch

Applies to Donor Units; Major Screen; Red Blood Cells Crossmatch; Transfusion; Whole Blood, Crossmatch

Test Commonly Includes ABO, Rh, antibody screen, major crossmatch. Serum, which must be from the correct patient, is tested against ABO and Rh compatible donor red cells with appropriate reagents, in order to detect ABO incompatibility and clinically significant unexpected antibodies that may cause decreased red cell survival in the recipient. The procedure includes ABO, Rh, and antibody screening test on the recipient's sample. This procedure is only required with components containing (or expected to contain) more than 5 mL of red cells. In general, selection of RBCs (or whole blood) is simple: select the same ABO and Rh type as the patient's. If this is not possible and transfusion cannot be postponed, see table.

Selection of Donor Blood for Transfusion to Recipients of Various ABO and Rh Types

Patient Blood Type	First Choice	Second Choice	Third Choice
O pos	O pos	O neg	None
O neg	O neg	None	O pos
A pos	A pos	A neg	O pos, O neg
A neg	A neg	None	O neg, O pos, A pos
B pos	B pos	B neg	O pos, O neg
B neg	B neg	None	O neg, O pos, B pos
AB pos	AB pos	AB neg, A pos, B pos, A neg, B neg	O pos, O neg
AB neg	AB neg	A neg, B neg	O neg, AB pos, A pos, B pos, O pos

Note: The technologist may always substitute Rh–negative donor RBC for Rh–positive patients, if supplies permit. Physician approval is required for third choice donor blood selection in the event that first and second choice are unavailable. In the case of using A or B for AB, it is either A or B for one patient, not both to the same patient, and before changing the blood type the Blood Bank physician must approve.

Patient Care PREPARATION: Patient should have wristband. Identification of specimens is critically important.

Specimen Blood CONTAINER: One red top tube and one lavender top (EDTA) tube COLLECTION: (Of sample from intended recipient): At the patient's bedside, ask the patient to give his or her name. Compare with the hospital wristband. Label the Transfusion Service wristband (if there is one) with the patient's full name, hospital number, date, and initials of collector. Label sample tube with the same information, including identification number from the wristband. Label requisition form with identification number. The collector signs the requisition, verifying the patient's identity with hospital wristband and Transfusion Service wristband. Some hospitals require additional information. It is always best to stamp the requisition with the patient's identification plate to avoid transcription errors. STORAGE INSTRUCTIONS: The sample used for crossmatching must be no more than 3 days old at the time of transfusion for patients who have been pregnant or transfused within the last 3 months or if the history is unknown. CAUSES FOR REJECTION: Gross hemolysis, sample placed in a serum separator tube, specimen tube not properly labeled TURNAROUND TIME: Detection of antibodies or incompatible reactions sometimes require significant time, to permit antibody identification and/or problem solving. The goal of type and crossmatch is the provision of blood safe for the intended recipient, without shortened survival of transfused RBCs. Remember that not all blood group antibodies are dangerous (see Antibody Identification, Red Cell). SPECIAL INSTRUCTIONS: Blood is usually held for a patient for only 24 hours.

Interpretive POSSIBLE PANIC RANGE: Incompatible crossmatch USE: Preparation for transfusion of blood. The major crossmatch detects ABO compatibility, and it or the antibody screening test detects antibodies in recipient serum that may be incompatible with donor red cells.[1] The crossmatch can detect unusual antigens in donor blood, which might be absent from screen-

(Continued)

Type and Crossmatch *(Continued)*

ing cells. **LIMITATIONS:** Does not assure normal red cell survival; will not detect all antibodies or incompatibilities; does not prevent all transfusion reactions; does not detect all errors in ABO grouping; does not detect Rh errors; does not prevent reactions to components of blood other than red cells. Clerical and technical competence is requisite. A great many pitfalls exist which may cause false-positive or false-negative reactions. **CONTRAINDICATIONS:** In emergencies, issue of uncrossmatched type O RBCs may be necessary. **METHODOLOGY:** Immediate spin, 37°C phase using RBCs suspended in saline, LISS (low ionic strength saline), or albumin, then indirect antiglobulin phase.

Alternative method: Since 1984, AABB Standards have allowed a crossmatch to be suitable for the detection only of ABO incompatibility (eg, only an immediate spin, without 37°C or antiglobulin phases). Such a crossmatch may be done only if:

- the antibody screen includes 37°C and antiglobulin
- the reagent red cells are not pooled
- the antibody screen has not detected a clinically significant antibody (see table in Antibody Identification, Red Cell)
- the patient has no record of previous detection of such antibodies[1]

Because brief delays in reading such crossmatches may permit hemolysis, which would be hard to see, it is probably wise to add EDTA to the saline used to suspend the donor RBCs.[2,3] Increasingly, larger hospitals are using this alternative system, because it greatly lessens the amount of laboratory work per unit at little or no increase in risk.[4] For example, crossmatching four units requires four immediate spins for the crossmatch and two or three indirect antiglobulins for the antibody screen by this alternative, as opposed to six or seven indirect antiglobulins the other way. So far, experience supports the safety of the simplified procedure. The real danger in transfusion is ABO incompatibility, not in missing an antibody to a low-incidence antigen that is absent from the screening cells.

ADDITIONAL INFORMATION: Additional preparation time should be allowed for patients known to be immunized to red cell antigens. Unanticipated problems (eg, positive antibody screen) will require antibody identification and selection of RBCs lacking the corresponding antigen. Patients receiving a series of RBC transfusions are at risk of forming red cell antibodies. For this reason, Standards[1] require a new sample and repeat antibody screen every 3 days.

Footnotes

1. Widmann FK, ed, *Standards for Blood Banks and Transfusion Services*, 15th ed, Bethesda, MD: American Association of Blood Banks, 1993, 24-7.
2. Shulman IA and Kent D, "Safety in Transfusion Practice. Is It Safe to Eliminate the Major Crossmatch for Selected Patients?" *Arch Pathol Lab Med*, 1989, 113(3):270-2.
3. Shulman IA and Calderon C, "Effect of Delayed Centrifugation or Reading on the Detection of ABO Incompatibility by the Immediate-Spin Crossmatch," *Transfusion*, 1991, 31(3):197-200.
4. Cordle DG, Strauss RG, Snyder EL, et al, "Safety and Cost-Containment Data That Advocate Abbreviated Pretransfusion Testing," *Am J Clin Pathol*, 1990, 94(4):428-31.

References

Oberman HA, "The Crossmatch, A Brief Historical Perspective," *Transfusion*, 1981, 21:645-51.

Perkins JT, Arruza M, Fong K, et al, "The Relative Utility of the Autologous Control and the Antiglobulin Test Phase of the Crossmatch," *Transfusion*, 1990, 30(6):503-7.

Plapp FV, "New Techniques for Compatibility Testing," *Arch Pathol Lab Med*, 1989, 113(1):262-9.

Type and Crossmatch for Exchange Transfusion of Newborn *see* Newborn Crossmatch and Transfusion *on page 1072*

Type and Rh *see* ABO Group and Rh Type *on page 1046*

Type and Screen

CPT *86880 (antiglobulin test, direct); 86886 (antiglobulin test, indirect); 86900 (ABO); 86901 (Rh(D))*

Related Information

Antiglobulin Test, Direct *on page 1049*
Antiglobulin Test, Indirect *on page 1051*
Prenatal Screen, Immunohematology *on page 1085*
Red Blood Cells *on page 1087*
Type and Crossmatch *on page 1100*

Test Commonly Includes ABO, Rh, and antibody screening test

Patient Care PREPARATION: Patient should have Transfusion Service wristband (mandatory in many institutions).

Specimen Blood CONTAINER: One red top tube and one lavender top (EDTA) tube COLLECTION: (Of sample from intended recipient): At the patient's bedside, ask the patient to give his or her name. Compare with the hospital wristband. Label the Transfusion Service wristband (if there is one) with the patient's full name, hospital number, date, and initials of the collector. Label sample tube with the same information, including identification number from the wristband. Label requisition form with identification number. The collector signs the requisition, verifying the patient's identity with hospital wristband and Transfusion Service wristband. Some hospitals require additional information. It is always best to stamp the requisition with the patient's identification plate, to avoid transcription errors. CAUSES FOR REJECTION: Gross hemolysis, sample placed in a serum separator tube, specimen tube not properly labeled TURNAROUND TIME: If blood should be needed for transfusion and a type and screen has been done, blood can be immediately available.

Some Operations for Which Routine Crossmatching Is Unnecessary and for Which a Type and Screen Can Usually Be Substituted Safely

General Surgery

- anal fissure or fistula repair*
- appendectomy*
- breast biopsy*
- cholecystectomy
- colostomy or closure
- exploratory laparotomy
- gastroenterostomy
- hemorrhoidectomy*
- inguinal, femoral or hiatal hernia repair*
- parathyroid excision or exploration
- pilonidal cystectomy
- polypectomy
- pyloroplasty
- sympathectomy
- thyroidectomy
- vein stripping

Urology

- ileal conduit
- Marshall-Marchetti procedure
- nephrostomy
- open biopsy of prostate
- penile prosthesis
- pyelolithotomy
- transurethral prostatectomy
- transurethral resection of bladder tumor
- ureterolithotomy

Plastic Surgery

- augmentation mammoplasty
- face lift*
- rhinoplasty*
- skin graft (excluding major burns)

Gynecology

- dilation and curettage, with or without conization
- exploratory laparotomy for infertility
- hysterectomy, abdominal or vaginal
- ovarian cystectomy
- tuboplasty
- vaginal plastic procedures

Obstetrics

- Cesarean section

Neurosurgery

- cordotomy
- hypophysectomy
- nerve repair
- shunt surgery
- sympathectomy

Orthopedics

- knee surgery
- leg amputation
- meniscectomy
- most open reductions
- osteotomy or biopsy of bone
- removal of hip pin
- shoulder reconstruction

*In these operations, even the type and screen is usually unnecessary.

From Huestis DW, Bove JR, and Busch S, *Practical Blood Transfusion,* 3rd ed, Boston, MA: Little, Brown and Co, 1981, 236, with permission.

(Continued)

Type and Screen *(Continued)*

Interpretive POSSIBLE PANIC RANGE: Screen positive, in a setting in which blood may be needed urgently USE: Determination of ABO, Rh, and possible presence of unexpected antibody, indicated for the preoperative patient undergoing a procedure in which transfusion is rarely needed.[1] See table. If a type and screen has been done in such a case and the antibody screen is negative, blood can be issued at once without waiting for a crossmatch in case of an unexpected need. On the other hand, when the procedure detects an antibody, the surgeon is forewarned that full crossmatching will be necessary. Prenatal screen for possible maternal-fetal blood incompatibility that may cause hemolytic disease of the newborn. LIMITATIONS: The type and screen is useful in hospitals that have good inventories of donor blood. The type and screen does not completely assure compatibility if blood is required before a crossmatch can be completed. Blood is **not** reserved or crossmatched if only a type and screen is ordered. The antibody screen does detect antibodies that are not clinically relevant or dangerous. AABB is currently proposing to replace the immediate spin crossmatch with a computer-monitored check on the ABO compatibility.[2] At this time, such a move seems premature. The crossmatch only rarely reveals clinically significant antibodies that may be missed by the antibody screen in the type and screen. The incidence of such antibodies, although extremely low, is not zero.[1] CONTRAINDICATIONS: Type and crossmatch should be ordered instead, if patient is likely to need transfusion within 24 hours, or is likely to need intraoperative transfusion, transfusion during imminent labor or delivery. Other contraindications, in which patients have a very high likelihood of needing transfusion, include shock and observed large blood loss.[1]

Footnotes

1. Mintz PD, Henry JB, and Boral LI, "The Type and Antibody Screen," *Clin Lab Med*, 1982, 2:169-80.
2. Meyer EA and Shulman IA, "The Sensitivity and Specificity of the Immediate Spin Crossmatch," *Transfusion*, 1989, 29(2):99-102.

References

Boral LI, Hill SS, Apollon CJ, et al, "The Type and Antibody Screen, Revisited," *Am J Clin Pathol*, 1979, 71:578-81.

Palmer RH, Kane JG, Churchill WH, et al, "Cost and Quality in the Use of Blood Bank Services for Normal Deliveries, Cesarean Sections, and Hysterectomies," *JAMA*, 1986, 256:219-23.

Uncrossmatched Blood, Emergency

***CPT** 36430*

Synonyms Emergency Blood; Emergency Transfusion; O Negative Blood; Type Specific Blood; Universal Donor Blood; Urgent Requirement for Blood

Applies to Emergency Issue of Uncrossmatched Blood; Exsanguinating Emergency; Massive Acute Blood Loss

Test Commonly Includes No testing before issued, but as soon as possible do ABO and Rh type, antibody screen, antibody identification if indicated, and crossmatch.

Specimen Venous or arterial blood CONTAINER: One or two red top tubes and one lavender top (EDTA) tube COLLECTION: (Of sample from intended recipient): Identify patient by wristband(s) or other system specially set up for identifying unconscious or noncommunicating patients in emergencies. Label tube specimen with the same information, including identification number from the wristband; label requisition form with identification number. Requisition should be signed by collector, indicating that patient's identity has been verified. Positive identification of patient sample is important, even in emergency. If it is impossible to get a blood sample, record this fact. CAUSES FOR REJECTION: Nonemergent situations TURNAROUND TIME: Although uncrossmatched O Rh-negative red blood cells can be issued immediately if available, ABO and Rh type can be done in only 5-10 minutes. As much as 1 hour may be needed for antibody screen and crossmatch, longer if antibodies are detected. Such time is significantly decreased if patient has already had a type and screen. SPECIAL INSTRUCTIONS: An emergency request for uncrossmatched blood should include name of physician requesting blood and signature of person authorized, name and location of patient, and nature of emergency. There should also be a statement that the situation was sufficiently urgent to require release of blood before completion of testing.[1]

Interpretive USE: Blood replacement in exsanguinating emergency, massive acute blood loss LIMITATIONS: Blood issued in life-threatening emergencies is clearly more dangerous than in controlled circumstances. All parties involved need to understand this. CONTRAINDICATIONS: Do not use group O whole blood even in emergencies, for patients of other types, because the anti-A and anti-B can cause hemolysis of the recipient's RBCs. In life-threatening trauma or bleeding when the patient is untyped, use O RBCs (packed cells).[2] Most of the antibodies have been removed from these. The risks of hemolytic transfusion reactions are real and should be carefully weighed against any benefits anticipated. **METHODOLOGY:** When issuing uncrossmatched blood, apply a label indicating uncrossmatched status.

EMERGENCY RELEASE
COMPATIBILITY TESTING
INCOMPLETE

ADDITIONAL INFORMATION: There is no such thing as a "universal donor." Type O blood lacks A and B but has antigens of other blood group systems, any of which may be a problem for a given patient. Blood can be ABO and Rh typed in 5-10 minutes, and the patient then should receive ABO-specific blood. **Volume can be made up temporarily with plasma expanders.** Type O Rh-negative red cells are not always available. Type O Rh-positive red cells (packed cells) are usually available. The risks of the Rh-positive cells include hemolytic transfusion reaction if the patient has anti-D, and immunization to D if the patient is D-negative but not previously immunized. Some trauma centers commonly use O Rh-positive red cells (packed cells) in emergencies[3] or uncrossmatched type-specific blood.[4] Pitfalls of fast ABO and Rh typing include: Blood sample must clot so that bits of fibrin are not mistaken for specific agglutination, or EDTA (lavender top) cells must be washed first. 5-10 minutes are consumed. Risk is greatly increased when antibody screen and crossmatch are not completed before blood is infused. See also Transfusions in Trauma and Other Emergencies in the introduction to this chapter.

Footnotes

1. Widmann FK, ed, *Standards for Blood Banks and Transfusion Services*, 15th ed, Bethesda, MD: American Association of Blood Banks, 1993, 29.
2. Walker RH, ed, *Technical Manual*, 10th ed, Arlington, VA: American Association of Blood Banks, 1990, 360-2.
3. Schmidt PJ, Leparc GF, and Samia CT, "Use of Rh Positive Blood in Emergency Situations," *Surg Gynecol Obstet*, 1988, 167(3):229-33.
4. Gervin AS and Fischer RP, "Resuscitation of Trauma Patients With Type-Specific Uncrossmatched Blood," *J Trauma*, 1984, 24:327-30.

References

Unkle D, Smejkal R, Snyder R, et al, "Blood Antibodies and Uncrossmatched Type O Blood," *Heart Lung*, 1991, 20(3):284-6.

Universal Donor Blood *see* Uncrossmatched Blood, Emergency *on previous page*

Urgent Requirement for Blood *see* Uncrossmatched Blood, Emergency *on previous page*

von Willebrand's Disease Therapy *see* Cryoprecipitate *on page 1058*

Warming, Blood

CPT 86999

Interpretive **USE:** For very rapid, massive transfusion (above 50 mL/minute) **LIMITATIONS:** Uncontrolled warming of donor blood can severely damage RBCs. Although red cells must be heated to 44°C or higher to be damaged, it is probably best not to allow warming above 38°C. **CONTRAINDICATIONS:** When moderate volumes of blood are given at ordinary rates, warming is unnecessary. It is probably unnecessary also in most patients with cold agglutinin disease or paroxysmal cold hemoglobinuria (warming the patient is more effective). **METHODOLOGY:** A considerable variety of hardware is available for blood warming (listed with commentary in Iserson and Huestis[1]). To be effective, an instrument should be able to warm blood efficiently at a flow rate of at least 150 mL/minute. A simple system, not needing expensive equipment, is to maintain a few 250 mL bags of isotonic saline at 70°C. Add this quantity rapidly to a unit of 4°C RBCs, and it immediately results in a temperature about 37°C, without hemolysis or other damage.[2] **ADDITIONAL INFORMATION:** Relatively large volumes of blood at refrigerator temperature, infused rapidly, can cause hypothermia and cardiac arrest. During transfusion of blood that is being warmed, the temperature of the blood warmer must be monitored. The

(Continued)

Warming, Blood *(Continued)*

temperature of the blood warmer should be recorded at 30 and 60 minutes from the start of the transfusion, if transfusion has not been completed. Blood subjected to excessive heat (ie, above 44°C) may be lethal. A quality assurance protocol is essential for all blood warmers.

Footnotes

1. Iserson KV and Huestis DW, "Blood Warming: Current Applications and Techniques," *Transfusion*, 1991, 31(6):558-71.
2. Iserson KV, Knauf MA, and Anhalt D, "Rapid Admixture Blood Warming: Technical Advances," *Crit Care Med*, 1990, 18(2):1138-41.

References

Mollison PL, Engelfriet CP, and Contreras M, *Blood Transfusion in Clinical Medicine*, 9th ed, Oxford, UK: Blackwell Scientific Publications, 1993, 699-700.

Washed Blood *see* Red Blood Cells, Washed *on page 1089*

Washed Cells *see* Red Blood Cells, Washed *on page 1089*

Weak D (D^u) *see* D^u *on page 1063*

White Cells, Transfusion *see* Granulocytes, Transfusion *on page 1069*

Whole Blood

***CPT** 36430 (transfusion); 36450 (exchange transfusion, newborn)*

Related Information

Donation, Blood *on page 1061*
Red Blood Cells *on page 1087*
Risks of Transfusion *on page 1093*

Applies to Complications of Transfusion; Fresh Blood; Massive Transfusions

Test Commonly Includes A unit of whole blood consists of about 450 mL (±10%) blood including plasma and about 63 mL of anticoagulant preservative such as citrate phosphate dextrose adenine solution (CPDA-1). A typical donor unit has a hematocrit of about 35% to 40%. The expiration date for CPDA-1 blood is 35 days after the date of collection if stored continuously at 1°C to 6°C, unless the seal has been broken. Anticoagulants in use have been recently tabulated.[1] ABO, Rh typing, and antibody screen of donor unit and of patient, and crossmatch are required.

Patient Care PREPARATION: The patient must be fully identified, preferably with a hospital identification band attached to the body, or with an alternative emergency identification. Measure blood loss if possible, as well as fluid intake and output. **Dosage and administration:** Give whole blood through a filter. It can be warmed, if warming is clinically indicated, as with rapid infusion of large volumes of blood at refrigerated temperature. The blood should not be warmed above 38°C. The rate of infusion depends on clinical conditions but should not be slower than 4 hours per unit. No medications or solutions should be added to blood. **Never give Ringer's lactate, hypotonic, or dextrose-containing solutions through the same tubing as blood.** AFTERCARE: Many of the important clinical manifestations of transfusion reaction occur during the administration of the first 50-100 mL of blood. Pay close attention to vital signs (ie, temperature, pulse, and blood pressure) before, after, and frequently during the transfusion. Reactions may occur up to several hours after transfusion, and delayed transfusion reactions can occur several days afterwards. Monitor electrolytes, hemoglobin/hematocrit.

Specimen Blood CONTAINER: One red top tube and one lavender top (EDTA) tube COLLECTION: (Of sample from intended recipient): At the patient's bedside, ask the patient to give his or her name. Compare with hospital wristband. Label the Transfusion Service wristband (if there is one) with the patient's name, hospital number, date, and initials of collector. Label sample tube with the same information, including identification number from the wristband. Label requisition form with identification number. The collector signs the requisition, verifying the patient's identity with hospital wristband and Transfusion Service wristband. Some hospitals require additional information. It is always best to stamp the requisition with the patient's identification plate, to avoid transcription errors. STORAGE INSTRUCTIONS: Stored in properly monitored Transfusion Service refrigerator at 1°C to 6°C until issue. If blood transfusion cannot be started immediately after blood is issued, blood must be returned to Transfusion Service/Blood Bank within approximately 20 minutes. Temperature must be kept between 1°C and 10°C during transportation. **Do not store blood in ward/nursing-station refrigerators.**

They are not monitored and are not safe. **CAUSES FOR REJECTION:** (Of patient sample): Gross hemolysis, sample placed in a serum separator tube, specimen tube not properly labeled **TURNAROUND TIME:** Because of required testing, the time from blood donation until the blood is available for transfusion varies from about 12-24 hours. **SPECIAL INSTRUCTIONS:** Request for blood must be legible and supply all appropriate identifying data including patient's first and last names and identification number. Other desirable information includes patient birthdate, room or bed number, physician's name, diagnosis, history of prior transfusion, and whether or not reaction occurred. Patient's sex and history of pregnancies, presence or absence of erythroblastosis fetalis are relevant. Blood crossmatched for a particular patient is usually cancelled automatically after 24 hours. Transfusion Service should be notified as soon as it is known that the patient will not need the transfusion, so blood can be used for another patient.

Interpretive **USE:** Nowadays, the principal use of whole blood is to serve as the raw material from which blood components are prepared. Replace red cell mass and plasma volume in patients in whom there is significant loss or depletion of both, improve oxygen transport (ie, treatment of acute blood loss). Acute bleeding, including massive transfusion in exsanguinating emergencies and some surgical cases. Exchange transfusion. Whole blood can be administered extremely rapidly. **LIMITATIONS:** Usually in short supply because of demand for blood components. Although whole blood provides plasma proteins, other sources of oncotic/coagulation proteins are available. Some components, eg, platelets, factor V, factor VIII (AHF), are labile and not present in sufficient quantity in whole blood to provide adequate replacement therapy. Coagulation factors are best replaced by appropriate components (eg, platelets, FFP, cryoprecipitate). Plasma potassium and ammonia increase in stored whole blood. Adenine, citrate, sodium, and antibodies are less in red blood cells, which are preferable to whole blood for patients with chronic renal or liver disease. Blood or components for immunosuppressed patients at risk for graft-versus-host disease, can be irradiated before elective transfusion. **CONTRAINDICATIONS:** Do not use whole blood when anemia can be corrected with specific, safer products (eg, iron, B_{12}, folic acid). Whole blood is contraindicated in patients with congestive heart failure, uremia or hepatic failure, or with other chronic decrease of red cell mass. Such patients should receive red cells rather than whole blood if they require transfusion. For exchange transfusion, whole blood should preferably not be more than 5 days old. Replace blood volume deficits more safely and adequately with other volume expanders (saline, Ringer's lactate, albumin, plasma protein fraction). Treat coagulation factor deficiencies with appropriate concentrates (eg, cryoprecipitate or factor VIII or IX). The infusion of large volumes of blood may cause additional bleeding due to dilution of clotting factors or platelets, and may expand blood volume such that therapy with appropriate fractions (eg, FFP) may become hazardous. IgA-deficient patients may have anaphylactic reaction. Donor and recipient should be ABO and Rh compatible, except in unusual, life-threatening emergencies. A crossmatch is necessary unless delay in provision of blood might result in death. **ADDITIONAL INFORMATION:** Whole blood is often not available. Red blood cells may be substituted. **Fresh blood** is impossible to define except by reference to whatever labile component is needed. Requests for "fresh" blood necessitate consultation and will usually be filled by issuing the appropriate components or fractions.

References

Circular of Information for the Use of Human Blood and Blood Components, American Red Cross, Council of Community Blood Centers, American Association of Blood Banks, 1992.

Sohmer PR, "Transfusion Therapy in Surgery," *Clinical Practice of Transfusion Medicine*, Petz LD and Swisher SN, eds, 2nd ed, New York, NY: Churchill-Livingston, 1989, 363-400.

Whole Blood, Crossmatch *see* Type and Crossmatch *on page 1100*

Whole Blood, Irradiated *see* Irradiated Blood Components *on page 1071*

Zygosity, Rh *see* Rh Genotype *on page 1090*

URINALYSIS AND CLINICAL MICROSCOPY

Glen R. Willie, MD
Wayne R. DeMott, MD
David S. Jacobs, MD

Analysis of urine dates to ancient times. Clinical microscopy has been practiced for several hundred years. Thus, many of the tests in this chapter are among the most enduring in medicine. Other more recently developed tests, such as dipstick screening procedures for urine glucose, protein, leukocyte esterase, and nitrite, yield significant clinical information rapidly and relatively inexpensively. Some of the other analyses performed on urine are listed in the Chemistry and Therapeutic Drug Monitoring/Toxicology/Drugs of Abuse chapters.

Urine color has been of interest for centuries. Its color is determined by its concentration, the presence of drugs, exogenous and endogenous compounds, and its pH. **Colorless** urine may be normal or secondary to diuretic use, high fluid intake, diabetes insipidus, or diabetes mellitus. **Cloudy or hazy** urine may reflect the presence of phosphates, pyuria, or bacteruria. On oxidation, development of a **black** color is evidence for alkaptonuria.[1] Increased indican may cause the urine to blacken on standing. **Dark** urine is the second most common sign of acute intermittent porphyria. Very rarely, dark urine may indicate the presence of malignant melanoma. **Green** urine may be produced by indigo carmine, methylene blue, phenol, and in some cases of iodochlorhydroxyquin (clioquinol)-induced subacute myelo-opticoneuropathy. Other causes of green urine are reported as *Pseudomonas* bacteremia, urinary bile pigments, amitriptyline hydrochloride or methocarbamol ingestion, and breath freshener abuse.[2] **Red** urine was described elegantly by Berman[3] and is described further in the listing, Blood, Urine. Red plasma and red urine indicate hemoglobin; clear plasma with red urine may indicate myoglobin, but may occur as well in congenital erythropoietic porphyria and cutanea tarda porphyria. **Purple** urine, after standing, may also be due to porphyrins.[4] **Yellow** to **orange** urine may contain bile and should be tested for the presence of bile. Other causes of darker yellow to orange urine include increased concentration of urine or the presence of riboflavin, quinacrine (Atabrine®), rifampin (Rifadin®, Rimactane®), phenazopyridine (Pyridium®), or salicylazosulfapyridine (Azulfidine®). Color and appearance of urine were outlined well by Bradley and Shumann,[5] and by Graff.[6] As in some examples above, **drugs** may cause unusual urine colors.[7] The plastic urine bag may discolor **purple** in the presence of the indican produced by *Providencia* or *Klebsiella* species.[8]

---

[1] Gaines JJ, "The Pathology of Alkaptonuric Ochronosis," *Hum Pathol*, 1989, 20:40-6.

[2] Norfleet RG, "Green Urine," *JAMA*, 1982, 247:29.

[3] Berman LB, "When the Urine is Red," *JAMA*, 1977, 237:2753-4.

[4] Forland M, "Urinalysis," *Internal Medicine*, 2nd ed, Chapter 85, Stein JH, ed, Boston, MA: Little, Brown and Company, 1987, 724-30.

[5] Bradley M and Schumann GB, "Examination of Urine," *Todd-Sanford-Davidsohn Clinical Diagnosis and Management by Laboratory Methods*, 17 ed, Henry JB, ed, Philadelphia, PA: WB Saunders Co, 1984, 380.

[6] Graff L, *Examination of Physical Characteristics, A Handbook of Routine Urinalysis*, Philadelphia, PA: JB Lippincott Co, 1982, 10-14.

[7] Lubran MM, "Effect of Drugs on Clinical Laboratory Tests," *Clinical Pathology in the Elderly*, Chapter 24, Rochman H, ed, Karger, 1988, 193-6.

[8] Dealler SF, Belfield PW, Belford M, et al, "Purple Urine Bags," *J Urol*, 1989, 142:769-70.

Acetoacetic Acid, Urine *see* Ketones, Urine *on page 1128*

Acetone, Semiquantitative, Urine *see* Ketones, Urine *on page 1128*

Addis Count, 12-Hour

***CPT** 81015*

Synonyms Urine Sediment, Quantitative

Test Commonly Includes Quantitation of casts, erythrocytes, and leukocytes

Interpretive USE: Primarily of historical interest LIMITATIONS: The Addis count is no longer in common clinical use because it is time consuming and is prone to technical inaccuracies. Semiquantitative urinalyses are now more commonly used. Note the dates of the publications listed in the following references. See Urinalysis test listing.

References

Addis T, "A Clinical Classification of Bright's Disease," *JAMA*, 1925, 85:163-7.

Addis T, "The Effect of Some Physiologic Variables on the Number of Casts, RBCs, WBCs, and Epithelial Cells in the Urine of Normal Individuals," *J Clin Invest*, 1926, 2:417-21.

Addis T, "The Number of Formal Elements in Urinary Sediment of Normal Individuals," *J Clin Invest*, 1928, 2:409-15.

Albumin, Urine *see* Protein, Semiquantitative, Urine *on page 1147*

Antispermatozoal Antibody Test *see* Infertility Screen *on page 1124*

Bacteria Screen, Urine *see* Leukocyte Esterase, Urine *on page 1131*

Bacteria Screen, Urine *see* Nitrite, Urine *on page 1137*

Beta-Hydroxybutyric Acid, Urine *see* Ketones, Urine *on page 1128*

Bile Fluid Examination

***CPT** 89050 (cell count, body fluid); 89060 (crystal identification, body fluid); 89100 (intubation, aspiration single specimen plus appropriate test procedure); 89105 (multiple fractional specimens with pancreatic or gallbladder stimulation)*

Related Information

Ova and Parasites, Stool *on page 836*

Synonyms Biliary Drainage Examination; Crystal Examination, Biliary Drainage; Duodenal Drainage Examination

Test Commonly Includes Identification of cholesterol, calcium bilirubinate, calcium carbonate crystals, bilirubin crystals, protozoan parasites (in particular, *Giardia lamblia*), tissue cells, and inflammatory cells

Abstract A variety of bile/duodenal content specimens obtained by tube aspiration or direct gallbladder puncture are studied for the presence of crystals/parasites indicative of gallbladder and/or pancreatic disease.

Patient Care PREPARATION: Specimen is obtained by use of a gastroduodenal tube or a fiberoptic endoscopy study, either by direct aspiration or into a trap. Patient must take nothing by mouth after midnight before the test.

Specimen Bile fluid, duodenal drainage specimen CONTAINER: Plastic container SAMPLING TIME: With tube in place and after a few minutes for a basal period Sincalide (Kinevac®-Squibb), a synthetic C-terminal octapeptide of cholecystokinin (CCK) is administered intravenously (I.V.) in a dose of 0.02 μg/kg of body weight and duodenal aspirate collected over the next 20-30 minutes. Alternatively, 100 units of cholecystokinin pancreozymin (the Boots Company, PLC, UK) may be given I.V. over a period of 1 minute. COLLECTION: Protocol for collection will vary with the institution and/or physician. The collection may be divided into multiple containers, usually three: "A" bile (yellow – common duct origin), "B" bile (viscous and green or green-brown – gallbladder bile), and "C" bile (lighter color – hepatic bile duct origin). Many physicians send only one specimen, either a "pool" or a collection of largely "B" bile. Such "B" bile (gallbladder origin) may have a volume of 30-50 mL. STORAGE INSTRUCTIONS: Method dependent (see below) TURNAROUND TIME: Method dependent (see below)

Interpretive REFERENCE RANGE: Normal bile should not include any significant number of cholesterin plates (cholesterol crystals), calcium bilirubinate or bilirubin crystals, parasites, or inflammatory cells. USE: Evaluate cholelithiasis and cholecystitis in cases where there is a high index of suspicion, but usual tests such as cholecystogram and ultrasound are negative; detect occult microlithiasis in cases of "idiopathic" acute pancreatitis;[1] a method for establishing

(Continued)

Bile Fluid Examination *(Continued)*

the presence of giardiasis. See also Ova and Parasites, Stool in the Microbiology chapter. **LIMITATIONS:** Specimen pH <4.5 may produce a false-positive bilirubin precipitate which may be confused with calcium bilirubinate. This diagnostic approach for identification of crystals and diagnosis of cholelithiasis is not widely used. **METHODOLOGY:** Variation in processing of duodenal bile specimens prior to microscopic examination has contributed to difficulty in comparison of results of published series. The technique used is usually that of Juniper and Burson.[2,3] Each bile fraction is centrifuged at 2000 rpm for 10 minutes and the sediment examined using transmitted and polarized light microscopy, and the number of crystals specified using a grading system of 1-4. Neoptolemos et al[4] centrifuged duodenal bile specimens at 3000 g for 10 minutes, examining the sediment at 20°C using direct and polarizing microscopy and examining a second sediment obtained by recentrifuging the supernatant after incubation at 37°C for 24 hours. Ramond et al,[5] studying gallbladder bile obtained by direct puncture at cholecystectomy, found sensitivity was increased by a second microscopic examination at 24 hours. They kept the bile samples at 37°C for at least 1 hour, centrifuged it at 12,000 rpm for 5 minutes, and examined the bile sample and pellet for crystals initially and after a 24-hour incubation at 37°C. **ADDITIONAL INFORMATION:** Microscopy of duodenal drainage bile may be useful in the investigation of cholelithiasis, "idiopathic" pancreatitis, and parasitism.[2,3,4,5,6] Analysis of aspirated stimulated "duodenal bile" can provide presumptive evidence of calculous biliary tract disease in patients with suggestive symptoms but negative gallbladder radiologic and ultrasonic studies.

In studies of gallbladder bile (obtained at cholecystectomy), presence of cholesterol crystals as an indication of cholesterol gallstones has a sensitivity approaching 90% and a specificity of nearly 100%.[5] Bilirubinate crystals alone as predictors of pigment stones have a lower level of sensitivity (about 70%) and specificity (slightly >90%).[5] Ramond et al found cholesterol crystals (in the absence of stones) in 4 of 11 patients with biliary stenosis, raising the possibility that bile stasis induces the formation of cholesterol crystals. As duodenal bile is diluted with variable amounts of gastric and small intestinal content, sensitivity of microscopy for crystals is likely somewhat decreased. Van Erpecum et al found the sensitivity (84%) of cholesterol crystals in fresh bile only slightly reduced in dilute gallbladder bile.[6] They note "...examination of fresh bile for cholesterol crystals is a specific and reasonably sensitive test for cholesterol gallstone disease."[6] Duodenal bile crystal analysis has been found useful in the investigation of "idiopathic" pancreatitis.[4] Microscopic examination of centrifuged duodenal bile in patients recovering from an episode of acute pancreatitis found cholesterol, bilirubinate, or calcium carbonate microspheroliths in 67% of cases while bile from postalcoholic pancreatitis patients was negative for crystals.[1] Study of gallbladder bile obtained at cholecystectomy (and/or serial GB ultrasonography) found biliary sludge or microlithiasis in 73% of patients.[1]

Bile cholesterol supersaturation with nearly all patients having cholesterol crystals in their bile has been reported in postcolectomy ulcerative colitis patients.[7] While a variety of protozoan, trematode, and nematode parasites have been found in duodenal specimens, *Giardia lamblia* is most frequently encountered.[2] In patients clinically suspected of opisthorchiasis, in whom stool specimens are negative for ova, bile microscopy may be of special importance in establishing the diagnosis.[8]

Nucleatian time (time required for the precipitation of cholesterol crystals in gallbladder bile) has been used in studies of the mechanism of gallstone dissolution by chenodeoxycholic acid versus ursodeoxycholic acid[9] and may be of use in predicting the formation of cholesterol gallstones.[10]

A sensitivity of 83% and specificity of 100% for recognition of cholelithiasis has been reported on the basis of microscopic examination of bile samples obtained at endoscopic retrograde cholangiography.[11]

Footnotes

1. Ros E, Navarro S, Bru C, et al, "Occult Microlithiasis in 'Idiopathic' Acute Pancreatitis: Prevention of Relapses by Cholecystectomy or Ursodeoxycholic Acid Therapy," *Gastroenterology*, 1991, 101(6):1701-9.
2. Juniper K and Burson EN Jr, "Biliary Tract Studies: II. The Significance of Biliary Crystals," *Gastroenterology*, 1957, 32:175-211.
3. Burnstein MJ, Vassal KP, and Strasburg SM, "Results of Combined Biliary Drainage and Cholecystokinin Cholecystography in 81 Patients With Normal Oral Cholecystograms," *Ann Surg*, 1982, 196:627-32.
4. Neoptolemos JP, Davidson BR, Winder AF, et al, "Role of Duodenal Bile Crystal Analysis in the Investigation of "Idiopathic" Pancreatitis," *Br J Surg*, 1988, 75(5):450-3.
5. Ramond MJ, Dumont M, Belghiti J, et al, "Sensitivity and Specificity of Microscopic Examination of Gallbladder Bile for Gallstone Recognition and Identification," *Gastroenterology*, 1988, 95(5):1339-43.

6. van Erpecum KJ, van Berge Henegouwen GP, Stoelwinder B, et al, "Cholesterol and Pigment Gallstone Disease: Comparison of the Reliability of Three Bile Tests for Differentiation Between the Two Stone Types," *Scand J Gastroenterol*, 1988, 23:948-54.
7. Harvey PR, McLeod RS, Cohen Z, et al, "Effect of Colectomy on Bile Composition, Cholesterol Crystal Formation, and Gallstones in Patients With Ulcerative Colitis," *Ann Surg*, 1991, 214(4):396-401.
8. Dao AH, Barnwell SF, and Adkins RB Jr, "A Case of Opisthorchiasis Diagnosed by Cholangiography and Bile Examination," *Am J Surg*, 1991, 57(4):206-9.
9. Sahlin S, Ahlberg J, Angelin B, et al, "Nucleation Time of Gallbladder Bile in Gallstone Patients: Influence of Bile Acid Treatment," *Gut*, 1991, 32(12):1554-7.
10. Marks JW, Broomfield P, Bonorris GG, et al, "Factors Affecting the Measurement of Cholesterol Nucleation in Human Gallbladder and Duodenal Bile," *Gastroenterology*, 1991, 101(1):214-9.
11. Buscail L, Escourrou J, Delvaux M, et al, "Microscopic Examination of Bile Directly Collected During Endoscopic Cannulation of the Papilla – Utility in Patients With Suspected Microlithiasis," *Dig Dis Sci*, 1992, 37(1):116-20.

References

Bockus HL, Shay H, Willard JH, et al, "Comparison of Biliary Drainage and Cholecystography in Gallstone Diagnosis: With Especial Reference to Bile Microscopy," *JAMA*, 1931, 96:311-17.

Janowitz P, Swobodnik W, Wechsler JG, et al, "Comparison of Gallbladder Bile and Endoscopically Obtained Duodenal Bile," *Gut*, 1990, 31(12):1407-10.

Magnuson TH, Lillemoe KD, Scheeres DE, et al, "Altered Bile Composition During Cholesterol Gallstone Formation: Cause or Effect?" *J Surg Res*, 1990, 48(6):584-9.

Paumgartner G and Sauerbruch T, "Secretions, Composition, and Flow of Bile," *J Clin Gastroenterol*, 1983, 12:3-23.

Priest RJ, "Tests Related to the Biliary Tract," *Bockus Gastroenterology*, Vol 1, 4th ed, Berk JE ed, Philadelphia, PA: WB Saunders Co, 1985, 29:402-9.

Shapiro HA, "Endoscopic Diagnosis and Treatment of Biliary Tract Disease," *Surg Clin North Am*, 1981, 61:843-64, (review).

Bile, Urine

CPT *81003*

Related Information

Bilirubin, Direct *on page 137*
Bilirubin, Total *on page 139*
Urobilinogen, 2-Hour Urine *on page 1167*

Synonyms Bilirubin, Urine

Abstract Screen for diseases characterized by increased serum conjugated bilirubin. Only conjugated bilirubin is passed into the urine.

Specimen Random urine **CONTAINER:** Plastic urine container **STORAGE INSTRUCTIONS:** If the specimen cannot be processed immediately by the laboratory, it should be refrigerated. **CAUSES FOR REJECTION:** Improper labeling, specimen not refrigerated

Interpretive **REFERENCE RANGE:** Negative **USE:** Detect the presence of bilirubin in urine; screen for some instances of liver disease. In obstructive disease of the biliary tract such as biliary calculi, carcinoma of the pancreas or of bile ducts, urine bilirubin is frequently positive. See table.

Differential Diagnosis Using Urine Bilirubin and Urobilinogen Tests

Type of Jaundice	Urine Bilirubin	Urine Urobilinogen
Normal	0	0 – trace
Hepatocellular jaundice (eg, hepatitis, chemical, or drug injury)	↑	↑
Biliary obstruction (extrahepatic and intrahepatic); obstructive jaundice	↑	0
Hemolytic jaundice	0	↑

0 = absent; ↑ = increased

LIMITATIONS: Occasional false-positives are seen, predominantly in elderly patients. They commonly represent stool contamination of the urine sample. Mefenamic acid administration and chlorpromazine therapy may result in false-positive reactions. Prolonged standing of the sample, especially at room temperature and in the light, may lead to false-negatives. Pyridium® (phenazopyridine) and Serenium® (ethoxazene hydrochloride) and local anesthetic metabo-

(Continued)

Bile, Urine *(Continued)*

lites give bright reddish orange colors which may mask the reaction of small amounts of bilirubin. Specific urine bile assays, even urine urobilinogen, provide substantial numbers of false-negatives when used as a screen for liver disease as determined by at least one abnormal serum liver function test abnormality. If just used to screen for the presence of raised serum bilirubin, the test is about 79% to 89% specific and has an 89% negative predictive value when used in an emergency room setting.[1] Indoxyl has been reported to interfere with dip-and-read testing for urine bilirubin sufficiently to mask a weak reaction. A more specific test such as the Ictotest® has been recommended when such dip-and-read results are inconclusive.[2] **METHODOLOGY:** Diazotization reaction in an acid medium **ADDITIONAL INFORMATION:** The method detects as little as 0.05-0.1 mg bilirubin/100 mL. The test is exquisitely sensitive for bilirubinuria. However, detection of bilirubinuria is not a sensitive indicator of hepatic disease. In uncomplicated hemolytic anemia serum bilirubin may be normal, or a minimal elevation of indirect bilirubin may be present; indirect (unconjugated) bilirubin does not readily pass through the glomerulus. Therefore, bile is not usually detectable in the urine in uncomplicated hemolytic anemia. Similarly, urine bilirubin may not be present with well advanced hepatic disease; serum total bilirubin is not always increased with advanced liver disease. If jaundice is severe, renal excretion becomes significant; and if renal function deteriorates, serum direct bilirubin levels may increase.[3] Urine bile, if positive, carries an implication of elevation of serum conjugated (direct) bilirubin and should be confirmed by measurement of total and direct bilirubin in serum, as well as liver-related enzymes. The liver cell conjugates bilirubin with glucuronic acid.

Footnotes

1. Binder L, Smith D, Kupka T, et al, "Failure of Prediction of Liver Function Test Abnormalities With the Urine Urobilinogen and Urine Bilirubin Assays," *Arch Pathol Lab Med*, 1989, 113(1):73-6.
2. Skjold AC, Freitag JF, and Stover LR, "Indoxyl Sulfate Interferes With Dip-and-Read Urinalysis," *Clin Chem*, 1980, 26(9):1368-9.
3. Fleischner G and Arias IM, "Recent Advances in Bilirubin Formation, Transport, Metabolism, and Excretion," *Am J Med*, 1970, 49:576-89.

Biliary Drainage Examination *see* Bile Fluid Examination *on page 1109*

Bilirubin, Urine *see* Bile, Urine *on previous page*

Blood, Occult, Stool *see* Occult Blood, Stool *on page 1138*

Blood, Occult, Urine *see* Blood, Urine *on this page*

Blood, Urine

CPT 89205

Related Information

Hemoglobin, Qualitative, Urine *on page 1122*
Hemosiderin Stain, Urine *on page 1123*
Kidney Stone Analysis *on page 1129*
Myoglobin, Qualitative, Urine *on page 1135*
Ova and Parasites, Urine *on page 839*
Urinalysis *on page 1162*
Urinalysis, Fractional *on page 1166*

Synonyms Blood, Occult, Urine; Hemoglobin, Urine; Occult Blood, Urine

Test Commonly Includes Dipstick method for occult blood is usually a part of urinalysis.

Abstract Positive dipstick usually indicates hematuria, hemoglobinuria, or myoglobinuria

Specimen Random urine **CONTAINER:** Plastic urine container **STORAGE INSTRUCTIONS:** If test not performed immediately, specimen should be refrigerated. **CAUSES FOR REJECTION:** Improper labeling. Standing for more than 2 hours at room temperature may be a reason to consider a specimen unacceptable.

Interpretive **REFERENCE RANGE:** Negative by dipstick; 2-3 red cells per high power field are generally accepted as normal by microscopy. **USE:** Detect myoglobin, hemoglobin, or red blood cells in urine (detect hematuria, microhematuria, hemoglobinuria, or erythrocyturia). See table. **LIMITATIONS:** Dipstick methods detect myoglobin as hemoglobin. Both intact erythrocytes and free hemoglobin give a positive reaction. Iodine solutions in urine, or applied to patient's skin, are reported to cause false-positives.[1] Certain oxidizing agents such as hypochlorite (bleach) may produce false-positive results if present in the collection vessel. Microbial

Blood, Urine

Causes of Hematuria	Causes of Hemoglobinuria

Renal diseases including:
  glomerulonephritis
  Goodpasture's syndrome
  lupus nephritis
  arteritis
  Wegener's granulomatosis
  stone
  tumor
  polycystic kidney
  infarct
  infection, including
    pyelonephritis
    necrotizing papillitis
  trauma
Blood diseases including:
  thrombocytopenia
  thrombotic thrombocytopenic purpura
  Henoch-Schönlein purpura
  infective endocarditis
  leukemia
  hemophilias
  sickle cell trait
Bladder diseases including:
  cystitis
  carcinoma
  papilloma
Prostatic diseases including:
  prostatitis
  BPH (benign nodular and glandular hyperplasia)
  prostatic adenocarcinoma
Urethral diseases including:
  urethritis
  tumor
Trauma
Drugs including:
  Coumadin®
  heparin
  salicylates
  many others
	Hemolysis associated with:
	  parasites (ie, malaria)
	  drugs
	  chemicals
	  antibodies
	March hemoglobinuria —
	  secondary to severe exercise
	Transfusion reactions
	  incompatible blood
	Burns
	Crush injury
	Poisoning
	  snake or spider bite
	Paroxysmal nocturnal hemoglobinuria
	Paroxysmal cold hemoglobinuria

peroxidase, associated with urinary tract infection and leukocyte peroxidase, may cause a false-positive reaction. Pyridium® (phenazopyridine) and Serenium® (ethoxazene hydrochloride) metabolites may mask the dipstick reaction. Large amounts of nitrite may delay reactions. The sensitivity of the occult blood test is reduced in urines with high specific gravity and/or high ascorbic acid content.[2] High urine protein and formalin are reported to cause false-negatives.[3] Prolonged air exposure of the dipstick (dipstick jar left uncapped) reduces the sensitivity of the dipstick for blood.[4] Transient hematuria can reflect menstruation, catheterization, and strenuous exercise. Urine sediment microscopy should be used to confirm a diagnosis of hematuria suggested by positive dipstick. **METHODOLOGY:** Dipstick is based on the pseudoperoxidase activity of hemoglobin. Microscopy is used for recognition of red blood cells and red cell casts. **ADDITIONAL INFORMATION:** The test will detect 0.03 mg/dL free hemoglobin or 10 intact red blood cells/μL. Further tests to work-up hematuria may include CBC, platelet count, urine culture, ESR, ANA, prothrombin time, PTT, serum BUN, creatinine, and other examinations as appropriate. More than 3 g of protein in a 24-hour urine collection provides indication of glomerular disease;[5] more than 1 g of protein is suggestive.

The number of red cells (grade of microhematuria) does not necessarily correlate with the degree or significance of urologic pathologic findings (ie, a patient with more than 5 unexplained red cells in urine may have an important urologic lesion). Additional studies (such as urine culture, cytology, excretory urography, cystoscopy) may be indicated. Patients on anticoagulants exhibiting gross or microscopic hematuria should be carefully evaluated. A recent review by Schuster and Lewis indicated the high likelihood (16 of 24 cases) of identifying significant pathologic findings in subjects with gross hematuria, which included carcinoma and calculi.[6] The use of nonsteroidal anti-inflammatory drugs including aspirin may be associated with a significant incidence of hematuria.[7]

(Continued)

Blood, Urine *(Continued)*

A positive dipstick test for blood without red cells in the urine sediment may indicate hemoglobinuria, myoglobinuria, or the presence of porphyrins. Drugs causing hematuria are listed.[5] Algorithms for diagnosis of hematuria are published for children[8] and adults.[9] Phenytoin does not cause urine to appear red, but uric acid and urate crystals in acid urine may cause a pink to red-brown color.[10] **See introduction to this chapter for further information on colored urine.**

Daum and coworkers studied correlation between dipsticks and microscopy in abdominal trauma. If the dipstick is positive, they decided that microscopy is needed to determine whether or not an IVP is indicated, although others have recommended urine microscopy in all cases of blunt abdominal traumas.[11] Kennedy et al report false-negatives and false-positives but conclude that the safety of dipsticks for hematuria in subjects sustaining blunt or penetrating abdominal trauma is acceptable.[12] Messing and coworkers found that hematuria, even in the presence of significant disease such as urinary tract malignancy, often was intermittent. They have proposed home dipstick screening based upon their study of asymptomatic men older than 50 years of age;[13] others disagree.[14]

An important response to the paper reporting inaccurate results of urine dipstick results[4] is that by Cadoff, who emphasizes the need for quality control and addresses the exemption of tests waivered under CLIA '88 by the Health Care Finance Administration. Cadoff perceives the need for laboratory testing to be performed by those well versed in good laboratory practice.[15]

Footnotes

1. Said R, "Contamination of Urine With Povidone-Iodine. Cause of False-Positive Test for Occult Blood in Urine," *JAMA*, 1979, 242:748-9.
2. Jaffe RM, Lawrence L, Schmid A, et al, "Inhibition by Ascorbic Acid (Vitamin C) of Chemical Detection of Blood in Urine," *Am J Clin Pathol*, 1979, 72:468-70.
3. Brown SH, MacDougall ML, and Wiegmann TB, "Microscopic Hematuria," *Kans Med*, 1986, 99-101.
4. Cohen HT and Spiegel DM, "Air-Exposed Urine Dipsticks Give False-Positive Results for Glucose and False-Negative Results for Blood," *Am J Clin Pathol*, 1991, 96(3):398-400.
5. Abuelo JG, "The Diagnosis of Hematuria," *Arch Intern Med*, 1983, 143:967-70.
6. Schuster GA and Lewis GA, "Clinical Significance of Hematuria in Patients on Anticoagulant Therapy," *J Urol*, 1987, 137:923-5.
7. Kraus SE, Siroky MB, Babayan RK, et al, "Hematuria and the Use of Nonsteroidal Anti-inflammatory Drugs," *J Urol*, 1984, 132:288-90.
8. Lieu TA, Grasmeder HM 3d, and Kaplan BS, "An Approach to the Evaluation and Treatment of Microscopic Hematuria," *Pediatr Clin North Am*, 1991, 38(3):579-92.
9. Restrepo NC and Carey PO, "Evaluating Hematuria in Adults," *Am Fam Physician*, 1989, 40(2):149-56.
10. Derby BM and Ward JW, "The Myth of Red Urine Due to Phenytoin," *JAMA*, 1983, 249:1723-4.
11. Daum GS, Krolikowski FJ, Reuter KL, et al, "Dipstick Evaluation of Hematuria in Abdominal Trauma," *Am J Clin Pathol*, 1988, 89(4):538-42.
12. Kennedy TJ, McConnell JD, and Thal ER, "Urine Dipstick vs Microscopic Urinalysis in the Evaluation of Abdominal Trauma," *J Trauma*, 1988, 28(5):615-7.
13. Messing EM, Young TB, Hunt VB, et al, "Urinary Tract Cancers Found by Homescreening With Hematuria Dipsticks in Healthy Men Over 50 Years of Age," *Cancer*, 1989, 64(11):2361-7.
14. Woolhandler S, Pels RJ, Bor DH, et al, "Dipstick Urinalysis Screening of Asymptomatic Adults for Urinary Tract Disorders – I. Hematuria and Proteinuria," *JAMA*, 1989, 262(9):1214-9.
15. Cadoff EM, "Inaccurate Results of Urine Dipstick Tests," *Am J Clin Pathol*, 1992, 98(2):269, (letter).

References

Abarbanel J, Benet AE, Lask D, et al, "Sports Hematuria," *J Urol*, 1990, 143(5):887-90.

Abuelo JG, "Evaluation of Hematuria," *Urology*, 1983, 21:215-25.

Bee DE, James GP, and Paul KL, "Hemoglobinuria and Hematuria: Accuracy and Precision of Laboratory Diagnosis," *Clin Chem*, 1979, 10:1696-9.

Bloom KJ, "An Algorithm for Hematuria," *Clin Lab Med*, 1988, 8:577-84.

Copley JC, "Isolated Asymptomatic Hematuria in the Adult," *Am J Med Sci*, 1986, 291:101-11, (review).

Mohr DN, Offord KP, and Owen RA, et al, "Asymptomatic Microhematuria and Urologic Disease," *JAMA*, 1986, 256:224-9.

Moore GP and Robinson M, "Do Urine Dipsticks Reliably Predict Microhematuria? The Bloody Truth!" *Ann Emerg Med*, 1988, 17:257-60.

Smith RF, Mohr DN, Torres VE, et al, "Renal Insufficiency in Community Patients With Mild Asymptomatic Microhematuria," *Mayo Clin Proc*, 1989, 64(4):409-14.

Yoshikawa N, Matsuyama D, Iijima K, et al, "Benign Familial Heamturia," *Arch Pathol Lab Med*, 1988, 112:794-7.

Calculus Analysis *see* Kidney Stone Analysis *on page 1129*

Casts, Urine *see* Urinalysis *on page 1162*

Cervical Mucus Interaction, Cross Hostility Tests *see* Sperm Mucus Penetration Test (Human or Bovine Cervical Mucus) *on page 1154*

Clinitest® for Sugar, Urine *see* Reducing Substances, Urine *on page 1150*

Colo-Rect® *see* Occult Blood, Stool *on page 1138*

Colo-Screen® *see* Occult Blood, Stool *on page 1138*

Concentrating Ability, Urine *see* Concentration Test, Urine *on this page*

Concentration Test, Urine

CPT 81002

Related Information

Calcium, Serum *on page 160*
Osmolality, Urine *on page 302*
Potassium, Blood *on page 330*

Synonyms Concentrating Ability, Urine; Fishberg Concentration Test; Urine Concentration Test

Applies to Vasopressin Concentration Test

Test Commonly Includes Assessment of concentrating ability of the kidney by determination of specific gravity or osmolality following water deprivation and/or after administration of vasopressin

Abstract Patients with polyuria are sometimes difficult to evaluate, as some have polydipsia with resulting polyuria and normal kidneys; others have polyuria with resultant mild or moderate hypernatremia and therefore polydipsia. To separate these groups, this test evaluates urine output and osmolality (and/or specific gravity) when water is deprived, sufficient to cause mild hypernatremia. Since the kidneys may abnormally excrete water in the face of hypernatremia or even hypovolemia, this test must be closely monitored to prevent patient injury (hyperosmolar state or dehydration).

Patient Care PREPARATION: The evening meal must be high in protein and contain not more than 200 mL of liquid. Patient is to consume no fluids after the evening meal. On awakening in the morning, the patient voids and saves the specimen in container #1. All further urine passed until 1 hour later is included in specimen #2. All further urine then until 2 hours later is collected as specimen #3. The volume of each voiding and the total volume of each collection is recorded. If urine specific gravity plateaus but a specific gravity of 1.027 or urine osmolality of 850 mOsm/kg is not achieved, vasopressin can be administered. AFTERCARE: Fluid restriction may decrease plasma volume and have an adverse effect on cardiac output in patients with compromised cardiac function. If diabetes insipidus is present, urine output may remain very high despite fluid deprivation. Body weight and blood pressure should be carefully followed throughout the procedure. If body weight is decreased by 5% or orthostatic hypotension occurs, the procedure should be terminated. The test should be supervised by the physician.

Specimen Urine CONTAINER: Three plastic urine containers STORAGE INSTRUCTIONS: Keep refrigerated

Interpretive REFERENCE RANGE: Normal: specific gravity of at least one specimen should be >1.026 or >850 mOsm/kg (SI: >850 mmol/kg); severe renal disease: <400 mOsm/kg (SI: <400 mmol/kg). A random urine collected without water restriction yielding a urine osmolality of ≥900 mOsm/kg (SI: ≥900 mmol/kg) or a specific gravity ≥1.027 virtually excludes a defect in concentrating ability, and thus, may be done as a screening procedure before more elaborate deprivation studies are undertaken.[1] USE: Evaluate renal concentrating ability, a test of tubular function; useful in the differential diagnosis of diabetes insipidus,[2] compulsive water drinking, and renal disease. LIMITATIONS: Protein and radiographic dyes can increase specific gravity despite decreased concentrating ability. The patient must not be taking diuretics. In polydipsic patients, the urine specific gravity may not rise to 1.026 until after many hours of deprivation. False-positive tests can be avoided by making sure serum sodium is 141-145 mmol/L before termination of the test. The test may have to be extended or adapted to the patient, and this is best done with a clear understanding of the physiology of vasopressin and of water metabolism. For details see reference by Robertson and Berl. CONTRAINDICATIONS: Glucosuria invalidates a concentration test by virtue of its diuretic effect; hypernatremia or orthostatic hypotension are contraindications. METHODOLOGY: Modified Fishberg procedure ADDITIONAL INFORMATION: Glomerular disorders causing proteinuria result in decreased concen-

(Continued)

Concentration Test, Urine *(Continued)*

trating ability by producing an osmotic diuresis in the functioning nephrons. Even subtle renal interstitial disorders may impair concentrating ability. Hypokalemia and hypercalcemia decrease renal medullary tonicity and inhibit tubular reabsorption of water. Sickle cell disease decreases medullary blood flow and interferes with loop of Henle sodium transport. Achievement of normal maximal urinary concentration requires a normal or near normal glomerular filtration rate.[1] In central diabetes insipidus, administration of vasopressin will raise urine osmolality. In nephrogenic diabetes insipidus, the urine osmolality will not increase with vasopressin or water deprivation.

Causes of Symptomatic (Polyuric) Deficiencies in Plasma Vasopressin

Decreased secretion

- Destruction of neurohypophysis (neurogenic diabetes insipidus)
  - Sporadic
    - Idiopathic
    - Trauma (surgical, accidental)
    - Malignancy
      - Primary (craniopharyngioma, dysgerminoma, meningioma, adenoma, glioma, astrocytoma)
      - Secondary (metastatic from lung or breast, lymphoma, leukemia, dysplastic pancytopenia)
    - Granuloma (sarcoid, histiocytosis, xanthoma disseminatum)
    - Infection (viral/bacterial meningitis, encephalitis)
    - Vascular (Sheehan's syndrome, carotid aneurysm, hematoma, aortocoronary bypass, ischemic brain death)
    - Autoimmune disease
    - Dysplasia (septo-optic, microcephaly, porencephaly, etc)
    - Metabolic (anorexia nervosa)
  - Familial (autosomal dominant)

Excessive water intake (primary polydipsia)

- Psychogenic (schizophrenia, ? neurosis)
- Dipsogenic (abnormal thirst)
  - Idiopathic
  - Trauma
  - Granuloma (neurosarcoid, tuberculous meningitis)
  - Autoimmune (multiple sclerosis)
  - Chemical (lithium)

Increased metabolism

- Gestational

From Robertson GL and Berl T, "Pathophysiology of Water Metabolism, "The Kidney, Brenner BM and Rector FC Jr, eds, Philadelphia, PA: WB Saunders Co, 1991, 695, with permission.

Causes of Defects in Antidiuretic Action of Vasopressin

Familial nephrogenic diabetes insipidus

- X-linked recessive

Sporadic nephrogenic diabetes insipidus

- Chemical (lithium, demeclocycline, methoxyflurane)
- Metabolic (hypokalemia, hypercalcemia)
- Mechanical (ureteral obstruction)
- Vascular (sickle cell disease or trait)
- Granulomatous (sarcoid)
- Dysplastic (polycystic disease)
- Infectious (pyelonephritis)
- Infiltrative (amyloid)
- Gestational
- Malignant (fibrosarcoma)

Solute diuresis

- Metabolic (glucosuria)
- Iatrogenic (mannitol, furosemide, radiocontrast dyes, saline loading)
- Mechanical (postureteral obstruction)

From Robertson GL and Berl T, "Pathophysiology of Water Metabolism, "The Kidney, Brenner BM and Rector FC Jr, eds, Philadelphia, PA: WB Saunders Co, 1991, 699, with permission.

Footnotes

1. Haycock GB, "Old and New Test of Renal Function," *J Clin Pathol*, 1981, 34:1276-81.
2. Price JD and Lauener RW, "Serum and Urine Osmolalities in the Differential Diagnosis of Polyuric States," *J Clin Endocrinol Metab*, 1966, 26:143-9.

References

Gupta AK, Kirchner KA, Nicholson R, et al, "Effects of α-Thalassemia and Sickle Polymerization Tendency on the Urine-Concentrating Defect of Individuals With Sickle Cell Trait," *J Clin Invest*, 1991, 88(6):1963-8.
Robertson GL and Berl T, "Pathophysiology of Water Metabolism," *Kidney*, Brenner BM and Rector FC Jr, eds, Philadelphia, PA: WB Saunders Co, 1991, 677-736.

Crystal Examination, Biliary Drainage *see* Bile Fluid Examination *on page 1109*

Crystals, Urine *see* Urinalysis *on page 1162*

Duodenal Drainage Examination *see* Bile Fluid Examination *on page 1109*

Eosinophils, Urine

***CPT** 85999*

Related Information

Ova and Parasites, Urine *on page 839*
Urinalysis *on page 1162*

Synonyms Eosinophiluria; Hansel's Stain of Urine; Urinary Eosinophils

Abstract A relatively new, nonspecific and poorly standardized marker for interstitial nephritis, eosinophilic cystitis, atheroembolic disease, and probably other entities.

Specimen Clean catch midstream urine specimen[1] **CONTAINER:** Plastic urine container **STORAGE INSTRUCTIONS:** Test should be done on a fresh specimen. **CAUSES FOR REJECTION:** Urine more than 3 hours old from time of collection

Interpretive **REFERENCE RANGE:** <100 eosinophils/mL; using Hansel's stain, <1% eosinophils[2] **USE:** Eosinophils are sought in urine to help confirm suspected cases of interstitial nephritis, eosinophilic cystitis, and renal atheroemboli (cholesterol emboli syndrome) **LIMITATIONS:** Eosinophiluria is not always present or prominent in interstitial nephritis and may be present in other disease entities. **METHODOLOGY:** Centrifuged clean catch, midstream urine, stained with Hansel's stain.[2] It is methylene blue and eosin Y in methanol (Lide Labs, Florissant, MO). Wright's stain is no longer recommended, as it is less sensitive, although still specific.

- Spin 10 mL of freshly voided urine at 2000 rpm, 5 minutes.
- Decant supernatant.
- Pipette sediment to a glass slide and air dry.
- Immerse slides in 95% methanol for 5 seconds.
- Apply Hansel's stain, 45 seconds.
- Add 20 drops of distilled water, allow to stand for 30 seconds.
- Remove excess stain with distilled water.
- Decolorize with four drops of methanol for 1-2 seconds.
- Rinse with distilled water.
- After drying, apply a coverslip with a drop of immersion oil.
- Following this protocol, 1% (or more) eosinophils is regarded as positive.[2]

ADDITIONAL INFORMATION: There is an uncertain relationship between eosinophiluria and peripheral blood eosinophilia. In only 33% of cases of drug-induced acute interstitial nephritis is the complete syndrome present. The complete syndrome includes fever, rash, eosinophiluria with acute renal failure.[2] Acute interstitial nephritis relates to penicillin derivatives, sulfa drugs, allopurinol, sulfinpyrazone, nitrofurantoin and erythromycin. Methicillin is frequently mentioned.[1] A recent report found eight of nine patients with biopsy proven atheroembolic renal failure with eosinophiluria by Hansel's stain. Six of eight of these patients had >5% of leukocytes as eosinophils.[3] Other diseases in which urinary eosinophilia is reported include contrast nephropathy, renal failure, glomerulonephritis, urinary tract infection,[4] and schistosomiasis.[5]

Footnotes

1. Sutton JM, "Urinary Eosinophils," *Arch Intern Med*, 1986, 146:2243-4.
2. Nolan CR III, Anger MS, and Kelleher SP, "Eosinophiluria – A New Method of Detection and Definition of the Clinical Spectrum," *N Engl J Med*, 1986, 315:1516-8.
3. Wilson DM, Salazer TL, and Farkouh ME, "Eosinophiluria in Atheroembolic Renal Disease," *Am J Med*, 1991, 91(2):186-9.
4. Corwin HL, Korbet SM, and Schwartz MM, "Clinical Correlates of Eosinophiluria," *Arch Intern Med*, 1985, 145:1097-9.

(Continued)

Eosinophils, Urine *(Continued)*

5. Eltoum IA, Ghalib HW, Sualaiman S, et al, "Significance of Eosinophiluria in Urinary Schistosomiasis – A Study Using Hansel's Stain and Electron Microscopy," *Am J Clin Pathol*, 1989, 92(3):329-38.

References

Corwin HL, Bray RA, and Haber MH, "The Detection and Interpretation of Urinary Eosinophils," *Arch Pathol Lab Med*, 1989, 113(11):1256-8.

Nolan CR III and Kelleher SP, "Eosinophiluria," *Clin Lab Med*, 1988, 8:577-84.

Eosinophiluria *see* Eosinophils, Urine *on previous page*

Esterase, Leukocyte, Urine *see* Leukocyte Esterase, Urine *on page 1131*

Fat, Semiquantitative, Stool

***CPT** 82705*

Related Information

Fecal Fat, Quantitative, 72-Hour Collection *on page 219*
Meat Fibers, Stool *on page 1133*
pH, Stool *on page 1143*

Synonyms Fatty Acid, Stool; Fecal Fat Stain; Neutral Fat, Stool; Sudan III Stain, Stool

Applies to Fecal Fat Analysis, 72-Hour

Abstract In this simple and low cost procedure, fecal fat is stained with Sudan III. The test is used as a screen for the presence of fecal neutral fat and fatty acids and may assist in the determination of the cause of steatorrhea.

Patient Care PREPARATION: Patient should be on diet containing at least 60 g of fat. The patient should not use suppositories or mineral oil before the specimen is collected. Oily material (eg, creams, lubricants, etc) should be avoided prior to collection of the specimen.

Specimen Fresh random stool CONTAINER: Plastic stool container TURNAROUND TIME: 1-2 hours

Interpretive REFERENCE RANGE: Neutral fat: <50 fat globules per high power field, reported as normal. Fatty acids: <100 fat globules per high power field is considered normal. USE: Screen for presence of fecal fatty acids and neutral fat. Increases in neutral fat are commonly associated with pancreatic exocrine insufficiency. Increase in stool fatty acids is likely to be associated with small bowel disease. LIMITATIONS: Castor oil or mineral oil droplets can mimic neutral fat. CONTRAINDICATIONS: Administration of barium, bismuth, Metamucil®, castor oil, or mineral oil within 1 week prior to collection of the specimen METHODOLOGY: Small amount of stool sample is mixed with two drops of water, two drops of 95% ethanol, and three to four drops of Sudan III stain. Increased yellow-orange refractile fat globules (direct Sudan III stain) identifies neutral fats. Fatty acids and fat soaps are detected utilizing hydrolysis by mixing stool sample with two to three drops each of Sudan III and glacial acetic acid, followed by heating before microscopic examination. ADDITIONAL INFORMATION: The test consists of determination of the presence of neutral fats and of total fats representing fatty acids. The results are reported semiquantitatively. In a comparison of screening tests for enteropathy in children, results of lactose breath hydrogen, 1-hour d-xylose absorption, and 72-hour fecal fat tests were compared with the results of jejunal biopsy. Only the d-xylose and fecal fat tests correlated significantly with biopsy results.[1] See listing for Meat Fibers, Stool.

Presence of steatorrhea can be established by the results of a 72-hour fecal fat analysis. Maldigestion or malabsorption may cause steatorrhea. Patients with maldigestion excrete excess triglyceride while patients with malabsorption excrete excess fatty acid. The 72-hour fecal fat determination involves saponification and does not usually provide for selective quantitation of triglyceride and fatty acid. The two-step Sudan III staining procedure (described above) has been considered capable of distinguishing triglyceride from fatty acid (and thereby maldigestion from malabsorption). However, there is evidence that in adults with pancreatic insufficiency, the fecal triglyceride content may be normal. At least, the fecal triglyceride expressed in mg/g of fecal weight is not increased in cases of pancreatic insufficiency.[2] One may not be able to differentiate maldigestion from malabsorption (pancreatic vs intestinal steatorrhea) by comparing fecal triglyceride/fatty acid or fecal fat concentration.[3,4,5,6] The influence of extrapancreatic lipase (eg, gastric lipase) must be considered.[7,8,9] Some experimental work has been performed toward a quantitative Sudan stain based procedure for fecal triglyceride and fatty acid.[10] Cholesterol absorption, in particular the serum level of high-density lipoprotein cholesterol, is decreased with pancreatic insufficiency and is increased as a result of exogenous pancreatic enzyme substitution.[9]

Footnotes

1. Levine JJ, Seidman E, and Walker WA, "Screening Tests for Enteropathy in Children," *Am J Dis Child*, 1987, 141:435-8.
2. Bernstein LH, "Old Insight Into a New Insight Into an Old Test," *Gastroenterology*, 1989, 97(2):552-3, (letter).
3. Khouri MR, Ng S-N, Huang G, et al, "Fecal Triglyceride Excretion Is Not Excessive in Pancreatic Insufficiency," *Gastroenterology*, 1989, 96(3):848-52.
4. Lembcke B, Grimm K, and Lankisch PG, "Raised Fecal Fat Concentration Is Not a Valid Indicator of Pancreatic Steatorrhea," *Am J Gastroenterol*, 1987, 82:526-31.
5. Bai JC, Andrüsh A, Matelo G, et al, "Fecal Fat Concentration in the Differential Diagnosis of Steatorrhea," *Am J Gastroenterol*, 1989, 84(1):27-30.
6. Kaunitz JD, "Dietary Fat Intake, 72-Hour Excretion, and Sudan Stain for Fecal Fat," *Gastroenterology*, 1989, 97(2):550-1, (letter).
7. DeNigris SJ, Hamosh M, Kasbekar DK, et al, "Secretion of Human Gastric Lipase From Dispersed Gastric Glands," *Biochim Biophys Acta*, 1985, 836:67-72.
8. Moreau H, Laugier R, Gargouri Y, et al, "Human Preduodenal Lipase Is Entirely of Gastric Fundic Origin," *Gastroenterology*, 1988, 95(5):1221-6.
9. Abrams CK, Hamosh M, Lee TC, et al, "Gastric Lipase: Localization in the Human Stomach," *Gastroenterology*, 1988, 95(6):1460-4.
10. Khouri MR, Huang G, and Shiau YF, "Sudan Stain of Fecal Fat: New Insight Into an Old Test," *Gastroenterology*, 1989, 96(2 Pt 1):421-7.

References

Ahnen DJ, "Disorders of Nutrient Assimilation," *Textbook of Internal Medicine*, 2nd ed, Chapter 80, Kelley WN, DeVita VT, Jr, Dupont HL, et al, eds, Philadelphia, PA: JB Lippincott Co, 1992, 479-80.

Roberts IM, Poturich C, Wald A, et al, "Utility of Fecal Fat Concentrations as Screening Test in Pancreatic Insufficiency," *Dig Dis Sci*, 1986, 10:1021-4.

Simko V, "Sudan Stain and Quantitative Fecal Fat," *Gastroenterology*, 1990, 98(6):1722-3, (letter; comment).

Vuoristo M, Väänänen H, and Miettinen TA, "Cholesterol Malabsorption in Pancreatic Insufficiency: Effects of Enzyme Substitution," *Gastroenterology*, 1992, 102(2):647-55.

Fatty Acid, Stool *see* Fat, Semiquantitative, Stool *on previous page*

Fat, Urine

CPT 89125

Related Information

Protein, Quantitative, Urine *on page 1145*
Urinalysis *on page 1162*

Synonyms Free Fat, Urine; Lipid, Urine

Test Commonly Includes Light and polarized microscopy of urine sediment and staining with Sudan III or IV

Abstract Oval fat bodies are lipid-laden, pathologic, renal tubular epithelial cells which bear a strong association with marked proteinuria.

Patient Care PREPARATION: Avoid contamination of the specimen with oils and lubricants from catheters and soaps. Avoid contamination with glove powder.

Specimen Random urine CONTAINER: Plastic urine container CAUSES FOR REJECTION: Contamination of specimen with oils, soaps, and lubricants

Interpretive REFERENCE RANGE: Negative USE: Evaluate nephrotic syndrome, renal tubular necrosis, mercury poisoning, ethylene glycol ingestion (which may produce oval fat bodies), and fatty casts in the urine; evaluate bone marrow and fat embolism, which may produce gross fat globules in the urine LIMITATIONS: Urinary fat globules, like air bubbles and yeasts, can be confused with erythrocytes if Sudan stain is not used. METHODOLOGY: Sudan III and IV staining of urine sediment. Microscopically fat globules appear as spherical or ovoid dark glistening bodies. Under polarized light they appear doubly refractile and give a Maltese cross pattern. Maltese cross patterns may also be seen with some crystals, in particular starch granules in some glove powders. Corn starch contamination can give rise to doubly refractile false urine lipid bodies.[1] These are not as regular and round as are free urine lipid bodies. With polarized light the conical configuration of false bodies tends to be off center, "French cross pattern."[2] True urine fat globules are usually seen in urines which also show heavy proteinuria. ADDITIONAL INFORMATION: Urinary doubly refractile lipid bodies usually occur with heavy proteinuria. Refractile lipid bodies have been found in nonglomerular renal disease at relatively low levels of proteinuria and, rarely, even in patients without renal disease. Frequency of urine lipid bodies in patients with nonglomerular renal diseases included chronic interstitial nephritis (26%), polycystic kidney disease (38%), prerenal azotemia (20%), acute tubular necrosis (15%), and

(Continued)

Fat, Urine *(Continued)*

acute interstitial nephritis (33%). Presence of refractile urine lipid bodies in numbers >5 per 20 high power microscopic fields may be required to differentiate glomerular from nonglomerular renal diseases.[3]

Footnotes

1. Senécal PE and Rochette J, "Misidentification of Urine Lipid Bodies Owing to Use of Starch-Powdered Gloves," *Clin Chem*, 1988, 34(9):1926-7.
2. Hudson JB, Dennis AJ, and Gerhardt RE, "Urinary Lipid and the Maltese Cross," *N Engl J Med*, 1978, 299:586.
3. Braden GL, Sanchez PG, Fitzgibbons JP, et al, "Urinary Doubly Refractile Lipid Bodies in Nonglomerular Renal Diseases," *Am J Kidney Dis*, 1988, 11(4):332-7.

References

Yager HM and Harrington JT, "Urinalysis and Urinary Electrolytes," *The Principles and Practice of Nephrology*, Chapter 28, Jacobson HR, Striker GE, and Klahr S, eds, Philadelphia, PA: BC Decker Inc, 1991, 167-77.

Fecal Chymotrypsin *see* Tryptic Activity, Stool *on page 1161*

Fecal Fat Analysis, 72-Hour *see* Fat, Semiquantitative, Stool *on page 1118*

Fecal Fat Stain *see* Fat, Semiquantitative, Stool *on page 1118*

Fecal Occult Blood Test *see* Occult Blood, Stool *on page 1138*

Fecal pH *see* pH, Stool *on page 1143*

Fecal Tryptic Activity *see* Tryptic Activity, Stool *on page 1161*

Fishberg Concentration Test *see* Concentration Test, Urine *on page 1115*

Franklin Dukes Test *see* Infertility Screen *on page 1124*

Free Fat, Urine *see* Fat, Urine *on previous page*

Glucose, Dipstick, Urine *see* Glucose, Semiquantitative, Urine *on next page*

Glucose, Qualitative, Urine *replaced by* Glucose, Semiquantitative, Urine *on next page*

Glucose, Quantitative, Urine

CPT 82947

Related Information

Fructosamine *on page 224*
Glucose, 2-Hour Postprandial *on page 237*
Glucose, Fasting *on page 238*
Glucose, Random *on page 240*
Glucose, Semiquantitative, Urine *on next page*
Glucose Tolerance Test *on page 241*
Glycated Hemoglobin *on page 244*
Ketone Bodies, Blood *on page 265*
Ketones, Urine *on page 1128*
Reducing Substances, Urine *on page 1150*

Synonyms Sugar, Quantitative, Urine; Urinary Sugar Test

Specimen 24-hour urine or other specific timed collections **CONTAINER:** Plain urine container, sodium fluoride preservative **STORAGE INSTRUCTIONS:** If the specimen cannot be processed immediately by the laboratory, it should be refrigerated. **CAUSES FOR REJECTION:** Improperly labeled container, specimen not kept cold **TURNAROUND TIME:** 24 hours

Interpretive **REFERENCE RANGE:** ≤100 mg/24 hours (SI: ≤5.6 mmol/day). Excretion <5% of total daily caloric intake has in the past been considered good diabetic control. Excretion >10% of total caloric intake is considered very poor control. Normal ranges are not available on random specimens. **USE:** Aid in the evaluation of glucosuria, renal tubular defects; management of diabetes mellitus **LIMITATIONS:** With the advent of home glucose monitoring and the usefulness of glycosylated hemoglobin in following the degree of glucose control in a diabetic subject, the measurement of quantitative urine glucose is no longer used for control of diabetic patients. **METHODOLOGY:** Glucose oxidase **ADDITIONAL INFORMATION:** Tests for ketones in serum and urine are useful adjuncts.

References

Knowles HC, "Evaluation of a Positive Urinary Sugar Test," *JAMA*, 1975, 234:961-3.

Glucose, Semiquantitative, Urine

CPT *81003*

Related Information

Glucose, 2-Hour Postprandial *on page 237*
Glucose, Fasting *on page 238*
Glucose, Quantitative, Urine *on previous page*
Glucose, Random *on page 240*
Glucose Tolerance Test *on page 241*
Glycated Hemoglobin *on page 244*
Ketone Bodies, Blood *on page 265*
Ketones, Urine *on page 1128*
Reducing Substances, Urine *on page 1150*
Urinalysis *on page 1162*

Synonyms Sugar, Qualitative, Urine; Urinary Sugar Test

Applies to Glucose, Dipstick, Urine; Glucose Tolerance Test Urines; Urines for Glucose Tolerance

Replaces Glucose, Qualitative, Urine

Test Commonly Includes Dipstick glucose is usually a part of urinalysis.

Specimen Random urine, double-void technique preferred **CONTAINER:** Plastic urine container **SAMPLING TIME:** Random or following a glucose load **STORAGE INSTRUCTIONS:** If the specimen cannot be processed immediately, it should be refrigerated. **CAUSES FOR REJECTION:** Improper labeling, specimen not refrigerated

Interpretive **REFERENCE RANGE:** None detected **USE:** Detect glucose (sugar) in the urine. Glycosuria may occur in situations, such as pregnancy, in which the increased filtered load may exceed renal tubular reabsorption capacity. Rarely corticosteroid therapy may cause a combination of mild hyperglycemia and increased renal glomerular filtration, producing glycosuria. Renal glycosuria due to a low renal threshold for glucose may occur. Because these causes of glucosuria are rare and glucosuria usually indicates significant hyperglycemia, a positive screening test for urine glucose is a significant sign and indicates a substantial likelihood of diabetes mellitus in the nonpregnant patient. In the pregnant patient, glucosuria had a 27% sensitivity and only a 7.1% predictive value for gestational diabetes. Its greatest value was to indicate which women should be screened with serum glucose after a 50 g oral glucose load **prior** to 24-28 weeks gestation, the usual recommended time of screening.[1] Urine glucose testing may be used as a monitor in diabetics in concert with plasma glucose and glycosylated hemoglobin. **LIMITATIONS:** Dipstick methods are limited in usefulness as quantitative methods.[2,3] Acquired color vision deficiency caused by diabetic retinopathy may cause erroneous reading of the strip by patients.[4] Each brand of commercial dipsticks lists interfering substances. Such package inserts should be reviewed. Home blood glucose testing has largely replaced qualitative and semiquantitative urine methods for long-term and outpatient monitoring of diabetic therapy.[5] Glucose in urine is detected later in time than the hyperglycemia it indirectly represents by approximately one-half the time between voidings. In renal failure, the time delay may become excessive due to oliguria. Excessive urinary bladder residual volume further limits the test as reflecting **current** hyperglycemia.

For diagnosis, fasting state urine glucose testing lacks sensitivity (17%) but provides 98% specificity. Postload glucosuria provides only moderate sensitivity and specificity, 70% to 80%.[6]

As a patient-based monitor of control in known diabetics, urine glucose determination does not provide reliable differentiation between current mild elevation, and normality or decrease of blood glucose. Urine glucose testing cannot detect hypoglycemia and lacks sufficient sensitivity for tight control. Urine glucose testing is considered inferior to self-monitoring of capillary glucose for type I diabetics.[6] Levels below the renal threshold of glucose are not subject to evaluation by urine glucose testing. The renal threshold for glucose is variable between different patients.[6]

Large quantities of ketones and ascorbic acid (eg, after ingestion of vitamin C tablets) may depress the color reaction. Contamination of the collection container by hypochlorite, chlorine or peroxide may cause false-positives. Pyridium® metabolites may mask the reaction.

The double enzyme (glucose-specific) method for urine sugar will not detect sugars in the urine other than glucose. For screening for other sugars, see the Reducing Substances, Urine test listing.

(Continued)

Glucose, Semiquantitative, Urine *(Continued)*

Urines negative for glucose with properly stored Multistix® (Miles Inc, Elkhart, IN) were trace positive following dipstick air exposure (jars left uncapped).[7]

METHODOLOGY: Double sequential enzyme analysis, specific for glucose (glucose oxidase/ peroxidase). Sensitivity is 50-100 mg glucose/dL (SI: 2.8-5.6 mmol/L) urine. **ADDITIONAL INFORMATION:** The renal threshold for glucose is 160-180 mg/dL (SI: 8.9-10.0 mmol/L). Thus, reasonable diabetic control can be maintained and the risk of hypoglycemia minimized if urine glucose screening tests are maintained at a trace to 1+ level. High urine specific gravity will decrease sensitivity.

Footnotes

1. Watson WJ, "Screening for Glycosuria During Pregnancy," *South Med J*, 1990, 83(2):156-8.
2. James GP and Bee DE, "Glycosuria: Accuracy and Precision of Laboratory Diagnosis by Dipstick Analysis," *Clin Chem*, 1979, 25:996-1001.
3. Dyerberg J, Pederson L, and Aagaard O, "Evaluation of a Dipstick Test for Glucose in Urine," *Clin Chem*, 1976, 22:205-10.
4. Bresnik GH, Groo A, Palta M, et al, "Urinary Glucose Testing Among Diabetic Patients. Effect of Acquired Color Vision Deficiency Caused by Diabetic Retinopathy." *Arch Ophthalmol*, 1984, 102:1489-96.
5. Miller PF, Stratton C, and Tripp JH, "Blood Testing Compared With Urine Testing in the Long-Term Control of Diabetes," *Arch Dis Child*, 1983, 58:294-7.
6. Singer DE, Coley CM, Samet JH, et al, "Tests of Glycemia in Diabetes Mellitus: Their Use in Establishing a Diagnosis and in Treatment," *Ann Intern Med*, 1989, 110(2):125-37.
7. Cohen HT and Spiegel DM, "Air-Exposed Urine Dipsticks Give False-Positive Results for Glucose and False-Negative Results for Blood," *Am J Clin Pathol*, 1991, 96(3):398-400.

References

Knowles HC, "Evaluation of a Positive Urinary Sugar Test," *JAMA*, 1975, 234:961-3.

McCarthy J, "Value of Urine Glucose Tests in the Management of Type II Diabetes Mellitus. Results of a Study of the Double-Void Technique." *Postgrad Med J*, 1984, 76:204-10.

Glucose Tolerance Test Urines *see* Glucose, Semiquantitative, Urine *on previous page*

Guaiac, Stool *see* Occult Blood, Stool *on page 1138*

Hamster (Human + Hamster) Test *see* Sperm Penetration Assay (Human Sperm-Hamster Oocyte) *on page 1155*

Hamster Test *see* Sperm Penetration Assay (Human Sperm-Hamster Oocyte) *on page 1155*

Hansel's Stain of Urine *see* Eosinophils, Urine *on page 1117*

Hema-Chek® *see* Occult Blood, Stool *on page 1138*

Hemizona Binding Assay *see* Infertility Screen *on page 1124*

Hemoccult® II, Stool *see* Occult Blood, Stool *on page 1138*

Hemoglobin, Qualitative, Urine

***CPT** 81003*

See Also Anemia Flowchart in the Hematology Appendix

Related Information

Blood, Urine *on page 1112*
Hemoglobin, Plasma *on page 559*
Hemosiderin Stain, Urine *on next page*
Kidney Biopsy *on page 68*
Myoglobin, Qualitative, Urine *on page 1135*
Ova and Parasites, Urine *on page 839*
Urinalysis *on page 1162*
Urinalysis, Fractional *on page 1166*

Test Commonly Includes Dipstick screening of urine for hemoglobin

Abstract Test for hemoglobin in urine. This also screens for blood in urine, which must be confirmed microscopically.

Specimen Random urine **CONTAINER:** Plastic urine container

Interpretive **REFERENCE RANGE:** Negative **USE:** Determine the presence of hemoglobinuria **LIMITATIONS:** Menstrual or other uterine bleeding may appear as a contaminant in the urine. False-positives to dipsticks occur with oxidizing contaminants or Betadine® (povidone-iodine).

False-negatives occur with large amounts of ascorbic acid. Formalin in urine can cause false-negative results.[1] Urine dipsticks for blood that are exposed to air lose sensitivity over time. To prevent this, keep dipstick jar tightly capped. **METHODOLOGY:** The peroxidase-like activity of hemoglobin catalyzes the reaction of cumene hydroperoxide and 3,3',5,5'-tetramethylbenzidine. **ADDITIONAL INFORMATION:** Hemoglobinuria, the presence of free hemoglobin in the urine, may result from hemolysis. It occurs if the serum haptoglobin binding capacity (100-200 mg/dL Hgb (SI: 1.0-2.0 g/L)) is exceeded and if the renal threshold for tubular reabsorption of hemoglobin (90-140 mg/dL Hgb (SI: 0.9-1.4 g/L)) is exceeded. Hemoglobin is catabolized in the renal tubular cells, and the iron is stored as hemosiderin. See Hemosiderin Stain, Urine listing. The urine in hemoglobinuria may be clear red, clear red-brown, or dark brown. Myoglobinuria also produces a dark or red-orange urine. Both hemoglobin and myoglobin produce positive dipstick tests for blood and must be identified by additional tests.[2] In hematuria, red cells or ghosts (lysed red cells) are observed microscopically. Algorithms for medical work-up of hematuria have been published.

Footnotes

1. Corwin HL and Silverstein MD, "Microscopic Hematuria," *Clin Lab Med*, 1988, 8:601-10.
2. Epstein M and Oster JR, "Renal and Electrolytes Disorder – General Considerations," *The Laboratory in Clinical Medicine: Interpretation and Application*, 2nd ed, Halsted JA and Halsted CH, eds, Philadelphia, PA: WB Saunders Co, 1981, 284.

Hemoglobin, Urine *see* Blood, Urine *on page 1112*

HemoQuant® *see* Occult Blood, Stool *on page 1138*

Hemosiderin Stain, Urine

CPT *83070 (qualitative); 83071 (quantitative)*

See Also Anemia Flowchart in the Hematology Appendix

Related Information

Blood, Urine *on page 1112*

Hemoglobin, Qualitative, Urine *on previous page*

Synonyms Iron Stain, Urine; Prussian Blue Stain, Urine

Specimen Random urine **CONTAINER:** Plastic urine container **STORAGE INSTRUCTIONS:** If the specimen cannot be processed promptly, it should be refrigerated. **TURNAROUND TIME:** About 8 hours

Interpretive **REFERENCE RANGE:** Negative **USE:** Determine the presence of hemosiderin in urine. Hemosiderinuria is an important clue in the diagnosis of unexplained anemia. Hemosiderinuria is a sign of recent intravascular hemolysis. Urine sediment stained for hemosiderin is a screen for increased iron excretion, which can be quantitated and is increased in hemochromatosis, hemolytic anemia, and nephrotic syndrome. **LIMITATIONS:** Hemosiderin is first shed in the urine a few days after hemolysis begins. Hemosiderinuria declines slowly after hemolysis stops. Quantitatively, iron excretion remains slightly elevated for months after replacement of a cardiac valve which has caused hemolytic anemia, although hemosiderinuria is usually absent after a few weeks. **METHODOLOGY:** Microscopic examination of slide stained for hemosiderin (Prussian blue reaction) **ADDITIONAL INFORMATION:** When haptoglobin is saturated, part of the hemoglobin in the plasma is filtered by the glomerulus and presented to the renal tubular cell. If tubular capacity is not exceeded, all hemoglobin in the urine may be absorbed by the proximal tubular cells where hemoglobin iron is converted to hemosiderin. When these cells are shed, hemosiderin appears in urine sediment. Hemosiderinuria with or without hemoglobinuria may be seen in chronic hemolytic anemia, paroxysmal nocturnal hemoglobinuria, hemochromatosis, multiple transfusions, and other conditions which result in deposition of iron in the renal parenchyma. Hemosiderinuria may occur when the degree of hemolysis is at such a low level that hemoglobinuria is not detected.[1] Hemosiderin may appear as a brown coarsely granular pigment in tubular epithelial cells, epithelial cell casts, or free in the urine sediment.

Footnotes

1. Pimstone NR, "Renal Degradation of Hemoglobin," *Physiology and Disorders of Hemoglobin Degradation*, Schmid R, Jaffé ER, eds, New York, NY: Grune and Stratton Inc, 1972, 32.

References

Lee GR, "Introduction to the Hemolytic Anemias," *Wintrobe's Clinical Hematology*, Lee GR, Bithell TC, Foerster J, et al, eds, Philadelphia, PA: Lea & Febiger, 1993, 1:944-64.

Tabbara IA, "Hemolytic Anemias. Diagnosis and Management," *Med Clin North Am*, 1992, 76(3):649-68.

Heterologous Ovum Penetration Test *see* Sperm Penetration Assay (Human Sperm-Hamster Oocyte) *on page 1155*

Immunoreactive Trypsin, Fecal Extracts *see* Tryptic Activity, Stool *on page 1161*

Indican, Semiquantitative, Urine

CPT 81005

Synonyms Indoxyl Sulfate, Urine

Applies to Purple Urine Bags

Abstract This simple test can be used to screen for intestinal bacterial overgrowth, malabsorption due to intestinal or biliary obstruction, or Hartnup disease. It can confirm indican as the etiology for a dark or black urine.

Specimen Fresh random urine **CONTAINER:** Plastic urine container **STORAGE INSTRUCTIONS:** The test must be run on fresh urine specimens. Transport specimen to the laboratory immediately upon collection. **CAUSES FOR REJECTION:** Improper labeling, delay in transport to the laboratory

Interpretive **REFERENCE RANGE:** Indican is normally present in urine in small amounts; <100 mg/day is normally excreted. It is detected by a semiquantitative color reaction and is reported as "positive" or "negative" (normal). **USE:** Evaluate intestinal integrity, absorption, and protein catabolism **LIMITATIONS:** Diurnal variation is described in urinary indican excretion.[1] Urine indican is rarely requested. **METHODOLOGY:** Detection of indican depends upon its decomposition and subsequent oxidation of the indoxyl to indigo blue and its absorption by chloroform. **ADDITIONAL INFORMATION:** Indole is produced by intestinal bacterial action on unabsorbed tryptophan. Although most indole is eliminated in the feces, a small amount is absorbed and detoxified to be excreted as indican (indoxyl potassium sulfate) in the urine. Urinary indican may be increased in biliary obstruction, intestinal obstruction, malabsorption syndromes, and syndromes associated with achlorhydria (eg, gastric carcinoma, pernicious anemia). Hartnup disease patients also have high urine indican. Increased indican may cause the urine to blacken on standing.

Purple urine drainage bags have been reported in a few chronically catheterized, elderly, female patients with urinary tract infection caused by *Providencia* or *Klebsiella*. Urine indican excretion in such subjects was increased.[2]

There is experimental animal evidence that saccharin can induce increase in urinary indican[3] and provide a noninvasive indicator of trypsin inhibitor activity.[4]

Indoxyl sulfate can alter the dip-and-read strip reaction for urinary bilirubin in urines positive for bilirubin, sufficiently to mask a weak reaction. A more specific test such as the Ictotest® has been recommended when dip-and-read bilirubin testing is inconclusive.[5]

Footnotes

1. Kirkland JL, Vargas E, and Lye M, "Indican Excretion in the Elderly," *Postgrad Med J*, 1983, 59:717-9.
2. Dealler SF, Belfield PW, Bedford M, et al, "Purple Urine Bags," *J Urol*, 1989, 142(3):769-70.
3. Sims J and Renick AG, "Diurnal Variation in the Excretion of Indican in Rats Fed Saccharin-Containing Diet," *Cancer*, 1984, 23:259-63.
4. Anderson RL, Maurer JK, Francis WR, et al, "Tryspin Inhibitor Ingestion-Induced Urinary Indican Excretion and Pancreatic Acinar Cell Hypertrophy," *Nutr Cancer*, 1986, 8:133-9.
5. Skjold AC, Freitag JF, Stover LR, et al, "Indoxyl Sulfate Interferes With Dip-and-Read Urinary Bilirubin Estimate," *Clin Chem*, 1980, 26(9):1368-9, (letter).

Indoxyl Sulfate, Urine *see* Indican, Semiquantitative, Urine *on this page*

Infertility Screen

CPT 89300 (semen analysis presence and/or motility of sperm); 89310 (semen analysis motility and count); 89320 (semen analysis complete; volume, count, motility and differential)

Related Information

Semen Analysis *on page 1151*
Sperm Mucus Penetration Test (Human or Bovine Cervical Mucus) *on page 1154*
Sperm Penetration Assay (Human Sperm-Hamster Oocyte) *on page 1155*

Applies to Antispermatozoal Antibody Test; Franklin Dukes Test; Hemizona Binding Assay; Sperm Agglutination and Inhibition; Sperm Antibodies; Sperm-Oolemma Binding Test

Test Commonly Includes Semen analysis

Abstract Extensive and sophisticated methodology for the evaluation of spermatozoa has been developed during the last decade. Expanding capabilities resulting from continuing growth in artificial insemination/*in vitro* fertilization has provided impetus for the study of sperm function, in particular by specialized andrology laboratories. The following is an overview of infertility evaluation, emphasis largely on the "male factor". It is hoped that the accompanying footnotes and references will provide entry to additional study and to the details of test methodology.

Patient Care PREPARATION: Follow physician's instructions. Ejaculation should be avoided for 2-3 days prior to collection of the specimen.

Specimen Serum (both partners) and semen CONTAINER: Blood: red top tube; semen: clean, dry, wide mouth glass or plastic container known to be free of detergent or other toxic agents COLLECTION: Semen: Postcoital or masturbation using condom-like Silastic seminal fluid collection device (see entry Semen Analysis). There is evidence that some seminal deficiency test parameters are improved by semen collection via intercourse using a seminal collection device as opposed to masturbation.[1] STORAGE INSTRUCTIONS: Tests should be started as soon as possible after collection of semen at least within 2-3 hours. CAUSES FOR REJECTION: Semen specimen more than 2 hours old, specimens with improper identification/label TURNAROUND TIME: 1-5 days SPECIAL INSTRUCTIONS: Semen, as with all blood, urine, and body fluid specimens, because of the risk of AIDS, should be received and handled with care to avoid contamination of laboratory personnel. Gloves must be worn during the handling and manipulation of sperm/semen-containing fluids. Persons with sores/open wounds of the skin must avoid contact with semen. Infertility screen testing is not offered by many routine clinical laboratories. Specialized infertility/andrology laboratories perform infertility testing, but there is not a standardized test menu.

Interpretive REFERENCE RANGE: Individual test and laboratory dependent USE: Evaluate infertility LIMITATIONS: While the existence of sperm antibodies relating to infertility seems firmly established, methodology of some early testing procedures has not proven to be highly technically reliable. Tests utilizing methanol-fixed spermatozoa may give unpredictable and nonreproducible results.[2] METHODOLOGY: Routine semen analysis protocols, semen function tests, computer-assisted sperm morphology/motility studies, Kibrick agglutination assay with or without the use gelatin, method of Franklin and Dukes[3], microagglutination tests, sperm immobilization/cytotoxicity tests (eg, Isojima assay), mixed antiglobulin reaction assay (MAR), enzyme-linked immunosorbent assay (ELISA) using as antigen glutaraldehyde-fixed spermatozoa, Immunobead™ binding assay[4,5], antisperm antibodies by indirect fluorescence using flow cytometry[6] ADDITIONAL INFORMATION: The possibility that a couple is infertile can be considered when there is failure to conceive after about 1 year of unimpaired intercourse. Approximately 95% of normal couples should conceive within 13-15 months.[7] Many factors may be responsible for infertility. These may be divided into "female factors" and "male factors". Common causes of infertility include endometriosis, tubal factors (often pelvic inflammatory disease), and ovulation and cervical/uterine factors. A "male factor" is responsible in some 20% of the cases.[7] Basic evaluation (American Fertility Society) includes history and examination of the female, postcoital test, evaluation of tubal patency (hysterosalpingogram), evaluation of hormonal factors, history and examination of the male, and semen analyses.[8] To overcome the effect of transient variables, multiple and/or periodic study of spermatozoa may be necessary. Immunologic factors are a potential important cause of infertility. It has been estimated that 7% to 14% of men attending a fertility clinic have sperm-bound antibodies (as compared to an incidence of 1% to 2% in fertile men without history of vasovasostomy).[9]

This text deals largely with tests that identify "male factor" causes of infertility. The past 15 years has seen increased interest in the evaluation of spermatozoa, reflecting increased understanding of sperm physiology and increased rate of new test development. Thus, the growing number and capability of fertility/andrology laboratories usually in support of assisted reproduction programs. The latter include such procedures as *in vitro* fertilization and embryonic transfer (IVF-ET) and gamete-intrafallopian tube transfer (GIFT). The American Fertility Society has published guidelines for human andrology laboratories including recognition of the National Committee for Clinical Laboratory Standards (NCCLS) specified format.[10] An example of a quality control and quality assurance program has been published.[11] An excellent current review presents relatively recently developed tests of human sperm function including:[12]

- resistance of sperm to decondensation in sodium dodecyl sulfate
- acidic aniline blue stain for immature sperm nuclei
- acridine orange stain for abnormal nuclear chromatin
- trypan blue or eosin Y membrane dye exclusion test

(Continued)

Infertility Screen *(Continued)*

- follicular fluid induction of acrosome reaction
- calcium ionophore A23187 induction of acrosome reaction
- acrosome assessment by *pisum sativum* agglutinin fluorescein stain
- measurement of acrosomal proteinase activity
- assessment of hyaluronidase activity
- sperm-oolemma binding test
- hypo-osmotic swelling test
- hemizona binding assay
- variety of tests for determination of antisperm antibodies (see below)

Presence of sperm antibodies has not been clearly associated with disease states. Sperm antibodies may be found in the circulation, free or as immune complexes, in seminal plasma, and/or attached to the sperm surface. Tests that measure immunoglobulin on the sperm surface have greater sensitivity than assays of serum antisperm antibodies. Some males may have blood negative for sperm antibodies but have demonstrable antibody on the surface of spermatozoa.[2] Sperm-bound antibody measured by ELISA has been found present in a greater percentage of infertile men with varicoceles than infertile men without varicoceles.[13] Results of a modification of the seminobead™ test (in which the beads are coated with MH61, a monoclonal antibody specific for acrosome-reacted sperm) have been shown to correlate with outcomes of sperm penetration assays (SPA) and IVF.[14]

Antibodies are found in some males with testicular disease. They are also seen in cases of autoimmune aspermatogenesis experimentally induced by immunization with semen, spermatozoa, or testicular homogenates. There may be a cause and effect relationship between spermatozoal antibodies in serum of females and unexplained infertility. Both members of the couple should have their serum tested. The use of a single type of test may not be adequate. Studies indicate that each test has a different incidence of positive results in an infertile population. Repeat of test procedure will at times give different results for a particular serum sample. A number of immunologic based methods for detection of antisperm antibodies have been developed. The Immunobead™ test is currently most commonly employed. Antisperm antibody tests are critiqued in the text by Glover et al including immunofluorescence; gelatin agglutination test (GAT), Kibrick method; tube-slide agglutination test (TSAT), Franklin Dukes method; tray agglutination test (TAT); slide agglutination test (SAT); modified slide agglutination test (MSAT); sperm immobilization test (SIT); mixed antiglobulin reaction (MAR); Immunobead™ test (IBT); enzyme-linked immunosorbent assay (ELISA).[15]

Electro-optical and computer assisted devices and systems are available for the semiautomated/automated study of sperm morphology and motility. These are in use by some andrology laboratories. Some aspects of their application and evaluation are detailed.[16,17,18,19,20,21,22] An editorial comment concerning the risk involved in hypertrophy of technology is especially noteworthy.[18]

A minimum level of extracellular ionized calcium is necessary to the maintenance of normal sperm motility. Spermatozoa appear to be dependent on intracellular translocation of calcium ions rather than on the extracellular concentration of ionized calcium.[23]

Evaluation of spermatozoal function has been approached by measuring surrogate cervical mucus penetration (see also entry Sperm Mucus Penetration Test) and the determination of sperm capacitation index, based on the degree of polyspermy in penetration of zona-free, pellucida-free hamster ova.[24] See also entry Sperm Penetration Assay.

A study involving 445 men found smoking correlated with decreased semen volume, and coffee drinking correlated with increase in sperm density and number of abnormal forms. Individuals consuming over four cups of coffee per day and who smoked over 20 cigarettes per day had a lower fraction of motile spermatozoa and more dead cells as compared to nonsmoker/coffee drinkers. Alcohol consumption, also studied, did not affect semen quality (by either univariate or multifactorial analysis).[25] A separate study has found use of cocaine associated with low sperm concentration, low sperm motility, and presence of abnormal morphology.[26]

It has been shown that antisperm antibodies will transfer from spermatozoa to immunobeads. It has been proposed that sperm processed using this technique may find application (intrauterine insemination) in the treatment of male immunologic infertility.[27]

Footnotes

1. Zavos PM and Goodpasture JC, "Clinical Improvements of Specific Seminal Deficiencies Via Intercourse With a Seminal Collection Device Versus Masturbation," *Fertil Steril*, 1989, 51(1):190-3.

2. Haas GG Jr, "Antibody-Mediated Causes of Male Infertility," *Urol Clin North Am*, 1987, 14:539-50.
3. Franklin RR and Dukes CD, "Further Studies on Sperm-Agglutinating Antibody and Unexplained Infertility," *JAMA*, 1964, 190:682.
4. Bronson R, Cooper G, Hjort T, et al, "Antisperm Antibodies Detected by Agglutination, Immobilization, Microcytotoxicity, and Immunobead™-Binding Assays," *J Reprod Immunol*, 1985, 8:279-99.
5. Clark GN, Elliott PJ, and Smaila C, "Detection of Sperm Antibodies in Semen Using the Immunobead™ Test: A Survey of 813 Consecutive Patients," *Am J Reprod Immunol*, 1985, 7:118-23.
6. Sinton EB, Riemann DC, and Ashton ME, "Antisperm Antibody Detection Using Concurrent Cytofluorometry and Indirect Immunofluorescence Microscopy," *Am J Clin Pathol*, 1991, 95(2):242-6.
7. Talbert LM, "Overview of the Diagnostic Evaluation," *Infertility – A Practical Guide for the Physician*, 3rd ed, Hammond MG and Talbert LM, eds, Boston, MA: Blackwell Scientific Publications, 1992, 1-10.
8. Taymor ML, *Infertility – A Clinician's Guide to Diagnosis and Treatment*, New York, NY: Plenum Medical Book Company, 1990, 12-3.
9. Glover TD, Barratt CLR, Tyler JPP, et al, "Seeking Possible Causes of Dysfunction," *Human Male Fertility and Semen Analysis*, San Diego, CA: Academic Press, 1990, 109.
10. Byrd W, Boldt JP, and Wolf DP, *Guidelines for Human Andrology Laboratories*, Birmingham, AL: The American Fertility Society, 1992, 58:11S.
11. Muller CH, "The Andrology Laboratory in an Assisted Reproductive Technologies Program – Quality Assurance and Laboratory Methodology," *J Androl*, 1992, 13(5):349-60.
12. Liu DY and Baker HWG, "Tests of Human Sperm Function and Fertilization *In Vitro*," *Fertil Steril*, 1992, 58(3):465-83.
13. Gilbert BR, Witkin SS, and Goldstein M, "Correlation of Sperm-Bound Immunoglobulins With Impaired Semen Analysis in Infertile Men With Varicoceles," *Fertil Steril*, 1989, 52(3):469-73.
14. Ohashi K, Saji F, Kato M, et al, "Evaluation of Acrosomal Status Using MH61-Beads Test and Its Clinical Application," *Fertil Steril*, 1992, 58(4):803-8.
15. Glover TD, Barratt CLR, Tyler JPP, et al, *Human Male Fertility and Semen Analysis*, San Diego, CA: Academic Press, 1990, 137-42.
16. Levine RJ, Mathew RM, Brown MH, et al, "Computer-Assisted Semen Analysis: Results Vary Across Technicians Who Prepare Videotapes," *Fertil Steril*, 1989, 52(4):673-7.
17. Aanesen A and Bendvold E, "Studies on Requirements for Trackpoints in CellSoft* Automated Semen Analysis," *Fertil Steril*, 1990, 54(5):910-6.
18. Williams M, Thompson L, Thomlinson M, et al, "Hypertrophy of Technology," *Fertil Steril*, 1990, 54(6):1188-91, (letter).
19. Bartoov B, Ben-Barak J, Mayevsky A, et al, "Sperm Motility Index: A New Parameter for Human Sperm Evaluation," *Fertil Steril*, 1991, 56(1):108-12.
20. Wang C, Leung A, Tsoi W-L, et al, "Computer-Assisted Assessment of Human Sperm Morphology: Comparison With Visual Assessment," *Fertil Steril*, 1991, 55(5):983-8.
21. Kruger TF, DuToit TC, Franken DR, et al, "A New Computerized Method of Reading Sperm Morphology (Strict Criteria) Is as Efficient as Technician Reading," *Fertil Steril*, 1993, 59(1):202-9.
22. Davis RO and Gravance CG, "Standardization of Specimen Preparation, Staining, and Sampling Methods Improves Automated Sperm-Head Morphometry Analysis," *Fertil Steril*, 1993, 59(2):412-7.
23. Aaberg RA, Sauer MV, Sikka S, et al, "Effects of Extracellular Ionized Calcium, Diltiazem and cAMP on Motility of Human Spermatozoa," *J Urol*, 1989, 141(5):1221-4.
24. Smith RG, Johnson A, Lamb D, et al, "Functional Tests of Spermatozoa: Sperm Penetration Assay," *Urol Clin North Am*, 1987, 14:451-8.
25. Marshburn PB, Sloan CS, and Hammond MG, "Semen Quality and Association With Coffee Drinking, Cigarette Smoking, and Ethanol Consumption," *Fertil Steril*, 1989, 52(1):162-5.
26. Bracken MB, Eskenazi B, Sachse K, et al, "Association of Cocaine Use With Sperm Concentration, Motility, and Morphology," *Fertil Steril*, 1990, 53(2):315-22.
27. "Abstracts – Scientific Papers to Be Presented at the Forty-Eighth Annual Meeting of the American Fertility Society, November 2-5, 1992, New Orleans, Louisiana," *Fertil Steril*, 1992, 57:S111.

References

Adelman MM and Cahill EM, *Atlas of Sperm Morphology*, Chicago, IL: ASCP Press, 1989.

Aitken RJ, Ross A, Hargreave T, et al, "Analysis of Human Sperm Function Following Exposure to the Ionophore A23187," *J Androl*, 1984, 5:321-9.

Amso NN and Shaw RW, "A Critical Appraisal of Assisted Reproduction Techniques," *Hum Reprod*, 1993, 8(1):168-74.

Bostofte E, Bagger P, Michael A, et al, "Fertility Prognosis for Infertile Couples," *Fertil Steril*, 1993, 59(1):102-7.

Brinsden PR and Rainsbury PA, *A Textbook of In Vitro* Fertilization and Assisted Reproduction, Park Ridge, NJ: The Parthenon Publishing Group, 1992.

Comhaire FH, "Sperm Antibodies – 'Gold Standard'?" *Fertil Steril*, 1993, 59(1):242-3, (letter).

Damjanov I, "Clinical Evaluation of the Infertile Couple," *Pathology of Infertility*, Chapter 2, St. Louis, MO: Mosby-Year Book Inc, 1993, 7-42.

Green DP, "Mammalian Fertilization as a Biological Machine: A Working Model for Adhesion and Fusion of Sperm and Oocyte," *Hum Reprod*, 1993, 8(1):91-6.

Gwatkin RBL, Collins JA, Jarrell JF, et al, "The Value of Semen Analysis and Sperm Function Assays in Predicting Pregnancy Among Infertile Couples," *Fertil Steril*, 1990, 53(4):693-9.

Haas GG Jr, "Antibody-Mediated Causes of Male Infertility," *Urol Clin North Am*, 1987, 14:539-50.

(Continued)

Infertility Screen *(Continued)*

Haas GG Jr and D'Cruz OJ, "Quantitation of Immunoglobulin G on Human Sperm," *Am J Reprod Immunol*, 1989, 20(2):37-43.

Hamamah S, Seguin F, Barthelemy C, et al, "[1]H Nuclear Magnetic Resonance Studies of Seminal Plasma From Fertile and Infertile Men," *J Reprod Fertil*, 1993, 97(1):51-5.

Hellstrom WJG, Overstreet IW, Samuels SJ, et al, "The Relationship of Circulating Antisperm Antibodies to Sperm Surface Antibodies in Infertile Men," *J Urol*, 1988, 140:1039-44.

Kjeldsberg CR and Knight JA, *Body Fluids: Laboratory Examination of Amniotic, Cerebrospinal, Seminal, Serous, and Synovial Fluids*, 3rd ed, Chicago, IL: ASCP Press, 1993, 255-64, 344-66.

Lähteenmäki A, "*In-Vitro* Fertilization in the Presence of Antisperm Antibodies Detected by the Mixed Antiglobulin Reaction (MAR) and the Tray Agglutination Test (TAT)," *Hum Reprod*, 1993, 8(1):84-8.

Liu DY and Baker HWG, "Morphology of Spermatozoa Bound to the Zona Pellucida of Human Oocytes That Failed to Fertilize *In Vitro*," *J Reprod Fertil*, 1992, 94(1):71-84.

Mackenna A, Barratt CLR, Kessopoulou E, et al, "The Contribution of a Hidden Male Factor to Unexplained Infertility," *Fertil Steril*, 1993, 59(2):405-11.

McClure RD, Tom RA, Watkins M, et al, "SpermCheck®: A Simplified Screening Assay for Immunological Infertility," *Fertil Steril*, 1989, 52(4):650-4.

McLendon WW, "The American Fertility Society – College of American Pathologists Collaborative Program for Accreditation of *In Vitro* Fertilization Laboratories: Building Bridges to Enhance Patient Care," *Arch Pathol Lab Med*, 1992, 116(4):317-8, (editorial).

Menge AC and Beitner O, "Interrelationships Among Semen Characteristics, Antisperm Antibodies, and Cervical Mucus Penetration Assays in Infertile Human Couples," *Fertil Steril*, 1989, 51(3):486-92.

Mortimer D, "The Male Factor in Infertility – Part I: Semen Analysis," *Current Problems in Obstetrics, Gynecology, and Fertility*, Chicago, IL: Year Book Medical Publishers Inc, 1985, 8:1-87.

Nagler HM and Zippe CD, "Varicocele: Current Concepts and Treatment," *Infertility in the Male*, 2nd ed, Chapter 15, Lipshultz LI and Howards SS, eds, St Louis, MO: Mosby-Year Book, 1991, 313-4.

Pedigo NG, Vernon MW, and Curry TE Jr, "Characterization of a Computerized Semen Analysis System," *Fertil Steril*, 1989, 52(4):659-66.

Rousseaux-Prevost R, De Almeida M, Arrar L, et al, "Antibodies to Sperm Basic Nuclear Proteins Detected in Infertile Patients by Dot-Immunobinding Assay and by Enzyme-Linked Immunosorbent Assay," *Am J Reprod Immunol*, 1989, 20(1):17-20.

Shulman S, "Human Sperm Antibodies and Their Detection," *Manual of Clinical Laboratory Immunology*, 3rd ed, Rose NR, Friedman H, and Fahey JL, eds, American Society for Microbiology, 1986, 771-7.

Strasinger SK, *Urinalysis and Body Fluids: A Self-Instructional Text*, Philadelphia, PA: FA Davis Co, 1985, 158-62.

Visscher RD, "Partners in Pursuit of Excellence: Development of an Embryo Laboratory Accreditation Program," *Arch Pathol Lab Med*, 1992, 116(4):318-9, (editorial).

Walker RH and McLendon WW, conference eds, "College of American Pathologists Conference XX on New Developments in Reproductive Biology: Foreward, August 21-23, 1991," *Arch Pathol Lab Med*, 1992, 116:323-43.

***In Vivo* Cervical Mucus Penetration (Postcoital) Test** *see* Sperm Mucus Penetration Test (Human or Bovine Cervical Mucus) *on page 1154*

Iron Stain, Urine *see* Hemosiderin Stain, Urine *on page 1123*

Joint Fluid Analysis *see* Synovial Fluid Analysis *on page 1158*

Ketones, Urine

CPT *81003*

Related Information

Anion Gap *on page 132*
Glucose, 2-Hour Postprandial *on page 237*
Glucose, Quantitative, Urine *on page 1120*
Glucose, Random *on page 240*
Glucose, Semiquantitative, Urine *on page 1121*
Ketone Bodies, Blood *on page 265*
Osmolality, Serum *on page 300*
Reducing Substances, Urine *on page 1150*
Urinalysis *on page 1162*
Volatile Screen *on page 1010*

Synonyms Nitroprusside Reaction for Ketones, Urine; Urine Ketones

Applies to Acetoacetic Acid, Urine; Acetone, Semiquantitative, Urine; Beta-Hydroxybutyric Acid, Urine

Specimen Random urine **CONTAINER:** Plastic urine container **STORAGE INSTRUCTIONS:** If sample cannot be tested immediately, it should be refrigerated. **SPECIAL INSTRUCTIONS:** Transport specimen to the laboratory promptly following collection.

Interpretive REFERENCE RANGE: Negative; in starvation diets or in other instances of abnormal carbohydrate metabolism, ketones appear in the urine in excessively large amounts before serum ketones are elevated USE: Semiquantitative test to evaluate ketonuria, detect acidosis, ketoacidosis of alcoholism and diabetes mellitus, fasting, starvation, high protein diets, and isopropanol ingestion. Remains useful as a monitor in known diabetics, in type I patients when ill and during marked hyperglycemia and in type II diabetics during acute illness. In pregnancy, the risk of ketosis is increased; all pregnant type I diabetics are advised to monitor urine for ketosis in first morning urine and when blood glucose is >150 mg/dL.[1] LIMITATIONS: Specimens containing large amounts of ascorbic acid or levodopa metabolites, valproic acid, phenazopyridine (Pyridium®), PSP dye, phenylketones, or phthalein compounds such as are administered for liver and kidney function tests may cause false-positives. Beta-hydroxybutyric acid (the third of the three ketone bodies) is not detected. N-acetylcysteine causes false-positive ketone results.[2] METHODOLOGY: Nitroprusside reaction, Ketostix® or Acetest®; acetoacetic acid and acetone react with nitroprusside to create a color change, especially the former. ADDITIONAL INFORMATION: In infants and children, ketonuria can occur with febrile illnesses, toxic states with marked vomiting or diarrhea. Genetic disorders resulting in ketonuria include propionyl CoA carboxylase deficiency, glycogen storage disease, branched chain ketonuria and methylmalonic aciduria. In adult healthy men, a fast of 18 hours or greater produces ketonemia at a level that would result in detectable ketonuria. Aging is associated with increased susceptibility to fasting-induced hyperketonemia.[3] Ketonuria may be noted in normal pregnancy.[4] Acetoacetic acid, beta-hydroxybutyric acid, and acetone are ketone bodies. In ketosis, usually 80% of total ketones are beta-hydroxybutyric acid. Acetoacetic acid comprises most of the remainder with acetone present in trace amounts. Urine ketones should generally be determined in patients with a positive urine test for urine glucose and followed during the management of diabetes mellitus and ketoacidosis.

Footnotes

1. Singer DE, Coley CM, Samet JH, et al, "Tests of Glycemia in Diabetes Mellitus – Their Use in Establishing a Diagnosis and in Treatment," *Ann Intern Med*, 1989, 110(2):125-37.
2. Poon R, Hinberg I, and Peterson RG, "N-Acetylcysteine Causes False-Positive Ketone Results With Urinary Dipsticks," *Clin Chem*, 1990, 36(5):818-9, (letter).
3. London ED, Margolin RA, Duara R, et al, "Effects of Fasting on Ketone Body Concentrations in Healthy Men of Different Ages," *J Gerontol* 1986, 41:599-604.
4. Chez RA and Curcio FD, 3d, "Ketonuria in Normal Pregnancy," *Obstet Gynecol*, 1987, 69:272-4.

References

Foster DW, "From Glycogen to Ketones and Back," *Diabetes*, 1984, 33:1188-99.
McGarry JD, "New Perspectives in the Regulation of Ketogenesis," *Diabetes*, 1979, 28:517-23.

Kidney Stone Analysis

***CPT** 82355 (qualitative chemical); 82360 (quantitative chemical); 82365 (infrared spectroscopy); 82370 (x-ray diffraction)*

Related Information

Alkaline Phosphatase, Serum *on page 109*
Blood, Urine *on page 1112*
Calcium, Ionized *on page 159*
Calcium, Serum *on page 160*
Calcium, Urine *on page 163*
Carbon Dioxide, Blood *on page 165*
Chloride, Serum *on page 182*
Creatinine Clearance *on page 201*
Creatinine, Serum *on page 202*
Cystine, Qualitative *on page 205*
Electrolytes, Blood *on page 212*
Electrolytes, Urine *on page 213*
Oxalate, Urine *on page 303*
Parathyroid Hormone *on page 311*
Phosphorus, Serum *on page 319*
Phosphorus, Urine *on page 322*
pH, Urine *on page 1144*
Potassium, Urine *on page 332*
Sodium, Urine *on page 351*
Thyroxine *on page 364*
(Continued)

Kidney Stone Analysis *(Continued)*

Urea Nitrogen, Blood *on page 376*
Uric Acid, Serum *on page 378*
Uric Acid, Urine *on page 380*
Urinalysis *on page 1162*
Urine Culture, Clean Catch *on page 881*
Vitamin D_3, Serum *on page 387*

Synonyms Calculus Analysis; Nephrolithiasis Analysis; Renal Calculus Analysis; Stone Analysis

Test Commonly Includes Analysis for calcium, carbonate, cystine, magnesium, oxalate, phosphates, and urates

Abstract Passage of a stone in the urinary tract is usually accompanied by hematuria and abrupt, severe, constant pain (acute renal colic). Infection may occur. About 80% of renal stones are calcium oxalate, of which about 30% include calcium phosphate (apatite); 10% are uric acid stones; only 1% are cystine; 15% to 17% are struvite (ammoniomagnesium phosphate).

Specimen Kidney stones **CONTAINER:** Glass bottle or plastic urine container **COLLECTION:** Specimen should be washed free of tissue and blood, and submitted in a clean, dry container. If necessary, urine should be filtered to recover gravel or stone. **STORAGE INSTRUCTIONS:** Do **not** apply any tape to stones. Adhesives interfere with infrared spectroscopy. **CAUSES FOR REJECTION:** Insufficient stone volume for complete analysis **TURNAROUND TIME:** Several days **SPECIAL INSTRUCTIONS:** Specify source of stone on requisition. Urinalysis can provide useful information including detection of crystalluria and presence of red blood cells. Urine culture is often indicated.

Interpretive USE: Evaluate stone composition; work up nephrolithiasis **LIMITATIONS:** Chemical analysis is generally available in most laboratories while x-ray diffraction and infrared spectroscopy are reference laboratory procedures. The relative merits of stone analysis techniques are subject to debate. Chemical analysis is less costly, more readily available, and is reported to correlate well with the more sophisticated techniques.[1] Chemical analysis requires 5 mg of stone. X-ray diffraction is able to separately determine the composition of the nidus as well as the major portion of the stone. **METHODOLOGY:** Chemical analysis, infrared spectroscopy, x-ray diffraction analysis, crystallographic analysis **ADDITIONAL INFORMATION: Twenty-four hour urine collections** for creatinine clearance, uric acid, oxalate, calcium, sodium, and phosphate should be delayed. Urine uric acid excretion reflects purine intake, usually from meats. Phosphate excretion reflects meat and dairy intake primarily. Sulfates reflect meat intake. Urine calcium is correlated with urine sulfate and urine sodium, giving clues to treatment. **Urine culture is needed.** Urine nitroprusside (for cystinuria), urine volume, and fasting morning urine pH (with electrolytes, for renal tubular acidosis) may be indicated.

Obtain a **serum chemistry panel** which includes calcium (for hyperparathyroidism), phosphorus, alkaline phosphatase (for Paget's disease of bone), uric acid, BUN, and creatinine. Serum sodium, potassium, chloride, and CO_2, and parathormone (PTH) levels, if indicated, may be useful additional investigations.

Cystinuria and xanthinuria are rare causes of renal calculi. See Cystine, Qualitative in the Chemistry chapter. Other uncommon causes of renal stones are sarcoidosis, Cushing's syndrome, excessive calcium or vitamin D ingestion, steroids, immobilization, bone disease, Paget's disease of bone, hyperthyroidism. An increasing but still low rate of triamterene stones has been noted.[2] Most calcium stones relate to idiopathic hypercalciuria and hyperuricosuria, which may coexist. Hyperoxaluria may also be a factor to be evaluated.[3] Males are two to three times more likely to develop stones than females. Whites are three to four times as likely as blacks to develop stones.[4] For a recent and comprehensive classification and review of nephrolithiasis, see paper by Coe and Favus.[5]

In subjects with hypercalciuria, it has been the practice in the past to restrict calcium intake, even though prospective studies had not established the efficacy of such advice. Many clinicians abandoned this approach except for those patients with obviously excessive calcium intakes. Currently, a higher intake of calcium is reported to be associated with a reduced risk of nephrolithiasis. Such inverse relationship between dietary calcium and kidney stone is probably caused by increased binding of oxalate by ingested calcium.[6] Urinary oxalate excretion falls by 1.1-1.8 mg/day for each increase of 100 mg in calcium ingestion.[7] The risk of calcium nephrolithiasis is related to the free ion concentration product of oxalate and calcium.

There are many urinary constituents which can complex calcium, but only calcium complexes and precipitates with oxalate. Potassium and fluid intake are also associated with reduced risk, but intake of animal protein is directly related to risk of kidney stones,[6] probably because sulfated amino acids increase calciuria.

Footnotes

1. Moriss RH, Bedir MF, and Freeman JA, *Urinary Stone Analysis in Laboratory Medicine/Urinalysis and Medical Microscopy*, 2nd ed, Philadelphia, PA: Lea & Febiger, 1983, 341-4.
2. Carr MC, Prien EL Jr, and Babayan RK, "Triamterene Nephrolithiasis: Renewed Attention Is Warranted," *J Urol*, 1990, 144(6):1339-40.
3. Robertson WG and Peacock M, "The Cause of Idiopathic Calcium Stone Disease: Hypercalciuria or Hyperoxaluria?" *Nephron*, 1980, 26:105-10.
4. Sarmina I, Spirnak JP, and Resnick MI, "Urinary Lithiasis in the Black Population: An Epidemiologic Study and Review of the Literature," *J Urol*, 1987, 138:14-7.
5. Coe FL and Favus MJ, "Nephrolithiasis," *Kidney*, Brenner BM and Rector FC, eds, Philadelphia, PA: WB Saunders Co, 1991, 1728-67.
6. Curhan GC, Willett WC, Rimm EB, et al, "A Prospective Study of Dietary Calcium and Other Nutrients and the Risk of Symptomatic Kidney Stones," *N Engl J Med*, 1993, 328(12):833-8.
7. Lemann J Jr, "Composition of the Diet and Calcium Kidney Stones," *N Engl J Med*, 1993, 328(12):880-2.

References

O'Brien WM, Rotolo JE, and Pahire JJ, "New Approaches in the Treatment of Renal Calculi," *Am Fam Physician*, 1987, 36:181-94.

Pak CY, "Medical Management of Nephrolithiasis in Dallas," *J Urol*, 1988, 140:461-7.

Preminger GM, "The Metabolic Evaluation of Patients With Recurrent Nephrolithiasis: A Review of Comprehensive and Simplified Approaches," *J Urol*, 1989, 141(3 Pt 2):760-3.

Shortliffe LM and Spigelman SS, "Infection Stones. Evaluation and Management." *Urol Clin North Am*, 1986, 13:717-26, (review).

Westbury EJ, "A Chemist's View of the History of Urinary Stone Analysis," *Br J Urol*, 1989, 64(5):445-50.

Ziyadeh FN and Goldfarb S, "XII Nephrolithiasis," *Sci Am*, 1993, 1-10.

Knee Fluid Analysis *see* Synovial Fluid Analysis *on page 1158*

Leukocyte Esterase, Urine

***CPT** 81003*

Related Information

Nitrite, Urine *on page 1137*
Urinalysis *on page 1162*
Urine Culture, Clean Catch *on page 881*

Synonyms Bacteria Screen, Urine; Esterase, Leukocyte, Urine

Test Commonly Includes Screening of urine for leukocyte esterase activity by dipstick, frequently a part of urinalysis

Abstract A rapid indirect test for detection of bacteriuria. It is a surrogate indicator for the presence of intact or lysed neutrophils.

Specimen Random clean catch urine; preferably midstream, clean catch collection **CONTAINER:** Plastic urine container **STORAGE INSTRUCTIONS:** If the specimen cannot be processed within 2 hours, it should be refrigerated. **CAUSES FOR REJECTION:** Improper labeling, specimen not refrigerated

Interpretive **REFERENCE RANGE:** Negative **USE:** Detect leukocytes in urine. It will detect either intact or lysed white blood cells and therefore can be positive when WBCs are not found on microscopic examination. The lysis of leukocytes that occurs when urine is allowed to stand intensifies the color reaction from release of esterase. It has been used to screen for urinary tract infections or, in males, urethritis. **LIMITATIONS:** False-positives may occur in specimens contaminated with vaginal secretions. Cephalexin, cephalothin or large amounts of oxalic acid (eg, iced tea drinkers) may lead to decreases. High glucose or specific gravity may lead to decreased results. The false-negative rate is low, but sensitivity decreases with urinary tract infections characterized by 10^3-10^4 colony forming units/mL. Albumin and ascorbic acid inhibit the method. Tetracycline may cause decreased reactivity or false-negatives. Neutropenia can cause false-negative results. Leukocyte esterase is unacceptable as a screen unless combined at least with nitrite testing. Leukocyte esterase, even combined with nitrite, should not replace microscopy and culture in symptomatic patients. Urine culture is indicated for subjects with symptoms of urinary tract infection. False-positive results from trichomonads have been controversial. **METHODOLOGY:** Indoxyl is released by leukocyte esterase if present in the urine specimen. The substrate on the strip is indoxyl carbonic acid ester. Indoxyl is oxidized

(Continued)

Leukocyte Esterase, Urine *(Continued)*

by atmospheric oxygen to indigo blue. The reaction time is 1 minute, but high sensitivity requires interpretation 5 minutes after immersion in the sample.[1] A package insert provides the following: "Granulocytic leukocytes contain esterases that catalyze the hydrolysis of the derivatized pyrrole amino acid ester to liberate 3-hydroxy-5-phenyl pyrrole. This pyrrole then reacts with a diazonium salt to produce a purple product," copyright Miles Inc. **ADDITIONAL INFORMATION:** Some institutions now perform microscopic urinalysis only on specific request or on the observation of an abnormal macroscopic finding. The principal advantage of the method is the ability to identify the presence of leukocyte esterase in dilute urine specimens and in specimens which have been subject to standing with lysis of the white cells. When combined with the nitrite test, it provides sensitivity for both tests of up to 85% and specificity of 65%, for infections with 10^5 colony forming units/mL. Of 750 obstetric patients, five had negative screening tests and positive cultures, each a gram-positive organism.[2] Some laboratories have established a screening protocol in which culture is only performed if screening with leukocyte esterase or nitrate is positive. Dipstick screening has been compared to Gram stains of unspun urine[3] and to urine sediment microscopy[4,5,6,7] and culture.[6,8] Some publications conclude that a role exists for screening without sediment microscopy on all urines. For instance, a 1988 proposal indicates that for screening, a clear yellow specimen negative for blood, leukocyte esterase, nitrite and with $\leq$30 mg/dL (SI: $\leq$0.3 g/L) of protein does not require microscopy, but even such samples should be examined by microscopy when from symptomatic subjects or persons with known renal disease.[7] Goldsmith and Campos found the leukocyte esterase comparable to urine sediment microscopy when negative but not positive with predictive accuracy for urines in the range of 10^4-10^5 bacteria/mL.[9] Others would not do away with urine microscopy based on normal dipstick tests.[10,11,12] Sensitivity and specificity of leukocyte esterase and nitrite screening have been criticized.[13] Leukocyte esterase has been used for detection of sexually transmitted disease.[14,15]

Footnotes

1. Shaw ST, Poon SY, and Wong ET, "Routine Urinalysis, Is the Dipstick Enough?" *JAMA*, 1985, 253:1596-1600.
2. Robertson AW and Duff P, "The Nitrite and Leukocyte Esterase Tests for the Evaluation of Asymptomatic Bacteriuria in Obstetric Patients," *Obstet Gynecol*, 1988, 71(6 Pt 1):878-81.
3. Sewell DL, Burt SP, Gabbert NJ, et al, "Evaluation of the Chemstrip 9™ as a Screening Test for Urinalysis and Urine Culture in Men," *Am J Clin Pathol*, 1985, 83:740-3.
4. Scheer WD, "The Detection of Leukocyte Esterase Activity in Urine With a New Reagent Strip," *Am J Clin Pathol*, 1987, 87:86-93.
5. Hamoudi AC, Bubis SC, and Thompson C, "Can the Cost Savings of Eliminating Urine Microscopy in Biochemically Negative Urines Be Extended to the Pediatric Population?" *Am J Clin Pathol*, 1986, 86:658-60.
6. Loo SY, Scottolini AG, Luangphinith S, et al, "Performance of a Urine Screening Protocol," *Am J Clin Pathol*, 1986, 85:479-84.
7. High SR, Rowe JA, and Maksem JA, "Macroscopic Physiochemical Testing for Screening Urinalysis," *Lab Med*, 1988, 19:174-6.
8. Gutman SI and Solomon RR, "The Clinical Significance of Dipstick-Negative, Culture-Positive Urines in a Veterans Population," *Am J Clin Pathol*, 1987, 88:204-9.
9. Goldsmith BM and Campos JM, "Comparison of Urine Dipstick, Microscopy, and Culture for the Detection of Bacteriuria in Children," *Clin Pediatr (Phila)*, 1990, 29(4):214-8.
10. Morrison MC and Lum G, "Dipstick Testing of Urine – Can It Replace Urine Microscopy?" *Am J Clin Pathol*, 1986, 85:590-4.
11. Nanji AA, Adam W, and Campbell DJ, "Routine Microscopic Examination of the Urine Sediment," *Arch Pathol Lab Med*, 1984, 108:399-400.
12. Propp DA, Weber D, and Ciesla ML, "Reliability of a Urine Dipstick in Emergency Department Patients," *Ann Emerg Med*, 1989, 18(5):560-3.
13. Wilkins EG, Ratcliffe JG, and Roberts C, "Leukocyte Esterase-Nitrite Screening Method for Pyuria and Bacteriuria," *J Clin Pathol*, 1985, 38:1342-5.
14. Sadof MD, Woods ER, and Emans SJ, "Dipstick Leukocyte Esterase Activity in First-Catch Urine Specimens: A Useful Screening Test for Detecting Sexually Transmitted Disease in the Adolescent Male," *JAMA*, 1987, 258:1932-4.
15. Shafer MA, Schacter J, Moscicki AB, et al, "Urinary Leukocyte Esterase Screening Test for Asymptomatic Chlamydial and Gonococcal Infections in Males," *JAMA*, 1989, 262(18):2562-6.

References

Hoffman GC, Green R, and Edinger CA, "Predicting a Positive Microscopic Examination of Urine," *Am J Clin Pathol*, 1990, 93(2):302-3.

Hurlbut TA, 3d and Littenberg B, "The Diagnostic Accuracy of Rapid Dipstick Tests to Predict Urinary Tract Infection," *Am J Clin Pathol*, 1991, 96(5):582-8.

Kusumi RK, Grover PJ, and Kunin CM, "Rapid Detection of Pyuria by Leukocyte Esterase Activity," *JAMA*, 1981, 245:1653-5.

Lachs MS, Nachamkin I, Edelstein PH, et al, "Spectrum Bias in the Evaluation of Diagnostic Tests: Lessons From the Rapid Dipstick Test for Urinary Tract Infection," *Ann Intern Med*, 1992, 117(2):135-40.

Leighton PM and Little JA, "Leukocyte Esterase Determination as a Secondary Procedure for Urine Screening," *J Clin Pathol*, 1985, 38:229-32.

Romero R, Emamian M, Wan M, et al, "The Value of the Leukocyte Esterase Test in Diagnosing Intra-Amniotic Infection," *Am J Perinatol*, 1988, 5:64-9.

Smalley DL, Kraus AP, and Baddour LM, "Clinical Use of the Leukocyte Esterase Test in Continuous Ambulatory Peritoneal Dialysis," *Lab Med*, 1988, 19:164-6.

White LV and Kunin CM, "Leukocyte Esterase Tests Detect Pyuria, Not Bacteriuria," *Ann Intern Med*, 1993, 118(3):230, (letter).

Yager HM and Harrington JT, "Urinalysis and Urinary Electrolytes," *The Principles and Practice of Nephrology*, Chapter 28, Jacobson HR, Striker GE, and Klahr S, eds, Philadelphia, PA: BC Decker Inc, 1992, 167-77.

Lipid, Urine *see* Fat, Urine *on page 1119*

Meat Fibers, Stool

CPT 89160

Related Information

Fat, Semiquantitative, Stool *on page 1118*
Fecal Fat, Quantitative, 72-Hour Collection *on page 219*
Reducing Substances, Stool *on page 1149*

Synonyms Muscle Fiber, Stool

Abstract A simple, low cost, nonspecific screen for malabsorption/pancreatic insufficiency

Patient Care **PREPARATION:** Patient is required to eat adequate amounts of red meat for 24-72 hours before testing. Specimens obtained with a warm saline enema or Fleet Phospho®-Soda are acceptable. Specimens obtained with mineral oil, bismuth, or magnesium compounds are unsatisfactory. Barium procedures or laxatives should be avoided for 1 week prior to collection of the specimen.

Specimen Stool **CONTAINER:** Plastic stool container **CAUSES FOR REJECTION:** Purgatives other than saline or Fleet®

Interpretive **REFERENCE RANGE:** Negative for muscle fibers **USE:** Evaluate malabsorption syndromes, pancreatic exocrine dysfunction, or gastrocolic fistula **METHODOLOGY:** Stool is mixed with a 10% solution of eosin in ethanol, stained on a slide for 3 minutes and coverslipped. Only rectangular-shaped fibers with identifiable cross striations are counted. **ADDITIONAL INFORMATION:** The presence of undigested muscle fibers in patient's stool implies impaired intraluminal digestion. There is good correlation with stool fat determinations. Study of stool for muscle fibers when a high meat intake has been maintained is a good and inexpensive but necessarily nonspecific test for malabsorption. The finding of fecal muscle fibers cannot differentiate pancreatic insufficiency from other causes of malabsorption.[1] More sophisticated tests of pancreatic exocrine function (secreting ability) include the pancreozymin secretin test, cerulein secretin test, NBT-PABA test, and pancreatic dual-label Schilling test.[2] Muscle fibers reported as present in urine are suggestive of fecal contamination of the specimen.[3]

Footnotes

1. Moore JG, Englert E Jr, Bigler AH, et al, "Simple Fecal Tests of Absorption – A Prospective Study and Critique," *Am J Dig Dis*, 1971, 16:97-105.
2. Chen WL, Morishita R, Eguchi T, et al, "Clinical Usefulness of Dual-Label Schilling Test for Pancreatic Exocrine Function," *Gastroenterology*, 1989, 96(5 Pt 1):1337-45.
3. Graff L Sr, *A Handbook of Routine Urinalysis*, Philadelphia, PA: JB Lippincott Co, 1982, 125.

References

Arvanitakis C and Cooke R, "Diagnostic Tests of Exocrine Pancreatic Function and Disease," *Gastroenterology*, 1978, 74:932-48.

Greenberger NJ and Isselbacher KJ, "Disorders of Absorption," Wilson JD, Braunwald E, Isselbacher KJ, et al, eds, *Harrison's Principles of Internal Medicine*, 12th ed, New York, NY: McGraw-Hill Inc, 1991, 1370, 1372.

Kao YS and Liu FJ, "Laboratory Diagnosis of Gastrointestinal Tract and Exocrine Pancreatic Disorders," *Clinical Diagnosis and Management by Laboratory Methods*, Chapter 23, Henry JB, ed, Philadelphia, PA: WB Saunders Co, 1991, 541.

Lankisch PG, Brauneis J, Otto J, et al, "Pancreolauryl and NBT-PABA Tests: Are Serum Tests More Practicable Alternatives to Urine Tests in the Diagnosis of Exocrine Pancreatic Insufficiency?" *Gastroenterology*, 1986, 90:350-4.

Microalbuminuria

CPT 82043 (quantitative); 82044 (semiquantitative)

Related Information

Glucose, 2-Hour Postprandial *on page 237*
Glucose, Fasting *on page 238*
Glycated Hemoglobin *on page 244*
Protein Electrophoresis, Urine *on page 737*
Protein, Quantitative, Urine *on page 1145*
Protein, Semiquantitative, Urine *on page 1147*
Urinalysis *on page 1162*

Test Commonly Includes Creatinine clearance may be advised from the same urine collection.

Abstract Test for early increase of proteinuria in diabetes and in pre-eclampsia, before proteinuria becomes evident by conventional urinalysis. "Microalbuminuria" is defined as albuminuria of 30-300 mg/24 hours.

Specimen 24-hour urine, timed overnight 10-hour collection, or spot AM urine after initial voiding **CONTAINER:** Plastic urine container **COLLECTION:** Instruct patient to void at 8 AM and discard the specimen. Then collect all urine including the final specimen voided at the end of the 24-hour collection period (ie, 8 AM the next morning). Label the container with the patient's name and date and time collection started and finished. **TURNAROUND TIME:** Commonly sent to reference laboratory

Interpretive **REFERENCE RANGE:** <20 mg/L (SI: <0.02 g/L) or ≤30 mg/24 hours (SI: ≤0.03 g/day). For spot AM samples, <.03 mg albumin/mg[1] creatinine **USE:** Attempted prediction of subsequent development of proteinuria, diabetic nephropathy, and early mortality in type I and/or II diabetes.[2,3]. This test may prove useful in the management of patients with relatively early diabetes mellitus to try to avoid or delay the onset of diabetic renal disease. Detect albuminuria in hypertension and systemic lupus erythematosus. **LIMITATIONS:** The appropriate clinical use of this test is still being determined. **METHODOLOGY:** Radioimmunoassay (RIA)[2], radial immunodiffusion (RID), enzyme-linked immunosorbent assay (ELISA), immunoturbidimetric methods.[4] Nephelometric and latex particle methods are described. For spot AM sample, determine simultaneous urine creatinine. **ADDITIONAL INFORMATION:** Normal albuminuria is <20 mg/L, much lower than the sensitivity of current urinalysis with dipstick (150-300 mg/L). Albumin:creatinine ratio ≥3.5 predicts an albumin excretion rate ≥30 μg/minute. A test strip for low concentrations of albumin in urine has been developed ("Micral-Test") and tested.[5] In insulin-dependent diabetes mellitus, detectable diabetic nephropathy begins with onset of microalbuminuria, 30-300 mg albumin in 24 hours. Such microalbuminuria may begin 5 years from onset of diabetes mellitus. The risk of cardiovascular disease is 30-40 times greater in those with nephropathy.[6]

Footnotes

1. Ellis D, Coonrod BA, Dorman JS, et al, "Choice of Urine Sample Predictive of Microalbuminuria in Patients With Insulin-Dependent Diabetes Mellitus," *Am J Kidney Dis*, 1989, 13(4):321-8.
2. Mogensen CE, "Microalbuminuria Predicts Clinical Proteinuria and Early Mortality in Maturity-Onset Diabetes," *N Engl J Med*, 1984, 310:356-60.
3. Gambino R, "Microalbuminuria and Renal Hyperfiltration," *Lab Report for Physicians*, 1984, 8:57-61.
4. Hindmarsh JT, "Microalbuminuria" *Clin Lab Med*, 1988, 8(3):611-6.
5. Jury DR, Mikkelsen DJ, Glen D, et al, "Assessment of Micral-Test Microalbuminuria Test Strip in the Laboratory and in Diabetic Outpatients," *Ann Clin Biochem*, 1992, 29(Pt 1):96-100.
6. Nathan, DM,"Long-Term Complications of Diabetes Mellitus," *N Engl J Med*, 1993, 328(23):1676-85.

References

Chase HP, Jackson WE, Hoops SL, et al, "Glucose Control and the Renal and Retinal Complications of Insulin-Dependent Diabetes," *JAMA*, 1989, 261(8):1155-60.

Chavers BM, Bilous RW, Ellis EN, et al, "Glomerular Lesions and Urinary Albumin Excretion in Type 1 Diabetes Without Overt Proteinuria," *N Engl J Med*, 1989, 320(15):966-70.

Shihabi ZK, Konen JC, and O'Connor ML, "Albuminuria vs Urinary Total Protein for Detecting Chronic Renal Disorders," *Clin Chem*, 1991, 37(5):621-4.

Townsend JC, "Increased Albumin Excretion in Diabetes," *J Clin Pathol*, 1990, 43(1):3-8.

Mucin Clot Test

CPT 83872

Synonyms Synovial Fluid Mucin Clot Test; Synovial Fluid Ropes Test; Synovial Fluid Viscosity

Applies to Synovial Fluid Hyaluronate Concentration

Abstract Qualitative test for the nature of hyaluronic acid in synovial fluid. In rheumatoid arthritis, clot is friable. This test lacks specificity.

Specimen Synovial fluid **CONTAINER:** Sterile tube or lavender top (EDTA) tube; avoid oxalate anticoagulants. **STORAGE INSTRUCTIONS:** Refrigerate if there is delay in analysis.

Interpretive **REFERENCE RANGE:** Mucin clot – positive (firm clot) **USE:** Useful in the differential diagnosis of joint disease. Findings are somewhat nonspecific and alone are not diagnostic of a single pathologic entity. **LIMITATIONS:** Results should be assessed with other cellular, chemical, and microscopic joint fluid characteristics as the mucin clot test lacks specificity (ie, not indicative of a single entity). Sibley et al[1] have argued that the mucin clot test should be excluded from the 11 criteria of rheumatoid arthritis by American Rheumatism Association. They feel the low specificity (49%) and positive predictive value (52%) make the test of little value. **METHODOLOGY:** Evaluate clot formed on reaction of synovial fluid with acetic acid. Quality of the clot may be graded as "good", "fair", or "poor". This test reflects the physical chemical status of hyaluronic acid in a qualitative manner. Inflammation degrades the quality of the mucin clot. Viscosity relates to mucin hyaluronate content and also can be evaluated by the quality of the string produced. Normal (noninflammatory) fluids produce long strings. Inflammatory fluids (low viscosity) produce short strings. **ADDITIONAL INFORMATION:** In osteoarthritis the clot is firm and the surrounding fluid remains clear even after agitation. In rheumatoid arthritis the clot is friable and the surrounding fluid is turbid. In acute rheumatic fever the clot is firm, and in lupus erythematosus the clot is firm (ie, normal). Synovial fluid hyaluronate concentration and degree of polymerization as determined by a high performance liquid chromatography (HPLC) procedure has been found to correlate with quality of the mucin clot.[2] It was considered that rheumatology units with HPLC analytic capability could use the more reproducible HPLC determinations to replace older mucin clot test/synovial fluid viscosity studies.

Footnotes

1. Sibley JT, Harth M, and Burns DE, "The Mucin Clot Test and the Synovial Fluid Rheumatoid Factor as Diagnostic Criteria in Rheumatoid Arthritis," *J Rheumatol*, 1983, 10:889-93.
2. Saari H and Konttinen YT, "Determination of Synovial Fluid Hyaluronate Concentration and Polymerisation by High Performance Liquid Chromatography," *Ann Rheum Dis*, 1989, 48(7):565-70.

References

Cheek KK and Neely AE, "Synovial Fluid," *Textbook of Urinalysis and Body Fluids*, Ross DL and Neely AE, eds, Norwalk, CT: Appleton-Century-Crofts, 1983, 253-66.

Krieg AF and Kjeldsberg CR, "Cerebrospinal Fluid and Other Body Fluids," *Clinical Diagnosis and Management by Laboratory Methods*, Chapter 18, Henry JB, ed, Philadelphia, PA: WB Saunders Co, 1991, 461.

McCarty DJ, ed, *Arthritis and Allied Conditions: A Textbook of Rheumatology*, 9th ed, Philadelphia, PA: Lea & Febiger, 1979.

Mucin Test for Hyaluronic Acid *see* Synovial Fluid Analysis *on page 1158*

Muscle Fiber, Stool *see* Meat Fibers, Stool *on page 1133*

Myoglobin, Qualitative, Urine

CPT 83874

Related Information

Blood, Urine *on page 1112*
Cocaine (Cocaine Metabolite), Qualitative, Urine *on page 955*
Coccidioidomycosis Antibodies *on page 664*
Creatine Kinase *on page 196*
Hemoglobin, Qualitative, Urine *on page 1122*
Muscle Biopsy *on page 75*
Myoglobin, Blood *on page 293*
Troponin *on page 375*

Synonyms Myoglobin Screen, Urine

Specimen Random urine **CONTAINER:** Clean, chemical-free, plastic (preferable) urine container

Interpretive **REFERENCE RANGE:** Negative **USE:** Determine the presence of myoglobinuria; investigate myositis and other entities which damage muscle. See table. **LIMITATIONS:** Urine tests for myoglobin may not be reliable. Presence of hypochlorite or microbial peroxidase or other oxidizing contaminants may cause false-positive reactions. Presence of ascorbic acid (high concentrations) may decrease sensitivity.[1] Serum testing is recommended. **METHODOLOGY:** Qualitative or screening methods are based on the oxidation of a chromogen (eg, orthotoluidine) with production of a colored compound. This reaction is catalyzed by hemoglobin or myoglobin. Test sensitivity is about 0.3 mg/dL (SI: 3 mg/L).[2] Specificity for myoglobin can be obtained by the ammonium sulfate test.[2] If initial testing is positive for blood (or myoglobin), preparation of an 80% saturated urine solution of ammonium sulfate will precipitate hemoglo-

(Continued)

Myoglobin, Qualitative, Urine *(Continued)*

Causes of Myoglobinuria

Metabolic — impaired substrate utilization for energy metabolism	Enzyme deficiencies (LD and others), substrate deficiency, hypokalemia, hypophosphatemia, hypomagnesemia
Excessive muscle use	Severe/unaccustomed exercise, seizures, march hemoglobinuria with myoglobinuria
Hyperpyrexia	Heat stroke, exertional hyperthermia, hyperthermia associated with drug use (eg, cocaine), heat injury
Postinfections	
viral	Influenza A, herpes simplex, Epstein-Barr, coxsackie
bacterial	Fever and sepsis, clostridial with gangrene
Primary muscle disease	Muscular dystrophy, McArdle's disease, polymyositis, dermatomyositis, familial paroxysmal myoglobinuria
Poisoning	
drug	Carbon monoxide, alcohol, barbiturate, cocaine, amphetamine, phencyclidine, neuroleptic malignant syndrome
animal	Hoff's disease (fish poisoning), sea snake bite (*Enhydrina schistosa*), trichinosis
Ischemia	Arterial occlusion, myocardial infarction, thromboembolism, infarction of large muscle, anterior tibial syndrome
Traumatic	Crush injury, wounds, surgical muscle trauma, beatings, electrocution, limb compression with prolonged immobilization due to sleep or coma

bin. On filtering or centrifugation myoglobin stays in solution. Color in the supernatant indicates presence of myoglobin pigment. Electrophoresis can provide definitive differentiation between hemoglobin and myoglobin. Immunoassays (immunodiffusion (ID), isoelectric focusing (IEF), radioimmunoassay (RIA), immunoprecipitation; immunonephelometric; hemagglutination inhibition (HAI)) can also be used in the determination of myoglobin. **ADDITIONAL INFORMATION:** Myoglobin (MW approximately 17,000) is released from cardiac/skeletal muscle, filtered by renal glomeruli and excreted in the urine. Resultant urine, depending upon the amount of excreted myoglobin varies in hue and intensity of red/brown/black color and is often referred to as cola colored. Myoglobin causes a false-positive reaction for urine hemoglobin on dipsticks. Serum myoglobin is not bound to haptoglobin and has a renal threshold of 2 mg/dL (SI: 20 mg/L). Muscle injury (metabolic or traumatic, see table) releases myoglobin into the circulation from which it is rapidly cleared into the urine.

Myoglobinuria has been associated with renal failure. Renal failure itself may cause high serum myoglobin level.[3] Myoglobinuric renal failure commonly complicates rhabdomyolysis of either traumatic and metabolic origin. The mechanism of renal injury is unknown but does not appear to be solely due to nephrotoxicity of myoglobin. The combined effects of toxic products released in rhabdomyolysis with dehydration, hypotension, and electrolyte imbalance may play a role in pathogenesis of the renal failure. Cases associated with the use of cocaine may develop as a result of cocaine-induced renal artery vasoconstriction, renal ischemia, and tubular damage.[4] Myoglobinuria may occur with myocardial infarction.[5] Myoglobin deposits in the kidney are demonstrable by immunofluorescent techniques.[6] There are a few reports of rhabdomyolysis-induced renal failure occurring in cases of child abuse.[7] Use of neuroleptic agents in individuals with or without predisposing factors (exhaustion, dehydration, others) may result in the neuroleptic malignant syndrome, a hyperpyrexic syndrome that may be fatal,[8] and associated with myoglobinuria. The dark urine color associated with myoglobinuria develops on standing or in the bladder at acid pH.

The pathophysiology of cocaine- (and other drugs of abuse) induced rhabdomyolysis is not clearly established. In addition to presence of serum and urine myoglobin, there is striking increase in serum CK and elevations of LD (LDH), AST (SGOT), and ALT (SGPT). Cocaine blocks presynaptic reuptake of neurotransmitters at postsynaptic receptor sites. In some cases, rhabdomyolysis subsequent to use of cocaine may relate to ischemia of arterial vasoconstriction, to muscle activity associated with dysphoric agitation, and/or to hyperthermia. The most common cause, however, of rhabdomyolysis related to use of abused drugs is limb compression during sleep or coma.[4] Serum CK is usually normal with hemolysis, in which serum LD is generally increased with high LD_1. With circulating myoglobin, serum CK is usually very high, serum LD may be moderately increased, but it is LD_5 that is usually elevated on LD isoenzyme electrophoresis.[9] An isomorphic pattern of LD isoenzymes may also be seen. When no specific cause of rhabdomyolysis is apparent, or when precipitating physical exercise was not extreme, or when CPK does not return to baseline, muscle biopsy with measurement of specific muscle enzymes may be indicated. In 77 such muscle biopsies, enzyme deficiencies were noted in 36 patients.[10]

Footnotes

1. Graff L, "Chemical Examination," *A Handbook of Routine Urinalysis*, Chapter 2, Philadelphia, PA: JB Lippincott Co, 1983, 52-5.
2. Race GJ and White MG, "Urinary Pigments," *Basic Urinalysis*, Chapter 12, Hagerstown, MD: Harper & Row Publishers, 1979, 50-1.
3. Feinfeld DA, Briscoe AM, Nurse HM, et al, "Myoglobinuria in Chronic Renal Failure," *Am J Kidney Dis*, 1986, 8:111-4.
4. Pogue VA and Nurse HM, "Cocaine-Associated Acute Myoglobinuric Renal Failure," *Am J Med*, 1989, 86(2):183-6.
5. Levine RS, Alterman H, Gubner RS, et al, "Myoglobinuria in Myocardial Infarction," *Am J Med Sci*, 1971, 262:179-83.
6. Kagan LJ, "Immunofluorescent Demonstration of Myoglobin in the Kidney," *Am J Med*, 1970, 48:649-53.
7. Mukherji SK and Siegel MJ, "Rhabdomyolysis and Renal Failure in Child Abuse," *AJR*, 1987, 148:1203-4.
8. Guzé BH and Baxter LR Jr, "Neuroleptic Malignant Syndrome," *N Engl J Med*, 1985, 313:163-6.
9. Faulkner WR, "Update on Myoglobinurias," *Lab Report for Physicians*, 1989, 11:91-2.
10. Tonin P, Lewis P, Servidei S, et al, "Metabolic Causes of Myoglobinuria," *Ann Neurol*, 1990, 27(2):181-5.

References

Engel AG, "Disease of Muscle (Myopathies) and Neuromuscular Junction," *Cecil Textbook of Medicine*, Wyngaarden JB and Smith LH Jr, eds, 18th ed, Philadelphia, PA: WB Saunders Co, 1988, 2282-3.

Penn AS, "Myoglobinuria," *Myology*, Engel AG and Banker BQ, eds, New York, NY: McGraw-Hill Inc, 1986, 1785-1803.

Schumann GB and Schweitzer SC, "Examination of Urine," *Clinical Diagnosis and Management by Laboratory Methods*, Chapter 17, Henry JB, ed, Philadelphia, PA: WB Saunders Co, 1991, 410-2.

Myoglobin Screen, Urine *see* Myoglobin, Qualitative, Urine *on page 1135*

Nephrolithiasis Analysis *see* Kidney Stone Analysis *on page 1129*

Neutral Fat, Stool *see* Fat, Semiquantitative, Stool *on page 1118*

Nitrite, Urine

***CPT** 81003*

Related Information

Leukocyte Esterase, Urine *on page 1131*
Urinalysis *on page 1162*
Urine Culture, Clean Catch *on page 881*

Synonyms Bacteria Screen, Urine

Applies to Urinary Tract Infection Screen; UTI Screen

Test Commonly Includes This test is usually part of a routine urinalysis.

Abstract A rapid method for detection of bacteriuria, reacting with those bacteria which reduce urinary nitrate to nitrite

Specimen Urine, first morning specimen is preferred; random urine is acceptable; preferably midstream, clean catch collection. **CONTAINER:** Plastic urine container **STORAGE INSTRUCTIONS:** If the specimen cannot be processed within 2 hours, it should be refrigerated.

Interpretive **REFERENCE RANGE:** Negative **USE:** Detect the presence of potentially significant bacteriuria; aid in the diagnosis of cystitis, pyelonephritis, urinary tract infection **LIMITATIONS:** The sensitivity of the nitrite test is decreased with high specific gravity and with high ascorbic acid content. False-negatives can occur when dipsticks are stored at ambient humidity.[1] False-negatives are relatively common and relate to varying retention times of urine in the bladder, varying urinary nitrate concentrations (diet dependent) and the presence and quantity of nitrate reducing organisms present. Storage of sample at room temperature for excessive periods (more than 2 hours) may lead to reduction of nitrite to nitrogen. Some urinary tract infections are caused by organisms which do not contain reductase to convert nitrate to ni-

(Continued)

Nitrite, Urine *(Continued)*

trite. These include infections caused by *Streptococcus faecalis* and other gram-positive cocci, *N. gonorrhoeae*, and *M. tuberculosis*. In addition, the urine may not have been retained in the bladder for 4 hours or more to allow adequate reduction of nitrate to occur. Negative results are found when infecting organisms do not convert nitrate to nitrite. **METHODOLOGY:** This reaction depends upon the conversion of nitrate to nitrite by the action of certain species of urinary bacteria. Nitrite from the urine reacts with *p*-arsanilic acid forming a diazonium compound. The diazonium compound couples with 1,2,3,4-tetrahydrobenzo(h)quinolin-3-ol. **ADDITIONAL INFORMATION:** A positive nitrite test is strongly suggestive of urinary tract infection (ie, $\geq 10^5$ organisms/mL). Therefore, when positive, a urine culture is recommended, but urine culture is indicated in any case if the patient is symptomatic. The use of nitrate and leukocyte esterase together is more extensively discussed in the listing Leukocyte Esterase, Urine.

Footnotes

1. Gallagher EJ, Schwartz E, and Weinstein RS, "Performance Characteristics of Urine Dipsticks Stored in Open Containers," *Am J Emerg Med*, 1990, 8(2):121-3.

References

Bartlett RC, Zern DA, Ratkiewicz MA, et al, "Screening for Urinary Tract Infection With the Yellow IRIS," *Lab Med*, 1992, 23(9):599-602.

Congdon DD and Fedorko DP, "Evaluation of Two Rapid Urine Screening Tests," *Lab Med*, 1992, 23(9):613-5.

Damato JJ, Garis J, Hawley RJ, et al, "Comparative Leukocyte Esterase-Nitrite and BAC-T-SCREEN Studies Using Single and Multiple Urine Volumes," *Arch Pathol Lab Med*, 1988, 112:533-5.

Hallander HO, Kallner A, Lundin A, et al, "Evaluation of Rapid Methods for the Detection of Bacteriuria (Screening) in Primary Healthcare," *Acta Pathol Microbiol Immunol Scand [B]*, 1986, 94:39-49.

Hurlbut TA, 3d and Littenberg B, "The Diagnostic Accuracy of Rapid Dipstick Tests to Predict Urinary Tract Infection," *Am J Clin Pathol*, 1991, 96(5):582-8.

Lachs MS, Nachamkin I, Edelstein PH, et al, "Spectrum Bias in the Evaluation of Diagnostic Tests: Lessons From the Rapid Dipstick Test for Urinary Tract Infection," *Ann Intern Med*, 1992, 117(2):135-40.

Nitroprusside Reaction for Ketones, Urine *see* Ketones, Urine *on page 1128*

Occult Blood, Semiquantitative, Urine *see* Urinalysis *on page 1162*

Occult Blood, Stool

CPT 82270

Related Information

^{51}Cr Red Cell Survival *on page 536*

Synonyms Blood, Occult, Stool; Colo-Rect®; Colo-Screen®; Fecal Occult Blood Test; Hema-Chek®; Hemoccult® II, Stool; HemoQuant®; Quick-Cult®

Applies to Guaiac, Stool; Stool Guaiac

Abstract Fecal occult blood screening is relatively insensitive as a screen for colorectal neoplasia and is even less sensitive for detection of polyps. False-positives, as well as, false-negatives occur. In spite of its shortcomings, annual fecal occult blood testing does diminish deaths from colorectal carcinomas. Successful detection and therapy of even a fraction of the approximately 160,000 new U.S. cases annually is meaningful.

Patient Care **PREPARATION:** Patient should not receive vitamin C (ascorbic acid) for 1-3 days prior to occult blood testing by guaiac. Vitamin C does not affect the HemoQuant® test. A high bulk, red meat free diet with restriction of peroxidase-rich vegetables (turnips, horseradish, artichokes, mushrooms, radishes, broccoli, bean sprouts, cauliflower, apples, oranges, bananas, cantaloupes, grapes) has been recommended for 72 hours prior to guaiac testing, and during testing, to decrease the incidence of false-positives. Ingestion of red meat or use of nonsteroidal anti-inflammatory drugs before or during the collection can affect results for Hemoccult® or HemoQuant®. Alcohol and aspirin, especially together, and other gastric irritants should also be avoided. Social use of ethanol alone is unlikely to cause false-positive HemoQuant® results but therapeutic doses of aspirin may do so.[1] Halogens and cimetidine can cause reactions with guaiac tests. Oral iron should not cause positive guaiac[2,3] or HemoQuant® stool assay results.[4] Positive stool reactions from subjects on therapeutic doses of oral iron should not be dismissed as false-positives.[4]

Specimen Stool **CONTAINER:** Plastic urine container **COLLECTION:** Stool collection has been offensive, unwieldy, and awkward under the best of circumstances. Mostly left to their own inspiration, some patients are unwilling or unable to comply. Up to 75% of blood leaches from the fecal surface into surrounding toilet water in 4-12 minutes. Many toilet sanitizers generate chlorine and are reported to cause false-positive reactions to guaiac tests. False-positives can be traced to toilet bowl water containing blood from menstruation or urine. A collection device is described.[5] Delay in examination can adversely affect Hemoccult® results. Delay does not affect HemoQuant® results. **SPECIAL INSTRUCTIONS:** Tests for stool occult blood are not appropriately applied to detection of blood in gastric juice by virtue of possible ingestion of drugs and the pH of gastric juice.

Interpretive **REFERENCE RANGE:** Guaiac: negative. (A positive report has much more significance than does a negative). No consistent fecal hemoglobin level exists above which guaiac tests are reliably positive or below which they are not.[6] HemoQuant®: <2 mg/g is considered normal, 2-4 mg/g is borderline. **USE:** Detect occult blood **LIMITATIONS:** Most methods lack sensitivity to small amounts of blood and might fail to detect slow rates of blood loss. Many adenomas and carcinomas do not bleed. When occult GI bleeding is suspected, at least three samples, preferably of separate bowel movements, should be submitted. Many substances and conditions interfere with guaiac tests. Vitamin C (ascorbic acid) and antacids may cause false-negatives to guaiac tests. False-positive results may be caused by excessive dietary intake of vegetable peroxidases, especially horseradish. Drugs shown to be associated with gastrointestinal blood loss in normal subjects include salicylates (aspirin), steroids, rauwolfia derivatives, all nonsteroidal anti-inflammatory drugs, and colchicine. The sensitivity of the slides is increased by rehydration prior to development. The increment in sensitivity provided by rehydration can be a useful adjunct to the use of the test,[7] but somewhat decreases its specificity; *vide infra*.

Ahlquist and Bakken quote Sherlock Holmes' observation that the old guaiacum test is very clumsy and uncertain and his lament of the lack of a reliable test ("A Study in Scarlet"). They describe the still current truth of Arthur Conan Doyle's criticism of guaiac false-positives and negatives,[8] which are outlined in the table. Guaiac tests present a number of other problems. Acid pH, heat, and dry stools lead to some false-negatives, while watery stools are more apt to test positive. **Intestinal converted fraction** is an expression which describes the fraction of heme converted to porphyrin during fecal transit, a phenomenon which leads to diminished guaiac sensitivity for carcinomas of the more proximal colon.[8,9,10]

Colorectal adenomas and carcinomas cause a minority of positive guaiac tests.[6] In a study of 12 unoperated patients with asymptomatic colorectal carcinoma, the mean cancer detection rate was only 57% for HemoQuant® and 25% for Hemoccult®. Testing three stools, reported detection rates improved moderately to 76% for HemoQuant® and 31% for Hemoccult®.[11] Others have not found HemoQuant® performance in carcinoma detection satisfactory.[12] A study of 485 persons who developed fatal colorectal carcinoma was reported, in which only 36% of Hemoccult® III tests done within a year of diagnosis were positive.[13] A multicenter study found Hemoccult® and HemoQuant® screening sensitivity each at 26% of all cancers with less sensitivity for polyps.[14] A 1993 *JAMA* editorial concludes that the real limit to occult blood stool testing is likely to be that many asymptomatic carcinomas do not lead to abnormal blood loss.[15]

METHODOLOGY: Guaiac is a leuko-dye. Commercially generated tests based on it include ColoScreen® (Helena Laboratories), Colo-Rect® (Roche Diagnostics), Hema-Chek® (Miles Laboratories), Quick-Cult® (Laboratory Diagnostics), and Hemoccult® II (SmithKline). The peroxidase-like activity of hemoglobin or nonspecific oxidants catalyze the reaction of peroxide and the chromogen ortho-toluidine to form blue oxidized orthotolidine. New methodology, based on heme-derived porphyrin fluorescence, is more expensive (HemoQuant®). It detects peroxidase-negative heme-derived porphyrins, peroxidase-positive hemoglobin, and free heme.[13] Immunologic tests have been developed, but enteric degradation of hemoglobin interferes with immunologic as well as guaiac tests. Immunologic tests do not react with drugs, red meats, or nonhemoglobin peroxidase compounds. See table.

When such paper slides impregnated with guaiac are not promptly processed, drying occurs, which may diminish sensitivity. Such slides may be rehydrated with a drop of deionized water, as was done in a major study.[16] Rehydration increased the number of positives but caused moderate diminution of specificity.[16,17] Rehydration is recommended.

ADDITIONAL INFORMATION: Methods for guaiac tests of stool for occult blood utilize peroxidation of a chromogen by stool peroxidases. Hemoglobin acts as a peroxidase, but stool may also contain meat, bacterial and plant peroxidases. Normal intestinal blood loss averages 2-2.5 mL. Hemoccult® begins to turn positive at about 5 mg hemoglobin/g feces, which is considered to be the upper limit of normal stool peroxidase activity. This method is capable of detection

(Continued)

Occult Blood, Stool *(Continued)*

Occult Blood, Stool[7]

	Guaiac	Heme-Derived Porphyrin Fluorescence	Immunoassays
Test	Hemoccult®	HemoQuant®	Antihemoglobin antibodies
Cost	Low	High (but indirect costs of false-positives and false-negatives are decreased)	Intermediate
Reliability	False-positives, false-negatives	Sensitive and more reliable	Intermediate
Specificity	Poor	Specific for heme	Improved over guaiac
Availability	Almost anywhere	Specimens must be sent to a reference laboratory, or application to SmithKline Beecham for a sublicense must be approved.	Limited availability
Recognition of porphyrin derived from heme	No	Yes	N/A
Recognition of bleeding from right colon (intestinal converted fraction)	Like immunologic tests, especially insensitive-enteric heme degradation	Sensitive	Similar to guaiac
Sensitivity deteriorates with time, fecal storage (eg, mailed in specimens)	Yes	No	Similar to guaiac
Such reducing substances as ascorbic acid cause false-negatives	Yes	No	No
Antacids cause false-negatives	Yes	No	No
Dietary (red meats) hemoglobin	Yes	Yes	No
Vegetable peroxidases	False-positives	Not affected	Not affected
Dietary hemoglobin	Yes	Yes	No
Detection adenomas 2 cm Detection colorectal cancer	17% 67% (11%-80%)	58% 97%	 65%
Ease of test performance	Not difficult	Complex	Complex – an enzyme immunoassay is available and counter immunoelectrophoresis is described.
Ship to laboratory performing test	Deliver promptly; do not mail.	Ship at 4°C or frozen	Probably best shipped at 4°C

of 6 mg of added hemoglobin/g feces in 90% of observations, but will fail 80% of the time to detect up to 1.5 mg/g feces. After ingestion of 8 oz of cooked red meat per day, reactions remain negative 95% of the time. The heme-derived porphyrin based method (HemoQuant®) has been shown to correlate closely with ^{51}Cr-labeled RBC radioisotope measurements of short term (12 day) quantitation of fecal blood loss.[18]

Recommendations for screening are recently published.[19]

Approximately 57,000 deaths occur in the U.S. annually from colorectal cancer.[16]

Footnotes

1. Fleming JL, Ahlquist DA, McGill DB, et al, "Influence of Aspirin and Ethanol on Fecal Blood Levels as Determined by Using the HemoQuant® Assay," *Mayo Clin Proc*, 1987, 62:159-63.
2. McDonnell WM, Ryan JA, Seeger DM, et al, "Effect of Iron on the Guaiac Reaction," *Gastroenterology*, 1989, 96(1):74-8.
3. Anderson GD, Yuellig TR, and Krone RE Jr, "An Investigation Into the Effects of Oral Iron Supplementation on *In Vivo* Hemoccult® Stool Testing," *Am J Gastroenterol*, 1990, 85(5):558-61.
4. Coles EF and Starnes EC, "Use of HemoQuant® Assays to Assess the Effect of Oral Iron Preparations on Stool Hemoccult® Tests," *Am J Gastroenterol*, 1991, 86(10):1442-4.
5. Ahlquist DA, Schwartz S, Isaacson J, et al, "A Stool Collection Device: The First Step in Occult Blood Testing," *Ann Intern Med*, 1988, 108(4):609-12.
6. Ahlquist DA, "Fecal Blood Testing: Demystifying the Occult," Annual Clinical Conference on Cancer, 30:Gastrointestinal Cancer: Current Approaches to Diagnosis and Treatment, University of Texas System Cancer Center, 1988.
7. Macrae FA, St John DJ, Caligiore P, et al, "Optimal Dietary Conditions for Hemoccult® Testing," *Gastroenterology*, 1982, 82:899-903.
8. Ahlquist DA and Bakken CL, "Fecal Blood Tests," *ASCP Check Sample®*, Chicago, IL: American Society of Clinical Pathologists, 1988.
9. Ahlquist DA, McGill DB, Schwartz S, et al, "HemoQuant®, A New Quantitative Assay for Fecal Hemoglobin," *Ann Intern Med*, 1984, 101:297-302.
10. Ahlquist DA, McGill DB, Schwartz S, et al, "Fecal Blood Levels in Health and Disease," *N Engl J Med*, 1985, 312:1422-8.
11. Ahlquist DA, Fleming JL, McGill DB, et al, "Patterns of Occult Bleeding in Asymptomatic Colorectal Cancer," *Cancer*, 1989, 63(9):1826-30.
12. St-John DJB, Young GP, McHutchison JG, et al, "Comparison of the Specificity and Sensitivity of Hemoccult® and HemoQuant® in Screening for Colorectal Neoplasia," *Ann Intern Med*, 1992, 117(5):376-82.
13. Selby JV, Friedman GD, Quesenberry CP Jr, et al, "Effect of Fecal Occult Blood Testing on Mortality From Colorectal Cancer," *Ann Intern Med*, 1993, 118(1):1-6.
14. Ahlquist DA, Wieand HS, Moertel CG, et al, "Accuracy of Fecal Occult Blood Screening for Colorectal Neoplasia – A Prospective Study Using Hemoccult and HemoQuant Tests," *JAMA*, 1993, 269(10):1262-7.
15. Selby JV, "How Should We Screen for Colorectal Cancer?" *JAMA*, 1993, 269(10):1294-6.
16. Mandel JS, Bond JH, Church TR, et al, "Reducing Mortality From Colorectal Cancer by Screening for Fecal Occult Blood," *N Engl J Med*, 1993, 328(19):1365-71.
17. Winawer SJ, "Colorectal Cancer Screening Comes of Age," *N Engl J Med*, 1993, 328(9):1416-7, (editorial).
18. Leahy MB, Pippard MJ, Salzmann MB, et al, "Quantitative Measurement of Faecal Blood Loss: Comparison of Radioisotopic and Chemical Analyses," *J Clin Pathol*, 1991, 44(5):391-4.
19. Levin B, "Colorectal Cancer Screening," *Cancer*, 1993, 72(3):1056-60.

References

Bahrt KM, Korman LY, and Nashel DJ, "Significance of a Positive Test for Occult Blood in Stools of Patients Taking Anti-inflammatory Drugs," *Arch Intern Med*, 1984, 144:2165-6.

Blebea J and McPherson RA, "False-Positive Guaiac Testing With Iodine," *Arch Pathol Lab Med*, 1985, 109:437-40.

Block GE, "Colon Cancer: Diagnosis and Prognosis in the Elderly," *Geriatrics*, 1989, 44(5):45-7, 52-3.

Doyle AC, "A Study in Scarlet," Philadelphia, PA: JB Lippincott Co, 1902.

Fleischer DE, Goldberg SB, Browning TH, et al, "Detection and Surveillance of Colorectal Cancer," *JAMA*, 1989, 261(4):580-5.

Klos SE, Drinka P, and Goodwin JS, "The Utilization of Fecal Occult Blood Testing in the Institutionalized Elderly," *J Am Geriatr Soc*, 1991, 39(12):1169-73.

Knight KK, Fielding JE, and Battista RN, "U.S. Preventive Services Task Force. Occult Blood Screening for Colorectal Cancer," *JAMA*, 1989, 261(4):587-93.

Losek JD and Fiete RL, "Intussusception and the Diagnostic Value of Testing Stool for Occult Blood," *Am J Emerg Med*, 1991, 9(1):1-3.

Pye G, Jackson J, Thomas WM, et al, "Comparison of ColoScreen Self-Test and Haemoccult Faecal Occult Blood Tests in the Detection of Colorectal Cancer in Symptomatic Patients," *Br J Surg*, 1990, 77(6):630-1.

Occult Blood, Urine *see* Blood, Urine *on page 1112*

Phenylalanine Test, Urine

CPT 81005

Related Information

Phenylalanine, Blood *on page 317*

Synonyms Phenylpyruvic Acid, Urine; PKU, Urine Test

Applies to Tyrosyluria

Specimen Freshly voided random urine **CONTAINER:** Plastic urine container **COLLECTION:** Transport specimen to the laboratory within 1 hour of collection. Container must state date and time of collection. **CAUSES FOR REJECTION:** Inadequate labeling, improper collection

Interpretive **REFERENCE RANGE:** Negative (level of detection with Phenistix® is 5-10 mg/100 mL) **USE:** Assist in the detection of hyperphenylalaninemia, including phenylalanine hydroxylase deficiency (phenylketonuria, PKU and non-PKU hyperphenylalaninemia), and tetrahydrobiopterin cofactor deficiency.[1] **Urine is not used as an initial screening test for PKU.** See entry Phenylalanine, Blood in the Chemistry chapter. **After birth, 2-6 weeks may pass before phenylpyruvic acid is excreted in the urine.**[2] After the diagnosis of PKU has been established, urine screening type tests may be employed to follow adequacy of dietary control including monitoring of dietary intake of pregnant women who lack phenylalanine hydroxylase. **LIMITATIONS:** Diluted urine may cause false-negatives. The urine screening tests may miss a significant number of cases due to interferences and insensitivity. Tyrosyluria, the result of transitory tyrosinemia in prematures due to immaturity of hepatic metabolism, may result in a positive ferric chloride test. **CONTRAINDICATIONS:** The ferric chloride method should not be used to screen newborns for PKU. Its primary use is to monitor dietary adherence in known cases. The level of phenylalanine in the blood is correlated with urine phenylpyruvic acid in older children.[3] **METHODOLOGY:** Screening tests:

- Ferric chloride method – green color
- Phenistix® urine reagent strips (a ferric chloride method) – a persistent blue-gray to gray-green color is produced with phenylpyruvic acid. (Salicylates or phenothiazine derivatives give pink to purple colors.) Tyrosyluria in the premature or newborn due to liver disease will produce a fading green color with ferric chloride screening tests.[2]

Confirmatory tests may be done by one of several methods:

- high voltage electrophoresis followed by chromatography
- cation exchange column chromatography
- Newer methods are more sensitive and specific, detecting phenylpyruvic acid in the urine by chemiluminescent or fluorometric techniques.[4] High performance liquid chromatography with fluorescent detection is also used, and can detect the low levels of phenylpyruvic acid in normal adults or newborns.

ADDITIONAL INFORMATION: The incidence of classic PKU varies considerably in different countries. It occurs in somewhat more than 1 of 11,000 births in the U.S. Mental retardation is the main finding clinically. There are some nine or more mutations at loci of chromosomes that encode components of the phenylalanine hydroxylation reaction.[1] This is the genetic basis for the heterogeneous phenotype of hyperphenylalaninemia. Many result in only transient or variable elevations in blood phenylalanine and presence of urine phenylalanine, tyrosine metabolites, or other amino acids. Phenylalanine hydroxylase deficient PKU (phenylketonuria) is characterized by impaired postnatal mental and physical development while non-PKU hyperphenylalaninemia is clinically benign. A blood level of 10-20 mg/dL of phenylpyruvic acid (phenylalanine metabolite) is required to produce a urine level ≥8 mg/dL which is the approximate threshold of the screening tests. The Guthrie bacterial inhibition test performed on blood is more sensitive and is the preferred and accepted screening procedure. Positive results of screening tests should be confirmed by a fluorometric method. The test should be performed after the newborn has had 24 hours of milk feeding. A metabolite of acetaminophen, has been reported to interfere with chromatographic analyses identifying phenylalanine.[5]

Monitoring of urinary excretion of phenylalanine metabolites (by gas chromatography/mass spectrometry) to avoid neurotoxic effects in children with PKU has been undertaken with the goal of identifying a range of blood phenylalanine that is associated with normal levels of excretion of such products.[6] The importance of controlling blood phenylalanine levels by diet during pregnancy in women with hyperphenylalaninemia (including those with diagnosed and undiagnosed phenylketonuria) has been emphasized in order to decrease the risk of maternal phenylketonuria syndrome.[7]

Footnotes

1. Scriver CR, Kaufman S, and Woo SLC, "The Hyperphenylalaninemias," *The Metabolic Basis of Inherited Disease*, 6th ed, Scriver CK, Beaudet AL, Sly WS, et al, eds, New York, NY: McGraw-Hill Inc, 1989, 495-546.

2. Strasinger SK, *Urinalysis and Body Fluids: A Self Instructional Text*, Philadelphia, PA: FA Davis Co, 1985, 116-9.
3. Langenbeck U, Behbehani A, Mench-Hoinowski A, et al, "Absence of a Significant Renal Threshold for Two Aromatic Acids in Phenylketonuric Children Over Two Years of Age," *Eur J Pediatr*, 1980, 134:115-8.
4. Sano A, Ogawa M, and Takitani S, "Fluorometric Determination of Phenylpyruvic Acid With 1,4-Dimethyl-3-Carbamoylpyridinium Chloride," *Chem Pharm Bull (Tokyo)*, 1987, 35:3746-9.
5. Shih VE, Nikiforov V, and Carney MM, "Acetaminophen Metabolite Interferes in Analysis for Amino Acids," *Clin Chem*, 1985, 31:148, (letter).
6. Michals K, Lopus M, and Matalon R, "Phenylalanine Metabolites as Indicators of Dietary Compliance in Children With Phenylketonuria," *Biochem Med Metab Biol*, 1988, 39:18-23.
7. Luder AS and Greene CL, "Maternal Phenylketonuria and Hyperphenylalaninemia: Implications for Medical Practice in the United States," *Am J Obstet Gynecol*, 1989, 161(5):1102-5.

References

American Academy of Pediatrics Committee on Genetics, "Newborn Screening Fact Sheets: Phenylketonuria (PKU)," *Pediatrics*, 1989, 83:461-2.

Hilton MA, Sharpe JN, Hicks LG, et al, "A Simple Method for Detection of Heterozygous Carriers of the Gene for Classic Phenylketonuria," *J Pediatr*, 1986, 109:601-4.

Holtzman C, Slazyke WE, Corders JF, et al, "Descriptive Epidemiology of Missed Cases of Phenylketonuria and Congenital Hypothyroidism," *Pediatrics*, 1986, 78:553-8.

Ponzone A, Guardamagna O, Ferraris S, et al, "Screening for Malignant Phenylketonuria," *Lancet*, 1987, 8531:512-3, (letter).

Phenylpyruvic Acid, Urine *see* Phenylalanine Test, Urine *on previous page*

pH, Stool

CPT 83986

Related Information

Fat, Semiquantitative, Stool *on page 1118*
Reducing Substances, Stool *on page 1149*
Tryptic Activity, Stool *on page 1161*

Synonyms Fecal pH; Stool pH

Patient Care PREPARATION: Barium procedures and laxatives should be avoided for 1 week prior to collection of the specimen.

Specimen Fresh random stool CONTAINER: Plastic stool container STORAGE INSTRUCTIONS: Refrigerate CAUSES FOR REJECTION: Specimen contaminated with urine, specimen improperly labeled.

Interpretive REFERENCE RANGE: Diet dependent; normal: neutral to slightly alkaline or acid. Stool pH is usually slightly acidic at pH 5-6. pH is increased with protein breakdown, decreased with carbohydrate or fat malabsorption. Breast-fed infants have slightly acid stools, bottle-fed infants, neutral or slightly alkaline. Acid stool is formed with fat malabsorption. In a South African population of control subjects, the mean stool pH of rural blacks was (pH 6.14) significantly lower than that in urban black individuals (pH 6.77) and in patients with chronic pancreatitis (pH 6.61).[1] USE: Screen for carbohydrate and fat malabsorption; evaluate small intestinal disaccharidase deficiencies LIMITATIONS: May have limited value in some cases due to dependence on stool volume and transit time. METHODOLOGY: Aqueous stool suspension measured with pH paper ADDITIONAL INFORMATION: Stool pH is dependent in part on fermentation of sugars. Colonic fermentation of normal amounts of carbohydrate sugars and production of fatty acids accounts for the normally slightly acidic pH. If disaccharide intolerance is suspect, simple screening tests may be performed. Slightly alkaline pH may occur in cases of secretory diarrhea without food intake, colitis, villous adenoma, and possibly with antibiotic usage (with resultant impaired colonic fermentation). A stool pH <6 (measured by pH paper) is suggestive evidence of sugar malabsorption. Children and some adults notice that their stools have a sickly sweet smell as the result of volatile fatty acids and the presence of undigested lactose. Low stool pH also contributes to excoriation of perianal skin which frequently accompanies diarrhea.[2] Determination of fecal reducing substances is a more reliable screening test for disaccharidase deficiency. See Reducing Substances, Stool and Fat, Semiquantitative, Stool listings.

High fecal pH may be a risk factor for colorectal cancer.[3,4,5,6,7] Intake of oat bran (75-100 g/day over a 14-day period) has been shown capable of reducing fecal pH by 0.4 units.[3] There is evidence, however, that high fecal pH may be secondarily rather than primarily related to cancer risk.[4]

(Continued)

pH, Stool *(Continued)*

Footnotes

1. Riedel L, Walker ARP, Segal I, et al, "Limitations of Faecal Chymotrypsin as a Screening Test for Chronic Pancreatitis," *Gut*, 1991, 32(3):321-4.
2. Cooper BT, "Lactose Deficiency and Lactose Malabsorption," *Dig Dis*, 1986, 4:72-82.
3. Kashtan H, Stern HS, Jenkins DJ, et al, "Manipulation of Fecal pH by Dietary Means," *Prev Med*, 1990, 19(6):607-13.
4. Kashtan H, Gregoire RC, Bruce WR, et al, "Effects of Sodium Sulfate on Fecal pH and Proliferation of Colonic Mucosa in Patients at High Risk for Colon Cancer," *J Natl Cancer Inst*, 1990, 82(11):950-2.
5. Thornton JR, "High Colonic pH Promotes Colorectal Cancer," *Lancet*, 1981, 1:1081-3.
6. Malhotra SL, "Faecal Urobilinogen Levels and pH of Stools in Population Groups With Different Incidence of Cancer of the Colon, and Their Possible Role in Its Aetiology," *J R Soc Med*, 1982, 75:709-14.
7. Walker ARP, Walker BF, and Walker AJ, "Faecal pH, Dietary Fibre Intake, and Proneness to Colon Cancer in Four South African Populations," *Br J Cancer*, 1986, 53:489-95.

References

Lebenthal E, "Small Intestinal Disaccharidase Deficiencies," *Pediatr Clin North Am*, 1975, 20:757-66.

Read NW, "Diarrhea, Chronic," *Difficult Diagnosis*, Taylor RB, ed, Philadelphia, PA: WB Saunders Co, 1985, 109-10.

pH, Urine

CPT 83986

Related Information

Kidney Stone Analysis *on page 1129*
pH, Blood *on page 315*
Urinalysis *on page 1162*

Test Commonly Includes pH is part of a routine urinalysis.

Specimen Random urine **CONTAINER:** Plastic urine container **STORAGE INSTRUCTIONS:** If the specimen cannot be processed promptly, it should be refrigerated. **CAUSES FOR REJECTION:** Improper labeling, specimen not refrigerated

Interpretive **REFERENCE RANGE:** 4.5-7.8; normal kidneys can produce urine with pH from 4.5-8.2, but with ordinary diet, urine pH is about 6.0. Urine becomes more alkaline after meals and is most acidic fasting in the morning. **USE:** Urine pH is a crude measure of the acid-base balance of the body. It may be helpful in determining subtle presence of distal renal tubular disease or pyelonephritis. Urine pH is useful for identifying crystals in urine and determining predisposition to form a given type of stone. See table. When an accurate pH assessment of

Conditions Associated With Acid Urine	Conditions Associated With Alkaline Urine	
Metabolic acidosis	Respiratory alkalosis	Postprandial alkaline tide (1 hour after meal)
Diabetes mellitus	Metabolic alkalosis	Fanconi's syndrome and Milkman's syndrome (increased urinary loss of bicarbonate)
Diarrhea	Urea-splitting bacteria (*Proteus* sp)	Alkali therapy (citrate, bicarbonate)
Starvation	Vegetable diet	
Respiratory acidosis	Gastric suction and vomiting	
Emphysema	Diuretic therapy	
Sleep		
Renal failure with lack of NH_3 buffer		

acid-base status and renal response is desired, the urine should be collected under circumstances more controlled than is usual. Attention is given to the time of day, the fasting status of the patient, and transfer of sample so as to prevent degassing of sample or growth of bacteria; rapid analysis by pH meter rather than dipstick is indicated. Usually simultaneous serum pH is then also ordered. **LIMITATIONS:** On standing urine becomes alkaline due to the action of urea splitting bacteria (*Proteus* sp). **METHODOLOGY:** Dipstick double indicator principle (methyl red and bromthymol blue) which gives a broad range of colors covering the urinary pH range 5-9 $\pm$0.5 pH units. A pH meter is the back-up and most accurate method. **ADDITIONAL INFORMATION:** Dietary factors affect urine pH. Alkaline urine is observed in persons who eat large quantities of citrus fruit and vegetables. Acid urine is observed with high meat intake. Pyridium® metabolites may mask the pH reaction. Urine pH $>$6.5 indicates presence of bicarbonate while pH $<$5.5 indicates absence of bicarbonate. Consistently acid urine, pH $<$5.5, is associated with xanthine, cystine, and uric acid stones. Calcium oxalate and apatite stones are not associated with any particular disturbance of urine pH. Alkaline urine (pH >7) is associated with calcium carbonate, calcium phosphate, and especially magnesium ammonium phosphate stones. In conjunction with serum pH and bicarbonate levels, urine pH may be applied to the study of renal tubular acidification.

References

Cogan MG and Rector FC Jr, "Acid-Base Disorders," *Kidney*, Chapter 18, Brenner BM and Rector FC Jr, eds, Philadelphia, PA: WB Saunders Co, 1991, 737-804.

Schumann GB and Schweitzer SC, "Examination of Urine," *Clinical Diagnosis and Management by Laboratory Methods*, Chapter 17, Henry JB, ed, Philadelphia, PA: WB Saunders Co, 1991, 398-400.

Ziyadeh FN and Goldfarb S, "XII Nephrolithiasis," *Sci Am*, 1993, 1-10.

PKU, Urine Test *see* Phenylalanine Test, Urine *on page 1142*

Protein, Quantitative, Urine

CPT *84155*

Related Information

Fat, Urine *on page 1119*
Immunoelectrophoresis, Serum or Urine *on page 706*
Immunofixation Electrophoresis *on page 707*
Kidney Biopsy *on page 68*
Microalbuminuria *on page 1134*
Protein Electrophoresis, Urine *on page 737*
Protein, Semiquantitative, Urine *on page 1147*
Protein, Total, Serum *on page 340*

Test Commonly Includes Concomitant creatinine clearance is often indicated. Total urine creatinine should be included to help assure that a complete 24-hour collection was tested.

Abstract Quantitation of urinary protein loss.

Specimen 24-hour urine **CONTAINER:** Plain urine container **COLLECTION:** Instruct patient to void at 8 AM and discard the specimen. Then collect all urine including the final specimen voided at the end of the 24-hour collection period (ie, 8 AM the next morning). Label the container with the patient's name and date and time collection started and finished. **STORAGE INSTRUCTIONS:** Refrigerate **TURNAROUND TIME:** 24 hours

Interpretive **REFERENCE RANGE:** 30-150 mg/24 hours (SI: 0.03-0.15 g/day) (method dependent) Proteinuria has been defined as 24-hour urine protein excretion >150 mg/24 hours (SI: >0.15 g/day).[1] In infants and children, different ranges apply and have been published; proteinuria >100 mg/day (SI: >0.10 g/day) in children younger than 10 years of age is regarded as abnormal.[2] **USE:** Evaluate proteinuria (eg, following urinalysis in which proteinuria is detected); evaluate renal diseases, including proteinuria complicating diabetes mellitus, the nephrotic syndromes (eg, lipoid nephrosis, membranous, proliferative glomerulopathies), metal poisoning (eg, gold, lead, and cadmium), renal vein thrombosis, systemic lupus erythematosus (SLE), constrictive pericarditis, and amyloidosis; work up other renal diseases including malignant hypertension, glomerulonephritis, Goodpasture's syndrome, Henoch-Schönlein purpura, thrombotic thrombocytopenic purpura, collagen diseases, cryoglobulinemia, toxemia of pregnancy, drug nephrotoxicity, hypersensitivity reactions, allergic reactions, and renal tubular lesions; management of myeloma and macroglobulinemia of Waldenström (Bence Jones proteinuria); evaluate hypoproteinemia; tubular proteinurias include Wilson's disease and Fanconi syndrome. Even in the table shown, some renal lesions are not easily categorized (eg, the glomerular lesions of chrysotherapy) and of toxemia of pregnancy. **LIMITATIONS:** Although evaluation for proteinuria may be the best single test to work up chronic renal disease, proteinuria may wax and wane. In toxemia of pregnancy (pre-eclampsia/eclampsia), magnesium sulfate is used therapeutically. This may result in high urine magnesium levels, which cause spurious Du Pont aca® urine protein levels by a method which otherwise seems excellent.[3] Toxemia is a state in which urine protein excretion is commonly measured. The standard for most methodologies is albumin. Different methods are more or less sensitive to globulin than to albumin. Thus, for nonselective proteinurias, in which a variety of proteins are present, different methodologies yield different results. Twenty-four hour urine collections are subject to collection errors. The laboratory method, depending on an aliquot and varying dilutions, is subject to calculation errors. When protein is determined by precipitation methods, x-ray contrast media, tolbutamide, penicillin or cephalosporin analogs, and sulfonamides may cause false-positives. Pyridium® interferes with the reaction by causing color interference. Function-

(Continued)

Outline of Causes of Proteinuria

Normal proteinuria		Albumin ≤35 mg/24 h
		Tamm–Horsfall ≤50 mg/24 h
Prerenal proteinuria		Congestive heart failure
		Orthostatic proteinuria
		Transient, associated with febrile illness, surgery, anemia, hyperthyroidism, stroke, exercise, seizures
		Bence Jones proteinuria associated with myeloma, Waldenström's macroglobulinemia, amyloidosis
		Lysozyme associated with myelocytic leukemia
Renal proteinuria		Renovascular hypertension
		Malignant hypertension of any cause
	Glomerular	Membranous nephropathy and proliferative glomerulonephritis
		Chronic pyelonephritis
		Polycystic disease
		Diabetic nephropathy
		Amyloidosis
		Lupus erythematosus (SLE)
		Goodpasture's syndrome
		Renal vein thrombosis
		Minimal change nephropathy
		Proteinuria >3.5 g/24 h usually reflects a glomerular lesion
		High molecular weight proteinuria
	Tubular	Fanconi syndrome
		Wilson's disease
		Renal tubular acidosis
		Heavy metal poisoning: lead, mercury, cadmium
		Galactosemia
		Low molecular weight (<60,000) proteinuria
		Beta$_2$-microglobulinemia (molecular weight 11,800)
		<1 g/24 h
	Interstitial	Bacterial pyelonephritis
		Uric acid, urate or calcium deposition
		Idiosyncratic drug reaction: methicillin, phenindione, sulfonamides, phenytoin, others
		Interstitial diseases generally reflected as tubular defects or mixed tubular interstitial
Postrenal		Tumors of the bladder or renal pelvis <1 g/24 h, IgM excretion significant marker, amount of proteinuria related to size and spread of tumor Cystitis, severe

al and postural proteinuria occur. **METHODOLOGY:** A number of methods are in use including trichloroacetic acid, sulfosalicylic acid precipitation, biuret method with phosphotungstic acid, and Coomassie blue dye binding. **ADDITIONAL INFORMATION:** Normal urine protein consists of albumin (up to 35 mg/24 hours), other plasma proteins (ie, globulins, haptoglobin, beta$_2$-microglobulin, and light chains), and Tamm-Horsfall glycoprotein secreted by renal tubular cells (may contribute up to 50 mg/24 hours). Urinary protein normally tends to increase with age, exercise, and standing posture.

Tests requiring a 24-hour urine collection with no preservative, such as creatinine, may also be performed on the same specimen. Although quantitative protein can be run on a random specimen or timed collections less than 24 hours, 24-hour collections are preferable for evaluation of the nephrotic states and inflammatory renal disorders. Creatinine, creatinine clearance, BUN, serum protein electrophoresis, ANA, anti-DNA antibodies, HIV, hepatitis C antibody, hepatitis B antigen, and complement levels (including total complement, C3, C4) are among useful tests to work up patients with proteinuria. Urine electrophoresis, immunofixation and immunoelectrophoresis are useful in patients older than 35 years of age to investigate possible diagnosis of amyloidosis, myeloma, and Waldenström's macroglobulinemia.

Some patients exhibit orthostatic proteinuria (ie, recumbent urine protein 100-180 mg in a 12-hour overnight urine collection and up to 1 g in the subsequent 12 hours while ambulatory). The presence of >200 mg of urinary protein in the overnight specimen or equally increased amounts of urine protein in both specimens indicates a need for further work-up.[4]

Nephrotic syndromes are the causes of the most severe urinary protein losses. Nephrotic syndrome is defined now usually by degree of proteinuria (ie, proteinuria >50 mg/kg/day). After time, additional signs and symptoms occur including hypoproteinemia, hypoalbuminemia, elevation of alpha$_2$-globulin with decreased gamma globulin on electrophoresis, hyperlipidemia, and edema. Urinary albumin is a more sensitive marker of progression and regression of renal disease than urine total protein, especially when urine total protein is <300 mg/g creatinine.[5] In most laboratories, urine albumin is available from protein electrophoresis following concentration procedures. However, this method is not sensitive to low concentrations of albumin.[5] For low concentrations, see listing, Microalbuminuria.

Footnotes

1. Epstein M and Oster JR, "Proteinuria," *The Laboratory in Clinical Medicine: Interpretation and Application*, 2nd ed, Halsted JA and Halsted CH, eds, Philadelphia, PA: WB Saunders Co, 1981, 318-23.
2. Kim MS, "Proteinuria," *Clin Lab Med*, 1988, 8(3):527-40.
3. Naccarato WF and Caffo AL, "The Performance Characteristics of the Urinary Protein Method for the Du Pont aca® Analyzer," *Technical Service Bulletin*, Clinical Systems, Du Pont, 1982.
4. Glassock RJ, "Postural (Orthostatic) Proteinuria: No Cause for Concern," *N Engl J Med*, 1981, 305:639-41.
5. Shihabi ZK, Konen JC, and O'Connor ML, "Albuminuria vs Urinary Tract Protein for Detecting Chronic Renal Disorders," *Clin Chem*, 1991, 37(5):621-4.

References

Burke EC and Stickler GB, "Proteinuria in Children. Review and Evaluation," *Clin Pediatr (Phila)*, 1983, 21:741-3.

Ginsberg JM, Chang BS, Matarese RA, and Garella S, "Use of Single Voided Urine Samples to Estimate Quantitative Proteinuria," *N Engl J Med*, 1983, 309:1543-6.

Glassock RJ, "The Nephrotic Syndrome: The Kidney in Health and Disease," *Hosp Pract*, 1979, 14:105-29.

Levey AS, Madaio MP, and Perrone RD, "Laboratory Assessment of Renal Disease: Clearance, Urinalysis, and Renal Biopsy," *Kidney*, Brenner BM and Rector FC Jr, eds, Philadelphia, PA: WB Saunders Co, 1991, 919-68.

Ward PCJ, "Renal Dysfunction, 2, Proteinuria," *Postgrad Med*, 1981, 69:91-9.

Protein, Screen, Urine *see* Protein, Semiquantitative, Urine *on this page*

Protein, Semiquantitative, Urine

CPT *84155*

Related Information

Microalbuminuria *on page 1134*
Protein Electrophoresis, Urine *on page 737*
Protein, Quantitative, Urine *on page 1145*
Urinalysis *on page 1162*

Synonyms Albumin, Urine; Protein, Screen, Urine; Protein, Urine, Sulfosalicylic Acid; Urine Screen for Albumin; Urine Screen for Protein

(Continued)

Protein, Semiquantitative, Urine *(Continued)*

Test Commonly Includes Screening for urine protein by dipstick and, in many laboratories, sulfosalicylic acid method for confirmation. This is part of a routine urinalysis.

Abstract Screening test for urinary protein loss. Dipstick methods are relatively insensitive to globulins such as light chains. They may be unreliable in unusually colored urines, when the specimen is highly alkaline or when a great deal of sediment is present. The precipitation methods include sulfosalicylic acid and trichloroacetic acid. These are more sensitive to globulins.

Specimen Random urine **CONTAINER:** Plastic urine container **COLLECTION:** Early morning specimen is recommended. This will provide maximally concentrated urine when Bence Jones urine protein (light chain) detection is important. For other renal disease, daytime urine is satisfactory or even preferred.[1,2] Transport specimen to the laboratory within 2 hours of collection. Container should state date and time of collection. **STORAGE INSTRUCTIONS:** If not run promptly, specimen should be refrigerated. **CAUSES FOR REJECTION:** Improper labeling, specimen not refrigerated

Interpretive **REFERENCE RANGE:** <20 mg/dL (SI: <0.2 g/L). The sensitivity of the dipstick is in the range of 150-300 mg/L. It is sensitive mostly for albumin. **USE:** Detect protein in the urine; screen for nephrotic syndromes, including complications of diabetes mellitus, glomerulonephritis, amyloidosis, and other renal diseases. Proteinuria is probably the single most important indicator of renal disease. **LIMITATIONS:** The dipstick method is sensitive to negatively charged proteins, but much less so to positively charged proteins and so commonly will not detect Bence Jones (light chain) or myeloma protein, to which sulfosalicylic acid procedures are usually sensitive. False-positive results may be obtained with highly alkaline (pH ≥7) urines on dipsticks, and false-negatives on such urines may be found with sulfosalicylic acid. Positive protein dipstick results, especially in very alkaline urines, should be confirmed by sulfosalicylic acid testing. Contaminating quaternary ammonium groups or chlorohexidine present in disinfectants may also give false-positive dipstick results. The test area on dipsticks is more sensitive to albumin than to globulin, hemoglobin, Bence Jones protein, or mucoprotein. A negative result, therefore, does not rule out the presence of these other proteins. Pyridium® metabolites may mask the reaction. X-ray contrast media, tolbutamide, nafcillin, massive doses of penicillin, sulfisoxazole (Gantrisin®), para-aminosalicylic acid, and high levels of cephalosporins may cause false-positive reactions with the sulfosalicylic acid method. The detection limit of Albustix® (Ames Division, Miles Laboratories) is reported as 300 mg/L or 500 mg/day protein. Since normal albuminuria is <20 mg/L, the screening dipstick lacks sensitivity for early detection of protein loss in diabetic nephropathy.[3] See listing for Microalbuminuria in this chapter. **METHODOLOGY:** Dipstick, and in some laboratories sulfosalicylic acid, are run on all urinalyses. The dipstick test is based on the color development of indicators. The sulfosalicylic acid test is based on the acid precipitation of protein. Immunofixation or immunoelectrophoresis is indicated when Bence Jones protein is suspected. **ADDITIONAL INFORMATION:** If the dipstick for protein is negative and the sulfosalicylic acid test is positive, Bence Jones proteinuria may be present. If clinically indicated, in this situation a urine for electrophoresis and immunoelectrophoresis for light chains or immunofixation should be considered. Normal newborns may have increased levels of proteinuria during first 3 days of life. Subclinical increased urinary albumin excretion is thought to be predictive of emergence subsequently of diabetic nephropathy.[1] A report suggests that in many situations, additional to diabetes, urine albumin by a specific method is much more sensitive to progressing renal disease than is urinary total protein (eg, hypertension, systemic lupus erythematosus). Urine albumin is easier to standardize and should be more sensitive to specific glomerular disease.[4] Following exercise, proteinuria relates more to intensity of exercise than to its duration.[5] Discrepancies between protein methods can be recognized in some settings by skilled microscopy of the urinary sediment.

Footnotes

1. Risdon P and Shaw AB, "Which Urine Sample for Detection of Proteinuria?" *Br J Urol*, 1989, 63(2):209-10.
2. Harrison NA, Rainford DJ, White GA, et al, "Proteinuria - What Value Is the Dipstick?" *Br J Urol*, 1989, 63(2):202-8.
3. Hindmarsh JT, "Microalbuminuria," *Clin Lab Med*, 1988, 8(3):611-6.
4. Shihabi ZK, Konen JC, and O'Connor ML, "Albuminuria vs Urinary Total Protein for Detecting Chronic Renal Disorders," *Clin Chem*, 1991, 37(5):621-4.
5. Poortmans JR, "Postexercise Proteinuria in Humans - Facts and Mechanisms," *JAMA*, 1985, 253:236-40.

References

Burke EC and Stickler GB, "Proteinuria in Children. Review and Evaluation," *Clin Pediatr (Phila)*, 1982, 21:741-3.

Schwab SJ, Christensen RL, Dougherty K, et al, "Quantitation of Proteinuria by the Use of Protein-to-Creatinine Ratios in Single Urine Samples," *Arch Intern Med*, 1987, 147:943-4.
Viberti G and Keen H, "The Patterns of Proteinuria in Diabetes Mellitus. Relevance to Pathogenesis and Prevention of Diabetic Nephropathy," *Diabetes*, 1984, 33:686-92, (review).

Protein, Urine, Sulfosalicylic Acid *see* Protein, Semiquantitative, Urine *on page 1147*

Prussian Blue Stain, Urine *see* Hemosiderin Stain, Urine *on page 1123*

Purple Urine Bags *see* Indican, Semiquantitative, Urine *on page 1124*

Quick-Cult® *see* Occult Blood, Stool *on page 1138*

Reducing Substances, Stool

CPT *81099*

Related Information

d-Xylose Absorption Test *on page 210*
Lactose Tolerance Test *on page 275*
Meat Fibers, Stool *on page 1133*
pH, Stool *on page 1143*

Test Commonly Includes Stool weight, stool pH, and total reducing substances

Abstract Test for fecal reducing substance (eg, sugars) as an indication of disaccharidase (sucrase, lactase) deficiency

Specimen Fresh random stool **CONTAINER:** Plastic stool container **COLLECTION:** Transport the specimen to the laboratory as soon as possible; delay may cause falsely low results. **STORAGE INSTRUCTIONS:** Freeze specimen if testing is delayed. **CAUSES FOR REJECTION:** Improper labeling, specimen collected in a diaper or other absorbent surface

Interpretive **REFERENCE RANGE:** Normal: <2 mg/g stool; borderline: between 2-5 mg/g stool; abnormal: >5 mg/g stool. Even though premature infants have relative lactase deficiency and pancreatic insufficiency, there is evidence that older (32 weeks gestation) prematures have insignificant fecal loss of intact carbohydrate. Comparison of fecal carbohydrate excretion in infants fed formulas of 50% lactose vs 50% lactose plus 50% glucose polymers found no significant difference. Mean excretion was <0.2 g/day (<1% of carbohydrate intake).[1] **USE:** Detect deficiency of intestinal border enzymes, primarily sucrase and lactase (disaccharidases) due to congenital deficiency or nonspecific mucosal injury **LIMITATIONS:** Bacterial fermentation may give falsely low results if specimen is not analyzed within 1 hour. In the neonatal period, high Clinitest® results may be observed. **METHODOLOGY:** Clinitest®[2] **ADDITIONAL INFORMATION:** Sugars should be rapidly absorbed in the upper small intestine. If not, however, they remain in the intestine and cause osmotic diarrhea by the osmotic pressure of the unabsorbed sugar in the intestine, drawing fluid and electrolytes into the gut. Carbohydrate malabsorption is a major cause of the watery diarrhea and electrolyte imbalance seen in patients with the short bowel syndrome. As a result of bacterial fermentation, the stools become acid with a high concentration of lactic acid. The pH measurement reflects this process. The unabsorbed sugars are measured as reducing substances. Although sucrose is not a reducing sugar, it is subjected to acid hydrolysis in the gut, and thus, is also measured as a reducing substance. Idiopathic lactase deficiency is common, occurring in 70% to 75% of Southern European Greeks and Italians, 70% of black adults, more than 90% of Oriental adults, and 5% to 20% of white American adults. Lactase activity declines with age in humans and is controlled genetically. It is influenced in its phenotypic expression as lactase malabsorption by several nongenetic factors (eg, adaption to nutritional intake of dairy products, biological (circadian) rhythm of enzyme activity, hormones and hormonal changes of the body and the brain, gastrointestinal functions such as motility and the nutritional components of digested food).[3] The breath hydrogen analysis test may provide more definitive information.[4,5] The $^{13}CO_2$ breath test is reportedly more sensitive and specific than the H_2 test in the detection of low jejunal lactase activity.[6] There is considerable variation in lactose tolerance between lactase deficient subjects. A 50 g lactose load has been reported to cause symptoms in 75% of lactase deficient adults whereas 10 g causes symptoms in only 50%.[7] A glass of milk has approximately 12 g of lactose. Classically, stools from patients with disaccharidase deficiency are liquid, acid, and frothy in appearance. The use of mucosal disaccharidase enzyme activity as an isolated diagnostic criterion may have limited value.[8]

Footnotes

1. Ameen VZ and Powell GK, "Quantitative Fecal Carbohydrate Excretion in Premature Infants," *Am J Clin Nutr*, 1989, 49(6):1238-42.

(Continued)

Reducing Substances, Stool *(Continued)*

2. Kerry KR and Anderson CM, "A Ward Test for Sugars in Feces," *Lancet*, 1964, 1:981.
3. Enck P and Whitehead WE, "Lactase Deficiency and Lactose Malabsorption. A Review," *Z Gastroenterol*, 1986, 24:125-34.
4. Rosado JL and Solomons NW, "Sensitivity and Specificity of the Breath Analysis Test for Detecting Malabsorption of Physiological Doses of Lactose," *Clin Chem*, 1983, 29:545-8.
5. Ostrander CR, Cohen RS, Hopper AO, et al, "Breath Hydrogen Analysis: A Review of the Methodologies and Clinical Applications," *J Pediatr Gastroenterol Nutr*, 1983, 2:525-33.
6. Hiele M, Ghoos Y, Rutgeerts P, et al, "$^{13}CO_2$ Breath Test Using Naturally ^{13}C-Enriched Lactose for Detection of Lactase Deficiency in Patients With Gastrointestinal Symptoms," *J Lab Clin Med*, 1988, 112(2):193-200.
7. Cooper BT, "Lactase Deficiency and Lactose Malabsorption," *Dig Dis*, 1986, 4:72-82.
8. Calvin RT, Klish WJ, and Nichols BL, "Disaccharidase Activities, Jejunal Morphology, and Carbohydrate Tolerance in Children With Chronic Diarrhea," *J Pediatr Gastroenterol Nutr*, 1985, 4:949-53.

References

Ameen VZ, Powell GK, and Jones LA, "Quantitation of Fecal Carbohydrate Excretion in Patients With Short Bowel Syndrome," *Gastroenterology*, 1987, 92:493-500.

Gray GM, "Congenital and Adult Intestinal Lactase Deficiency," *N Engl J Med*, 1976, 294:1057-8.

Hammer HF, Fine KD, Santa Ana CA, et al, "Carbohydrate Malabsorption. Its Measurement and Its Contribution to Diarrhea," *J Clin Invest*, 1990, 86(6):1936-44.

Lloyd ML and Olsen WA, "A Study of the Molecular Pathology of Sucrase-Isomaltase Deficiency: A Defect in the Intracellular Processing of the Enzyme," *N Engl J Med*, 1987, 316:438-42.

Reducing Substances, Urine

***CPT** 81005*

Related Information

Glucose, 2-Hour Postprandial *on page 237*
Glucose, Fasting *on page 238*
Glucose, Quantitative, Urine *on page 1120*
Glucose, Random *on page 240*
Glucose, Semiquantitative, Urine *on page 1121*
Glucose Tolerance Test *on page 241*
Ketone Bodies, Blood *on page 265*
Ketones, Urine *on page 1128*

Synonyms Clinitest® for Sugar, Urine

Test Commonly Includes Clinitest® testing of urine

Specimen Random urine **CONTAINER:** Plastic urine container **STORAGE INSTRUCTIONS:** If the specimen cannot be processed promptly by the laboratory, it should be refrigerated. **CAUSES FOR REJECTION:** Improper labeling, specimen not refrigerated

Interpretive **REFERENCE RANGE:** None detected **USE:** Semiquantitative determination of reducing substances (usually glucose) in urine; detect glycosuria, galactosuria; screen for overt diabetes mellitus; screen for pentosuria; detect renal glycosuria. With the widespread availability and low cost of specific glucose-oxidase test strips for the detection of glucosuria, this test remains useful for the screening of sick newborns and children for various errors of sugar metabolism.[1] Positive urine samples that are negative for glucose should be further confirmed by sugar chromatography. In this setting, even trace positive Clinitest® results should be recognized as abnormal. **LIMITATIONS:** Clinitest® is not specific for glucose and will react with sufficient quantities of **any** reducing substance in the urine. Glucose, lactose, fructose, galactose and pentose all cause positive Clinitest®. Large quantities of salicylates, penicillin, ascorbic acid, nalidixic acid, cephalosporins, glucuronic acid, creatinine, uric acid, formaldehyde, and probenecid may cause false-positives.[2] Low specific gravity urines may give slightly elevated results. **METHODOLOGY:** Copper sulfate reacts with reducing substances in urine, converting cupric sulfate to cuprous oxide. The lower limit of glucose detection by Clinitest® is 200 mg glucose/dL (SI: 11.1 mmol/L). Semiquantitation is accomplished by comparison of the color generated with a reference chart. Semiquantitation of urine glucose is also readily accomplished by urine dipstick. This reaction is also utilized in detection of reducing substances in stool.

Footnotes

1. Wannmacher CMD, Wajner M, Buchalter MS, et al, "Detection of Inborn Errors of Metabolism in Unselected Patients From Pediatric Intensive Care Units in Porto Alegre, Brazil: Evaluation of Screening Techniques," *Braz J Med Biol Res*, 1987, 20:11-23.
2. McCue JD, Gal P, and Pearson RC, "Interference of New Penicillins and Cephalosporins With Urine Glucose Monitoring Tests," *Diabetes Care*, 1983, 6:504-5.

Refractive Index, Urine *see* Specific Gravity, Urine *on next page*

Renal Calculus Analysis *see* Kidney Stone Analysis *on page 1129*

Semen Analysis

CPT 89320

Related Information

Infertility Screen *on page 1124*
Sperm Mucus Penetration Test (Human or Bovine Cervical Mucus) *on page 1154*
Sperm Penetration Assay (Human Sperm-Hamster Oocyte) *on page 1155*

Synonyms Seminal Cytology; Sperm Count; Sperm Examination; Sperm Morphology Study

Test Commonly Includes A variety of parameters may be included in a "standard" semen analysis, generally an assessment of number, motility, and morphology of the spermatozoa. More specifically, volume of the semen specimen, concentration of sperm, total count, liquefaction status, viscosity, color, odor, assessment of motility, determination of viability, and detection of abnormal morphologic forms. Direct microscopy of wet preparations and/or a modified Papanicolaou method may be utilized.

Abstract Analysis usually consists of a number of measurements including the physical characteristics of the semen and the functional ability of its constituent spermatozoa.

Patient Care **PREPARATION:** Ejaculation should be avoided for 2-3 days prior to collection.

Specimen Semen from ejaculate specimen **CONTAINER:** Clean, dry, wide mouth glass or plastic bottle maintained warm and known to be free of detergent or other toxic compounds **COLLECTION:** Physician will usually provide instruction for collection. Specimen quality is enhanced when collected in physician's office or laboratory obviating delay in testing and exposure to extremes of temperature occasioned by transportation. Alternately, specimen may be obtained at patient's house by coitus interruptus or masturbation and delivered to the laboratory as soon as possible.[1] Collection of semen during intercourse using a seminal collection device may yield a specimen of higher quality as compared to collection by masturbation.[2,3] Use of such a Silastic condom-type seminal pouch (with a small pencil lead-size perforation) to obtain a specimen for analysis in overcoming human infertility is acceptable to and falls within the principles of the Catholic Church.[4] Patient should be instructed to bring specimen to the laboratory within 30-60 minutes after collection maintaining warmth (37°C) during transport. Patient should be instructed to transport specimen in a pocket close to the skin. **CAUSES FOR REJECTION:** Specimen more than 2 hours old, error or problem with identification/labeling **SPECIAL INSTRUCTIONS:** Requisition should specify infertility study or postvasectomy study. Semen, as with all blood, urine, and body fluid specimens, because of the risk of AIDS, should be received and handled with attention to cleanliness. Gloves must be worn during the handling and manipulation of sperm/semen containing fluids. Persons with sores/open wounds of the skin must avoid contact with semen.

Interpretive **REFERENCE RANGE:** Volume: 2-5 mL; appearance: white, viscid, opaque; clotting and liquefaction: complete in 20-30 minutes; pH: 7.12-8; sperm count: 50-150 million/mL; motility: at least 60% mobile; morphology: at least 70% normal oval-headed forms **USE:** Infertility studies, postvasectomy studies; diagnose azoospermia, oligospermia **LIMITATIONS:** Low temperature during transport may decrease motility of sperm; lack of standardization of many test parameters **METHODOLOGY:** Macroscopic and microscopic analysis; direct observation, enumeration, and description; systems for computer-assisted study of morphology and motility are available commercially. **ADDITIONAL INFORMATION:** In a series of seven patients, there is suggestive evidence that sperm counts may be some 30% reduced in patients taking cimetidine.[5] The mechanism for sperm count reduction is unknown. LH response to LHRF was reduced and plasma testosterone levels were increased. Other drugs that may be responsible for decrease in sperm count include cyclophosphamide, nitrogen mustard, procarbazine, vincristine, methotrexate, and possibly other chemotherapeutics. Estrogens and methyltestosterone may suppress spermatogenesis. Orchitis, testicular atrophy (as after mumps), varicocele testicular failure, obstruction of vas deferens (as after vasectomy), and hyperpyrexia may be associated with hypospermia or azoospermia and/or morphologically aberrant forms of spermatozoa. The motility of spermatozoa is dependent upon the level of ionized calcium, in particular the intracellular translocation of calcium ions.[6] Cigarette smoking is associated with decrease in volume of semen; coffee drinking with increase in sperm density and percentage of abnormal forms.[7] There is evidence that alcohol consumption does not affect sperm function as measured at semen analysis.[7] In some cases of infertility, cytologically abnormal spermatocytes or spermatogonia may be seen. A number of associations and known

(Continued)

Semen Analysis *(Continued)*

etiologies not withstanding the cause of oligospermia in most infertile men will remain unknown. Fertility correlates most closely with the parameters of sperm motility and morphology. For high volume testing, automated computer-assisted semen analysis has been introduced.[8]

Footnotes

1. Cannon DC and Henry JB, "Seminal Fluid," *Clinical Diagnosis and Management by Laboratory Methods*, 18th ed, Henry JB, ed, Philadelphia, PA: WB Saunders Co, 1991, 497-503.
2. Zavos PM, "Seminal Parameters of Ejaculates Collected From Oligospermic and Nonspermic Patients Via Masturbation and at Intercourse With the Use of a Silastic Seminal Fluid Collection Device," *Fertil Steril*, 1985, 44:517-20.
3. Zavos PM and Goodpasture JC, "Clinical Improvements of Specific Seminal Deficiencies Via Intercourse With a Seminal Collection Device Versus Masturbation," *Fertil Steril*, 1989, 51(1):190-3.
4. Griese ON, Rev Msgr, *Catholic Identity in Healthcare: Principles and Practice*, The Pope John Center, 1987, 51-3.
5. Fuentes RJ Jr and Dolinsky D, "Endocrine Function After Cimetidine," *N Engl J Med*, 1979, 301:501-2, (letter).
6. Aaberg RA, Sauer MV, Sikka S, et al, "Effects of Extracellular Ionized Calcium, Diltiazem, and cAMP on Motility of Human Spermatozoa," *J Urol*, 1989, 141(5):1221-4.
7. Marshburn PB, Sloan CS, and Hammond MG, "Semen Quality and Association With Coffee Drinking, Cigarette Smoking, and Ethanol Consumption," *Fertil Steril*, 1989, 52(1):162-5.
8. Johnson JE, Boone WR, and Shiparo SS, "Determination of the Precision of an Automated Semen Analyzer," *Lab Med*, 1990, 21:33-8.

References

Adelman MM and Cahill EM, *Atlas of Sperm Morphology*, Chicago, IL: ASCP Press, 1989.

Ginsburg KA, Sacco AG, Ager JW, et al, "Variation of Movement Characteristics With Washing and Capacitation of Spermatozoa. II. Multivariate Statistical Analysis and Prediction of Sperm Penetrating Ability," *Fertil Steril*, 1990, 53(4):704-8.

Glover TD, Barratt CLR, Tyler JPP, et al, *Human Male Fertility and Semen Analysis*, San Diego, CA: Academic Press Inc, 1990, 123-45.

Kjeldsberg CR and Knight JA, *Body Fluids: Laboratory Examination of Amniotic, Cerebrospinal, Seminal, Serous, and Synovial Fluids: A Textbook Atlas*, 2nd ed, Chicago, IL: ASCP Press, 1986, 117-27.

Overstreet JW and Katz DF, "Semen Analysis," *Urol Clin North Am*, Philadelphia, PA: WB Saunders Co, 1987, 14:441-9.

Van Thiel DH, Gavaler JS, Smith WI Jr, et al, "Hypothalamic-Pituitary-Gonadal Dysfunction in Men Using Cimetidine," *N Engl J Med*, 1979, 300:1012-5.

World Health Organization, *WHO Laboratory Manual for the Examination of Human Semen and Semen-Cervical Mucus Interaction*, New York, NY: Cambridge University Press, 1987.

Zamboni L, "Clinical Relevance of Evaluation of Sperm and Ova," *Pathology of Reproductive Failure*, Kraus FT, Damjanov I, and Kaufman N, eds, *Intl Acad Pathol Monograph*, Baltimore, MD: Williams & Wilkins, 1991, 10-31.

Seminal Cytology *see* Semen Analysis *on previous page*

SG, Urine *see* Specific Gravity, Urine *on this page*

SPA, Hamster Zona-Free Ovum Test *see* Sperm Penetration Assay (Human Sperm-Hamster Oocyte) *on page 1155*

Specific Gravity, Body Fluid *see* Specific Gravity, Urine *on this page*

Specific Gravity, Urine

CPT 81003

Related Information

Osmolality, Urine *on page 302*

Urinalysis *on page 1162*

Synonyms Refractive Index, Urine; SG, Urine

Applies to Specific Gravity, Body Fluid

Test Commonly Includes Specific gravity is usually part of Urinalysis.

Specimen Random void urine or body fluid **CONTAINER:** Plastic urine container **COLLECTION:** First morning specimen is recommended, unless part of complete urinalysis. Transport specimen to the laboratory within 2 hours of collection. **STORAGE INSTRUCTIONS:** If not run promptly, specimen should be refrigerated. **CAUSES FOR REJECTION:** Improper labeling, specimen not refrigerated **SPECIAL INSTRUCTIONS:** Container should state date and time of collection.

Interpretive **REFERENCE RANGE:** Range: 1.003-1.029; adult on normal fluid intake: 1.016-1.022; specific gravity decreases with increasing age **USE:** Evaluate concentrating and excretory

Specific Gravity, Urine

Increased **>1.020**	**Decreased** **<1.009**	**Fixed** **1.010**
Water restriction Dehydration Fever Sweating Vomiting Diarrhea Diabetes mellitus (glycosuria) Proteinuria Congestive heart failure X-ray dyes Adrenal insufficiency Inappropriate antidiuretic hormone secretion syndrome Tumors secreting antidiuretic hormone	Excess water ingestion Excess I.V. fluids Diuresis Hypothermia Impaired renal concentrating ability pyelonephritis glomerulonephritis diabetes insipidus	Severe renal damage, urine concentration fixed at 1.010, the value of glomerular filtrate

power of the kidneys. See table. The urine specific gravity test strips have been effective in home use to help stone formers drink enough water to reduce stone formation risk. **LIMITATIONS:** Radiographic dyes in urine increase the specific gravity by hydrometer or refractometer.[1] Glucose or protein also increase specific gravity out of proportion to osmolality, as measured by hydrometer or refractometer. **Strip method urine specific gravity** was reported as having a significant positive bias at urine pH ≤6 and negative bias at pH >7 compared to specific gravity by refractometer.[2] Urine osmolality is considered preferable in some settings. Benitez et al suggest that osmolality is the only accurate measure of urine concentration in newborn infants.[3] **METHODOLOGY:** Refractometer and colorimetric (reagent strip). **Dipstick method** responds to the ionic strength of urine (linear relation to osmolality due to electrolytes). The strip provides a polyionic polymer with binding sites saturated with hydrogen ions that with urine testing are replaced by sodium or potassium cations, consequent release of hydrogen ions (change of pH) affecting an indicator color change; apparent pKa change. Albumin and glucose osmotic effects are not measured, and as such a true specific gravity measurement may not be obtained.[4] **ADDITIONAL INFORMATION:** The specific gravity of urine indicates the relative proportions of dissolved solid components to the total volume of the specimen. It reflects the relative degree of concentration or dilution of the specimen. Knowledge of the specific gravity is needed in interpretation of results of most tests in urinalysis. Specific gravity must be interpreted in light of presence or absence of glycosuria and/or proteinuria. Measurement of urine specific gravity is easier and more convenient than direct measurement of osmolality. The two methods correlate well. However, measured osmolality in newborns is generally lower than would be expected by refractometer specific gravity. In newborns, an elevated specific gravity should be confirmed by direct measurement of osmolality when the state of hydration and water balance are being assessed.[3]

Reagent **strip methods** for the determination of urine specific gravity employ a colorimetric method and are sensitive to ions but not undissociated solutes such as urea. The strip method requires a corrected reading for pH ≥6.5 and protein increases the reading.[4] Critical clinical decisions should be based on the more definitive methods. The strip methods are reported to be suitable for urine screening purposes, but not uniformly so. Strip methods are not described as showing a high degree of correlation with refractometer or urinometer methods.[5] Their additional cost as well as bias leads Adams to conclude that strip specific gravity methods are neither cost-effective nor clinically useful[2] and Assadi and Fornell to conclude that the magnitude of observed discrepancies places important limitations on strip test SG measurement.[4]

When using the refractometer, cloudy urines or those with visible particles should be centrifuged, and the supernatant used for refractometer specific gravity determination.

Footnotes

1. Smith C and Arbogast PR, "Effects of X-Ray Contrast Media on the Results for Relative Density of Urine," *Clin Chem*, 1983, 29:730-8.
2. Adams LJ, "Evaluation of Ames Multistix® SG for Urine Specific Gravity Versus Refractometer Specific Gravity," *Am J Clin Pathol*, 1983, 80:871-3.

(Continued)

Specific Gravity, Urine *(Continued)*

3. Benitez OA, Benitez M, Stijnen T, et al, "Inaccuracy of Neonatal Measurement of Urine Concentration With a Refractometer," *J Pediatr*, 1986, 108:613-6.
4. Assadi FK and Fornell L, "Estimation of Urine Specific Gravity in Neonates With a Reagent Strip," *J Pediatr*, 1986, 108:995-6.
5. Ciulla AP, Newsome B, and Kaster J, "Reagent Strip Method for Specific Gravity: An Evaluation," *Lab Med*, 1985, 16:38-40.

References

Schumann GB and Schweitzer SC, "Examination of Urine," *Clinical Diagnosis and Management by Laboratory Methods*, Chapter 17, Henry JB, ed, Philadelphia, PA: WB Saunders Co, 1991, 396-7.

Sperm Agglutination and Inhibition *see* Infertility Screen *on page 1124*

Sperm Antibodies *see* Infertility Screen *on page 1124*

Sperm Count *see* Semen Analysis *on page 1151*

Sperm Examination *see* Semen Analysis *on page 1151*

Sperm Morphology Study *see* Semen Analysis *on page 1151*

Sperm Mucus Penetration Test (Human or Bovine Cervical Mucus)

CPT 89330

Related Information

Infertility Screen *on page 1124*
Semen Analysis *on page 1151*
Sperm Penetration Assay (Human Sperm-Hamster Oocyte) *on next page*

Applies to Cervical Mucus Interaction, Cross Hostility Tests; *In Vivo* Cervical Mucus Penetration (Postcoital) Test

Patient Care PREPARATION: Follow physician's instructions. Ejaculation should be avoided for 2-3 days prior to collection.

Specimen Liquefied semen. Normal seminal fluid should be liquefied by about 30 minutes after collection (at 37°C). Test should be started within 2-3 hours after collection of the sample. CONTAINER: Clean, dry, wide mouth glass or plastic bottle known to be free of detergent or substances toxic to spermatozoa COLLECTION: Postcoital or masturbation using condom-like Silastic seminal fluid collection device (see Semen Analysis listing) or directly into sterile glass jar. STORAGE INSTRUCTIONS: Samples should be tested as soon as possible after collection. Time between ejaculation and start of test should not be over 2-3 hours. Human cervical mucus (obtained during time of ovulation) may be stored for some hours at 4°C in the refrigerator. CAUSES FOR REJECTION: Specimen more than 2 hours old, improper identification TURNAROUND TIME: 1 day SPECIAL INSTRUCTIONS: Semen, as with all blood, urine, and body fluid specimens, because of the risk of AIDS, should be received and handled with close attention to cleanliness. Gloves must be worn during the handling and manipulation of sperm/semen containing fluids. Persons with sores/open wounds of the skin must avoid contact with semen.

Interpretive REFERENCE RANGE: ≥30 mm penetration by the "vanguard sperm" (Penetrak™ test) USE: Evaluate interaction between spermatozoa and cervical mucus LIMITATIONS: Test provides information additional to other semen tests (sperm count, motility, morphology; see Semen Analysis) and is not intended for use as a sole diagnostic indicator of male fertility potential.[1] METHODOLOGY: Miller and Kurzrok, in 1932, developed and made clinical application of a semen-mucus phase boundary test. A 3 mm-sized fragment of cervical mucus and a similar sized drop of semen were placed 3 mm from each other on a glass slide. A coverslip was applied with minimal motion and the events occurring at the semen-mucus interface were studied by microscopy.[2] In 1965 Kremer described the construction of a "sperm penetration meter" and its use in a cervical mucus sperm penetration test.[3] In the commercially available "Penetrak™" test, bovine cervical mucus is kept frozen in flat sealed capillary tubes. Using a standardized technique, sperm migration through the mucus over a 90-minute period is measured. The distance traveled by the sperm the furthest down the tube (the "vanguard sperm") is measured and reported. The average of duplicate values is reported. If values differ by more than 15 mm, it is recommended that the test be repeated on a different specimen. ADDITIONAL INFORMATION: In a study published in 1981, the bovine CMPT identified a group of individuals with inadequate penetration (<15 mm) who had mean sperm density of $53.8 \pm 6.8 \times 10^6$/mL (sperm counts within normal limits).[4] Significant numbers of individuals (5%, 10%, and 15% of different groups) had inadequate penetration, but adequate to high sperm counts or levels of motility. Results of *in vitro* tests of sperm penetration have been found to correlate with fertility (pregnancy). Cervical mucus penetration testing has been found of value in assessment of fertility prognosis, in particular when modified to produce a crossmatching penetrability test. The latter study compares results of penetration using cervical mucus of the patient's wife by subject's spermatozoa and additionally with use of semen from fertile donors.[5] The use of hormonally standardized human cervical mucus from female partners has been considered superior to bovine cervical mucus as a penetration medium and as to ability to provide information about sperm function.[6] There are data to suggest that the ability of cervical mucus to accept spermatozoa is dependent upon the carbohydrate composition of mucus glycoproteins.[7] See Sperm Penetration Assay (SPA) entry. The SPA uses the zona-free hamster egg, 100% penetration can be achieved by human spermatozoa. Techniques for optimizing and standardizing sperm and ovum preparation have been established. Correlation of SPA test results with human *in vitro* fertilization showed a very low incidence of individuals whose sperm penetrated zona-free hamster ova but did not efficiently penetrate human eggs.[8]

Footnotes

1. Serono Diagnostics Inc, Norwell, MA, 1987, (package insert).
2. Miller EG Jr and Kurzrok R, "Biochemical Studies of Human Semen. III. Factors Affecting Migration of Sperm Through the Cervix," *Am J Obstet Gynecol*, 1932, 24:19-26.
3. Kremer J, "A Simple Sperm Penetration Test," *Int J Fertil*, 1965, 10:209-15.
4. Alexander NJ, "Evaluation of Male Infertility With an *In Vitro* Cervical Mucus Penetration Test," *Fertil Steril*, 1981, 36:201-8.
5. Eggert-Kruse W, Gerhard I, Tilgen W, et al, "Clinical Significance of Crossed *In Vitro* Sperm-Cervical Mucus Penetration Test in Infertility Investigation," *Fertil Steril*, 1989, 52(6):1032-40.
6. Eggert-Kruse W, Leinhos G, Gerhard I, et al, "Prognostic Value of *In Vitro* Sperm Penetration Into Hormonally Standardized Human Cervical Mucus," *Fertil Steril*, 1989, 51(2):317-23.
7. Morales P, Roco M, and Vigil P, "Human Cervical Mucus: Relationship Between Biochemical Characteristics and Ability to Allow Migration of Spermatozoa," *Hum Reprod*, 1993, 8(1):78-83.
8. Smith RG, Johnson A, Lamb D, et al, "Functional Tests of Spermatozoa: Sperm Penetration Assay," *Urol Clin North Am*, 1987, 14:451-8.

References

Adelman MM and Cahill EM, *Atlas of Sperm Morphology*, Chicago, IL: ASCP Press, 1989, 99.

Sperm-Oolemma Binding Test *see* Infertility Screen *on page 1124*

Sperm Penetration Assay (Human Sperm-Hamster Oocyte)

***CPT** 89329*

Related Information

Infertility Screen *on page 1124*
Semen Analysis *on page 1151*
Sperm Mucus Penetration Test (Human or Bovine Cervical Mucus) *on previous page*

Synonyms Hamster (Human + Hamster) Test; Hamster Test; Heterologous Ovum Penetration Test; SPA, Hamster Zona-Free Ovum Test

Abstract The SPA is an *in vitro* test that can provide an important measure of the fertilizing capacity of human spermatozoa. The test measures the ability of human sperm to penetrate zona-free hamster oocytes. The test thus reflects the ability of sperm to capacitate, acrosome react, fuse with the oolemma and decondense (within zona-free hamster oocytes).

Patient Care **PREPARATION:** Abstinence for a period of at least 48 hours prior to test; less than 48 hours (12 or 24 hours) is associated with reduced penetration potential even though sperm count or motility may not be decreased.[1]

Specimen Semen **CONTAINER:** Clean, wide mouth glass or plastic container; condom-like device (Silastic seminal fluid collection device – available commercially) placed in a clean jar. Containers should be known free of detergent or other toxic compounds. **COLLECTION:** Proper collection and handling of the semen specimen is critically necessary to obtain representative results. Semen collection by masturbation in a special room within or adjacent to the laboratory performing the analysis is ideal for some patients. This allows for direct transfer to the laboratory of a fresh specimen without risking degradation of spermatozoa by aging or temperature extremes incurred during transportation.[2] Patient preference, however, may dictate the use of a coital specimen (collected during intercourse) using a Silastic seminal fluid collection device. Commercial sources for such devices include (but may not be limited to) Male-Factor Pak manufactured by Apex Medical Technologies Inc, available from Fertility Technologies Inc, Natick, Massachusetts; HDC Corporation, Mountain View, California. There is evidence

(Continued)

Sperm Penetration Assay (Human Sperm-Hamster Oocyte) *(Continued)*

that semen quality is improved when collected during intercourse using such a device.[3,4,5] Specimen must be delivered to the laboratory within 30-60 minutes after collection. Avoid exposure to extremes of heat or cold during transport (patient should be instructed to carry specimen in a pocket close to the skin). **STORAGE INSTRUCTIONS:** Specimen is maintained in the laboratory at room temperature, allowed to liquefy (usually occurs within 30 minutes, abnormal if not liquefied by 60 minutes), standard semen analysis is commonly initiated, and specimen is buffered (see below) and incubated at 4°C for 18 hours or longer. **CAUSES FOR REJECTION:** Question concerning authenticity of specimen identification (label, content), exposure to extreme of temperature, specimen more than 1 hour old (sperm should not stay in contact with seminal fluid for more than 1-2 hours prior to processing) **TURNAROUND TIME:** Results usually available within 36 hours (dependent upon preincubation time which in current procedures may be as long as 18-22 hours). **SPECIAL INSTRUCTIONS:** Semen, as with all blood, urine, and body fluid specimens, because of the risk of AIDS, should be received and handled with close attention to cleanliness. Gloves must be worn during the handling and manipulation of sperm/semen containing fluids. Persons with sores/open wounds of the skin must avoid contact with semen specimens.

Interpretive **REFERENCE RANGE:** Penetration of 21% to 100% – ("good category");[6] penetration index of over 0.2. The terms "penetration index,"[6] "fertilization index,"[7] and "sperm capacitation index,"[8] are a measure of polyspermy (the average number of penetrations per ovum). Earlier procedural protocols found the lower limit of the penetration range for fertile men to vary from 11% to 25%.[7] **USE:** Evaluate fertilizing capability of human spermatozoa;[8] application to the study of effect that environmental factors have on male fertility; a clinical test of sperm function in conjunction with semen analysis and other studies as a screen for *in vitro* fertilization. The SPA measures components of sperm penetration including capacitation (see below), acrosome reaction, chromatin decondensation, and ability to fuse with oolemma. **LIMITATIONS:** SPA does not assess all functions of human spermatozoa. The test does not measure the ability of sperm to penetrate human ova with granulosa cells and zona pellucida intact. Ability of spermatozoa to bind the zona pellucida is species specific. Thus, semen with a positive SPA result may not necessarily have sperm with normal penetrating ability (false-positive result). Rarely, a patient with a score of zero on SPA will subsequently initiate a pregnancy (false-negative result).[9] The test suffers from lack of standardization and is relatively expensive. Cumulus and zona-free hamster oocytes are not true physiologic models. Extensive experience with the SPA used in conjunction with *in vitro* fertilization, however, indicates that in the great majority of individuals, sperm capable of penetrating zona-free hamster ova can also penetrate intact human eggs.[10] **METHODOLOGY:** The original method of Yanagimachi et al utilized a modified Krebs-Ringer's culture medium developed by Biggers, Whitten, and Whittingham (BWW medium) supplemented with human serum albumin.[11] Ova were obtained from superovulated hamsters and prepared by treatment with bovine testicular hyaluronidase (divests the surrounding cumulus cells). The zona pellucida was removed by treatment with bovine pancreatic trypsin. Human semen, after liquification was diluted with BWW medium, filtered, washed, resuspended, and incubated at 37°C for up to 7.5 hours in air or 5% CO_2. A drop of sperm suspension was placed with ova in BWW medium and examined periodically using phase contrast microscopy for evidence of sperm penetration. Evidence of penetration (fertilization) was presence of swollen sperm heads within the cytoplasm of an oocyte.

The need for maintenance of a hamster colony with production and harvesting of ova on demand and subsequent considerable manipulation and processing places this procedure beyond the capability of most general routine clinical laboratories. The assay has undergone continuing improvement and simplification. Sperm function, (capacitation) has been enhanced by use of TES and TRIS (TEST)-yolk-extender buffer (TYB) system, cooling slowly and incubating for 22-42 hours (may be kept up to 96 hours).[6,12,13] The TYB system has increased SPA sensitivity and has allowed specimens to be sent to a reference laboratory. In addition, cryopreserved hamster ova have become commercially available (Cryotech™ hamster ova, Charles River Laboratories, Wilmington, Massachusetts; sales agent Fertility Technologies, Natick, Massachusetts). These are provided in straws, frozen at -150°C (requires liquid nitrogen). Availability of frozen ova simplifies the SPA procedure, logistically allows for ova on demand (can be prepared for use in about 7 minutes) and provides a baseline for use in quality control procedures. The ova (15 per straw) are suspended in propylene glycol (cryoprotectant) in an isotonic salt solution. A sucrose solution, isosmotic to the propylene glycol, is also present in the straw. It acts as an osmotic buffer during dilution of the cryoprotectant out of the ova. The frozen ova were found to be statistically equivalent (% penetration and penetration index) to unfrozen ova in a study of the SPA using 547 frozen hamster ova.[14]

A modification of the SPA uses 10 μL wells of Teraski tissue-typing plates allowing the study of very small numbers of spermatozoa as they interact with single hamster ova. This modification may be of value clinically in cases of severe abnormality when few motile spermatozoa can be recovered.[15]

ADDITIONAL INFORMATION: There is a lack of consensus and a surprisingly wide variety of opinion concerning the value of the sperm penetration assay in the study of fertility. The 1992 review by Liu and Baker[8] indicates that "the clinical significance of the SPA in predicting male fertility is still disputed" but that "the SPA has been widely used as a clinical test of sperm function." Correlation with the results of *in vitro* fertilization (IVF) has been variable.[6] Over 200 publications dealt with the SPA from 1981-1985.[7] Lack of standardized test parameters, small sample size, and/or variable, often poorly defined parameters of the patient test population characterize many of these reports. Comparisons and conclusions are problematic.

There is unanimity of opinion that the SPA does assess sperm capacitation, acrosome reaction, ability to fuse with oolemma, and chromatin decondensation with head swelling in cytoplasma of the ovum.[6,8] These are major physiologic events necessary to fertilization. The acrosome is a double- layered membrane, an envelope covering the anterior two-thirds of the sperm head. The acrosome contains hydrolytic enzymes including acrosin and hyaluronidase. With the acrosome reaction there is fusion and vesiculation of membranes, formation of pores, and eventual loss of sperm, and outer acrosomal membranous envelope anterior to the equator of the sperm head. The acrosome reaction must occur before the sperm can penetrate the zona pellucida. Round headed spermatozoa (without acrosomes) are thus not capable of fertilization. Before ejaculated spermatozoa are functional, they require a period of time (within the female tract or *in vitro*) before they can fertilize. This process is termed "capacitation" and is followed by an influx of calcium ions leading to the acrosome reaction. Capacitation is not associated with a recognizable morphologic change, thus, the important role of functional based assays such as the SPA.

A large study (241 couples) published in 1992 compared the results of SPA under conditions that enhance sperm capacitation (use of TYB system and cool incubation as detailed in methodology above) with outcome of *in vitro* fertilization.[6] A significant correlation was found between SPA penetration category (poor: 0% to 20%; good: 21% to 100%), and pregnancy rate after IVF. No pregnancy occurred (among eight embryo transfers) in the 31 cases falling into the "poor SPA" category. On the other hand there were 73 pregnancies (34.8%) in the 210 cases falling into the "good SPA" category. Sperm quality (count, motility, and morphology) were all significantly higher in "good SPA" versus the "poor SPA" categories. The authors concluded that the SPA "is a useful screening assay before IVF together with sperm morphology."[6]

Findings from computer-assisted semen analysis have been compared with SPA penetration rates. A study published in 1993 used total motile oval count (TMO), compared to concentration, motility, and technician determined morphology considered independently in predicting the outcome of SPA.[16] TMO was defined as the product of total count, percent motility, and percent normal (oval) forms in the semen specimen. TMO was a greater risk factor than percent sperm with oval morphology in relation to the outcome of SPA. Below 20% penetration in the SPA assay, both TMO and percent oval sperm were comparable predictive factors.

Footnotes

1. Rogers BJ, Perreault SD, Bentwood BJ, et al, "Variability in the Human-Hamster *In Vitro* Assay for Fertility Evaluation," *Fertil Steril*, 1983, 39:204-11.
2. Overstreet JW and Katz DF, "Semen Analysis," Male Infertility, *Urol Clin North Am*, 1987, 14:441-9.
3. Zavos PM, "Characteristics of Human Ejaculates Collected Via Masturbation and a New Silastic Seminal Fluid Collection Device," *Fertil Steril*, 1985, 43:491-2.
4. Zavos PM, "Seminal Parameters of Ejaculates Collected From Oligospermic and Normospermic Patients Via Masturbation and at Intercourse With the Use of a Silastic Seminal Fluid Collection Device," *Fertil Steril*, 1985, 44:517-20.
5. Zavos PM and Goodpasture JC, "Clinical Improvements of Specific Seminal Deficiencies Via Intercourse With a Seminal Collection Device Versus Masturbation," *Fertil Steril*, 1989, 51(1):190-3.
6. Soffer Y, Golan A, Herman A, et al, "Prediction of *In Vitro* Fertilization Outcome by Sperm Penetration Assay With TEST-Yolk Buffer Preincubation," *Fertil Steril*, 1992, 58(3):556-62.
7. Rogers BJ, "The Sperm Penetration Assay: Its Usefulness Reevaluated," *Fertil Steril*, 1985, 43:821-40.
8. Liu DY and Baker HWG, "Tests of Human Sperm Function and Fertilization *In Vitro*," *Fertil Steril*, 1992, 58(3):465-83.

(Continued)

Sperm Penetration Assay (Human Sperm-Hamster Oocyte) *(Continued)*

9. Kuzan FB, Muller CH, Zarutaskie PW, et al, "Human Sperm Penetration Assay as an Indicator of Sperm Function in Human *In Vitro* Fertilization," *Fertil Steril*, 1987, 48:282-6.
10. Smith RG, Johnson A, Lamb D, et al, "Functional Tests of Spermatozoa: Sperm Penetration Assay," *Urol Clin North Am*, 1987, 14:451-8.
11. Yanagimachi R, Yanagimachi H, and Rogers BJ, "The Use of Zona-Free Animal Ova as a Test-System for the Assessment of the Fertilizing Capacity of Human Spermatozoa," *Biol Reprod*, 1976, 15:471-6.
12. Johnson AR, Syms AJ, Lipshultz LI, et al, "Conditions Influencing Human Sperm Capacitation and Penetration of Zona-Free Hamster Ova," *Fertil Steril*, 1984, 41:603-8.
13. Veeck LL, "TES and TRIS (TEST)-Yolk Buffer Systems, Sperm Function Testing, and *In Vitro* Fertilization," *Fertil Steril*, 1992, 58(3):484-6.
14. Leibo SP, Giambernardi TA, Meyer TK, et al, "The Efficacy of Cryopreserved Hamster Ova in the Sperm Penetration Assay," *Fertil Steril*, 1990, 53(5):906-12.
15. Bronson RA, Oula L, and Bronson SK, "A Microwell Sperm Penetration Assay," *Fertil Steril*, 1992, 58(5):1078-80.
16. Brandeis VT, "Importance of Total Motile Oval Count in Interpreting the Hamster Ovum Sperm Penetration Assay," *J Androl*, 1993, 14(1):53-9.

References

Glover TD, Barratt CLR, Tyler JPP, et al, *Human Male Fertility and Semen Analysis*, San Diego, CA: Academic Press Inc, 1990, 123-45.

Lipshultz LI and Witt MA, "Infertility in the Male," *Infertility: A Practical Guide for the Physician*, 3rd ed, Hammond MG and Talbert LM, eds, Boston, MA: Blackwell Scientific Publications, 1992, 26-55.

Mao C and Grimes DA, "The Sperm Penetration Assay: Can It Discriminate Between Fertile and Infertile Men?" *Am J Obstet Gynecol*, 1988, 159:279-86.

Paulson RJ, Sauer MV, Francis MM, et al, "A Prospective Controlled Evaluation of TEST-Yolk Buffer in the Preparation of Sperm for Human *In Vitro* Fertilization in Suspected Cases of Male Infertility," *Fertil Steril*, 1992, 58(3):551-5.

Zamboni L, "Clinical Relevance of Evaluation of Sperm and Ova," *Pathology of Reproductive Failure*, Kraus FT, Damjanov I, and Kaufman N, eds, *Intl Acad Pathol Monograph*, Baltimore, MD: Williams & Wilkins, 1991, 10-31.

Stone Analysis *see* Kidney Stone Analysis *on page 1129*

Stool for Trypsin *see* Tryptic Activity, Stool *on page 1161*

Stool Guaiac *see* Occult Blood, Stool *on page 1138*

Stool pH *see* pH, Stool *on page 1143*

Stool Tryptic Activity *see* Tryptic Activity, Stool *on page 1161*

Sudan III Stain, Stool *see* Fat, Semiquantitative, Stool *on page 1118*

Sugar, Qualitative, Urine *see* Glucose, Semiquantitative, Urine *on page 1121*

Sugar, Quantitative, Urine *see* Glucose, Quantitative, Urine *on page 1120*

Synovial Fluid Analysis

CPT *87070 (culture bacterial); 88104 (cytopathology, smears with interpretation); 89051 (cell count with differential); 89060 (crystal identification)*

Related Information

Biopsy or Body Fluid Aerobic Bacterial Culture *on page 778*
Biopsy or Body Fluid Anaerobic Bacterial Culture *on page 778*
Biopsy or Body Fluid Fungus Culture *on page 780*
Biopsy or Body Fluid Mycobacteria Culture *on page 782*
Body Fluid Glucose *on page 148*
Body Fluid Lactate Dehydrogenase *on page 149*
Body Fluids Analysis, Cell Count *on page 523*
Body Fluids Cytology *on page 482*
Gram Stain *on page 815*
Rheumatoid Factor *on page 740*

Synonyms Joint Fluid Analysis; Knee Fluid Analysis

Applies to Mucin Test for Hyaluronic Acid

Test Commonly Includes May vary between laboratories but generally includes cell count and differential, cultures for pathogens, cytology, analysis to include clot lysis and viscosity, microscopic examination, uric acid, and rheumatoid factor

Abstract Analysis of joint fluid usually includes multiple studies (eg, cell count, microscopic exam, culture) to determine if joint pathology is present and to assess its nature and severity. Analyses are particularly helpful in differentiating traumatic arthritis from the immune-based and crystal-induced arthritides.

Patient Care PREPARATION: As per physician's usual aseptic aspiration technique

Specimen Joint fluid; simultaneously drawn venous blood in red top tube often helpful, especially with order for serum chemistry profile CONTAINER: Capped syringe or three sterile tubes, one with heparin and two red top tubes for joint fluid; one to two red top tubes of venous blood desirable; Thayer-Martin agar is best inoculated with joint fluid at bedside if gonococcal (GC) infection is suspected. COLLECTION: An experienced physician, using sterile technique, obtains the specimen (arthrocentesis). Media appropriate for culture of *N. gonorrhoeae*, *M. tuberculosis*, and other organisms should be available if indicated. STORAGE INSTRUCTIONS: Testing should be initiated, in most cases, shortly after receipt of the specimen. CAUSES FOR REJECTION: Some constituent tests of the analysis may not be performed if gross contamination has occurred. TURNAROUND TIME: From hours to days (eg, culture results) SPECIAL INSTRUCTIONS: Specimens should be delivered immediately to the laboratory and placed in the hands of a technologist. **Physician should indicate clinical impression and indicate tests he/she feels are necessary.**

Interpretive REFERENCE RANGE: When synovial fluid can be aspirated, abnormality is probably evident. Normal synovial fluid does not clot spontaneously, because it lacks fibrinogen. Clotting bears an implication of inflammation. There should be <200 WBCs/mm^3, 0% to 25% neutrophils, protein should be ≤ 3.0 g/dL (SI: ≤ 30 g/L), uric acid should be <8.0 mg/dL (SI: <476 μmol/L) and fluid LD (LDH) should be the same or less than that of the patient's serum drawn at the same time. Glucose is significantly abnormal in the nonfasting subject when it is <40 mg/dL (SI: <2.2 mmol/L). There should be a long string produced normally when synovial fluid is poured from a container and the mucin clot test is normally positive (ie, a firm mucin clot is formed in the presence of acetic acid). USE: Aid the diagnosis of rheumatic disease and diseases which cause joint symptoms, pain, increase in joint fluid or destruction of joint space, including rheumatoid arthritis, joint infection, gout, and pseudogout LIMITATIONS: Appropriate work-up may not be accomplished unless there is discussion between physician and analyst. Oxalate anticoagulants may lead to problems in crystal identification. If laboratory is unaware of possible gonococcal arthritis, it may not inoculate specimen on Thayer-Martin medium. If GC is possible, ideally the physician should plate out the Thayer-Martin medium at the bedside at time of aspiration. Limited sensitivity and specificity exist overall for synovial fluid analysis. Save for further analysis for possible bacterial and crystal-induced disease entities. METHODOLOGY: Includes polarizing as well as conventional microscopy. Laboratory notes color and presence of clot in centrifuged specimen. Cultures are made from centrifuged sediment and media inoculated for acid-fast bacteria, fungus, routine culture, and Gram stain smear. Rheumatoid factor titer is desirable in suspected cases of rheumatoid arthritis. Other testing methodologies may be applied as indicated or ordered. ADDITIONAL INFORMATION: Normal fluid is rarely obtained because of its small volume; therefore, any fluid which is aspirated is a potential diagnostic specimen. When the analysis is combined with the clinical impression of the physician, a high rate of accurate diagnosis is obtained. Some diagnoses cannot be made without the analysis. Heparinized tube is needed for cell count and differential. A red cell count is not necessary, but if grossly bloody, a hematocrit should be ordered. Joint fluid and/or serum uric acid may be helpful in cases of possible gout. Joint fluid uric acid significantly higher than serum uric acid may be diagnostic of gout. Other chemistries are usually of little value with the occasional exception of protein, LD (LDH), and glucose. Decreased fluid glucose indicates inflammation, but the result should be compared to that of serum or plasma. High synovial LD but normal serum LD suggests RA, infectious arthritis, or gout. Synovial LD is normal in degenerative joint disease.

Sediment or fluid may be given to Cytology mainly for examination for cartilage. The presence of cartilage cells supports diagnosis of traumatic arthritis or osteoarthritis. While involvement of joints by malignancy is uncommon, both primary and metastatic tumors should be included in the differential consideration.[1] Cytologic examination may support diagnosis of pigmented villonodular synovitis or Reiter's syndrome. While rhomboid cholesterol crystals have been reported in chronic joint effusions of rheumatoid arthritis and osteoarthritis, birefringent lipid bodies (lipid microspherules, liposomes, smectic mesophases, lipid liquid crystals), intra- and extracellular, at least partly formed of cholesterol ester, have been found in fluids from acute and chronic arthritis, traumatic arthritis, and pigmented villonodular synovitis.[2,3] Liposomes

(Continued)

Synovial Fluid Analysis *(Continued)*

(smectic mesophases, lipid liquid crystals), birefringent multilamellated (by EM) lipid microspherules have phospholipid characteristics and have been reported in cases of unexplained acute monoarthritis.[4]

Phase microscopy is used to look for intracellular inclusions in pus cells. These are "RA cells" only if the rheumatoid titer is positive. Synovial fluid in pseudogout, traumatic arthritis and osteoarthritis rarely also may contain intraleukocytic cytoplasmic inclusions. Polarizing microscopy is done to identify crystals of urate and pyrophosphate, the causes of gout and pseudogout. Calcium pyrophosphate dihydrate (CPPD) crystal deposition disease does not equate exclusively with a diagnosis of pseudogout (chondrocalcinosis). It is important to recognize that CPPD disease encompasses an array of disorders occurring largely in the aged.[5] These include asymptomatic chondrocalcinosis, acute pseudogout, and chronic pyrophosphate arthropathy. Cases of CPPD disease may be sporadic, familial, or secondary to metabolic disease.[5] Hyperparathyroidism and hemochromatosis may be associated with CPPD deposition. Pyrophosphate salt deposition usually occurs in those of advanced age. As an example, asymptomatic chondrocalcinosis occurs in 10% to 15% in 65-75 years of age and in 30% to 60% of those older than 80 years of age.[5] Cholesterol crystals occur occasionally, indicating RA, and steroid crystals after injection may be found. LE cells may be noted in fluid.

Test for viscosity and mucin test for hyaluronic acid measure the character of the synovial fluid. Abnormality in either of these tests indicates dilution or inflammation. The viscosity can be evaluated by the quality of stringing; inflammatory fluids of low viscosity produce very short strings, but normal or noninflammatory fluids produce long strings. Viscosity is generally equivalent to mucin hyaluronate content.

The finding of amyloid in synovial fluid (using Congo red stained sections of 10% formol saline fixed, paraffin-embedded, centrifuged sediment) has been considered a sufficient finding to establish a diagnosis of amyloid arthropathy.[6]

More than 2% eosinophils in synovial fluid may be a clue to presence of Lyme disease. Rheumatoid factor negative patients with oligoarthritis of unknown etiology were tested for *Chlamydia trachomatis* utilizing antigen specific synovial T-cell response and detection of bacterial antigen. Antigen specific lymphocyte proliferation was found in the synovial fluid of 34% of such patients. *C. trachomatis* was the most frequent single agent detected. Only chlamydial antigen was found in synovial fluid cells by monoclonal antibody technique.[7]

A variety of cytokines have been found in synovial fluid. Some (IL-6 and IL-8) are increased in cases of inflammatory arthritis (RA) as compared with cases of osteoarthritis.[8]

Individual laboratories may not be proficient in the identification of crystals in synovial fluid.[9] Artifacts and unexplained birefringent materials may be present. Patients with hemarthrosis may develop solid and angular birefringent crystals of two different types. Rectangular hemoglobin- like crystals within red cells are weakly birefringent. Golden brown rhomboid crystals (likely hematoidin) are intensely birefringent with positive or negative elongation. These red cell-derived crystals may be confused with pathogenic crystals.[10]

Footnotes

1. Chakravarty KK and Webley M, "Monarthritis: An Unusual Presentation of Renal Cell Carcinoma," *Ann Rheum Dis*, 1992, 51(5):681-2.
2. Ugai K, Kurosaka M, and Hirohata K, "Lipid Microspherules in Synovial Fluid of Patients With Pigmented Villonodular Synovitis," *Arthritis Rheum*, 1988, 31(11):1442-6.
3. Baer AN and Wright EP, "Lipid Laden Macrophages in Synovial Fluid: A Late Finding in Traumatic Arthritis," *J Rheumatol*, 1987, 14:848-51.
4. Reginato AJ, Schumacher HR, Allan DA, et al, "Acute Monoarthritis Associated With Lipid Liquid Crystals," *Ann Rheum Dis*, 1985, 44:537-43.
5. Bonafede RP, "Evaluating CPPD Crystal Deposition, An Important Disease of Aging," *Geriatrics*, 1988, 43(11):59-68.
6. Muñoz-Gómez J, Gómez-Pérez R, Solé-Arques M, et al, "Synovial Fluid Examination for the Diagnosis of Synovial Amyloidosis in Patients With Chronic Renal Failure Undergoing Haemodialysis," *Ann Rheum Dis*, 1987, 46:324-6.
7. Sieper J, Braun J, Brandt J, et al, "Pathogenetic Role of *Chlamydia*, *Yersinia*, and *Borrelia* in Undifferentiated Oligoarthritis," *J Rheumatol*, 1992, 19(8):1236-42.
8. Remick DG, DeForge LE, Sullivan JF, et al, "Profile of Cytokines in Synovial Fluid Specimens From Patients With Arthritis – Interleukin 8 (IL-8) and IL-6 Correlate With Inflammatory Arthritides," *Immunol Invest*, 1992, 21(4):321-7.
9. McGill NW and York HF, "Reproducibility of Synovial Fluid Examination for Crystals," *Aust N Z J Med*, 1991, 21(5):710-3.

10. Tate GA, Schumacher HR Jr, Reginato AJ, et al, "Synovial Fluid Crystals Derived From Erythrocyte Degradation Products," *J Rheumatol*, 1992, 19(7):1111-4.

References

Brommer EJ, Dooijewaard G, Dijkmans BA, et al, "Plasminogen Activators in Synovial Fluid and Plasma From Patients With Arthritis," *Ann Rheum Dis*, 1992, 51(8):965-8.

Kerolous G, Clayburne G, and Schumacher HB Jr, "Is It Mandatory to Examine Synovial Fluids Promptly After Arthrocentesis?" *Arthritis Rheum*, 1989, 32(3):271-8.

Johnson KD, "Synovial Fluid," *Body Fluids: Laboratory Examination of Amniotic, Cerebrospinal, Seminal, Serous, and Synovial Fluids*, 3rd ed, Chapter 6, Kjeldsberg CR and Knight JA, eds, Chicago, IL: ASCP Press, 1993, 265-301.

Krieg AF and Kjeldsberg CR, "Cerebrospinal Fluid and Other Body Fluids," *Clinical Diagnosis and Management by Laboratory Methods*, Chapter 18, Henry JB, ed, Philadelphia, PA: WB Saunders Co, 1991, 457-63.

Pascual E, Tovar J, and Ruiz MT, "The Ordinary Light Microscope: An Appropriate Tool for Provisional Detection and Identification of Crystals in Synovial Fluid," *Ann Rheum Dis*, 1989, 48(12):983-5.

Ridderstad A, Abedi-Valugerdi M, Ström H, et al, "Rheumatoid Arthritis Synovial Fluid Enhances T-Cell Effector Functions," *J Autoimmun*, 1992, 5(3):333-50.

Sorsa T, Konttinen YT, Lindy O, et al, "Collagenase in Synovitis of Rheumatoid Arthritis," *Semin Arthritis Rheum*, 1992, 22(1):44-53.

Swan AJ, Heywood BR, and Dieppe PA, "Extraction of Calcium Containing Crystals From Synovial Fluids and Articular Cartilage," *J Rheumatol*, 1992, 19(11):1764-73.

Teloh HA, "Clinical Pathology of Synovial Fluid," *Ann Clin Lab Sci*, 1975, 5:282-7.

Synovial Fluid Hyaluronate Concentration *see* Mucin Clot Test *on page 1134*

Synovial Fluid Mucin Clot Test *see* Mucin Clot Test *on page 1134*

Synovial Fluid Ropes Test *see* Mucin Clot Test *on page 1134*

Synovial Fluid Viscosity *see* Mucin Clot Test *on page 1134*

Three Glass Test, Urine *see* Urinalysis, Fractional *on page 1166*

Tryptic Activity, Feces *see* Tryptic Activity, Stool *on this page*

Tryptic Activity, Stool

CPT 84488 (qualitative); 84490 (quantitative, 24-hour)

Related Information

Chloride, Sweat *on page 183*
Cystic Fibrosis DNA Detection *on page 903*
pH, Stool *on page 1143*

Synonyms Fecal Chymotrypsin; Fecal Tryptic Activity; Immunoreactive Trypsin, Fecal Extracts; Stool for Trypsin; Stool Tryptic Activity; Tryptic Activity, Feces

Test Commonly Includes Evaluation of the ability of aqueous stool suspension at dilutions of 1:5, 1:10, 1:20, 1:40, 1:80 to digest (or clear) x-ray film

Patient Care PREPARATION: Avoid barium procedures and laxatives for 1 week prior to specimen collection.

Specimen Fresh random stool CONTAINER: Plastic stool container COLLECTION: Deliver specimen to the laboratory promptly after collection. CAUSES FOR REJECTION: Specimen more than 2 hours in transit to the laboratory, specimen contaminated with urine and/or water, specimen containing interfering substances (ie, castor oil, barium)

Interpretive REFERENCE RANGE: Pediatrics: infants younger than 1 year of age, activity at >1:80 dilution; older children, activity at >1:40 dilution; children with cystic fibrosis, activity at <1:10 dilution USE: Screen for pancreatic exocrine function, malabsorption syndromes LIMITATIONS: Diagnosis of pancreatic insufficiency should not be made until at least three separate stool specimens have been reported to have no tryptic activity. This test is most useful in evaluating malabsorption in children younger than 4 years of age. In older children and adults, the test is unreliable because of trypsin inactivation by intestinal flora. Bacterial proteases may produce positive reactions when no pancreatic trypsin is present; thus, caution in interpreting both positive and negative results is indicated.[1] METHODOLOGY: X-ray film method, kinetic, potentiometric methods utilizing synthetic substrates[2] ADDITIONAL INFORMATION: Fecal chymotrypsin measurements in children (including some with cystic fibrosis) have been shown to correlate with apparent chymotrypsin secretion rates after stimulation with pancreozymin and nasoduodenal tube sampling.[2] RIA immunologic based methods for the pancreatic endoproteases trypsin, chymotrypsin, and elastase have been developed and applied to the study of

(Continued)

Tryptic Activity, Stool *(Continued)*

normal levels of these endoproteases in the feces.[3] Fecal chymotrypsin analysis may show loss of specificity (as an indirect measure of pancreatic function) in some postgastrectomy patients.[4] There is evidence that fecal chemotrypsin values in some rural (South African) populations are lower than those in urban controls as well as those in patients with chronic pancreatitis. This may relate to a lower fecal pH in rural than in urban individuals. It has been recommended that if a low fecal chymotrypsin level is found, fecal pH be determined.[5] The use of enzyme biochemical tests may have limited application to the diagnosis of pancreatic carcinoma (see reference by Schmidt and Schmidt). Elastase 1 and chymotrypsin B activity in stool (and in pancreatic secretion) have been found to reflect pancreatic function.[6] Cystic fibrosis DNA detection is addressed in the Molecular Pathology chapter.

Footnotes

1. Ammann RW, Tagwecher E, Kashiwagi H, et al, "Diagnostic Value of Fecal Chymotrypsin and Trypsin Assessment for Detection of Pancreatic Disease. A Comparative Study," *Am J Dig Dis*, 1968, 13:123-46.
2. Brown GA, Sule D, Williams J, et al, "Faecal Chymotrypsin: A Reliable Index of Exocrine Pancreatic Function," *Arch Dis Child*, 1988, 63(7):785-9.
3. Bohe M, Borgström A, Genell S, et al, "Determination of Immunoreactive Trypsin, Pancreatic Elastase and Chymotrypsin in Extracts of Human Feces and Ileostomy Drainage," *Digestion*, 1983, 27:8-15.
4. Heptner G, Domschke S, and Domschke W, "Exocrine Pancreatic Function After Gastrectomy. Specificity of Indirect Test," *Gastroenterology*, 1989, 97(1):147-53.
5. Riedel L, Walker ARP, Segal I, et al, "Limitations of Faecal Chymotrypsin as a Screening Test for Chronic Pancreatitis," *Gut*, 1991, 32(3):321-4.
6. Sziegoleit A, Krause E, Klör H-U, et al, "Elastase 1 and Chymotrypsin B in Pancreatic Juice and Feces," *Clin Biochem*, 1989, 22(2):85-9.

References

De Pedro C, Codoceo R, and Vazquez P, "Fecal Chymotrypsin Levels in Children With Pancreatic Insufficiency," *Clin Biochem*, 1986, 19:338-40.

Schmidt E and Schmidt FW, "Advances in the Enzyme Diagnosis of Pancreatic Diseases," *Clin Biochem*, 1990, 23(5):383-94.

Two Glass Test, Urine *see* Urinalysis, Fractional *on page 1166*

Tyrosyluria *see* Phenylalanine Test, Urine *on page 1142*

UA *see* Urinalysis *on this page*

Urinalysis

CPT *81000*

Related Information

Anion Gap *on page 132*
Blood, Urine *on page 1112*
Cystine, Qualitative *on page 205*
Eosinophils, Urine *on page 1117*
Ethylene Glycol *on page 965*
Fat, Urine *on page 1119*
Glucose, Semiquantitative, Urine *on page 1121*
Hemoglobin, Qualitative, Urine *on page 1122*
Ketones, Urine *on page 1128*
Kidney Biopsy *on page 68*
Kidney Profile *on page 268*
Kidney Stone Analysis *on page 1129*
Leukocyte Esterase, Urine *on page 1131*
Microalbuminuria *on page 1134*
Nitrite, Urine *on page 1137*
Osmolality, Urine *on page 302*
pH, Urine *on page 1144*
Protein, Semiquantitative, Urine *on page 1147*
Specific Gravity, Urine *on page 1152*
Tests for Uncommon Inherited Diseases of Metabolism and Cell Structure *on page 605*
Urinalysis, Fractional *on page 1166*

Synonyms UA

Applies to Casts, Urine; Crystals, Urine; Occult Blood, Semiquantitative, Urine; Urine Crystals

Test Commonly Includes Opacity, color, appearance, specific gravity, pH, protein, glucose, occult blood, ketones, bilirubin, and in some laboratories, urobilinogen and microscopic examination of urine sediment. Some laboratories include screening for leukocyte esterase and nitrite and do not perform a microscopic examination unless one of the chemical screening (macroscopic) tests is abnormal or unless a specific request for microscopic examination is made.

Abstract The examination of urine is one of the oldest practices in medicine. A carefully performed urinalysis still provides a wealth of information about the patient, both in terms of differential diagnosis, and by exclusion of many conditions when the urinalysis is "normal."

Patient Care PREPARATION: Instructions should be given in method of collection. Both males and females need instruction in cleansing the urethral meatus. "Midstream collections" are performed by initiating urination into the toilet, then bringing the collection device into the urine stream to catch the midportion of the void.

Specimen Urine CONTAINER: Plastic urine container COLLECTION: A voided specimen is usually suitable. If the specimen is likely to be contaminated by vaginal discharge or hemorrhage, a clean catch specimen is desirable. If the specimen is collected by catheter, it should be so labeled. The timing of urine collection will vary with the purpose of the test. To check for casts or renal concentration ability, a first voided morning specimen may be preferred. For screening purposes, this is also the best time, as a later and more dilute specimen may make small increases in protein, RBC, or WBC excretion harder to detect. The upright position increases protein excretion by hemodynamic factors. Mid-morning urine is likely to give the highest albumin excretion, but early morning urine is best when attempting to detect Bence Jones protein. STORAGE INSTRUCTIONS: Transport specimen to the laboratory as soon as possible after collection. If the specimen cannot be processed immediately by the laboratory it should be refrigerated. Refrigeration preserves formed elements in the urine, but may precipitate crystals not originally present. CAUSES FOR REJECTION: Specimen delayed in transport, fecal contamination, decomposition, or bacterial overgrowth

Interpretive REFERENCE RANGE: See table. **Crystals** are interpreted by the physician. Warm, freshly voided urine sediment from normal subjects almost never contains crystals, despite maximal concentration. Xanthine, cystine, and uric acid crystal (and stone) formation is favored by a consistently acid urine (pH <5.5-6). Calcium oxalate and apatite stones are associated with no particular disturbance of urine pH. Calcium carbonate, calcium phosphate, and especially magnesium ammonium phosphate stones are associated with pH >7. Urine pH >7.5 may briefly follow meals (alkaline tide) but more commonly indicate systemic alkali intake ($NaHCO_3$, etc) or urine infected by bacteria which split urea to ammonia. POSSIBLE PANIC RANGE: The presence of massive amounts of oxalate crystals in fresh urine should be reported promptly to the physician, as this finding may represent ethylene glycol intoxication. USE: Screen for abnormalities of urine; diagnose and manage renal diseases, urinary tract infection, urinary tract neoplasms, systemic diseases, and inflammatory or neoplastic diseases adjacent to the urinary tract LIMITATIONS: Insufficient volume, less than 2 mL, may limit the extent of procedures performed. Metabolites of Pyridium® may interfere with the dipstick reactions by producing color interference. High vitamin C intake may cause an underestimate of glucosuria, or a false-negative nitrate test. Survival of WBCs is decreased by low osmolality, alkalinity, and lack of refrigeration. Formed elements in the urine including casts disintegrate rapidly, therefore the specimen should be analyzed as soon as possible after collection. Specific gravity is affected by glucosuria, mannitol infusion, or prior administration of iodinated contrast material for radiologic studies (IVP dye). Some brands of test strips give a "trace positive" protein indication if not stored in dry atmosphere (cap of test strip bottle not on tight). Ambient humidity exposure of the test strips over time also causes some reduction of sensitivity for occult blood and nitrate and increased sensitivity for glucose (false-

Urinalysis

Test	Reference Range
Specific gravity	1.003–1.029
pH	4.5–7.8
Protein	Negative
Glucose	Negative
Ketones	Negative
Bilirubin	Negative
Occult blood	Negative
Leukocyte osterase	Negative
Nitrite	Negative
Urobilinogen	0.1–1.0 EU/dL
WBCs	0–5/hpf
RBCs	male: 0–3/hpf female: 0–5/hpf
Casts	0–4/lpf hyaline
Bacteria	Negative

hpf = high power field
lpf = low power field
EU = Ehrlich units

(Continued)

Urinalysis *(Continued)*

positive). This can be detected by using tap water as a negative control. False-positive tests for protein can also be due to contamination of the urine by an ammonium-containing cleansing solution. Problems relevant to the sensitivity of protein detection have led to development of methods described in the listing Microalbuminuria. **METHODOLOGY:** The chemical portion of the urinalysis is done by test strip, with confirming chemical method for protein (sulfosalicylic acid precipitation). See individual test entries for further information. **ADDITIONAL INFORMATION:**

MICROSCOPY:

Crystalluria is frequently observed in urine specimens stored at room temperature or refrigerated. Such crystals are diagnostically useful when observed in warm, fresh urine by a physician evaluating microhematuria, nephrolithiasis, or toxin ingestion.

In abundance, **calcium oxalate** and/or **hippurate crystals** may suggest ethylene glycol ingestion (especially if known to be accompanied by neurological abnormalities, appearance of drunkenness, hypertension, and a high anion gap acidosis.) Urine is usually supersaturated in calcium oxalate, often in calcium phosphate, and acid urine is often saturated in uric acid. Yet crystalluria is uncommon (in warm, fresh urine) because of the normal presence of crystal inhibitors, the lack of available nidus, and the time factor. When properly observed in fresh urine, crystals may provide a clue to the composition of renal stones even not yet passed, the nidus for such stones, or, as such, have been associated with microhematuria.

Uric acid crystals are reddish brown, rectangular, rhomboidal, or flower-like structures of narrow rectangular petals. **Ammonium urates,** in alkaline urine, are irregular blobs and crescents, sometimes resembling fragmented red cell shapes.

Calcium oxalate crystals are fairly uniform small double pyramids, base to base, which under the microscope look like little crosses on a square.

Calcium phosphate crystallizes in urine as flowers of narrow rectangular needles.

Cystine crystals, uniquely in urine, form large irregular hexagonal plates, which may dissolve if alkalinized. They occur only in the urine of subjects with cystinuria. (See the listing Cystine, Qualitative).

Calcium magnesium ammonium phosphate, or "triple phosphate," forms unique "coffin lid" angularly domed rectangles which may be present in massive quantities in alkaline urine. They usually are associated with urine infected by urea splitting bacteria which cause "infection," or "triple phosphate" stones.

Leukocyturia may indicate inflammatory disease in the genitourinary tract, including bacterial infection, glomerulonephritis, chemical injury, autoimmune diseases, or inflammatory disease adjacent to the urinary tract such as appendicitis[1] or diverticulitis.

White cell casts indicate the renal origin of leukocytes, and are most frequently found in acute pyelonephritis. White cell casts are also found in glomerulonephritis such as lupus nephritis, and in acute and chronic interstitial nephritis. When nuclei degenerate, such leukocyte casts resemble renal tubular casts.

Red cell casts indicate renal origin of hematuria and suggest glomerulonephritis, including lupus nephritis. Red cell casts may also be found in subacute bacterial endocarditis, renal infarct, vasculitis, Goodpasture's syndrome, sickle cell disease, and in malignant hypertension. Degenerated red cell casts may be called **"hemoglobin casts"**. Orange to red casts may be found with myoglobinuria as well.

Dysmorphic red cells are observed in glomerulonephritis. "Dysmorphic" red cells refer to heterogeneous sizes, hypochromia, distorted irregular outlines and frequently small blobs extruding from the cell membrane. Phase contrast microscopy best demonstrates RBC and WBC morphology. Nonglomerular urinary red blood cells resemble peripheral circulating red blood cells.[2] Schramek et al have used the presence or absence of dysmorphic red cells to direct the degree of work-up for hematuria and for follow-up.[3]

Crenated RBCs provide no implication regarding RBC source.

Dark brown or smoky urine suggests a renal source of hematuria.

A **pink or red urine** suggests an extrarenal source.

Hyaline casts occur in physiologic states (eg, after exercise) and many types of renal diseases. They are best seen in phase contrast microscopy or with reduced illumination.

Renal tubular (epithelial) casts are most suggestive of tubular injury, as in acute tubular necrosis. They are also found in other disorders, including eclampsia, heavy metal poisoning, ethylene glycol intoxication, and acute allograft rejection.

Granular casts: Very finely granulated casts may be found after exercise and in a variety of glomerular and tubulointerstitial diseases.; coarse granular casts are abnormal and are present in a wide variety of renal diseases.

"Dirty brown" granular casts are typical of acute tubular necrosis.

Waxy casts are found especially in chronic renal diseases, and are associated with chronic renal failure; they occur in diabetic nephropathy, malignant hypertension, and glomerulonephritis, among other conditions. They are named for their waxy or glossy appearance. They often appear brittle and cracked.

Fatty casts are found in the nephrotic syndromes generally, diabetic nephropathy, other forms of chronic renal diseases, and glomerulonephritis. The fat droplets originate in renal tubular cells when they exceed their capacity to reabsorb protein of glomerular origin. Their inclusions have the features and significance of oval fat bodies. See Fat, Urine listing.

Broad casts originate from dilated, chronically damaged tubules or the collecting ducts. They can be granular or waxy. **Broad waxy casts** are called "renal failure casts."

Spermatozoa may be seen in male urine related to recent or retrograde ejaculation. In female urine, the presence of spermatozoa may provide evidence of vaginal contamination following recent intercourse.

Automation of the urinalysis is routine in many laboratories.[4,5] Some authors wish to abandon microscopic evaluation of the urine, which is not easily automated, on urine samples testing "normal" by dipstick screening. A urine sample that is normal to inspection and dipstick will be normal to microscopic exam 95% of the time.[6]

One instrument for automating the entire urinalysis, the Yellow IRIS®, includes a module that automates the microscopic sediment exam. This has been found to be more consistent than the manual method for routine urinalysis and has increased the number of abnormal urines detected.[4,5,7]

Tests for **inherited diseases of metabolism** involve blood as well as urine. These subjects are summarized in the listings, Tests for Uncommon Inherited Diseases of Metabolism and Cell Structure in the Hematology chapter.

Footnotes

1. Scott JH, "Abnormal Urinalysis in Appendicitis," *J Urol*, 1983, 129:1015.
2. Rizzoni G, Braggion F, and Zacchello G, "Evaluation of Glomerular and Nonglomerular Hematuria by Phase Contrast Microscopy," *J Pediatr*, 1983, 103:370-4.
3. Schramek P, Schuster FX, Georgopoulos M, et al, "Value of Urinary Erythrocyte Morphology in Assessment of Symptomless Microhaematuria," *Lancet*, 1989, 2(8675):1316-9.
4. Roe CE, Carlson DA, Daigneault RW, et al, "Evaluation of the Yellow IRIS®. An Automated Method for Urinalysis," *Am J Clin Pathol*, 1986, 86:661-5.
5. Wargotz ES, Hyde JE, Karcher DS, et al, "Urine Sediment Analysis by the Yellow IRIS® Automated Urinalysis Workstation," *Am J Clin Pathol*, 1987, 88:746-8.
6. Wenz B and Lampasso JA, "Eliminating Unnecessary Urine Microscopy – Results and Performance Characteristics of an Algorithm Based on Chemical Reagent Strip Testing," *Am J Clin Pathol*, 1989, 92(1):78-81.
7. Carlson D and Statland BE, "Automated Urinalysis," *Clin Lab Med*, 1988, 8(3):449-61.

References

Cohen HT and Spiegel DM, "Air-Exposed Urine Dipsticks Give False-Positive Results for Glucose and False-Negative Results for Blood," *Am J Clin Pathol*, 1991, 96(3):398-400.

Freeman JA and Beeler MF, *Laboratory Medicine/Urinalysis and Medical Microscopy*, 2nd ed, Philadelphia, PA: Lea & Febiger, 1983.

Haber MH, "Quality Assurance in Urinalysis," *Clin Lab Med*, 1988, 8:431-47.

Haber MH, *Urinary Sediment: A Textbook Atlas*, American Society of Clinical Pathologists, 1981.

Kiel DP and Moskowitz MA, "The Urinalysis: A Critical Appraisal," *Med Clin North Am*, 1987, 71:607-24.

Mariani AJ, Luangphinith S, Loo S, et al, "Dipstick Chemical Urinalysis: An Accurate Cost-Effective Screening Test," *J Urol*, 1984, 132:64-6.

Schumann GB, "Cytodiagnostic Urinalysis for the Nephrology Practice," *Semin Nephrol*, 1986, 6:308-45.

Schumann GB, *Urine Sediment Examination*, Baltimore, MD: Williams and Wilkins, 1980.

Segasothy M, Lau T, Birch DF, et al, "Immunocytologic Dissection of the Urine Sediment Using Monoclonal Antibodies," *Am J Clin Pathol*, 1988, 90:691-6.

Sheets C and Lyman JL, "Urinalysis," *Emerg Med Clin North Am*, 1986, 4:263-80.

Shenoy UA, "Current Assessment of Microhematuria and Leukocyturia," *Clin Lab Med*, 1985, 5:317-29, (review).

(Continued)

Urinalysis *(Continued)*

Yager HM and Harrington JT, "Urinalysis and Urinary Electrolytes," *The Principles and Practice of Nephrology*, Chapter 28, Jacobson HR, Striker GE, and Klahr S, eds, Philadelphia, PA: BC Decker Inc, 1991, 167-77.

Urinalysis, Fractional

***CPT** 81000 (each fraction)*

Related Information

Blood, Urine *on page 1112*
Hemoglobin, Qualitative, Urine *on page 1122*
Urinalysis *on page 1162*

Synonyms Three Glass Test, Urine; Two Glass Test, Urine

Test Commonly Includes Microscopic examination of each fraction

Abstract Sequential urinalysis is performed on the initial urine voided, the midstream urine, and the final passage of urine to gain information regarding the anatomic source of cellular elements in the urine.

Specimen Urine **CONTAINER:** Plastic urine container **COLLECTION:** Patient voids and the specimen is collected in two or three containers without interrupting the flow of urine. If three containers are ordered, small amounts of urine are collected in the first and third while the second has the largest volume. Sometimes this method is modified by stopping the flow of urine after the second glass and the third glass is collected after prostatic massage. The exact collection procedure followed should be recorded on the requisition so that the results can be interpreted properly. **CAUSES FOR REJECTION:** Improper labeling

Interpretive **REFERENCE RANGE:** RBCs: 2-3 cells per high power field; WBCs: 0-5 cells per high power field **USE:** Define the location of the source of red blood cells and white blood cells present in the urine of male patients. The primary use is in the differential diagnosis of urethritis vs cystitis and pyelonephritis. The test may also contribute to the differentiation of renal vs nonrenal hematuria. **ADDITIONAL INFORMATION:** Initial hematuria, red blood cells in the first specimen, implies hematuria of urethral origin. Total hematuria, red cells in all three samples, implicates the upper urinary tract. Terminal hematuria, red cells in the last specimen, implies hematuria of prostatic or bladder neck origin. Recently, phase contrast microscopy of urinary red blood cells has been used to differentiate hematuria of glomerular vs nonglomerular origin.[1] Glomerular hematuria is characterized by "dysmorphic" urinary RBCs while red cells of nonglomerular origin are "eumorphic." Dysmorphic cells have irregular outlines, granular inhomogeneous cytoplasm (with phase microscopy), uneven cytoplasmic staining and hypochromia (with Wright's stain), and often have small blob-like membrane extrusions (phase microscopy). Eumorphic cells have uniform size and are similar to normal circulating red cells. Nonglomerular hematuria may also be characterized by the presence of red cell "ghosts" (empty membranous sacks which have lost their hemoglobin).[2] Glomerular hematuria is likely when 10% of all urinary RBCs are dysmorphic.[1] If additional evidence of glomerulonephritis is present (edema, proteinuria, renal cellular casts), the glomerular nature of hematuria is essentially established. If all urine red cells are eumorphic, clinical evaluation for extraglomerular sources of hematuria is indicated. Glomerular hematuria does not exclude, in addition, bladder or prostate pathology or malignancy.

Footnotes

1. Stapleton FB, "Morphology of Urinary Red Blood Cells: A Simple Guide in Localizing the Site of Hematuria," *Pediatr Clin North Am*, 1987, 34:561-9.
2. Fairley KF and Birch DF, "Hematuria: A Simple Method for Identifying Glomerular Bleeding," *Kidney Int*, 1982, 21:105-8.

Urinary Eosinophils *see* Eosinophils, Urine *on page 1117*

Urinary Sugar Test *see* Glucose, Quantitative, Urine *on page 1120*

Urinary Sugar Test *see* Glucose, Semiquantitative, Urine *on page 1121*

Urinary Tract Infection Screen *see* Nitrite, Urine *on page 1137*

Urine Concentration Test *see* Concentration Test, Urine *on page 1115*

Urine Crystals *see* Urinalysis *on page 1162*

Urine Ketones *see* Ketones, Urine *on page 1128*

Urine Screen for Albumin *see* Protein, Semiquantitative, Urine *on page 1147*

Urine Screen for Protein *see* Protein, Semiquantitative, Urine *on page 1147*

Urine Sediment, Quantitative *see* Addis Count, 12-Hour *on page 1109*

Urines for Glucose Tolerance *see* Glucose, Semiquantitative, Urine *on page 1121*

Urobilinogen, 2-Hour Urine

***CPT** 84580 (quantitative, timed); 84583 (semiquantitative)*

Related Information

Bile, Urine *on page 1111*
Bilirubin, Direct *on page 137*
Bilirubin, Total *on page 139*
Porphobilinogen, Qualitative, Urine *on page 325*

Synonyms Urobilinogen, Quantitative, Urine

Replaces Urobilinogen, 24-Hour Urine

Abstract This urine screening test detects some but not all instances of hemolytic anemia and liver diseases such as hepatitis and cirrhosis. It is not widely used.

Patient Care **PREPARATION:** Alkalinization of the urine by sodium bicarbonate administration increases excretion of urobilinogen. A marked diurnal peak in excretion occurs; therefore an afternoon collection ideally should be scheduled.

Specimen 2-hour urine **CONTAINER:** Dark urine container or foil wrapped container **COLLECTION:** Have patient void at 2 PM and discard urine. Give patient 500 mL of water to be ingested at once. Collect all urine from 2 PM - 4 PM. Transport promptly to the laboratory. Urobilinogen is sensitive to room temperature and light. **STORAGE INSTRUCTIONS:** Refrigerate specimen, protect from light. **CAUSES FOR REJECTION:** Completed 2-hour specimen not received, specimen exposed to light or not refrigerated

Interpretive **REFERENCE RANGE:** Male: 0.3-2.1 mg/2 hours (SI: 0.5-3.6 μmol/2 hours); female: 0.1-1.1 mg/2 hours (SI: 0.2-1.9 μmol/2 hours). Results are sometimes expressed in Ehrlich units, 1 mg urobilinogen = 1 EU. **USE:** Screen for biliary and liver disease, obstructive jaundice; increased in hemolytic anemia, hepatitis, liver damage with or without jaundice (eg, cirrhosis, congestive heart failure) **LIMITATIONS:** Antibiotics supressing intestinal flora may cause very low levels. Levels may be normal with incomplete obstructive jaundice. Patients with acute porphyria may have an increased value because porphobilinogen also gives a positive result with Ehrlich's aldehyde reagent, as does para-aminosalicylic acid. The absence of or low urobilinogen cannot be determined by dipsticks, a serious drawback, since detection of decreased urine urobilinogen would enhance diagnosis of common duct obstruction. Drugs containing azo dyes may mask the reaction. Like urine bile detection, screen for urobilinogen in urine has fairly good specificity. However, the two tests lack great sensitivity when compared with a variety of serum tests related to liver disease.[1] **METHODOLOGY:** Urobilistix®, Watson's method, Ehrlich's aldehyde reagent; para-diethylaminobenzaldehyde reacts with urobilinogen with a color enhancer **ADDITIONAL INFORMATION:** Urobilinogen is formed in the intestine by the action of bacteria on excreted conjugated (direct) bilirubin. A portion of the urobilinogen is absorbed from the gastrointestinal tract into the bloodstream. It returns to the liver where some is re-excreted in bile (enterohepatic circulation), and the rest (via the general circulation) is excreted into the urine. Urine urobilinogen can be increased as an early indicator of moderate hepatic parenchymal damage. Early toxic injury or hepatitis may also cause increased urine urobilinogen. However, if no bilirubin enters the bile no urobilinogen will be produced; thus, with complete common bile duct obstruction, both urine and fecal urobilinogen will be decreased. Collection time is important because of diurnal variation in urobilinogen excretion. Alkaline pH of urine increases clearance of urobilinogen and increases reliability of results.

Footnotes

1. Binder L, Smith D, Kupka T, et al, "Failure of Prediction of Liver Function Test Abnormalities With the Urine Urobilinogen and Urine Bilirubin Assays," *Arch Pathol Lab Med*, 1989, 113(1):73-6.

Urobilinogen, 24-Hour Urine *replaced by* Urobilinogen, 2-Hour Urine *on this page*

Urobilinogen, Quantitative, Urine *see* Urobilinogen, 2-Hour Urine *on this page*

UTI Screen *see* Nitrite, Urine *on page 1137*

Vasopressin Concentration Test *see* Concentration Test, Urine *on page 1115*

VIROLOGY

Larry D. Gray, PhD
Rebecca T. Horvat, PhD

Clinical (diagnostic) virology is the most rapidly advancing component of clinical microbiology. In the past, tests to isolate and identify specific viruses were offered only by specialized laboratories, usually located in large cities or major medical centers. In addition, clinicians were accustomed to long turnaround times, to relying on viral serology rather than virus isolation, and to determining if the delays and limited choice of tests were of any real value, especially considering the fact that few, if any, antiviral therapeutic agents were available. Clinicians can now submit specimens suspected of containing viruses to hospital virology laboratories and, in many cases, receive results in less than 1 day. Furthermore, several antiviral therapeutic agents (eg, acyclovir, amantadine, ganciclovir, ribavirin, and zidovudine) are now available for the treatment of specific viral infections (see Table and Figure 1 in the Virology Appendix).

Viruses, viral antigens, and antibodies to viruses in clinical specimens can be detected by several methods, all of which are presented in this chapter. Many of the methods or variations of these methods are rapid, reliable, inexpensive, technically simple, and continually being developed to make clinical virology increasingly more relevant and available to physicians.

Virus Isolation/Cell Culture: Specimens are inoculated onto appropriate cell culture lines, the cultures are incubated, virus-specific cytopathic effect (CPE) is observed, and viruses are identified by methods such as hemadsorption, characteristic CPE, and the use of labeled virus-specific monoclonal antibody.

Shell Vial Technique: Specimens are centrifuged onto cell cultures in small vials, the vials are incubated (usually overnight), and labeled virus-specific monoclonal antibody is applied to the infected cell cultures.

Direct Detection: Specimens or histological sections of specimens are placed onto microscope slides and are treated with labeled virus-specific monoclonal antibody. In addition, enzyme-linked immunoabsorbent assays are available to detect viral antigens in cell cultures and clinical specimens.

Nucleic Acid Hybridization: Nucleic acid probes for the direct detection of viral genomes in specimens and for confirmation of viruses in cell culture are beginning to be commercially available and will continue to be developed into valuable diagnostic reagents.

Viral Serology: Measurement and comparison of virus-specific antibody in acute and convalescent sera has been and continues to be useful in the diagnosis of many viral infections.

See also Rabies listing in the Anatomic Pathology chapter and the multiple hepatitis listings in the Immunology and Serology chapter, as well as Hepatitis B DNA Detection in the chapter Molecular Pathology. Other tests relevant to viral disease are to be found in the Immunology and Serology, and Molecular Pathology chapters.

For reference, the Virology Appendix contains:

- a list of antiviral agents and their target viruses
- molecular structures of antiviral agents (Figure 1)
- brief current classification schemes for major viruses (Figures 2 and 3)
- representations of the structures of major viruses (Figure 4)

Adenovirus Culture

CPT *87252 (tissue culture, inoculation and observation); 87253 (tissue culture, additional studies, each isolate)*

Related Information

Adenovirus Antibody Titer *on page 629*
Adenovirus Culture, Rapid *on next page*
Conjunctival Culture *on page 803*
Viral Culture, Respiratory Symptoms *on page 1204*
Viral Culture, Urine *on page 1207*

Test Commonly Includes Culture for adenovirus only; adenovirus is usually detected in a routine/general virus culture.

Specimen Midstream urine, stool or rectal swabs, nasopharyngeal secretions, eye exudates, throat swab or tissue, cerebrospinal fluid **CONTAINER:** Sterile container. Swabs should be placed into cold viral transport medium. **STORAGE INSTRUCTIONS:** Keep specimens cold and moist. Adenoviruses are more stabile than are most other viruses; however, specimens should not be stored or refrigerated for long periods of time. Specimens should be delivered immediately to the clinical laboratory. **CAUSES FOR REJECTION:** Dry specimen, specimen not in proper viral transport medium, specimen not refrigerated during transport, specimen fixed in formalin **TURNAROUND TIME:** Variable (1-14 days) and depends on culture method used and amount of virus in the specimen

Interpretive **REFERENCE RANGE:** No virus isolated **USE:** Aid in the diagnosis of disease caused by adenovirus (eg, conjunctivitis, cystitis, gastroenteritis, pneumonia, and pharyngoconjunctivitis) **LIMITATIONS:** Rule out or identify adenovirus **only** **METHODOLOGY:** Inoculation of specimen into cell cultures, incubation of cell cultures, observation for characteristic cytopathic effect (CPE), and identification by fluorescent monoclonal antibody **ADDITIONAL INFORMATION:** Adenoviruses are spread directly by oral transmission or infectious aerosols. Infections with adenoviruses occur throughout the year, especially in people who are grouped together such as those in schools, day care centers, nursing home facilities, and hospitals.[1] Adenoviruses can be the etiologic agent of respiratory infections in children up to 6 years of age and of ocular infections in both children and adults. Adenovirus respiratory infections can mimic pertussis.

Adenoviruses type 40 and 41 can cause gastroenteritis in young children and infants. These types are usually not associated with respiratory illness. Diarrhea can persist for up to 14 days, and during this period virus can be shed.[2] However, culture of type 40 and 41 is more difficult than culture of other adenoviruses and may not be isolated. Stool specimens can be examined for adenovirus type 40 and 41 using an enzyme immunoassay or electron microscopy.[3,4]

Serology to detect adenovirus antibodies is available and is often helpful in establishing a diagnosis; see listings in the Immunology and Serology chapter.

Footnotes

1. Foy HM, "Adenoviruses," *Viral Infections of Humans, Epidemiology and Control*, 3rd ed, Evans AS, ed, New York, NY: Plenum Publishing, 1989, 17-36.
2. Kotloff KL, Losonsky GA, Morris JG Jr, et al, "Enteric Adenovirus Infection and Childhood Diarrhea: An Epidemiologic Study in Three Clinical Settings," *Pediatrics*, 1989, 84(2):219-25.
3. Bhisitkul DM, Todd KM, and Listernick R, "Adenovirus Infection and Childhood Intussusception," *Am J Dis Child*, 1992, 146(11):1331-3.
4. Van R, Wun CC, O'Ryan ML, et al, "Outbreaks of Human Enteric Adenovirus Types 40 and 41 in Houston Day Care Centers," *J Pediatr*, 1992, 120(4 Pt 1):516-21.

References

Christensen ML, "Human Viral Gastroenteritis," *Clin Microbiol Rev*, 1989, 2(1):51-89.

Hierholzer JC, "Adenoviruses," *Manual of Clinical Microbiology*, 5th ed, Balows A, Hausler WJ Jr, Herrmann KL, et al, eds, Washington, DC: American Society for Microbiology, 1991, 896-903.

Hierholzer JC, "Adenoviruses – A Spectrum of Human Diseases," *Clin Microbiol Newslet*, 1992, 14(15):113-20.

Kowalski RP and Gordon YJ, "Comparison of Direct Rapid Tests for the Detection of Adenovirus Antigen in Routine Conjunctival Specimens," *Ophthalmology*, 1989, 96(7):1106-9.

Martin AL and Kudesia G, "Enzyme-Linked Immunosorbent Assay for Detecting Adenoviruses in Stool Specimens: Comparison With Electron Microscopy and Isolation," *J Clin Pathol*, 1990, 43(6):514-5.

Wingand R, "Pitfalls in the Identification of Adenovirus," *J Virol Methods*, 1987, 16:161-9.

Adenovirus Culture, Rapid

CPT *87252 (tissue culture, inoculation and observation); 87253 (tissue culture, additional studies, each isolate)*

Related Information

Adenovirus Antibody Titer *on page 629*
Adenovirus Culture *on previous page*
Conjunctival Culture *on page 803*
Viral Culture, Eye or Ocular Symptoms *on page 1202*
Viral Culture, Respiratory Symptoms *on page 1204*
Viral Culture, Urine *on page 1207*
Virus, Direct Detection by Fluorescent Antibody *on page 1208*

Synonyms Adenovirus Shell Vial Method

Test Commonly Includes Inoculation of cell cultures in shell vials, 2-day and 5-day incubations, and immunofluorescence staining of adenovirus antigens with specific monoclonal antibodies

Specimen Midstream urine, stool or rectal swabs, nasopharyngeal secretions, eye exudates, throat swab, or tissue **CONTAINER:** Sterile container. Swabs should be placed into cold viral transport medium. **STORAGE INSTRUCTIONS:** Keep specimens cold and moist. Adenoviruses are more stabile than are most other viruses; however, specimens should not be stored or refrigerated for long periods of time. Specimens should be delivered immediately to the clinical laboratory. **CAUSES FOR REJECTION:** Dry specimen, specimen not in proper viral transport medium, specimen not refrigerated during transport, specimen fixed in formalin **TURNAROUND TIME:** 2-5 days, depending on method and capability of laboratory

Interpretive **USE:** Aid in the diagnosis of disease caused by adenovirus (eg, conjunctivitis, cystitis, pneumonia, and pharyngoconjunctivitis). This method provides a more rapid detection of adenovirus than does routine culture. **METHODOLOGY:** Specimens are centrifuged onto cell cultures grown on coverslips in the bottoms of 1-dram shell vials. Centrifugation greatly accelerates virus attachment and penetration. After incubation for 2 and/or 5 days, fluorescein-labeled monoclonal antibodies are applied to the infected cells to detect viral antigens that are expressed in the membranes of the cells. Characteristic fluorescent foci indicate the presence of virus. **ADDITIONAL INFORMATION:** The sensitivity of this rapid culture technique has been reported to be 52% and 97% after 1 and 2 days of incubation, respectively.[1]

Footnotes

1. Espy MJ, Hierholzer JC, and Smith TF, "The Effect of Centrifugation on the Detection of Adenovirus in Shell Vials," *Am J Clin Pathol*, 1987, 88:358-60.

References

Hughes JH, "Physical and Chemical Methods for Enhancing Rapid Detection of Viruses and Other Agents," *Clin Microbiol Rev*, 1993, 6(2):150-75.

Olsen MA, Shuck KM, Sambol AR, et al, "Isolation of Seven Respiratory Viruses in Shell Vials: A Practical and Highly Sensitive Method," *J Clin Microbiol*, 1993, 31(2):422-5.

Adenovirus Culture, Stool *see* Viral Culture, Stool *on page 1205*

Adenovirus Shell Vial Method *see* Adenovirus Culture, Rapid *on this page*

AIDS Virus Culture *see* Human Immunodeficiency Virus Culture *on page 1185*

Blood Culture for CMV *see* Viral Culture, Blood *on page 1197*

Blood Culture for Enterovirus *see* Viral Culture, Blood *on page 1197*

Body Fluid Viral Culture *see* Viral Culture, Body Fluid *on page 1198*

Buffy Coat Culture for CMV *see* Viral Culture, Blood *on page 1197*

Cerebrospinal Fluid Virus Culture *see* Viral Culture, Central Nervous System Symptoms *on page 1199*

Cervical *Chlamydia* Culture *see Chlamydia trachomatis* Culture *on next page*

Cervical Culture for T-Strain *Mycoplasma* *see* Genital Culture for *Ureaplasma urealyticum on page 1180*

Cervical Culture for *Ureaplasma urealyticum* *see* Genital Culture for *Ureaplasma urealyticum on page 1180*

Chickenpox Culture *see* Varicella-Zoster Virus Culture *on page 1193*

Chlamydia trachomatis Culture

CPT *87110*

Related Information

Cervical/Vaginal Cytology *on page 491*
Chlamydia Group Titer *on page 663*
Chlamydia trachomatis Direct FA Test *on page 1173*
Chlamydia trachomatis DNA Probe *on page 897*
Conjunctival Culture *on page 803*
Endometrium Culture *on page 811*
Genital Culture *on page 814*
Lymphogranuloma Venereum Titer *on page 722*
Urine Culture, Clean Catch *on page 881*
Viral Culture, Eye or Ocular Symptoms *on page 1202*
Viral Culture, Urogenital *on page 1207*

Synonyms Lymphogranuloma Venereum Culture; TRIC Agent Culture

Applies to Cervical *Chlamydia* Culture; Eye Swab *Chlamydia* Culture; Urethral *Chlamydia* Culture

Test Commonly Includes Cell culture for evaluation of *Chlamydia*

Specimen *Chlamydia* is an intracellular pathogen. Obtain swab specimens containing columnar epithelial cells of urethra, cervix, rectum, conjunctiva, posterior nasopharynx, or throat. **CONTAINER:** Culturette® (dacron) swabs should be used and placed in *Chlamydia* transport medium. **COLLECTION:** **Urethra:** Remove mucous/pus. The swab should be inserted 2-4 cm into the urethra. Use firm pressure to scrape cells from the mucosal surface. If possible repeat with second swab. Patient should not urinate within 1 hour prior to specimen collection.

Cervix: Remove mucous/pus with a Culturette® and use firm and rotating pressure to obtain specimen with another swab. May be combined with a urethral swab into same transport medium. This two-swab method is highly recommended.

Rectum: Sample anal crypts with a Culturette®.

Conjunctiva: Remove mucous and exudate. Use a Culturette® and firm pressure to scrape away epithelial cells from upper and lower lids.

Posterior nasopharynx or throat: Collect epithelial cells by using a Culturette®.

STORAGE INSTRUCTIONS: Deliver inoculated transport medium **immediately** to the laboratory. **Specimens must be refrigerated** if stored or transported for 2 days. Specimen must be frozen at -70°C if stored more than 2 days. **TURNAROUND TIME:** Cultures with no growth usually will be reported after 7 days. Rapid culture methods for detection of *Chlamydia* require a minimum of 48 hours. **SPECIAL INSTRUCTIONS:** Availability and specific specimen collection requirements for *Chlamydia* cultures vary. Consult the laboratory for specific instructions, swabs, and transport materials prior to collection of the specimen.

Interpretive **REFERENCE RANGE:** No *Chlamydia* isolated **USE:** Aid in the diagnosis of infections caused by *Chlamydia* (eg, cervicitis, trachoma, conjunctivitis, pelvic inflammatory disease, pneumonia, urethritis, nongonococcal urethritis, pneumonitis, and sexually transmitted diseases) **LIMITATIONS:** Culture may be negative in presence of *Chlamydia* infection. Culture is probably not the gold standard for the detection of *C. trachomatis*. The sensitivity of culture probably is only 70% to 90% because *C. trachomatis* does not always survive transit to the laboratory and because of often inadequate sampling with (multiple) swabs.[1] **METHODOLOGY:** Inoculation of specimen onto McCoy cell, HeLa-229, or Buffalo green monkey cell culture and subsequent detection of *Chlamydia*-infected cells by monoclonal antibody and immunofluorescence **ADDITIONAL INFORMATION:** This organism infects the endocervical columnar epithelial cells and will not be found in the inflammatory cells. In obtaining the specimen, clean the area of inflammatory cells and then attempt to scrape epithelial cells for culturing. The results of cytological diagnosis of chlamydial infection of the female genital tract have been disappointing. Papanicolaou-stained cervical smears are not reliable enough to help establish or exclude the presence of *Chlamydia*. Direct immunofluorescence techniques and enzyme immunoassays are available to detect *Chlamydia* in clinical specimens. These methods usually provide reliable results in high-prevalence populations and detect both viable and nonviable organisms. *Chlamydia* can now be detected by using a DNA probe chemiluminescence test.[2] This test appears to be as sensitive as immunoassays and more sensitive than culture. Selection of the most efficient method for recovery of *Chlamydia* depends upon the incidence in the patient population and the local availability of the various methods. Urine culture for *Chlamydia* is not a sensitive procedure and generally should not be done.[3] Urine samples can be tested for *Chlamydia* using an immunoassay rather than culture.[4]

(Continued)

Chlamydia trachomatis Culture *(Continued)*

Genital infections due to *C. trachomatis* are the most frequent reportable bacterial sexually transmitted disease in the United States. There are more than 4 million infections reported annually.[5] Many of the cases are asymptomatic or minimally symptomatic. Many will eventually progress to produce serious infections including pelvic inflammatory disease, ectopic pregnancy, and infertility in women.[6,7] Infection with *Chlamydia* during pregnancy places the newborn infant at risk of pneumonia and conjunctivitis.[7]

Culture should be the test-of-choice in cases of child abuse, ascending pelvic infections, rectal and throat infections, and when a test-for-cure is desired.

Chlamydia is a single genus and consists of the following:

- *C. trachomatis* (serotypes A-K): inclusion conjunctivitis, trachoma, and genital infections
- *C. trachomatis* (serotypes L1-L3): lymphogranuloma venereum
- *C. psittaci*: psittacosis
- *C. pneumoniae* (TWAR): respiratory infections

Serology to detect antibodies to all three species of *Chlamydia* is available.

Laboratory diagnosis of *C. pneumoniae* infections is not widely available; commercial tests for *C. pneumoniae* are not available. *C. pneumoniae* is responsible for approximately 10% of community-acquired pneumonias. The cells (McCoy) usually used to culture *C. trachomatis* will not reliably support the growth of *C. pneumoniae*. Recent studies have shown that other cell lines (H 292 and HEp-2) are more appropriate.[8] An alternate, widely used method for the laboratory diagnosis of *C. pneumoniae* infection is serology by microimmunofluorescence. Currently, this serological test is the most sensitive and specific laboratory test for *C. pneumoniae*.

Footnotes

1. Harper M and Johnson R, "The Predictive Value of Culture for the Diagnosis of Gonorrhea and *Chlamydia* Infections," *Clin Microbiol Newslet*, 1990, 12:54-6.
2. Iwen PC, Blair TMH, and Woods GL, "Comparison of the Gen-Probe PACE2® System, Direct Fluorescent Antibody, and Cell Culture for Detecting *Chlamydia trachomatis* in Cervical Specimens," *Am J Clin Pathol*, 1991, 95(4):578-82.
3. Schachter J, "Urine as a Specimen for the Diagnosis of Sexually Transmitted Disease," *Am J Med*, 1983, 75:93-7.
4. Leonardi GP, Seitz M, Edstrom R, et al, "Evaluation of Three Immunoassays for Detection of *Chlamydia trachomatis* in Urine Specimens From Asymptomatic Males," *J Clin Microbiol*, 1992, 30(11):2793-6.
5. Centers for Disease Control, "False-Positive Results With the Use of *Chlamydia* Tests in the Evaluation of Suspected Sexual Abuse – Ohio," *MMWR Morb Mortal Wkly Rep*, 1990, 39:932-5.
6. Stamm WE, "Diagnosis of *Chlamydia trachomatis* Genitourinary Infections," *Ann Intern Med*, 1988, 108(5):710-7.
7. Department of Health and Human Services, Sexually Transmitted Disease Branch, NIH, "Pelvic Inflammatory Disease: Research Directions in the 1990s," *Sex Transm Dis*, 1991, 18(1):46-64.
8. Wong KH, Skelton SK, and Chan YK, "Efficient Culture of *Chlamydia pneumoniae* With Cell Lines Derived From the Human Respiratory Tract," *J Clin Microbiol*, 1992, 30(7):1625-30.

References

Barnes RC, "Laboratory Diagnosis of Human Chlamydial Infections," *Clin Microbiol Rev*, 1989, 2(2):119-36.

Chirgwin K, Roblin PM, Gelling M, et al, "Infection With *Chlamydia pneumoniae* in Brooklyn," *J Infect Dis*, 1991, 163(4):757-61.

Fraiz J and Jones RB, "Chlamydial Infections," *Annu Rev Med*, 1988, 39:357-70.

Grayston JT, "*Chlamydia pneumoniae*, Strain TWAR," *Chest*, 1989, 95(3):664-9.

Grayston JT, "Infections Caused by *Chlamydia pneumoniae* Strain TWAR," *Clin Infect Dis*, 1992, 15(5):757-61.

Grayston JT, Campbell LA, Kuo CC, et al, "A New Respiratory Tract Pathogen: *Chlamydia pneumoniae* Strain TWAR," *J Infect Dis*, 1990, 161(4):618-25.

Le Scolea LJ Jr, "The Value of Nonculture Chlamydial Diagnostic Tests," *Clin Microbiol Newslet*, 1991, 13(3):21-4.

Lombardo JM and Gadol CL, "*Chlamydia trachomatis*: A Perfect Test?" *Clin Microbiol Newslet*, 1990, 12(13):100-2.

Roblin PM, Dumornay W, and Hammerschlag MR, "Use of HEp-2 Cells for Improved Isolation and Passage of *Chlamydia pneumoniae*," *J Clin Microbiol*, 1992, 30(8):1968-71.

Chlamydia trachomatis Direct FA Test

***CPT** 87206*

Related Information

Cervical/Vaginal Cytology *on page 491*
Chlamydia Group Titer *on page 663*
Chlamydia trachomatis Culture *on page 1171*
Chlamydia trachomatis DNA Probe *on page 897*
Conjunctival Culture *on page 803*
Genital Culture *on page 814*
Lymphogranuloma Venereum Titer *on page 722*
Ocular Cytology *on page 506*
Viral Culture, Eye or Ocular Symptoms *on page 1202*

Synonyms MicroTrak®

Test Commonly Includes Examination of specimen, specifically for *Chlamydia trachomatis*

Patient Care PREPARATION: For urogenital specimens, patient should not urinate 1 hour prior to collection.

Specimen Direct smear CONTAINER: Single well (8 mm) glass slide, dacron swabs (one large, one small), one cytobrush, methanol fixative (0.5 mL vial). These items are contained in a commonly used direct detection kit (collection pack) known as MicroTrak®. COLLECTION: **Endocervical with cytology brush:** Nonpregnant women. Use large swab to remove exudate or mucous from exocervix. Insert cytobrush into cervical os past the squamocolumnar junction. Rest 2-3 seconds, rotate brush 360 degrees to gather columnar cells and withdraw brush. Do not touch vaginal walls with brush, and prepare slides immediately by rotating and twisting brush back and forth across center of slide well.

Endocervical with swab: Pregnant women. Use large swab to remove exudate or mucous from exocervix. Insert another large dacron swab until tip is no longer visible, rotate swab 5-10 seconds, and withdraw swab. Do not touch vaginal walls and prepare slides immediately. Firmly roll one side of swab over top half of well. Turn swab over and roll other side over bottom half of slide well.

Urethral: Males. Patient should not urinate 1 hour before sampling. Remove pus or exudate, insert small swab with wire shaft 2-4 cm into penis. Gently rotate swab to dislodge cells, rest swab 2 seconds, withdraw swab, and prepare slide immediately as above.

Rectal: Symptomatic patients only. Use large swab. Insert approximately 3 cm into anal canal. Move swab from side to side to sample crypts. If fecal contamination occurs, discard swab and obtain another specimen. Prepare slide immediately as above.

Conjunctival: Neonates, symptomatic only. Use large swab to gently remove pus or discharge and discard. If both eyes are sampled, swab less affected eye first. Swab inside of lower, then upper lid, and prepare slide immediately as above.

Nasopharyngeal: Neonates, symptomatic only. Use small swab or nasal aspirator. Collect specimen from posterior nasopharynx using standard collection method. If swab was used, prepare slide immediately. If nasal aspirate was collected, deliver to the laboratory technician immediately for slide preparation.

All specimens: Write patient name and date on slip and outside of collection pack. Allow specimen to air dry. Lay slide flat and flood with methanol fixative. Let entire quantity evaporate. Refold pack without touching fixed specimen.

The direct detection of *Chlamydia* in specimens depends largely on the preparation of the cell smear. Smears that are too thick or lumpy can cause false-positive results. Contamination with red blood cells makes the smears difficult to interpret. Smears with too few cells can cause false-negative results.

STORAGE INSTRUCTIONS: Refrigerate slides at 2°C to 8°C or at room temperature (20°C to 30°C) until taken to the laboratory. Slides must be stained within 7 days of collection. CAUSES FOR REJECTION: Specimen not labeled, slide received broken, less than 10 columnar or cuboidal epithelial cells on slide, slide more than 7 days old TURNAROUND TIME: The time required to stain and examine the specimen is generally less than 1 hour. Turnaround time depends on staffing within the laboratory. SPECIAL INSTRUCTIONS: Specify specimen origin. Include all pertinent information, label slide and collection pack.

Interpretive REFERENCE RANGE: Negative for *Chlamydia* USE: Aid in the diagnosis of disease caused by *Chlamydia* (eg, pneumonitis, sexually transmitted disease, inclusion conjunctivitis,

(Continued)

Chlamydia trachomatis Direct FA Test *(Continued)*

trachoma, and pneumonia) **LIMITATIONS:** The direct detection of *C. trachomatis* is a useful tool in screening high-risk populations and in clinical situations where rapid positive results may be useful. However, the direct fluorescent antibody procedure is considerably less sensitive than the cell culture procedure. The number of cells on the slide can be too low for diagnosis. **METHODOLOGY:** The *Chlamydia trachomatis* direct test uses fluorescein-conjugated monoclonal antibodies (reactive with all 15 known serotypes of *C. trachomatis*) to detect elementary bodies in clinical smears. The fluorescein-labeled monoclonal antibody is allowed to react with cell smears. After washing away the unbound antibodies, the specimen is examined under a fluorescent microscope. This test detects only *Chlamydia trachomatis* major outer membrane protein (MOMP). The test does not distinguish between living and dead organisms. Therefore, the test does not necessarily serve as a test-of-cure. **ADDITIONAL INFORMATION:** *Chlamydia trachomatis*, primarily a human pathogen, has been implicated in neonatal/infantile conjunctivitis and afebrile pneumonia. Thirty-three percent to 50% of babies born vaginally to mothers with chlamydial infection of the cervix will be infected; the majority of these neonates will develop inclusion conjunctivitis and/or a respiratory tract infection that can lead to the distinctive (afebrile) pneumonia syndrome.

Conjunctivitis: Conjunctivitis in infected neonates usually occurs between the 5th and 12th day after birth. In neonates born to mothers with premature rupture of the membranes, *C. trachomatis* has been detected, in rare cases, as early as the first day following birth.

Afebrile pneumonia: Many neonatal chlamydial infections also involve the respiratory tract. Respiratory infections usually occur secondarily to inclusion conjunctivitis. Rhinitis is often a prodrome for severe lower respiratory tract involvement. Signs of chlamydial pneumonia include cough, tachypnea, inspiratory rales, and, in more severe cases, vomiting and periods of apnea.

References

Barnes RC, "Laboratory Diagnosis of Human Chlamydial Infections," *Clin Microbiol Rev*, 1989, 2(2):119-36.

Clarke LM, Sierra MF, Daidone BJ, et al, "Comparison of the Syva MicroTrak® Enzyme Immunoassay and Gen-Probe PACE2® With Cell Culture for Diagnosis of Cervical *Chlamydia trachomatis* Infection in a High-Prevalence Female Population," *J Clin Microbiol*, 1993, 31(4):968-71.

Schwebke JR, Stamm WE, Handsfield HH, et al, "Use of Sequential Enzyme Immunoassay and Direct Fluorescent-Antibody Tests for the Detection of *Chlamydia trachomatis* Infections in Women," *J Clin Microbiol*, 1990, 28(11):2473-6.

Stamm WE, "Diagnosis of *Chlamydia trachomatis* Genitourinary Infections," *Ann Intern Med*, 1988, 108:710-7.

CMV Culture *see* Cytomegalovirus Culture *on next page*

CMV Culture *see* Viral Culture, Blood *on page 1197*

CMV Culture, Urine *see* Viral Culture, Urine *on page 1207*

CMV Early Antigen FA Method *see* Cytomegalovirus Isolation, Rapid *on page 1176*

CMV Isolation, Rapid *see* Cytomegalovirus Isolation, Rapid *on page 1176*

CMV Shell Vial Method *see* Cytomegalovirus Isolation, Rapid *on page 1176*

Comprehensive Viral Culture *see* Viral Culture *on page 1195*

Coxsackie A Virus Culture *see* Enterovirus Culture *on page 1178*

Coxsackie B Virus Culture *see* Enterovirus Culture *on page 1178*

Coxsackie Virus Culture, Stool *see* Viral Culture, Stool *on page 1205*

CPE *see* Viral Culture *on page 1195*

Culture, EBV *see* Epstein-Barr Virus Culture *on page 1179*

Culture, HSV *see* Herpes Simplex Virus Culture *on page 1182*

Culture, HSV Only *see* Herpes Simplex Virus Isolation, Rapid *on page 1184*

Culture, RSV *see* Respiratory Syncytial Virus Culture *on page 1190*

Culture, VZV *see* Varicella-Zoster Virus Culture *on page 1193*

Cytomegalovirus Culture

CPT *87252 (tissue culture, inoculation and observation); 87253 (tissue culture, additional studies, each isolate)*

Related Information

Bronchial Washings Cytology *on page 485*
Bronchoalveolar Lavage Cytology *on page 487*
Cervical/Vaginal Cytology *on page 491*
Cytomegalic Inclusion Disease Cytology *on page 496*
Cytomegalovirus Antibody *on page 672*
Cytomegalovirus Isolation, Rapid *on next page*
Sputum Cytology *on page 510*
Urine Cytology *on page 513*
Viral Culture, Blood *on page 1197*
Viral Culture, Urine *on page 1207*

Synonyms CMV Culture; Viral Culture, Cytomegalovirus

Test Commonly Includes Culture for CMV only; CMV also is usually detected in a routine/general virus culture

Abstract Cytomegalovirus is a DNA herpes virus which infects up to 90% of the adult population, usually asymptomatically. It is a major problem in immunocompromised patients after renal and other organ transplantation, in allogeneic bone marrow transplantation patients, and in patients with AIDS. Transmission of CMV to neonates can occur and is known to cause illness and death in infants.

Specimen Urine, throat, bronchoalveolar lavage, bronchial washings, lung biopsy, whole blood, stool **CONTAINER:** Sterile container; cold viral transport medium for swabs **COLLECTION: Urine:** A first morning clean catch urine should be submitted in a sterile screw-cap container.

Throat: Rotate swab in both tonsillar crypts and against posterior oropharynx. Place swab in tube of viral transport medium, break off end of swab and tighten cap.

Blood: Collect in a green top Vacutainer® tube containing free heparin.

STORAGE INSTRUCTIONS: Do **not** freeze. Keep specimens cold and moist. Specimens should be delivered to the laboratory and handed to a technologist within 30 minutes of collection. If freezing is absolutely necessary, most specimens can be frozen by adding an equal amount of 0.4M sucrose-phosphate to the specimen before freezing. White blood cells should be isolated from blood specimens before freezing. **CAUSES FOR REJECTION:** Dry specimen, specimen not refrigerated during transport, specimen fixed in formalin, unlabeled specimen **TURNAROUND TIME:** Variable (1-14 days) and depends on culture method used and amount of virus in the specimen. Negative cultures are usually not reported for 28 days. **SPECIAL INSTRUCTIONS:** Obtain viral transport medium from the laboratory prior to collecting the specimen.

Interpretive **REFERENCE RANGE:** No virus isolated **USE:** Aid in the diagnosis of disease caused by CMV (eg, viral pneumonia and gastrointestinal tract involvement in organ transplant-related disease).[1] Clinical manifestations of CMV disease include fever, malaise, arthralgias, hematologic abnormalities, hepatitis, chorioretinitis, skin lesions, Guillain-Barré syndrome, and allograft dysfunction.[1] **LIMITATIONS:** CMV culture may be positive in the absence of obvious clinical disease.[2] **METHODOLOGY:** Inoculation of specimen into cell cultures, incubation of cultures, observation for characteristic cytopathic effect (CPE), and identification by fluorescent monoclonal antibody **ADDITIONAL INFORMATION:** CMV infections are very common in normal individuals and are usually asymptomatic. However, CMV infections are frequently severe and life-threatening in immunocompromised patients, including organ recipients and AIDS patients. CMV is the major viral pathogen following renal transplantation. Blood cultures positive for CMV predict progression.[1] Knowledge of CMV infection is of utmost importance so that ganciclovir can be started as soon as possible.

CMV is the most frequent cause of congenital viral infections in humans and occurs in about 1% of all newborns. Approximately 90% have no clinical symptoms at birth. Ten percent to 20% of these infants will develop complications before school age. Congenital infection may occur as a result of either primary or recurrent maternal infection.

Serology for the detection of cytomegalovirus is available, but the results usually are of limited value. Cytomegalovirus inclusions are recognizable microscopically, and are characterized as owl's eye intranuclear inclusions (Cowdry A inclusions). Cytoplasmic inclusions are found as well.[3]

Footnotes

1. Farrugia E and Schwab TR, "Subspecialty Clinics: Nephrology – Management and Prevention of Cytomegalovirus Infection After Renal Transplantation," *Mayo Clin Proc*, 1992, 67(9):879-90.

(Continued)

Cytomegalovirus Culture *(Continued)*

2. Zurlo JJ, O'Neill D, Polis MA, et al, "Lack of Clinical Utility of Cytomegalovirus Blood and Urine Cultures in Patients With HIV Infection," *Ann Intern Med*, 1993, 118(1):12-7.
3. Schwartz DA and Wilcox CM, "Atypical Cytomegalovirus Inclusions in Gastrointestinal Biopsy Specimens From Patients With the Acquired Immunodeficiency Syndrome: Diagnostic Role of *In Situ* Nucleic Acid Hybridization," *Hum Pathol*, 1992, 23(9):1019-26.

References

Ayala E, Martinez EM, Enghardt MH, et al, "An Improved Cytomegalovirus Immunostaining Method," *Lab Med*, 1993, 24:39.

Drew WL, "Nonpulmonary Manifestations of Cytomegalovirus Infection in Immunocompromised Patients," *Clin Microbiol Rev*, 1992, 5(2):104-10.

Griffiths PD and Grundy JE, "The Status of CMV as a Human Pathogen," *Epidemiol Infect*, 1988, 100:1-15.

Jiwa M, Steenbergen RDM, Zwaan FE, et al, "Three Sensitive Methods for the Detection of Cytomegalovirus in Lung Tissue of Patients With Interstitial Pneumonitis," *Am J Clin Pathol*, 1990, 93(4):491-4.

Mazzulli T, "Improved Diagnosis of Cytomegalovirus Infection by Detection of Antigenemia or Use of PCR Methods," *Clin Microbiol Newslet*, 1993, 15:97-100.

Cytomegalovirus Isolation, Rapid

CPT *87252 (tissue culture, inoculation and observation); 87253 (tissue culture, additional studies, each isolate)*

Related Information

Bronchial Washings Cytology *on page 485*
Bronchoalveolar Lavage Cytology *on page 487*
Cervical/Vaginal Cytology *on page 491*
Cytomegalic Inclusion Disease Cytology *on page 496*
Cytomegalovirus Antibody *on page 672*
Cytomegalovirus Culture *on previous page*
Sputum Cytology *on page 510*
Urine Cytology *on page 513*
Viral Culture, Blood *on page 1197*
Viral Culture, Urine *on page 1207*

Synonyms CMV Early Antigen FA Method; CMV Isolation, Rapid; CMV Shell Vial Method

Test Commonly Includes Inoculation of cell cultures in shell vials, 16-hour incubation, and immunofluorescence staining of CMV early nuclear antigen with monoclonal antibodies; conventional cell culture inoculation

Specimen Urine, bronchoalveolar lavage, blood, tracheal aspirates, appropriate autopsy and biopsy specimens **CONTAINER:** Sterile container; cold viral transport medium for swabs **COLLECTION:** See viral culture, specific specimen. **TURNAROUND TIME:** Overnight to 2 days depending on method and capability of laboratory

Interpretive **REFERENCE RANGE:** No CMV detected **USE:** Aid in the diagnosis of disease caused by CMV (eg, viral infections, pneumonia, and organ transplant-related disease) **LIMITATIONS:** Requires highly skilled, specialized laboratory personnel, often not available in many clinical laboratories. **METHODOLOGY:** Specimens are centrifuged onto cell cultures grown on coverslips in the bottoms of 1-dram shell vials. Centrifugation greatly accelerates virus attachment and penetration. After incubation, fluorescein-labeled monoclonal antibodies are applied to the infected cells to detect viral antigens that are expressed in the membranes of the cells. Characteristic fluorescent foci indicate the presence of virus. *In situ* DNA hybridization is also available for CMV.[1] **ADDITIONAL INFORMATION:** The rapid shell vial method for the detection of CMV has been reported to be more sensitive than and as specific as conventional tube cell culture.[2] The sensitivity of viral culture depends greatly on the type and age of host cells which may vary between laboratories. Several modifications of the shell vial method have been reported to enhance sensitivity.[3] Quantitative results of shell vial procedures sometimes are used to determine the level of viremia in organ and bone marrow transplant recipients.[4,5]

Footnotes

1. Schwartz DA and Wilcox CM, "Atypical Cytomegalovirus Inclusions in Gastrointestinal Biopsy Specimens From Patients With the Acquired Immunodeficiency Syndrome: Diagnostic Role of *In Situ* Nucleic Acid Hybridization," *Hum Pathol*, 1992, 23(9):1019-26.
2. Gleaves CA, Smith TF, Shuster EA, et al, "Comparison of Standard Tube and Shell Vial Cell Culture Techniques for the Detection of Cytomegalovirus in Clinical Specimens," *J Clin Microbiol*, 1985, 21:217-21.
3. Li SB and Fong CK, "Detection of Human Cytomegalovirus Early and Late Antigen and DNA Production in Cell Culture and the Effects of Dimethyl Sulfoxide, Dexamethasone, and DNA Inhibitors on Early Antigen Induction," *J Med Virol*, 1990, 30(2):97-102.

4. Slavin MA, Gleaves CA, Schoch HG, et al, "Quantification of Cytomegalovirus in Bronchoalveolar Lavage Fluid After Allogeneic Marrow Transplantation by Centrifugation Culture," *J Clin Microbiol*, 1992, 30(10):2776-9.
5. Buller RS, Bailey TC, Ettinger NA, et al, "Use of a Modified Shell Vial Technique to Quantitate Cytomegalovirus Viremia in a Population of Solid-Organ Transplant Recipients," *J Clin Microbiol*, 1992, 30(10):2620-4.

References

Smith TF, "Rapid Methods for the Diagnosis of Viral Infections," *Lab Med*, 1987, 18:16-20.
Woods GL and Thiele GM, "Rapid Detection of Cytomegalovirus by 24-Well Plate Centrifugation With the Use of a Monoclonal Antibody to an Early Nuclear Antigen," *Am J Clin Pathol*, 1989, 91(6):695-700.

Cytopathic Effect *see* Viral Culture *on page 1195*

Direct Detection of Virus *see* Virus, Direct Detection by Fluorescent Antibody *on page 1208*

Direct Fluorescent Antibody Test for Virus *see* Virus, Direct Detection by Fluorescent Antibody *on page 1208*

EBV Culture *see* Epstein-Barr Virus Culture *on page 1179*

Echovirus Culture *see* Enterovirus Culture *on next page*

Echovirus Culture, Stool *see* Viral Culture, Stool *on page 1205*

Electron Microscopic Examination for Viruses, Stool

CPT 88348

Related Information

Electron Microscopy *on page 45*
Histopathology *on page 57*
Rotavirus, Direct Detection *on page 1191*
Rotavirus Serology *on page 742*
Skin Biopsies *on page 84*
Stool Culture *on page 858*
Viral Culture, Stool *on page 1205*

Synonyms Enteric Viruses by EM; Gastrointestinal Viruses by EM

Applies to Rotavirus Detection by EM; Skin Viral Disease; Viral Disease in Tissue

Test Commonly Includes Use of the electron microscope to visualize viruses directly in stool

Specimen Stool from the acute, diarrheal phase of disease; skin lesions; tissues (biopsy/autopsy) **CONTAINER:** Sterile vial, tube, Petri dish, or stool container **SAMPLING TIME:** As soon as possible after the onset of disease **TURNAROUND TIME:** Less than 1 day **SPECIAL INSTRUCTIONS:** Laboratory must be notified prior to requesting examination of any specimen by EM.

Interpretive **REFERENCE RANGE:** Viruses not observed **USE:** Demonstrate viral particles (eg, rotavirus, Norwalk virus, calcivirus, astrovirus, and coronavirus) in stool specimens from patients with suspected viral gastroenteritis; examination of tissue from biopsy or autopsy in which immunofluorescent and immunoperoxidase staining is negative. **LIMITATIONS:** Generally, EM visualization of virus particles is not as sensitive as is cell culture, except for detecting nonculturable viruses such as rotavirus. EM can detect viruses if they are present in quantities of 10^6 to 10^7 particles/mL. This sensitivity is appropriate for agents causing diarrhea but is not sufficiently sensitive for the detection of other potential pathogens.[1] It is often difficult to differentiate (by EM) the aforementioned viruses. Very few clinical microbiology/virology laboratories have access to electron microscopes. **METHODOLOGY:** Diluted stool (either with or without being mixed with patient serum) is mixed with an electron-opaque heavy metal solution such as phosphotungstic acid. The stool solution is placed onto an electron-lucent grid support and examined by electron microscopy. Virions or virions agglutinated by specific antibodies (if present in serum) appear as a negative image against a black surrounding background.[1] **ADDITIONAL INFORMATION:** The electron microscopic observation of viruses is the basis for identification Electron microscopy is a useful procedure in cases where identification of viruses suspected of causing disease have not been identified by other methods.

Footnotes

1. Drew WL, "Diagnostic Virology," *Clin Lab Med*, 1987, 7:721-40.

References

Christensen ML, "Human Viral Gastroenteritis," *Clin Microbiol Rev*, 1989, 2(1):51-89.
Gray LD, "Novel Viruses Associated With Gastroenteritis," *Clin Microbiol Newslet*, 1991, 13(18):137-44.

(Continued)

Electron Microscopic Examination for Viruses, Stool *(Continued)*

Herrmann JE, Taylor DN, Echeverria P, et al, "Astroviruses as a Cause of Gastroenteritis in Children," *N Engl J Med*, 1991, 324(25):1757-60.

Hedberg CW and Osterholm M, "Outbreaks of Foodborne and Waterborne Viral Gastroenteritis," *Clin Microbiol Rev*, 1993, 6:199-210.

Johnson PC, "Small Round Gastroenteritis Viruses," *Inf Dis Newslet*, 1988, 7:25-7.

Lew JF, Moe CL, Monroe SS, et al, "Astrovirus and Adenovirus Associated With Diarrhea in Children in Day Care Settings," *J Infect Dis*, 1991, 164(4):673-8.

Miller SE, "Diagnostic Virology by Electron Microscopy," *Am Soc Microbiol News*, 1988, 54:475-81.

Enteric Viruses by EM *see* Electron Microscopic Examination for Viruses, Stool *on previous page*

Enterovirus Culture

CPT *87252 (tissue culture, inoculation and observation); 87253 (tissue culture, additional studies, each isolate)*

Related Information

Coxsackie A Virus Titer *on page 668*
Coxsackie B Virus Titer *on page 668*
Ova and Parasites, Stool *on page 836*
Poliomyelitis I, II, III Titer *on page 733*
Stool Culture *on page 858*
Viral Culture, Blood *on page 1197*
Viral Culture, Central Nervous System Symptoms *on page 1199*
Viral Culture, Stool *on page 1205*
Viral Culture, Urine *on page 1207*

Applies to Coxsackie A Virus Culture; Coxsackie B Virus Culture; Echovirus Culture; Poliovirus Culture

Test Commonly Includes Culture for Coxsackie A virus, Coxsackie B virus, echovirus, and poliovirus

Specimen Stool (best specimen), rectal swab, cerebrospinal fluid, upper and lower respiratory tract specimens, whole blood, throat swab, various organs and tissues **CONTAINER:** Sterile container **SAMPLING TIME:** It is important to obtain specimens very early in the disease; however, virus is shed in the stool for weeks. **STORAGE INSTRUCTIONS:** Enteroviruses are rather hardy; however, specimens should be refrigerated or placed into cold virus transport medium and delivered immediately to the clinical laboratory. **CAUSES FOR REJECTION:** Dry specimen, specimen not in proper viral transport medium, specimen not refrigerated during transport, specimen fixed in formalin, unlabeled specimen **TURNAROUND TIME:** Variable (1-4 days) and depends on culture method used and amount of virus in specimen. Negative cultures often are reported after 2 weeks.

Interpretive **REFERENCE RANGE:** No virus isolated **USE:** Aid in the diagnosis of disease caused by enteroviruses (eg, polio, congenital viral infections, viral pericarditis, and meningitis, aseptic) **LIMITATIONS:** Cell culture generally does not support the growth of certain Coxsackie A enteroviruses. Infrequently, aseptic meningitis is caused by Coxsackie A virus types which require animal inoculation for isolation. **METHODOLOGY:** Inoculation of specimens into cell culture, incubation of cultures, and observation for characteristic cytopathic effect (CPE). Enteroviruses are stable at pH 3; rhinoviruses are unstable at this pH. Specimens suspected of containing Coxsackie A virus are inoculated into suckling mice which are then observed for flaccid paralysis without encephalitis.

Clinical Diseases Caused By Enteroviruses

Cardiovascular	Myocarditis Pericarditis
Neurologic	Aseptic meningitis Encephalitis Poliomyelitis
Respiratory	Common cold Stomatitis Hand-foot-mouth syndrome Pharyngitis Tonsillitis Rhinitis
Miscellaneous	Febrile, exanthematous illness Acute hemorrhagic conjunctivitis (enterovirus 70, Coxsackie A24)

From Rotbart HA, "Nucleic Acid Detection Systems for Enteroviruses," *Clin Micro Rev*, 1991, 4:156-8, with permission.

Some (usually reference) laboratories can identify specific enteroviruses by using a battery of specific enterovirus-neutralizing antibodies. These antibodies are useful in identifying and typing Coxsackie A, Coxsackie B, echovirus, and poliovirus.

ADDITIONAL INFORMATION: Enteroviruses cause a wide variety of clinical diseases in humans (see table).[1] Humans are the only known reservoir for enteroviruses. Infection occurs by direct contact, the oral-fecal route or the respiratory route. Enteroviral infections most commonly occur from July to September. Children are more likely to become infected than are adults.

The detection of enteroviral nucleic acid directly from specimens seems promising but is not currently used in clinical laboratories.[1,2]

Footnotes

1. Rotbart HA, "Nucleic Acid Detection Systems for Enteroviruses," *Clin Microbiol Rev*, 1991, 4(2):156-8.
2. Chapman NM, Tracy S, Gauntt CJ, et al, "Molecular Detection and Identification of Enteroviruses Using Enzymatic Amplification and Nucleic Acid Hybridization," *J Clin Microbiol*, 1990, 28(5):843-50.

References

Dowsett EG, "Human Enteroviral Infections," *J Hosp Infect*, 1988, 11:103-15.

Menegus M, "Enteroviruses," *Manual of Clinical Microbiology*, 5th ed, Balows A, Hausler WJ Jr, Herrmann KL, et al, eds, Washington, DC: American Society for Microbiology, 1991, 943-7.

Modlin JF and Kinney JS, "Perinatal Enterovirus Infections," *Adv Pediatr Infect Dis*, 1987, 2:57-78.

Enterovirus Culture, Stool *see* Viral Culture, Stool *on page 1205*

Epstein-Barr Virus Culture

CPT *87252 (tissue culture, inoculation and observation); 87253 (tissue culture, additional studies, each isolate)*

Related Information

Epstein-Barr Virus Serology *on page 676*
Heterophil Agglutinins *on page 694*
Infectious Mononucleosis Screening Test *on page 713*
Lymph Node Biopsy *on page 72*
Viral Culture, Blood *on page 1197*

Synonyms Culture, EBV; EBV Culture

Applies to Lymph Node Culture for EBV; Lymphocyte Culture for EBV; Spleen Cell Culture for EBV

Test Commonly Includes Culture for EBV only

Abstract Epstein-Barr virus (EBV) is a herpesvirus. It was originally isolated from Burkitt's lymphomas. The geographic distribution of Burkitt's lymphoma is similar to that of yellow fever.

Specimen Whole blood, lymph node, spleen, tumor biopsies, throat garglings (for isolation of excreted virus) **CONTAINER:** Green top (heparin) tube for blood; sterile container for other specimens **STORAGE INSTRUCTIONS:** Blood specimen can be maintained at room temperature but should be immediately transported to the laboratory. Biopsy specimen should be sent to the Virology Laboratory immediately after collection. **CAUSES FOR REJECTION:** Dry specimen, specimen not refrigerated during transport, specimen fixed in formalin, unlabeled specimen, specimen not received in sterile container, excessive delay in transit to the laboratory **TURNAROUND TIME:** Cultures often are observed for 6 weeks before being reported as negative. **SPECIAL INSTRUCTIONS:** The laboratory always should be notified prior to receipt of specimen.

Interpretive **REFERENCE RANGE:** No growth of EBV in lymphocyte culture **USE:** Aid in the diagnosis of disease caused by EBV (eg, infectious mononucleosis, undifferentiated nasopharyngeal carcinoma, post-transplantation, and Burkitt's lymphomas) **LIMITATIONS:** Cell culture for EBV is not routinely available and not diagnostically practical because EBV proliferate only in B cells, which often are difficult to obtain and process. In addition, many asymptomatic individuals can shed virus orally. Cell culture requires at least 4 weeks to detect EBV infection. EB virus culture is unnecessary for most cases of infectious mononucleosis (IM). **The diagnosis of IM is based on three pillars: clinical appearance, CBC with differential, and conventional serology.** **METHODOLOGY:** Virus is given opportunity to grow for 4 weeks in a lymphocyte culture. Virus-infected cells will proliferate; if virus is not present, lymphocytes will die. Positive cultures are confirmed for EBV antigens using monoclonal antibodies. **ADDITIONAL INFORMATION:** Viral serology (usually immunofluorescence) is the preferred diagnostic method.[1,2] EBV persists regularly in the lymphoreticular system of EBV-infected individuals. EBV-positive lymphoblast lines can be established frequently from peripheral leukocytes and lymph node cells from those individuals.

(Continued)

Epstein-Barr Virus Culture *(Continued)*

EBV is closely associated with Burkitt's lymphoma and with nasopharyngeal carcinomas. The virus is often identified in these samples by DNA amplification techniques, *in situ* hybridization, and immunohistochemical detection.[3,4]

See the comparison listings, Epstein-Barr Virus Serology, Heterophil Agglutinins, and Infectious Mononucleosis Screening Test.

Footnotes

1. Straus SE, "Epstein-Barr Virus and Human Herpesvirus-6," *Practical Diagnosis of Viral Infections*, Galasso GJ, Whitley RJ, Merigan TC, eds, New York, NY: Raven Press, 1993, 253-67.
2. Okano M, Thiele EM, Davis JR, et al, "Serologic and Molecular Diagnosis of Epstein-Barr Virus Infection," *Clin Immunol Newslet*, 1988, 9:94-6.
3. Tyan YS, Liu ST, Ong WR, et al, "Detection of Epstein-Barr Virus and Human Papillomavirus in Head and Neck Tumors," *J Clin Microbiol*, 1993, 31(1):53-6.
4. Borisch B, Finke J, Hennig F, et al, "Distribution and Localization of Epstein-Barr Virus Subtypes A and B in AIDS-Related Lymphomas and Lymphatic Tissue of HIV-Positive Patients," *J Pathol*, 1992, 168(2):229-36.

References

Chang KL, Chen Y-Y, and Weiss LM, "Lack of Evidence of Epstein-Barr Virus in Hairy Cell Leukemia and Monocytoid B-Cell Lymphoma," *Hum Pathol*, 1993, 24(1):58-61.

Gratama JW, Oosterveer MA, Lepoutre JM, et al, "Serological and Molecular Studies of Epstein-Barr Virus Infection in Allogeneic Marrow Graft Recipients," *Transplantation*, 1990, 49(4):725-30.

Lennette E, "Epstein-Barr Virus," *Manual of Clinical Microbiology*, 5th ed, Balows A, Hausler WJ Jr, Herrmann KL, et al, eds, Washington, DC: American Society for Microbiology, 1991, 847-52.

Okano M, Thiele GM, Davis JR, et al, "Epstein-Barr and Human Diseases: Recent Advances in Diagnosis," *Clin Microbiol Rev*, 1988, 1:300-12.

Exanthems and Lesions of the Skin *see* Viral Culture, Dermatological Symptoms *on page 1201*

Eye Swab *Chlamydia* Culture *see Chlamydia trachomatis* Culture *on page 1171*

Gastrointestinal Viruses by EM *see* Electron Microscopic Examination for Viruses, Stool *on page 1177*

General Viral Culture *see* Viral Culture *on page 1195*

Genital Culture for *Mycoplasma* T-Strain *see* Genital Culture for *Ureaplasma urealyticum on this page*

Genital Culture for *Ureaplasma urealyticum*

CPT *87081*

Related Information

Endometrium Culture *on page 811*
Genital Culture *on page 814*
Neisseria gonorrhoeae Culture *on page 831*
Viral Culture, Central Nervous System Symptoms *on page 1199*

Synonyms Genital Culture for *Mycoplasma* T-Strain; *Mycoplasma* T-Strain Culture, Genital; *Ureaplasma urealyticum* Culture, Genital

Applies to Cervical Culture for T-Strain *Mycoplasma*; Cervical Culture for *Ureaplasma urealyticum*; Urethral Culture for T-Strain *Mycoplasma*

Test Commonly Includes Culture and identification of *Ureaplasma urealyticum* from genital specimens

Abstract The class Mollicutes includes the genera *Mycoplasma* and *Ureaplasma*.

Specimen Culturette® swab of urethra or cervix **CONTAINER:** Culturette® swab **STORAGE INSTRUCTIONS:** Keep specimen refrigerated. **Organism is remarkably sensitive to drying**. Swab must be placed promptly into Culturette® and hand delivered to the Microbiology Laboratory. If stored longer than 24 hours, the specimens should be frozen at -70°C. **TURNAROUND TIME:** 8 days if negative, up to 2 weeks if positive **SPECIAL INSTRUCTIONS:** *Ureaplasma* and *Mycoplasma* are sensitive to delays in processing and storage. Consult the laboratory prior to collecting the specimen for optimal handling instructions.

Interpretive **REFERENCE RANGE:** Frequently isolated from asymptomatic individuals **USE:** Establish the diagnosis of *Ureaplasma urealyticum* infection in suspected cases of nongonococcal urethritis and cervicitis. It is associated with chorioamnionitis and with perinatal morbidity and mortality. It can be isolated from the central nervous system and the lower respiratory tract of infected neonates. **LIMITATIONS:** Culture can be negative in the presence of infection, and the presence of *Ureaplasma urealyticum* or *Mycoplasma hominis* does not always indicate infection, although there is a significant association with symptomatic disease. **METHODOLOGY:** Culture on selective media[1] **ADDITIONAL INFORMATION:** *Ureaplasma* and *Mycoplasma* can be isolated from urethral and genital swabs and from urine of sexually active individuals. Sixty percent or more of all women asymptomatically carry *U. urealyticum* in their genital tract. Usual prevalence of these organisms in patients with urethral symptoms also is high; thus, conclusions regarding the etiologic role of an isolate in a given patient are difficult to make. *U. urealyticum* is usually associated with cases of nongonococcal urethritis.

Footnotes

1. Al-Zahawi MF, Kearns AM, Sprott MS, et al, "A Study of Three Blood Culture Media for Isolating Genital Mycoplasmas From Obstetrical and Gynaecological Patients," *J Infect*, 1990, 21(2):143-50.

References

Carey JC, Blackwelder WC, Nugent RP, et al, "Antepartum Cultures for *Ureaplasma urealyticum* Are Not Useful in Predicting Pregnancy Outcome," *Am J Obstet Gynecol*, 1991, 164(3):728-33.

Cassell GH, Waites KB, Watson HL, et al, "*Ureaplasma urealyticum* Intrauterine Infection: Role in Prematurity and Disease in Newborns," *Clin Microbiol Rev*, 1993, 6(1):69-87.

Gray DJ, Robinson HB, Malone J, et al, "Adverse Outcome in Pregnancy Following Amniotic Fluid Isolation of *Ureaplasma urealyticum*," *Prenat Diagn*, 1992, 12(2):111-7.

Genital Culture, Virus *see* Viral Culture, Urogenital *on page 1207*

German Measles Culture *see* Rubella Virus Culture *on page 1192*

Hemadsorbing Virus *see* Influenza Virus Culture *on page 1186*

Hemadsorbing Virus *see* Mumps Virus Culture *on page 1187*

Hemadsorbing Virus *see* Parainfluenza Virus Culture *on page 1189*

Herpes Culture *see* Herpes Simplex Virus Culture *on next page*

Herpes Simplex 1 and 2 Culture *see* Herpes Simplex Virus Culture *on next page*

Herpes Simplex Virus Antigen Detection

CPT *87206*

Related Information

Conjunctival Culture *on page 803*
Genital Culture *on page 814*
Herpes Cytology *on page 502*
Herpes Simplex Antibody *on page 692*
Herpes Simplex Virus Culture *on next page*
Herpes Simplex Virus Isolation, Rapid *on page 1184*
Herpesvirus Antigen *on page 693*
Oral Cavity Cytology *on page 507*
Skin Biopsies *on page 84*
Urine Cytology *on page 513*
Viral Culture, Dermatological Symptoms *on page 1201*

Synonyms Herpes Simplex Virus by DFA; Herpes Simplex Virus, Direct Immunofluorescence; HSV Antigen Detection, Direct

Test Commonly Includes Direct (nonculture) detection of HSV-infected cells in smears of specimens

Specimen Basal cells of a freshly unroofed lesion rolled onto a clean microscope slide **SAMPLING TIME:** Preferably within 3 days of lesion eruption. Specimens taken after 5 days are less likely to contain viral particles. **COLLECTION:** Make a preparation of cells taken from the suspected herpetic lesion onto a plain 1" x 3" glass slide. Cells from the bottom of an ulcer or vesicle should be scraped with a swab, scalpel, or curette. Swabs should be **rolled** (**not** smeared) across a small area of the slide several times, and cells scraped with a scalpel should be gently dabbed onto the slide. The best specimen is a collection of the cells at the base of an intact vesicle. Cells from a diseased cornea can also be used. **The smear should be air dried at room temperature**. The success of direct detection procedures depends on the careful preparation of cell smears. **STORAGE INSTRUCTIONS:** Do not store the specimen. Send it to the laboratory immediately. **CAUSES FOR REJECTION:** Insufficient quantity of specimen on slide, poorly prepared or labeled slides **TURNAROUND TIME:** Less than 1 day **SPECIAL INSTRUCTIONS:** Make more than one slide preparation.

(Continued)

Herpes Simplex Virus Antigen Detection *(Continued)*

Interpretive REFERENCE RANGE: No herpes simplex virus-infected cells detected USE: Rapid detection of herpes simplex virus in oral or genital lesions LIMITATIONS: Some of the variables in this test include proper collection of specimens, stage and location of lesion, and community prevalence of the disease. The efficiency of detection of HSV material depends in great part on the collection of a sufficiently large number of intact infected cells from the lesion. Specimen smears that are too thick can retain or trap the fluorescent reagent and make the test difficult to interpret. If at all possible, it is important to obtain cells from the base of an intact vesicle. The presence of infected cells decreases as the lesion heals, and crusted lesions may have little or no herpes antigenic material remaining. METHODOLOGY: The specimen smear is fixed and then directly overlaid with a fluorescein-labeled monoclonal antibody specific for HSV 1 and/or 2. After the excess antibody is removed, the specimen is examined by fluorescent microscopy for the presence of HSV-infected cells. ADDITIONAL INFORMATION: In certain situations, this direct antigen detection test can be more sensitive than cell culture; however, and in general, this test is only approximately 70% as sensitive as cell culture. In critical situations, clinicians should consider using both methods.[1] Air-dried preparations on slides can also be stained with Giemsa or Diff-Quik™ stains (Tzanck). Fixed preparations (usually 95% ethanol) can also be stained with the Papanicolaou or immunoperoxidase methods. Smears fixed with hairspray and subsequently stained with the Papanicolaou stain usually are excellent preparations.

Footnotes

1. Rawls WE, "Herpes Simplex Viruses: Types 1 and 2," *Laboratory Diagnosis of Viral Infections*, Lennette EH, ed, New York, NY: Morcel Dekker Inc, 1992, 443-61.

References

Drew WL, "Diagnostic Virology," *Clin Lab Med*, 1987, 7:721-40.
Smith TF, "Rapid Diagnosis of Viral Infections," *Adv Exp Med Biol*, 1990, 263:115-21.

Herpes Simplex Virus by DFA *see* Herpes Simplex Virus Antigen Detection *on previous page*

Herpes Simplex Virus Culture

CPT *87140 (culture typing, fluorescent method); 87252 (tissue culture, inoculation and observation); 87253 (tissue culture, additional studies, each isolate)*

Related Information

Conjunctival Culture *on page 803*
Genital Culture *on page 814*
Herpes Cytology *on page 502*
Herpes Simplex Antibody *on page 692*
Herpes Simplex Virus Antigen Detection *on previous page*
Herpes Simplex Virus Isolation, Rapid *on page 1184*
Herpesvirus Antigen *on page 693*
Neisseria gonorrhoeae Culture *on page 831*
Oral Cavity Cytology *on page 507*
Viral Culture, Central Nervous System Symptoms *on page 1199*
Viral Culture, Dermatological Symptoms *on page 1201*
Viral Culture, Eye or Ocular Symptoms *on page 1202*

Synonyms Culture, HSV; Herpes Culture; Herpes Simplex 1 and 2 Culture; HSV 1 and 2 Culture; HSV Culture

Applies to Viral Culture, Eye; Viral Culture, Genital; Viral Culture, Skin

Test Commonly Includes Culture for HSV only; HSV also is usually detected in a routine/general virus culture

Specimen Specimen depends on type of infection:

- genital – vesicle fluid, lesion, endocervical
- conjunctivitis – conjunctival
- congenital – throat, vesicle, cerebrospinal fluid
- encephalitis – brain biopsy, cerebrospinal fluid
- meningitis – cerebrospinal fluid , genital
- respiratory/oral – throat, vesicle

CONTAINER: Sterile container; cold viral transport medium for swabs COLLECTION: All specimens should be kept cold and moist. As for most viral cultures, specimens should be collected in the acute stage of the disease, preferably within 3 days and no longer than 7 days after the onset of illness. Spinal fluid specimens should be submitted in the usual sterile tube; no special transport medium is necessary. All other specimens should be collected on a sterile swab as described and the swab should be placed into cold viral transport medium immediately after collection.

Endocervical: Swab cervix with a rolling/scraping motion to assure obtaining epithelial cells.

Vesicular lesion: Wash vesicles with sterile saline. Carefully open several vesicles and soak up vesicular fluid with swab. If vesicles are absent, vigorously swab base of lesion (specimen should be collected during first 3 days of eruption, because specimens collected later in the course of disease rarely yield virus).

Conjunctival: Using a moistened swab, firmly rub conjunctiva using sufficient force to obtain epithelial cells.

Throat, respiratory, oral: Rotate swab in both tonsillar crypts and against posterior oropharynx.

STORAGE INSTRUCTIONS: Specimens should be delivered to the laboratory and handed to a technologist within 30 minutes of collection. Outpatient specimens: If transport is to be delayed more than 30 minutes after collection, specimen **must** be refrigerated (held at 4°C to 8°C) until it can be transported to the laboratory. If inoculation onto cell cultures is not possible within 48 hours, specimens should be frozen at -70°C. Do not freeze at -20°C. **CAUSES FOR REJECTION:** Dry specimen, specimen not refrigerated during transport, specimen fixed in formalin, unlabeled specimen **TURNAROUND TIME:** Variable (1-14 days) and depends on culture method used and amount of virus in specimen **SPECIAL INSTRUCTIONS:** Special viral transport medium must be obtained from the laboratory prior to collection of specimen.

Interpretive **REFERENCE RANGE:** No virus isolated **USE:** Aid in the diagnosis of disease caused by HSV **METHODOLOGY:** Inoculation of specimen into cell cultures, incubation of cultures, observation for characteristic cytopathic effect (CPE), and identification of HSV by fluorescein-labeled monoclonal antibodies specific for type 1 or 2.[1] **ADDITIONAL INFORMATION:** HSV can only rarely be isolated from the CSF of patients with HSV 1 encephalitis. The virus is occasionally isolated from spinal fluid of patients with HSV 2 meningitis and of neonates with congenital herpes. Virus can also be isolated from urine in patients with primary genital HSV infections concurrent with cystitis.

Serology for the detection of herpes simplex virus is available, but the results usually are of value only in the diagnosis of primary HSV infections. There is much cross reaction between the antibodies to HSV 1 and HSV 2.

Immunocompromised patients can develop disseminated HSV infections. These infections are characterized by a persistent, severe mucocutaneous infection involving the mouth, face, genital, or perianal areas. Sometimes these infections spread to organs such as the liver, lungs, adrenal glands, and bone marrow. Genital herpes infection has been suggested to be a possible risk factor for HIV-1 infection.[2] At the present time, it is unclear whether this relationship is biological or due to the sexual habits of the individual.

Footnotes

1. Corey L, "Laboratory Diagnosis of Herpes Simplex Virus Infections: Principles Guiding the Development of Rapid Diagnostic Tests," *Diagn Microbiol Infect Dis*, 1986, 4:111S-19S.
2. Hook EW 3d, Cannon RO, Nahmias AJ, et al, "Herpes Simplex Virus Infection as a Risk Factor for Human Immunodeficiency Virus Infection in Heterosexuals," *J Infect Dis*, 1992, 165(2):251-5.

References

Arvin AM and Prober CG, "Herpes Simplex Viruses," *Manual of Clinical Microbiology*, 5th ed, Balows A, Hausler WJ Jr, Herrmann KL, et al, eds, Washington DC: American Society for Microbiology, 1991, 822-8.

Brown ZA, Benedetti J, Ashley R, et al, "Neonatal Herpes Simplex Virus Infection in Relation to Asymptomatic Maternal Infection at the Time of Labor," *N Engl J Med*, 1991, 324(18):1247-52.

Dawkins BJ, "Genital Herpes Simplex Infections," *Prim Care*, 1990, 17(1):95-113.

Drew WL, "Laboratory Diagnosis of HSV Infections," *Clin Lab Med*, 1987, 7:721-91.

Forbes BA, "Perinatal Viral Infections," *Clin Microbiol Newslet*, 1992, 14(22):169-72.

Koelle DM, Benedetti J, Langenberg A, et al, "Asymptomatic Reactivation of Herpes Simplex Virus in Women After the First Episode of Genital Herpes," *Ann Intern Med*, 1992, 116(6):433-7.

Mertz GJ, Benedetti J, Ashley R, et al, "Risk Factors for the Sexual Transmission of Genital Herpes," *Ann Intern Med*, 1992, 116(3):197-202.

Solomon AR, "New Diagnostic Tests for Herpes Simplex and Varicella-Zoster Infections," *J Am Acad Dermatol*, 1988, 18:218-21.

Herpes Simplex Virus, Direct Immunofluorescence *see* Herpes Simplex Virus Antigen Detection *on page 1181*

Herpes Simplex Virus Isolation, Rapid

CPT *87140 (culture typing, fluorescent method); 87252 (tissue culture, inoculation and observation); 87253 (tissue culture, additional studies, each isolate)*

Related Information

Conjunctival Culture *on page 803*
Herpes Cytology *on page 502*
Herpes Simplex Antibody *on page 692*
Herpes Simplex Virus Antigen Detection *on page 1181*
Herpes Simplex Virus Culture *on page 1182*
Herpesvirus Antigen *on page 693*
Oral Cavity Cytology *on page 507*
Viral Culture, Dermatological Symptoms *on page 1201*
Viral Culture, Eyė or Ocular Symptoms *on page 1202*

Synonyms HSV Isolation, Rapid; HSV Shell Vial Method, Spin Amplification

Applies to Culture, HSV Only; HSV, Rapid Isolation; Skin Culture for HSV

Test Commonly Includes Inoculation of cell cultures in shell vials, 16-hour incubation, and immunofluorescence staining for HSV 1 and 2

Specimen Swab of genital, lip, or mucous membrane lesion; vesicular fluid; biopsy **CONTAINER:** Sterile container; cold viral transport medium for swabs **COLLECTION:** See viral culture, specific specimen. **TURNAROUND TIME:** Overnight to 2 days depending on method and capability of laboratory

Interpretive **REFERENCE RANGE:** No HSV detected **USE:** Rapid culture and detection of HSV in clinical specimens **LIMITATIONS:** The rapid shell vial culture technique for the detection of HSV 1 and 2 has been reported to be as sensitive as conventional cell culture methods.[1] However, some workers reported that shell vial methods are less sensitive than are tube cultures.[2] The procedure requires an experienced technician to interpret results. **METHODOLOGY:** Shell vial isolation technique with direct immunofluorescent staining for HSV 1 and HSV 2. Specimens are centrifuged onto cell cultures grown on coverslips in the bottoms of 1-dram shell vials. Centrifugation greatly accelerates virus attachment and penetration. After incubation, fluorescein-labeled monoclonal antibodies are applied to the infected cells to detect viral antigens that are expressed in the membranes of the cells. Characteristic fluorescent foci indicate the presence of virus. **ADDITIONAL INFORMATION:** The rapid detection of HSV in clinical specimens is increasingly becoming more sensitive and more practical for use in clinical laboratories. A new method of infecting cells with HSV in suspension has been studied and seems to be promising.[3,4] The detection of HSV-specific DNA is also under investigation.[5,6]

Footnotes

1. Gleaves CA, Wilson DJ, Wald AD, et al, "Detection and Serotyping of Herpes Simplex Virus in MRC-5 Cells by Use of Centrifugation and Monoclonal Antibodies 16-Hour Postinoculation," *J Clin Microbiol*, 1985, 21:29-32.
2. Johnston SL and Siegal CS, "Comparison of Enzyme Immunoassay, Shell Vial Culture, and Conventional Cell Culture for the Rapid Detection of Herpes Simplex Virus," *Diagn Microbiol Infect Dis*, 1990, 13(3):241-4.
3. Johnson FB and Visick EM, "A Rapid Culture Alternative to the Shell-Vial Method for the Detection of Herpes Simplex Virus," *Diagn Microbiol Infect Dis*, 1992, 15(8):673-8.
4. Luker G, Chow C, Richards DF, et al, "Suitability of Infection of Cells in Suspension for Detection of Herpes Simplex Virus," *J Clin Microbiol*, 1991, 29(7):1554-7.
5. Aurelius E, Johansson B, Skoldenborg B, et al, "Rapid Diagnosis of Herpes Simplex Encephalitis by Nested Polymerase Chain Reaction Assay of Cerebrospinal Fluid," *Lancet*, 1991, 337(8735):189-92.
6. Cone RW, Hobson AC, Palmer J, et al, "Extended Duration of Herpes Simplex Virus DNA in Genital Lesions Detected by the Polymerase Chain Reaction," *J Infect Dis*, 1991, 164(4):757-60.

References

Espy MJ, Wold AD, Jespersen DJ, et al, "Comparison of Shell Vials and Conventional Tubes Seeded With Rhabdomyosarcoma and MRC-5 Cells for the Rapid Detection of Herpes Simplex Virus," *J Clin Microbiol*, 1991, 29(12):2701-3.

Forbes BA, "Perinatal Viral Infections," *Clin Microbiol Newslet*, 1992, 14:169-72.

Solomon AR, "New Diagnostic Tests for Herpes Simplex and Varicella-Zoster Infections," *J Am Acad Dermatol*, 1988, 18:218-21.

HIV Culture *see* Human Immunodeficiency Virus Culture *on next page*

Human Immunodeficiency Virus Culture

CPT *87252 (tissue culture, inoculation and observation); 87253 (tissue culture, additional studies, each isolate)*

Related Information

HIV-1/HIV-2 Serology *on page 696*
Human Immunodeficiency Virus DNA Amplification *on page 915*
Lymphocyte Subset Enumeration *on page 720*
p24 Antigen *on page 727*
Polymerase Chain Reaction *on page 927*
Zidovudine *on page 1012*

Synonyms AIDS Virus Culture; HIV Culture; HTLV-III Culture

Test Commonly Includes Isolation of HIV from clinical specimens

Specimen Whole blood (20-40 mL), cerebrospinal fluid (10 mL), other body fluids, biopsies.[1] See special precautions in Specimen Collection chapter. All specimens **must** be labeled with the patient's name or code and **must** be transported to the laboratory in a **sealed** plastic bag with the request form attached. Some laboratories will not accept patient names associated with HIV specimens. **CONTAINER:** Green top (heparin) tube for blood, sterile container for CSF and other fluids **COLLECTION:** Routine venipuncture. Invert the tubes several times after drawing the blood to be sure the blood is thoroughly mixed with the heparin. **STORAGE INSTRUCTIONS:** Do not store the specimen. Send it to the laboratory immediately. Some laboratories require that the specimen be received in the laboratory the same day the specimen is obtained. **CAUSES FOR REJECTION:** Specimen not refrigerated during transport, specimen fixed in formalin, unlabeled specimen **TURNAROUND TIME:** Positive cultures are usually reported after two consecutive positive reverse transcriptase assays. Blood cultures are usually incubated 4 weeks and some laboratories incubate CSF cultures 8 weeks before reporting as negative. **SPECIAL INSTRUCTIONS:** Request form must be complete with type of specimen and site of specimen if applicable.

Interpretive **REFERENCE RANGE:** No virus isolated **USE:** Aid in the diagnosis of disease caused by HIV **LIMITATIONS:** A negative culture cannot be assumed to rule out the presence of the virus. Fresh human lymphocytes are needed for growth of HIV. These cells are costly and more difficult to maintain than are cell lines. Many laboratories do not have the capability of HIV culture. Culture of HIV poses a risk to laboratory personnel. **METHODOLOGY:** Growth of virus in lymphocyte culture and subsequent (indirect) testing for presence of virus in culture supernatant fluids by enzyme immunoassay (EIA) or reverse transcriptase assay **ADDITIONAL INFORMATION:** Serology for the detection of HIV antibodies is widely available.[2] Detection of antibodies to HIV is the most common method of HIV testing. It is better suited for routine use in screening patients for exposure to HIV.[3] DNA amplification for detection of HIV (either proviral DNA or viral RNA) is useful in diagnosing HIV in infants of HIV-seropositive mothers[4] and for individuals at high risk for HIV infection.[5]

Footnotes

1. Clarke JR, Williamson JD, Mitchell DM, "Comparative Study of the Isolation of Human Immunodeficiency Virus From the Lung and Peripheral Blood of AIDS Patients," *J Med Virol*, 1993, 39(3):196-9.
2. Abb J, "Diagnostic and Prognostic Significance of Testing for HIV Antigen," *Clin Immunol Newslet*, 1988, 9:85-7.
3. Weniger BG, Quinhões EP, Sereno AB, et al, "A Simplified Surveillance Case Definition of AIDS Derived From Empirical Clinical Data," *J Acquir Immune Defic Syndr*, 1992, 5(12):1212-23.
4. Rogers MF, Ou C-Y, Rayfield M, et al, "Use of the Polymerase Chain Reaction for Early Detection of the Proviral Sequences of Human Immunodeficiency Virus in Infants Born to Seropositive Mothers," *N Engl J Med*, 1989, 320(25):1649-54.

(Continued)

Human Immunodeficiency Virus Culture *(Continued)*

5. Loche M and Mach B, "Identification of HIV-Infected Seronegative Individuals by a Direct Diagnostic Test Based on Hybridization to Amplified Viral DNA," *Lancet*, 1989, 2(8608):418-21.

References

Erice A, Sannerud KJ, Leske VL, et al, "Sensitive Microculture Method for Isolation of Human Immunodeficiency Virus Type 1 From Blood Leukocytes," *J Clin Microbiol*, 1992, 30(2):444-8.

Forbes BA, "Perinatal Viral Infections," *Clin Microbiol Newslet*, 1992, 14(22):169-72.

Jackson JB, "Human Immunodeficiency Virus Type 1 Antigen and Culture Assays," *Arch Pathol Lab Med*, 1990, 114(3):249-53.

Jackson JB and Balfour HH, "Practical Diagnostic Testing for Human Immunodeficiency Virus," *Clin Microbiol Rev*, 1988, 1:124-38.

Khan NC, Chatterjee S, and Nielson LN, "Pathogenesis of HIV Infection," *Clin Microbiol Newslet*, 1990, 12(23):177-84.

Markham PD and Salahuddin SZ, "*In Vitro* Cultivation of Human Leukocytes: Methods for the Expression and Isolation of Human Retroviruses," *BioTechniques*, 1987, 5:432-43.

Influenza Virus Culture

CPT *87140 (culture typing, fluorescent method); 87252 (tissue culture, inoculation and observation); 87253 (tissue culture, additional studies, each isolate)*

Related Information

Influenza A and B Titer *on page 713*

Viral Culture, Respiratory Symptoms *on page 1204*

Virus, Direct Detection by Fluorescent Antibody *on page 1208*

Applies to Hemadsorbing Virus

Test Commonly Includes Culture for influenza A and B. Also includes concurrent culture for other respiratory viruses (parainfluenza and respiratory syncytial virus).

Specimen Throat or nasopharyngeal swab, sputum, bronchial washings, bronchoalveolar lavage **CONTAINER:** Sterile container; cold virus transport medium for swabs **SAMPLING TIME:** Specimens should be collected within 3 days of the onset of illness. **STORAGE INSTRUCTIONS:** Specimens should be placed into viral transport medium and kept cold at all times. Specimens should be delivered immediately to the laboratory. Do not freeze specimens. **CAUSES FOR REJECTION:** Dry specimen, specimen not refrigerated during transport, specimen fixed in formalin, unlabeled specimen **TURNAROUND TIME:** Variable (5-14 days) and depends on culture method used and the amount of virus in the specimen. Negative cultures usually are reported after 2 weeks.

Interpretive **REFERENCE RANGE:** No virus isolated **USE:** Isolate and identify influenza virus as an etiologic agent in cases of influenza and viral pneumonia **METHODOLOGY:** Inoculation of specimens into cell cultures, incubation of cultures, observation for characteristic cytopathic effect (CPE), and identification/speciation by methods such as hemadsorption and fluorescent monoclonal antibodies specific for influenza virus A or B **ADDITIONAL INFORMATION:** Influenza is very contagious and is usually transmitted from person to person by inhalation of aerosols, especially in crowded conditions.[1] The peak incidence of influenza infection is between December and March. Both influenza A and influenza B have been implicated in epidemics every 3-6 years.[2]

The shell vial technique to rapidly (within 24 hours) detect viruses has been adopted to detect influenza A and B viruses.[3,4] Serology for the detection of influenza antibodies is available. Antibody levels usually peak 4-6 weeks after infection. A single high antibody titer in convalescent serum is suggestive of a recent infection. However, the recommended procedure for a diagnostic antibody titer is comparison of acute and convalescent titers.[5] A commercial and rapid (less than 15 minutes) enzyme immunoassay for the detection of influenza A virus in patient specimen is also available.[6]

Footnotes

1. Leigh MW, Carson JL, and Denny FW Jr, "Pathogenesis of Respiratory Infections Due to Influenza Virus: Implications for Developing Countries," *Rev Infect Dis*, 1991, 13(Suppl 6):S501-8.
2. Kendal AP, "Epidemiologic Implication of Changes in the Influenza Virus Genome," *Am J Med*, 1987, 82:S4-14.
3. Espy M, Smith TF, and Harmon MV, "Rapid Detection of Influenza Virus by Shell Vial Assay With Monoclonal Antibodies," *J Clin Microbiol*, 1986, 24:677-9.
4. Guenthner SH and Linneman CC, "Indirect Immunofluorescence Assay for Rapid Diagnosis of Influenza Virus," *Lab Med*, 1988, 581-3.
5. Harmon MW, Rota PA, Walls HH, et al, "Antibody Response in Humans to Influenza Virus Type B Host-Cell-Derived Variants After Vaccination With Standard (Egg-Derived) Vaccine or Natural Infection," *J Clin Microbiol*, 1988, 26:333-7.

6. Waner JL, Todd SJ, Shalaby H, et al, "Comparison of Directigen FLU-A With Viral Isolation and Direct Immunofluorescence for the Rapid Detection and Identification of Influenza A Virus," *J Clin Microbiol*, 1991, 29(3):479-82.

References

Couch RB, "Respiratory Diseases," *Practical Diagnosis of Viral Infections*, Galasso GJ, Whitley RJ, Merigan TC, eds, New York, NY: Raven Press, 1993, 143-8.

Harmon MW and Kendal AP, "Influenza Viruses," *Manual of Clinical Microbiology*, 5th ed, Balows A, Hausler WJ Jr, Herrmann KL, et al, eds, Washington, DC: American Society for Microbiology, 1991, 868-77.

Shaw MW, Arden NH, and Maassab HF, "New Aspects of Influenza Viruses," *Clin Microbiol Rev*, 1992, 5(1):74-92.

Influenza Virus, Direct Detection *see* Virus, Direct Detection by Fluorescent Antibody *on page 1208*

Lumbar Puncture Hazards *see* Viral Culture, Central Nervous System Symptoms *on page 1199*

Lymph Node Culture for EBV *see* Epstein-Barr Virus Culture *on page 1179*

Lymphocyte Culture for EBV *see* Epstein-Barr Virus Culture *on page 1179*

Lymphogranuloma Venereum Culture *see Chlamydia trachomatis* Culture *on page 1171*

Measles Culture, 3-Day *see* Rubella Virus Culture *on page 1192*

Measles Virus, Direct Detection *see* Virus, Direct Detection by Fluorescent Antibody *on page 1208*

MicroTrak® *see Chlamydia trachomatis* Direct FA Test *on page 1173*

Mumps Virus Culture

CPT *87252 (tissue culture, inoculation and observation); 87253 (tissue culture, additional studies, each isolate)*

Related Information

Mumps Serology *on page 726*
Viral Culture, Central Nervous System Symptoms *on page 1199*
Viral Culture, Urine *on page 1207*

Applies to Hemadsorbing Virus

Test Commonly Includes Culture for the presence of mumps virus in clinical specimens; mumps virus is isolated from routine viral cultures

Specimen Saliva, urine, cerebrospinal fluid **CONTAINER:** Sterile container for urine and CSF; tube with cold viral transport medium for swabs **SAMPLING TIME:** At or within 5 days of the onset of illness **COLLECTION:** It is desirable to collect specimens as early in the disease as possible. Saliva, days one and two after onset; spinal fluid of patients with meningoencephalitis within 6 days after onset. Virus is also excreted in urine for as long as 14 days after the onset of illness. In young patients, saliva is collected by a suitable suction device or by swabbing, especially the area around the orifices of the Stensen duct. The swabs must immediately be placed into cold viral transport medium. Spinal fluid is obtained in the usual manner and put into a sterile tube. For urine specimens, preferably the first voided morning urine is collected in a sterile container. All specimens must immediately be placed on ice and sent to the laboratory. **STORAGE INSTRUCTIONS:** Do **not** freeze at -20°C. Storage at -20°C rapidly inactivates the mumps virus. If inoculation is delayed by more than 48 hours, specimens should be frozen at -70°C. **CAUSES FOR REJECTION:** Dry specimen, specimen not refrigerated during transport, specimen fixed in formalin, unlabeled specimen **TURNAROUND TIME:** Variable (5-14 days) and depends on methods used and amount of virus in the specimen. Negative cultures usually are reported at 2 weeks.

Interpretive **REFERENCE RANGE:** No virus isolated **USE:** Aid in the diagnosis of disease caused by mumps virus, especially meningitis **METHODOLOGY:** Inoculation of specimen into cell cultures, incubation of cultures, observation for characteristic cytopathic effect (CPE), and identification by methods such as hemadsorption and fluorescent monoclonal antibodies **ADDITIONAL INFORMATION:** Although virus isolation is the most certain means for establishing the laboratory diagnosis, serologic methods are also useful and technically easier. Demonstration of IgM antibodies in acute serum is diagnostic of primary infection. The incidence of mumps infections has dramatically declined since the introduction of the mumps vaccine in 1967. However, there still remains a significant population of individuals that are unvaccinated or without prior exposure.[1]

(Continued)

Mumps Virus Culture *(Continued)*

Footnotes

1. Cochi SL, Preblud SR, and Orestein WA, "Perspective on the Relative Resurgence of Mumps in the United States," *Am J Dis Child*, 1988, 142(5):499-507.

References

Kleiman MB, "Mumps Virus," *Laboratory Diagnosis of Viral Infections*, Lennette EH, ed, New York, NY: Marcel Dekker Inc, 1992, 549-66.

Swierkosz EM, "Mumps Virus," *Manual of Clinical Microbiology*, 5th ed, Balows A, Hausler WJ Jr, Herrmann KL, et al, eds, Washington, DC: American Society for Microbiology, 1991, 912-7.

Mumps Virus Culture, Urine *see* Viral Culture, Urine *on page 1207*

Mumps Virus, Direct Detection *see* Virus, Direct Detection by Fluorescent Antibody *on page 1208*

Mycoplasma pneumoniae Diagnostic Procedures

CPT 86738 (antibodies); 87109 (culture)

Related Information

Mycoplasma pneumoniae DNA Probe Test *on page 923*
Mycoplasma Serology *on page 727*
Sputum Culture *on page 849*

Synonyms *Mycoplasma pneumoniae* Culture

Test Commonly Includes Culture and identification of *Mycoplasma pneumoniae*

Abstract *Mycoplasma pneumoniae* commonly causes respiratory infections. Most involve the upper respiratory tract, but pneumonia and other manifestations can occur as well.

Specimen Throat or nasopharyngeal swabs **COLLECTION:** Throat or nasopharyngeal swabs should be placed **immediately** in transport medium and sent immediately to the laboratory. **TURNAROUND TIME:** 2-3 weeks

Interpretive **REFERENCE RANGE:** No *Mycoplasma pneumoniae* identified **USE:** Aid in the diagnosis of pneumonia caused by *Mycoplasma pneumoniae* **LIMITATIONS:** The culture procedure is not often used because it is slow and somewhat insensitive; 2-3 weeks or more are often required for isolation and definitive identification of positive cultures. **METHODOLOGY:** Isolates are cultured in special broth and on special agar media and are identified by biochemical tests and ability to hemolyze erythrocytes. However, the most commonly used and currently recommended method of diagnosis is serology to measure acute and convalescent antibody levels to *M. pneumoniae*. **ADDITIONAL INFORMATION:** *Mycoplasma pneumoniae* infection is acquired via the respiratory route from small-particle aerosols or large droplets of secretions. The organism can penetrate the mucociliary barrier of respiratory epithelium and produce cellular injury and ciliostasis which may account for the prolonged cough observed clinically. Most infections are observed in older children and young adults. Early infection in infancy or childhood may increase the severity of subsequent infections. The recently described *M. genitalium* might play a role in the pathogenesis of *M. pneumoniae* disease.[1] Cold agglutinins and *Mycoplasma pneumoniae* complement fixation serology have been the mainstays of diagnosis because of the limitations and long turnaround time for cultures. However, immunofluorescence techniques and immunoassays to detect antibodies to *M. pneumoniae* are available and are the recommended diagnostic methods. Detection of *Mycoplasma pneumoniae* DNA is being evaluated for use as a rapid diagnostic tool.[2] However, these tests are not yet available for routine testing. Consult the laboratory for availability of specific tests and specific instructions for specimen collection. See table on following page.

Footnotes

1. Tully JG, "The Current Enigma of *Mycoplasma genitalium*: New Findings That Affect *Mycoplasma* Identification in the Clinical Microbiology Laboratory," *Clin Microbiol Newslet*, 1989, 11:4-6.
2. Buck GE, O'Hara LC, and Summersgill JT, "Rapid, Sensitive Detection of *Mycoplasma pneumoniae* in Simulated Clinical Specimens by DNA Amplification," *J Clin Microbiol*, 1992, 30(12):3280-3.

References

Lee SH, Charoenying S, Brennan T, et al, "Comparative Studies of Three Serologic Methods for the Measurement of *Mycoplasma pneumoniae* Antibodies," *Am J Clin Pathol*, 1989, 92(3):342-7.

Mansel JK, Rosenow EC 3d, Smith TF, et al, "*Mycoplasma pneumoniae* Pneumonia," *Chest*, 1989, 95(3):639-46.

"The Changing Role of Mycoplasmas in Respiratory Disease and AIDS," *Clin Infect Dis*, 1993, 17(Suppl 1).

Wijnands GJ, "Diagnosis and Interventions in Lower Respiratory Tract Infections," *Am J Med*, 1992, 92(4SA):91S-7S.

Mycoplasma pneumoniae **Clinical Manifestations of Infection**

Respiratory	Pneumonia Pharyngitis Otitis media Bullous myringitis Sinusitis Laryngotracheobronchitis Bronchiolitis Nonspecific upper respiratory symptoms
Neurologic	Meningoencephalitis Encephalitis Transverse myelitis Cranial neuropathy Poliomyelitis-like syndrome Psychosis Cerebral infarction Guillain-Barré syndrome
Cardiac	Pericarditis Myocarditis Complete heart block Congestive heart failure Myocardial infarction
Gastrointestinal	Hepatic dysfunction Pancreatitis
Hematologic	Autoimmune hemolytic anemia Bone marrow suppression Thrombocytopenia Disseminated intravascular coagulation
Musculoskeletal	Myalgias Arthralgias Arthritis
Genitourinary	Glomerulonephritis Tubulointerstitial nephritis Tubo-ovarian abscess
Immunologic	Depressed cellular immunity and neutrophil chemotaxis

From Broughton RA, "Infections Due to *Mycoplasma pneumoniae* in Childhood," *Pediatr Infect Dis J*, 1986, 71-85, with permission.

Mycoplasma **T-Strain Culture, Genital** *see* Genital Culture for *Ureaplasma urealyticum on page 1180*

Parainfluenza 1, 2, and 3 Virus Culture *see* Parainfluenza Virus Culture *on this page*

Parainfluenza Virus Culture

CPT *87140 (culture typing, fluorescent method); 87252 (tissue culture, inoculation and observation); 87253 (tissue culture, additional studies, each isolate)*

Related Information

Parainfluenza Viral Serology *on page 728*
Viral Culture, Respiratory Symptoms *on page 1204*
Virus, Direct Detection by Fluorescent Antibody *on page 1208*

Synonyms Parainfluenza 1, 2, and 3 Virus Culture

Applies to Hemadsorbing Virus

Test Commonly Includes Culture and identification of parainfluenza viruses. Concurrent culture for other respiratory viruses (influenza, adenovirus, and respiratory syncytial viruses)

Specimen Throat or nasopharyngeal swab, nasopharyngeal washes and secretions **CONTAINER:** Sterile container; cold viral transport medium for swabs **COLLECTION:** Place swabs into cold viral transport medium and keep cold. Infants and small children: soft catheters and suction devices (syringes and suction bulbs) can be used to collect nasal secretions from far back in the nose (best specimens). Another excellent method is to introduce 3-7 mL of sterile saline into the child's posterior nasal cavity and immediately aspirate the fluid. **Note**: Do not use

(Continued)

Parainfluenza Virus Culture *(Continued)*

cold sterile saline when aspirating samples. Warm to room temperature. **STORAGE INSTRUCTIONS:** Keep specimens ice cold after collection, but **do not freeze specimens at -20°C**. Specimens that cannot be inoculated into cell culture within 72 hours should be frozen at -70°C. **CAUSES FOR REJECTION:** Dry specimen, specimen not refrigerated during transport, specimen fixed in formalin, unlabeled specimen **TURNAROUND TIME:** Variable (5-14 days), depending on culture method and amount of virus in specimen. Negative cultures are usually reported after 2 weeks.

Interpretive **REFERENCE RANGE:** No virus isolated **USE:** Aid in the diagnosis of disease caused by parainfluenza virus **METHODOLOGY:** Inoculation of specimens into cell cultures, incubation of cultures, observation for hemadsorption or characteristic cytopathic effect (CPE), and identification/speciation by fluorescent monoclonal antibodies specific for types 1, 2, or 3 or by virus neutralization **ADDITIONAL INFORMATION:** Most virology laboratories hemadsorb all viral (especially respiratory) cultures at 14 days (prior to discarding the culture) to detect hemadsorbing viruses that have not produced cytopathic effect (CPE) by that time. Positive hemadsorption tests are often reported as "hemadsorbing virus present." This result suggests the presence of influenza, parainfluenza, measles, and/or mumps virus.

Serology for the detection of parainfluenza antibodies is available, but the results are often difficult to interpret. Studies are underway to investigate a rapid shell vial assay for detection of several respiratory viruses. This test will detect influenza A and B virus, respiratory syncytial virus, and parainfluenza virus 1, 2, and 3.[1]

Footnotes

1. Schirm J, Luijt DS, Pastoor GW, et al, "Rapid Detection of Respiratory Viruses Using Mixtures of Monoclonal Antibodies on Shell Vial Cultures," *J Med Virol*, 1992, 38(2):147-51.

References

Costello MJ, Smernoff NT, and Yungblath M, "Laboratory Diagnosis of Viral Respiratory Tract Infections," *Lab Med*, 1993, 24:150-7.

Waner JL, "Parainfluenza Viruses," *Manual of Clinical Microbiology*, 5th ed, Balows A, Hausler WJ Jr, Herrmann KL, et al, eds, Washington, DC: American Society for Microbiology, 1991, 878-82.

Parainfluenza Virus, Direct Detection *see* Virus, Direct Detection by Fluorescent Antibody *on page 1208*

Poliovirus Culture *see* Enterovirus Culture *on page 1178*

Poliovirus Culture, Stool *see* Viral Culture, Stool *on page 1205*

Rabies Virus, Direct Detection *see* Virus, Direct Detection by Fluorescent Antibody *on page 1208*

Respiratory Syncytial Virus Culture

CPT *87140 (culture typing, fluorescent method); 87252 (tissue culture, inoculation and observation); 87253 (tissue culture, additional studies, each isolate)*

Related Information

Respiratory Syncytial Virus Serology *on page 739*
Viral Culture, Respiratory Symptoms *on page 1204*
Virus, Direct Detection by Fluorescent Antibody *on page 1208*

Synonyms Culture, RSV; RSV Culture

Test Commonly Includes Culture for respiratory syncytial virus (RSV) as well as concurrent culture for other respiratory viruses (influenza and parainfluenza viruses)

Specimen Throat or nasopharyngeal swab, nasopharyngeal washes and secretions **CONTAINER:** Sterile container; cold viral transport medium for swabs **COLLECTION:** Place swabs into cold viral transport medium and keep cold. Infants and small children: soft catheters and suction devices (syringes and suction bulbs) can be used to collect nasal secretions from far back in the nose (best specimens). Another excellent method is to introduce 3-7 mL of sterile saline into the child's posterior nasal cavity and immediately aspirate the fluid. Do not use **cold** sterile saline when aspirating samples. Warm to room temperature. **STORAGE INSTRUCTIONS:** Respiratory syncytial virus is extremely labile. **Do not freeze specimens at -20°C.** Send specimens to the laboratory **as soon as possible**. Although less than optimal conditions, specimens can be stored up to 48 hours at 4°C. If necessary specimen can be quickly frozen at -70°C, but freezing will cause loss of infectivity. **CAUSES FOR REJECTION:** Dry specimen, specimen not refrigerated during transport, specimen fixed in formalin, unlabeled specimen **TURNAROUND TIME:** Variable (1-14 days) depending on culture method and amount of virus in specimen. Negative results are usually reported after 2 weeks.

Interpretive **REFERENCE RANGE:** No virus isolated **USE:** Aid in the diagnosis of respiratory disease caused by respiratory syncytial virus **LIMITATIONS:** RSV is a very thermolabile virus and may not survive transport to the laboratory or extreme conditions. Thus, false-negative cultures occur. **METHODOLOGY:** Inoculation of specimen into cell cultures, incubation of cultures, observation for characteristic cytopathic effect (CPE) in 2-7 days, and identification by fluorescent monoclonal antibodies specific for respiratory syncytial virus. The use of a rapid shell viral culture technique is reported to yield positive culture results overnight.[1] **ADDITIONAL INFORMATION:** Serology is available to detect antibodies to respiratory syncytial virus. Many laboratories offer enzyme immunoassay (EIA) tests for the direct detection of RSV in patient specimens. In general, these tests are very rapid, sensitive, and specific.[2]

Footnotes

1. Mathey S, Nicholson D, Ruhs S, et al, "Rapid Detection of Respiratory Viruses by Shell Vial Culture and Direct Staining by Using Pooled and Individual Monoclonal Antibodies," *J Clin Microbiol*, 1992, 30(3):540-4.
2. Bruner TA and Fedorko DP, "Opportunities for Rapid Viral Diagnosis," *Clin Microbiol Newslet*, 1993, 15(9):65-9.

References

Takimoto CH, Cram DL, and Root RK, "Respiratory Synctial Virus Infections on an Adult Medical Ward," *Arch Intern Med*, 1991, 151(4):706-8.

Toms GL, "Respiratory Syncytial Virus: Virology, Diagnosis, and Vaccinaton," *Lung*, 1990, 168 (Suppl):388-95.

Welliver RC, "Detection, Pathogenesis, and Therapy of Respiratory Syncytial Virus Infections," *Clin Microbiol Rev*, 1988, 1:27-39.

White JM, Poupard JA, Knight RA, et al, "Evaluation of Two Commercially Available Test Methods to Determine the Feasibility of Testing for Respiratory Syncytial Virus in a Community Hospital Laboratory," *Am J Clin Pathol*, 1988, 90(2):175-80.

Rotavirus Detection by EM *see* Electron Microscopic Examination for Viruses, Stool *on page 1177*

Rotavirus, Direct Detection

CPT *83518 (immunoassay); 86403 (particle agglutination)*

Related Information

Electron Microscopic Examination for Viruses, Stool *on page 1177*
Ova and Parasites, Stool *on page 836*
Rotavirus Serology *on page 742*
Stool Culture *on page 858*
Viral Culture, Stool *on page 1205*

Synonyms Rotavirus Rapid Detection

Applies to Viral Antigen Detection, Direct, Stool

Test Commonly Includes Direct (nonculture) detection of rotavirus in stool specimens

Specimen Stool from the acute, diarrheal phase of disease; rectal swab **CONTAINER:** Plastic stool container **SAMPLING TIME:** As soon as possible after onset of disease, preferably 3-5 days after onset **COLLECTION:** Several specimens during the course of illness should be submitted in an attempt to eliminate false-negative results. **CAUSES FOR REJECTION:** Excessive transit time to the laboratory, unlabeled specimen **TURNAROUND TIME:** Less than 1 day

Interpretive **REFERENCE RANGE:** No virus detected **USE:** Detect rotavirus in stools of patients suspected of having viral gastroenteritis **LIMITATIONS:** Quality of specimens cannot be evaluated, and specimens are collected randomly. **METHODOLOGY:** Several commercially available (and often automated) enzyme immunoassays (EIA) are the preferred diagnostic methods. However, these kits were not developed according to standardized procedures and reagents.[1] In general, these assays detect the highly conserved internal capsid protein of the rotavirus group. **ADDITIONAL INFORMATION:** Rotavirus is a common cause of pediatric gastroenteritis. The illness is most likely to occur in winter, is highly contagious, involves 5-8 days of diarrhea, and is rarely fatal.[2] Patients should also be evaluated for possible bacterial gastroenteritis. If available, electron microscopy is a useful technique for detection of rotavirus in stool specimens.

Footnotes

1. Christensen ML and Howard C, "Viruses Causing Gastroenteritis," *Manual of Clinical Microbiology*, 5th ed, Balows A, Hausler WJ Jr, Herrmann KL, et al, eds, Washington DC: American Society for Microbiology, 1991, 950-8.
2. Blacklow NR and Greenberg HB, "Viral Gastroenteritis," *N Engl J Med*, 1991, 325(4):252-64.

(Continued)

Rotavirus, Direct Detection *(Continued)*

References

Christensen ML, "Human Viral Gastroenteritis," *Clin Microbiol Rev*, 1989, 2(1):51-89.
Gray LD, "Novel Viruses Associated With Gastroenteritis," *Clin Microbiol Newslet*, 1991, 13(18):137-44.

Rotavirus Rapid Detection *see* Rotavirus, Direct Detection *on previous page*
Routine Viral Culture *see* Viral Culture *on page 1195*
RSV Culture *see* Respiratory Syncytial Virus Culture *on page 1190*

Rubella Virus Culture

CPT *87252 (tissue culture, inoculation and observation); 87253 (tissue culture, additional studies, each isolate)*

Related Information

Rubella Serology *on page 743*

Synonyms German Measles Culture; Measles Culture, 3-Day

Test Commonly Includes Isolation and identification of rubella virus in cell culture

Specimen Two throat swabs, 10 mL urine, cerebrospinal fluid, tissues, amniotic fluid **CONTAINER:** Sterile urine container **SAMPLING TIME:** Virus is more likely to be isolated if specimen is collected within 5 days after onset of illness. **STORAGE INSTRUCTIONS:** Specimens should not be stored. Specimens should be delivered immediately to the laboratory. If unavoidable delays occur the specimen can be stored at 4°C for up to 3 days, but there is a loss of infectivity when culture is delayed. **CAUSES FOR REJECTION:** Dry specimen, specimen not refrigerated during transport, specimen fixed in formalin, unlabeled specimen **TURNAROUND TIME:** Positive cultures are detected in 3-7 days. Negative cultures are usually reported after 3 weeks.

Interpretive **REFERENCE RANGE:** No virus isolated **USE:** Aid in the diagnosis of disease caused by rubella virus (eg, congenital viral infection) **LIMITATIONS:** Isolation of rubella virus is usually of little help in the diagnosis of rubella except in cases of severe rubella complications, epidemiological purposes, and fatality. Serological diagnosis is much more useful. **METHODOLOGY:** Cell culture, isolation, and confirmation/identification by antibody-specific neutralization **ADDITIONAL INFORMATION:** The incidence of rubella has been reduced dramatically by the wide use of immunization in children. However, rubella can still occur in older people who were not vaccinated or people who have immigrated to the United States from countries where vaccination for rubella is not common.[1] Pregnant women, who become infected with rubella, have a very high chance of the virus crossing the placenta and infecting the fetus. Congenital rubella infections have disastrous effects, causing fetal death, premature delivery, and severe congenital defects including deafness and congenital heart disease. Neonates with congenital rubella excrete rubella virus in nasopharyngeal secretions and urine for many months after birth. These children pose a risk to susceptible pregnant women.[2] Serology is available for diagnostic purposes. Usually immune status can be determined by examining a single serum sample.

Footnotes

1. Centers for Disease Control, "Increase in Rubella and Congenital Rubella Syndrome – United States, 1988-1990," *MMWR Morb Mortal Wkly Rep*, 1991, 40(6):93-9.
2. Herrman KL, "Rubella Virus," *Laboratory Diagnosis of Viral Infections*, Lennette EH, ed, New York, NY: Marcel Dekker Inc, 1992, 731-47.

References

Chernesky MA and Mahony JB, "Rubella Virus," *Manual of Clinical Microbiology*, 5th ed, Balows A, Hausler WJ Jr, Herrmann KL, et al, eds, Washington, DC: American Society for Microbiology, 1991, 918-23.

Shingles Culture *see* Varicella-Zoster Virus Culture *on next page*
Skin Culture for HSV *see* Herpes Simplex Virus Isolation, Rapid *on page 1184*
Skin Viral Disease *see* Electron Microscopic Examination for Viruses, Stool *on page 1177*
Spleen Cell Culture for EBV *see* Epstein-Barr Virus Culture *on page 1179*
TRIC Agent Culture *see Chlamydia trachomatis* Culture *on page 1171*
***Ureaplasma urealyticum* Culture, Genital** *see* Genital Culture for *Ureaplasma urealyticum on page 1180*
Urethral *Chlamydia* Culture *see Chlamydia trachomatis* Culture *on page 1171*

Urethral Culture for T-Strain *Mycoplasma* *see* Genital Culture for *Ureaplasma urealyticum on page 1180*

Varicella-Zoster Virus Culture

CPT *87140 (culture typing, fluorescent method); 87252 (tissue culture, inoculation and observation); 87253 (tissue culture, additional studies, each isolate)*

Related Information

Skin Biopsies *on page 84*
Varicella-Zoster Virus Culture, Rapid *on next page*
Varicella-Zoster Virus Serology *on page 761*
Viral Culture, Dermatological Symptoms *on page 1201*
Virus, Direct Detection by Fluorescent Antibody *on page 1208*

Synonyms Chickenpox Culture; Culture, VZV; Shingles Culture; VZV Culture

Applies to Viral Culture, Rash; Viral Culture, Skin

Test Commonly Includes Culture for VZV only; VZV also is usually detected in a routine/general virus culture

Specimen Swab specimens of the base of fresh, unroofed lesions, vesicle fluid, vesicle scrapings; blood or bronchial washings (immunocompromised patients); cerebrospinal fluid. In addition, acute and convalescent sera should be collected at appropriate times to document a clinically significant rise in antibody titer. **CONTAINER:** Cold viral transport medium for swab specimens; green top (heparin) tube for blood; sterile CSF tube for CSF **SAMPLING TIME:** Specimens should be collected during the acute phase of the disease (within 3 days of lesion eruption). **COLLECTION:** Unroofed lesions should be cleaned before specimens are taken. Vesicle fluid from several vesicles can be pooled and added to viral transport medium. Alternatively, the bases of several freshly unroofed lesions can be vigorously sampled with a sterile swab which subsequently should be placed into cold viral transport medium and sent to the laboratory as soon as possible. **STORAGE INSTRUCTIONS:** Keep specimens cold and moist. **Do not freeze specimens at -20°C**. VZV is extremely labile. If immediate inoculation onto cell cultures is not possible, specimens should be frozen quickly at -70°C. Freezing at -70°C will reduce infectivity 10% to 30%. **CAUSES FOR REJECTION:** Dry specimen, specimen not refrigerated during transport, specimen fixed in formalin, unlabeled specimen, specimen delayed by more than 2 days in transit to the laboratory **TURNAROUND TIME:** Variable (1-14 days) and depends on cell culture method used and amount of virus in the specimen. Negative cultures are usually reported after 4 weeks.

Interpretive **REFERENCE RANGE:** No virus isolated **USE:** Aid in the diagnosis of disease caused by varicella-zoster virus (ie, chickenpox and shingles) **LIMITATIONS:** VZV is extremely labile and many times cannot be isolated from specimens which have been transported and/or stored in adverse conditions. **METHODOLOGY:** Inoculation of specimens into cell cultures, incubation of cultures, observation for characteristic cytopathic effect (CPE), and identification by fluorescent monoclonal antibody **ADDITIONAL INFORMATION:** Varicella-zoster virus is a single virus which causes two diseases: **chickenpox** (varicella) in children and, after reactivation from latency, **shingles** (zoster) in adults. Disease caused by VZV is usually self-limited. However, the disease can be life-threatening in pregnant persons, immunocompromised persons, children who receive cancer therapy, and in fetuses exposed during pregnancy. Congenital chickenpox can result in neonatal systemic disease and/or congenital malformations. People suffering from AIDS can have prolonged reactivated VZV infections.[1,2]

Serology for the detection of VZV antibodies is available. Rapid turnaround time of serological tests can be especially important in detecting the presence of antibody (prior exposure) in pregnant women who have been exposed to individuals with chickenpox. In these cases VZV-specific immunoglobulin should be given within 3 days (maximum) of exposure.

Cell culture of VZV often has been reported to be less sensitive than direct antigen detection of VZV by immunofluorescence.[3]

Footnotes

1. Hoppenjans WB, Bibler MR, Orme RL, et al, "Prolonged Cutaneous Herpes Zoster in Acquired Immunodeficiency Syndrome," *Arch Dermatol*, 1990, 126(8):1048-50.
2. LeBoit PE, Límouá M, Yen TS, et al, "Chronic Verrucous Variella-Zoster Virus Infection in Patients With the Acquired Immunodeficiency Syndrome (AIDS). Histologic and Molecular Biologic Findings," *Am J Dermatopathol*, 1992, 14(1):1-7.
3. Rawlinson WD, Dwyer DE, Gibbons V, et al, "Rapid Diagnosis of Varicella-Zoster Virus Infection With a Monoclonal Antibody Based Direct Immunofluorescence Technique," *J Virol Methods*, 1989, 23(1):13-8.

(Continued)

Varicella-Zoster Virus Culture *(Continued)*

References

Solomon AR, "New Diagnostic Tests for Herpes Simplex and Varicella-Zoster Infections," *J Am Acad Dermatol*, 1988, 18:218-21.

Strommen GL, Pucino F, Tight RR, et al, "Human Infection With Herpes Zoster: Etiology, Pathophysiology, Diagnosis, Clinical Course, and Treatment," *Pharmacotherapy*, 1988, 8:52-68.

Varicella-Zoster Virus Culture, Rapid

CPT *87140 (culture typing, fluorescent method); 87252 (tissue culture, inoculation and observation); 87253 (tissue culture, additional studies, each isolate)*

Related Information

Varicella-Zoster Virus Culture *on previous page*
Varicella-Zoster Virus Serology *on page 761*
Viral Culture, Central Nervous System Symptoms *on page 1199*
Viral Culture, Dermatological Symptoms *on page 1201*
Virus, Direct Detection by Fluorescent Antibody *on page 1208*

Synonyms VZV Centrifugation Culture; VZV Culture, Rapid; VZV Shell Vial Method

Test Commonly Includes Inoculation of cell cultures in shell vials, (usually) 2- and 5-day incubations, and immunofluorescence staining of VZV antigens with specific monoclonal antibody

Specimen Swab specimens from the base of fresh, unroofed lesions; vesicle fluid; vesicle scrapings; blood or bronchial washings; cerebrospinal fluid. In addition, acute and convalescent sera should be collected at appropriate times to document a clinically significant rise in antibody titer. **CONTAINER:** Cold viral transport medium for swab specimens; green top (heparin) tube for blood; sterile container for washings or CSF **COLLECTION:** Lesions should be cleaned before specimens are taken. Vesicle fluid from several vesicles can be pooled and added to viral transport medium. Alternatively, the bases of several freshly unroofed lesions can be vigorously sampled with a sterile swab which subsequently should be placed into cold viral transport medium and sent to the laboratory as soon as possible. **STORAGE INSTRUCTIONS:** VZV is extremely labile. Specimen should be kept on ice or cold during shipment to the laboratory. **Do not freeze at -20°C**. Specimens can be quickly frozen at -70°C for longer storage, but this will reduce infectivity. **TURNAROUND TIME:** 2-5 days (usually) depending on method and capability of laboratory. Negative cultures are usually reported after 5 days.

Interpretive **REFERENCE RANGE:** No virus isolated **USE:** Aid in the diagnosis of disease caused by varicella-zoster virus (ie, chickenpox and shingles) **LIMITATIONS:** VZV is very labile and often does not grow in cell culture if the specimen is transported and/or stored in adverse conditions. **METHODOLOGY:** Specimens are centrifuged onto cell cultures grown on coverslips in the bottoms of 1-dram shell vials. Centrifugation greatly accelerates virus attachment and penetration. After incubation, fluorescein-labeled monoclonal antibodies are applied to the infected cells to detect viral antigens that are expressed in the membranes of the cells. Characteristic fluorescent foci indicate the presence of virus. **ADDITIONAL INFORMATION:** The sensitivity of this rapid culture technique has been reported to be greater than that of conventional cell culture.[1]

Footnotes

1. Schirm J, Meulenberg JJ, Pastoor GW, et al, "Rapid Detection of Varicella-Zoster Virus in Clinical Specimens Using Monoclonal Antibodies on Shell Vials and Smears," *J Med Virol*, 1989, 28:1-6.

References

Hughes JH, "Physical and Chemical Methods for Enhancing Rapid Detection of Viruses and Other Agents," *Clin Microbiol Rev*, 1993, 6(2):150-75.

Varicella-Zoster Virus, Direct Detection *see* Virus, Direct Detection by Fluorescent Antibody *on page 1208*

Vesicle Viral Culture *see* Viral Culture, Dermatological Symptoms *on page 1201*

Viral Antigen Detection, Direct, Stool *see* Rotavirus, Direct Detection *on page 1191*

Viral Culture

CPT *87252 (tissue culture, inoculation and observation); 87253 (tissue culture, additional studies, each isolate)*

Related Information

Biopsy or Body Fluid Anaerobic Bacterial Culture *on page 778*
Blood Culture, Aerobic and Anaerobic *on page 784*
Bone Marrow *on page 524*
Conjunctival Culture *on page 803*
Skin Biopsies *on page 84*
Viral Culture, Blood *on page 1197*
Viral Culture, Body Fluid *on page 1198*
Viral Culture, Central Nervous System Symptoms *on page 1199*
Viral Culture, Dermatological Symptoms *on page 1201*
Viral Culture, Eye or Ocular Symptoms *on page 1202*
Viral Culture, Stool *on page 1205*
Viral Culture, Tissue *on page 1206*
Viral Culture, Urine *on page 1207*

Synonyms Comprehensive Viral Culture; General Viral Culture; Routine Viral Culture; Virus Culture; Virus Isolation

Applies to CPE; Cytopathic Effect

Test Commonly Includes Inoculation of specimen onto appropriate cell cultures; isolated viruses are identified using specific monoclonal antibodies, neutralization, or hemadsorption

Viruses Typically Isolated From Clinical Specimens

Specimen	Virus*
Blood	CMV, enteroviruses†,#, HSV, VZV
CSF and CNS tissues	Enteroviruses, mumps virus, HSV, CMV
Dermal lesions	HSV, VZV, adenovirus, enteroviruses
Eye	HSV, VZV, adenovirus, enteroviruses, CMV, *Chlamydia*
Genital	HSV, CMV, *Chlamydia*
Mucosal	HSV, VZV
Oral	HSV, VZV
Rectal	HSV, VZV, enterovirus
Respiratory tract upper	Adenovirus, rhinovirus, influenza, parainfluenza, enteroviruses, RSV, reovirus, HSV
lower	Adenovirus, influenza, parainfluenza, RSV, CMV•
Stool	Enteroviruses, adenoviruses
Tissues	CMV, HSV, enteroviruses
Urine	CMV, adenovirus, enteroviruses, mumps

*Abbreviations:
HSV — herpes simplex virus
CMV — cytomegalovirus
VZV — varicella-zoster virus
RSV — respiratory syncytial virus
†Enteroviruses: coxsackie virus, poliovirus, echovirus, and enterovirus.
#Occasionally isolated.
•Usually in immunocompromised hosts.

Specimen Whole blood, cerebrospinal fluid, dermal, ocular, genital, mucosal, respiratory, oral, stool, rectal, urine, tissue, biopsy. See table. Whenever a viral etiology is suspected and whenever appropriate, acute and convalescent serum should be collected for viral serology tests. **CONTAINER:** Viral transport medium (available from clinical laboratory) for swabs; sterile screw-cap tube or container for fluids, feces, nasal washings, urine, or biopsy (without preservative); green top (heparin) tube for blood, bone marrow, and buffy coat. **Keep all specimens cold and moist. COLLECTION:** Always consult the laboratory for specific details prior to collecting specimen. Specimen should be collected during the acute phase of the disease, as follows.

(Continued)

Viral Culture *(Continued)*

Blood: Collect 5 mL whole blood into a heparinized tube. Consult laboratory to which specimen will be sent for specific recommendations.

Cerebrospinal fluid: Collect 1 mL CSF aseptically in a sterile dry screw-cap vial. **Keep cold and bring to the laboratory immediately.**

Skin lesions: Open the vesicle and absorb exudate into a dry swab, and/or vigorously scrape base of freshly exposed lesion with a swab to obtain cells which contain viruses. If enough vesicle fluid is available, aspirate the fluid with a fine-gauge needle and tuberculin syringe, and place the fluid into cold viral transport medium. Use Virocult® or Culturette® swabs for specimen collection. **Keep cold and bring to the laboratory immediately.**

Eye swab or scraping: Use a Virocult® or Culturette® swab to collect conjunctival material or take conjunctival scrapings with a fine sterile spatula and transfer the scraping to a viral transport medium. **Keep cold and bring to the laboratory immediately.**

Genital swab: See skin. **Keep cold and bring to the laboratory immediately.**

Throat swab: Carefully rub the posterior wall of the nasopharynx with a dry, sterile swab. Avoid touching the tongue or buccal mucosa. Use Virocult® or Culturette® swabs for specimen collection. **Keep cold and bring to the laboratory immediately.**

Feces: Collect 4-8 g of feces (about the size of a thumbnail), and place in a clean, leakproof container. Do **not** dilute the specimen (into virus transport medium) or use preservatives. **Keep cold and bring to the laboratory immediately.**

Rectal swab: Insert a sterile swab 2-4 inches into the rectum and rub the mucosa. Use Virocult® or Culturette® swabs for specimen collection. **Keep cold and bring to the laboratory immediately.** Swab may be placed into cold virus transport medium.

Urine: Collect clean-catch, midstream urine in a leakproof, sterile, plastic container. **Keep cold and bring to the laboratory immediately.**

Tissue: Use a fresh set of sterile instruments to collect each tissue. Place each specimen in its own dry, sterile nontoxic leakproof container. Identify each tissue with patient's name, type of tissue, and date collected. **Keep cold and bring tissue to the laboratory immediately.**

Calcium alginate swabs are toxic to *Chlamydia* and many enveloped viruses. **Do not use calcium alginate swabs for viral or chlamydial isolation.**

STORAGE INSTRUCTIONS: Specimen must be kept cold and moist, and must be delivered to the laboratory as soon as possible. If a longer period is required, specimen should be stored or transported according to the laboratory that will receive the specimen. **Do not freeze specimens at -20°C**; if absolutely necessary store specimens at 4°C to 6°C or freeze quickly at -70°C. Specimens to be cultured for influenza virus and cytomegalovirus should be sent on wet ice or with an ice pack. **CAUSES FOR REJECTION:** Dry specimen, specimen not refrigerated during transport, specimen fixed in formalin, unlabeled specimen **TURNAROUND TIME:** The presence of viruses is usually suggested by the characteristic cytopathic effect (CPE) they cause when they infect cell cultures. CPE (and, therefore, positive results) can be observed as soon as 1 day and as late as 28 days postinoculation of the cell culture.[1] **SPECIAL INSTRUCTIONS:** Culture and serological tests for certain specific viruses are available. When possible, the serological tests should be requested at same time as culture. Acute and convalescent blood samples (5 mL) are required for serologic studies. Requisition **must** state specific virus(s) suspected, source of specimen, age of patient, current antibiotic therapy, relevant vaccinations, and pertinent clinical history.

Interpretive **REFERENCE RANGE:** No virus isolated **USE:** Aid in the diagnosis of viral diseases (eg, AIDS, conjunctivitis, congenital viral infections, keratitis, chickenpox, shingles, viral pneumonia, and diseases characterized by skin vesicles and rashes) **LIMITATIONS:** For all practical purposes, many common viruses are not culturable: Coxsackie A viruses, hepatitis viruses, arboviruses, parvoviruses, human papillomaviruses, reoviruses, measles virus, and gastrointestinal viruses (rota, corona, calici, astro, and Norwalk). Isolation of virus may not be related to the patient's disease. Some positive cultures are sent to State Health Laboratory for specific virus identification. **METHODOLOGY:** Inoculation of specimen into cell cultures, incubation of cultures, observation for characteristic cytopathic effect (CPE), and identification by methods such as hemadsorption and fluorescent monoclonal antibodies. If specific viruses such as HSV, CMV, VZV, influenza, or adenovirus are suspected, the laboratory might be able to use rapid (1-2 days) culture (shell vial) methods to detect these viruses. **ADDITIONAL INFORMATION:**

Serological tests:[2] Give date of onset of illness, date of collection of sera and either a brief clinical description or the provisional diagnosis. It is helpful to the laboratory to know such things as does the patient have a rash, a respiratory illness, or neurological symptoms? The acute serum (5 mL clotted blood or 2 mL serum) should be collected as early as possible, and the second or convalescent serum should be drawn 2-4 weeks later. The paired sera **should** be run in parallel, and a **fourfold rise** in antibody titer is suggestive of a current infection. The ordering physician should see that both specimens are obtained. **Viral cultures:** Specimens should be collected in the acute stage of the illness, kept moist, and refrigerated immediately. Whenever possible, specimens should be shipped so they will not arrive in the laboratory over the weekend. Stool specimens should not be placed into viral transport medium or frozen. Spinal fluid and throat washings must be kept cold and must not be frozen. Swabs of lesions or of throat should be rinsed immediately into 1 or 2 mL of viral transport medium; preferably, the swab should be broken off into the medium and sent in the medium to the laboratory. Autopsy material should be collected in sterile containers. Urine specimens for CMV culture **must not** be frozen; they should be packed with an ice pack or snow gel, but not with dry ice.

Footnotes

1. Yolken RH, "Laboratory Diagnosis of Viral Infections," *Practical Diagnosis of Viral Infections*, Galasso GJ, Whitley RJ, Merigan TC, eds, New York, NY: Raven Press, 1993, 17-67.
2. Bryan JA, "The Serologic Diagnosis of Viral Infections," *Arch Pathol Lab Med*, 1987, 111:1015-23.

References

Drew WL, "Controversies in Viral Diagnosis," *Rev Infect Dis*, 1988, 8:814-24.

Forbes BA, "Perinatal Viral Infections," *Clin Microbiol Newslet*, 1992, 14:169-72.

Korones SB, "Uncommon Virus Infections of the Mother, Fetus, and Newborn: Influenza, Mumps, and Measles," *Clin Perinatol*, 1988, 15:259-72.

Lennette DA, "Preparation of Specimens for Virological Examination," *Manual of Clinical Microbiology*, 5th ed, Balows A, Hausler WJ Jr, Herrmann KL, et al, eds, Washington, DC: American Society for Microbiology, 1991, 818-21.

Viral Culture, Amniotic Fluid *see* Viral Culture, Body Fluid *on next page*

Viral Culture, Biopsy *see* Viral Culture, Tissue *on page 1206*

Viral Culture, Blood

CPT 87252 (tissue culture, inoculation and observation); 87253 (tissue culture, additional studies, each isolate)

Related Information

Blood Culture, Aerobic and Anaerobic *on page 784*
Coxsackie A Virus Titer *on page 668*
Coxsackie B Virus Titer *on page 668*
Cytomegalovirus Culture *on page 1175*
Cytomegalovirus Isolation, Rapid *on page 1176*
Enterovirus Culture *on page 1178*
Epstein-Barr Virus Culture *on page 1179*
Viral Culture *on page 1195*

Synonyms Blood Culture for CMV; Blood Culture for Enterovirus; Buffy Coat Culture for CMV; CMV Culture

Test Commonly Includes Usually includes both rapid shell vial isolation technique (to detect CMV early) and conventional cell culture for all major viruses

Patient Care PREPARATION: Cleanse skin with 70% isopropyl alcohol. Apply povidone-iodine in concentric circles. **Note:** Iodine should remain in contact with skin for at least 1 minute prior to venipuncture to ensure complete antisepsis. Remove iodine with 70% isopropyl alcohol in concentric circles after venipuncture. Obtain 3-6 mL of blood.

Specimen Whole blood CONTAINER: Green top (heparin) tube. Some laboratories request that blood be collected in citrate anticoagulant. Alternatively, a blood specimen can be obtained in a (previously) heparinized syringe. The heparin should be sterile and free of preservative. SAMPLING TIME: Collect blood during early acute phase of infection. COLLECTION: Strict aseptic technique is essential. STORAGE INSTRUCTIONS: **Do not store specimen.** Send to the laboratory immediately. CAUSES FOR REJECTION: Specimen improperly collected, inadequate volume, improperly labeled specimen, excessively long delay in transit to the laboratory TURNAROUND TIME: Shell vial rapid isolation: 1-2 days; conventional culture: 2 days to 4 weeks SPECIAL INSTRUCTIONS: Requisition should specify organism suspected, clinical diagnosis, and date and time collected.

(Continued)

Viral Culture, Blood *(Continued)*

Interpretive USE: Aid in the diagnosis of systemic viral infections (eg, transplantation-associated viral diseases, infectious mononucleosis, and congenital viral diseases) LIMITATIONS: Blood (serum in particular) is generally not a good specimen from which to recover viruses. METHODOLOGY: Inoculation of peripheral blood cells or serum onto cell cultures (either shell vials or tube cultures); identification of virus by cytopathic effect (CPE) and monoclonal antibodies ADDITIONAL INFORMATION: White blood cells can be a source of CMV, and serum has been reported to be a source of enterovirus.[1] See table in Viral Culture test listing.

Footnotes

1. Hughes JH, "Physical and Chemical Methods for Enhancing Rapid Detection of Viruses and Other Agents," *Clin Microbiol Rev*, 1993, 6(2):150-75.

References

Jacobson MA and Mills J, "Serious Cytomegalovirus Disease in the Acquired Immunodeficiency Syndrome (AIDS). Clinical Findings, Diagnosis, and Treatment," *Ann Intern Med*, 1988, 108:585-94.

Lennette DA, "Preparation of Specimens for Virological Examination," *Manual of Clinical Microbiology*, 5th ed, Balows A, Hausler WJ Jr, Herrmann KL, et al, eds, Washington, DC: American Society for Microbiology, 1991, 818-21.

Viral Culture, Body Fluid

CPT 87140 (culture typing, fluorescent method); 87252 (tissue culture, inoculation and observation); 87253 (tissue culture, additional studies, each isolate)

Related Information

Biopsy or Body Fluid Anaerobic Bacterial Culture *on page 778*
Body Fluid *on page 145*
Body Fluids Cytology *on page 482*
Bone Marrow *on page 524*
Viral Culture *on page 1195*
Viral Culture, Central Nervous System Symptoms *on next page*

Synonyms Body Fluid Viral Culture

Applies to Viral Culture, Amniotic Fluid; Viral Culture, CSF; Viral Culture, Joint Fluid; Viral Culture, Normally Sterile Body Fluid; Viral Culture, Peritoneal Fluid

Test Commonly Includes Isolation and identification of virus

Patient Care PREPARATION: Aseptic preparation of the aspiration site

Specimen Body fluids (eg, cerebrospinal fluid, pleural fluid, pericardial fluid, amniotic fluid) CONTAINER: Sterile tube or container COLLECTION: Specimens obtained aseptically. **Do not place fluids into virus transport medium.** Keep specimens cold (2°C to 8°C) because viruses isolated from body fluids are often labile. Transport to the laboratory as soon as possible. CAUSES FOR REJECTION: Dry specimen, specimen not refrigerated during transport, specimen fixed in formalin, unlabeled specimen TURNAROUND TIME: Variable (1-28 days) and depends on culture methods and amount and type of virus in specimen SPECIAL INSTRUCTIONS: Requisition must be completed with patient's name, hospital number, birth date, physician, date of collection, site of specimen, and clinical findings. Continuing communications between the virology laboratory and the physician is essential. If a specific virus is suspected, please write this on the request form.

Interpretive REFERENCE RANGE: No virus isolated USE: Aid in the diagnosis of systemic viral diseases (eg, pericarditis) LIMITATIONS: If bacteria are suspected, a separate specimen must be submitted. Often, only a few virus-infected cells are present in fluids. Therefore, larger amounts of fluid are most productive, and specimens should be placed onto cell cultures as soon as possible. METHODOLOGY: Inoculation of specimen into cell cultures, incubation of cultures, observation for characteristic cytopathic effect (CPE), and identification/speciation by methods such as hemadsorption and fluorescent monoclonal antibodies. If specific viruses such as HSV, CMV, VZV, or adenovirus are suspected, the laboratory might be able to use rapid (1-2 days) culture (shell vial) methods to detect these viruses. ADDITIONAL INFORMATION: See table in Viral Culture test listing.

References

Smith TF, "Rapid Diagnosis of Viral Infections," *Adv Exp Med Biol*, 1990, 263:115-21.

Yolken RH, Coutlee F, and Viscidi RP, "New Prospects for the Diagnosis of Viral Infections," *Yale J Biol Med*, 1989, 62(2):131-9.

Viral Culture, Brain *see* Viral Culture, Central Nervous System Symptoms *on next page*

Viral Culture, Brain *see* Viral Culture, Tissue *on page 1206*

Viral Culture, Bronchial *see* Viral Culture, Tissue *on page 1206*

Viral Culture, Bronchial Wash *see* Viral Culture, Respiratory Symptoms *on page 1204*

Viral Culture, Central Nervous System Symptoms

CPT *87140 (culture typing, fluorescent method); 87252 (tissue culture, inoculation and observation); 87253 (tissue culture, additional studies, each isolate)*

Related Information

Bacterial Antigens, Rapid Detection Methods *on page 775*
California Encephalitis Virus Titer *on page 651*
Cerebrospinal Fluid Anaerobic Culture *on page 797*
Cerebrospinal Fluid Analysis *on page 527*
Cerebrospinal Fluid Culture *on page 798*
Cerebrospinal Fluid Fungus Culture *on page 800*
Cerebrospinal Fluid Glucose *on page 176*
Cerebrospinal Fluid Lactic Acid *on page 178*
Cerebrospinal Fluid Mycobacteria Culture *on page 801*
Cerebrospinal Fluid Protein *on page 659*
Coxsackie A Virus Titer *on page 668*
Coxsackie B Virus Titer *on page 668*
Enterovirus Culture *on page 1178*
Genital Culture for *Ureaplasma urealyticum on page 1180*
Herpes Simplex Virus Culture *on page 1182*
Mumps Serology *on page 726*
Mumps Virus Culture *on page 1187*
Rabies *on page 82*
St Louis Encephalitis Virus Serology *on page 749*
Varicella-Zoster Virus Culture, Rapid *on page 1194*
Viral Culture *on page 1195*
Viral Culture, Body Fluid *on previous page*

Synonyms Cerebrospinal Fluid Virus Culture

Applies to Lumbar Puncture Hazards; Viral Culture, Brain; Viral Culture, CSF

Test Commonly Includes Isolation and identification of virus

Abstract Viral meningitis is by far the most important cause of aseptic meningitis, a condition which has several clinical presentations and which has both infectious and noninfectious etiologies. Most cases of aseptic meningitis are caused by viruses, especially enteroviruses, most often in the late summer. Patients are usually children and young adults. Enteroviruses include polioviruses, coxsackie viruses, and echoviruses. Ratzan provides a definition of viral meningitis as part of an aseptic meningitis syndrome characterized by acute disease with signs and symptoms of meningeal inflammation, pleocytosis (usually mononuclear), variable increase in protein content, normal glucose level, and no demonstrable organism by smear and culture of the cerebrospinal fluid.[1] By definition, the cerebrospinal fluid in aseptic meningitis will show a pleocytosis of white blood cells and will be culture-negative.[2]

Specimen Cerebrospinal fluid (do not put into virus transport medium), brain biopsy, lesions, throat or throat washings, stool, urine **CONTAINER:** Sterile CSF tube; sterile screw-cap container for biopsy, tissue, urine, or throat washing; sterile viral transport medium for swab specimens **SAMPLING TIME:** As soon as possible after the onset of symptoms. Many viruses are more likely to be cultured when samples are obtained early. **COLLECTION:** Always consult the laboratory for specific details prior to collecting specimen. Specimen should be collected during the acute phase of the disease, as follows.

Cerebrospinal fluid: Collect 1 mL CSF aseptically in a sterile dry screw-cap vial. **Keep cold and bring to the laboratory immediately.**

The following specimens may be useful for diagnosis of CNS viral infection:

Eye swab or scraping

Skin lesions: Vigorously scrape base of freshly exposed lesion with a swab to obtain cells which contain viruses. Alternatively, open the vesicle and absorb exudate into a dry swab. If enough vesicle fluid is available, aspirate the fluid with a fine gauge needle and tuberculin sy-

(Continued)

Viral Culture, Central Nervous System Symptoms *(Continued)*

ringe, and place the fluid into cold viral transport medium. Use Virocult® or Culturette® swabs for specimen collection. **Keep cold and bring to the laboratory immediately.** The clinical appearance of herpes zoster or the vesicles of herpes simplex may suggest the diagnosis.

Throat swab: May be useful for identification of coxsackie, mumps, adenovirus, herpes type 1. Epstein-Barr virus may be recovered from throat washings.

Feces: Enterovirus, adenovirus, cytomegalovirus, herpes simplex, measles, and varicella-zoster virus may be recovered.

Urine: Mumps virus and cytomegalovirus may be recovered.

Genital swab

STORAGE INSTRUCTIONS: Keep all specimens cold and moist. Transport to the laboratory immediately. Enteroviruses are relatively stable from -70°C to 4°C but are labile if allowed to dry or to be at room temperature for several hours. Specimens suspected of having varicella-zoster virus should never be frozen at -20°C or left at room temperature. Freezing at -20°C for 24 hours results in 99% reduction in viral isolation. **CAUSES FOR REJECTION:** Dry specimen, specimen not refrigerated during transport, specimen fixed in formalin, unlabeled specimen **TURNAROUND TIME:** Variable (1-14 days) and depends on type of virus, culture method used, and amount of virus in specimen

Interpretive **REFERENCE RANGE:** No virus isolated **USE:** Determine etiological agent of viral CNS diseases (eg, aseptic meningitis, meningoencephalitis, polio, and encephalitis) **LIMITATIONS:** The CSF findings in tuberculous meningitis may simulate those of viral meningitis, especially herpes simplex and mumps. **METHODOLOGY:** Inoculation of specimen into cell cultures, incubation of cultures, observation for characteristic cytopathic effect (CPE), and identification/speciation by methods such as hemadsorption and fluorescent monoclonal antibodies. If specific viruses such as HSV, CMV, VZV, or adenovirus are suspected, the laboratory might be able to use rapid (1-2 days) culture (shell vial) methods to detect these viruses. Suckling mice are usually inoculated with the specimen if group A Coxsackie virus is suspected. The mice are observed for the development of flaccid paralysis. Bacterial culture, Gram stain, cell count, glucose, and protein are needed to rule out bacterial meningitis, with antigen agglutination when indicated. **ADDITIONAL INFORMATION:** Arthropod-borne (arbo) viruses and reoviruses are not considered culturable and may be detected indirectly by viral serology.

The seasonal peak of viral meningitis in late summer is widely recognized and clinically significant in differential diagnosis.[1,3] The significance of seasonal curves for viral meningitis (more frequent in summer) versus bacterial meningitis is greater than most physicians recognize.[3] Meningitis caused by HIV, Epstein-Barr virus, CMV, or herpes simplex lacks seasonal variation.

Mumps meningitis is usually self limited and benign.[1] As with lymphocytic choriomeningitis and herpes simplex meningoencephalitis, hypoglycorrhachia may be found.

In the differential diagnosis between viral and bacterial meningitis, much higher CSF WBC count (>1180/mm^3) and protein (>220 mg/dL) are found in many cases of bacterial meningitis. Spanos' reported that in one group of studied patients no patient with acute viral meningitis had glucose <30.6 mg/dL but 43% of the patients with acute bacterial meningitis had glucose levels this low.[3] Although aseptic meningitis is usually characterized by mononuclear cells, PMNs may predominate early in the disease.[4,5,6] Hammer and Connolly summarized the typical CSF laboratory test profile in viral aseptic meningitis as one with WBC count <500/mm^3 with lymphocyte predominance, protein <100 mg/dL, and normal glucose.[6] Blood cultures are desirable because they are usually positive in infants and children with bacterial meningitis.[7] Five patients with mixed viral-bacterial meningitis of 276 patients with viral and/or bacterial culture proven meningitis have been described.[8] Many negative lumbar punctures in babies presenting with fever but without other specific findings have been reported.[9] In a study of 171 children with febrile convulsions, only one child had bacterial meningitis, and four children had aseptic meningitis.[9]

Complications of lumbar puncture (LP) are between 0.19% and 0.43%, reaching up to 35.5% when minor complications are included. Instances of meningitis and local infection are described following LP in subjects with bacteremia, who may be at risk for meningeal seeding during the puncture.[9,10] Repeat lumbar puncture may fail to identify patients who require further therapy.[10]

Nonviral causes of aseptic meningitis include meningeal carcinomatosis, collagen diseases, sarcoidosis, drugs (including antineoplastic agents and immunosuppressants, and materials used in radiology units), Mollaret's meningitis and many other entities.[5,11]

See table in Viral Culture test listing for the appropriate specimen that should be collected based on the suspected viral infection.

Footnotes

1. Ratzan KR, "Viral Meningitis," *Med Clin North Am*, 1985, 69:399-411.
2. Polito JM 2d and Stollerman GH, "Aseptic Meningitis: A Case for Clinical Experience," *Hosp Pract Off Ed*, 1992, 27(5A):27-39.
3. Spanos A, Harrell FE Jr, and Durack DT, "Differential Diagnosis of Acute Meningitis – An Analysis of the Predictive Value of Initial Observations," *JAMA*, 1989, 262(19):2700-7.
4. Amir J, Harel L, Frydman M, et al, "Shift of Cerebrospinal Polymorphonuclear Cell Percentage in the Early Stage of Aseptic Meningitis," *J Pediatr*, 1991, 119(6):938-41.
5. Rubeiz H and Roos RP, "Viral Meningitis and Encephalitis," *Semin Neurol*, 1992, 12(3):165-77.
6. Hammer SM and Connolly KJ, "Viral Aseptic Meningitis in the United States: Clinical Features, Viral Etiologies, and Differential Diagnosis," *Curr Clin Top Infect Dis*, 1992, 12:1-25.
7. Sáez-Llorens X and McCracken GH Jr, "Bacterial Meningitis in Neonates and Children," *Infect Dis Clin North Am*, 1990, 4(4):623-44.
8. Sferra TJ and Pacini DL, "Simultaneous Recovery of Bacterial and Viral Pathogens From Cerebrospinal Fluid," *Pediatr Infect Dis J*, 1988, 7:552-6.
9. Levy M, Wong E, and Fried D, "Diseases That Mimic Meningitis. Analysis of 650 Lumbar Punctures," *Clin Pediatr (Phila)*, 1990, 29(5):254-5, 258-61.
10. Fishman RA, *Cerebrospinal Fluid in Diseases of the Nervous System*, 2nd ed, Philadelphia, PA: WB Saunders Co, 1992, 266, 277-343.
11. Connolly KJ and Hammer SM, "The Acute Aseptic Meningitis Syndrome," *Infect Dis Clin North Am*, 1990, 4(4):599-622.

References

Behrman RE, Kliegman RM, Nelson WE, et al, *Nelson Textbook of Pediatrics*, 14th ed, Philadelphia, PA: WB Saunders Co, 1992, 664-6.

Chonmaitree T, Baldwin CD, Lucia HL, et al, "Role of the Virology Laboratory in Diagnosis and Management of Patients With Central Nervous System Disease," *Clin Microbiol Rev*, 1989, 2(1):1-14.

Greenlee JE, "Approach to Diagnosis of Meningitis – Cerebrospinal Fluid Evaluation," *Infect Dis Clin North Am*, 1990, 4(4):583-98.

Lennette DA, "Preparation of Specimens for Virological Examination," *Manual of Clinical Microbiology*, 5th ed, Balows A, Hausler WJ Jr, Herrmann KL, et al, eds, Washington, DC: American Society for Microbiology, 1991, 818-21.

Walsh-Kelly C, Nelson DB, Smith DS, et al, "Clinical Predictors of Bacterial Versus Aseptic Meningitis in Childhood," *Ann Emerg Med*, 1992, 21(8):910-4.

Viral Culture, Cervical *see* Viral Culture, Urogenital *on page 1207*

Viral Culture, Conjunctiva *see* Viral Culture, Eye or Ocular Symptoms *on next page*

Viral Culture, CSF *see* Viral Culture, Body Fluid *on page 1198*

Viral Culture, CSF *see* Viral Culture, Central Nervous System Symptoms *on page 1199*

Viral Culture, Cytomegalovirus *see* Cytomegalovirus Culture *on page 1175*

Viral Culture, Dermatological Symptoms

CPT *87140 (culture typing, fluorescent method); 87252 (tissue culture, inoculation and observation); 87253 (tissue culture, additional studies, each isolate)*

Related Information

Herpes Simplex Virus Antigen Detection *on page 1181*
Herpes Simplex Virus Culture *on page 1182*
Herpes Simplex Virus Isolation, Rapid *on page 1184*
Skin Biopsies *on page 84*
Varicella-Zoster Virus Culture *on page 1193*
Varicella-Zoster Virus Culture, Rapid *on page 1194*
Viral Culture *on page 1195*
Viral Culture, Urogenital *on page 1207*

Synonyms Vesicle Viral Culture; Viral Culture, Lesion; Viral Culture, Pustule; Viral Culture, Rash; Viral Culture, Skin/Dermatological Specimen; Viral Culture, Skin Scrapings; Viral Culture, Ulcer

(Continued)

Viral Culture, Dermatological Symptoms *(Continued)*

Applies to Exanthems and Lesions of the Skin

Test Commonly Includes Isolation and identification of virus

Patient Care PREPARATION: **Do not prep skin with alcohol, iodine, or Betadine® prior to collection.**

Specimen Lesion scraping, swab, fluid CONTAINER: Viral transport medium (available from Microbiology Laboratory) for swabs SAMPLING TIME: Preferably within 3 days of dermatological symptoms COLLECTION: Consult the laboratory for specific details prior to collecting specimen. Specimen should be collected during the acute phase of the disease, as follows. **Skin lesions:** Open the vesicle and absorb exudate into a dry swab, and/or vigorously scrape base of freshly exposed lesion with a swab to obtain cells which contain viruses. If enough vesicle fluid is available, aspirate the fluid with a fine-gauge needle and tuberculin syringe, and place the fluid into cold viral transport medium. Use Virocult® or Culturette® swabs for specimen collection. **Keep cold and bring to the laboratory immediately.** STORAGE INSTRUCTIONS: Specimens should be kept cold and transported to the laboratory immediately especially if varicella-zoster virus is suspected. CAUSES FOR REJECTION: Dry specimen, specimen not refrigerated during transport, specimen fixed in formalin, unlabeled specimen TURNAROUND TIME: Variable (1-14 days) and depends on culture method and amount of virus in specimen

Interpretive REFERENCE RANGE: No virus isolated USE: Determine etiological agent of viral dermatological infections (eg, chickenpox, shingles, herpes, and other viral diseases characterized by skin lesions and rashes) LIMITATIONS: Virus cannot always be cultured from skin lesions. Crusted lesions do not contain viral particles. METHODOLOGY: Inoculation of specimen into cell cultures, incubation of cultures, observation for characteristic cytopathic effect (CPE), and identification/speciation by fluorescent monoclonal antibodies. If specific viruses such as HSV, VZV, or adenovirus are suspected, the laboratory might be able to use rapid (1-2 days) culture (shell vial) methods to detect these viruses. ADDITIONAL INFORMATION: Virus shedding often diminishes rapidly after the onset of illness; therefore, it is important to collect specimens as early as possible after onset of symptoms. For all practical purposes, measles virus is not culturable from patients.

Usually, only dermatological specimens are collected if rash is not associated with systemic disease (eg, HSV, VZV, and some enteroviruses). If systemic disease is associated with the rash, throat swab, rectal swab, stool, or serum can be taken for the isolation of other viruses (eg, enteroviruses, mumps virus, measles virus, and rubella virus). See table in Viral Culture test listing.

References

Siegel CS, "Measles – A Review of the Virological and Serolgoical Methods for Early Detection," *Clin Microbiol Newslet*, 1991, 13(23):177-84.

Straus S, "Clinical and Biological Differences Between Recurrent Herpes Simplex Virus and Varicella-Zoster Virus Infections," *JAMA*, 1989, 262(24):3455-8.

Viral Culture, Endocervical *see* Viral Culture, Urogenital *on page 1207*

Viral Culture, Eye *see* Herpes Simplex Virus Culture *on page 1182*

Viral Culture, Eye *see* Viral Culture, Eye or Ocular Symptoms *on this page*

Viral Culture, Eye or Ocular Symptoms

CPT *87140 (culture typing, fluorescent method); 87252 (tissue culture, inoculation and observation); 87253 (tissue culture, additional studies, each isolate)*

Related Information

Adenovirus Culture, Rapid *on page 1170*
Chlamydia trachomatis Culture *on page 1171*
Chlamydia trachomatis Direct FA Test *on page 1173*
Chlamydia trachomatis DNA Probe *on page 897*
Conjunctival Culture *on page 803*
Herpes Simplex Virus Culture *on page 1182*
Herpes Simplex Virus Isolation, Rapid *on page 1184*
Ocular Cytology *on page 506*
Viral Culture *on page 1195*

Synonyms Viral Culture, Conjunctiva; Viral Culture, Eye; Viral Culture, Sclera

Test Commonly Includes Isolation and identification of virus

Patient Care **PREPARATION:** Local anesthesia might be necessary. Corneal and sclera specimens should be taken only by an ophthalmologist or other properly trained physician.

Specimen Conjunctival scrapings or swabs, eye exudate, vitreous washings, corneal biopsy **CONTAINER:** Cold and sterile viral transport medium for swabs; sterile container for washings or biopsy **COLLECTION:** Pus should be removed with a sterile swab. Do not submit this exudate. Obtain conjunctival scrapings with a sterile spatula. Collect eye exudate by rubbing palpebral conjunctiva with sterile moist swab. Place swab into cold viral transport medium. Conjunctivitis due to *Chlamydia trachomatis* should be collected with a swab and media specific for chlamydial infections; see *Chlamydia* listings. **STORAGE INSTRUCTIONS:** Specimen should be kept cold and transported to the laboratory immediately. **CAUSES FOR REJECTION:** Dry specimen, specimen not refrigerated during transport, specimen fixed in formalin, unlabeled specimen **TURNAROUND TIME:** Variable (1-14 days) and depends on culture method and amount of virus in specimen

Interpretive **REFERENCE RANGE:** No virus isolated **USE:** Determine etiological agent of viral ocular infections (eg, conjunctivitis and keratitis) **METHODOLOGY:** Inoculation of specimen into cell cultures, incubation of cultures, observation for characteristic cytopathic effect (CPE), and identification/speciation by fluorescent monoclonal antibodies. If specific viruses such as HSV, CMV, VZV, or adenovirus are suspected, the laboratory might be able to use rapid (1-2 days) culture (shell vial) methods to detect these viruses; see appropriate listings. **ADDITIONAL INFORMATION:** Adenovirus, VZV, and HSV are the most common viral etiological agents that cause eye infection. Viral serology can be helpful in establishing a diagnosis. See table in Viral Culture test listing.

References

Kowalski RP and Gordon YJ, "Comparison of Direct Rapid Tests for the Detection of Adenovirus Antigen in Routine Conjunctival Specimens," *Ophthalmology*, 1989, 96(7):1106-9.

Liesegang TJ, "Diagnosis and Therapy of Herpes Zoster Ophthalmicus," *Ophthalmology*, 1991, 98(8):1216-29.

Martin AL and Kudesia G, "Enzyme-Linked Immunosorbent Assay for Detecting Adenoviruses in Stool Specimens: Comparison With Electron Microscopy and Isolation," *J Clin Pathol*, 1990, 43(6):514-5.

Pavan-Langston D, "Major Ocular Viral Infections," *Practical Diagnosis of Viral Infections*, Galasso GJ, Whitley RJ, Merigan TC, eds, New York, NY: Raven Press, 1993, 69-108.

Viral Culture, Fallopian Tube *see* Viral Culture, Urogenital *on page 1207*

Viral Culture, Genital *see* Herpes Simplex Virus Culture *on page 1182*

Viral Culture, Genital *see* Viral Culture, Urogenital *on page 1207*

Viral Culture, Heart *see* Viral Culture, Tissue *on page 1206*

Viral Culture, Joint Fluid *see* Viral Culture, Body Fluid *on page 1198*

Viral Culture, Kidney *see* Viral Culture, Tissue *on page 1206*

Viral Culture, Labial *see* Viral Culture, Urogenital *on page 1207*

Viral Culture, Lesion *see* Viral Culture, Dermatological Symptoms *on page 1201*

Viral Culture, Lung *see* Viral Culture, Tissue *on page 1206*

Viral Culture, Muscle *see* Viral Culture, Tissue *on page 1206*

Viral Culture, Nasopharyngeal *see* Viral Culture, Respiratory Symptoms *on next page*

Viral Culture, Normally Sterile Body Fluid *see* Viral Culture, Body Fluid *on page 1198*

Viral Culture, Peritoneal Fluid *see* Viral Culture, Body Fluid *on page 1198*

Viral Culture, Prostate *see* Viral Culture, Urogenital *on page 1207*

Viral Culture, Pulmonary Biopsy *see* Viral Culture, Respiratory Symptoms *on next page*

Viral Culture, Pustule *see* Viral Culture, Dermatological Symptoms *on page 1201*

Viral Culture, Rash *see* Varicella-Zoster Virus Culture *on page 1193*

Viral Culture, Rash *see* Viral Culture, Dermatological Symptoms *on page 1201*

Viral Culture, Respiratory Symptoms

CPT *87140 (culture typing, fluorescent method); 87252 (tissue culture, inoculation and observation); 87253 (tissue culture, additional studies, each isolate)*

Related Information

Adenovirus Antibody Titer *on page 629*
Adenovirus Culture *on page 1169*
Adenovirus Culture, Rapid *on page 1170*
Bronchial Washings Cytology *on page 485*
Bronchoalveolar Lavage *on page 793*
Bronchoalveolar Lavage Cytology *on page 487*
Coxsackie A Virus Titer *on page 668*
Coxsackie B Virus Titer *on page 668*
Influenza Virus Culture *on page 1186*
Parainfluenza Viral Serology *on page 728*
Parainfluenza Virus Culture *on page 1189*
Pneumocystis carinii Preparation *on page 508*
Respiratory Syncytial Virus Culture *on page 1190*
Respiratory Syncytial Virus Serology *on page 739*
Sputum Culture *on page 849*
Sputum Cytology *on page 510*
Sputum Fungus Culture *on page 853*
Sputum Mycobacteria Culture *on page 855*
Virus, Direct Detection by Fluorescent Antibody *on page 1208*
Viscosity, Serum/Plasma *on page 611*

Synonyms Viral Culture, Bronchial Wash; Viral Culture, Nasopharyngeal; Viral Culture, Pulmonary Biopsy; Viral Culture, Throat Swab

Test Commonly Includes Isolation and identification of virus most likely to cause respiratory disease

Patient Care PREPARATION: Local anesthesia might be necessary

Specimen Throat swab; throat washing; nasopharyngeal washing, aspirates, or secretions; sputum; bronchial washings or lavage; lung biopsy CONTAINER: Cold and sterile viral transport medium for swabs; sterile container for washings, aspirates, and sputum SAMPLING TIME: As soon as possible after onset of illness COLLECTION: Methods are the same as those used for collecting most respiratory specimens (see specimen). If respiratory syncytial virus or parainfluenza virus is suspected, see collection techniques for these viruses. STORAGE INSTRUCTIONS: Keep specimen cold and moist. Transport to the laboratory immediately. Can be stored at 4°C up to 48 hours. If longer storage is required freeze quickly at -70°C. **Do not freeze at -20°C**. CAUSES FOR REJECTION: Dry specimen, specimen not refrigerated during transport, specimen fixed in formalin, unlabeled specimen TURNAROUND TIME: Variable (1-14 days) and depends on culture method and amount of virus in specimen

Interpretive REFERENCE RANGE: No virus isolated USE: Determine etiological agent of viral respiratory infections (eg, pneumonia, pneumonitis, croup, and influenza) LIMITATIONS: Presence of nonculturable, disease-causing virus (eg, encephalitis, hepatitis, and gastroenteritis viruses); invasive procedures. Many asymptomatic persons carry and shed viruses which might not be related to illness. METHODOLOGY: Inoculation of specimen into cell cultures, incubation of cultures, observation for characteristic cytopathic effect (CPE), and identification/speciation by methods such as hemadsorption and the use of fluorescent monoclonal antibodies. If specific viruses such as HSV, CMV, VZV, RSV, influenza, or adenovirus are suspected, the laboratory might be able to use rapid (1-2 days) culture (shell vial) methods to detect these viruses. Most laboratories use hemadsorption to help determine the presence of a respiratory virus in cell culture and usually will report "hemadsorbing virus present." Some laboratories are capable of using specific virus-neutralizing antibodies to determine the particular type of virus which caused the observed hemadsorption. This final identification can require as many as several days and often is done only by reference laboratories. ADDITIONAL INFORMATION: Viruses to be considered as causes of viral respiratory illness include the following: influenza virus, parainfluenza virus, rhinovirus, RSV, adenovirus, CMV, and reovirus. Immunocompromised patients can also have respiratory illness due to HSV or VZV. See table in Viral Culture test listing. Contact the Virology Laboratory and inform the staff if influenza or parainfluenza is suspected. Rapid detection of several respiratory viruses by using mixtures of monoclonal antibodies and shell vial cultures are under investigation.[1,2]

Footnotes

1. Schrim J, Luijt DS, Pastoor GW, et al, "Rapid Detection of Respiratory Viruses Using Mixtures of Monoclonal Antibodies on Shell Vial Cultures," *J Med Virol*, 1992, 38(2):147-51.

2. Olsen MA, Shuck KM, Sambol AR, et al, "Isolation of Seven Respiratory Viruses in Shell Vials: A Practical and Highly Sensitive Method," *J Clin Microbiol*, 1993, 31(2):422-5.

References

Costello MJ, Smernoff NT, and Yungbluth M, "Laboratory Diagnosis of Viral Respiratory Tract Infections," *Lab Med*, 1993, 24:150-7.

Takimoto S, Grandien M, Ishida MA, et al, "Comparison of Enzyme-Linked Immunosorbent Assay, Indirect Immunofluorescence Assay, and Virus Isolation for Detection of Respiratory Viruses in Nasopharyngeal Secretions," *J Clin Microbiol*, 1991, 29(3):470-4.

Viral Culture, Sclera *see* Viral Culture, Eye or Ocular Symptoms *on page 1202*

Viral Culture, Skin *see* Herpes Simplex Virus Culture *on page 1182*

Viral Culture, Skin *see* Varicella-Zoster Virus Culture *on page 1193*

Viral Culture, Skin/Dermatological Specimen *see* Viral Culture, Dermatological Symptoms *on page 1201*

Viral Culture, Skin Scrapings *see* Viral Culture, Dermatological Symptoms *on page 1201*

Viral Culture, Stool

CPT *87140 (culture typing, fluorescent method); 87252 (tissue culture, inoculation and observation); 87253 (tissue culture, additional studies, each isolate)*

Related Information

Electron Microscopic Examination for Viruses, Stool *on page 1177*
Entamoeba histolytica Serological Test *on page 675*
Enterovirus Culture *on page 1178*
Poliomyelitis I, II, III Titer *on page 733*
Rotavirus, Direct Detection *on page 1191*
Stool Culture *on page 858*
Viral Culture *on page 1195*
Yersinia enterocolitica Antibody *on page 765*
Yersinia pestis Antibody *on page 766*

Applies to Adenovirus Culture, Stool; Coxsackie Virus Culture, Stool; Echovirus Culture, Stool; Enterovirus Culture, Stool; Poliovirus Culture, Stool

Test Commonly Includes Isolation and identification of viruses

Specimen Stool or rectal swab. Freshly passed stool is much more preferable than a rectal swab. **CONTAINER:** Stool: plastic screw-cap container, do not use cardboard or waxed containers; swab: cold viral transport medium **COLLECTION:** Collect stools into a clean and dry container. Insert swab gently into rectum and hold there for 10-15 seconds, moisten with contents of Culturette® bulb, and send to the laboratory. **STORAGE INSTRUCTIONS:** Keep specimens cold. **CAUSES FOR REJECTION:** Dry specimen, specimen not refrigerated during transport, specimen fixed in formalin, unlabeled specimen **TURNAROUND TIME:** Variable (usually 1-14 days) and depends on cell culture methods and amount of virus in the specimen

Interpretive **REFERENCE RANGE:** No virus isolated **USE:** Identify carriage or excretion of a virus in stool; isolate and identify an enterovirus which could be the cause of meningitis **LIMITATIONS:** Cannot detect the presence of nonculturable, disease-causing virus (eg, Norwalk group, calicivirus, and gastroenteritis viruses). Some bacterial toxins in fecal specimens, such as *Clostridium difficile* toxin A, can mimic viral cytopathic effect (CPE) in many cell lines. **METHODOLOGY:** Inoculation of specimen into cell cultures, incubation of cultures, observation for characteristic cytopathic effect (CPE), and identification/speciation by methods such as hemadsorption and fluorescent monoclonal antibodies **ADDITIONAL INFORMATION:** Isolation of virus from stool specimens may be helpful diagnostically. It is important to be aware of viral shedding to avoid transmission to other people. Children recently vaccinated against polio can shed poliovirus in the stool for months after vaccination. Children convalescing from upper respiratory illness or aseptic meningitis can shed virus in the stool for weeks. See table in Viral Culture test listing for viruses most likely to be isolated from stool specimens. The viruses most likely to be isolated from stool specimen are those which are extremely hardy and which do not have a lipid membrane envelope (ie, adenovirus, enterovirus, polio, coxsackie, and echoviruses). Many viruses responsible for diarrhea can be detected with immunoassays or electron microscopy.

References

Bhan MK, Raj P, Bhanduri N, et al, "Role of Enteric Adenoviruses and Rotaviruses in Mild and Severe Acute Enteritis," *Pediatr Infect Dis J*, 1988, 7:320-3.

(Continued)

Viral Culture, Stool *(Continued)*

Blacklow NR and Greenberg HB, "Viral Gastroenteritis," *N Engl J Med*, 1991, 325(4):252-64.

Viral Culture, Throat Swab *see* Viral Culture, Respiratory Symptoms *on page 1204*

Viral Culture, Tissue

CPT 87140 (culture typing, fluorescent method); 87252 (tissue culture, inoculation and observation); 87253 (tissue culture, additional studies, each isolate)

Related Information

Hepatitis B DNA Detection *on page 913*
Histopathology *on page 57*
Human Immunodeficiency Virus DNA Amplification *on page 915*
Human Papillomavirus DNA Probe Test *on page 916*
Viral Culture *on page 1195*

Applies to Viral Culture, Biopsy; Viral Culture, Brain; Viral Culture, Bronchial; Viral Culture, Heart; Viral Culture, Kidney; Viral Culture, Lung; Viral Culture, Muscle; Viral Culture, Trachea

Test Commonly Includes Isolation and identification of virus

Specimen Biopsy, swab, brush, or scrape specimen from any suspect organ, site, lesion, or tissue **CONTAINER:** Sterile, screw-cap container **SAMPLING TIME:** As soon as possible after onset of illness **COLLECTION:** Always consult the laboratory for specific details prior to collecting specimen. Specimen should be collected during the acute phase of the disease, as follows.

Tissue: Use a fresh set of sterile instruments to collect each tissue. Place each specimen in its own dry, sterile nontoxic leakproof container. Identify each tissue with patient's name, type of tissue, and date collected. **Keep cold and bring tissue to the laboratory immediately.**

Biopsy, lung, kidney, heart muscle, brain: Specimens should be placed into a sterile container and kept cold.

Tracheal or bronchial tissue or brushings: If possible, brushes should be placed into cold viral transport medium.

STORAGE INSTRUCTIONS: Specimens should be kept cold and moist. If specimen is to be stored longer than 48 hours it should be frozen at -70°C. **Do not freeze at -20°C**. **CAUSES FOR REJECTION:** Dry specimen, specimen not refrigerated during transport, specimen fixed in formalin, unlabeled specimen **TURNAROUND TIME:** Variable (usually 1-14 days) and depends on culture method and amount of virus in specimen

Interpretive **REFERENCE RANGE:** No virus isolated **USE:** Aid in the diagnosis of disseminated viral diseases (eg, encephalitis and meningitis) **LIMITATIONS:** Presence of nonculturable, disease-causing virus (eg, encephalitis, hepatitis, and gastroenteritis viruses); invasive procedures **METHODOLOGY:** Inoculation of specimen into cell cultures, incubation of cultures, observation for characteristic cytopathic effect (CPE), and identification/speciation by methods such as hemadsorption and fluorescent monoclonal antibodies. If specific viruses such as HSV, CMV, VZV, or adenovirus are suspected, the laboratory might be able to use rapid (1-2 days) culture (shell vial) methods to detect these viruses. **ADDITIONAL INFORMATION:** See table in Viral Culture test listing for the viruses most likely to be isolated from clinical specimens. Generally, tissues should be stored and transported in sterile, screw-cap container. Tissues should not be put into viral transport medium. Viral DNA can now be detected using nucleic acid amplification procedures or *in situ* hybridization. These techniques are very sensitive and specific. In some viral diseases, such tests can be diagnostically useful (eg, hepatitis). However, other viruses can reside in the host in a latent form without causing disease (CMV, HSV, VZV). Such latent viruses can produce false-positive results if amplification of DNA in these viruses is used in a diagnostic test.

References

Hughes JM, "Physical and Chemical Methods for Enhancing Rapid Detection of Viruses and Other Agents," *Clin Microbiol Rev*, 1993, 6(2):150-75.

Wiedbrauk DL and Johnston SLG, "Specimen Collection and Processing," *Manual of Clinical Virology*, New York, NY: Raven Press, 1993, 22-32.

Viral Culture, Trachea *see* Viral Culture, Tissue *on this page*

Viral Culture, Ulcer *see* Viral Culture, Dermatological Symptoms *on page 1201*

Viral Culture, Urethra *see* Viral Culture, Urogenital *on this page*

Viral Culture, Urine

CPT *87140 (culture typing, fluorescent method); 87252 (tissue culture, inoculation and observation); 87253 (tissue culture, additional studies, each isolate)*

Related Information

Adenovirus Culture *on page 1169*
Adenovirus Culture, Rapid *on page 1170*
Cytomegalovirus Culture *on page 1175*
Cytomegalovirus Isolation, Rapid *on page 1176*
Enterovirus Culture *on page 1178*
Mumps Virus Culture *on page 1187*
Urine Culture, Clean Catch *on page 881*
Urine Cytology *on page 513*
Viral Culture *on page 1195*

Applies to CMV Culture, Urine; Mumps Virus Culture, Urine

Test Commonly Includes Isolation and identification of viruses

Specimen Urine **CONTAINER:** Sterile screw-cap container **SAMPLING TIME:** Shedding of CMV can be intermittent. Therefore, several specimens should be collected, if possible. **COLLECTION:** Clean catch, midstream urine in sterile, screw-cap container **STORAGE INSTRUCTIONS:** Refrigerate if delay of more than 1 hour in transit to the laboratory. Specimen may be stored up to 72 hours at 4°C before inoculation onto cell culture. **Do not freeze specimens at -20°C**. Some viruses are inactivated by freezing at -20°C. Specimens that need to be stored longer than 72 hours can be frozen at -70°C or below in the presence of 30% sorbitol.[1] **CAUSES FOR REJECTION:** Specimen not refrigerated during transport, specimen fixed in formalin, unlabeled specimen **TURNAROUND TIME:** Variable (1-14 days) and depends on cell culture method and amount of virus in specimen. Routine CMV cultures usually are observed for up to 4 weeks before final results are issued.

Interpretive **REFERENCE RANGE:** No virus isolated **USE:** Aid in the diagnosis of viral diseases (eg, cytomegalovirus disease, mumps, and cystitis) **LIMITATIONS:** Urine can be toxic for cell cultures and can result in inconclusive results **METHODOLOGY:** Inoculation of specimen into cell cultures, incubation of cultures, observation for characteristic cytopathic effect (CPE), and identification/speciation by hemadsorption and/or fluorescent monoclonal antibodies. If specific viruses such as CMV or adenovirus are suspected, the laboratory might be able to use rapid (1-2 days) culture (shell vial) methods to detect these viruses. **ADDITIONAL INFORMATION:** The viruses most frequently isolated from urine are CMV, mumps, and adenoviruses. See table in Viral Culture test listing.

Footnotes

1. Fedorko DP, Ilstrup DM, and Smith TF, "Effect of Age of Shell Vial Monolayers on Detection of Cytomegalovirus From Urine Specimens," *J Clin Microbiol*, 1989, 27(9):2107-9.

References

Lennette DA, "Preparation of Specimens for Virological Examination," *Manual of Clinical Microbiology*, 5th ed, Balows A, Hausler WJ Jr, Herrmann KL, et al, eds, Washington, DC: American Society for Microbiology, 1991, 818-21.

Wiedbrauk DL and Johnston SLG, "Specimen Collection and Processing," *Manual of Clinical Virology*, New York, NY: Raven Press, 1993, 22-32.

Viral Culture, Urogenital

CPT *87140 (culture typing, fluorescent method); 87252 (tissue culture, inoculation and observation); 87253 (tissue culture, additional studies, each isolate)*

Related Information

Cervical/Vaginal Cytology *on page 491*
Chlamydia trachomatis Culture *on page 1171*
Chlamydia trachomatis DNA Probe *on page 897*
Genital Culture *on page 814*
Human Papillomavirus DNA Probe Test *on page 916*
Viral Culture, Dermatological Symptoms *on page 1201*

Synonyms Genital Culture, Virus; Viral Culture, Genital

Applies to Viral Culture, Cervical; Viral Culture, Endocervical; Viral Culture, Fallopian Tube; Viral Culture, Labial; Viral Culture, Prostate; Viral Culture, Urethra

(Continued)

Viral Culture, Urogenital *(Continued)*

Test Commonly Includes Isolation and identification of virus

Specimen Cervical, urethral, and genital lesions, surgical and biopsy tissue **CONTAINER:** Sterile and cold viral transport medium **SAMPLING TIME:** As soon as possible after the eruption of vesicles or lesions, preferably within 3 days of lesion eruption. Only occasionally can HSV be isolated as late as 7-10 days after onset. **COLLECTION:** Disinfection of site prior to collection is generally not recommended. Use a Culturette® swab, spatula, or scalpel blade to scrape away cells from the base of freshly unroofed lesions, and place the swab or collected cells immediately into cold viral transport medium. Vesicular fluid is an excellent specimen, and can be collected by using a tuberculin syringe and a 26-gauge needle. Rinse contents of syringe into cold viral transport medium. **STORAGE INSTRUCTIONS:** Keep all specimens cold and moist. Specimens which cannot be inoculated onto cell cultures within 48 hours should be frozen at -70°C. **CAUSES FOR REJECTION:** Dry specimen, specimen not refrigerated during transport, specimen fixed in formalin, unlabeled specimen **TURNAROUND TIME:** Variable (1-14 days), depends on culture methods and amount of virus in specimen

Interpretive **REFERENCE RANGE:** No virus isolated **USE:** Aid in the diagnosis of viral diseases (eg, sexually transmitted diseases and herpes infection) **LIMITATIONS:** Some laboratories use methods which detect only HSV in genital specimens; presence of nonculturable, disease-causing virus (eg, papillomavirus); invasive procedures **METHODOLOGY:** Inoculation of specimen into cell cultures, incubation of cultures, observation for characteristic cytopathic effect (CPE), and identification/speciation by fluorescent monoclonal antibodies. If specific viruses such as HSV, CMV, or adenovirus are suspected, the laboratory might be able to use rapid (1-2 days) culture (shell vial) methods to detect these viruses. **ADDITIONAL INFORMATION:** Urogenital, dermal, oral, and mucosal specimens often yield the same viruses. See table in Viral Culture test listing. The detection of virus such as HSV or CMV in pregnant women is important in preventing the complications of neonatal infections.[1,2] Infants are at risk of infection during delivery even if the mother is asymptomatic. Human papillomavirus (HPV) causes genital warts. Certain strains of HPV are associated with cervical cancer. This virus can be detected using *in situ* hybridization, Southern blot analysis, or DNA amplification.[3]

Footnotes

1. Prober CG, Corey L, Brown ZA, et al, "The Management of Pregnancies Complicated by Genital Infections With Herpes Simplex Virus," *Clin Infect Dis*, 1992, 15(6):1031-8.
2. Pass RF, Little EA, Stagno S, et al, "Young Children as a Probable Source of Maternal and Congenital Cytomegalovirus Infection," *N Engl J Med*, 1987, 316:1366-71.
3. Schiffman MH, Bauer HM, Lorincz AT, et al, "Comparison of Southern Blot Hybridization and Polymerase Chain Reaction Methods for the Detection of Human Papillomavirus DNA," *J Clin Microbiol*, 1991, 29(3):573-7.

References

Arvin AM and Alford CA, "Chronic Intrauterine and Perinatal Infections," *Practical Diagnosis of Viral Infections*, Galasso GJ, Whitley RJ, Merigan TC, eds, New York, NY: Raven Press, 1993, 211-42.

Gibbs RS, Amstey MS, Sweet RL, et al, "Management of Genital Herpes Infection in Pregnancy," *Obstet Gynecol*, 1988, 71:779-80.

Moscicki AB, "Human Papillomavirus Infections," *Adv Pediatr*, 1992, 39:257-79.

Viral Disease in Tissue *see* Electron Microscopic Examination for Viruses, Stool *on page 1177*

Virus Culture *see* Viral Culture *on page 1195*

Virus, Direct Detection by Fluorescent Antibody

CPT *87206*

Related Information

Adenovirus Antibody Titer *on page 629*
Adenovirus Culture, Rapid *on page 1170*
Bronchial Washings Cytology *on page 485*
Bronchoalveolar Lavage Cytology *on page 487*
Frozen Section *on page 54*
Histopathology *on page 57*
Influenza A and B Titer *on page 713*
Influenza Virus Culture *on page 1186*
Parainfluenza Virus Culture *on page 1189*
Rabies *on page 82*

Respiratory Syncytial Virus Culture *on page 1190*
Respiratory Syncytial Virus Serology *on page 739*
Sputum Cytology *on page 510*
Varicella-Zoster Virus Culture *on page 1193*
Varicella-Zoster Virus Culture, Rapid *on page 1194*
Varicella-Zoster Virus Serology *on page 761*
Viral Culture, Respiratory Symptoms *on page 1204*

Synonyms Direct Detection of Virus; Direct Fluorescent Antibody Test for Virus; Virus Fluorescent Antibody Test

Applies to Influenza Virus, Direct Detection; Measles Virus, Direct Detection; Mumps Virus, Direct Detection; Parainfluenza Virus, Direct Detection; Rabies Virus, Direct Detection; Varicella-Zoster Virus, Direct Detection

Test Commonly Includes Direct (nonculture) detection of virus-infected cells

Specimen Impression smears of tissues, lesion scrapings and swabs, frozen sections, cell suspensions, upper respiratory tract swabs **CAUSES FOR REJECTION:** Insufficient material, slides broken or badly scratched, fixative used on slide preparation. **TURNAROUND TIME:** Less than 1 day **SPECIAL INSTRUCTIONS:** Make at least four impression smears or place four frozen sections on four separate slides. Cell suspensions should be centrifuged, resuspended to slight turbidity, and applied to prewelled slides.

Interpretive **REFERENCE RANGE:** No virus detected **USE:** Useful in the rapid diagnosis of HSV, VZV, RSV, parainfluenza, influenza, and rabies infections **LIMITATIONS:** It is possible for the test to be negative in the presence of viral infection. Expertly trained and experienced personnel, excellent quality reagents, and adequate numbers of cells are required. **Contact laboratory prior to requesting test to determine if laboratory offers this/these tests.** **METHODOLOGY:** Monoclonal antibody reagents and immunofluorescence microscopy are used to detect viruses/viral antigens in specimen cells. **ADDITIONAL INFORMATION:** Several viruses (adenovirus, CMV, HSV, VZV, RSV, influenza, parainfluenza, measles, mumps, and rabies virus) can be detected in this manner. However, generally this test is not as sensitive as cell culture. Direct detection of viruses in respiratory secretions can be diagnostically helpful because cell culture results often take several days to weeks.[1]

Footnotes

1. McIntosh K, Halonen P, and Ruuskanen O, "Report of a Workshop on Respiratory Viral Infections: Epidemiology, Diagnosis, Treatment, and Prevention," *Clin Infect Dis*, 1993, 16(1):151-64.

References

Costello MJ, Smernoff NT, and Yungbluth M, "Laboratory Diagnosis of Viral Respiratory Tract Infections," *Lab Med*, 1993, 24:150-7.
Smith TF, "Rapid Diagnosis of Viral Infections," *Adv Exp Med Biol*, 1990, 263:115-21.

Virus Fluorescent Antibody Test *see* Virus, Direct Detection by Fluorescent Antibody *on previous page*

Virus Isolation *see* Viral Culture *on page 1195*

VZV Centrifugation Culture *see* Varicella-Zoster Virus Culture, Rapid *on page 1194*

VZV Culture *see* Varicella-Zoster Virus Culture *on page 1193*

VZV Culture, Rapid *see* Varicella-Zoster Virus Culture, Rapid *on page 1194*

VZV Shell Vial Method *see* Varicella-Zoster Virus Culture, Rapid *on page 1194*

VIROLOGY APPENDIX

Antiviral Agents and Their Target Virus(es)

Antiviral Agent	Target Virus(es)
Nucleoside Analogs	
Acyclovir*	HSV, VZV, EBV, CMV
Bromovinyldeoxyuridine (BVDU)	Some herpesviruses
Buciclovir	HSV
Didanosine (ddl)	HIV
Dideoxoycytidine (Ddc)*	HIV
Dideoxyinosine (Ddi)*	HIV
Fluoroiodoaracytosine (FIAC)	Some herpesviruses
Ganciclovir (DHPG)*	CMV
Idoxuridine (IDU)*	HSV
Trifluridine (TFT)*	HSV
Vidarabine (ara-A)*	HSV, VZV
Zalcitabine (ddc)	HIV
Zidovudine (AZT)*	HIV
Nucleoside-like Analogs	
Ribavirin*	Influenza virus, parainfluenza virus, HSV, Lassa fever virus, hepatitis A virus, respiratory syncytial virus
Other Antiviral Agents	
Amantadine*/rimantadine	Influenza virus
Antimoniotungstate (HPA-23)	Retroviruses
Castanospermine	Retroviruses
Disoxaril (Win 51711)	Rhinoviruses, enteroviruses
Phosphonoformate (foscarnet)*	Retroviruses, influenza virus, HSV, CMV
Suramin	Retroviruses
Immunomodulators	
Ampligen	Retroviruses
Interferons	Several viruses

*Agent is FDA-approved for clinical use but not necessarily for use in disease(s) caused by all of the viruses given for that agent. Consult pharmacist and package inserts for indications.

Figure 1

Molecular Structures of Representative Antiviral Agents

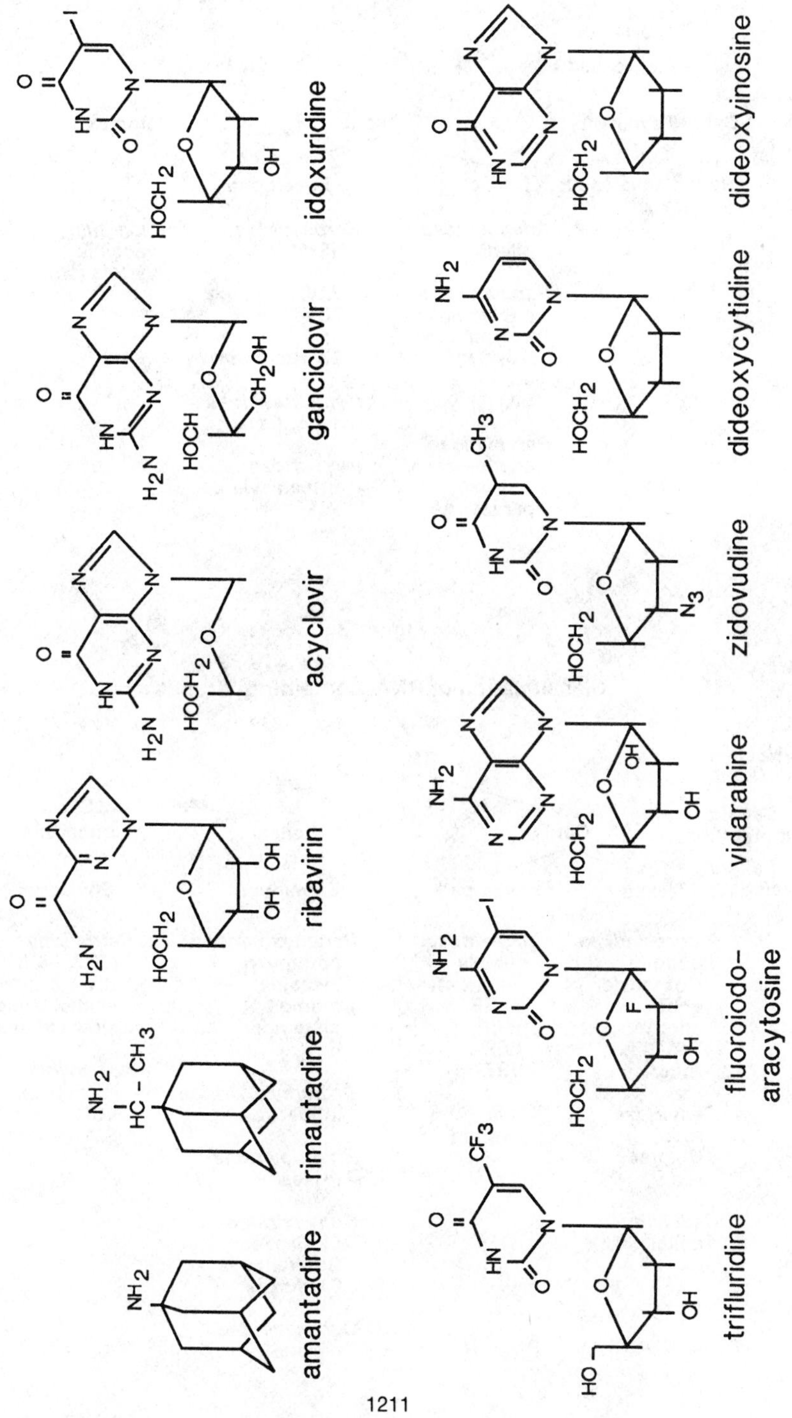

idoxuridine

ganciclovir

acyclovir

ribavirin

rimantadine

amantadine

dideoxyinosine

dideoxycytidine

zidovudine

vidarabine

fluoroiodo-aracytosine

trifluridine

Figure 2

Classification of DNA-Containing Viruses

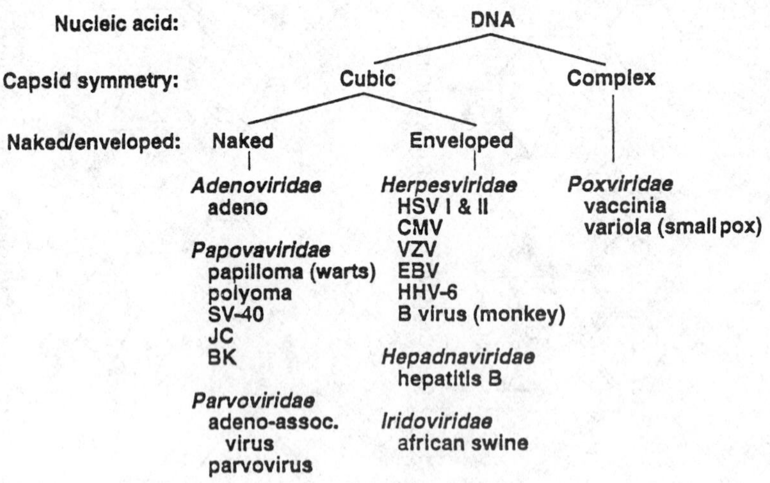

Figure 3

Classification of RNA-Containing Viruses

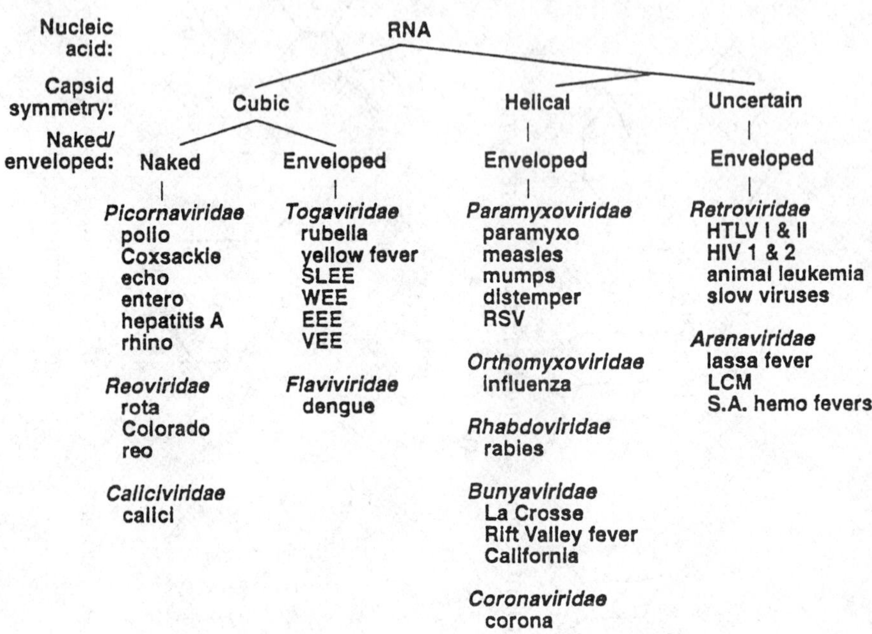

Figure 4

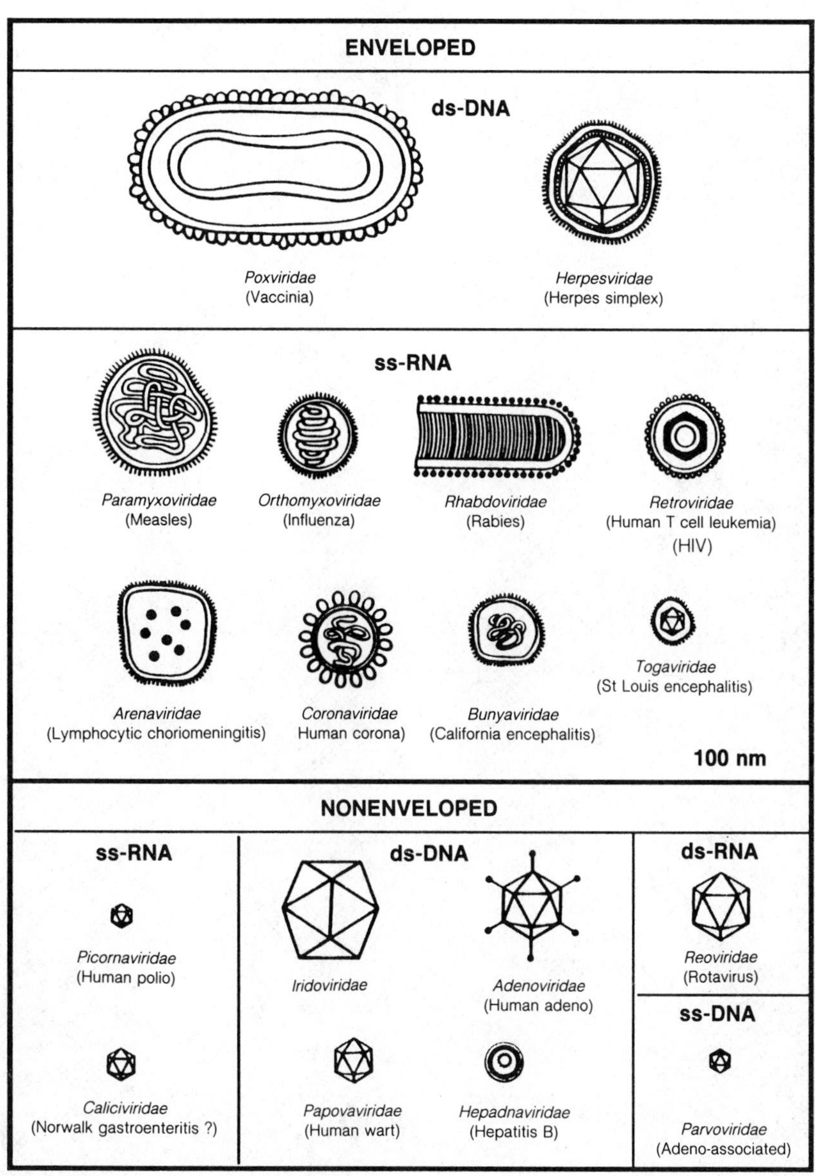

Diagram illustrating the shapes and relative sizes of animal viruses of the major families (bar = 100 nm). Representative members that infect humans are listed in parentheses. Iridoviridae are not known to infect humans. From Melnick JL, "Structure and Classification of Viruses," *Textbook of Human Virology*, Belshe RB, ed, Chicago, IL: Yearbook Medical Publishers, 1984, 1-28, with permission.

ACRONYMS AND ABBREVIATIONS GLOSSARY

This glossary provides a useful listing of many acronyms and abbreviations commonly associated with laboratory medicine. We offer this glossary not as an exhaustive authoritative list, but more as a guide to assist in interpreting frequently used terminology.

ACRONYMS AND ABBREVIATIONS GLOSSARY

A . . . . apical; artery
A_1 . . . . blood group antigen
A1AT . . . . alpha$_1$ antitrypsin
A_2 . . . . aortic second sound; blood group antigen
aa . . . . of each (ana)
AABB . . . . American Association of Blood Banks
AAC . . . . antibiotic associated colitis
AACC . . . . American Association of Clinical Chemistry
AaG . . . . alveolar arterial gradient
AAL . . . . anterior axillary line
AAP . . . . American Academy of Pediatrics
AAPCC . . . . American Association of Poison Control Centers
AAS . . . . acute abdominal series; atomic absorption spectrometry
AAT . . . . alpha antitrypsin
Ab . . . . antibody
AB . . . . abort; antibiotic
ABC . . . . avidin-biotin complex
ABE . . . . acute bacterial endocarditis
ABG . . . . arterial blood gas
ABL . . . . abetalipoprotein
ABLB . . . . alternate binaural loudness balance
ABO . . . . ABO blood group
ABPA . . . . allergic bronchopulmonary aspergillosis
ABR . . . . auditory brainstem response
ABS . . . . alkylbenzene sulfonate
ac . . . . before meals (ante cibum)
Ac . . . . actinium
AC . . . . air conduction; alternating current
ACA . . . . anticardiolipin antibody; Du Pont chemistry analyzer
ACC . . . . amylase creatinine clearance
ACD . . . . acid-citrate-dextrose
ACE . . . . angiotensin converting enzyme
AChR . . . . acetylcholine receptor antibody
ACLS . . . . advanced cardiac life support
ACOG . . . . American College of Obstetrics and Gynecology
AcP . . . . acid phosphatase
ACT . . . . activated clotting time
ACTH . . . . adrenocorticotropic hormone
ad . . . . right ear; up to (ad)
ADCC . . . . antibody-dependent cell-mediated cytotoxicity
ADH . . . . alcohol dehydrogenase; antidiuretic hormone
ADL . . . . active daily living
ad lib . . . . as desired (ad libitum)
ADM . . . . admission
ADNase . . . . anti-DNAse
ADP . . . . adenosine 5-diphosphate
ADT . . . . adenosine triphosphate; alternate-day treatment
AED . . . . anticonvulsant drugs
AEP . . . . average evoked potential
AF . . . . acid-fast; amniotic fluid; artrial fibrillation
AFB . . . . acid-fast bacillus
AFP . . . . alphafetoprotein
Ag . . . . antigen; silver
A/G . . . . albumin/globulin ratio
AGA . . . . accelerated growth area
AGN . . . . acute glomerular nephritis
$AgNO_3$ . . . . silver nitrate
AGS . . . . adrenogenital syndrome
AH . . . . antihyaluronidase
A-H . . . . atrial-HIS
AHA . . . . acquired hemolytic anemia; autoimmune hemolytic anemia
AHBC . . . . hepatitis B core antibody

AHF . . . . antihemophilic factor
AHFS . . . . American Hospital Formulary Service
AHG . . . . antihemophilic globulin
AHT . . . . antihyaluronidase titer
AI . . . . allergy index; aortic insufficiency
AICC . . . . anti-inhibitor coagulant complex
AIDS . . . . acquired immune deficiency syndrome
AIHA . . . . autoimmune hemolytic anemia
AIP . . . . acute intermittent porphyria; average intravascular pressure
AJ . . . . ankle jerk
AK . . . . adenylate kinase; above the knee
Al . . . . aluminum
ALA . . . . aminolevulinic acid
alb . . . . albumin
alk . . . . alkaline
AlkP . . . . alkaline phosphatase
ALL . . . . acute lymphoblastic leukemia; acute lymphocytic leukemia
$Al(OH)_3$ . . . . aluminum hydroxide
AlP . . . . alkaline phosphatase
ALPI . . . . alkaline phosphatase isoenzymes
ALS . . . . advanced life support; amyotrophic lateral sclerosis; antilymphocyte serum
ALT . . . . alanine aminotransferase
Am . . . . americium
AM . . . . morning
AMA . . . . against medical advice; American Medical Association; antimitrochondrial antibody
AMI . . . . acute myocardial infarction
AML . . . . acute myeloblastic leukemia; acute myelogenous leukemia
AMP . . . . adenosine monophosphate
AMPS . . . . acid mucopolysaccharide
ANA . . . . antinuclear antibody
ANCA . . . . antineutrophil cytoplasmic antibodies
ANF . . . . antinuclear factor
ANLL . . . . acute nonlymphocytic leukemia
ANP . . . . atrial natriuretic peptide
A & O . . . . alert and oriented
AODM . . . . adult onset diabetes mellitus
AOS . . . . acridine orange staining
AP . . . . antepartum; anteroposterior
A & P . . . . anterior and posterior; assessment and plans
APCA . . . . antiparetial cell antibody
APhA . . . . American Pharmaceutical Association
APP . . . . alum-precipitating pyridine
APTT . . . . activated partial thromboplastin time
APUD . . . . amine precursor uptake and decarboxylation
aq . . . . water (aqua)
Ar . . . . argon
ARA . . . . antireticulin antibody
ARD . . . . antimicrobial removal device; acute respiratory distress
ARDS . . . . adult respiratory distress syndrome
ARF . . . . acute renal failure
Ars . . . . arylsulfatase
ART . . . . arterial line
as . . . . left ear
As . . . . arsenic
AS . . . . anal sphincter; ankylosing spondylitis; aortic stenosis
AsA . . . . arylsulfatase A
ASA . . . . acetylsalicylic acid
ASAP . . . . as soon as possible
AsB . . . . arylsulfatase B
ASCP . . . . American Society of Clinical Pathologists
ASCVD . . . . arteriosclerotic cardiovascular disease

ASD . . . . atrial septal defect
ASHD . . . . arteriosclerotic heart disease
ASHP . . . . American Society of Hospital Pharmacists
ASK . . . . antistreptokinase
ASKA . . . . antiskeletal antibody
ASLO . . . . antistreptolysin O
ASMA . . . . antismooth muscle antibody
ASO . . . . antistreptolysin O; arterioselerosis obliterans
AST . . . . aspartate aminotransferase
ASVD . . . . arteriosclerotic vascular disease
At . . . . astatine
AT III . . . . antithrombin III
ATN . . . . acute tubular necrosis
ATP . . . . adenosine triphosphate
ATPase . . . . adenosine triphosphatase
ATS . . . . American Thoracic Society
au . . . . each ear (auris utro)
Au . . . . gold
^{198}Au . . . . radioisotope of gold
A-V . . . . arteriovenous; atrioventricular; audiovisual
AVA . . . . availability
AVM . . . . arteriovenous malformation
AVP . . . . arginine vasopressin
A & W . . . . alive and well
Ax . . . . axillary
AZT . . . . zidovudine

B . . . . boron
Ba . . . . barium
BA . . . . Bachelor of Arts
BAC . . . . blood alcohol concentration
BAE . . . . barium enema
BAEP . . . . brainstem auditory evoked potential
BAER . . . . brainstem auditory evoked response
BAL . . . . bronchial alveolar lavage
BAO . . . . basal acid output
BB . . . . Blood Bank
BBB . . . . blood brain barrier; bundle branch block
BBPRL . . . . big big prolactin
BBT . . . . basal body temperature
BC . . . . bone conduction
BCG . . . . bacillus Calmette-Guérin
BCM . . . . bovine cervical mucus
BCP . . . . birth control pills; blood cell profile
bcr . . . . breakpoint cluster region
BD . . . . bronchodilators
Be . . . . beryllium
BE . . . . bacterial endocarditis; barium enema
BEP . . . . brainstem evoked potential
BERA . . . . brainstem evoked response auditory
BF . . . . black female
BFT . . . . bentonite flocculation test
BGP . . . . bone GLA protein
BHB . . . . beta-hydroxybutyrate
BHI . . . . brain heart infusion
Bi . . . . bismuth
bid . . . . twice a day (bis in die)
BJ . . . . Bence Jones; biceps jerk; bone and joint
Bk . . . . berkelium
BK . . . . below knee
Bl Obs . . . . bladder observation

BLS .... basic life support
BM .... black male; bone marrow; bowel movement; breast milk
BMR .... basal metabolic rate
BMT .... bone marrow transplant
BNO .... bladder neck obstruction
BP .... blood pressure
BPD .... biparietal diameter
BPH .... benign prostatic hyperplasia
Br .... bromine; bromide
BR .... bathroom; bedrest
BrdU 5-bromodeoxyuridine
BRP .... bathroom privileges
BRU .... bromide urine
BS .... Bachelor of Science; blood sugar; bowel sounds; breath sounds
bsa .... body surface area
BSEP .... brainstem evoked potential
BSO .... bilateral salpingo-oophorectomy
BSP .... bromsulfophthalein
BTG .... beta thromboglobulin
BTL .... bilateral tubal ligation
BUN .... blood urea nitrogen
BVL .... bilateral vas ligation
BW .... birth weight; body weight
Bx .... biopsy

c .... with (cum)
C .... carbon
C_2 .... second cervical vertebra
Ca .... calcium
CA .... cancer antigen; cardiac arrest; chronological age
CA 15-3 .... tumor marker antigen
CA 19-9 .... tumor marker antigen
CA 50 .... tumor marker antigen
CA 125 .... tumor marker antigen
CAB .... coronary artery bypass
CABG .... coronary artery bypass graft
CAC .... circulating anticoagulant
CaCl .... calcium chloride
$CaCO_3$ .... calcium carbonate
CAD .... coronary artery disease
CaEDTA .... calcium disodium edetate
CAH .... chronic active hepatitis
CALLA .... common acute lymphoblastic leukemia antigen
cAMP .... cyclic AMP
CAPD .... chronic ambulatory peritoneal dialysis
CASA .... computer-assisted semen analysis
CAT .... computed axial tomography
CBAT .... Coag battery; Coulter battery
CBC .... complete blood count
CBD .... common bile duct
CBF .... cerebral blood flow
CBG .... capillary blood gases
CBIL .... conjugated bilirubin
CBS .... chronic brain syndrome
CBT .... computerized body tomography
CC .... chief complaint; closing capacity
CCI .... corrected count increment
CCK .... cholecystokinin
CCK-OP .... cholecystokinin-octapeptide
CCU .... cardiac care unit; coronary care unit
Cd .... cadmium

CDA . . . . congenital dyserythropoietic anemia
CDC . . . . Centers for Disease Control
CDP . . . . continuous distending pressure; cytidine diphosphate
CDU . . . . cumulative dose unit
Ce . . . . cerium
CEA . . . . carcinoembryonic antigen
Cf . . . . californium
CF . . . . cardiac failure; caucasian female; complement fixation; cystic fibrosis
CFU . . . . colony forming units
CGL . . . . chronic granulocytic leukemia
CH . . . . congenital hypothyroidism
CHBHA . . . . congenital Heinz body hemolytic anemia
CHD . . . . congenital heart disease
CHF . . . . congestive heart failure
CI . . . . cardiac index; color index; confidence intervals
CIC . . . . circulating immune complexes
CIE . . . . counterimmunoelectrophoresis
CIF . . . . clone-inhibiting factor
CIN . . . . cervical intraepithelial neoplasia
CIP . . . . cellular immunocompetence profile
CIPD . . . . chronic inflammatory demyelinating polyradiculoneuropathy
CJD . . . . Creutzfeldt-Jakob disease
CK . . . . creatine kinase
Cl . . . . chlorine
CLA . . . . certified laboratory assistant
CLL . . . . chronic lymphocytic leukemia
CLS . . . . clinical laboratory science
cm . . . . centimeter
cm^2 . . . . square centimeter
Cm . . . . curium
CM . . . . caucasian male; contrast media; culture media
CMG . . . . cystometrogram
CML . . . . cell mediated lysis; chronic myelogenous leukemia
cmm . . . . square centimeter cm^2
CMP . . . . cardiomyopathy; cervical mucus penetration
CMPT . . . . cervical mucous penetration test
CMV . . . . cytomegalovirus
CMVS . . . . culture midvoid specimen
CN . . . . cyanogen
CNS . . . . central nervous system
CNSHA . . . . congenital nonspherocytic hemolytic anemia
Co . . . . cobalt
^{57}Co . . . . radioisotope of cobalt
^{60}Co . . . . radioisotope of cobalt
CO . . . . carbon monoxide; cardiac output
CO_3 . . . . carbonate
C/O . . . . complaint of
coag . . . . coagulation
COHb . . . . carboxyhemoglobin
COLD . . . . chronic obstructive lung disease
COP . . . . chronic obstructive pulmonary
COPD . . . . chronic obstructive pulmonary disease
C & P . . . . cystoscopy and pyelogram
CPA . . . . carotid phonoangiography
CPAP . . . . continuous positive airway pressure
CPB . . . . cardiopulmonary bypass
CPD . . . . cyst disease protein; citrate phosphate dextrose
CPDA . . . . citrate phosphate dextrose adenine
CPE . . . . cytopathogenic effects
CPI . . . . coronary prognostic index
CPK . . . . creatine phosphokinase
cpm . . . . counts per minute

CPP . . . . cerebral perfusion pressure
CPPB . . . . continuous positive pressure breathing
CPPD . . . . calcium pyrophosphate dihydrate
CPR . . . . cardiopulmonary resuscitation
CPS . . . . Compendium of Pharmaceuticals and Specialties
cps . . . . cycles per second
CPT . . . . chest physiotherapy
Cr . . . . chromium
^{51}Cr . . . . radioisotope of chromium
CRA . . . . central retinal artery
Cre . . . . creatinine
creat . . . . creatinine
CRF . . . . chronic renal failure; corticotropin releasing factor
CRM . . . . cross reacting material
CRP . . . . C-reactive protein
CRS . . . . catheter related sepsis
CRST . . . . calcinosis, Raynaud's phenomenon, sclerodactylia, telangiectasis
CRT . . . . cathode ray tube
Cs . . . . cesium
CS . . . . cesarean section; coronary sclerosis
C & S . . . . culture and sensitivity
CS & CC . . . . culture, sensitivity and colony count
CSF . . . . cerebrospinal fluid
CSP . . . . chemistry screening profile
CSR . . . . corrected sedimentation rate
CT . . . . circulation time; clotting time; computerized tomography
CTA . . . . Committee on Thrombolytic Agents
CTAB . . . . cetyltrimethylammonium bromide
CTD . . . . carpal tunnel decompression; congenital thymic dysplasia
CTM . . . . *Chlamydia* transport media
CTT . . . . computerized transaxial tomography
Cu . . . . copper
CUC . . . . chronic ulcerative colitis
CV . . . . cardiovascular; coefficient of variation; conjugata vera
CVA . . . . cerebrovascular accident
CVD . . . . cardiovascular disease
CVE . . . . cerebrovascular evaluation
CVI . . . . cerebral vascular insufficiency; continuous venous infusion
CVP . . . . central venous pressure
CVS . . . . cardiovascular system; clean voided specimen
Cx . . . . cervical; cervix
CXR . . . . chest x-ray

D_5W . . . . 5% dextrose in water solution
DALA . . . . delta aminolevulinic acid
DAT . . . . direct antiglobulin test
db . . . . decibel
DB . . . . deep breath
DBI . . . . development at birth index
DBP . . . . diastolic blood pressure
DC . . . . direct current
D & C . . . . dilatation and curettage
DCG . . . . dynamic electrocardiogram
DCH . . . . delayed and cutaneous hypersensitivity
DD . . . . differential diagnosis
DDD . . . . degenerative disc disease
DDT . . . . dichloro-diphenyltrichloroethane
DDX . . . . differential diagnosis
DEA . . . . Drug Enforcement Agency
DEAE . . . . diethylaminoethyl
DER . . . . dermatome evoked response

DFA . . . . direct fluorescent antibody
dg . . . . decigram
DH . . . . dermatitis herpetiformis
DHA . . . . dehydroepiandrosterone
DHEA . . . . dehydroepiandrosterone
DHEA-S . . . . dehydroepiandrosterone sulfate
DHL . . . . diffuse histiocytic lymphoma
DHS . . . . duration of hospital stay
DHT . . . . dihydrotestosterone
DI . . . . diabetes insipidus
DIC . . . . disseminated intravascular coagulation
diff . . . . differential
DIP . . . . dichlorophenolindophenol
DISIDA . . . . diisopropyl-iminodiacetic acid
DJD . . . . degenerative joint disease
DKA . . . . diabetic ketoacidosis
dL . . . . deciliter
D-L . . . . Donath-Landsteiner
DLCO . . . . diffusing capacity of the lung for carbon monoxide
DLE . . . . discoid lupus erythematosus
DLF . . . . digoxin-like factors
dm . . . . decimeter
DM . . . . diabetes mellitus; diastolic murmur
DMO . . . . dimethyloxazolidinedione
DMSO . . . . dimethylsulfoxide
DNA . . . . deoxyribonucleic acid
DNase . . . . deoxyribonuclease
DNBT . . . . dinitroblue
DNPH . . . . dinitrophenylhydrazine
DOA . . . . date of admission; dead on arrival
DOB . . . . date of birth
DOC . . . . deoxycorticosterone
DOE . . . . dyspnea on exertion
DOI . . . . date of injury
dos . . . . dose (dosis)
DP . . . . diastolic pressure
DPG . . . . diphosphoglycerate
DPH . . . . diphenylhydantoin
DPT . . . . diphtheria toxoid, pertussis vaccine, tetanus toxoid
DQ . . . . developmental quotient
Dr . . . . doctor
DR . . . . donor related
DRG . . . . diagnostic related group(s)
DSA . . . . digital subtraction angiography
DSD . . . . discharge summary dictated; dry sterile dressing
ds-DNA . . . . double stranded DNA
DSF . . . . disulfiram
DST . . . . dexamethasone suppression test
DT . . . . delirium tremons; duration tetany; dye test
dtd . . . . let such doses be given (dentur tales doses)
DTM . . . . dermatophyte test medium
DTR . . . . deep tendon reflex
dU . . . . deoxyuridine
DVT . . . . deep vein thrombosis
dw . . . . dry weight
Dx . . . . diagnosis
Dy . . . . dysprosium

EA . . . . early antigen
EAC . . . . external auditory canal
EACA . . . . epsilon-aminocaproic acid

EB ....Epstein-Barr
EBEA..........Epstein-Barr early antigen
EBNA..........Epstein-Barr nuclear antigen
EBV ....Epstein-Barr virus
EBVCA ....Epstein-Barr viral capsid antigen
EBVEA.........Epstein-Barr virus, early antigen
EBVNA ....Epstein-Barr virus, nuclear antigen
EC ....*Escherichia coli*; extracellular
ECA ....external carotid artery
ECG...........electrocardiogram
ECT ....emission computed tomography
EDTA..........ethylenediaminetetraacetic acid
EDX ....electrodiagnosis
EEG ....electroencephalogram
EENT ....eyes, ears, nose, throat
EF ....ejection fraction; extended-field
EFA ....essential fatty acids
EFM ....external fetal monitoring
eg ....example
EGA ....estimated gestational age
EGD...........esophagogastroduodenoscopy
EGFR..........epidermal growth factor receptor
EH ....enlarged heart; essential hypertension
EHEC..........enterohemorrhagic *E. coli*
EIA ....enzyme immunoassay
EID ....electroimmunodiffusion
EIEC...........enteroinvasive *E. coli*
EKG ....electrocardiogram
ELISA..........enzyme-linked immunosorbent assay
ELT ....euoglobulin lysis time
EM ....electron microscopy
EMA ....endomysial antibody
EMG ....electromyogram
EMIT ....enzyme-multiplied immunoassay technique
EMS...........eosinophil myalgia syndrome
ENA ....extractable nuclear antigen
ENG ....electronystagmography
ENT ....ear, nose and throat
EOG...........electro-oculogram
eos ....eosinophil
EPA ....Environmental Protection Agency
EPBI...........exercise penile-brachial index
EPEC ....enteropathogenic *E. coli*
EPIS...........episiotomy
EPS ....electrophysiologic studies
Eq ....equivalent
Er ....erbium
ER ....emergency room; estrogen receptors
ERA ....estrogen receptor assay; evoked response audiometry
ERCP..........endoscopic retrograde cholangiopancreatography
ERG ....electroretinogram
ERPF ....effective renal plasma flow
ERV ....expiratory reserve volume
Es ....Einsteinium
ES ....electrical stimulation
ESP ....extrasensory perception
ESR ....erythrocyte sedimentation rate
ESRD..........end-stage renal disease
EST ....electroshock therapy
et ....and (et)
ETEC ....enterotoxigenic *E. coli*
EtOH ....ethyl alcohol

ETT . . . . extrathyroidal thyroxine
EU . . . . Ehrlich unit
EVI . . . . endocardial, vascular, and interstitial

F . . . . fluorine
FA . . . . fatty acid; filterable agent; fluorescent antibody
FAB . . . . French-American-British
FACP . . . . Fellow of the American College of Physicians
FAD . . . . flavin adenine dinucleotide
FAMA . . . . fluorescent antibody to membrane antigen
FANA . . . . fluorescent antinuclear antibody
FAS . . . . fetal alcohol syndrome
FB . . . . finger breadths; foreign bodies
FBC . . . . functional bactericidal concentration
FBP . . . . fibrin breakdown product
FBS . . . . fasting blood sugar
Fc . . . . portion of antibody molecule bound by membrane receptors
FDA . . . . Federal Drug Administration
FDP . . . . fibrin degradation product; fructose diphosphate
Fe . . . . iron
$FeCl_3$ . . . . ferric chloride
FEF . . . . forced expiratory flow
FENa . . . . fractional excretion of sodium (Na)
FEP . . . . free erythrocyte protoporphyrin
FES . . . . functional electrical stimulation
FETI . . . . fluorescent energy transfer immunoassay
FEV . . . . forced expiratory volume
FF . . . . filtration fraction; force fluids
FFA . . . . free fatty acids
FFP . . . . fresh frozen plasma
fg . . . . femtogram
FH . . . . family history
FHH . . . . familial hypocalciuric hypercalcemia
FHR . . . . fetal heart rate
FHS . . . . fetal heart sounds
FIC . . . . functional inhibitory concentration
FIF . . . . forced inspiratory flow
FITC . . . . fluorescein isothiocyanate
FIVC . . . . forced inspiratory vital capacity
fL . . . . femtoliter; fluid
Fm . . . . fermium
fmol . . . . femtomole
FMULC . . . . free monoclonal urinary light chains
FNA . . . . fine needle aspiration
FOB . . . . fiberoptic bronchoscopy
FOS . . . . fiberoptic sigmoidoscopy
FP . . . . false-positive
FPIA . . . . fluorescence polarization immunoassay
Fr . . . . francium
FRA . . . . fluorescent rabies antibody
FRC . . . . functional residual capacity
FS . . . . frozen section
FSH . . . . follicle stimulating hormone
FSI . . . . foam stability index
FSP . . . . fibrin split products
ft . . . . make (fiat, fiant)
FTA . . . . fluorescent treponemal antibody
FTA-ABS . . . . fluorescent treponemal antibody absorption
FTI . . . . free thyroxine index
FTND . . . . full-term normal delivery
FUO . . . . fever of undetermined origin

FVC . . . . forced vital capacity
Fx. . . . . fracture
FX . . . . factor X

g . . . . gram
G-6-PD . . . . glucose 6-phosphate dehydrogenase
Ga . . . . gallium
GABA . . . . gamma-aminobutyric acid
GAL . . . . galactosemia
GAW . . . . airway conductance
GAZT . . . . glucuronide derivative of azidothymidine
GB . . . . gallbladder
GBM . . . . glomerular basement membrane
GC . . . . geriatric chair; gonorrhea culture; gas chromatography
GC/MS . . . . gas chromatography/mass spectrometry
Gd . . . . gadolinium
g/dL . . . . gram percent
gdw . . . . gram dry weight
Ge . . . . germanium
GE . . . . gastroesophageal
GFR . . . . glomerular filtration rate
GGCT . . . . ground glass clotting time
GGT . . . . gamma-glutamyltransferase
GH . . . . growth hormone
GHB . . . . glycohemoglobin
GI . . . . gastrointestinal
GIH . . . . gastric inhibitory hormone
GIP . . . . gastric inhibitory polypeptide
GIS . . . . gastrointestinal series
GK . . . . galactokinase
GLC . . . . gas-liquid chromatography
GM . . . . geometric mean
GMS . . . . Grocott-Gomori methenamine-silver
GnRH . . . . gonadotropin releasing hormone
GOT . . . . glutamic-oxaloacetic transaminase
GP . . . . glycoprotein
GPK . . . . guinea pig kidney
GPT . . . . glutamic-pyruvic transaminase
GPUT . . . . glactose phosphate uridyl transferase
GR . . . . glutathione reductase
GSD . . . . glycogen storage disease
GSH . . . . glutathione; growth stimulating hormone
GSR . . . . galvanic skin response; generalized Schwartzman reaction
GSSR . . . . generalized Sandarelli-Shwartzman reaction
GT . . . . gait training; gamma-glutamyltransferase
GTP . . . . glutamyl transpeptidase
GTT . . . . glucose tolerance test
gtt(s) . . . . drop(s) (gutta)
GU . . . . genitourinary; gastric ulcer; gonococcal urethritis
GVHD . . . . graft versus host disease
GXT . . . . graded exercise test
gyn . . . . gynecological

h. . . . . hour (hora)
H . . . . hydrogen
Ha . . . . hahnium
HA . . . . headache; hemagglutination
HAA . . . . hepatitis-associated antigen
HABA. . . . . hydroxybenzeneazobenzoic acid
HAI. . . . . hemagglutination inhibition
HANE . . . . hereditary angioneurotic edema
HAV . . . . hepatitis A virus

HAVAB .... hepatitis A virus antibody
Hb .... hemoglobin
HBAB .... hepatitis B antibody
HB_c .... hepatitis B core
HBD .... hydroxybutric dehydrogenase
HBDH .... hydroxybutyrate dehydrogenase
HB_eAg .... hepatitis B e antigen
HBP .... high blood pressure
HB_sAg .... hepatitis B surface antigen
HBV .... hepatitis B virus
HC .... homocystinuria
HCFA .... Health Care Financing Administration
hCG .... human chorionic gonadotropin
HCl .... hydrochloric acid
HCO_3 .... bicarbonate
HCS .... human chorionic somatomammotropin
Hct .... hematocrit
HD .... Hodgkin's disease
HDL .... high density lipoprotein
HDLC .... high density lipoprotein cholesterol
HDN .... hemolytic disease of the newborn
HDP .... hydroxydimethylpyrimidine
He .... helium
HEMPAS .... here. erythroblastic multinuclearity with positive acidified serum
HEp .... human epithelial cells
HES .... acute hypereosinophilic syndrome
Hf .... hafnium
HFI .... hereditary fructose intolerance
Hg .... mercury
^{197}Hg .... radioisotope of mercury
^{203}Hg .... radioisotope of mercury
HG .... herpes gestationis
HGA .... homogentisic acid
Hgb .... hemoglobin
HGG .... human gamma globulin
HGH .... human growth hormone
HGPRT .... hypoxanthine guanine phosphoribosyl transferase
HHC .... home health care
HHD .... hypertensive heart disease
HHH .... hyperornithinemia, hyperammonemia-homocitrullinuria
HHM .... humoral hypercalcemia of malignancy
HHT .... head holter traction
HI .... hydriodic acid
HIAA .... hydroxyindoleacetic acid
HIB .... *Haemophilus influenzae* B
HIDA .... acetanilidoiminodiacetic acid
HIP .... humoral immunocompetence profile
HIV .... human immunodeficiency virus
HK .... hexokinase
HL .... hearing level
HLA .... human leukocyte antigen
HMO .... Health Maintenance Organization
HMS .... hexose monophosphate shunt
HMW .... high molecular weight
HMWK .... high molecular weight kininogen
HN .... head nurse
Ho .... holmium
HO .... house officer
H/O .... history of
HOB .... head of bed
HP .... hot packs
H & P .... history and physical

hpf . . . . high power field
HPFH . . . . hereditary persistence of fetal hemoglobin
HPI . . . . history of present illness
HPL . . . . human placental lactogen
HPLC . . . . high-performance liquid chromatography
HPN . . . . home parenteral nutrition
HPP . . . . human pancreatic polypeptide
HPPH . . . . hydroxyphenyl-phenylhydantoin
HPT . . . . hyperparathyroidism
HPV . . . . human papillomavirus
HR . . . . heart rate; hospital record
HRANA . . . . histone reactive ANA
HRLM . . . . high resolution light microscopy
hs . . . . at bedtime (hora somni)
HS . . . . herpes simplex; hereditary spherocytosis
HSV . . . . herpes simplex virus
HT . . . . hypertension; hypodermic tablet
HTLV . . . . human T-lymphotropic virus
HTN . . . . hypertension
HTP . . . . hydroxytrytophan
HTVD . . . . hypertensive vascular disease
HUS . . . . hemolytic-uremic syndrome; hyaluronidase unit for semen
H-V . . . . HIS-ventricular
HVA . . . . homovanillic acid
Hx . . . . history
Hz . . . . hertz

I . . . . iodine
^{125}I . . . . radioisotope of iodide
^{131}I . . . . radioisotope of iodide
I-3-AA . . . . indole-3-acetic acid
Ia . . . . antigen
IAA . . . . indole acetic acid
IABP . . . . intra-aortic balloon pump
IADH . . . . inappropriate antidiuretic hormone
IAT . . . . indirect antiglobulin test
Ib . . . . a glycoprotein
IBC . . . . iron binding capacity
IC . . . . immune complexes; inspiratory capacity
ICA . . . . internal carotid artery
ICD . . . . isocitrate dehydrogenase
ICDH . . . . isocitrate dehydrogenase
ICF . . . . intracellular fluid
ICG . . . . indocyanine green
ICN . . . . intensive care neonatal
ICS . . . . intercostal space
ICSH . . . . interstitial cell stimulating hormone
ICT . . . . indirect Coombs' test
ICU . . . . intensive care unit
ID . . . . identification; immunodiffusion; infectious disease; intradermal(ly)
IDA . . . . iron deficiency anemia; image display and analysis
IDAT . . . . indirect antiglobulin test
IDDM . . . . insulin dependent diabetes mellitus
IDL . . . . intermediate-density lipoprotein
IEF . . . . isoelectric focusing
IEM . . . . inborn errors of metabolism
IEP . . . . immunoelectrophoresis
IF . . . . immunofluorescence; inspiratory force; interstitial fluid; intrinsic factor
IFA . . . . indirect fluorescent antibody
IFIX . . . . immunofixation
Ig . . . . immunoglobulin

IGT . . . . impaired glucose tolerance
IHA . . . . indirect hemagglutination
IIb-IIIa . . . . glycoproteins found on platelet membranes
IIF . . . . indirect immunofluorescence
I.M. . . . . intramuscular
IMD . . . . inherited metabolic disorders
IMP . . . . impression
IMV . . . . intermittent mandatory ventilation
In . . . . indium
INH . . . . isonicotinic acid hydrazide; isoniazid
INR . . . . international normalized ratio
IOFNA . . . . intraoperative fine needle aspiration
IOL . . . . intraocular lens
IOP . . . . intraocular pressure
IOT . . . . intraocular tension
IP . . . . intraperitoneal(ly)
I-PAO . . . . insulin induced peak acid output
IPF . . . . idiopathic pulmonary fibrosis
IPG . . . . impedence phlebograph
IPPB . . . . intermittent positive pressure breathing
Ir . . . . iridium
IR . . . . infrared
IRDS . . . . infant respiratory distress syndrome
IRG . . . . immunoreactive glucose
IRGH . . . . immunoreactive growth hormone
IRI . . . . immunoreactive insulin
IRMA . . . . immunoradiometric assay
IRT . . . . immunoreactive trypsinogen
ISD . . . . isosorbide dinitrate
ISE . . . . ion-selective electrode
IT . . . . inhalation therapy; intrathecal(ly)
ITP . . . . idiopathic thrombocytopenic purpura
ITT . . . . insulin tolerance test
IU . . . . International unit
IUD . . . . intrauterine device
IUGR . . . . intrauterine growth retardation
IUP . . . . intrauterine pregnancy
I.V. . . . . intravenous
IVAC . . . . I.V. infusion control device
IVAD . . . . implanted vascular access device
IVC . . . . inferior vena cava; intravenous cholangiography
IVP . . . . intravenous push; intravenous pyelogram
IVPB . . . . intravenous piggyback
IVSD . . . . intraventricular septal defect

JVD . . . . jugular-venous distenion
JVP . . . . jugular venous pressure; jugular venous pulse

K . . . . potassium
K-B . . . . Kleihauer-Betke
kcal . . . . kilocalorie
KCl . . . . potassium chloride
KCN . . . . potassium cyanide
kg . . . . kilogram
KGS . . . . ketogenic steroids
kL . . . . kiloliter
km . . . . kilometer
KO . . . . keep open
KOH . . . . potassium hydroxide
Kr . . . . krypton
KS . . . . ketosteroids; Kaposi's sarcoma
KU . . . . Karmen units

KUB . . . . kidney and urinary bladder
KVO . . . . keep vein open
KW . . . . Keith-Wagener

L . . . . left; liter; lumbar
L_2 . . . . second lumbar vertebra
La . . . . lanthanum
LA . . . . latex agglutination; left artrium; local anesthetic
LAD . . . . left anterior descending (artery)
LAI . . . . labioincisal
LAO . . . . left anterior oblique
LAP . . . . leucine aminopeptidase; leukocyte alkaline phosphatase
Lap . . . . laparotomy
LASA . . . . lipid associated sialic acid
LATS . . . . long-acting thyroid stimulating hormone
LBBB . . . . left bundle branch block
LBM . . . . lean body mass
LBW . . . . low birth weight
LC . . . . lethal concentration
LCI . . . . lung clearance index
LCIS . . . . lobular carcinoma *in situ*
LCM . . . . lymphocytic choriomeningitis
LCS . . . . Leydig cell stimulation
LD . . . . lactate dehydrogenase; lethal dose; light difference
LD_1 . . . . lactate dehydrogenase fraction 1
LDH . . . . lactate dehydrogenase
LDHI . . . . LDH isoenzymes
LDL . . . . low density lipoprotein
LDLC . . . . low density lipoprotein cholesterol
LDT . . . . lactate dehydrogenase total
LDV . . . . lactate dehydrogenase virus
Le . . . . Lewis antigen
LE . . . . lower extremity; lupus erythematosus
LEA . . . . lower extremity arterial
LES . . . . lower esophageal sphincter
LEV . . . . lower extremity venous
LFT . . . . liver function test
LGV . . . . lymphogranuloma venereum
LH . . . . luteinizing hormone
LHRF . . . . luteinizing hormone releasing factor
LHRH . . . . luteinizing hormone releasing hormone
LHV . . . . left ventricular hypertrophy
Li . . . . lithium
LISS . . . . low ionic strength saline
L-J . . . . Löwenstein-Jensen
LKM . . . . liver/kidney microsomes
LKS . . . . liver, kidneys, spleen
LLA . . . . lupus like anticoagulant
LLDH . . . . liver lactate dehydrogenase
LLL . . . . left lower lobe
LLQ . . . . left lower quadrant
LM . . . . light microscopy
LMN . . . . lower motor neuron
LMP . . . . last menstrual period
LMWH . . . . low molecular weight heparin
LOA . . . . left occipital anterior
LOM . . . . limitation of motion
LOS . . . . length of stay
LP . . . . light perception; lumbar puncture
LPC . . . . leukocyte-poor cells (leukocyte depleted)
lpf . . . . low power field

LPO .... left posterior oblique
LPRBC .... leukocyte-poor red blood cells
LRC .... Lipid Research Clinic
L/S .... lecithin/sphingomyelin ratio
LSD .... lysergic acid diethylamide
LSG .... labial salivary gland
LTC .... long-term care
LTCPs .... L-tryptophan-containing products
LTT .... lymphocyte transformation test
Lu .... lutetium
LUL .... left upper lobe
LUQ .... left upper quadrant
LV .... lung volume
LVET .... left ventricular ejection time
LVH .... left ventricular hypertrophy
LVOT .... left ventricular outflow tract
LVW .... lateral vaginal wall
Lw .... lawrencium
L & W .... living and well
Lytes .... electrolytes

m .... meter
m^2 .... square meter
m^3 .... cubic meter
M .... mix (misce)
mA .... milliampere
MA .... Master of Arts
M/A .... mood and/or affect
MA-1 .... a type of respirator
MAA .... microaggregatedalbumin
MAI .... *Mycobacterium avium-intracellulare*
MAO .... maximal acid output; monoamine oxidase
MAR .... medication administration record; mixed antiglobulin reaction
MB .... a fraction of creatine kinase
MBA .... Master of Business Administration
MBC .... minimum bactericidal concentration; maximum breathing capacity
MBD .... maximum bactericidal dilution
MBP .... myelin basic protein
mc .... millicurie
MC-Ab .... monoclonal antibody
MCAD .... medium chain ACYL CO-A dehydrogenase
MCH .... mean corpuscular hemoglobin
MCHC .... mean cell hemoglobin concentration
mCi .... millicurie
MCL .... midclavicular line; midcostal line
MCT .... medium chain triglycerides
MCTD .... mixed connective tissue disease
MCV .... mean corpuscular volume
Md .... mendelevium
MD .... medical doctor
MDM .... minor determinant mixture
MDP .... mentodextra posterior
MDR .... minimum daily requirement
MDS .... materials distribution system
MDV .... multiple dose vial
MEA .... mercaptoethylamine; multiple endocrine adenomatosis
MED .... minimal erythemal dose
MEET .... multistage exercise electrocardiographics test
MEIA .... microparticle enzyme immunoassay
MEN .... multiple endocrine neoplasia
mEq .... milliequivalent

METS .... metastases
MF .... mycosis fungoides
MFC .... minimum fungicidal concentration
mg .... milligram
Mg .... magnesium
$MgCl_2$ .... magnesium chloride
$MgCO_3$ .... magnesium carbonate
MGP .... methyl green pyronine
$MgSO_4$ .... magnesium sulfate
MH .... malignant hyperthermia; marital history; menstrual history; mental health
MHA .... microhemagglutination
MHA-TP .... microhemagglutination *Treponema pallidum*
MHPG .... methoxyhydroxyphenylglycol
MHz .... megahertz
MI .... myocardial infarction; maturation index
MIC .... minimum inhibitory concentration
μL .... microliter
μm^3 .... cubic micrometer
μ .... micron
μg .... microgram
μm .... micrometer
μmol/L .... micromolar
μmol .... micromole
μOsm .... micro-osmolar
μU .... microunit
MID .... maximum bactericidal dilution
MIF .... merthiolate-iodine-formalin; migration inhibitory factor
MIT .... migration inhibition test
mIU .... milli International unit
mL .... milliliter
MLC .... mixed leukocyte culture; mixed lymphocyte culture
MLD .... metachromatic leukodystrophy; minimum lethal dose
MLR .... mixed lymphocyte reaction
MLT .... medical laboratory technician
MLV .... monitored live voice
mm .... millimeter
mm^2 .... square millimeter
mm^3 .... cubic millimeter
MMA .... methylmalonic acid
MMC .... minimal medullary concentration
MMEF .... mean midexpiratory flow
MMF .... maximal midexpiratory flow rate
mm Hg .... millimeters of mercury
mmol .... millimole
mmol/L .... millimolar
MMPI .... Minnesota multiple personality inventory
MMR .... measles, mumps, rubella
MMT .... manual muscle test
Mn .... manganese
MNS .... MNS blood group
Mo .... molybdenum
MO .... mesio-occlusal
mol .... mole
mol/L .... molar
mOsm .... milliosmole
mph .... miles per hour
MPH .... Master of Public Health
MPHD .... methoxyhydroxphenolglycerol
MPS .... mucopolysaccharidosis
MPV .... mean plasma volume; mean platelet volume
MR .... moderately resistant
mrad .... millirad

MRI . . . . magnetic resonance imaging
MRSA . . . . methicillin-resistant *S. aureus*
MS . . . . mental status; mitral stenosis; multiple sclerosis
MSAFP . . . . maternal serum alpha fetoprotein
MSD . . . . metabolic screening disorders
msec . . . . millisecond
MSH . . . . melanocyte stimulating hormone
MSL . . . . midsternal line
MSLT . . . . multiple sleep latency test
MSUD . . . . maple syrup urine disease
mt . . . . send of such (mitte talis)
MT . . . . medical technologist
MTB . . . . mycobacterium tuberculosis
^{99m}Tc . . . . radioisotope of technetium Tc 99m
MTRX . . . . methotrexate
MTX . . . . methotrexate
mU . . . . milliunit
MUGA . . . . multiple gated scan
MUP . . . . monitor unit potential
MV . . . . minute volume
MVP . . . . mitral valve prolapse
MVV . . . . maximum voluntary ventilation
MW . . . . molecular weight
MZ . . . . monozygotic

N . . . . nitrogen; normal
Na . . . . sodium
NA . . . . not applicable; nursing assistant
Na_2CO_3 . . . . sodium carbonate
NACI . . . . National Advisory Committee on Immunization
NaCl . . . . sodium chloride
NAD . . . . nicotinamide adenine dinucleotide; no acute distress; no apparent distress
NADH . . . . reduced form of NAD
NADP . . . . nicotinamide adenine dinucleotide phosphate
NADPH . . . . reduced form of NADP
NaF . . . . sodium fluoride
NaOH . . . . sodium hydroxide
NAPA . . . . n-acetylprocainamide
NAS . . . . no added salt
NATP . . . . neonatal autoimmune thrombocytopenic purpura
Nb . . . . niobium
NBIL . . . . neonatal bilirubin
NBT . . . . nitro blue tetrazolium
NC . . . . nerve conduction
NCA . . . . National Certification Agency; nonspecific cross reacting antigen
NCCLS . . . . National Committee for Clinical Laboratory Standards
NCEP . . . . National Cholesterol Education Program
NCI . . . . National Cancer Institute
NCS . . . . nerve conduction study
NCV . . . . nerve conduction velocity
Nd . . . . neodymium
Ne . . . . neon
ng . . . . nanogram
NGU . . . . nongonococcal urethritis
NH_4Cl . . . . ammonium chloride
NH_4OH . . . . ammonium hydroxide
Ni . . . . nickel
NICU . . . . neonatal intensive care unit
NIH . . . . National Institutes of Health
NK . . . . natural killer

NKA . . . . no known allergies
nL . . . . nanoliter
NL . . . . normal
nm . . . . nanometer
NMJ . . . . neuromuscular junction disease
nmol. . . . . nanomole
nmol/L . . . . millimicromolar
NMR. . . . . nuclear magnetic resonance
No . . . . nobelium
noc. . . . . in the night (nocturnal)
non rep . . . . do not repeat; no refills
Np . . . . neptunium
NP . . . . nasopharynx
NPO . . . . nothing by mouth
NPT . . . . nocturnal penile tumescence
NPTM. . . . . nocturnal penile tumescence monitoring
nr . . . . do not repeat (non repetatur)
NRBCs. . . . . nucleated red blood cells
NRC . . . . National Research Council; Nuclear Regulatory Commission
NS . . . . normal saline; not seen; not significant
NSA . . . . no salt albumin
NSE . . . . neuron specific enolase
NSR . . . . normal sinus rhythm
NST . . . . nonstress test
NSU . . . . nonspecific urethritis
NSVD. . . . . normal spontaneous vaginal delivery
NT . . . . nasotracheal
N & T . . . . nose and throat
NTI . . . . nonthyroidal illness; nonthyroidal index
N & V . . . . nausea and vomiting
NVD . . . . nausea, vomiting, diarrhea
NYD . . . . not yet diagnosed

O . . . . oxygen
OB . . . . obstetrics; occult blood
OBS . . . . organic brain syndrome
OC . . . . on call; oral contraceptive
OCG . . . . oral cholecystogram
OCT . . . . ornithine carbamyl transferase
od . . . . right eye (oculus dexter)
OD . . . . overdose
ODC . . . . oxygen dissociation curve
ODE . . . . O-desmethylencainide
ODm . . . . ophthalmodynamometry
O/E . . . . on examination
OGTT. . . . . oral glucose tolerance test
OH . . . . hydroxide; hydroxyl
17-OHCS 17-hydroxycorticosteroids
OHCS . . . . hydroxycorticosteroid
OIF . . . . oil immersion field
OKT . . . . a group of monoclonal antibodies for typing lymphocytes
OM . . . . otitis media
OOB . . . . out of bed
OPG . . . . ocular plethysmography
OPV . . . . out patient visit; oral polio vaccine
O.R. . . . . operating room
os . . . . left eye (oculus sinister)
Os . . . . osmium
OT . . . . old tuberculin
OTC . . . . ornithine transcarbamylase
ou. . . . . each eye (oculus uterque)

ov . . . . ovarian

p24 . . . . antigen in HIV infection
p50 . . . . half saturation (oxygen)
P . . . . phosphorus; pulse
^{32}P . . . . radioisotope of phosphorus
Pa . . . . protactinium
PA . . . . phenylalinine; platelet associated; pernicious anemia; physician's assistant
P & A . . . . percussion and auscultation
PABA . . . . para-aminobenzoic acid
PAC . . . . premature atrial contraction
PAH . . . . phenylalanine hydroxylase
PAI . . . . plasminogen activator inhibitor
PAO . . . . peak acid output
Pap . . . . Papanicolaou's stain
PAP . . . . peroxidase antiperoxidase; pri. atypical pneum.; prostate acid phosphatase
PAR . . . . pulmonary arteriolar resistance
PAS . . . . para-aminosalicylic acid; periodic acid Schiff stain
PAT . . . . paroxysmal atrial tachycardia; preadmission testing
Pb . . . . lead
PBC . . . . primary biliary cirrhosis
PBG . . . . porphobilinogen
PBI . . . . protein-bound iodine
PBL . . . . peripheral blood lymphocytes
PBS . . . . peripheral blood smear
pc . . . . after meals (post cibum)
PC . . . . porto-caval; present complaint
pc1 . . . . platelet count pretransfusion
pc2 . . . . platelet count post-transfusion
PCA . . . . parietal cell antibody; percutaneous coronary angioplasty
PCB . . . . polychlorinated biphenyls
PCE . . . . pseudocholinesterase
PCG . . . . pneumocardiogram
PCH . . . . paroxysmal cold hemoglobinuria
PCHE . . . . pseudocholinesterase
PCI . . . . prothrombin consumption index
pCO_2 . . . . carbon dioxide partial pressure (tension)
PCP . . . . phencyclidine
PCR . . . . polymerase chain reaction
PCT . . . . prothrombin consumption test
PCU . . . . patient care unit
PCV . . . . packed cell volume
Pd . . . . palladium
PD . . . . postural drainage
PDR . . . . *Physician's Desk Reference*
PDW . . . . platelet distribution width
PE . . . . physical examination; pleural effusion; pulmonary embolism
PEEP . . . . positive end-expiratory pressure
PEF . . . . peak expiratory flow
PEFR . . . . peak expiratory flow rate
PEFT . . . . peak expiratory flow time
PEG . . . . polyethylene glycol
PEP . . . . phosphoenolpyruvate
PERLA . . . . pupils equal, reactive to light and accommodation
PET . . . . positron emission tomography; pre-eclamptic toxemia
PF . . . . platelet factor; preservative free
PFK . . . . phosphofructoaldolase
PFS . . . . penile flow study; prefilled syringe
PFT . . . . pulmonary function test
pg . . . . picogram

PG . . . . phosphatidyl glycine
PGD . . . . phosphogluconate dehydrogenase
PGI . . . . phosphoglucose isomerase
PGK . . . . phosphoglycerokinase
PgR . . . . progesterone receptor
pH . . . . measurement of acidity or alkalinity
pHa . . . . arterial blood pH
PHA . . . . phytohemagglutinin activation
PhD . . . . Doctor of Philosophy
PHI . . . . phosphohexoseisomerase
PHP . . . . persistent hyperphenylalaninemia
PHT . . . . peroxide hemolysis test
pi . . . . platelet count increment
PI . . . . phosphatidylinositol; protamine insulin; pulmonary infarction
PID . . . . pelvic inflammatory disease
PIV . . . . parainfluenza virus
PK . . . . pyruvate kinase
PKU . . . . phenylketonuria
Plt . . . . platelet
Pm . . . . promethium
PM . . . . afternoon
PMD . . . . primary myocardial disease; progressive muscular dystrophy
PMH . . . . past medical history
PM-I . . . . platelet membrane antigen
PMN . . . . polymorphonuclear neutrophil
pmol . . . . picomole
PMP . . . . previous menstrual period
PM & R . . . . physical medicine and rehabilition
PMS . . . . premenstrual syndrome
PNH . . . . paroxysmal nocturnal hemoglobinuria
PNP . . . . nonprotein nitrogen
pNPP . . . . paranitrophenylphosphate
Pnx . . . . pneumothorax
po . . . . by mouth (per os)
Po . . . . polonium
pO_2 . . . . oxygen partial pressure (tension)
POA . . . . pancreatic oncofetal antigen
POMR . . . . problem oriented medical record
POR . . . . problem oriented record
PP . . . . postprandial
PPBS . . . . postprandial blood sugar
PPD . . . . purified protein derivative
PPF . . . . plasma protein fraction
PPG . . . . photoplethysmography
PPLO . . . . pleuropneumonia-like organisms
ppm . . . . parts per million
ppt . . . . precipitate
Pr . . . . praseodymium; presbyopia
PR . . . . per rectum
PRA . . . . plasma renin activity; progesterone receptor assay
PRBCs . . . . packed red blood cells
PRG . . . . phleborheography
PRL . . . . prolactin
prn . . . . as needed (pro re nata)
PROM . . . . premature rupture of membranes; prolonged rupture of membranes
PRP . . . . polyribophosphate
PRSM . . . . peripheral smear
PSA . . . . prostate specific antigen
PSG . . . . polysomnography
PSIS . . . . posterior/superior iliac spine
PSP . . . . phenolsulfonphthalein
PSRO . . . . Professional Standards Review Organization

PSS . . . . progressive systemic sclerosis
PS-VER . . . . pattern shift – visual evoked response
Pt . . . . platinum
PT . . . . physical therapy; prothrombin time
P & T . . . . Pharmacy & Therapeutics
PTA . . . . platelet thromboplastin antecedent; prothrombin activity
PTAH . . . . phosphotungstic acid hematoxylin
PTC . . . . phenylthiocarbamide; plasma thromboplastin component
PTH . . . . parathyroid hormone
PTP . . . . prothrombin-proconvertin
PTS . . . . pneumatic tube system
PTT . . . . partial thromboplastin time
Pu . . . . plutonium
PU . . . . peptic ulcer
PUD . . . . peptic ulcer disease
pulv . . . . a powder (pulvis)
PV . . . . plasma volume
PVA . . . . polyvinyl alcohol
PVC . . . . premature ventricular contraction
PVD . . . . peripheral vascular disease
PVR . . . . pulse volume recording
PVT . . . . paroxysmal ventricular tachycardia
PWM . . . . pokeweed mitogen
Px . . . . physical
PYP . . . . pyrophosphate

q . . . . every (quaque)
QBCA . . . . quantitative buffy coat analysis
qd . . . . every day (quaque die)
qh . . . . every hour (quaque hora)
qhr . . . . every hour (quaque hora)
qid . . . . four times a day (quarter in die)
QNS . . . . quantity not sufficient
qod . . . . every other day
qs . . . . sufficient quantity (quantum sufficiat)
qs ad . . . . sufficient quantity to make (quantum sufficiat ad)
QTC . . . . quantitative tip culture
qv . . . . as much as you will (quam volveris)

R . . . . respiration; right
Ra . . . . radium
RA . . . . rheumatoid arthritis; right atrium
RAC . . . . right atrial catheter
RAD . . . . radiation absorbed dose
RAF . . . . rheumatoid arthritis factor
RAI . . . . radioactive iodine
RAO . . . . right anterior oblique
RAP . . . . rheumatoid arthritis precipitins
RAW . . . . airway resistance
Rb . . . . rubidium
RBC . . . . red blood cell
RBP . . . . retinol binding protein
RC . . . . red cell; retrograde cystogram
RCM . . . . radiographic contrast media; right costal margin
RCMI . . . . red cell morphology index
rd . . . . rutherford
RDS . . . . respiratory distress syndrome
RDW . . . . red cell distribution width
Re . . . . rhenium
REM . . . . rapid eye movement
repet . . . . to be repeated (repetatur)
Rf . . . . rutherfordium

RF . . . . renal failure; rheumatoid factor
Rh . . . . antigen; rhodium; rhesus
RhIG . . . . $Rh_o(D)$ immune globulin
$Rh_o(D)$ . . . . red cell antigen
RI . . . . reticulocyte index
RIA . . . . radioimmunoassay
RID . . . . radial immunodiffusion
RIPA . . . . radioimmunoprecipitation
RISA . . . . radioiodinated serum albumin
RK . . . . radial keratotomy
RLL . . . . right lower lobe
RLQ . . . . right lower quadrant
RMSF . . . . Rocky Mountain spotted fever
Rn . . . . radon
RN . . . . registered nurse
RNA . . . . ribonucleic acid
RNP . . . . ribonucleoprotein
RO . . . . routine order
R/O . . . . rule out
RODAC . . . . replicate organism detection and counting
ROM . . . . range of motion
ROS . . . . review of symptoms; review of systems
RPBI . . . . resting penile-brachial index
RPF . . . . renal plasma flow
RPGN . . . . rapidly progressive glomerulonephritis
RPI . . . . reticulocyte production index
rpm . . . . revolutions per minute
RPO . . . . right posterior oblique
RPR . . . . rapid plasma reagin
RPT . . . . right occipital transverse
RQ . . . . respiratory quotient
RR . . . . recovery room; respiratory rate
RRA . . . . right renal artery
RSV . . . . respiratory syncytial virus
RTA . . . . renal tubular acidosis
Ru . . . . ruthenium
RUG . . . . right upper quadrant
RUL . . . . right upper lobe
RUQ . . . . right upper quadrant
RV . . . . reserve volume
RVH . . . . right ventricular hypertrophy
RVVT . . . . Russell viper venom test
Rx . . . . a recipe

s . . . . without (sine)
S . . . . sulfur
S_1 . . . . first heart sound
S_2 . . . . second heart sound
SA . . . . surface area; sinoatrial
SACE . . . . serum angiotensin converting enzyme
SAH . . . . subarachnoid hemorrhage
SAL . . . . suction assisted lipectomy
Sb . . . . antimony
SBB . . . . small bowel biopsy; specialist in Blood Bank technology
SBE . . . . subacute bacterial endocarditis
SBL . . . . serum bactericidal level
SBP . . . . systemic blood pressure; systolic blood pressure
Sc . . . . scandium
SC . . . . sickle cell; subclavian; subcutaneous
SCAT . . . . sheep cell agglutination test
SCC . . . . squamous cell carcinoma

SCE . . . . sister chromatid exchange
SCID . . . . severe combined immunodeficiency
Scl . . . . scleroderma; scleroderma antibody
SD . . . . senile dementia; spontaneous delivery; standard deviation
S-D . . . . strength duration
SDA . . . . same day admission
SDAS . . . . same day admission for surgery
SDFP . . . . single donor frozen plasma
SDS . . . . same day surgery
Se . . . . selenium
SEM . . . . scanning electron microscopy; standard error of the mean
SEP . . . . serum electrophoresis; somatosensory evoked potential
SER . . . . somatosensory evoked response
SF-EMG . . . . single fiber electromyography
SG . . . . specific gravity
SGOT . . . . serum glutamic oxaloacetic transaminase
SGPT . . . . serum glutamic pyruvic transaminase
SH . . . . serum hepatitis
SHBG . . . . sex hormone binding globulin
Si . . . . silicon
SI . . . . Système International (SI) units
SIADH . . . . syndrome of inappropriate antidiuretic hormone
SIDS . . . . sudden infant death syndrome
Sig . . . . mark, write (signa)
SISI . . . . short increment sensitivity index
SK . . . . streptokinase
SKAB . . . . skeletal antibody
SKSD . . . . streptokinase-streptodornase
SL . . . . sublingual(ly)
SLCG . . . . sulfolithoecholylglycine
SLE . . . . systemic lupus erthyematosus
Sm . . . . samarium; Smith antigen
SMA . . . . sequential/serial multiple analysis; smooth muscle antibody
Sn . . . . tin
SNF . . . . skilled nursing facility
SOAP . . . . subjective, objective, assessment and plans
SOB . . . . short of breath
SOD . . . . superoxide dismutase
sos . . . . if there is need (si opus sit)
SPC . . . . standard plate count
SPCA . . . . serum prothrombin conversion accelerator
SPECT . . . . single-photon emission tomography
SPEP . . . . serum protein electrophoresis
SPI . . . . selective protein index
SPL . . . . sound pressure level
SPS . . . . sodium polyanetholsulfonate; sulfite polymyxin sulfadiazine
SQ . . . . subcutaneous(ly)
Sr . . . . strontium
SR . . . . sedimentation rate; sustained release; systems review
SRAW . . . . specific airway resistance
SRIF . . . . somatotropin releasing inhibiting factor
SRT . . . . speech reception threshold
ss . . . . one-half (semis)
SS . . . . *Salmonella-Shigella*; saturated solution; subaortic stenosis
SS-A . . . . Sjögren's syndrome A antibody
SS-B . . . . Sjögren's syndrome B antibody
SS-DNA . . . . single stranded DNA
SSEP . . . . somatosensory evoked potential
SSKI . . . . saturated solution of potassium iodide
SSPE . . . . subacute sclerosing panencephalitis
stat . . . . at once (statim); immediately
STD . . . . skin test dose; sexually transmitted disease

STH .... somatotropic hormone
STI .... systolic time intervals
STIC .... serum trypsin inhibitory capacity
STP .... standard temperature and pressure
STS .... serologic test for syphillis
supp .... suppository (suppositorium)
SVC .... slow vital capacity
SVR .... systemic vascular resistance
SW .... short wave
Sx .... signs; symptom(s)
syr .... syrup (syrupus)

T .... temperature
T_3 .... tri-iodothyronine
T_4 .... thyroxine
Ta .... tantalum
TA .... thyroglobulin autoprecipitins
T & A .... tonsillectomy and adenoidectomy
tab .... tablet (tabella)
TAb .... therapeutic abortion
TAD .... tricyclic antidepressant drug
TAH .... total abdominal hysterectomy
tal .... such
tal dos .... such doses
TAT .... thematic apperception test; toxin-antitoxin; turnaround time
Tb .... terbium
TB .... tuberculosis
TBA .... to be administered; to be admitted
TBG .... thyroxine binding globulin
TBGI .... thyroid binding globulin index
TBI .... thyroid binding index; thyroxine binding index
TBM .... tuberculous meningitis
TBPA .... thyroxine binding prealbumin
TBW .... total body water
Tc .... technetium
TC .... throat culture; total cholesterol
T & C .... type and crossmatch
TCA .... trichloracetic acid
TCBS .... thiosulfate citrate bile salts sucrose
TCM .... tissue culture medium
TCT .... thrombin clotting time
TDM .... therapeutic drug monitoring
TdT .... terminal deoxynucleotidyl transferase
Te .... tellurium
TEAC .... tetraethylammonium chloride
TeBG .... testosterone-estradiol-binding globulin
TEE .... transesophageal echocardiography
TENS .... transcutaneous electrical nerve stimulation
TET .... treadmill exercise test
TG .... triglyceride
TGT .... thromboplastin generation test
TGV .... thoracic gas volume
th .... thoracic
Th .... thorium
THA .... transient hemispheric attack
THb .... total hemoglobin
THC .... tetrahydrocannabinol
Ti .... titanium
TI .... total iron
TIA .... transient ischemic attack
TIBC .... total iron binding capacity

tid .... three times a day (ter in die)
TIUV .... total intrauterine volume
TK .... transketolase
TKO .... to keep open
Tl .... thallium
TL .... tubal ligation
TLA .... translumbar aortogram
TLC .... thin-layer chromatography; total lung capacity
Tm .... thulium
TMB .... transient monocular blindness
TMJ .... temporomandibular joint
TMP .... trimethoprim
TMP-SMX ...... trimethoprim-sulfomethoxazole
TNS .... transcutaneous nerve stimulation
TOS .... thoracic outlet syndrome
TP .... total protein
TPA .... tissue plasminogen activator; *Treponema pallidum* agglutination
TPC .... telescoping plugged catheter
TPI .... *Treponema* immobilization test; triose phosphate isomerase
TPN .... total parenteral nutrition
TPP .... thiamine pyrophosphate
TPR .... temperature, pulse, respiration
TRAP .... tartrate resistance leukocyte acid phosphatase
TRH .... thyroid releasing hormone
TRIC .... trachoma inclusion conjunctivitis
trig .... triglycerides
TRIS .... tris(hydroxymethyl)aminomethane
trit .... triturate (tritura)
TRP .... tubular reabsorption of phosphorus
TS .... total solids
TSB .... trypticase soy broth
TSH .... thyroid stimulating hormone
TSI .... thyroid stimulating immunoglobulin; total serum iron
tsp .... teaspoon
TT .... thrombin time
TTP .... thrombotic thrombocytopenic purpura
TU .... thiouracil; Todd unit; toxic unit; tuberculin unit
TUR .... transurethral resection
TURP .... transurethral resection of prostate
TV .... tidal volume; total volume
TVC .... triple voiding cystogram
Tx .... therapy; treatment

U .... uranium
UA .... uric acid; urinalysis
UAO .... upper airway obstructions
UB12BC .... unsaturated B_{12} binding capacity
UBBC .... unsaturated vitamin B_{12} binding capacity
UBBST .... universal blood and body substance technique
UBC .... unsaturated binding capacity
UCG .... urinary chorionic gonadotropin
ud .... as directed (ut dictum)
UDP .... uridine diphosphate
UDPG .... uridinediphosphoglucose
UEA .... upper extremity arterial
UES .... upper esophageal sphincter
UFC .... urinary free cortisol
UGI .... upper GI
UIBC .... unbound iron binding capacity
U-I-S .... uroporphyrinogen-I-synthetase
UK .... urokinase

UMN .... upper motor neuron
ung .... ointment (unguentum)
UP .... universal precautions
URI .... upper respiratory infection
US .... ultrasound
U.S. .... United States
USAN .... United States Adopted Names
USP .... United States Pharmacopeia
ut dict .... as directed (ut dictum)
UTI .... urinary tract infection
UUN .... urine urea nitrogen
UV .... ultraviolet

V .... vanadium
VA .... visual activity
VAD .... vascular access device; venous admixture
VBG .... venous blood gases
VC .... vena cava; vital capacity
VCA .... viral capsid antigen
VCA-EB .... viral capsid antigen, Epstein-Barr
VCG .... vectorcardiogram
VCT .... venous clotting time
VCU .... voiding cystourethrogram
VCUG .... voiding cystourethrogram
VD .... venereal disease
VDRL .... Venereal Disease Research Laboratory; test for syphilis
VE .... visual efficiency
VEP .... visual evoked potential
VER .... visual evoked response
VF .... ventricular fibrillation; vision field
VIP .... vasoactive intestinal polypeptide
VLDL .... very low density lipoprotein
VLM .... visceral larva migrans
VMA .... vanillylmandelic acid
vo .... verbal order
VP .... venous pressure
VS .... vital signs
VSD .... ventricular septal defect
VSS .... vital signs stable
VSV .... vesicular stimatitis virus
VT .... ventricular tachycardia
VTM .... virus transport media
VU .... voltage unit
vW .... von Willebrand
vWD .... von Willebrand's disease
vWF .... von Willebrand factor
V-Z .... varicella-zoster
VZIG .... varicella-zoster immune globulin
VZV .... varicella-zoster virus

W .... tungsten
wa .... while awake
WB .... weight bearing; whole blood
WBC .... white blood cell
WD .... well developed
WDHA .... watery diarrhea-hypokalemia-achlorhydria
WDHH .... watery diarrhea-hypokalemia-hypochlorhydria
WF .... white female
W-F .... Weil-Felix
WM .... white male
WN .... well nourished
WNL .... within normal limits

WP . . . . whirlpool
WPW . . . . Wolff-Parkinson-White syndrome
WSR . . . . Westergren sedimentation rate

Xe . . . . xenon
XO . . . . gonadal dysgenesis of Turner type

y . . . . year
Y . . . . yttrium
YAG . . . . yttrium-argon-garnet - a type of laser
Yb . . . . ytterbium

Z-E . . . . Zollinger-Ellison
ZIG . . . . zoster immune globulin
ZIP . . . . zoster immune plasma
Zn . . . . zinc
ZPP . . . . zinc protophorhyrin
Zr . . . . zirconium
ZSR . . . . zeta sedimentation rate

KEY WORD INDEX

The Key Word Index is not intended in any way to suggest patterns of physicians' orders, nor is it complete. Rather, it is the intent of the authors and editors to make the information easier to find and utilize in order to support better patient care.

The Key Word Index provides a reference to the test name based on a diagnostic property, disease entity, organ system, or syndrome for which the test is useful. It lists descriptions of specific tests. Some may support possible clinical diagnoses or rule out other diagnostic possibilities.

Each laboratory test relevant to the indexed diagnosis is listed and weighted. Two symbols (••) indicate that the test is diagnostic, that is, it documents the diagnosis if the expected result is found. A single symbol (•) indicates a test frequently used in the diagnosis or management of the particular disease. The other listed tests are useful on a selective basis with consideration of clinical factors and specific aspects of the case.

Diagnoses with *International Classification of Disease—Ninth Revision—Clinical Modification* (ICD-9-CM) codes are indicated within the [ ] symbol.

(Continued)

(Continued)

(Continued)

(Continued)

(Continued)

(Continued)

(Continued)

(Continued)

(Continued)

(Continued)

(Continued)

(Continued)

(Continued)

(Continued)

(Continued)

(Continued)

(Continued)

(Continued)

(Continued)

(Continued)

(Continued)

(Continued)

(Continued)

(Continued)

(Continued)

(Continued)

(Continued)

(Continued)

(Continued)

(Continued)

(Continued)

(Continued)

(Continued)

(Continued)

(Continued)

(Continued)

(Continued)

(Continued)

(Continued)

(Continued)

(Continued)

(Continued)

CPT-4 INDEX

CPT-4 codes are provided with each test for reference, as a basis for documentation of diagnostic procedures performed and to facilitate financial and patient record keeping. The codes are current. Applications of codes may vary by region of the country and in some instances the application of a specific code to a given procedure is a matter of individual interpretation.

CPT is a listing of descriptive terms and five-digit numeric identifying codes and modifiers for reporting medical services performed by physicians. This presentation includes only CPT descriptive terms, numeric identifying codes and modifiers for reporting medical services, and procedures that were selected by Lexi-Comp Inc for inclusion in this publication.

The most current CPT is available from the American Medical Association.

No fee schedules, basic unit values, relative value guides, conversion factors or scales or components thereof are included in CPT.

Lexi-Comp has selected certain CPT codes and service/procedure descriptions and assigned them to various specialty groups. The listing of a CPT service or procedure description and its code number in this publication does not restrict its use to a particular specialty group. Any procedure or service in this publication may be used to designate the services rendered by any qualified physician.

The AMA assumes no responsibility for the consequences attributable to or related to any use or interpretation of any information or views contained in or not contained in this publication.

ALPHABETICAL INDEX

The most expedient method for locating a given test is the Alphabetical Index in the last section of this handbook. Test names and synonyms are listed and the page number on which the test description may be found is indicated.

NOTES

NOTES
